Principles and Practice of Pain Medicine

Notice

Principles and Practice of Pain Medicine

Second Edition

Edited by

Carol A. Warfield, MD

Chairman, Department of Anesthesia and Critical Care
Beth Israel Deaconess Medical Center
Edward Lowenstein Professor of Anesthesia
Harvard Medical School
Boston, Massachusetts

Zahid H. Bajwa, MD

Assistant Professor of Anesthesia and Neurology
Harvard Medical School
Director, Education and Clinical Pain Research
Beth Israel Deaconess Medical Center
Boston, Massachusetts

McGraw-Hill
Medical Publishing Division

New York / Chicago / San Francisco / Lisbon
London / Madrid / Mexico City / Milan / New Delhi
San Juan / Seoul / Singapore / Sydney / Toronto

The McGraw·Hill Companies

Principles and Practice of Pain Medicine, Second Edition

1234567890 KGPKGP 0987654

ISBN: 0-07-144349-5

This book was set by Matrix Publishing.
The editors were James Shanahan, Michelle Watt, and Karen G. Edmonson.
The production supervisor was Richard Ruzycka.
The cover designer was Janice Bielawa.
The indexer was Nancy Newman.
Quebecor World Kingsport was printer and binder.

This book is printed on acid-free paper.

Cataloging-in-Publication Data is on file with the Library of Congress.

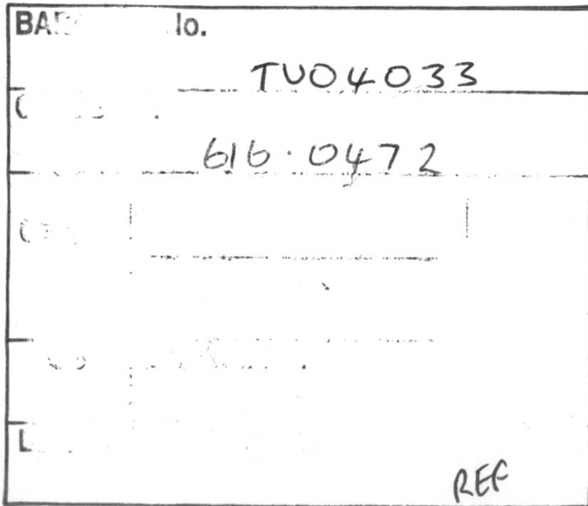

This book is dedicated to my husband Gordon,
and children Rick, Chris, and Alex

CAW

This book is dedicated to my wife Fatima
and children, Ahmad, Tania, and Sarah

ZHB

Contents

PART V PAIN SYNDROMES 379

A. NEUROPATHIC PAIN

B. ACUTE AND PERIOPERATIVE PAIN

C. PAIN IN THE TERMINALLY ILL

D. PAIN ASSOCIATED WITH MEDICAL ILLNESS

Contributors

Salahadin Abdi, MD, PhD
Professor and Chief
University of Miami Pain Center
Department of Anesthesiology, Perioperative Medicine, and Pain Management
Jackson Memorial Hospital
University of Miami School of Medicine
Miami, Florida

Vimal K. Akhouri, MD
Instructor in Anesthesia
Harvard Medical School
Arnold Pain Management Center
Beth Israel Deaconess Medical Center
Boston, Massachusetts

Moris M. Aner, MD
Instructor in Anesthesia
Harvard Medical School
Arnold Pain Management Center
Beth Israel Deaconess Medical Center
Boston, Massachusetts

Gerald M. Aronoff, MD
Carolina Pain Associates, Presbyterian Hospital
Charlotte, North Carolina

Joseph F. Audette, MD
Medical Director, Harvard Medical School
Division of Complementary & Alternative Medicine
Director, Outpatient Pain Services
Spaulding Rehabilitation Hospital
Spaulding-Medford Outpatient Center
Medford, Massachusetts

Zahid H. Bajwa, MD
Assistant Professor of Anesthesia and Neurology
Harvard Medical School
Director, Education and Clinical Pain Research
Beth Israel Deaconess Medical Center
Boston, Massachusetts

Charles B. Berde, MD, PhD
Professor of Anesthesia
Harvard Medical School
Director, Pain Treatment Service
Children's Hospital
Boston, Massachusetts

Harvey J. Blumenthal, MD
Neurological Associates of Tulsa, Inc.
Tulsa, Oklahoma
Saint Francis Hospital
Vice Head, Department of Neurology
Clinical Professor of Neurology
University of Oklahoma
College of Medicine
Tulsa, Oklahoma

René Cailliet, MD
Professor Emeritus
University of Southern California
Pacific Palisades, California

Daniel B. Carr, MD
Saltonstall Professor of Pain Research
Vice Chairman for Research
Department of Anesthesia
Tufts-New England Medical Center
Professor of Anesthesiology and Medicine
Tufts University School of Medicine
Tufts-New England Medical Center
Boston, Massachusetts

Gretchen A. Case, MPH
Director, The Bioethics Program
Saint John's Health Center
Santa Monica, California

Margaret Caudill-Slosberg, MD, PhD
Adjunct Professor of Anesthesiology
Dartmouth Medical School
Hanover, New Hampshire

Robert I. Cohen, MD
Instructor of Anesthesia
Harvard Medical School
Beth Israel Deaconess Medical Center
Boston, Massachusetts

Steven P. Cohen
Associate Professor of Anesthesia
New York University Medical Center
New York, New York

Stephen A. Cohen, MD, MBA
Instructor in Anesthesia
Harvard Medical School
Director of Ambulatory Anesthesia
Beth Israel Deaconess Medical Center
Boston, Massachusetts

JOSEPH CONDON, MD
Division of Pain Medicine
Department of Anesthesiology and Pain Medicine
Associate Professor of Anesthesiology
University of California, Davis
Sacramento, California

F. MICHAEL CUTRER, MD
Director, Headache
Department of Neurology
Mayo Clinic
Rochester, Minnesota

MILES DAY, MD
Assistant Professor of Anesthesiology
Department of Anesthesia
Texas Tech University Health Sciences Center
Lubbock, Texas

RICHARD DERBY, MD
Spinal Diagnostics and Treatment Center
Daly City, California

JOHN M. DESIO, MD
Medical Director
The De Sio Pain Institute
Toms River, New Jersey

RANJAN DEY, MD
Assistant Professor
Pain Management Services
Department of Anesthesiology
Medical College of Virginia Hospitals and Physicians
Richmond, Virginia

DAVID DUBUISSON, MD, PHD
Palmetto Neurosurgery & Spine Center
Columbia, South Carolina

ANNA R. DU PEN, MN, ARNP
Bainbridge Island, Washington

STUART L. DU PEN, MD
Bainbridge Island, Washington

PAUL J. DURAN, MD
The Richeimer Institute at Saint John's Health Center
Santa Monica, California

JOHN H. EICHHORN, MD
Professor of Anesthesiology
Lexington, Kentucky

JENNIFER A. ELLIOTT, MD
Assistant Professor
Department of Anesthesiology
University of Missouri-Kansas City School of Medicine
Staff Pain Physician
St. Luke's Hospital of Kansas City
Kansas City, Missouri

GILBERT J. FANCIULLO, MD
Associate Professor of Anesthesia
Dartmouth Medical School
Director, Section of Pain Medicine & Palliative Care
Department of Anesthesiology
Dartmouth Hitchcock Medical Center
Lebanon, New Hampshire

HILARY J. FAUSETT, MD
Medical Director
The Foothill Center for Wellness and Pain Management
Glendale, California

HONGHUI FENG, MD
Attending Physician
Anesthesia Associates of New London, Connecticut
Lawrence and Memorial Hospital
New London, Connecticut

SCOTT M. FISHMAN, MD
Chief, Division of Pain Medicine
Departments of Anesthesiology and Pain Medicine
Professor of Anesthesiology
University of California, Davis
Sacramento, California

B. LACHLAN FORROW, MD
Associate Professor of Medicine
Harvard Medical School
Director, Palliative Care Programs
Division of General Medicine and Primary Care
Beth Israel Deaconess Medical Center
Boston, Massachusetts

JILLIAN B. FRANK, PHD
Clinical Psychologist
Brookline, Massachusetts
Instructor in Psychiatry
Department of Psychiatry
Harvard Medical School
Beth Israel Deaconess Medical Center
Boston, Massachusetts

WALTER R. FRONTERA, MD, PHD
Earle P. and Ida S. Charlton Associate Professor
and Chairman
Harvard Medical School
Physiatrist-in-Chief
Department of Physical Medicine & Rehabilitation
Spaulding Rehabilitation Hospital
Boston, Massachusetts

RICHARD L. GILBERT, MD
Department of Anesthesiology
Carolinas Medical Center
Charlotte, North Carolina

GISELE J. GIRAULT, MD
Department of Anesthesiology
Dartmouth Hitchcock Medical Center
Lebanon, New Hampshire

Richard T. Goldberg, PhD
Associate Clinical Professor of Psychology
Department of Psychiatry
Harvard Medical School
Senior Clinical Psychologist
Spaulding Rehabilitation Hospital
Boston, Massachusetts

Jeremy Goodwin, MD
Clinical Assistant Professor
Departments of Neurology, Neurosurgery, and Pediatrics
Past Chief, Division of Pain Medicine (Neurosurgery)
Past Director, Adult & Pediatric Headache Clinics (Neurology & Pediatrics)
The Oregon Health & Science University
Portland, Oregon

Leonidas C. Goudas, MD, PhD
Assistant Professor of Anesthesiology
Tufts University School of Medicine
Special and Scientific Staff
New England Medical Center
Boston, Massachusetts

Martin Grabois, MD
Professor and Chairman
Department of Physical Medicine and Rehabilitation
Baylor College of Medicine
Houston, Texas

Daniel P. Gray, MD
Academic Anesthesiology and Pain Medicine
Edmonton, Canada

Christine D. Greco, MD
Co-Director, Pain Management Service
Department of Anesthesiology
The Children's Hospital
Boston, Massachusetts

Sandra W. Hamelsky, PhD, MPH
New Jersey School of Public Health
University of Medicine and Dentistry of New Jersey
Piscataway, New Jersey

Sarah H. Hines, MD
University of Mississippi
Jackson, Mississippi

Mark Holtsman, PharmD
Associate Clinical Professor
Department of Pharmacy
Associate Professor of Anesthesiology
University of California, Davis
Sacramento, California

Charles Ho, MD
Department of Anesthesia
Beth Israel Deaconess Medical Center
Boston, Massachusetts

Stuart W. Hough, MD
Anesthesiologist
Comprehensive Pain Management Center, Ltd
Rockville, Maryland

Kenneth C. Jackson II, PharmD
Texas Tech University Health Sciences Center
Lubbock, Texas

Ronald M. Kanner, MD
Chairman, Department of Neurology
Long Island Jewish Hospital
Professor of Neurology
Albert Einstein College of Medicine
New Hyde Park, New York

David A. Keith, DMD
Associate Professor of Surgery
Department of Oral Surgery
Massachusetts General Hospital
Boston, Massachusetts

Laura R. Kenderes, BS
Spinal Diagnostics and Treatment Center
Daly City, California

Jonathan Kleefield, MD
Associate Professor of Radiology
Harvard Medical School
Department of Radiology
Beth Israel Deaconess Medical Center
Boston, Massachusetts

Galit Kleiner-Fisman, MD
Department of Neurology
Beth Israel Deaconess Medical Center
Boston, Massachusetts

Anastasia Kucharski, MD
Staff Psychiatrist
Harvard Medical School
Boston, Massachusetts

Tim J. Lamer, MD
Chair, Department of Anesthesiology
Chair, Division of Pain Services
Mayo Clinic Jacksonville
Jacksonville, Florida

Alyssa A. LeBel, MD
Clinical Pain Service
Allegheny University of the Health Sciences
MCP/Hahnemann School of Medicine
Philadelphia, Pennsylvania

Matthew Lefkowitz, MD
Formerly, Clinical Associate
Professor of Anesthesiology
State University of New York Health Sciences Center
Brooklyn, New York

Lance J. Lehmann, MD
Director, Pain Consultants of Florida
Hollywood, Florida

Eric D. Leskowitz, MD
Assistant Professor of Psychiatry
Harvard Medical School
Spaulding Rehabilitation Hospital
Boston, Massachusetts

Morris Levin, MD
Assistant Professor of Medicine (Neurology)
Dartmouth Medical School
Hanover, New Hampshire

Seth H. Lichtenstein, MD
Department of Neurosurgery
Beth Israel Deaconess Medical Center
Boston, Massachusetts

Dwight Ligham, MD
Staff Physician
Yale Center for Pain Management
Yale University School of Medicine
New Haven, Connecticut

Yuan-Chi Lin, MD, MPH
Assistant Professor of Anesthesia and Pediatrics
Harvard Medical School
Director, Medical Acupuncture Service
Associate Director, Pain Treatment Services
Department of Anesthesiology,
Perioperative and Pain Medicine
The Children's Hospital
Boston, Massachusetts

Arthur G. Lipman, PharmD
Professor, College of Pharmacy
Director of Clinical Pharmacology, Pain Management and Research Centers
University of Utah Health Sciences Center
Salt Lake City, Utah

Richard B. Lipton, MD
Professor of Neurology
Departments of Neurology, Epidemiology and Social Medicine
Albert Einstein College of Medicine
Bronx, New York

Elizabeth Loder, MD, FACP
Assistant Professor of Medicine
Harvard Medical School
Director, Pain and Headache Management Programs
Spaulding Rehabilitation Hospital
Boston, Massachusetts

Edward Lowenstein, MD
Henry Isaiah Dorr Professor of Research and Teaching in Anaesthesia
Professor of Medical Ethics
Harvard Medical School
Provost
Department of Anesthesia and Critical Care
Massachusetts General Hospital
Boston, Massachusetts

Steven Macres, MD
Associate Professor of Anesthesiology
Department of Anesthesiology
UC Davis Medical Center
University of California, Davis
Sacramento, California

Atif B. Malik, MD
Beth Israel Deaconess Medical Center
Harvard Medical School
Boston, Massachusetts

Natalie Moryl, MD
Clinical Affiliate, Pain and Palliative Care Service
Department of Neurology
Memorial Sloan-Kettering Cancer Center
New York, New York

Jyotsna Nagda, MD
Instructor in Anesthesia
Harvard Medical School
Department of Anesthesia and Critical Care
Beth Israel Deaconess Medical Center
Boston, Massachusetts

Thorkild Vad Norregaard, MD
Assistant Professor of Surgery
Harvard Medical School
Boston, Massachusetts

Amy O'Donnell, MD
Partners Headache Center
Massachusetts General Hospital-Brigham and Women's Hospital
Harvard Medical School
Boston, Massachusetts

Akiko Okifuji, PhD
Associate Professor of Anesthesiology
University of Utah School of Medicine
Salt Lake City, Utah

Conor O'Neill, MD
Spinal Diagnostics and Treatment Center
Daly City, California

Richard Payne, MD
Chief, Pain & Palliative Care Service
Memorial Sloan-Kettering Cancer Center
Professor of Neurology and Pharmacology
Weill Medical College at Cornell University
New York, New York

Christine G. Peeters-Asdourian, MD
Instructor in Anesthesia
Harvard Medical School
Director, Arnold Pain Management Center
Beth Israel Deaconess Medical Center
Boston, Massachusetts

Russell Portenoy, MD
Chairman, Department of Pain Medicine and Palliative Care
Beth Israel Medical Center
New York, New York

P. Prithvi Raj, MD, FACPM
Professor of Anesthesia
Texas Tech University Health Sciences Center
Lubbock, Texas

Somayaji Ramamurthy, MD
Director, Pain Management Clinic
Professor, Department of Anesthesiology
University of Texas Health Science Center
San Antonio, Texas

Alan M. Rapoport, MD
Director, The New England Center for Headache
Stamford, Connecticut

Elizabeth M. Raynor, MD
Assistant Professor of Neurology
Harvard Medical School
Director, Electromyography Laboratory
Department of Neurology
Beth Israel Deaconess Medical Center
Boston, Massachusetts

Daniel Ricciardi, MD
Director of Medical Education
Long Island College Hospital
Brooklyn, New York

Steven H. Richeimer, MD
Medical Director
USC Pain Management Center
Clinical Associate Professor
University of Southern California
Los Angeles, California

Daniel Rockers, PhD
Administrative Director
Center for Pain Medicine
Department of Anesthesiology and Pain Medicine
University of California, Davis Medical Center
Sacramento, California

Mark E. Romanoff, MD
Director of Acute Pain Service
Southeast Anesthesiology Consultants
Charlotte, North Carolina

Edgar L. Ross, MD
Assistant Professor of Anesthesia
Harvard Medical School
Director of the Pain Management Center
Brigham and Women's Hospital
Boston, Massachusetts

John C. Rowlingson, MD
Professor of Anesthesiology
Director/Pain Medicine Services
Department of Anesthesiology
University of Virginia Health System
Charlottesville, Virginia

Seward B. Rutkove, MD
Associate Professor of Neurology
Harvard Medical School
Department of Neurology
Beth Israel Deaconess Medical Center
Boston, Massachusetts

Lloyd Saberski, MD
Medical Director
Advanced Diagnostic Pain Treatment Centers
New Haven, Connecticut

D. Sara Sangha, PhD
Regional Scientific Services Manager
Allergan Medical Affairs—BOTOX Division
Irvine, California

Samuel C. Sayson, MD
San Antonio, Texas

Michael Schaufele
Department of Physical Medicine and Rehabilitation
Harvard Medical School
Spaulding Rehabilitation Hospital
Boston, Massachusetts

Donna Schramm-Bloodworth, MD
Assistant Professor
Baylor College of Medicine
Houston, Texas

Craig L. Shalmi, MD
Attending Physician
Department of Pain and Palliative Care
Beth Israel Medical Center
New York, New York
Assistant Professor
Albert Einstein College of Medicine
Bronx, New York

Lee S. Simon, MD
Associate Professor of Medicine
Harvard Medical School
Director of Clinical Rheumatology Research
Department of Rheumatology
Beth Israel Deaconess Medical Center
Boston, Massachusetts

Thomas T. Simopolous, MD
Instructor in Anesthesia
Harvard Medical School
Director of Acute Pain Services
Beth Israel Deaconess Medical Center
Boston, Massachusetts

Gerald W. Smetana, MD
Division of General Medicine and Primary Care
Beth Israel Deaconess Medical Center
Associate Professor of Medicine
Harvard Medical School
Boston, Massachusetts

Howard S. Smith, MD
Director, Pain Fellowship Program
Albany Medical Center
Albany, New York

Egilius L.H. Spierings, MD, PhD
Associate Professor of Neurosurgery
Harvard Medical School
Boston Clinical Research Center
Wellesley Hills, Massachusetts

Michael J. Stabile, MD
Senior Anesthesiologist
Centennial Medical Center
Nashville, Tennessee

Milan Stojanovic, MD
Division of Pain Management
Massachusetts General Hospital
Boston, Massachusetts

Michael Stanton-Hicks, MD
Professor of Anesthesiology
Department of Anesthesia
Cleveland Clinic Foundation
Cleveland, Ohio

Alicja Soczewko Steiner, MD
Assistant Professor of Anesthesia
University of California-San Diego Medical Center
San Diego, California

Walter F. Stewart, PhD, MPH
Director
Outcomes Research Institute
Geisinger Health Systems
Danville, Pennsylvania

Scott Strassels, PharmD, BCPS
Pharmaceutical Outcomes Research and Policy Program
Department of Pharmacy
University of Washington
Seattle, Washington

Ronald R. Tasker, MD, FRCS(C)
Division of Neurosurgery
Western Division, The Toronto Hospital
Toronto, Ontario Canada

Edwin M. Todd, MD
Clinical Professor of Neurosurgery
University of Southern California
Los Angeles, California
Co-sponsor Todd-Wells Chair in Neurosurgery
University of Southern California, Los Angeles, California

Dennis C. Turk, PhD
John & Emma Bonica Professor of Anesthesiology and Pain Research
Department of Anesthesiology
University of Washington
Seattle, Washington

Steven D. Waldman, MD
Clinical Professor of Anesthesiology
Southland Pain Management Center
Lakewood, California

Thomas N. Ward, MD
Associate Professor of Medicine (Neurology)
Section of Neurology
Dartmouth Medical School
Lebanon, New Hampshire

Carol A. Warfield, MD
Chairman, Department of Anesthesia and Critical Care
Beth Israel Deaconess Medical Center
Edward Lowenstein Professor of Anaesthesia
Harvard Medical School
Boston, Massachusetts

Ursula Wesselmann, MD
Associate Professor of Neurology, Neurological Surgery and Biomedical Engineering
Johns Hopkins University School of Medicine
Department of Neurology
Blaustein Pain Treatment Center
Baltimore, Maryland

Harriët Wittink, PhD, PT
Vrije Universiteit Medical Center
Amsterdam, The Netherlands

Aida Won, MD
Instructor in Medicine
Harvard Medical School
Hebrew Rehabilitation Center for Aged
Boston, Massachusetts

R. Joshua Wootton, PhD
Instructor of Psychology
Department of Psychiatry
Harvard Medical School
Director of Pain Psychology
Arnold Pain Management Center
Beth Israel Deaconess Medical Center
Boston, Massachusetts

Tony L. Yaksh, PhD
Professor of Anesthesiology and Pharmacology
University of California, San Diego
La Jolla, California

PREFACE TO THE FIRST EDITION

Pain is an almost universal aftermath of injury. In this context, it serves a useful purpose as a warning system, alerting the individual to seek treatment of the underlying pathology. It is now well accepted that pain can occur without any discernable trauma at all, or can persist beyond the expected healing period. This knowledge prompted the taxonomy committee of the International Association for the Study of Pain to define pain as "an unpleasant sensory and emotional experience associated with actual or potential tissue damage, or described in terms of such damage."

Pain takes its toll, not only in human suffering, but also causes relationship and job disruption and has a tremendous economic impact on society. In 1980, it was estimated that approximately 65,000,000 Americans suffered from chronic pain and that of these, 50,000,000 were partially or totally disabled. Their pain resulted in over 70,000,000 lost work days and cost Americans nearly 60 billion dollars annually.[1] In 1991, Frymoyer[2] estimated that 50–100 billion dollars were spent each year on the direct and indirect costs of low back pain alone and that 75 percent of these costs could be attributed to the 5 percent of patients who become disabled because their pain has not been adequately treated.

Despite these startling statistics, pain still remains inappropriately or inadequately treated. Although tremendous scientific and technological advances have been made in recent years, the knowledge and techniques available are widely underutilized. This is due in great part to a lack of dissemination of information to clinicians. Formal medical education and training has long considered pain treatment a discipline of little importance. This is evidenced by the lack of formal training in pain management in most residency programs today, even in such disciplines as anesthesiology, neurology, neurosurgery, psychiatry, and orthopedic surgery.

On the other hand, anesthesiologists in particular are called upon more and more frequently to treat chronic painful syndromes.[3] Since the first pain clinics were established in the 1940s, the number of pain clinics has risen dramatically. Today there are hundreds of pain clinics in the United States, over 60 percent of which are directed by anesthesiologists.[4] The field of pain management is finally gaining recognition as a subspecialty as is evidenced by the International Association for the Study of Pain's publication of standards for physician fellowships in pain management.[5] In addition, the American Board of Anesthesiology is making plans for the first examination to grant anesthesiologists board certification in pain management.

In the 1960s, the idea of a multidisciplinary approach to pain management was born. Although many pain clinics today are multidisciplinary in nature, many others rely upon one type of treatment or discipline and yet others treat only a particular type of pain (such as headaches).

For most, however, it has become obvious that pain specialists cannot practice pain management in a vacuum. They must rely upon their colleagues in other disciplines to lend their expertise and in this regard must have a solid knowledge of the other techniques available to treat pain and their physiological and pharmacological basis.

Most anesthesiologists have been trained to deal exclusively with acute pain. Once its function as a warning system has served its purpose to define the underlying pathology, acute pain should be swiftly and aggressively treated to prevent the untoward physiological and emotional effects of pain. Chronic pain, however, is not the same as acute pain and should not be treated as such. Not only is the pathophysiology distinct, but the patient will experience different physiological and psychological responses to chronic pain than to acute pain.

Chronic pain has often been arbitrarily defined as pain persisting for longer than six months. This distinction is not always correct, however, and chronic pain can better be defined as pain persisting for longer than the expected time for an injury to heal. Chronic pain may be caused by chronic somatic or visceral pathology, by a dysfunction of the peripheral or central nervous system, or by psychological or environmental factors. The physiological changes associated with acute pain (tachycardia, diaphoresis, etc.) are often lacking and in their place affective disorders are more common.

The clinician must learn to make the distinction between acute and chronic pain before embarking upon treatment. The skills of proper pain management lie not in the ability to perform technically difficult nerve blocks but in the determination of appropriate diagnostic and therapeutic modalities.

In recent years several texts have been written on the subject of

---

[1] Bonica JJ. Pain research and therapy: Past and current status and future needs. In: Ng LKY and Bonica JJ, eds. *Pain, Discomfort and Humanitarian Care.* New York: Elsevier; 1980:1–46.

[2] Frymoyer JM. Cata-Baril WL: An overview of the incidences and costs of low back pain. *Orthop Clin North Am* 1991; 22(2):263–271.

[3] Carron H. The changing role of the anesthesiologist in pain management. *Reg Anesth* 1989: 14(1):4–9.

[4] American Society of Anesthesiologists. *Pain Center/Clinic Directory.* Park Ridge, IL: American Society of Anesthesiologists; 1979.

[5] International Association for the Study of Pain Newsletter; January–February 1991:1.

pain management. This text is intended specifically for the pain specialist who is called upon to manage painful syndromes. Part I provides the basic knowledge needed for initial diagnostic approach to the patient. Part II deals with pain by anatomic location, since most patients will present to the clinician with a complaint of pain in some general location. This section is intended to provide the physician with a differential diagnosis of potential causes of pain in the area of the patient's complaints. In Part III, a comprehensive discussion of the diagnosis and treatment of common painful syndromes is presented. Part IV includes a detailed explanation of the mechanisms of action and indications for the various treatments used in pain management. The last chapter deals with the clinician's legal obligations and rights in the practice of pain management.

Since this text was not intended as an atlas of regional anesthesia, techniques of specific nerve blocks were not included in the chapters. The Appendix include guidelines and illustrations of the technical aspects of blocks commonly utilized in pain management. It also contains an example of a pain unit chart that has incorporated space for recording anesthetic procedures. A table of commonly used local anesthetics is also included.

The glossary provides definitions of some of the confusing terminology associated with pain treatment. It also contains a listing of commonly used abbreviations.

I hope the readers find this text a useful guide in their treatment of pain.

PREFACE

During the past decade, since the publication of the first edition of *Principles and Practice of Pain Management*, the field of pain medicine has matured even further as a multidisciplinary specialty with a broad and informative knowledge base. This second edition seeks to capture the essentials of this knowledge in a comprehensive review of pain medicine. Since the topic of analgesia is the domain of no single discipline, the content of this book is authored by leaders who represent the many disciplines that comprise the field. One could easily write entire volumes about the topic of each of the chapters in this text, but the task of the authors and editors here was to assimilate this large body of information on pain medicine and condense it into a useful textbook of manageable size. Each chapter represents a careful distillation of theory, associated concepts, and, where applicable, clinical treatments of the subject at hand into an accessible format. For those readers seeking to expand their horizons further, the authors have prepared extensive lists of references at the end of each chapter to provide the reader with further details.

This second edition discusses the fundamental dimensions of pain, the various diseases and disorders in which pain poses a major problem, and the methods employed in its management, with special emphasis on the use of analgesic block as an aid to diagnosis, prognosis, and therapy. It covers the history of pain, its biology, and the principles of physical and psychological evaluation of chronic pain. It goes on to discuss pain categorized by anatomic location, as well as by syndromes, such as acute and perioperative pain, neuropathic pain, pain in the terminally ill, and pediatric and geriatric pain. The authors have been careful to incorporate vivid illustrations depicting the physical symptoms and anatomy of each site, as well as key imaging findings from MRI, CT, and conventional radiography. The next group of chapters discusses pain therapies and includes detailed attention to pharmacologic treatments, interventional therapies, and complementary and physical treatments for pain. Lastly, as pain medicine has now grown beyond its clinical bounds, we have introduced chapters covering the new areas of pain and law, ethics, and business administration.

The breadth and rapidity of change in this specialty has prompted the publication of this second edition to the original version, with the new edition reflecting the expansion of pain medicine with every chapter updated. We have even modified the name of the original text, *Principles and Practice of Pain* ***Management,*** to *Principles and Practice of Pain* ***Medicine*** as the specialty has matured to develop its own identity in the panopoly of medical practice. We have also attempted to be comprehensive in our consideration of pain medicine from a multidisciplinary perspective, with the idea that, regardless of the reader's background and training—whether anesthesiology, neurology, physical medicine and rehabilitation, neurosurgery, psychology, or other specialties—a picture of pain medicine as a multifaceted and continually evolving field emerges as with the first edition. We welcome comments, suggestions, and constructive criticism from all our readers.

Carol A. Warfield, MD
Zahid H. Bajwa, MD

PRINCIPLES AND PRACTICE OF PAIN MEDICINE

PAIN: HISTORICAL PERSPECTIVES

Anastasia Kucharski and Edwin M. Todd

For more than 50,000 years, pain has been part of the human experience. Pain has had different meanings for different people. Likewise theories about the causes and mechanisms of pain reflect the state of knowledge of the societies devising the theories. In all ages pain has been a very real and immediate concern, but always the attitudes and responses of people have been shaped by magical, demonological, theological, philosophical, and practical influences in varying degrees and with shifting emphasis. It is our purpose to capture and examine some of these changing interpretations of pain through time.

Pain as a specific object of scientific inquiry was unrecognized until the early modern era. Attention was paid instead to illnesses and cures, anatomy and physiology. Until recently scientists sought a *sensorium commune,* an undetermined site somewhere in the body where the nature of pain would be revealed. However, in every language more than one word can refer to pain. Awareness of pain and suffering has been part of the feelings of compassion, sympathy, and forgiveness that serve to bond us with each other. Now, instead of looking for a locus for pain we are developing explanatory models that take into account contemporary knowledge of physiology, psychology, and technology.

As the hunter-gatherers migrated from northern African to Asia, Europe, and eventually the Americas, their small communities found ways to deal with the illnesses and accidents that occurred to people subject to environmental stress and human frailty. Wars and conflicts led to the development of curative potions and surgical techniques, some of which remain in use to this day. By performing rituals the communities appealed to their gods for help against their enemies, whether human or natural. The people appointed members of their groups to become proficient in the ways that would satisfy their gods and help individuals feel less pain. These early communities used heat and cold, mud packs and poetics, intoxicants and analgesics, simple techniques of extracting foreign bodies, and bone-setting procedures to deal with pain. They also had trephinations and ceremonial mutilations such as circumcisions, castrations, and piercing operations that suggest well established surgical skills.[1]

Evidence of their practice remains in fossils, carvings and cave paintings, and primitive tools. In the fertile crescent of land between the Euphrates and Tigris rivers known as Mesopotamia, a practical system of writing was first invented. The Code of Hammurabi portrays the expectations for a stable and organized society in which medical practice relied on omens, divination, and astrology. It was eminently safer to diagnose and treat in accordance with revelations conjured out of livers and other entrails of sacrificed animals than to rely on surgical skills, for it was expressly stated in the Code: "If a surgeon has opened an eye infection with a bronze instrument and so saved the man's eye, he shall take ten shekels. If a surgeon has opened an eye infection with a bronze instrument and thereby destroyed the man's eye, they shall cut off his hand." Scientific medicine was a descriptive art that designated the heart as the seat of intelligence; the liver, of emotion; the uterus, of compassion; and the stomach, of cunning.[2] Disease was a punishment for bad behavior. Sacrifice and prayer were required to atone for these transgressions. Pain therefore was a sign with multiple meanings. It indicated that a person was suffering, yet may or may not deserve sympathy and assistance, depending on the cause of the pain. Injuries were treated, whereas internal pain might be a result of the "intrusion" of spirits or the "withdrawal" of life-sapping forces.[3]

ANCIENT CIVILIZATIONS

As people migrated throughout the world, they settled in fertile valleys at the mouths of great waterways. Their small groups evolved into civilized societies. Under the growing stimulus of accumulating knowledge and technology, medicine flourished in early settlements along the Nile, Indus, and Yangtze and Hwang Ho rivers.

Egypt

Because of their ability to transform reeds into papyri and make stable dyes and inks, the Egyptians were able to pass on their medical practices, as seen in the Beers, Berlin, and Edwin Smith papyri. These writings give only a fragmented glimpse, but clearly reveal little cameos of medical practice.[4] A rational empiricism is exhibited in the therapeutic decisions of the Edwin Smith papyrus, copied by scribes in the sixteenth century BC from earlier medical writings ascribed to the era of Imhotep of the Third Dynasty. Imhotep built pyramids and was the "blameless physician" whose apotheosis later served as the prototype for the Greek deification of Asclepios.[5]

Unfortunately the high level of clinical competence shown by the Smith papyrus and the amazing spectrum of pharmaceutical knowledge of the Ebers manuscript were not sustained in later periods as Egyptian medicine declined under the growing influence of religious mysticism and demonology.[6] The Egyptians' concept of pain was a complex elaboration of the beliefs of early societies. Anthropomorphic spirits of the dead with sinister intent to cause pain were dispatched by the gods and other forces of darkness into human orifices or through pores to wreck havoc within. The left nostril was a favorite portal of entry.

Despite the mystical explanations for pain, the Egyptians attempted to develop anatomical and physiological models as well. Their society did not forbid human dissection, which reached its highest expression in the masterful works of morticians rather than physicians. The former were a secretive group who did not broadcast their techniques but left only their products for our edification. Nevertheless, there are numerous references in the papyri from which we may draw reasonable assumptions.

The brain was totally ignored as a vital organ, although paresis of the opposite side of the body resulting from head injury is described in the Smith papyrus.[6] The brain was the one organ destroyed or discarded in the embalming process, which more or less signifies the esteem it engendered. The Egyptians elevated the heart to a state of preeminence over all organs. With its vessels reaching out into all areas, the heart was credited with being the seat of all motor and sensory activity. There was no knowledge of a nervous system. The heart and its vessels were believed to serve these functions, which included the appreciation of pain from obvious causes such as gross injury, although the anatomic references are often intermingled with confusing mystical associations.[7]

India

Unlike ancient civilizations that enjoyed a prominent moment in history and then faded into obscurity, those that arose along the waters of the Indus and in the river valleys of China have endured and have projected many of their ancient medical practices into the present. In both countries, anesthetic techniques and analgesics were old when western practices were new.

The oldest of the sacred books of India, the *Rig-Veda,* reputedly written as far back as 4000 BC, describes hundreds of methods deriving from mineral, plant, and animal sources, including anesthetics and analgesics still in use. Practical healing and vigorous therapeutic measures ranging through a versatile surgical repertory culminated in Susruta, the great physician and surgeon who lived about 600 BC. It was a time when disease had a locus in anatomy, and physiologic explanations aided in the diagnosis of disturbed function. A crude concept of the nervous system centered on the heart, from which ducts radiated to all sensory organs and all excitable parts. Susruta's writings reflect some awareness of pain pathways connected with this misconceived center.[8] The advent of buddhism in the fifth century BC cast a pall over scientific discovery and directed medical thinking into spiritual channels. Physiologic phenomena were unreal and pain was denied existence. The slow, steady crawl of scientific progress in anatomic matters was abruptly arrested by religious dogma just as it seemed poised on the threshold of new adventure, and the creative energies of Indian medicine were diverted to other interests.[9]

China

From very early times the Chinese viewed the human predicament as a microcosm of the harmonious universe. Harmony prevailed in life when the polarity of yang and yin was in proper balance. *Nei Ching,* the Chinese canon of medicine, reflects the very ancient concern with maintaining a state of equilibrium between opposing forces. There is no clear distinction between mythology and historical reality in these writings, and mystical numerology, remindful of Pythagorean precepts, strongly influences an oversystematized medical taxonomy.[10] Yang represents maleness, light, heat, aggressiveness, and strength, whereas yin exemplifies femaleness, darkness, cold, passivity, and weakness. There are five elements in nature (earth, water, fire, wood, and metal), five organs in the body (heart, lungs, liver, spleen, and kidneys), and five winds that inhabit the arteries. Natural laws regulating the universe also participate in the functioning of human physiology as reflected in the forces of yang and yin. The brain is simply the marrow of the skull, playing no part in vital activities. The heart is the major organ because it is the storehouse of the blood and airs. It contains the vital energy and intelligence that circulate to all areas, announcing the state of health of the body in a variety of pulses. Clinical practice depends on an astute appreciation of subtle messages conveyed in these pulsations. There are 365 parts of the body, and each has a precise focal representation so important to the therapeutic arts of moxibustion and acupuncture.

Pain has no particular center, but disturbance in yang or yin, especially excesses of heat or cold, usually relate to the heart and vessels. Emotional overindulgence upsets yang or yin and begets pain in the particular organ allotted the psychologic function involved. Rage upsets yin in the liver, and violent joy is hurtful to yang in the heart. Excessive grief disturbs the lung, and evil thoughts provoke the spleen. "Moderation in all things" obviously was as important to yang and yin as it was to healthy coexistence of mind and body in Hellenic Greece.[7] The anatomy of pain had a situational, multifocal orientation for ancient China, leading to therapeutic responses practiced today throughout the world.

CLASSICAL GREECE AND ROME

Greek ideas in medicine, as in art, architecture, astronomy, literature, and philosophy, still excite and exalt us. Pain-relieving drugs and healing arts are woven into the fabric of Homeric legend and Greek mythology, from which Greek medicine originated. Mythology and legend provided a strong base for early medical practice in other ancient societies as well, but the Greek emphasis on individual achievement allowed creative thinkers to emerge from anonymity.[7]

Greek tragedy of the fifth century BC teaches us not only about pain but also about suffering in the most physical and blunt way. The presence of a person in pain, badly wounded and shattered, added to the truth of the story. Euripedes had Hippolytus come back on stage suffering after his frenzied attempts to escape a bull that had risen from the sea. Greek society participated in theater as a matter of course that was both civil and religious. It accepted pain as an explicit part of everyday life.[11]

Greek science began at about the same time in the sixth century BC in Ionia. As in the Greek theater, the line between mythology and history became more distinct. In science, myth and religious dogma yielded to rational natural laws. The legacy of Thales (624–545 BC) and his philosophical colleagues was a new, open-minded world view that filtered down from philosophy to science and ignited an intellectual explosion that reverberated through time and space into every aspect of human inquiry. The first great medical figure was Alcmaeon (c. 500 BC) of Croton. Alcmaeon was a student and disciple of Pythagoras (566–497 BC), the mystic numerologist and patron saint of theoretical science. Pythagoras had already established a brotherhood and center for the arts and science in this ancient Greek colony at the southern tip of the Italian peninsula, when Alcmaeon added his medical school. Relying on the findings of animal dissection, Alcmaeon elaborated a theory of sensation that had the brain as its center. He postulated a mechanism of consciousness dependent on variations in cerebral circulation for sleep and wakefulness. His concept of the nervous system consisted of a network of ducts and vessels carrying sensation in the form of particles of elements that invaded the body through several sensory organs to the sensorium in the brain.[9] The views of Alcmaeon, an early empiricist, were neglected by the rationalist society that preferred the more noble mental gymnastics of Plato and Aristotle in physiology to the results of vulgar dissection.

However, there were other empiricists practicing in the fourth century BC. Democritus (460–362 BC), who taught that all matter was composed of ever-changing atoms of the elements of fire, air, earth, and water, applied this theory to sensation and pain. Sensation was a state of awareness of the soul occasioned when elementary particles invaded the body's pores and ducts. The size, shape, and movement of particles determined the nature of the perception. Thus, pain was an intrusion of sharp-hooked particles in a state of agitated motion disturbing the normal calm of the soul atoms. Democritus scattered body and soul atoms over a universe in which life and death did not exist, where everything was always changing and only the total quality of matter remained constant. He did concede that the center of reason and consciousness was in the brain; emotions, in the heart; and lust, in the liver.[3]

The Hippocratic Corpus reflects the medical spirit and methods of the physician Hippocrates (c. 460–360 BC) of Cos. Hippocratic medicine was practical and rational, stressing an expectant attitude while trusting in the marvelous healing power of nature.[2] Anatomy was rudimentary, and physiology was based on a proper balance of the four elements, the four qualities (hot, cold, moist, dry), and the four humors present in every body. Pain was a manifestation of conditions disturbing the natural state of equilibrium in the healthy body. The brain was considered some sort of gland that excreted mucous matter that played a part in regulating body heat. With his disciples, Hippocrates paid considerable attention to the problem of pain, continually seeking effective measures for easing human suffering at the clinical level. They experimented with drugs, including opium, mandrake, and hemlock, and actively employed cooling techniques and physiotherapy. To ease the pain of surgery, they sometimes produced unconsciousness by compressing the carotid arteries, the name *carotid* deriving from *Karoun,* the Greek word for deep sleep. Always stressing moderation, Hippocrates cautioned his students and colleagues to observe carefully, proceed slowly, and exercise restraint in treatment, a philosophy expounded in his aphorism "First do no harm."[7,12,13]

In contrast to the pragmatic and empirical approach of Hippocrates, who used methods that remain familiar, the speculative physiology of Plato (427–347 BC), lacking the necessary substratum of anatomy, as with all Greeks since Alcmaeon, frequently appears obscure to the contemporary reader. In *Timaeus,* Plato presents a model of the brain and mind. The fundamental blending of mortal body with immortal soul entails a rather complicated commotion of atoms and elements in relation to a percipient soul scattered among a multiplicity of organs.[7] Pain is perceived by the soul in its several sites from the intrusion of the four elements, streaming into the body from without in disharmonious and violent motions.

Aristotle (384–322 BC), son of a physician, was uninterested in medicine but nevertheless able to write on biology. There is no reference to human dissection in his works, which deal exclusively with the comparative anatomy of animals. A teleological point of view permeates his thinking on structure and function. *De Partibus Animalius,* his major physiological treatise, reiterates the premise that everything has a design or purpose. It sometimes is difficult to reconcile the exquisitely detailed differentiations of form and function in his comparative anatomy with this mistaken ideas concerning the brain and heart. For Aristotle the heart was the seat of intelligence, emotion, and sensation; the brain was a thermostatic sponge that cooled the heart to prevent overheating. Vital heat in the heart's blood controlled sensitivity to pain. Flesh was the end organ from which pain sensation was conveyed by blood vessels to the heart, where it was perceived and dealt with in accordance with the heart's enormous proclivities for regulating reception and response. Aristotle compounded his mistake about the function of the heart and brain by coining the term *sensorium commune,* which implied a unitary theory and site for pain.

Aristotle died in 322 BC. His theories influenced the Romans, including Galen, as well as religious philosophers of the Middle Ages such as Aquinas. The powerful effect of his prodigious output in all fields of knowledge gave his works a force of dogma that misdirected physiologic research for 2,000 years.[3,7,9]

Alexandria

Alexander the Great was Aristotle's most famous student. He died in 323 BC, a year before his teacher, at the age of 35. In 322 BC, he founded the city of Alexandria on the Nile River delta. Under the suzerainty of Ptolemy, a spirit of free inquiry drew scholars from all over the world. Ptolemy's successors became the new dynasty of Egypt. They built museums and a library, which in the early second century BC had over 500,000 volumes, the largest collection in the ancient world. Mind and technical skills were united for intensive study of the human body in health and disease. The practice of human dissection in preconfucian China and prebuddist India had never progressed to a level of fruitful revelation. Meaningful study of pain and discovery of a functioning nervous system were not possible under conducive circumstances.[11]

Drawn to Alexandria by the inviting intellectual climate, Herophilus (315–280 BC) of Chalcedon was the first great talent to address these problems. His extensive anatomic dissections on human cadavers identified the brain as the seat of motor and sensory function. He clearly distinguished between nerves and arteries and traced the course of nerves to and from the brain and spinal cord. Moreover, he recognized the function of these nerves in motor and sensory activities. His laboratory findings led him to speculate on the site of the soul; he placed it in the fourth ventricle.[13–15] These original observations were first challenged, then brilliantly expanded, a generation later by Erasistratus (310–250 BC) of Cheos. Erasistratus went into great detail describing and differentiating the cerebrum and cerebellum with their deep-lying system of ventricles and connecting foramina. He differed with Herophilus on the proper dwelling for the soul, placing it somewhere in the cerebellum. He commented on the rich convolutions seen in the development of the human brain and hypothesized as an association with intellectual capacity. He noted the constant tripartite company of artery, vein, and nerve along pathways to subservient organs and other discrete anatomic parts. He identified the heart as a central pump propelling blood and air to all parts of the body and discredited it as a sensory organ.[3,9,15]

After Cleopatra's death in 31BC, the Roman Emperor Augustus took over Alexandria. The city soon competed with Constantinople for the trade of the eastern Roman Empire. The major museum and most of the library was burned in AD 270 in a civil disturbance. In 391, the Roman Emperor Theodosius I ordered the library to be sacked again. Any remaining parts were destroyed in 640 by the Muslims under Caliph Umar I.[11]

All the original texts of these great contributors have disappeared. Fragmentary accounts from Galen and other diverse sources have justified the recognition of Herophilus as the father of human anatomy and of Erasistratus as the founder of experimental physiology. Celsus, the encyclopedist of the early Empire recounted their practical interests in pain:[3,9]

> Moreover, as pain and also various kinds of disease arise in the internal parts, they hold that no one can apply remedies for these who

> are ignorant of the parts themselves: hence it becomes necessary to lay open bodies of the dead and to scrutinize their viscera and intestines . . . for when pain occurs internally, it is not possible for one to learn what hurts the patient unless he has acquainted himself with the position of each organ or intestine; nor can a diseased portion of the body be treated by one who does not know what that part is.

Centuries would pass before these ideas would gain any significant recognition.

Rome

During the early years of Rome, people appeared to be unimpressed by the development of medical science in other parts of the world. Pain was something to be borne with magnanimity and stoic indifference, as is usually characteristic of the warrior mentality. For hundreds of years, ancient herbal lore and prayers or incantations to a variety of household gods served the Romans' unpretentious medical requirements. As the Roman legions spread out over the known world, the culture and finer representations of the conquered were preserved and absorbed. Greek medical arts were part of the bounty, and although the Romans never exhibited an enthusiasm to participate, they did often encourage and actively patronize some of the more gifted Greek practitioners. In a long poem, "De Rerum Natura," Lucretius (97–54 BC), an Epicurean disciple, brought a wide spectrum of Greek science to the attention of literate Romans. His physiology of pain, based on the atomic theories of Democritus, stimulated considerable interest despite the Romans' preference for pragmatic action.[15] They were also content with compilation and commentary as so admirably demonstrated by the works of Celsus (AD ?–100) and Pliny the elder (23–79). It remained for Galen (130–200), a Greek physician from Pergamon, to rescue the grand achievements of the Alexandrians and to restore the concept of a central nervous system to explain the physiology of sensation.

Animal dissection supplemented by practical observations in his role as surgeon to the gladiators led Galen to much personal theorizing about psychological mechanisms. It is not possible to distinguish his own opinions from the knowledge he acquired from Herophilus and Erasistratus, but his systematized organization of data had a compelling ring of authority that appealed to church fathers, who later attached the stamp of dogma to his work. Galen's experiments on the spinal cord and peripheral nerves were richly rewarding in providing new information about motor and sensory enervation. He concluded that pain was the lowest form of conscious sensation, caused either by dissolution of continuity in tissues (cuts, burns, overdistention of hollow viscera) or by sudden violent commotion in the humors (pressure and tension). Unfortunately, Galen's physiology was contaminated by Aristotelian teleological influences. Instead of attempting to ascertain how organs and systems functioned, he sought to determine why, and this led his reasoning off in unusual directions. His doctrine of Vitalism, his belief in the transmission of blood from right to left heart through invisible pores, and his concept of suppuration as an essential part of healing sent medical theory off in a centuries-long digression, yet his fruitful experimental physiology, his excellent anatomic descriptions, and his encyclopedic records of the knowledge of his time far outweighed his errors. Roman medicine died with Galen.[12,15,16]

THE MIDDLE AGES

The Roman Empire in the west ended in 476 when a mercenary army sacked the city of Rome, setting up centuries of political and economic chaos, wars, and famine.[17] From its establishment in 330 to its fall in 1453, Constantinople served as a junction between Graeco-Roman culture and the civilizations of the east. Christian beliefs about pain supplanted classical views in the west, while in the cities of Baghdad, Antioch, and Gunde-Shapur in Persia, Islam influenced Arab medicine.

After all the invasions of the barbarian hordes, famine, plagues, and economic chaos, the people of western Europe made Christianity the rallying force that restored some promise of salvation, but its triumph was a defeat for science. Physiologic experimentation died under the force of church dogma that brooked no threat of challenge or contradiction. Pain was perceived in Christian doctrine as a means of purification and redemption; the sufferings of Christ had endowed it with a touch of divinity. Mystical attitudes toward pain promoted martyrdom and gave voluntary suffering an exalted aura of spiritual beauty.[18] Nature could never be questioned for its secrets. Medieval philosophers were restricted under the ban of authority to seek truth through logical deduction. The monastic library replaced the laboratory as the source of discovery. Individual monks could make up their own herbal remedies for the patients treated in the villages and towns near the monasteries and cathedrals.[19–22]

To Gunde-Shapur and other cities in Persia fled refugee scholars attracted by an enthusiastic climated for learning and the generous patronage of the ruling class. Hindu, Chinese, and Persian influences blended with surviving vestiges of ancient Near Eastern cultures gathered by Jewish and Syrian scholars. This selective corpus of knowledge was richly expanded by Greek and Roman remnants brought by the Nestorians after they were expelled from Edessa in 489. In 529, the year of the founding of the Benedictine Monte Cassino monastery, the Greek Academy was closed by the Emperor Justinian because of its pagan teachings. Many of its teachers escaped to Persia with priceless treasures of Greek learning that would otherwise most certainly have been destroyed. Much of the basic knowledge of the anatomy and physiology of pain was preserved because of the fortuitous coincidence of time and place that made such a magnificent reservoir possible. The miracle is compounded by the subsequent series of events.

After the death in 632 of Mohammed, Muslim armies poured out of the Saudi Arabian desert and conquered all before them in the name of Allah. These religious warriors carried their message triumphantly into Persia and India, and paradoxically exhibited a merciful regard for preserving the culture and properties of the conquered in deference to the veneration for knowledge and learning that their prophet preached. The true greatness of Mohammed is best exemplified in the Islamic doctrine: "Science lights the path to paradise. Take ye knowledge even from the lips of the infidel. The ink of the scholar is more holy than the blood of the martyr." This statement was the grounding precept for the preservation of antiquity. Islamic centers of learning gathered scholars of all faiths and ethnic backgrounds. The school of medicine founded by the Nestorians in Gunde-Shapur was the first of many spread out over the Arab world, and science flourished. Ancient Greek and Latin texts were translated by Jewish and Syriac philologists into Syriac and Hebrew, and later into Arabic.

Persian centers dominated in the early years of Islam with new developments in chemistry and pharmacology and with the emergence of great medical writers. Al Rhazi (860–932) wrote extensively, elaborating on ancient ideas and contributing new ones. The most influential physician was another Persian: Avicenna, or Ibn Sina (980–1063). His medical textbook, the *Canon,* exercised a persuasive influence over medical practice for centuries. Avicenna's notions of pain were drawn from his encyclopedic knowledge of Hippocrates, Aristotle, Galen, and Nemesius, a fourth-century Syrian. He recognized 15 varieties of pain produced by humoral changes that disturbed the natural state of things in the body. Not satisfied with the vague cerebral sensory centers of Galen, he followed the lead of Herophilus, who advocated a fourth-ventricle localization, but Avicenna distributed the sites more generously through the ventricles as suggested by Nemesius. From an extensive Arab pharmaceutical lore he extracted three groups of medicinals for relief of pain: those contrary to the cause, those that exert a soothing effect, and those that have anesthetic properties. Opium, herbage, and mandrake were liberally prescribed.[23]

By the eleventh century, the scientific and medical leadership had shifted westward to the Moorish capitals on the Iberian peninsula, now Spain. It was largely dominated by Jewish scholars who reached great heights in medicine and philosophy under Islam. Jewish medicine, and pain treatment in particular, was basically rational, practical, and highly effective. With the creative energies of Islam exhausted, the decline of Moorish capitals coincided with a corresponding reawakening of long-dormant cultural interests in western Europe, initially in Italy.[3,9,24,25]

THE EARLY MODERN ERA

The fourteenth and fifteenth centuries were a pivotal period in the development of Western civilization. Italian merchants and bankers had long traded with merchants from Persia and Constantinople despite their religious differences. Surrounding the cosmopolitan Mediterranean cities were the feudal states of northern Europe and the Mongol hordes of western Asia. Encouraged by the medieval popes, feudal princes led Crusades to Jerusalem to prevent its takeover by Moslems. Although the Crusaders failed in their goal, they did strengthen the authority and organization of the secular states. Meanwhile, the papacy's authority was weakened by a series of schisms and rivalries.[26] Some Christians appeared to become more interested in sanctity and piety, and in finding ways in which they could ensure their place in heaven. Others found the practice of acquiring indulgences offensive. In 1517 Martin Luther, a priest who was professor of theology at the University of Wittenberg, published his Ninety-five Theses. He allegedly nailed them on the door of the Castle Church in Wittenberg.

Instead of looking for miracles and good works, Luther believed that people had it within themselves to achieve goodness. Luther's doctrines and the subsequent Reformation are relevant to the history of pain because they helped to change peoples' orientation about themselves. Individuals became objects worthy of study.

Luther noted in his Theses that people were buying indulgences to help finance the construction of St. Peter's in Rome. Italian Renaissance artists were not only painting religious frescoes and designing cathedrals, they also were changing how they were painting by adding a harmonious coordination of perspective, movement, and color. The people of the Renaissance were living in a period of excitement, for they had survived the plague that swept through Italy in the fourteenth century.[27,28]

While the Chinese fleet was retreating from the Indian and Pacific oceans, explorers from western Europe sailed the Atlantic. The invention of printing most advantageously facilitated communication, as navigation broadened geographic perspectives. After the fall of Constantinople in 1453, fleeing Greek scholars fanned out over Europe to give the humanist movement the necessary impetus. A closer intermingling of the arts and sciences provided mutual benefits. Interest of the legal profession in autopsies spurred the revival of human dissection, which in turn was raised to a higher plane by the involvement of physicians in art and of artists in dissection. Berengarius, Vesalius, and Eustachious were notable anatomists with uncommon artistic skills, and of course Leonardo da Vinci was a skilled dissector whose great original anatomic discoveries and physiologic speculations were mislaid for centuries. Leonardo's extensive dissections on cadavers were conducted in secrecy for a very practical reason: survival. The specter of heresy still muted the creative urge. Leonardo's dissections focused on the ventricles, brainstem, and spinal cord. He also left voluminous notes on peripheral nerves and their functions. He described but did not recognize the significance of the sympathetic nervous system or the reflex arc. Experimenting with frogs, he found persisting sensations and motion after decerebration, but almost instant death when he pithed the medulla. He concluded that it must be the site of the soul. He regarded pain as a component or particularly intense aspect of the sensation of touch. His animal experiments included sensory mapping of anesthetic areas produced by cutting specific nerves. From these investigations he was motivated to speculate on the selective protectiveness of pain in vital areas.[3,19,29,30]

A more open and audacious anatomist was Vesalius, a Belgian lured to Padua by its superior facilities and academic opportunities, whose masterful technique and original, inquiring mind unmasked the absurdities of Galenic animal dissections. His great work, *De Humani Corporis Fabrica* (1543), brilliantly illustrated by woodcuts of Von Kalcar and superbly printed by Oporinus at Basle, is one the priceless treasures of the Renaissance. He brazenly refuted many established anatomic misconceptions and paid the price in character assassination and exile. No less beautiful in design or accurate in detail are the exquisite copper plates of Eustachius, which, possibly because of the fate of Vesalius, remained unprinted until recovered from the Vatican library 162 years later.[20]

Religious proscriptions put an effective damper on the employment of pain-relieving drugs, although sporadic accounts of their use appear in the literature. Paracelsus rediscovered ether, the "sweet vitriol" of Ramon Lullus, when he mixed sulfuric acid and alcohol, and he was aware of its sleep-inducing qualities. Surgeons were known to use soporific sponges, and physicians were well acquainted with the narcotic effects of opium, but these were the dangerous times of the Inquisition and Counter-Reformation. Pain was considered an instance of God's will, and the stake loomed as a threat to those who would ally themselves with the devil's work. Kings could "lay on hands" to accomplish miraculous cures; the lowly practitioner had to avoid the inquisitors of witchcraft and heresy.[31] Nevertheless, carotid compression anesthesia was used by Ambroise Pare. Snow packs and other cold applications were used for local anesthesia, and a small rebellious group, taking courage from the writings and example of Paracelsus, used atropine, belladonna, mandrake, and a host of medicinals for pain, as described in the splendid pharmaceutical books of Cordus and others.[3,9]

In the seventeenth century the chain of events initiated by Copernicus and substantially implemented by Kepler and Galileo culminated in the synthesis of Newton to complete the scientific revolution. A rash of attempts to systematize all fields of knowledge then appeared. Efforts to demonstrate a system of medicine reflecting the same order as Newton's universe approached the ludicrous. The mysteries of the central nervous system remained unresolved, but contributions of enormous consequence were made in anatomy and physiology. However, it was not until 1800,when Bell and Magendie defined the roles of the anterior and posterior nerve roots, that pain physiology could step beyond the advances made by the ancient Alexandrians. Meanwhile the foundation was established as scientific methodology and equipment were invented.

Francis Bacon has been credited with devising the experimental method, and criticized for emphasizing the mechanical and technical over the theoretical parts of science. The Royal Society in England and other scientific societies were founded and journals printed. In 1628 William Harvey's (1578–1657) *De Motu Cordis* was published. It was as important for physiology as the *Fabrica* was for anatomy. Not only was the circulation of the blood proven by morphologic, experimental, and mathematical arguments, but physiology itself was elevated on the strengths of this discovery to the status of a dynamic science. Harvey's genius for inductive reasoning did not sustain him when he ventured into the realm of sensation, where his Aristotelian indoctrination misled him to view the circulating blood as the abode of the soul and the heart as the center of sensation and the seat of all natural motion.

Medieval mysticism continued to exert a crippling influence on scientific thought well into the next century. Iatrochemists made notable contributions to physiology and added to our comprehension of pain while introducing considerable confusion with their mysterious archeus, or spirit forces that governed bodily functions. Von Helmont (1577–1649), a follower of Paracelsus, was so fascinated by the stomach in his original studies on digestion that he made it the dominant organ of the body and resting place of the soul, holding dominion over consciousness, emotion, and pain. Despite the confusing superimposition of the spirits on physiologic systems, the iatrochemists were the first to introduce the idea of a physical transmission of nerve impulses in motor and sensory processes.[3]

By deducing *cogito, ergo sum* Rene Descartes (1596–1650) introduced the mind-body controversy that has bedeviled philosophers and scientists for over 300 years. In 1644, he suggested that the pain system resembled an alarm-bell mechanism. For example, a flame sets particles in the foot into activity, and the motion is sent up the leg and back into the head, where some sort of signal is set off. The person then feels the pain and responds to it. Descartes thus proposed what became the traditional theory of pain, or scientific theory. In *De Homine* (1662), he demonstrated a physiology derived from Galen. Impressed by the delicately poised central position of the pineal gland, he made it the site of the soul and had his sensory-motor response mechanism operate from it.[32] Cartesian dualism has led to models of the mind that compete with the theoretical constructs of neurophysiology to explain how we experience pain.

THE AGE OF INDUSTRY

Until the end of the eighteenth century, scientists continued the work of their predecessors. They incorporated Newtonian concepts of energy and momentum into their theoretical models, which tended to follow the system proposed by Descartes. Meanwhile Descartes, through his meditations, came to devalue the senses and to attribute all thought and creativity to the mind. His viewpoint came to be debated well into the twentieth century. British empiricists, including John Locke and David Hume, questioned whether any knowledge could be accepted on the basis of introspective evidence. Sensory ideas were the only reliable source of knowledge. Locke described the process of how words came to stand for ideas, which grew out of sensory experience. He then posited a person who could, through reason and reflection, generalize from these ideas rather than from a simple comparison with experience, as had Descartes.

Hume was skeptical about whether there was any causal link between ideas and generalizations; he could only assume that in the future the same pattern would repeat. For Hume the mind was an abstract name for a series of ideas. Before long the central premise of epistemological discussions was that our conceptual apparatus was built up from qualities perceived in the outside world, just as models for pain were set up.

Kant, in his *Critique of Pure Reason* (1781), attempted to synthesize the empiricist and rationalist schools by suggesting that there was knowledge that existed *a priori* and was only waiting to be discovered. The person coordinated sensations and ideas into a coherent body of knowledge. Kant doubted that a science of psychology was possible because the mind was affected by studying itself, was impossible to map, and could not have a mathematical basis. His viewpoint was seriously challenged in the next century by developments in statistics and mathematical logic. Russell and the British school of analytical philosophy attempted to clarify how we perceive and use our senses; Wittgenstein challenged them in his *Philosophical Investigations* of language.[33–35]

Meanwhile Willis, Borelli, Malpighi, von Haller, and others made significant progress in researching the central nervous system, while Winslow and others described the anatomy and physiology of the autonomic nervous system. By the end of the eighteenth century, new methods of analgesia were started with Priestley's discovery of nitrous oxide and Sir Humphrey Davy's observation of the analgesic properties of the gas. In 1806, Serturner isolated morphine from crude opium. Refining the technique of getting pure crystalline drugs from crude mixtures led to the isolation of codeine in 1832. In 1828, Leroux reported the isolation of saline, and Wohler the synthesis of urea. By 1897, Bayer chemist Felix Hoffman developed a stable form of this compound found in willow tree bark or meadow grasses, which was called acetylsalicylic acid.[30]

Ether, made from sulfuric acid and alcohol, had long been used as a sedative in the treatment of tuberculosis, asthma, and whooping cough, and as a remedy for toothache. William T.G. Morton (1819–1868), a dentist interested in new ideas, revolutionized surgical and medical practice by demonstrating surgery under ether anesthesia at the Massachusetts General Hospital in Boston in 1846. Seeking to find an alternative to ether, which had an unpleasant smell and occasionally needed to be used in large amounts especially in prolonged labor, James Young Simpson (1811–1870), a professor of midwifery at Edinburgh, found chloroform to be efficacious and relatively safe. After Queen Victoria was anesthetized in 1853 for the birth of Prince Leopold and in 1857 for Princess Beatrice, the practice became common among the upper and middle classes. In the 1850s Charles Gabriel Pravaz (1791–1853), a French surgeon, and Alexander Wood (1817–1884) of Edinburgh independently invented the syringe. Injections of morphine were used for local pain. In 1884, Karl Koller demonstrated the local anesthetic efficacy of cocaine.[36]

By the 1880s, anesthesia with aseptic technique was standard practice in American and European operating rooms. Middle-class patients who usually had been treated at home now sought admission to hospitals for operations. Hospitals were transformed from charitable asylums for the poor into service institutions that were also teaching resources. Neurologists and psychiatrists now had patients whom they could observe for the clinical validity of the theories of pain developed during the century.

In the early nineteenth century the work of Charles Bell and Francois Magendie showed that the posterior roots of the spinal nerves responded to sensations, whereas the anterior roots were associated with motor responses. This idea of specific neural pathways for pain was elaborated in 1839 by Johannes Muller's theory of "specific nerve energies." Muller (1801–1858), a professor at Berlin, suggested that the same cause, such as electricity, could simultaneously affect all sensory organs, yet the kind of sensation would be different in each. Muller at first was uncertain if the sensation was owing to energy inherent in the sensory nerves themselves or to special properties at the site of termination in the brain. By the end of the century, it was concluded that the quality of sensation was given by the termination of the nerves in the brain.[32]

Each sensory nerve then was assumed to have a distinct brain center. Between 1894 and 1895, Max von Frey published a series of articles about a theory of cutaneous senses that became the basis for contemporary specificity theory. He expanded Muller's concept to four major cutaneous modalities: touch, warmth, cold, and pain. His work was based on Schiff's experiments in animals in 1858. Schiff noted that the effects of incisions in the spinal cord suggested that pain and touch were independent. Experiments by Funk in 1879 and by Blix, Goldscheider, and Donaldson in 1882 found separate spots for warmth, cold, and touch.[23,32]

Eventually a search for the "pain pathway" in the spinal cord was made. Experiments with animal subjects suggested that the anterolateral quadrant of the spinal cord was critically important for pain sensation. Spiller observed that a man with a lesion in this area was analgesic in part of his body below the level of the lesion, and persuaded Martin, a neurosurgeon, to cut the anterolateral spinal cord in patients who suffered pain. Anterolateral cordotomy for pain relief appeared successful, and the spinothalamic trace came to be known as the "pain pathway." Head in 1920 proposed that the "pain center" was located in the thalamus because cortical lesions or excisions rarely abolish pain and can make it worse. Critics of the specificity theory pointed to pathologic pain states such as phantom limb, causalgia, and the neuralgias as phenomena not covered by the theory.[32,37]

An alternative to the specificity theory was the intensive (summation) theory that Erb explicitly formulated in 1874. He maintained that every sensory stimulus could produce pain if it reached sufficient intensity. The theory was supported by Wundt, Blix, and especially Goldscheider. Goldscheider at first favored specificity, but by 1894, he thought that stimulus intensity and central summation were the critical determinants of pain. Pain occurs when either the total output of cells exceeds a critical level because of the excessive stimulation of nonnoxious thermal or tactile stimuli or by pathologic conditions that enhance the summation of impulses produced by normally nonnoxious stimuli. Abnormally prolonged time periods of summation produced the long delays and persistent pain seen in pathologic pain states. The "summation path" that transmitted the signal to the brain consisted of slowly conducting, multisynaptic fiber chains, and the large fibers that project up the dorsal column pathways carried the tactile discrimination properties of cutaneous sensation.[23,32,38]

Goldscheider's summation or pattern theory led to several modifications, which emphasize either peripheral or central mechanisms. In the peripheral pattern theory, pain is considered to be caused by excessive peripheral stimulation that produces a pattern of nerve impulses interpreted centrally as pain. Weddell and Sinclair, in 1955, based their theory on Nafe's suggestion, in 1934, that all cutaneous qualities are produced by spatial and temporal patterns of nerve impulses rather than by separate, modality-specific transmission routes. The theory assumes that all fiber endings are alike, so that the pattern for pain is produced by intense stimulation. However, the physiologic evidence is that there is a high degree of receptor-fiber specialization.[32,39–41]

These peripheral-based theories still fail to account for the pathologic pain states, which suggest that some of their underlying mechanisms may be found in the central nervous system. Livingston first suggested specific central nervous system mechanisms to account for the summation phenomena in these pain syndromes. He proposed that pathologic stimulation of sensory nerves that occurs after peripheral nerve damage initiates activity in reverberatory circuits in neuron pools in the spinal cord. This abnormal activity, triggered by nonnoxious inputs, can then generate volleys of nerve impulses that are interpreted centrally as pain.[42]

Livingston's general summation theory is especially powerful in explaining phantom limb pain. Amputation initiates abnormal firing patterns in closed, self-exciting neuron loops in the dorsal horns of the spinal cord, which send volleys of nerve impulses to the brain, giving rise to pain. Moreover, the reverberatory activity may spread to adjacent neurons in the lateral and ventral horns and produce autonomic and muscular manifestations in the limb, such as sweating and jerking movements of the stump. In turn these produce further sensory input, creating a "vicious cycle" between central and peripheral processes that maintain the abnormal spinal cord activity. Stress reactions and minor irritations near the site of the operation can then feed into the active site, keeping it in an abnormal, disturbed state over periods of years. Impulse patterns that would normally be interpreted as touch would trigger these neuron pools into greater activity, thus sending more messages to the brain to produce pain. Emotional activity could also trigger these neuron pools into greater activity and more pain. In 1951, Gerard proposed an alternative mechanism for the theory in which a peripheral nerve lesion could lead to a temporary loss of sensory control of firing in spinal cord neurons, which would then start to fire in synchrony, possibly due to the spread of electrical fields, and would recruit additional units as the group moved into gray matter.[43]

The theory could not account for the fact that surgical lesions in the dorsal horns should stop the pain. However, White and Sweet reported the return of phantom limb pain after cordotomy in 7 of 18 lower limb and 3 of 4 upper limb cases. Even bilateral cordotomy could fail.[32] Efforts were made to find a leak in the pain projection system; a multisynaptic propriospinal system was suggested as an alternative by Noordenbos in 1959. Hebb, in 1949, proposed a central summation mechanism in which synchronized firing in the thalamocortical neural circuits provided the signal for pain. The loss of sensory control of the synchronized activities would lead to excessive synchronous firing in brain cells that would distort the normal cognitive and perceptual patterns. The distortion was pain.[32,44,45]

Similar to the central summation theories is sensory interaction theory, which holds that a specialized input-controlling mechanism that normally prevents summation from occurring can lead to pathologic pain states when it is destroyed. Melzack and Wall, in 1965, noted that this theory, which is derived from Goldscheider's original concept, proposed the existence of a rapidly firing system that inhibited transmission in a more slowly conducting system that carried the signal for pain. These two systems were identified as the epicritic and protopathic (Head, 1920), fast and slow (Bishop, 1946), phylogentically old and new (Bishop, 1959), and myelinated and unmyelinated (Noordenbos, 1959) fiber systems.[46] Noordenbos suggested a shift in the ratio of large to small fibers, arranged in a multisynaptic afferent system, which was a significant departure from the traditional direct system from peripheral neuron to brain.[32]

As the neurophysiologic research progressed, the philosophers were joined by other neurologists, psychologists, and psychiatrists who were exploring the affective and cognitive dimensions of pain. Freud set up a structural theory of the mind that incorporated the language of nineteenth-century science (i.e., instincts, drives, and energy). He proposed a pleasure principle as the driving force for human activity. Dreams expressed their dreamers' wishes. When faced with examples of self-destructive or unpleasant experiences, he modified his theory so that there were two competing forces, eros and thanatos. Thanatos represented death, pain, and suffering.[47,48] Later psychoanalysts replaced his drive theory for the structural theory of ego, superego, and id. Anna Freud proposed a number of defenses, such as sublimation and repression, that the ego used to deal with unacceptable feelings and thoughts.[49] Repression could block a feeling from conscious awareness. Unconscious guilt then would be expressed through self-destructive behavior. Conversion pain symbolized a repressed, probably traumatic, incident. By the 1930s repressed affect was thought to underly psychosomatic illnesses. The pain of arthritis, colitis, and headaches was believed to be caused, in part, by the patient's inability to express what was unacceptable, such as anger and anxiety. The task of therapy was to explore the basis for these unacceptable affects and then assist the patient to express, tolerate, and master them.[50,51]

Just as philosophy had empirical and rationalist schools, psychology had a behavioral alternative to psychoanalysis. Pavlov in Russia and then Skinner in proposed models of conditioning based on animal experiments that suggested that pain was accompanied by behaviors and thoughts that reinforced the pain. Because these were learned behaviors, treatment could help people in pain by providing them with ways of acting that were less likely to aggravate the pain.

Sherrington, in 1900, acknowledged that pain was composed of sensory and affective dimensions. He suggested that "mind rarely, probably never, perceives any object with absolute indifference, that is, without 'feeling' . . . affective tone is an attribute of all sensation, and among the attribute tones of skin sensation was skin pain." Pain was a primary sensation that had cognitive and emotional reactions.[32,52] Hardy, Wolff, and Goodell, in the 1940s, called this model the fourth theory of pain. The perception of pain, like other sensations, was accomplished through "relatively simple and primitive" neural receptive and conductive mechanisms, whereas the "reaction pain threshold" was a complex physiopsychologic process involving the cognitive functions of the individual and influenced by past experience, culture, and psychological factors.[53]

In 1965, Melzack and Wall proposed the gate control theory, which would take into account the evidence of physiologic specialization, central summation, or patterning, and modulation of input, and the influence of psychological factors. A spinal gating mechanism in the dorsal horn was thought to modulate the transmission of nerve impulses from afferent fibers to the spinal cord T cells. Activity in larger diameter fibers tended to inhibit transmission; it closed the gate. Small fibers opened the gate. A "central control trigger" activated selective cognitive processes that influenced, by way of descending fibers, the spinal gating mechanism. This system carries precise information so rapidly that it not only could affect the receptivity of cortical neurons for subsequent afferent volleys but also, through the descending fibers, influence the sensory input at the segmental gate control system and at other levels of the neuraxis. The rapid transmission enables the brain to evaluate and codify the sensory input before the action system was activated. When the output of the spinal transmission (T) cells exceeded a critical level, the action system was activated. The action system was the complex sequence of behavior and experience characteristic of pain.

Melzack and Wall modified the theory three years later to take into account neural systems beyond the gate. They suggested that the neospinothalamic projecting system in the brain processed sensory discriminative information about the location, intensity, and duration of the stimulus, while impulses from the paleospinothalamic tract and paramedial ascending system activated reticular and limbic structures that provoke the aversive drive and unpleasant affect that triggers action in the organism. Neocortical central nervous system processes, such as evaluation of input based on past experience, exert control over discriminative and motivational systems.[46] The gate control theory was a sophisticated mechanical model that reflected the legacy of Newtonian physics and suggested the limits of that system, because pathways could only account for part of the pain experience.

CONCLUSION

Improvement in the resolution capacity of electron microscopes and the development of advanced imaging techniques in radiology such as magnetic resonance imaging (MRI) signaled the transition from sequential models of pain such as the gate theory to concurrent and simultaneous models, which are based on neurotransmitters, reciprocal pathways, and the images of positron emission tomography (PET) and MRI scans. Wall modified the gate control theory in 1999 by suggesting that the brain analyses its sensory input in terms of the possible action that would be appropriate to the event that triggered the whole nocioceptive process. No action actually needs to take place.[54]

In the thirty years since the gate control theory was introduced, research has proceeded on the neuronal level. Enkephalins in the spinal cord and endorphins in the brain were discovered in the mid-1970s. Stimuli that elicited pain were thought to do so by releasing chemicals into the tissues. These chemical substances include histamine, bradykinin, prostaglandins, and potassium and sodium ions. In the dorsal horn, pain transmission occurs through the release of substance P, an 11-amino-acid peptide, present in dense core granules in the synaptic terminals of primary afferents in the dorsal horn. Substance P functions as a sensory neurotransmitter for the relay of pain signals to second-order neurons of the spinothalamic system. Enkephalin, an endogenous opioid peptide, is found in neurons of lamina II of the spinal cord dorsal horn and in the trigeminal nuclei of the brainstem. Electron microscopic studies showed that substance P neurons terminated on enkephalin-containing cells. The enkephalins and β-endorphin inhibit substance P release and thus block pain transmission at the level of the spinal cord and brainstem. Opiate receptors have also been found in the periaqueductal gray matter of the brainstem and in the medial thalamus, amygdaloid nuclei, caudate nuclei, and frontotemporal cortex. This distribution can account for the affective and antinocioceptive effects of opioid compounds.

Electrically stimulating the periaqueductal region can inhibit pain transmission by both ascending and descending effects. Descending pathways from large neurons of the brainstem reticular formation also modulate pain transmission at the dorsal horn. The descending pathways contain enkephalin, serotonin, and dopamine and terminate in laminae I and V of the dorsal horn. Other peptides, including angiotensin II and somatostatin, and the inhibitory neurotransmitters, γ-aminobutyric acid (GABA) and glycine, are also found in sensory neurons of the dorsal root ganglia and substantia gelatinosa.[54,55]

Many of these same neurotransmitters are found to be deficient in depression, anxiety, and psychotic states. Antidepressants act by increasing the cortical levels of neurotransmitters. The early excitement encouraged by the effectiveness of these medications on mood as well as on neuropathic pain has been tempered by the realization that there is no simple pathway to account for depression—just as pain is not the result of nocioceptive stimulation later interpreted by the cortex. However, as seen in patients who underwent prefrontal lobotomies to modify their affective behavior, response to pain was also changed. Patients displayed minimal concern and were not apparently troubled by painful stimuli, although they were able to report on the severity of the stimuli.

Advanced imaging techniques such as PET scanning highlight the simultaneous response to sensory stimuli. Among the earliest studies were those of the anterior cingulate gyrus, where activity was detected on the right side regardless of the site of the pain, including a single nerve neuropathy. This area also is active in directed visual and auditory attention, precise eye and hand movements, and complex speech. Cingulotomies have been performed on patients with treatment-refractory depression.

With the passage of time, the knowledge of pain and effective means for its alleviation increased quantitatively. A mass of overlapping data now await unscrambling and reorganization into a coherent theoretical structure for debate and application to our era. The puzzle is far from solved, especially now that the number of pieces has multiplied exponentially. To cast a glance at the past refreshed and assures us that we are not alone in our frustration. The task has always been arduous, and it is part of a tradition that has attracted the great minds of the past.

REFERENCES

1. Gurdjian ES. *Head Injury from Antiquity to Present with Special Reference to Penetrating Head Wounds.* Springfield, Ill: Charles C Thomas; 1973.
2. Agneu LRC. Medicine, History of. In: *The New Catholic Encyclopedia.* New York, NY: McGraw-Hill; 1967.
3. Keele KD. *Anatomies of Pain.* Springfield, Ill: Charles C Thomas; 1957.
4. Porter R. *The Greatest Benefit to Mankind.* New York, NY: WW Norton; 1997.
5. Camac CNB. *From Imhotep to Harvey.* New York, NY: Paul B Hoeber; 1931.
6. Breasted JH. *The Edwin Smith Surgical Papyrus.* Chicago, Ill: University of Chicago Press; 1930.
7. Sarton G. *A History of Science: Ancient Science through the Golden Age of Greece.* New York, NY: WW Norton; 1952.
8. Methu DC. *The Antiquity of Hindu Medicine and Civilization.* New York, NY: Paul B Hoeber; 1931.
9. Seeman B. *Man Against Pain.* Philadelphia, Pa: Chilton; 1962.
10. Morse WR. *Chinese Medicine.* New York, NY: Paul B Hoeber; 1929.
11. Rey R. *The History of Pain.* Cambridge, Mass: Harvard University Press; 1993.
12. Gordon BL. *Medicine Throughout Antiquity.* Philadelphia, Pa: FA Davis; 1949.
13. Singer CJ. *Greek Biology and Greek Medicine.* London, England: Oxford University Press; 1922.
14. Asimov IA. *A Short History of Biology.* Garden City, NY: The Natural History Press; 1964.
15. Sarton G. *A History of Science: Hellenistic Science and Culture in the Last Three Centuries BC.* New York, NY: Norton; 1959.
16. Cumston CG. *An Introduction to the History of Medicine.* London, England: Dawson of Pall Mall; 1968.
17. Clark K. *Civilization: A Personal View.* New York, NY: Harper & Row; 1969.
18. Morris DB. *The Culture of Pain.* Berkeley, CA: University of California Press; 1993.
19. Ackerknecht EH. *A Short History of Medicine.* New York, NY: The Ronald Press; 1968.
20. Garrison FH. *An Introduction to the History of Medicine.* 4th ed. Philadelphia, Pa: WB Saunders; 1929.
21. Reisman D. *The Story of Medicine in the Middle Ages.* New York, NY: Paul B Hoeber; 1935.
22. Walsh JJ. *Medieval Medicine.* New York, NY: Macmillan; 1920.
23. Bonica JJ. *The Management of Pain.* Vol. I. Philadelphia, Pa: Lea & Febiger; 1990.
24. Browne EG. *Arabian Medicine.* Cambridge, England: Cambridge University Press; 1921.
25. Simpson MWH. *Arab Medicine and Surgery.* London, England: Oxford University Press; 1922.
26. Weinstein D, Bell RM. *Saints and Sinners: The Two Worlds of Western Christendom, 1000–1700.* Chicago, Ill: University of Chicago Press; 1982.
27. Meiss M. *Painting in Florence and Siena after the Black Death.* New York, NY: Harper & Row; 1951.
28. Burckhardt J. *The Civilization of the Renaissance in Italy.* Vol. II. New York, NY: Harper & Row; 1958.
29. Boas M. *The Scientific Renaissance, 1450–1630.* New York, NY: Harper & Row; 1962.
30. Castiglione A. *The Renaissance of Medicine in Italy.* Baltimore, Md: Johns Hopkins Press; 1934.
31. Daniel-Rops H. *The Catholic Reformation.* Vol. II. Garden City, NY: Doubleday; 1962.
32. Melzack R. *The Puzzle of Pain.* New York, NY: Basic Books; 1973.
33. Scarry E. *The Body in Pain: The Making and Unmaking of the World.* New York, NY: Oxford University Press; 1985.
34. Chappell VC, ed. *The Philosophy of Mind.* Englewood Cliffs, NJ: Prentice-Hall; 1962.
35. Shaffer JA. *The Philosophy of Mind.* Englewood Cliffs, NJ: Prentice-Hall; 1968.
36. The relief of pain and suffering. Symposium at the John C Liebeskind History of Pain Collection at the Louise M Darling Biomedical Library, UCLA; 1968. Available at: http://www.library.ucla.edu/libraries/biomed/his/Pain Exhibit/index.html.
37. Head H. *Studies in Neurology.* London, England: Kegan Paul; 1920.

38. Goldscheider A. *Ueber den Schmerz in Physiologischer und Klinischer Hinsicht.* Hirschwald; 1894.
39. Weddell G. Somethesis and the Clinical Senses. *Annu Rev Psychol.* 1955;6:119.
40. Sinclair DC. *Cutaneous Sensations.* London, England: Oxford University Press; 1967.
41. Nafe JP. The pressure, pain and temperature senses. In: Murchison CA, ed. *Handbook of General Experimental Psychology.* Worcester, Mass: Clark University Press; 1934.
42. Livingston WK. *Pain Mechanisms.* New York, NY: Macmillan; 1943.
43. Gerard RW. The physiology of pain: Abnormal neuron states in causalgia and related phenomena. *Anesthesiology.* 1951;12:1.
44. Hebb DO. *The Organization of Behavior.* New York, NY: Wiley; 1949.
45. Noordenbos W. *Pain.* New York, NY: Elsevier Press; 1959.
46. Melzak R, Wall PD. Pain mechanisms: A new theory. *Science.* 1959;150:971.
47. Gedo JE, Goldberg A. *Models of the Mind.* Chicago, Ill: University of Chicago Press; 1973.
48. Freud S. *Beyond the Pleasure Principle,* standard edition. Vol. 17. London, England: Hogarth Press; 1920:7–64.
49. Freud A. *Ego and the Mechanisms of Defense.* New York, NY: International Universities Press; 1949.
50. Deutsch F. *Applied Psychoanalysis.* New York, NY: Grune & Stratton; 1949.
51. Zetzel E. The theory of therapy in relation to a developmental model of the psychic apparatus. *Int J Psycho-analysis.* 1965;46:39–52.
52. Sherrington CS. Cutaneous sensations. In: Schafer EA, ed. *Textbook of Physiology.* Pentland; 1900.
53. Hardy JD, Wolff HG, Goodell H. *Pain Sensations and Reactors.* New York, NY: Williams & Wilkins; 1952.
54. Wall PD, Melzack R. *Textbooks of Pain.* 4th ed., Edinburgh, Scotland: Churchill Livingstone; 1999.
55. Adams RD, Martin JB. Acute and chronic pain: Pathophysiology and management. In: *Harrison's Principles of Internal Medicine.* 10th ed. New York, NY: McGraw-Hill; 1983.

PART I

PAIN: BIOLOGY, ANATOMY AND PHYSIOLOGY

CHAPTER 1 MOLECULAR BIOLOGY OF PAIN

Tony L. Yaksh

"Stimuli become adequate as excitants of pain when they are of such intensity as threatens damage to the skin."
SHERRINGTON (1906)[1]

OVERVIEW

The acute activation of small sensory afferent axons by high-intensity thermal and mechanical stimuli evokes locally organized spinal motor reflexes (nociceptive reflexes), autonomic responses, and pain behavior in animals and humans. This effect is mediated by the local encoding of afferent input at the level of the dorsal horn and the activation of spinofugal projection neurons. These projection systems travel both ipsilaterally and contralaterally in the ventrolateral aspect of the spinal cord, projecting supraspinally into the medulla, mesencephalon, and diencephalon. Medullary projections serve to activate spinobulbospinal reflexes that influence autonomic tone. Other projections into the mesencephalon and thalamus are assumed to contribute to the perceptual and complex emotive and discriminative components of the pain state. It is important to appreciate that the encoding by the sensory afferent and the spinal dorsal horn of the nociceptive stimulus is the first step in nociceptive processing, and this encoding process contributes properties that are important to the understanding of the behavioral correlates of nociception. The following sections consider aspects of the mechanisms whereby injury leads to an ongoing pain state from the perspective of the organization of the sensory afferents and the spinal dorsal horn. Of particular importance is the appreciation that these linkages have distinct pharmacologies and that these systems can be regulated to display prominent increases (hyperalgesia) and decreases (analgesia) in the input-output function.

PRIMARY AFFERENTS

Morphology

Sensory afferents represent the first link between the nervous system and the peripheral milieu. Whether they are enteroceptive organs such as viscera or blood vessels, the meninges, deep structures such as muscle or joint, or the skin, all surfaces are innervated by axons that transduce the local milieu to generate action potentials that provide input to the neuraxis. These primary afferent axons are constituted of the central (root) and peripheral (nerve) projections and the dorsal root ganglion cell body that is connected to the root by a sinuous glomerulus. With the exception of several cranial nerves, all axons have their primary cell body in the dorsal root ganglia that lie outside of the neuraxis proper.[2]

Normal Sensory Afferent Activity

Classification of Sensory Afferents These axons may be classified according to the nature of the peripheral terminals, their size (large or small), state of myelination (myelinated or unmyelinated), and, functionally, according to their conduction velocity (large axons are rapid; small axons are slower) and to the modality of stimulation that most effectively results in activity in the associated axon.

Sensory Nerve Endings It is important to emphasize that the peripheral afferent terminal is an exceedingly specialized region. The terminal provides the transduction properties that convert stimulus of a given modality into a local sodium channel–mediated depolarization that leads to activity in the afferent axon.[3] This degree of depolarization leads to activation of the axon, the frequency of which is proportional to the stimulus intensity. Large axons typically display complex, specialized structures, such as pacinian corpuscles or stretch sensitive organs, that transduce mechanical stimuli and define the nature of the afferent response; for example, a rapidly adapting response in which a continued stimulus may evoke an output when the stimulus is applied and then again when it is removed (i.e., rapidly adapting, as compared with slowly adapting). Small afferents may not display evident specialization and, hence, are commonly referred to as being "free" nerve endings. These free nerve endings are, however, extremely complex, providing a transduction of different modalities and various chemical stimuli.[4]

Effective Stimuli Under normal conditions, the cardinal observation is that sensory afferents show minimal, if any, spontaneous activity. However, the brief application of a peripheral mechanical or thermal stimulus will often evoke intensity-dependent increases in firing rates. As outlined in Table 1-1, recording from fibers identified according to their conduction velocity reveals that large Aβ (group II) fibers are typically activated by low thresholds (i.e., mechanoreceptors). Small, lightly myelinated axons A∂ (group III) fibers that conduct at a lower velocity may belong to populations that are heterogeneous, responding to low or high thresholds, mechanical or thermal. Thus, low-threshold afferents may begin firing at temperatures that are not noxious (30°C) and increase their firing rate monotonically as the temperature rises. Other populations of A∂ fibers may begin to fire at temperatures that are mildly noxious and increase their firing rates up to very high temperatures (52°–55°C). These would be referred to as thermal nociceptors. Small, unmyelinated, slowly conducting afferents (C fiber or group IV) constitute the largest population of sensory axons. The large majority of these small afferents are activated by high-threshold thermal, mechanical, and chemical stimuli and are, therefore, called C-polymodal nociceptors.[5] Accordingly, the afferent input from a given stimulus will reflect on (1) the modality of the stimulus (e.g., thermal, mechanical, or chemical); and (2) the coactivation of several populations of afferents, which transduce that stimulus energy

TABLE 1-1 **Primary Afferents Classed by Conduction Velocity and Physical Nature of the Effective Stimulus**

Fiber Class*	Velocity	Effective Stimuli
Aβ (myelinated) (12–20 μ dia)	Group II (> 40–50 m/sec)	Low-threshold mechanoreceptors Specialized nerve endings (pacinian corpuscles)
Aδ (myelinated) (1–4 μ dia)	Group III (10 < x < 40 m/sec)	Low-threshold mechanical or thermal High-threshold mechanical or thermal Specialized nerve endings
C (unmyelinated) (0.5–1.5 μ dia)	Group IV (< 2 msec).	High threshold thermal, mechanical, and chemical Free nerve endings

*Aβ/Aδ/C is the Erlanger-Gasser classification and refers to axon size; II/III/IV is the Lloyd-Hunt classification and is defined on conduction velocity in muscle afferents. Because of the relationship between size and state of myelination with conduction velocity, these designations are often used interchangeably.

and a discharge frequency that covaries with stimulus intensity over a range reflecting a low versus high stimulus-intensity threshold (Fig. 1-1).

Psychophysical Correlates of Afferent Activity In normal, uninjured tissue, stimuli that give rise to activity in small sensory afferents evoke a psychophysical report of pain sensation in humans and a somatotopically organized escape response in animals (e.g., withdrawal of the stimulated limb). The intensity of the report and the vigor of the escape is typically monotonically correlated with stimulus intensity and, hence, with the frequency of discharge in a given sensory axon. Conversely, electrical activation of Aδ nociceptors produces a short-lasting pricking sensation (first pain), whereas activation of C fibers results in a poorly localized burning sensation (second pain). In the absence of tissue injury, the removal of the stimulus leads to rapid abatement of the afferent input and disappearance of the pain sensation.

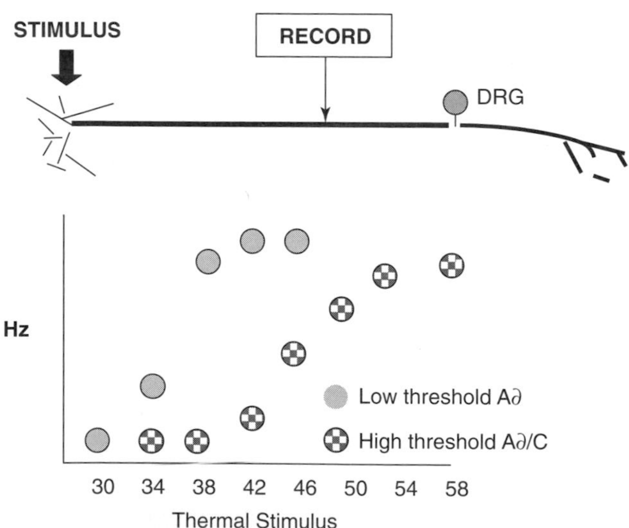

Figure 1-1 (**Top**) Schematic of sensory axon fiber with peripheral nerve ending. (**Bottom**) It is indicated that two types of fibers—low-threshold A∂ and high-threshold A∂ and C fibers—typically show little, if any, spontaneous activity, but show a monotonic increase in response to increasing stimulus intensities. For the high-threshold afferents, the triggering threshold usually reflects temperatures that would correspond to a temperature at which a pain report would be elicited.

Afferent Activity After Tissue Injury

Afferent Response After Tissue Injury If a stimulus produces a local injury, as in a tissue crush or incision, two events are observed to occur.

1. The normally silent sensory afferent begins to display a persistent bursting discharge that continues for an extended interval (minutes to hours) after the injuring stimulus is removed (Fig. 1-2).
2. The stimulus intensity required for activating the otherwise high-threshold afferent may fall significantly, such that otherwise moderately intense stimuli will be highly effective. In effect, this serves to shift the relationship between response (frequency of discharge) and stimulus intensity up, to the left, and increases its slope. The extreme example of this peripheral sensitization is the population of afferent C fibers referred to as silent nociceptors. These afferents are normally only poorly activated by even extreme mechanical stimuli. In the presence of tissue injury or inflammation, these previously silent afferents may develop spontaneous activity and a low mechanical threshold.

Origin of Persistent Afferent Activity The ongoing activity observed after injury originates from the terminal region of the sensory afferent and appears to have two sources:

1. Afferent terminals that are in the vicinity of the injury may develop spontaneous activity, in part because of local damage to the terminal that may result in an increase in local sodium channel activation.
2. A tissue-injuring stimulus will lead to the release of local factors that (a) directly activate the local terminals of afferents (that are otherwise silent), and (b) facilitate the discharge of the afferent in response to otherwise submaximal stimuli (Fig. 1-3). Some of these local factors are enumerated in Table 1-2.

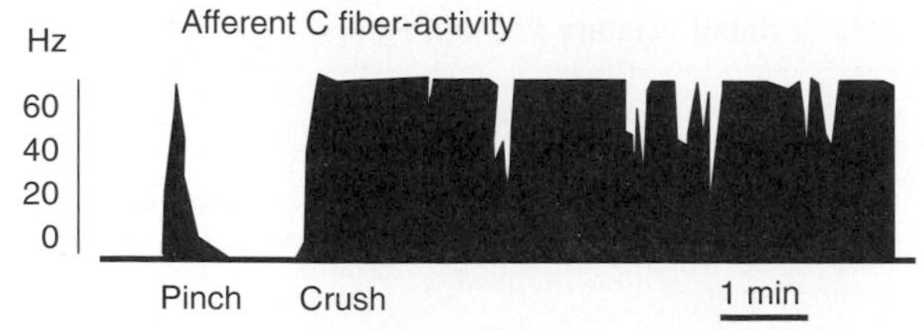

Figure 1-2 Schematic presenting the firing rate to pinch and to tissue crush of a single, small, cutaneous afferent axon. Note that in the absence of stimulation, there is no spontaneous activity in this small afferent axon. After a brief pinch, there is a brief stimulus-linked discharge. Creation of tissue injury by a mechanical crush leads to a prolonged, ongoing discharge.

Importantly, exogenous administration of these products has been shown to directly excite C fibers and facilitate C-fiber firing, resulting in a shift to the left and increased slope of its frequency response curve.[6] For the substances in which it has been examined, these agents, when applied to the skin of humans and animals, usually evoke pain behavior and increase the magnitude of the reported pain response evoked by a given stimulus (hyperalgesia) (Fig. 1-4).[7,8]

In short, peripheral mechanical and thermal stimuli will evoke intensity-dependent increases in firing rates of small afferents, and this response corresponds to the psychophysical report of pain sensation in humans and the vigor of the escape response in animals. Such stimuli may result in local injury and the subsequent elaboration of active products that directly activate the local terminals of afferents (which are otherwise essentially silent) innervating the injury region and facilitate their discharge in response to otherwise submaximal stimuli.

SPINAL SYSTEMS ENCODING SENSORY INPUT EVOKED BY INJURY

Sensory afferents project into the spinal dorsal horn and make synaptic contact with dorsal horn neurons. Two issues pertinent to our understanding of spinal organization should be considered: (1) the organization of the afferent termination in the dorsal horn, and (2) the classes of neurons that receive these projections.

General Organization of the Spinal Dorsal Horn

The spinal cord is divided into several broad anatomic regions (dorsal root entry zone, dorsal horn, and ventral horn; gray and white matter). These regions are further divided on the basis of descriptive anatomy into spinal lamina (Rexed)[9,10] (Fig. 1-5).

Spinal Terminals of Primary Afferents

Spinal Trajectory of Afferent Axons In the peripheral nerve, afferents are anatomically intermixed. As the sensory root approaches the spinal dorsal root entry zone, large afferents tend to move medially, and these displace smaller, unmyelinated afferents laterally.

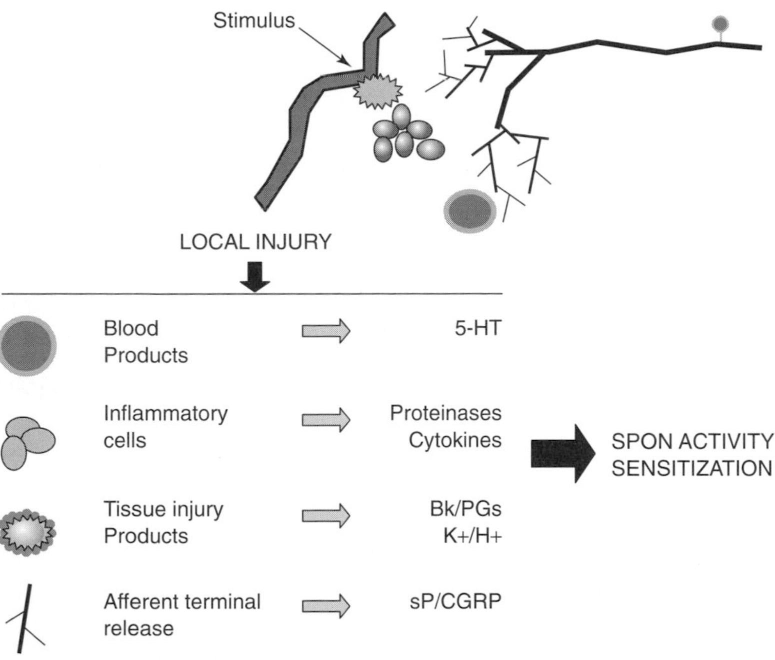

Figure 1-3 Schematic of local organization causing changes in the chemical milieu in the region of a local injury that lead to afferent activation and sensitization. Primary afferent terminal A: Local damaging stimulus leads to activation of the fine sensory afferent (C fiber). Activity proceeds orthodromically to the spinal cord and antidromically to invade local peripheral collaterals. This antidromic activity can depolarize the peripheral terminals and locally release their peptide content. The orthodromic traffic reaches the spinal cord and may serve to produce sufficient local depolarization in the dorsal horn that an antidromic action potential is generated in the terminals of an adjacent sensory axon. The antidromic activity generated by a local axon reflex and by the spinal component invades the distal terminal region locally to release neuropeptides (substance P [sP], calcitonin gene related peptide [CGRP]). Local injury and the released hormones serve to activate local inflammatory cells. Hormones, such as bradykinin, prostaglandins, and cytokines, or K^+/H^+ released from inflammatory cells and plasma extravasation products result in stimulation and sensitization of free nerve endings.

TABLE 1-2 **Classes of Agents Released after Tissue Injury That Influence Activity in Small Primary Afferent Fibers***

Agents	Action
Amines	Histamine (granules of mast cells, basophils, and platelets) and serotonin (mast cells and platelets) are released by a variety of stimuli, including mechanical trauma, heat, radiation, certain byproducts of tissue damage, thrombin, collagen, epinephrine, and members of the arachidonic acid cascade, leukotrienes, and prostanoids.
Kinin	A variety of kinins, notably bradykinin, are released by physical trauma. Peptide is synthesized by a cascade that is triggered by the activation of factor XII by agents such as kallikrein and trypsin. Bradykinin acts by specific bradykinin receptors (B1/B2) to activate free nerve endings.
Lipid acids	Agents are synthesized by lipoxygenase or cyclooxygenase (prostanoids) upon the release of cell membrane–derived arachidonic acid secondary to the activation of phospholipase A_2. A number of prostanoids, including PGE_2, can directly activate C fibers. Others such as PGI_2 and TXA_2, and several leukotrienes, can markedly facilitate the excitability of C fibers. These effects are also mediated by specific membrane receptors.
Cytokines	Cytokines such as the interleukins are formed as part of the inflammatory reaction involving macrophages and have been shown to exert powerful sensitizing effects on C fibers. Interleukins such as Il-1 may sensitive C fibers via a prostaglandin intermediary.
Primary afferent peptides	CGRP and sP are found in and released from the peripheral terminals of C fibers and will produce local cutaneous vasodilation, plasma extravasation, and sensitization in the region of skin innervated by the stimulated sensory nerve.
[H]/[K]	Elevated H^+ (low pH) and high K^+ are found in injured tissue. These ions can directly stimulated C fibers and facilitate the discharge produced by a given stimulus (e.g., hyperalgesia activates the local axon reflex and results in the local release of CGRP, a potent vasodilator and modulator of plasma extravasation). A population of C nociceptors sensitive to noxious intensities of mechanical and thermal stimuli also respond in a stimulus-released fashion to solutions of increasing proton concentration injected into their receptive fields. These receptors develop a lower threshold and enhanced response to mechanical stimuli. Similar injections in humans induce a sustained graded pain and hyperalgesia. Increasing evidence suggests that agents such as capsaicin may interact directly with peripheral terminal membranes to increase proton conductance.
Proteinases	Thrombin or trypsin, among others, are released from inflammatory cells and can cleave tethered peptide ligands that exist on the surface of small primary afferents. These tethered peptide act upon adjacent receptors (PARs) that can serve to depolarize the terminal, causing an orthodromic input and the local release of sP and CGRP into the injured tissues.

CGRP, calcitonin gene–related peptide; PAR, proteinase-activated receptor; PGE_2, prostaglandin E_2; PGI_2, prostaglandin I_2; sP, substance P; TXA_2, thromboxane A_2.
*(6–8).

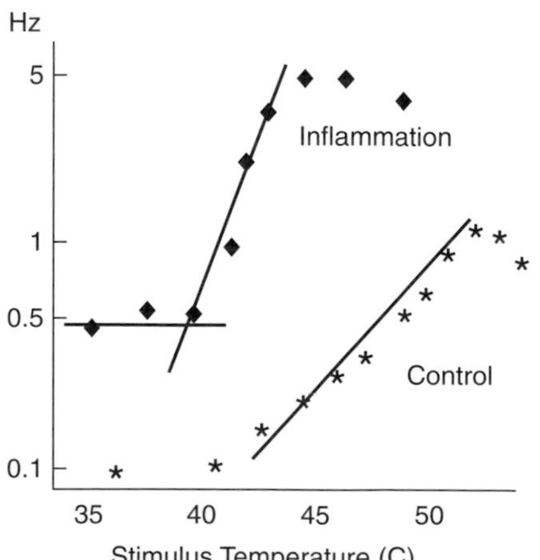

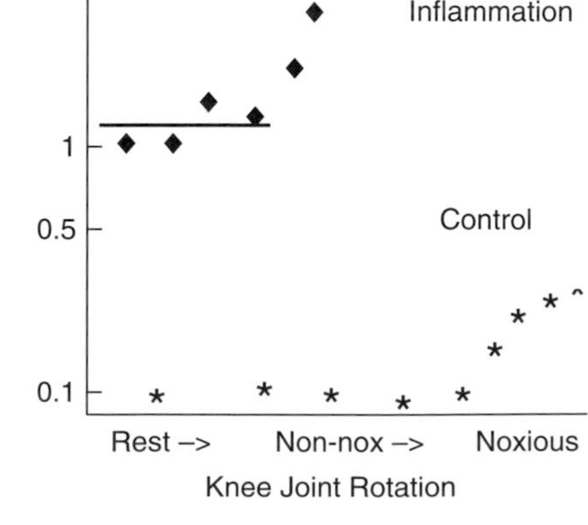

Figure 1-4 Representation of the response of small axons innervating the skin to thermal stimuli before and after the injection of a local inflammatory substance (**left**) and the activity in an afferent to a range of knee joint motion before and after inflammation of the knee joint (**right**). Following the initiation of cutaneous inflammation, the afferent shows increasing spontaneous activity, a left shift, and an increase in the slope in the stimulus-response curve, indicating a facilitated response to the thermal stimulus. In the knee, the articular afferent shows little response to normal rotation and only fires in response to extreme rotation. After the initiation of joint inflammation, even mild rotation results in a significant discharge.

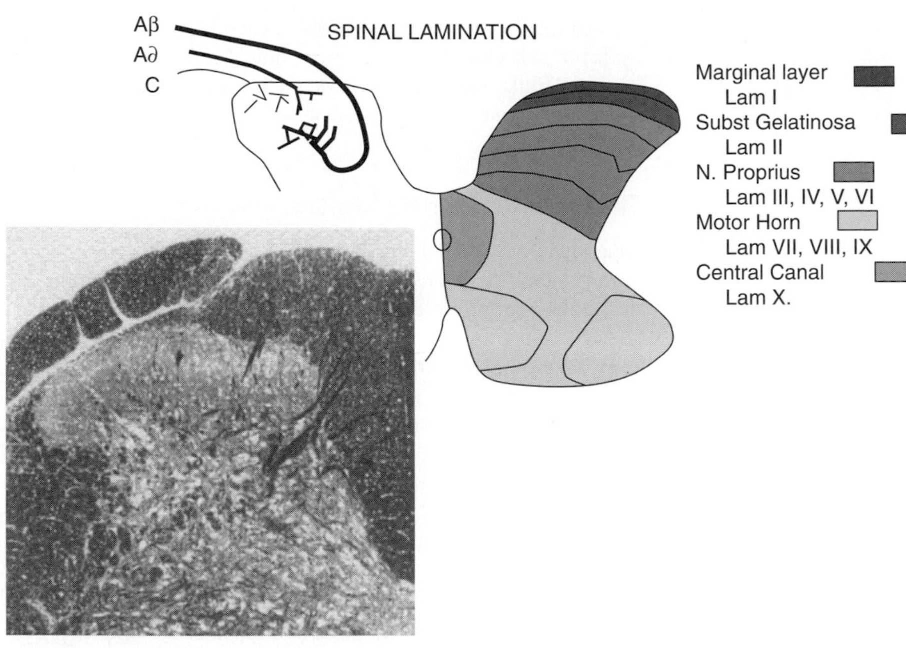

Figure 1-5 Schematic showing the Rexed lamination (**right**) and the approximate organization of the approach of the afferent to the spinal cord (**left**) as they enter at the dorsal root entry zone and then penetrate into the dorsal horn to terminate in laminae I and II (A/C) or penetrate more deeply to loop upward to terminate as high as the dorsum of lamina III (Aβ). Inset in lower left shows histologic appearance of the left dorsal quadrant. Note root entry zone, substantia gelatinosa, and large, myelinated axons.

Upon entering the spinal cord at the dorsal root entry zone, the central processes of the afferents collateralize, sending fibers rostrally and caudally up to several segments in Lissauer's tract (small, C fiber afferents) or in the dorsal columns (large afferents) and into the segment of entry. Upon penetrating into the parenchyma, the terminal fields ramify rostrally and caudally for several millimeters[10] (Fig. 1-6).

Spinal Terminals of Afferent Axons In the spinal cord, terminals from the large, myelinated afferents are found in the deeper laminae (Rexed III–VI). Smaller myelinated fibers terminate in the marginal zone (Rexed lamina I), the ventral portion of lamina II, and throughout lamina III. Small-diameter, unmyelinated fibers (C fibers) largely terminate throughout lamina II and in lamina X around the central canal.

From a functional standpoint, this ramification emphasizes that neurons that lie distal to the segment of entry of the afferent will receive excitatory input. Electrophysiologic studies have shown that whereas the strongest excitation is observed in neurons in the segment of entry, excitation from the L5 root may be observed in cells as far as five to seven segments rostrally. As discussed later in this chapter, factors that alter the excitability of these distant neurons may thus increase the apparent size of the receptive field for a given neuron.[11,12]

Primary Afferent Transmitters

Activation of primary afferents typically induces a postsynaptic excitation. Excitation is mediated by the release of neurotransmitters from the afferent terminal. Considerable effort has been directed at establishing the identity of the excitatory neurotransmitters in the primary afferent. Some of these are listed in Table 1-3.[13]

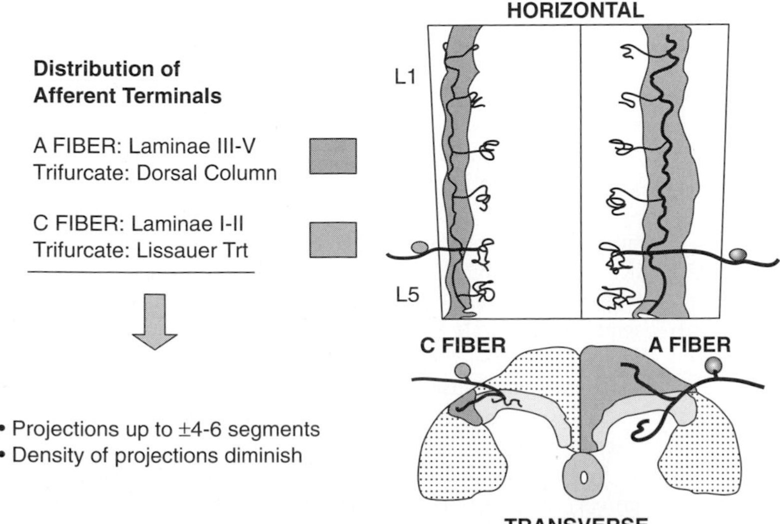

Figure 1-6 Schematic displaying the ramification of C fibers (**left**) into the dorsal horn and collateralization into Lissauer's tract and of Aβ fibers (**right**) into the dorsal columns and into the dorsal horn. Note that the densest terminations are within the segment of entry, and that there are less-dense collateralizations into the dorsal horns at the more distal spinal segments. This density of collateralization corresponds to the potency of the excitatory drive into these distal segments.

TABLE 1-3 **Summary of Several Products Contained and Released from Small Primary Afferents**

Peptides	Excitatory Amino Acids	Other
Substance P	Glutamate	Purines (ATP)
Calcitonin gene–related peptide	Aspartate	
Galanin		
Vasoactive intestinal polypeptide		
Somatostatin		

ATP, adenosine triphosphate.

Characteristics of Primary Afferent Transmitters A number of properties characterize the transmitters that are contained in and released from the primary afferent. Peptides and glutamate have been shown to exist within subpopulations of small, type B dorsal root ganglion cells (giving rise to C fibers) and are in laminae I and II of the dorsal horn of the spinal cord, where the majority of primary afferent terminals are found (Fig. 1-7). These levels in the dorsal horn are reduced by rhizotomy or ganglionectomy, or both, or by treatment with the small afferent neurotoxin, capsaicin.

Many peptides present in large dense core vesicles (e.g., substance P and calcitonin gene–related peptide) as well as excitatory amino acids in small, clear core synaptic vesicles (glutamate) are present in and released from the same terminal. Iontophoretic application onto the dorsal horn of the several amino acids and peptides found in primary afferents has been shown to produce excitatory effects. Amino acids produce a very rapid, short-lasting depolarization. Peptides produce a delayed and long-lasting depolarization. Local spinal administration of several agents, such as substance P and glutamate, does yield pain behavior, suggesting their possible role as transmitters in the pain process.[14]

A large proportion of nociceptive dorsal horn neurons are contacted by substance P–containing terminals. Administration of noxious, but not innocuous, stimulation to the tissue results in release of several of these peptides into the spinal dorsal horn. With regard to the excitatory amino acids, their release has been evoked by acute and chronic nociceptive stimuli, including joint inflammation. Unlike the peptides, amino acids are also present in large primary afferents, and their spinal release can also be induced by activation of Aβ fibers.

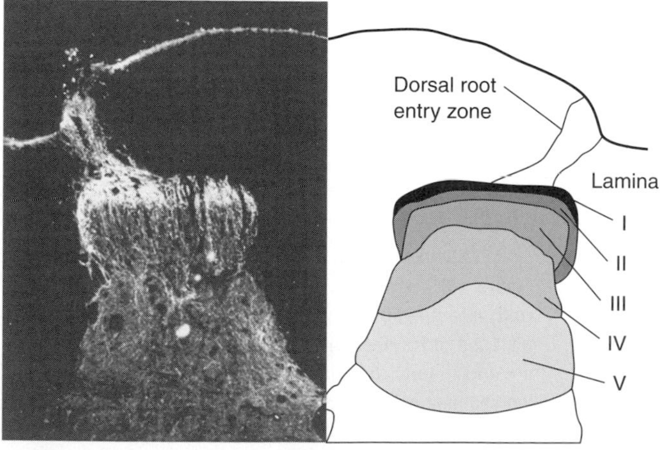

Figure 1-7 Histochemistry showing distribution of substance P immunoreactivity in laminae I and II (substantia gelatinosa) of the dorsal horn.

Classes of Dorsal Horn Neurons

Anatomically, dorsal horn neurons may be broadly described in terms of their location (marginal layer, substantia gelatinosa, and the nucleus proprius), size (small, magnocellular), and functional response properties and neurochemistry. The complexity of this region accordingly cannot be overstated. For practical purposes related to nociceptive processing, it is reasonable to consider the functional properties of two principal classes of neurons. Electrophysiologic recording from single neurons in the spinal dorsal horn reveals several populations that are activated by high-intensity stimuli: nociceptive-specific (marginal cells) and wide-dynamic range (lamina V neurons) (Fig. 1-8).

Nociceptive-specific Neurons Marginal neurons, located in lamina I of the dorsal horn, are large neurons that are oriented transversely across the cap of the dorsal gray matter and receive input from small unmyelinated and lightly myelinated afferents (see Fig. 1-5). Some project to the thalamus via ipsilateral and contralateral ascending pathways, and others project intra- and intersegmentally along the dorsal and dorsolateral white matter. Populations of these neurons respond selectively to intense cutaneous and muscle stimulation. Whereas some are modality specific (e.g., firing in response only to thermal or mechanical stimuli), others respond to both types of stimuli. Activity in these subpopulations of neurons provides an unambiguous message that nociceptors have activated. Other prominent cell types in lamina I include (1) thermoreceptive "cool" cells that are activated and inhibited by innocuous cooling and warming, respectively, and (2) heat, pinch, and cold cells that are similar to traditional marginal cells but also are excited by noxious cold.[15]

Wide-dynamic-range (WDR) Neurons The cell bodies of lamina V cells are located in the nucleus proprius of the dorsal horn and send their apical dendrites up into laminae II and III (see Fig. 1-8). An important property of these cells is that they receive convergent input from a variety of functionally distinct primary afferents.[16] Practically, there are three kinds of convergence.

1. Fiber response properties. As indicated schematically in Figure 1-8, WDR-type cells receive input both from large, typically low-threshold afferents that project deep into the dorsal horn and from small, typically high-threshold afferents that project only into laminae I and II. As suggested schematically, some of this input, particularly that which is superficial, is mediated by excitatory interneurons. These WDR cells accordingly display a graded increase in the frequency of response to stimuli that are progressively more intense and recruit increasingly higher threshold populations of afferents Aβ to A∂ and C. This convergence thus permits these single cells to integrate input activated by a wide range of stimuli that vary in intensity, with higher frequency firing being noted as stimulus intensity rises.

2. Spatial convergence. As outlined in Figure 1-6, earlier, primary afferents entering a specific segment have their primary excitatory input on dorsal horn neurons in that segment of entry. Still, it is clear that such axons can collateralize and mediate an

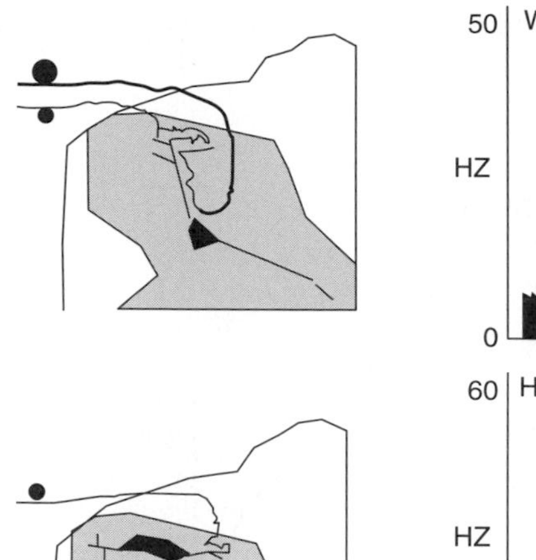

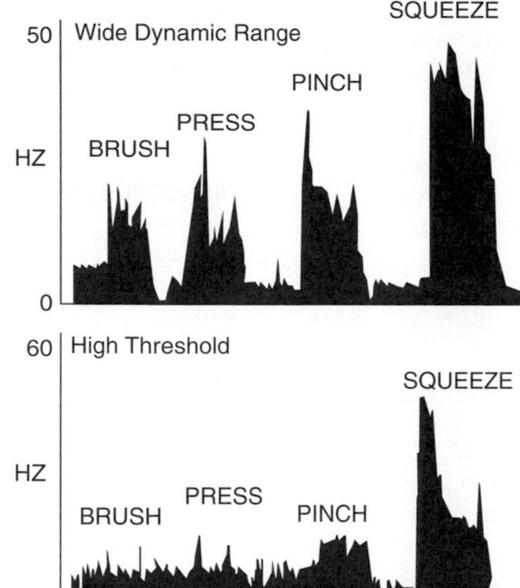

Figure 1-8 Schematic representing the morphology and dendritic pattern (**left**) of a lamina V – wide-dynamic-range neuron (**top**) and a lamina I, marginal neuron (**bottom**). The firing patterns of the respective classes of neurons are indicated in the representation on the right, in which a post-stimulus time histogram shows the frequency of firing in response to four, graded, mechanical stimuli ranging from innocuous (brush/press) to noxious (pinch/squeeze).

excitatory effect on cells that lie in distal dermatomes. Accordingly, the size of the dermatome of that segment is actually larger than the peripheral distribution of the afferents in the root of that respective segment. As noted later in this discussion, it is likely that the size of the receptive field of a given neuron may be increased by conditions that lead to an enhancement of its excitability as inputs that are relatively weak become able to drive activity in that now "sensitized" spinal neuron.

3. Organ convergence. Depending on the spinal level, a WDR neuron can be activated by input traveling with the sympathetics (e.g., as activated by distention of hollow viscera [bladder, small intestine, and gallbladder), injection of bradykinin into the mesenteric artery, close intraarterial administration of bradykinin or the injection of hypertonic saline into muscle/tendon, or group III afferent stimulation from the gastrocnemius. The same WDR neuron can thus be excited by cutaneous or deep (muscle and joint) input applied within the dermatome that coincides with the segmental location of these spinal cells. Thus, stimulation of the skin and muscles of the left shoulder and upper arm (T_1–T_5 dermatome) activates WDR neurons that are also excited by coronary artery occlusion. These results indicate that the phenomenon of *referred* visceral pain, for example, has its substrate in the anatomic convergence of input from viscera, muscle, and skin onto the same populations of dorsal horn neurons.[17]

Ascending Spinal Tracts

Clinical experience based on local spinal lesions of the ventrolateral quadrant suggests that pain is a "crossed" pathway with relevant projections traveling in the contralateral ventrolateral white matter. Midline myelotomies that destroy fibers crossing the midline at the levels of the cut produce bilateral pain deficits. These observations suggest that the relevant pathways for nociception are predominantly crossed. Similarly, stimulation of the ventrolateral tracts in awake subjects undergoing percutaneous cordotomies results in reports of contralateral warmth and pain. In accord with these observations, tract-tracing studies and electrophysiologic investigations emphasize that activity evoked in the spinal cord by high-threshold stimuli reaches supraspinal sites by several long and tract systems that travel within the ventrolateral quadrant[18] (Fig. 1-9).

Spinoreticular Fibers Spinoreticular axons originating in laminae V through VIII terminate ipsilaterally and contralaterally to

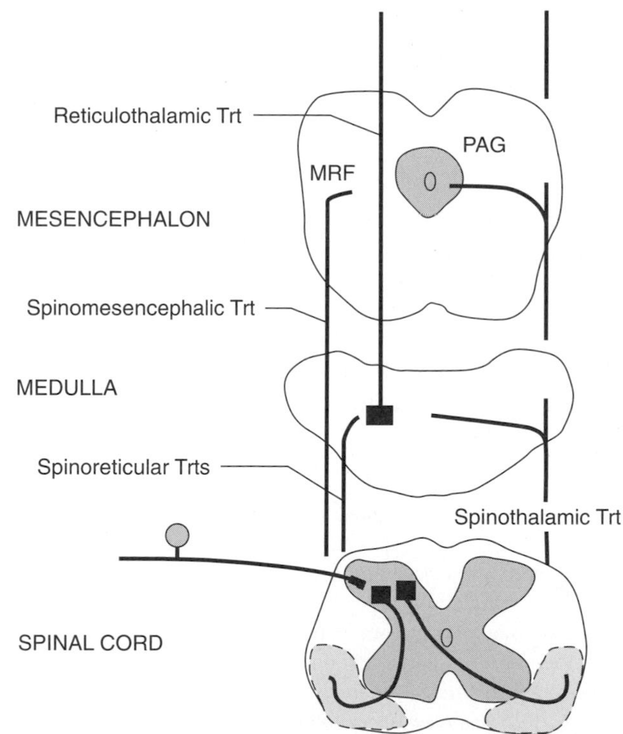

Figure 1-9 Schematic demonstrating the ascending crossed projections from dorsal horn neurons into the brainstem (spinoreticular) and into the thalamus (spinothalamic). The ventrobasal thalamus receives somatically mapped input from the spinal cord and projects this input into the somatosensory cortex, where the somatotopy is preserved. Other projections go to the medial thalamus and, from there, to a variety of limbic forebrain sites.

their spinal site or origin. In the medulla, the fibers aggregate laterally, and collaterals of these fibers terminate in the more medially situated brainstem reticular nuclei. Reticulothalamic afferents excited by this input then project to the thalamus.

Spinomesencephalic Fibers Spinomesencephalic tracts originate primarily in lamina I, with a smaller component from laminae VI through VIII and X. They project into the mesencephalic reticular formation and the lateral periaqueductal gray matter.

Spinothalamic Fibers The cells of origin of this tract, the most extensively studied of the ventrolateral tract systems, are not limited to the dorsal gray matter, but are found throughout laminae I through VII and X of the spinal gray matter. Axons originating in the marginal layer and the neck of the nucleus proprius ascend predominantly in the contralateral ventral quadrant. Spinothalamic axons differentiate into a lateral and medial component in the posterior portion of the thalamus: the medial component passes through the internal medullary lamina to terminate in the nucleus parafascicularis, and the intralaminar and paralaminar nuclei. The majority of fibers pass laterally to terminate throughout the nucleus ventralis posterolateralis, the medial aspect of the posterior nucleus complex, and the intralaminar nuclei. A significant proportion of the neurons projecting laterally in the thalamus (ventral posterior lateral complex) also project to the medial (central lateral nucleus or dorsal medial nucleus) portion (Fig. 1-10).

Suprathalamic Projection Projections to higher centers include specific mapping of input from the ventrobasal complex into the somatosensory cortex and multiple outputs particularly from the medial and intralaminar nuclei projects diffusely to wide areas of the cerebral cortex, including the frontal, parietal, and limbic regions. Positron emission tomographic (PET) scanning studies in humans have confirmed that noxious stimuli will activate the appropriate cortical regions in the somatosensory cortex and limbic regions such as the anterior cingulate gyrus[19] (see Fig. 1-10).

Significance of Ascending Pathways: Sensory-discriminative and Affective-motivational

Early thinking made the useful conjecture that pain could be considered in terms of two principal components: the sensory-discriminative and the affective-motivational components.[20] An important question is whether this functional distinction finds parallels in the underlying physiology and connectivity of the substrates thus far examined as being relevant to nociceptive processing.

At present, it is appreciated that the WDR neurons typically project into the ventrobasal thalamus, where their input is mapped precisely onto a sensory homunculus. These cells then project rostrally to the somatosensory cortex, where that input is similarly mapped onto a sensory homunculus.

In this system, each site on the body surface is faithfully mapped, and this map is maintained to the cortex. This system is uniquely able to preserve anatomic information and information regarding the intensity of the stimulus (as initially provided by the frequency response characteristics of the WDR neuron). This system is able to provide the information necessary for mapping the *sensory-discriminative* dimension of pain.

On the other hand, it has become evident that marginal, nociceptive-specific neurons also project contralaterally into the thalamus. This input thus provides one aspect of a circuit that appears to be activated by only particularly intense stimuli. This input function is defined by the response properties of the spinal marginal cell. It might be speculated that this circuit may underlie the *affective-motivational* component of the pain pathway.

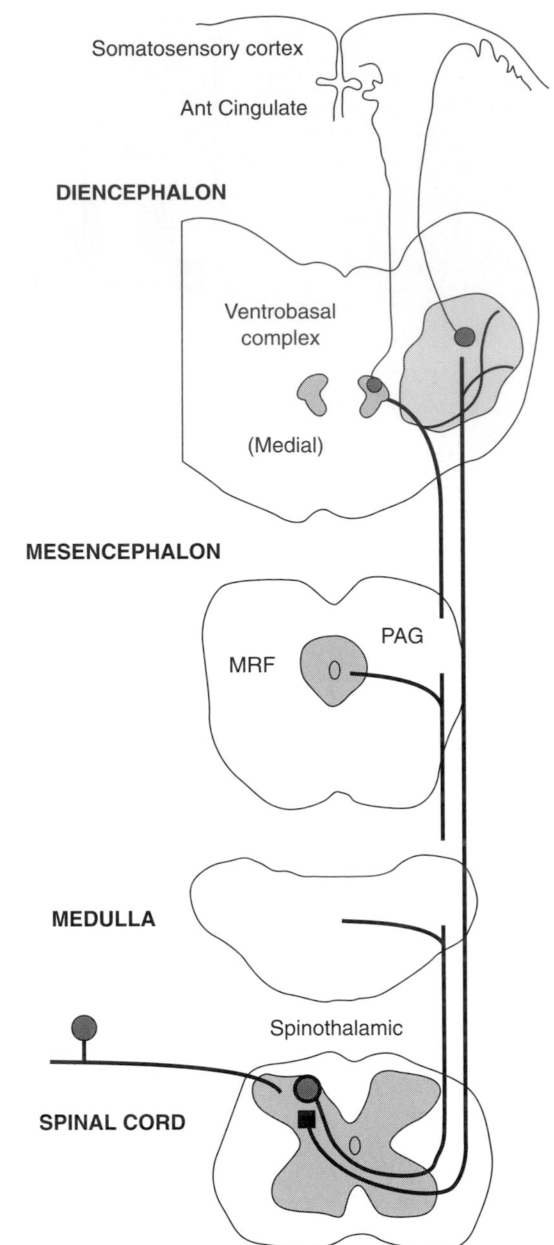

Figure 1-10 Sensory input into the spinal cord leads to the local activation of complex linkages that eventually project rostrally in the contralateral-ventrolateral pathways to medullary and diencephalic structures. In this schematic organization, it is emphasized that these ascending projections provide input in the lateral thalamus, which is somatotopically organized and projects from there into the somatosensory cortex. Importantly, a significant portion of the ascending traffic travels medially and makes synaptic contact in these medial regions with ascending projections that travel to the limbic cortex, such as the anterior cingulate cortex. Organizationally, it has been suggested that these different projection targets reflect upon substrates that underlie the "sensory-discriminative" and "affective-motivational" aspects of the pain experience.

The preceding recitation of the pathways through which afferent information evoked by high-threshold information travels reflects what traditionally is known as the pain pathway. In fact, this schematic, although correct, vastly oversimplifies the true organization. At every synapse, the transmission through the dorsal horn and brainstem is subject to significant modulation.

In some instances, it is believed that the modulation may serve to diminish the pain message (i.e., endogenous analgesic systems). However, as subsequently discussed, there are several circumstances in which repetitive afferent drive results in the involvement of an active facilitation of the message. In other cases, the non-aversive nature of large afferent stimulation (Aβ) is non-noxious, because of the continued presence of small inhibitory interneurons that have no effect on activity in C fibers.

DYNAMIC ASPECTS OF ENCODING OF INJURY-GENERATED INPUT

The preceding section emphasized that tissue injury yielded activity in small primary afferents and that small afferent input resulted in monosynaptic and polysynaptic excitation of dorsal horn neurons that projected to the brainstem and higher centers. Importantly, the pathway appears to preserve several properties of the stimulus, the anatomic sign (localization), and intensity. Thus, input from an area of skin might be expected to activate a given population of spinal neurons that received afferent input from that part of the body surface, and the intensity of the stimulus was mirrored either by the specific neuronal population activated (e.g., nociceptive specific cells) or by the frequency of the discharge (as with the WDR neurons), or both. This linkage, even in its simplest form, would be described as the "pain pathway," as it reflects the connectivity by which afferent traffic generated by tissue injury reaches higher centers and the conscious state. This afferent substrate, in fact, represents only one component of the system that is essential to the processing of nociceptive input. The excitation of dorsal horn neurons evoked by small afferent input is subject to modulation by a number of receptor systems within the spinal cord. Technically, this modulation may be thought of in terms of those systems that increase or decrease the efficacy of synaptic connections of the afferent pathway.

Plasticity of the Encoding of Persistent Afferent Input

Acute activation of small afferents by high-intensity mechanical or thermal stimuli will result in a clearly defined pain behavior in humans and animals. This event is believed to be mediated by the release of the excitatory afferent transmitters outlined earlier and, consequently, the depolarization of projection neurons. The magnitude of the response of a dorsal horn neuron, either WDR or nociceptive specific, is related to the frequency (and identity) of the afferent input.

The frequency of the afferent input is proportional to the magnitude of the acutely applied stimulus. The organization of this system's response to an acute stimulus is thus typically modeled in terms of a monotonic (linear) relationship between activity in the peripheral afferent and the activity of neurons that project out of the spinal cord to the brain.

As previously noted, in the face of tissue injury, the afferent input is characterized by a persistent afferent barrage. As discussed subsequently, such input reveals the initiation of a variety of inhibitor and facilitatory processes that lead to a nonlinear increase in spinal output.

Intrinsic Inhibitory Processes

The activation of dorsal horn neurons by afferent input can be attenuated by several discrete systems.

Large Afferent Axon Interactions Dorsal horn WDR neurons can be inhibited by transient activation of large primary afferents. Such inhibition is mediated by a local spinal circuit that produces primary afferent depolarization (PAD), which exerts an inhibitory effect on the terminals of adjacent afferents. This serves to reduce the amount of neurotransmitter released from the afferent fibers in response to a fixed input. PAD is mediated by release from local interneurons in the substantia gelatinosa of the inhibitory amino acids, γ-aminobutyric acid (GABA) and glycine.[21] In human psychophysical studies, vibratory stimuli applied to a painful area served to activate large myelinated fibers and reduced perception of chronic musculoskeletal pain. Dorsal column stimulation by antidromically activating collaterals of large primary afferent fibers would also induce PAD, and this mechanism may account for some of the antinociceptive actions of dorsal column stimulation.

It is important to appreciate that the presence of these small inhibitory interneurons is important for the ongoing encoding of large afferent input. Thus, the spinal action of $GABA_A$ and glycine receptor inhibitors will induce a potent tactile allodynia. These results suggest that the nonaversive characteristics of large afferent stimulation depend on this ongoing modulation. Studies in nerve injury–induced pain states have suggested that there is a loss of glycine or GABAergic inhibition secondary to the loss of dorsal horn neurons. The reduction in such inhibition may provide a partial explanation of the potent allodynia that accompanies such nerve injury states.

Bulbospinal and Spinal Modulation Considerable evidence indicates that a variety of spinal terminal systems may serve to attenuate small, afferent-evoked excitation. Early work demonstrated that activation of bulbospinal pathways would suppress spinal nociceptive processing and produce a behaviorally defined analgesia by the release of noradrenaline and the activation of dorsal horn α_2 receptors. Evidence that small afferent activation could indirectly activate systems that mediated the spinal release of hormones, such as enkephalin or noradrenaline, which could act at such modulatory receptors supported the perspective that nociceptive processing was under a tonic endogenous inhibition. In spite of the observation that activating these receptors (e.g., spinal injection of opiate and α_2 agonists) could yield a powerful analgesia by an action pre- and postsynaptic to the small afferent terminal, the delivery of antagonists for these receptors has surprisingly modest effects on spontaneous pain thresholds. This suggests that however potent a modulatory system these several receptors represent, these endogenous systems are not in a tonically active mode, and downregulation of small afferent input is not a pervasive component of the ongoing processing of input generated by tissue injury.[22]

Intrinsic Facilitatory Processes: Repetitive Small Afferent Input

WDR neurons in the spinal and medullary dorsal horn display a stable response to the discrete, periodic activation of afferent C fibers. However, repetitive stimulation of C (but not A) fibers at a moderately faster rate results in a progressively facilitated discharge. This facilitated response is called "wind-up" (see Fig. 1-9). This condition has three properties:

1. The conditioning serves to enhance the response of the dorsal horn neuron to subsequent input, such that a given stimulus yields a greater response that would otherwise be anticipated from that stimulus.
2. The conditioning of the spinal cord with repetitive small afferent stimulation has the additional effect of increasing the receptive field size of the neuron. Thus, afferent input from dermatomal areas that previously did not activate the WDR neuron being studied now evokes a prominent response. The anatomic substrate for this increased receptive field size is believed to reflect the otherwise weak excitatory input that comes from collaterals of afferents innervating the skin areas adjacent to the injury. In the face of the induction of a facilitated state in the specific neuron under study, this otherwise ineffective excitatory drive becomes adequate to drive depolarization. Intracellular recording reveals that the facilitated state reflects a progressive and sustained partial depolarization of the cell, rendering the membrane increasingly susceptible to afferent input.
3. Low-threshold tactile stimulation also becomes increasingly effective in driving these neurons. This facilitation by repetitive C fiber input, therefore, increases the subsequent neuronal response to low-threshold afferent input, and enhances the response generated by a given noxious afferent input. These mechanisms are discussed further in the next sections.

Wind-up and Central Facilitation

In animal studies, WDR neurons in the dorsal horn display a stimulus-dependent response to discrete activation of afferent C fibers. Repetitive stimulation of C (but not A) fibers at a moderately faster rate results in a progressively facilitated discharge.

The exaggerated discharge was dubbed wind-up by Mendell[23] (Fig. 1-11). Intracellular recording has indicated that the facilitated state is represented by a progressive and long-sustained partial depolarization of the cell, rendering the membrane increasingly susceptible to afferent input.[24]

Given the likelihood that WDR discharge frequency contributes to the encoding of a high-threshold stimulus as aversive, and that many of these WDR neurons project through the ventrolateral quadrant of the spinal cord (i.e., spinobulbar or spinothalamic projections), this augmented response is believed to be an important component of the pain message. In addition, the conditioning of the afferent input as described has the added effect of increasing the receptive field size of the neurons, such that afferent input from dermatomal areas that previously did not activate the WDR neuron now evokes a prominent response. Moreover, low-threshold tactile stimulation also becomes increasingly effective in driving these neurons.

This facilitation by repetitive C-fiber input, therefore, increases the subsequent neuronal response to low-threshold afferent input, enhances the response generated by a given noxious afferent input, and increases the size of the receptive field at which a stimulus can evoke activity in that neuron. Given the likelihood that WDR discharge frequency is part of the encoding of the intensity of a high-threshold stimulus, and that many of these WDR neurons project in the ventrolateral quadrant of the spinal cord (i.e., spinobulbar projections), this augmented response is believed to be an important component of the pain message.

The enhanced responsiveness reflects an augmented sensitization of the neuronal membrane leading to an enhanced response for a given depolarization. The pharmacology leading to this sensitization is examined in the discussion that follows. The enlarged receptive field is believed to reflect, in part, on the collateral input from distal segments (see Fig. 1-6). In the presence of sensitization, these distal inputs that exert a degree of excitation that is otherwise inadequate to activate the neuron will become sufficient. This combination of spinal events results in an apparent increase in the size of the neuronal receptive field.

Functional Correlates of Injury-evoked Central Facilitation

Protracted pain states, such as those that may occur with inflamed or injured tissue (leading to the peripheral release of active factors), would routinely result in such an augmented afferent drive of the WDR neuron and, thence, to the ongoing facilitation. Such observations are consistent with the speculation that the afferent C-fiber burst may initiate long-lasting events, resulting in changes in spinal processing that will alter the response to subsequent input. The preceding observations regarding this dorsal horn system have been shown to have behavioral consequences. This phenomenon has clear functional correlates.

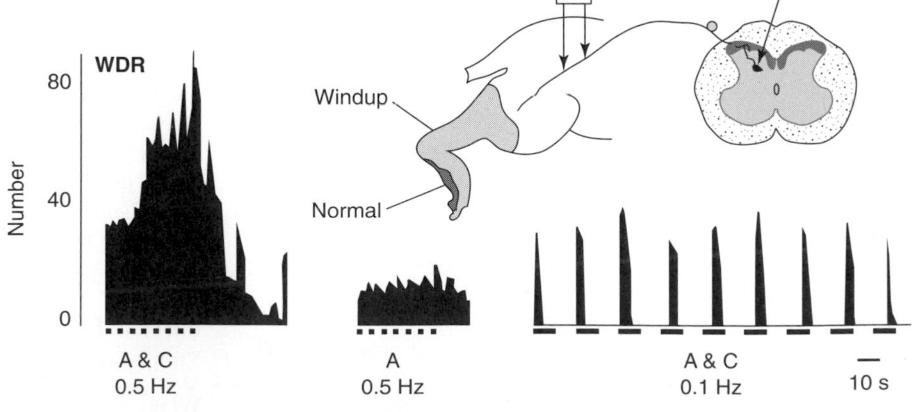

Figure 1-11 Schematic showing a single unit recording from wide-dynamic-range neurons in response to an electrical stimulus delivered at 0.1 Hz (**right**). A very reliable, stimulus-linked response is evoked at this frequency. In contrast, when the stimulation rate is increased to 0.5 Hz, there is a progressive increase in the magnitude of the response generated by the stimulation (**left**). This facilitation results from the C-fiber input and not an A-fiber input (**middle**) and is called "wind-up."

Studies in animals have shown that the acute injection of an irritant such as formalin will induce an acute afferent barrage followed by a prolonged low level of afferent activity. During this later period after formalin injection, WDR dorsal horn neurons show an unexpected level of activity, given the modest afferent input (e.g., a central facilitation). Finally, examination of behavior has shown that the animal displays an exaggerated response (flinching) during the second phase, consistent with the activity in dorsal horn neurons but, again, greater than might be anticipated based on the afferent traffic[25] (Fig. 1-12).

The role of this afferent-evoked facilitation in the postinjury pain state cannot be minimized. After tissue injury, in animals and in humans, inflammation and cellular/vascular injury lead to the local peripheral release of active factors. Such active factors will produce a prolonged activation of C fibers that evoke a facilitated state of processing in WDR neurons, and, thence, an ongoing facilitation of nociceptive perception. Such observations are consistent with the speculation that the afferent C-fiber burst may initiate long-lasting events, resulting in changes in spinal processing, which will alter the response to subsequent input.

The relevance of this C-fiber–evoked facilitation to humans has been emphasized by psychophysical studies. To observers, the activation of C fibers by the intradermal injection of capsaicin will lead to an initial pain state followed for an extended period of time by a large region of profoundly enhanced mechanical and thermal sensitivity.[26] This phenomenon is referred to as secondary hyperesthesia (Fig. 1-13). Thus, in humans, following local injury where C-fibers are similarly activated, there is every reason to believe that similar processes apply and that important components of the post-injury pain state are the events consequent to the afferent barrage and not, strictly speaking, the input present in the post-injury phase.

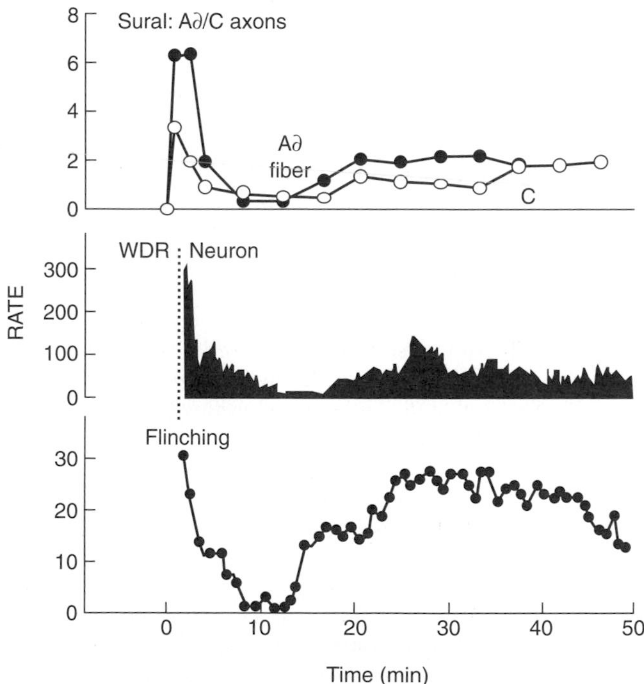

Figure 1-12 C-fiber activity (firing rate/sec; **top**) measured in the sural nerve of the anesthetized rat; firing of wide dynamic range neuron (anesthetized rat; **middle**) and number of flinches in the unanesthetized rat (**bottom**) measured before and after the ipsilateral subcutaneous injection of formalin into the hind paw at the time indicated by the vertical dashed line. Note the low level of input during the second phase, in which behavior suggestive of pain is particularly high. Importantly, the second phase of the formalin test persists in spite of the animal being deeply anesthetized during the first phase.

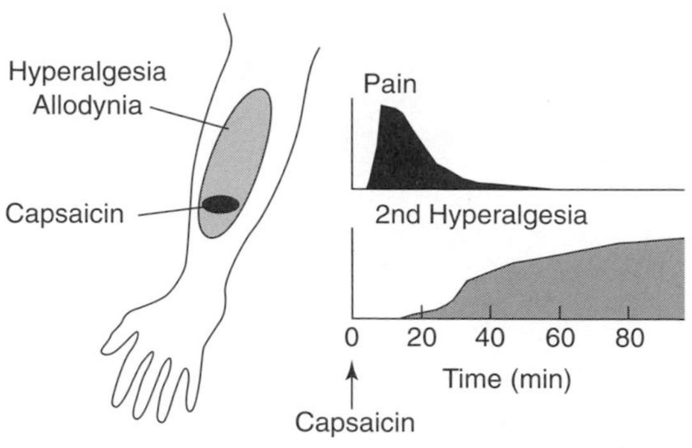

Figure 1-13 Schematic illustrating the effects of injecting the C-fiber stimulant, capsaicin, under the skin. This generates an intense local pain sensation that persists for about 20 to 30 minutes. This sensation diminishes, and it is possible to demonstrate that the patient/observer reports a large area of secondary hyperalgesia that persists for hours. Importantly, if the area of the injection is anesthetized with local anesthetic prior to capsaicin delivery, then when the initial capsaicin effect is gone and the local anesthesia reverses, the observer reports no secondary allodynia.

Pharmacology of Central Facilitation

The pharmacology of this central facilitation suggests that the wind-up state reflects more than simply the repetitive activation of a simple excitatory system. The first real demonstration of this unique pharmacology was presented by showing that the phenomenon of spinal wind-up was prevented by the spinal delivery of antagonists for the *N*-methyl-D-aspartate (NMDA) receptor[27] (Fig. 1-14). Importantly, this agent had no effect on acute evoked activity, but reduced the wind-up. Subsequent behavioral work demonstrated that such drugs had no effect on acute pain behavior, but reduced the facilitated states induced after tissue injury.

Protracted pain states, such as those that may occur with inflamed or injured tissue (leading to the peripheral release of active factors), will routinely result in such an augmented afferent drive of the WDR neuron and, thence, to an ongoing facilitation (such as the wind-up described in Fig. 1-14, for example). Such observations are consistent with the speculation that the afferent C-fiber burst may initiate longer lasting events, resulting in changes in spinal processing that will alter the response to subsequent input. The pharmacology of the central facilitation suggests that the state of central facilitation reflects more than the repetitive activation of a simple excitatory system. Based on studies examining the spinal pharmacology of the electrophysiologic and behavioral response to the postinjury stimulus state, it has become apparent that the arrival of the first small afferent barrage appears to trigger a cascade of events that serve to facilitate the response to subsequent peripheral stimuli.

Aspects of the complex pharmacology of central facilitation in the dorsal horn are presented in Fig. 1-15. The following points may be made that define components of spinal systems involved in the postinjury pain state. For review purposes, the cascade may be thought of in terms of primary and secondary systems.

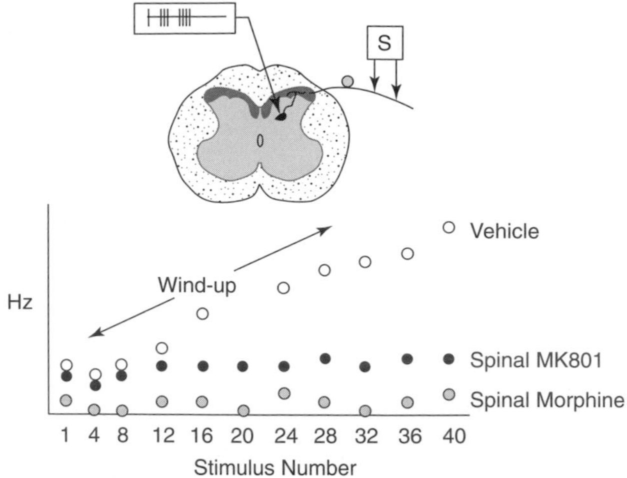

Figure 1-14 Repetitive C-fiber stimulation was repeated 40 times at 2 Hz, and the response of a spinal wide-dynamic-range (WDR) neuron was counted. As indicated under control conditions, there was a progressive increase in the number of discharges counted with each subsequent stimulus. Addition of morphine resulted in a block of the initial C-fiber–evoked discharge, and there was no subsequent increase. In contrast, the delivery of *N*-methyl-D-aspartate (NMDA) antagonists resulted in no change in the initial discharge, but prevented the subsequent wind-up.

Primary Systems The initial activation generated by small afferent input is mediated by specific primary afferent transmitters. Primary afferent C fibers release peptide (e.g., substance P, calcitonin gene–related peptide, and others) and excitatory amino acid (glutamate) products. These substances evoke excitation in second-order neurons.

Substance P Receptors The spinal delivery of substance P results in a mild acute "pain behavior" and a subsequent reduced response latency to thermal stimuli (thermal hyperalgesia). These effects are believed to be mediated by neurokinin 1 (NK-1) receptors that are located in the superficial dorsal horn on second-order neurons. Blockade of the NK-1 receptor by intrathecal antagonists or downregulation of NK-1 receptor expression by intrathecal treatment with NK-1 receptor mRNA antisense has little effect on acute nociceptive thresholds, but reduces the facilitated state and behaviorally defined hyperalgesia (as in the second phase of the formalin test) induced by peripheral injury.[29]

Glutamate Receptors For glutamate, direct monosynaptic excitation of the second-order neuron is believed to be mediated by the ionotrophic non-NMDA (AMPA) receptors (i.e., acute primary afferent excitation of dorsal horn neurons is not mediated by the NMDA receptor). The spinal delivery of agonists for the alpha-amino-3-hydroxy-5-methyl-4-isoxazole propionic acid and NMDA receptors will evoke a potent spontaneous pain behavior and a subsequent hyperalgesia and tactile allodynia.[30]

Opiates targeted at the spinal cord serve to block the release of transmitter from C fibers by acting presynaptically on the terminals of C fibers to prevent the opening of voltage-sensitive calcium channels responsible for the depolarization-evoked release of terminal transmitters. Opioid receptors have been demonstrated to be present on small afferent terminals, with the highest density of opioid binding present in the substantia gelatinosa.

Secondary Systems Following the initial excitation, it is appreciated that the spinal dorsal horn displays a prominent facilitation of its input-output function. This central facilitation represents a cascade that is initiated by the ongoing afferent drive.

Glutamate As indicated earlier, wind-up as evoked by repetitive small afferent input is diminished by NMDA receptor antagonists. Repetitive small afferent input (as occurs after tissue injury) will evoke spinal glutamate release (see Fig. 1-14). Blockade of spinal AMPA receptors by intrathecal antagonists will elevate acute nociceptive thresholds, as well as the first and second phase of the formalin test. In contrast, intrathecal NMDA antagonists have little effect on acute nociception, but diminish facilitated states of processing. It is appreciated that the channel associated with the NMDA receptor is blocked by normal resting physiologic levels of magnesium, and so no change in excitability of the neurons possessing NMDA receptors can occur until this is removed (Fig. 1-16). The magnesium block is only removed by a shift in the membrane voltage toward depolarization. Thus, the binding of glutamate to the receptor alone is insufficient to activate the channel. The receptor channel complex is unique because of this dual requirement: the channel is gated by both ligand binding to the receptor, and by the membrane voltage. An added degree of complexity is that glycine is a required coagonist with glutamate for activation of the receptor, acting at a strychnine-insensitive site closely associated with the NMDA receptor. Thus, for the NMDA receptor channel to operate, certain conditions need to be met: the release and binding of glutamate and the binding of glycine at the strychnine-insensitive site on the NMDA ionophore are needed, together with a non-NMDA–induced depolarization to remove the tonic magnesium block. C-fiber stimulation will induce the release of glutamate but also with excitatory peptides, and the latter may provide the required depolarization. Hence, as noted in the discussion that follows, the events mediated by NMDA-receptor activation occur secondary to an initial conditioning input. Mechanistically, the NMDA receptor is a Ca^{2+} ionophore that, when activated, will lead to a significant increase in intracellular Ca^{2+}. As emphasized later, it is in part due to this increase in intracellular Ca^{2+} that the cascade initiated by repetitive afferent input is initiated.[31]

Prostaglandins Cyclooxygenase is found in the spinal dorsal horn and inhibitors, and prostaglandin-receptor antagonists given intrathecally will diminish hyperalgesia induced in the postinjury pain state. This reaction reflects on the important role of prostaglandins released from the spinal cord. Dialysis of the spinal cord has emphasized that in the postinjury pain state, there is an increase in prostaglandin E_2 release. Prostanoids will facilitate release of C-fiber transmitters such as substance P. Consistent with the observation that NMDA antagonists can block a hyperalgesic state, spinal NMDA agonists evoke a hyperalgesic state, and this hyperalgesia is blocked by spinal cyclooxygenase inhibitors. Such observations suggest that spinal NMDA-receptor occupancy can evoke the release of prostanoids that, in turn, augments spinal nociceptive processing.[32]

It is currently appreciated that there are two cyclooxygenase enzymes. The present data emphasizes that the cyclooxygenase-2 (COX-2) isozyme is constitutively in the spinal cord, and it is

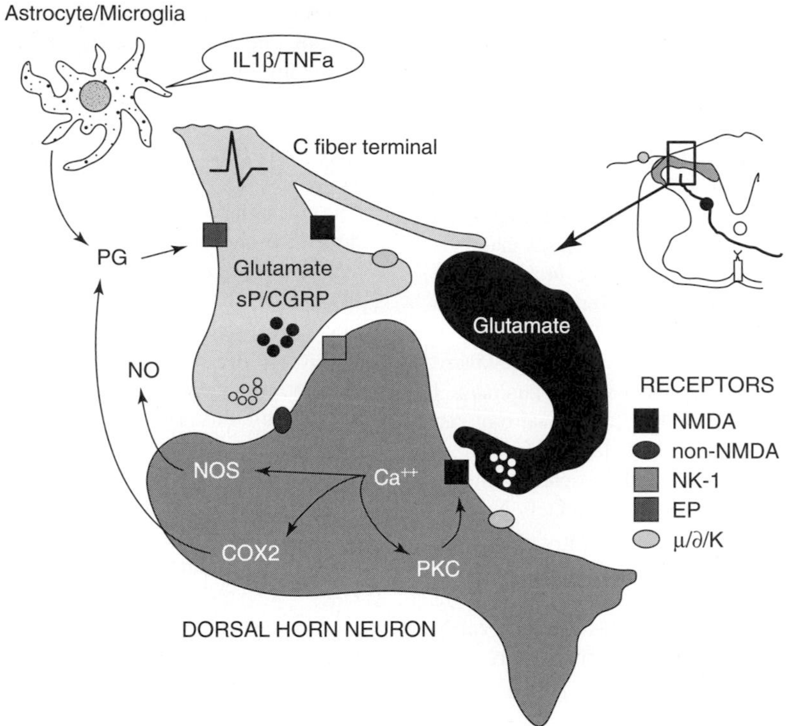

Figure 1-15 Schematic summarizing the organization of dorsal horn systems that contribute to the processing of nociceptive information. (1) Primary afferent C fibers release peptide (e.g., substance P [sP], calcitonin gene–related peptide [CGRP], and so on) and excitatory amino acid (glutamate) products. Small dorsal root ganglion (DRG) cells, as well as some postsynaptic elements contain nitric oxide synthase (NOS) and are able, upon depolarization, to release NO (nitric oxide). (2) Peptides and excitatory amino acids evoke excitation in second-order neurons. For glutamate, direct monosynaptic excitation is mediated by non–*N*-methyl-D-aspartate (NMDA) receptors (i.e., acute primary afferent excitation of WDR neurons is not mediated by the NMDA or neurokinin 1 [NK-1] receptor). (3) Interneurons excited by afferent barrage induce excitation in second-order neurons via an NMDA receptor. This leads to a marked increase in intracellular Ca^{2+} and the activation of kinases and phosphorylating enzymes. Prostaglandins (PG) generated by cyclooxygenase-2 (COX-2) and NO by NOS are formed and released. These agents diffuse extracellularly and facilitate transmitter release (retrograde transmission) from primary and nonprimary afferent terminals, either by a direct cellular action (e.g., NO) or by an interaction with a specific class of receptors (e.g., EP receptors for prostanoids). (4) Non-neuronal sources of prostaglandins may include activated astrocytes and microglia that are stimulated by circulating cytokines, which are lease secondary to peripheral injury and inflammation. Terminal excitability can be altered by activation of a variety of receptors located on the sensory terminal, including those for μ, ∂, and κ opioids. See text for other details.[28]

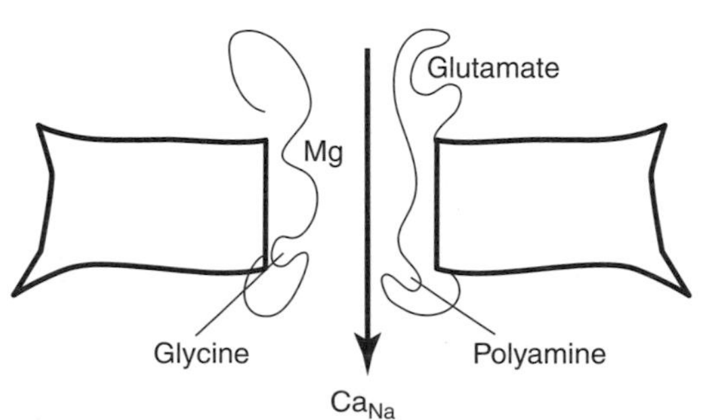

Figure 1-16 As indicated in the text, the *N*-methyl-D-aspartate (NMDA) receptor is a Ca^{2+} ionophore that, when activated, results in an influx of Ca^{2+}. To be activated, the receptor requires the occupancy by glutamate, the removal of the Mg block by a mild membrane depolarization, and the occupancy of the "glycine site," along with several allosterically coupled elements, including the "polyamine site." Together, these events permit the ionophore to be activated.

COX-2 that is primarily responsible for the prostaglandin E_2 release generated by small afferent input.

An additional interesting variant, suggested in Figure 1-15, is that COX-2 (and likely other proteins) expression may be elevated by circulating factors, released by inflammation and septic process, such as interleukin-1β, tumor necrosis factor-α, and lipopolysaccharide, that activate spinal astrocytes and microglia. Such activation may lead to an enhanced expression of a variety of enzymes (such as COX-2), channels, and receptors. The relevance of this non-neuronal expression in the central nervous system is not certain, but these cells may serve as a source of neuraxial prostaglandins. Such material would likely result in an enhanced release from neuronal terminals. It suggests an additional and intriguing role played by the central COX-2 isozyme and its selective inhibitors. Interestingly, these factors are believed to work on terminals that may lie distant from the site of synthesis and release. As such, they are referred to as volume transmitters.[33]

Nitric Oxide (NO) Small dorsal root ganglion cells as well as some postsynaptic elements contain NO synthase (NOS). NOS inhibitors given intrathecally will diminish hyperalgesia induced by intrathecal NMDA and by the postinjury pain state. Increased citrulline (a product of NO formation) is released from the spinal cord in the postinjury pain state. NO has been shown to facilitate terminal release of glutamate.[34]

Kinases and Phosphorylation Increasing intracellular $Ca^{2+}{}_I$ — through the inositol 1,4,5-triphosphate (IP_3) pathway by neurokinin receptor or by the influx of Ca^{2+} through voltage-gated Ca^{2+} channels or ionophores (NMDA receptor)—activates kinases that phosphorylate and phosphatases that dephosphorylate local proteins. Phosphorylating enzyme systems consist of several classes of kinases that are distinguished by the structure and pharmacology of their inhibitors. In the spinal dorsal horn, mitogen-activated kinases (e.g., MAP kinases), cAMP-dependent kinase, and camkinase II have been observed in the spinal dorsal horn and dorsal root ganglia. Protein kinase C (PKC) consists of a large family of isozymes. Although some or all of the previously noted phosphorylating enzymes may play a role, the use of inhibitors for protein kinase A (PKA) and PKC have shown the particular importance of this family of kinases in regulating spinal facilitation. Many hyperalgesic states are mediated by a spinal NMDA receptor. The NMDA receptor is multiply phosphorylated by PKA and PKC. Intrathecal delivery of PKC inhibitors has been shown stereospecifically to diminish injury induced-hyperalgesia.[35,36]

System Interaction

After local tissue injury, the components of posttissue injury pain reflect an increased receptive field and a left shift in the stimulus response curve for spinal dorsal horn neurons that is evoked initially and then sustained in part by persistent small afferent input. The contribution of these changes in spinal function to the behaviorally relevant nociceptive state is substantiated by comparing the pharmacology associated with the effects on the behavior of the unanesthetized animal with the effects of the drugs on the underlying electrophysiology. Based on such observations, it is possible to formulate a heuristic picture of the organization of several pharmacologically defined spinal systems that mediate the response of the animal to a strong and tissue-injurious stimulus. Thus, repetitive afferent input increases excitatory amino acid and peptide release from primary afferents that serve initially to depolarize dorsal horn neurons. Persistent depolarization serves to increase intracellular calcium, activating a variety of intracellular enzymes (COX-2, NOS) and various kinases (PKC). Prostaglandins and nitric oxide are released spinally and serve acutely to enhance the subsequent release of afferent peptides and glutamate. Activation of local kinases serves to phosphorylate membrane receptors and channels. As an example, the NMDA receptor when phosphorylated displays an enhanced calcium flux (see Fig. 1-5). The role of these system-level changes in spinal nociceptive processing in "pain behavior" is supported by the analgesic effects of spinally delivered agents known (1) to reduce small afferent transmitter release (μ, ∂ opioid, and α_2-adrenergic agonists) and the antihyperalgesic actions of spinally delivered neurokinin-1 and NMDA-receptor antagonists, as well as inhibitors of spinal COX-2, NOS, and PKC.

It is important to note that the WDR-wind-up studies discussed earlier are carried out in animals that are under 1 minimum alveolar concentration anesthesia. The relevance of the observations to the performance of surgery on volatile "anesthetized" patients is clear. The implication of the afferent-evoked facilitation is that it is better to prevent small afferent input than to deal with its sequelae. This is believed to represent the basis of the consideration of the use of preemptive analgesics.[37]

CONCLUSION

The preceding comments have provided a general overview of components of the neuraxis that contribute to the encoding of the pain state. It is clear that there are a number of discrete substrates through which such information generated by a high-intensity stimulus may travel. It is equally clear that the process of encoding is plastic and the through-put function at every level is subject to alteration, which can significantly modify the message generated by a given stimulus. The developing appreciation of this complex biology has been briefly touched on here, but it can be appreciated that this complex pharmacology provides an increasing number of venues whereby afferent input can be regulated. This basic concept provides particular hope that the selective regulation of pain states may be achieved.

REFERENCES

1. Sherrington CS. *The Integrative Action of the Nervous System.* New Haven, Conn: Yale University Press; 1906.
2. Myers RR, Olmarker K. Anatomy of DRG, intrathecal nerve roots, and epidural nerves with emphasis on mechanisms of neurotoxic injury. In: Yaksh TL, ed. *Spinal Drug Delivery.* Amsterdam, Netherlands: Elsevier Science BV; 1999.
3. Waxman SG, Cummins TR, Dib-Hajj S, et al: Sodium channels, excitability of primary sensory neurons, and the molecular basis of pain. *Muscle Nerve* 1999;22:1177–1187.
4. Myers RR. Morphology of the peripheral nervous system and its relationship to neuropathic pain. In: Yaksh TL, Lynch C III, Zapol WM, et al, eds. *Anesthesia: Biologic Foundations.* Philadelphia, Pa: Lippincott-Raven; 1997.
5. Raja SN, Meyer RA, Campbell JN. Transduction properties of the sensory afferent fibers. In: Yaksh TL, Lynch C III, Zapol WM, et al, eds. *Anesthesia: Biologic Foundations.* Philadelphia, Pa: Lippincott-Raven; 1997.
6. Dray A. Pharmacology of peripheral afferent terminals. In: Yaksh TL, Lynch C III, Zapol WM, et al, eds. *Anesthesia: Biologic Foundations.* Philadelphia, Pa: Lippincott-Raven; 1997.
7. Schaible HG, Grubb BD. Afferent and spinal mechanisms of joint pain. *Pain* 1993;55:5–54.
8. Watkins LR, Wiertelak EP, Goehler LE, et al. Characterization of cytokine-induced hyperalgesia. *Brain Res* 1994;654:15–26.
9. Rexed B. The cytoarchitectonic organization of the spinal cord in the cat. *J Comp Neurol* 1952;96:415–495.
10. Kerr FW. Neuroanatomical substrates of nociception in the spinal cord. *Pain* 1975;1:325–356.
11. Shortland P, Wall PD. Long-range afferents in the rat spinal cord. II. Arborizations that penetrate grey matter. *Philos Trans R Soc Lond B Biol Sci* 1992;337:445–455.
12. Wall PD, Shortland P. Long-range afferents in the rat spinal cord. 1. Numbers, distances and conduction velocities. *Philos Trans R Soc Land B Biol Sci* 1991;334:85–93.
13. Sorkin LS, Carlton SM. Spinal anatomy and pharmacology of afferent processing. In: Yaksh TL, Lynch C III, Zapol WM, et al, eds. *Anesthesia: Biologic Foundations.* Philadelphia, Pa: Lippincott-Raven; 1997.
14. Yaksh TL, Malmberg AB. Central pharmacology of nociceptive transmission. In: Wall P, Melzack R, eds. *Textbook of Pain.* 4th ed. Edinburgh, Scotland: Churchill Livingstone; 1999.
15. Craig AD, Krout K, Andrew D. Quantitative response characteristics

of thermoreceptive and nociceptive lamina I spinothalamic neurons in the cat. *J Neurophysiol* 2001;86:1459–1480.

16. Willis WD, Westlund K. Neuroanatomy of the pain system and of the pathways that modulate pain. *J Clin Neurophysiol* 1997;14:2–31.
17. Cervero F. Mechanisms of acute visceral pain. *Br Med Bull* 1991;47: 549–560.
18. Hodge CJ Jr, Apkarian AV. The spinothalamic tract. *Crit Rev Neurobiol* 1990;5:363–397.
19. Schnitzler A, Ploner M. Neurophysiology and functional neuroanatomy of pain perception. *J Clin Neurophysiol* 2000;17:592–603.
20. Melzack R, Casey KL. Sensory, motivational, and central control determinants of pain: A new conceptual model. In: Kenshalo D, ed. *The Skin Senses.* Springfield, Ill: Charles C Thomas; 1968:423–443.
21. Rudomin P, Schmidt RF. Presynaptic inhibition in the vertebrate spinal cord revisited. *Exp Brain Res* 1999;129:1–37.
22. Fields HL. Pain modulation: Expectation, opioid analgesia and virtual pain. Review. *Prog Brain Res* 2000;122:245–253.
23. Mendell LM, Wall PD. Responses of single dorsal cord cells to peripheral cutaneous unmyelinated fibers. *Nature* 1965;206:97–99.
24. Woolf CJ, Thompson SW. The induction and maintenance of central sensitization is dependent on *N*-methyl-D-aspartic acid receptive activation; implications for the treatment of post-injury pain hypersensitivity states. *Pain* 1991;44:293–299.
25. Yaksh TL, Ozaki G, McCumber D, et al. An automated flinch detecting system for use in the formalin nociceptive bioassay. *J Appl Physiol* 2001;90:2386–2402.
26. LaMotte RH, Torebjork HE, Robinson CJ, et al. Time-intensity profiles of cutaneous pain in normal and hyperalgesic skin: A comparison with C-fiber nociceptor activities in monkey and human. *J Neurophysiol* 1984;51:1434–1450.
27. Dickenson AH, Sullivan AF. Evidence for a role of the NMDA receptor in the frequency dependent potentiation of deep rat dorsal horn nociceptive neurones following C fibre stimulation. *Neuropharmacology* 1987;26:1235–1238.
28. Yaksh TL, Hua X-Y, Kalcheva I, et al. The spinal biology in humans and animals of pain states generated by persistent small afferent input. *Proc Natl Acad Sci USA* 1999;96:7680–7686.
29. Saria A.The tachykinin NK1 receptor in the brain: Pharmacology and putative functions. *Eur J Pharmacol* 1999;375:51–60.
30. Madsen U, Stensbol TB, Krogsgaard-Larsen P. Inhibitors of AMPA and kainate receptors. *Curr Med Chem* 2001;8:1291–1301.
31. Klein RC, Castellino FJ. Activators and inhibitors of the ion channel of the NMDA receptor. *Curr Drug Targets* 2001;2:323–329.
32. Svensson CI, Yaksh TL. The spinal phospholipase-cyclooxygenase-prostanoid cascade in nociceptive processing. *Annu Rev Pharmacol Toxicol* 2002;42:553–583.
33. Watkins LR, Milligan ED, Maier SF. Glial activation: A driving force for pathological pain. *Trends Neurosci* 2001;24:450–455.
34. Sorkin LS. NMDA evokes an L-NAME sensitive spinal release of glutamate and citrulline. *Neuroreport* 1993;4:479–482.
35. Akinori M. Subspecies of protein kinase C in the rat spinal cord. *Prog Neurobiol* 1998;54:499–530.
36. Zhuo M. Silent glutamatergic synapses and long-term facilitation in spinal dorsal horn neurons. *Prog Brain Res* 2000;129:101–113.
37. Wilder-Smith OH. Pre-emptive analgesia and surgical pain. *Prog Brain Res* 2000;129:505–524.

CHAPTER 2 ANATOMY AND PHYSIOLOGY OF PAIN

Hilary J. Fausett

Understanding the anatomy and physiology of pain transmission systems is important for the pain management specialist. Injuries to these areas may cause the common pain syndromes for which patients seek help (e.g., diabetic neuropathy, postherpetic neuralgia). Interventions at distinct anatomic sites may provide the relief the patient seeks (nerve blocks, implantable devices). And ongoing research may reveal new modalities or pharmaceutical agents to provide relief, such as the cyclooxygenase-2 (COX-2) inhibitors. This chapter is designed as an overview for the clinician and not as a comprehensive review of the anatomy and physiology of the nervous system, about which textbooks have been written.

This chapter reviews the transmission of a nociceptive or pain impulse from the site of stimulus in the periphery to the central nervous system. The basic anatomic pathways of nociceptive transmission and of descending nociceptive modulations are described. Some of the basics of physiology also are discussed, with the assumption that the reader is knowledgeable about the fundamentals of neuronal transduction, such as action potential propagation and the relationship of the cell body to the dendrites and axon. Although some mention of pathophysiology and disease states is made, for further discussion, please see the specific chapters in this book.

This chapter focuses on the ability of the nervous system to transmit and modulate nociceptive stimuli. The studies reviewed here likely apply more to acute pain than to chronic pain. Although there is intense interest in developing an animal model of chronic pain, most of the experimental paradigms used are more closely analogous to the injury of acute pain than chronic pain. The latter is both a physical and emotional entity and may result from plasticity in the nervous system.[1] The complexities of chronic pain syndromes, including such theories as chronic pain as a variant of depressive disorders,[2] are discussed elsewhere.

Knowledge of nociceptive transmission has advanced considerably since Descartes outlined his concept of the nerve as tubes with delicate threads to convey a painful impulse.[3] It is now widely believed that stimulation of a primary afferent neuron in the peripheral nervous system results in activation of neurons in the dorsal horn of the spinal cord and then in transmission rostrally to the brain.

PRIMARY AFFERENTS

Sensory neurons, called primary afferents, have a cell body in the dorsal root ganglia (DRG) of the spinal cord or in the ganglia of the cranial nerves. Cranial nerves V, VII, IX, and X receive inputs from primary afferents and, thus, sensory information from the head, face, and throat. Cells in the DRG are a heterogenous population of size and function; a reflection of the heterogeneity of the sensory inputs processed by the central nervous system.[4]

This heterogeneity is reflective of the multiple functions of the peripheral sensory nervous systems, as well as the supportive function of the glial system. The classic nomenclature of peripheral neurons relies on the size of the axon and presence or absence of myelin as distinguishing characteristics. This taxonomy is referred to as the Erlanger-Gasser classification.[5] There are three major groups, A, B, and C, in order of diminishing axonal diameter. Group A is further divided into four subgroups: Aα, or primary muscle spindle and motor to skeletal muscles; Aβ, which are cutaneous touch and pressure afferents; Aγ, motor to muscle spindle; and Aδ, which are mechanoreceptors, nociceptors, thermoreceptors, and sympathetic postganglionic fibers. Group B is sympathetic preganglionic fibers. Group C refers to mechanoreceptors, nociceptors, and thermoreceptors, as well as sympathetic postganglionic fibers.

Classification of primary afferents on the basis of size and morphology is convenient for scientific experimentation, and thus there has been interest in refining the Erlanger-Gasser classification.[4] Most pain management practitioners are familiar with the traditional classification and are acquainted with the terms *A*δ and *C fibers* as pain transmission fibers. Neuronal fibers have also been classified, again on the basis of the size of the cross-section of the axon, as type Ia/b, II, III, and IV, from large myelinated to smaller and more slowly conducting fibers. Because this more recent terminology is used less often by clinicians, in this chapter the terminology more familiar to clinicians is used.

Thus, the sensory neurons of greatest interest to the pain clinician are the Aδ and C fibers, which have cell bodies in the DRG and which project from the periphery to the dorsal horn of the spinal cord (or the equivalent area for the cranial nerves).[6] The morphology of the peripheral termination of the axon is a reflection of the neuron's function: mechanoreceptors end in specialized structures, whereas nociceptors have free endings. Although the majority of Aδ fibers respond to low-intensity mechanical, chemical, or thermal stimuli, the free nerve endings of the Aδ and C-type neurons likely allow the specialized response to hazardous, potentially dangerous, and damaging stimuli.[7] It may be an evolutionary protective mechanism to have fibers respond to the threat of damage and thus avoid the possibility of permanent injury.[8] There is evidence that chronic pain may be related to central nervous system changes.[9] This chapter focuses primarily on the anatomy and physiology of acute pain in the undamaged nervous system.

The nociceptive primary afferents supply all the areas of the body: skin and subcutaneous tissue; muscle, joints, and periosteum; and the viscera. The skin, subcutaneous tissue, and fascia are supplied by mechanical nociceptors (Aδ high-threshold mechanoreceptors,) polymodal nociceptors (C-fiber nociceptors), and myelinated mechanothermal nociceptors (Aδ heat nociceptors).[10] The latter respond to both noxious heat and intense mechanical stimuli. It is likely that these Aδ fibers are responsible for the first pain perceived after heat stimulation.[4,6,7] This is in contrast to the high-threshold Aδ mechanoreceptors, which respond to repeated stimuli and not to the initial noxious stimulus of heat or cold. These fibers are likely responsible for sensitization.[11] The C-polymodal nociceptors, which also respond to high-intensity stimuli, whether mechanical or heat, respond by sensitizing to heat but, interestingly, the response to mechanical stimuli is fatigue.[9,12]

The unique properties of these neurons account for the variety of responses seen to noxious stimuli, both clinically and experimentally. Brief noxious input results in an immediate but transient sensation that is mediated by Aδ fibers. The same stimulus also evokes a slow-onset burning pain sensation that is C-fiber dependent.[9,13] Following injury, endogenous nerve growth factor and impulse-sensitive neuronal mechanisms are needed to regulate collateral sprouting of sensory axons in rats.[14] Microneurography allows studies to be conducted in humans.[15] Thus, the properties postulated from animal studies are now being shown experimentally in humans, and the potential for further diagnostic applications is intriguing.[16]

Muscle, fascia, and tendons are innervated by Aδ and C fibers. Activation of these neurons by noxious stimulation produces diffuse, aching pain that is poorly localized. Ischemic contraction of muscle may result in C-fiber activation. The muscle nociceptors are also activated by chemical stimulation.[17] Joints are innervated by Aδ and C fibers, which, when activated in a normal joint, result in deep aching pain. In an arthritic joint or during acute inflammation, however, even normal and minimal activities result in pain. There is significant interest in the pathogenesis of arthritis and the interaction between inflammatory changes and the development of chronic pain.[18]

The periosteum of bone is acutely sensitive to noxious stimuli, whereas the marrow and cortex of the bone are not pain responsive under normal conditions.[16] Teeth are innervated by nociceptive and mechanical afferents. Both the inner and outer aspects of the tooth are innervated. The tooth pulp has a mixed population of afferents and responds to chemical, thermal, and mechanical stimuli.[19,20]

The viscera are innervated by nociceptors as well as parasympathetic and sympathetic fibers. In contrast to cutaneous innervation, visceral structures are sparsely innervated so that few fibers respond to stimuli over a large area.[21] Whether specific organs have specifics nociceptors is still controversial.[7] Clinically, patients are likely to complain of diffuse discomfort or poorly localized pain except under conditions of extremes (e.g., appendicitis, pleurisy). Very often, even extreme perturbations are interpreted as discomfort rather than pain (e.g., acute myocardial infarction). There is evidence of convergence of deep somatic (muscle, joints) and visceral nociceptive information at higher midbrain structures.[22] This finding may also contribute to the poor localization of noxious stimuli.

The heart has Aδ fibers (and some C fibers), which appear to be responsive to stretch but function primarily as part of the cardiovascular reflex responsiveness, more than as an early warning sign of potential damage. The classic pain of myocardial ischemia, angina, is postulated to be mediated via chemical sensitization of afferents by substances released by the damaged cells (potassium, hydrogen ions) as well as humoral factors (bradykinin and prostaglandins).[10,12]

The lungs and bronchi are also innervated by Aδ and C fibers. These fibers play a diverse role, serving to warn of irritants in the airway that are either mechanical or chemical. Furthermore, such distinct stimuli as pulmonary edema, embolism, and changes in oxygen tension may give rise to the sensation of dyspnea.

The abdominal viscera include such diverse structures as the stomach and intestines, gallbladder, and urinary bladder. These structures have sympathetic and parasympathetic innervation. Mechanoreceptors also innervate these hollow viscera. The mechanoreceptors transmit changes such as distention and contractions associated with pain. There is currently a great deal of interest in understanding visceral nociception.[21,22] Controversy abounds in the clinical realm of pain management as to the etiology of visceral pain states. For example, the innervation of the viscera includes sympathetic and parasympathetic fibers, but whether certain chronic abdominal pain syndromes are sympathetically maintained pain syndromes is not proven. (See Chapters 34 and 39.)

Chronic pelvic pain and interstitial cystitis are two common clinical manifestations of visceral pain states. Both syndromes may be disabling to patients and are frustratingly difficult to treat. The urinary system has both nociceptive and sympathetic innervation. Distention may lead to C-fiber activation as well as Aδ involvement.[23] These stimuli, such as with a renal stone entering a ureter, may lead to intense cramping and pain. The reproductive system is highly innervated with slowly adapting mechanoreceptors and more sparsely innervated by Aδ and C fibers.[23] Mechanisms do exist, however, so that repeated noxious stimuli may result in sensitization. (See subsequent chapters for more details and for discussion of clinical pain states and therapies.)

The primary afferents, which have their cell bodies in the DRG, extend from the periphery to terminate centrally in the dorsal horn. The fibers that enter the dorsal horn are segregated by size as they form small bands or rootlets and approach the dorsal horn. Lissauer observed that the smaller fibers are segregated laterally and then terminate in the first layers of the dorsal horn. This area has come to be known as Lissauer's tract. There are clinical applications of knowledge of the anatomy of the dorsal horn and dorsal root entry zone. Neurosurgeons may perform a selective posterior rhizotomy in the hopes of ablating otherwise intractable, unrelenting chronic pain. These techniques are discussed further in the chapters on clinical pain management.

It is important to note that many cells in the DRG have more than one process.[24] Thus, a fiber may receive input from two distinct areas, such as the dura mater and part of the face. The connections that appear to subserve sensory processing during migraine, for example, are complex.[25] The terminal connections may also branch and innervate multiple spinal levels.[26] There is also evidence that sensory fibers may travel in the ventral roots, as well. There are certainly small unmyelinated fibers in ventral tracts. Thus, the anatomy is more complex than a simple schema can represent. These complexities may explain why selective posterior rhizotomy is rarely successful clinically in providing complete relief of unrelenting pain. But as understanding of the peripheral nervous system grows, so does an appreciation of its complexity. Injury to peripheral nerves may result in chronic changes. Initial injury and acute changes may develop into chronic ectopic inputs, which may induce a state of central sensitization and structural reorganization of dorsal horn synapse.[11] Thus, there are profound physiologic reasons why a surgical anatomic approach to pain management may not be sufficient.

The majority of primary afferents terminate in the ipsilateral dorsal horn. The process of the spinal neurons bifurcates into an ascending and a descending branch, thus innervating the spinal cord over several spinal segments. Some processes travel dorsal to the central canal to end in the contralateral dorsal horn. The terminus of each primary afferent is the reflection of its function, as the dorsal horn neurons are segregated by physiology. Rexed divided the gray matter of the spinal cord into ten laminae.[27] This classic cytoarchitectural segregation yields six subdivisions of the dorsal horn (laminae I through VI) and three subdivisions of the ventral horn (laminae VII through IX.) Lamina X describes the column of cells around the central canal.

The dorsal laminae of the spinal cord run its entire length and in the medulla become the medullary dorsal horn. The marginal layer of the dorsal horn refers to lamina I. Lamina II, or the substantia gelatinosa, is subdivided into outer and inner areas (IIo and IIi). The substantia gelatinosa is of interest to clinicians and researchers.[28] Laminae III through V are referred to as the nucleus proprius or the magnocellular layer.

Dorsal horn neurons, which process nociceptive information, are a heterogenous population. Laminae I and V have nociceptive specific neurons. There are two populations of nociceptive-specific neurons. One type receives inputs from Aδ fibers, both high-threshold mechanoreceptors and temperature-sensitive receptors and from polymodal C fibers. The second type of nociceptive-specific neuron appears to receive inputs only from high-threshold Aδ mechanoreceptors. The other neuron type that processes nociceptive input is the wide-dynamic-range neuron. Found predominantly in lamina V (and to a lesser degree in lamina I,) the wide-dynamic-range neuron receives input from Aδ fibers of both high-threshold mechanoreceptors and temperature-sensitive neurons and also from polymodal C fibers as well as Aβ low-threshold mechanoreceptors.[25]

The physiology of the dorsal horn explains the heterogeneity of function. Lamina I cell projection pathways have been shown to be concerned with long-latency, long-duration reactions to prolonged events, rather than to brief stimuli.[26] Lamina I neurons, which project via the spinothalamic tract, are an integral component of the central representation of pain and temperature. These nociceptive-specific neurons, both the high-threshold mechanoreceptors and the temperature-sensitive polymodal C fibers, are inhibited by morphine in a dose-dependent manner.[29,30] This suggests that opiate-modulation of nociceptive transmission is functionally organized. Both substance P and neurokinin A are released by neurons in the substantia gelatinosa when a noxious impulse is transmitted.[31] Somatostatin is released following noxious thermal but not noxious mechanical stimuli, which implies some encoding of information by the dorsal horn.[11]

The fibers of greatest interest to pain clinicians are Aδ and C fibers. The Aδ nociceptors terminate in laminae I and IIo and have collateral branches that terminate in laminae V and X. Similarly, the C fibers, which enter the spinal cord via the lateral aspect of Lissauer's tract, also terminate in laminae I and IIo, as well as lamina V. The termination of the large, myelinated Aβ fibers is in laminae III and IV, as well as lamina V.[27] Following an injury, however, there may be marked alterations in the cytoarchitecture of the dorsal horn. Woolf and colleagues have reported that following nerve injury, large-diameter fibers may invade laminae I and IIo.[11] This may provide a mechanism to explain the clinical finding of allodynia and the physiologic alterations in neuropathic pain syndromes.[32–34] This subject is discussed in detail in subsequent chapters.

The information conveyed by the primary afferents travels first to the dorsal horn and then from the dorsal horn rostral via the ascending tracts.[35] A variety of neurotransmitters is used to convey noxious information.[29,36] There are distinct areas of dopamine-containing neurons.[37] The peptide substance P is found in the dorsal horn.[38,39] There is evidence that glutaminergic neurons are also involved, as well as neurons that respond to γ-aminobutyric acid (GABA), although these neurons are not as prevalent.[40] A segmental chronic pain syndrome can be induced in rats by an intrathecal infusion of *N*-methyl-D-aspartate (NMDA).[41] The possibility of targeting a specific receptor to provide relief has generated a great deal of excitement from clinicians. And, indeed, medications that target a variety of receptors are used by clinicians to modulate pain transmission.[1] Although the neurons that carry noxious stimuli are in many ways distinct and segregated from those that carry innocuous stimuli, there remains an amount of interspersion of these distinctive fibers in the ascending systems.[42,43]

The spinothalamic tract (STT) and the trigeminothalamic tract transmit primarily pain and temperature information.[44,45] Neither tract, however, transmits exclusively noxious stimuli: the tracts are heterogenous and transmit some innocuous stimuli such as light touch, as well.[43] Furthermore, it is now accepted that other ascending tracts convey noxious information, as well.[46–48]

The lateral and ventral STTs travel in the anterior lateral quadrant of the spinal cord. The spinomesencephalic tract (SMT) is located in the anterior lateral quadrant and in the dorsolateral funiculus.[45] The dorsal column postsynaptic spinomedullary system is a second-order dorsal column pathway that is located appropriately in the dorsal column.[49,50] The propriospinal multisynaptic ascending system is a more complicated network of short chains of neurons, which may play a role in nociceptive transmission.[49,51]

A lesion of the anterior lateral quadrant (which disrupts the STT, and the SMT) results in the abolition of pain sensation on the side contralateral to the lesion, below the spinal segment.[52] There is also some mild decrease in responsiveness to noxious stimuli on the ipsilateral side. The neurons of the STT are located throughout the dorsal horn, but with the greatest concentration in lamina I.[53] As it ascends, the STT widens as fibers are added along the anteromedial border. Thus, the STT has somatotropic organization, with axons originating in the sacral region lateral to those of the lumbar region and so forth, and with the cervical region representing the most medial aspect in the spinal cord but the facial area being the most medial in the medulla. As the STT travels rostrally it divides, at the mesencephalon, into a medial component that innervates the medial thalamic region and a lateral component that projects to the ventrobasal and posterior thalamus. The ventroposterolateral (VPL) nucleus of the thalamus is somatotropically organized, in contrast to the other thalamic nuclei, and receives the majority of the lamina I projections.[53]

The SRT conveys impulses from the spinal cord to the reticular formation. The reticular formation triggers arousal, and so the SRT likely conveys information that becomes the affective aspect of pain. The SRT may be important for the motivational and emotional aspect of pain (and of autonomic and somatic motor reflexes). The SMT projects to the midbrain reticular formation. Its function, therefore, is likely similar to that of the SRT. These tracts, the SRT and the SMT, are likely to be involved in the perpetuation of chronic pain in many individuals. White and Sweet, in their classic neurosurgery text,[52] report that lesioning medial to the STT in the midbrain resulted in relief of chronic pain.

Evidence exists of alternative ascending pathways that convey nociceptive impulses. A small percentage of neurons in the dorsal column postsynaptic system respond to noxious stimuli.[46] The spinocervical tract (SCT) has neurons that respond to tactile stimuli as well as noxious stimuli. Although the SCT appears to play a role in the transmission of nociceptive impulses in the cat, its role in the transduction of pain in humans is unclear.[43] In cats, there is a convergence of visceral and somatic inputs in the medulla.[47] The propriospinal multisynaptic ascending system is composed of neurons with short axons that make multiple synaptic contacts with other short-axon neurons. Basbaum proposed a role for this multisynaptic ascending system in the maintenance of chronic pain.[49]

The anatomy and physiology of the neurons that serve the head and face are similar to the systems that transmit impulses from the body.[54] The nerves that transmit noxious stimuli are those of the cranial nerves; specifically, the trigeminal nerve (CN V,) the fascial nerve (CN VII,) the glossopharyngeal nerve (CN IX,) and the vagus nerve (CN X.) The area of the medulla that receives these inputs is often referred to as the medullary dorsal horn. Because the trigeminal system is the one most important to pain clinicians, it is the system reviewed here.

The trigeminal nerve system is of particular interest to pain clinicians because of a number of chronic pain states, such as tic douloureux and postherpetic neuralgia. The trigeminal ganglion divides into three branches: the ophthalmic, maxillary, and mandibular nerves. Each division carries information about proprioception, touch and pressure, and pain and temperature. The gasserian ganglion has somatotropic organization, and this is preserved as the fibers course to their unique terminations. The somatotropic laminar organization is true for both myelinated and unmyelinated fibers. The large-diameter fibers terminate in the main sensory nucleus, whereas the Aδ and C fibers terminate in the subnucleus caudalis.[55]

The trigeminal subnucleus caudalis can be subdivided by its cytoarchitecture into three layers. These three layers have been termed the marginal layer, the substantia gelatinosa, and the magnocellular layer. These areas correlate with their dorsal horn counterparts in both form and function.[55,56] Thus, this area is appropriately called the medullary dorsal horn. This is not meant to imply that the trigeminal system is a separate entity from the dorsal horn. There is evidence that central neurons may send collateral projections to both the sensory trigeminal nuclei and the spinal cord.[57]

The ascending trigeminal systems that convey sensory information from the face are similar to the spinal systems. Neurons in the subnucleus caudalis (which receives the projections from the nociceptors, the A and C fibers) travel in the ventral trigeminothalamic tract to the thalamus and the cortex.[58] There is also a tract that is likely analogous to the neospinothalamic tract: the neotrigeminothalamic system (nTTS.) The nTTS is somatotropically organized and conveys information about pain and temperature to the ventroposteromedial thalamic nucleus.

There is also a paleotrigeminothalamic system (pTTS.) Some fibers from the subnucleus caudalis project to a variety of terminations, thus, having both ipsilateral and contralateral connections to the brainstem reticular formation, as well as to the periaqueductal gray matter, hypothalamus, and medial and intrathalamic nuclei. As these structures project diffusely, including to the limbic system, the pTTS likely plays a role in the affective qualities of pain.[56]

The parabrachial region may be an important relay station for further processing of nociceptive information from trigeminal afferents.[59] There is interest in the parabrachial region as an area that may modulate pain and tonic immobility.[60] In certain species, analgesia may reinforce immobility as an adaptation of defense mechanisms during predator-prey confrontation.[59] It is uncertain if an analogous function exists in humans.

Supraspinal Systems: Thalamus

The thalamus is both an end point and the transition area for the sensory input traveling to the sensory cortex.[61,62] The medial and intralaminar nuclei of the thalamus receive input from the spinal cord and the reticular formation but are not somatotropically organized. The nuclei receive input from the ascending spinal (and trigeminal) systems and the reticular formation and innervate a wide area of the brain.[63] In contrast, the ventrobasal complex of the thalamus is somatotropically organized. The ventrobasal thalamus receives input from the neospinothalamic tract and the neotrigeminothalmic tract and projects to the primary somatosensory (SI) and secondary somatosensory (SII) region of the somatosensory cortex, allowing localization and sensory discrimination.[62,64]

The ventrobasal complex of the thalamus refers to the region composed of the ventral and the posterior thalamic nuclei. It is subdivided in the lateral division (the ventroposterolateral nucleus) and a medial division (the ventroposteromedial nucleus). The neurons respond primarily to stimuli on the contralateral surfaces of the body or face.[65] The thalamus may have a modulatory role on nociceptive transmission during varied states of arousal.[66] White and Sweet[52] reported that the lesions in this area of the thalamus produced transient analgesia but a marked interference of a patient's ability to perceive spatial discrimination. In patients with spinal cord transection, somatotropic organization and spontaneous neuronal activity in thalamic nuclei has been described.[67]

RETICULAR FORMATION

The reticular formation is involved with the affective component of pain. The aversive response and the motivational aspect of pain are modulated via reticular activation. Similarly, the motor, autonomic, and sensory functions that are a response to noxious stimuli are mediated by the pathways through the reticular formation. It is possible that the reticular formation is involved in pain behavior.[64] Casey proposes that one way in which opiates may relieve suffering without altering an individual's ability to recognize a stimulus as noxious is via the reticular formation.[68,69]

Hypothalamus

The hypothalamus has a role in both the autonomic nervous system and the neuroendocrine response. The hypothalamus probably plays a role in the response both to somatic and visceral tissue damage and to pain.[70] Thus, the emotional response and autonomic arousal elicited by pain is likely mediated, at least in part, by the hypothalamus. There are STT neurons that provide nociceptive input to the many areas that are involved in producing the multifaceted response to pain, which is familiar to clinicians.[71]

Limbic System

The limbic system refers to a wide array of structures that are part of the telencephalon, diencephalon, and mesencephalon. The parts of the telencephalon that contribute to the limbic system are the amygdala, hippocampus, nucleus accumbens, and preoptic regions. In the diencephalon, the hypothalamus and parts of the thalamus contribute to the limbic system. The limbic area also encompasses the ventral tegmental area, the dorsal tegmental nucleus, and parts of the midbrain raphe nuclei and the periaqueductal gray matter. The interconnections between these areas and wider areas of the cortex are complex and diverse.[72] This organization explains the allowable diversity of response to painful stimuli.

Cerebral Cortex

The human cortex has two main areas that receive sensory inputs: SI and SII. SI, on the postcentral gyrus, receives direct somatotropically organized input from the ipsilateral ventrobasal complex of the thalamus (the ventroposterolateral and the ventroposteromedial nuclei). The SII area is smaller than the SI area and is located on the parietal lobe of the cortex. The somatosensory cortex allows the discrimination of sensation. The somatotropic organization of the somatosensory cortex was mapped in the first half of this century by Penfield and Rasmussen.[73] The illustrated representation of this mapping, the homunculus, is familiar to any medical student.

The role of the sensory cortex in nociceptive processing is the subject of renewed research and debate. Although early studies revealed that many SI neurons respond to noxious stimuli, these responses were putatively only localizing in nature. Further investigation suggested that the SI neurons actually have an integrative function whereby the intensity of a stimulus is encoded and processed.[74,75] The nitric oxide–cyclic guanosine monophosphate pathway appears to play a role in cortical nociceptive processing.[76]

Descending Pathways

The descending nociceptive modulatory system is of interest to researchers and clinicians. Melzack and Wall proposed the existence of a nociceptive modulating system in their seminal article in *Science* in 1965.[3] The gate-control hypothesis of pain proposed that dorsal horn processing could be modified not only by stimulation that arrived from the periphery, but also from putative descending pathways. A few years later, Reynolds demonstrated the effect of electrical stimulation in the periaqueductal gray matter (PAG) on the nocifensive responses of the rat.[77] It is now widely believed that descending antinociceptive mechanisms are an important part of an animal's defense system.[78]

The remarkable effect of PAG electrical stimulation is to diminish or ablate the animal's response to a noxious stimulus while preserving the sensation of light touch.[79] During PAG electrical stimulation, the animal maintains normal motor control and the ability to eat. Electrical stimulation of the PAG completely inhibits the nocifensive response of an animal to a variety of noxious stimuli, not limited to somatic stimuli, but including visceral and tooth pulp stimulation. The analgesic response endures for a brief time following termination of the stimulation. Electrical stimulation of the PAG results in analgesia that is naloxone reversible, implying an opiate-mediated response.[80] Stimulation of the PAG has been shown to provide pain relief to humans with a variety of pain diagnoses, although it remains an experimental therapy.[81,82] There remains tremendous interest in providing some type of pain relief to patients with neuropathic pain. In animal models, PAG stimulation appears to provide an antinociceptive effect.[83] The result in humans, however, is more difficult to ascertain.

The electrical stimulation and, thus, the activation of neurons in the PAG results in suppression of activity of dorsal horn neurons.[84] Basbaum and Fields have published extensively both together and independently on the putative descending nociceptive modulatory systems and have elucidated the anatomic and physiologic pathways of descending inhibition of nociception.[85,86] The PAG has connections to the nucleus raphe magnus in the medulla, as well as to the parabrachial nucleus, a proposed site of behavior modification.[87] Subsequent studies revealed that the function of the nucleus raphe magnus was served by a group of nearby structures within the rostral ventromedial medulla (RVM). The information from these rostral areas is conveyed to the dorsal horn by way of the dorsal lateral funiculus. If any of these structures or their connections are ablated, so is the inhibition of nocifensive reflexes.[88]

The PAG and the RVM are also involved in opiate analgesia.[89] Microinjection of morphine or of selective μ-opioid agonists into the PAG or RVM results in potent naloxone-reversible antinociception. Lesioning the dorsal lateral funiculus unilaterally diminishes the opiate analgesia produced by PAG microinjection; and bilateral lesions of the dorsal lateral funiculus ablate the opiate effect on nocifensive reflexes. Thus, a system of descending endogenous opioid analgesia can be elucidated, and a pathway from the PAG to the dorsal horn, by way of the RVM and the dorsal lateral funiculus, has been demonstrated in a variety of animal species; this pathway seems likely to exist in humans, as well.[90] The connections of the neurons in the medulla are complex, but it appears as if serotonergic cell projections to brainstem sites may contribute to the integration of sensory, autonomic, and motor modulation at the brainstem level.[91] There are other loci, such as the nucleus cuneiformis, which may also play a role in sensory and motor integration of responses to noxious stimuli.[92]

Fields and colleagues noted that the electrophysiologic responses of neurons in the RVM to microinjection or iontophoresis of opiates was mixed: some neurons became less active and others became more active.[93] Electrical stimulation has the effect of activating neurons, whereas μ-opioid agonists inhibit neuronal response. Thus, the disparate responses of neurons to two stimuli that elicit the same analgesic response in animals could be rectified: a heterogenous population of neurons was described.

Certain neurons in the RVM are activated by noxious stimuli. Called "on-cells," these neurons fire more rapidly during noxious stimuli, and if these cells are spontaneously firing and a noxious stimulus is applied, the nocifensive reflex time is shortened. μ-Opioid agonists diminish or ablate the firing of on-cells. The second cell population stops firing before a nocifensive reflex response occurs. These "off-cells" are activated by opiates, and if a noxious stimulus is applied during the spontaneous firing of an off-cell, the nocifensive reflex time is lengthened.[93]

The circuitry of the RVM involves excitatory amino acids, GABA and opioids, as well as serotonergic and noradrenergic neurons.[94] Neurotensin microinjected into the RVM has either a facilitatory or an inhibitory effect on the response of spinal neurons to noxious thermal stimulation, depending on the dose of the neurotensin.[95] During conditions of analgesia, the removal of the RVM predictably lessens the analgesic response of the animal. During conditions of hyperalgesia, the temporary blocking of the RVM with local anesthetic actually attenuates the hyperalgesic response.[96] Thus, the RVM contains a heterogenous population of neurons that has the potential to either ameliorate or facilitate nociceptive transmission. This descending modulatory system occurs in a number of species and is likely to exist in humans, as well. And, whereas the electrophysiologic classification of neurons in humans is likely to remain elusive, the ability to modulate hyperalgesia and chronic pain is the goal of every pain clinician.

REFERENCES

1. Russo CM, Brose WG. Chronic pain. *Annu Rev Med.* 1998;49:123.
2. Blumer D, Heilbronn M. Chronic pain as a variant of depressive disease: The pain-prone disorder. *J Nerv Ment Dis.* 1982;170:381.
3. Melzack R, Wall PD. Pain mechanisms: A new theory. *Science.* 1965; 150:971.
4. Yaksh TL, Hammond DL. Peripheral and central substrates in the rostral transmission of nociceptive information. *Pain.* 1982;13:1.
5. Gasser HS. Pain-producing impulses in peripheral nerves. *Proc A. Res Nerv Ment Dis.* 1943;23:44.

6. Wilkinson SV, Neary MT, Jones RO, Sunshein KF. The neuroanatomy of pain. *Clin Podiatr Med Surg.* 1994;11:1.
7. Adriaensen H, Gybels J, Handwerker HO, Van Hees J. Presonse properties of thin myelinated (A-delta) fibers in human skin nerves. *Pain.* 1981;1:S89.
8. Georgopoulos AP. Stimulus-response relations in high-threshold mechanothermal fibers innervating primate glaborous skin. *Brain Res.* 1977;128:547.
9. Hallin RG, Torebjork HE, Wiesenfeld Z. Nociceptors and warm receptors innervated by C fibers in human skin. *J Neurrol Neurosurg Psychiat.* 1981;44:313.
10. Diamond J, Holmes M, Coughlin M. Endogenous NGF and nerve impulses regulate the collateral sprouting of sensory axons in the skin of the adult rat. *J Neurosci.* 1992;12:1454.
11. Woolf CJ. The pathophysiology of peripheral neuropathic pain—abnormal peripheral input and abnormal central processing. *Acta Neurochir Suppl (Wien).* 1993;58:125.
12. Van Hees J, Gybels JM. C nociceptor activity of human nerve during painful and nonpainful skin stimulation. *J Neurol Neurosurg Psychiat.* 1981;44:600.
13. Price DD, Hu JW, Dubner R, Gracely RH. Peripheral suppression of first pain and central summation of second pain evoked by noxious heat pulses. *Pain.* 1977;3:57.
14. Greer KR, Hoyt JW. Pain: Theory, anatomy, and physiology. *Crit Care Clin.* 1990;6:227.
15. Helme RD, Gibson S, Khalil Z. Neural pathways in chronic pain. *Med J Aust.* 1990;153:400.
16. LaMotte RH, Campbell JN. Comparison of responses of warm and nociceptive C fiber afferents in monkey with human judgments of thermal pain. *J Neurophysiol.* 1978;41:509.
17. Kniffiki KD, Menses S, Schmidt RF. Responses of group IV afferent units from skeletal muscle to stretch, contraction, and chemical stimulation. *Exp Brain Res.* 1978;31:511.
18. Coggeshall RE, Hong KA, Langford LA, Schaible HG, Schmidt RF. Discharge characteristics of fine medial articular afferents at rest and during passive movements of inflamed knee joints. *Brain Res.* 1983;272:185.
19. Byers MR. Dental sensory receptors. *Int Rev Neurobiol.* 1984;25:39.
20. Yokota T, Nishikawa Y, Koyama N, Fujino Y. Differential distribution of four types of tooth pulp neurons in the caudal medulla oblongata of the cat. *Brain Res.* 1996;715:230.
21. Melzack R, Wall PD. *The Challenge of Pain.* New York, NY: Basic Books; 1982.
22. Keay KA, Clement CI, Owler B, Depaulis A, Bandler R. Convergence of deep somatic and visceral nociceptive information onto a discrete ventrolateral midbrain periaqueductal gray region. *Neuroscience.* 1994; 61:727.
23. Kumazawa T, Mizumura K. Mechanical and thermal responses of polymodal receptors recorded from the superior spermatic nerve of dogs. *J Physiol.* 1980;259:233.
24. Langerford LA, Coggeshall RE. Branching of sensory axons in the peripheral nerve of the rat. *J Comp Neurol.* 1981;203:745.
25. Goadsby PJ, Zagami AS, Lambert GA. Neural processing of craniovascular pain: A synthesis of the central structures involved in migraine. *Headache.* 1991;31:365.
26. Strassman AM, Raymond SA, Burstein R. Sensitization of menigeal sensory neurons and the origin of headaches. *Nature.* 1996;384:560.
27. Rexed B. A cytoarchitectonis atlas of the spinal cord in the cat. *J Comp Neurol.* 1954;100:297.
28. Strassman AM, Potrebic S, Maciewicz RJ. Anatomical properties of brainstem trigeminal neurons that respond to electrical stimulation of dural blood vessels. *J Comp Neurol.* 1994;346:349.
29. Iggo A, Steedman WM, Fleetwood-Walker S. Spinal processing: Anatomy and physiology of spinal nociceptive mechanisms. *Philos Trans R Soc Lond B Biol Sci.* 1985;308:235.
30. Craig AD, Serrano LP. Effects of systemic morphine on lamina I spinothalamic tract neurons in the cat. *Brain Res.* 1994;636:233.
31. Cervero F, Iggo A. The substantia gelatinosa of the spinal cord: A critical review. *Brain.* 1980;103:717.
32. Wall PD, Bery J, Saade N. Effects of lesions to rat spinal cord lamina I cell projection pathways on reactions to acute and chronic noxious stimuli. *Pain.* 1988;35:327.
33. Woolf CJ, Shortland P, Coggeshall RE. Peripheral nerve injury triggers central sprouting of myelinated afferents. *Nature.* 1992;355:75.
34. Aminoff MJ. Sensory modulation and the spinal cord [editorial]. *Ann Neurol.* 1993;34:511.
35. Coggeshall RE, Chung K, Chung JM, Langford LA. Primary afferent axons in the tract of Lissauer in the monkey. *J Comp Neurol.* 1981; 196:431.
36. Bennet GJ, Abelmoumene M, Hayashi H, Dubner R. Physiology and morphology of substantia gletanisoa neurons intracellularly stained with horseradish peroxidase. *J Comp Neurol.* 1980;194:809.
37. Lindvall O, Bjorklund A, Skagerberg G. Dopamine-containing neurons in the spinal cord: Anatomy and some functional aspects. *Ann Neurol.* 1983;14:255.
38. Duggan AW, Furmidge LJ. Probing the brain and spinal cord with neuropeptides in pathways related to pain and other functions. *Front Neuroendocrinol.* 1994;15:275.
39. Ding YQ, Takada M, Shigemoto R, Mizumo N. Spinoparabrachial tract neurons showing substance P receptor–like immunoreactivity in the lumbar spinal cord of the rat. *Brain Res.* 1995;674:336.
40. Lekan HA, Carlton SM. Glutamatergic and GABAergic input to rat spinothalamic tract cells in the superficial dorsal horn. *J Comp Neurol.* 1995;361:417.
41. Zochodne DW, Murray M, Nag S, Riopelle RJ. A segmental chronic pain syndrome in rats associated with intrathecal infusion of NMDA: Evidence for selective action in the dorsal horn. *Can J Neurol Sci.* 1994;21:24.
42. Almeida A, Tavares I, Lima D. Projection sites of superficial or deep dorsal horn in the dorsal reticular nucleus. *Neuroreport.* 1995;6: 1245.
43. Willis WD. Nociceptive pathways: Anatomy and physiology of nociceptive ascending pathways. *Philos Trans R Soc Lond B Biol Sci.* 1985; 308:253.
44. Brodal A. *Neurological Anatomy in Relation to Clinical Medicine.* 3rd ed. New York, NY: Oxford University Press; 1981.
45. Young PA. The anatomy of the spinal cord pain paths: A review. *J Am Paraplegia Soc.* 1986;9:28.
46. Ekerot CF, Garwicz M, Schouenborg J. The postsynaptic dorsal column pathway mediates cutaneous nociceptive information to cerebellar climbing fibres in the cat. *J Physiol (Lond).* 1991;441:275.
47. Roy JC, Bing Z, Villanueva L, Le Bars D. Convergence of visceral and somatic inputs onto subnucleus reticularis dorsalis neurones in the rat medulla. *J Physiol (Lond).* 1992;458:235.
48. Ness TJ. Evidence for ascending visceral nociceptive information in the dorsal midline and lateral spinal cord. *Pain.* 2000;87:83.
49. Basbaum AI. Conduction of the effects of noxious stimulation by short fiber multisynaptic systems of the spinal cord in rat. *Exp Neurol.* 1973; 40:699.
50. Bennett GJ, Nishikawa N, Lu GW, Hoffert MJ, Dubner R. The morphology of dorsal column post-synaptic spinomedullary neurons in the cat. *J Comp Neurol.* 1984;224:568.
51. Basbaum AI. Anatomical substrates of pain and pain modulation and their relationship to analgesic drugs. In: Kuhar M, Pasternak C, eds. *Analgesics: Neurochemical, Behavioral and Clinical Perspective.* New York, NY: Raven Press; 1984.
52. White JC, Sweet WH. *Pain and the Neurosurgeon.* Springfield, Ill: Charles C Thomas; 1963.
53. Ralston HR. Synaptic organization of the spinothalamic tract projection to the thalamus with special reference to pain. In: Kruger L, Liebeskind JC, eds. *Advances in Pain Research and Therapy.* Vol. 6. New York, NY: Raven Press; 1984.
54. Sessle BJ. Neural mechanisms of oral and facial pain. *Otolaryngol Clin North Am.* 1989;22:1059.
55. Price DD, Dubner R, Hu JW. Trigeminothalamic neurons in nucleus caudalis responsive to tactile, thermal, and nociceptive stimulation of monkey's face. *J Neurophysiol.* 1976;39:936.

56. Hayashi H. Morphology of terminations of small and large myelinated trigeminal primary afferent fibers in the cat. *J Comp Neurol.* 1985;204:71.
57. Li YQ, Takada M, Shinonaga Y, Mizuno N. Collateral projections of single neurons in the nucleus raphe magnus to both the sensory trigerminal nuclei and spinal cord in the rat. *Brain Res.* 1993;602:331.
58. Young RF. Effect of trigeminal tractotomy on dental sensation in humans. *J Neurosurg.* 1982;56:812.
59. Menescal-de-Oliveira L, Hoffmann A. The parabrachial region as a possible region modulating simultaneously pain and tonic immobility. *Behav Brain Res.* 1993;56:127.
60. Wang LG, Li HM, Li JS. Formalin induced FOS-like immunoreactive neurons in the trigeminal spinal caudal subnucleus project to contralateral parabrachial nucleus in the rat. *Brain Res.* 1994;649:62.
61. Penny GR, Itoh K, Diamond IT. Cells of different sizes in the ventral nuclei project to different layers of the somatic cortex in the cat. *Brain Res.* 1982;242:55.
62. Martin RJ, Apkarian AV, Hodge CJ Jr. Ventrolateral and dorsolateral ascending spinal cord pathway influence on thalamic nociception in cat. *J Neurophysiol.* 1990;64:1400.
63. Hsu MM, Shyu BC. Electrophysiological study of the connection between medial thalamus and anterior cingulate cortex in the rat. *Neuroreport.* 1997;8:2701.
64. Morrow TJ, Casey KL. Suppression of bulboreticular unit responses to noxious stimuli by analgesic mesencephalic stimulation. *Somatosens Res.* 1983;1:151.
65. Desbois C, Villanueva L. The organization of lateral ventromedial thalamic connections in the rat: A link for the distribution of nociceptive signals to widespread cortical regions. *Neuroscience.* 2001;102:885.
66. Morrow TJ, Casey KL. Modulation of the spontaneous and evoked discharges of ventral posterior thalamic neurons during shifts in arousal. *Brain Res Bull.* 1988;21:433.
67. Lenz FA, Kwan HC, Martin R, Tasker R, Richardson RT, Dostrovsky JO. Characteristics of somatotopic organization and spontaneous neuronal activity in the region of the thalamic principal sensory nucleus in patients with spinal cord transection. *J Neurophysiol.* 1994;72:1570.
68. Casey KL, Morrow TJ. Effect of medial bulboreticular and raphe nuclear lesions on the excitation and modulation of supraspinal nocifensive behaviors in the cat. *Brain Res.* 1989;501:150.
69. Casey KL, Svensson P, Morrow TJ, Raz J, Jone C, Minoshima S. Selective opiate modulation of nociceptive processing in the human brain. *J Neurophysiol.* 2000;84:525.
70. Bester H, Menendez L, Besson JM, Bernard JF. Spino (trigemino) parabrachiohypothalamic pathway: Electrophysiological evidence for an involvement in pain processes. *J Neurophysiol.* 1995;73:568.
71. Kostarczyk E, Zhang X, Giesler GJ Jr. Spinohypothalamic tract neurons in the cervical enlargement of rats: Locations of antidromically identified ascending axons and their collateral branches in the contralateral brain. *J Neurophysiol.* 1997;77:435.
72. Romanski LM, Clugnet MC, Bordi F, LeDoux JE. Somatosensory and auditory convergence in the lateral nucleus of the amygdala. *Behav Neurosci.* 1993;107:444.
73. Penfield W, Rasmussen T. *The Cerebral Cortex of Man.* New York, NY: Macmillan; 1950.
74. Kenshalo DR, Iwata K, Sholas M, Thomas DA. Response properties and organization of nociceptive neurons in area 1 of monkey primary somatosensory cortex. *J Neurophysiol.* 2000;84:719.
75. Ploner M, Schmitz F, Freund HJ, Schnitzler A. Differential organization of touch and pain in human primary somatosensory cortex. *J Neurophysiol.* 2000;83:1770.
76. Salter M, Strijbos PJ, Neale S, Duffy C, Follenfant RI, Garthwaite J. The nitric oxide–cyclic GMP pathway is required for nociceptive signalling at specific loci within the somatosensory pathway. *Neuroscience.* 1996;73:649.
77. Reynolds DV. Surgery in the rat during electrical analgesia induced by focal brain stimulation. *Science.* 1969;164:444.
78. Harris JA. Descending antinociceptive mechanisms in the brainstem: Their role in the animal's defensive system. *J Physiol Paris.* 1996;90:15.
79. Reichling DB, Kwiat GC, Basbaum AI. Anatomy, physiology and pharmacology of the periaqueductal gray contribution to antinociceptive controls. *Prog Brain Res.* 1988;77:31.
80. Thorn BE, Applegate L, Johnson SW. Ability of periaqueductal gray subdivisions and adjacent loci to elicit analgsia and ability of naloxone to reverse analgesia. *Behav Neurosci.* 1989;103:1335.
81. Meyerson BA, Boethius J, Carlsson AM. Percutaneous central gray stimulation for cancer pain. *Appl Neurophysiol.* 1978;41:57.
82. Hosobuchi Y. Subcortical electrical stimulation for control of intractable pain in humans. Report of 122 cases (1970–1984). *J Neurosurg.* 1986;64:543.
83. Lee BH, Park SH, Won R, Park YG, Sohn JH. Antiallodynic effects produced by stimulation of the periaqueductal gray matter in a rat model of neuropathic pain. *Neurosci Lett.* 2000;291:29.
84. Willis WD Jr. Anatomy and physiology of descending control of nociceptive responses of dorsal horn neurons: Comprehensive review. *Prog Brain Res.* 1988;77:1.
85. Basbaum AI, Fields HL. The origin of descending pathways in the dorsolateral funiculus of the spinal cord of the cat and rat: Further studies on the anatomy of pain modulation. *J Comp Neurol.* 1979;187:513.
86. Fields HL, Basbaum AI. Brainstem control of spinal pain-transmission neurons. *Annu Rev Physiol.* 1978;40:217.
87. Krout KE, Jansen AS, Loewy AD. Periaqueductal gray matter projection to the parabrachial nuelcus in rat. *J Comp Neurol.* 1998;401:437.
88. Basbaum AI, Clanton CH, Fields HL. Opiate and stimulus-produced analgesia: Functional anatomy of a medullospinal pathway. *Proc Natl Acad Sci USA.* 1976;73:4685.
89. Fields HL, Anderson SD, Clanton CH, Basbaum AI. Nucleus raphe magnus: A common mediator of opiate- and stimulus-produced analgesia. *Trans Am Neurol Assoc.* 1976;101:208.
90. Basbaum AI, Fields HL. Endogenous pain control systems: Brain spinal pathways and endorphin circuitry. *Annu Rev Neurosci.* 1984;7:309.
91. Gao K, Mason P. Somatodendritic and axonal anatomy of intracellularly labeled serotonergic neurons in the rat medulla. *J Comp Neurol.* 1997;389:309.
92. Zemlan FP, Behbehani MM. Nucleus cuneiformis and pain modulation: Anatomy and behavioral pharmacology. *Brain Res.* 1988;453:89.
93. Fields HL, Heinricher MM. Anatomy and physiology of a nociceptive modulatory system. *Philos Trans R Soc Lond B Biol Sci.* 1985;308:361.
94. Heinricher MM, McGaraughty S. Analysis of excitatory amino acid transmission within the rostral ventromedial medulla: Implications for circuitry. *Pain.* 1998;75:247.
95. Urban MO, Gebhart GE. Characterization of biphasic modulation of spinal nociceptive transmission by neurotensin in the rat rostral ventromedial medulla. *J Neurophysiol.* 1997;78:1550.
96. Kaplan HJ, Fields HL. Hyperalgesia during acute opioid abstinence: Evidence for a nociceptive facilitating function of the rostral ventromedial medulla. *J Neurosci.* 1991;11:1433.

BIBLIOGRAPHY

Hylden JLK, Hayashi H, Bennett GJ. Lamina I spinomesencephalic neurons in cat ascend via the dorsolateral funiculi. *Somatosens Mot Res.* 1986;4:31.

Levitt M. The theory of chronic deafferentation dysesthesias. *J Neurosurg Sci.* 1990;34:71.

Mizumura K, Sugiura Y, Kumazawa T. Spinal termination patterns of canine identified A-delta and C spermatic polymodal receptors traced by intracellular labeling with *Phaseolus vulgaris*-leucoagglutinin. *J Comp Neurol.* 1993;335:460.

CHAPTER 3 PATHOPHYSIOLOGY OF PAIN

Stephen A. Cohen

After great pain, a formal feeling comes—
The Nerves sit ceremonious, like Tombs—
EMILY DICKINSON (1862)

Acute, nociceptive pain results from the complex convergence of many signals traveling up and down the neuraxis and serves to warn us of impending harm. The painful sensations ultimately leave the periphery and travel centrally, carried by the axons of the primary sensory neurons, the dorsal root ganglia (DRG), which are relatively quiescent unless specifically stimulated by sensory input. Unlike the "tombs" that the Belle of Amherst describes, however, if inflammation or injury damages the neural structures, pain sensation (neuropathic pain) may continue long after the noxious stimuli subside. The pain response can then harm rather than help the individual. Injured DRG may become hyperexcitable and display considerable spontaneous electrical activity. Such increased activity results from the expression of a dramatically different constellation of many cell-specific molecules in injured cells compared with normal ones. Ultimately, the operation of complex neuronal circuits may be markedly altered. Chronic pain sensation can result from such injury.

Considerable advances have been made in the last decade, which have given some insight into the mechanisms responsible for the development of chronic pain. Understanding the changes that follow injury at a cellular and molecular level may help lead to new therapeutic interventions. In this chapter I focus on neuropathic pain and highlight, rather than exhaustively chronicle, these findings. I first describe peripheral sensitization changes seen in inflammatory pain, then central mechanisms of sensitization, followed by the role of neurotrophic factors, the effects on neuronal ionic channels, and higher neural mechanisms, concluding with a brief word on central pain.

PERIPHERAL SENSITIZATION

Unmyelinated C or thinly myelinated Aδ afferent fibers convey pain sensation. Minor irritation of tissue in a neuron's receptive field results in the release of inflammatory mediators, which is often accompanied by a reduction in the nociceptor threshold. Such a change, called peripheral sensitization, renders the nerve ending responsive to weak, normally nonpainful stimuli (allodynia). Stronger stimuli typically provoke exaggerated pain (hyperalgesia). Sensitization involves not only normal nociceptive fibers but also the recruitment of so-called silent nociceptors, which are not usually sensitive to painful stimuli or inflammatory substrates such as prostaglandins or bradykinin.

Bradykinin can sensitize C and Aδ fibers to prostaglandins, protons, serotonin, heat, and mechanical stimuli.[1–4] Because its algesic effect displays considerable tachyphylaxis, however, bradykinin alone cannot account for the hyperalgesia seen in inflammation.[3] Bradykinin also appears to facilitate the production of prostaglandins.[5] Similarly, prostaglandins sensitize nerve afferents to bradykinin action.[6] Blockade of such sensitization accounts for the clinical efficacy of antiinflammatory drugs such as aspirin and cyclooxygenase-1 and -2 inhibitors.

Some light has been shed on cellular transduction mechanisms that may be involved in the development of this type of sensitization. For example, the afterhyperpolarization of primary afferent fibers decreases, which renders the cell more likely to fire repetitive action potentials in response to subsequent stimuli. The process appears to involve adenyl cyclase and the second messenger cyclic adenosine monophosphate (cAMP). The latter provokes the phosphorylation of potassium (K) channels, which is catalyzed by protein kinase A (PKA). Excitability increases as K conductance decreases. Some investigators have proposed a universal role for cAMP in producing sensitization in response to multiple physical and chemical noxious stimuli.[7–9] Some evidence suggests the role of cAMP-PKA in decreasing the activation threshold and increasing the size and rate of activation of a tetrodotoxin-resistant sodium (Na) channel in nociceptive neurons, too.[10] The decrease in inflammatory pain seen in mice that have a point mutation in a PKA subunit supports the importance of this cAMP-PKA mechanism.[8]

Phospholipase C induction by the activation of bradykinin or neurokinin (NK) receptors can ultimately lead to increased electrical activity of primary afferent nerve terminals. Intracellular calcium (Ca) increases, which may increase adenyl cyclase activity and cAMP levels. Phosphorylation of specific cation channels and their subsequent increased activity results.[11]

Primary afferent nerve fibers have many 5-HT_{2A} receptors,[12] the activation of which produces a G protein–mediated decrease in K currents.[13,14] Hence, 5-HT_{2A} receptor blockade can antagonize this component of inflammatory pain.[13] Prostaglandins may also provoke a separate type of decrease in outward K current, mediated by cAMP-PKA.[8]

Inflammation leads to an upregulation of nitric oxide (NO) synthetase in DRG and other cells. Ultimately, neuropeptides may be released from nociceptive nerve terminals, which can produce inflammatory hyperalgesia.[4] Whereas subcutaneous injection of NO produces pain,[15] interruption of NO synthetase blocks the hyperalgesia.[16] These findings oversimplify the role of NO in peripheral sensitization, however, because some data suggest an antinociceptive role for NO.[4,17,18] Although NO generates cyclic guanosine monophosphate (cGMP) as an intracellular second messenger, the cyclic nucleotide does not seem to contribute to the sensitization of the nerve terminals.[7,19] Recent data suggest that NO may exert its action on peripheral nerve terminals indirectly. Moreover, NO synthetase may be involved early in the inflammatory response, but NO itself does not participate in chronic inflammation.[20] This indirect action, which may be mediated by its effect on blood vessels, coupled with its direct action on nerve terminals has led some investigators to postulate a role for NO in triggering migraine headaches.[21]

Considerable evidence exists for the role of neurotrophic factors in the long-term development of neuropathic pain (see later discussion). Recent data have suggested that neurotrophins can also affect neuronal function in the short term. Although not studied directly in C-fiber terminals, changes in ionic current flow, intracellular Ca level, and protein phosphorylation have been shown to lead to altered neuronal excitability, neurotransmitter release, receptor distribution, and synaptic efficacy in other systems.[4,22–26]

The recruitment of previously mechanically silent nerve fibers that become sensitive to mechanical or thermal stimuli after exposure to inflammatory mediators such as bradykinin suggests another mechanism of peripheral sensitization.[27,28] Investigators have proposed that primary afferent substance P–containing neurons are involved in developing hyperalgesia. The demonstration that prostaglandins can increase the number of bradykinin-responsive, substance P–containing fibers is consistent with this finding.[29]

In summary, multiple mechanisms modulate the functioning of primary afferent nerve terminals. The final common pathway appears to involve the increase in intracellular Ca and protein kinase levels. Both Ca and protein kinases exert a profound influence on the control of gene transcription (see later discussion).

CENTRAL SENSITIZATION

Central sensitization refers to the plasticity displayed by central neural structures involved in pain perception. Some of these physiologic neuronal changes can occur within a few minutes. These may not be maintained once the stimulus is removed. Still other changes remain long after the noxious stimuli are removed and may reflect irreversible processes. Two prominent features of peripheral tissue injury include pain and an exaggerated response to noxious stimuli, such as heat. However, the hallmark of clinical pain, mechanical allodynia, cannot easily be explained without invoking central neuronal plasticity. Central mechanisms must also be considered in describing referred pain.[4]

One clinical example of central sensitization is seen in amputees who exhibit phantom limb pain, which is similar to that experienced prior to the amputation. The pain can remain long after the inciting peripheral stimulus is removed. Surgical patients who have derived benefit from preemptive analgesia constitute another example. In these patients, the short- and long-term central neural structure changes that might lead to sensitization are blocked.

Considerable experimental data support the concept that mechanical allodynia results from the activation of Aβ nerve fibers, which normally subserve light touch or vibration, not pain. Some of the evidence is indirect but includes the following.[4] Primary afferent nerve fiber injury leads to abnormal electrical excitability of both small and large fibers, including Aβ fibers. The latter exhibit exquisite sympathetic sensitivity after injury, and pharmacologic or surgical sympathectomy can ameliorate mechanical allodynia.[30,31] High-threshold C or Aδ fibers do not seem responsible for the allodynia, because the transduction sensitivity of these single fibers remains stable before and after injury.[30,32] The time course of onset of allodynia correlates with the more rapid conduction velocity of the larger fibers.[30] Blockade of only Aβ fibers extinguishes allodynia.[33] Aβ fibers activate AMPA (DL-α-amino-2,3-dihydro-5-methyl-3-oxo-4-isoxazolepropanoic acid)/kainic acid receptors in the dorsal horn (DH) of the spinal cord. Such receptors have not been found on C fibers, and their specific antagonism reduces allodynia.[34] The time course of the appearance of allodynia following nerve injury corresponds to that of the upregulation of AMPA receptors.[4] Finally, without inflammation, normal touch does not lead to changes in gene expression.[35] In summary, although some of the evidence is indirect, Aβ fibers appear to play a powerful role in the mediation of mechanical allodynia.

Recent reports have demonstrated secondary hyperalgesia to only mechanical stimuli. The investigators suggested that independent peripheral mechanisms accounted for the evoked pain and central sensitization.[36] The involvement of Aβ fibers in mechanical allodynia, as noted earlier, also suggests that central, rather than peripheral, mechanisms must be operative.[4]

Data suggest that maintained pain can result from several specific processes that converge on the DH of the spinal cord. They include neuronal sensitization, reduction in inhibitory interneuron activity, and a modulation of descending pathway activity.[4] Brief descriptions of each follow.

Neuronal Sensitization

DH neuron changes resembling long-term potentiation and long-term depression can result from high-frequency stimulation of C fibers or low-frequency stimulation of Aδ fibers, respectively.[37–39] Intense electrical or noxious stimulation of C fibers can promote wide-dynamic-range (WDR) neuron hyperexcitability in the DH. *N*-methyl-D-aspartate (NMDA) receptors and levels of intracellular Ca and protein kinases play a crucial role in this sensitization.[37,40] Sensitization may involve two qualitatively different actions at synapses. At one type of synapse, transmission efficacy increases in a graded fashion. At the other, so-called silent synapses switch to active ones.[41,42]

Sensitization can be demonstrated in DH neurons even after short periods of electrical or noxious stimulation. For example, repetitive electrical stimulation provokes increased excitability lasting about an hour. Such action potential "windup" has been used to model pain at the cellular level. Windup refers to the slow, prolonged depolarization and ultimate burst of action potentials seen with stimulation.[43] It can be demonstrated in only a few cells, which suggests a cell-specific mechanism of generation.[40] During such hyperexcitability several neuronal changes occur, with presumptive clinical correlates. First, subsequent stimuli evoke a longer and more intense period of action potential firing, which qualitatively resembles hyperalgesia. Second, receptive fields increase in size, which is consistent with secondary hyperalgesia. Finally, the threshold for firing action potentials is decreased and responses to Aβ fibers appear, which resembles allodynia.[4]

Temporal and spatial summation of fast and slow synaptic potentials and action potential windup can explain the period of DH neuronal hyperexcitability. Heterosynaptic facilitation also develops whereby the increased excitability derived from one synaptic input increases the response amplitude from a second, separate input.[37]

Most of the recent work on unraveling the molecular mechanisms of WDR neuron sensitization has focused on three classes of agents: excitatory amino acids, tachykinins, and calcitonin gene–related peptide (CGRP). Other compounds have been less well studied. These transmitters and neuromodulators affect DH neuron activity by directly increasing cation fluxes, impinging on intracellular transduction mechanisms, and modulating receptor and transmitter gene transcription. Synaptic transmission augmentation at NMDA receptors is the final common pathway.[4,44–46]

Because the central role of the NMDA receptor in sensitization cannot be overemphasized, its following properties may lend some insight.[4] Magnesium (Mg) blocks the ionic channel at rest but can be displaced by adequate depolarization.[47,48] Ca readily permeates its ionic channel; hence its activation increases intracellular Ca levels.[49] Increased intracellular Ca levels augment protein kinase activity.[50] Phosphorylation antagonizes the Mg-channel blockade, which then can function at hyperpolarized levels.[51] Bursts of action potentials can result from NMDA receptor activation, which greatly increases transmitter release at higher levels in the nervous system. Activation of presynaptic NMDA receptors causes increased release of excitatory amino acids and substance P.[52] Hence, several mechanisms serve to amplify signals transmitted through NMDA receptors.

AMPA, NK, metabotropic glutamate (mGlu), and CGRP receptors also play roles in the sensitization of DH neurons.[4] Activation of AMPA receptors leads to increased intracellular Ca and depolarization. In other areas of the nervous system, AMPA and NMDA receptors reciprocally activate one another. With a time course of 10 to 15 minutes, the AMPA receptors are ultimately phosphorylated, which increases their responsiveness. Some investigators have proposed a role for them in maintaining long-term potentiation.[53,54]

Substance P and neurokinin A (NKA), which are released by stimulation of C fibers, exert their actions at neurokinin-1 (NK-1) and neurokinin-2 (NK-2) receptors, respectively.[55] Activation of these receptors supplements DH neuron sensitization. Moreover, NK-1 receptors appear to strengthen the sensitizing actions mediated by NMDA receptors. Consequently, administering specific antagonists of both receptors can ameliorate certain painful states.[56,57]

Subtypes of mGlu receptors are coupled to phospholipase C, which suggests that their activation increases intracellular Ca levels. In the cerebral cortex, evidence exists that mGlu receptors augment the sensitizing actions of NMDA receptors.[58,59] They also augment AMPA receptor excitability.[60] Their appearance at high density in lamina II of the DH indirectly suggests a role for them in pain transmission. The action of CGRP in the spinal cord remains poorly understood, but investigators have suggested that it potentiates NMDA and NK-1 receptor opening.[61]

The preceding cell-surface receptor actions suggest that intracellular Ca levels, Ca influx, and protein kinase activation play an important intracellular role in DH neuron sensitization.[4] Different intracellular stores of Ca may promote different events in the neurons. On balance, the increased levels of intracellular Ca generate sensitization but suitable negative feedback mechanisms are activated to minimize the likelihood of cell death resulting from toxic intracellular levels of free Ca. Ca levels induce protein kinase activity in the neuronal soma, which leads to phenotypic and ultimately genotypic changes. For example, under the influence of high intracellular Ca, protein kinase C phosphorylates NMDA receptors, which promotes long-term potentiation.[50,62] Activation of nuclear transcription factors and gene transcription also occurs.[63,64]

Reduction in Inhibitory Interneuron Activity

Diminution of the inhibitory influences supplied by inhibitory interneurons results in increased WDR neuron excitability consistent with clinical hyperalgesia and mechanical allodynia.[65] The loss of γ-aminobutyric acidergic (GABAergic) and glycinergic activity in the DH produces a state of neuronal hyperexcitability. Such inhibitory loss amplifies the excitability of WDR projections.[66,67] As would be expected, pharmacologic antagonism of GABAergic and glycinergic receptors with bicuculline and strychnine produces a functional state resembling clinical allodynia. Conversely, the allodynia produced by injury is ameliorated by GABA agonist administration.[68]

Considerable research has addressed the possible mechanisms responsible for the reduction in inhibitory interneuron activity.[4] If a decrease in GABAergic and glycinergic activity can mimic allodynia, does such a diminution actually cause chronic pain? Although the final verdict is not yet in, it appears that primary afferent fiber injury leads not only to NMDA receptor activation, with consequent sensitization of WDR neurons, but also to a huge outpouring of excitatory amino acid neurotransmitters at inhibitory interneuron NMDA synapses. Such release has been postulated to cause massive accumulation of intracellular Ca and NO, which ultimately leads to cell death.[69,70] Other speculation attributes the decrease in inhibitory interneuron activity to loss of neurotrophic factors from injured primary afferent fibers.[71] In this regard, the role of GABA attracts attention, because primary afferent terminal degeneration provokes a biphasic response of GABAergic neurons, which suggests a trophic role for GABA itself in the reorganization of spinal networks.[72]

Modulation by Descending Pathways

For some time, neuroscientists have envisaged a role for descending input from supraspinal pathways in controlling nociceptive signaling in the DH of the spinal cord.[73] Signals transmitted to higher centers depend on tremendous afferent and efferent integration of information processing at lower centers.[74] Recently, investigators have examined the role of supraspinal structures in the development of secondary allodynia.[75] Blocking allodynia with precisely localized microinjections of lidocaine, they concluded that brainstem pathways immediately adjacent to the raphe magnus contribute to the development of secondary allodynia.

Several neurotransmitter systems appear to be involved in the increases or decreases in descending facilitation or inhibition, respectively.[4,76] Recent data suggest that augmentation of serotonergic systems contributes to DH neuron sensitization. Primary afferent nerve terminals, excitatory interneurons, and projection neurons exhibit multiple types of 5-HT receptors over their plasmalemmae. Evidence suggests that the 5-HT_3 receptor subtype accounts for the facilitatory action of 5-HT on the evoked release of substance P–like immunoreactive materials. NO mediates the intracellular signal transduction by promoting an increase in cGMP production.[77] Stimulation of the 5-HT_{1A} subtype enhances K currents and suppresses Ca currents.[78] These data have led to the suggestion that inhibition of inhibitory interneuron 5-HT_{1A} receptors reinforces DH neuron sensitization and, therefore, allodynia.[76]

Descending dopaminergic systems also play a role in regulating spinal neuron excitability. Two families of dopamine receptors have been defined based on their properties. One includes dopaminergic receptors that are D_1-like, which consists of D_1 and D_5, and another that are D_2-like, which consists of D_2, D_3, and D_4. Stimulation of members of the first group increases adenyl cyclase and potentiates neuronal excitability.[79] Stimulation of members of the second group inhibits neuronal excitability by inhibiting adenyl cyclase and Ca currents and augmenting K currents. Such changes may play a role in the sensitization of WDR neurons. D_1 agonists provoke release of CGRP and substance P from the spinal cord, which correlates with their ability to increase nociception at the level of the projection neurons.[80]

Inhibition of nociception involves mesolimbic, mesocortical, and nigrostriatal dopaminergic circuits.[81–83] An understanding of how these functionally impinge on lower centers remains incomplete.[84,85]

Descending adrenergic pathways innervating the spinal cord derive primarily from the locus ceruleus, subceruleus, and medullary raphe nuclei.[86–89] They exert descending inhibitory and facilitatory influence on spinal neurons by action on specific adrenoreceptors. The three major classes of such receptors, α_1, α_2, and β, can be further divided into ten subtypes, which are designated α_{1A}, α_{1B}, α_{1D}, α_{2A}, α_{2B}, α_{2C}, β_1, β_2, β_3, and β_4. The first three promote mobilization of intracellular Ca by coupling to phospholipase C and voltage-dependent Ca channels. The α_2 class inhibits adenyl cyclase, facilitates K currents, and inhibits Ca currents, and the β class stimulates adenyl cyclase and, hence, neuronal excitability.

Under normal conditions, descending noradrenergic pathways display little spontaneous activity. Various events can provoke considerable change in their activity, which plays a significant role in the modulation of descending inhibition.[76,90] For example, noxious stimuli activate release of noradrenaline in the DH of the spinal cord, which excites α_2 receptors to effect "pain-induced analgesia." Some investigators have developed a model of allodynia in which locus ceruleus neurons become activated.[91] Such activation also potentiates descending noradrenergic inhibitory circuits.

Evidence exists for the facilitation of efferent antinociceptive adrenergic systems provoked by acute and chronic noxious stimuli. Much of this research has focused on the inhibition of nociception mediated by α_{2A} receptors, which are negatively coupled to adenyl cyclase.[87] Contrariwise, data also suggest that higher nervous centers cause hyperexcitation of spinal neurons by increasing intracellular Ca, an effect that is mediated by the activation of α_1 adrenoreceptors.[87,92] Recent data corroborate these findings. Destruction of p75 nerve growth factor (NGF) receptor afferents (see later discussion) does not interfere with the hypersensitivity to mechanical stimuli that results from nerve injury. Such injury does disrupt the inhibitory action of descending α_2 circuits, however, which exerts net reinforcement of hypersensitivity and neuropathic pain states.[93]

Descending facilitation also plays an important role in the pathophysiology of pain. For example, diminished cerebral GABAergic tone such as may occur with direct brain injury can lead to the disinhibition of descending facilitation.[94] The rostromedial area of the ventral medulla seems to be involved, because blocking electrical transmission there with lidocaine ameliorates experimental allodynia.[4]

NEUROTROPHIC INTERACTIONS

In addition to the rapid (msec time course) electrical signaling that occurs in the nervous system, neuron-neuron and neuron-muscle communication also occurs over a much longer time course. This has been perhaps most apparent at the skeletal neuromuscular junction, where disruption of the nerve innervating the muscle not only causes absence of voluntary movement but also leads to profound changes in the muscle cell. We say that the nerve exerts a "trophic," or nourishing effect, on the muscle. Without activity and the so-called "neurotrophic" influences of the nerve, the muscle loses many specialized features and becomes "atrophic." Profound molecular changes occur in, for example, the muscle membrane's electrical properties; the number, type, and distribution of acetylcholine receptors over the surface of the muscle fiber; and the proteins of the contractile mechanism in the sarcomeres.

Another large body of information exists about the mechanisms and actions of NGF. More than 50 years ago, the requirement of NGF for the development of sensory and sympathetic neurons was described.[95–97] According to the theory, the neurotrophic factors made by target postsynaptic cells are transported retrogradely to the presynaptic neuronal soma where they are required for the survival, development, and differentiation of the presynaptic neurons. Over the last half-century, many lines of research have tended to support Levi-Montalcini's seminal theory.

Developmental biologists have performed many of the studies that contribute to our knowledge of neurotrophic factors. Many factors besides NGF have been identified as playing a role in the integrity of nerve and muscle cells. More recently, investigators have realized the importance of such factors not only in the growth and development of immature cells, but also in the maintenance of differentiated properties of mature cells. Hence, our definition of neurotrophic factors in the sensory nervous system has been broadened to include those factors that permit the long-term growth, survival, or differentiation of neurons. Our current knowledge of factors important in sensory nerve integrity focuses on the neurotrophin (NT) family and the glial cell line–derived neurotrophic factor (GDNF) family of factors.

The NT family consists of NGF, brain-derived neurotrophic factor (BDNF), neurotrophin-3 (NT3), neurotrophin-4/5 (NT4/5), and, in teleost fish *Xiphophorus*, neurotrophin-6 (NT6). The factors are basic proteins of about 120 amino acids and weigh about 13 kDa. Family members display considerable (~50%) homology of amino acids and exist as homodimers. The GDNF family of trophic factors belongs to the transforming growth factor-β (TGF-β) superfamily and includes GDNF, neurturin, persephin, and artemin. They signal by way of a complex composed of a tyrosine kinase transduction domain (RET) and a ligand-binding domain, the GDNF family receptor-α (GFR-α).[98]

All neurotrophins bind specifically, selectively, and with high affinity to one or more of the three known tyrosine kinase (Trk) receptors: TrkA, TrkB, and TrkC. NGF binds preferentially to TrkA, NT3 binds to all three Trks but exerts its effects mainly through TrkC, and both BDNF and NT4/5 bind preferentially to TrkB. In general, high-affinity binding ($K_d \sim 10^{-11}$ M) constitutes only 10% to 30% of the total binding to Trk receptors, with the remainder being low affinity. Moreover, all members of the family bind with low affinity ($K_d \sim 10^{-8}$–10^{-9} M) and somewhat different characteristics to a so-called low-affinity nerve growth factor receptor (LNGFR) or p75, which is also a member of the tumor necrosis factor receptor family.[98,99]

Structurally, Trk receptors consist of four main regions: one, which is extracellular for ligand binding; a second, which is immunoglobulin G–like; a third, which spans the membrane (transmembrane domain); and a fourth, which is the kinase domain.[99–101] Different isoforms can be distinguished on the basis of different amino acid residues of the extracellular domain.[99,101] Still other isoforms have been identified that lack the kinase domain.[99] The significance of these differences remains to be determined.

Nerve Growth Factor

Based largely on studies of the action of NGF on PC-12 cells (a pheochromocytoma cell line), some of the steps of signal transduction following Trk activation have been described. Neurotrophin-receptor interaction activates multiple pathways. After ligand binding, receptor autophosphorylation of tyrosine residues occurs, which is likely mediated by dimerization as an obligatory step in the activation process.[102,103] Other substrates such as phospholipase C (PLC-γ) are also phosphorylated.[98] Interaction between phosphatidylinositol-3 kinase and the Trk domain occurs, but its significance is not clear.

The p75 receptor spans the cell membrane and contains both an intracellular region and an extracellular glycoprotein moiety. It appears to act, at least in part, to facilitate high-affinity neurotrophin-Trk binding. Although some investigators refute the role of p75 alone in neurotrophin signaling, others suggest that it may mediate NGF signal transduction through TrkA receptors.[99,100] In cultured Schwann cells, the induction of NF-κB nuclear staining by NGF depends on the presence of the p75 receptor.[104] NF-κB is a transcription factor, which translocates to the nucleus and regulates gene transcription after suitable activation.[105] Such activation also enables NF-κB to bind particular DNA chains.[104] It has also been hypothesized that NGF-p75-NF-κB activation is involved in the generation of hyperalgesia.[104,106]

Neurotrophin receptors are distributed widely and specifically throughout the nervous system. For example, so-called small, dark DRG, which display the neuropeptide marker CGRP, express predominantly TrkA receptors. So-called large, light DRG, which stain with the neurofilament antibody RT97, express TrkC. TrkB receptors appear only on certain types of DRG, which are not distinguishable by any histochemical staining property. For the most part, DRG expressing a Trk also express a p75. About one third of DRG do not express either a Trk or a p75.

More recent investigation has promoted the concept that NGF also plays an important role in persistent pain states. Some studies suggest that NGF not only can modulate the sensitivity of sensory neurons, but also can mediate inflammatory pain. The precise mechanisms remain unclear, but some of the data are presented in the discussion that follows.

Different neurotrophins affect functionally different groups of DRG. Small-diameter DRG require NGF for survival. Two methods have been used to eliminate NGF during development: gene deletion and in utero antibody application.[107,108] The resultant absence of NGF during development renders animals virtually devoid of small-diameter DRG, which express the nociceptive mediators CGRP and substance P. Such animals display significant hypoalgesia.[98]

Adult DRG do not possess the developmental requirement of NGF for survival. However, they are still exquisitely sensitive to NGF. For example, exogenous NGF added to cultured DRG elicits prolific neurite outgrowth[109] and regulates the expression of both CGRP and substance P as well as the chemosensitivity of the ganglion cells.[24] Interestingly, in the absence of NGF, capsaicin sensitivity, a specific proton-evoked current, and GABA sensitivity were diminished, but adenosine triphosphate (ATP) sensitivity was unaffected. NGF has recently been shown to increase selectively the expression of bradykinin-binding sites on cultured DRG mediated by a mechanism, which requires the p75 receptor.[110] Such an increase has been associated with the increased excitability of nociceptors seen in chronic pain.[11]

Injection of minute amounts of NGF can produce pain and hyperalgesia at the site of injection.[106,111] Because of the localization of these effects, some investigators have suggested that the NGF exerts its actions on the peripheral terminals of nociceptors.[111]

Nerve activity regulates both neurotrophin synthesis and release from dendrites. Neurotrophins also promote transmitter release, which is mediated by the specific Trk receptor, from corresponding neurons. Hence, the suggestion has been made that neurotrophins act as retrograde messengers and regulate synaptic efficacy and neuronal plasticity.[112]

An interaction between NGF and sympathetic neurons during inflammation has been proposed. Sympathectomy leads to reduction of the short latency hyperalgesia produced by NGF.[113,114] NGF may also cause peripheral sensitization by activating 5-lipoxygenase to generate leukotrienes. Martin[115] showed that leukotriene B_4 sensitizes pain afferents to thermal and mechanical stimuli. Conversely, inhibition of 5-lipoxygenase prevents NGF-injection–produced hyperalgesia.[116] Curiously, indomethacin does not prevent such hyperalgesia.[117]

Although systemically administered NGF does not penetrate the spinal cord, it does appear to affect central pain pathways.[98] NGF may also produce increased neurotransmitter release from nociceptive afferents.[118] Finally, NGF appears able to upregulate BDNF synthesis in some pain sensory cells. Hence, NGF seems to induce central sensitization in resetting the sensitivity of spinal processing of painful stimuli.

Nerve injury as modeled by axotomy provokes a multitude of biochemical responses. Although traumatic plexus and root lesions do constitute serious clinical problems, frank nerve section does not account for many of the clinical syndromes seen. Some, but not all, of the neuronal changes provoked by axotomy are also seen in other neuropathies. For example, normal retrograde flow of neurotrophic substances ceases. About 30% of sensory neurons degenerate and die.[119] C-*jun* gene expression increases[120] but can be blocked by NGF treatment.[121] Substance P and CGRP levels are reduced and vasoactive intestinal peptide and galanin levels are increased.[122] Neurofilament production is reduced. Axon diameter and conduction velocity decrease. DRG produce more of the phosphoprotein, GAP-43, which is important in neuronal development and plasticity.[123] Some of these changes can be partly ameliorated by the exogenous administration of NGF. Other axotomy induced effects such as downregulation of isolectin B4 binding, thiamine monophosphatase activity, and somatostatin expression can be reversed by GDNF, but not NGF, administration.[98,124]

Because the most commonly seen clinical neuropathies do not involve overt transection of the peripheral nerve, axotomy may not provide a suitable model for studying the mechanisms of chronic pain development. Rather, diabetic neuropathy is the most common neuropathy seen clinically and is usually seen as a distal symmetric sensorimotor neuropathy. It progresses by a nerve terminal dying-back phenomenon. Recently, investigators have studied the actions of trophic factors in both animal models and human clinical trials of diabetic neuropathy. Streptozotocin treatment of rats to produce a model of diabetic neuropathy provokes a number of neuronal changes such as elevation of tail-flick threshold (thermal hypoalgesia), increase in compound action potential latency, decrement in C-fiber conduction velocity, and fall in substance P, CGRP, and CGRP mRNA levels.[125] NGF can at least partially reverse some of these changes.[98]

Some researchers have begun administering neurotrophic factors in clinical trials for the treatment of diabetic neuropathy. One such phase II trial using recombinant human NGF (rhNGF) showed improvement in the sensory component of the neurologic examination, two quantitative sensory tests, and the subjective impression of the patients who received rhNGF compared to those subjects who received placebo.[126] Efficacy of rhNGF failed statistical significance, however, in a large phase III trial.[127] In this trial, subjects received 0.1 μg/kg of rhNGF subcutaneously three times a week. Doses reported to be effective in animal studies ranged from 3 to 5 mg/kg. Moreover, the serum half-life of NGF has been calculated to be only 7.2 minutes. Hence, it has been suggested that the lack of effect shown in the phase III trial might be the result of inadequate dose. In this context, the recent publication using genomic virus-mediated gene transfer of neurotrophin to protect against pyridoxine neuropathy in the rat elicits optimism.[128] Such gene transfer of the coding sequences for specific trophic substances may circumvent the dose and delivery problem and enable the factors' therapeutic abilities.

Two strategies have been used to elucidate the role of endogenous NGF in the pathophysiology of pain. One involves genetic manipulation to eliminate either NGF or its receptor ("knock-out"), and the other involves inhibiting the actions of NGF by adding selective blockers. For example, blocking NGF for 10 to 12 days leads to fewer nociceptors responding to heat and to a right-shifted, flatter stimulus-response curve generated by measuring the neural firing to intracutaneous heat application. The mechanical stimulus threshold remained unchanged.[129] Taken together, the two kinds of experiments support the notion that native NGF modulates pain sensitivity.[98]

Considerable experimental evidence supports the hypothesis that NGF plays an important role acting as a mediator in inflammatory pain. In both human and animal studies, data suggest that inflammation generally causes increased NGF levels and consequent hyperalgesia.[130,131] Such increase appears to depend on the synthesis and release of NGF *de novo* in the affected cells.[132]

How NGF may play a role in the development of neuropathic pain, however, remains speculative. In many neuropathic conditions, abnormal sympathetic nerve sprouting creates basketlike arborizations around large-diameter DRG, which resemble the connections that develop in animals exposed to excessive NGF.[133–135] Hence, one hypothesis suggests that such NGF abundance, per se, can produce maintained pain.[134,136–138] In axotomy, however, NGF levels are reduced, which has led to the hypothesis that merely an imbalance of NGF can produce chronic pain.[98] Wallerian degeneration of injured nerves appears to be linked to both pain development and sympathetic sprouting. Ramer and colleagues have speculated that NGF serves as a mediator for both processes.[139]

Decreased NGF levels seen after nerve injury have been reputed to be responsible for changes in spinal cord connectivity, too.[98] Normally, only unmyelinated C fibers, many of which are nociceptors, terminate on lamina II of the DH and myelinated A fibers terminate exclusively on laminae I, III, IV, and V. However, after nerve injury, myelinated nerve fibers sprout into lamina I and II.[140,141] Investigators have suggested that this anatomic reorganization may play a role in pain mediated by A fibers.[141] NGF administration prevents such sprouting.[142,143]

Brain-derived Neurotrophic Factor

BDNF levels also increase in small DRG during inflammation.[98] Unlike NGF, its transport away from the neuronal soma occurs in the anterograde direction.[144–146] In this regard, BDNF resembles prototypal neurotrophic factors collectively called neuregulins, which are seen in the motor, rather than sensory, system.[147] It has been suggested that the binding of BDNF to TrkB, which activates NMDA receptor phosphorylation, may ultimately lead to central neuronal hyperexcitability.[148,149] Such heightened excitability might play a role in the maintenance of pain. To test this idea, a molecular tool has been synthesized, a TrkB-IgG complex, that specifically binds BDNF and effectively renders it inactive. The probe was shown to have binding characteristics similar to intact Trks. When the complex is applied to the spinal cord after inflammation, the hyperexcitability subsides,[98,150] thus implicating BDNF as a mediator of central sensitization.

Neurotrophin-3 and Neurotrophin-4/5

Less information exists regarding the roles of NT3 and NT4/5 in the development of chronic pain. In inhibiting the electrically evoked release of substance P–like immunoreactivity from isolated rat spinal cords, investigators have recently suggested that NT3 displays antinociceptive properties.[118] They further argued that enkephalins in DH neurons mediate such NT3-induced hypoalgesia because the effect can be blocked by naloxone. Indeed, injected NT3 can transiently reverse experimentally induced inflammatory hyperalgesia.[151] NT3 also increased substance P release from high-threshold (C) fibers in rat spinal cord by electrical stimulation and capsaicin superfusion. Such release was not associated with the development of thermal hyperalgesia.[118,152] Electrophysiologic and behavioral studies in intact rats confirmed that only the TrkB agonists NGF, BDNF, and NT4/5 induced thermal hyperalgesia, whereas the TrkC agonist NT3 had no effect.[153] Hence, investigators have tested and found that NT3 can reverse some injury-induced neuronal changes.[154] Systemic administration of NT3 did produce mechanical hyperalgesia acutely, however, which the authors attributed to autonomic nervous system activation mediated by a relatively nonspecific action on TrkA receptors caused by a transient high concentration.[118,152] They speculated that neurotrophic factor application may have some efficacy in treating nerve root avulsion injuries.[152]

Another recent report has claimed that DRG satellite cells synthesize NT3, which contributes to the sprouting of the sympathetic baskets mentioned earlier around injured neurons.[155] Blocking NT3 with a specific antibody reduces the sprouting by more than 50%.

Glial Cell Line–derived Neurotrophic Factor

GDNF has been recently shown to exert an effect on adult sensory neurons, at least some of which is mediated by purinergic receptors. These receptors are important in the activation of peripheral nociceptors[147,156] by nucleotides and nucleotide phosphates. The two different subtypes of purinoreceptors, P1 and P2, display differential sensitivity to adenosine and adenosine triphosphate/adenosine diphosphate (ATP/ADP), respectively. The P2 receptors can be further divided into P2X, which are agonist-induced ionic channels, and P2Y families. P2X receptors are usually distributed widely in the central nervous system. One subtype, however, called $P2X_3$, can be found only on small, nociceptive, peripheral sensory neurons that bind isolectin B4.[157,158] At low doses, adenosine selectively modulates prejunctional nociceptive transmission. At high doses it appears to act synergistically with the $P2X_3$ ATP receptor to stimulate pain.[147]

GDNF plays an important role in the regulation of $P2X_3$ receptors and, hence, in the development of pain. After axotomy, $P2X_3$ expression decreases by at least 50%. Intrathecal GDNF administration reverses this downregulation of $P2X_3$ receptors[159] and prevents, as well, the decrease of isolectin B4 binding, the number of cells showing thiamine monophosphatase activity, and somatostatin expression. It also prevents the sprouting of A fibers into lamina II of the spinal cord and the slowing of conduction velocity.[142]

IONIC CHANNELS

The dramatic changes in electrical properties of primary sensory neurons seen after injury have led researchers to investigate the role that various neuron-specific ionic channels might play in the development of chronic pain.

Sodium Channels

In one line of inquiry, the importance of Na channels in the development of the hyperexcitability seen after nerve injury has been evaluated. Recent data suggest that at least ten distinct subtypes of Na channels exist.[160–163] These channels have been classified on the basis of their differential sensitivity to the Na channel–blocking drug tetrodotoxin (TTX), their voltage dependence, and their kinetics. Primary sensory neurons express at least six of these channel types, and DRG and trigeminal ganglion cells express three. A single DRG can express more than one type of Na channel. Discrete genes encode for each type. Using reverse transcription-polymerase chain reaction (RT-PCR) or hybridization technologies, α-subunit mRNAs for ten different Na channels have been demonstrated.[162] Large and medium-size DRG produce two TTX-sensitive (TTX-S) channels, which are denoted $Na_V1.6$ and Na_x. Another TTX-S channel called $Na_V1.7$ is found near DRG terminals.[164] DRG also show TTX-resistant (TTX-R) channels, which have been designated $Na_V1.9$ and $Na_V3.1$. Small, nociceptive DRG also express $Na_V1.8$ and $Na_V3.1$channels.

The various Na channels are distributed differently over different populations of DRG. Because they also have different voltage dependencies and kinetics, they confer markedly different electrophysiologic properties on the various populations of neurons that express them. Axotomy has been shown to modulate DRG electrogenesis considerably.[165] The demonstration of abnormal collections of Na channels on injured axons and the partial efficacy of Na channel blockers in ameliorating experimental models of neuropathic pain have led to the suggestion that Na channel activation plays a role in the hyperexcitability seen in chronic pain.[160]

Recent studies have shown that $Na_V1.8$ (formerly denoted SNS/PN3)[166] and $Na_V1.9$ (formerly denoted NaN)[167] channel genes are downregulated after axotomy, and a normally silent $Na_V1.3$ (formerly denoted α-III)[168] gene is upregulated. Hence, there is a decrease in TTX-R Na channels, but an increase in TTX-S currents that recover much more rapidly from inactivation (the $Na_V1.3$ channel).[169] The net effect has been postulated to produce abnormal action potential activity with a lower threshold for firing.[160]

Neurotrophins mediate at least some of the changes in Na channel expression. For example, *in vitro* application of NGF promotes downregulation and upregulation of $Na_V1.3$ and $Na_V1.8$ mRNA expression, respectively.[170] The meaning of the apparent opposing effects of NGF on the membrane excitability of small DRG remains yet unexplained. *In vivo,* NGF effects an incomplete rescue of the $Na_V1.8$ mRNA downregulation seen after axotomy.[171] GDNF appears to at least partly reverse the fall in $Na_V1.9$ mRNA levels seen after axotomy.[172] BDNF appears to have little effect on Na channel expression in DRGs, but does play a role in GABA receptor expression.[173]

Inflammatory pain states also demonstrate abnormal Na channel expression. For example, in such models $Na_V1.8$ mRNA levels increase dramatically in the DRG projecting to the affected extremity.[174] Correlative electrophysiologic studies revealed an increase in both the amplitude and current density of TTX-R Na currents. $Na_V1.9$ mRNA levels also increase.[175]

Some of these changes seem likely mediated by neurotrophins, but the precise sequence of events has not yet been determined. Recently, GDNF and NGF have been shown to reverse the changes seen in repriming of TTX-S Na currents after axotomy.[176] As previously suggested, intact, noninjured DRG normally display two TTX-R Na channel genes ($Na_V1.8$ and $Na_V1.9$) and a silent TTX-S one ($Na_V1.3$). The TTX-R currents inactivate slowly and the TTX-S ones inactivate rapidly. The TTX-R and TTX-S channels also have different kinetics, which allows analysis of recovery from inactivation of Na currents, so-called repriming. The different repriming kinetics permit separation of the TTX-R and TTX-S Na channel currents. The rapidly repriming TTX-S Na currents predominate after axotomy. Both NGF and GDNF can partially ameliorate this shift in repriming current kinetics. Coadministration of NGF and GDNF resulted in complete restoration of the Na channel repriming kinetics.

Potassium Channels

Using human DRG cells obtained from trauma patients and dissociated cultured rat DRG, reports have recently shown changes in specific types of K channels after injury, too.[177] Ca-activated K channels can be divided into three main classes, which display a small (SK), intermediate (IK), or "big" (BK) conductance. The classes can be further divided into different subtypes.[178] Intracellular Ca gates all of them. SK channel activation partly causes the prolonged membrane hyperpolarization that is called the slow afterhyperpolarization, which inhibits or limits action potential generation.

Using immunohistochemical techniques, investigators have demonstrated the presence of a human SK type 1 (hSK1) and a human IK type 1 (hIK1) on the soma of small-to-medium-sized DRG. The hSK1 immunoreactivity decreased in traumatically avulsed DRG. The hIK1 reactivity decreased mostly in large DRG acutely and all-sized DRG chronically. NGF increased the number of hSK1-positive cells in the cultured neurons, whereas NT3 and GDNF did not. NGF also stimulated the expression of the voltage-gated Na channel ($Na_V1.8$). NT3 stimulated the expression of hIK1, but NGF and GDNF did not. The authors suggest that the decreased retrograde transport of the neurotrophic factors that may be seen with injury significantly contribute to the reduced expression of these specific ionic channels and, hence, increased neuronal excitability. They further speculate that novel K channel opener molecules may prove to have therapeutic benefit. Along these lines, the facilitation of K currents by drugs such as mexiletine has been postulated to account for its role in diminishing neuropathic pain.[179,180]

Calcium Channels

Ca channels have been variously classified as L-, P/Q-, N-, R-, and T-type depending on their different α subunit composition.[181] N-type Ca channels mediate excitation-secretion coupling at sensory, sympathetic, and central neurons.[182,183] Specific Ca channel blockers can partially relieve neuropathic pain and decrease ectopic electrical activity in DRG, hence implicating a role for the channel's overactivity in chronic pain states.[184] However, blocking L-type Ca channels appears not to ameliorate nociceptive pain. The clinical efficacy of anticonvulsants such as carbamazepine and gabapentin in the treatment of neuropathic pain has been related to their interactions with Ca channels.[185–187]

HIGHER NEURAL MECHANISMS

In addition to the changes seen in peripheral neural structures, nociceptive and neuropathic pain can modulate neuronal function in supraspinal centers such as the thalamus and somatosensory cortex.[4] For example, Faggin and colleagues[188] recently demonstrated extensive reorganization of the nervous system in response to reversible peripheral sensory deactivation by making concurrent recordings of ventroposteromedial thalamic nuclei and somatosensory cortical neurons. They could not attribute their results to plasticity of cortical circuits alone, but rather needed to invoke the changes in the thalamus as necessary to the cortical reorganization. Other investigators have emphasized the importance of both thalamocortical and corticothalamic signaling in the modulation of supraspinal centers important in the sensation of pain.[189–191] The picture that emerges suggests considerable bidirectional processing of information rather than simply a relay mechanism as nociceptive impulses ascend the neuraxis.[192]

In a strychnine-induced rat model of allodynia, Sherman and colleagues[193] demonstrated alterations in receptive fields and sensory modalities of ventroposterolateral thalamic neurons. After intrathecal strychnine administration, innocuous tactile stimuli elicited painful responses, the spinal afferent neuron cutaneous receptive fields expanded, and the nociceptive-specific ventroposterolateral neurons displayed lower threshold responsiveness. Because strychnine antagonizes glycine action, their data implicate glycinergic inhibitory interneurons as important mediators of allodynia.

Recently, the activity state of rats has been shown to affect tactile stimuli signal processing in the thalamus.[194] Thalamic neurons in rats display low-pass filter characteristics in quiescent animals so that stimulation above frequencies of 2 Hz are cut off and not transmitted to the somatosensory cortex. The same neurons in active animals pass frequencies at up to 40 Hz.

Clinical experience has led to insight about the pathophysiology of thalamic pain signal processing. For example, using single-unit microelectrode recordings of human sensory thalamic neurons in a variety of patients, Hua and colleagues[195] have recently shown the alteration of receptive fields in limb amputation victims. Their studies document the plasticity of the human thalamus in processing both painful and nonpainful stimuli.

Basal ganglia also appear to play a role in nociception. Clinicians have noticed that patients with basal ganglionic disorders such as Parkinson's or Huntington's diseases display abnormal pain sensation. Ganglionic neurons appear to encode stimulus intensity well but not stimulus location. Hence, investigators have proposed that the basal ganglia function in the sensory-discriminative, affective, and cognitive dimensions of pain.[196]

Some somatosensory cortical neurons display variable integration of pain signaling. It has been known for some time that firing patterns characteristic of sensitization, such as paroxysmal bursts seen in the thalamus, are not seen in somatosensory neurons.[197] More recently, some somatosensory cells have been shown to display much less sensitization to sustained application of heat stimuli than heat-responsive neurons in the thalamus. Some somatosensory thermal nociceptive cortical neurons encode the magnitude of heat intensity by continuously varying their mean discharge frequency. Significant numbers of high-threshold and wide-range thermoreceptive neurons, however, do not display such encoding.[198] Still other reports have documented sensitization that is more marked in the cortex than in the thalamus.[199] Finally, in a rat model of chronic arthritis, both sensitized thalamic and somatosensory cortical neurons displayed activation to non-nociceptive stimulation. Clearly, we have only just begun to unravel the complexity of supraspinal pain signal processing and modulation.

GABAergic, NMDA, excitatory amino acid, and glutamatergic neurotransmitter systems have been implicated in supraspinal pain sensation neuronal modulation.[4] For example, recent data have demonstrated the prevention of an extreme type of neuronal hyperexcitability, kainic acid–induced seizures, by the $GABA_A$ agonist, muscimol.[200] Kao and colleagues[201] showed corticothalamic excitatory postsynaptic currents, which displayed electrophysiologic and pharmacologic properties of NMDA-receptor mediated currents; moreover, an NMDA antagonist antagonized them. They also found inhibitory postsynaptic currents, components of which showed sensitivity to bicuculline and a $GABA_B$ antagonist. Because at least some thalamocortical sensory transmission seems to be mediated by NMDA receptors, investigators have proposed that NMDA plays a significant role in the sensitization of the thalamus and somatosensory cortex seen in pain states.[41] Data suggest that the NMDA system maintains the hyperalgesia seen from inflammation, which is perhaps mediated by NO.[202] Researchers have proposed other potential candidates, such as neuropeptides, neurotrophins, or cytokines, that might exert a neuromodulatory action on higher pain sensation centers, but further study remains.

CENTRAL PAIN

Damage to the central nervous system itself can lead to so-called central pain. In such cases, rather than diminishing pain, injury to central pain processing centers often exacerbates the pain sensation, which can be exceedingly difficult to treat. Disease processes such as cerebrovascular ischemia, malignancies, and neurodegenerative disorders can all lead to the development of a central pain syndrome.[4]

For a long time, neuronal events such as proliferation, maturation, neurite outgrowth, and apoptosis have been known to be critical during the formation and development of the brain. These processes were not thought to be significant in the adult. Recent studies have emphasized, however, that central nervous system plasticity continues in the adult and plays a role in the development of central pain. After brain injury, neuronal connections change and form new synapses to occupy the empty places left by degenerating synaptic boutons. Moreover, axonal sprouting may lead to entirely new sites of synaptic contact being made.[203] Indeed, a balance is struck between certain kinds of axonal sprouting being promoted and other types being repelled. The authors speculate that reactive astrocytes may elaborate extracellular matrix molecules such as tenascin-C, proteoglycans, neurocan, or brevican to guide the process.[203] Mechanistically, such injury elicits a response of neurotrophins, adhesion molecules, glia, and many other cellular mediators, which is qualitatively similar to that seen in the periphery.

Brain injury stimulates cytokine production in intrinsic neuroglial cells as well as extrinsic migrating inflammatory macrophages and mast cells.[203] The roles of NGF, BDNF, and tumor necrosis factor (TNF-α) in the development of central pain have drawn attention, but precise mechanisms have not yet been worked out.

Investigators have also focused on the role of the neuronal growth associated phosphoprotein, GAP-43 (neuromodulin), in regulating nerve terminal growth. Experimentally induced excess of GAP-43 provokes *de novo* synaptogenesis and more profuse axonal sprouting after injury.[204] It seems to exert a powerful influence in particular on the neuron's cytoskeleton. Protein kinase C phosphorylation appears to mediate the transduction of intra- and extracellular signals regulating nerve terminal sprouting and long-term potentiation in response to injury. Moreover, it has been shown that radiolabeled phosphate incorporation into GAP-43 correlates with the extent of synaptic enhancement.[205] An NMDA receptor antagonist that blocks long-term potentiation has been shown to inhibit the increase in phosphorylation.[206] Thus, it appears that some postsynaptic event requiring NMDA-receptor activation leads to GAP-43 phosphorylation and then to a retrograde signal, which modulates presynaptic GAP-43.[207]

CONCLUSION

During the so-called decade of the brain, the 1990s, scientists made considerable advances in our understanding the pathophysiology of chronic pain. The research that has lead to a better understanding of the operative cellular and molecular mechanisms has continued into the new millennium. Much has been learned that will, it is hoped, lead to the development of therapeutic interventions to treat these conditions. Much remains to be discovered.

REFERENCES

1. Khan AA, Raja SN, Manning DC, Campbell JN, Meyer RA. The effects of bradykinin and sequence-related analogs on the response properties of cutaneous nociceptors in monkeys. *Somatosens Mot Res* 1992;9:97–106.
2. Lang E, Novak A, Reeh PW, Handwerker HO. Chemosensitivity of fine afferents from rat skin in vitro. *J Neurophysiol* 1990;63:887–901.
3. Manning DC, Raja SN, Meyer RA, Campbell JN. Pain and hyperalgesia after intradermal injection of bradykinin in humans. *Clin Pharmacol Ther* 1991;50:721–729.
4. Millan MJ. The induction of pain: An integrative review. *Prog Neurobiol* 1999;57:1–164.
5. Prado GN, Taylor L, Polgar P. Effects of intracellular tyrosine residue mutation and carboxyl terminus truncation on signal transduction and internalization of the rat bradykinin B2 receptor. *J Biol Chem* 1997;272:14638–14642.
6. Coleman RA, Smith WL, Narumiya S. International Union of Pharmacology classification of prostanoid receptors: Properties, distribution, and structure of the receptors and their subtypes. *Pharmacol Rev* 1994;46:205–229.
7. Kress M, Rodl J, Reeh PW. Stable analogues of cyclic AMP but not cyclic GMP sensitize unmyelinated primary afferents in rat skin to heat stimulation but not to inflammatory mediators, in vitro. *Neuroscience* 1996;74:609–617.
8. Malmberg AB, Brandon EP, Idzerda RL, Liu H, McKnight GS, Basbaum AI. Diminished inflammation and nociceptive pain with preservation of neuropathic pain in mice with a targeted mutation of the type I regulatory subunit of cAMP-dependent protein kinase. *J Neurosci* 1997;17:7462–7470.
9. Levine JD, Reichling DB. Peripheral mechanisms of inflammatory pain. In: Wall PD, Melzack R, eds. *Textbook of Pain.* 4th ed, New York, NY: Churchill Livingstone; 1999:59–84.
10. Gold MS, Reichling DB, Shuster MJ, Levine JD. Hyperalgesic agents increase a tetrodotoxin-resistant Na+ current in nociceptors. *Proc Natl Acad Sci U S A* 1996;93:1108–1112.
11. Dray A, Perkins M. Bradykinin and inflammatory pain. *Trends Neurosci* 1993;16:99–104.
12. Carlton SM, Coggeshall RE. Immunohistochemical localization of 5-HT2A receptors in peripheral sensory axons in rat glabrous skin. *Brain Res* 1997;763:271–275.
13. Abbott FV, Hong Y, Blier P. Persisting sensitization of the behavioural response to formalin-induced injury in the rat through activation of serotonin2A receptors. *Neuroscience* 1997;77:575–584.
14. Todorovic SM, Scroggs RS, Anderson EG. Cationic modulation of 5-HT2 and 5-HT3 receptors in rat sensory neurons: the role of K+, Ca2+, and Mg2+. *Brain Res* 1997;765:291–300.
15. Holthusen H, Arndt JO. Nitric oxide evokes pain in humans on intracutaneous injection. *Neurosci Lett* 1994;165:71–74.
16. Lawand NB, Willis WD, Westlund KN. Blockade of joint inflammation and secondary hyperalgesia by L-NAME, a nitric oxide synthase inhibitor. *Neuroreport* 1997;8:895–899.
17. Duarte ID, dos Santos IR, Lorenzetti BB, Ferreira SH. Analgesia by direct antagonism of nociceptor sensitization involves the arginine-nitric oxide-cGMP pathway. *Eur J Pharmacol* 1992;217:225–227.
18. Kawabata A, Manabe S, Manabe Y, Takagi H. Effect of topical administration of L-arginine on formalin-induced nociception in the mouse: A dual role of peripherally formed NO in pain modulation. *Br J Pharmacol* 1994;112:547–550.
19. Holthusen H, Kindgen-Milles D, Ding ZP. Substance P is not involved in vascular nociception in humans. *Neuropeptides* 1997;31:445–448.
20. Fletcher DS, Widmer WR, Luell S, et al. Therapeutic administration of a selective inhibitor of nitric oxide synthase does not ameliorate the chronic inflammation and tissue damage associated with adjuvant-induced arthritis in rats. *J Pharmacol Exp Ther* 1998;284:714–721.
21. Fozard JR. The 5-hydroxytryptamine-nitric oxide connection: The key link in the initiation of migraine? *Arch Int Pharmacodyn Ther* 1995;329:111–119.
22. Berninger B, Garcia DE, Inagaki N, Hahnel C, Lindholm D. DNF and NT-3 induce intracellular Ca2+ elevation in hippocampal neurones. *Neuroreport* 1993;4:1303–1306.
23. Berninger B, Poo M. Fast actions of neurotrophic factors. *Curr Opin Neurobiol* 1996;6:324–330.
24. Bevan S, Winter J. Nerve growth factor (NGF) differentially regulates the chemosensitivity of adult rat cultured sensory neurons. *J Neurosci* 1995;15(pt 1):4918–4926.
25. Winter J. Brain derived neurotrophic factor, but not nerve growth factor, regulates capsaicin sensitivity of rat vagal ganglion neurones. *Neurosci Lett* 1998;241:21–24.
26. Sherwood NT, Lesser SS, Lo DC. Neurotrophin regulation of ionic currents and cell size depends on cell context. *Proc Natl Acad Sci U S A* 1997;94:5917–5922.
27. Handwerker HO, Kilo S, Reeh PW. Unresponsive afferent nerve fibres in the sural nerve of the rat. *J Physiol* 1991;435:229–242.
28. Meyer RA, Davis KD, Cohen RH, Treede RD, Campbell JN. Mechanically insensitive afferents (MIAs) in cutaneous nerves of monkey. *Brain Res* 1991;561:252–261.
29. Stucky CL, Thayer SA, Seybold VS. Prostaglandin E2 increases the proportion of neonatal rat dorsal root ganglion neurons that respond to bradykinin. *Neuroscience* 1996;74:1111–1123.
30. Handwerker HO, Kobal G. Psychophysiology of experimentally induced pain. *Physiol Rev* 1993;73:639–671.
31. Treede RD, Davis KD, Campbell JN, Raja SN. The plasticity of cutaneous hyperalgesia during sympathetic ganglion blockade in patients with neuropathic pain. *Brain* 1992;115(pt 2):607–621.

32. Gracely RH, Lynch SA, Bennett GJ. Painful neuropathy: Altered central processing maintained dynamically by peripheral input. *Pain* 1992;51:175–194.
33. Koltzenburg M. Stability and plasticity of nociceptor function and their relationship to provoked ongoing pain. *Semin Neurosci* 1995;7: 199–210.
34. Sang CN. NDMA-receptor antagonists in neuropathing pain: Experimental methods to clinical trials. *J Pain Symptom Manage* 2000; 19(suppl S21–25).
35. Ma Z-P, Woolf CJ. Basal and touch-evoked fos-like immunoreactivity during experimental inflammation in the rat. *Pain* 1996;67:307–316.
36. Ali Z, Meyer RA, Campbell JN. Secondary hyperalgesia to mechanical but not heat stimuli following a capsaicin injection in hairy skin. *Pain* 1996;68:401–411.
37. Woolf CJ. A new strategy for the treatment of inflammatory pain. Prevention or elimination of central sensitization. *Drugs* 1994;47(suppl 5):1–9; 46–47.
38. Gozariu M, Bouhassira D, Willer JC, Le Bars D. The influence of temporal summation on a C-fibre reflex in the rat: Effects of lesions in the rostral ventromedial medulla (RVM). *Brain Res* 1998;792:168–172.
39. Guirimand F, Dupont X, Brasseur L, Chauvin M, Bouhassira D. The effects of ketamine on the temporal summation (wind-up) of the R(III) nociceptive flexion reflex and pain in humans. *Anesth Analg* 2000; 90:408–414.
40. Baranauskas G, Nistri A. Sensitization of pain pathways in the spinal cord: Cellular mechanisms. *Prog Neurobiol* 1998;54:349–365.
41. Isaac JT, Crair MC, Nicoll RA, Malenka RC. Silent synapses during development of thalamocortical inputs. *Neuron* 1997;18:269–280.
42. Malenka RC, Nicoll RA. Silent synapses speak up. *Neuron* 1997;19: 473–476.
43. King AE, Thompson SWN. Brief and prolonged changes in spinal excitability following peripheral injury. *Semin Neurosci* 1995;7:233–243.
44. Lin Q, Peng YB, Wu J, Willis WD. Involvement of cGMP in nociceptive processing by and sensitization of spinothalamic neurons in primates. *J Neurosci* 1997;17:3293–3302.
45. Sluka KA, Milton MA, Willis WD, Westlund KN. Differential roles of neurokinin 1 and neurokinin 2 receptors in the development and maintenance of heat hyperalgesia induced by acute inflammation. *Br J Pharmacol* 1997;120:1263–1273.
46. Sluka KA, Rees H, Chen PS, Tsuruoka M, Willis WD. Capsaicin-induced sensitization of primate spinothalamic tract cells is prevented by a protein kinase C inhibitor. *Brain Res* 1997;772:82–86.
47. Chizh BA, Cumberbatch MJ, Herrero JF, Stirk GC, Headley PM. Stimulus intensity, cell excitation and the N-methyl-D-aspartate receptor component of sensory responses in the rat spinal cord in vivo. *Neuroscience* 1997;80:251–265.
48. Sharma G, Stevens CF. A mutation that alters magnesium block of N-methyl-D-aspartate receptor channels. *Proc Natl Acad Sci U S A* 1996;93:9259–9263.
49. Reichling DB, MacDermott AB. NMDA receptor-mediated calcium entry in the absence of AMPA receptor activation in rat dorsal horn neurons. *Neurosci Lett* 1996;204:17–20.
50. Zheng X, Zhang L, Wang AP, Bennett MV, Zukin RS. Ca2+ influx amplifies protein kinase C potentiation of recombinant NMDA receptors. *J Neurosci* 1997;17:8676–8686.
51. Lerea LS. Glutamate receptors and gene induction: Signalling from receptor to nucleus. *Cell Signal* 1997;9:219–226.
52. Coggeshall RE, Carlton SM. Receptor localization in the mammalian dorsal horn and primary afferent neurons. *Brain Res Brain Res Rev* 1997;24:28–66.
53. Barria A, Muller D, Derkach V, Griffith LC, Soderling TR. Regulatory phosphorylation of AMPA-type glutamate receptors by CaM-KII during long-term potentiation. *Science* 1997;276:2042–2045.
54. Lisman J, Malenka RC, Nicoll RA, Malinow R. Learning mechanisms: The case for CaM-KII. *Science* 1997;276:2001–2002.
55. Abbadie C, Trafton J, Liu H, Mantyh PW, Basbaum AI. Inflammation increases the distribution of dorsal horn neurons that internalize the neurokinin-1 receptor in response to noxious and non-noxious stimulation. *J Neurosci* 1997;17:8049–8060.
56. Chapman V, Buritova J, Honore P, Besson JM. Physiological contributions of neurokinin 1 receptor activation, and interactions with NMDA receptors, to inflammatory-evoked spinal c-Fos expression. *J Neurophysiol* 1996;76:1817–1827.
57. Clayton JS, Gaskin PJ, Beattie DT. Attenuation of Fos-like immunoreactivity in the trigeminal nucleus caudalis following trigeminovascular activation in the anaesthetised guinea-pig. *Brain Res* 1997; 775:74–80.
58. Huber KM, Sawtell NB, Bear MF. Effects of the metabotropic glutamate receptor antagonist MCPG on phosphoinositide turnover and synaptic plasticity in visual cortex. *J Neurosci* 1998;18:1–9.
59. Vickery RM, Morris SH, Bindman LJ. Metabotropic glutamate receptors are involved in long-term potentiation in isolated slices of rat medial frontal cortex. *J Neurophysiol* 1997;78:3039–3046.
60. Budai D, Larson AA. The involvement of metabotropic glutamate receptors in sensory transmission in dorsal horn of the rat spinal cord. *Neuroscience* 1998;83:571–580.
61. Miletic V, Tan H. Iontophoretic application of calcitonin gene-related peptide produces a slow and prolonged excitation of neurons in the cat lumbar dorsal horn. *Brain Res* 1988;446:169–172.
62. Rostas JA, Brent VA, Voss K, Errington ML, Bliss TV, Gurd JW. Enhanced tyrosine phosphorylation of the 2B subunit of the N-methyl-D-aspartate receptor in long-term potentiation. *Proc Natl Acad Sci U S A* 1996;93:10452–10456.
63. Bito H, Deisseroth K, Tsien RW. Ca2+-dependent regulation in neuronal gene expression. *Curr Opin Neurobiol* 1997;7:419–429.
64. Deisseroth K, Heist EK, Tsien RW. Translocation of calmodulin to the nucleus supports CREB phosphorylation in hippocampal neurons. *Nature* 1998;392:198–202.
65. Lin Q, Peng YB, Willis WD. Inhibition of primate spinothalamic tract neurons by spinal glycine and GABA is reduced during central sensitization. *J Neurophysiol* 1996;76:1005–1014.
66. Malcangio M, Bowery NG. GABA and its receptors in the spinal cord. *Trends Pharmacol Sci* 1996;17:457–462.
67. Todd AJ, Watt C, Spike RC, Sieghart W. Colocalization of GABA, glycine, and their receptors at synapses in the rat spinal cord. *J Neurosci* 1996;16:974–982.
68. Hwang JH, Yaksh TL. The effect of spinal GABA receptor agonists on tactile allodynia in a surgically-induced neuropathic pain model in the rat. *Pain* 1997;70:15–22.
69. Gu ZZ, Pan YC, Cui JK, Klebuc MJ, Shenaq S, Liu PK. Gene expression and apoptosis in the spinal cord neurons after sciatic nerve injury. *Neurochem Int* 1997;30:417–426.
70. Nishio E, Watanabe Y. NO induced apoptosis accompanying the change of oncoprotein expression and the activation of CPP32 protease. *Life Sci* 1998;62:239–245.
71. Oliveira AL, Risling M, Deckner M, Lindholm T, Langone F, Cullheim S. Neonatal sciatic nerve transection induces TUNEL labeling of neurons in the rat spinal cord and DRG. *Neuroreport* 1997;8: 2837–2840.
72. Dumoulin A, Alonso G, Privat A, Feldblum S. Biphasic response of spinal GABAergic neurons after a lumbar rhizotomy in the adult rat. *Eur J Neurosci* 1996;8:2553–2563.
73. Basbaum AI, Fields HL. Endogenous pain control systems: Brainstem spinal pathways and endorphin circuitry. *Annu Rev Neurosci* 1984;7:309–338.
74. Melzack R, Wall PD. Pain mechanisms: A new theory. *Science* 1965;150:971–979.
75. Mansikka H, Pertovaara A. Supraspinal influence on hindlimb withdrawal thresholds and mustard oil-induced secondary allodynia in rats. *Brain Res Bull* 1997;42:359–365.
76. Millan MJ. Descending control of pain. *Prog Neurobiol* 2002;66: 355–474.

77. Inoue A, Hashimoto T, Hide I, Nishio H, Nakata Y. 5-Hydroxytryptamine-facilitated release of substance P from rat spinal cord slices is mediated by nitric oxide and cyclic GMP. *J Neurochem* 1997;68:128–133.
78. Yang SW, Guo YQ, Kang YM, Qiao JT, Laufman LE, Dafny N. Different gaba-receptor types are involved in the 5-ht induced antinociception at the spinal level: A behavioral study. *Life Sci* 1998;62:PL143–PL148.
79. Vallone D, Picetti R, Borrelli E. Structure and function of dopamine receptors. *Neurosci Biobehav Rev* 2000;24:125–132.
80. Bourgoin S, Pohl M, Mauborgne A, et al. Monoaminergic control of the release of calcitonin gene-related peptide- and substance P-like materials from rat spinal cord slices. *Neuropharmacology* 1993;32:633–640.
81. Gao K, Mason P. Serotonergic raphe magnus cells that respond to noxious tail heat are not ON or OFF cells. *J Neurophysiol* 2000;84:1719–1725.
82. Gear RW, Aley KO, Levine JD. Pain-induced analgesia mediated by mesolimbic reward circuits. *J Neurosci* 1999;19:7175–7181.
83. Gilbert AK, Franklin KB. Characterization of the analgesic properties of nomifensine in rats. *Pharmacol Biochem Behav* 2001;68:783–787.
84. Ciliax BJ, Nash N, Heilman C, et al. Dopamine D(5) receptor immunolocalization in rat and monkey brain. *Synapse* 2000;37:125–145.
85. Kitahama K, Nagatsu I, Geffard M, Maeda T. Distribution of dopamine-immunoreactive fibers in the rat brainstem. *J Chem Neuroanat* 2000;18:1–9.
86. Hokfelt T, Arvidsson U, Cullheim S, et al. Multiple messengers in descending serotonin neurons: Localization and functional implications. *J Chem Neuroanat* 2000;18:75–86.
87. Millan MJ. The role of descending noradrenergic and serotoninergic pathways in the modulation of nociception: focus on receptor multiplicity. In: Dickenson A, Besson JM, eds. *The Pharmacology of Pain: Handbook of Experimental Pharmacology* vol. 130. Berlin, Germany: Springer-Verlag; 1997:385–446.
88. Schreihofer AM, Guyenet PG. Identification of C1 presympathetic neurons in rat rostral ventrolateral medulla by juxtacellular labeling in vivo. *J Comp Neurol* 1997;387:524–536.
89. Simpson KL, Altman DW, Wang L, Kirifides ML, Lin RC, Waterhouse BD. Lateralization and functional organization of the locus coeruleus projection to the trigeminal somatosensory pathway in rat. *J Comp Neurol* 1997;385:135–147.
90. Martin WJ, Gupta NK, Loo CM, Rohde DS, Basbaum AI. Differential effects of neurotoxic destruction of descending noradrenergic pathways on acute and persistent nociceptive processing. *Pain* 1999;80:57–65.
91. Milne B, Hall SR, Sullivan ME, Loomis C. The release of spinal prostaglandin E2 and the effect of nitric oxide synthetase inhibition during strychnine-induced allodynia. *Anesth Analg* 2001;93:728–733.
92. Jones SL. Noradrenergic modulation of noxious heat-evoked fos-like immunoreactivity in the dorsal horn of the rat sacral spinal cord. *J Comp Neurol* 1992;325:435–445.
93. Paqueron X, Li X, Eisenach JC. P75-expressing elements are necessary for anti-allodynic effects of spinal clonidine and neostigmine. *Neuroscience* 2001;102:681–686.
94. Hammond DL. Inhibitory neurotransmitters and nociception: Role of GABA and glycine. In: Dickenson A, Besson J-M, eds. *The Pharmacology of Pain: Handbook of Experimental Pharmacology* vol. 130 Berlin, Germany: Springer-Verlag; 1997:361–384.
95. Levi-Montalcini R. The nerve growth factor: Its mode of action on sensory and sympathetic nerve cells. *Harvey Lect* 1966;60:217–259.
96. Levi-Montalcini R. The saga of the nerve growth factor. *Neuroreport* 1998;9:R71–R83.
97. Levi-Montalcini R, Dal Toso R, della Valle F, Skaper SD, Leon A. Update of the NGF saga. *J Neurol Sci* 1995;130:119–127.
98. McMahon SB, Bennett DLH. Trophic factors and pain. In: Wall PD, Melzack R, eds. *Textbook of Pain* 4th ed. New York, NY: Churchill Livingstone; 1999:105–128.
99. Chao MV. The p75 neurotrophin receptor. *J Neurobiol* 1994;25:1373–1385.
100. Barbacid M. The Trk family of neurotrophin receptors. *J Neurobiol* 1994;25:1386–1403.
101. Barbacid M. The Trk family of neurotrophin receptors: Molecular characterization and oncogenic activation in human tumors. In: Levine AJ, Schmidek HH, eds. *Molecular Genetics of Nervous System Tumors* New York, NY: Wiley and Sons;1993:123–135.
102. Clary DO, Weskamp G, Austin LR, Reichardt LF. TrkA cross-linking mimics neuronal responses to nerve growth factor. *Mol Biol Cell* 1994;5:549–563.
103. Ibanez CF, Ilag LL, Murray-Rust J, Persson H. An extended surface of binding to Trk tyrosine kinase receptors in NGF and BDNF allows the engineering of a multifunctional pan-neurotrophin. *EMBO J* 1993;12:2281–2293.
104. Carter BD, Kaltschmidt C, Kaltschmidt B, et al. Selective activation of NF-kappa B by nerve growth factor through the neurotrophin receptor p75. *Science* 1996;272:542–545.
105. Baeuerle PA, Henkel T. Function and activation of NF-kappa B in the immune system. *Annu Rev Immunol* 1994;12:141–179.
106. Lewin GR, Ritter AM, Mendell LM. Nerve growth factor-induced hyperalgesia in the neonatal and adult rat. *J Neurosci* 1993;13:2136–2148.
107. Crowley C, Spencer SD, Nishimura MC, et al. Mice lacking nerve growth factor display perinatal loss of sensory and sympathetic neurons yet develop basal forebrain cholinergic neurons. *Cell* 1994;76:1001–1011.
108. Ruit KG, Elliott JL, Osborne PA, Yan Q, Snider WD. Selective dependence of mammalian dorsal root ganglion neurons on nerve growth factor during embryonic development. *Neuron* 1992;8:573–587.
109. Lindsay RM, Harmar AJ. Nerve growth factor regulates expression of neuropeptide genes in adult sensory neurons. *Nature* 1989;337:362–364.
110. Petersen M, von Banchet S, Heppelmann B, Koltzenburg M. Nerve growth factor regulates the expression of bradykinin binding sites on adult sensory neurons via the neurotrophin receptor p75. *Neuroscience* 1998;83:161–168.
111. Petty BG, Cornblath DR, Adornato BT, et al. The effect of systemically administered recombinant human nerve growth factor in healthy human subjects. *Ann Neurol* 1994;36:244–246.
112. Thoenen H. Neurotrophins and neuronal plasticity. *Science* 1995;270:593.
113. Andreev NY, Dimitrieva N, Koltzenburg M, McMahon SB. Peripheral administration of nerve growth factor in the adult rat produces a thermal hyperalgesia that requires the presence of sympathetic post-ganglionic neurones. *Pain* 1995;63:109–115.
114. Woolf CJ, Ma QP, Allchorne A, Poole S. Peripheral cell types contributing to the hyperalgesic action of nerve growth factor in inflammation. *J Neurosci* 1996;16:2716–2723.
115. Martin HA, Basbaum AI, Goetzl EJ, Levine JD. Leukotriene B4 decreases the mechanical and thermal thresholds of C-fiber nociceptors in the hairy skin of the rat. *J Neurophysiol* 1988;60:438–445.
116. Amann R, Schuligoi R, Lanz I, Peskar BA. Effect of a 5-lipoxygenase inhibitor on nerve growth factor-induced thermal hyperalgesia in the rat. *Eur J Pharmacol* 1996;306:89–91.
117. Bennett G, al-Rashed S, Hoult JRS, Brain SD. Nerve growth factor induced hyperalgesia in the rat hind paw is dependent on circulating neutrophils. *Pain* 1998;77:315–322.
118. Malcangio M, Garrett NE, Cruwys S, Tomlison DR. Nerve growth factor- and neurotrophin-3-induced changes in nociceptive threshold and the release of substance P from the rat isolated spinal cord. *J Neurol Sci* 1997;17:8459–8467.
119. Rich KM, Luszczynski JR, Osborne PA, Johnson EM Jr. Nerve growth factor protects adult sensory neurons from cell death and atrophy caused by nerve injury. *J Neurocytol* 1987;16:261–268.
120. Mulderry PK, Dobson SP. Regulation of VIP and other neuropeptides by c-Jun in sensory neurons: implications for the neuropeptide response to axotomy. *Eur J Neurosci* 1996;8:2479–2491.

121. Gold BG, Storm-Dickerson T, Austin DR. Regulation of aberrant neurofilament phosphorylation in neuronal perikarya. IV. Evidence for the involvement of two signals. *Brain Res* 1993;626:23–30.
122. Hokfelt T, Zhang X, Wiesenfeld-Hallin Z. Messenger plasticity in primary sensory neurons following axotomy and its functional implications. *Trends Neurosci* 1994;17:22–30.
123. Woolf CJ, Reynolds ML, Molander C, O'Brien C, Lindsay RM, Benowitz LI. The growth-associated protein GAP-43 appears in dorsal root ganglion cells and in the dorsal horn of the rat spinal cord following peripheral nerve injury. *Neuroscience* 1990;34:465–478.
124. Bennett DLH, Michael GJ, Ramachandran N, et al. A distinct subgroup of small DRG cells express GDNF receptor components and GDNF is protective for these neurons after nerve injury. *J Neurol Sci* 1998;18:3059–3072.
125. McMahon SB, Priestley JV. Peripheral neuropathies and neurotrophic factors: Animal models and clinical perspectives. *Curr Opin Neurobiol* 1995;5:616–624.
126. Apfel SC, Kessler JA, Adornato BT, Litchy WJ, Sanders C, Rask CA. Recombinant human nerve growth factor in the treatment of diabetic polyneuropathy. NGF Study Group. *Neurology* 1998;51:695–702.
127. Apfel SC, Schwartz S, Adornato BT, et al. Efficacy and safety of recombinant human nerve growth factor in patients with diabetic polyneuropathy: A randomized controlled trial. rhNGF Clinical Investigator Group. *JAMA* 2000;284:2215–2221.
128. Chattopadhyay M, Wolfe D, Huang S, et al. In vivo gene therapy for pyridoxine-induced neuropathy by herpes simplex virus-medicated gene transfer of neurotrophin-3. *Ann Neurol* 2002;51:19–27.
129. Bennett DL, Koltzenburg M, Priestley JV, Shelton DL, McMahon SB. Endogenous nerve growth factor regulates the sensitivity of nociceptors in the adult rat. *Eur J Neurosci* 1998;10:1282–1291.
130. Aloe L, Tuveri MA, Carcassi U, Levi-Montalcini R. Nerve growth factor in the synovial fluid of patients with chronic arthritis. *Arthritis Rheum* 1992;35:351–355.
131. Lowe EM, Anand P, Terenghi G, Williams-Chestnut RE, Sinicropi DV, Osborne JL. Increased nerve growth factor levels in the urinary bladder of women with idiopathic sensory urgency and interstitial cystitis. *Br J Urol* 1997;79:572–577.
132. Bennett DLH, McMahon SB, Rattray M, Shelton D. Nerve growth factor and sensory nerve function. In: Brain SD, Moore PK, eds. *Pain and Neurogenic Inflammation* Berlin, Germany: Springer-Verlag; 1999.
133. Deng YS, Zhong JH, Zhou XF. Effects of endogenous neurotrophins on sympathetic sprouting in the dorsal root ganglia and allodynia following spinal nerve injury. *Exper Neurol* 2000;164:344–350.
134. Ramer MS, Kawaja MD, Henderson JT, Roder JC, Bisby MA. Glial overexpression of NGF enhances neuropathic pain and adrenergic sprouting into DRG following chronic sciatic constriction in mice. *Neurosci Lett* 1998;251:53–56.
135. Ramer MS, Thompson SWN, McMahon SB. Causes and consequences of sympathetic basket formation in dorsal root ganglia. *Pain Supp* 1999;6:S111–S120.
136. Davis BM, Albers KM, Seroogy KB, Katz DM. Overexpression of nerve growth factor in transgenic mice induces novel sympathetic projections to primary sensory neurons. *J Comp Neurol* 1994;349:464–474.
137. Davis BM, Goodness TP, Soria A, Albers KM. Over-expression of NGF in skin causes formation of novel sympathetic projections to trkA-positive sensory neurons. *Neuroreport* 1998;9:1103–1107.
138. Jones MG, Munson JB, Thompson SW. A role for nerve growth factor in sympathetic sprouting in rat dorsal root ganglia. *Pain* 1999 Jan;79(1):21–29.
139. Ramer MS, French GD, Bisby MA. Wallerian degeneration is required for both neuropathic pain and sympathetic sprouting into the DRG. *Pain* 1997;72:71–78.
140. Shortland P, Woolf CJ. Chronic peripheral nerve section results in a rearrangement of the central axonal arborizations of axotomized A beta primary afferent neurons in the rat spinal cord. *J Comp Neurol* 1993;330:65–82.
141. Woolf CJ, Shortland P, Coggeshall RE. Peripheral nerve injury triggers central sprouting of myelinated afferents. *Nature* 1992;355: 75–78.
142. Bennett DL, French J, Priestley JV, McMahon SB. NGF but not NT-3 or BDNF prevents the A fiber sprouting into lamina II of the spinal cord that occurs following axotomy. *Mol Cell Neurosci* 1996; 8:211–220.
143. Eriksson NP, Aldskogius H, Grant G, Lindsay RM, Rivero-Melian C. Effects of nerve growth factor, brain-derived neurotrophic factor and neurotrophin-3 on the laminar distribution of transganglionically transported choleragenoid in the spinal cord dorsal horn following transection of the sciatic nerve in the adult rat. *Neuroscience* 1997; 78:863–872.
144. Cho HJ, Kim JK, Zhou XF, Rush RA. Increased brain-derived neurotrophic factor immunoreactivity in rat dorsal root ganglia and spinal cord following peripheral inflammation. *Brain Res* 1997;764: 269–272.
145. Cho HJ, Kim SY, Park MJ, Kim DS, Kim JK, Chu, MY. Expression of mRNA for brain-derived neurotrophic factor in the dorsal root ganglion following peripheral inflammation. *Brain Res* 1997;749:358–362.
146. Michael GJ, Averill S, Nitkunan A, et al. Nerve growth factor treatment increases brain-derived neurotrophic factor selectively in TrkA-expressing dorsal root ganglion cells and in their central terminations within the spinal cord. *J Neurosci* 1997;17:8476–8490.
147. Burnstock G, Wood JN. Purinergic receptors: Their role in nociception and primary afferent neurotransmission. *Curr Opin Neurobiol* 1996;6:526–532.
148. Levine ES, Crozier RA, Black IB, Plummer MR. Brain-derived neurotrophic factor modulates hippocampal synaptic transmission by increasing N-methyl-D-aspartic acid receptor activity. *Proc Natl Acad Sci U S A* 1998;95:10235–10239.
149. McMahon SB, Lewin GR, Wall PD. Central hyperexcitability triggered by noxious inputs. *Curr Opin Neurobiol* 1993;3:602–610.
150. Shelton DL, Sutherland J, Gripp J, et al. Human trks: Molecular cloning, tissue distribution, and expression of extracellular domain immunoadhesins. *J Neurosci* 1995;15(pt 2):477–491.
151. Watanabe M, Endo Y, Kimoto K, Katoh-Semba R, Arakawa Y. Inhibition of adjuvant-induced inflammatory hyperalgesia in rats by local injection of neurotrophin-3. *Neurosci Lett* 2000;282:61–64.
152. Ramer MS, Priestley JV, McMahon SB. Functional regeneration of sensory axons into the adult spinal cord. *Nature* 2000;403:312–316.
153. Shu XQ, Llinas A, Mendell LM. Effects of trkB and trkC neurotrophin receptor agonists on thermal nociception: a behavioral and electrophysiological study. *Pain* 1999;80:463–470.
154. Ohara S, Tantuwaya V, DiStefano PS, Schmidt RE. Exogenous NT-3 mitigates the transganglionic neuropeptide Y response to sciatic nerve injury. *Brain Res* 1995;699:143–148.
155. Zhou XF, Deng YS, Chie EC, et al. Satellite-cell-derived nerve growth factor and neurotrophin-3 are involved in noradrenergic sprouting in the dorsal root ganglia following peripheral nerve injury in the rat. *Eur J Neurosci* 1999;11:1711–1722.
156. Bland-Ward PA, Humphrey PP. Acute nociception mediated by hindpaw P2X receptor activation in the rat. *Br J Pharmacol* 1997;122: 365–371.
157. Chen CC, Akopian AN, Sivilotti L, Colquhoun D, Burnstock G, Wood JN. A P2X purinoceptor expressed by a subset of sensory neurons. *Nature* 1995;377:428–431.
158. Lewis C, Neidhart S, Holy C, North RA, Buell G, Surprenant A. Coexpression of P2X2 and P2X3 receptor subunits can account for ATP-gated currents in sensory neurons. *Nature* 1995;377:432–435.
159. Bradbury EJ, Burnstock G, McMahon SB. The expression of P2X3 purinoreceptors in sensory neurons: Effects of axotomy and glial-derived neurotrophic factor. *Mol Cell Neurosci* 1998;12:256–268.

160. Waxman SG, Cummins RR, Dib-Hajj S, Fjell J, Black JA. Sodium channels, excitability of primary sensory neurons, and the molecular basis of pain. *Muscle Nerve* 1999;22:1177–1187.
161. Goldin AL. Diversity of mammalian voltage-gated sodium channels. *Ann N Y Acad Sci* 1999;868:38–50.
162. Goldin AL. Resurgence of sodium channel research. *Annu Rev Physiol* 2001;63:871–894.
163. Goldin AL, Barchi RL, Caldwell JH, et al. Nomenclature of voltage-gated sodium channels. *Neuron* 2000;28:365–368.
164. Toledo-Aral JJ, Moss BL, He ZJ, et al. Identification of PN1, a predominant voltage-dependent sodium channel expressed principally in peripheral neurons. *Proc Natl Acad Sci U S A* 1997;94:1527–1532.
165. Gurtu S, Smith PA. Electrophysiological characteristics of hamster dorsal root ganglion cells and their response to axotomy. *J Neurophysiol* 1988;59:408–423.
166. Dib-Hajj S, Black JA, Felts P, Waxman SG. Down-regulation of transcripts for Na channel alpha-SNS in spinal sensory neurons following axotomy. *Proc Natl Acad Sci U S A* 1996;93:14950–14954.
167. Dib-Hajj SD, Black JA, Cummins TR, Kenney AM, Kocsis JD, Waxman SG. Rescue of alpha-SNS sodium channel expression in small dorsal root ganglion neurons after axotomy by nerve growth factor in vivo. *J Neurophysiol* 1998;79:2668–2676.
168. Waxman SG, Kocsis JD, Black JA. Type III sodium channel mRNA is expressed in embryonic but not adult spinal sensory neurons, and is reexpressed following axotomy. *J Neurophysiol* 1994;72:466–470.
169. Cummins TR, Waxman SG. Downregulation of tetrodotoxin-resistant sodium currents and upregulation of a rapidly repriming tetrodotoxin-sensitive sodium current in small spinal sensory neurons after nerve injury. *J Neurosci* 1997;17:3503–3514.
170. Black JA, Langworthy K, Hinson AW, Dib-Hajj SD, Waxman SG. NGF has opposing effects on Na+ channel III and SNS gene expression in spinal sensory neurons. *Neuroreport* 1997;8:2331–2335.
171. Dib-Hajj SD, Tyrrell L, Black JA, Waxman SG. NaN, a novel voltage-gated Na channel, is expressed preferentially in peripheral sensory neurons and down-regulated after axotomy. *Proc Natl Acad Sci U S A* 1998;95:8963–8968.
172. Fjell J, Cummins TR, Dib-Hajj SD, Fried K, Black JA, Waxman SG. Differential role of GDNF and NGF in the maintenance of two TTX-resistant sodium channels in adult DRG neurons. *Brain Res Mol Brain Res* 1999;67:267–282.
173. Oyelese AA, Rizzo MA, Waxman SG, Kocsis JD. Differential effects of NGF and BDNF on axotomy-induced changes in GABA(A)-receptor-mediated conductance and sodium currents in cutaneous afferent neurons. *J Neurophysiol* 1997;78:31–42.
174. Tanaka M, Cummins TR, Ishikawa K, Dib-Hajj SD, Black JA, Waxman SG. SNS Na+ channel expression increases in dorsal root ganglion neurons in the carrageenan inflammatory pain model. *Neuroreport* 1998;9:967–972.
175. Tate S, Benn S, Hick C, et al. Two sodium channels contribute to the TTX-R sodium current in primary sensory neurons. *Nat Neurosci* 1998;1:653–655.
176. Leffler A, Cummins TR, Dib-Hajj SD, Hormuzdiar WN, Black JA, Waxman SG. GDNF and NGF reverse changes in repriming of TTX-sensitive Na+ currents following axotomy of dorsal root ganglion neurons. *J Neurophysiol* 2002;88:650–658.
177. Boettger MK, Till S, Chen MX, et al. Calcium-activated potassium channel SK1- and IK1-like immunoreactivity in injured human sensory neurones and its regulation by neurotrophic factors. *Brain* 2002; 125(pt 2):252–263.
178. Vergara C, Latorre R, Marrion NV, Adelman JP. Calcium-activated potassium channels. *Curr Opin Neurobiol* 1998;8:321–329.
179. Khandwala H, Hodge E, Loomis CW. Comparable dose-dependent inhibition of AP-7 sensitive strychnine-induced allodynia and paw pinch-induced nociception by mexiletine in the rat. *Pain* 1997;72: 299–308.
180. Sato T, Shigematsu S, Arita M. Mexiletine-induced shortening of the action potential duration of ventricular muscles by activation of ATP-sensitive K+ channels. *Br J Pharmacol* 1995;115:381–382.
181. Fisher TE, Bourque CW. The function of Ca(2+) channel subtypes in exocytotic secretion: New perspectives from synaptic and non-synaptic release. *Prog Biophys Mol Biol* 2001;77:269–303.
182. Diaz A, Dickenson AH. Blockade of spinal N- and P-type, but not L-type, calcium channels inhibits the excitability of rat dorsal horn neurones produced by subcutaneous formalin inflammation. *Pain* 1997;69:93–100.
183. Wright CE, Angus JA. Effects of N-, P- and Q-type neuronal calcium channel antagonists on mammalian peripheral neurotransmission. *Br J Pharmacol* 1996;119:49–56.
184. Bowersox SS, Gadbois T, Singh T, Pettus M, Wang YX, Luther RR. Selective N-type neuronal voltage-sensitive calcium channel blocker, SNX-111, produces spinal antinociception in rat models of acute, persistent and neuropathic pain. *J Pharmacol Exp Ther* 1996;279: 1243–1249.
185. Field MJ, Oles RJ, Lewis AS, McCleary S, Hughes J, Singh L. Gabapentin (neurontin) and S-(+)-3-isobutylgaba represent a novel class of selective antihyperalgesic agents. *Br J Pharmacol* 1997;121: 1513–1522.
186. Todorovic SM, Lingle CJ. Pharmacological properties of T-type Ca2+ current in adult rat sensory neurons: Effects of anticonvulsant and anesthetic agents. *J Neurophysiol* 1998;79:240–252.
187. Todorovic SM, Perez-Reyes E, Lingle CJ. Anticonvulsants but not general anesthetics have differential blocking effects on different T-type current variants. *Mol Pharmacol.* 2000;58:98–108.
188. Faggin BM, Nguyen KT, Nicolelis MA. Immediate and simultaneous sensory reorganization at cortical and subcortical levels of the somatosensory system. *Proc Natl Acad Sci U S A* 1997;94:9428–9433.
189. Castro-Alamancos MA, Calcagnotto ME. Presynaptic long-term potentiation in corticothalamic synapses. *J Neurosci* 1999;19:9090–9097.
190. Gil Z, Amitai Y. Adult thalamocortical transmission involves both NMDA and non-NMDA receptors. *J Neurophysiol* 1996;76:2547–2554.
191. Gil Z, Amitai Y. Properties of convergent thalamocortical and intracortical synaptic potentials in single neurons of neocortex. *J Neurosci* 1996;16:6567–6578.
192. Sherman SM, Guillery RW. Functional organization of thalamocortical relays. *J Neurophysiol* 1996;76:1367–1395.
193. Sherman SE, Luo L, Dostrovsky JO. Altered receptive fields and sensory modalities of rat VPL thalamic neurons during spinal strychnine-induced allodynia. *J Neurophysiol* 1997;78:2296–2308.
194. Castro-Alamancos MA. Different temporal processing of sensory inputs in the rat thalamus during quiescent and information processing states *in vivo*. *J Physiol Soc* 2002;539:567–578.
195. Hua SE, Garonzik IM, Lee JI, Lenz FA. Microelectrode studies of normal organization and plasticity of human somatosensory thalamus. *J Clin Neurophysiol* 2000;17:559–574.
196. Chudler EH, Dong WK. The role of the basal ganglia in nociception and pain. *Pain* 1995;60:3–38.
197. Lamour Y, Guilbaud G, Willer JC. Altered properties and laminar distribution of neuronal responses to peripheral stimulation in the SmI cortex of the arthritic rat. *Brain Res* 1983;273:183–187.
198. Dong WK, Chudler EH, Sugiyama K, Roberts VJ, Hayashi T. Somatosensory, multisensory, and task-related neurons in cortical area 7b (PF) of unanesthetized monkeys. *J Neurophysiol* 1994;72:542–564.
199. Guilbaud G, Benoist JM. Thalamic and cortical processing in rat models of clinical pain. In: Besson J-M, Guilbaud G, Ollat H, eds. *Forebrain Areas Involved in Pain Processing* Paris, France: John Libbey Eurotext; 1995:79–92.
200. Zhang X, La Salle G, Ridoux V, Yu PH, Ju G. Prevention of kainic acid-induced limbic seizures and Fos expression by the GABA-A receptor agonist muscimol. *Eur J Neurosci* 1997;9:29–40.

201. Kao CQ, Coulter DA. Physiology and pharmacology of corticothalamic stimulation-evoked responses in rat somatosensory thalamic neurons in vitro. *J Neurophysiol* 1997;77:2661–2676.
202. Shaw PJ, Salt TE. Modulation of sensory and excitatory amino acid responses by nitric oxide donors and glutathione in the ventrobasal thalamus of the rat. *Eur J Neurosci* 1997;9:1507–1513.
203. Deller T, Frotscher M. Lesion-induced plasticity of central neurons: Sprouting of single fibres in the rat hippocampus after unilateral entorhinal cortex lesion. *Prog Neurobiol* 1997;53:687–727.
204. Benowitz LI, Routtenberg A. GAP-43: An intrinsic determinant of neuronal development and plasticity. *Trends Neurosci* 1997;20:84–91.
205. Ramakers GM, De Graan PN, Urban IJ, et al. Temporal differences in the phosphorylation state of pre- and postsynaptic protein kinase C substrates B-50/GAP-43 and neurogranin during long-term potentiation. *J Biol Chem* 1995;270:13892–13898.
206. Linden DJ, Wong KL, Sheu FS, Routtenberg A. NMDA receptor blockade prevents the increase in protein kinase C substrate (protein F1) phosphorylation produced by long-term potentiation. *Brain Res* 1988;458:142–146.
207. Linden DJ, Routtenberg A. The role of protein kinase C in long-term potentiation: A testable model. *Brain Res Brain Res Rev* 1989;14:279–296.

PART II

PAIN: GENERAL PRINCIPLES AND EVALUATION

CHAPTER 4

DEFINITIONS AND CLASSIFICATION OF PAIN

Jyotsna Nagda and Zahid H. Bajwa

"For all the happiness
Mankind can gain;
Is not in pleasure,
But in rest from pain."
JOHN DRYDEN (1631–1701)

Relief of pain is one of the great objectives of medicine. Pain is the most common symptom reported to physicians; more than 80% of all patients who see physicians do so because of pain. It has been a predominant concern of humankind since the beginning of recorded history. Chronic pain affects hundreds of millions of people worldwide, altering their physical and emotional functioning, decreasing their quality of life, and impairing the ability to work. It affects general health, psychological health, and social and economic well-being. Patients in chronic pain use health services up to five times more frequently than the rest of the population. The cost of unrelieved chronic pain in the United States is more than $50 billion per year (more than $80 billion per year if lost wages from work are counted) and in the age of steady cost-cutting in a managed care environment, we can no longer afford it. More than 550 million workdays are lost every year because of chronic pain. Yet 40% of all cancer patients, 50% of nursing home patients, 55% of postoperative patients, and 70% of patients with acquired immunodeficiency syndrome (AIDS) have unrelieved or inadequately relieved pain.

In October 2000, the 106th U.S. Congress passed HR 3244, which was then signed into law. Title VI, Sec. 1603, provides for the "Decade of Pain Control and Research," to begin January 2001. It follows the "Decade of the Brain" and is only the second congressionally declared, medically related decade. Pain is now designated as a public health problem of national significance. Beginning in 2001, the Joint Commission on Accreditation of Healthcare Organizations (JCAHO) implemented new standards to assess and treat pain. To qualify for accreditation, all facilities, including rehabilitation centers, outpatient surgical centers, hospitals, and nursing homes, must recognize the right of patients to appropriate assessment and management of pain. All health care facilities must identify pain in patients during initial assessment and, where required, during ongoing periodic assessments and must educate patients and their families about pain management.

The word *pain* is derived from the Latin *poena,* meaning punishment. The International Association for the Study of Pain (IASP) defines pain as "an unpleasant sensory and emotional experience associated with actual or potential tissue damage, or described in terms of such damage."[1] This definition may appear somewhat convoluted, but it clearly states that pain is subjective. It is both a physiologic sensation and an emotional reaction to that sensation. Viewed from an evolutionary prospective, pain has is perceived as a threat or damage to one's biological integrity and has three components: sensory-discriminative, motivational-affective, and cognitive-evaluative.

The concepts of pain and suffering are frequently mixed and sometimes confused in the dialogue between patient and physician, especially because pain is commonly used as if it were synonymous with suffering. However, pain and suffering are distinct phenomena. Suffering is loosely defined as a "state of severe distress associated with events that threaten the intactness of person." Not all pain causes suffering, and not all suffering expressed as pain or coexisting with pain, stems from pain.

Pain has a protective role. It warns us of imminent or actual tissue damage. If tissue damage is unavoidable, a set of excitability changes in the peripheral and central nervous systems establish profound but reversible pain hypersensitivity in inflamed and surrounding tissue. This process avoids further damage until wound healing has occurred. In contrast, chronic pain syndromes offer no biologic advantage and cause suffering and distress.

DEFINITIONS

Acute pain Acute pain signifies the presence of a noxious stimulus that produces actual tissue damage or possesses the potential to do so. The presence of acute pain implies the presence of an intact nervous system and is associated with autonomic hyperactivity: hypertension, tachycardia, sweating, and vasoconstriction. A common definition of acute pain is "the normal, predicted physiologic response to an adverse chemical, thermal, or mechanical stimulus . . . associated with surgery, trauma, and acute illness." Acute pain is short lived.

Allodynia Implies pain caused by a stimulus, which does not normally provoke pain. *Allo* means "other" in Greek and is a common prefix for medical conditions that diverge from the expected. *Odynia* is derived from the Greek word "odune" or "odyne," which is used in "pleurodynia" and "coccydynia" and is similar in meaning to the root from which we derive words with –algia or –algesia in them. Allodynia is common in many neuropathic conditions, such as postherpetic neuralgia, chronic regional pain syndromes, and certain peripheral neuropathies. Allodynia can be produced in two ways: by the action of low-threshold myelinated Aβ fibers on an altered central nervous system, and by a reduction in the threshold of nociceptor terminals in the periphery. As allodynia is used in the terms of clinical diagnosis, it can be also used to subclassify the broader symptoms of hyperalgesia, which may help identify the mechanisms causing it.

Analgesia Implies absence of pain in response to stimulation, which would normally be painful. Analgesia can be produced peripherally (at the site of tissue damage, receptor, or nerve) or centrally (in the spinal cord or brain).

Anesthesia dolorosa Implies pain in an area or region, which is anesthetic. Anesthesia dolorosa is more common after lesions that totally denervate a region. It is most commonly noted after surgery for atypical facial pain but can occur after surgery for tic douloureux or after traumatic nerve injury.

Central pain Pain initiated or caused by a primary lesion or dysfunction in the central nervous system. Any type of vascular, demyelinating, infectious, inflammatory, or traumatic lesion in the brain or spinal cord can produce central pain syndrome.

Chronic pain Defining when a pain becomes chronic is always difficult. Pain that is unlikely to resolve or pain that lasts longer than the usual healing time is defined as chronic pain. From a temporal perspective, pain is deemed to be chronic when it persists beyond 3 months. Function of the nervous system becomes reorganized (neuroplasticity) with the potential for spontaneous and atopic nerve excitation.

Complex regional pain syndrome Used to describe the painful syndromes that formerly were described under the title of reflex sympathetic dystrophy and causalgia. The term *reflex sympathetic dystrophy* was a misnomer, because not all cases have sympathetically maintained pain and not all were dystrophic. Thus, in 1993, a consensus group of pain medicine experts (a special consensus workshop of the IASP) gathered with the task of redefining causalgia and reflex sympathetic dystrophy. The diagnostic criteria proposed are purely clinical, with no laboratory test or diagnostic blocks. The consensus group divided the disorders based on the type of injury that initiated the disorder: type I, following a soft tissue injury, similar to reflex sympathy dystrophy (RSD), and type II, following well-defined nerve injury.

The criteria for complex regional pain syndrome, type I, are as follows:

1. The presence of an initiating noxious event or a cause for immobilization.
2. Continuing pain, allodynia, or hyperalgesia in which the pain is disproportionate to any known or inciting event.
3. Evidence at some time of edema, changes in the skin blood flow, or abnormal sudomotor activity in the region of pain.
4. The diagnosis is excluded by the existence of other conditions that would otherwise account for the degree of dysfunction.

Complex regional pain syndrome, type II, has the same clinical features as type I except for the clinical signs and history consistent with a specific nerve injury.

Dysesthesia An unpleasant abnormal sensation, whether spontaneous or evoked. Examples include the burning feet that may be felt in alcoholic neuropathy.

Hyperalgesia An increased response to a stimulus that is normally painful. It is the result of abnormal processing of nociceptor input. Stimulus-evoked hyperalgesias are commonly classified into subgroups on the basis of modality (i.e., mechanical, thermal, or chemical). Mechanical hyperalgesias are further classified as brush-evoked (dynamic), pressure-evoked (static), and punctuate hyperalgesia. Brush-evoked (dynamic) hyperalgesia is a consequence of increased central response to Aβ fiber input.

Hyperesthesia Increased sensitivity to stimulation, excluding special senses.

Hyperpathia A painful syndrome characterized by an abnormally explosive painful reaction to a stimulus, especially a repetitive stimulus, as well as an increased threshold. Faulty identification and localization of the stimulus, delay, radiating sensation, and after sensation may occur.

Hypoalgesia Diminished response to a normally painful stimulus.

Hypoesthesia Decreased sensitivity to stimulation, excluding the special senses.

Neuralgia Pain in the distribution of a peripheral nerve, typically described as lancinating or electric shock–like sensation

Neuritis A special type of neuropathy; the term is reserved primarily for describing inflammatory process affecting nerves.

Neurogenic pain Pain initiated or caused by a primary lesion or dysfunction, or by transitory perturbation in the peripheral or central nervous system.

Neuropathic pain Pain initiated or caused by a primary lesion or dysfunction in the nervous system. Neuropathic pain syndromes can originate at any point or points along the somatosensory pathways, from the most distal nerve endings in the skin to the somatosensory cortex in the parietal lobe.

Neuropathy A disturbance of function or pathologic change in nerves. It may be in a single nerve (mononeuropathy), in several nerves (mononeuropathy multiplex), or symmetric and bilateral (polyneuropathy).

Nociceptor A receptor preferentially sensitive to a noxious stimulus or to a stimulus that would become noxious if prolonged.

Noxious stimulus A stimulus that is damaging to normal tissues.

Pain threshold The least experience of pain that a subject can recognize.

Pain tolerance level The greatest level of pain a subject is prepared to tolerate.

Paresthesia An abnormal sensation, whether spontaneous or evoked. The most common paresthesia is the sense of "pins and needles."

Peripheral neurogenic pain Pain initiated or caused by a primary lesion or dysfunction, or by transitory perturbation in the peripheral nervous system.

Peripheral neuropathic pain Pain initiated or caused by a primary lesion or dysfunction in the peripheral nervous system.

Phantom pain Pain in a part of the body that has been surgically removed or is congenitally absent. Although best described after limb amputations, phantom pain can occur after a wide variety of amputations, including mastectomy, dental extraction, and removal of visceral organs such as the rectum.

Referred pain Pain localized not to the site of its cause but to an area that may be adjacent to or at a distance from such a site. An example is shoulder pain caused by diaphragmatic irritation.

CLASSIFICATION OF PAIN

The most recognized categories of classification are based on neurophysiologic mechanism, temporal aspects, etiology, or region affected.

Neurophysiologic

The neurophysiologic classification is based on inferred mechanism of pain. There are essentially two types of pain: nociceptive pain and non-nociceptive pain.

The term *nociceptive* is applied to pain that is presumed to be maintained by continual tissue injury. Nociceptive pain results from the activation or sensitization of nociceptors in the periphery, which transduce noxious stimulus into electrochemical impulses. These impulses are then transmitted to the spinal cord and higher rostral centers within the central nervous system. Arthritic, acute postoperative, and postoperative pain fall into this category.

Nociceptive pain is further subdivided into somatic and visceral pain, which can be distinguished by the quality of the pain and associated clinical features. Somatic pain results from excitation and sensitization of nociceptors in tissues such as bone, periarticular soft tissue, joints, and muscles. Four physiologic processes are involved in the somatic nociception: (1) transduction, (2) transmission, (3) modulation, and (4) perception. Somatic pain is characterized as being well localized topographically, intermittent, or constant and is described as "aching, stabbing, gnawing, or throbbing."

Visceral pain has five important clinical characteristics:

1. It is not evoked from all visceral organs, such as liver; kidney, most solid viscera, and lung parenchyma are not sensitive to pain.
2. It is not always linked to visceral injury (cutting the intestine causes no pain, whereas stretching of the bladder causes pain).
3. It is diffuse and poorly localized, owing to organization of visceral nociceptive pathways in the central nervous system, particularly the absence of a separate visceral sensory pathway and the low proportion of the visceral afferent nerve fibers.
4. It is referred to other locations.
5. It is accompanied by motor and autonomic reflexes, such as the nausea, vomiting, and lower back muscle tension that occur in renal colic. Discrete nociceptors in the cardiovascular, respiratory, gastrointestinal, and genitourinary systems mediate visceral pain. Although its neural pathways are less well defined than those of somatic pain, the visceral pathways share some of the features with somatic pathways. Visceral pain is less topographically distinct and is described as diffuse. It may be intermittent or constant and is often described as "dull, colicky, or squeezing."

Non-nociceptive pain can be subdivided into neuropathic and idiopathic pain. Neuropathic pain results from injury to neural structures within the peripheral or central nervous system. It is believed to be sustained by aberrant somatosensory processing in the periphery or central nervous system. Neuropathic pain is typically described as "sharp or burning." There are three subsets of neuropathic pain. Peripherally generated neuropathic pain involves such entities as cervical or lumbar radiculopathy, spinal nerve lesions, and brachial or lumbosacral plexopathies. Centrally generated pain involves injury to the central nervous system at the level of the spinal cord or above. Sympathetically maintained pain may be generated peripherally or centrally and is characterized by localized autonomic dysregulation in the affected area, with vasomotor or sudomotor changes, edema, sweating, and atrophy. It is referred to as reflex sympathetic dystrophy, causalgia, or, more recently, complex regional pain syndrome.

The term *idiopathic pain* has been used interchangeably with the term *psychogenic pain*. Idiopathic pain is probably the more appropriate term because it implies a wider spectrum of poorly understood pain states. Myofascial pain syndrome and somatoform pain disorder are examples of idiopathic pain. In some patients, there is no evidence of an associated organic cause, whereas in others, pain and associated symptoms are grossly out of proportion to identifiable organic pathology.

Finally, it is worth emphasizing that all pain has a psychological component. Psychological factors, which are often not obvious, as well as cultural and environmental factors, must be taken into consideration when evaluating a patient with chronic pain. For example, emotional arousal can enhance nociception at the periphery. Heightened sympathetic activity with the release of norepinephrine at the sympathetic terminals can sensitize or directly activate nociceptors; similarly, reflex muscle spasm caused by anxiety can contribute to a positive feedback loop in which nociception fosters increased muscle tone in the area near the site of injury, eventually activating the muscle nociceptors. Patients in clinical practice often exhibit more than one type of pain. One example is patients with cancer pain who may have neuropathic, nociceptive, and myofascial pain.

Temporal

The temporal classification is based on the duration of symptoms and is usually divided into acute and chronic categories. The major shortcoming is that distinction between acute and chronic is arbitrary. Cancer pain includes pain associated with the disease progression, treatment, and concurrent conditions. Hence, the pain associated with cancer may be acute or chronic. Some clinicians advocate cancer pain as a third category, distinct from acute and chronic pain.

Mechanism-based

In 1998, Woolf and his colleagues suggested implementation of a mechanism-based classification of pain. They believed it could have profound implications: drugs could be developed that target distinct mechanisms, basic scientists could have new guidelines for experimental design, and clinicians could be armed with more reliable and valid diagnostic tools for treatment and clinical investigation.

Etiologic

The etiologic classification pays more attention to the primary disease process in which the pain occurs, rather than to the neurophysiologic basis. Examples include cancer pain, arthritis pain, and pain in sickle cell disease. Therapeutically, it is less useful than the neurophysiologic classification.

Regional

The regional classification is strictly topographic and does not infer pathophysiology or etiology. It is defined by the part of the body affected.

Multiaxial

An alternative to the one-dimensional approach is the multidimensional approach. The IASP has published an expert-based multiaxial classification of chronic pain with the goals of standardization and provision of a point of reference. The published taxonomy classifies chronic pain patients according to five axes based on the best-published information and consensus:

a. Region of the body affected (axis I)
b. System whose abnormal functioning could conceivably produce pain (axis II)
c. Temporal characteristics of pain and pattern of occurrence (axis III)
d. Patient's statement of intensity and time since the onset of pain (axis IV)
e. Presumed etiology (axis V)

CONCLUSION

Pain management is a rapidly advancing field. Many concepts and terminologies that were a source of confusion in the past have now been more clearly defined. However, more work clearly needs to be done in classification and taxonomy to simplify the communication and meet the objectives of basic scientists, researchers, and clinicians providing patient care.

REFERENCES

Bonica JJ. *Pain Terms and Taxonomies of Pain. The Management of Pain.* 3rd ed. Philadelphia, Pa: John D Loeser; 2001.

Cervero F, Laid J. Visceral pain. *Lancet.* 1999;353:2145–2148.

Melzack R. The short McGill Pain Questionnaire. *Pain.* 1987;30:191–197.

Merskey H, Bogduk N. *International Association for the Study of Pain (IASP): Classification of Chronic Pain.* 2nd ed. Seattle, Wash: IASP Press; 1994

Raja SN, Grabow TS. Complex regional pain syndrome I (reflex sympathetic dystrophy). *Anesthesiology.* 2002;96:1254–1260.

Todd M, Raja SN, Eisenach J. International Association for the Study of Pain, 9th World Congress on Pain. *Anesthesiology.* 2000;92:292–294.

Woolf C, Max Ml. Mechanism-based pain diagnosis: Issues for analgesic drug development. *Anesthesiology.* 2001:95:241–249.

Woolf CJ, Bennett GJ, Doherty M, et al: Towards a mechanism based classification of pain? *Pain.* 1998;77:227–229.

Woolf CJ, Mannion RJ. Neuropathic pain: Etiology, symptoms, mechanisms, and management. *Lancet.* 1999;353:1959–1964.

CHAPTER 5

UNDERSTANDING THE PATIENT WITH CHRONIC PAIN

Jeremy Goodwin and Zahid H. Bajwa

"It is not suffering that diminishes man, but suffering without meaning."
VICTOR FRANKL

Asked to describe their pain, especially chronic pain, patients often appear perplexed, stating, "I don't know. It just hurts." Pain is a subject of deceptive complexity. It means different things to different people. Algology is the study of pain, and this chapter discusses a number of important points relevant to its clinical application, pain medicine.

CLASSIFICATION OF PAIN

Before we focus on the patient with chronic pain and a general approach to pain management, basic nosology and terminology need clarification.

There are a number of ways to classify pain. Some pain specialists separate it into malignant (cancer) and nonmalignant pain. Others divide it into acute, recurrent acute, and chronic pain. Acute pain is short-lived and follows injury or near injury to tissue. Recurrent acute pain is similar in duration but tends to recur. It need not involve injury. Examples are migraine headache and sickle cell vasoocclusive episodes. Depending on the injury, chronic pain is variably defined as that persisting 1 to 6 months after the tissue has healed. One example of chronic pain is postherpetic neuralgia.

Pain can also be classified in terms of mechanism. *Nociceptive pain* denotes pain arising from tissue injury, and the degree of pain is usually somewhat proportional to the degree of injury. Nociceptive pain itself may be subcategorized into visceral pain, a dull, crampy, and poorly localizable discomfort—as might be experienced in gastroenteritis—or somatic pain, a sharper and more localizable sensation of the body wall, as might be felt after a laceration. Each type of pain may be mild or intense.

Neuropathic pain is not nociceptive, and the degree of pain is not proportional to the degree of injury; it is caused by disordered sensory processing of the nervous system and is a pathologic persistence of a normal sensitizing mechanism that can be useful in the setting of acute pain. Neuropathic pain can be subcategorized into *central neuropathic pain*, which can originate at any level of the central nervous system, and *peripheral neuropathic pain*, which is generated at the level of a nerve or nerve root. The most famous example of central pain is poststroke thalamic pain; common examples of peripheral neuropathic pain are neuromas, diabetic neuropathy, and complex regional pain syndrome, types 1 and 2 (previously known as reflex sympathetic dystrophy and causalgia). As with central pain, a number of different mechanisms may be involved. Even when the damage occurs in the periphery, such as injury to a nerve, the constant bombardment of sensory neurons in the spinal cord with pain signals from the periphery renders the neurons hypersensitive to all input, even to non-noxious stimuli. Neurons then almost continuously "fire up" the pain pathway. Although this is a normal sequence of events in acute injury (i.e., sensitizing injured areas so that they may be protected from further harm), when it fails to abate with healing, it becomes pathologic. This process is called central sensitization of pain and is related to the concept of windup.

Other relevant terminology includes:

- Hyperpathia, an elevated sensory threshold above which is generated an abnormally intense and prolonged response to pain
- Hyperalgesia, which is secondary to a lowered threshold to pain
- Allodynia, a painful response to a nonpainful stimulus
- Hyperesthesia, caused by a lowered threshold to any stimuli
- Hypoesthesia, the opposite of hyperesthesia
- Analgesia, without pain
- Anesthesia, without sensation

Incident pain is generated by mechanical factors characteristic of movement and position. Incident pain commonly occurs in cancer patients in whom, for example, metastatic spread of the cancer involves the skeleton. Such pain may be neuropathic or nociceptive, depending on the structures involved. For example, a pathologic or metastatic rib fracture results in nociceptive bone pain and neuropathic pain in the distribution of the rib's intercostal nerve.

SPECIAL POPULATIONS AFFECTED BY MISCONCEPTIONS ABOUT PAIN

Infants and Children

Patients within certain age groups are often subjected to unnecessary pain and suffering, which may have long-term consequences. Children are still relatively undermedicated compared with adults, and although the situation is improving, there continues to be room for improvement. Surgeons were operating on infants who were only partially anesthetized as late as the early 1980s.

Misconceptions about pain and the consequences of its treatment continue to impede patient care. For example, nurses concerned about the risk of addiction may read a physician's "prn" order to mean "as little as possible" rather than "as needed." Or they may rely too much on changes in vital signs, such as quickened heart rate or increased blood pressure, to decide if a child's complaint of pain is "real" or not and may thus withhold "prn" medications inappropriately. We are aware of no evidence that appropriate opioid use in pediatric pain management leads to addiction in childhood or adulthood. And we now know that there is great variability in individual pain thresholds and ability to cope with pain, so that *vital signs may not correlate as well with the level of pain as previously thought*. In infants and children, fluctuating levels in vital signs may be a better indicator of pain than absolute levels. It is, therefore, wise to combine several methods of pain evaluation, no matter what the patient's age. Verbal or visual analog pain scores (from 0 to 10), a developmentally sensitive analysis of general behavior and body language, and facial expression can provide valuable information for the assessment of pain.

Some practitioners believe that infants feel little pain because their nervous systems are immature. The anatomic, biochemical, and physiologic apparatus necessary for the perception of pain is present 2 to 3 months before term, but because the descending inhibitory modulating system is immature, and because of a higher than adult level of cutaneous pain receptor density, infants may, in fact, be hyperalgesic. They may have a lower average threshold to pain than adults. The main consequence of immature central and peripheral myelination is poorly coordinated nocifensive (defensive) behavior, which is reflexive but modified by experience. Newborns quickly learn to squirm and kick during a heelstick blood draw. Facial grimacing and fluctuating vital signs belie their experience of pain. There is even growing evidence that infants subjected to long and painful treatments without pain management in intensive care units are more likely to develop problems of somatization in school compared with those given intermittent or constant infusions of carefully adjusted opioid medications.[1]

Elderly Patients

Geriatric patients also suffer from caregivers who have been misinformed about pain management. Although those aged 70 or older may in general be more susceptible to medication side effects, it does not mean that they should be left untreated for pain.

Careful dose adjustment is key to good pain management, as is awareness of the various delivery systems that might minimize systemic side effects. Patients who experience intolerable side effects from high-dose oral narcotics for persistent malignant or nonmalignant pain may benefit from the implantation of an intrathecal opioid pump, through which relatively tiny amounts of medication are placed directly into the cerebrospinal fluid. It then enters the spinal cord and brain quickly and efficiently, minimizing spread to other systems. Similarly, a well-placed epidural catheter may provide better short-term postoperative analgesia with fewer side effects than intermittent nurse-given intravenous narcotics or boluses delivered by a patient-controlled analgesia (PCA) device. And even when dementia is of concern, one needs simply to titrate more carefully and to employ adjuvant medications and techniques that might prove opioid sparing. However, it must be remembered that in this group of patients, even normally well-tolerated medications may have adverse effects on mentation as well as on the gastrointestinal and cardiovascular systems.

EFFECTIVE APPROACHES TO CHRONIC PAIN

It is a little appreciated but important concept that chronic pain is *not* merely a protracted form of acute pain, and it is often preventable. Chronic pain is not a symptom; it is a disease and should be treated as such. There is now a general consensus that an interdisciplinary or multidisciplinary approach to pain management is most effective. But prevention is still the key to avoiding the consequences of chronic pain. In addition to the effect that chronic pain has on the sufferer and his or her immediate family, it affects the greater community. The financial burden to society from lost productivity resulting from recurrent acute and chronic pain is staggering. Estimates range from $50 billion to $100 billion yearly for headache and low back pain alone. But the problem is wider and more serious than that. Failure to alleviate unnecessary suffering creates distrust between clinicians and patients, and this, in turn, diminishes the efficacy of our medical system. If patients feel forced to seek alternative and more caring treatments, they may fail to seek appropriate care for other serious conditions when it is needed. More people than ever before are seeking alternatives to allopathic medicine, but not necessarily always to their advantage. Missing the opportunity for early cancer detection, for example, may have tragic consequences.

The public's trust must be regained. What causes this distrust? On both sides, much of it results from a feeling of lack of control. Patients become anxious and distraught as their pain persists and become frustrated with the inability of medical professionals to alleviate it. Clinicians become frustrated with their own lack of understanding of pain and their inability to control it. Sometimes these feelings of frustration and inadequacy are turned against the patient in the form of "there is nothing more that can be done" or "obviously something else is going on, so I'm sending you to a psychiatrist." At such times, it may be more appropriate (and less destructive for the patient) to state that "there is little more that *I* am able to do," or preferably, "your situation is quite complex and involves suffering beyond that of the physical pain alone, so we need to have it assessed more fully to formulate a better plan for pain management." This last comment, of course, needs expansion and explanation because a common interpretation of this is that "the doctor thinks it is all in my head." Trust takes considerable effort and risk on both sides. It requires empathy: the adage "to hear about pain is to have doubt, but to experience it is to have certainty" is true.

WHAT IS CHRONIC PAIN IF NOT PROTRACTED ACUTE PAIN?

There are certain concepts that need emphasis to answer this question. The first of these is that *pain and suffering are not synonymous*. Although pain has been described as an unpleasant sensory and emotional experience arising from actual or potential damage to tissue, only when the consequences of pain—usually prolonged—begin to interfere negatively with the physical and emotional experience of life is suffering said to occur. In this way, pain may be likened to stress. A little pain is not necessarily a terrible thing. It may serve to focus attention on a stimulus and foster an appropriate reaction to it, but too much pain may prove overwhelming, exhausting, and demoralizing. It may lead to depression, which may intensify the experience. And depression is not benign. With little warning, it may lead to suicide. Saying that "there is nothing more that can be done" may take away the only hope that keeps the patient going.

Continuing the analogy to stress, pain is difficult to study. It is not easily monitored or objectively assessed, nor are its effects predictable from one individual to another. Indeed, pain thresholds may vary, not only between people, but also within the individual person over time according to mood, previous experience, and expectations. This complexity, fortunately, provides multiple levels or points at which pain management may prove successful. Appropriate interventions may be pharmacologic, invasive (i.e., surgery or nerve block), behavioral, or a combination of all three.

What, then, is the difference between pain and suffering? To answer this question, it must be understood that pain may affect a person's life in different ways according to their general state of well-being. Someone who is tired, hungry, anxious, or depressed reacts to an unpleasant sensation differently from someone who is well rested, in excellent shape, and in high spirits. When pain persists and overwhelms a person's coping mechanisms, it is likely to be seen as insurmountable and may take on a life of its own. Eventually, the tail wags the dog, as the saying goes. With this loss of control and autonomy and a growing feeling of helplessness, the person begins to experience a downward spiraling of emotional and physical well-being, in which severe deconditioning threatens normal functioning at home, work, and play. The consequence is a state of suffering of which only a portion is physical pain. This is why pain management clinicians do not advocate simply prescribing the strongest medication possible when the patient states, "if you just give me something to kill the pain, I will go back to work and everything will be OK." If only it were so simple! The wise practitioner tries to convince the patient that going back to work first—in graded increments—may offer a useful distraction from the pain and explains why a concurrent and multifaceted approach to pain management is needed. Although no single physician is capable of all aspects of care, in a multidisciplinary setting, there needs to be one clinician in overall charge of each patient's regimen to avoid processing patients "by committee."

Clinical Example: The Downward Spiral That Turns Pain Into Suffering

To illustrate how a fairly minor event may lead to catastrophic results if early warning signs of chronic pain are not recognized and responded to appropriately, one may use the common scenario of a 50-year-old citizen sitting in a stationary car, hit from behind. There is no apparent injury at the time. Over the next few days, the patient experiences tightening up of muscles and low back pain, described as "spasms." These get worse over time. The patient is reassured by the family's practitioner that it is only a muscular problem. Although the patient is willing to accept this for a while, a friend suggests initiating a lawsuit just in case something is more seriously wrong. This philosophy is reinforced by an attorney who states that he has seen many patients settle a case too early only to find out later that they have a lifelong disability for which they have no financial coverage.

The driver now sues and becomes hypervigilant about symptoms, becoming anxious every time pain is felt. The family physician reasserts that there is no neurologic dysfunction and states that x-ray studies fail to show any skeletal injury. The patient disagrees. The pain is prolonged and is seemingly becoming intensified. He or she seeks a second opinion and, not satisfied with it, seeks a third, fourth, and so on until somebody is found who echoes his or her concerns and who is willing to order a magnetic resonance imaging (MRI) scan. MRI then reveals degenerative changes not apparent on x-ray films, but probably consistent with age, such as "bulging discs" that do not clearly impinge a nerve root or the spinal cord but nonetheless are read correctly as just "touching" a nerve root. The consulting surgeon, wanting to help the patient, offers to operate and see if he or she can remove the tissue that "might" be touching a nerve and setting off the pain. The patient agrees, giving consent, but doesn't hear the qualification "might."

As often happens, the surgery does not ameliorate the pain, and within a few months, a new pain begins. Subsequent MRI reveals evidence of scarring about the nerve root, one of the possible complications of invasive surgery. As the scar contracts, it pulls and irritates the nerve root, causing radicular pain in the dermatomal distribution of the corresponding peripheral nerve. The patient becomes frustrated, despondent, and depressed. The family physician then prescribes antidepressants for pain, but they seem to negatively affect the patient's ability to think clearly at work. The patient now no longer trusts the family physician's judgment (or prescriptions) and begins to take multiple over-the-counter drugs or uses "alternative" therapy that may be expensive and of dubious value. The pain persists.

Eventually, the family physician is forced to prescribe a mild narcotic for ongoing and worsening pain. This is taken over the next few months, with escalating dose requirements because the patient has developed tolerance to the drug, leading to stronger medications, a pattern to which the clinician responds with concern, stating that he or she is not going to prescribe these medicines any more "because you are becoming addicted to them." They argue, and the patient is forced to seek care elsewhere. By now, having missed work so often and failing as well in personal relationships, the patient is fired at work and unhappy at home. The patient becomes more depressed and cannot sleep well, escalating the pain.

Having been physically inactive now for several months, the patient is physically deconditioned and the ensuing poor posture and ill-functioning musculature (some muscles are chronically contracted to minimize painful movements; others are weak and flaccid from disuse) induces myofascial (soft-tissue) pain, worsening the situation. The patient is no longer able to go out with friends or to visit family because of neck and back pain that prohibit driving. Sitting or standing in any one place for too long brings on the pain. The family withdraws, unable to console the patient and feeling inadequate. The patient ends up at a multidisciplinary pain management clinic, diagnosed with failed back surgery syndrome complicated by depression and severe deconditioning. A fairly long and expensive treatment program is now required to help the patient pick up the pieces. *The pain has become a state of suffering.*

Without analyzing this scenario step-by-step, it is clear that a fairly innocuous event initiated a domino effect, resulting in biologic, psychological, and social disruption of the patient's life. This is why a biopsychosocial approach to pain management is necessary. Early recognition of this downward spiral might have helped the patient if a brief period of pain management–oriented counseling or relaxation-based cognitive therapy was initiated to help the patient look at the pain from a different perspective. Furthermore, the likelihood of successful pain management might have been increased by incorporating physical therapy early to prevent a deconditioning process. Short-term use of nonsteroid antiinflammatory drugs (NSAIDs), tricyclic antidepressants, or muscle relaxants might have decreased pain and improved sleep, minimizing the potential for depression.

Close communication between the clinician and patient is needed to develop mutual trust. Limits need to be specified with regard to medication refill requests and self-adjustments of dose to avoid misunderstandings that might lead to suspicion of addictive behavior. *Prescribing medications without adequate thought and discussion and then abruptly stopping them simply generates patient frustration, bewilderment, and resentment.* Setting limits early and paying firm attention to them fosters the patient's respect and trust. With the rules established at the outset, perhaps in the form of a signed agreement, the chance for misunderstanding is minimized. Such an agreement amounts to informed consent.

PSYCHIATRIC COMORBIDITY AND CHRONIC PAIN

A common misconception is that chronic pain is the result of psychiatric disease. No doubt the two often coexist, but psychiatric illness is more often a reaction to the pain. The prevalence and incidence of psychiatric comorbidity in patients with chronic pain is probably no greater than that seen in other patients with chronic medical disorders (e.g., epilepsy). A history of sexual, physical, or emotional abuse, with the resultant psychological ramifications, is astonishingly prevalent in a wide range of clinical settings, if one takes the time to look. These issues may have special relevance to patients for whom invasive treatments are being contemplated, and this is one of the reasons that such histories are pursued (and found to exist) in the pain clinic.

Poor coping skills and mood disorders may affect the experience of pain, but the decision that depression, for example, is causing a person's pain should be made with the help of a trained mental health professional. Even somatoform pain is real pain; it is simply treated from a more behavioral perspective. Assuming somatization without the assistance of a mental health professional may prove incorrect and result in invalidation of the patient's complaint. Worse, somatization may be confused with malingering and may unjustly and significantly influence legal and disability compensation issues. Thus, one must be careful in using terms such as "psychogenic" or "somatoform pain."[2] According to the *Diagnostic and Statistical Manual of Mental Disorders* (DSM-IV), the former term is no longer acceptable and the latter is relatively uncommon. The current terminology is "pain disorder associated with psychological factors." When a medical condition also affects the patient's experience of pain, it is termed "pain disorder associated with both psychological factors and a general medical condition."

Evaluating pain as physical ("real") or psychological ("unreal") is a simplistic and a limited approach that serves no useful purpose: "absence of evidence is not evidence of absence." For example, when MRI and a nerve conduction test fail to reveal a cause of a person's chronic low back pain, it is often assumed that there is no observable lesion. The problem is then usually treated with physical therapy and often with psychotherapy. Recent work has demonstrated that focal pathology may, in fact, exist but be out of the reach of the technology used to find it. For example, although MRI of a disk may appear normal, this technology cannot evaluate the inside of the disk: it will not reveal internal disk disruption, a painful tear. Thus, some specialists inject disks with a contrast agent (provocative diskography), pressurizing it to determine if the pain induced is concordant with the clinical complaint. A normal disk is not painful during this procedure; however, whereas this is true of the lumbar region, it is controversial in the cervical spine. Specially guided computed tomographic (CT) scans of these contrast-injected disks may then reveal fissures within the disk, some grades of which correlate well with the pain, and may prove predictive of success with further intervention. Elimination of the pain might be achieved (rarely) by corticosteroid injection into the disk; ablation of the sensory nerves subserving the disk; stiffening the disk by intradiskal electrothermal therapy (IDET), sometimes referred to as intradiskal electrothermal annuloplasty (IDEA); or disk removal with fusion of the vertebrae. IDET was approved by the Food and Drug Administration (FDA) in 1998 and was found useful in worker's compensation and non–worker's compensation patients in a controlled study.[3] Similarly, facet joint–mediated spine pain may be missed without precision spine injections, because there is a relatively poor correlation between the reported symptoms, physical examination, and electrodiagnostic and imaging test results. Currently, there is renewed interest in this controversial approach to the diagnosis and treatment of spine pain, because improvements in patient selection and procedure technique have begun to help a significant number of those with "whiplash" and other so-called minor strain injuries.[4,5]

To summarize, *one need not attribute a patient's pain to organic pathology in order to validate it as real.* Pain is what the patient says it is. And if psychological factors are found to be important in a patient's experience of pain, their importance should not be underestimated. Depression kills. Conversely, unless the diagnostic workup is well thought out, important physical pain generators may be missed; centralization of pain, however, may still prove problematic. Therefore the question should not be, "Is this person's pain real (physical) or unreal (psychological)?" but, "Will this person's pain most likely respond to medical, invasive, or psychological intervention?"

ARE PLACEBOS USEFUL IN THE DIAGNOSIS OF PAIN?

The systematic use of placebo control is important in clinical research, but it is controversial in diagnostic medicine. This is another deceptively complex topic, fraught with misunderstanding. The placebo response has no bearing on whether pain is real or unreal, it merely defines the sufferer as a placebo responder or nonresponder. It neither confirms a psychogenic cause nor rules out physical pathology. And there is no clear correlation of personality type with the likelihood of placebo response. A person may respond to placebo on one occasion but not on another. There may even be a spectrum of responses. And contrary to popular belief, the placebo response does not predictably occur one third of the time or in one third of the subjects. This notion stems from a paper in the *Journal of the American Medical Association* in which the author averaged the results of 11 studies to come up with 35.2%.[6] More recent studies estimate the rate to vary between 0% and 100%.[7] Placebo response varies widely between and within groups according to the expectations of both examiners and examinees. Its mechanism is controversial and incompletely understood, although it may, in part, result from the release of endorphins. The use of placebo may, under some circumstances, prove damaging. When used without consent, it may be seen by the patient as trickery. It can undermine the patient-clinician relationship, resulting in loss of trust. We have already established that trust is necessary for a good therapeutic outcome. Using a placebo may even violate the spirit of informed consent, if the placebo-controlled part of a procedure is not disclosed. Disclosure will not necessarily interfere with the placebo's usefulness. One simply explains to the patient that response to treatment is complicated and may be influenced by patient expectation. The patient should be reassured that the medicine will be given, but in a manner and timing of which the patient will be unaware. The reassurance that they *will* receive the medication (not just placebo) is important. And as Patrick Wall has noted, the power of suggestion is a tool that may be employed benevolently and appropriately: "Mummy will kiss it better" is a wonderfully effective remedy.[8]

WHAT ABOUT NARCOTICS AND SUBSTANCE ABUSE?

The use of opioid medications in the management of nonmalignant pain remains controversial, despite more than a decade of active debate. Here, too, there is much prejudice and misunderstanding. Contrary to popular belief, narcotic medications have a lower risk for addiction than previously thought, if used appropriately in the management of pain. This is especially true in patients without a history of substance abuse and applies to infants, children, and adults.

Tolerance is defined as an increasing dose requirement to maintain the same therapeutic effect. This may or may not occur in an individual on opioid therapy, but when it does, it does not necessarily equate with addiction. *Physical dependence* is another confusing term that is often misapplied as a synonym for addiction. It merely describes the potential for developing a physical state of withdrawal if the medication is weaned too quickly. Patients can usually be weaned successfully from drug therapy without inducing symptoms of withdrawal. Furthermore, tolerance and physical dependence together do not make for addiction. *Psychological dependence*, however, is equivalent to addiction. It may be present long after the weaning process and, therefore, long after tolerance and physical dependence abate.

Psychological dependence is defined as a psychological fixation on a drug; the behavioral manifestation is continued use of it, despite potential harm to the patient. This problem is estimated to occur less than one tenth of 1% of the time in short-term treatment with strong narcotics (when there is no history of substance abuse). Even in long-term treatment, the addiction rate is probably between 3% and 16%; the vast majority of those addicted have a history of substance abuse.[9,10] This means that there is unlikely to be a problem with addiction 84% to 97% of the time. The role of cigarette smoking is unknown, but it is not generally considered to be an indicator of potential medication abuse problems. A history of addiction does not mean that patients in pain should go untreated or be denied opioids. The clinician must simply monitor the patient more closely than usual for signs of addictive behavior. In general, it is good advice to have the patient sign a contract or an agreement that outlines the parameters within which the relationship of prescriber to prescribee may operate smoothly. Breaking this agreement is grounds for dissolution of the relationship. If this happens, there is an ethical obligation on the part of the physician to reasonably help the patient find care elsewhere.

Drug-seeking behavior is *not* synonymous with pain avoidance behavior (otherwise known as pseudoaddiction). The main difference between the two is that a person who is initially undermedicated and protests such treatment as though he or she is drug-seeking will likely stop such demands once the pain is controlled. His or her protests and pain behaviors are rational. The psychologically dependent (addicted) person may never seem to be appeased. When there is concern over patient behavior, it is appropriate to ask for help from a pain specialist or an addictionologist to evaluate and interpret the situation.

MEDICATIONS, ALTERNATIVE DELIVERY SYSTEMS, AND SURGERY

Pharmacotherapy is one of the mainstays of treatment of pain. Only brief mention of it is made here. The reader is directed to Fields and Liebeskind[11] for a detailed overview. In addition to the anti-inflammatory agents and narcotics, certain antidepressant and antiepilepsy medications may prove useful for a variety of painful conditions. Those agents that elevate serotonin *and* norepinephrine in the brain, primarily the tricyclic and several atypical antidepressants, may activate a descending pain modulatory system, thereby diminishing some forms of pain. Antidepressants may also diminish anxiety and improve sleep, reducing irritability and the negative affective ramifications of chronic pain. Pain relief with antidepressants usually occurs independent of the drug's effect on mood; antidepressants attenuate pain more quickly and at lower doses than is commonly needed for depression. Of the selective serotonin reuptake inhibitors (SSRIs), only paroxetine hydrochloride (Paxil), venlafaxine hydrochloride (Effexor), and citalopram hydrobromide (Celexa) have clinically demonstrable effects on neuropathic pain. It is not clear why the effects should differ from those of fluoxetine hydrochloride (Prozac) or sertraline hydrochloride (Zoloft).

Some antiepilepsy medications (and tricyclic antidepressants) act as membrane-stabilizing agents, elevating the threshold for neuronal firing. They, too, may help diminish neuropathic pain. Whether or not membrane stabilization is the mechanism for their analgesic effect is controversial (each drug may have multiple mechanisms of action). And, although it is often taught that tricyclic depressants are best for treatment of burning neuropathic pain and anticonvulsants are best for paroxysmal or shooting pain, either class can be used with some efficacy and should be selected on the basis of cost, effect and side-effect profile, and likelihood of compliance. Antidepressants are commonly tried first because of their potential effect on problems other than pain. The only clear indication for a specific medication for neuropathic pain is that for the antiepilepsy drug carbamazepine (Tegretol) to treat trigeminal neuralgia. In this case, there is well-documented evidence for its superiority over other agents. Likewise, the majority of the literature supports the use of tricyclic antidepressants over other agents for treatment of postherpetic neuralgia, although a number of viable options exist. These include opioids, gabapentin (Neurontin), and topical lidocaine (Lidoderm 5% patches).

There are many other medications for which anecdotal evidence for efficacy in pain control exists. The skillful practitioner should be able to use combinations of some of these agents to minimize pain and suffering in patients for whom single agents have proven ineffective. It also pays to be aware of different delivery systems available for these agents. Epidural and subarachnoid catheters, PCA devices, and the use of oral, rectal, sublingual, buccal, subcutaneous, intravenous, and intramuscular routes of administration all have their place in pain management.

Added to these modes of delivery is the neurosurgical approach to pain management. Under appropriate circumstances, pain pathways may be cut or neurostimulatory devices used with considerable efficacy at the level of the peripheral nerve, spinal cord, and subcortical and neocortical brain regions. Even ablation of the pituitary gland may significantly diminish the whole-body pain of metastatic cancer. Implanted intrathecal medication pumps and intraventricular catheters are useful modes of treatment in selected cases. Pain-oriented neurosurgery may prove valuable to multidisciplinary pain management teams. And, because some of the procedures are reversible (e.g., spinal cord stimulation), neurosurgical intervention is not necessarily a "last resort." Use of it early in the course may preclude medication side effects and toxicity. Surgical treatment of pain is thoroughly addressed elsewhere.[12]

BRINGING IT ALL TOGETHER

What we have discussed here is a multimodal and interdisciplinary approach to the patient with chronic pain. A biopsychosocial approach (however fuzzy that sounds) is useful to analyze and effectively manage the physical, emotional, and social aspects of patients' pain and suffering. Reasonable goals should be set with respect to diminution of pain and improvement in function. At a minimum, a good interdisciplinary team should include (1) one or two physicians well-versed in pharmacologic and interventional procedures; (2) a counselor, psychologist, or psychiatrist to diagnose and treat psychiatric conditions that may result from, cause, or exacerbate the pain; (3) a physical therapist or rehabilitation specialist to assess physical conditioning requirements; and (4) nurses knowledgeable about how these approaches may be applied to the specific patient.

Nurses help move clinics along efficiently and allay patient anxiety by being able to return calls promptly and expertly. Their skill in patient triage and procedure and postprocedural evaluation may prove invaluable to successful pain management. From the patient's perspective, the quality and responsiveness of the nursing staff may make the difference between an overall positive or negative clinical experience.[13]

Pain management teams that have frequent multidisciplinary meetings to discuss individual patients and their diagnoses and progress are more likely to be effective in carrying out a reasonable plan. But there are too many patients with chronic pain to expect pain specialists alone to care for them. Primary care physicians are also well suited to the task and can be highly successful if some of the principles discussed in this chapter are followed. Note, however, that success does not always mean cure. If an approach to pain management diminishes a person's pain score by 1 point out of 10, then applying three or four approaches in concert may drop a person's pain score from 8 to 4, making the difference between a state of suffering and one of simple pain. If this allows that person to return to school or to work with an improved level of function, then the pain management program may be called a success.

Acknowledgment

The authors wish to express their gratitude to Julie A. Brady, RN, whose experience and comments proved invaluable to the production of this manuscript.

REFERENCES

1. McGrath PA, et al. Controlling children's pain: A practical approach to assessment and management. 8th World Congress of Pain. Refresher course syllabus, 157–170. International Association for the Study of Pain (IASP), Vancouver, Canada; 1996.
2. Covington EC. Psychogenic pain—what it means, why it does not exist, and how to diagnose it. *Pain Med* 2000;1:287–294.
3. Karasek M, Bogduk N. Twelve-month follow-up of a controlled trial of intradiscal electro thermal annuloplasty for the treatment of low back pain due to internally disrupted discs. *Spine* 2000;25:2601–2607.
4. Bogduk N, et al. Precision diagnosis of spinal pain. 8th World Congress of Pain. Refresher course syllabus, 313–323. International Association for the Study of Pain (IASP), Vancouver, Canada; 1996.
5. Goodwin JLR. Current concepts in the neurologic assessment of spinal pain: Cancer and noncancer pain. In: Burchiel KJ, ed. *Surgical Management of Pain*. New York, NY: Thieme Medical Publishers; 2002:98–127.
6. Beecher HK. The powerful placebo. *JAMA*. 1955;159:1602–1606.
7. Wall PD. The placebo and the placebo response. In: Wall PD, Melzack R, eds. *Textbook of Pain*. 4th ed. Philadelphia, Pa: Churchill Livingstone; 1999:1419–1430.
8. Wall PD. The placebo and the placebo response. In: Wall PD, Melzack R, eds. *Textbook of Pain*. 3rd ed. Philadelphia, Pa: Churchill Livingstone; 1994:1297–1308.
9. Portenoy RK. Chronic opioid therapy in nonmalignant pain. In Fields: HL, Liebeskind JC, eds. *Pharmacological Approaches to the Treatment of Chronic Pain: New Concepts and Critical Issues*. Seattle, Wash: International Association for the Study of Pain (IASP) Press; 1994.
10. Fishbain DA, et al. Drug abuse, dependence, and addiction in chronic pain patients. *Clin J Pain* 1992;8:77–85.
11. Fields HL, Liebeskind JC, eds. *Pharmacological Approaches to the Treatment of Chronic Pain: New Concepts and Critical Issues*. Seattle, Wash: International Association for the Study of Pain (IASP) Press; 1994.
12. Burchiel KJ, ed. *Surgical Management of Pain*. New York, NY: Thieme Medical Publishers; 2002.
13. Brady JA, Jeffreys LK. Role of the nurse clinician. In: Burchiel KJ, ed. *Surgical Management of Pain*. New York, NY: Thieme Medical Publishers; 2002:246–256.

BIBLIOGRAPHY

Ballantyne J, Fishman SM, Abdi S (eds) Philadelphia, Lippincott Williams & Wilkins, 2002.

Borsook D, et al, eds. *The Massachusetts General Hospital Handbook of Pain Management,* 2nd edition. New York, NY: Little, Brown; 1996.

A useful manual giving special attention to selected procedures, headache, and pediatric and AIDS-related pain.

Burchiel KJ, ed. *Surgical Management of Pain*. New York, NY: Thieme Medical Publishers; 2002.

The most current and wide-ranging textbook on medical and surgical approaches to pain management. A number of chapters pertain to issues discussed in this chapter.

Diagnostic and Statistical Manual of Mental Disorders (DSM-IV). Washington, DC: American Psychiatric Association; 1994.

Ferrell BR, Terrell BA. Pain in the elderly. In: *Task Force on Pain in the Elderly*. Seattle, Wash: International Association for the Study of Pain (IASP) Press; 1996:1–130.

Fields HL, Liebeskind JC, eds. *Pharmacological Approaches to the Treatment of Chronic Pain: New Concepts and Critical Issues*. Seattle, Wash: International Association for the Study of Pain (IASP) Press; 1994.

Goodwin JLR. Current concepts in the neurologic assessment of spinal pain: Cancer and noncancer pain. In Burchiel KJ, ed. *Surgical Management of Pain*. New York, NY: Thieme Medical Publishers; 2002: 98–127.

Loeser J, ed. *Bonica's Management of Pain*. 3rd ed. Philadelphia, Pa: Lippincott Williams & Wilkins; 2001.

One of the most comprehensive and resourceful textbooks on pain.

McGrath PA, et al. Controlling children's pain: A practical approach to assessment and management. 8th World Congress of Pain. Refresher course syllabus, 157–170. International Association for the Study of Pain (IASP), Vancouver, Canada; 1996.

Schecter NL, Berde CB, Yaster M, eds. Pain in infants, children, and adolescents. Philadelphia, Pa: Lippincott Williams & Wilkins, 2003.

The definitive textbook of pain management pertaining to the pediatric and adolescent years.

Wall PD, Melzak R, eds. *Textbook of Pain*. 4th ed. New York, NY: Churchill Livingstone; 1999.

Another comprehensive and resourceful textbook on pain.

CHAPTER 6 EVALUATING THE PATIENT WITH CHRONIC PAIN

Jeremy Goodwin and Zahid H. Bajwa

Pain is a complex multidimensional symptom. It is determined not only by actual or potential tissue injury and normal and abnormal activity of the nervous system, but also by the patient's personal beliefs, mood, previous painful experiences, psychosocial stressors, coping mechanisms, and motivational factors. Evaluation of a patient with chronic pain should take into consideration all of these factors. Unfortunately, there is no single test or scale that can measure pain comprehensively, reliably, or objectively. Thus, assessment of pain requires a thorough history and physical examination in combination with other diagnostic tools. Several visits may be required to elucidate relevant medical and pyschosocial factors. The patient's motivation for the evaluation must be clarified early (i.e., whether there are issues of litigation or disability affecting the patient's pain, and whether he or she perceives the potential to control pain as coming from without or within). To do this, it is important to listen well and not overly structure the interview. Chronic pain patients need validation. Without it, they cannot offer their trust, and trust is vital for treatment compliance and a successful outcome.

Pain assessment is a dynamic process that evolves with the pain management plan. The pain evaluation should be used to localize the source of pain; to determine its quality, pattern, and intensity; to define exacerbating and attenuating factors; and to assess how environmental and behavioral influences affect the pain. Clinicians should always try to make a diagnosis before implementing a treatment plan, recognizing that jumping to a premature conclusion might result in inappropriate treatment or harm to the patient. It is also necessary, at times, to rethink the diagnosis, despite previous and thorough workups.

DEFINING THE TYPE OF PAIN

Pain should be broadly defined as nociceptive (somatic or visceral), neuropathic, or idiopathic. Toward this end, pain *location* is of utmost importance to accurate diagnosis. It may be well localized, as in entrapment neuropathy (e.g., carpal tunnel syndrome), widespread and diffuse (e.g., fibromyalgia), or regional (e.g., musculoskeletal pain). Patterns of *radiation* may help determine the site of pathology, such as in cervical or lumbar radiculopathy. Radicular pain (along a dermatome) implies involvement of a nerve root. Pain may also be *referred*, as in visceral pain, when it is felt over a particular area of skin that is embryologically associated with but anatomically distant from the source of irritation. Accurate characterization of the pain's location and pathophysiology provides the rationale for treatment. Tables 6-1, 6-2, and 6-3 provide examples of referred pain contrasted with clinical findings associated with nerve root versus peripheral nerve pathology.

TAKING THE HISTORY

Detailed history taking at the first visit and a focused history (with emphasis on response to recent intervention) on subsequent visits is extremely beneficial. In many pain centers, the physician obtains a history after reviewing forms (see Appendix B) completed by the patient before the first interview. Some of the important points to be covered in this part of the evaluation are:

1. Location of pain
2. Character of pain
3. How and when the pain started
4. Is it continuous or intermittent?
5. Exacerbating and relieving factors
6. Effect of certain positions and activities on pain
7. Effect of stress on the pain
8. Effect of alcohol and other substances on pain
9. Is there an associated sleep disturbance?
10. Is there an associated mood disturbance?
11. Effect of pain on functioning at work or school
12. Effect of pain on quality of life, including social, sexual, and family interactions
13. Effect of pain *treatment* on cognitive, social, and sexual function
14. Motivation: issues of secondary gain (i.e., disability or psychological attention from partner, parents, or spouse)
15. Is a lawsuit involved?
16. Who, if anyone, does the patient blame for the pain?

Beware of attributing new pain to an already defined process. For example, someone with ankylosing spondylitis can still develop a herniated disk, and cancer pain may change or worsen because of disease spread, tolerance to medications, side effect of treatment, or a new psychosocial stressor.

PHYSICAL EXAMINATION

The physical examination starts with the first clinical interaction between the patient and clinician. It begins with how the patient responds to the initial greeting: getting up, walking, sitting down, and posture during these activities. Appearance (general health, weight, muscle bulk, and grooming), attitude and behavior (degree of distress and reactions to specific examination maneuvers), and gait (ataxia, walking with a limp, or requiring a cane or walker) can provide important information. The presence or absence of masses or lesions, signs of injury or trauma, and limb asymmetry regarding skin, hair, nails, or temperature changes should be noted. Alignment of the spine (scoliosis, kyphosis, loss of curvature) and range of motion (ROM) should be noted. Pain-exacerbating maneuvers, such as the straight-leg raising test, Spurling's maneuver

TABLE 6-1 **Patterns of Referred Pain**

Origins of Pain	Region of Pain Referral
Heart	Chest, left arm, jaw, epigastrium (C8–T8)
Esophagus	Substernal region
Diaphragm/liver capsule	Shoulder (C4)
Kidney	Lower thorax and back (T11–L1)
Ureter (upper)	Groin, testes, or ovary
Ureter (terminal)	Scrotum, labia
Prostate	Lower back (T10–T12)
Uterus	Lower back (T10–T12)
Ovary	Anterior thigh
Upper cervical facets	Occiput, vertex, and toward frontal region of head
Lower cervical facets	Shoulder, neck, and scapulae
Lumbar facets	Groin, buttocks, anterior and posterior thighs, calves; can be felt above L5, midline
Sacroiliac joints	Groin, buttocks, anterior and posterior thighs, calves; should not refer above L5, midline

of the neck, Patrick's test of the hip, and spinal ROM tests, may yield important diagnostic information. Joint shape, swelling, redness, and tenderness should be noted. Measurement of vital signs may prove useful in evaluating stress, pain (which alters vital signs in young children), and side effects of medication.

PERTINENT NEUROLOGIC AND PSYCHIATRIC EXAMINATIONS

Focused neurologic and psychiatric examinations also start with the first clinic visit. If the patient is able to give a clear and adequate history, a formal mental status examination is usually unnecessary, but range of affect (facial expression) and its congruency with language content and mood can provide important clues to the presence or absence of depression or anxiety. The effect of analgesics on higher intellectual function should be documented to help with future medication trials and to interpret problems of mental status. And unless the patient suffers from a headache or cranial nerve pain or dysfunction (i.e., trigeminal neuralgia or trigeminal neuropathy), the cranial nerve examination can generally be simplified by checking facial symmetry and eye movements (for a detailed outline, see Table 6-4). Experience best guides the clinician in the directed examination; however, subtle and sometimes significant findings may be missed by using a screening technique.

Results of the motor, sensory, and deep tendon reflex examination should be viewed together. Patients with lumbar or cervical radiculopathy may have more than one measurable objective sign or abnormality, although pain in a nerve root distribution may be the only symptom. If a single nerve or nerve root is involved, motor, sensory, and reflex abnormalities should coincide with and not contradict one another (see Tables 6-2, 6-3, 6-5, and 6-6). If a nerve plexus is involved, the situation is more complex and may require more extensive neurologic or electrodiagnostic evaluation. It is helpful to know that the boundaries of sensory-motor deficits are less clear in plexopathies than they are in peripheral nerve injury and that pain can occur without such deficits. Progression of sensory dysfunction, even outside of the originally involved area (i.e., allodynia), may indicate centralization of pain or disordered sensory processing in the spinal cord and not necessarily psychiatric overlay, as is often supposed.

We recommend *functional* motor assessment as an initial evaluative tool for the motor system, followed by a more focused examination of any abnormal findings (Tables 6-2 through 6-7). For example, if patients with back pain can rise from a chair without using their arms and can easily walk on tip-toes and heels, they are unlikely to have lower extremity weakness on manual-motor testing.

Some tests are more nerve root–specific than others. Great toe extension is mostly controlled by the L5 nerve root, whereas dorsiflexion of the foot involves nerve roots L4 through S1. It is vital to distinguish true muscle weakness from pain-limited strength and lack of effort. "Giveway" weakness may be indicative of either. Feigned unilateral weakness, an uncommon problem, is harder to maintain when both limbs are assessed at the same time. Table 6-7 summarizes some likely "nonorganic" signs and symptoms that are referred to as "illness or pain behavior."

The sensory examination should include response to light touch, light pressure, pinprick or cold (i.e., metal object or alcohol swab because pain and temperature are carried in the same pathway), and vibration and assessment of proprioception or joint position sense. If the patient's Romberg stance is stable, significant loss of vibratory and position sense is unlikely, but still possible. The affected skin area, which almost always manifests hyperesthesia, should be tested at the end of the examination. Allodynia should be sought in terms of light touch, light tapping, mechanical movement, and cold stimuli. Hyperpathia is elicited by fairly rapidly applying pinpricks to the focal area. What at first appears to be a diminution in pain sensation suddenly becomes an abnormally intense and prolonged discomfort lasting beyond the time of stimulation. When pain has become chronic and local tissue injury has healed, the persistence of allodynia, with or without hyperpathia, points to a neuropathic rather than nociceptive pain process. This may have important implications for further workup and treatment. Nociceptive pain, on the other hand, is generally associated with hyperesthesia that resolves with healing.

Examination of gait is not only helpful in screening for motor, sensory, or balance dysfunction, but it can also help evaluate the toxicity of some analgesic medications (high levels of some antiseizure medications used for pain may cause a broad-based gait and loss of balance, otherwise known as truncal ataxia). Conversely, the *absence* of a widely based gait in a patient complaining of difficulty balancing raises the question of astasia-abasia or functional sway. If present, the latter does not negate a physical basis for pain, but raises the question as to whether psychologic factors influence the degree of patient suffering.

ELECTRODIAGNOSTIC TESTING, SPINAL INJECTIONS, AND NEURAL BLOCKADE

Methods of evaluation may not be as equivalent as they first appear. Electromyography and neural blockade is a case in point.

TABLE 6-2 **Clinical Manifestations of Root Versus Nerve Lesions in the Arm**

Roots	C5	C6	C7	C8	T1
Sensory supply	Lateral border of upper arm	Lateral forearm, including finger 1	Over triceps, midforearm, and finger 3	Medial forearm to finger 5	Axilla down to elbow
Reflex affected	Biceps reflex	None	Triceps reflex	None	None
Motor loss	Deltoid	Biceps	Latissimus dorsi	Finger extensors	Intrinsic hand muscles (in some thenar muscles through C8)
	Infraspinatus	Brachialis	Pectoralis major	Finger flexors	
	Rhomboids	Brachioradialis	Triceps	Flexor carpi ulnaris	
	Supraspinatus		Wrist extensors	Wrist flexors	
Nerves	Axillary (C5, C6)	Axillary (C5, C6)	Radial (C5–C8)	Median (C6–C8, T1)	Ulnar (C8, T1)
Sensory supply	Over deltoid	Lateral forearm to wrist	Lateral dorsal and back of thumb and finger 2	Lateral palm and lateral fingers 1, 2, 3, and half of 4	Medial palm and fingers and medial half of finger 4
Reflex affected	None	Biceps reflex	Triceps reflex	None	None
Motor loss	Deltoid	Biceps brachialis	Brachioradialis	Abductor pollicis brevis	Intrinsic hand muscles
			Finger extensors	Long flexors of fingers 1, 2, 3	Flexor carpi ulnaris
			Forearm supinator		
			Triceps	Pronators of forearms	Flexors of fingers 4 and 5
			Wrist extensors	Wrist flexors	

From Patten J. *Neurological Differential Diagnosis.* New York, NY: Springer-Verlag; 1977.

Electromyography, including the electromylogram (EMG) and nerve conduction tests (NCT), can help rule in or out a myopathy, neuropathy, radiculopathy, or plexopathy accompanying a painful condition. It can also help determine chronicity. Several spinal and nerve root levels may be tested in a single session. Reflex arcs of the spinal cord can be evaluated and peripheral neurologic findings on the physical examination confirmed, but EMG cannot measure pain. EMG cannot measure small-fiber dysfunction (i.e., as caused by diabetes) and should not be attempted until 2 to 3 weeks after the onset of symptoms. This minimizes the chance of false-

TABLE 6-3 **Clinical Manifestations of Root Versus Nerve Lesions in the Leg**

Roots	L2	L3	L4	L5	S1
Sensory supply	Across upper thigh	Across lower thigh	Across knee to medial malleolus	Side of leg to dorsum and sole of foot	Behind lateral malleolus to lateral foot
Reflex affected	None	None	Patellar reflex	None	Achilles tendon reflex
Motor loss	Hip flexion	Knee extension	Inversion of foot	Dorsiflexion of toes and foot	Plantar flexion and eversion of foot
Nerves	Obturator (L2–L4)	Femoral (L2–L4)	Peroneal division of sciatic nerve (L4, L5, S1–S3)	Tibial division of sciatic nerve (L4, L5, S1–S3)	
Sensory supply	Medial thigh	Anterior thigh to medial malleolus	Anterior leg to dorsum of foot	Posterior leg to sole and lateral aspect of foot	
Reflex affected	None	Patellar reflex	None	Achilles tendon reflex	
Motor loss	Adduction of thigh	Extension of knee	Dorsiflexion, inversion, and eversion of foot	Plantar flexion and inversion of foot	

From Patten J. *Neurological Differential Diagnosis.* New York, NY: Springer-Verlag; 1977.

TABLE 6-4 **Clinical Evaluations of Cranial Nerve Function**

Cranial Nerve	Name	Evaluation Procedures
I	Olfactory	Test ability to identify familiar aromatic odors (e.g., coffee grounds, vanilla extract), one naris at a time and with eyes closed. Not routinely tested.
II	Optic	Test vision with Snellen chart or Rosenbaum near-vision chart. Perform ophthalmoscopic examination of fundi. Recognize papilledema and retinal hemorrhages. Test fields of vision using confrontation and double simultaneous stimulation. Is color vision equal for both eyes?
III, IV	Oculomotor, trochelar	Inspect eyelids for drooping (ptosis). Inspect pupil reactivity and size for equality (direct and consensual response) and rule out paradoxical dilation or afferent pupillary defect with swinging flashlight test (optic neuritis). Check for nystagmus of immediate, delayed, and attenuating type. Assess basic fields of gaze. Note asymmetric extraocular movements. Test ability to bury sclera when right or left eye looks toward nose.
V	Trigeminal	Test corneal reflex. Test superficial pain and touch sensation in each branch: V_1, V_2, V_3.
VI	Abducent	Test ability to bury sclera when right or left eye looks to side.
VII	Facial	Palpate jaw muscles for tone and strength while patient clenches teeth. Inspect symmetry of facial features. Test adequacy of closed-eye strength. Have patient smile, frown, puff cheeks, wrinkle forehead to test symmetry. Watch for spasmodic, jerking movements of face.
VIII	Acostic	Test sense of hearing with watch or rubbing fingers 6 in. from ear. Compare bone and air conduction of sound (Weber's and Rinne tests).
IX X	Glossopharyngeal Vagus	Test gag reflex and ability to swallow. Inspect palate for symmetry of evaluation when patient says "ahhhh." Observe for swallowing difficulty. Have patient take small sip of water. Watch for nasal or hoarse quality of speech. Can patient make a quick, clear "cough"?
XI	Spinal accessory	Test trapezius strength (have patient shrug shoulders against resistance). Test sternocleidomastoid muscle strength (have patient turn head against resistance).
XII	Hypoglossal	Inspect tongue in mouth and while protruded for symmetry, fasciculations, and atrophy. Test tongue strength with index fingers when tongue is pressed against cheek.

Note: Taste, like smell, is not routinely assessed. When necessary, it should probably be assessed by a neurologist.

Modified from Donohoe CD. Targeted history and physical examination. In: Waldman SD, ed. *Interventional Pain Management.* 2nd ed. Philadelphia, Pa: WB Saunders; 2001:90.

negative results. EMG and NCT are extremely operator dependent, in terms of both technique and interpretation.

Selective nerve root blockade and spinal injection into vertebral disks (diskograms) and zygahypophyseal (facet) joints or the epidural space may prove diagnostic or therapeutic but offer no clues to chronicity. Except for diskography, multiple levels of testing are not easily or wisely done during a single visit, because specificity is lost. Although the usefulness of EMG, NCT, and selective nerve root blockade may overlap, information obtained through one does not necessarily negate the need for the other. If in doubt about which diagnostic test is most appropriate, ask a colleague with advanced understanding of that particular field.

IMAGING STUDIES

Choosing the appropriate mode of imaging can be difficult, the consequence of which may hasten or slow the time to accurate diagnosis. A general guide to the commonly used techniques is presented in Table 6-8. Advice should be sought from knowledgeable colleagues for specific case applications.

PAIN MEASUREMENT TOOLS

No single tool or instrument can measure pain fully and objectively in a clinical setting. But several measurement instruments have

TABLE 6-5 **Deep Tendon Reflex Scale**

0	No response
1+	Sluggish
2+	Active or normal
3+	More brisk than expected, slightly hyperactive
4+	Abnormally hyperactive, with intermittent clonus

From Seidel HM, et al. *Mosby's Guide to Physical Examination.* 3rd ed. St. Louis, Mo: Mosby-Yearbook; 1995.

been developed to assess the most clinically relevant aspects of pain and ways in which it affects the patient's life. These tools are either easily used but limited in what they measure (unidimensional scales) or require time to apply and psychological expertise to interpret (multidimensional scales).

Unidimensional Instruments, Scales, and Indices

In clinical practice, unidimensional and self-report scales offer a simple, useful, and valid method for assessment and monitoring of a patient's pain. Unidimensional scales measure only the intensity of pain.

Numeric Rating Scale (NRS) or Verbal Rating Scale (VRS) This is the simplest and most commonly used scale to evaluate pain. On a scale of 0 to 10, where 0 represents "no pain" and 10 the "worst imaginable pain," the patient chooses a number to describe the pain intensity. Advantages of this scale are that it is simple and reproducible, it is easily understood by most patients, and small changes in pain can be measured. Its major disadvantage is its inability to reflect anything more than the intensity of pain. Ramifications of pain on mood (or vice versa) are not so easily measured.

Visual Analog Scale (VAS) The VAS is very similar to the NRS or VRS except that the patient puts a mark on a *nongradated* 10-cm line, with one end labeled as "no pain" and the other as "worst pain imaginable." Using the VAS, pain can be evaluated on a 0 to 10 scale and can be described as such. The advantages and disadvantages are very similar to the NRS, but the VAS is used more commonly in clinical pain research. VAS results do not always match, but the discrepancy itself can prove useful, since it stimulates a more in-depth evaluation.

Verbal Descriptor Scales With verbal descriptor scales, patients are asked to describe their pain by choosing descriptors from a list of adjectives reflecting pain intensity. One example is a five-word scale denoting pain as *mild, uncomfortable, distressing, horrible,* or *excruciating*. A major limitation of this scale is that patients often select moderate descriptors rather than extremes to appear more "reasonable" or may select extremes rather than more moderate descriptors when their level of distress is very high. This should prompt a search for confounding factors, such as anxiety or fear, which can greatly affect the level of pain or suffering.

Faces Pain Rating Scale Evaluating pain in children younger than 8 years old is extremely challenging because of their inability to fully describe pain or understand pain assessment forms. The Faces Pain Rating Scale depicts sketches of facial expression, ranging from a happy, smiley face to a very distressed and teary face. Several versions are in common use. In evaluating children in pain, their cognitive-developmental level, pain self-support, pain behavior, and physiologic parameters, such as variation in blood pressure and heart rate, must also be taken into account. The Faces Pain Rating Scale may also be useful in developmentally disabled patients, cognitively impaired geriatric patients, and sometimes in patients who do not speak English (when no interpreter is available).

Multidimensional Instruments, Scales, or Indices

These instruments provide more detailed information about the patient's pain than do unidimensional scales. They are especially useful in the evaluation of complex pain in patients whose suffering is likely multifactoral in origin. However, these tools are relatively cumbersome and time-consuming, requiring expert interpretation. They are usually reserved for use in clinical research or in-depth multidisciplinary evaluations at comprehensive pain management centers. Pain psychologists often employ a battery of such tests in conjunction with the psychiatric interview. Only a few are mentioned here for the purpose of illustration.

It is important to reemphasize that no single assessment tool can fully evaluate a person's pain. Just as magnetic resonance imaging cannot replace the acumen of the clinician, so these mea-

TABLE 6-6 **Grading of Muscle Strength**

Clinical Finding	Grade	% of Normal Response
No evidence of contractility	0	0
Slight contractility, no movement	1	10
Full range of motion with gravity eliminated	2	25
Full range of motion with gravity	3	50
Full range of motion against gravity, some resistance	4	75
Full range of motion against gravity, full resistance	5	100

From Chipps EM, et al. *Neurologic Disorders.* St. Louis, Mo: Mosby-Yearbook; 1992.

TABLE 6-7 **Chronic Low Back Pain: Symptoms and Signs of Physical Disease Versus Abnormal Illness Behavior**

	Physical Disease	Abnormal Illness Behavior
Symptoms		
Pain	Anatomic distribution	Whole leg pain
Numbness	Dermatomal	Whole leg numbness
Weakness	Myotomal	Whole leg giving way
Time pattern	Varies with time	Never free of pain
Response to treatment	Variable benefit	Intolerance of treatments
Signs		
Tenderness	Anatomic distribution	Superficial Widespread, nonanatomic
Axial loading	No lumbar pain	Lumbar pain
Simulated rotation	No lumbar pain	Lumbar pain
Straight-leg raising	Limited on distraction	Improves with distraction
Sensory	Dermatomal	Regional, but patchy numbness may indicate spinal cord lesion
Motor	Myotomal	Regional, jerky, giving way

Modified from Waddell G, et al. Clinical evaluation of disability in low back pain. In: Frymoyer JW, et al, eds. *The Adult Spine: Principles and Practice.* 2nd ed. Philadelphia, Pa: Lippincott-Raven; 1997:171–184.

surement tools are limited to an adjunctive role in evaluation of the neuropsychologic pain. The value of these tests lies in their appropriate use by trained individuals.

Minnesota Multiphasic Personality Inventory (MMPI) This instrument is a long and complex questionnaire that requires caution in interpretation (its scales are based on the general population, not a chronic pain patient population). A number of scales are generated, which may lead to a false sense of confidence in the ability of the test to assess pain. The ability to predict outcome of treatment is variable. The test is better at predicting who is not likely to return to work than who is. Thus, the degree to which this tool is helpful depends greatly on the application, knowledge, and skill of the clinician using it. Many pain centers use an abbreviated and modified version called the MMPI-2.

McGill Pain Questionnaire (MPQ) Historically, this is one of the most commonly used multidimensional instruments. Patients select descriptive terms from groups of words ranked in order of severity. Pain location is also sketched on a human figure drawing. Present and previous pain experiences are noted, and all of this is integrated into a general analysis of the patient's pain experience. The MPQ requires some patient sophistication in the use of language, reducing the valuc of the test considerably if applied indiscriminately.

Brief Pain Inventory (BPI) The BPI asks patients to rate the pain at its worst, least, and average intensity, as experienced at the time of evaluation. It also asks patients to present the location of their pain on a schematic diagram of the body. The BPI is a cross-cultural instrument and is particularly useful in clinical pain research.

TWO MODELS OF PAIN ASSESSMENT AND MANAGEMENT

As we have discussed, no single scale or test is able to fully evaluate a patient with chronic pain, but a combination of the patient's history and physical examination, diagnostic tests, and some of the assessment tools can be very helpful. Each pain center or clinician can develop a pain assessment form dictated by the type of pain problems most often encountered in their referral group. Appendix A is the pain assessment form used by the pain management center at the Beth Israel-Deaconess Medical Center (BIDMC) in Boston. Patients complete the center's assessment form before their first appointment. This approach is a classic consultative model. Referral is made by primary care or treating clinician, via a referral letter or form provided by the BIDMC pain center. Once the referral is received, a pain management specialist reviews the information and decides on the best line of action, based on the nature of the pain and urgency of the situation. Urgent appointments are scheduled with patients for whom immediate interventions may prevent chronic pain and disability, such as patients in the early stages of reflex sympathetic dystrophy (recently renamed complex regional pain syndrome, type 1) or postherpetic neuralgia.

All patients are required to complete the assessment form before their first visit. Some patients are selected for a "comprehensive pain evaluation" based on the chronicity and complexity of their pain, response to previous interventions, and complicating factors, such as substance abuse, psychiatric illness, or factors associated with possible secondary gain. The comprehensive pain evaluation requires completion of modified versions of the Beck Depression Inventory (BDI), the MMPI, and other behavior assessment tools before the first visit. These patients are then scheduled to see a team composed of one or two physicians, a nurse, a psychologist, and a physical or occupational therapist, all on the

TABLE 6-8 **Imaging Procedures With Best Diagnostic Value by Body Region**

Body Region	Recommended Procedure(s)*
Head and brain	**MRI**
	CT scan
	Angiography
	Plain films
Neck and spine	**MRI**
	Plain films
	Myelography
	CT scan
Extremities, soft tissues (including muscle, excluding bone)	**MRI**
	Plain films
	Ultrasonography
	CT scan
	Venography
Bone	**Plain films**
	Bone scintigraphy
	CT scan
	MRI
Joint	**MRI**
	Plain films
	Arthrography
Chest	**Plain films**
	CT scans
	MRI
	Radionuclide studies
	Coronary arteriography
	Aortography
Abdomen	**Ultrasonography**
	CT scan
	Contrast studies (barium meal or enema, IV pyelography)
	Plain films
	MRI
	Radionuclide studies
Pelvis	**Ultrasonography**
	MRI
	CT scan

*Boldface indicates procedure of choice. CT, computed tomography; MRI, magnetic resonance imaging.

Modified from Banitzky S, et al. Radiologic testing in patient evaluation. In: Waldman SD, ed. *Interventional Pain Management,* 2nd ed. Philadelphia, Pa: WB Saunders; 2001:129.

same day. Then, the full multidisciplinary team (i.e., clinicians who have personally seen the patient plus those who have not) discusses the evaluation team's findings and impressions and arrives at a realistic, practical, and long-term plan.

The cornerstone of this model is that pain specialists act as *consultants* in coordinating short-term and long-term care of a variety of patients with chronic pain. Once the patient is stabilized on a certain regimen or has reached a medical end point, patient management is taken over by the referring clinician. The patient must have a primary care clinician to be seen. The pain specialist does not "take over" responsibility of the patient's care but may be heavily involved in it, at least initially. Where possible, the primary care clinician should prescribe the pain medications, once the dose has been stabilized. This allows closer monitoring of a patient's health over time and minimizes the chance of accidental drug-drug interactions. The fewer people prescribing for a patient, the better.

A modification of this approach (used where state health plans or insurance coverage is more restrictive) begins with the pain physician's initial evaluation on referral by another clinician. The pain physician then refers to other clinicians (not necessarily in his or her clinic) as necessary and as authorized by the third-party payer. As the third-party payer milieu continues to evolve, more pain centers may have to adopt this potentially less expensive and slower approach. One of the authors (Goodwin) and Kim J. Burchiel, MD, Chairman of the Department of Neurological Surgery at the Oregon Health and Science University, believe that a potentially successful means of doing this is via a coordinated network of persons, clinicians, and services who are financially independent of each other yet complementary in terms of skills, philosophy, and training. Such interdisciplinary or interdepartmental cooperation could provide a depth and breadth of resources unlikely to be available in a smaller, single department–funded multidisciplinary pain center. If alternative medicine is specifically and *openly* included in interdisciplinary patient care and not just used as an adjunctive complementary or alternative approach, the care can then rightly be referred to as *integrative* pain medicine.

Finally, in some states, such as Oregon, patient evaluation by a pain specialist, or an expert on the physiologic or anatomic system that is painful (e.g., urologist, orthopedist, gastroenterologist), is required by law so that a primary care provider can prescribe long-term opioids for the management of nonmalignant pain without concern of criticism by the medical board of examiners. This particular type of evaluation may or may not require a team approach, depending on the complexity of the situation.

PUTTING IT ALL TOGETHER

Evaluating a patient with chronic pain can be time-consuming and frustrating, because clinicians must rely greatly on the patient's subjective report and the somewhat limited results of objective tests. An understanding of central and peripheral neuroanatomy and pathophysiology, visceral innervation, and musculoskeletal function is essential for interpretation of findings by review of the history, physical examination, and other diagnostic tools. If done correctly, the evaluation alone can prove therapeutic; just having a diagnosis can alleviate stress. It is the first step in building the physician-patient relationship and therapeutic alliance. It is important always to listen to and believe in your patients and involve them in the decision-making process. The clinician should be empathic, supportive, and honest, neither promising too much nor removing all hope. There is a big difference between stating, "There is nothing I can do," and, "There is nothing more that can be done." The suffering patient is a human being in distress, not a disease. Tests and measurement tools aid in diagnosis and treatment but cannot replace a thorough history and physical examination. Several visits may be necessary before the picture becomes clear. If the preceding approach is followed, especially within a multidisciplinary or interdisciplinary setting, then there is a reasonable chance that a correct diagnosis will be followed by appropriate management.

BIBLIOGRAPHY

Aprill C. Diagnostic disc injections I (cervical) and II(lumbar). In: Frymoyer JW, ed. *The Adult Spine*. Philadelphia, Pa: Lippincott-Raven; 1997:523–562.

Cipriano JJ. *Photographic Manual of Regional Orthopaedic and Neurological Tests*. 3rd ed. Baltimore, Md: Williams & Wilkins; 1997.

Donohoe CD. Targeted history and physical examination. In: Waldman SD, ed. *Interventional Pain Management.* 2nd ed. Philadelphia: WB Saunders; 2001:83–94.

Finley GA, McGrath PJ, eds. *Measurement of Pain in Infants and Children. Progress in Pain Research and Management.* Vol IV. Seattle, Wash: International Association for the Study of Pain (IASP) Press; 1998.

Gagliese L, Melzack R. The assessment of pain in the elderly. In: Mostofsky DI, Lomranz J, eds. *Handbook of Pain and Aging*. New York, NY: Plenum Press; 1997:69–96.

Goodwin JLR. Current concepts in the neurologic assessment of spinal pain: Cancer and noncancer pain. In: Burchiel KJ, ed. *Surgical Management of Pain*. New York, NY: Thieme Medical Publishers; 2002:98–127.

Karasek M, Bogduk N. Twelve-month follow-up of a controlled trial of intradiscal electro thermal annuloplasty for the treatment of low back pain due to internally disrupted discs. *Spine.* 2000;25:2601–2607.

Klein JD, Garfin SR. Clinical evaluation of patients with suspected spine problems. In: Frymoyer JW, ed. *The Adult Spine: Principles and Practice*. 2nd ed. Philadelphia, Pa: Lippincott-Raven; 1997:319–340.

Menses S, Simons DG, eds. *Muscle Pain: Understanding Its Nature, Diagnosis, and Treatment*. Philadelphia, Pa: Lippincott Williams & Wilkins; 2001.

Waldman SD, ed. *Interventional Pain Management*. 2nd ed. Philadelphia, Pa: WB Saunders; 2001.

CHAPTER 7 OUTCOME MEASUREMENTS IN PAIN MEDICINE

Harriët Wittink, Leonidas C. Goudas, Scott Strassels, and Daniel B. Carr

Central to the evaluation of health care is the measurement of health. Until the first part of the twentieth century, health was defined as the absence of disease and was measured in terms of morbidity and mortality. This simple approach to health status was rejected in 1948 with the expansion of the concept of health by the World Health Organization (WHO), which defined health as, "A state of complete *physical*, *mental* and *social* well being and not merely the absence of disease or infirmity."[1] This definition reflected the multidimensionality of health and considered not only biologic markers, but also the ability to perform physically, psychologically, and socially in the everyday environment.

This change in the definition of health gave rise to the current outcomes movement. Other factors, such as the reversal of the proportion of care rendered for acute illnesses versus chronic diseases, technological advancements in health care, rising health care costs, the emerging concept of quality of care, and increased recognition of the importance of patients' views about their care and health, have further fostered the growth of this movement. Outcomes research seeks to define which treatments are effective, at which point in the natural history of medical conditions these interventions should be provided, for which patients, and at what cost, thus providing objective evidence to guide treatment.

Conscientious health care providers use both individual clinical expertise and the best available objective, external evidence for treatment. The best available external evidence for treatment is defined as clinically relevant research, often from the basic sciences of medicine, but especially from patient-based clinical research into the accuracy and precision of diagnostic tests (including the clinical examination), the power of prognostic markers, and the efficacy and safety of therapeutic, rehabilitative, and preventive regimens.[2] The integration of clinical expertise and best available external evidence for treatment is the practice of evidence-based medicine. With the plethora of current and relevant literature, it is impossible for most clinical care providers to keep abreast of the latest developments in their field. Because of this problem, structured approaches to literature synthesis, such as that organized by the Cochrane Collaboration, have arisen to summarize, with the least possible bias, the best available research on a specific topic (see later discussion). The goal is to make relevant information widely available, and evidence-based practice unencumbered for all health care providers.

This chapter focuses on common terminology used in outcomes assessment, and on outcomes measurement tools used in research on and treatment of patients with chronic noncancer pain, as they are part of the foundation of what will become evidence-based practice and perhaps eventually guidelines for treatment. Although the comprehensiveness and validity of outcome measures for the treatment of all types of pain lags behind those of equally high-impact conditions that affect the public's health, this lag is even more pronounced for cancer pain than for noncancer pain.[3] Much more research has addressed functional assessment, and how pain management influences function, in patients with acute or chronic noncancer pain than in those whose pain results from malignancy.[4]

OUTCOMES RESEARCH

We, as health care providers, treat patients to make them "better." How is "better" defined, and by whom? "Better" from the point of view of the practitioner, the patient, or society? Does "better" equate to less pain, increased physical functioning, decreased disability (as judged by the physical therapist), improved quality of life (as judged by the patient), or decreased cost of worker's compensation charges and fewer health care visits (as judged by payers)? Does the same intervention that benefits one patient benefit a group of patients with similar conditions? How do we know whether it does? These are questions that the outcomes assessment movement is trying to address.

Outcomes research studies the results of medical care.[5] It involves "the rigorous determination of what works in medical care and what does not" and states that "outcomes research, by informing the content of policy positions, payment rules, and practice guidelines, presumably solves both the problems of quality and cost that beset health care and does so by scientific rather than political means" (p. 1268).[6] Outcomes research is the foundation of evaluation of the quality and costs of health care delivery. Adoption of an evidence-based approach to health care, exemplified by the Cochrane Collaboration,[2,7,8] has been accompanied by a shift towards emphasis on patient-centered health outcomes.[9] This broadened perspective has heightened the need for tools to monitor and adjust treatment and to approach clinical decision making from a viewpoint that is evidence based and patient centered.[10] The pressing need to know which treatments reduce chronic pain, which improve functional status (including return to work and social activities), whether or not they change pain intensity, and, in particular, which treatments are worth paying for, has fueled the development of a number of instruments. These instruments are intended to capture in a simple, speedy, and robust fashion the health status of patients.[11]

HEALTH STATUS ASSESSMENT: DEFINITIONS AND TERMS

This section discusses common terminology used in outcomes assessment and provides several examples of assessment tools used in measuring outcomes during the treatment of patients with chronic noncancer pain. Health assessments focus on three broad categories of measures: traditional biologic, general (or generic), and disease specific.[12] Traditional biologic measures may be primary, such as morbidity and mortality, or surrogate, such as a decrease in blood pressure in patients given an antihypertensive drug. Measures used for patient-centered outcomes generally estimate persons' health-related quality of life (HRQOL) and their ability to function and to do the things they want to do. These measures may be generic, evaluating overall health status, or disease-specific, focusing on the effect of a given condition on a person's life.

HRQOL assessment is the measurement or evaluation of the health of an individual or a patient. HRQOL may include biologic markers, but it emphasizes indicators of physical functioning, mental health, social functioning, and other health-related concepts, such as pain, fatigue, and perceived well-being.[13] Concepts included in some commonly applied HRQOL instruments are presented in Table 7-1.

Quality of life includes HRQOL, but is a broader term that includes nonmedical aspects of life that reflect the aggregate impact of food, shelter, safety, living standards, and social and physical environmental factors.[13]

Patient based outcome measures are indicators of patients' evaluations of both changes in patient health status, including HRQOL and mortality, and the quality of health care. The importance of patients' views has been increasingly recognized in health care.[14] One might even argue that the increased interest in palliative care and pain control in recent years is the direct result of a power shift in which patients and their families—the consumers of health care—have much greater autonomy and power than under the previous disease-centered model of care.[15] Clinicians' taking the patient's view into account is associated with greater patient satisfaction with care,[16] better compliance with treatment programs,[17] and an increased likelihood of maintaining a continuous relationship during health care.[18]

The distinction between disease-based clinical investigation and patient-centered outcomes research is analogous to that between measures of efficacy and measures of effectiveness. In an ideal setting, such as a randomized, controlled clinical trial, the *efficacy* of a treatment may be derived as the dose-response relationship for a given physiologic effect assessed under well-controlled conditions. In controlled trials, the end points of interest are usually biologic measures, such as changes in blood glucose levels or blood pressure. However, equally important to practitioners and patients is the *effectiveness* of a treatment, which refers to the outcomes of this treatment when applied in typical practice settings, measured over the course of disease, and including measures that matter most to patients (patient-centered outcomes).[19] Outcomes research is more likely to be generalizable to typical medical practice than are controlled clinical trials. Terminology commonly employed in outcomes research is presented in Table 7-2.

CHOICE OF INSTRUMENTS

Because the purpose of this overview is to present a few widely applied outcomes measurement tools and the context in which they are used, we next describe the criteria used to select one from among available instruments rather than how to create a new questionnaire.

Selection of a specific outcomes tool will depend on the population of interest and the ability of the measurement tool to detect changes within the domain of interest. The selection of an instrument consists of two phases. The first has to do with the condition(s) for which this instrument will be used; the second has to do with the psychometric properties of the instrument.

Choosing a domain-specific, condition-specific, or generic instrument depends on the aim of the study. If one specific domain is of interest, such as pain intensity or depression, a domain-specific instrument can be used (e.g., the McGill Pain Questionnaire or the Beck Depression Inventory). In general, a condition- (or disease-) specific instrument will have a narrow focus but will provide considerable detail in the area of interest. If the interest is in general HRQOL, comparison with different conditions, or with healthy people, a generic instrument can be used. Generic and condition-specific HRQOL instruments can be used together to sup-

TABLE 7-1 **Domains Used in Health-related Quality-of-Life Measurements**

Domains	QWB	SIP	NHP	QLI	COOP	EQ-5D	DUKE	MOS SF-36
Physical functioning	X	X	X	X	X	X	X	X
Social functioning	X	X	X	X	X	X	X	X
Role functioning	X	X	X	X	X	X	X	X
Psychological distress		X	X	X	X	X	X	X
Health perceptions (general)			X	X	X	X	X	X
Pain (bodily)		X	X		X	X	X	X
Energy/fatigue	X		X				X	X
Psychological well-being							X	X
Sleep		X	X				X	
Cognitive functioning		X				X		
Quality of life					X			
Reported health transition					X			

COOP, Darthmouth Function Charts; DUKE, Duke Health Profile; EQ-5D, European Quality of Life; MOS SF-36, Medical Outcomes Study 36-item Short-Form Health Survey; NHP, Nottingham Health Profile; QLI, Quality of Life Index; QWB, Quality of Well-Being Scale; SIP, Sickness Impact Profile Index.

Modified from Ware J. The status of health assessment 1994. *Ann Rev Public Health.* 1995;16:327–354.

TABLE 7-2 **Terms and Definitions Commonly Employed in Outcomes Assessment**

Term	Definition
Item	A single question (such as, "In general, how would you say your health is?")
Scale	A range of available responses to an item Can be categorical (e.g., excellent, very good, good, fair, poor), numerical, or consist of a visual analog scale
Domain	Identifies a particular focus of attention (e.g., physical functioning, mental or general health, patient satisfaction with care) and may comprise the response to a single item or responses to several related items May consist of one scale (a collection of related items) or multiple scales
Instrument	A group of items used for the collection of desired data May contain a single item or multiple items that may or may not be divided into domains
Domain- or dimension-specific instrument	A one-scale instrument (e.g., the McGill Pain Questionnaire)
Ceiling or floor effect	Indicates the lack of sensitivity of an instrument to discriminate differences at the higher or lower end of a scale used to measure this effect (e.g., a ceiling effect may be a 10/10 pain intensity that is now reported as a 12/10 by a patient)
Disease- or condition-specific tools	Instruments used exclusively for assessment of the health status of populations with a specific disease or condition (e.g., back pain, post-herpetic neuralgia)
Generic HRQOL tools	Instruments that estimate an individual's overall health status that can be used to compare HRQOL between groups of patients with different diseases

HRQOL, health-related quality of life.

plement the information collected.[20] Using a condition-specific survey or module together with a generic scale may provide more insight into aspects of health that are not well measured by either type of instrument.[21–23] Comparison of the impact of pain on health status with the impact of other chronic illnesses on general health status, for example, allows researchers to conduct trials of various treatments so as to make clinical decisions in medical practice and inform health care policy.[12]

Important psychometric properties to consider include the following[24–26]:

- *Test-retest reliability:* the extent to which the measure generates consistent results. How closely do the results of repeated applications agree with each other?
- *Internal reliability:* (quantitated by Cronbach α) the sensitivity of the number of items that make up the measure and the degree of intercorrelation between the items. A Cronbach α of 0.9 or higher is generally preferred for measurement in a single person, whereas Cronbach α of 0.7 or higher is preferred for group measurement.[27]
- *Validity:* the extent to which the instrument actually measures what it claims (i.e., the correspondence between what the instrument reports and reality).
- *Responsiveness:* the ability of an instrument to detect changes, particularly clinically important changes, over time in individuals or in groups of subjects.
- *Applicability:* the appropriateness of the instrument's use in the specific study population.
- *Practicality:* the likelihood that an instrument can be applied readily, without excessive burden to patient or investigator, and produce data that can be easily analyzed and applied.

Cronbach alpha = a coefficient of reliability (or consistency) used to measure how well a set of items (or variables) measures a single unidimensional latent construct. It ranges from 0 to 1. (For details see: http://www.ats.ucla.edu/stat/spss/fqq/alpha.html.

DESCRIPTIONS OF SELECTED GENERIC HEALTH-RELATED QUALITY-OF-LIFE INSTRUMENTS

Of the many generic instruments available to assess HRQOL, four validated, widely used questionnaires stand out. Brief descriptions of these instruments are given in Table 7-3.

PAIN-SPECIFIC OUTCOMES MEASUREMENT

Pain, in general, and chronic and persistent pain, specifically, is a unique challenge to outcomes research because of the importance of subjective information. Unlike the majority of other medical conditions, chronic pain may not involve a distinct organ system, pathophysiologic process, or specific discipline. Although pain is

TABLE 7-3 **Generic Outcomes Assessment Tools**

Name of Instrument	Internal Reliability (Cronbach α)	Cross-validation instruments	Number of Items	Number of Domains	Time to Complete (min)	References
Nottingham Health Profile (NHP)	Cronbach α was reported as 0.77–0.85 for the first section and 0.44–0.86 for the second section in a sample of patients with osteoarthritis	SIP SF-36 COOP WONCA EQ-5D	37	Six plus: Physical abilities, pain, sleep, social isolation, emotional reactions, and energy level A second section includes optional questions about work, social and sex life, interests and hobbies, and holidays	10–15	Hunt and McEwen,[28] Hunt et al,[29] Essink-Bot et al.[30,31]
Medical Outcomes Study 3d-item Short-Form Health Survey (SF-36)	Cronbach α in both general and chronic disease populations ranges from 0.78–0.93	Oswestry Disability Index SIP NHP EQ-5D Social Maladjustment Schedule WOMAC Osteoarthritis Index Chronic Pain Grade Questionnaire	36	Eight scales of general health and functioning: physical functioning, role—physical (limitations in physical roles due to health problems), bodily pain, general health, vitality, social functioning, role—emotional (limitations in emotional roles due to health problems), and mental health	10–15	Tarlov et al,[32] Stewart,[33] Ware,[34] McHorney et al,[35] Stansfeld et al,[36] Grevitt et al[37] See also http://www.rand.org/health/totalsnav.html
Sickness Impact Profile (SIP)	Cronbach $\alpha = 0.94$ Test-retest reliability r = 0.92	NHP SF-36 EQ-5D MMPI	136	12	20–30	Bergner et al[38–40]
European Quality of Life (EQ-5D, Euro-QoL)	Test-retest reliability in stroke patients: κ 0.63–0.80	SF-36 NHP COOP WONCA	15	Five dimensions: mobility, self care, usual activities, pain/discomfort, and depression/anxiety The sixth item is a global evaluation of one's own health using a visual analog scale of 0–100 (worst imaginable health to best imaginable health)	Few	Essink-Bot et al[30,31] See also http://www.euroqol.org

COOP, Dartmouth Function Tests; ED-5D, European Quality of Life; MMPI, Minnesota Multiphasic Personality Inventory; NHP, Nottingham Health Profile; SF-36, Short-Form Health Survey; SIP, Sickness Impact Profile; WOMAC, Western Ontario and McMaster Universities Arthritis; WONCA, World Organization of Family Doctors.

characterized as a symptom, it is, in fact, a subjective experience, a perception.[41] This perception not only depends on nociceptive transmission and modulation within the CNS, but is integrated with psychological, social, and other environmental factors.[42] Physical functioning, work, family, and social relationships are usually impaired by chronic pain. Comorbid conditions, such as depression or anxiety, often accompany chronic pain.[43] For these reasons, it is argued that the assessment of patients with chronic pain should be accomplished within a multidimensional framework.[44] Assessment of chronic pain should provide clinicians with relevant information to formulate a treatment plan, and also allow for measurement of the outcome of treatment interventions. The generic HRQOL instruments discussed earlier are mostly epidemiologic tools and as such are able to measure change in large samples of patients. By design they are not intended, nor are they sufficiently sensitive, to measure changes in a single subject. Furthermore, these instruments do not provide information on items frequently assessed in pain management, such as solicitous responses,[45,46] coping ability,[47,48] fear avoidance,[49–51] and the extent of disablement from pain.

Many instruments are used to assess the impact of pain on patients' lives. Ideally the instrument should provide relevant information to all clinicians within an inter- or multidisciplinary team, have a low respondent burden, and be sensitive enough to detect changes at both group and individual levels. Widely used methods to assess pain and its influence range from domain to condition specific. Some of the most frequently used tools are presented next.

Domain-specific Measurements

Pain Intensity (or Pain Relief) The three most commonly used methods to assess pain intensity are the verbal rating scales, visual analog scales, and numerical rating scales (Table 7-4). Von Korff[52] cautions that multiple factors influence patients' pain reports, including time of day. Aggregated pain measures have, therefore, been shown to be more reliable and more sensitive to treatment effects than single items.[53] Aggregated pain measures are scores that are created from multiple measures. For instance, the average of three concurrent responses to a 100-mm visual analog scale of pain intensity ratings of current, average, and best pain can be taken.[54] A composite measure shown in cancer pain patients to have high internal consistency (Cronbach $\alpha > 0.8$) consists of an average of ratings on a 0-to-10 scale of current, least, and average pain.[55] Jensen and colleagues[56] report that individual 0-to-10 pain intensity ratings have sufficient psychometric strength to be used in chronic pain research, especially in studies with large sample sizes, but composites of 0-to-10 ratings may be more useful when maximal reliability is necessary (i.e., in studies with small sample sizes or in the monitoring of an individual patient).

Verbal Rating Scales (VRSs) These scales are positively and significantly related to other measures of pain intensity.[26] Jensen and colleagues[57] reported on the potential clinical utility of classifying pain as mild, moderate, or severe based on the impact of pain on quality of life. There is a nonlinear relationship between pain intensity and pain interference. Pain intensity begins to have a serious impact on functioning when it reaches a specific threshold; about 5 on a 0-to-10 scale in patients with cancer pain.[55] To explore in greater detail the relationship between pain severity and interference in patients with cancer pain, Serlin and colleagues[55] administered the Brief Pain Inventory to a total of 1897 patients from numerous sites in the United States, France, China, and the Phillippines. In this classic study, they gathered self-reported data on pain severity as well as interference by pain with enjoyment of life, activity, walking, mood, sleep, work and relations with others. These four diverse populations had "fairly consistent patterns relating pain severity to pain interference." Statistical analyses showed that pain severity on a 0–10 verbal numerical rating scale could be stratified according to the degree of interference it produced as mild (1–4), moderate (5–6), and severe (7–10).

TABLE 7-4 **Pain Intensity Scales**

Scale	Description
Verbal rating scale (VRSs)	A list of adjectives describing different levels of pain intensity (e.g., 0 = no pain, 1 = slight pain, 2 = moderate pain, 3 = severe pain)
Visual analog scales (VASs)	Lines that are usually 100-mm long and represent the continuum of the symptom being rates, with labels at either end to represent the extremes of the symptom (e.g., 0 = "no pain," 100 = "pain as bad as it could be")
Numerical rating scales (NRSs)	Ascending sequences of numbers, each representing increasing levels of pain intensity (e.g., 11-point scale in which 0 = no pain, 10 = worst possible pain).

Visual Analog Scales (VASs) These are simple tools to assess intensity and other dimensions of pain, such as anxiety, efficacy of treatment, and emotional responses[26,58,59] (Fig. 7-1). Patients mark the scale at a point that represents the severity of their pain at a specified time point, or within a well-defined interval (e.g., the past 24 hours). Variations of these techniques request that patients circle a number from 0 to 10, or place a mark through one of these numbers. VASs are more sensitive and precise than descriptive scales. They are also easy to use and interpret; however, they are limited to expressing only one dimension of the complex experience of pain. It may be difficult for patients to imagine the worst pain imaginable, or they might report their pain as being outside the 0-to-10 limits, saying that it is a 20, for example.

The validity of VASs is supported by their positive relations to other measures of pain intensity.[24,60] They are sensitive to treatment effect and are distinct from measures of other subjective components of pain.[52]

Numerical Rating Scales (NRSs) These scales were demonstrated to provide sufficient levels of discrimination for patients with chronic pain to describe their pain intensity.[61] Like VRSs and VASs, NRSs demonstrate positive and significant correlations with other measures of pain intensity.[26,60]

Pain Affect

The McGill Pain Questionnaire (MPQ) The questionnaire provides estimates of the sensory, affective, and evaluative dimensions of pain.[62] It is one of the most frequently used instruments for pain measurement and is considered useful for evaluating pain treatments and as a diagnostic aid.[26,63–66] In addition to collecting information about diagnosis, drug therapy, pain and medical history, and other symptoms and modifying features, the MPQ also contains a list of words that describe pain, divided into groups pertaining to the sensory, affective, and evaluative dimensions of the pain experience.

The MPQ is available in several languages, as well as extended (Dartmouth Pain Questionnaire, McGill Comprehensive Pain Questionnaire) and shortened versions. Components of the MPQ have been incorporated into other instruments.[26] Although the MPQ is one of the leading pain assessment tools, and is considered the gold standard of pain assessment tools, it has some limitations.[67] For the purposes of this discussion, clinicians should keep in mind that it may be difficult to discriminate between types of pain syndromes in persons who are very anxious or who have other psychological morbidity.

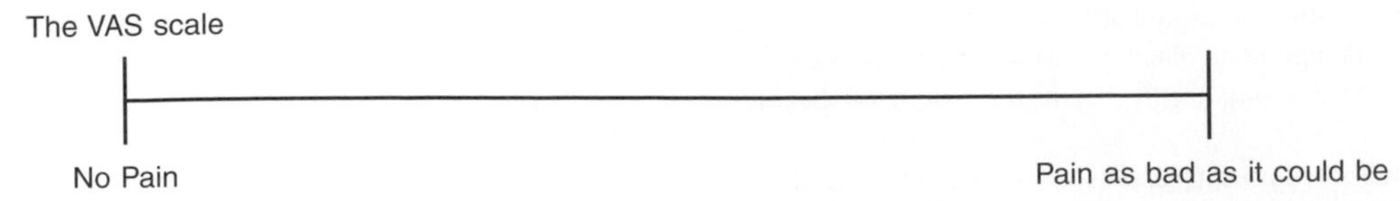

Figure 7-1 The visual analog scale.

Pain Distress Scales The Acute Pain Management Guideline Panel[68] recommends, among other tools, the use of the scales shown in Figure 7-2.

MULTIDIMENSIONAL MEASUREMENTS

Brief Pain Inventory (BPI)

The BPI was originally developed for use in persons with cancer, although it is also used to assess pain in people with other diseases.[26] The purpose of the BPI is to assess the severity of pain and the impact of pain on daily functions. Assessment areas include severity of pain, impact of pain on daily function, location of pain, pain medications, and the amount of pain relief in the past 24 hours or the past week.[69] The internal consistency ranges from Cronbach α 0.77 to 0.91. The form takes about 10 minutes to complete. It is valid for use in Chinese (Mandarin),[70] Filipino, French, Hindi,[71] Italian,[72] Japanese, and Vietnamese, among other languages. It is also available in a shortened form, the BPI-SF[73,74] that takes 5 minutes to complete. When applying the BPI to persons with chronic noncancer pain, the clinician should keep in mind that interpretation may be difficult if the questions asked do not reflect the patient's experience. Furthermore, questions about functioning are subject to both floor and ceiling effects. The BPI is copyrighted, but permission to use it is routinely granted at no cost after providing a short description of intended use. (Samples of the form, both the short and the long version, can be found at http://prg.mdanderson.org/bpicopy.htm.)

Multidimensional Pain Inventory (MPI)

The MPI (formerly the West Haven-Yale Multidimensional Pain Inventory, or WHYMPI) was developed by Kerns and colleagues.[45] It is a 64-item, self-report questionnaire comprising three parts and 12 subscales. The first two parts are related to patients' appraisals of pain and its impact on different domains of their lives, and patients' perceptions of the responses of significant others to their distress and suffering. The third part assesses how frequently patients perform 18 common daily activities. Internal consistency ranges from Cronbach α 0.70 for outdoor activities to 0.90 for interference.

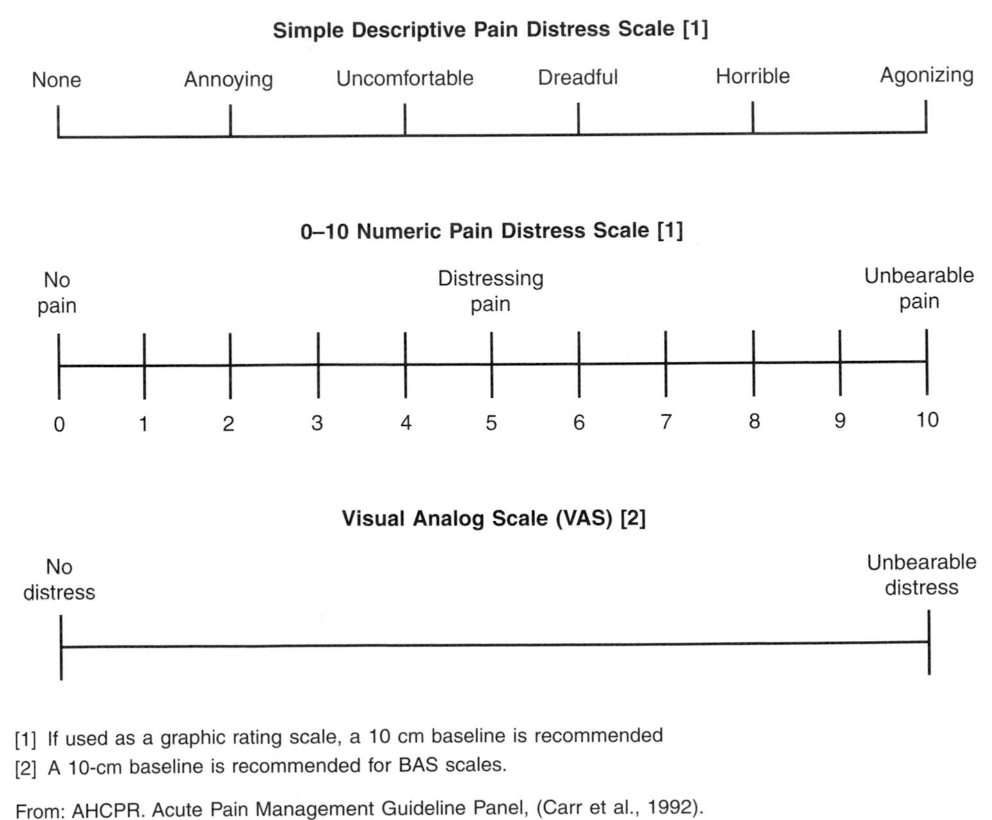

Figure 7-2 Examples of pain distress tools.

Using cluster-analytic and multivariate classification methods, three homogeneous subgroups of patients with chronic pain have been identified and replicated across a wide range of medical diagnoses (back pain, temporomandibular disorders, headache). The three groups' distinct profiles were labeled "dysfunctional," "interpersonally distressed," and "adaptive coper."

Burton and colleagues[75] suggested that a psychometric battery consisting of the MPI and the BPI[76] was useful for both identifying problem areas that might impede treatment of patients with chronic pain and assessing treatment outcome. Moreover, the MPI has been shown to be predictive of chronicity of pain following acute symptom onset.[77,78] The MPI has demonstrated reliability and validity in patients with chronic low back pain.[79]

A recent study compared the redundancy, reliability, validity, and sensitivity to change among the Short-Form Health Survey (SF-36), Oswestry Disability Index (ODI, see later in this chapter), and MPI on a cross-sectional sample of N = 424, with a follow-up sample of N = 87 of patients with chronic pain, seen in an interdisciplinary pain clinic.[80] The Cronbach αranged from 0.69 to 0.92 for the MPI, from 0.79 to 0.91 for the SF-36, and was 0.86 for the ODI. Three concepts overlapped between the SF-36 and the MPI: pain, interference/social functioning, and mental health. Both the SF-36 and the MPI contributed unique scales (e.g., the MPI "significant other" scales; R^2 range 0.03–0.16). Significant changes following treatment were observed for the MPI pain severity, interference and outdoor work activities; the SF-36 physical and social functioning, bodily pain; and the ODI. The MPI is used widely, and has been translated into Spanish, Portuguese, French, Swedish, Dutch, and Italian.[44,81,82]

Treatment Outcomes of Pain System (TOPS)

Because, when applied to individual patients, the SF-36 lacked measurement reliability for assessment of treatment outcomes, lacked sensitivity to upper extremity or facial pathology, and failed to separate limitations of work versus everyday activity, two of us (Wittink and Carr) and colleagues conducted a two-part study to develop an outcomes instrument suitable for measurement of change in individual patients with chronic pain. A novel group of scales derived from responses to 61 questions (which include the SF-36) proved sufficiently reliable for routine follow-up of individual patients during treatment for chronic pain. This new instrument, the TOPS, allows assessment of individual patient outcomes and aggregate or individual clinician performance during interdisciplinary treatment of chronic pain.[22,23]

In addition to the SF-36, this instrument contains demographic data and 14 scales of which 7 fit into the Nagi framework.[83] The remaining 7 scales are considered to be mediating factors between the domains of pain, functional limitation, and disability. The 7 main scales include pain symptom, perceived and objective family disability, work limitations, objective work disability, and upper and lower body limitations. The Cronbach α of these scales ranges from 0.70 for objective work disability to 0.92 for lower body functioning and 0.93 for perceived family/social disability. The mediating scales include fear-avoidance, passive coping, life control, and solicitous responses. In addition, two scales measure patient satisfaction with care and outcomes. The final scale is the total pain experience scale, which is a composite of pain intensity, pain interference, physical functioning, and disability.

For evaluating a single patient, the TOPS pain symptom, perceived family/social disability, and total pain experience scales are considerably more sensitive to individual change than the SF-36 bodily pain (BP) scale. Their increased sensitivity can be attributed to their greater measurement reliability. For example, the Cronbach α equals 0.93 for total pain experience compared with 0.84 for the SF-36 BP scale. The TOPS scales also provide a clearer and more clinically relevant set of concepts for the pain clinician who may have objectives apart from a simple reduction in pain intensity, such as the reduction of suffering or the reduction of disability in spite of pain. This high internal consistency allows for the measurement of change during treatment of an individual patient.[22]

Pain clinic normative values were established based on a sample of 1230 administrations of the tool in interdisciplinary pain clinics in Boston and Salt Lake City. The instrument was translated and validated in French Canadian and 8 European languages.[84] The TOPS takes10 to 15 minutes to complete.

INSTRUMENTS MEASURING MENTAL HEALTH AND COGNITIONS

Many patients with chronic pain learn to function normally despite their pain, continue to work productively, and rarely seek medical care. Factors such as coping ability,[85–87] fear avoidance,[49,88] self efficacy[89,90] and catastrophizing[90–92] have been associated with adjustment differences in patients with chronic pain. The beliefs or cognitions that patients have regarding their pain problem are hypothesized to have a direct impact on mood. For instance, negative thoughts about pain are strongly related to depressive symptomatology.[93] Depression has been associated with high health care utilization and costs[94] and is prevalent in patients with chronic pain. Patients with chronic pain may develop a variety of psychological problems, including depression, anxiety, sleep disorders, and disruptions in family life. Because of the importance of psychological factors in the experience of chronic pain, adding an assessment of mental health and cognitive factors to generic and condition-specific HRQOL may help patients and health care providers work together more effectively toward their common goals of pain relief and improved functioning. Some commonly used mental health assessment tools are listed in Table 7-5.

TABLE 7-5 **Selected Mental Health Assessment Tools**

Beck Depression Inventory (BDI)
Carroll Rating Scale for Depression
Center for Epidemiologic Studies Depression Scale (CES-D)
Depression Adjective Checklists
Geriatric Depression Scale
Hamilton Rating Scale for Depression
Millon Behavioral Health Inventory
Minnesota Multiphasic Personality Inventory (MMPI)
Montgomerysberg Depression Rating Scale
Multidimensional Health Locus of Control Scale
Self-Rating Depression Scale (Zung)
Symptom Checklist-90 (SL-90)

Moderate to strong associations have been identified between coping responses, pain severity, psychological well-being, and physical functioning.[95,96] Fear avoidance beliefs correlated significantly with self-reported disability in activities of daily living and work loss[49] and were shown to be a significant predictor of chronic pain[40,97] in patients with musculoskeletal disorders. Catastrophizing was shown to predict depression,[86,90,91] perception of pain,[87,98] lower self-efficacy for pain, lower spousal ratings of self-efficacy for control of fatigue or mood symptoms,[99] and disability.[100] Patients' beliefs and self-appraisals thus play a large part in shaping the outcome of treatment. Many instruments exist that measure patient beliefs; here, we limit ourselves to discussing a few widely used tools.

Coping Strategies Questionnaire (CSQ)

Questionnaires that address cognitive factors include the widely used CSQ and the Pain Beliefs and Perceptions Inventory (PBPI). The CSQ was designed to help identify methods of coping used by persons with chronic low back pain.[101] It contains six types of cognitive strategies, two types of behavioral mechanisms, and two effectiveness ratings. The CSQ was found to be internally reliable when used to assess pain coping strategies. The authors also found that praying, hoping, and coping self-statements were used frequently, while others such as reinterpretation of pain sensations, were not. Overall, cognitive coping and suppression, helplessness, and diverting attention or praying explained much of the variance in coping strategies. The CSQ has been studied widely to better describe its factor structure, its utility in persons with low back pain or cancer pain, and its utility for prediction of patient and spouse ratings of patients' self-efficacy.[87,99, 102–106]

Pain Beliefs and Perceptions Inventory (PBPI)

The PBPI assesses three aspects of pain beliefs: self-blame, perception of pain as mysterious in origin, and beliefs about pain duration.[107] These authors found that the belief that pain will last is associated with greater pain intensity and decreased compliance with psychological and physical therapies. The PBPI contains only 16 items; thus, respondent burden is very low. Like the CSQ, the PBPI has also been used widely and has been translated for use in the United Kingdom.[108–110]

Fear Avoidance Beliefs Questionnaire (FABQ)

The FABQ is a 16-item instrument developed by Waddell and colleagues.[49] Within the 16 items are two fear-avoidance scales. The first scale (7 items) concerns fear-avoidance beliefs about work and the second scale (4 items) concerns fear-avoidance beliefs about physical activity. The internal consistencies (Cronbach α values) for these two scales were 0.88 and 0.77, respectively. Test-retest reliability had a κ equal to 0.74.

Pain Catastrophizing Scale (PCS)

The PCS is a 13-item instrument developed in 1995 at the Dalhousie University Pain Research Centre to facilitate research on the mechanisms by which catastrophizing has an impact on the pain experience.[111] The items on the PCS were drawn from previous experimental and clinical research on catastrophic thinking in relation to pain experience.[101,112,113]

The PCS yields a total score and three subscale scores assessing rumination ("I can't stop thinking about how much it hurts"), magnification ("I worry that something serious might happen"), and helplessness ("There is nothing I can do to reduce the intensity of the pain").[114] A total PCS score of 38 represents a clinically relevant level of catastrophizing.[114]

The Cronbach α for the total PCS is 0.87; for rumination, 0.87; for magnification, 0.66; and for helplessness, 0.78. Test-retest reliability across a 6-week period was r = 0.75.[111] The PCS takes about 5 minutes to complete. Support for good internal consistency and validity of the PCS was provided by others.[115,116]

DISEASE-SPECIFIC OUTCOMES MEASURES

Disease-specific instruments reflect particular limitations or restrictions associated with specific disease states. These instruments are designed to be sensitive in determining the effects of treatment on or the spontaneous longitudinal course of a single disease or condition. Disease-specific measures have been developed for almost each imaginable condition. For an overview of pain specific tools, see Table 7-6.

A few further examples of disease-specific instruments are instruments that measure the impact of migraine,[117] shoulder pain,[118–120] knee pain[121] (KOOS, a knee injury and osteoarthritis outcome tool, and Lysholm scales),[122] neck pain,[123] and back pain. Two of the most commonly used disease-specific tools for back pain are the Oswestry Disability Index (ODI)[124] and the Roland-Morris Disability Questionnaire (RDQ).[125] The ODI and RDQ scores are highly correlated, with similar test-retest reliability and internal consistency. Floor and ceiling effects determine the choice of instruments. A greater proportion of patients score in the top half of the distribution of RDQ sores than in the top half of the ODI scores. The ODI is, therefore, recommended in patients who are likely to have persistent severe disability and the RDQ in patients who are likely to have relatively little disability.[126]

Oswestry Disability Index (ODI)

The ODI[124] is one of the most frequently used tools in back pain research. It consists of ten sections that include pain intensity, personal care, lifting, walking, sitting, standing, sleeping, sex, social life, and traveling. Each section is scored on a 6-point scale (0–5), with 0 representing no limitation and 5 representing maximal limitation. The subscales combined add up to a maximum score of 50. The score is then doubled and interpreted as a percentage of patient perceived disability (the higher the score, the greater the disability).

The ODI has excellent test-retest reliability (r = 0.99,[124] ICC = 0.83,[127]) and clinical face validity. The internal reliability, Cronbach α, was found to be 0.71 for version 1.0.[128] Two studies that determined Cronbach α of version 2.0 found it to be 0.76[14] and 0.87.[129]

Roland-Morris Disability Questionnaire (RDQ)

The RDQ[125] was derived from the Sickness Impact Profile (SIP). The generic SIP was modified to become disease-specific by adding "because of my back pain" to each item. Twenty-four items were selected from the SIP by the original authors because they related specifically to physical functions that were likely to be affected by low back pain. These items include walking, bending over, sitting, lying down, dressing, sleeping, self-care, and activities of daily living. The Cronbach α for the scale has been estimated to be between 0.84 and 0.93.[126] The RDQ correlates well

TABLE 7-6 **Selected Pain-specific Health-related Quality-of-Life Instruments**

Arthritis Impact Measurement Scales (AIMS-2)	Neck Disability Index (NDI)
Back Pain Classification Scale (BPCS)	Neuropathic Pain Scale (NPS)
Brief Pain Inventory (BPI, BPI-SF; formerly Wisconsin Brief Pain Inventory)	Oswestry Low Back Pain Disability Questionnaire
Biobehavioral Pain Profile	Pain and Distress Scale (PAD)
Catastrophizing Scale	Pain Disability Index (PDI)
Family Pain Questionnaire	Pain Distress Scales
Fear Avoidance Beliefs Questionnaire (FABQ)	Pain and Impairment Relationship Scale (PAIRS)
Fibromyalgia Impact Questionnaire (FIQ)	Pain Perception Profile (PPP)
Graded Chronic Pain Scale (GCPS)	Patient Pain Questionnaire
Illness Behavior Questionnaire	Roland-Morris Disability Questionnaire (RDQ)
Low Back Pain Rating Scale	Somatic Input, Anxiety, and Depression (SAD) Index for the Clinical Assessment of Pain
McGill Pain Questionnaire (MPQ, MPQ-SF)	Treatment Outcomes of Pain System (TOPS)
Medical Outcomes Study Pain Measures	Visual Analog Pain Rating Scales
Multidimensional Pain Inventory (MPI; formerly West Haven-Yale Multidimensional Pain Inventory)	Work Limitations Questionnaire (WLQ)

with the SF-36 physical subscales, the SIP,[130] and pain ratings.[131] It is available in 12 languages, and translations are available from the author (mroland@man.ac.uk).

Work Limitations Questionnaire (WLQ)

The WLQ was developed by Lerner and Amick with support from GlaxoWellcome, Inc. The WLQ is a 25-item, self-administered questionnaire that evaluates the degree to which health problems interfere with ability to perform job roles. It was designed to assess groups of individuals who are currently employed. The WLQ indicates the degree to which health problems interfere with specific aspects of job performance (on-the-job disability), and the impact of these limitations on workers' productivity.

The WLQ items ask respondents to rate their level of difficulty (or, on one scale, their level of ability) to perform 25 specific job demands. These demands have four defining features: (1) a wide range of jobs in the United States include these demands; (2) a wide variety of physical and emotional health problems can make it difficult to perform these demands effectively; (3) the demands are considered important to their jobs by workers who hold these jobs; and (4) losses in individual work productivity are frequently related to the degree to which these job-related demands are not met.

Responses to the 25 items are combined into four work limitation scales: the Time Management scale (Question 1), the Physical Demands scale (Question 2), the Mental/Interpersonal Demands scale (Questions 3 and 4) and the Output Demands scale (Question 5). The Cronbach α ranged from 0.88 for Output Demands to 0.91 for Mental/Interpersonal Demands. The WQL was shown to have high reliability and validity.[132] The instrument takes 5 to 10 minutes to complete. (For more information, contact wlq@lifespan.org.)

EVIDENCE-BASED RESEARCH AND GUIDELINES

The gold standard of current evidence-based literature synthesis is the Cochrane Collaboration. The Cochrane Collaboration was developed in response to a call by Archie Cochrane, a British epidemiologist, for systematic, up-to-date reviews of all randomized controlled trials on health care. Several centers have been established throughout the world, and collaborative review groups prepare and maintain systematic reviews. At the beginning of 1997, the existing and planned review groups (more than 40) cover most of the important areas of health care. Relevant to this chapter, Cochrane collaborative review groups have been formed to assess spine problems, musculoskeletal pathology, and pain (palliative and supportive care).[8] The Cochrane group aims are "preparing, maintaining and disseminating systematic reviews of the effects of health care" to provide reliable, unbiased, up-to-date information to health care providers worldwide to permit informed decisions about the specific effects of health care interventions.[8] As stated earlier, in making decisions about the care of individual patients, the results of these reviews must be integrated with the clinician's expertise, which has been acquired through experience and practice. The results of the reviews must also be integrated with patients' understanding and preferences, which derive from their knowledge of their condition (particularly if it is a chronic or recurrent health problem), the treatments offered, and the responsiveness or otherwise of the former to the latter (http://www.cochrane.org/cochrane/cc-broch.htm#GDAHC). The integration of the results of the reviews, clinician expertise, and patient feedback and participation is considered evidence-based practice.

Methods for scoring the quality of research reviewed have been established.[133] If studies are combinable, a meta-analysis can be performed. A meta-analysis is a synthesis, usually understood to be quantitative, of the results of several studies.[2] The precision of such a meta-analysis is greater than any one of its component studies because of the aggregation of patient numbers. Cumulative meta-analysis recalculates aggregate treatment effects and confidence intervals as each new relevant study is published. This technique of ongoing recalculation permits early decisions as to whether a treatment is efficacious or not, thereby averting the need for subsequent unneeded, costly, time-consuming (and some would say, unethical) clinical trials. Cumulative meta-analysis has documented that it may take years for statistically significant conclusions from randomized controlled trials to diffuse into textbooks and narrative review articles.[134]

One meta-analysis published outside of the Cochrane library identified published studies of treatment in multidisciplinary pain clinics (MPCs) between 1960 and 1990.[135] These authors identified 65 studies that met inclusion criteria. They concluded that multidisciplinary pain treatment resulted in large effect sizes that were maintained for more than 6 months, that MPCs were efficacious, and that the effects were not limited to patients' perceptions but also extended to objective behavior, such as return to work or decreased use of health care resources. One analysis evaluated whether return to work could be predicted after MPC treatment.[136] These authors concluded that although prediction of return to work is an increasingly important topic, few of the studies they evaluated met appropriate design and statistical criteria. They were unable to clearly identify which variables were useful predictors of return to work.

One of the challenges unique to evaluating treatment at MPCs is that the criteria used to define success are often not uniform.[137] Despite this problem, Turk and colleagues[137] found that reported pain reduction ranged from 14% to 60%, and that reductions appeared to be well maintained at follow-up, although some studies reported no improvement during treatment. Treatment was reported to result in decreased opioid use in nearly three fourths of persons, whereas untreated people generally reported no change. Treatment was also noted to improve activity levels and return to work, lower use of the health care system (including hospitalization and surgery), and increase the percentage of disability claims that were settled. This last point suggests that many persons with chronic noncancer pain can return to work, even after an extended period of being disabled.

Finally, one group of researchers performed a meta-analysis of meta-analyses.[138] These researchers concluded that MPC treatment is consistently effective for most outcomes, including return to work, although many different outcome variables were assessed in individual meta-analyses and ultimately, it was "unclear what combination of treatments is necessary for an effective [treatment] package." Meta-analytic results depend, however, on the studies included within the analysis. Thus, owing to a variety of methodologic problems that affect pain treatment studies, the results of this literature synthesis should be interpreted cautiously. Indeed, some experts have argued that a single meta-analysis of heterogeneous trials of a single intervention applied to diverse groups of patients with a complex clinical condition may be frankly misleading.[139]

The College of Physicians and Surgeons of Ontario, Canada, was the first to publish guidelines on the treatment of chronic, noncancer pain based on the best available evidence in November 2000. (A PDF file of the entire guide is available at http://www.cpsbc.bc.ca/physician/documents/pain.htm.) Clinical practice guidelines have been defined as "systematically developed statements to assist practitioner and patient decisions about appropriate health care for specific clinical circumstances." In the establishment of guidelines, levels of evidence generally are stratified as follows:

Level I	Strong evidence from at least one systematic review of multiple well-designed randomized controlled trials.
Level II	Strong evidence from at least one properly designed randomized controlled trial of appropriate size.
Level III	Evidence from well-designed trials without randomization, single group pre-post, cohort, time series, or matched case-controlled studies.
Level IV	Evidence from well-designed nonexperimental studies from more than one center or research group.
Level V	Opinions from respected authorities, based on clinical evidence, descriptive studies, or reports of expert committees.

Often, guideline committees will add a second dimension that documents not only the nature of the evidence that forms the basis of the recommendations, but also the strength and consistency of the evidence. Guidelines thus incorporate Cochrane or other systematic reviews when available, but go one step further by making specific recommendations with the definite intent to influence what clinicians do. (Evidence reports and clinical practice guidelines can be found on http://www.ahrq.gov.)

CONCLUSION

In this chapter, we have presented an overview of the terminology used in HRQOL outcomes assessment and examples of instruments that can be applied in clinical practice. Systematic measurement and documentation of HRQOL is a useful, clinically relevant approach to incorporate patient preferences into front-line medical decision making. Doing so is expected to improve overall patient satisfaction with care.[10] No tool will be used if it is too burdensome (too long or too difficult to understand). Instruments must be easily understood, administered, and interpreted by both clinicians and patients. No instrument is ideal for all intended uses; questionnaires are available in a variety of forms and many of these can be readily incorporated into clinical care and research. Outcomes assessment is a dynamic area, particularly as it stands at the interface between routine practice and new standards for pain assessment and treatment applied by the Joint Commission for the Assessment of Healthcare Organizations. The dissemination of ever-simpler and more powerful means to capture data electronically in everyday health care opens new opportunities for understanding which treatments are effective, and for whom, and may provide irrefutable evidence that we who treat pain add patient-centered value to the health care enterprise.

Web Sites to Visit for Measurement Tools

http://www.stat.washington.edu/TALARIA/talaria0/LS2.2.html: measurement of pain in children and patients with cancer pain
http://www.outcomes-trust.org/instruments/
http://www.york.ac.uk/inst/crd/welcome.htm
http://eircae.net/testcol.htm: test locator site

Web Sites to Visit for Evidence-based Research

http://www.cochrane.org: main site for the Cochrane Collaboration
www.med.unr.edu/medlib/netting.html: Web site containing evidence-based Web sites
http://www.herts.ac.uk/lis/subjects/health/ebm.htm: Web sites and databases
http://www.jr2.ox.ac.uk/bandolier/: bandolier EBM
htt://www.jr2.ox.ac.uk/bandolier/painres/painres.html: pain research at Bandolier EBM

http://www.iwh.on.ca/home.htm: Institute for Work and Health, Canada

http://www.ahcpr.gov/: Agency for Healthcare Research and Quality

Web Sites to Visit for Guidelines on Managing Pain

http://www.ampainsoc.org/pub/bulletin/nov00/clin1.htm

http://www.guideline.govhttp://www.nlm.nih.gov/nichsr/hsrsites.html: research on health care in general

REFERENCES

1. World Health Organization. *Constitution of the WHO, Basic Documents*. Geneva, Switzerland: WHO;1948.
2. Sackett DL, Haynes RB, Rosenberg W, Richardson WS. *Evidence-Based Medicine: How to Practice and Teach EBM.* Orlando, Florida: WB Saunders; 1997.
3. Goudas L, Carr DB, Bloch R, et al. Management of cancer pain. In: *Evidence Report/Technology Assessment No. 35*. Rockville, Md: Agency for Healthcare Research and Quality; 2001. AHRQ Publication No. 02-E002.
4. McQuay H, Moore A. *An Evidence-based Resource for Pain Relief.* Oxford, England: Oxford University Press; 1998.
5. Foundation for Health Services Research. Health outcomes research: A primer [Association for Health Services Research Web site]. 1994. Available at: http://www.ahsr.org. Accessed April 17, 2002.
6. Tanenbaum SJ. What physicians know. *N Engl J Med* 1993;329: 1268–1271.
7. Mulrow CD, Oxman A, eds. Cochrane Collaboration Handbook [updated September 1997]. In: The Cochrane Library [database on disk and CDROM]. The Cochrane Collaboration. Oxford, England: Update software, issue 4; 1997.
8. Carr DB, Wiffen P, Fairman F, LeMaitre M. The Cochrane Collaboration and its Pain, Palliative, and Supportive care review group. In: Max M, ed. *Pain 1999—An Updated Review.* Refresher course syllabus. Seattle, Wash: IASP; 1999:399–410.
9. Gerteis M, Edgman-Levitan S, Daley J, Delbanco TL, eds. *Through the Patient's Eyes: Understanding and Promoting Patient-Centered Care.* San Francisco, Calif: Jossey-Bass; 1993.
10. Marvel MK, Epstein RM, Flowers K, Beckman HB. Soliciting the patient's agenda: Have we improved? *JAMA* 1999;281:283-287.
11. Rucker KS, Metzler HM, Kregel J. Standardization of chronic pain assessment: A multiperspective approach. *Clin J Pain* 1996;12:94–110.
12. Ware J. The status of health assessment 1994. *Ann Rev Public Health* 1995;16:327–354.
13. Greenfield S, Nelson EC. Recent developments and future issues in the use of health status assessment measures in clinical settings. *Med Care* 1992;30:MS23–MS41.
14. Fisher K, Johnson M. Validation of the Oswestry low back pain disability questionnaire, its sensitivity as a measure of change following treatment and its relationship with other aspects of the chronic pain experience. *Physiother Theory Pract* 1992;13:67–80.
15. Carr DB. The development of national guidelines for pain control: Synopsis and commentary. *Eur J Pain* 2001;5(suppl A):91–98.
16. Hall JA, Roter DL, Katz NR. Meta-analysis of correlates of provider behavior in medical encounters. *Med Care* 1988;26:657–675.
17. Becker MH. Patient adherence to prescribed therapies. *Med Care* 1985;23:539–555.
18. Kaplan SH, Greenfield S, Ware JE. Assessing the effects of physician-patient interactions on the outcomes of chronic disease. *Med Care* 1989;7(suppl):S110–S127.
19. Pransky G, Himmelstein J. Outcomes research; implications for occupational health. *Am J Ind Med* 1996;29:573–583.
20. Ware JE Jr. Conceptualizing and measuring generic health outcomes. *Cancer* 1991;67(suppl):774–779.
21. Wagner AK, Rogers WH, Sukiennik A, et al. Outcomes assessment in chronic pain treatment: The need to supplement the SF-36. American Pain Society, 1995 Annual Meeting Program; A-66
22. Rogers W, Wittink HM, Wagner A, Cynn D, Carr DB. Assessing individual outcomes during outpatient, multidisciplinary chronic pain treatment by means of an augmented SF-36. *Pain Med* 2000;1:44–54.
23. Rogers WH, Wittink HM, Ashburn MA, Cynn D, Carr DB. Using the "TOPS": An outcomes instrument for multidisciplinary outpatient pain treatment. *Pain Med* 2000;1:55–67.
24. Jensen MP, Karoly P, Braver S. The measurement of clinical pain intensity: A comparison of six methods. *Pain* 1986;27:117–126.
25. Wood-Dauphinee S, Troidl H. Endpoints for clinical studies: Conventional and innovative variables. In: Troidl H, Spitzer WO, McPeek B, et al, eds. *Principles and Practice of Research: Strategies for Surgical Investigators.* 2nd ed. New York, NY: Springer-Verlag; 1991:151–168.
26. McDowell I, Newell C. *Measuring Health: A Guide to Rating Scales and Questionnaires.* New York, NY: Oxford University Press; 1996.
27. Nunnally J. *Psychometric Theory.* New York, NY: McGraw-Hill; 1978.
28. Hunt SM, McEwen J. The development of a submissive health indicator. *Social Health Illness* 1980;2:231–246.
29. Hunt SM, McKenna SP, Williams J. Reliability of a population survey tool for measuring perceived health problems: A study of patients with osteoarthrosis. *J Epidemiol Community Health* 1981;35:297–300.
30. Essink-Bot ML, Krabbe PF, van Agt HM, Bonsel GJ. NHP or SIP—a comparative study in renal insufficiency associated anemia. *Qual Life Res* 1996;5:91–100.
31. Essink-Bot ML, Krabbe PF, Bonsel GJ, Aaronson NK. An empirical comparison of four generic health status measures. The Nottingham Health Profile, the Medical Outcomes Study 36-item Short-Form Health Survey, the COOP/WONCA charts, and the EuroQol instrument. *Med Care* 1997;35:522–537.
32. Tarlov AR, Ware JE Jr, Greenfield S, Nelson EC, Perrin E, Zubkoff M. The Medical Outcomes Study. An application of methods for monitoring the results of medical care. *JAMA* 1989;262:925–930.
33. Stewart AL, Hays RD, Ware JE Jr. The MOS short-form general health survey. Reliability and validity in a patient population. *Med Care* 1988;26:724–735.
34. Ware JE Jr, Sherbourne CD. The MOS 36-item Short-Form Health Survey (SF-36). I. Conceptual framework and item selection. *Med Care* 1992;30:473–483.
35. McHorney CA, Ware JE, Raczek AE. The MOS 36-Item Short-Form Health Survey (SF-36): II. Psychometric and clinical tests of validity in measuring physical and mental health constructs. *Med Care* 1994; 31:247–263.
36. Stansfeld SA, Roberts R, Foot SP. Assessing the validity of the SF-36 General Health Survey. *Qual Life Res* 1997;6:217–224.
37. Grevitt M, Khazim R, Webb J, Mulholland R, Shepperd J. The short form-36 health survey questionnaire in spine surgery. *J Bone Joint Surg Br* 1997;79:48–52.
38. Bergner M, Bobbitt RA, Carter WB, Gilson BS. The Sickness Impact Profile: Development and final revision of a health status measure. *Med Care* 1981;19:787–805.
39. Bergner M, Bobbitt RA, Kressel S, Pollard WE, Gilson BS, Morris JR. The sickness impact profile: Conceptual formulation and methodology for the development of a health status measure. *Int J Health Serv* 1976;6:393–415.
40. Bergner M, Bobbitt RA, Pollard WE, Martin DP, Gilson BS. The Sickness Impact Profile: Validation of a health status measure. *Med Care* 1976;14:57–67.
41. Chapman CR, Gavrin J. Suffering: The contributions of persistent pain. *Lancet* 1999;353:2233–2237.
42. Brown J, Klapow J, Doleys D, Lowery D, Tutak U. Disease-specific and generic health outcomes: A model for the evaluation of long-term

intrathecal opioid therapy in noncancer low back pain patients. *Clin J Pain* 1999;15:122–131.
43. Rudy TE, Kerns RD, Turk DC. Chronic pain and depression: Towards a cognitive-behavioral mediation model. *Pain* 1988;35:129–140.
44. Lousberg R, Van B, Groenman NH, Schmidt AJ, Arntz A, Winter FA. Psychometric properties of the Multidimensional Pain Inventory, Dutch language version (MPI-DLV). *Behav Res Ther* 1999;37:167–182.
45. Kerns RD, Turk DC, Rudy TE. The West Haven-Yale Multidimensional Pain Inventory (WHYMPI). *Pain* 1985;23:345–356.
46. Romano JM, Turner JA, Jensen MP, et al. Chronic pain patient-spouse behavioral interactions predict patient disability. *Pain* 1995;63:353–360.
47. Tan G, Jensen MP, Robinson-Whelen S, Thornby JI, Monga TN. Coping with chronic pain: A comparison of two measures. *Pain* 2001; 90:127–133.
48. Nielson WR, Jensen MP, Hill ML. An activity pacing scale for the chronic pain coping inventory: Development in a sample of patients with fibromyalgia syndrome. *Pain* 2001;89:111–115.
49. Waddell G, Newton M, Henderson I, Somerville D, Main CJ. A Fear-Avoidance Beliefs Questionnaire (FABQ) and the role of fear-avoidance beliefs in chronic low back pain and disability. *Pain* 1993;52: 157–168.
50. Vlaeyen JW, Linton SJ. Fear-avoidance and its consequences in chronic musculoskeletal pain: A state of the art [review]. *Pain* 2000; 85:317–332.
51. Al Obaidi SM, Nelson RM, Al Awadhi S, Al Shuwaie N. The role of anticipation and fear of pain in the persistence of avoidance behavior in patients with chronic low back pain. *Spine* 2000;25:1126–1131.
52. Von Korff M, Jensen MP, Karoly P. Assessing global pain severity by self-report in clinical and health services research. *Spine* 2000;25: 3140–3151.
53. Jensen MP, McFarland CA. Increasing the reliability and validity of pain intensity measurement in chronic pain patients. *Pain* 1993;55: 195–203.
54. Dworkin SF, Von Korff M, Whitney CW, LeResche L, Dicker BG, Barlow W. Measurement of characteristic pain intensity in field pain research. *Pain* 1990;(suppl 5):S290.
55. Serlin RC, Mendoza TR, Nakamura Y, Edwards KR, Cleeland CS. When is cancer pain mild, moderate or severe? Grading pain severity by its interference with function. *Pain* 1995;61:277–284.
56. Jensen MP, Turner JA, Romano JM, Fisher LD. Comparative reliability and validity of chronic pain intensity measures. *Pain* 1999;83: 157–162.
57. Jensen MP, Smith DG, Ehde DM, Robinsin LR. Pain site and the effects of amputation pain: Further clarification of the meaning of mild, moderate, and severe pain. *Pain* 2001;91:317–322.
58. Scott J, Huskisson EC. Graphic representation of pain. *Pain* 1976;2: 175–184.
59. Huskisson EC. Measurement of pain. *Lancet* 1974;2:1127–1131.
60. Kremer E, Atkinson JH, Ignelzi RJ. Measurement of pain: Patient preference does not confound pain measurement. *Pain* 1981;10:241–248.
61. Jensen MP, Turner JA, Romano JM. What is the maximum number of levels needed in pain intensity measurement? *Pain* 1994;58: 387–392.
62. Melzack R. The McGill pain questionnaire: Major properties and scoring methods. *Pain* 1975;1:275–299.
63. Graham C, Bond SS, Gerkousch MM, Cook MR. Use of the McGill Pain Questionnaire in the assessment of cancer pain: Replicability and consistency. *Pain* 1980;8:377–387.
64. Keefe FJ, Wilkins RH, Cook WA, Crisson JE, Muhlbaier LH. Depression, pain, and pain behavior. *J Consult Clin Psychol* 1986;54: 665–669.
65. Melzack R. The McGill pain questionnaire. In: Melzack R, ed. *Pain Measurement and Assessment.* New York, NY: Raven Press; 1983:41–47.
66. Sternbach RA, Murphy RW, Timmermans G, Greenhoot JH, Akeson WH. Measuring the severity of clinical pain. In: Bonica JJ, ed. *Advances in Neurology.* vol 4. New York, NY: Raven Press; 1974:281–288.
67. Turk DC, Melzack R, eds. *Handbook of Pain Assessment.* New York, NY: Guilford Press; 1992.
68. Carr DB, Jacox AK, Chapman CR, et al. *Acute Pain Management: Operative or Medical Procedures and Trauma. Clinical Practice Guideline No. 1.* Rockville, Md: Agency for Health Care Policy and Research, Public Health Service, US Department of Health and Human Services; February 1992. AHCPR Pub. NO 92-0032.
69. Cleeland CS. Pain assessment in cancer. In: Osoba D, ed. Effect of Cancer on Quality of Life. Boca Raton, Fla: CRC Press; 1991:293–305.
70. Uki J, Mendoza TR, Gao SZ, Cleeland CS. The Chinese version of the Brief Pain Inventory (BPI-C): Its development and use in a study of cancer pain. *Pain* 1996;67:407–416.
71. Saxena A, Mendoza T, Cleeland CS. The assessment of cancer pain in north India: The validation of the Hindi Brief Pain Inventory—BPI-H. *J Pain Symptom Manage* 1999;17:27–41.
72. Caraceni A, Mendoza TR, Mencaglia E, et al. A validation study of an Italian version of the Brief Pain Inventory (Breve Questionario per la Valutazione del Dolore). *Pain* 1996;65:87–92.
73. Cleeland CS, Ryan KM. Pain assessment: Global use of the Brief Pain Inventory. *Ann Acad Med Singapore* 1994;23:129–138.
74. Cleeland CS, Syrjala KL. How to assess cancer pain. In: Turk D, Melzack R, eds. *Pain Assessment.* New York, NY: Guilford Press; 1992:360–387.
75. Burton HJ, Sline SA, Hargadon R, Cooper BS, Shick RD, Ong-Lam MC. Assessing patients with chronic pain using the basic personality inventory as a complement to the multidimensional pain inventory. *Pain Res Manage* 1999;4:131–129.
76. Jackson DN. *The Basic Personality Inventory: The BPI Manual.* Port Huron, MI, USA: Research Psychologists Press; 1989.
77. Epker J, Gatchel RJ. Prediction of treatment-seeking behavior in acute TMD patients: Practical application in clinical settings. *J Orofacial Pain* 2000;14:303–309.
78. Olsson I, Bunketorp O, Carlsson SG, Styf J. Prediction of outcome in whiplash-associated disorders using West Haven-Yale Multidimensional Pain Inventory. *Clin J Pain* 2002;18(4):238–244.
79. Turk DC, Rudy TE. The robustness of an empirically derived taxonomy of chronic pain patients. *Pain* 1990;43:27–35.
80. Wittink H, Turk DC, Carr DB, Sukiennik A, Rogers W. Assessing Chronic Pain Treatment Outcomes: Comparison of the SF-36, ODI, and MPI. *Clin J Pain* 2003 (in press).
81. Walter L, Brannon L. A cluster analysis of the Multidimensional Pain Inventory. *Headache* 1991;31:476–479.
82. Bergström G, Jensen IB, Bodin L, Linton SJ, Nygren AL, Carlsson SG. Reliability and factor structure of the Multidimensional Pain Inventory–Swedish language version (MPI-S). *Pain* 1998;75:101–110.
83. Nagi S. Disability concepts revisited: Implications for prevention. In: Pope AM, Tarlov A, eds. *Disability in America: Toward a National Agenda for Prevention.* Committee on a National Agenda for the Prevention of Disabilities, Division of Health Promotion and Disease Prevention, Institute of Medicine. Washington DC: National Academy Press; 1991:309–327.
84. Nadjar A. Personal communication. Lyon, France: MAPI Research Institute; 2002.
85. Nicassio PM, Schoenfeld-Smith K, Radojevic V, Schuman C. Pain coping mechanisms in fibromyalgia: Relationship to pain and functional outcomes. *J Rheumatol* 1995;22:1552–1558.
86. Turner JA, Jensen MP, Romano JM. Do beliefs, coping, and catastrophizing independently predict functioning in patients with chronic pain? *Pain* 2000;85:115–125.
87. Geisser ME, Robinson ME, Henson CD. The Coping Strategies Questionnaire and chronic pain adjustment: A conceptual and empirical reanalysis. *Clin J Pain* 1994;10:98–106.

88. Lethem J, Slade PD, Troup JDG, Bentley G. Outline of a fear-avoidance model of exaggerated pain perceptions. *Behav Res Ther* 1983; 21:401–408.
89. Geisser ME, Robinson ME, Keefe FJ, Weiner ML. Catastrophizing, depression and the sensory, affective and evaluative aspects of chronic pain. *Pain* 1994;59:79–83.
90. Keefe FJ, Lefebvre JC, Egert JR, Affleck G, Sullivan MJ, Caldwell DS. The relationship of gender to pain, pain behavior, and disability in osteoarthritis patients: The role of catastrophizing. *Pain* 2000;87: 325–334.
91. Keefe FJ, Brown GK, Wallston KA, Caldwell DS. Coping with rheumatoid arthritis pain: Catastrophizing as a maladaptive strategy. *Pain* 1989;37:51–56.
92. Buckelew SP, Parker JC, Keefe FJ, et al. Self-efficacy and pain behavior among subjects with fibromyalgia. *Pain* 1994;59:377–384.
93. Geisser ME, Roth RS, Theisen ME, Robinson TE, Riley TL. Negative affect, self-report of depressive symptoms, and clinical depression: Relation to the experience of chronic pain. *Clin J Pain* 2000; 16:110–120.
94. Engel CC, Von K, Katon WJ. Back pain in primary care: Predictors of high health-care costs. *Pain* 1996;65:197–204.
95. Jensen MP, Karoly P. Control beliefs, coping efforts, and adjustment to chronic pain. *J Consult Clin Psychol* 1991;59:431–438.
96. Jensen MP, Turner JA, Romano JM, Karoly P. Coping with chronic pain: A critical review of the literature. *Pain* 1991;47:249–283.
97. Klenerman L, Slade PD, Stanley IM, et al. The prediction of chronicity in patients with an acute attack of low back pain in a general practice setting. *Spine* 1995;20:478–484.
98. Hassett AL, Cone JD, Patella SJ, Sigal LH. The role of catastrophizing in the pain and depression of women with fibromyalgia syndrome. *Arthritis Rheum* 2000;43:2493–2500.
99. Keefe FJ, Kashikar-Zuck S, Robinson E, et al. Pain coping strategies that predict patients' and spouses' ratings of patients' self-efficacy. *Pain* 1997;73:191–199.
100. Martin MY, Bradley LA, Alexander RW, et al. Coping strategies predict disability in patients with primary fibromyalgia. *Pain* 1996;68: 45–53.
101. Rosenstiel AK, Keefe FJ. The use of coping strategies in chronic low back pain patients: Relationship to patient characteristics and current adjustment. *Pain* 1983;17:33–44.
102. Riley JL, Robinson ME. CSQ: Five factors or fiction? *Clin J Pain* 1997;13:156–162.
103. Robinson ME, Riley JL, Myers CD, et al. The Coping Strategies Questionnaire: A large sample, item level factor analysis. *Clin J Pain* 1997; 13:43–49.
104. Swartzman LC, Gwadry FG, Shapiro AP, Teasell RW. The factor structure of the Coping Strategies Questionnaire. *Pain* 1994;57:311–316.
105. Dozois DJA, Dobson KS, Wong M, Hughes D, Long A. Predictive utility of the CSQ in low back pain: Individual vs. composite measures. *Pain* 1996;66:171–180.
106. Lin CC. Comparison of the effects o perceived self-efficacy on coping with chronic cancer pain and coping with chronic low back pain. *Clin J Pain* 1998;14:303–310.
107. Williams DA, Thorn BE. An empirical assessment of pain beliefs. *Pain* 1989;36:351–358.
108. Williams AC, Richardson PH. What does the BDI measure on chronic pain? *Pain* 1993;55:259–266.
109. Herda CA, Siegeris K, Basler H-D. The Pain Beliefs and Perceptions Inventory: Further evidence for a 4-factor structure. *Pain* 1994;57:85–90.
110. Morley S, Wilkinson L. The pain beliefs and perceptions inventory: A British replication. *Pain* 1995;61:427–433.
111. Sullivan MJL, Bishop SR, Pivik J. The Pain Catastrophizing scale: Development and validation. *Psychol Assess* 1995;7:524–532.
112. Chaves JF, Brown JM. Spontaneous cognitive strategies for the control of clinical pain and stress. *J Behav Med* 1987;10:263–276.
113. Spanos NP, Perlini AH, Robertson LA. Hypnosis, suggestion, and placebo in the reduction of experimental pain. *J Abnorm Psychol* 1989;98:285–293.
114. Sullivan MJL. *The Pain Catastrophizing Scale Manual.* Halifax, Nova Scotia: Dalhousie University, Pain Research Centre; 2000.
115. Osman A, Barrios FX, Gutierrez PM, Kopper BA, Merrifield T, Grittmann L. The Pain Catastrophizing Scale: Further psychometric evaluation with adult samples. *J Behav Med* 2000;23:351–365.
116. Osman A, Barrios FX, Kopper BA, Hauptmann W, Jones J, O'Neill E. Factor structure, reliability, and validity of the Pain Catastrophizing Scale. *J Behav Med* 1997;20:589–605.
117. Patrick DL, Hurst BC, Hughes J. Further development and testing of the migraine-specific quality of life (MSQOL) measure. *Headache* 2000;40:550–560.
118. Beaton DE, Richards RR. Measuring function of the shoulder. A cross-sectional comparison of five questionnaires. *J Bone Joint Surg Am* 1996;78:882–890.
119. Roddey TS, Olson SL, Cook KF, Gartsman GM, Hanten W. Comparison of the University of California-Los Angeles Shoulder Scale and the Simple Shoulder Test with the shoulder pain and disability index: Single-administration reliability and validity. *Phys Ther* 2000; 80:759–768.
120. van der Heijden GJ, van der Windt DA, de Winter AF, Koes BW, Deville W, Bouter LM. The responsiveness of the Shoulder Disability Questionnaire. *Ann Rheum Dis* 1998;57:82–87.
121. Roos EM, Roos HP, Lohmander LS, Ekdahl C, Beynnon BD. Knee Injury and Osteoarthritis Outcome Score (KOOS)—development of a self-administered outcome measure. *J Orthop Sports Phys Ther* 1998;28:88–96.
122. Lysholm J, Gillquist J. Evaluation of knee ligament surgery results with special emphasis on use of a scoring scale. *Am J Sports Med* 1982;10:150–154.
123. Vernon H, Mior S. The Neck Disability Index: A study of reliability and validity. [erratum appears in J Manipulative Physiol Ther 1992; 15]. *J Manipulative Physiol Ther* 1991;14:409–415.
124. Fairbank J, Couper J, Davies J, O'Brien J. The Oswestry Low Back Pain Disability Questionnaire. *Physiotherapy* 1980;66:271–273.
125. Roland M, Morris R. A study of the natural history of back pain. Part I: Development of a reliable and sensitive measure of disability in low-back pain. *Spine* 1983;8:141–144.
126. Roland M, Fairbank J. The Roland-Morris Disability Questionnaire and the Oswestry Disability Questionnaire. *Spine* 2000;25:3115–3124.
127. Gronblad M, Hupli M, Wennerstrand P, et al. Intercorrelation and test-retest reliability of the Pain Disability Index (PDI) and the Oswestry Disability Questionnaire (ODQ) and their correlation with pain intensity in low back pain patients. *Clin J Pain* 1993;9:189–195.
128. Strong J, Ashton R, Large RG. Function and the patient with chronic low back pain. *Clin J Pain* 1994;10:191–196.
129. Kopec JA, Esdaile JM, Abrahamowitz ED, et al. The Quebec back pain disability scale: Conceptualization and development. *J Clin Epidemiol* 1996;49:151–161.
130. Jensen MP, Strom SE, Turner JA, Romano JM. Validity of the Sickness Impact Profile Roland scale as a measure of dysfunction in chronic pain patients. *Pain* 1992;50:157–162.
131. Beurskens AJ, de Vet HC, Koke AJ. Responsiveness of functional status in low back pain: A comparison of different instruments. *Pain* 1996;65:71–76.
132. Lerner D, Amick BC, Rogers WH, Malspeis S, Bungay K, Cynn D. The Work Limitations Questionnaire. *Med Care* 2001;39:72–85.
133. Jadad AR, McQuay HJ. Meta-analyses to evaluate analgesic interventions: A systematic qualitative review of their methodology. *J Clin Epidemiol* 1996;49:235–243.
134. Lau J, Antman EM, Jimenez-Silva J, Kupelnick B, Mosteller F, Chalmers TC. Cumulative meta-analysis of therapeutic trials for myocardial infarction. *New Engl J Med* 1992;327:248–254.

135. Flor H, Fydrich T, Turk DC. Efficacy of multidisciplinary pain treatment centers: A meta-analytic review. *Pain* 1992;49:221–230.
136. Fishbain DA, Rosomoff HL, Goldberg M, et al. The prediction of return to the workplace after multidisciplinary pain center treatment. *Clin J Pain* 1993;9:3–15.
137. Turk DC. Efficacy of multidisciplinary pain centers in the treatment of chronic pain. In: Cohen MJM, Campbell JN, eds. *Pain Treatment Centers at a Crossroads: A Practical and Conceptual Reappraisal.* vol 7. Seattle, Wash: IASP Press; 1996:257–272.
138. Fishbain DA, Cutler RB, Rosomoff HL, Rosomoff RS. Status of chronic pain treatment outcomes research. In: Aronoff GM, ed. *Evaluation and Treatment of Chronic Pain.* 3rd ed. Baltimore, Md: Williams & Wilkins; 1999:655–670.
139. Lau J, Ioannides JPA, Schmid CH. Summing up evidence: One answer is not always enough. *Lancet* 1998;351:123–127.

BIBLIOGRAPHY

Fischer D, Stewart AL, Bloch DA, Lorig K, Laurent D, Holman H. Capturing the patient's view of change as a clinical outcome measure. *JAMA* 1999;282:1157–1162.

Galer BS, Jensen MP. Development and preliminary validation of a pain measure specific to neuropathic pain: The Neuropathic Pain Scale. *Neurology* 1997;48:332–338.

Gill TM, Feinstein AR. A critical appraisal of the quality of quality-of-life measurements. *JAMA* 1994;272:619–626.

Hunt SM, McKenna SP, McEwen J, Backett EM, Williams J, Papp E. A quantitative approach to perceived health status: A validation study. *J Epidemiol Community Health* 1980;34:281–286.

Meenan RF, Mason J, Anderson JJ, Guccione AA, Kazis L. The content and properties of a revised and expanded Arthritis Impact Measurement Scales Health Status Questionnaire. *Arthritis Rheum* 1992;35:1–10.

Stewart AL, Greenfield S, Hays RD, et al. Functional status and well-being of patients with chronic conditions. Results from the Medical Outcomes Study [published erratum appears in *JAMA* 1989;262:2542]. *JAMA* 1989;262:907–913.

Turk DC, Rudy TE. Toward an empirically derived taxonomy of chronic pain patients: Integration of psychological assessment data. *J Consult Clin Psychol* 1988;56:233–238.

World Health Organization. *International Classification of Impairments, Disabilities and Handicaps (ICIDH).* Geneva, Switzerland: WHO; 1980.

CHAPTER 8 RADIOLOGIC EVALUATION OF SPINAL DISEASE

Jonathan Kleefield

TECHNICAL CONSIDERATIONS

As the millennium has just passed, it is appropriate to review the significant advances in spinal imaging that have occurred in the preceding quarter century. Before then, plain film radiography, conventional tomography, and myelography with either gas or oily material as contrast agents had been the only methods available for imaging abnormalities involving the vertebrae, intervertebral disks, spinal cord, or cauda equina.

By 1975, a nonionic intrathecal contrast agent, metrizamide, was approved for clinical use. Unlike oily agents, nonionic contrast carried negligible risk for arachnoiditis, was absorbable, and thus eliminated the need for its removal from the thecal sac. Secondly, its neurotoxicity was minimal, compared with ionic water-soluble media, which never achieved widespread acceptance in the United States.

In 1977, the introduction of whole-body computed tomography (CT) permitted direct cross-sectional imaging of both spinal and paraspinal structures. However, the margins of the spinal cord could only be reliably demonstrated after the intrathecal administration of water-soluble contrast. This procedure is known as CT myelography (CTM). Because of the greater contrast sensitivity of CT, as compared with plain film myelographic technique, a smaller, less potentially neurotoxic dose of contrast agent could be administered for CTM. Nevertheless, this procedure still requires a lumbar puncture, with its attendant hazards to the patient.

By 1982, magnetic resonance imaging (MRI) became clinically feasible. MRI has proven to be superior to CT because the spinal cord and nerve roots could be visualized directly without the requirement for intrathecal contrast material. Most significantly, the parenchyma of the spinal cord could now be imaged and assessed for intrinsic pathology, such as multiple sclerosis plaques. These lesions may not alter the shape of the spinal cord, and, therefore, would be undetectable by CTM. Secondly, MRI provides multiplanar imaging, including sagittal and coronal orientations, with spatial and contrast resolution equivalent to the axial plane. Lastly, MRI poses no known health risk as it uses only radiofrequency energy, not ionizing radiation as is the case with CT.

Sagittal plane MRI is ideal for extended, rapid evaluation of the entire vertebral column, a procedure facilitated because the spine is arranged in a sagittal plane. Recent improvements in MRI receiver coil design (phased array coil) have provided the capacity to image the entire spine with excellent detail in less than 10 minutes (Fig. 8-1). This is especially helpful in the evaluation for spinal metastases, as these patients are often in pain, and thus have difficulty in remaining motionless for MRI. Newer pulse sequences, including half-Fourier turbo-spin echo (HASTE), can provide interpretable scans in less than 10 seconds, albeit with reduced spatial resolution compared with conventional magnetic resonance studies. HASTE imaging can also suppress some metal-induced artifacts arising from surgical hardware (Fig. 8-2), allowing improved visibility of anatomy or pathology otherwise obscured by these artifacts.

Although CT is capable of producing sagittal plane spinal scans, these can only be obtained by reformatting the data from prior axial plane scans, as positioning the patient for direct sagittal spine scanning within the gantry aperture is not physically feasible. Moreover, the number and thickness of the axial scans limits the longitudinal coverage and spatial resolution of the reformatted sagittal CT images (Fig. 8-3). Such restrictions do not apply to sagittal plane MRI, which acquires data in any selected plane with equivalent, selectable spatial and contrast resolution. Moreover, MRI can image pathology not apparent on CT. Intrinsic spinal cord disease, including syringomyelia or multiple sclerosis plaques, is uniquely observable by MRI. MRI is performed by subjecting the patient to a sequence of radiofrequency (RF) pulses while he or she is positioned within a strong, fixed magnetic field. By the use of various combinations of these RF pulses, known as pulse sequences, images can be created that are, in effect, a map of the differing energy-releasing characteristics of tissues, known as the T1 and T2 relaxation constants, within a selected plane of anatomy. In general, scans emphasizing T1 characteristics (i.e. T1 "weighted") clearly define the outline of an anatomic structure, such as the spinal cord, whereas so-called T2-weighted images are more sensitive in distinguishing a region of pathology, including edema surrounding a tumor, gliosis, demyelination, or hemorrhage.

In the past few years, helical (spiral) CT scanners have been introduced into clinical practice. This machine, as compared with a conventional CT scanner, employs continuous x-ray tube rotation while the patient is moved by the motor-driven scanning table through the aperture in the scanner gantry. This volumetric data acquisition scheme is more flexible than so-called single slice scanning, because it allows multiplanar reconstructions of adjustable *spatial* resolution. However, *contrast* resolution, which is most important for delineating the thecal sac and other neurologic structures is, if anything, inferior to conventional single slice scanning. Therefore, helical spinal CT is most helpful in imaging intrinsically high-contrast bony structures and their related pathologic processes (e.g., fractures or degenerative arthritic osteophytic spurs). Helical CT scanning should not be viewed as a substitute for MRI. Nevertheless, if plain films are inconclusive, patients suspected of having acute spinal fractures are examined by helical CT, as opposed to MRI, because CT provides optimum bone detail and permits very rapid scanning of these patients. An even faster CT scanner has now been introduced, using multiple x-ray beams and detectors that create simultaneous, staggered helical scans. Such a device is capable of scanning the entire spine in about 20 seconds, albeit with the limited spatial and contrast resolution issues noted previously.

At present, nearly all patients with back pain requiring diagnostic imaging are most efficaciously studied by MRI. MRI should be obtained when patients either have failed a period of conserva-

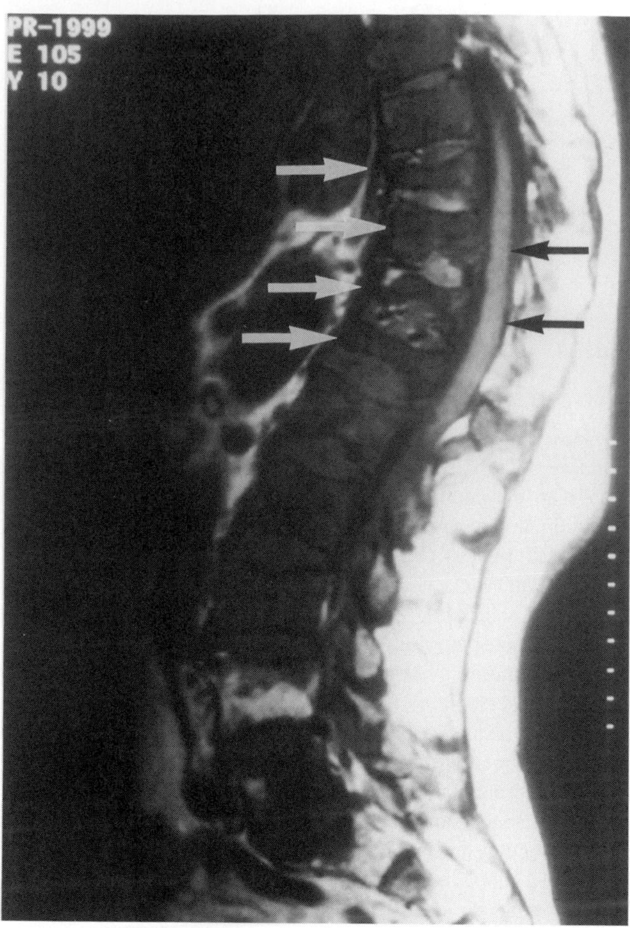

Figure 8-1 Midline sagittal T1-weighted image of the spine. This single image encompasses the spine from T6 to the sacrum. Scanning time was 3 minutes, because of implementation of phased array coil. Patient has a number of pathologic compression fractures (*white arrows*) from metastatic breast cancer. Spinal cord is clearly imaged (*black arrows*). Total examination of the spine can now be rapidly accomplished using magnetic resonance imaging, eliminating the need for invasive myelography.

tive treatment for back pain, or are suspected of having an illness needing urgent treatment (these would include spinal cord compression from a tumor or an infection such as osteomyelitis, diskitis, or epidural abscess). If an acute fracture is clinically suspected, plain films are first obtained. If they are not diagnostic, helical CT with sagittal and coronal reformatted images is used to provide maximum bony detail. However, intrinsic spinal cord injury, including a contusion or hemorrhage, is best depicted by MRI. From this discussion, it should be apparent that it is my opinion that plain film spinal radiography is overused as a screening tool, especially in light of its considerable insensitivity in delineating neoplasms and infections. Other than as an imaging "triage" for acute spinal trauma, plain film examination of the spine should be curtailed, using logic analogous to the abandonment of skull radiographs for evaluation of most neurologic disease. These imaging recommendations have been formulated into an algorithm.

Supplementary CT may be helpful when MRI is equivocal. This situation can occur particularly in the postsurgical spine, where metallic internal fixation devices may severely degrade or even preclude MRI, despite the use of the aforementioned HASTE sequences. With CT, usable images may still be obtainable, obviating myelography or CTM. Additionally, CT can more reliably detect calcific or ossific lesions than MRI. For example, cases of ossification of the posterior longitudinal ligament can be difficult to visualize on MRI, but are clearly depicted by CT (Fig. 8-4). MRI, however, shows the relationship of the spinal cord to the ligamentous ossification more clearly than CT. As such, I view CT and MRI as being complementary techniques.

In my experience, it is now rarely necessary to perform CTM. CTM is reserved for those patients who are unable to undergo MRI (Table 8-1) or in whom MRI and plain CT are nondiagnostic. In the unoperated patient, conventional myelography or CTM is rarely a primary diagnostic imaging study at the medical center where I practice. Only severely scoliotic patients may be requested to undergo myelography for orthopedic surgical planning, but this requirement is by no means universally applied at this institution. Myelography or CTM carries the risks of a potentially fatal anaphylactic contrast reaction, introduction of septic material into the subarachnoid space, as well as disabling post-lumbar puncture headache. It is my contention that MRI, as compared with myelography or CTM, offers superior imaging of both extra- and intradural structures with no known patient morbidity. Both MRI and CT *directly* visualize the extradural space, which harbors the most frequent pathologic processes: disk disease and facet joint arthropathy. Myelography, which fills the intradural compartment (thecal sac) with contrast, at best provides indirect evidence of extradural pathology by virtue of indentations on the sac or nerve root sleeves. Lesions in the extradural space that do not adjoin the thecal sac or the nerve root sleeves will be undetectable by myelography. No such limitation applies to MRI or CT. MRI pulse sequences have been developed that permit the rapid acquisition of heavily T2-weighted images with high spatial resolution. These are called fast spin echo or turbo spin –echo. With strong T2 weighting, the cerebrospinal fluid appears bright, and essentially identical in appearance to intrathecal contrast used in CTM (Fig. 8-5). Thus, the CTM image equivalent is achieved *noninvasively* by MRI, which, in my opinion, usually renders CTM superfluous.

As noted previously, T2 signal abnormalities in the spinal cord can represent several pathologic processes, including gliosis, edema, or tumor. The differentiation between these entities has been refined through the use of the MRI contrast agent, gadolinium diethylenetriamine pentaacetic acid (DTPA). Gadolinium, a rare earth metal, is a paramagnetic element, causing shortening of the T1 relaxation time of tissues that accumulate it. T1 shortening translates into brightening on a magnetic resonance image that is T1 weighted. Moreover, in humans, the transport kinetics of gadolinium are identical to those of iodinated radiographic contrast agents.

This means that both gadolinium and iodinated contrast material cause enhancement primarily through accumulation of either substance in the extravascular soft tissues. For delivery of gadolinium, the metal is chelated to a carrier molecule, DTPA, and this pharmaceutical is injected intravenously. Formerly, dosage recommendations were 0.1 mmol/ kg body weight. Presently, most patients are satisfactorily imaged with a 10-mL dose. Gadolinium carries almost no patient risks, with only extremely rare instances of anaphylaxis, far fewer than with iodinated contrast used for CT. Even patients with hepatic and renal compromise can tolerate gadolinium DTPA more readily than iodinated contrast. Nevertheless, it is prudent to administer gadolinium with discretion, particularly in these debilitated patients. Gadolinium will cause enhancement of most spinal tumors, as well as postoperative granulation tissue and many inflammatory processes.

A

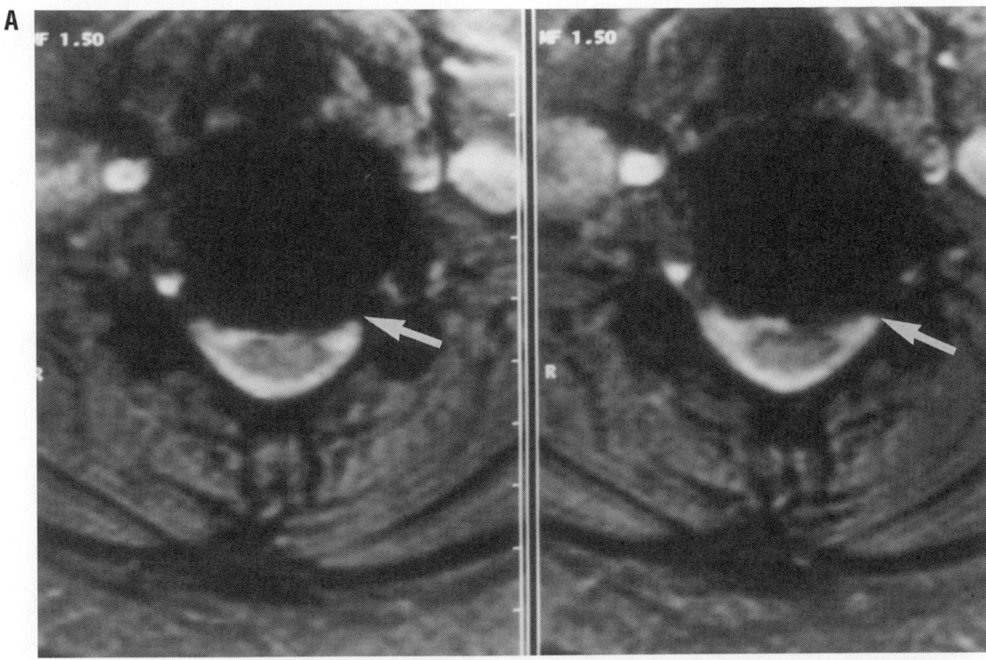

B

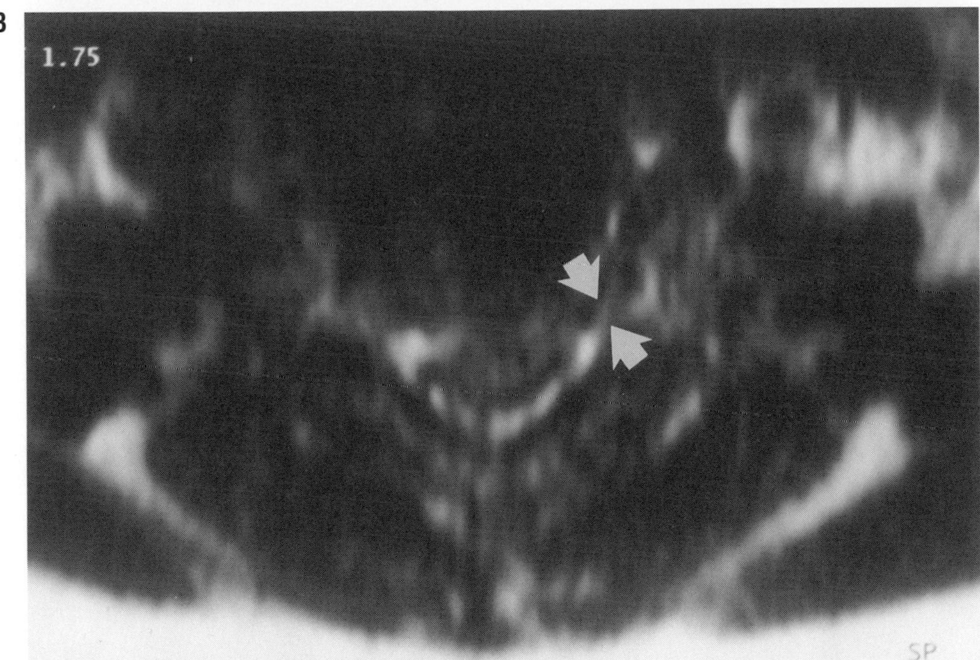

Figure 8-2 **(A)** Axial gradient echo magnetic resonance (MR) image of cervical spine. Left neural foramen (*arrows*) obscured by dark scan artifact arising from metallic internal fixation device (plates and screws). **(B)** Axial half-Fourier turbo spin echo (HASTE) MR image, obtained in 18 seconds, suppresses the artifact. Image is blurred, but of sufficient resolution to show that the left neural foramen (*arrows*) is not stenotic.

Low back pain is often a nonspecific symptom that may relate to paraspinal pathology involving retroperitoneal structures, including tumors. Therefore, when imaging the spine with either CT or MRI, it is recommended that at least some coverage of the paraspinal region be provided, particularly in the axial sections. Pathology such as aortic aneurysms, infections, and retroperitoneal tumors can be demonstrated via either technique.[1] Secondly, it is extremely important that the radiologist be provided with pertinent clinical history, particularly with regard to any localization, especially lateralization of pain, weakness, or other neurologic symptomatology. The imaging facility with which I am affiliated has patients note their perception of pain on an anatomic diagram (Fig. 8-6), as well as answer a series of questions concerning their symptoms. This is a procedure that I have found very useful on a number of occasions, as it is well known that many imaging abnormalities may have no correlative clinical significance.

In recent years, there has been a proliferation of so-called open magnet imaging devices. These machines have great marketing appeal, and they are often billed as being "patient friendly" and capable of accommodating even those who are claustrophobic or morbidly obese. These claims are not unwarranted. However, it should be recognized that even recently designed open systems cannot deliver image quality commensurate with that of high-field systems. This is readily explained when it is understood that the open system magnet field strengths range from one fifth to one tenth those of a high-field imager. The lower field strength means that the re-

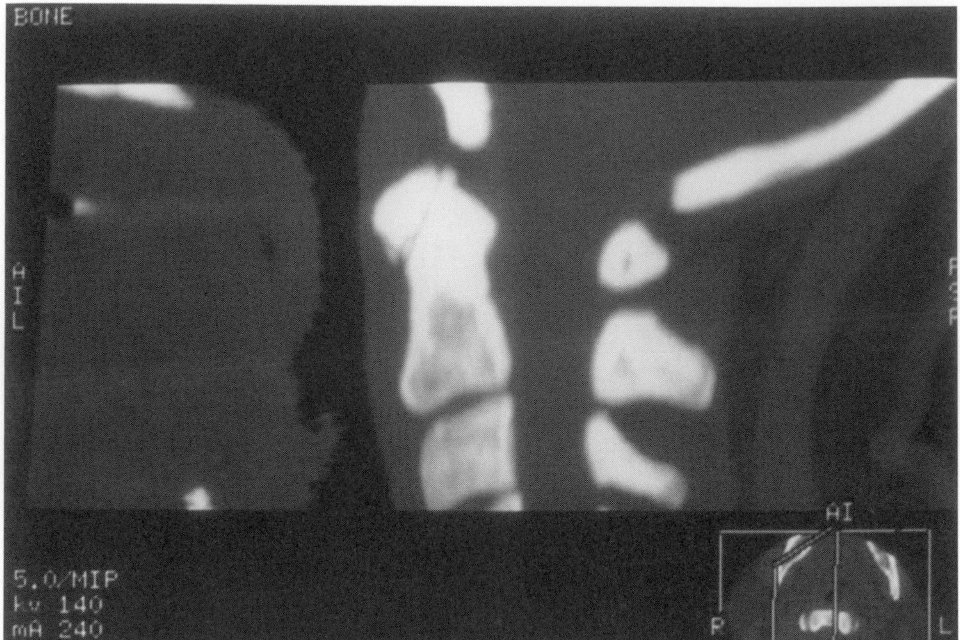

Figure 8-3 Midline sagittal reconstructed cervical spine image obtained by helical CT scanning with 1-mm-thick sections. Spatial resolution (image sharpness) is excellent, but longitudinal coverage is limited to C1 through C3 vertebral segments. Greater longitudinal coverage can be achieved at the expense of diminished spatial resolution. Newer, multidetector scanners, noted in text, can extend longitudinal coverage without sacrificing spatial resolution.

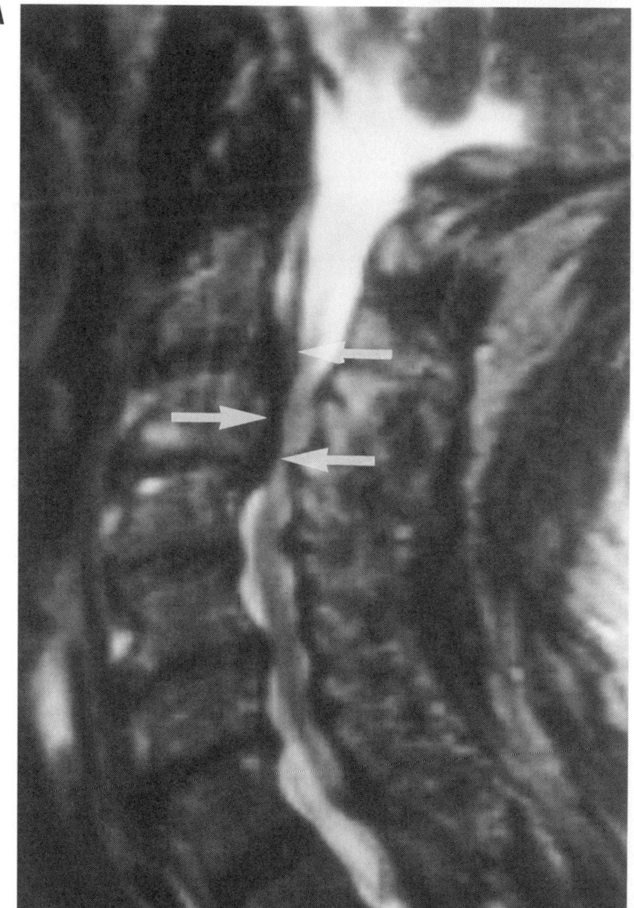

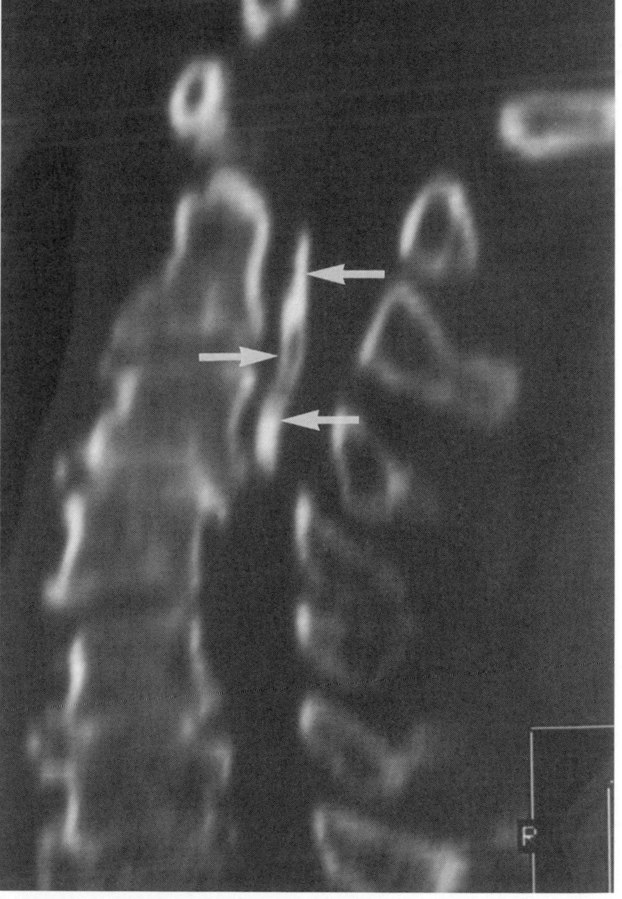

Figure 8-4 **(A)** Ossification of the posterior longitudinal ligament. Parasagittal T2-weighted image shows the abnormality (a linear dark area) to some extent (*arrows*) but distinction from the adjacent vertebral bodies is limited. **(B)** Same case as in A, with sagittal reconstructed computed tomography (CT) scan. Clear definition and more comprehensive imaging of the ossified ligament is now obtained (*arrows*) due to superior bone resolution using CT. Ossification of the posterior longitudinal ligament can cause myelopathic symptoms, which were present in this patient's neurologic examination.

TABLE 8-1 **Contraindications to Magnetic Resonance Imaging**

Ferromagnetic aneurysm clip
Cardiac pacemaker
Metallic foreign body in the globes
Starr Edwards cardiac valve
Certain stapes and cochlear prostheses
Recent (<24 hours) coronary bypass surgery

sultant images will be derived from proportionately weaker radio signals coming from the patient. Although novel pulse sequences such as constructive interference in the steady state (CISS) can help to alleviate this problem, as is usually the case in MRI, this comes at a price: reduced T2 sensitivity (Fig. 8-7). However, low-field scanners can produce excellent cervical spine scans, as this region of the body is relatively diminutive. The small diameter of most necks permits the receiving coil to be close to the region of interest (cervical spine), maximizing the ability to detect signals arising from the spinal tissues. Additionally, low-field units are less susceptible to artifacts arising from vascular pulsation or respiration, both of which can degrade neck images. Nevertheless, in general, low-field scanners require more time to scan the patients, again a function of their operating with weaker magnets. Longer scan times may not be tolerated by a patient as a result of pain, with resultant artifacts secondary to patient motion. Low-field imagers really cannot compete with their high-field brethren in the production of thin section scans, where signals are at a premium. Therefore, it is my opinion that "all imagers are not created equal." Whenever possible, I prefer to scan patients with high-field machines to guarantee optimal image quality. Newer high-field units have a so-called short (magnet) bore, with flared ends of the scanning aperture, soft lighting, and abundant ventilation. Such amenities significantly diminish the patient's perception of confinement. Where necessary, the nursing staff can provide either oral or intravenous conscious sedation, which usually makes it possible to scan even the most anxious individual.

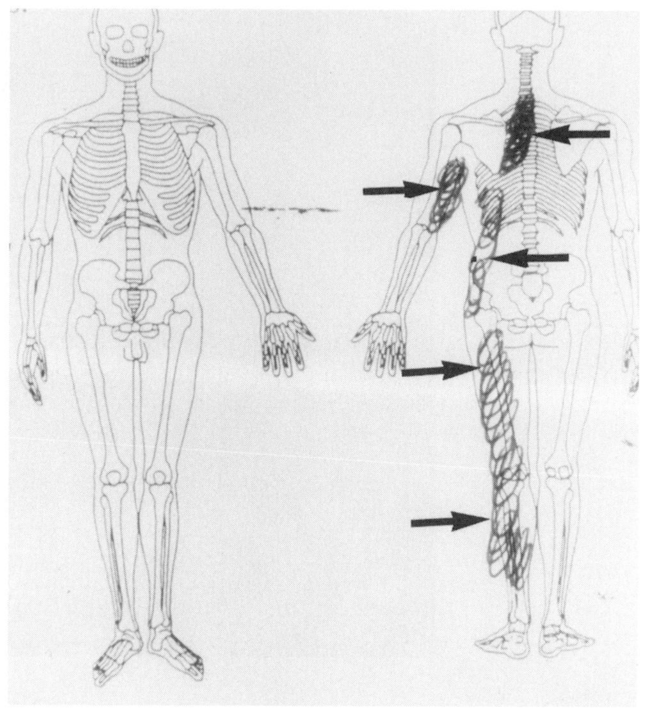

Figure 8-6 Anatomic diagram noted on a magnetic resonance imaging intake sheet. Patient notes areas of pain or paresthetic sensations (*arrows*), ensuring radiologist has pertinent lateralizing signs, if present. Such information supplements that derived from requisition. Additional questions on this intake sheet provide pertinent past medical history, such as prior spinal surgery.

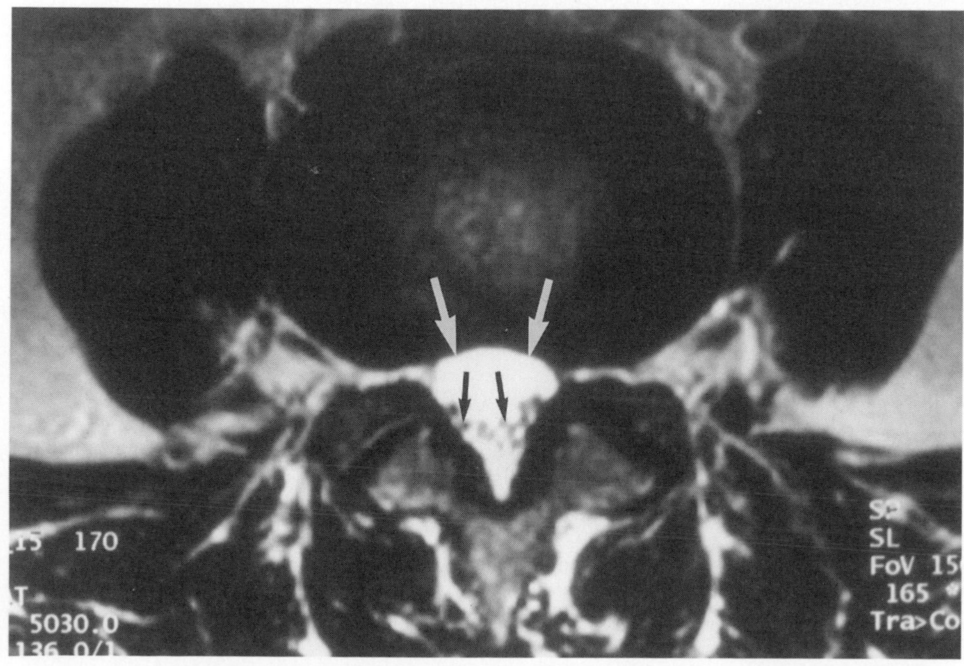

Figure 8-5 Axial T2-weighted fast spin echo image of the lumbar spine. Note excellent delineation of bright spinal fluid within thecal sac. Each rootlet of the cauda equina (*small black arrows*) is clearly distinguishable. Also noted is excellent contrast between normal, dark, kidney-shaped posterior disk margin (*white arrows*) and spinal fluid. CT myelography is now superfluous.

A

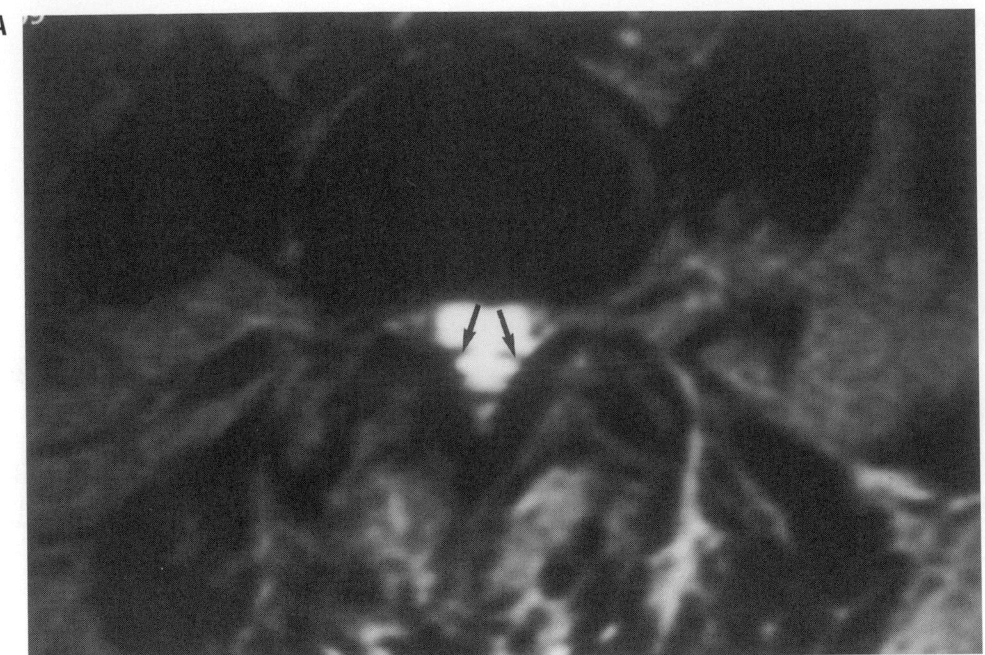

B

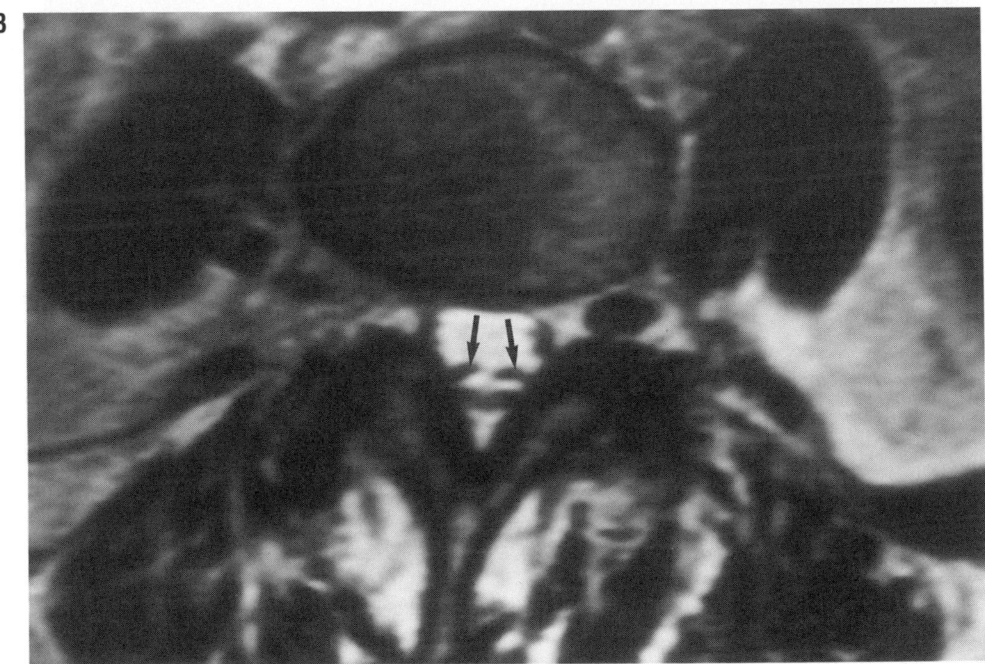

Figure 8-7 **(A)** Conventional axial T2-weighted fast spin echo image of the lumbar spine obtained on low-field "open" magnet. Image noise blurs the cauda equina (*arrows*). **(B)** Axial constructive interference in the steady state (CISS) image at same level as in A. Note improved clarity of the cauda equina (*arrows*). This image was obtained on the same open system as part A. Unfortunately, CISS images take considerable scanning time to acquire.

DISK DISEASE

The most common causes of neck and back pain that can be imaged are intervertebral disk disease and facet joint degeneration. Disk disorders are more prevalent in adulthood, whereas facet degeneration is more frequent in the elderly. However, the two disease processes are often concurrent. Although MRI depicts disk pathology with great sensitivity, recent publications have noted the detection of disk abnormalities in asymptomatic individuals.[2,3] Therefore, any *radiologic* finding of disk disease must be viewed in the context of *clinical* symptomatology before it should be deemed significant. Furthermore, some types of disk pathology occur more frequently in the asymptomatic patient. For example, Jensen and colleagues[3] observed that a bulging disk, defined as a

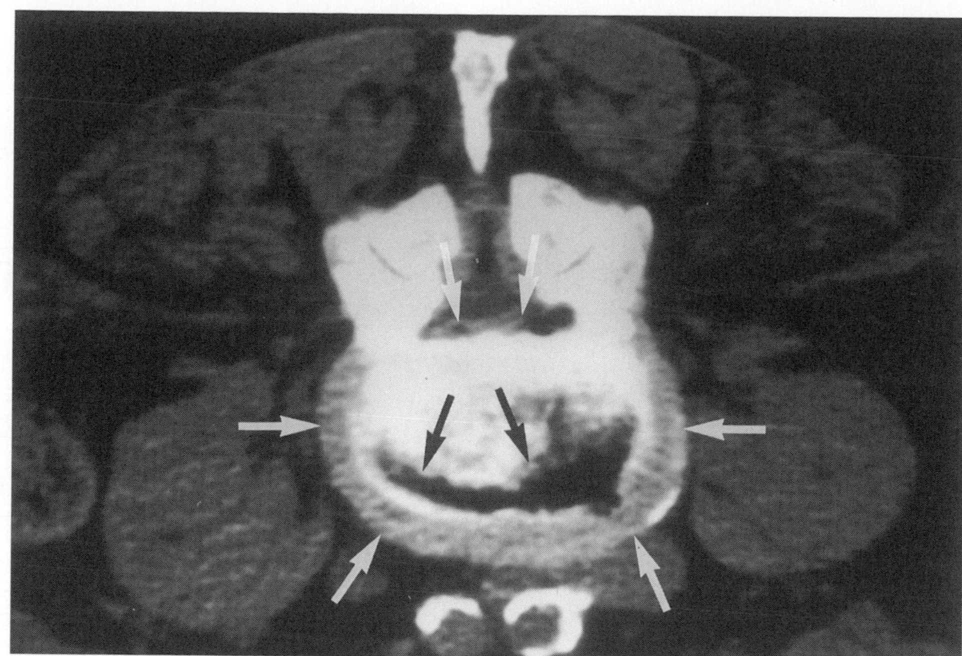

Figure 8-8 Axial computed tomography scan of bulging disk. Note disk margins extend beyond the vertebral body (*white arrows*) in a uniform, circumferential fashion. Dark areas in disk (*black arrows*) indicate vacuum degeneration of the disk material. This can be seen on a plain lumbar spine film, as well.

concentric, uniform expansion of disk material (Fig. 8-8), was more frequently asymptomatic than what was termed an extruded disk. (These authors grouped herniated disks in the category of extruded disk. This apparent terminologic variation underscores the need for a more standardized nomenclature of disk abnormalities, to predictably assign clinical significance.) A protruding disk is a focal deformity of the outer disk margin, with a broad base relative to the anteroposterior (AP) extent of the lesion (Fig. 8-9). This may also be associated a tear of the outer disk material, the anulus, and thus is referred to as an anular tear (Fig. 8-10). The pathology of an anular tear is analogous to a tear of a meniscal cartilage. It usually presents as an area of increased T2 signal in the anulus, highlighted from the dense collagen of the normal anulus, which is dark on T2-weighted scans. A herniated disk is a focal distortion of disk margin, in which the AP extent of the deformity approaches or exceeds its width (Fig. 8-11). Extruded disks, as defined here, remain connected to the "parent" disk while progressing cephalad, caudad, or bidirectionally relative to the plane of the disk space (Fig. 8-12). Finally, a free disk fragment is separable from the parent disk (Fig. 8-13).

In the cervical spine, midline posterior disk protrusions or herniations are clearly defined by sagittal MRI scan series (Fig. 8-14)

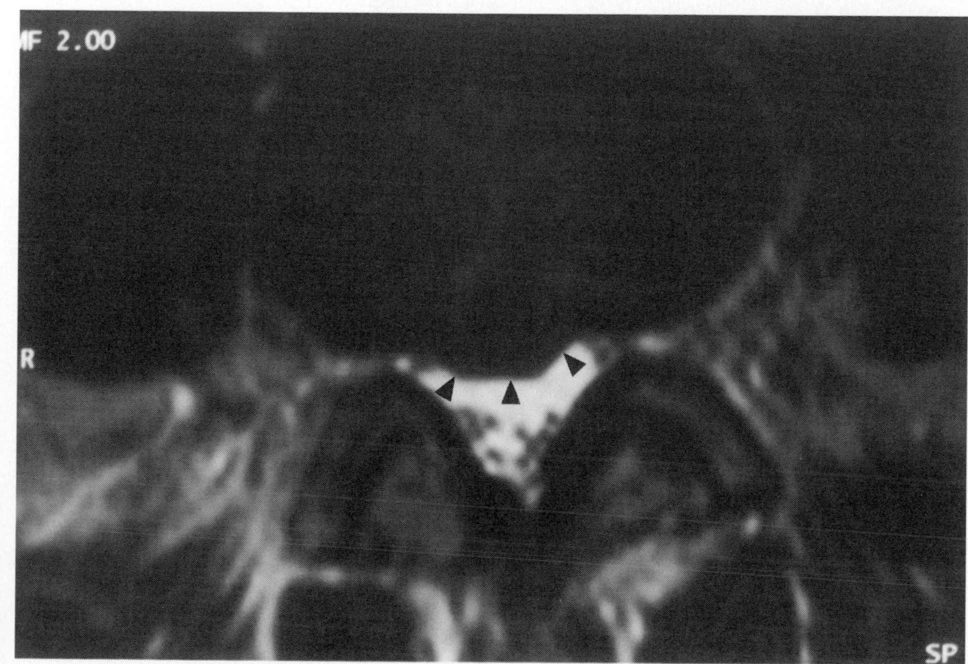

Figure 8-9 Axial T2-weighted fast spin echo magnetic resonance image of protruding lumbar disk. Note disk protrusion (*arrowheads*) seen as a focal deformity, whose base of attachment to the "parent" disk is wider than its anteroposterior diameter.

A

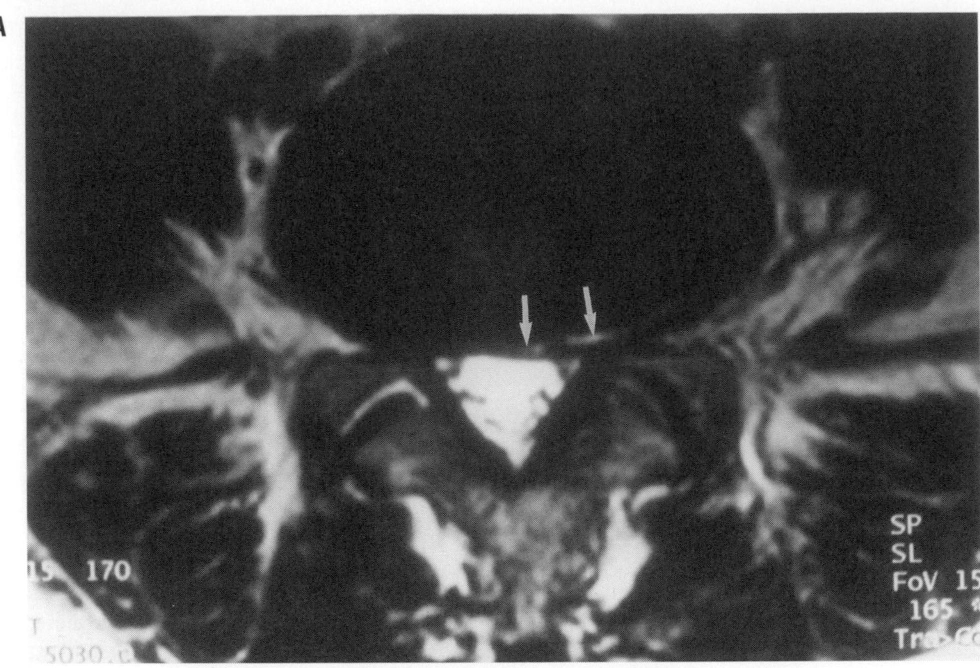

B

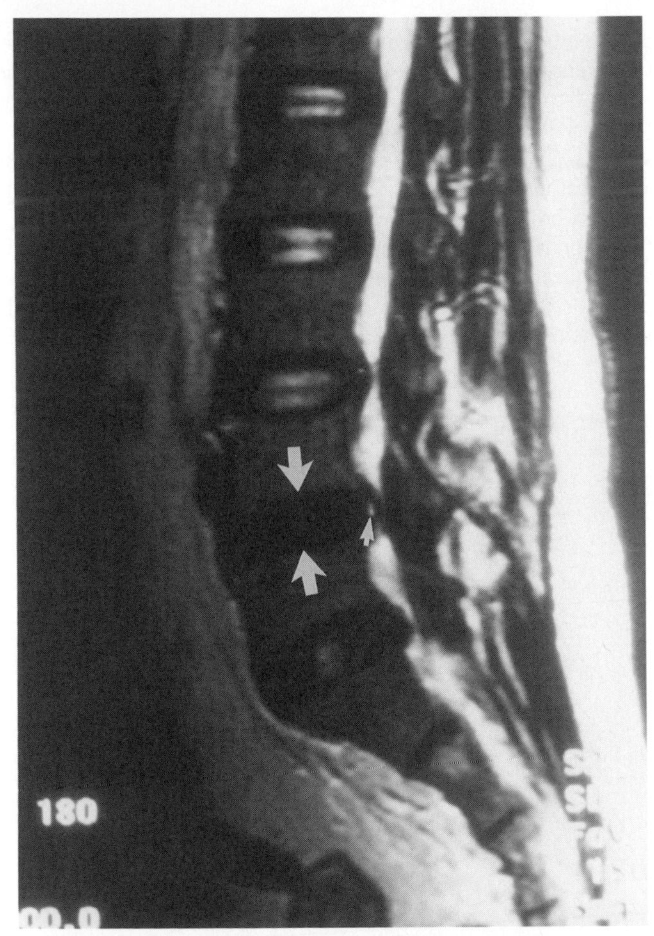

Figure 8-10 **(A)** Axial T2-weighted fast spin echo magnetic resonance (MR) image of an anular tear. This tear (*arrows*) has curvilinear shape, brighter than the adjacent disk material, along the periphery (anulus) of the disk. More commonly, anular tears are radially oriented. **(B)** Sagittal T2-weighted fast spin echo MR image of anular tear (same patient as in A). Note punctate area (*small arrow*) of hyperintensity, representing a cross-sectional view of the anular tear. The remainder of the disk (*large arrows*) is dark, representing disk desiccation. This is an early form of disk degeneration, presumably resulting from loss of water-binding capacity of chondroitin sulfate, found within the disk itself.

A

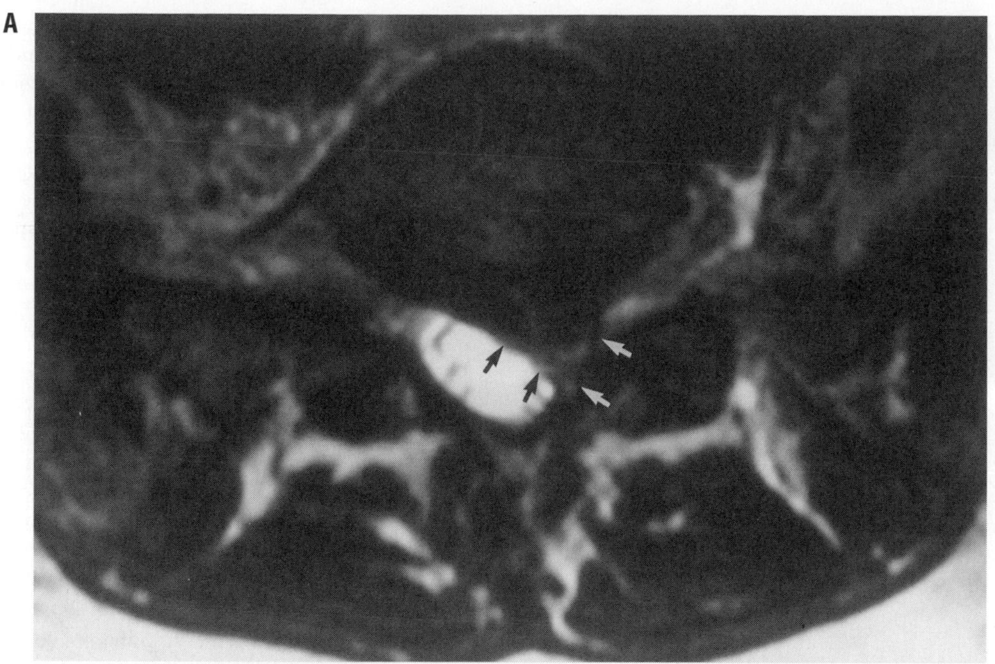

B

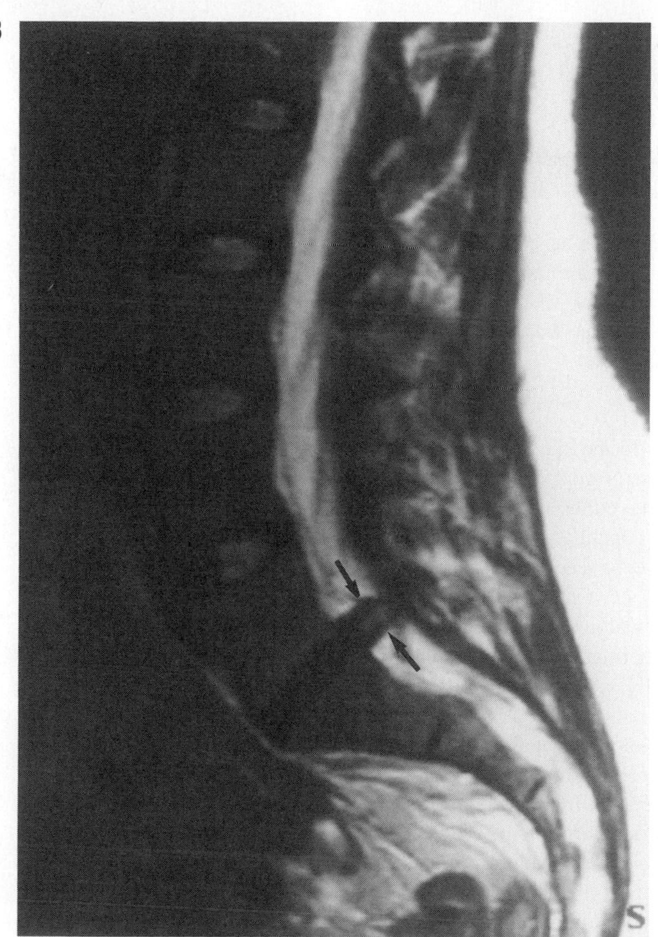

Figure 8-11 **(A)** Axial T2-weighted fast spin echo magnetic resonance (MR) image of a large herniated disk. Note the anvil shape of the left-sided disk herniation (*black and white arrows*) obliterating the left root sleeve and causing considerable deformity of the left ventrolateral aspect of the thecal sac. **(B)** Sagittal T2-weighted fast spin echo MR image (same patient as in A). Disk herniation (*arrows*) extends far posterior to the "parent" disk but remains attached to it.

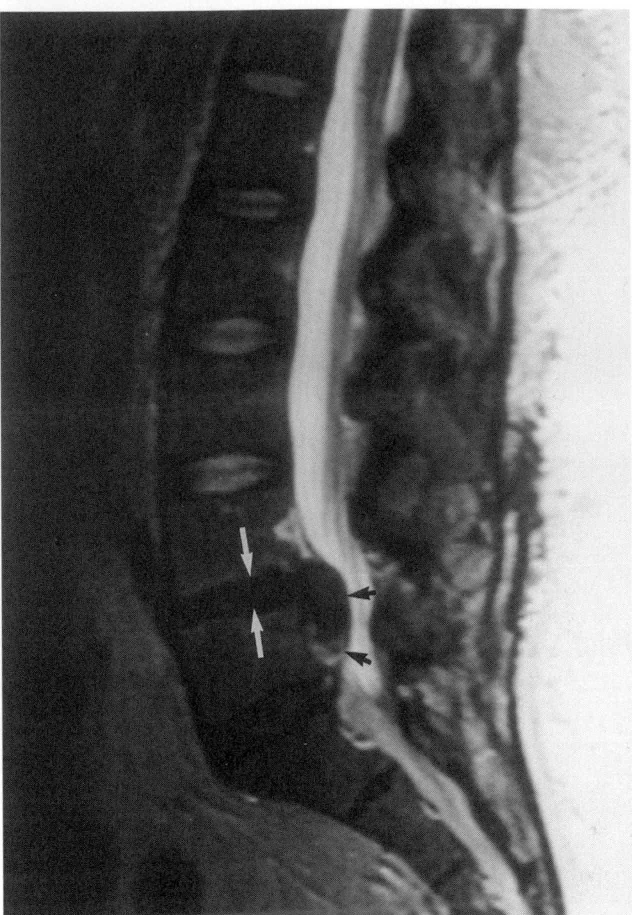

Figure 8-12 Sagittal T2-weighted fast spin echo magnetic resonance image of a caudally extruded L4-5 disk (*small black arrows*). Extruded disk extends caudal to the plane of the "parent" L4-5 disk, which is narrowed and desiccated (*white arrows*). However, the extrusion remains attached to the parent disk.

as the section plane is perpendicular to the site of the pathology. T2-weighted images can show increased signal intensity within the compressed spinal cord, representing either edema or gliosis.[4] (High T2 signal could also occur in a concurrent abnormality, such as a spinal cord tumor. Gadolinium-enhanced MRI scanning has improved the detectability of spinal cord neoplasms. Typically, these lesions enhance whereas the edematous component does not.) A laterally situated cervical disk herniation, typically causing radiculopathic symptoms, is optimally visualized by MRI in the axial plane (Fig. 8-15). The parasagittal images are not as revealing in this location because of the oblique orientation of the cervical neural foramina. However, a lateral, intraforaminal lumbar disk herniation can also be clearly seen with either axial or sagittal MRI, owing to the parasagittal orientation of the plane of the lumbar neural foramina. As previously noted, a portion of disk can separate from the parent disk, producing a free fragment.[5] Virtually all free fragments remain extradural in location. Rare cases of fragments perforating the posterior longitudinal ligament and dura and, thus, lodging intradurally have been reported,[6] but almost always diagnosed retrospectively at surgery (Fig. 8-16). The conus medullaris is well delineated on routine sagittal scans, permitting exclusion of a tumor at that site. On occasion, a conus medullaris tumor can symptomatically mimic a disk herniation.

Although MRI provides superlative depiction of disk disease, axial CT is often just as effective, particularly when there are associated osteophytic spurs. As previously noted, CT provides excellent delineation of bone. Clinical localization is helpful in directing the CT examination to the appropriate levels of the spine because it is impractical to scan the entire spine axially by CT. "Surveys" of this sort are best handled by MRI. However, the more directed an examination of any type can be, the more likely it is to provide useful clinical information.

Thoracic disk pathology was formerly thought to be much less prevalent than those involving lumbar disks. However, the incidence was underestimated because of low imaging sensitivity of plain films and myelography, particularly in the thoracic spine owing to the typical hyphotic curvature, which limited pooling of myelographic contrast agent along the posterior disk margins. The ease of comprehensive thoracic spine imaging by MRI and its abundant use has altered our perception of thoracic disk disease (Fig. 8-17). Thoracic disks have a higher frequency of dystrophic calcification than disks in other regions of the spine. As a result, CT may be able to delineate the disk abnormality, as this modality is quite sensitive to calcification.

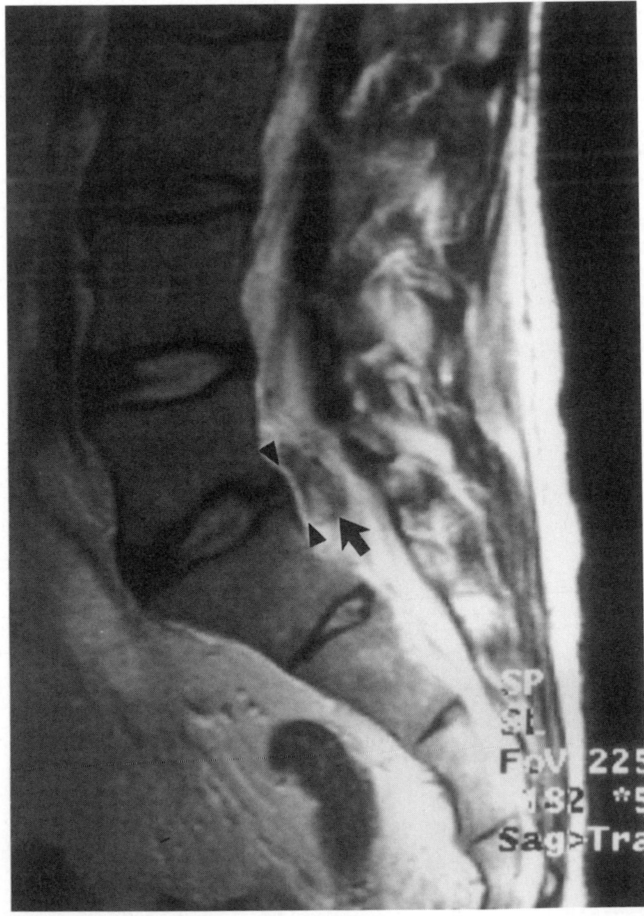

Figure 8-13 Sagittal T2-weighted fast spin echo magnetic resonance image of a free disk fragment (*arrow*). Note clear separation of the free disk fragment (*arrowheads*) from the "parent" disk. Both extruded disks and free fragments are typically subligamentous in location.

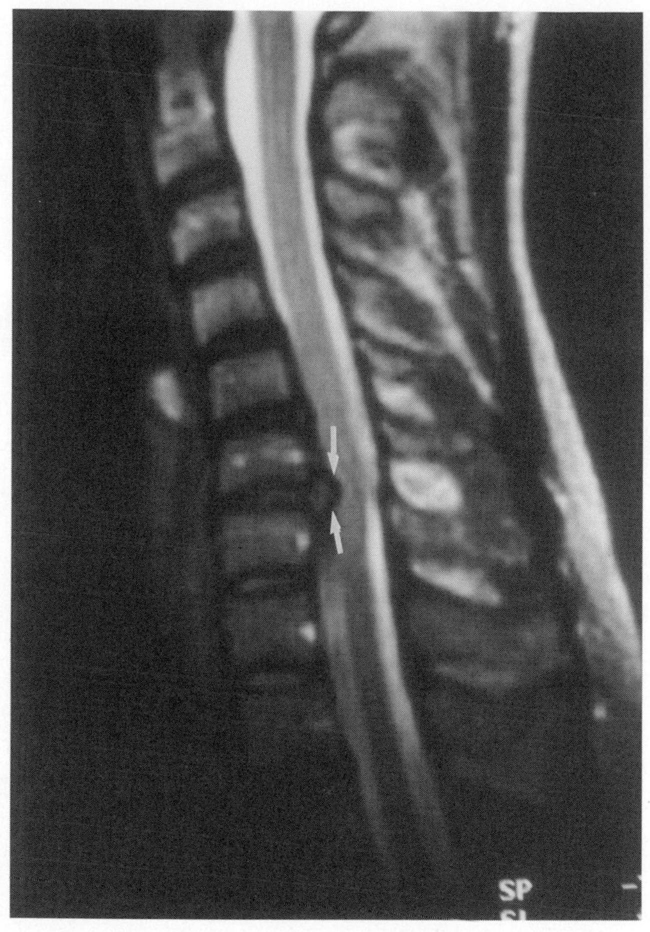

Figure 8-14 Sagittal T2-weighted fast spin echo magnetic resonance image of a moderate-sized C6-7 disk protrusion (*arrows*). This disk protrusion deforms the spinal cord.

In recent years, serial spinal MRI has validated the merit of conservative treatment strategies. Disk herniations, particularly those that are large, can occasionally regress over time without surgical intervention (Fig. 8-18). Yock[7] has offered the explanation that the herniation may have associated hemorrhagic elements, which could be progressively resorbed and thus account for the apparent reduction in size. Spontaneous epidural fibrosis, which would contain the herniation, likely plays a role in the healing process, promoting reduction in size of the herniation.

In the past, some of the most difficult issues to be resolved have related to postoperative cases. The determination of whether there is a recurrent or residual disk herniation, or both, has been simplified with gadolinium-enhanced MRI.[8] Gadolinium will enhance postoperative scar tissue, because of the presence of vasa vasorum within the fibrosis. Disk material, not possessing this vascular component, will not undergo enhancement, provided scanning is accomplished promptly after gadolinium is injected. Otherwise, the disk material may "imbibe" the contrast agent. Obviously, differentiation of scar from residual or recurrent disk disease is critical in the surgeon's decision as to whether reoperation would be beneficial. I have also found that supplemental axial T2-weighted imaging can be of help in distinguishing a disk fragment from an entrapped nerve root sleeve (Fig. 8-19). Ross and colleagues[9] noted that over a period of a year, postoperative epidural scar underwent little change in morphology. In another paper, Ross and associates[10] found that there was a correlation between the intensity of postoperative radiculopathic symptoms and the quantity of scar. Lastly, Ross and coauthors[11] described a pattern of gadolinium enhancement of the endplates typical of benign fibrosis in the post-diskectomy patient. This pattern of enhancement was not indicative of postoperative diskitis, an important differential consideration when reviewing MRI scans of this patient population.

Over the past few decades, diskography has been advocated, principally by the orthopedic surgical community as a methodology for detecting and characterizing disk pathology via injection

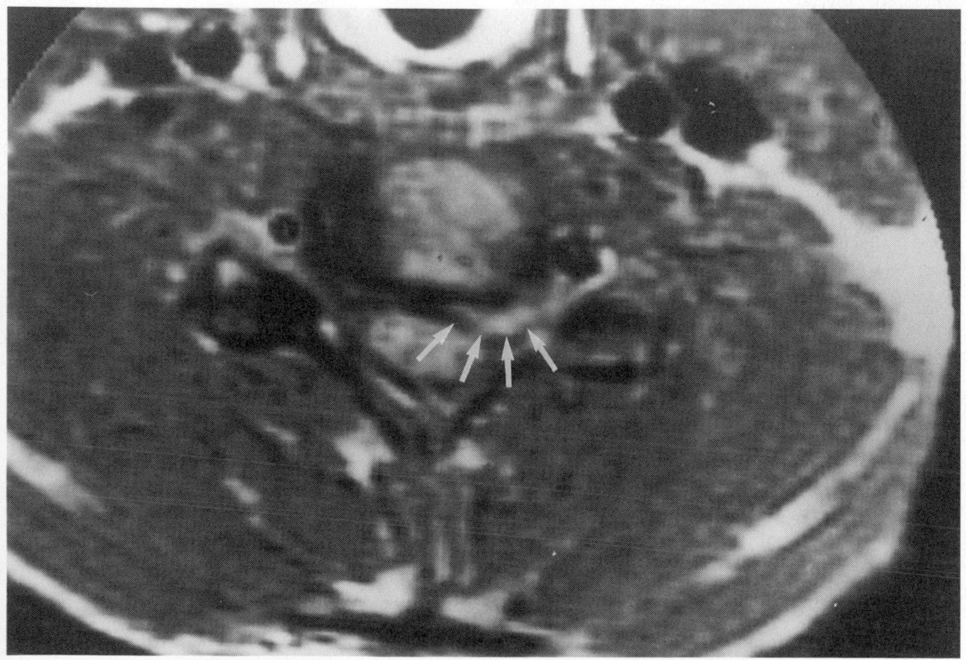

Figure 8-15 Axial T1-weighted magnetic resonance imaging scan (low-field "open" magnet image) of left lateral intraforaminal disk herniation (*arrows*). Intraforaminal disk abnormalities in the cervical region are not clearly discernible on parasagittal scans, because of oblique orientation of the cervical neural foramina. In contrast, lumbar foraminal disk abnormalities are well shown on parasagittal scans.

A

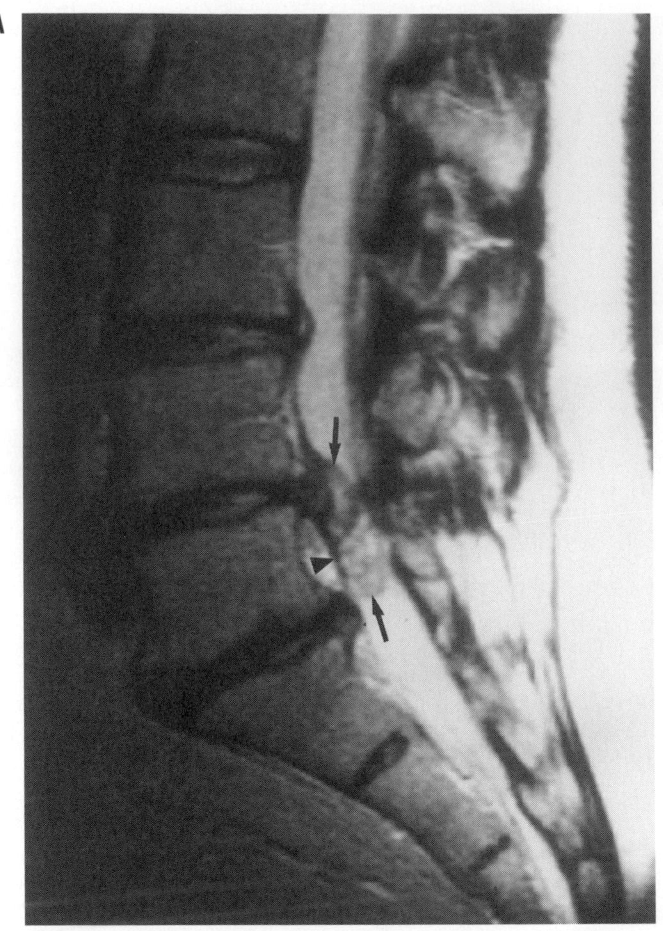

B

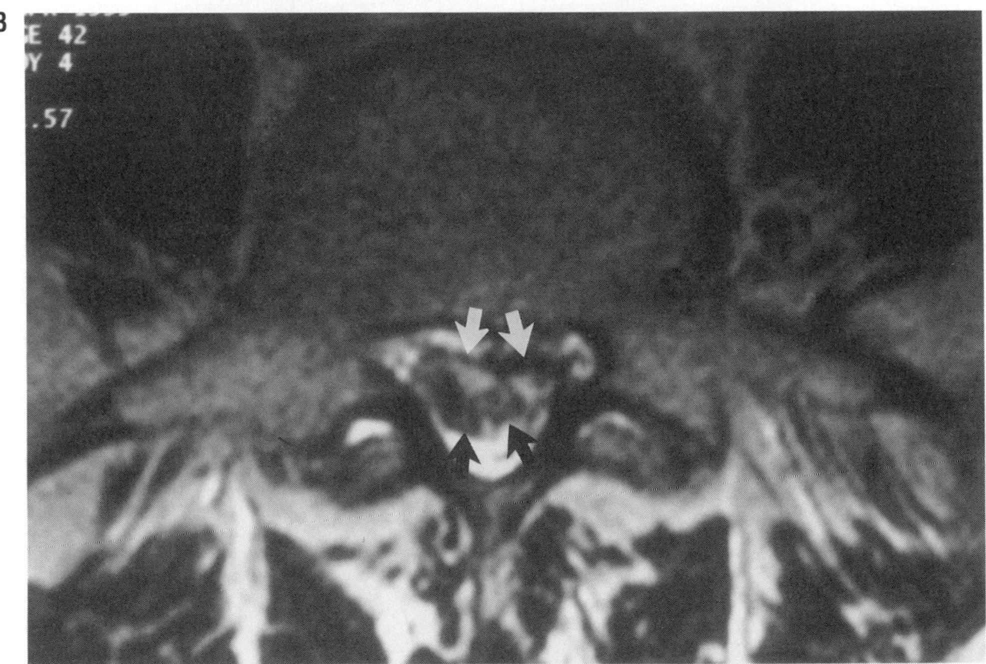

Figure 8-16 **(A)** Sagittal T2-weighted fast spin echo magnetic resonance (MR) image of a large, lobulated intradural disk herniation (*arrows*). Dark line (*arrowhead*) shows anterior dural margin of the thecal sac in front of the disk abnormality, implying an intradural location of the herniation. This very rare form of disk herniation was proven at surgery. **(B)** Axial T2-weighted fast spin echo MR image (same patient as in A). Intradural disk fragment (*black and white arrows*) is well shown. Distinction from tumor is possible. Most tumors enhance whereas disk abnormalities, including that seen in this case, do not.

A

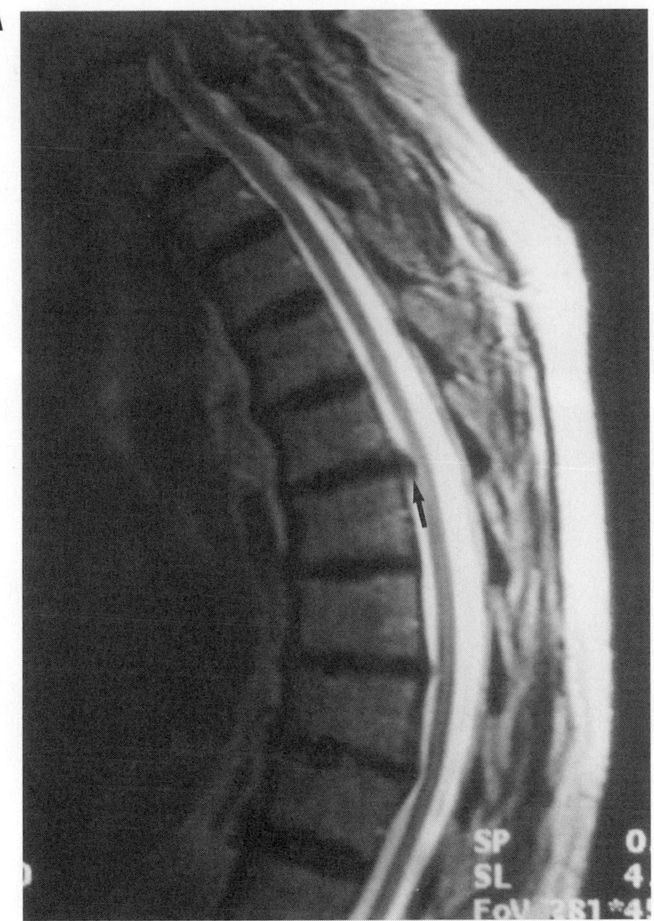

B

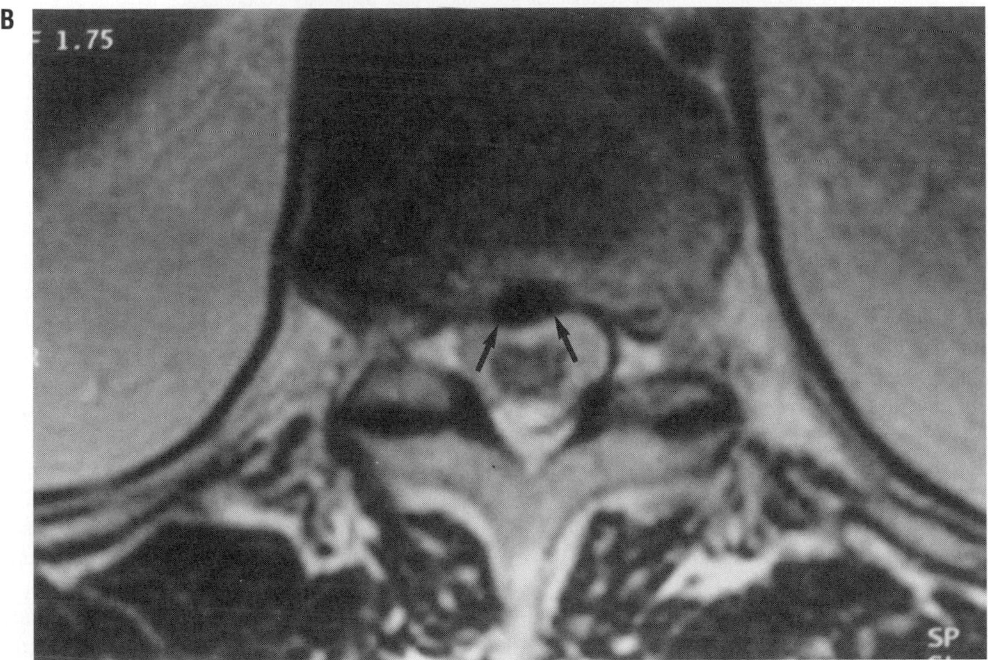

Figure 8-17 **(A)** Sagittal T2-weighted fast spin echo magnetic resonance (MR) image of tiny midthoracic disk protrusion (*arrow*). This disk abnormality was an incidental finding. **(B)** Axial T2-weighted fast spin echo MR image (same patient as in A). Small disk protrusion (*arrows*) is shown as a dark region along the posterior disk margin. No cord deformity is seen.

A

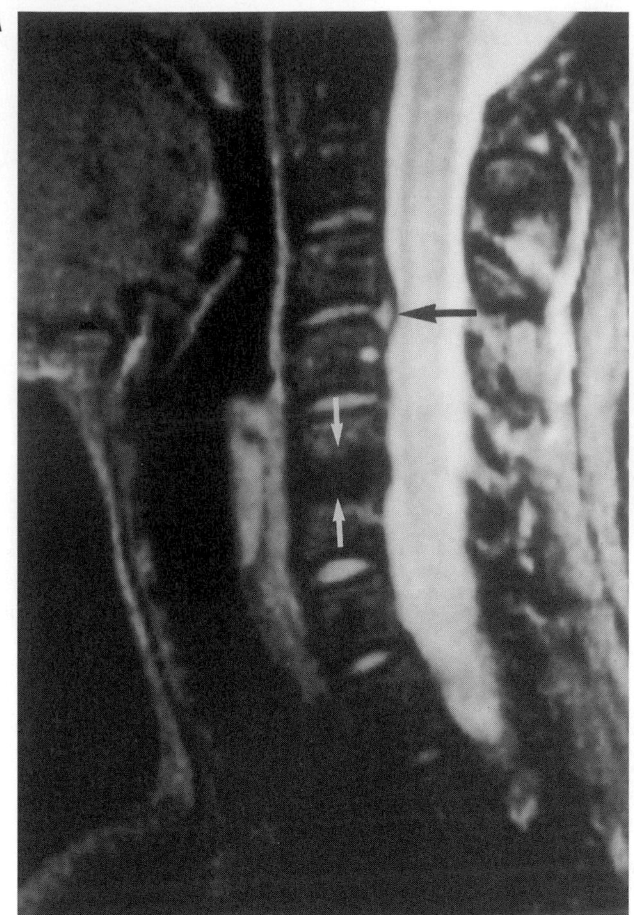

B

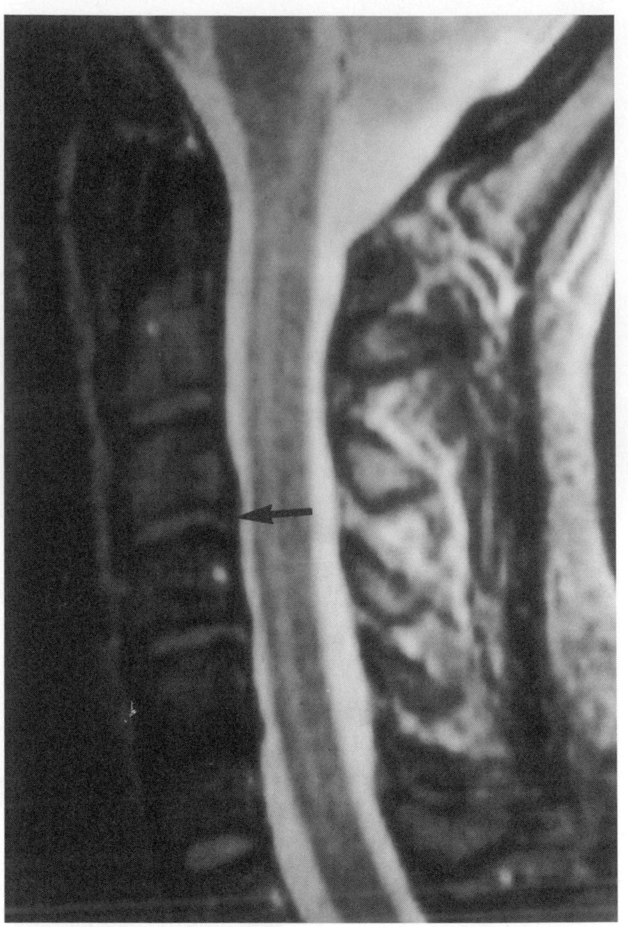

Figure 8-18 **(A)** Sagittal T2-weighted fast spin echo magnetic resonance (MR) image of C3-4 disk protrusion (black arrow). Note the C5-6 anterior cervical fusion (*white arrows*) shown as a dark region. The fixation of this interspace likely altered the spinal biomechanics, facilitating the development of the more cephalad disk protrusion at C3-4. In the unfused cervical spine, most disk pathology occurs at the regions of maximum normal mobility (C5-6 and C6-7 interspaces). **(B)** Sagittal T2-weighted fast spin echo MR image (same patient as in A), 4 months later. Note spontaneous regression of the C3-4 disk protrusion (*arrow*).

of contrast material into the disk and imaging with plain radiography or CT. It has also been used as a provocative test (diskomanometry) to observe whether injecting the disk with saline reproduces the patient's symptoms, implying causation. Publications endorsing the utility of diskography have appeared, again mostly in the orthopedic literature.[12–14] However, contrary opinions concerning the efficacy of diskography have been cited.[15] There has been limited endorsement of diskography by radiologists, particularly in view of the large accumulated experience with MRI and CT, which are noninvasive techniques. Diskography carries the risk of introduction of infection into the disk and adjacent bone (Fig. 8-20), as well as potentially life-threatening allergic reaction to the contrast agent.

FACET DEGENERATION

Facet joint degeneration occurs most commonly in the lumbar and cervical portion of the spinal column and least commonly in the thoracic region. Presumably, this is because of the limited mobility within the thoracic spine, compared with cervical and lumbar sites. Degenerative arthritis leads to facet joint space narrowing and eburnation. Bony spurs may produce thecal sac or nerve root sleeve compression, secondary to central spinal canal or neural foraminal stenosis. This spinal stenosis can be aggravated by thickening of the ligamentum flavum posteriorly, an abnormality that frequently accompanies facet joint degeneration. Moreover, facet arthropathy often accompanies degenerative disk disease. The two pathologic processes together may cause spinal stenosis, the extent of which can be accurately demonstrated by MRI (Fig. 8-21). CT is an excellent alternative imaging study, provided the clinical examination can serve to accurately direct the placement of the axial scans to the suspected interspace level.

As facet joint degeneration intensifies, spondylolisthesis can occur, with the resultant malaligned vertebrae aggravating the spinal stenosis. In nearly all cases, the vertebral segment that displaces does so anteriorly relative to the contiguous, caudal segment. The spondylolisthesis can be visualized by plain radiographs, MRI, or CT (Fig. 8-22). Degenerative spondylolisthesis should be distinguished from spondylolisthesis with an accompanying pars defect,

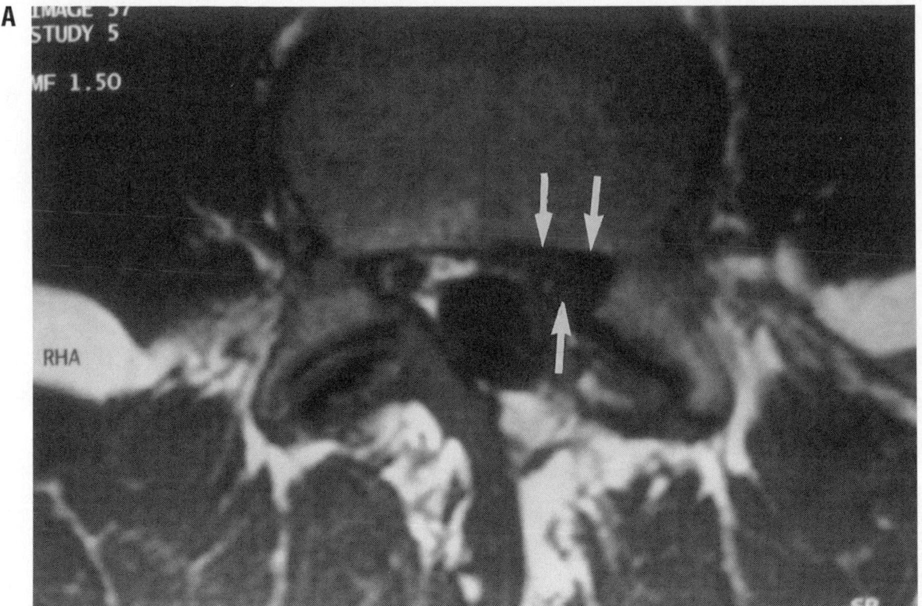

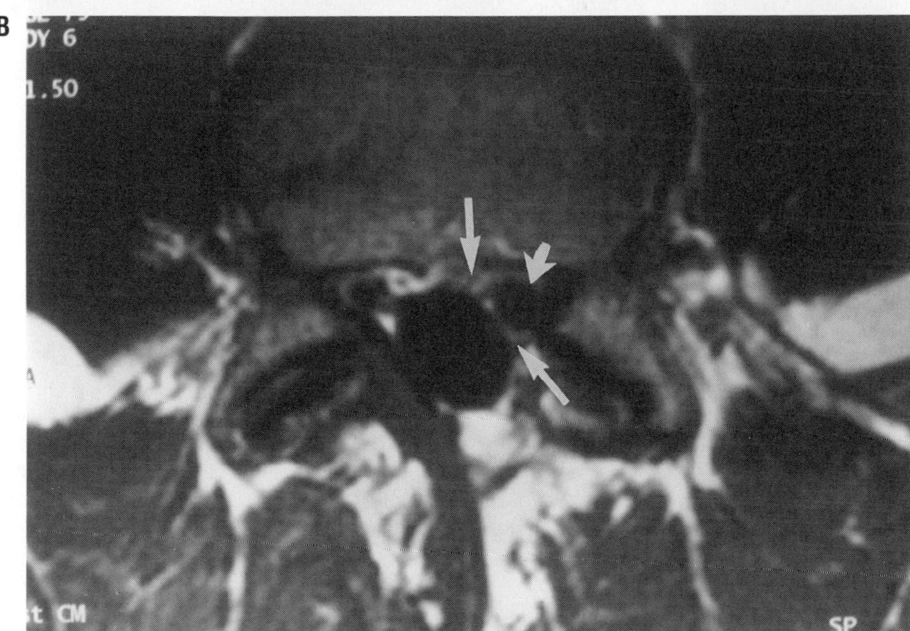

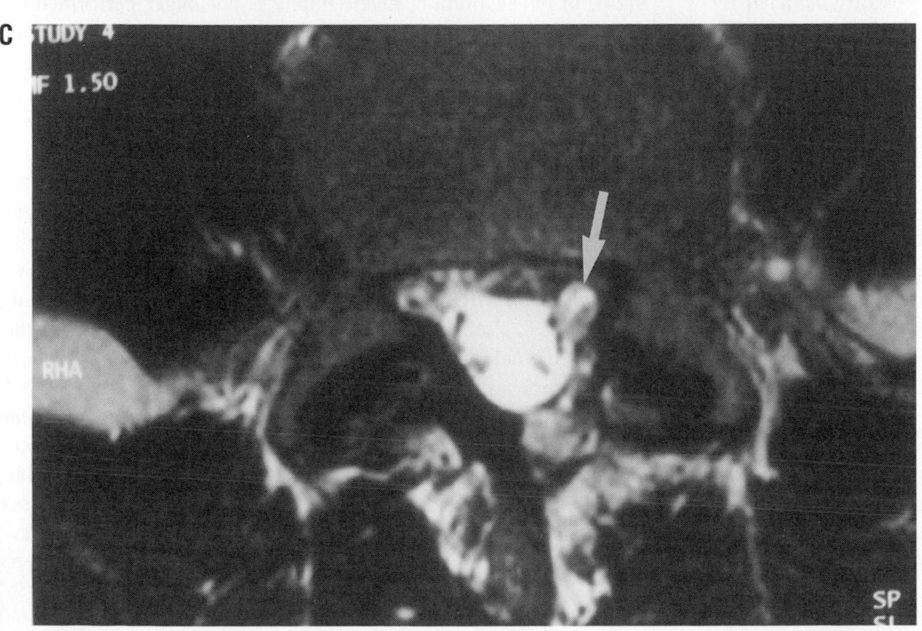

Figure 8-19 **(A)** Axial T1-weighted magnetic resonance imaging (MRI) scan of L4-5 disk space. Status is post–left hemilaminectomy and diskectomy. Dark soft tissue region obscures left L5 nerve root sleeve region (*arrows*). **(B)** Axial T1-weighted MRI scan of L4-5 disk space following gadolinium administration. Note enhancement of scar tissue (*arrows*) surrounding residual dark region (*short arrow*). Is this latter region recurrent disk fragment or nerve root sleeve? **(C)** Axial T2-weighted MRI scan of same patient at same site as in A and B. Formerly dark area turns bright (*arrow*), making this area a water-filled nerve root sleeve and not a disk fragment, which would usually remain darker than spinal fluid.

A

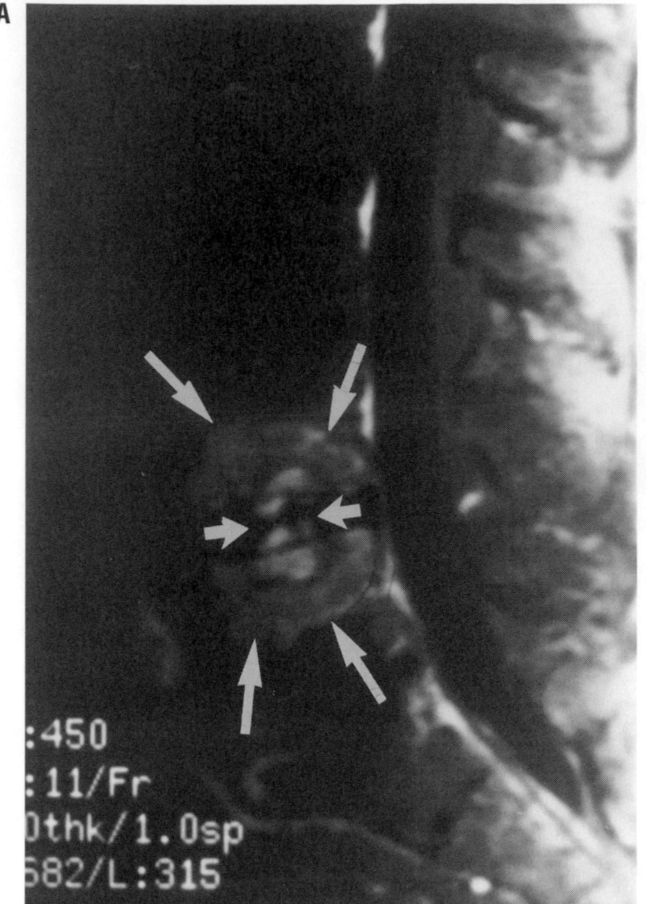

B

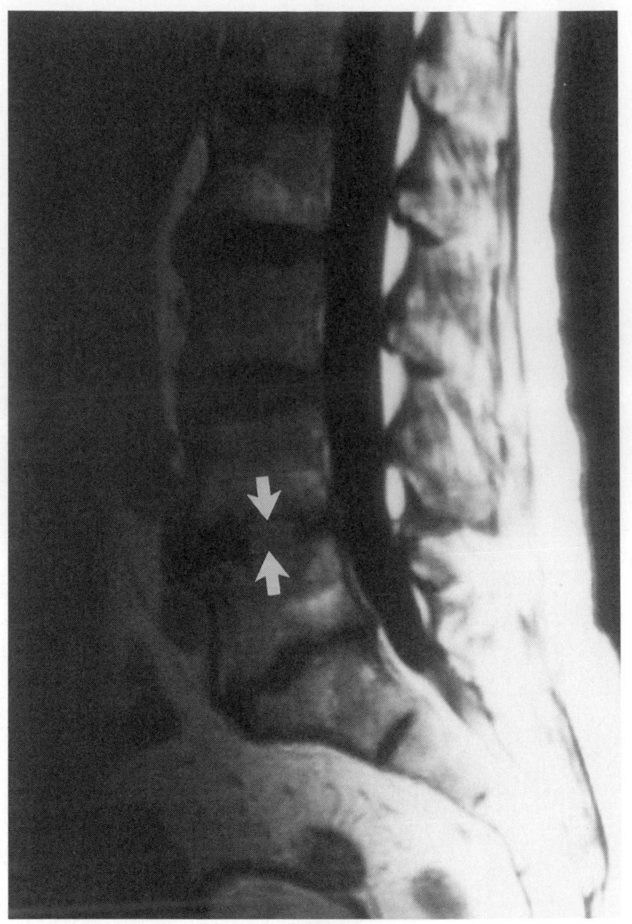

Figure 8-20 **(A)** Sagittal T2-weighted inversion recovery magnetic resonance (MR) image of lumbar spine. Status is postdiskography, with fever and low back pain. This heavily T2-weighted scan shows high signal in the center of the disk (*small arrows*) as well as the adjacent vertebral bodies (*larger arrows*). *Staphylococcus aureus* diskitis and osteomyelitis resulted from introduction of septic material during diskography. This was proven at subsequent percutaneous computed tomography–guided disk aspiration. **(B)** Sagittal T1-weighted gadolinium-enhanced MR image of the lumbar spine (same patient as in A), 2 weeks after first study. Enhancement in center of disk (*arrows*) is seen at the proven septic site resulting from prior diskography.

known as spondylolysis. The defect is most readily depicted by sagittally reformatted CT, and is most commonly seen at the L5 level (Fig. 8-23). Spondylolisthesis can occur secondary to spondylolysis. In this case, the greatest stenosis is seen at the neural foramina, secondary to the pars above the defect being displaced into the foramen. The central spinal canal, if anything, is elongated in its AP dimension owing to the effective break in the neural arch secondary to the spondylolysis. However, some central canal stenosis can ensue as a result of encroachment by eburnated bone arising from the pseudoarthrosis created by the spondylolysis. Nearly always, the spondylolysis is bilateral.

NEOPLASTIC SPINAL DISEASE

Neoplastic disease in the spine usually presents with back pain. The most common tumor is a metastasis from a breast or lung carcinoma. MRI is exquisitely sensitive to the presence of bony vertebral metastatic disease[16–21] and any associated epidural tumor extension that is causing spinal cord or nerve root compression (Fig. 8-24). In my institution, myelography is no longer performed on patients to exclude cord compression from metastatic disease, because MRI provides superior delineation of this pathologic process noninvasively, and with a degree of precision more than sufficient to plan radiotherapy. Metastatic disease involving the leptomeninges can also be detected on MRI, particularly with gadolinium enhancement (Fig. 8-25). However, even with enhancement, MRI is only about one third as sensitive as serial lumbar punctures in detecting leptomeningeal spread of tumor.[22]

Patients with suspected metastatic disease who are unable to be examined with MRI for technical or medical reasons can be evaluated by CT, after directing the study to a specific region of the spine by the aid of the clinical findings, plain radiographs, and, if time permits, a radionuclide bone scan. This latter study is still a very sensitive and inexpensive method of surveying the vertebral column for the presence of bony malignancy, although purely lytic metastases may not be detectable. As helical scanning has become more readily available, more extended CT scans of the spinal column are now possible, although with limited spatial and contrast resolution as compared with MRI.

A

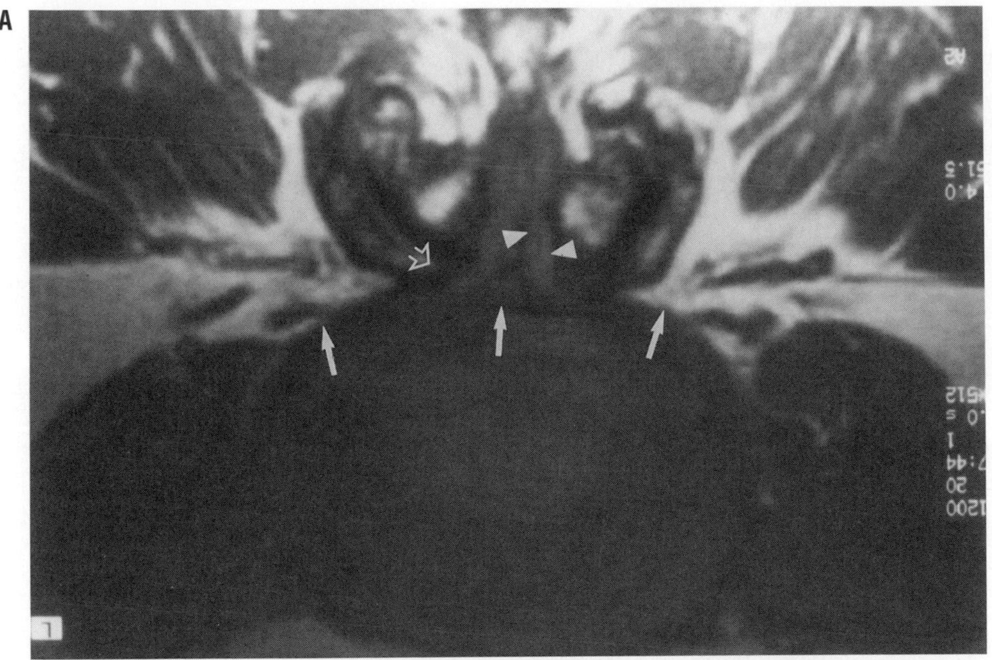

B

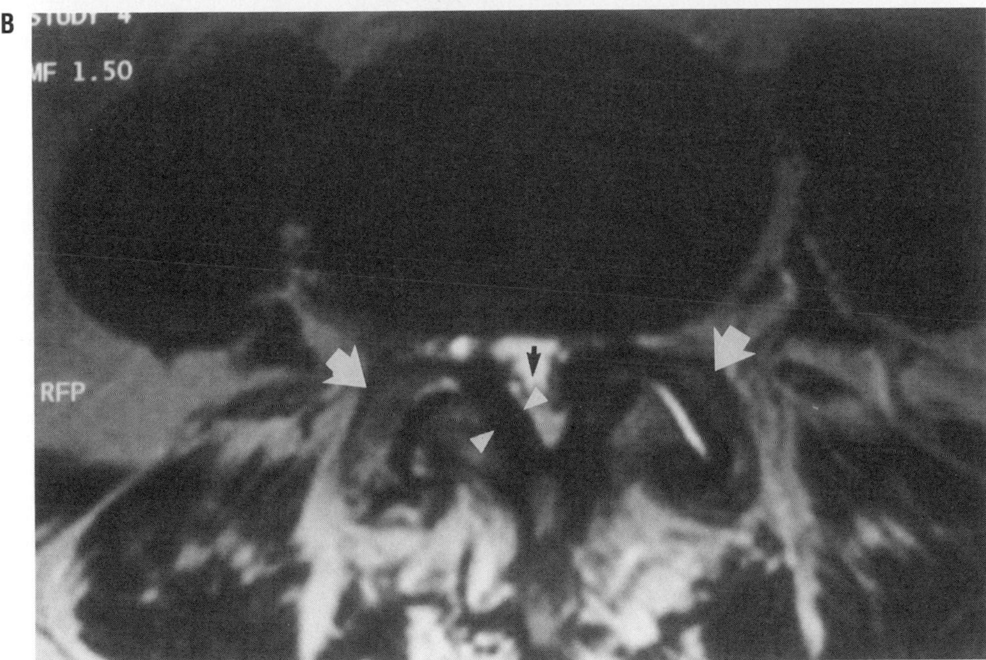

Figure 8-21 **(A)** Axial T1-weighted magnetic resonance (MR) image shows severe spinal stenosis resulting from a combination of facet joint degeneration (*hollow arrow*), thickening of the ligamenta flava (*arrowheads*), and bulging disk (*arrows*). However, distinction of thecal sac itself is poor secondary to using a T1-weighted scan, rather T2-weighted imaging. As noted in the text, T2-weighted scans make spinal fluid bright, and therefore easily distinguishable from disk and ligamentous margins. **(B)** Axial T2-weighted fast spin echo MR image of another patient with spinal stenosis. The bright spinal fluid in the thecal sac (*tiny black arrow*) permits ready distinction of this structure being stenosed by the darker degenerated facets (*large white arrows*) and thickened ligamentum flavum (*white arrowheads*). Therefore, fast spin echo T2-weighted imaging is the preferred technique for imaging thecal sac deformation from a multitude of pathologic processes, including degenerative disk and facet joint disease. Such imaging clarity renders computed tomographic myelography superfluous, in the author's opinion.

A

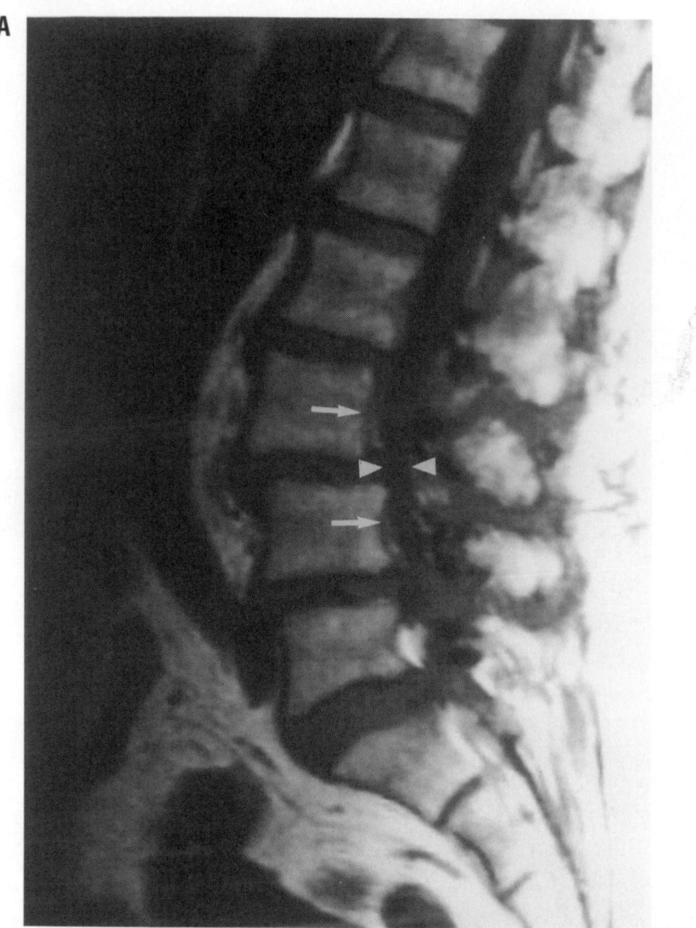

B

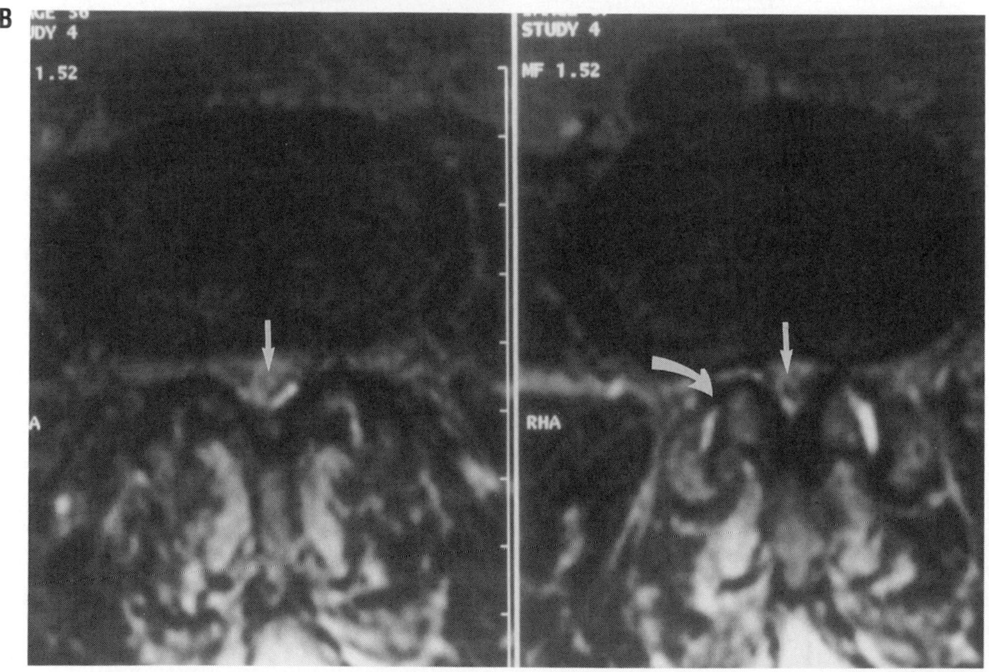

Figure 8-22 **(A)** Sagittal T1-weighted magnetic resonance (MR) image of degenerative spondylolisthesis of L3 on L4. Note forward displacement of L3 body relative to L4 (*arrows*). Narrowed central spinal canal (*arrowheads*) results from this malalignment of the component vertebrae. **(B)** Axial T2-weighted fast spin echo MR images of same patient as in A. Composite of two adjacent scan levels. Central spinal stenosis is evident on both images (*arrows*), with malalignment of facets (*curved arrow*) seen as a consequence of the subluxation noted in degenerative spondylolisthesis.

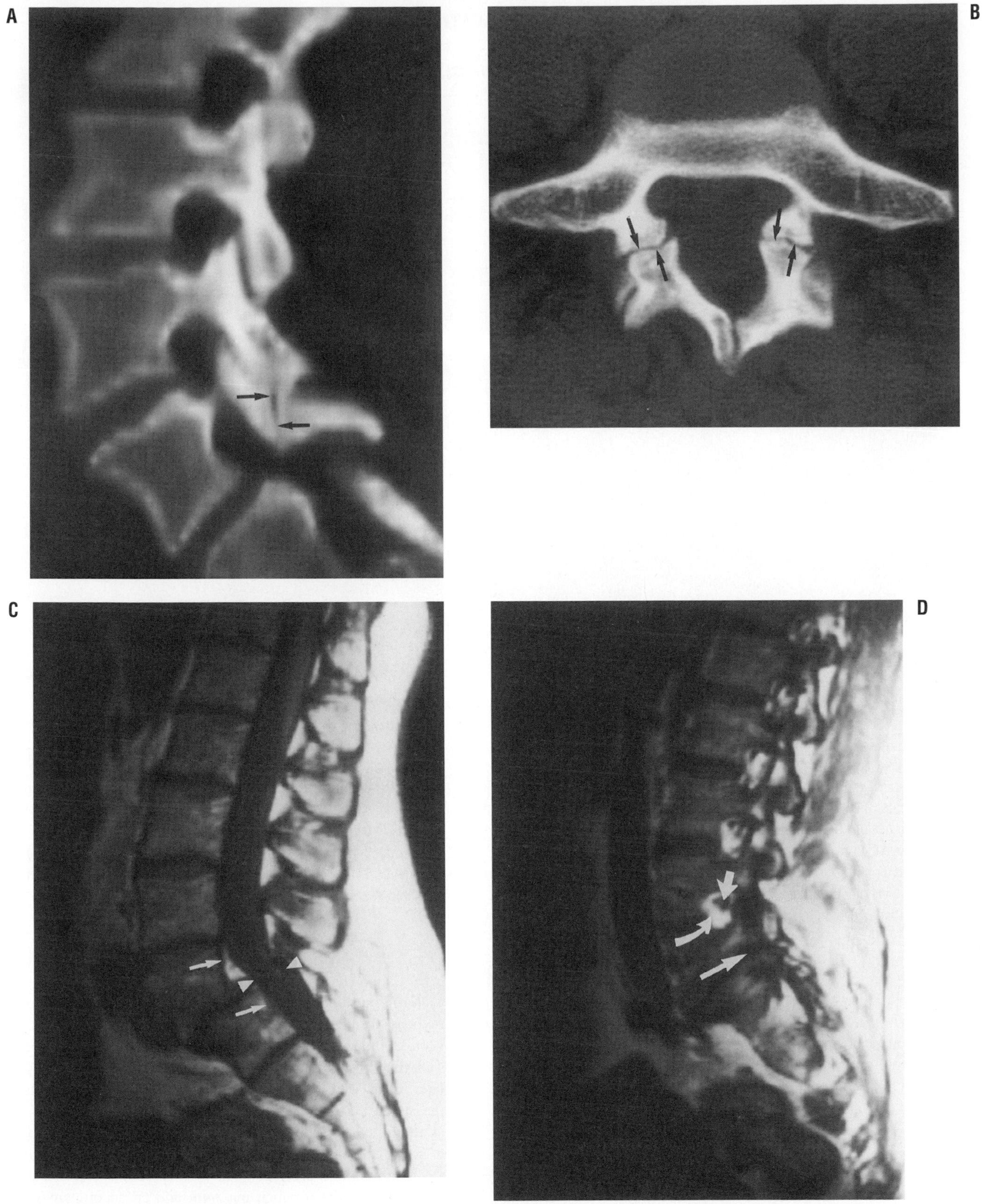

A

B

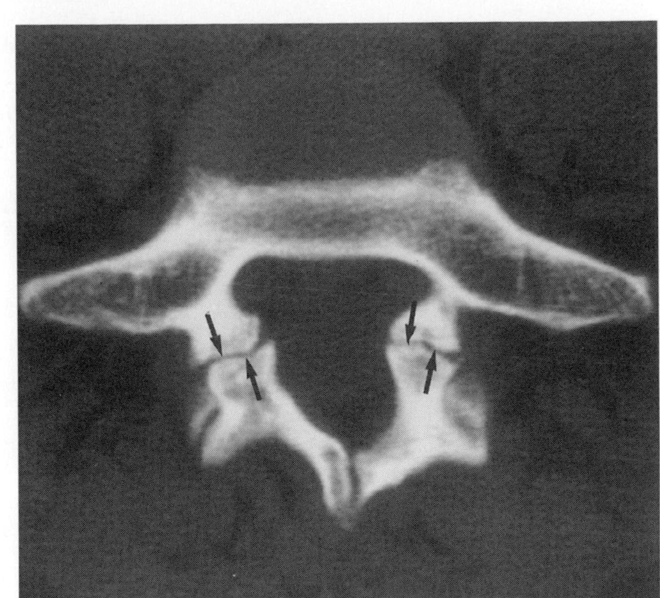

C

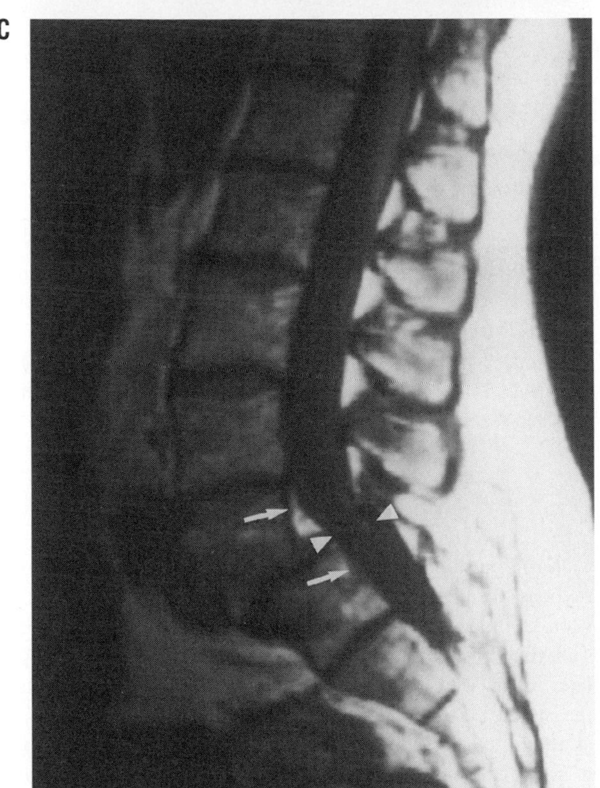

D

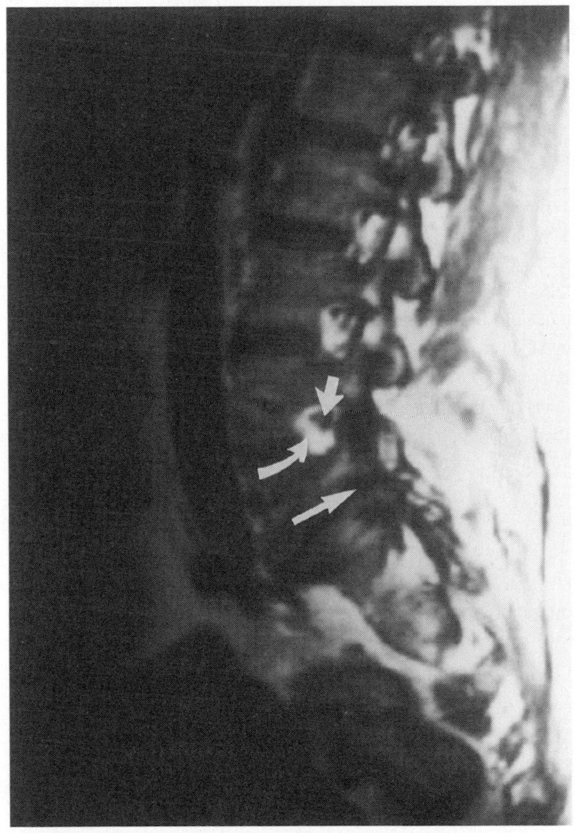

Figure 8-23 **(A)** Parasagittal reconstructed computed tomographic (CT) image shows pars defect (*arrow*) in L5, pathognomonic of spondylolysis. There was no accompanying spondylolisthesis in this case. **(B)** Axial CT scan shows bilateral pars defects (*arrows*), seen in spondylolysis. Unilateral pars defects are much less commonly observed. CT is the preferred method for visualizing pars defects. **(C)** Sagittal T1-weighted magnetic resonance (MR) image of a patient with spondylolysis with spondylolisthesis. Note forward displacement of L4 on L5 (*arrows*), with only mild central canal narrowing (*arrowheads*), caused by break in the neural arch from accompanying spondylolysis at L4. **(D)** Parasagittal T1-weighted MR image of same patient as in B. Pars defect is not clearly seen (a typical problem in MRI versus ease of depiction with CT). However, there is clear demonstration of complete effacement of the L5-S1 neural foramen (*arrow*) caused by the pars above the spondylolytic defect encroaching on the foramen. Note patent foramina above this level, visible by virtue of normally bright foraminal fat (*curved arrow*) outlining the exiting root sleeve (*short arrow*).

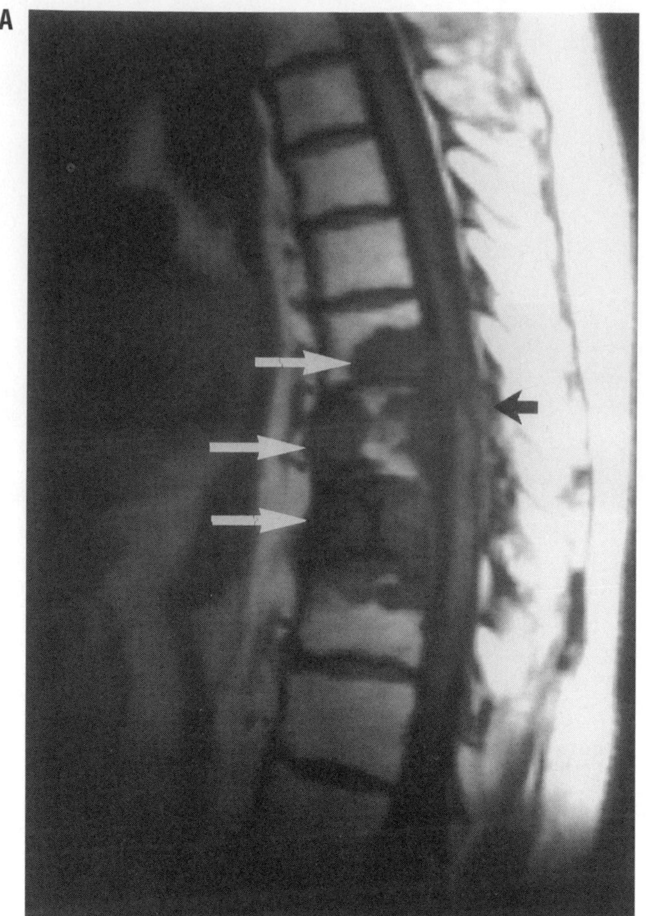

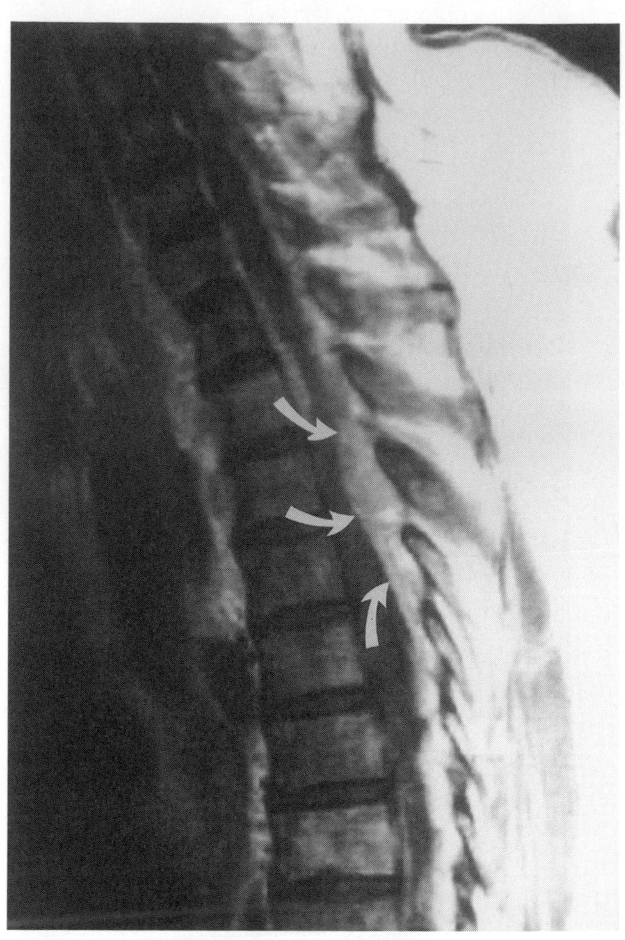

Figure 8-24 **(A)** Sagittal T1-weighted magnetic resonance (MR) image of thoracic spine showing multiple areas of metastatic lung cancer (*white arrows*). Tumor T1 signal is lower (darker) than normal marrow fat, making the tumor clearly discernible. Dorsal tumor deposit (*black arrow*) compresses spinal cord. Tumor within bone is less conspicuous on T2-weighted images, as contrast between fleshy tumor and marrow fat is reduced. **(B)** Sagittal T1-weighted gadolinium-enhanced MR image of the thoracic spine shows enhancing epidural tumor deposit (*arrows*) secondary to multiple myeloma causing extensive cord compression. An epidural abscess can have an identical radiographic appearance. Gadolinium-enhanced T1-weighted images diminish the contrast between tumor within bone and normal marrow fat. This is caused by gadolinium uptake by tumor increasing its signal to nearly that of the normally brighter fat. Therefore, a spinal MR study directed to exclude bony metastases should always include a noncontrast T1-weighted scan.

Intradural neoplasms can be classified as intramedullary or extramedullary. Intramedullary tumors are most commonly low-grade astrocytomas or ependymomas. Spinal cord gliomas can involve virtually the entire extent of the spinal cord. Again, MRI is the imaging modality of choice. These neoplasms usually expand the spinal cord and alter its signal intensity, making their visualization easy. However, it is often possible to differentiate the tumor margins from accompanying cysts or edema by using gadolinium-DTPA[23] (Fig. 8-26). Most extramedullary intradural tumors are meningiomas or schwannomas. These neoplasms may compress both the spinal cord and nerve roots (Fig. 8-27), findings easily delineated by MRI. However, distinction between meningioma and schwannoma can sometimes be accomplished with CT, which can better demonstrate calcification seen occasionally but almost exclusively with meningioma. Spinal schwannomas can occur as solitary lesions or as a manifestation of neurofibromatosis I, an inherited neurocutaneous disorder, or phakomatosis.[24]

Some intramedullary tumors may be associated with syringomyelia.[25] If the detection of one pathologic process in the spine has been facilitated by MRI, it is syringomyelia (Fig. 8-28). Formerly, such time-consuming, invasive procedures as gas myelography and, later, CTM were the only methods for demonstrating cysts within the spinal cord. CTM was not universally successful in demonstrating a syrinx, as this necessitated progressive imbibition of contrast agent into the central cystic cavity. Chiari malformations of the hindbrain and cervical spine with cerebellar tonsillar displacement through the foramen magnum and an accompanying syrinx are optimally demonstrated by MRI.[26] The syrinx can extend the length of the entire spinal cord. In the lumbar spine, dysraphic states, such as meningoceles or tethering of the spinal cord with an associated lipoma, are best imaged by MRI[27] (Fig. 8-29).

Demyelination in the spinal cord can present as a radiculopathy[28] clinically mimicking disk herniation, particularly in the cervical region. Before MRI, there was no method capable of directly

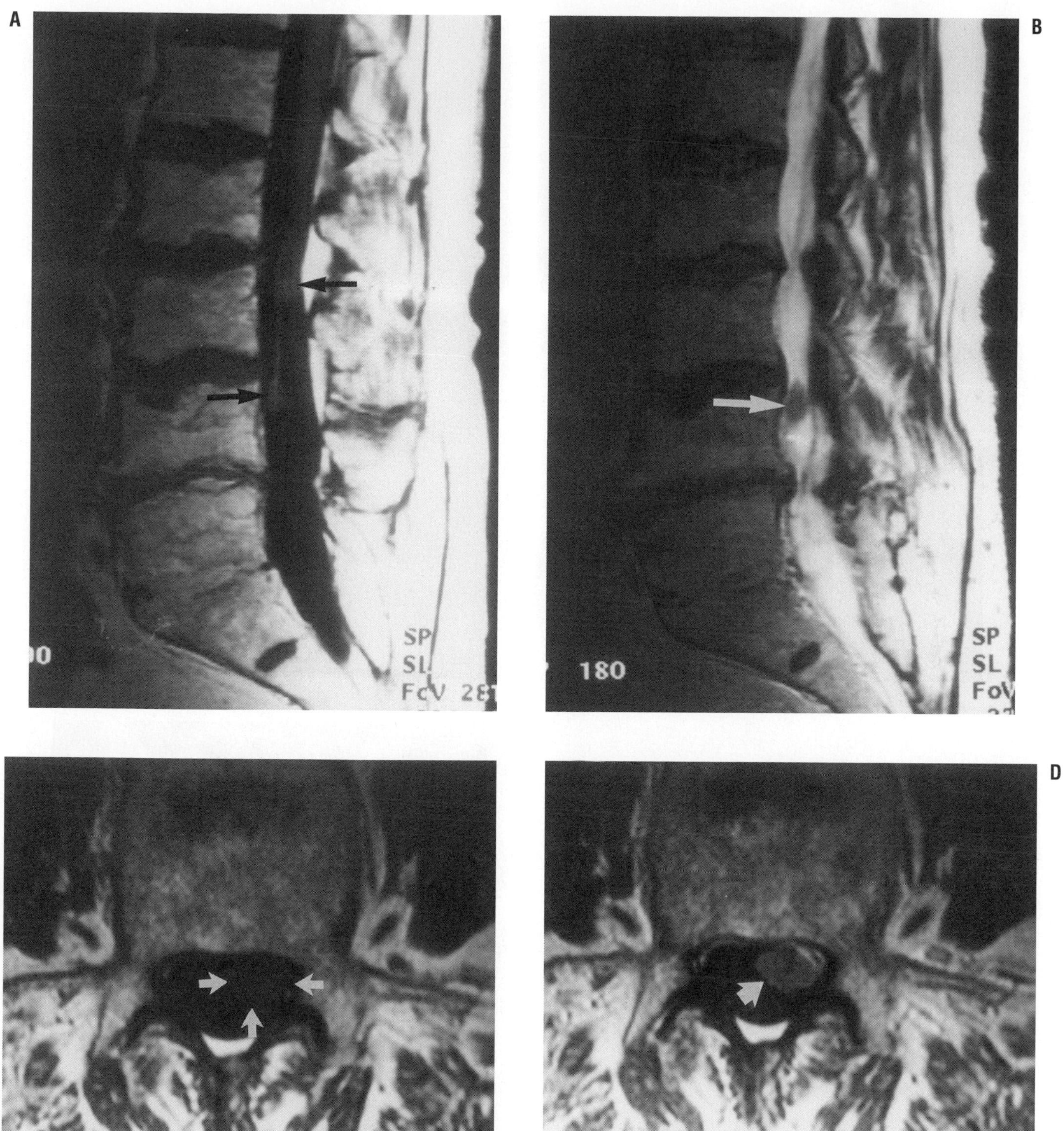

Figure 8-25 **(A)** Sagittal T1-weighted lumbar spine magnetic resonance (MR) image shows barely discernible intradural nodules (*arrows*). **(B)** Sagittal T2-weighted fast spin echo MR image (same patient as in A) shows one nodule (*arrow*) darker than surrounding spinal fluid. Appearance is nonspecific. **(C)** Axial T1-weighted MR image through nodule (*arrows*); lesion is essentially invisible. **(D)** Axial T1-weighted gadolinium-enhanced MR image at same level as in C shows the lesion (*arrow*) enhancing and now clearly defined. Diagnosis: leptomeningeal spread of metastatic lung cancer.

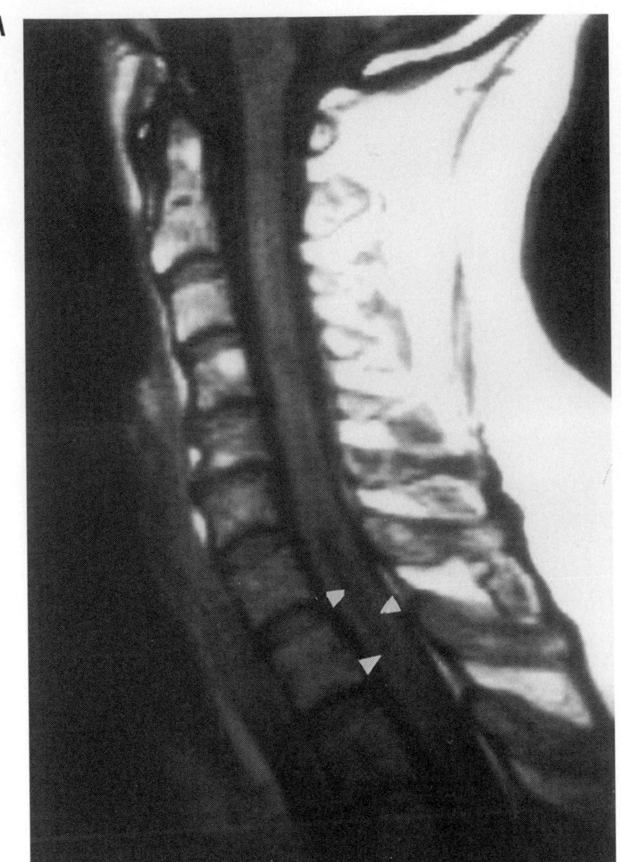

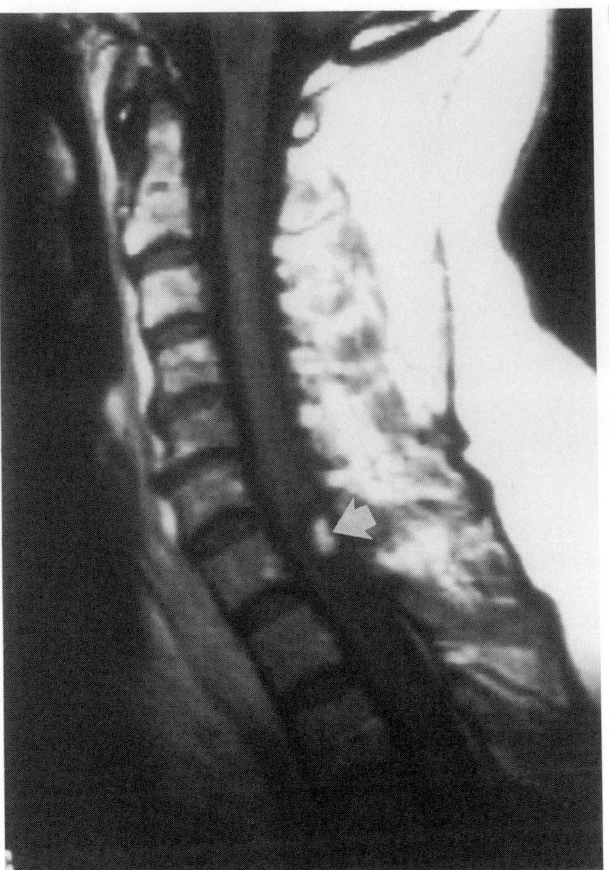

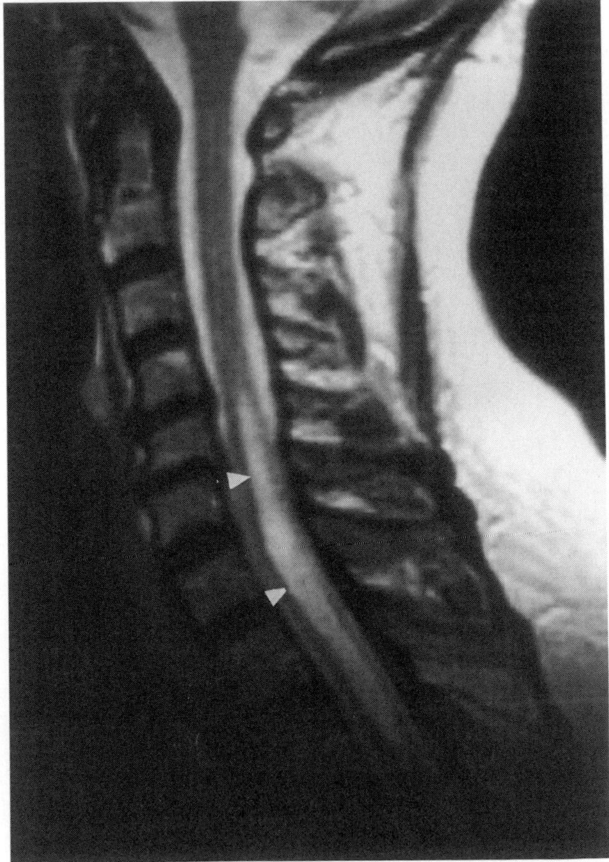

Figure 8-26 **(A)** Sagittal T1-weighted cervical spine magnetic resonance (MR) image shows mild dilation of the upper thoracic cord and slight internal hypointensity (*arrowheads*). **(B)** Sagittal T1-weighted gadolinium-enhanced MR image (same patient as in A) shows superficially situated enhancing tumor nodule (*arrow*) at level of C7. **(C)** Sagittal T2-weighted MR image (same patient as in B) shows extensive edema (*arrowheads*) associated with the tumor. Diagnosis: hemangioblastoma. Hemangioblastomas can occur as isolated entities or as a component of von Hippel-Lindau disease, one of the phakomatoses.

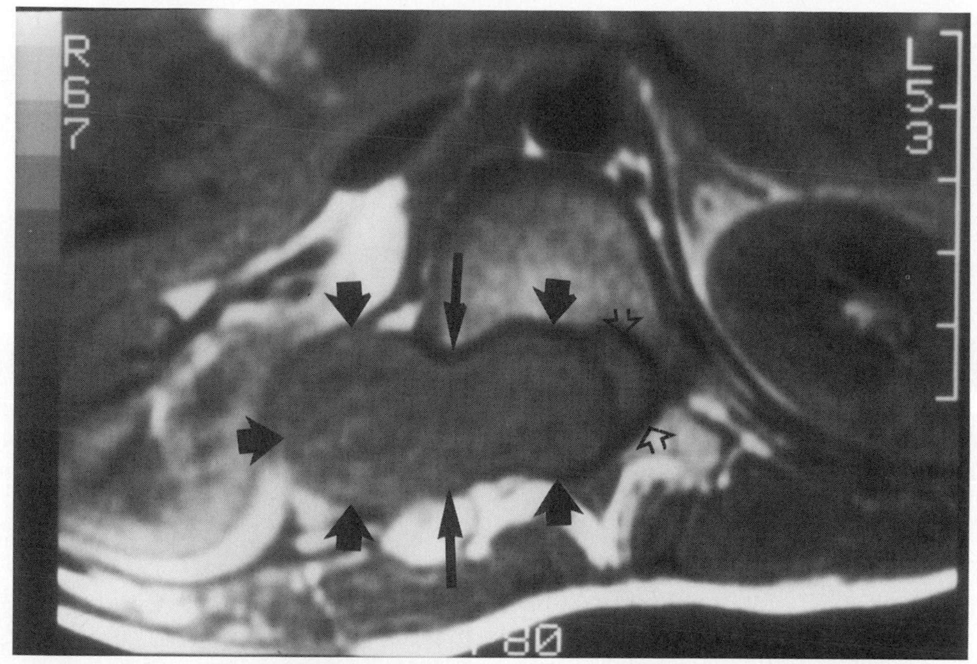

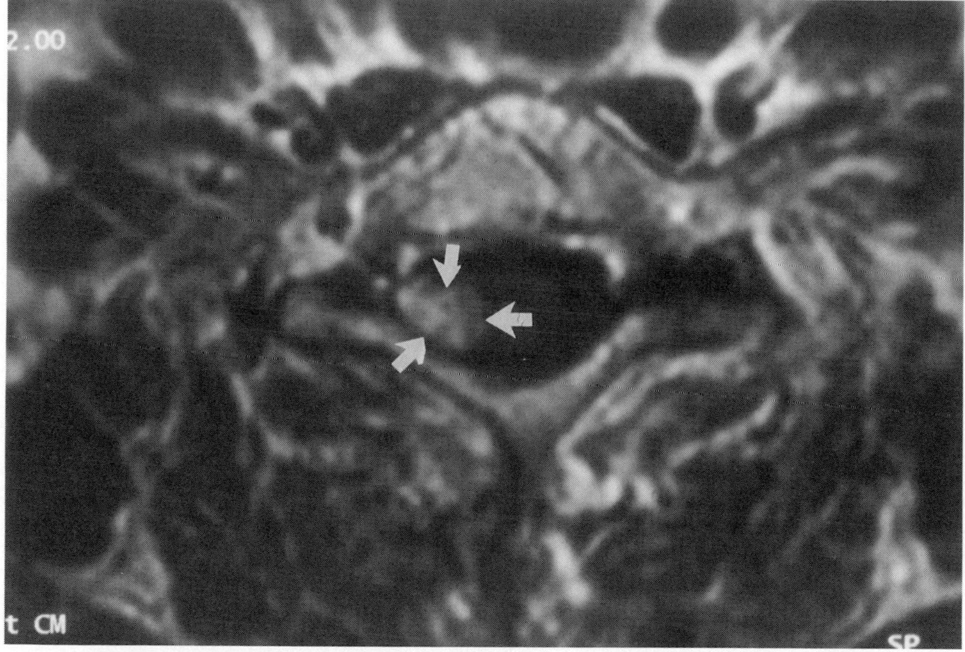

Figure 8-27 **(A)** Axial T1-weighted magnetic resonance imaging scan at level of L1 lumbar vertebra shows large dumbbell-shaped tumor (*short arrows*) markedly widening the right neural foramen (*long arrows*) and compressing the spinal cord (*hollow arrows*). Diagnosis: extradural and intradural schwannoma. **(B)** Axial T1-weighted gadolinium-enhanced scan shows a right-sided enhancing intradural tumor (*arrows*) at the level of C7 vertebra. Diagnosis: meningioma.

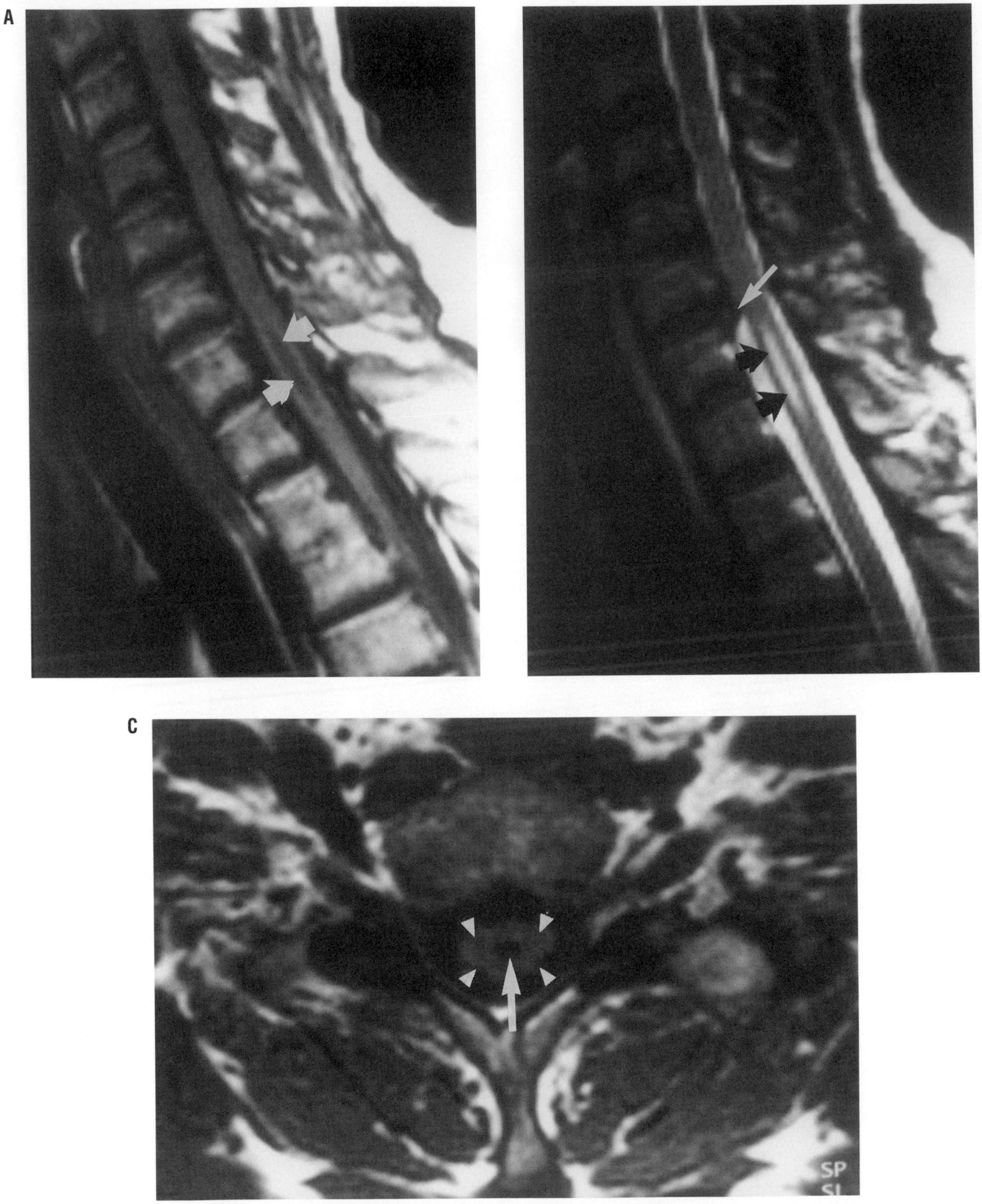

A

B

C

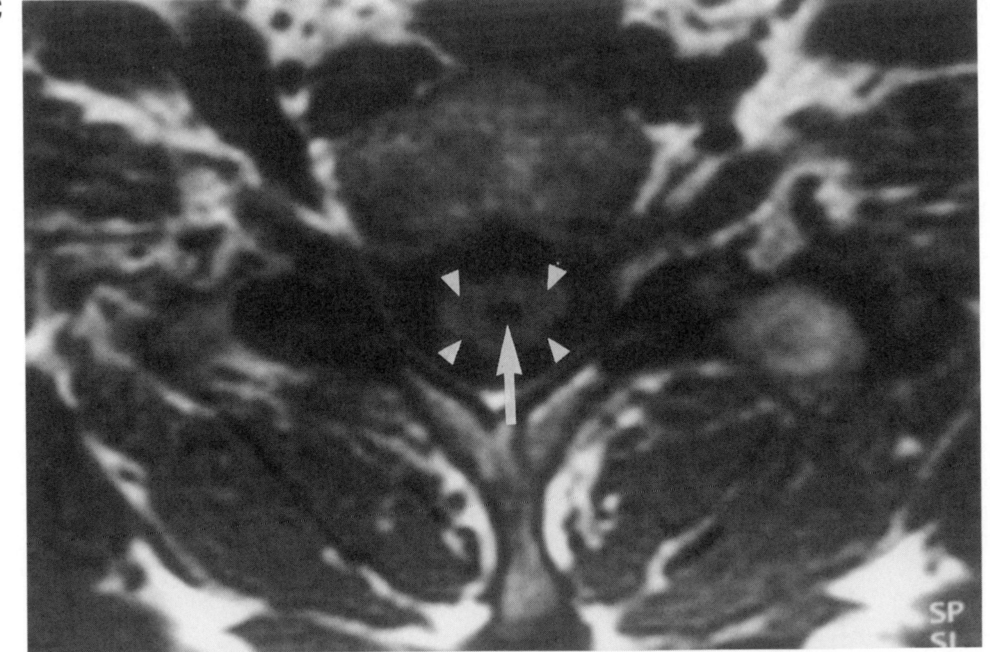

Figure 8-28 **(A)** Sagittal T1-weighted magnetic resonance imaging (MRI) scan of cervical and upper thoracic spine shows sharply demarcated linear area of low T1 signal within spinal cord (*arrows*). **(B)** Sagittal T2-weighted MRI scan (same patient as in A) shows linear, high T2 signal (*black arrows*) at same location as low T1 signal. Diagnosis: syringomyelia. Note disk herniation (*white arrow*), which potentially is causative of the syrinx. **(C)** Axial T1-weighted MRI scan (same patient as in B) shows syrinx cavity in cross section as circular area of low T1 signal (*arrow*) in the center of the spinal cord. The margins of the cord are indicated (*arrowheads*).

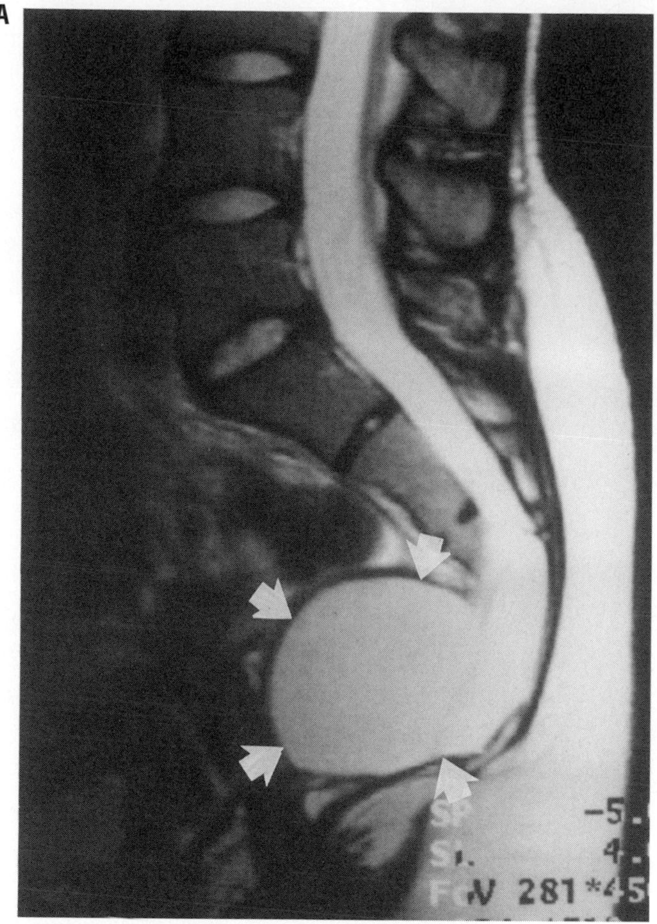

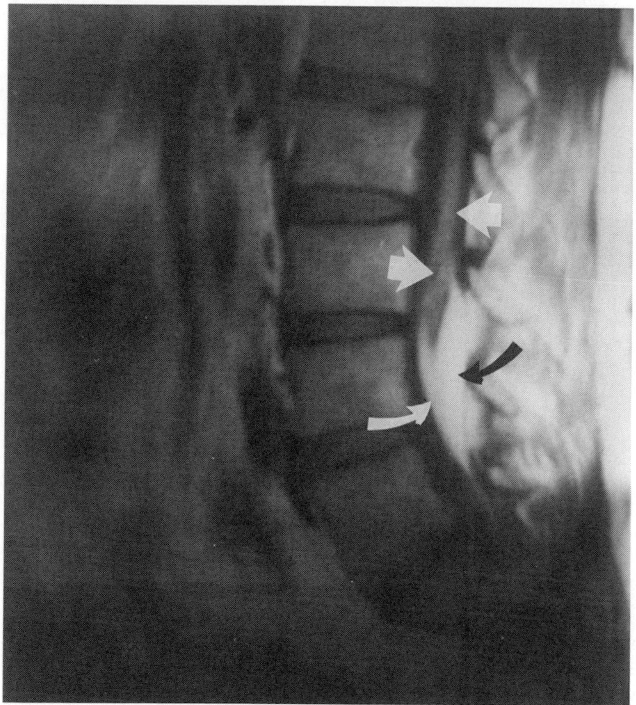

Figure 8-29 **(A)** Sagittal T2-weighted magnetic resonance imaging (MRI) scan of lumbosacral spine shows large, spinal fluid-filled mass (*arrows*) extending in continuity with distal thecal sac into the pelvis. Diagnosis: anterior sacral meningocele. These lesions can cause symptoms of a pelvic mass, including bowel and bladder dysfunction, as well as dyspareunia. An anterior sacral meningocele is a lesion within the spectrum of spinal dysraphism. **(B)** Sagittal T1-weighted MRI scan of tethered spinal cord (*thick white arrows*). The spinal cord terminates at the level of L4, much lower than normal (at T12-L1) and is surrounded by the bright fat of an associated lipoma (*curved black and white arrows*).

identifying demyelinating plaques within the spinal cord, although frequently such lesions could be demonstrated in the brain by CT. Typically, demyelination produces one or more discrete foci of elevated T2 signal intensity within the spinal cord, at times with cord expansion if the lesion is acute (Fig. 8-30). Besides the clinical features, confirmation that the signal abnormalities in the cord may be caused by a demyelinating process can be obtained by MRI of the brain, demonstrating additional foci of T2 hyperintensity in the periventricular white matter.[29]

TRAUMA

Trauma to the spine traditionally has been initially imaged with plain x-ray films. These studies often serve to guide subsequent CT scanning, which provides excellent imaging of the extent of most fractures. MRI provides superior definition of soft tissue injuries, especially if there is an associated spinal hematoma or cord contusion.[4,30] However, in the acutely traumatized patient who may be in traction or on external life-support systems, it is often physically impractical to employ MRI. The recent introduction of wide-bore, so-called open magnet systems may facilitate scanning of these patients by granting support personnel greater access to the patient. Nevertheless, as previously noted, image quality issues may outweigh ease of access (Fig. 8-31).

INFECTIONS

An increasingly common cause of back pain is spinal osteomyelitis and epidural abscess, which are now being seen with greater frequency because of larger numbers of intravenous drug abusers and generally debilitated patients. Vertebral and intervertebral disk destruction is the critical observation in diskitis or osteomyelitis, yet such abnormalities occur late in the course of the disease. With epidural abscess, plain films will be unrevealing. Therefore, plain films should not be relied on to rule out an infectious process. MRI is the preferred technique for imaging both osteomyelitis or diskitis and epidural abscess[31,32] (Fig. 8-32). Because epidural abscesses may extend in a discontinuous fashion, it is recommended that the

A

B

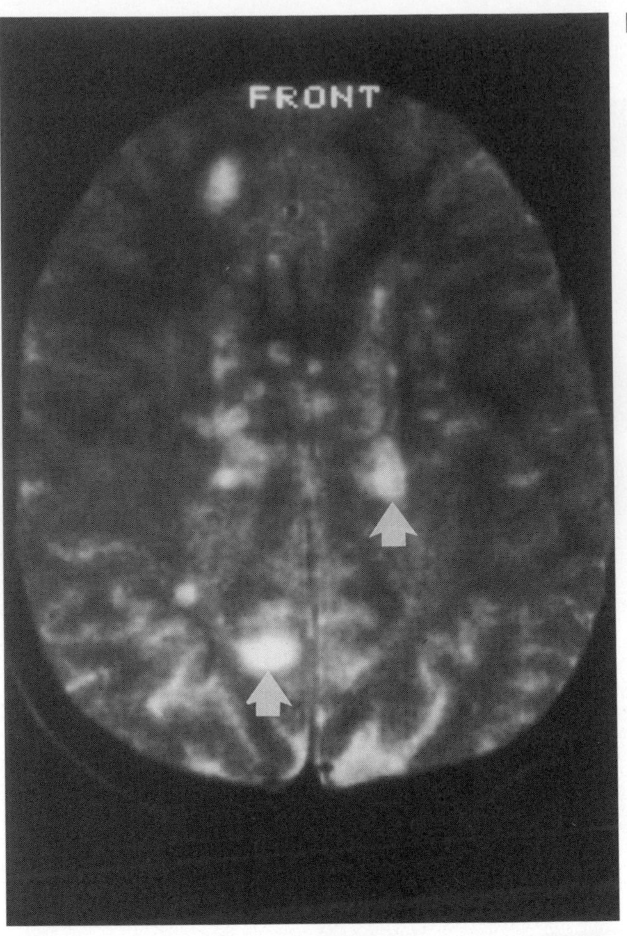

Figure 8-30 **(A)** Sagittal T2-weighted fast spin echo magnetic resonance (MR) image of the midthoracic spinal cord, showing small area of T2 hypertensity (*arrow*) slightly expanding the cord. **(B)** Axial T2-weighted MR image of brain of this patient shows innumerable T2 hyperintense foci in the periventricular white matter, with the largest lesions demarcated (*arrows*). The combination of periventricular brain and spinal lesions is virtually pathognomonic of a demyelinating disorder, in this case, multiple sclerosis.

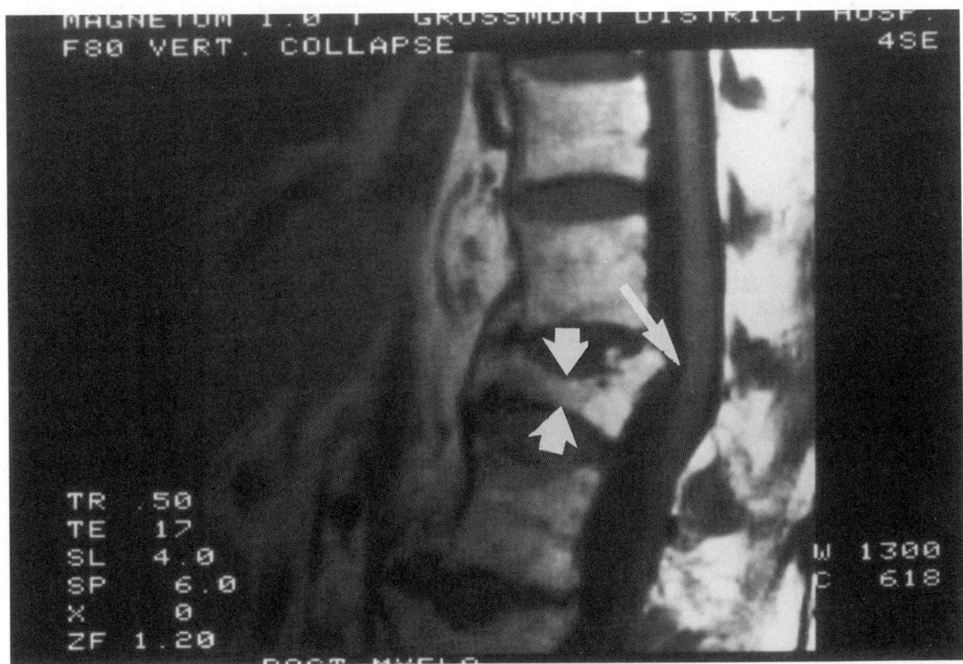

Figure 8-31 Sagittal T1-weighted magnetic resonance (MR) image of a midthoracic compression fracture (*thick arrows*), secondary to osteoporosis in an elderly patient. The signal within the marrow of the compressed bone is similar to that of adjacent normal vertebrae. This pattern is consistent with a chronic benign fracture. Note fracture causing focal angulation of the spinal cord (*thin arrow*).

A

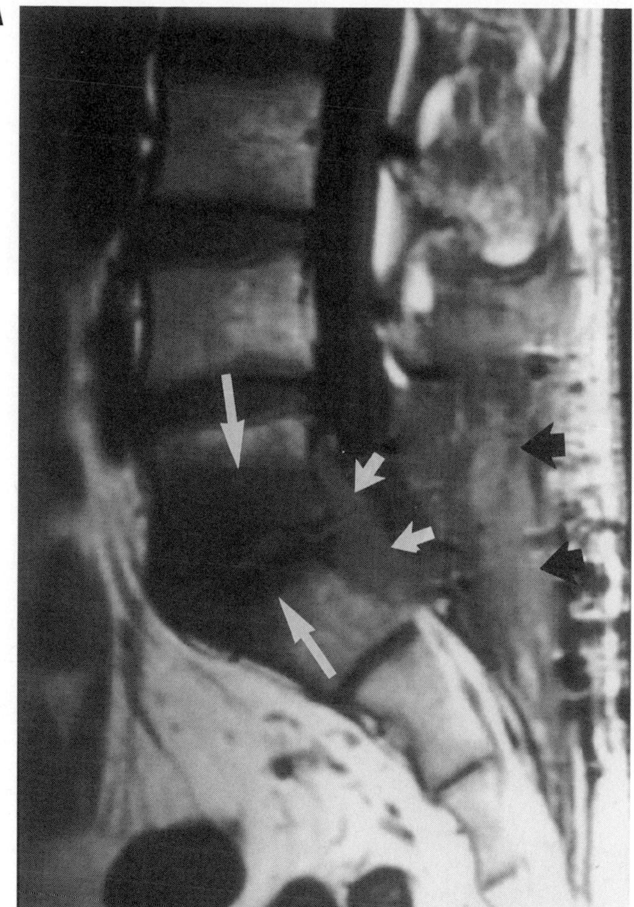

B

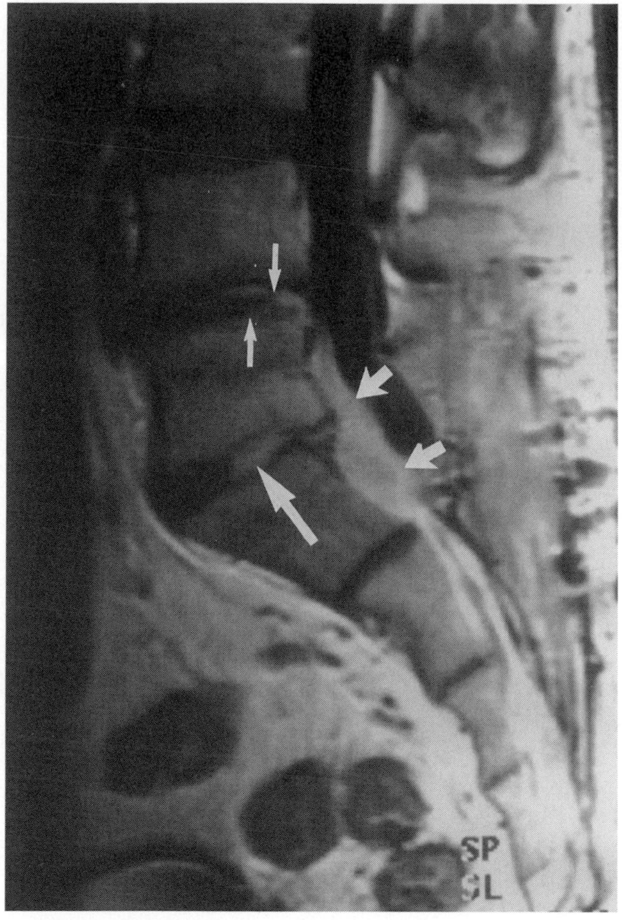

Figure 8-32 **(A)** Sagittal T1-weighted magnetic resonance (MR) image of lumbosacral junction of a patient with low back pain and fever, status is post-laminectomy and diskectomy at L4-5 and L5-S1. Epidural soft tissue mass (*short white arrows*) is noted posterior to the L5-S1 disk space, with soft tissue (*black arrows*) spanning the laminectomy defect. Note edema within bone marrow of L4 and L5 vertebral bodies, shown as dark regions (*long white arrows*). The edema is a manifestation of osteomyelitis. **(B)** Sagittal T1-weighted MR image (same patient as in A) shows gadolinium enhancing the epidural mass (*arrows*) as well as extensively within the L5-S1 disk itself (*small arrows*) and within the laminectomy defect. Diagnosis: L5-S1 diskitis, osteomyelitis, and epidural abscess. Enhancement within laminectomy defect was sterile scar tissue. Note wishbone-shaped enhancement (*tiny arrows*) within the L4-5 disk space, a pattern that is indicative of normal postoperative enhancement within an operated disk space, as compared with the more global disk enhancement suggesting diskitis (at L5-S1 in this case). Finally, note that the marrow edema (marked by *long white arrows* in A) exhibits enhancement. This finding is nonspecific and can be seen in noninfected marrow degenerative change resulting from fibrovascular infiltration of the marrow itself. Such marrow abnormality is a result of disk degeneration. However, in this case, there was surgically proven osteomyelitis.

entire spine be imaged, at least in sagittal plane, with supplemental multiplanar sequences in the area of clinical symptomatology. An epidural abscess may take the form of a pus-filled cavity. In this case, the membrane delimiting the cavity will enhance, whereas the liquefied center will not. Another form of abscess, known as a phlegmon, tends to enhance more uniformly.

VASCULAR ABNORMALITIES

Perhaps the rarest cause of back pain that can mimic symptoms of spinal stenosis is a vascular malformation involving the spinal cord or surrounding dura mater.[33–37] In preparation for either surgical resection or therapeutic embolization of a vascular malformation, selective spinal angiography is an essential diagnostic and therapeutic procedure. However, MRI has supplanted myelography in detection of intramedullary vascular malformations and, often, dural-based arteriovenous fistulas (Fig. 8-33). Formerly thought to be a rare phenomenon, the dural arteriovenous fistula can mimic the symptoms of spinal stenosis. It is imperative to search for such a lesion, particularly in the middle-aged patient, as failure to detect and treat this lesion can lead to progressive para- or quadriplegia secondary to venous infarction of the spinal cord.

CONCLUSION

In most patients suffering from back pain, MRI is the preferred spinal imaging procedure. Nevertheless, this powerful, but expensive tool should be used with discretion, with both reasonable clinical indications for obtaining the study and, where possible, only after failure of conservative treatment strategies. Remembering that

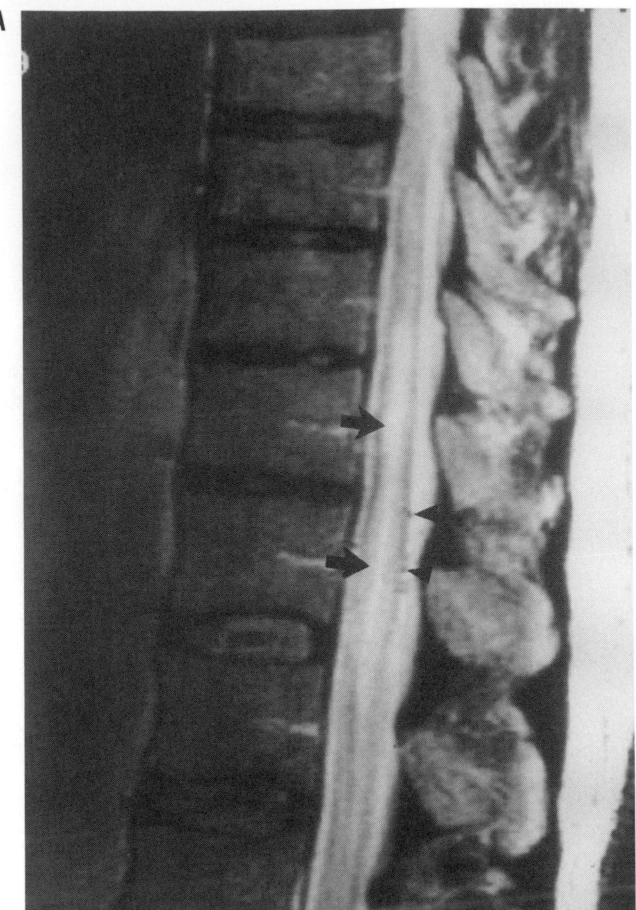

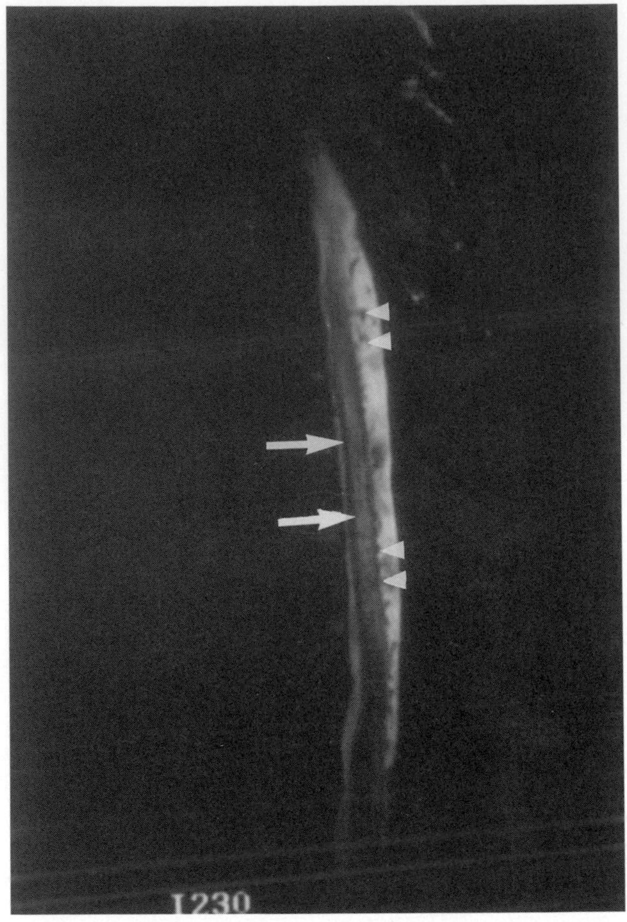

Figure 8-33 **(A)** Sagittal T2-weighted fast spin echo magnetic resonance (MR) image of distal thoracic spine shows edema within the spinal cord *(arrows)* as well as tiny dark regions along the dorsal cord surface (*arrowheads*). The latter finding represents cross-sectional depiction at several turns of a serpiginous draining vein accompanying a dural arteriovenous fistula. The fistula itself is not visualized on this MR study and cannot be seen on MR studies in general, because of its small size and location, generally near a root sleeve. The fistula is thought to cause venous congestion and spinal cord edema as secondary manifestations. The result can be a myelopathy or symptom complex resembling spinal stenosis. These lesions should be searched for in patients who have these symptoms without evidence for typical structural stenosis. Localization and treatment of the fistula itself necessitates selective spinal angiography. **(B)** Sagittal T2-weighted fast spin echo image of distal thoracic spine of another patient showing findings similar to those shown in A, but with a more prominent draining vein dorsal to the cord (*arrowheads*). Spinal cord edema is seen in this case as well (*arrows*). Diagnosis: dural arteriovenous fistula. Although generally found at the thoracolumbar junction of the spine, fistulae can occur anywhere in the spine, even along the clivus, and often far away from the area of venous congestion and spinal cord edema. Therefore, the diagnostic spinal angiogram cannot be considered a complete "search" until all potential feeding vessels, including the vertebral arteries, thyrocervical and costocervical trunks, are injected.

most back pain resolves over time will save many patients an unnecessary imaging study and society at large a considerable savings of valuable health care resources.

REFERENCES

1. Olson PM, Wong WHM, Hesselink JR. Extraspinal abnormalities detected on MR images of the spine. *AJR Am J Roentgenol.* 1994;162: 679–684.
2. Boden SD, Davis DO, Dina TJ. Abnormal magnetic resonance scans of the lumbar spine in asymptomatic subjects. *J Bone Joint Surg Am.* 1990;72:403–408.
3. Jensen MC, Brant-Zawadksi MN, Obuchowski N, et al. Magnetic resonance imaging of the lumbar spine in people without back pain. *N Engl J Med.* 1994;331:69–73.
4. Hackney DB, et al. Hemorrhage and edema in acute spinal cord compression: Demonstration by MR imaging, *Radiology.* 1986;161:387–390.
5. Masaryk T, Ross JS, Modic MT, et al. High resolution MR imaging of sequestered lumbar intervertebral disks. *AJNR Am J Neuroradiol.* 1988; 9:351–358.
6. Snow RD, Williams TP, Weber ED, et al. Enhancing transdural lumbar disc herniation. *Clin Imaging.* 1995;19:12–16.
7. Yock D. *Magnetic Resonance Imaging of the CNS: A Teaching File.* 3rd ed. St. Louis, Mo: CV Mosby; 1994:515.
8. Modic M, Masaryk TJ, Ross JS. *Magnetic Resonance Imaging of the Spine.* 2nd ed. St. Louis, Mo: CV Mosby; 1994:151–190.

9. Ross JS, Obuchowski N, Zepp R. The postoperative lumbar spine: Evaluation of epidural scar over a 1 year period. *AJNR Am J Neuroradiol.* 1998;19:183–186.
10. Ross JS, Robertson JT, Frederickson RL, et al. Association between peridural scar and recurrent radiculopathy after lumbar discectomy: Magnetic resonance evaluation. *Neurosurgery.* 1996:38:885–861.
11. Ross JS, Zepp R, Modic MT. The postoperative lumbar spine: Enhanced MR evaluation of the intervertebral disc. *AJNR Am J Neuroradiol.* 1996;17:323–331.
12. Osti OL, Fraser RD. MRI and discography in anular tears and intervertebral disc degeneration. A prospective clinical comparison. *J Bone Joint Surg Br.* 1992;74:431–435.
13. Linson MA, Crowe CH. Comparison of magnetic resonance imaging and lumbar discography in the diagnosis of disc degeneration. *Clin Orthop.* 1990;250:160–163.
14. Min K, Leu HJ, Perrenoud A. Discography with manometry and discographic CT; their value in patient selection for percutaneous lumbar nucleotomy. *Bull Hosp Jt Dis.* 1996;54:153–157.
15. Gibson MJ, Buckley J, Mawhinney R, et al. Magnetic resonance imaging and discography in the diagnosis of disc degeneration. A comparative study of 50 discs. *J Bone Joint Surg Br.* 1986;68:369-673.
16. Algra PR, Bloem JL, Tissing H, et al. Detection of vertebral metastases: Comparison between MR imaging and bone scintigraphy. *Radiographics.* 1991;11:219–232.
17. Carmody RF, Yang PJ, Seeley GW, et al. Spinal cord compression due to metastatic disease: Diagnosis with MR imaging versus myelography. *Radiology.* 1989;173:225–229.
18. Smoker WRK, et al. Role of MR imaging in evaluating metastatic spinal disease. *AJNR Am J Neuroradiol.* 1987;8:901–908.
19. Williams MP, Cherryman GR, Husband JE. Magnetic resonance imaging in suspected metastatic spinal cord compression. *Clin Radiol.* 1989;40:186–290.
20. Lien HH, Blomlie V, Heimdal KL. Magnetic resonance imaging of malignant extradural tumors with acute spinal cord compression. *Acta Radiol.* 1990;31:187–190.
21. Avrahami E, Tadmor R, Dally O, et al. Early MR demonstration of spinal metastases in patients with normal radiographs and radionuclide bone scans. *J Comput Assist Tomogr.* 1989;13:598–602.
22. Yousem DM, Patrone PM, Grossman RI. Leptomeningeal metastases: MR evaluation. *J Comput Assist Tomogr.* 1990;14:255–261.
23. Dillon WP, et al. Intradural spinal cord lesions: Gd-DTPA-enhanced MR imaging. *Radiology.* 1989;170:229–238.
24. Elster AD. Radiologic screening in the neurocutaneous syndromes: Strategies and controversies. *AJNR Am J Neuroradiol.* 1992;13:1078–1082.
25. Poser CM. The relationship between syringomyelia and neoplasm. In: *American Lecture Series No. 262. American Lectures in Neurology.* Springfield, Ill: Charles C Thomas; 1956.
26. Wolpert SM, et al. Chiari II malformation: MR imaging evaluation. *AJNR Am J Neuroradiol.* 1987;8:783–792.
27. Barnes PD, Lester PD, Yamanashi WS, Prince JR. Magnetic resonance imaging in infants and children with spinal dysraphism. *AJNR Am J Neuroradiol.* 1986;7:465–472.
28. Matthews WB. Clinical symptoms and signs. In: Matthews WB, Acheson ED, Batchelor JR, Weller RO, eds. *McAlpine's Multiple Sclerosis.* Edinburgh, Scotland: Churchill Livingstone; 1985.
29. Edwards MK, Farlow MR, Stevens JC. Cranial MR in spinal cord MS: Diagnosing patients with isolated spinal cord symptoms. *AJNR Am J Neuroradiol.* 1986;7:1003–1006.
30. Schweitzer ME, Cervilla V, Resnick D. Acute cervical trauma: correlation of MR imaging findings with neurologic deficit. *Radiology.* 1991:179:287–288.
31. Post MJD, Sze G, Quencer RM, et al. Gadolinium-enhanced MR in spinal infection. *J Comput Assist Tomogr.* 1990:14:721–729.
32. Angtuaco EJC, McConnell JR, Chaddock WM, et al. MR imaging of spinal epidural sepsis. *AJNR Am J Neuroradiol.* 1987;8:879–883.
33. Rosenblum B, Oldfield EH, Doppman JL, et al. Spinal arteriovenous malformations: A comparison of dural arteriovenous fistulas and intradural AVMs in 81 patients. *J Neurosurg.* 1987;67:795–802.
34. Symon L, Kuyama H, Kendall B. Dural arteriovenous malformations of the spine: Clinical features and surgical results in 55 cases. *J Neurosurg.* 1984;60:238–247.
35. Masaryk TJ, Ross JS, Modic MT, et al. Radiculomeningeal vascular malformations of the spine: MR imaging. *Radiology.* 1987:164:845–849.
36. Terwey B, Becker H, Thron AK, Vahldiek G. Gadolinium DTPA enhanced MR imaging of spinal dural arteriovenous fistulas. *J Comput Assist Tomogr.* 1989:13:30–37.
37. Larsson E-M, Desai P, Hardin CW, et al. Venous infarction of the spinal cord resulting from dural arteriovenous fistula: MR imaging findings. *AJNR Am J Neuroradiol.* 1991:12:739–743.

CHAPTER 9

ROLE OF ELECTRODIAGNOSTICS IN PAIN ASSESSMENT

Seward B. Rutkove and Seth H. Lichtenstein

Electrodiagnosis can play a crucial role in identifying the underlying problem in a patient presenting with a pain disorder. Although electrodiagnostic testing is older than some radiologic modalities such as magnetic resonance imaging (MRI), it provides unique functional information about the integrity of both the central and peripheral nervous systems. In addition to localizing the problem, electrodiagnostic testing can give insight into its chronicity and severity, while often also providing helpful prognostic information. Although minor structural abnormalities may be readily identified on MRI, their clinical significance may be uncertain. For example, disk bulges at multiple levels are routinely found on MRI studies of the lumbar spine. Electrodiagnostic testing has the unique ability to determine whether one of these bulges is actually producing nerve damage. Moreover, such testing may also demonstrate abnormalities in patients with inflammatory lesions, where neuroimaging is often normal.

In general, electrodiagnostic testing encompasses nerve conduction studies (NCSs) and electromyography (EMG), which together provide information about the peripheral nerves and muscles, and evoked potentials, which are used predominantly for evaluation of the central nervous system. Other tests, including intraoperative monitoring, autonomic function testing, and analysis of movement disorders, also fall under the rubric of electrodiagnostic testing, but generally have a limited role in the evaluation of pain disorders.

In the first part of this chapter, we review the methodology and interpretation of electrodiagnostic studies in general. As only a limited summary is provided, additional information regarding this complex topic may be obtained from several excellent texts.[1–3] In the second part of the chapter, we examine the usefulness of electrophysiologic testing in specific neurologic disorders associated with pain.

ELECTRODIAGNOSTIC STUDIES: METHODS AND INTERPRETATION

Nerve Conduction Studies

NCSs and EMG are usually performed at the same session because the procedures are complementary, each providing unique information about the peripheral nerves and muscles. Generally, NCSs are performed before EMG, with the results of the NCSs used to guide the needle electrode examination. NCSs provide quantitative information, whereas EMG, as performed in its standard fashion, is more subjective.

Only a few nerves are routinely studied. In the arms, these nerves include the median, radial, and ulnar, and in the legs, posterior tibial, deep peroneal, and sural. The facial and trigeminal nerves can also be studied. All of these nerves are easily accessible to stimulation and are commonly involved in neurogenic illness. A number of additional nerves, including musculocutaneous, superficial peroneal, and saphenous, are studied less often but are sometimes helpful in localizing a lesion.

Motor Nerve Conduction Studies When performing motor studies, an active recording electrode is placed over a muscle belly and a referential recording electrode is placed over the tendon insertion of that muscle. The nerve is then stimulated at a fixed distance from the muscle (Fig. 9-1). The electrical response represents the depolarization of the muscle beneath the active electrode relative to the referential electrode (Fig. 9-2). Stimulus intensity is gradually increased until the motor response (the compound motor action potential [CMAP]) no longer increases in amplitude. Stimulation is then performed at a second, more proximal site.

Latencies and amplitudes are identified for each stimulation site. By subtracting the latency of the distal stimulation site from that of the proximal and dividing by the distance between them, a conduction velocity for that nerve segment is obtained. A conduction velocity for the distal segment (between distal stimulation site and muscle) cannot be obtained because of delays inherent to the neuromuscular junction and the depolarization of the muscle fibers.

F responses are also recorded during motor studies. F responses (named for the foot, where they were first identified) are after discharges that occur normally in motor nerves. When the nerve is stimulated as described earlier, depolarization of the axon actually progresses both distally and proximally. Whereas the distal depolarization produces the motor response described earlier, the proximal depolarization reaches the spinal cord, producing a backfiring of a few motor neurons and resulting in a new descending nerve depolarization. Eventually, this small depolarization reaches the muscle, producing the F response. F-response testing allows for the integrity of the entire motor nerve to be evaluated.

Sensory Nerve Conduction Studies In antidromic sensory studies, active and reference electrodes are placed over a distal nerve segment and the nerve is stimulated proximally (Fig. 9-3). Alternatively, the distal portion of the nerve may be stimulated with proximal recording (orthodromic studies). Similar to motor recordings, stimulation intensity is gradually increased until maximal sensory response amplitude is obtained (Fig. 9-4). Unlike motor studies, stimulation at a second site is usually not performed because a distal conduction velocity can be calculated using the first site alone. Also, for complex reasons, when recording over longer segments of nerve, sensory response amplitudes decrease profoundly, making them difficult to record with proximal stimulation. Even with distal stimulation only, sensory responses are about 100 to 1000 times smaller than motor responses, necessitating the use of digital averaging.

Reflex Studies Reflex studies refer to electrical tests in which sensory nerve fibers are stimulated and motor responses are

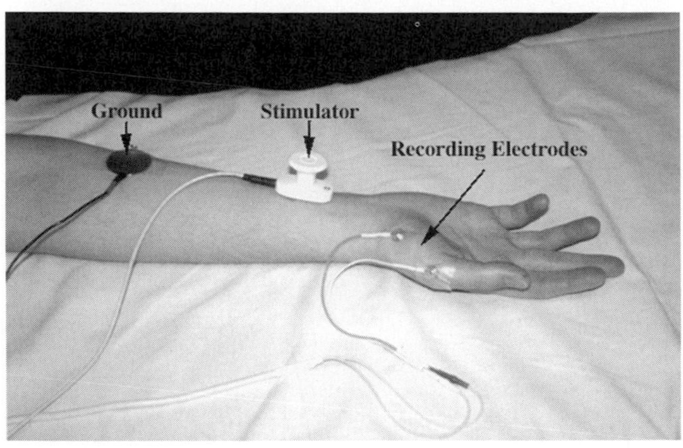

Figure 9-1 Standard setup for median motor nerve conduction study, with stimulator at the wrist and recording electrodes over abductor pollicis brevis.

recorded. The two most frequently performed are the soleus H-reflex and the blink reflex. The soleus H-reflex (named after Hoffman, who first described it) is essentially the electrical equivalent of the ankle jerk. To obtain this reflex, *sub*maximal stimulation in the popliteal fossa is used to depolarize selectively the large IA afferent fibers of the posterior tibial nerve. The sensory neurons depolarize to the level of the dorsal horn, which in turn produce a depolarization in the motor neurons of the anterior horn and a contraction of the soleus muscle that is recorded.

In the blink reflex, stimulation of the first division of the trigeminal nerve (supraorbital nerve) is performed while recording simultaneously from bilateral orbicularis oculi muscles. Two responses are recorded: a local monosynaptic one and, later, one produced through more diffuse, bilateral polysynaptic connections. This test allows for the integrity of the fifth and seventh cranial nerves, including their central connections, to be evaluated.

Electromyography

As with NCSs, EMG requires reference and active electrodes to record electrical signals. In the case of concentric needles, the active electrode is at the tip while the barrel makes up the reference. Monopolar needles, in which the active tip of the needle is referenced against a separate skin electrode, are also used. Both are usually of small diameter, corresponding to about a 27-gauge phlebotomy needle. The needle is attached to an oscilloscope with an amplifier, allowing the electromyographer to evaluate the muscle by both observing waveforms and listening to their characteristic sounds.

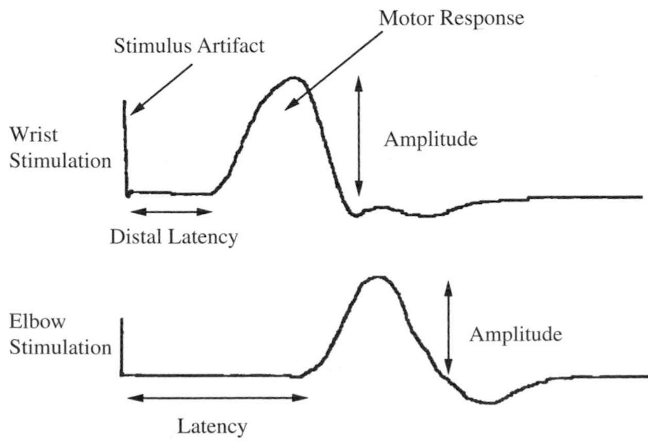

Figure 9-2 Median motor responses recording from both wrist and elbow.

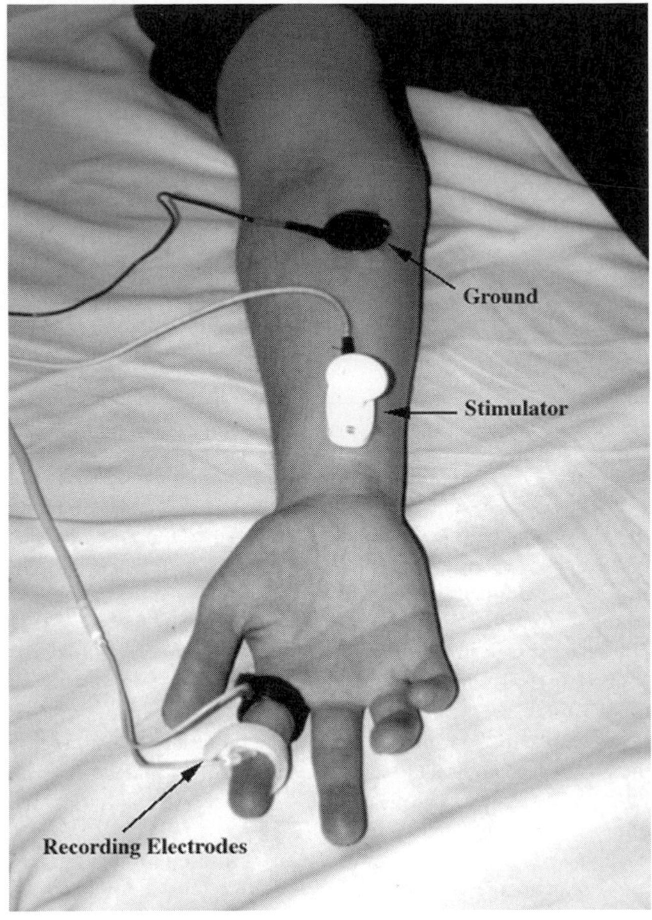

Figure 9-3 Standard setup for median antidromic sensory conduction study, with stimulator at the wrist and recording electrodes on digit 2.

There are two basic parts to EMG: evaluation of spontaneous activity and evaluation of the motor unit action potentials (MUAPs). To evaluate spontaneous activity, the patient is asked to keep the limb as relaxed as possible. The physician then makes small movements with the needle. Normal muscle should remain stable and silent after needle movement. If the muscle fiber membrane is electrically unstable, fibrillation potentials or positive sharp waves may be present (Fig. 9-5). Occasionally, other abnormal discharges may be identified.

After evaluating for spontaneous activity, the patient is asked to perform a gentle isometric muscle contraction. The electromyographer observes and listens to the MUAPs, which are produced by the electrical firing of groups of muscle fibers innervated by single motor axons (motor units). Abnormally enlarged MUAPs suggest chronic neurogenic disease, whereas small ones most frequently suggest a primary muscle disorder (Fig. 9-6). In addition to these basic abnormalities, the electromyographer evaluates the "recruitment" of motor units. Normally, with increasing effort, ad-

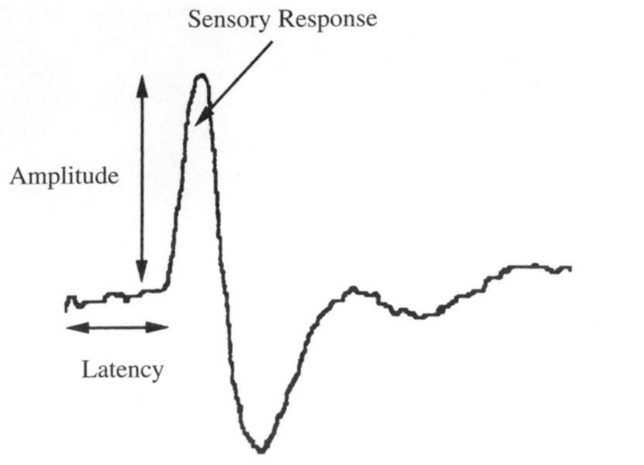

Figure 9-4 Antirdomic median sensory response recording from digit 2.

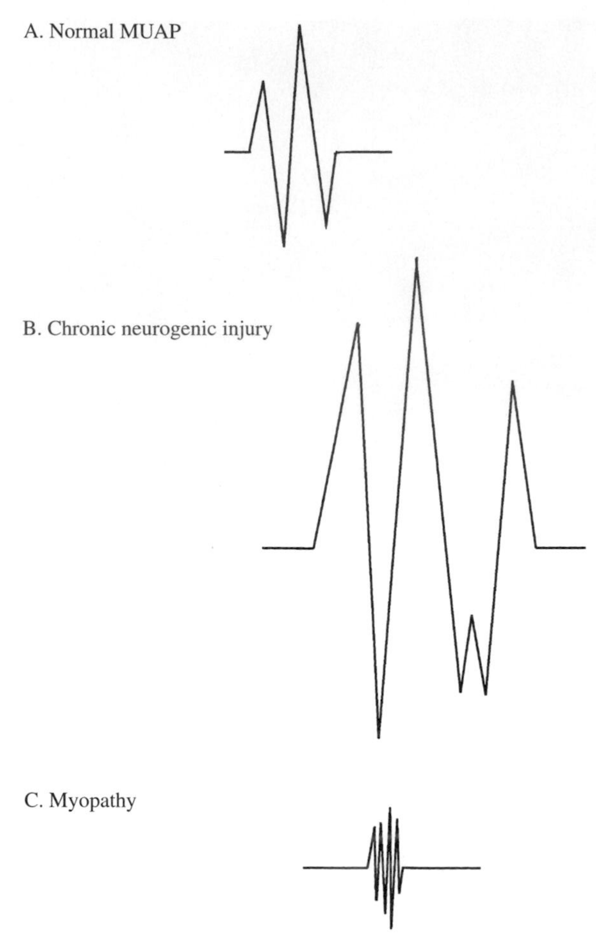

Figure 9-6 Motor unit action potential (MUAP) morphology. (**A**) Normal MUAP. (**B**) Loss of neighboring motor neurons resulting from neurogenic injury has caused the remaining MUAPs to increase in size over normal, with increased amplitude, duration, and phases. (**C**) Loss and injury to muscle fibers in a myopathy produces MUAPs with reduced amplitude, duration, and increases phases.

ditional motor units are "recruited" into the contraction until the oscilloscope screen fills up with dozens of motor units (Fig. 9-7). In patients with neurogenic disease, fewer motor units are present, so that with increasing effort, the functioning units fire faster than normal, compensating for their missing counterparts. This is described as reduced recruitment. In extreme cases, only one motor unit may remain, firing up to five times as fast as normal. In patients with a primary muscle disease, the opposite occurs, because the number of motor units is relatively normal, but their size is reduced as a result of muscle fiber loss. Hence, with only minimal effort, many motor units fire.

Finally, activation is also examined. Activation is the term used to describe the central nervous system drive involved in contracting a muscle. This drive, whether reduced by true central pathology or simply poor effort, will look identical on EMG: only a few motor units fire no matter how hard the patient seems to try. Unlike reduced recruitment, however, the firing rate for a given motor unit does not increase above normal.

Somatosensory Evoked Potentials

Somatosensory evoked potentials (SSEPs) are one of several electrophysiologic tests that can be used to evaluate central nervous system function. Brainstem auditory evoked potentials and visual evoked potentials are the other two routine studies, but have minimal relevance in the evaluation of pain disorders.

Although still performed regularly in many clinical sittings, with the advent of MRI scanning over the past 10 to 15 years, the utility of these SSEPs has decreased significantly. For example, previously in patients with symptoms of possible cervical myelopathy (e.g., secondary to a demyelinating plaque from multiple sclerosis), SSEPs may have been the only means for detecting an abnormality in the region. Today, however, MRI scanning is so sensitive and specific that even small areas of demyelination can be detected within the spinal cord.

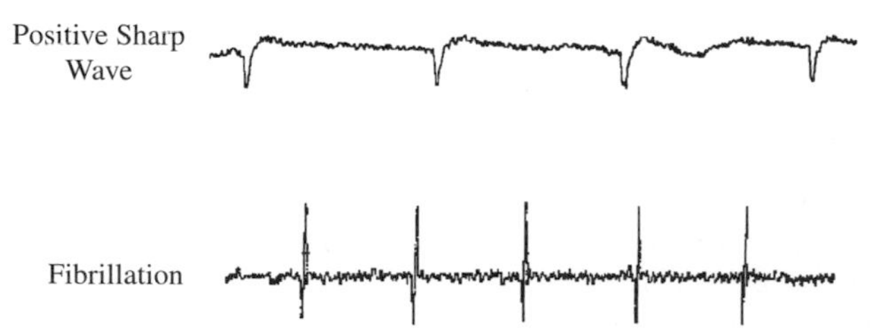

Figure 9-5 Positive sharp waves and fibrillations.

SSEPs are performed by electrically stimulating nerves in the upper or lower extremities (generally median or ulnar nerves in the arm and tibial nerve in the leg) and recording responses over the lumbar spine, cervical spine, Erb's point, and over the scalp. Electrical responses can be detected at these different sites (Fig. 9-8). As the responses are very small, hundreds of individual recordings are digitally averaged. Generally, these responses should have relatively fixed latencies. If the latency prolongs significantly between two recording sites, a structural or demyelinating lesion may be present. For example, after stimulating the tibial nerve, an N22 peak (negative peak with a latency of 22 milliseconds) may be identified in the lumbar spine and an N30 peak in the cervical spine. Normally these should be about 8 msec apart (N30–N22). However, if the N30 peak falls at 36 msec, then a delay is present. This would suggest a lesion somewhere between the cervical and

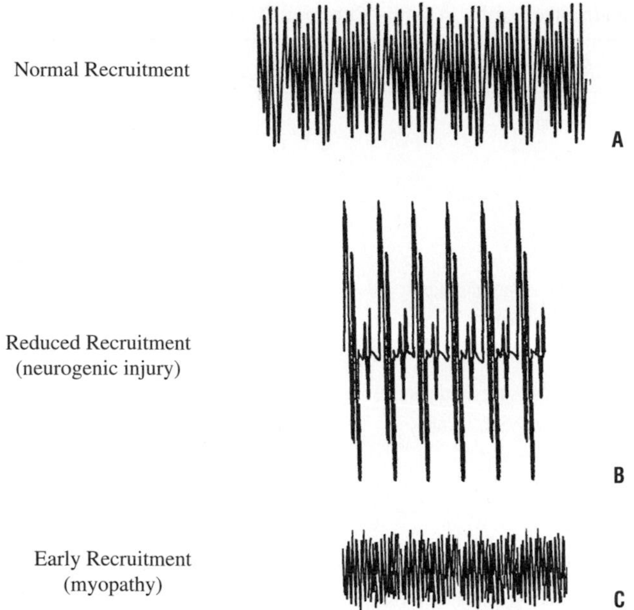

Figure 9-7 Recruitment of MUAPs. (**A**) Normal recruitment. (**B**) Reduced recruitment, as seen in neurogenic injury. Because fewer motor units are present, to produce a muscle contraction with the greatest force, the remaining motor units muscle fire more rapidly. In this case, two motor units remain. (**C**) Early recruitment. In this example, the patient's muscles are minimally contracting, yet many small motor units are brought into the contraction to produce some force.

lumbar spine. Similarly radiculopathies, plexopathies, or more rostral problems, such as brainstem tumor, can be identified by prolongation of latency. Amplitudes may also decrease if abnormalities are severe.

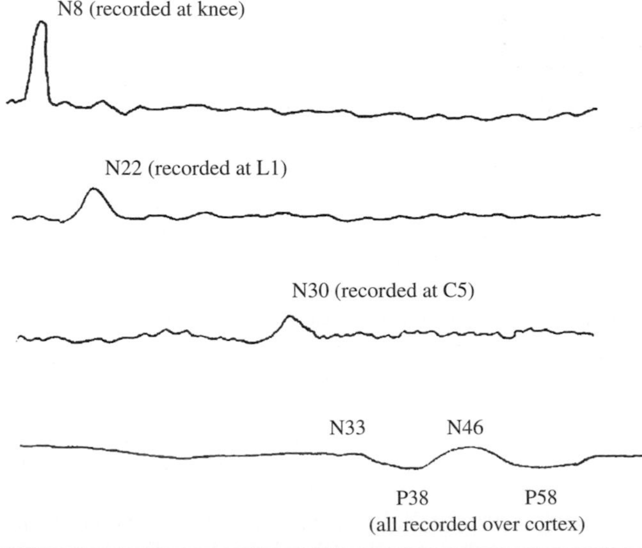

Figure 9-8 Tibial somatosensory evoked potentials, recording from popliteal fossa, lumbar spine, cervical spine, and brain.

ELECTRODIAGNOSIS OF SPECIFIC DISORDERS

Radiculopathy

One of the most frequent reasons for referring a patient to the electrodiagnostic laboratory is for the evaluation of radiculopathy. In addition to identifying which root or roots are the most likely involved, electrodiagnostic testing will also provide insight into the severity and chronicity of the lesion (Table 9-1). Although the sensitivity of EMG in the diagnosis of radiculopathy is less than that of MRI, its specificity is significantly better.[4–6]

In general, NCSs play a limited role in the electrodiagnosis of radiculopathy. Rather, they are used to exclude other processes, such as compression mononeuropathy or plexopathy. In radiculopathy, sensory NCSs are normal, as compression of the nerve root occurs proximal to the dorsal root ganglion. Although motor NCSs may show mild reductions in response amplitude and distal conduction velocity if radiculopathy is severe, these studies are often normal as well, because a given muscle contains contributions from multiple roots, obscuring disease at only one level. F-response prolongation and, in S1 radiculopathy, H-reflex prolongation are also helpful, though nonspecific, findings.

The diagnosis of radiculopathy relies primarily on the electromyographic examination. In a subacute, single nerve root lesion, fibrillations and positive waves will be present in multiple muscles of that myotome. Sampling of additional muscles both proximally and distally in the extremity as well as those innervated by other nerve roots is also performed in order to "frame" the lesion while excluding other possible etiologies, such as mononeuropathy or polyneuropathy. Paraspinal muscles are also routinely examined; abnormalities in these muscles help confirm the presence of a root lesion.

There is a well-described time course for the development of abnormalities after a root injury. Immediately at the time of injury, the only abnormality identifiable on EMG is reduced recruitment of motor units in muscles innervated by that root. By the end of the first week after injury, positive waves and fibrillations will begin to appear in adjacent paraspinal muscles. It may take 3 to 4 more weeks before fibrillation potentials and positive waves are identified in the most distal extremity muscles. Once present, these abnormalities will persist until reinnervation is complete, which can take up to 2 years.

There are a number of important limitations to the electrophysiologic evaluation of radiculopathy. Firstly, not all muscles may be equally affected by a nerve root compression; if the electromyographer happens to study one or two that are relatively uninvolved, the lesion may be missed. Another limitation occurs from the fact that myotomes often overlap in muscles, preventing exact localization of the nerve root level. For example, it may be difficult to differentiate a C5 radiculopathy from a C6, given that most of the muscles typically studied, including deltoid and biceps, are supplied by both nerve roots. In addition, preferential compression and inflammation of the dorsal root with associated pain may produce few EMG abnormalities, as the diagnosis of radiculopathy depends on loss of motor neurons in the ventral root. This is sometimes the case in patients who present with exquisitely painful diabetic radiculopathies. Finally, in very mild radiculopathy where there is no axonal loss and only demyelination at the level of the root, few abnormalities will be identified.

TABLE 9-1 **Summary of Abnormalities on Nerve Conduction Studies and Electromyography in Some Common Disorders**

Disorder	Motor Studies	F and H Responses	Sensory Studies	EMG
Radiculopathy	Usually normal; occasional reduction in amplitude if severe and muscle studied is derived from affected root	Mild to moderate prolongation of F and H response latencies	Normal	Reinnervation and PSWs and fibrillations in muscles supplied by that root
Axonal polyneuropathy	Reduced amplitude in distal muscles of feet	Mild to moderate prolongation of F and H responses	Reduced amplitude of distal nerves (e.g., sural)	Reinnervation and PSWs and fibrillations in distal muscles
Demyelinating polyneuropathy	Variable amplitude reduction; severe slowing of conduction velocity; prolongation of distal latency	Severe prolongation; absence of F and H responses from multiple nerves	Reduced amplitude and conduction velocity	Variable degrees of chronic reinnervation and fibrillations and PSWs; reduced recruitment of motor units
Compression neuropathy	Focal conduction velocity slowing across affected segment if mild; reduction in amplitude if severe	Mild prolongation in F responses	Slowing of conduction velocity across affected segment; reduction in amplitude if severe	Reinnervation and PSWs and fibrillations in muscles supplied by that nerve
Plexopathy	Reduced amplitude in muscles supplied by affected fibers	Mild to moderate prolongation of F and H response latencies	Reduced amplitude in sensory nerves traversing affected part of plexus	Reinnervation and PSWs and fibrillations in muscles supplied by affected fibers
Mononeuropathy multiplex	Focal "axonal" lesions of multiple nerves with markedly decreased amplitude	Mild prolongation or absence of F and H responses	Reduced or absent responses in affected nerves	Marked abnormalities in muscles supplied by affected nerve

EMG, electromyography; PSWs, positive sharp waves.

SSEPs are theoretically useful in the diagnosis of radiculopathy. Prolongation of latency when recording from the lower back in lumbosacral radiculopathy and from the neck in cervical radiculopathy may suggest root disease. However, compared with EMG/NCS, SSEPs usually serve only a minor role in evaluating this diagnostic possibility.[7]

Polyneuropathy

Electrodiagnostic testing, especially NCSs, is especially helpful in accurately diagnosing polyneuropathy. These studies can help determine the pathology of the process, whether both sensory and motor nerves are involved, and its severity and chronicity (see Table 9-1).

The electrical abnormalities generally fall into two broad categories: axonal and demyelinating injury. Demyelination reduces the effectiveness of saltatory conduction, prolonging distal latencies and F responses and causing profound slowing of conduction velocity. Temporal dispersion, the abnormal broadening of the responses, also occurs as the conduction velocity of individual fibers variably slows. In addition, with severe demyelination, neuronal conduction may actually be completely impeded. Termed *conduction block*, this finding represents the ultimate result of myelin injury. Although demyelinating polyneuropathies are uncommon and pain more mild, these disorders are usually treatable with immune-modulating therapies.

Axonal polyneuropathy occurs when there is primary injury to the axon itself, rather than the myelin sheath. In this situation, the predominant abnormality on NCSs is reduction in response amplitudes. Nerves of the lower extremities tend to be preferentially affected in most axonal polyneuropathies given the length-dependent nature of the process.[8] As the fastest conducting fibers are often lost, there is usually a mild prolongation of distal latency and slowing of conduction velocity, although not to the degree of that seen with demyelinating injury. With increasing severity of axonal injury, the response can become undetectable. This process is often more prominent on sensory conduction studies than motor, because sensory amplitudes are much smaller than motor responses at baseline. Axonal polyneuropathies are often associated with diabetes mellitus, alcohol use, late-stage human immunodeficiency virus (HIV) infection, and chemotherapy.[9]

On EMG examination of an axonal polyneuropathy, a gradient of abnormalities, with distal musculature being more affected than proximal, is usually found. EMG may show fibrillations and positive waves as well as enlarged motor units, depending on its time course. In demyelinating polyneuropathies, abnormalities may be present in many muscles, and a distal-to-proximal gradient is usually less evident.

Although electrodiagnostic testing is extremely important in the evaluation of polyneuropathy, it has limitations. First, a specific etiology for the process cannot be identified; instead, only the type of process (i.e., axonal versus demyelinating) can be described. In addition, standard NCSs only examine the largest, myelinated nerve fibers. Patients with painful neuropathies that affect predominantly small, thinly myelinated and unmyelinated fibers may have entirely normal NCSs. The sympathetic skin response can get at this problem by measuring autonomic function in the hand and foot.[10] Unfortunately, however, this is a rather crude test that is not well quantified. Additional autonomic testing, including the quantitative sudomotor axon reflex test (QSART), may be helpful but may not be routinely available. More recently, intraepidermal nerve fiber counts have become available to also evaluate these small neurons.

Compression Neuropathy

Compression neuropathies occur when a segment of nerve is compressed at an anatomically vulnerable site, producing focal demyelination and, if severe enough, axonal degeneration. These nerve lesions are usually accompanied by pain, with symptoms that may be severe despite only mild nerve irritation. NCSs and EMG are generally extremely effective in characterizing this form of nerve injury (see Table 9-1).

Carpal tunnel syndrome, caused by entrapment of the median nerve as it traverses through a bony tunnel in the wrist, is by far the most common compression neuropathy. The predominant abnormalities in this disorder include slowing of the sensory conduction velocity and prolongation of the distal motor latency. When these results are not clearly abnormal, studying a shorter segment of median nerve across the wrist, only, and comparing it with the same region of ulnar nerve can be extremely helpful. This approach helps eliminate other variables that may slow velocity, such as mild polyneuropathy or reduced hand temperature. EMG of the extremity can be very helpful, in both assessing severity of the lesion (by looking for abnormalities in abductor pollicis brevis) and excluding a superimposed cervical radiculopathy.[11]

Ulnar neuropathy usually occurs at the elbow, with focal demyelination at either the humeral epicondylar groove or slightly more distally in the cubital tunnel, as the nerve passes through the flexor carpi ulnaris muscle. The ulnar motor nerve conduction study is the most important part of this investigation, because focal slowing of motor conduction velocity across the elbow segment, occasionally with conduction block, may be demonstrated. In more severe cases, a reduction in distal ulnar sensory and motor response amplitudes may also occur as axonal loss ensues. Identifying the exact area of entrapment within the elbow segment is usually difficult, and, because the treatments are similar, not generally attempted. EMG of ulnar-innervated muscles may show fibrillations and positive waves, as well as enlarged motor units. As with carpal tunnel syndrome, in very mild cases all studies may be normal, often disproportionate to the patient's symptoms. Near-nerve studies, incorporating the use of needle electrodes proximal and distal to the presumed site of compression, can demonstrate abnormalities when standard surface studies are entirely normal.[12]

The two most common sites of entrapment of the radial nerve occur at the spiral groove of the humerus and in the upper forearm at the arcade of Frohse ("Saturday night palsy" and the posterior interosseous syndrome, respectively). Compression at the spiral groove produces wrist drop, weakness of finger extension, and sensory loss over the dorsum of the hand. NCSs may demonstrate conduction velocity slowing with or without associated conduction block across the spiral groove. Entrapment of the posterior interosseous nerve at the arcade of Frohse is often accompanied by prominent, poorly localized forearm pain. If the lesion is severe enough, slowing of conduction velocity across the arcade can be demonstrated.

In the lower extremity, the most common compression neuropathy is a peroneal neuropathy at the fibular head, usually presenting as foot drop and numbness or paresthesias in the dermatomal distribution of the peroneal nerve. Motor NCSs generally reveal slowing of conduction velocity with or without conduction block across the fibular neck. EMG helps to localize the process by excluding L5 radiculopathy or sciatic neuropathy as the source of symptoms.

In patients with foot pain, especially when associated with plantar paresthesias and sensory loss, the possibility of tarsal tunnel syndrome is often raised. This rarely diagnosed malady occurs when the tibial nerve is compressed under the flexor retinaculum at the medial malleolus. Electrophysiologic evaluation includes demonstration of a prolonged tibial motor distal latency and slowing of conduction velocity on additional studies, such as recording at the ankle when stimulating the medial and lateral plantar nerves in the midsole.[13] If only one foot is affected, comparisons can be made with the unaffected side. If pain is present in both feet, convincingly identifying entrapment at the tarsal tunnel becomes much more difficult because mild polyneuropathy may also produce similar electrophysiologic abnormalities. EMG in the affected foot musculature is useful only when compared with the unaffected side, because enlargement of motor units and positive sharp waves are present even in most normal feet.

A controversial cause of pain, the piriformis syndrome, may be considered in patients presenting with complaints of pain and paresthesias in the gluteal region that radiate in a sciatic distribution. Pain can be reproduced by applying pressure over the sciatic notch, where the nerve is thought to be compressed by the piriformis muscle.[14] H-reflex latency has been found to be prolonged in some individuals with this disorder[15]; however, definite electrophysiologic abnormalities are rare. EMG is helpful in excluding other processes (namely L5 or S1 radiculopathies).

Plexopathy

Common causes of plexopathy include compression due to mass lesion, inflammation, radiation-induced injury, and, in the upper extremities, traction injury. Electrodiagnostic studies can be especially helpful in localizing the lesion to a particular region of the plexus and assessing its severity and chronicity[16] (see Table 9-1).

In evaluation of a plexus injury, intimate knowledge of the anatomy of myotomes, dermatomes, and peripheral nerve distribution is required to exclude other processes, such as a radiculopathy or proximal neuropathy. In an investigation of brachial plexopathy, a combination of NCSs and EMG is performed to localize the lesion to a particular cord or trunk. Although motor response amplitudes may drop in plexopathy, reductions in sensory response amplitudes are especially helpful because they demonstrate that the lesion is distal to the dorsal root ganglion, hence, helping to exclude a root lesion. Both routine and less commonly performed studies can help localize a lesion. For example, in an upper trunk lesion, the musculocutaneous sensory nerve response may have reduced amplitude whereas in a lower trunk injury, reduction in the ulnar and medial antebrachial cutaneous sensory responses is common. Careful comparisons to the contralateral, uninvolved arm are also extremely helpful, because amplitudes should remain at least 40% to 50% of the normal side. When evaluating the lumbosacral plexus, along with routine studies, the saphenous and superficial peroneal sensory nerves are studied.

EMG further localizes the lesion by looking for abnormalities in muscles supplied by a particular branch or cord of the plexus. Needle examination can exclude a distal peripheral nerve injury by documenting abnormalities in muscles supplied by more than one nerve. In addition, evaluation of shoulder muscles can be very helpful in distinguishing an upper trunk or lateral cord injury from a C5-6 radiculopathy. In some situations, such as stretch injury with root avulsion, the findings may support simultaneous radiculopathy and plexopathy. Severity of the lesion can also be judged by the profusion of fibrillation potentials and positive sharp waves and the number of motor units that can be recruited. Finally, an unusual spontaneous discharge on EMG, called a myokymic discharge, may help support the diagnosis of a radiation-induced injury.[17]

Although SSEPs can be used in the evaluation of plexopathy, as with radiculopathy, the combination of NCSs with EMG generally is more helpful.

One special case of brachial plexopathy is thoracic outlet syndrome. In neurogenic thoracic outlet syndrome, a fibrous band from a cervical rib to the first thoracic rib impinges on the lower trunk of the plexus. This produces an unusual constellation of abnormalities, including reduced ulnar sensory and median and ulnar motor responses.[18] EMG generally demonstrates abnormalities most severe in abductor pollicis brevis. In patients with vascular thoracic outlet syndrome (generally diagnosed in patients with chronic arm and shoulder pain, reduced radial pulse with external rotation and abduction of the arm [Wright maneuver], with or without a cervical rib, but no neurologic signs), electrophysiologic testing is normal.

Mononeuropathy Multiplex

This disorder, which is usually associated with vasculitic conditions such as Churg-Strauss syndrome and polyarteritis nodosa, is associated with multiple acute painful mononeuropathies. In addition to weakness and sensory loss, pain can be severe in affected limbs. NCSs and EMG generally demonstrate abnormalities consistent with multiple severe axonal mononeuropathies (see Table 9-1). Rather than slowing across a site of entrapment, complete loss of the motor and sensory responses for that nerve with marked fibrillation potentials and positive waves in affected muscles is usually found.[19] In long-standing cases, multiple mononeuropathies in the legs may become confluent, producing the picture of a severe axonal polyneuropathy.

Myopathy

Most muscle diseases have only limited pain associated with them.[20] However, in some disorders, such as the metabolic myopathies (including McArdle's disease and phosphofructokinase deficiency) pain can be brought on with exercise. Generally, NCSs reveal minimal abnormalities in myopathies. Occasionally, if severe, reductions in motor response amplitude may occur. On EMG, short-duration, low-amplitude motor units with early recruitment are observed. Spontaneous activity, including fibrillation potentials and positive waves, is also common in many inflammatory, toxic, and congenital myopathies. Finally, the presence of myotonia can limit the diagnostic possibilities to one of the myotonic disorders, such as myotonic dystrophy.

Disorders of the Perineal Region

Occasionally, patients present with neuropathic pain involving the perineal region. A number of possible diagnoses are often raised, including lumbar radiculopathy, with pain referred into the distribution of the ilioinguinal nerve; ilioinguinal or genitofemoral neuropathies; S2 to S4 radiculopathy, with pain referred to the genitalia; and pudendal neuropathy, occasional secondary to trauma (such as repeated bike riding in men).[21,22]

Although not often pursued, neurophysiologic testing in this region can be helpful in reaching a diagnosis. Standard studies of the lower extremities can help identify a lumbar or S1-2 radiculopathy; in a low sacral radiculopathy (e.g., S2–S4), fibrillation potentials in the associated paraspinal muscles and in the anal sphincter may be found. Unfortunately, ilioinguinal and genitofemoral neuropathies are extremely difficult to evaluate. Pudendal nerve integrity can be examined using the electrical bulbocavernosus reflex.[23,24] In this uncomfortable study, the glans of the penis in men or the clitoris in women is electrically stimulated while recording with needle electrodes placed in the external anal and urethral sphincters. Prolonged latency of this reflex with normal paraspinal muscle EMG, suggests pudendal neuropathy.

Disorders of the Thoracic and Abdominal Regions

Unfortunately, neurophysiologic tests have a limited role in the evaluation of thoracic or abdominal pain. In these regions, most neurologic problems stem from spinal nerve root or intercostal nerve compression, trauma, or inflammation. Although intercostal NCSs can be performed,[25] they are technically difficult, have few good normal controls, and are unlikely to be definitively diagnostic. Needle EMG of paraspinal muscles can help determine if a problem is occurring at the root level. EMG of intercostal muscles is usually not performed secondary to the potential for pneumothorax. Needle examination of the rectus abdominis muscle is generally safe, providing information about the T8 to T11 intercostal nerves. SSEPs can also be helpful in evaluating the thoracic spinal cord itself (see later discussion).

Herpes Zoster

The painful recrudescence of varicella zoster with associated rash in a limited dermatomal distribution produces herpes zoster (shingles). Although pain is the predominant complaint, on careful examination some sensory loss in the region of the rash may also be identified. If zoster occurs in a dermatome of either the leg or arm, sensory NCSs of that involved segment may demonstrate reduced sensory response amplitudes secondary to destruction of sensory nerve cell bodies in the dorsal root ganglia.[26] In some patients, the associated radiculitis is so widespread as to involve the anterior motor root as well, producing reductions in motor response amplitude and abnormalities on needle EMG.[26,27]

Syndromes of Excessive Muscle Activity

Several painful neurologic disorders are associated with generalized or focal excess muscle activity. These unusual disorders include cramps and fasciculation syndrome, stiff-person syndrome, tetanus, and Isaac's syndrome.

Cramps and Fasciculation Syndrome The syndrome of cramps and fasciculations is an unusual neuromuscular disorder in which patients complain of painful cramping in the legs with associated muscle twitching.[28] Exercise and caffeine may worsen symptoms. Repetitive stimulation at 5 Hz can produce cramping in these individuals, with associated muscle contraction that can be measured with surface electrodes.[28] Cramp potentials (rapidly firing motor units) may also be observed on EMG. Also, isolated fasciculation potentials are prominent in affected muscles.

Stiff-Person Syndrome In stiff-person syndrome, patients develop intermittent painful stiffness of one or more limbs. Serum antibodies to glutamic acid decarboxylase (one of the enzymes participating in the synthesis of gamma-aminobutyric acid [GABA]) may be identified, suggesting an autoimmune disorder. Generally, the stiffness is episodic, but can progress over time to become protracted and generalized. Although EMG will only demonstrate normally firing motor units without any other pathology, blink reflex studies may be abnormal in some of these patients.[29]

Tetanus In tetanus, the organism *Clostridium tetani* produces tetanus toxin, which interferes with the inhibitory synapses in the spinal cord and brain, producing excessive muscular activity. Although the diagnosis can usually be reached historically and clinically, electrophysiologic testing may reveal subtle abnormalities using specialized tests.[30]

Isaac's Syndrome In Isaac's syndrome, often a paraneoplastic phenomenon, antibodies are produced against ion channels in motor neurons, producing spontaneous firing of motor units. Unique discharges (termed *neuromyotonic*) are identified on EMG in this disorder.[31]

Dystonia Patients with dystonia occasionally present with pain as the predominant complaint rather than incoordination of movement. NCS can be helpful in excluding an underlying nerve lesion, whereas EMG of dystonic muscles, usually normal in idiopathic dystonia, can demonstrate reinnervation if nerve damage has occurred.

Reflex Sympathetic Dystrophy

Reflex sympathetic dystrophy, a syndrome characterized by skin changes, bone loss, and pain, usually occurs after trauma to an extremity, with or without associated nerve damage. Sympathetic nerve dysfunction has been suggested as causative. This causation is supported by the fact that patients may show improvement with sympathetic blockade or neurolysis.

Despite the presumed involvement of the sympathetic nerves, electrophysiologic studies do not reveal specific abnormalities in this disorder, unless an associated nerve injury (e.g., compression neuropathy) can be identified. Sympathetic nerve fiber function itself is difficult to test, relatively limited to the sympathetic skin response. One study has suggested relative reductions in the amplitude of this response in the affected as compared with the unaffected extremity.[32]

Fibromyalgia and Myofascial Pain Syndromes

Although presumably a disease of muscle, this disorder also has no definite electrophysiologic correlate. As noted earlier, muscle diseases may have pain components, including polymyositis and metabolic myopathies. However, generally, these disorders have limited pain associated with them, and weakness and other symptoms are prominent. In patients in whom the complaint of painful muscles is widespread, a diagnosis of fibromyalgia and myofascial pain may be considered. Although increased insertional activity at trigger points has been suggested,[33] other studies have not confirmed any abnormality in multiple aspects of muscle function and electrophysiology.[34–36] Ultimately, the diagnosis of fibromyalgia and myofascial pain syndrome remains a clinical one.

Polymyalgia Rheumatica

A sometimes overlooked diagnosis, polymyalgia rheumatica often is associated with complaints of proximal pain and aching in the arms and legs, especially in the morning, with improvement in symptoms as the day progresses. Although there have been reported cases of EMG abnormalities suggestive of inflammatory myopathy,[37,38] in general, electrophysiologic studies are normal. This leaves the overall clinical picture and an associated elevation in sedimentation rate as the usual diagnostic modalities.

Facial and Cranial Pain

In idiopathic trigeminal neuralgia, electrophysiologic testing is usually normal.[20] However, in patients with trigeminal nerve pain secondary to another process, such as that associated with brainstem demyelination or infarcts, blink reflex testing will be abnormal. In addition, brainstem evoked potentials may show prolongation of latencies or reductions in response amplitudes.

Other forms of facial or cranial pain, including glossopharyngeal neuralgia and occipital neuralgia, cannot be readily assessed with electrophysiologic testing. In patients with retroorbital pain secondary to optic neuritis, visual evoked potentials may be helpful in diagnosis.

Central Pain Syndromes

Again, since the advent of MRI, the utility of electrodiagnostic testing in the evaluation of central pain has been greatly reduced. Nonetheless, in certain situations, evoked potentials can be helpful in finding the site of a lesion. For example, in a patient presenting with pain affecting a specific limb and in whom peripheral electrophysiologic testing is normal, SSEPs can be used to localize the problem to a region of the central nervous system. In such a case, testing may reveal a prolonged latency in the thoracic cord, hence localizing the problem to that region. Directed MRI scanning of that region may then reveal the cause of the problem.

REFERENCES

1. Aminoff MJ. *Electrodiagnosis in Clinical Neurology*. 3rd ed. New York, NY: Churchill-Livingstone; 1992.
2. Kimura J. *Electrodiagnosis in Diseases of Nerve and Muscle: Principles and Practice*. 2 ed. Philadelphia, Pa: FA Davis; 1989.
3. Preston DC, Shapiro BE. *Electromyography and Neuromuscular Disorders: Clinical-Electrophysiologic Correlations*. Boston, Mass: Butterworth-Heinemann; 1998.
4. Dvorák J. Neurophysiologic tests in diagnosis of nerve root compression caused by disc herniation. *Spine*. 1996;21:39S–44S.
5. Robinson LR. Electromyography, magnetic resonance imaging, and

radiculopathy: It's time to focus on specificity. *Muscle Nerve.* 1999; 22:149–150.

6. Nardin RA, Patel MR, Gudas TF, et al. Electromyography and magnetic resonance imaging in the evaluation of radiculopathy. *Muscle Nerve.* 1999;22:151–155.
7. Lomen-Hoerth C, Aminoff MJ. Clinical neurophysiologic studies: Which is test is useful and when? *Neurol Clin.* 1999;17:65–74.
8. Albers JW. Clinical neurophysiology of generalized polyneuropathy. *J Clin Neurophysiol.* 1993;10:149–166.
9. Chalk CH. Acquired peripheral neuropathy. *Neurol Clin.* 1997;15:501–528.
10. Shahani BT, Halperin JJ, Boulu P, Cohen J. Sympathetic skin response—a method of assessing unmyelinated axon dysfunction in peripheral neuropathies. *J Neurol Neurosurg Psychiatry.* 1984;47:546–542.
11. Gnatz SM. The role of needle electromyography in the evaluation of patients with carpal tunnel syndrome: Needle EMG is important. *Muscle Nerve.* 1999;22:282–283.
12. Rosenfalck A. Early recognition of nerve disorders by near-nerve recording of sensory action potentials. *Muscle Nerve.* 1978;1:360–367.
13. Oh SJ, Sarala PK, Kuba T, Elmore R. Tarsal tunnel syndrome: Electrophysiological study. *Ann Neurol.* 1979;5:327–330.
14. Solheim LF, Siewers P, Paus B. The piriformis muscle syndrome: Sciatic nerve entrapment treated with section of the piriformis muscle. *Acta Orthop Scand.* 1981;52:73–75.
15. Fishman LM, Zybert PA. Electrophysiologic evidence of piriformis syndrome. *Arch Phys Med Rehab.* 1992;73:359–364.
16. Parry GJ. Electrodiagnostic studies in the evaluation of peripheral nerve and brachial plexus injuries. *Neurol Clin.* 1992;4:921–934.
17. Albers JW, Alan AA, Bastron JA, et al. Limb myokymia. *Muscle Nerve.* 1981;4:494–504.
18. Forestier N Le, Moulonguet A, Maisonobe T, et al. True neurogenic thoracic outlet syndrome: Electrophysiological diagnosis in six cases. *Muscle Nerve.* 1998;21:1129–1134.
19. Parry GJG. AAEM Case Report #11: Mononeuropathy multiplex. *Muscle Nerve.* 1985;8:493–498.
20. Griggs RC, Mendell JR, Miller RG. *Evaluation and Treatment of Myopathies*. Philadelphia, Pa: FA Davis; 1995.
21. Oberpenning F, Roth S, Leusmann DB, et al. The Alcock syndrome: Temporary penile insensitivity due to compression of the pudendal nerve within the Alcock canal. *J Urol.* 1994;151:423–425.
22. Silbert PL, Dunne JW, Edis RH, et al. Bicycling induced pudendal nerve pressure neuropathy. *Clin Exp Neurol.* 1991;28:191–196.
23. Bilkey WJ, Awad EA, Smith AD. Clinical application of sacral reflex latency. *J Urol.* 1983;129:1187–1189.
24. Tackmann W, Porst H, Ahlen HV. Bulbocavernosus reflex latencies and somatosensory evoked potentials after pudendal nerve stimulation in the diagnosis of impotence. *J Neurol.* 1988;235:219–225.
25. Pradham S, Taly A. Intercostal nerve conduction study in man. *J Neurol Neurosurg Psychiatry.* 1989;52:763–766.
26. Merchut MP, Gruener G. Segmental zoster paresis of limbs. *Electromyogr Clin Neurophysiol.* 1996;36:369–375.
27. Sachs GM. Segmental zoster paresis: An electrophysiological study. *Muscle Nerve.* 1996;19:784–786.
28. Tahmoush AJ, Alonso RJ, Tahmoush GP, et al. Cramp-fasciculation syndrome: A treatable hyperexcitable peripheral nerve disorder. *Neurology.* 1991;41:1021–1024.
29. Meinck H-M, Ricker K, Conrad B. The stiff-man syndrome: New pathophysiological aspects from abnormal exteroceptive reflexes and the response to clomipramine, clonidine, and tizanidine. *J Neurol Neurosurg Psychiatry.* 1984;47:280–287.
30. Struppler A, Struppler E, Adams RD. Local tetanus in man: Its clinical and neurophysiological characteristics. *Arch Neurol.* 1963;8:162–178.
31. Lütschg J, Jerusalem F, Ludin HP. The syndrome of "continuous muscle fiber activity." *Arch Neurol.* 1978;35:198–205.
32. Drory VE, Korczyn AD. The sympathetic skin response in reflex sympathetic dystrophy. *J Neurol Sci.* 1995;128:92–95.
33. Hubbard DR, Berkoff GM. Myofascial trigger points show spontaneous needle EMG activity. *Spine.* 1993;18:1803–1807.
34. Durette MR, Rodriquez AA, Agre JC, et al. Needle electromyographic evaluation of patients with myofascial or fibromyalgic pain. *Am J Phys Med Rehabil.* 1991;70:154–156.
35. Simms RW. Is there muscle pathology in fibromyalgia syndrome? *Rheum Dis Clin North Am.* 1996;22:245–266.
36. Zidar J, Backman E, Bengtsson A, et al. Quantitative EMG and muscle tension in painful muscles in fibromyalgia. *Pain.* 1990;40:249–254.
37. Bromberg MB, Donofrio PD, Segal BM. Steroid-responsive electromyographic abnormalities in polymyalgia rheumatica. *Muscle Nerve* 1990;13:138–141.
38. Radhamanohar M. An unusual presentation of polymyalgia rheumatica with severe muscle weakness. *Br J Clin Pract.* 1992 Autumn; 46(3):213–214.

CHAPTER 10

Measuring Pain With Functional Magnetic Resonance Imaging

Milan Stojanovic

Pain is recognized as a sensory and emotional experience in humans. Unfortunately, there is no objective test for measuring pain. This has hampered both the clinical management and the scientific understanding of pain. In the clinical setting, physicians daily encounter difficulties in diagnosing chronic pain conditions. The findings of commonly used testing modalities (magnetic resonance imaging [MRI], computed tomography, electromyography) are frequently normal. History and physical examination are highly subjective tests and prone to examiner bias. Complaints of chronic pain patients are frequently labeled "psychogenic" in origin. The majority of chronic pain patients suffer from depression; however, it is difficult to determine if depression is a consequence of chronic pain or vice versa. Indeed, emotional and pain brain networks share similar anatomic structures.

Most of the limited knowledge of central nervous system (CNS) pain processing is derived from animal research using electrophysiologic recordings. The animal data do not provide adequate insight into human aspects of pain processing, such as the affective component of pain. There is need for a better understanding of the following aspects of human pain networks: (1) chronic pain states in which altered CNS processing is taking place; (2) effects of various drugs on brain activation in acute and chronic pain; and (3) perception of pain in altered states of conciousness.

The initial findings that provided an insight into human CNS pain networks were accomplished by functional brain imaging using positron emission tomography (PET) technology, followed by studies using functional magnetic resonance imaging (fMRI). Although still in their infancy, these tools are extremely valuable in bridging the gap between clinical practice and animal research in understanding pain.

Functional brain imaging techniques are based on similar methods of measuring brain neuronal activity. Glucose is the main energy source for human brain metabolism. The coupling between regional cerebral blood flow and local cerebral glucose use has been established and supported by experimental data. Glucose metabolism reflects the brain neuronal synaptic and presynaptic activity needed for maintenance of membrane potentials and restoration of ion gradients. Functional brain imaging, by measuring the regional blood flow, provides indirect data on regional brain neuronal activity, be it local activation or inhibition.

POSITRON EMISSION TOMOGRAPHY

PET is an instrument that allows accurate measurements of small concentrations of radioactivity in living tissue. Positron-emitting isotopes have been incorporated as tracers into a wide range of molecules to provide information about various biologic processes after inhalation or intravenous administration. By using this technique, the whole brain metabolic activity in pain states can be measured. The ability to overlap brain metabolic activity data acquired by PET with structural magnetic images of brain (MRI) enhanced the effective spatial resolution of PET. There are numerous studies using this technology in medicine.

The first brain mapping study focusing on pain used PET. This study demonstrated that painful heat produced activation in multiple brain areas, including cortical and subcortical structures.[1] Since then, PET with various experimental paradigms has helped provide a better understanding of the brain circuitry involved in pain processing.[2–5] In these studies, noxious stimulation produced activation in multiple brain regions, most commonly the cingulate gyri, somatosensory cortex, thalamus, insula, frontal lobes, and cerebellum. The fact that hypnosis can modulate subjective pain perception in anterior cingulate gyri was also shown using PET technology.[6] Recently, fMRI studies have replicated results previously accomplished by PET technology. Taking into consideration its advantages over PET, fMRI has become a promising tool for brain mapping in pain states. However, PET may remain the gold standard for receptor-binding imaging.

FUNCTIONAL MAGNETIC RESONANCE IMAGING

Essentially, fMRI is the "ultrafast" MRI. Similar to PET methodology, fMRI is based on the tight relationship among neuronal synaptic activity, metabolism, and blood circulation. Conventional MRI was first performed in the 1940s, and today its principle is used routinely in the clinical setting in the form of the MRI scanner. When a patient is placed in the MRI scanner, hydrogen nuclei from water molecules are oriented along the magnetic fields of the scanner. By administering radiofrequency pulses to these nuclei, their alignment can be disturbed. After the radiofrequency pulse ceases, the nuclei realign themselves by transmitting a radiofrequency signal that can be detected in a receiver coil placed around the patient's body. Different structures in the human body have different water content, and, therefore, reflect different intensities of radiofrequency signal. The map of these transmitted signals represents a magnetic resonance image. However, obtaining each slice of the magnetic resonance image requires a new radiofrequency pulse to be transmitted and new excitation of water molecules to occur. For that reason, it may take a long time to obtain a magnetic resonance image of the human brain, containing multiple slices.

The slow acquisition of a signal through conventional MRI hampered the development of functional imaging. This problem was overcome by the development of echo planar imaging (EPI). EPI enables the spatial information of an object to be efficiently sampled after a single excitation of the water molecules. In this way, sampling an image can take less than 100 msec as opposed to the several tens of seconds required when using conventional MRI. By using ultrafast MRI with EPI, the brain can be visualized in almost real time. This rapid acquisition of data led to the development of fMRI.[7]

The first fMRI study using EPI principles was accomplished by injecting a bolus of paramagnetic contrast agent, gadolinium, into the bloodstream and comparing images of blood volumes before and after visual stimulation with flashing light. The results revealed an increase in the primary visual cortex blood volume during stimulation.[8]

Difficulties with injecting contrast medium have been overcome by using the blood oxygen level–dependent (BOLD) technique in all recent studies. BOLD fMRI relies on the different magnetic properties of oxyhemoglobin and deoxyhemoglobin. In active brain regions, an increase in the regional blood flow causes an increased ratio of oxyhemoglobin to deoxyhemoglobin, which is detected by fMRI as increased activity.[9]

BOLD fMRI has demonstrated good correlation with PET studies. There are multiple advantages of fMRI over PET, in particular: (1) fMRI does not require injection of radiotracers and, therefore, does not expose patients to radiation; (2) fMRI provides better spatial and temporal resolution than PET; (3) fMRI can be studied in individuals; and (3) every conventional MRI scanner can be converted to fMRI and potentially used for clinical purposes.

The scanners that are often used in hospitals for clinical purposes use 1.5 tesla (T) MRI. It has been demonstrated that magnetic fields higher than 1.5 T result in an improved contrast and elevated sensitivity to the BOLD technology used in fMRI. Recently developed magnetic fields of up to 4 T can provide even better fMRI results.

Many areas in medicine can potentially benefit from fMRI imaging. There are already many reports of fMRI use in brain mapping during auditory, olfactory, visual, somatosensory, and motor tasks. Furthermore, fMRI has been used to study brain activity during complex mental tasks and in people with psychiatric disease and addiction. fMRI could be used for presurgical mapping, to identify certain brain functions to be spared, or in patients with seizure disorders as a way of mapping epileptic foci.

FUNCTIONAL MAGNETIC RESONANCE IMAGING STUDIES IN PAIN STATES

Although there are far more published PET reports on regional brain activity in pain states, recent developments in fMRI provide excellent insight into brain functioning, with even better spatial and temporal resolution than PET.

A study comparing warm (41°C) and noxious heat (46°C) stimuli applied on the dorsum of the hand in human volunteers revealed increased activity in multiple brain regions.[10] Positive activation was found in the anterior and posterior cingulate gyri, thalamus, motor cortex, somatosensory cortex (SI and SII), insula, cerebellum, frontal gyri, and supplemental motor area. Negative activation was observed in hypothalamus and amygdala. All areas activated by 41°C were activated by 46°C; however, significantly more activation was found with the 46°C stimulus, except for the thalamus and SI brain regions. With both temperatures, four stimuli were delivered, dispersed by stimuli-free intervals. A significant attenuation of the signal change was observed over the four stimuli at 46°C, but not at 41°C. The signal attenuation concurs with previous studies on time courses of peripheral nociceptor sensitization to noxious heat. The study results showed involvement of somatotopic and limbic brain areas in pain processing. They also revealed an integrative role of various brain areas in pain, as well as the adaptive nature of the pain system to noxious stimuli.

In another study, brain activation was produced by noxious electrical stimuli at two frequencies (5 Hz and 250 Hz) in six human volunteers.[11] Both stimuli produced similar subjective levels of pain intensity, but later psychophysical measurements demonstrated a significant difference in pain unpleasantness between the two frequencies. An increased fMRI signal was observed in multiple brain areas, including anterior and posterior cingulate gyri, insulae, and frontal gyri, after stimulation by both frequencies. In these regions, the 5-Hz stimulation produced larger volumes of significant signal change. Other brain areas, such as medial thalamus, brainstem, precentral gyrus, and temporal gyrus, demonstrated significant fMRI signal change only by 5-Hz stimulation. A significant decrease in the fMRI signal was observed in similar brain regions by both 5-Hz and 250-Hz stimuli. These findings suggest that different neural networks are involved in processing sensory-discriminative and affective components of pain, and that the subjective experience of pain unpleasantness is subserved by qualitative and quantitative changes in CNS activation patterns.

Using fMRI , brain activation was measured during the thermal painful task and its overlap compared to cortical areas activated during vibrotactile and motor tasks in ten healthy volunteers.[12] Predictor functions were generated from fMRI impulse response function, the time courses of thermal stimuli, and associated pain ratings. The correlation between these predictor functions and cortical activations in the painful thermal task indicated a gradual transition of information processing anteroposteriorly in the parietal cortex. The region best related to the thermal stimulus was the insular cortex at the level of the anterior commissure, and Brodmann's area 5/7 was the region best related to the pain perception.

Hypersensitivity of the skin to non-noxious stimuli (allodynia) and increased sensitivity to noxious stimuli (hyperalgesia) are commonly found in states of central sensitization and in chronic neuropathic pain states. Capsaicin-induced secondary hyperalgesia in healthy volunteers presents a form of experimentally induced central sensitization. One fMRI study compared brain activation patterns between light touch stimuli and hyperalgesia in healthy volunteers.[13] Nonpainful mechanical stimulation of the skin resulted in activation of contralateral somatosensory cortex (SI) and bilateral secondary somatosensory cortex (SII). To the contrary, hyperalgesia induced activation of contralateral prefrontal cortex, along with the middle (Brodmann's areas 6, 8, and 9) and inferior frontal gyri. Prefrontal activation is thought to result from cognitive evaluation, attention, and planning of motor behavior in response to pain.

A study designed to compare activation of thalamic nuclei, insula, and SII to noxious and tactile stimuli was performed using fMRI.[14] Painful thermal stimuli activated regions within the lateral and medial thalamus, predominantly anterior insula, and the contralateral SII in half of the subjects. The innocuous thermal stimuli did not activate SII in any of the subjects but activated the thalamus and posterior insula in 50% of subjects. The innocuous tactile stimulation consistently activated SII bilaterally and the contralateral lateral thalamus. These results indicate different pathways involved in processing somatotopic and emotional aspects of pain. They also demonstrate good spatial resolution of fMRI, enabling researchers to study specific brain nuclei involved in pain processing. Similar fMRI studies[15,16] focus on somatosensory cortex and insula.

Spinal cord stimulation is used routinely in the treatment of chronic neuropathic pain, with success rates exceeding 50%. The exact mechanism of pain relief is unclear, but it is thought to result from stimulation of sensory tracts in the dorsal column and inhibition of nociceptive pathways, as described by Melzack and Wall's gate control theory. Other putative mechanisms for pain relief might be an increase in spinal cord concentration of γ-aminobutyric acid (GABA), an inhibitory neurotransmitter. An fMRI study that investigated brain activation in three patients with chronic lower extremity pain during spinal cord stimulation[17] found significant activation of contralateral somatosensory cortex in all patients and of anterior cingulate gyrus in one patient. These findings correlated with patients' pain relief. Although a case study, this report sheds some light on the mechanisms of action of spinal cord stimulation for the relief of intractable pain.

Visceral pain is transmitted to the brain via slightly different neural networks. The main difference between somatic pain and visceral pain is poor representation of visceral organs in somatosensory brain areas. For this reason, visceral pain is often poorly localized, hampering its diagnosis and treatment. Commonly, visceral pain is referred to the distant site as a result of convergence of somatic and visceral neurons. In another fMRI study, esophageal stimulation was performed by intraesophageal perfusion of 0.1N HCl (1 mL/min), and the results of brain activation were compared with those of saline infusion and balloon distention. Both balloon distention and acid perfusion resulted in significant brain activation, but there was no increase of brain metabolic activity with saline perfusion.[18]

Leão spreading depression provides a possible explanation for the development of visual migraine headache attacks. These attacks were thought to be associated with decreased cerebral blood flow in affected brain regions. Occipital cortex activation was measured during visual stimulation using fMRI in patients with migraine and in healthy volunteers.[19] In 50% of the patients with migraine, the onset of headache or visual change was preceded by suppression of brain activation that propagated into the occipital cortex. Initial suppression was accompanied by signal increase, indicating vaso dilation. The vasodilation that follows the initial stage of hypoperfusion may be responsible for the onset of headache in migraine attacks.

Phantom pain following amputation of the extremity is a good example of the CNS role in chronic pain. An fMRI case study of a patient after arm amputation reveals a striking example of acute CNS plasticity following amputation.[20] The patient's phantom limb pain was activated by tactile stimulation of the ipsilateral corner of the mouth 24 hours after amputation. fMRI findings 1 month later revealed contralateral activation of the somatosensory (SII) area in the vicinity where the hand is thought to be represented. These findings were accomplished by tactile stimulation of the ipsilateral corner of the mouth, producing phantom pain in the ipsilateral hand.

Because they process affective and sensory experience, brain pain pathways are complex, changing, and often influenced by psychophysical settings. Only an anticipation of pain produces brain activation in the medial frontal lobe, insular cortex, and cerebellum, as measured by fMRI.[21] These areas are distinct but close to the brain regions activated by pain, which indicates that they share similar CNS networks.

CENTRAL NERVOUS SYSTEM PAIN PROCESSING: THE ROLE OF FUNCTIONAL IMAGING

Before the era of functional brain imaging, all information about the CNS role in pain processing was derived from animal studies. It was assumed that nociceptive signals made their way to the dorsal horn of the spinal cord, were transmitted to the thalamus, and reached the somatosensory cortex, finally entering the mind through an unclear process.[22] Many theories proposed before the advent of functional brain imaging focused on a specific "brain center" responsible for pain. Somatosensory cortex (SI) was thought to have such a role. In the last decade, functional brain imaging studies revealed many brain regions responsible for pain perception (Table 10-1), a scenario known as distributed pain processing.[23]

Because pain is an emotional experience, brain regions involved in emotions are also involved in pain processing. The best example of these areas is the anterior cingulate gyrus. Cingulotomies have been performed for the treatment of obsessive-compulsive disorder, severe depression, and pain. Indeed, postcingulotomy patients reported sensation of pain but no emotional response attached to it. Medial and lateral thalamic nuclei were thought to have a role in processing affective and somatotopic components of pain, respectively, based on animal experiments. Those data were partially replicated in fMRI studies.[14] Several studies have supported the role of insula in affective and motivational aspects of pain.[24]

Somatosensory cortex has been visualized in some studies but not in others. The SI activation can be highly modulated by factors that alter pain perception. On the other hand, inter- and intra-

TABLE 10-1 **Brain Areas Commonly Activated by Pain as Demonstrated by Functional Brain Imaging**

Somatotopic Regions	Limbic Affective Regions	Other Regions	Descending Areas
Primary somatosensory cortex (SI)	Anterior cingulate gyrus	Frontal cortex	Periaqueductal gray
Secondary somatosensory cortex (SII)	Posterior cingulate gyrus	Parietal gyrus	
Thalamus	Putamen	Supplementary motor area	
	Insula	Prefrontal cortex	
	Cerebellum		
	Lentiform nucleus		
	Amygdala		

subject anatomic variations can lead to variable SI activation. Besides having a somatotopic role, the other functions of SI region in pain processing remain to be discovered.

Multiple other brain areas are activated by pain. The pattern of activation varies across the studies and subjects. There are several explanations for these phenomena, but the major reason probably lies in the fact that pain is a complex experience and multiple psychophysical factors modulate perception of pain. Future functional brain imaging studies will gradually explain the complex brain circuitry involved in pain processing.

Functional brain imaging is a new and exciting field that enables clinicians to better understand higher CNS functions in pain states. It is hoped that this methodology will gradually evolve into a useful clinical tool, enabling practitioners to better diagnose and treat painful conditions in everyday practice.

REFERENCES

1. Talbot JD, Marrett S, Evans AC, Meyer E, Bushnell MC, Duncan GH. Multiple representations of pain in human cerebral cortex. *Science.* 1991;251:1355–1358.
2. Casey KL, Minoshima S, Berger KL, Koeppe RA, Morrow TJ, Frey KA. Positron emission tomographic analysis of cerebral structures activated specifically by repetitive noxious heat stimuli. *J Neurophysiol.* 1994;71:802–807.
3. Hsieh JC, Stahle-Backdahl M, Hagermark O, Stone-Elander S, Rosenquist G, Ingvar M. Traumatic nociceptive pain activates the hypothalamus and periaqueductal gray: A positron emission tomography study. *Pain.* 1996;64:303–314.
4. Iadarola MJ, Max MB, Berman KF, et al. Unilateral decrease in thalamic activity observed with positron emission tomography in patients with chronic neuropathic pain. *Pain.* 1995;63:55–64.
5. Jones AK, Brown WD, Friston KJ, Qi LY, Frackowiak RS. Cortical and subcortical localization of response to pain in man using positron emission tomography. *Proc R Soc Lond B Biol Sci.* 244:39–44.
6. Rainville P, Duncan GH, Price DD, Carrier B, Bushnell MC. Pain encoded in human anterior cingulate but not somatosensory cortex. *Science.* 1997;277:968–971.
7. Le Bihan D, Jezzard P, Haxby J, Sadato N, Rueckert L, Mattay V. Functional magnetic resonance imaging of the brain. *Ann Intern Med.* 1995; 122:296–303.
8. Belliveau JW, Kennedy DN Jr, McKinstry RC, et al. Functional mapping of the human visual cortex by magnetic resonance imaging. *Science.* 1991;254:716–719.
9. Kwong KK. Functional magnetic resonance imaging with echo planar imaging. *Magn Reson Quart.* 1995;11:1–20.
10. Becerra LR, Breiter HC, Stojanovic M, et al. Human brain activation under controlled thermal stimulation and habituation to noxious heat: An fMRI study. *Magn Reson Med.* 1999;41:1044–1057.
11. Stojanovic M, Becerra L , Breiter HC, et al. fMRI Analysis of Human CNS Activation Following Noxious Electrical Stimulation at 5 Hz and 250 Hz. New Orleans, La: American Pain Society; 1997:16.
12. Apkarian AV, Darbar A, Krauss BR, Gelnar PA, Szeverenyi NM. Differentiating cortical areas related to pain perception from stimulus identification: Temporal analysis of fMRI activity. *J Neurophysiol.* 1999;81: 2956–2963.
13. Baron R, Baron Y, Disbrow E, Roberts TP. Brain processing of capsaicin-induced secondary hyperalgesia: A functional MRI study. *Neurology.* 1999;53:548–557.
14. Davis KD, Kwan CL, Crawley AP, Mikulis DJ. Functional MRI study of thalamic and cortical activations evoked by cutaneous heat, cold, and tactile stimuli. *J Neurophysiol.* 1998;80:1533–1546.
15. Disbrow E, Buonocore M, Antognini J, Carstens E, Rowley HA. Somatosensory cortex: A comparison of the response to noxious thermal, mechanical, and electrical stimuli using functional magnetic resonance imaging. *Hum Brain Mapping.* 1998;6:150–159.
16. Oshiro Y, Fuijita N, Tanaka H, Hirabuki N, Nakamura H, Yoshiya I. Functional mapping of pain-related activation with echo-planar MRI: Significance of the SII-insular region. *Neuroreport.* 1998;9:2285–2289.
17. Kiriakopoulos ET, Tasker RR, Nicosia S, Wood ML, Mikulis DJ. Functional magnetic resonance imaging: A potential tool for the evaluation of spinal cord stimulation: Technical case report. *Neurosurgery.* 1997; 41:501–504.
18. Kern MK, Birn RM, Jaradeh S, et al. Identification and characterization of cerebral cortical response to esophageal mucosal acid exposure and distention. *Gastroenterology.* 1998;115:1353–1362.
19. Cao Y, Welch KM, Aurora S, Vikingtad EM. Functional MRI-BOLD of visually triggered headache in patients with migraine. *Arch Neurol* 1999;56:548–554.
20. Borsook D, Becerra L, Fishman S, et al. Acute plasticity in the human somatosensory cortex following amputation. *Neuroreport.* 1998;9: 1013–1017.
21. Ploghaus A, Tracey I, Gati JS, et al. Dissociating pain from its anticipation in the human brain. Science. 1999;84:1979–1981.
22. Chapman CR, Nakamura Y. Pain and consciousness. *Pain Forum.* 1999;8:113–123.
23. Coghill RC, Talbot JD, Evans AC, et al. Distributed processing of pain and vibration by the human brain. *J Neurosci.* 1994;14:4095–4108.
24. Greenspan JD, Lee RR, Lenz FA. Pain sensitivity alterations as a function of lesion location in the parasylvian cortex. *Pain.* 1999;81:273–282.
25. Bushnell MC, et al. 1999.

CHAPTER 11 DIAGNOSTIC INJECTIONS FOR SPINE PAIN

Conor W. O'Neill, Richard Derby, and Laura R. Kenderes

Identifying the specific pathology responsible for spinal pain is often difficult. This is particularly true given the high incidence of anatomic abnormalities in asymptomatic individuals, and the presence of normal anatomy in some painful individuals, at least as demonstrated on conventional imaging studies.[1,2] The primary purpose of diagnostic injections for chronic spinal pain is to identify which anatomic structure of the spine is causing pain and what is the pathologic disorder affecting it. Before performing these injections, the clinical utility of making an anatomic diagnosis should be well established.

Whether or not it is important to make an anatomic diagnosis in patients with spinal pain is a matter of some debate.[3,4] While some would argue that in the majority of patients, attempts at making an anatomic diagnosis are contraindicated, others feel that at a minimum, making a diagnosis will help patients to heal by providing them with a clear understanding of their problem.[5] The most important reason to make an anatomic diagnosis, however, is if there are treatments that can be directed toward specific pathology, leading to good outcomes. Many patients with spinal pain can be treated with interventional pain management procedures. The success of these procedures may depend on an accurate anatomic diagnosis; however, typically little harm will come to the patient if the procedure fails. Traditionally, the indications for surgery have been felt to be neurologic loss. Increasingly, however, surgery is being performed for pain without neurologic loss, essentially becoming a pain management procedure. Although surgery may help some patients with chronic pain, the tissue injury that necessarily accompanies surgery may potentially lead to devastating consequences. If surgery is being considered for patients with chronic pain, an accurate diagnosis is essential. In this chapter, we focus on the role of diagnostic injections in presurgical decision making.

SPINAL PAIN

There are two types of spinal pain: radicular pain and axial pain.[6] Radicular pain results from mechanical compression or chemical irritation of a nerve root, or both. Establishing an anatomic diagnosis for patients with radicular pain is important, as surgical treatments have excellent outcomes in well-selected patients. The source of radicular pain, typically either a herniated nucleus pulposus or spinal stenosis, can be definitively diagnosed at surgery; therefore, there is a gold standard that can be used to assess the validity of diagnostic studies. Consequently, the ability of both clinical findings and imaging studies to diagnose the site of pathology is well defined. A diagnostic injection may be indicated when imaging studies suggest that more than one nerve root may be responsible for a patient's symptoms. In that circumstance, a selective epidural injection may be useful.

In contrast to radicular pain, the relationship between spinal pathology and axial pain is uncertain. There are a number of anatomic structures that are potential sources of pain, including myofascial tissues, synovial joints, and the intervertebral discs. Although discogenic pain is felt by many to be an indication for surgical fusion, outcome studies have demonstrated variable results.[7–16] As there is no gold standard for diagnosing the tissue source of axial pain, it is not possible to rigorously validate diagnostic studies.[17] Discography is frequently performed on patients with axial pain, but its use remains controversial.[18,19]

Complicating the diagnosis and treatment of spinal pain is the influence of psychosocial factors on pain. Pain is a complex phenomenon, with components secondary to both tissue injury and the emotional reaction to tissue injury. Although there is considerable controversy regarding the relative importance of psychosocial and biologic factors in causing spinal pain,[20–22] there is evidence to suggest that the level of psychological distress can affect the results from diagnostic injections[23] as well as the outcomes from treatment.[24] It is important to recognize the potential importance of psychosocial factors in diagnosing and treating patients with spinal pain.

If surgery is being considered for a patient with spinal pain—and the source of pain is unclear despite a clinical evaluation, imaging studies, and, potentially, electrodiagnostics—a diagnostic injection may be indicated. Either discography or a selective epidural injection may be considered, depending on whether the patient has radicular pain or axial pain.

LUMBAR DISCOGRAPHY

Overview

The lumbar intervertebral disc can be injected with contrast, local anesthetic, or other substances. Although observing the effect of a local anesthetic injection on pain and function (analgesic discography) can potentially provide useful information, the clinical utility of this has not been well defined. However, the effect of an applied mechanical or chemical stimulus on pain (provocative discography) has demonstrated clinical utility.

In addition to provoking pain that can be compared with the patient's clinical symptoms, injecting contrast into the disc may demonstrate pathology that is not otherwise revealed on conventional imaging studies. Prior to the introduction of sophisticated imaging studies such as computed tomography (CT) and magnetic resonance imaging (MRI), lumbar discography was often used primarily as a radiologic imaging study to complement myelography.[25] Several studies have confirmed the accuracy of lumbar discography as a radiologic test in demonstrating both disc herniations and disc degeneration.[2,26–31] With the advent of MRI scanning, and in particular the use of gadolinium enhancement in evaluating postoperative patients, the utility of lumbar discography purely as a radiologic study has diminished. However, both cadaver and clinical studies have demonstrated that discography is more sensitive than MRI in detecting disc degeneration, particularly when postdiscography CT scanning is added.[2,28,31–33]

The purpose of discography is to determine whether the intervertebral disc is a source of clinical symptoms. Although interpretation of the radiologic images obtained at the time of discography is important, in contemporary practice discography is primarily a provocative clinical test, rather than a radiologic imaging procedure.

Provocative Discography

A variety of pathologic processes affect the intervertebral disc, potentially causing noxious stimulation of nerve endings. A precision injection of contrast dye into the disc nucleus also stimulates nerve endings. The stimulus applied with discography has two components: a chemical stimulus resulting from contact between contrast dye and sensitized tissues, and a mechanical stimulus resulting from a fluid-distending stress. The underlying premise of discography is that this applied stimulus replicates the clinical noxious stimulus responsible for the patient's symptoms, and that reproduction of the patients clinical symptoms during the injection confirms the disc as the source of pain.

As with any diagnostic test, it is important to know the false-positive and false-negative rates associated with provocative discography, which are used to calculate sensitivity and specificity. Defining the false-positive and false-negative rates requires comparing the test results against a gold standard.[17,34,35] A gold standard is a method for definitively establishing a diagnosis and is typically obtained from biopsy, surgery, or long-term follow-up.[17] Unfortunately, in contrast to radicular pain, there is no absolute method to determine the tissue origin of lumbar axial pain, and, therefore, no way to determine the sensitivity and specificity of discography.

A variety of factors can lead to both false-positive and false-negative results from provocative discography. One possible source of both false-positive and false-negative injections is that the stimulus applied with the injection may not be selective for the nerve endings in the disc being studied. The nerve endings in the lumbar disc are in the end plates and middle and outer annulus. Although pathologic processes involving the end plate can occur,[36,37] the innervated portion of the disc most often affected by pathologic processes is the annulus. For the provocative discography construct to be valid, the injection must selectively affect the nerve endings in the annulus of the disc being studied, which is the presumed site of the clinical noxious stimulus. A number of authors have suggested alternate sources for the pain of discography, other than stimulation of annular nerve endings.[38] Postulated pain mechanisms include increased pressure at the end plates or within the vertebral body,[39] increased substance P and VIP in the dorsal root ganglion,[40] or transmission of mechanical stimulation to the facet joints. Despite these hypotheses, there is good evidence that the provocative response resulting from discography is related to stimulation of nerve endings in the outer annulus, rather than other factors.[41–43] Although relatively unusual, painful end-plate disruptions can also occur.[36]

The complex nature of anatomic structures can also lead to inaccurate results from discography. Anatomic structures are typically composed of several different types of tissues. A pathologic process can potentially affect just one component of a structure, which may not be the same component targeted by a precision injection. For example, discogenic pain is commonly felt to be a result of annular fissures originating in the nucleus and extending to the outer annulus, which is where the majority of the disc nerve endings reside. During discography, contrast is injected into the nucleus. If there are not fissures, the contrast will be confined to the nucleus. However, histologic studies have demonstrated that there can be middle or outer annular abnormalities that are not contiguous with the nucleus.[28] In such cases, an injection into the nucleus could lead to a false-negative result.

Another potential source of inaccurate results from discography is the change in central nervous system (CNS) nociceptive processing that occurs with chronic pain. The neuroanatomic pathways mediating acute pain behave as a hard-wired system, with a pure stimulus-response relationship.[44] However, these neuroanatomic pathways are plastic, as they change with the development of chronic pain. With chronic pain, central sensitization occurs and dorsal horn cell activity no longer depends on peripheral tissue injury.[44,45] A pure stimulus-response relationship no longer exists. Both previously innocuous stimuli to the dorsal horn and stimuli from outside the original receptive field cause pain. As a result, the interpretation of diagnostic injections based on an acute pain paradigm may be inaccurate.[45] In the presence of chronic pain, it is possible that an anesthetic injection of an injured nerve or structure may not produce complete pain relief, anesthetizing an adjacent normal nerve or structure may relieve pain, and provoking a normal structure or nerve may reproduce a patient's clinical pain.

Finally, psychological factors are important sources of false-positive results with discography. There are two components to pain. The first is the nociceptive process initiated by tissue injury, and the second is the psychological and emotional reaction to nociception. A patient with chronic pain should always be seen in the context of these interacting factors. Measuring the response to a diagnostic injection, and in particular to provocative discography, always relies, to some extent, on a patients' self-reports of pain. Therefore, psychological factors can clearly affect the measurement of the response to a diagnostic injection. As a result, when assessing patients' responses to diagnostic injections, the relative contribution of nociception and psychological factors should be considered and the reliability of patients' self-reports of pain estimated.

Clearly, there are a number of potential sources of both false-positive and false-negative responses with discography. In an effort to study the potential for false-positive results, several studies have investigated the ability of discography to provoke back pain in asymptomatic subjects.

Holt, in 1968, reported a 36% rate of positive discography in asymptomatic subjects, leading him to discredit the use of the test.[46] However, there were several methodologic flaws with this study. The most notable flaws were that all of the subjects were prisoners, a highly irritating contrast medium was used, and, most importantly, Holt did not include a positive pain response as a criterion for a positive injection (i.e., the criteria for a positive result were based primarily on radiologic images).

Holt's findings were subsequently refuted in a well-designed study by Walsh and colleagues, who demonstrated a 0% rate of positive discography in asymptomatic volunteers.[47] Walsh and colleagues studied ten asymptomatic subjects and seven patients with chronic low back pain. The criteria for a positive result differed between the two groups. For both groups, a positive result required a 3-out-of-5 pain intensity (using a pain thermometer), two types of pain behavior (as assessed by videotape review), and structural degeneration. For the patients with chronic low back pain, a positive result also required that the provoked pain be similar to their usual pain. Obviously, it was not possible to evaluate the similarity of pain in asymptomatic subjects, as they had no pain prior to the injection. Among the asymptomatic subjects, five of ten had at least one structurally abnormal disc; however, none satisfied the criteria for a positive test. Thus, the false-positive rate in these asymptomatic volunteers was 0%. Among the chronic low back pain patients, all seven had at least one structurally abnormal disc, and six of seven patients had at least one disc that satisfied the criteria for a positive result. Overall, 13 discs were structurally abnormal, with 7 being positive and 6 negative. Of note, two of the seven had at least one disc that was structurally abnormal and was associated with intense, but atypical, provoked pain, as well as pain behaviors. In each case the test result was considered to be negative, given that the provoked pain was different from the patient's typical pain.

The Walsh study was important for several reasons. Firstly, using strict criteria for a positive test, including postinjection review of videotaped responses, there was excellent interrater reliability. Diagnostic tests that rely on an observer's interpretation are not clinically useful unless there is good interobserver reliability (i.e., the same test applied to the same patient should always produce the same result).[77] Thus, Walsh and colleagues' study established reproducible criteria for a positive result from discography. Secondly, by demonstrating a 0% false-positive rate in asymptomatic subjects, Walsh and colleagues effectively refuted Holt's assertion that the false-positive rate of discography was so high as to make it useless. Thirdly, Walsh and colleagues demonstrated that patients suffering from chronic low back pain were capable of developing different types of pain in response to provocation discography. According to their criteria, only provoked pain that was similar to the patients typical symptoms constituted a positive test. Atypical provoked pain, even if intense and accompanied by pain behaviors, constituted a negative test.

The asymptomatic subjects studied by Walsh and colleagues were all healthy volunteers, with an average age of 23. Caragee and colleagues recently expanded on the Walsh study of asymptomatic subjects, by studying a cohort of subjects who did not have low back pain, but whose clinical characteristics more closely matched those of patients with low back pain who typically present for discography.[23] Thirty subjects with no history of low back pain were recruited: ten had previous cervical surgery with good results, ten had the same surgery but had persistent chronic pain, and ten had primary somatization disorders. Lumbar discography was performed and interpreted according to the Walsh protocol. Four somatization patients dropped out before beginning the study and two stopped the study after only one or two discs were injected, and, therefore, were not included in the study analysis.

Among the subjects with good results from previous cervical surgery, seven of ten had at least one disc that had an outer annular rupture (10 of 30 discs, total), while only one of ten had a positive result. The patient with a positive test had a high Zung depression score. Of the subjects with chronic pain, five of ten patients had at least one disc that had an outer annular rupture (11 of 32 discs, total), with four of ten having at least one positive disc. Of the 11 discs with significant structural abnormalities, 7 were positive and four were negative. Among the subjects with somatization disorder three quarters had at least one disc that had an outer annular rupture (6 of 13 discs, total), with three quarters having at least one positive disc. Of the six discs with significant structural abnormalities, two were positive and four were negative. Based on these data, Caragee and colleagues concluded that in individuals with normal psychometrics and without chronic pain, the rate of false-positives is very low if strict criteria are applied, and that the false-positive rate increases with increased annular disruption.

The study by Caragee and colleagues is important for a number of reasons. Firstly, it confirms the finding by Walsh and colleagues that in subjects without a history of low back pain, and without psychosocial risk factors, provocation of a significant pain response with discography is unusual, with an incidence of 0% in the Walsh study and 10% in the Caragee study. It also confirms the Walsh finding that although discs in this population are often structurally abnormal (combining the studies, 12 of 20 subjects had at least one structurally abnormal disc) they are no more likely to be positive than a structurally normal disc. More importantly, the Caragee study reveals that in subjects without a history of low back pain, but with a history of chronic pain or a somatization disorder, provocation of a significant pain response with discography is common, with an incidence of 40% in the chronic pain group and 75% in the somatization disorder group. Furthermore, the more disrupted the annulus, the greater is the chance of a positive response.

Caragee and colleagues' study is a powerful reminder of the importance of psychosocial factors in modulating pain, while also demonstrating the potential of false-positive responses with discography. However, in assessing the importance of this information, it is necessary to reconsider the premise of discography.

The premise of discography is that reproduction of a patients' clinical symptoms during the injection identifies the disc as the source of pain. The rationale for its use is that the results can help discriminate among the various structures that may be responsible for axial pain. Therefore, to establish its validity, the criteria for a true positive disc must be determined in the relevant population, which is back pain sufferers. The Walsh data on patients with chronic low back pain demonstrated that it is common for patients undergoing discography to have intense pain that is very different in location and character from their clinical symptoms. In the Walsh study, the criteria for a positive test in the chronic low back pain population required that provoked pain be similar to the patient's clinical symptoms. Unfortunately, without a gold standard for axial pain, the validity of incorporating measures of familiarity of pain into the criteria for a positive test cannot be precisely defined.[17]

Caragee and colleagues clearly demonstrated the potential for false-positive responses with discography. However, given the premise of discography, and the fact that patients with chronic low back pain frequently have intense but atypical pain during discography, it is difficult to know the significance of any pain response in an asymptomatic subject.

Although the sensitivity and specificity of provocative discography cannot be precisely defined, it is important to remember that the ultimate criterion for a diagnostic test is whether the patient is better off as a result. If a test can predict the response to treatment, and is reliable and reproducible, then it may be clinically useful,[17,34,35] even without a defined sensitivity and specificity. The primary indication for provocative discography is to determine whether a patient with chronic spinal pain, who has failed aggressive efforts at conservative care, can be helped with spinal fusion.

In contrast to the surgical treatment of radiculopathy, the surgical treatment of axial pain is controversial, as studies have demonstrated a wide disparity in outcomes.[7–15,48] This disparity has been attributed to a number of factors, including type of fusion (interbody versus intertransverse, instrumented versus noninstrumented), approach (anterior versus posterior versus 360 degree), surgeon variability, and methodologic differences. The results from discography have been an important part of the preoperative evaluation in most of these studies, but typically, the criteria for a positive test have not been strictly defined. The validity of the criteria used to define a positive discogram is another variable that could potentially affect surgical outcome.

Pressure-controlled Discography

In an effort to develop criteria for discography that can be used to predict surgical outcome, Derby and colleagues reported on a cohort of patients who underwent provocative discography under pressure monitoring.[41] Although the pathophysiology of lumbar discogenic pain is still uncertain, there is presumptive evidence that it results from both mechanical stimulation of nociceptors in the annulus as well as by chemical irritation by enzymes and breakdown products involved in the degradative process.[41]

Physiologic loading of the disc creates horizontal and vertical stresses within the nucleus, annulus, and end plates of the disc that are directly related to the weight of the body above the segment and any added moment stresses resulting from body position. The relationship between intradiscal pressure and body position has been quantified by several investigators.[19,49] Derby and colleagues hypothesized that some discs were more sensitive to chemical stimuli than mechanical stimuli. Pain at discography which occurred at low pressures, below the typical weighted values, would result from chemical stimulation of the outer annulus by contact with contrast dye. Pain occurring at higher pressures would result from mechanical stimulation of the annulus by the fluid-distending stress of discography.

In order to establish the criteria for chemical and mechanical stimulation, Derby and colleagues used data from a preliminary study on disc pressure measurements at the time of discography.[41] In a preliminary study, they combined provocative discography with measurement of intradiscal pressure, comparing results from discography performed in the lying position with results from discography performed in the sitting position. The criteria for a positive result was 6-out-of-10 concordant pain. In normal discs, the average opening pressure, representing the intrinsic pressure of the disc, was 27 pounds per square inch (psi) in the side-lying position and 85 psi in the sitting position. As the degree of degeneration increased, the opening pressure decreased in both positions. However, the threefold difference between the opening pressure in the sitting position versus the lying position was maintained between equally degenerated discs. In the majority of discs, concordant pain provocation occurred when contrast first reached the outer annulus, with the maximal pain response usually occurring at pressures only 10 to 30 psi above the opening pressure. From these findings, Derby and colleagues concluded that in degenerated discs with annular disruption, pain provocation during discography is usually caused by low-pressure stimulation of an irritable outer annulus by a chemical stimulus.

Based on this information, the authors created a protocol for grading the sensitivity of the disc annulus that could be used to predict surgical outcome. Four categories of discs were defined. In chemical discs, pain is provoked at minimal pressure; 15 psi above opening pressure was chosen as the threshold for a chemical disc, as this is well below the mechanical load resulting from sitting. In mechanical discs, pain is provoked at pressures between standing and lying; that is, between 15 and 50 psi above opening pressure. In indeterminate discs, pain occurs between 51 and 90 psi above opening pressure, and in normal discs, there is no pain.

This classification system was applied to a consecutive series of patients referred for lumbar discography prior to potential fusion surgery. Following discography, patients were returned to the care of their referring surgeons, who independently decided whether surgery was indicated, and if so, whether it should be an intertransverse or interbody fusion. The disc classification was not reported to the surgeon.

The subjects were contacted at two follow-up intervals, at a mean time of 16 and 32 months, with the overall outcome classified as favorable or unfavorable depending on the results from three different outcome tools. Looking at all surgical cases combined, there was no significant difference in outcome between patients undergoing interbody versus intertransverse fusion, with both groups having approximately a 50% favorable outcome.

However, among patients classified as having a chemically sensitive disc, there was a highly significant difference in outcome between patients undergoing interbody versus intertransverse fusion. Within that group, 89% of the interbody fusion patients had a favorable outcome, while only 20% of the intertransverse fusion patients had a favorable outcome. Patients with chemically sensitive discs who did not have surgery of any kind had an 88% unfavorable outcome. There was no significant difference in patient demographics, including the percentage of patients with worker's compensation claims, between the patients with favorable outcomes and unfavorable outcomes. Other than workers' compensation status, psychosocial risk factors were not assessed.

Until now, the clinical significance of degenerative disc disease in a patient with axial pain was uncertain, as treatments directed specifically at the disc (i.e., fusion) led to variable outcomes. Based on the data of Derby and colleagues, it now appears that there is a subset of patients with degenerative disc disease who have chemically sensitive discs, and who have outcomes with surgery that rival those of patients undergoing partial disc excision for herniated nucleus pulposus. The surgery performed must be an interbody fusion, presumably because the disc is completely excised, therefore removing the source of the noxious stimulus. If these results stand up to long-term follow-up, and are replicated by other investigators, then the use of pressure-controlled discography as a diagnostic test to predict patients who will benefit from surgical fusion will be validated.

In addition to potentially having the ability to predict outcome, adding pressure monitoring to provocative discography improves interobserver reliability and, therefore, reproducibility. Assessing the response to discography requires measuring pain before and after the injection. There are three components to pain: its intensity, location, and character. If the location and character of the pain provoked at discography is similar to or exactly the same as the patient's clinical symptoms, it satisfies the criteria for concordant pain. The intensity of pain is measured both by the patient's self-report (e.g., using a numerical rating) and by observed pain behaviors. However, the intensity of provoked pain is dependent on the intensity of the stimulus. In simple terms, the harder one pushes on the syringe the more likely the disc is to hurt. By measuring intradiscal pressures, the intensity of the stimulus can be quantified, allowing more reliable comparisons between patients and discographers. Although it is possible to estimate injection pressures manually, using a controlled inflation syringe with digital pressure readout provides a precise value.

Technique

There are two approaches to the lumbar disc: posterior and lateral.[50] The posterior approach necessitates a dural puncture, and therefore should be avoided. Disc puncture is typically performed with a 22- or 25-gauge needle). There is some evidence that using an introducer needle can reduce the risk of infection, although this is not a universal practice.[51] Although rarely encountered, a variety of complications are possible with discography, including neural injury, bleeding, and intradural leakage of injected substances.[38,52,53] There have been case reports of disc herniations resulting from discography.[54,55] Canine studies have had conflicting results on the potential for disc injury during discography; however, the weight of evidence in humans suggests that this is not a significant problem.[55–58]

The most significant risk associated with discography is infection. The rate of discitis reported in the literature is as high as 1.3% per disc, and serious morbidity has resulted.[51,59,60] However, practice audits at centers performing a large volume of discography have demonstrated infection rates as low as 0 out of 10,000 (R. Derby, personal communication). There is experimental evidence that prophylactic antibiotics, both intravenous and intradiscal, can prevent discitis.[61–64] As a result, many practitioners routinely administer prophylactic antibiotics, particularly to high-risk patients such as diabetics.

Summary of Lumbar Discography

The primary utility of discography is as a provocative clinical test for the evaluation of axial spinal pain. The usefulness of any diagnostic study is critically dependent on the critical diagnosis and the pretest probability that a particular disorder is present.[17,34,35] Therefore, the results from discography must always be interpreted in the context of the patient's clinical presentation. In particular, prior to discography there should be a careful assessment of psychosocial risk factors.

An underlying assumption of the rationale for diagnostic injections, including provocative discography, is that it is possible to accurately measure pain. Measuring the change in pain after an injection relies to a large extent on a patient's self-report. Psychosocial factors affect the reaction to changes in nociceptive input, and, therefore, self-reports of pain. If patients are psychologically distressed the rationale for the injection may be invalid. This can potentially lead to both false-positive and false-negative responses. In assessing patients' responses to diagnostic injections, the relative contribution of nociception and psychological factors should be considered, and the reliability of patients' self-reports of pain estimated. Caragee and associates demonstrated the potential for psychological factors to affect the results from discography. Although more study is needed in this area, at a minimum it is important to be aware of psychosocial risk factors and understand how they might affect interpretation of the results from diagnostic injections. Moreover, the implications of psychosocial risk factors on eventual treatment, regardless of any results on diagnostic injections, should be considered. As an example, patients with somatization disorders are probably not good candidates for spinal fusion for axial pain. Therefore, discography is not a clinically useful test in those individuals and should only be performed in exceptional circumstances.

If a patient is being considered for surgical fusion for axial pain, pressure-controlled discography is indicated to determine whether they have chemically sensitized discs, in which case the data of Derby and colleagues suggests a high likelihood of success with an anterior interbody fusion.[41] At present it is not clear what the appropriate treatment should be for discs falling into either the mechanically sensitive or the indeterminate category. Preliminary information suggests that intertransverse fusion alone may be effective for mechanically sensitive discs.[41] Future research should focus on validating the disc classification system proposed by Derby and colleagues, and, in particular, further studying the predictive value of the mechanically sensitive and indeterminate categories.

Although not the primary focus of discography, it is important to assess the radiologic findings. The images should be reviewed to confirm that the needle was placed into the nucleus and that the subsequent dye injection fills the nucleus. Annular injections, injections into the space between the annulus and the nuclear cavity, and venous uptake are all possible and may invalidate the results.[65,66]

Several classification schemes have been developed to describe annular pathology as visualized by discography.[25,33,67–70] Regardless of the exact classification scheme used, it is important to note the degree of annular degeneration, the presence of annular fissures, and whether the annulus is competent or incompetent. If a patient has a convincing pain response but no evidence of a radial annular fissure on discography, postdiscography CT scanning should be considered, as some discs that appear normal on discography are found to be disrupted on CT discography.[33] In addition to annular pathology, both Schmorl's nodes and end-plate disruptions should be noted, as they may be clinically significant.[36,37]

If a patient has at least one disc that is both normal structurally and does not elicit a pain response, that is considered by some surgeons to serve as a control disc. A control injection may be helpful in deciding whether a pain response at another disc is a true positive result or reflects an exaggerated reaction to nociception. However, a more valid control would probably be a structurally abnormal disc. Although the significance of the results from control injections has not been formally validated, clinical experience suggests that if at least one structurally abnormal disc does not hurt, then pain provoked at another disc is more likely to be a true positive.

As a final note, there are some surgeons who do not believe that discography is necessary prior to fusion, as they feel that the diagnosis of discogenic pain can be made by clinical and radiographic criteria. There are substantial data suggesting that the clinical examination is of minimal use in discriminating between potential axial pain generators.[71,72] A possible exception to this is a McKenzie mechanical assessment, which may be able to predict the results from discography.[73] There have been several studies demonstrating that MRI cannot reliably predict which discs are painful on discography, at least to the level of confidence required to rely solely on MRI for surgical decision making.[2,31,74] A high-intensity zone in the posterior annulus, as visualized on MRI, has recently been proposed as a marker for painful discs.[75,76] Although highly specific, the sensitivity of this finding is only 26%, which limits the usefulness of the high-intensity zone in selecting patients for surgery.[33] If a patient undergoes a fusion for lumbar axial pain without preoperative discography, both the patient and the surgeon should be aware that the level adjacent to the planned fusion may be a source of clinical symptoms, regardless of the findings on MRI scan.

LUMBAR SELECTIVE EPIDURAL INJECTION

As is the case with the intervertebral disc, spinal nerves can be injected with contrast, local anesthetic, or other substances. Both the provocative response (pain occurring in response to a mechanical or chemical stimulus, or both) and the analgesic response provide clinically useful information.

Nerve root blocks were first developed to diagnose the source of radicular pain when imaging studies suggested possible compression of several roots.[20,77–84] Early studies on selective nerve root injections described an extraforaminal approach, in which a needle is advanced at right angles to the spinal nerve outside the neural foramen. Localization of the needle adjacent to the nerve relies on leg pain provocation, presumably resulting from penetration of the nerve by the needle.[20,81,82,84]

A selective epidural injection is a variation of the selective nerve root injection. As the nerve roots leave the dura to enter the foramen and form the spinal nerve, they carry an extension of the dura with them, which becomes the epineurium of the spinal nerve. The epineurium is, in turn, enveloped by an epiradicular membrane, which is an extension of the anterior and posterior epidural membranes.[85] Injection of contrast into the epiradicular membrane will outline the nerve root, dorsal root ganglion, spinal nerve, and ventral ramus. Proximally, contrast will flow around the dural sac at the takeoff of the nerve root. If injected outside the epiradicular membrane, contrast will spread diffusely in the epidural fat and, therefore, be of limited diagnostic value.

A selective epidural injection differs from a selective nerve root injection in that the goal is to inject into the epiradicular tissues. The spread of injected solutions will depend on the anatomy of the epiradicular membrane, which is an extension of the epidural space, leading to the term *selective epidural injection*. There are two major advantages of a selective epidural technique over a selective nerve root technique. Firstly, with a selective epidural injection, a foraminal approach is used and contact with the nerve is avoided, minimizing the potential for neural injury. Rather than relying on leg pain provocation from needle contact, needle localization is confirmed with contrast-enhanced images demonstrating an outline of the nerve. Secondarily, a selective epidural approach ensures that the injection incorporates all the sites where pathology can affect the nerve, from the disc level in the subarticular zone out lateral to the extraforaminal zone. If the pathology causing a patient's symptoms is a paramedian disc herniation, but the nerve is injected in the extraforaminal zone, as with a classic selective nerve root injection, the portion of the nerve from which the pain is coming may not be anesthetized, potentially leading to a false-negative result.

A selective epidural injection anesthetizes not only the spinal nerve itself but also all its branches. Two important branches of the spinal nerve are the sinuvertebral nerve and the medial branch of the dorsal primary ramus. The sinuvertebral nerve forms just lateral to the foramen from the ventral ramus and the grey ramus communicans.[6] Once formed, the nerve reenters the foramen, where it runs across the back of the vertebral body just below the upper pedicle. Two branches arise from the nerve, one ascending branch supplying the PLL and the next higher disc, and one descending, innervating the disc and PLL at the level of entry of the parent nerve.[6] Each sinuvertebral nerve is also distributed to the dura mater, with descending branches up to two segments caudally and an ascending branch up to one segment. The dorsal primary ramus from each spinal nerve divides into three branches, the medial, lateral, and intermediate (except at L5, which has only a medial and a lateral branch).[6] The most important of these branches is the medial branch, which hooks medially around the base of the SAP at the inferior most aspect of the intervertebral foramen, supplying the Z joints just above and below it's course. Thus, a selective epidural injection will partially anesthetize the dura (including the dural nerve root sleeves) up to two segments caudally and one segment rostrally, the PLL and intervertebral disc at the same level as the nerve and one segment rostrally, and the Z joints at the same level of the nerve and one segment below.

If a selective epidural injection is being performed for radicular pain, the fact that these structures are also anesthetized is irrelevant because they are sources of axial pain, not radicular pain. However, if an injection is being performed for axial pain, it is important to realize that pain relief after an injection can occur with pathology in any of the structures innervated by the nerve.

A selective epidural injection can potentially be helpful in diagnosing axial pain.[86] Any lesion that affects a nerve root also necessarily affects its dural sleeve and, therefore, is a potential cause of axial pain. In the case of herniated nucleus pulposus, disc material in the epidural space has been demonstrated to elicit an inflammatory response not only in the nerve root but also the dura. Relief of both axial and radicular pain with a selective epidural injection suggests that the same lesion is responsible for both. However, one cannot be certain that the axial component of the pain is arising from structures above or below the injected level. In patients with predominantly axial pain, fully characterizing the source of pain may require synovial joint or disc injections, or both, depending on the clinical situation.

A selective epidural injection has two components. The first is the provocative pain response resulting from contrast injection, and the second is the analgesic response resulting from injection of local anesthetic or corticosteroid, or both. In evaluating provoked pain, it is important to compare the location and character of the provoked response to the patient's typical symptoms. Furthermore, the onset of provoked pain should be related to the location of the leading edge of the contrast solution when pain begins.[86] Normal epidural tissue is not painful when gently stimulated by contrast solution. In the absence of scar tissue, pain provocation indicates that the tissue being stimulated is irritated. For example, early provocation of pain, when contrast is still in the foramen, suggests foraminal stenosis or a foraminal disc herniation. Late pain provocation when the contrast approaches the disc above is consistent with a paramedian disc herniation.

Immediately after the injection, the effect of the local anesthetic injected on the patient's symptoms should be assessed, both at rest and in response to mechanical stimulation. Studies on selective nerve root injections have used the criterion for a positive analgesic response to be from 80% (1) to 100% (2) relief.[77,86] The significance of lesser degrees of pain relief in response to an injection is uncertain. If corticosteroid is included in the injection, the patient should be reevaluated 1 week afterward, because the degree of pain relief at that interval can provide important information (see later discussion).

As is the case with provocative discography, a number of factors can lead to both false-positive and false-negative results from selective epidural injections. These factors include changes in CNS nociceptive processing that occur with chronic pain, psychological factors, and placebo responses.[44,45] However, in contrast to provocative discography, selective epidural injections are performed primarily for radicular pain. Therefore, there is a well-established gold standard—surgical exploration—against which diagnostic tests can be compared.

Several studies have evaluated the clinical utility of selective epidural and selective nerve root injections. Individual studies have investigated the predictive value of pain provocation, immediate pain relief from local anesthetic injection, and prolonged pain relief from corticosteroid in evaluating patients with radiculopathy.[77,83,86,87] A synthesis of the results from the studies on clinical utility suggests that the following protocol should be used to interpret the response to selective nerve root injections:

- If a patient has concordant or exact provoked pain in response to injection of contrast, complete pain relief following injection of local anesthetic, and a prolonged steroid response (>1 week), the injected nerve root is mediating the patient's symptoms and a good result can be expected from surgical decompression, assuming a correctable lesion is demonstrated on imaging studies.
- If a patient has discordant pain, incomplete immediate pain relief, and no prolonged steroid response, the injected nerve is probably not mediating the patient's symptoms and an alternate pain generator should be searched for.
- If an intermediate response occurs, a number of different possibilities exist. The patient may still have symptoms arising from a single nerve root, he or she may have symptoms from multiple roots, or he or she may not have radicular pain. If the clinical situation is highly suggestive of radiculopathy, it may be reasonable to repeat the selective nerve root injection, potentially with a control injection at an adjacent nerve. If the control injection is negative, the result from the active injection is more likely to be a true positive, particularly if there are multiple factors supporting a clinical significant response. If the control injection is positive or intermediate, and there is evidence of nerve root compression at both levels, it may be reasonable to perform a multilevel decompression, depending, of course, on the many clinical variables that may exist.

As with any diagnostic injection, if patients are psychologically distressed, the criteria used to interpret the test may be invalid. Recent data from Caragee and colleagues on lumbar discography reinforces the effect that psychosocial risk factors have on pain responses. Although more study is needed in this area, at a minimum it is important to note these risk factors and understand how they might affect interpretation of the result.

The usefulness of a selective epidural injection is primarily related to the associated provocative and analgesic pain responses. However, the contrast-enhanced images from the injection can reveal pathologic findings.[77,86] Two examples of this are a perpendicular nerve root sign, resulting from up-down foraminal stenosis, and obstruction to proximal flow of contrast, which can occur with foraminal stenosis, disc herniations, and scar tissue. The primary utility of findings such as these is to confirm findings evident on advanced imaging studies.

CERVICAL DISCOGRAPHY

Overview

Cervical discography is comparable in many ways to lumbar discography. The underlying premise of both is the same: Injection of the disc replicates the clinical noxious stimulus responsible for the patient's symptoms, and reproduction of the patients clinical symptoms during the injection confirms the disc as the source of pain. Both are subject to the confounding variables of nervous system plasticity and psychological factors. Similar to lumbar discography, the primary utility of cervical discography is as a clinical test, rather than a radiologic imaging test.

A major difference between lumbar and cervical discography is the relationship between pain provocation and disc morphology. In the lumbar spine, discs have varying degrees of disruption of the outer annulus. The pain resulting from lumbar discography has been shown to be directly related to the degree of fissuring of the outer annulus.[42,43] This finding provides a link between disc pathology and provoked pain, supporting circumstantial evidence suggesting that internal disc disruption is an important cause of axial low back pain.[6] Obviously, it would not have been possible to make this observation if all lumbar discs had the same degree of annular disruption.

Morphologically, cervical discs are very different from lumbar discs. Although both have a peripheral annulus fibrosus and a central nucleus, the cervical disc also has posterolateral uncovertebral joints. These are not true joints but are clefts in the annulus that communicate with the nucleus in the majority of individuals by early adulthood.[88] As a result of these clefts, if contrast is injected into cervical discs, the majority of them will demonstrate "annular tears."[89] Some cervical discs hurt when injected; others do not. Because they all have annular disruption, however, it is not possible to correlate provoked pain with underlying pathology.[89]

At present, the mechanisms responsible for cervical discogenic pain are unknown. Therefore, although a positive discogram in the lumbar spine can be used to diagnose a specific pathologic syndrome, a positive discogram in the cervical spine cannot. Ideally a diagnostic test will reveal the underlying target disorder that is responsible for pain.[17] The fact that cervical discography cannot do so compromises its clinical utility and constitutes a significant difference between cervical and lumbar discography.

Validity of Cervical Discography

Several studies have cast doubt on the validity of cervical discography.[90–92] Holt, in 1964, reported a 100% rate of positive discography in asymptomatic subjects. As in his study on lumbar discography, all the subjects were prisoners and he used a highly irritating contrast medium. In contrast to his lumbar study, a positive pain response, rather than a radiologic abnormality, was the criterion for a positive result.[91] Shinomaya and colleagues reported a 50% rate of positive discography in patients without neck pain. However, this was a group of patients with spondylitic myelopathy, therefore constituting a very different group than the one in which the test is typically performed.[92]

Bogduk and Aprill studied patients who had axial neck pain, only (i.e., without neurologic symptoms), with both Z-joint injections and discography. Using 100% pain relief as the criteria for a positive Z joint, they discovered that 41% had a positive disc and a positive Z joint at the same level. If Z-joint blocks were both highly sensitive and specific, this result would be an indication that there is a high false-positive rate associated with discography; that is, if the Z-joint block is a true positive, the disc must be a false-positive. However, the Z-joint blocks in this study were not controlled, which in other studies has been shown to have a false-positive rate of 27%.[93] This would suggest a 14% false-positive rate for discography, if the response to Z-joint blocks was used as the gold standard by which to judge discography.[90]

Schellhas and colleagues, in a well-designated study, used a nonirritating contrast medium to perform cervical discography on a group of volunteers recruited from the community as well as on a series of patients with chronic neck pain. They found that the majority of discs in both subjects and patients, including those that appeared normal on MRI, had annular tears on discography. However, discs from asymptomatic subjects, even if morphologically abnormal, were associated with low level pain responses. Among patients with chronic neck pain, however, there was a group that had intense pain with disc injection.[89]

The results from this study refutes the findings of Holt and Shimomaya, which suggested that the degree of pain provocation with discography was unrelated to whether or not the patient had neck pain. The Schellhas findings demonstrated that most cervical discs are morphologically abnormal and are associated with some discomfort on injection, but there is a definite, severe, concordant pain response in symptomatic patients that does not occur in asymptomatic subjects. The Schellhas study complements the Walsh study in the lumbar spine, demonstrating that although pain can occur during injection of discs in asymptomatic subjects, it occurs at low levels of intensity. Schellhas and colleagues evaluated interobserver reliability for the morphologic evaluation of MRI and discograms but did not assess the interobserver reliability of the pain response, as did Walsh. The importance of psychosocial factors was not addressed in the Schellhas study, but presumably they are as important with cervical discography as in lumbar discography.

Regardless of these studies on the sensitivity and specificity of cervical discography, it is important to remember that the ultimate criterion for a diagnostic test is whether the patient is better off as a result.[17] The primary indication for provocative discography is to determine whether a patient with chronic spinal pain, who has failed aggressive efforts at conservative care, can be helped with spinal fusion. As in the lumbar spine, the surgical treatment of axial neck pain is controversial. However, there is evidence that patients selected for anterior spinal fusion on the basis of discography can achieve outcomes in some studies ranging from 70% to 80%.[94–96]

Although the results from discography played an important part in surgical decision making in these studies, the criteria for a positive test were not strictly defined. Unlike the lumbar spine, pressure-controlled discography has not been used in the cervical spine. There is abundant evidence regarding the role of mechanical and chemical factors in causing lumbar spinal pain; however, there is little equivalent information in the cervical spine. While there is some information on the normative values for intradiscal pressures in the cervical spine,[97] for technical reasons it is difficult to measure pressures accurately at the time of cervical discography. Therefore, at present there is no way to reproducibly measure the stimulus applied to the cervical disc.

Technique

The cervical disc is approached via a right anterolateral approach.[50] As a result, a number of potential complications can occur.[98–101] As the needle is advanced to the disc, puncture of the carotid artery or deeper vessels of the neck can lead to bleeding complications and possible airway compromise. If the needle is advanced too far in a posterior direction, it may puncture vessels in the anterior epidural space, potentially resulting in hematoma formation and spinal cord compression. Puncture of the spinal cord itself is possible, with obvious consequences, particularly if contrast is injected into the cord. Acute quadriplegia has been reported following cervical discography, presumably related to posterior displacement of disc tissue with injection and resultant spinal cord compression.[99]

In addition to the risks associated with needle placement, infectious complications related to cervical discography are potentially devastating. In addition to the risk of introduction of skin organisms, there is a potential for enteric organisms to be introduced into the disc if the needle passes through the hypopharynx or esophagus. Discitis may lead to epidural abscess, with resultant quadriplegia.[97] Because of the potentially catastrophic adverse effects associated with discitis in the cervical spine, some consider diabetes mellitus to be an absolute contraindication to cervical discography. Prophylactic antibiotics, either intravenous or intradiscal, should be strongly considered for all patients.

Summary of Cervical Discography

At this time cervical discography must be considered primarily an art rather than a science. We do not really know the underlying disorder we are diagnosing with this test, nor can we predict with confidence the results from surgery. Given the potential complications associated with cervical discography, it should only be performed by individuals who have a detailed understanding of the anatomy of the cervical spine and are skilled in performing and interpreting diagnostic spinal injections of other structures, most notably the lumbar disc. As virtually all cervical discs contain annular tears, the role of CT discography in the cervical spine is limited. There are no published data suggesting that postdiscography CT provides clinically useful information.

Retrospective studies suggest that anterior interbody fusion may be an effective treatment for discogenic neck pain; however, at present, there are no discographic criteria that can be used reliably to predict outcome from surgery. Understanding that clinically useful criteria for interpreting cervical provocative discography have not been defined, experienced discographers consider the following characteristics to suggest a symptomatic disc: concordant or exact pain (exact more significant), intensity greater than 6-out-of-10, pain 1 minute after injection at least 50% of the maximum intensity, two or more pain behaviors in response to injection, low intradiscal pressure at pain provocation (as estimated by manual pressure), and a negative control injection.

CERVICAL SELECTIVE EPIDURAL STEROID INJECTION

As in the lumbar spine, the epineurium of each cervical spinal nerve root is enveloped by an epiradicular membrane, which is an extension of the anterior and posterior epidural membranes.[84] As a result, selective epidural injections may be performed in the cervical spine, and given the analogous innervation of the cervical and lumbar spines,[30] may be used to accomplish the same goal; that is, to determine the nerve root responsible for radicular pain.

Cervical selective nerve root injections are performed using an anterolateral approach, with the radiologic landmark being the base of the superior articular process as viewed in an oblique projection of the spine, and the midpoint of the lateral mass as viewed in the anteroposterior projection. Care must be taken to keep the needle tip posterior to the vertebral artery at all times during insertion.

Unlike the lumbar spine, there is no information on the predictive value of pain provocation, immediate pain relief from local anesthetic injection, and prolonged pain relief from corticosteroid in evaluating patients with cervical radiculopathy. Nonetheless, the responses to these injections are commonly interpreted using the same criteria as in the lumbar spine. There have been no studies correlating pathology with the contrast-enhanced images from selective cervical epidural injections; therefore, the primary clinical utility of these images is to ensure that injectate is confined to the target nerve root.

REFERENCES

1. Boden SD, Davis DO, Dina TS, et al. Abnormal magnetic-resonance scans of the lumbar spine. In: Asymptomatic subjects. A prospective investigation. *J Bone Joint Surg Am* 1990;72A:403–408.
2. Zucherman J, Derby R, Hsu K, et al. Normal magnetic resonance imaging with abnormal discography. *Spine* 1988;13:1355–1359.
3. Borkan JM, Koes B, Reis S, et al. A report from the Second International Forum for Primary Care Research on Low Back Pain. Reexamining priorities. *Spine* 1998;23:1992–1996.
4. Hadler NM. Back pain in the workplace. What you lift or how you lift matters far less than whether you lift or when [editorial]. *Spine* 1997;22:935–940.
5. Cherkin DC. Primary care research on low back pain. The state of the science. *Spine* 1998;23:1997–2002.
6. Bogduk N. *Clinical Anatomy of the Lumbar Spine and Sacrum.* 3rd ed. New York: Churchill Livingstone; 1997.
7. Colhoun E, McCall IW, Williams L, et al. Provocation discography as a guide to planning operations on the spine. *J Bone Joint Surg Br* 1988;70B:267–271.
8. Gill K, Blumenthal S: Functional results after anterior lumbar fusion at L5-S1 in patients with normal and abnormal MRI scans. *Spine* 1992;17:940–942.
9. Greenough C, Peterson M, Taylor L, et al. Lumbar spinal fusion: A comparison of anterior and instrumented posterolateral technique. In: International Society for the Study of the Lumbar Spine; June 1996; Vermont; Abstracts.
10. Knox BD, Chapman TM. Anterior lumbar interbody fusion for discogram concordant pain. *J Spinal Disord* 1993;6:242–244.
11. Lee CK, Vessa P, Lee JK. Chronic disabling low back pain syndrome caused by internal disc derangements: The results of disc excision and posterior lumbar interbody fusion. *Spine* 1995;20:356–361.
12. Newman MH, Grinstead GL. Anterior lumbar interbody fusion for internal disc disruption. *Spine* 1992;17:831–833.
13. Parker LM, Murrell SE, Boden S, et al. The outcome of posterolateral fusion in highly selected patients with discogenic low back pain [see comments]. *Spine* 1996;21:1909–1916; discussion 1916–1917.
14. Simmons EH, Segil CM. An evaluation of discography in the localization of symptomatic levels in discogenic disease of the spine. *Clin Orthop* 1975;108:57–69.
15. Vamvanji V, Fredrickson BE, Thorpe JM, et al. Outcome and intertransverse fusion in internal disc disruption. In: International Society for the Study of the Lumbar Spine; June 25–29, 1996; Burlington, Vermont; Abstracts.
16. Wetzel FT, LaRocca SH, Lowery GL, et al. The treatment of lumbar spinal pain syndromes diagnosed by discography. Lumbar arthrodesis [see comments]. *Spine* 1994;19:792–800.
17. Sackett D. Clinical epidemiology. A basic science for clinical medicine. 2nd ed. Boston, Ma: Little Brown; 1991.
18. Caragee E, Vittum D, Tanner C, et al. The deceptive discogram: Positive provocative discography as a misleading finding in the evaluation of back pain. In: North American Spine Society, 12th annual meeting; October 22–25, 1997; New York, NY.
19. Nachemson A. Lumbar discography—where are we today? [see comments]. *Spine* 1989;14:555–557.
20. Hansen FR, Biering-Sorensen F, Schroll M. Minnesota Multiphasic Personality Inventory profiles in persons with or without low back pain. A 20-year follow-up study [see comments]. *Spine* 1995;20: 2716–2720.
21. Sullivan M. The problem of pain in the clinicopathological method. *Clin J Pain* 1998;14:197–201.
22. Wallis BJ, Lord SM, Barnsley L, et al. Pain and psychologic symptoms of Australian patients with whiplash [see comments]. *Spine* 1996;21:804–810.
23. Caragee E, Tanner C, Norbash A, et al. The rates of false positive discography in select patients without low back complaints. *Spine* [in press].
24. Schofferman J, Anderson D, Hines R, et al. Childhood psychological trauma correlates with unsuccessful lumbar spine surgery. *Spine* 1992;17:138–144.
25. Lindblom K. Diagnostic puncture of intervertebral disks in sciatica. *Acta Orthop Scand* 1948;17:237–238.
26. Bernard TN Jr. Using computed tomography/discography and enhanced magnetic resonance imaging to distinguish between scar tissue and recurrent lumbar disc herniation. *Spine* 1994;19:2826–2832.
27. Brodsky AE, Binder WF. Lumbar discography—its value in diagnosis and treatment of lumbar disc lesions. *Spine* 1979;4:110–120.
28. Gunzburg R, Parkinson R, Moore R, et al. A cadaveric study comparing discography, magnetic resonance imaging, histology, and mechanical behavior of the human lumbar disc. *Spine* 1992;17:417–426.
29. Jackson RP, Glah JJ. Foraminal and extraforaminal lumbar disc herniation: Diagnosis and treatment. *Spine* 1987;12:577–585.
30. Mendel T, Wink CS, Zimny ML. Neural elements in human cervical intervertebral discs. *Spine* 1992;17:132–135.
31. Simmons JW, Emery SF, McMillin JN, et al. Awake discography. A comparison study with magnetic resonance imaging. *Spine* 1991; 16(suppl):S216–S221.
32. Bernard TN Jr. Lumbar discography followed by computed tomography—refining the diagnosis of low-back pain. *Spine* 1990; 15:690–707.
33. Sachs BL, Vanharanta H, Spivey MA, et al. Dallas discogram description. A new classification of CT/discography in low-back disorders. *Spine* 1987;12:287–294.
34. Jaeschke R, Guyatt G, Sackett DL. Users' guides to the medical literature. III. How to use an article about a diagnostic test. A. Are the results of the study valid? The Evidence-Based Medicine Working Group. *JAMA* 1994;271:389–391.
35. Jaeschke R, Guyatt GH, Sackett DL. Users' guides to the medical literature. III. How to use an article about a diagnostic test. B. What are the results and will they help me in caring for my patients? The Evidence-Based Medicine Working Group. *JAMA* 1994;271:703–707.
36. Hsu KY, Zucherman JF, Derby R, Goldthwaite N, Wynne G. Painful lumbar endplate disruptions: A significant discographic finding. *Spine* 1988;13:76–78.
37. Malmivaara A, Videman T, Kuosma E, et al. Plain radiographic, discographic, and direct observations of Schmorl's nodes in the thoracolumbar junctional region of the cadaveric spine. *Spine* 1987;12: 453–457.

38. Guyer RD, Ohnmeiss DD. Lumbar discography. Position statement from the North American Spine Society Diagnostic and Therapeutic Committee [see comments]. *Spine* 1995;20:2048–2059.
39. Heggeness MH, Doherty BJ. Discography causes end plate deflection. *Spine* 1993;18:1050–1053.
40. Weinstein J, Claverie W, Gibson S. The pain of discography. *Spine* 1988;13:1344–1348.
41. Derby R, Howard M, Grant J, et al. The ability of pressure controlled discography to predict surgical and non-surgical outcome. *Spine* 1999;24:364–371.
42. Moneta GB, Videman T, Kaivanto K, et al. Reported pain during lumbar discography as a function of anular ruptures and disc degeneration. A re-analysis of 833 discograms. *Spine* 1994;19:1968–1974.
43. Vanharanta H, Sachs BL, Spivey MA, et al. The relationship of pain provocation to lumbar disc deterioration as seen by CT/discography. *Spine* 1987;12:295–298.
44. Siddall PJ, Cousins MJ. Spinal pain mechanisms. *Spine* 1997;22:98–104.
45. North RB, Kidd DH, Zahurak M, et al. Specificity of diagnostic nerve blocks: A prospective, randomized study of sciatica due to lumbosacral spine disease. *Pain* 1996;65:77–85.
46. Holt EP Jr. The question of lumbar discography. *J Bone Joint Surg Am* 1968;50:720–726.
47. Walsh TR, Weinstein JN, Spratt KF, et al. Lumbar discography in normal subjects. A controlled, prospective study. *J Bone Joint Surg Am* 1990;72:1081–1088.
48. Fluke MM. The treatment of lumbar spine pain syndromes diagnosed by discography: lumbar arthrodesis [letter; comment]. *Spine* 1995;20: 501–504.
49. Quinnell RC, Stockdale HR, Willis DS. Observations of pressures within normal discs in the lumbar spine. *Spine* 1983;8:166–169.
50. Aprill C. Diagnostic disc injection. In: Fyrmoyer JW, ed. *The Adult Spine* New York, NY: Raven; 1991:403–442.
51. Fraser RD, Osti OL, Vernon-Roberts B. Discitis after discography. *J Bone Joint Surg Br* 1987;69B:26–35.
52. MacMillan J, Schaffer JL, Kambin P. Routes and incidence of communication of lumbar discs with surrounding neural structures. *Spine* 1991;16:167–171.
53. Troisier O. An accurate method for lumbar disc puncture using a single channel intensifier. *Spine* 1990;15:222–228.
54. Gill K. New-onset sciatica after automated percutaneous discetomy. *Spine* 1994;19:466–467.
55. Grubb S, Lipscomb H, Guilford W. The relative value of lumbar roentgenograms metrizamide myelography, and discography in the assessment of patients with chronic low-back syndrome. *Spine* 1987; 12:282–286.
56. Inufusa A, Hasegawa T, Fuse K, et al. Effect of annular puncture on the adolescent canine intervertebral disc. In: North American Spine Society, 12th annual meeting; October 22–25, 1997; New York, NY.
57. Johnson RG. Does discography injure normal discs? An analysis of repeat discograms. *Spine* 1989;14:424–426.
58. Kahanovitz N, Arnoczky SP, Sissons HA, et al. The effect of discography on the canine intervertebral disc. *Spine* 1986;11:26–27.
59. Guyer RD, Collier R, Stith WJ, et al. Discitis after discography. *Spine* 1988;13:1352–1354.
60. Junila J, Niinimaki T, Tervonen O. Epidural abscess after lumbar discography—a case report. *Spine* 1997;22:2191–2193.
61. Fraser RD, Osti OL, Vernon-Roberts B. Iatrogenic discitis: The role of intravenous antibiotics in prevention and treatment. An experimental study. *Spine* 1989;14:1025–1032.
62. Jamrich E, Fabian H, Raabe T. Antibiotic penetration into the adult human nucleus pulposus. In: North American Spine Society, 12th annual meeting; Oct 22–25, 1997; New York, NY.
63. Lang R, Folman Y, Ravid M, et al. Penetration of ceftriaxome into the intervertebral disc. *J Bone Joint Surg Br* 1994;76A:689–691.
64. Osti OL, Fraser RD, Vernon-Roberts B. Discitis after discography—the role of prophylactic antibiotics. *J Bone Joint Surg Br* 1990;72: 271–274.
65. Quinnell RC, Stockdale HR. An investigation of artefacts in lumbar discography. *Br J Radiol* 1980;53:831–839.
66. Schellhas K. Venous opacification during discography: Therapeutic implications. In: International Spinal Injection Society, 4th annual meeting; August 16, 1996; Vancouver, Canada.
67. McCutcheon ME, Thompson WC. CT scanning of lumbar dicography. A useful diagnostic adjunct. *Spine* 1986;11:257–259.
68. Ninomiya M, Muro T. Pathoanatomy of lumbar disc herniation as demonstrated by computed tomography/discography. *Spine* 1992;17: 1316–1322.
69. Quinnell RC, Stockdale HR. The use of in vivo lumbar discography to assess the clinical significance of the position of the intercrestal line. *Spine* 1983;8:305–307.
70. Videman T, Malmivaara A, Mooney V. The value of the axial view in assessing discograms. An experimental study with cadavers. *Spine* 1987;12:299–304.
71. Schwarzer AC, Aprill CN, Bodguk N. The sacroiliac joint in chronic low back pain. *Spine* 1995;20:31–37.
72. Schwarzer AC, Aprill CN, Derby R, et al. The relative contributions of the disc and zygapophyseal joint in chronic low back pain. *Spine* 1994;19:801–806.
73. Donelson R, Aprill C, Medcalf R, et al. A prospective study of centralization of lumbar and referred pain. A predictor of symptomatic discs and anular competence. *Spine* 1997;22:1115–1122.
74. Osti OL, Fraser RD. MRI and discography of annular tears and intervertebral disc degeneration. A prospective clinical comparison [published erratum appears in J Bone Joint Surg Br 1992;74:793] [see comments]. *J Bone Joint Surg Br* 1992;74:431–435.
75. Aprill C, Bodguk N. High-intensity zone: A diagnostic sign of painful lumbar disc on magnetic resonance imaging. *Br J Radiol* 1992;65: 361–369.
76. Schellhaus K, Heithoff K, Pollei S. Lumbar disc high intensity zone: Pain managment with intradiscal steroids. In: North American Spine Society, 11th annual meeting; October 23–26, 1996; Vancouver, Canada.
77. Dooley JF, McBroom RJ, Taguchi T, et al. Nerve root infiltration in the diagnosis of radicular pain. *Spine* 1988;13:79–83.
78. Haueisen DC, Smith BS, Myers SR, et al. The diagnostic accuracy of spinal nerve injection studies. Their role in the evaluation of recurrent sciatica. *Clin Orthop* 1985;198:179–183.
79. Herron LD. Selective nerve root block in patient selection for lumbar surgery: Surgical results. *J Spinel Disord* 1989;2:75–79.
80. Hoppenstein R. A new approach to the failed back syndrome. *Spine* 1980;5:371–379.
81. Kikuchi S, Hasue M, Nishiyama K, et al. Anatomic and clinical studies of radicular symptoms. *Spine* 1984;9:23–30.
82. Krempen JF, Smith BS. Nerve-root injection: A method for evaluating the etiology of sciatica. *J Bone Joint Surg Am* 1974;56:1435–1444.
83. Stanley D, McLaren MI, Euinton HA, et al. A prospective study of nerve root infiltration in the diagnosis of sciatica. A comparison with radiculography, computed tomography, and operative findings. *Spine* 1990;15:540–543.
84. Tajima K. [Selective radiculography and block (author's translation)]. *Nippon Seikeigeka Gakkai Zasshi* 1982;56:71–90.
85. Kikuchi S. Anatomical and experimental studies of nerve root infiltration. *Nippon Seikeigeka Gakkai Zasshi* 1982;56:605–614.
86. Derby R, Kine G, Saal J, et al. Precision percutaneous blocking procedures for localizing spinal pain. Part 2: The lumbar neuraxial compartment. *Pain Digest* 1993;3:175–188.
87. Derby R, Kine G, Saal JA, et al. Response to steroid and duration of radicular pain as predictors of surgical outcome. *Spine* 1992; 17(suppl):S176–S183.

88. Oda J, Tanaka H, Tsuzuki N. Intervertebral disc changes with aging of human cervical vertebra. From the neonate to the eighties. *Spine* 1988;13:1205–1211.
89. Schellhas KP, Smith MD, Gundry CR, et al. Cervical discogenic pain. Prospective correlation of magnetic resonance imaging and discography in asymptomatic subjects and pain sufferers. *Spine* 1996;21:300–311, discussion 311–312.
90. Bogduk N, Aprill C. On the nature of neck pain, discography, and cervical zygapophysial joint blocks. *Pain* 1993;54:213–217.
91. Holt E Jr. Fallacy of cervical discography. *JAMA* 1964;188:799–801.
92. Shinomiya K, Nakao K, Shindoh S, et al. Evaluation of cervical diskography in pain origin and provocation. *J Spinal Disord* 1993;6:422–426.
93. Lord SM, Barnsley L, Bogduk N. The utility of comparative local anesthetic blocks versus placebo-controlled blocks for the diagnosis of cervical zygapophysial joint pain. *Clin J Pain* 1995;11:208–213.
94. Kikuchi S, Macnab I, Moreau P. Localisation of the level of sympatomatic cervical disc degeneration. *J Bone Joint Surg Br* 1981;63B: 272–277.
95. Riley LH Jr, Robinson RA, Johnson KA, et al. The results of anterior interbody fusion of the cervical spine. Review of ninety-three consecutive cases. *J Neurosurg* 1969;30:127–133.
96. Whitecloud TSD, Seago RA. Cervical discogenic syndrome. Results of operative intervention in patients with positive discography. *Spine* 1987;12:313–316.
97. Pospiech J, Stolke D, Wilke HJ, et al. Intradiscal pressure recordings in the cervical spine. *Neurosurgery* 1999;44:379–384.
98. Connor PM, Darden BVD. Cervical discography complications and clinical efficacy. *Spine* 1993;18:2035–2038.
99. Guyer RD, Ohnmeiss DD, Mason SL, et al. Complications of cervical discography: Findings in a large series. *J Spinal Disord* 1997; 10:95–101.
100. Laun A, Lorenz R, Agnoli AL. Complications of cervical discography. *J Neurosurg Sci* 1981;25:17–20.
101. Zeidman SM, Thompson K, Ducker TB. Complications of cervical discography: Analysis of 4400 diagnostic disc injections. *Neurosurgery* 1995;37:414–417.

PART III

Psychological Evaluation and Treatment of Chronic Pain

CHAPTER 12 PSYCHOLOGICAL ASPECTS OF PAIN

Dennis C. Turk and Akiko Okifuji*

It is important to consider how we conceptualize pain. Our views of pain will influence our evaluations of patients who report pain and the nature of the interventions that we use to treat them. The way in which we conceptualize pain depends largely on the nature of the information acquired and the models we were exposed to during our training. In the first section of this chapter, we review the traditional conceptualizations of pain. Although these models are not necessarily inaccurate, they are incomplete. We propose that a broader, multidimensional perspective is required to understand pain and to treat patients appropriately. We describe the role of behavioral, cognitive, and affective factors that have been shown to be relevant to the experience of pain, disability, and response to treatment. We provide data demonstrating that these psychological factors may have an effect on both patients' behavior and physiology. Finally, we raise the issue of the "patient uniformity myth" and describe the subgroups of pain patients based on psychosocial and behavioral characteristics. We provide preliminary data suggesting that knowledge of such patient subgroups may serve as a basis for matching patients to treatments based on their characteristics.

UNIDIMENSIONAL SENSORY MODEL

Historically, pain has been understood from the perspective of Cartesian dualism wherein pain was viewed as purely sensory, reflecting the degrees of incoming noxious sensory stimuli. This perspective assumes that there are two ends to a pain pathway. At the periphery are sensory receptors where noxious information is received; at the other end, regions located in the brain where information is registered passively. From this perspective, noxious stimulation inevitably results in the sensation of pain, as if pulling a string at the periphery activates a bell located in the brain. Variations of this model have been prominent since first proposed by Aristotle.

A central belief of sensory models is that the amount of pain experienced is a direct result of the amount, degree, or nature of sensory input or physical damage and is explained in terms of specific physiologic mechanisms. Clinically, it is expected that the report of pain will be directly proportional to the amount of pathology. This model dictates that assessment should focus on identifying the cause of the pain. Once identified, treatment should involve removal of the cause or severing the specific pain pathways by surgical or pharmacologic means.

* Preparation of this manuscript was supported by grants from the National Institute of Child Health and Development (P01 HD33989) and the National Institute of Arthritis and Musculoskeletal and Skin Diseases (R01 AR 44724) awarded to the first author and the National Institutes of Health/Shannon Director's Award (R55 AR44230) awarded to the second author.

Sensory models continued to maintain a prominent position in medicine despite the inability of this model to account for a number of observations. For example:

- Patients with equivalent degrees and types of objectively determined tissue pathology vary widely in their reports of pain severity.
- Patients with only minimal objectively determined pathology may report severe pain.
- Asymptomatic individuals often reveal significant amount of physical pathology on imaging procedures that might be expected to produce pain.
- Surgical procedures designed to inhibit pain transmission by severing neurologic pathways believed to be underlying the reported pain may fail to alleviate pain.
- Patients with equivalent degrees of tissue pathology who are treated with identical treatments respond in widely differently ways.
- There are only modest associations among impairment, pain, and disability.

Thus, we see a number of paradoxes in clinical practice: patients who report severe pain with limited physical pathology and, conversely, individuals who have significant physical pathology but no pain; pain pathway ablated but continued pain; and identical treatments provided for the same diagnosis with different outcomes.

Unfortunately, for many chronic pain sufferers, the underlying causes for their pain frequently remain unknown despite the development and use of sophisticated diagnostic imaging procedures such as computed tomography (CT) scan or magnetic resonance imaging (MRI). For example, objective evidence of physical pathology is only identified in about 15% of the cases of back pain.[1] In some conditions, such as recurrent headaches, diagnostic procedures do not reveal any biologic problem that is sufficient to account for the pain reported. Obviously, something other than identifiable physical pathology is influencing patients' reports.

How can such paradoxes be understood? As is frequently the case in medicine, when objective physical evidence and explanations prove inadequate to explain symptoms, psychological alternatives are proposed. If the pain reported by a patient is believed to be *disproportionate* to objectively determined physical pathology or if the complaint is recalcitrant to so-called appropriate treatment, then it is assumed that psychological factors must be involved, even if not causal. Thus, there appears to be a somatogenic-psychogenic dichotomy in how pain is construed.

PSYCHOGENIC PERSPECTIVE

It is important to realize that determination of whether the reported pain is disproportionate is subjective. There is no objective way to determine how much pain is *proportionate*. How much should a given amount of tissue pathology hurt? Similarly, determination of appropriate treatment is not totally objective. Different health care providers might recommend widely different treatments for patients with the same presenting symptoms. For example, treatments for patients with temporomandibular disorders range from surgery to psychotherapy.

The somatogenic-psychogenic dichotomy forms the basis for the distinction underlying attempts to identify "functional" versus "organic" pain, as well as references to a "functional overlay." The American Psychiatric Association[2] created two psychiatric diagnoses associated with pain in the 4th edition of the *Diagnostic and Statistical Manual of Mental Disorders*—pain associated with psychological factors either with or without a diagnosed medical condition. The specific diagnosis of "Pain Disorder Associated with Psychological Factors and a General Medical Condition" is characterized by the fact that both psychological and a general medical conditions have important roles in the onset, severity, exacerbation, and maintenance of pain. This set of diagnoses is so broadly defined, however, that virtually all patients who have persistent pain could be diagnosed as suffering from a psychiatric disorder.

MOTIVATIONAL VIEW

A variation of the dichotomous somatic-psychogenic views is a conceptualization that is ascribed to by many insurance carriers and other third-party payers. They suggest that if physical pathology is insufficient to support the claim of pain, then the complaint is invalid. Instead, pain is assumed to result from symptom exaggeration or outright malingering. The assumption is that reports of pain without adequate biomedical evidence are motivated primarily by desire for financial gain. This belief has resulted in a number of attempts to *catch* malingerers using surreptitious observation methods and the use of sophisticated biomechanical machines geared toward identifying inconsistencies in functional performance. There is, however, very little empirical support for this belief. No studies, for example, have demonstrated dramatic improvement in pain reports subsequent to receiving disability awards (i.e., no further need to exaggerate symptoms).

The conceptualizations previously described view physical and psychological factors as if they are mutually exclusive. Next, we examine the nature of the psychological processes and factors that have been demonstrated to play an important role in pain perception, disability, and response to treatment.

PSYCHOLOGICAL FACTORS AFFECTING PAIN EXPERIENCE

A number of psychological principles based in leaning theory have been extended to pain. These principles provide helpful explanations for many clinical observations. Moreover, a number of cognitive and affective factors have been demonstrated to influence expressions of pain and participation in rehabilitation. We can consider the major psychological, sociocultural, and behavioral principles and factors studied and then consider how they can be integrated to create a comprehensive model of pain that can serve as a guide for assessment and, ultimately, treatment.

Operant Learning Mechanisms

As long ago as the early part of the twentieth century, the effects of environmental factors in shaping the experience of pain were acknowledged. A new era in thinking about pain began in 1976 when Fordyce[3] extended the principles of operant conditioning to chronic pain and disability.

In the operant conditioning formulation, behavioral manifestations of pain rather than pain per se are central. When a person experiences noxious sensation, the initial response is a withdrawal or escape response. This may be accomplished by avoidance of activity believed to cause or exacerbate pain, help-seeking to reduce symptoms, and so forth. These behaviors are observable and, consequently, subject to the principles of operant conditioning, namely, reinforcement and avoidance learning.

The operant view proposes that pain behaviors, such as avoidance of activity to protect a wounded limb from producing additional noxious input, may come under the control of external contingencies of reinforcement (responses increase or decrease as a function of their reinforcing consequences). It is these reinforcement contingencies that contribute to the maintenance of the problems associated with chronic pain and disability. Pain behaviors (e.g., limping, grimacing, and inactivity) are conceptualized as overt expressions of pain, distress, and suffering. These behaviors may be positively reinforced directly, for example, by attention from a spouse or from health care providers. Pain behaviors also may be maintained by the escape from noxious stimulation through the use of drugs or rest, or the avoidance of undesirable activities such as work. In addition "well behaviors" (e.g., activity, working) may not be positively reinforcing, and the more rewarding pain behaviors may, therefore, be maintained.

We can illustrate the role of operant factors in a case of chronic back pain. When a woman with a painful back has a flare-up, she may lie down on the floor and hold her back. Her husband will notice these behaviors and infer that she is in pain. The husband's behavioral response is influenced by his observation of her behavior. He typically responds to her pain complaints by spending extra time and massaging her back. In this case, her lying down has resulted in the pain sufferer receiving attention from her husband, a positive consequence. According to the laws of operant learning, behaviors that result in a positive consequence are more likely to recur.

Another powerful way the husband reinforces his wife's pain behaviors is by permitting her to avoid undesirable activities. When observing his wife lying on the floor, the husband suggests that they cancel their plans to get together with his brother that evening. If the pain sufferer would prefer not to spend time with her husband's brother, then the avoidance of the undesirable activity is reinforced and may contribute to reports of pain whenever activities with her husband's brother are planned. In this situation, her pain reports and behaviors are rewarded both by her husband providing her with extra attention and support, and by the opportunity to avoid an undesirable social obligation.

It is important to clarify that the operant learning does not require the pain sufferer's intentional and conscious efforts to elicit a desirable outcome. It results from a gradual learning process that neither the sufferer nor others recognize. One should not assume pain behaviors are synonymous with malingering. Malingering involves the patient consciously and purposely faking a symptom such as pain for some gain, usually financial. In the case of pain behaviors, there is no suggestion of conscious deception; rather, the unintended performance of pain behaviors results from laws of learning based on environmental reinforcement contingencies. Typically, there is little awareness that these behaviors are being displayed or that the patient is consciously motivated to obtain a positive reinforcement from the behaviors. The pain behavior in response to initial injury may encounter reinforcing events, thereby determining probability of that behavior recurring in the future. Once the behavior is learned, the presence of initial pain is no longer needed for that behavior to recur.

The operant conditioning formulation does not concern itself with the initial cause of pain. Rather, it considers pain an internal subjective experience that can only be indirectly assessed and may be maintained even after an initial physical basis of pain has resolved. Because of the consequences of specific behavioral responses, it is proposed that pain behaviors may persist long after the initial cause of the pain is resolved or greatly reduced. Thus, in one sense, the operant conditioning model can be viewed as analogous to the psychogenic models described earlier. That is, psychological factors are treated as secondary, reactions to sensory stimulation, rather than directly involved in the perception of pain per se.

The operant view has generated what has proven to be an effective treatment for select samples of patients with chronic pain.[4] Treatment focuses on eliminating pain behaviors by withdrawal of attention and increasing "well behaviors" (e.g., activity) by positive reinforcement. Although operant factors undoubtedly play a role in the maintenance of disability, exclusive reliance on the operant conditioning model to explain the experience of pain may not be appropriate. It has been criticized for its exclusive focus on motor pain behaviors, failure to consider the emotional and cognitive aspects of pain, and failure to treat the subjective experience of pain.[5]

Respondent Learning Mechanisms

Factors contributing to chronicity that have previously been conceptualized in terms of operant learning may also be initiated and maintained by classical or so-called respondent conditioning.[6,7] If an aversive stimulus is paired with a neutral stimulus several times, the neutral stimulus will come to elicit aversive experience in the individual. The patient leans to anticipate negative consequences even in the absence of the noxious stimulus. This process has been observed frequently in cancer patients receiving chemotherapy. Patients have been observed to report nausea, even before any cytotoxic medication has been administered, when they enter the room where they have received chemotherapy. Similarly, a patient with back pain who received a painful treatment from a physical therapist may become conditioned to experience a negative emotional response to the presence of the physical therapist, to the treatment room, and to any stimulus associated with the nociceptive stimulus (e.g., exercise equipment). The negative emotional reaction may lead to tensing of muscles and this, in turn, may exacerbate pain, thereby reinforcing the association between the presence of the physical therapist and pain.

The most relevant emotional conditioning in pain probably is anxiety. Anxiety is often the affect underlying avoidance of activities. Pain patients often experience temporary aggravation of pain following physical activities. Avoiding such activities leads to no pain exacerbation, thus reinforcing inactivity and maintaining anxiety for activity. In other words, the persistence of avoidance of specific activities reduces disconfirmations that could provide corrective feedback.[8] Insofar as avoidance does not produce disconfirmation, the behaviors will persist.[9] By contrast, when the anticipated consequence does not occur (disconfirmation), modification of learning also takes place. Thus, the physical therapist may have to encourage the patient to exercise to provide disconfirmation of the anticipation that exercise will hurt and lead to increased injury. The therapist has to emphasize that hurt and harm are not the same things. Both respondent conditioning and operant learning may contribute to the development and maintenance of dysfunctional behavioral patterns in patients with chronic pain. Over time, more and more activities, people, and physical locations may be seen as eliciting or exacerbating pain and will be avoided (stimulus generalization). Fear of pain and avoidance may become conditioned to an expanding number of situations (response generalization). In addition to the avoidance learning, pain may be exacerbated and maintained in these encounters with potentially pain-increasing situations because of the anxiety-related increases in sympathetic activation and muscle tension that may occur in anticipation of pain and, also, as a consequence of pain. Thus, as we emphasize later in this chapter, psychological factors may directly affect nociceptive stimulation and need not be viewed as only reactions to pain.

Social Learning Mechanisms

Social learning has received some attention in the study of acute pain and the development and maintenance of chronic pain states. From this perspective, how we experience pain is shaped and influenced by what we have observed, so-called observational learning. That is, individuals can acquire responses that were not previously in their behavioral repertoire by watching others perform these activities. Children acquire attitudes about health, health care, and the perceptive style for recognizing and understanding bodily symptoms from their parents and social environment. They also learn how injuries and diseases should be attended. As they grow older, the learning emerges as their tendency to ignore or over-respond to symptoms they experience. The culturally acquired interpretations of symptoms determine how people deal with illness.

There is ample experimental evidence of the role of social learning from controlled laboratory pain studies and some evidence based on observations of patients' behaviors in field and clinical settings. Physiologic responses to pain stimuli may be conditioned during observation of others in pain. For example, patients on a burn unit have sufficient opportunity to observe the responses of other burn patients.[10] Each patient's response to his or her situation is affected by observations of other patients. In one study, children of chronic pain patients chose more pain-related responses to scenarios presented to them than did children of healthy or diabetic parents. Moreover, teachers rated the children of pain patients as displaying more illness behaviors (e.g., complaining, absences from school, visits to the school nurse) than the children of healthy controls.[11] Expectancies as well as actual behavioral responses to noxious stimuli are based, at least partially, on prior social leaning history. This situation may contribute to the marked variability in response to objectively similar degrees of physical pathology noted by health care providers.

ROLE OF COGNITIVE FACTORS IN PAIN

A great deal of research has been directed toward explicating the role of cognitive factors in pain. These studies have consistently demonstrated that patients' attitudes, beliefs, and expectancies about their situation, themselves, their coping resources, and the health care system affect the reports of pain, activity, disability, and response to treatment.[12,13]

Beliefs about Pain

Clinicians working with patients who have chronic pain are aware that patients having similar pain histories and expressions of pain may differ greatly in their beliefs about their pain.[14] Behavior and emotion are influenced by how one interprets events, rather than by objective characteristics of the events. Thus, pain, when interpreted as signifying ongoing tissue damage or a progressive disease, is likely to elicit considerably more suffering and behavioral dysfunction than when it is viewed as being the result of a transient problem that eventually will improve. Consider the case of an individual who wakes up one morning with a headache. Very different responses would be expected if he attributed the headache to excessive alcohol consumption the night before than would be the case if he interpreted the headache as a signal of a brain tumor. Thus, although the amount of nociceptive input in the two cases may be equivalent, the emotional and behavioral responses would vary in nature and intensity.

Certain beliefs may lead to maladaptive coping, increased suffering, and greater disability. Patients who believe that there is nothing they can do to control pain may be passive in their coping efforts and fail to make use of available resources to cope with pain. Patients who consider their pain to be an unexplainable mystery feel helpless and clueless as to how to cope with the situation. The sense of helplessness contributes to negative evaluations of one's own abilities and coping strategies as effective in controlling and decreasing pain.[15] Once beliefs and expectancies about a disease are formed, they become stable and are very difficult to modify. Patients tend to avoid experiences that could invalidate their beliefs (disconfirmation), and they guide their behavior in accordance with these beliefs (confirmation), even when the beliefs are no longer valid. Consequently, as noted earlier when the role of respondent conditioning was described, they do not obtain corrective feedback. For example, feeling muscular pain following activity may be caused by lack of muscle strength and general deconditioning and not by additional tissue damage.

Patients with chronic low back pain generally demonstrate poor behavioral persistence in various exercise tasks, and their performance on these tasks is independent of physical exertion or actual self-reports of pain, but rather is related to previous pain reports.[16] These patients appear to have a negative view of their abilities and expect increased pain if they perform physical exercises. Thus, the rationale for their avoidance of exercise is not the presence of pain but their learned expectation of heightened pain and accompanying physical arousal that might exacerbate pain and reinforce their beliefs regarding the pervasiveness of their disability. If patients view disability as an expected consequence of their pain, that activity is dangerous, and the pain is an acceptable excuse for neglecting responsibilities, they are likely to experience prolonged disability. Patients' negative perceptions of their capabilities for physical performance form a vicious circle, with the failure to perform activities reinforcing the perception of helplessness and incapacity. Once again, avoidance of activity prevents disconfirmation.

The strong influence by one's belief system can also be associated with pain resulting from serious diseases. Spiegel and Bloom[17] reported that the pain severity of cancer patients could be predicted by the use of analgesics, affective state, and assumed pathology of pain. Patients who attributed their pain to a progression of their underlying disease experienced more pain despite comparable levels of disease than did patients with more benign interpretations.

In addition to beliefs about capabilities to function despite pain, beliefs about pain per se appear to be of importance in understanding response to treatment, adherence to self-management activities, and disability.[15] When successful rehabilitation occurs, there appears to be an important cognitive shift from beliefs about helplessness and passivity to resourcefulness and ability to function regardless of pain.[12,13]

Clearly, it is essential for patients with chronic and recurrent pain to develop adaptive beliefs and to emphasize the importance of maintaining functionality despite pain. In fact, changes in pain levels do not necessarily parallel changes in other variables of interest, including activity level, medication use, return to work, rated ability to cope with pain, and pursuit of further treatment.[18]

Self-Efficacy

Another important cognitive factor related to beliefs about pain is the belief about one's ability to cope with pain, referred to as self-efficacy.[19] A self-efficacy expectation is defined as a personal conviction that one can successfully execute a course of action (perform required behaviors) to produce a desired outcome in a given situation. This variable has been demonstrated as a major mediator of therapeutic change. Given sufficient motivation to engage in a behavior, it is a person's self-efficacy beliefs that determine the choice of activities he or she will initiate, the amount of effort that will be expended, and how long the person will persist in the face of obstacles and aversive experiences. Efficacy judgments are based on four sources of information regarding one's capabilities, listed in descending order of impact:

- One's own past performance at the task or similar tasks
- The performance accomplishments of others who are perceived to be similar to oneself
- Verbal persuasion by others that one is capable
- Perception of one's own state of physiologic arousal, which is in turn partly determined by prior efficacy estimation[19]

Experience of performance mastery is critical in developing adequate self-efficacy belief. It can be achieved by starting patients at a modest level with graded activities added gradually. From this perspective, the occurrence of coping behaviors is conceptualized as being mediated by people's beliefs that situation demands do not exceed their coping resources. Council and colleagues[20] asked patients to rate their self-efficacy as well as expected level of pain related to performing movement tasks. Patients' performance levels were highly related to their self-efficacy expectations, which, in turn, appeared to be determined by their expectancy of pain levels.

Catastrophizing

So-called catastrophizing—extremely negative thoughts about one's plight and interpretation of even minor problems as major catastrophes—appears to be a particularly potent way of thinking that greatly influences pain and disability. Several lines of research, including experimental laboratory studies of acute pain with normal volunteers and field studies with clinical patients suffering clinical pain, have indicated that catastrophizing and adaptive coping strategies are important in determining reactions to pain.[21] Individuals who spontaneously use catastrophizing self-statements reported more pain than those who did not catastrophize in several acute and chronic pain studies. Turk and colleagues concluded that "what appears to distinguish low from high pain tolerant individuals is their cognitive processing, catastrophizing thoughts and feelings that precede, accompany, and follow aversive stimulation" (p. 197).[22]

Coping

Self-regulation of pain management depends on the individual's specific ways of dealing with pain, adjusting to pain, and reducing or minimizing pain and distressed caused by pain—coping strategies. Coping is manifested spontaneously; coping action is employed purposefully and intentionally, and it can be assessed in terms of overt and covert behaviors.[13] Overt behavioral coping strategies include rest, medication, and use of relaxation. Covert coping strategies include various means of distracting oneself from pain, reassuring oneself that the pain will diminish, seeking information, and problem solving. Coping strategies are thought to alter both the perceived pain intensity and one's ability to manage or tolerate pain and to continue everyday activities.

Coping can be beneficial or detrimental in management of pain. Studies have found active coping strategies (e.g., efforts to function in spite of pain or to distract oneself from pain, such as engaging in activity, ignoring pain) to be associated with adaptive functioning. Passive coping strategies (e.g., depending on others for help in pain control and restriction on activities) were related to greater pain and depression.[21] In a number of studies, it has been demonstrated that if participants are instructed in the use of adaptive coping strategies, the pain intensity decreases and tolerance of pain increases.[14] The most prominent factor in poor coping appears to be the presence of catastrophizing rather than differences in the nature of specific strategies.

INDIRECT EFFECTS OF COGNITIVE FACTORS ON PAIN

Cognitive factors may act indirectly on pain and disability by reducing physical activity, and, consequently reducing muscle flexibility, strength, and tone. Fear of re-injury, fear of losing disability compensation, and low level of job dissatisfaction can also adversely influence return to work.

Pain sufferers can develop ways of coping that in the short run seem adaptive but in the long run serve to maintain the chronic pain condition and result in greater disability. As noted earlier, one of these ways of coping is avoidance of activities because of the fear of pain or injury. For example, following an accident in which a man hurts his back, he learns that certain movements make his pain worse. In response, he may stop engaging in activities that exacerbate his pain and restrict his movements in an attempt to avoid pain. As a result, he may lose muscle strength, flexibility, and endurance. Here a vicious circle can begin, for as the muscles became weaker, more and more activities caused pain. As individuals with back pain remain inactive and become more physically deconditioned, they may not allow themselves the opportunity to be rehabilitated by identifying the activities that build flexibility, endurance, and strength without the risk of pain or injury. In addition, the distorted movements and postures that individuals use to protect themselves from pain may cause further pain unrelated to the initial injury. For example, when a woman who has hurt her leg limps, she protects muscles on one side of her back but the muscles on the other side of her back may become overactive and can develop into painful conditions of their own. Thus, avoidance of activity, although it is a seemingly rationale way to manage a pain problem, can actually play a large role in maintaining the chronic pain condition and increasing disability. In addition to contributing to the maintenance of the pain condition, the use of avoidant-coping strategies has other negative consequences.

After having limited success in controlling pain, the chronic pain sufferers may perceive pain and the factors that influence the pain to be outside of their personal control. Individuals who feel pain is uncontrollable are not likely to attempt new strategies to manage their pain. Instead, pain sufferers feel increasingly frustrated and demoralized when *uncontrollable* pain interferes with participation in rewarding recreational, occupational, and social activities. It is common for pain sufferers to resort to passive coping strategies, such as inactivity, self-medication, or alcohol, to reduce emotional distress and pain.

Pain sufferers who feel little personal control over their pain are also likely to catastrophize about the impact of situations that trigger or exacerbate their pain and about pain flare-ups. In contrast, individuals who believe in their own ability to control the situations contributing to flare-ups are more resourceful and are more likely to develop self-management strategies that are effective in limiting the impact of the pain episodes or flare-ups, and thus are able to limit the impact of the pain problem.

Whereas maladaptive cognition can worsen pain, adaptive cognition can have a positive effect. Individuals who feel they have a number of successful methods for coping with pain may suffer less then those who feel helpless and hopeless. Psychological interventions such as relaxation, contingency management, and coping skills training have been shown to be effective in helping people with persistent pain to either eliminate their pain or, if pain cannot be eliminated, reduce their pain, distress, and suffering. These interventions are designed not only to decrease pain, but also to improve physical and psychological functioning.

DIRECT EFFECTS OF PSYCHOLOGICAL FACTORS ON PAIN

Several studies have suggested that psychological factors may actually have a direct effect on physiologic parameters associated more directly with the production or exacerbation of nociception.[23] Cognitive interpretations and relevant arousal may have a direct effect on physiology by increasing sympathetic tones, endogenous opioid (endorphins) production, and levels of muscle tension.

Effects of Thoughts on Autonomic Arousal

Circumstances that are appraised as potentially threatening to safety or comfort are likely to generate strong physiologic reactions. In a sample of patients suffering from recurrent migraine headaches, Jamner and Tursky[24] observed an increase in skin conductance, indicating autonomic arousal, in response to seeing words describing migraine headaches simply displayed on a screen. Prolonged autonomic arousal might contribute to headaches.

Chronic increases in sympathetic nervous system activation are known to decrease skeletal muscle tone and, thus, may set the stage for hyperactive muscle contraction and possibly for the persistence of a contraction following conscious muscle activation. Excessive sympathetic arousal is viewed as the immediate precursor of muscle hypertonicity, hyperactivity, and persistence. These responses, in turn, are the proximate causes of muscle spasm and pain. In is not usual for someone in pain to amplify the significance of the problem and needlessly *turn on* the sympathetic nervous system. In this way, thought processes may influence sympathetic arousal and predispose the individual to further pain or otherwise complicate the process of recovery.

The direct effect of thoughts on muscle tension response was demonstrated by Flor and colleagues.[23] These investigators interviewed patients with back pain disorders, patients with other pain disorders, and healthy individuals. Muscle tension sensors were placed on the surface of the lower back, forearm, and forehead. During the monitoring of muscle activity, patients were asked to recall and describe in as much detail as possible the last time they experienced extreme pain and the last time they experienced severe stress. The study found that when discussing their pain or stress, the patients with back pain had significantly elevated muscle tension in their back, but not in their forehead or forearm. However, when these patients with back pain were resting and not discussing their pain or stress, their back muscle tension level was no higher than the non–back pain patients or the healthy individuals. Neither the non–back pain patients nor the healthy individuals showed elevations in muscle tension when discussing severe stresses. Thus, patients with back pain showed pain site–specific muscular arousal simply by talking about their pain and stress. Similar results have been observed in studies with patients who had chronic arm and shoulder pain[25] and those with temporomandibular disorders.[26]

Effects of Thoughts on Biochemistry

Bandura and colleagues[27] directly examined the role of central opioid activity in cognitive control of pain. They trained subjects to use various coping strategies for alleviating pain, including attention diversion from pain sensations to other matters, engaging imagery, imaginal separation (dissociation) of the limb in pain from the rest of the body, transformation of pain as nonpain sensations, and self-encouragement of coping efforts. They demonstrated that (1) self-efficacy increased with cognitive training, (2) self-efficacy predicted pain tolerance, and, importantly, (3) naloxone (an opioid antagonist) blocked the effects cognitive coping. The latter result specifically implicates the direct effects of thoughts on endogenous opioids. Bandura and colleagues concluded that the physical mechanism by which self-efficacy influences pain perception might at least be partially mediated by the endogenous opioid system.

O'Leary and colleagues[28] provided stress management treatment to patients with rheumatoid arthritis. Degree of self-efficacy (expectations about the ability to control pain and disability) enhancement was correlated with treatment effectiveness. Patients with higher self-efficacy and greater self-efficacy enhancement displayed greater numbers of suppressor T cells. Significant effects were also obtained for self-efficacy, pain, and joint impairment. Increased self-efficacy for functioning was associated with decreased disability and joint impairment.

EFFECTS OF AFFECTIVE FACTORS ON PAIN

The International Association for the Study of Pain specifies that "[Pain] is unquestionably a sensation in a part or parts of the body but it is also always unpleasant and therefore also an emotional experience."[29] The affective factors associated with pain include many different emotions, but they are primarily negative in quality. Anxiety and depression have received the greatest amount of attention in patients with chronic pain; however, anger has recently received considerable interest as an important emotion in these patients.

Depression and Anxiety

Research suggests that from 40% to 50% of patients with chronic pain suffer from depression.[30] There has been extensive debate concerning the causal relationship between depression and pain. In the majority of cases, depression appears to be patients' reaction to their plight.[31]

Given the chronicity and impact, it should not surprise us that a large number of patients with chronic pain are depressed. It is interesting to ponder the other side of the coin. How is it that all such patients are *not* depressed? Turk and colleagues examined this question and determined that patients' appraisals of the impact of the pain on their lives and of their ability to exert any control over the pain and their lives mediated the pain-depression relationship.[31,32] We have also recently noted that pain severity and sensitivity do not differentiate depressed from nondepressed chronic pain patients.[33]

Anger

Anger has been widely observed in individuals with chronic pain. Pilowsky and Spence[34] reported an incidence of "bottled-up anger" in 53% of patients with chronic pain. Kerns and colleagues[35] noted that the internalization of angry feelings was strongly related to measures of pain intensity, perceived interference, and reported frequency of pain behaviors. Anger and hostility are closely associated with pain in persons with spinal cord injuries.[36]

Frustrations related to persistence of symptoms, limited information on etiology, and repeated treatment failures along with anger toward employers, the insurance carrier, the health care system, family members, and themselves, all contribute to the general dysphoric mood of these patients. The impact of anger and frustration on exacerbation of pain and treatment acceptance has not received adequate attention. It would be reasonable to expect that the presence of anger may serve as an aggravating factor, associated with increasing autonomic arousal and blocking motivation and acceptance of treatments oriented toward rehabilitation and disability management rather than cure, which are often the only treatments available for chronic pain.

PATIENT UNIFORMITY MYTH

The importance of psychological factors has been widely recognized and many pain treatment programs include interventions designed to address cognitive, affective, and behavioral components of the pain experience. One consistent finding seems to be that each treatment seems to work for some patients but no treatment works for everyone. Thus, clinicians must be careful not to be trapped in the "patient homogeneity myth." Although characterization of patient populations may help classify patients and direct treatment plans, research has shown that any populations that are defined by pain diagnoses demonstrate heterogeneity in their cognitive-affective-behavioral dimensions.

To address the heterogeneity of pain patients, Kerns and colleagues[37] developed a comprehensive inventory, the Multidimensional Pain Inventory (MPI). The MPI was designed to assess the cognitive, affective, and behavioral responses of patients with chronic pain to their symptoms. The MPI focuses on patients' interpretation of their plight, effects of interpersonal relationships, and functional limitations. Using a statistical procedure (i.e., cluster analysis), Turk and colleagues[38] identified three distinct profiles of patients with chronic pain. They were labeled as: (1) *"dysfunctional"* (DYS), characterized by high levels of pain, life interference, emotional distress, and functional limitations; (2) *"interpersonally distressed"* (ID), similar to the DYS but further characterized by low level of support from their significant others; and (3) *"adaptive copers"* (AC), characterized by low levels of pain, functional limitations, and emotional distress. The classification system has been replicated in several studies conducted in Finland,[39] the Netherlands,[40] and in a large, multi-centered study in the United States.[41]

Research using the MPI has demonstrated that the majority of patients with diverse chronic pain disorders (e.g., low back pain, temporomandibular disorder, headaches, fibromyalgia, and metastatic disease) can be classified into one of the three empirically derived profiles.[38,42,43] Although the percentage of patients classified within each of the profiles varies across pain disorders, patients' styles of adaptation to pain are very consistent within a profile regardless of their medical diagnosis, suggesting the relative independence of psychosocial dimension of chronic pain from biomedical factors (Fig. 12-1). The results from these studies suggest that a dual-diagnostic approach may be useful, whereby two diagnoses are assigned concurrently—physical and psychosocial-behavioral—and treatment plans can be developed within each of the diagnostic frames.[44]

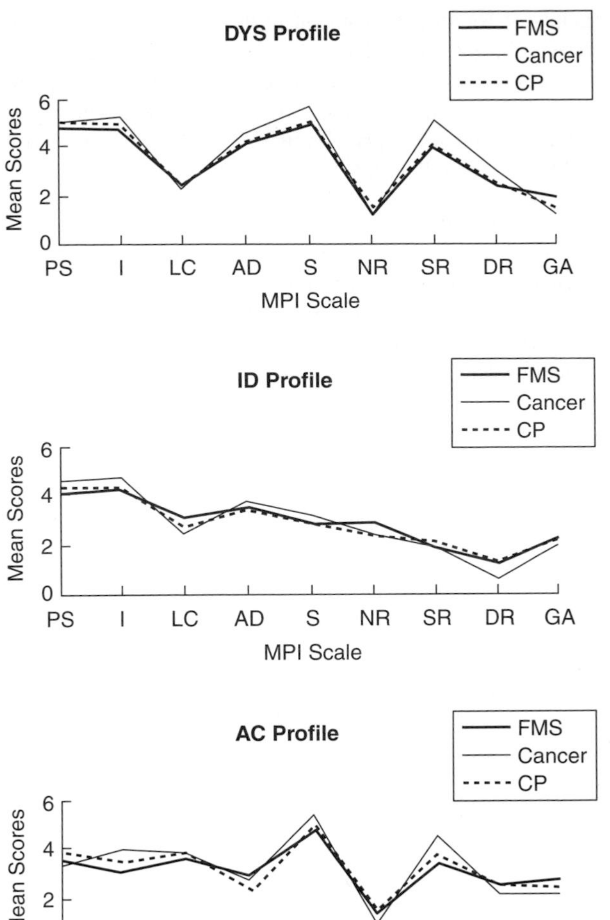

Figure 12-1 Mean multidimensional pain inventory (MPI) scale scores in three groups of pain patients, by MPI profile. DYS, dysfunctional; ID, interpersonally distressed; AC, adaptive copers.

	DYS	ID	AC
Treatment 1: Focusing on maladaptive thoughts and coping skills			
Treatment 2: Focusing on interpersonal and communication skills			
Treatment 3: Focusing on supportive counseling			

Matched treatment

Potential "overtreatment"

Undertreatment

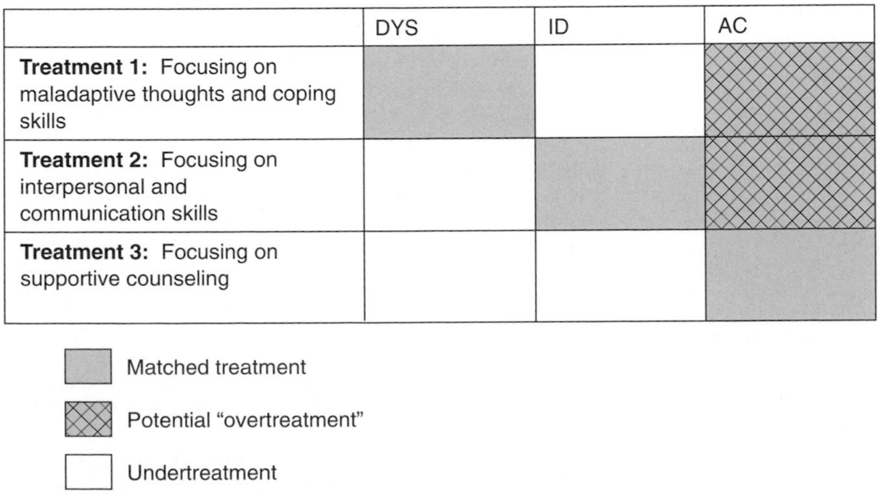

Figure 12-2 Sample treatment-matching chart. DYS, dysfunctional; ID, interpersonally distressed; AC, adaptive copers.

Example of Treatments Matched to Psychosocial and Behavioral Characteristics We would hypothesize that providing a treatment plan that specifically addresses psychosocial needs of each profile should show superior outcome to unmatched treatment. A basic cognitive-behavioral approach, including cognitive restructuring and behavioral skill training for pain management, is the most widely practiced method by pain psychologists.[45] Our previous trials showed that although, as a group, patients with chronic pain show significant treatment gains from this approach, the three profile groups differentially responded to the treatment.[46] Most notably, patients who fit into the interpersonally distressed profile did not show significant improvement.[46]

Instead of the "one-size-fits-all" method, we need to address the "what-treatment-works-for-whom" question. One example can be seen in Fig. 12-2. Three specific plans may be developed on the basis of the profile characteristics of the MPI classification. In this matrix, dysfunctional patients should benefit most from treatment 1, whereas interpersonally distressed patients should show improvement when they undergo treatment 2, over and beyond the improvement expected from the nonspecific effects of treatment. Treatment 3 can be considered as minimal psychological intervention, because adaptive copers are adjusting reasonably well, this minimal approach may be sufficient for these patients to achieve beneficial effects from the overall therapy. Elimination of inappropriate treatments should save cost as well as time, effort, and frustration for patients and treating clinicians.

SUMMARY

Understanding of the role of psychological factors has greatly increased since the first edition of this volume was published. Research efforts have confirmed that pain is a multifactorial phenomenon. In particular, several psychological factors, learning principles, cognitive factors, and affective components have been found to significantly influence how people experience pain, cope with pain, and recover from pain. In this chapter, we described different perspectives on pain and suggested that the unidimensional models (biomedical, psychogenic, motivational, behavioral) are inadequate both to explain chronic pain and as the basis for treatment. We examined the range of psychological factors that play an intricate role in pain perception, disability, and response to treatment. We raised a concern about the patient homogeneity myth and described one effort to subdivide patients based on a set of psychosocial and behavioral factors. Finally, we provided some preliminary evidence demonstrating that patients with different characteristics respond quite differently to the same treatment. Additional studies are needed to confirm these results, and studies are needed to evaluate the potential of a specific treatment-matching strategy.

Although we focused in this chapter on the role of psychological factors in chronic pain, we believe that these same factors may play a role in acute pain states as well. We believe that physical, psychosocial, and behavioral factors are all important in the experience of pain, per se. The relative weight of these factors may vary, however, with physical factors making a larger contribution in acute pain states than chronic pain states and psychological factors making a more significant contribution in chronic pain than acute pain. In each of these instances, however, attention should be given to the range of factors that contribute to the total experience of pain.

REFERENCES

1. Deyo RA. Early diagnostic evaluation of low back pain. *J Gen Intern Med* 1986;1:328–338.
2. American Psychiatric Association. *Diagnostic and Statistical Manual.* vol. IV. Washington, DC: American Psychiatric Association; 1994.
3. Fordyce W. *Behavioral Methods in Chronic Pain and Illness.* St. Louis, Mo: CV Mosby; 1976.
4. Vlaeyen J, Haazen I, Schuerman J, et al. Behavioural rehabilitation of chronic low back pain: Comparison of an operant treatment, an operant-cognitive treatment and an operant-respondent treatment. *Br J Clin Psychol* 1995;34:95–118.
5. Turk DC, Flor H. Pain is > than pain behaviors: The utility and limitations of the pain behavior construct. *Pain* 1987;31:277–295.
6. Turk DC, Okifuji A, Sherman J. Psychological aspects of back pain: Implications for physical therapists. In: Twomey L, Taylor J, eds. *Physical Therapy of the Low Back.* 3rd ed. New York, NY: WB Saunders; 2000:353–383.
7. Turk DC, Flor H. Chronic pain: A biobehavioral perspective. In: Gatchel R, Turk DC, eds. *Psychological Factors in Pain.* New York, NY: Guilford Press; 1999:18–34.
8. Schmidt A, Brands A. Persistence behavior of chronic low back pain patients in an acute pain situation. *J Psychosom Res* 1986;30:339–346.
9. Arntz A, Vaneck M, DeJong P. Avoidance of pain of unpredictable intensity. *Behav Res Ther* 1991;29:197–202.
10. Fagerhaugh S. Pain expression and control on a burn care unit. *Nursing Outlook* 1974;22:645–650.
11. Richard K. The occurrence of maladaptive health-related behaviors and teacher-related conduct problems in children of chronic low back pain patients. *J Behav Med* 1988;11:107–116.
12. Tota-Faucette ME, Gil KM, Williams DA, et al. Predictors of response to pain management treatment. The role of family environment and changes in cognitive processes. *Clin J Pain* 1993;9:115–123.
13. Jensen MP, Turner JA, Romano JM, et al. Coping with chronic pain: A critical review of the literature. *Pain* 1991;47:249–283.
14. DeGood D, Shutty M. Assessment of pain beliefs, coping and self-efficacy. In: Turk DC, Melzack R, eds. *Handbook of Pain Assessment.* New York, NY: Guilford Press; 1992:214–234.
15. Williams D, Thorn B. An empirical assessment of pain beliefs. *Pain* 1989;36:185–190.
16. Arntz A, Peters M. Chronic low back pain and inaccurate predictions of pain: Is being too tough a risk factor for the development and maintenance of chronic pain? *Behav Res Ther* 1995;33:49–53.
17. Spiegel D, Bloom JR. Pain in metastatic breast cancer. *Cancer* 1983;52:341–345.
18. Turk DC, Okifuji A, Sinclair JD, et al. Interdisciplinary treatment for fibromyalgia syndrome: Clinical and statistical significance. *Arthritis Care Res* 1998;11:186–195.
19. Bandura A, Cioffi D, Taylor CB, et al. Perceived self-efficacy in coping with cognitive stressors and opioid activation. *J Pers Soc Psychol* 1988;55:479–488.
20. Council J, Ahern D, Follick M, et al. Expectancies and functional impairment in chronic low back pain. *Pain* 1988;33:323–331.
21. Keefe FJ, Brown GK, Wallston KA, et al. Coping with rheumatoid arthritis pain: Catastrophizing as a maladaptive strategy. *Pain* 1989;37:51–56.
22. Turk DC, Meichenbaum M, Genest M. *Pain and Behavioral Medicine: A Cognitive-Behavioral Perspective.* New York, NY: Guilford Press; 1983.
23. Flor H, Turk DC, Birbaumer N. Assessment of stress-related psychophysiological reactions in chronic back pain patients. *J Consult Clin Psychol* 1985;53:354–364.
24. Jamner L, Tursky B. Discrimination between intensity and affective pain descriptors: A psychophysiological evaluation. *Pain* 1987;30:271–283.
25. Moulton B, Spence S. Site-specific muscle hyper-reactivity in musicians with occupational upper limb pain. *Behav Res Ther* 1992;30:375–386.

26. Flor H, Birbaumer N, Schugens MM, et al. Symptom-specific psychophysiological responses in chronic pain patients. *Psychophysiology* 1992;29:452–460.
27. Bandura A, O'Leary A, Taylor CB, et al. Perceived self-efficacy and pain control: Opioid and nonopiod mechanisms. *J Pers Soc Psychol* 1987;53:563–571.
28. O'Leary A, Shoor S, Lorig K, et al: A cognitive-behavioral treatment for rheumatoid arthritis. *Health Psychol* 1988;7:527–544.
29. International Association for the Study of Pain. Classification of chronic pain. Descriptions of chronic pain syndromes and definitions of pain terms. *Pain* 1986;3:S1–226.
30. Romano JM, Turner JA. Chronic pain and depression: Does the evidence support a relationship? *Psychol Bull* 1985;97:18–34.
31. Rudy TE, Kerns RD, Turk DC. Chronic pain and depression: Toward a cognitive-behavioral mediation model. *Pain* 1988;35:129–140.
32. Turk DC, Okifuji A, Scharff L. Chronic pain and depression: Role of perceived impact and perceived control in different age cohorts. *Pain* 1995;61:93–101.
33. Okifuji A, Turk DC, Sherman J. Fibromyalgia syndrome and depression: Why are not all fibromyalgia patients depressed? 2000;27: 212–219.
34. Pilowsky I, Spence N. Pain, anger, and illness behaviour. *J Psychosom Res* 1976;20:411–416.
35. Kerns R, Rosenberg R, Jacob M. Anger expression and chronic pain. *J Behav Med* 1994;17:57–67.
36. Summers JD, Rapoff MA, Varghese G, et al. Psychosocial factors in chronic spinal cord injury pain. *Pain* 1991;47:183–189.
37. Kerns RD, Turk DC, Rudy TE. The West Haven–Yale Multidimensional Pain Inventory (WHYMPI). *Pain* 1985;23:345–356.
38. Turk DC, Rudy TE. Toward an empirically derived taxonomy of chronic pain patients: Integration of psychological assessment data. *J Consult Clin Psychol* 1988;56:233–238.
39. Talo S, Rytokoski U, Puukka P. Patient classification, a key to evaluate pain treatment: A psychological study in chronic low back pain patients. *Spine* 1992;17:998–1011.
40. Lousberg R, Schmidt AJ, Groenman NH, et al. Validating the MPI-DLV using experience sampling data. *J Behav Med* 1997;20:195–206.
41. Jamison RN, Rudy TE, Penzien DB, et al. Cognitive-behavioral classifications of chronic pain: Replication and extension of empirically derived patient profiles. *Pain* 1994;57:277–292.
42. Turk DC, Okifuji A, Sinclair JD, et al. Pain, disability, and physical functioning in subgroups of patients with fibromyalgia. *J Rheumatol* 1996;23:1255–1262.
43. Turk DC, Sist TC, Okifuji A, et al. Adaptation to metastatic cancer pain, regional/local cancer pain and noncancer pain: Role of psychological and behavioral factors. *Pain* 1998;74:247–256.
44. Turk DC. Customizing treatment for chronic pain patients: Who, what, and why. *Clin J Pain* 1990;6:255–270.
45. Turk DC, Okifuji A. A cognitive-behavioral approach to pain management. In: Wall P, Melzack R, eds. *Textbook of Pain.* 4th ed. London, England: Churchill-Livingstone; 2000:1431–1444.
46. Turk DC, Okifuji A, Starz T, et al. Differential responses by psychosocial subgroups of fibromyalgia syndrome patients to an interdisciplinary treatment. *Arthritis Care Res* 1998;11:397–404.

CHAPTER 13 PSYCHOSOCIAL ASSESSMENT OF CHRONIC PAIN

R. Joshua Wootton

Why does one patient develop chronic pain and face disability, while another—with seemingly the same injuries, extent of tissue damage, and quality of medical care—recovers and returns to normal activity following a brief convalescence? Arguably, there may be biologic variables between the two that are difficult to discern medically, but a comparison, in most cases, is likely to reveal that the greater portion of the variance consists of psychosocial differences. When pain physicians wonder why a patient fails to respond to procedures and medications that have proven efficacious for many others with the same medical presentation, it is frequently the pain psychologist who can offer the most reasonable and, more importantly, functional set of hypotheses.

Although nociceptive or purely physiologic factors may instigate pain, how it is expressed by the individual, over time, suggests that what might have begun as a simple picture can become considerably more complicated and intricate through the influence of psychological and social factors. Melzack and Wall's gate control theory emphasizes that pain cannot be fully understood without an assessment of the motivational-affective, sensory-discriminative, and cognitive-evaluative processes of the individual. Adherents to the biopsychosocial, mind-body, and behavioral medicine approaches to pain all affirm that, whereas the origin of pain may not be psychological, how one *responds* to it *is*. Assessing this response expediently and accurately may redirect the focus of a patient's treatment, highlighting the psychosocial dimension of the patient's experience as essential to diagnosis and successful outcome. Chronic pain may not lead to adjustment difficulties, mental disorder, and disability, but when it does, psychosocial assessment may offer the only helpful perspective on why, as well as the best hope for recovery.

COMPREHENSIVE EVALUATION OF PAIN AND DISABILITY

Social policy and, in some instances, medical practice have lagged behind science in operationalizing the comprehensive approach to pain management. Psychological services, for example, are a requirement for pain treatment centers seeking accreditation by the Commission on Accreditation of Rehabilitation Facilities (CARF)[1]; yet many health insurance carriers balk at the idea of reimbursing for psychological evaluation and treatment, and there are no uniformly endorsed standards in the private sector. In medical practice, physicians who do not see their patients in a multidisciplinary setting may not involve psychological evaluation in cases of chronic pain, until considerable frustration and the question of *functional versus organic origin* has arisen. Ironically, by that time, the interpretation of the patient's pain has often passed from a medical to a wholly psychological one, and the wish not to affront or unduly alarm the patient is well past consideration.

When patients are asked to see a psychologist or to complete a battery of psychological tests and questionnaires, many indeed respond defensively and, sometimes, even hostilely. For many, referral to a psychologist is tantamount to confrontation with their worst fear: "My doctor doesn't believe me." How the physician approaches the patient, therefore, frequently becomes the first crucial step toward putting together a comprehensive picture of what the patient is experiencing. It may prove helpful to remind patients that their chronic pain is likely one of the biggest problems in their lives—if not indeed *the* biggest—and that it would be surprising if it did not affect their relationships and usual ways of coping. The principal goal of psychosocial assessment in chronic pain is not, as some patients fear, to determine whether or how much pain can be attributed to psychological sources but rather to identify the emotional, behavioral, and social factors that may be complicating the experience of pain—prolonging it beyond its organic usefulness, rendering it less tractable to treatment, and moving the patient toward physical and psychological disability. The development of a successful plan for treatment often depends on identifying these influences and strategizing how to address them expediently, sensitively, and thoroughly.

In this comprehensive approach to chronic pain, the question of disability becomes more complex than one of straightforward injury and tissue damage. How the patient responds to his or her pain raises questions about the contributions of temperament, personality, coping style, psychopathology, and the dominant beliefs or explanatory model through which he or she tries to make sense of his or her pain. If these dimensions of the patient's experience are not carefully and thoughtfully evaluated, then the risk of missing a critical piece of information relevant to planning treatment is greatly increased. A misstep can set the patient back, physically and emotionally, at once contributing to the needlessly increased cost of care and the frustration of providers, families, employers, and health insurance carriers.

Although successful treatment is the designated end of psychosocial assessment, psychologists may be asked to evaluate a range of secondary issues, including estimated course of health care utilization, probability of returning to previous employment, and probability of re-injury.[2] Depending on the setting, they may also be asked to screen patients for the appropriateness of medical and surgical interventions, to evaluate the risk of substance abuse or suicide, to assess the likelihood of compliance with medical recommendations, and to render an opinion in the determination of whether a patient is partially or totally, temporarily or permanently disabled.[3,4] Especially when the question of disability is raised, psychological evaluation may move to the foreground—not only as an assessment of those psychosocial factors contributing to disability, but as a vehicle for cross-validating the available medical findings.

Unfortunately, whether from the medical or the psychological perspective, there are few objective clinical or empirical measures with any reliability or predictive validity where the determination of disability based on chronic pain is concerned. Clinical data from physical examinations are often notoriously at variance with patients' reports of their distress; and, to date, there are no laboratory measures available to quantify the experience of pain or even establish whether pain is present. What physicians have at their disposal in cases of chronic pain is frequently little better than their patients' self-report and their own informed observation, whereas what they are usually asked to provide are "objective" findings. The use of clinical "signs" to establish the presence of nonorganic factors in pain is a well-established tradition,[5] but such examinations are frequently skewed by patients' attempts to draw attention to their plight by endorsing a broad range of sometimes contradictory symptoms.

When insurance carriers and disability determination boards ask for objective indications of disability, there is enormous potential for equivocating on the term *objective,* because many clinically important findings from physical examination are "semi-objective," at best.[6] The result is a growing dissatisfaction with health care for chronic pain by all concerned and a renewed emphasis on the need for a comprehensive approach to the problem.[7] With so much at stake for the patient with chronic pain, a disservice is done, when diagnosis and treatment are undertaken haphazardly, fragmentarily, or even sequentially, by providers working independently without adequate cross-consultation. A comprehensive evaluation, involving a team of providers—pain physicians, pain psychologists, physical therapists, nurses, and complementary specialists—working toward an interdisciplinary synthesis of all the available data, may be the only means of ensuring the likelihood of an accurate, useful, and fair assessment of chronic pain.

PSYCHOSOCIAL RISK FACTORS IN CHRONIC PAIN

Frustration in arriving at a reliable and predictively valid means of medically determining disability based on chronic pain, as well as numerous cases of failure prominently displayed in the media, has historically led to speculation that the causes of chronic pain may be primarily or wholly psychogenic and that only particular types of personality are affected. The search for the so-called pain-prone personality, however, never produced a satisfying or useful model and never received much empirical support.[8,9] Given the array of variables, it would be surprising if a unified theory were to emerge. The combination of temperament, traits, coping style, influential beliefs, and a host of environmental factors is expressed uniquely in the personality of each patient. Furthermore, there is evidence suggesting that chronic pain unfolds according to a developmental course, in which each of the preceding variables may present differently, according to the level of psychological distress.[8]

If profiling offers few answers, there is nevertheless a valuable model proposed by the current heuristic approach to pain, which suggests that a range of factors may be associated with the subjective experience of pain, each of which can exert an influence on the individual's unique interpretation of nociception. As chronic pain emerges over time, the interaction of psychological, social, and environmental factors with physical pathology tends to influence the patient's perception of pain, as well as his or her interpretation of its impact on life, sometimes leading to disability and the adoption of the sick role.[10] These psychosocial factors have been found to be even more influential than medical factors in the development and report of disability across cultures.[11]

Comparatively recent efforts to delineate those psychosocial influences with the greatest and most consistent impact on the development of disability have led to the identification of a number of largely independent risk factors associated with poor recovery from injury and the development of chronic pain. When these risk factors are present premorbidly or develop comorbidly with injury, they may complicate the patient's subjective experience of pain, moving him or her toward a state of learned helplessness out of which chronic pain and disability can develop. One exhaustive review of the literature proposes a list of eight risk factors, documented as obstacles to the recovery from acute pain and as predisposing influences in the development of chronic pain.[12] To these eight factors, the author has added one, *(j),* which has received much recent scientific scrutiny, and divided another into two *(b* and *c).* The resulting list of ten psychosocial factors can be further divided into comorbid and premorbid influences.

The only factor that may be considered exclusively comorbid is *(a) pain duration.* As pain endures, the likelihood increases that a chronic pain syndrome and disability have developed. Pain of 2 years' duration is often cited as the decisive threshold, when multiple courses of medical or surgical intervention have failed to produce relief. When the criterion shifts to that of a successful return to work, however, much shorter durations of pain become actuarially significant. The likelihood of a patient's returning to his or her old job, after 6 months of unemployment resulting from chronic pain, is only 50%; and, after a year, there is only a 10% chance of a successful return.

Two risk factors that may exert either a premorbid or comorbid influence are *(b) a history of major psychopathology* and *(c) a history of substance abuse or dependence.* Both of these factors may predispose an individual toward the development of chronic pain, but either may emerge from within the context of chronic pain, as well (see Chap. 14). The presence of premorbid mood, anxiety, psychotic, or personality disorder places an additional burden on the patient and may mean that he or she faces a new problem, such as injury and pain, with already compromised or maladaptive coping skills. Mood, anxiety, and adjustment disorders can also develop comorbidly, as expressions of the pain-stress cycle, contributing a new and, where the patient is concerned, often unprecedented burden. Somatoform disorders may have existed previously, with the focus on pain or other physical symptoms, or they may coalesce around the advent of a new constellation of symptoms. Premorbid problems with substance abuse can similarly predispose patients toward maladaptive coping strategies, leading to over-reliance on medications and noncompliance with medical recommendations. Substance abuse problems may also develop comorbidly in treatment, through the impulsive or injudicious use of opioid and anxiolytic medications.

The remaining psychosocial risk factors are generally considered to exert a premorbid influence on the development of chronic pain and disability. When patients report *(d) job dissatisfaction,* one of the principal motivations for recovery may be absent. When there is *(e) a history of prolonged recovery from previous experiences of pain,* the expectation that any injury or illness may require extended convalescence is already established. When there is *(f) a pattern of reduced activity, coupled with excessive pain behaviors, supported by family and other social contacts who are either too solicitous or inconsistent or too harsh and punitive in their responses,* the resulting struggles around secondary gain may completely derail treatment, giving disability a firm foothold. As factors predisposing patients toward the development of chronic pain, all three may severely inhibit the frequently necessary transition of the patient from passive recipient of care to active participant in care.

In cases where there is *(g) a history of psychological or physical trauma* or *(h) a history of emotional, physical, or sexual abuse,* chronic pain may represent a means of psychologically symbolizing and organizing an unbearable, traumatic event or series of events. When a patient's focus on chronic pain and disability serves to defend against the experience of overwhelming affects by displacing emotional conflict onto the somatic sphere, the motivation to recover may be inhibited or removed. The high correlation between a history of childhood physical and sexual abuse, for example, and the development of chronic pain syndromes later in life is a well-documented phenomenon.[13–15]

The presence of *(i) negative or anxiety-provoking beliefs about the meaning of pain* suggests that—whether through misinformation, superstition, or distortion—the patient has acquired a set of maladaptive but nevertheless predisposing beliefs about his or her pain that are neither physiologically accurate nor psychologically realistic. One of the more persistent and insidious of these negative beliefs about chronic pain is that hurt means harm: "If it hurts, I must be injuring myself." Other negative beliefs tend to lead to the premature conclusion of disability: "I'll never be able to work again, if I can't get rid of this pain!" This risk factor may not be prominent, until the advent of serious injury and pain; but it tends to reflect long-standing patterns of maladaptive coping and pessimistic thinking.

One last predisposing factor has been the focus of increasing attention in the past few years; namely, the patient's *(j) explanatory model of pain* and how he or she interprets the meaning of pain in the context of his or her relationship to the world or to God.[16] There is a growing body of surprisingly rigorous empirical studies suggesting that an affirmative outlook and an essentially optimistic philosophy can make a positive contribution to recovery from illness and the restoration of health. By contrast, patients who feel that their suffering represents a punishment or that they are being persecuted or victimized by pain often have an arduous path to recovery and may contribute to the poor tractability of their pain by assuming a passive, helpless role.

Although the presence of any of these ten risk factors *(a–j)* in a patient's life predisposes toward the onset of chronic pain and disability, five psychosocial factors have been identified as predictors of negative outcome in the treatment of chronic pain.[12] These include three of the factors already discussed—*job dissatisfaction, reduced activity, and negative beliefs*—coupled with *a sustained attitude of hostility, anger, and alienation* and a reliance on *maladaptive coping strategies.* Anger and hostility are disruptive of treatment and destructive of the alliance between physician and patient, often perpetuating the pain-stress cycle and thwarting intervention,[17] whereas the maintenance of defective strategies for coping tends to disclose an inflexibility of psychological defenses. In both cases, psychotherapeutic intervention and management may prove necessary adjuncts to recovery. When one or more of these five factors is present, the course of treatment will almost certainly involve frustration for both patient and providers.

READINESS FOR CHANGE IN CHRONIC PAIN

The influence of any psychosocial risk factor may signal reluctance on the part of the patient to give up his or her pain and suffering and relinquish the refuge of disability. Whether the motivation for this reluctance is unconscious conflict, primary or secondary gain, inflexibility associated with a personality disorder, psychopathology, deficits in education, or simply poor coping skills, investigators have found that patients vary considerably regarding how prepared they are to make changes in their behavior around the management of pain. The prevailing paradigm for understanding change in this context is the transtheoretical model, which proposes a series of stages that must be progressively negotiated, if change in behavior is to occur and endure.[18,19] Although initially developed in the context of addictive behaviors and habit management, the model has been applied successfully to chronic pain in several settings and even across national boundaries.[20–22]

Assessing *readiness for change* may prove essential to understanding why some patients never seem to improve, as well as to the planning of interventions to promote behavioral change, active participation in care, and increased self-management of chronic pain. One way of assisting patients toward a greater acceptance of responsibility in the management of their pain is to help them see that changing or not changing is up to them and that they can *choose* to change. Cognitive therapy often begins with two questions that establish the cognitive framework within which change is possible: (1) What do you want (to change)? (2) What are you willing to do to get it?[23] The first question is easy for most patients with chronic pain, but the second implies work and sacrifice and is not so easy when patients are preoccupied with their own suffering and deprivation. Assessing how ready patients are to do the work and make the sacrifice in their own behalf is a first and necessary step in deciding which interventions, both medical and psychological, are most likely to succeed and which are likely to fail or even cause harm.

The first stage in the transtheoretical model is *precontemplation.* It represents the point at which patients are highly resistant to change and disinterested in making any accommodation or adjustment in their own behavior, even for the sake of treatment. Such patients usually arrive at pain clinics with the attitude that only medical interventions will make any positive impact and that there is little they can do on their own to influence their pain. Patients in this stage are often characterized as helpless, passive, and highly distressed, and they typically challenge any suggestion that psychological factors can have any bearing on their pain.

Patients who are willing to consider the possibility that stress may affect their pain and that there may be steps they can take toward managing their stress and pain, even though they are not yet sure or committed, are in the *contemplation* stage. Such patients have begun to entertain and nurture the idea of change but are not sure how or whether they can do it. They have acknowledged that they are stuck, but they have no firm ideas about how to move forward. Much of the effort of psychoeducation in pain management programs is directed toward nurturing the appeal of change by challenging patients' resistances and offering reasonable alternative explanations for what they are experiencing–in effect, moving them from the precontemplation to the contemplation stage of readiness for change.

Patients in the third or *preparation* stage have progressed to the point where they understand that change will offer them a route to more successful pain management, but they are not yet sure of what to change or how to begin changing. This stage often represents the time during which patients are considering their options and developing plans to make changes—whether adding new wellness behaviors, such as relaxation exercises, or dropping maladaptive behaviors, such as isolating themselves. The fourth or *action* stage represents the point at which the decision to change is translated into action. Patients endeavor to inhibit, reduce, or extinguish behaviors that cast them in the "sick" role and to promote and increase behaviors that give them a measure of control in managing their stress and pain. The fifth or *maintenance* stage sees them working to sustain the changes they have made, even through exacerbations and relapses. The motivation has shifted to the rewards of mastery and self-efficacy and the understanding that, not only is change possible, but it is desirable and even necessary, if pain is to continue to be successfully managed.

Because psychotherapeutic management in chronic pain encourages change in both behavior and attitude, it becomes critical to assess accurately where patients are in their readiness to make these changes. Recommending a course in relaxation techniques to a patient in the precontemplation stage will likely prove a futile and thankless intervention. Psychotherapy and, indeed, the efforts of all the members of a multidisciplinary team must respect and work within the context of the patient's current stage of readiness if frustration is to be minimized and progress achieved. Clues regarding readiness for change can be gathered through the clinical interview of the patient, as well as by reviewing the medical record and interviewing the family; but a psychometric instrument has recently been developed with an already promising body of research behind it.

The Pain Stages of Change Questionnaire (PSOCQ) is a comparatively new entry in the panoply of measures devoted to the assessment of chronic pain.[21] The PSOCQ applies the transtheoretical model of behavioral change, linked to a cognitive-behavioral perspective on chronic pain, in a 30-item, self-report format characterizing the patient's stage of readiness on a continuum of four scales: Precontemplation, Contemplation, Action, and Maintenance. More research is needed to confirm the instrument's predictive validity; however, the value of a measure that provides a means of cross-validating a patient's simple profession of willingness to adopt a self-management approach to chronic pain may prove to be of enormous value in the selection of patients for particular approaches to treatment.

THE CLINICAL INTERVIEW IN PSYCHOSOCIAL ASSESSMENT

Evaluating which psychosocial risk factors may be influential in the life of a patient, as well as how committed that patient is to being an active, cooperative participant in his or her own care, are the objectives of psychosocial assessment in a multidisciplinary setting. The pain physician, like the psychologist, structures his or her time in discussion and examination of the patient, not only in the service of diagnosing pathology, but in an attempt to learn more about the patient's experience and his or her responses to pain and illness. When one or more of the previously discussed psychosocial risk factors is identified as influential in the patient's life, a referral for a more psychosocially based evaluation is indicated. In pain management centers and clinic or hospital-based practices, the psychosocial assessment of patients is usually coordinated by a psychologist, psychiatrist, clinical social worker, or psychiatric nurse practitioner.

The evaluation of the patient by the pain psychologist begins with a careful review of the available records in preparation for the clinical interview. When time and resources allow, the process may be extended to include (1) consultation with other providers, including the primary care physician; (2) ancillary interviews with family members; and (3) psychometric assessment. What happens during the time of the clinical interview is critical, not only because of the importance of the observations and data gathered by the psychologist, but because of the impression developed by the patient concerning the purpose and meaning of the visit. It is, therefore, essential to structure the time well and to make the patient feel comfortable and safe by allaying any fears and addressing any distortions he or she may harbor regarding how the information will be used. To overcome any initial defensiveness on the patient's part, it is frequently helpful to begin by stating that the purpose of the interview is to find out more about the impact of the patient's pain on his or her circumstances and level of functioning—how pain has affected his or her work, livelihood, family, relationships with friends, and personal goals.

Structured and Semistructured Pain Interviews

There are few structured interviews developed specifically for use with the pain patient, but one of the more widely used of these is the Psychosocial Pain Inventory (PSPI).[24] This instrument guides the psychologist in gathering information from the patient and a family member through a series of 25 open-ended questions, all reflecting a psychosocial dimension of the patient's experience of pain. The items included in the inventory explore major stressful life events, pain-related stressors, pain behavior at home, previous painful or disabling medical problems, and models of chronic pain in the patient's family. An additional feature is that each of the 25 items can be scored according to a standardized system, with the goal of identifying those factors that are most influential in the patient's pain. A drawback of the PSPI is that a careful administration often stretches into 1½ to 2 hours, sometimes taxing the patient and introducing a cost-effectiveness variable into practice management.

Semistructured interviews enjoy a wider use and broader application than structured interviews, but there is little standardization of format or administration among them. Many clinicians choose to adapt them still further to the needs of their settings. One attempt to describe the field of inquiry of the semistructured interview, regardless of format, suggests the necessary inclusion of seven objectives: (1) recording a careful pain history, (2) identifying the events that precede and follow exacerbations in pain perception and pain behavior, (3) evaluating daily activities and limitations, (4) determining whether there are family models of chronic pain and disability, (5) determining whether the patient has suffered physical or sexual abuse, (6) evaluating the degree of affective disturbance, and (7) determining the degree to which the patient is experiencing sexual dysfunction.[25] Using these objectives as a guide, a useful semistructured interview can be developed for almost any setting or population of patients.

Psychiatric Interviews

Although not developed specifically for use with pain patients, structured and semistructured psychiatric interviews are administered routinely in many pain management centers, as well as in chronic pain research. The format of the psychiatric interview is designed to assess psychosocial history in depth and to juxtapose this "life story" with a patient's current symptomatologic profile. The interview itself may be thought of as a tool for systematically disclosing the dynamic relationship between the two—history and symptoms. Two widely used, structured formats for the psychiatric interview are based on the current edition of the *Diagnostic and Statistical Manual of Mental Disorders* (DSM-IV). The National Institute of Mental Health Diagnostic Interview Schedule for DSM-IV (DIS-IV)[26] and the Structured Clinical Interview for DSM-IV (SCID)[27] were developed to assess not only current psychiatric symptoms and disorders but lifetime histories of psychiatric diagnoses, as well. Both instruments require a brief course of training, and either may be administered by nonclinician assistants; but the SCID offers greater latitude to supplement the structured interview with spontaneous questions for clarification and challenges to inconsistent responses. The DIS-IV also is offered in a computerized version, which can be interviewer-administered or self-administered.

Despite the advantages of a standardized and structured format, many pain psychologists prefer the greater latitude offered by the generic psychiatric interview adapted to the situation of chronic pain. Although there are essential elements to the psychiatric interview, there is no standard or established structure. Its strength, when administered by a skilled clinician, lies in its flexibility and interactive freedom. It is frequently organized along progressive sections, which minimally include (1) presenting problem, (2) history of presenting problem, (3) psychiatric history, (4) substance abuse history, (5) medical history, (6) developmental and social history, and (7) the mental status examination. Each of these broad components can be modified to pose questions relevant to the patient's experience of pain; or, the entire format can be shifted to make chronic pain the presenting problem and focus of the interview.[28,29]

Table 13-1 presents an example of how the format of the general psychiatric interview can be altered to shift the focus to a psychosocially based clinical interview for chronic pain. All of the previously discussed, essential objectives of the semistructured pain interview can easily be incorporated into this format; and its inherent flexibility facilitates the investigation of the broad range of psychosocial issues and risk factors that may be associated with the patient's particular situation of chronic pain.[25] When the results of psychological testing are available, it is often revealing to discuss them, in brief, with the patient; and when the data gathered during the interview are at variance with his or her responses on the psychometric measures, it is usually a good idea to call attention to the discrepancy and to wonder aloud with the patient what it might mean—that is, to discuss it without drawing or presenting conclusions. Many patients may deny feeling depressed during the interview, for example, but may nevertheless endorse a number of items reflecting mood disturbance and neurovegetative difficulties on the Beck Depression Inventory (BDI) or Minnesota Multiphasic Personality Inventory (MMPI-2).

TABLE 13-1 **Concise Format of the Psychosocially-based Clinical Pain Interview**

Presenting pain complaint
History of presenting pain complaint
Current level of functioning
Current identifiable stressors
Medical history
Psychiatric history
Substance abuse history
Developmental and social history
Mental status examination
Review and discussion of psychological testing results
Review of patient's questions and goals for treatment

In the psychosocially based clinical pain interview, the pain psychologist has the opportunity to develop lines of inquiry sequentially or organically, in a purposeful manner, fashioning each successive question to the immediate verbal and affective responses of the patient. This is especially important when reviewing the patient's questions and goals for treatment at the conclusion of the session. It is here that the patient's beliefs about pain and explanatory model of pain can be discussed in comparatively greater depth. It is here, as well, that the first indications of his or her readiness for change may be revealed. The pain psychologist's questions should be formulated to elicit additional information and elaboration, not to convey judgment or sabotage future plans for psychoeducation by attempting prematurely to correct distortions or offer more logical explanations. At this first encounter, understanding the patient's experience should be the guiding principle.

PSYCHOMETRIC MEASURES IN PSYCHOSOCIAL ASSESSMENT

The interview is an indispensable feature of psychosocial assessment; however, developing diagnostic and prognostic impressions and a treatment plan based solely on the patient's verbal self-report can prove a problematic enterprise. Even in casual conversation, people are likely to forget, editorialize, distort, and defensively censor themselves—both consciously and unconsciously—when disclosing personal information; and the situation of the clinical interview, as a sample of human behavior, is no different. One study even suggests that patients with chronic pain who wish to appear socially conventional—the response bias of *social desirability*—typically report less depression and anxiety but higher levels of pain.[30] Although it is not feasible to test the veracity of every statement, it is nevertheless possible to improve on the likelihood of arriving at an accurate appreciation of an individual patient's experience and story. Comparing data gathered by other providers, reviewing the available records, interviewing family members, and administering one or more psychometric instruments are all ways of cross-validating the data from the clinical interview of the patient.

The point is not to catch patients in the act of consciously or unconsciously misleading their providers but to gain as accurate an assessment as possible of the impact of pain on their lives. When a patient denies having used opioid medications while a previous medical report refers to "drug-seeking behavior"; when a family member contradicts what a patient has said; when a testing report characterizes a patient as severely depressed and anxious, even though he or she insists otherwise—these are all inconsistencies that require elucidation, if the patient's situation is to be understood. The addition of psychometric instruments elicits one more sampling of the patient's behavior; and patients frequently react differently to the situation of completing a questionnaire or computerized test or inventory than they do to the direct questions of psychologists and physicians. Furthermore, because the methods of test construction sometimes obscure the intention of certain questions, the point or interpretation of any particular item or trend is not always immediately discernible, sometimes resulting in a less defensive response. Especially when preparing forensic reports or documentation for outside agencies, having an actuarial or statistically meaningful basis for cross-validating a patient's verbal self-report makes psychometric measures an important addition to psychosocial assessment.

Measures Developed for Use in Chronic Pain

Of the literally thousands of psychometric measures available for use in clinical settings and research, hundreds have been created or adapted specifically for application to patients with chronic pain or chronic illness. Most of these are pencil-and-paper, self-report instruments, but some are available in software editions; and the computerized pain testing battery is becoming increasingly popular in pain management centers. A few of these measures are multidimensional in scope; however, most were designed to assess one dimension of the experience of pain, with the categories of assessment being generally defined as (1) pain intensity, (2) pain beliefs and coping, and (3) functional capacity.

Measures of Pain Intensity Measures of pain intensity provide quantitative estimates of a patient's pain. The simplest of these are unidimensional scales—numerical rating scales (NRSs) and visual analog scales (VASs)—which ask patients to depict the severity of their pain as a number on a scale of "0 to 10" or "0 to 100" or to represent it on a line or continuum with bipolar attributes, such as "no pain" to "worst pain." These are often used as clinical or bedside measures, because they provide a basis for longitudinal comparison of the patient's progress. A "5," today, is better than an "8," yesterday. Verbal rating scales (VRSs) present lists or continua of adjectives or descriptors and ask the patient to select the word or words that best describe his or her pain. VRSs typically add a sensory and even a reactive dimension to the assessment of intensity, because many words describing pain are typically affect-laden (e.g., "annoying," "excruciating," "unbearable"). The application of these unidimensional measures is widespread, and they are generally held to be useful as indicators of pain intensity, but they offer no valid basis for comparison between patients.

One of the most comprehensive measures of pain intensity, the McGill Pain Questionnaire (MPQ),[31] is also one of the oldest and most widely used and cited pencil-and-paper instruments developed for pain. The MPQ presents three classes of pain-related adjectives—sensory, affective, and evaluative—in 20 subclasses or groupings and instructs patients to endorse those words that accurately describe their pain. Scores are then derived for the sensory, affective, and evaluative dimensions of pain, along with a score of intensity from a five-item VRS. Line drawings depicting the front and back views of the body are also presented with instructions to portray the spatial distribution of pain. The MPQ has been criticized for requiring a comparatively high level of reading ability and intelligence, for lacking a consistent scoring technique, for the lengthy administration time, and for problems with construct validity; but it possesses a high content validity and is the measure of pain intensity most widely applied to research. A shorter form of the instrument (SF-MPQ)[32] has been developed that correlates highly with the longer version and has a greater ease of administration.

Measures of Coping and Beliefs About Pain A second category of measures developed for use in chronic pain consists of those instruments devoted to assessing (1) the ways in which patients attempt to cope with pain, as well as the relative success of their coping strategies; and (2) what patients believe about their pain and the ways in which their beliefs influence their responses to pain. The prevailing model of coping, based on the transactional model of stress, suggests that coping is a continuous process in which external and internal demands are managed through constantly changing cognitive and behavioral efforts.[33] In effect, patients are always attempting to control or manage stressors, including the experience of their pain, by appraising their situations, reacting, and then reappraising their situations, based on the results of their actions.

Coping is both a conscious and an unconscious process, the characteristic patterns of which may be called a patient's coping techniques or strategies. Not all of these techniques and strategies are effective, however, and learning more about the ways in a patient is trying to cope with pain can be a critical feature of psychosocial assessment and the planning of interventions. Similarly, what patients believe about their pain—whether deeply rooted philosophical assumptions or dominant attitudes or uncritically accepted superstitions—can contribute greatly to their ongoing experience of pain. Unrealistic or negative thinking can lead to intensified pain perception, increased distress, and a greater sense of suffering and disability. When a patient believes, for example, that further diagnostic procedures will eventually enable clinicians to arrive at an answer for his or her pain, then the idea of effective self-management can be postponed indefinitely. When a patient believes that he or she cannot function productively with his or her pain, then the motivation to become an active participant in treatment is reduced.

There are many available self-report measures of coping and beliefs about pain, including the Coping Strategies Questionnaire (CSQ),[34] the Vanderbilt Pain Management Inventory (VPMI),[35] the Chronic Pain Coping Inventory (CPCI),[36] the Behavioral Assessment of Pain Questionnaire (BAP)[37] the Survey of Pain Attitudes (SOPA),[38] the Pain Beliefs and Perceptions Inventory (PBAPI),[39] the Cognitive Risk Profile (CRP), [40] the Inventory of Negative Thoughts in Response to Pain (INTRP),[41] and the already mentioned Pain Stages of Change Questionnaire (PSOCQ).[21] Three of the more versatile and widely applied of these measures are summarized in Table 13-2.

Measures of Functional Capacity One of the most important objectives of pain management is the increase of functional capacity. Is a reduction in pain meaningful if there is no noticeable change in the patient's level of activity or ability to work or social involvement? Patients with pain describe considerable variation in the degree of interference they experience from distress and impairment; and it is usually a good idea to assess a patient's perceived level of disability, from the outset of treatment, as well as

TABLE 13-2 **Selected Measures of Coping and Pain Beliefs**

Instrument	Format	Features
Coping Strategies Questionnaire (CSQ)	50 items, each rated on a 7-point scale depicting frequency of use, assessing 6 cognitive and 1 behavioral coping strategies: diverting attention, reinterpreting pain, coping self-statements, ignoring pain, praying and hoping, catastrophizing, and increased activity	Widely applied in research on coping and adjustment, with a number of additional composite measures or scales—such as active and passive coping dimensions and coping flexibility—having been developed through factor analysis and other techniques
Vanderbilt Pain Management Inventory (VPMI)	19 items, assessing active (self-management) and passive (helpless or dependent) coping strategies relevant to chronic pain	Evaluates patients' reported efforts at coping, with less effort—passive coping—being associated with higher levels of pain, distress, and disability
Survey of Pain Attitudes (SOPA)	57 items, each rated on a 5-point scale, assessing subscales of control, disability, medical cures, solicitude, medication, emotion, and harm	The most frequently studied and widely used measure of pain beliefs, with multiple revisions and two abbreviated versions

longitudinally to mark his or her progress. A reliable measure of functional capacity can serve to quantify and cross-validate a patient's self-report of changes in what he or she can do, as a result of treatment. A number of measures can be used to assess functional capacity, including the West-Haven Yale Multidimensional Pain Inventory (WHYMPI),[42] the Chronic Illness Problem Inventory (CIPI),[43] the Illness Behavior Inventory (IBI),[44] the Sickness Impact Profile (SIP),[45] the Short-Form Health Survey (SF-36),[46] and the Pain Disability Index (PDI).[47] Three of these measures are summarized in Table 13-3.

Measures of Psychopathology Applied to Chronic Pain

Most patients with chronic pain do not present with histories of major psychiatric disorder. Assessing psychopathology and its po-

TABLE 13-3 **Selected Measures of Functional Capacity**

Instrument	Format	Features
Pain Disability Index (PDI)	7 questions, assessing degree of interference with functioning in the areas of home responsibilities, recreation, social activities, occupation, sexual behavior, self-care, and life support activity	Brief and easy to administer, but the PDI has been criticized because of its too-obvious face validity and resulting potential for systematic response biases
Sickness Impact Profile (SIP)	136-item checklist, assessing 12 dimensions of functioning: ambulation, mobility, body care and movement, social interaction, communication, alertness, emotional behavior, sleep and rest, eating, work, home management, and recreation	Comprehensively tested and revised; dimensions may be combined to form broader scales of physical, psychosocial, and total disability; may be administered as an interview or as a self-report, pencil-and-paper instrument
West Haven–Yale Multidimensional Pain Inventory (WHYMPI)	52 items, each related on 7-point scale depicting frequency of use, assessing 12 dimensions of chronic pain in 3 sections: 5 dimensions of pain experience: interference in functioning, support from others, pain severity, life control, and affective distress 3 dimensions of perceptions of others' responses: negative, solicitous, and distracting 4 categories of common daily activities: household chores, outdoor work, activities away from home, and social activities	Developed specifically for use with chronic pain patients; based on a cognitive-behavioral model; classifies patients into three types (dysfunctional, interpersonally distressed, and adaptive copers); widely used in both clinical and research settings

TABLE 13-4 **Measures of Psychopathology Applied to Chronic Pain**

Instrument	Format	Features
Beck Depression Inventory (BDI)	21 items, each rated on a 4-point scale of intensity, assessing mood and neurovegetative dimensions of depression	Easy to administer and quick to score; used in many settings as a screening device
Millon Behavioral Health Inventory (MBHI)	150 true-false items, assessing 20 subscales clustering around (1) styles of relating to providers, (2) psychosocial stressors, and (3) response to illness	Emphasizes medical rather than emotional concerns; capable of assessing mood and personality; normalized on medical, not psychiatric patients
Minnesota Multiphasic Personality Inventory (MMPI-2)	567 true-false items, distributed across 7 validity scales, 10 basic clinical scales, 15 content scales, 27 content component scales, 18 supplementary scales, 3 social introversion scales, and 28 Harris-Lingoes subscales	Most widely used objective test of personality in the United States and abroad; applied more often to the assessment of chronic pain than any other instrument; criticized for the length of administration (60–90 minutes)

tential influence on the development and maintenance of pain is, nevertheless, critical for three reasons: (1) chronic pain is far more prevalent among psychiatric populations, (2) the incidence of patients developing comorbid psychiatric symptoms is high, and (3) major psychopathology is associated with poor prognosis in the treatment of chronic pain and disability (see Chap. 14). Some of the more useful measures of psychopathology applied to patients with chronic pain include the Beck Depression Inventory (BDI),[48] the Pain Patient Profile (P3),[49] the Millon Behavioral Health Inventory (MBHI),[50] the Minnesota Multiphasic Personality Inventory (MMPI-2),[51] and the Symptom Checklist 90 (SCL-90R).[52] Three of these measures are summarized in Table 13-4.

FROM A MULTI- TO AN INTERDISCIPLINARY APPROACH TO PAIN

The existence of such a broad array of techniques and measures employed in the psychosocial assessment of chronic pain is compelling evidence of the complexity of the problem. No single approach to diagnosis can discern all that we need to consider about a patient's experience of pain. Cross-validating clinical impressions with other sets of data from multiple providers is, therefore, critical to the accurate diagnosis and effective treatment of chronic pain. The addition of a psychosocial approach to evaluation can ensure the likelihood of not missing a critical piece of the pain picture. When psychosocial factors are identified as influential in the patient's history and presentation, a comprehensive evaluation, involving a multidisciplinary team of providers working toward an interdisciplinary synthesis of all the available data, may be the only means of ensuring a sensitive, accurate, and, above all, useful assessment of the patient's problem.

REFERENCES

1. Commission on Accreditation of Rehabilitation Facilities (CARF): The Rehabilitation Commission. *Quality Through Accreditation: Interdisciplinary Pain Rehabilitation Programs.* Available at: http://www.carf.org. Accessed February 10, 2002.
2. Turk DC, Rudy TE, Sorkin BA. Neglected topics in chronic pain treatment outcome studies: Determination of success. *Pain* 1993;53:3–16.
3. DeGood DE, Dane JR. The psychologist as a pain consultant in outpatient, inpatient, and workplace settings. In: Gatchel RJ, Turk DC, eds. *Psychological Approaches to Pain Management: A Practitioner's Handbook.* New York, NY: Guilford Press; 1996;403–437.
4. Massie MJ, Chertkov L, Fleishman SB, et al. Pain rounds: The experts comment. In: Oldham JM, Riba MB, series eds. Review of Psychiatry Series, vol. 19, no. 2: Massie MJ, ed. *Pain: What Psychiatrists Need to Know.* Washington, DC: American Psychiatric Press; 2000;133–173.
5. Waddell G, McCulloch JA, Kummel E, et al. Nonorganic physical signs in low-back pain. *Spine* 1980;5:117–125.
6. Robinson JP. Disability evaluation in painful conditions. In: Turk DC, Melzack R, eds. *Handbook of Pain Assessment.* 2nd ed. New York, NY: Guilford Press; 2001;248–272.
7. Waddell G. Low back pain: A twentieth century health care enigma. *Spine* 1996;21:2820–2825.
8. Gatchel RJ, Weisberg JM. Introduction. In: Gatchel RJ, Weisberg JM, eds. *Personality Characteristics of Patients with Pain.* Washington, DC: American Psychological Association; 2000;3–22.
9. Turk DC, Melzack R. The measurement of pain and the assessment of people experiencing pain. In Turk DC, Melzack R, eds. *Handbook of Pain Assessment.* 2nd ed. New York, NY: Guilford Press; 2001;3–11.
10. Turk DC. Biopsychosocial perspectives on chronic pain. In: Gatchel RJ, Turk DC, eds. *Psychological Approaches to Pain Management: A Practitioner's Handbook.* New York, NY: Guilford Press; 1996;3–32.
11. Ormel J, Voncorff M, Ustun TB, et al. Mental disorders and disability across cultures. *JAMA* 1994;272:1741–1748.
12. Eimer BN, Freeman A. *Pain Management Psychotherapy: A Practical Guide.* New York, NY: John Wiley & Sons; 1998.
13. Glod CA. Long-term consequences of childhood physical and sexual abuse. *Arch Psychiatr Nurs* 1993;7:163–173.
14. Goldberg RT. Childhood abuse, depression, and chronic pain. *Clin J Pain* 1994;10:277–281.
15. Linton SJ, Larden M, Gillow A-M. Sexual abuse and chronic musculoskeletal pain: Prevalence and psychological factors. *Clin J Pain* 1996; 12:215–221.
16. Benson H. *Timeless Healing: The Power and Biology of Belief.* New York, NY: Scribner; 1996.
17. Fernandez E, Turk DC. The scope and significance of anger in the experience of chronic pain. *Pain* 1995;61:165–175.
18. Prochaska JO, DiClemete CC. The transtheoretical approach. In: Norcross JC, Goldfried MR, eds. *Handbook of Psychotherapy Integration.* New York, NY: Basic Books; 1992;300–334.

19. Prochaska JO, DiClemente CC, Norcross JC. In search of how people change: Applications to addictive behaviors. *Am Psychol* 1992;47: 1102–1114.
20. Keefe FJ, Lefebvre JC, Kerns RD, et al. Understanding the adoption of arthritis self-management: Stages of change profiles among arthritis patients. *Pain* 2000;87:303–313.
21. Kerns RD, Rosenberg R, Jamison RN, et al. Readiness to adopt a self-management approach to chronic pain: The pain stages of change questionnaire (PSOCQ). *Pain* 1997;72:227–234.
22. Jensen MP, Nielsen WR, Romano JM, et al. Further evaluation of the pain stages of change questionnaire: Is the transtheoretical model of change useful for patients with chronic pain? *Pain* 2000;86:255–264.
23. Wessler R, Hankin S, Stern J. *Succeeding with Difficult Clients: Applications of Cognitive Appraisal Therapy.* San Diego, Calif: Academic Press; 2001.
24. Heaton RK, Getto CJ, Lehman RAW, et al. A standardized evaluation of psychosocial factors in chronic pain. *Pain* 1982;12:165–174.
25. Bradley LA, McKendree-Smith NL. Assessment of psychological status using interviews and self-report instruments. In: Turk DC, Melzack R, eds. *Handbook of Pain Assessment.* 2nd ed. New York, NY: Guilford Press; 2001;292–319.
26. *The Diagnostic Interview Schedule for DSM-IV (DIS-IV).* August 4, 2000. Available at: http://epi.wustl.edu/DIS/dishisto.htm. Accessed February 11, 2002.
27. *Welcome to the SCID Web Page.* November 6, 2001. Available at: http://cpmcnet.columbia.edu/dept/scid. Accessed February 11, 2002.
28. Fishbain DA, Cutler RB, Rosomoff RS, et al. The problem-oriented psychiatric examination of the chronic pain patient and its application to the litigation consultation. *Clin J Pain* 1994;10:28–51.
29. Wootton J. Psychological evaluation of chronic pain. In: Warfield CA, Fausett HJ, eds. *Manual of Pain Management.* 2nd ed. Philadelphia, Pa: Lippincott Williams & Wilkins; 2002;25–31.
30. Deshields TL, Tait RC, Gfeller JD, et al. Relationship between social desirability and self-report in chronic pain patients. *Clin J Pain* 1995;11:189–193.
31. Melzack R. The McGill Pain Questionnaire: Major properties and scoring methods. *Pain* 1975;1:277–299.
32. Melzack R. The short-form McGill Pain Questionnaire. *Pain* 1987;30: 191–197.
33. Lazarus RS, Folkman S. *Stress, Appraisal, and Coping*. New York, NY: Springer; 1984.
34. Rosenstiel AK, Keefe FJ. The use of coping strategies in chronic low back pain patients: Relationship to patient characteristics and current adjustment. *Pain* 1983;17:34–44.
35. Brown GK, Nicassio PM, Wallston KA. Pain coping strategies and depression in rheumatoid arthritis. *J Consult Clin Psychol* 1989;37: 652–657.
36. Jensen MP, Turner JA, Romano JM, et al. The Chronic Pain Coping Inventory: Development and preliminary validation. *Pain* 1995;60: 203–216.
37. Tearnan BH, Lewandowski MJ: The Behavioral Assessment of Pain Questionnaire: The development and Validation of a comprehensive self-report instrument. *Am J Pain* 1992;2:181–191.
38. Jensen MP, Karoly P, Huger P. The development and preliminary validation of an instrument to assess patients' attitudes toward pain. *J Psychosom Res* 1987;31:393–400.
39. Williams DA, Thorn BE. An empirical assessment of pain beliefs. *Pain* 1989;36:351–358.
40. DeGood DE, Kiernan BD, Cundiff G, et al. Development of a patient self-report inventory for predicting pain treatment response: The Cognitive Risk Profile. Poster presented at the Eighth World Congress on Pain; 1996; Vancouver, British Columbia, Canada (August 17–22, 1996).
41. Gil K, Williams DA, Keefe F, et al. The relationship of negative thoughts to pain and psychological distress. *Behav Ther* 1990;21:349–362.
42. Kerns RD, Turk DC, Rudy TE. The West Haven–Yale Multidimensional Pain Inventory. *Pain* 1985;23:345–356.
43. Kames LD, Naliboff BD, Heinrich RL, et al. The Chronic Illness Problem Inventory: Problem-oriented psychosocial assessment of patients with chronic illness. *Int J Psychiatr Med* 1984;14:65–75.
44. Turkat ID, Pettigrew LS. Development and validation of the Illness Behavior Inventory. *J Behav Assess* 1983;5:35–47.
45. Bergner M, Bobbit RA, Carter WB, et al. The Sickness Impact Profile: Development and final revision of a health status measure. *Med Care* 1981;19:787–805.
46. Ware JE, Sherbourne CD. The MOS 36-item Short-Form Health Survey (SF-36). *Med Care* 1992;30:473–483.
47. Pollard CA. Preliminary validity study of the Pain Disability Index. *Percept Mot Skills* 1984;59:974–984.
48. Beck AT, Steer RA. *Beck Depression Inventory Manual.* New York, NY: Psychological Corp; 1987.
49. Tollison CD, Langley JC. *Pain Patient Profile Manual.* Minneapolis, Minn: National Computer Systems; 1995.
50. Millon T, Green JC, Meagher, RB Jr. The MBHI: A new inventory for the psychodiagnostician in medical settings. *Professional Psychol* 1979;10:529–539.
51. Butcher JN, Dahlstrom WG, Graham JR, et al. *MMPI-2: Manual for Administration and Scoring.* Minneapolis, Minn: University of Minnesota Press; 1989.
52. Derogatis LR. *The SCL-90-R Manual II: Administration, Scoring, and Procedures.* Towson, Md: Clinical Psychometric Press; 1983.

CHAPTER 14 PSYCHOTHERAPEUTIC MANAGEMENT OF CHRONIC PAIN

R. Joshua Wootton, Margaret A. Caudill-Slosberg, and Jillian B. Frank

When the International Association for the Study of Pain (IASP) arrived at a definition of pain that included the "emotional experience," as well as the "unpleasant sensory experience associated with actual or potential tissue damage,"[1] they were acknowledging the impact of pain on our human capacity for sentience and reflection and, by extension, suffering. By the time pain has become chronic in an individual's life, it has almost certainly achieved the status of a major source of stress. More than merely an unpleasant sensory stimulus, chronic pain can come to affect the whole individual by becoming, itself, the source of a broad range of psychosocial stressors. The following case report illustrates the extent to which this is possible.

Case 1 A 42-year-old married man was referred to a pain management center, 8 months after suffering a work-related, crush-type injury to his hand. His pain, which had been diagnosed as complex regional pain syndrome, type 1 (CRPS-1), had remained intractable to conservative measures and surgical intervention. According to the patient, several trials of medications had left him with uncomfortable mental status changes, and a reparative surgery and several procedures had exacerbated his pain considerably. He reported his distress as "worse than ever" and indicated that he was unable to work or pursue any of his previous recreational outlets. Although his primary care physician and surgeon supported his claim to disability, his worker's compensation carrier's representatives insisted that he should be able to return to light duty at his previous job. As a result, the patient had entered a lengthy and frustrating process of litigation, which had proved exhausting and overwhelming. As his anxiety escalated concerning his loss of income, mounting legal fees, and inability to resume work and provide for his family, he became increasingly withdrawn, irritable, and depressed. His marriage and relationships with his children and friends suffered; and, by the time he arrived at the pain management center, he reported feeling angry, helpless, hopeless, and suicidal.

Cases such as this are familiar to everyone who specializes in the treatment of chronic pain. The challenge, where successful medical resolution is concerned, is to maintain the focus on the whole of the individual's experience, both sensory and affective, because the development and course of chronic pain represents a progressive series of complex interactions among the biologic, psychological, and social dimensions of an individual's life. Purely physiologic explanations cannot account for its impact.[2] Nor can an exclusive reliance on the interventions that spring from such a limited understanding ordinarily bring the enduring relief and solace sought by many patients with chronic pain.[3]

The quality, intensity, and duration of pain are influenced by a myriad of psychological and social factors, which—while they may have arisen in the context of pain—are by no means less influential or consequential than the unpleasant sensory experience arising from actual or potential tissue damage.[4] Such factors may, indeed, play a critical role in the etiology, severity, exacerbation, and maintenance of pain, suffering, and disability.[5] The experience of chronic pain ultimately comes to be the product of conflict between a sensory stimulus and the entire individual. It will always require some level of adaptation and adjustment, but it can, in many cases, interfere with one's work and livelihood, recreational pursuits, relationships with family and friends, and even sexual intimacy. Through the introduction of more enduring affective changes, it can also influence one's self-esteem and the ways in which one views oneself as a man or woman, husband or wife, father or mother, friend, member of society, and spiritual being.

WHY A MULTIDISCIPLINARY APPROACH IS NEEDED

With so much at stake for the patient with chronic pain, it is not surprising that psychological evaluation is a required or highly recommended feature of comprehensive evaluation in many pain management centers.[6] For many patients, some form of psychological intervention is also recommended as part of the comprehensive treatment plan. Such interventions are usually prescribed to run concurrently with medical treatment and other therapies and may include one or more of many available modes of individual or group psychotherapy. When offered as part of a multidisciplinary package, psychotherapeutic approaches to managing chronic pain have demonstrated their efficacy repeatedly, and there is considerable evidence to suggest that the more effectively such interventions are integrated into a comprehensive or team approach, the greater are the chances of improvement for health and quality of life.[7]

With the IASP reporting an incidence of chronic pain in the United States of 70 million, and with more than 50 million being partially or totally disabled for periods ranging from a few days to a few months, a concerted multidisciplinary effort becomes even more critical to the effective marshaling of available medical resources.[8] Especially for patients whose chronic pain has remained initially intractable to medical and surgical interventions, a careful plan of treatment coordinated by a team of providers can ultimately result in greatly reducing the costs of health care, as well as raising the quality of that care—improving patients' response to treatment, level of functioning, and satisfaction—and enhancing the morale of all the providers concerned.[9] Psychotherapeutic management, in this context, necessarily involves not only a multidisciplinary approach, but an interdisciplinary effort in which the interventions of each member of the team—physicians, nurses, physical therapists, medical and complementary specialists, and mental health providers—can be seen as having a psychotherapeutic impact on the patient and must be directed toward having a complementary effect on the interventions of all other members of the team.

Psychological Factors in Chronic Pain

It is, by now, a generally accepted, if not always carefully considered tenet, that stress is influential in the development, expression, and tractability of chronic pain.[10] Because stress is also influential in the development and expression of somatization and other psychological symptoms, associations among chronic pain, stress, and psychiatric disorder are frequently observed and well-documented in the literature of both pain and psychiatry.[11] Attempting to parse or separate these influences prematurely for the sake of treatment is frequently tantamount to disregarding the often-volatile interactions among these factors and the cyclically reinforcing relationship between chronic pain and stress.

When such a unilateral approach is taken, it often represents the attempt of physicians adhering to too strict a medical model to establish the extent to which a patient's problem may be *mental*, as opposed to *physical*. As a result, both physician and patient may be left wondering why a clearly prescribed nerve block or medication has not achieved the expected relief. It may also lead to the premature and potentially harmful conclusion by the physician and the patient's health insurance carrier that nothing further can be done medically or surgically to assuage the patient's pain and that the problem is no longer a medical one but strictly a psychological one, now unrelated to a precipitating injury or historical tissue damage. What is being overlooked is the individual patient's stress-reactivity and the enduring influence of the pain-stress cycle on the development and maintenance of chronic pain.

Stress-reactivity and the Pain-stress Cycle The term *stress-reactive* is suggestive of a continuum of the degree to which any individual reacts to external or internal stressors, including the stressors of pain and its psychosocial sequelae. We are all on this continuum, but highly stress-reactive individuals are likely to develop a broader spectrum of more severe psychological and social concomitants or consequences, as well as to experience their pain with greater affective involvement and suffering. Less stress-reactive individuals may still experience the need to accommodate to their pain, psychologically, socially, and occupationally, but their adjustment to living with chronic pain is typically more successful and their adaptation to their limitations, more enduring.

The term *pain-stress cycle* is indicative of the unfolding neuropsychosocial matrix in which (1) pain tends to amplify the impact of stress while (2) stress magnifies the subjective experience of suffering associated with pain. The former occurs when a patient's experience of pain facilitates the development of new and secondary psychosocial stressors, as in Case 1, earlier; but it may also be evident in the patient's tendency to rely on or resort to maladaptive coping strategies, such as self-medication, social withdrawal, and the development of generalized, reactive pain behaviors. The latter refers more specifically to the contributions of heightened autonomic arousal and musculoskeletal tension in the maintenance and intensity of the experience of pain.

We have only an inchoate appreciation of how these mechanisms work and interact, but advances in our understanding of the neurophysiology and molecular biology of our perception and experience of pain strongly suggest that the influence of psychosocial factors and emotions is translated neurophysiologically into the realm of perception and behavior.[12] Stress, regardless of its origin, can result in physiologic deterioration and the exacerbated experience of pain through a variety of mechanisms. Neurosignature patterns can be modulated or altered destructively by stress of psychological origin, no less than by sensory input. Because any stressor, whether external or internal, physical or psychological, can affect stress-regulation systems adversely, the resulting lesions or tissue damage can influence the neurosignature patterns that originate chronic pain.[13]

Seen from this perspective, the distinction between stresses of psychological versus physical origin tends to assume less importance, and a multidisciplinary or comprehensive approach to treatment becomes paramount. All models of chronic pain acknowledge the neuropsychosocial relationship and interaction between stress and pain; however, it is yet a further step to begin to understand and appreciate how this works in the life of a particular patient or how to incorporate this approach into a successful plan of treatment. In a multidisciplinary approach to treating chronic pain, therefore, making an assessment of the degree to which any patient is stress-reactive and addressing the nature of his or her unique expression of the pain-stress cycle become primary objectives of intervention in pain management.

There is a tendency to regard this as the special province or purview of the psychologist, psychiatrist, or clinical social worker, but, in a team approach, all interventions may be seen as having a psychotherapeutic action. The reassurances of the physician or nurse that a patient's pain is being taken seriously, the verbal reinforcement to the patient by all providers that progress in pain relief and management can be achieved, and even the comforting touch of physicians, nurses, and physical therapists during examinations, procedures, or exercises—all may possess a powerful psychotherapeutic dimension. What is shared in team meetings and clinical rounds can also prove critical to all providers in assessing a patient's progress and determining the extent to which he or she remains stress-reactive, as well as how the pain-stress cycle continues to unfold in the context of his or her family, social relationships, work, and livelihood.

Influence of Psychopathology As the ongoing evaluation and treatment of chronic pain proceeds, one area in which psychologists, psychiatrists, and clinical social workers can be especially valuable lies in determining the extent to which psychopathology is present and influential. As psychological intervention begins, the first important consideration—one that will likely have implications for both prognosis and treatment—concerns the juxtaposition of psychological factors affecting the patient's pain experience, especially with regard to the order, magnitude, and relative duration of influence. In some cases, psychopathology occurs as a complicating feature in the diagnosis and treatment of chronic pain and existed prior to the development of the pain syndrome. In these instances, some delineation of the premorbid or existing psychopathology becomes critical to understanding the role and meaning of pain from the patient's perspective. In other cases, psychopathology is reactive to and arises within the context of the patient's experience of pain, and special care may be needed to introduce the idea of and address the disorder without the patient's feeling that the focus has been removed from his or her pain.

Chronic pain is far more prevalent among the psychiatrically disordered than in the general population, and there is considerable evidence that alterations in pain experience occur in conjunction with some psychiatric disorders, including mood disorders, anxiety disorders, and psychotic disorders.[14] Prevalence rates for depression among chronic pain sufferers in clinic-based samples vary in the literature from 30% to 54%,[15] with significant depressive symptoms ranging from 60% to as high as 100% in some samples.[16] The question of which came first—the depression or the pain—remains controversial,[17] and clinical evaluation can certainly reveal depressive symptomatology to be a premorbid or disposing influence in the development of chronic pain, as well as a comorbid one. That depression might be a consequence of chronic pain is acknowledged by many patients; but that pain might constitute the somatized expression of premorbid but unacknowledged depression or intrapsychic conflict typically meets with resistance from some patients and their families, who may find a psychiatric diagnosis both less accessible and less acceptable than a medical one.

Case 2 A 52-year-old married woman with a previous lumbar laminectomy and a well-documented history of mild, episodic, but well-managed low back pain developed an exacerbation shortly after the last of her three children left home to enter college. Her pain did not resolve as easily as it had in the past, and 2 months later, she presented to a pain management center, tearful, agitated, and in obvious distress, having exhausted her primary care physician's ordinarily effective armamentarium of conservative treatments. Her husband reported that she had become increasingly withdrawn from her friends and previously busy schedule and now stayed mostly in bed, watching television or sleeping. With a diagnostic workup and clinical examination devoid of any findings except a few mild trigger points, the patient's pain physicians prescribed an antidepressant, which they were careful to explain is also considered a "pain medication," and referred her to a structured group psychotherapy program, emphasizing the importance of learning techniques for greater musculoskeletal relaxation. One month later, the patient presented for follow up, excitedly discussing her cognitive-behavioral assignments for stress management from her group and chatting with the nurses about the success of her children, with whom she had developed a frequent e-mail correspondence. She complained of occasional, mild residual pain but was not allowing this to impede the gradual resumption of her daily schedule.

In this case, the patient had little insight into the development of her reactive depression or its relationship to her worsening pain. Considering her history of surgery and episodic low back pain, it is difficult to ascribe her distress solely to somatization; but instances of pure somatization are usually difficult to document convincingly. As in most cases, this woman's exacerbation of pain appears to stem from both physiologic and psychological factors; and, especially when discussing her experience with the patient herself, it is important not to become distracted by questions of primacy. When there is a clear, established history of a premorbid psychiatric disorder, it becomes critical to understand how such psychological factors may have contributed to the development of chronic pain and how they shape the patient's experience of chronic pain. When there is little to suggest premorbid psychiatric influences, however, it is far more important to maintain a clinical focus on the relationship between psychological and physical factors, as a whole, as well as their ongoing interaction.

For this reason, a model reflecting the influence of stress-reactivity and the pain-stress cycle is probably more versatile and more efficacious in such cases, because it promotes a view of health that takes into account the interaction of psychological and physical factors, without the need or presumptive burden of trying to establish causal direction—an enterprise that, despite our best efforts and intentions, might easily result in harm to the patient. With such a model, psychological factors can be viewed as both amplifying pain and inhibiting successful adjustment to it, whereas chronic pain itself can be viewed as a potent psychological stressor in its own right and one that can easily give rise to other psychosocial stressors.[18]

The disposing premorbidity, for example, of personality disorders, depression, and posttraumatic stress in the development of chronic pain is often accepted uncritically in the clinical arena. That they are found in significantly greater proportion comorbidly is indisputable.[19,20] Yet, when viewed according to a diathesis-stress model, even personality disordered and posttraumatic stress disordered behaviors may emerge for the first time and coalesce around chronic pain.[21] So the question becomes less a chicken-or-egg issue of, "Which came first, the chronic pain or the psychiatric disorder?" but rather, "What approach is more helpful to the patient in understanding and assisting in the resolution, both psychologically and physically, of his or her pain?"

Somatization, according to this model, can be seen as an immature psychological defense capable either of giving rise to pain in the apparent absence of organic pathology or of complicating and magnifying pain in the established presence of organic pathology. As a defense, it simply represents the symbolic displacement of intrapsychic conflict onto the somatic sphere in an unconscious attempt to avoid distressing affects associated with psychosocial stress. All stress-reactive individuals tend to somatize, when under sustained or escalating stress; and, because we are all on a stress-reactive continuum, we all tend to express affects through our bodies to some degree. Highly stress-reactive patients may have well-documented histories of somatization and physical complaints at many sites, but any tendency toward somatization can magnify a patient's suffering well beyond what is expectable, given the nature and extent of actual tissue damage.

Alexithymia can be a predisposing, complicating, and exacerbating feature of somatization,[22] because patients who are unable to articulate their emotions and affective states in words may have few outlets, other than bodily expression, for their intrapsychic pain and discomfort. For those who have come to regard the experience of psychological distress or displays of affect as signs of weakness or occasions for shame, displacing intrapsychic conflict onto the body may also allow them to feel that they have more legitimate claims to others' attention and the fulfillment of their needs—a phenomenon or symptom also known as *secondary gain*. Such constructs as alexithymia and secondary gain, in turn, raise the question of whether the phenomenologic focus of the interaction between pain and stress is more appropriately placed on psychiatric disorder or on temperament, personality traits, coping attributes, and even environmental factors, such as availability of support.[23] Shifting the clinical focus too quickly to that of psychiatric disorder can discourage the patient further or even lead to the termination of treatment.

The dangers of prematurely settling on a psychiatric diagnosis are especially apparent in the case of the somatoform disorders, the common feature of which is the presence of physical symptoms suggesting a general medical condition but which cannot be completely attributed to such a condition or the effects of a substance or another mental disorder.[24] The category of somatoform disorders—conversion disorder, somatization disorder, pain disorder, and hypochondriasis—may be both descriptive of a patient's symptoms and representative of clinical observation, but too often such diagnoses represent the closing of the door to continued medical attention and intervention. So, too, the coincidence of mood, anxiety, and personality disorders should not be considered a medical end point, but rather should highlight the need for multidisciplinary approaches to the treatment of chronic pain. Psychiatric diagnosis in chronic pain is valuable only insofar as it develops a deeper and richer understanding of the patient and promotes multidisciplinary options for treatment, including that of psychotherapeutic intervention.

Preparing for Psychotherapeutic Intervention

Not all patients with chronic pain exhibit significant psychopathology, of course, or experience the complicating influences of the range of psychological factors that can affect the course of physical symptoms. Many individuals adjust well to the limitations imposed by their pain and continue to work productively and to enjoy satisfying relationships and rewarding personal interests. Most of them have no histories of premorbid psychopathology; and, by virtue of resilient temperaments, adaptive personality traits, and successful coping skills, they manage to avoid the comorbid development of psychological distress and psychiatric symptoms that can become associated with chronic pain.

Those who are less fortunate, however, include among them the most memorable and challenging patients in any primary care practice or pain management center. Their suffering is often dramatic and, even when their numbers are few, their drain on resources is considerable, when calculated in terms of time, money, and the morale of staff. Their families, other physicians, employers, and even health insurance carriers frequently become demanding agents in their behalf, even as their pain remains puzzling and intractable to an ever-lengthening list of interventions; while their escalating sense of urgency continually reminds us of our limitations as health care providers. When all else appears to have failed and all available resources have been tapped, it is a small step toward collusion with the patient's own escalating sense of urgency to make one more referral to yet another specialist or to raise the level of pain medication, one more time; to consider one more improbable intervention or, as is often the case, to simply close the door, abandoning the patient to begin the process all over again.

It is under such circumstances that psychologists and psychiatrists frequently find the chronic pain patient at their doors. Having been told that there is nothing further that can be done, that there is no hope of further surgical or medical palliation, patients can be left to begin the process of psychologically adjusting to their pain and its sequelae in the most angry, anxious, and despairing of states. For these individuals, pain may already have become an organizing principle, and the enterprise of psychotherapeutic management is no longer only that of addressing transiently reactive mood or anxiety or difficulties with adjustment, but that of attempting to alter a way of life or effecting change at the level of personality. Chronic pain of this nature continues to call for a multidisciplinary approach, often just at a time when patients are most discouraged by or disillusioned with their medical care; and it is often a long road back to successful pain management, made far more arduous for having been consigned to being undertaken in pieces.

When psychological factors are influential in the development or maintenance of chronic pain, the greatest progress is likely to be achieved most expediently when there is not only interdisciplinary cooperation but an integrated, comprehensive plan of treatment in which all providers are working together, with the same goals in sight. Undertaking medical and psychotherapeutic approaches to chronic pain separately—or worse, sequentially—greatly reduces the chances of making global progress in patients' adjustment to their pain, while increasing the chances that interventions from different disciplines may compete or contradict one another, leaving patients feeling confused and helpless. It can also leave physicians and psychotherapists feeling alone and unassisted in their attempts to help their patients and more likely, as a result, to communicate their own anxiety and sense of helplessness about the slowness or lack of progress back to the patient.

The patient's developing stability and success with managing chronic pain may well depend on an abiding trust that his or her physicians are doing everything possible to offer appropriate relief and comfort through medical means, while his or her psychotherapist is doing everything possible to assist with the adjustment to what the patient sees as the emotional impact and consequences of pain. This does not mean that there is a strict division of labor, however; and patients often will turn to their physicians and nurses for emotional support and ask their psychotherapists for reassurance about medical decisions. Patients with chronic pain often ask their providers, without respect to discipline, for *validation*—the reassurance that their physicians, nurses, physical therapists, and psychotherapists have heard their concerns and understand their experience. Many have gone from provider to provider, encountering repeated disappointments in their search for answers, and their often challenging and sometimes provocative presentations may reflect the defensiveness, hypersensitivity, and hypervigilance of the scars, both physical and psychological, they have sustained in their search for relief and solace.

Establishing a good working *alliance* is, therefore, critical for all members of a multidisciplinary team. Patients' compliance with directives and interventions and their cooperation with a plan of treatment often depend on their perception that all members of the team are working together in their behalf. When patients lose trust in their providers or sense that providers are not fully engaged in the process of helping them in their search for answers and relief, the alliance deteriorates, sometimes irredeemably. Patients' complaints of feeling rushed, dismissed, or devalued may result, not surprisingly, in an increase in pain behaviors and dependency, as well as tendencies toward the expression of retaliatory impulses. In a multidisciplinary approach to treatment, the responsibility for maintaining the integrity of the alliance is shared among all providers, with the result that the patient's urgency is experienced by all as less demanding or overwhelming.

When the psychologist, psychiatrist, or clinical social worker enters the scene, patients frequently need the reassurance of the rest of the team that their pain has not suddenly been relegated to the uncertain status of being purely psychological in origin, or "all in the head." Especially in the initial psychological interview, it is reassuring to patients to be able to focus on what they know best—namely, the emotional impact of pain on their lives—and not to feel as if their beliefs and psychological defenses are being challenged or threatened. When the patient feels secure that his or her story has been heard and fully appreciated, the direction of the psychotherapist's inquiry can turn toward a consideration of the psychological and behavioral antecedents, correlates, and sequelae of pain—all of the factors influencing the pain-stress cycle. Once the patient is willing to acknowledge and discuss the possibility that stress may contribute to his or her subjective experience of pain, the way is prepared for psychotherapeutic intervention.

It is, nevertheless, critical not to presume too much or too quickly here. A final, essential question to consider in preparing for psychotherapeutic intervention concerns the range of variables in individual temperament and personality that make psychological adjustment possible: Is the patient disposed toward making the changes necessary to facilitate more adaptive coping? Because patients vary widely in their receptiveness to making the behavioral changes that lead to more successful adjustment, their readiness for change[20,25] may require continual monitoring and nurturing in psychotherapy (see Chap. 13). Suggesting to someone who is waiting for his or her physician to "fix the problem" that relaxation exercises might assist in the management of pain is unlikely to result in anything but frustration. Accurately assessing and nurturing the patient's readiness for change, therefore, becomes one of the principal prerequisites for the successful psychotherapeutic management of chronic pain.

INDIVIDUAL PSYCHOTHERAPY

The psychotherapeutic treatment of pain disorder or chronic pain accompanying other psychiatric disorders may have more than one goal, including the relief of pain itself, the decrease of disability and illness-related or "pain behaviors," the restoration of activity and the increase in functional quality of life, as well as the decrease in reliance on opioid and other analgesic or anxiolytic medications.[26] Individual psychotherapy may prove to be of great benefit in achieving these goals, but it must be noted from the outset that structured group programs, whether inpatient or outpatient, have been studied more widely and demonstrated to be of greater efficacy in their application to chronic pain populations.[27]

The hallmark of such programs has been the successful integration of multidisciplinary approaches into a unified interdisciplinary perspective, with greater coordination of services and frequent communication among all providers. Progress in individual psychotherapy, by itself, is frequently hamstrung by a less unified, more piecemeal approach to the patient's concerns, which may change from session to session. As a result, more structured forms of individual treatment, such as cognitive-behavioral therapy, have been developed specifically for pain patients. But individual treatment, whether combined with structured group psychotherapy or undertaken on its own, tends to work best when its approach is eclectic and includes a number of components,[20] each of which may appeal to a different or succeeding stage in the patient's receptivity or readiness for change.[25]

Keeping in mind that psychotherapeutic management is the concern of the entire treatment team, any intervention may, broadly speaking, have a psychotherapeutic impact on the patient. The beginning of formal psychotherapeutic intervention, however, is usually marked by a clinical interview and anamnesis administered by the psychologist, psychiatrist, or clinical social worker. Psychological testing may also be included as a means of evaluating the current level of functioning, symptoms of psychopathology, presence of psychosocial risk factors affecting prognosis, and other cultural, educational, and attitudinal indicators warranting consideration in the planning of treatment. Psychopharmacologic evaluation may be included at this stage, as well, but many pain physicians are conversant with the use of psychotropics in pain management and referral to a specialist is often considered redundant, unless the initial interventions have proven unsuccessful. Once a picture of the patient's presenting baseline of coping and functioning emerges, ongoing and longitudinal assessments provide a measure of psychotherapeutic progress, as well as indications for appropriate changes in the treatment plan.

Psychodynamic Psychotherapy

Psychodynamic or insight-oriented and supportive psychotherapies are not usually considered treatments of choice for the chronic pain patient, precisely because their approach is less structured and more patient-directed; but they may be the logical starting point for patients whose pain and disability are sustained or exacerbated by intrapsychic conflict or unconscious motives, such as trauma or secondary gain.[28] The high correlation between the history of physical or sexual abuse and the subsequent development of chronic pain is well documented in the literatures of psychiatry and pain.[29–31] In patients who have suffered abuse as children or as adults or who have experienced or witnessed situations in which either death or serious injury was real or threatened, chronic pain may come to represent a means of psychologically symbolizing and organizing an unbearable traumatic event or series of events. Nor is the situation of childhood or adult abuse the only form of trauma associated with chronic pain and disability. The development of comorbid posttraumatic stress disorder is also prevalent in work-related injuries and motor vehicle accidents.[32,33]

Whether premorbid or comorbid, posttraumatic stress disorder remains a powerful confounding factor in many cases of chronic pain; and, for those patients with such a background, a frequently necessary step in the development of their readiness for change is the experience of making a conscious connection between their trauma and their pain. In cases in which premorbid psychopathology has contributed to the development of chronic pain and disability, an understanding of the relationship between the patient's history and the development of his or her symptoms may prove essential in assisting him or her toward a more active role in treatment.

Case 3 A 28-year-old, recently married woman was referred to a pain management center with a 6-month history of chronic abdominal and pelvic pain of uncertain etiology. She reported having a history of episodically severe "stomach aches and cramps," as a child, but felt that these had long since been resolved. Although similar to these early episodes, her current pain had become more intense and urgent, even to the point where walking was sometimes difficult, literally necessitating her husband's support to get down the stairs in their home. Her anxiety had also escalated, interfering with the couple's sexual intimacy, despite her husband's obvious concern and willingness to assist her in whatever ways she asked. The patient agreed to enter psychotherapy but denied the impact of any stress in her life, beyond that of her pain. During the course of treatment, she disclosed to her psychotherapist that she had endured sexual abuse from her father as a child, but, again, placed no significance on its enduring influence. When asked how and when the abuse stopped, she indicated that her father typically became more solicitous of her and less likely to molest her, when she became ill. Over time, she made the connection that her pain had begun in the weeks immediately following her wedding, when the couple's sexual intimacy had greatly increased in frequency. Wondering whether there might be a relationship between her pain and her feelings and attitudes about sex, she eventually came to the realization that her developing sexual relationship with her husband was, through no fault of her own or her husband's, recapitulating her childhood trauma. Once she recognized that this recapitulation might have contributed to the onset of her pain, she became motivated to address the complete range of issues both influencing and influenced by her pain. Several months later, following the addition of couples therapy and a cognitive-behavioral component to her individual treatment, her pain was largely resolved, and she and her husband were reporting the mutually satisfying reintroduction of sexual intimacy to their relationship.

This case illustrates how an instance of primary somatization can become a defensive process around which a personality can coalesce unconsciously. If the impact of such a process goes unacknowledged and its possible influence, unrecognized, then the motivation for change is likely to remain insufficient. In this patient's case, not only did she need to examine her immediate situation, but she had to recognize and accept the connections between her emotional experience and her chronic pain before she could accept a more active role in her own recovery and rehabilitation. Similarly, when the trauma of a work-related injury or motor vehicle accident triggers and recapitulates an earlier, unresolved emotional trauma, such as childhood abuse, then what appears to be a straightforward physical injury can easily become complicated by premorbid psychological factors, making pain more tenacious and less tractable. It is not unreasonable to think that many individuals suffering such injuries, but without a history of trauma in their backgrounds, might experience a few days or weeks of discomfort but otherwise emerge essentially unscathed, having put the experience behind them.

Another problem often adversely affecting a patient's adjustment to and recovery from injury and pain is that of *secondary gain*, an unconscious motivation to maintain a symptom in order to gain some advantage.[11] In secondary gain, the advantage is derived from symptoms that have already formed and so could not have been foreseen or sought, even unconsciously, at the time of the original injury and development of pain and other symptoms. The gain did not contribute to the formation of the symptoms, therefore, but now contributes to the maintenance of the illness and potentially to resistance toward treatment. In psychoanalytic theory, *primary gain*, by contrast, relates to the intrapsychic motivation that led to symptom formation in the first place, such as the need or wish to assume the sick role and to feel both cared for and taken care of, thereby keeping an internal conflict, such as fear of inadequacy or failure, out of awareness.[11]

Secondary gain refers to those interpersonal gratifications that, once enjoyed through the sick role, make recovery less appealing. The sympathy and concern of family and friends, preferential treatment, disability benefits, drugs, interpersonal domination, the increased comfort of a socially sanctioned change in role, and the avoidance of certain activities may all be considered forms of secondary gain. Primary gain unfolds intrapsychically, whereas secondary gain tends to manifest in an interpersonal context. A third complication is frequently the presence of *tertiary gain*, which is wholly external to the patient but consists of the benefits derived by family or other caretakers from reinforcing the patient's pain behaviors.[34] The suppression of familial conflict, material benefit, and the reallocation of power within the family are among the more frequently cited tertiary gains in the economy of family dynamics. Because these unconscious motives on the part of family members can have a huge impact on the treatment of the patient and because family members can often be enlisted as allies in treatment, family meetings or, in some cases, ongoing family therapy may prove necessary to the successful psychotherapeutic management of the patient with chronic pain.[35]

According to the strict psychoanalytic scheme, secondary gain follows primary gain, which makes it more accurately applied to instances of somatoform disorders, such as conversion and somatization. In reality, the individual obtains certain gains with any illness, and unconscious secondary gain can develop in the aftermath of actual physical injury or disease, just as easily. Identifying what a patient gains and loses—secondary losses, such as loss of a satisfying job, livelihood, and prestige—can be critical, both to diagnosis and to treatment and recovery.[11] For this reason, the medical and legal scrutiny of secondary gain is frequently given great emphasis in cases of chronic pain, and it is frequently left to a psychiatric evaluation and a psychodynamic approach to treatment to attempt to discern conscious from unconscious motivations and to distinguish instances of malingering, factitious disorder, and primary somatization from the more expectable somatizing complications occurring around physical injury or illness.[36]

Where the medical and legal determination of disability is concerned, strong evidence of primary gain can, nevertheless, point toward a disabling condition but may change the focus of diagnosis and treatment from medical to psychological. In some cases, the effect of this shift is to exculpate employers, insurance carriers, and other litigants from any legal responsibility for compensation or even treatment. For this reason, evidence of premorbid psychopathology is often of as great an interest, legally, as whether the sum total of secondary gains outweighs the apparent secondary losses. As with the problem of measuring pain itself, there is no empirically verifiable method of accurately and reliably determining the presence or influence of primary or secondary gain in any individual's case, but the domain of inquiry can often be approached only through psychodynamic and supportive interventions, when the patient's welfare is the prime concern.

A number of difficulties with the traditional concept of secondary gain have called both the concept and its utility into question. Given the obvious problem of trying to discern what is conscious from what is unconscious, some clinical researchers favor definitions of secondary gain that do away with the distinction and focus instead on behaviors that *appear* as if the patient is seeking some expression of gain.[34] This promotes a more operational definition and opens the way to empirical investigation, but it begs the clinical question of how to approach secondary gain that is genuinely unconsciously motivated. For patients who cannot seem to make significant progress in managing their pain through behavioral and cognitive-behavioral psychotherapy and techniques, an insight-oriented approach may prove the only avenue open to influencing their level of motivation.

Supportive Psychotherapy

Although psychodynamic psychotherapy tends to place the reward on insight and interpretation of unconscious conflicts, the emphasis in supportive psychotherapy is on the strengthening of ego functions and improved adaptation.[37] The psychotherapist's understanding of the patient remains psychodynamic, but the interventions are crafted to improve the patient's level of functioning in at least two critical dimensions: firstly, to enhance the patient's capacity for reality testing—in effect, to anticipate what others see, when they encounter him or her, and to develop a self-observing capacity for monitoring his or her own reactions and motivations—and, secondly, to bolster the patient's healthiest psychological defenses and emotional and intellectual resources in the service of adjusting to a new set of circumstances.

The first and often necessary step in this process for many patients with chronic pain is the experience of feeling understood, usually achieved through the opportunity to tell their story to a sympathetic listener whom they perceive to be in the helping role. What patients know best and typically wish to discuss most urgently is the social, emotional, and behavioral impact of their pain on their lives. Even when they make no connection or outright deny any influence of these factors on the development and maintenance of their physical symptoms, patients need to feel that their suffering is validated and the circumstances of their misfortune are fully appreciated by their providers. Once the patient begins to trust this inchoate alliance, often made possible by the supportive efforts of psychotherapeutic management by the entire team, the collaborative development of a rationale for psychotherapy may ensue.

The major shift enabled by supportive psychotherapy, and the reason why it is frequently a necessary prerequisite step to any other psychotherapeutic intervention, lies in its approach to moving patients from a purely mechanistic understanding of their dilemma to one in which they can consider assuming an active role in their own recovery and rehabilitation. Patients whose explanatory models of pain are deterministic or who are unaware of the influence of secondary gain, often insist on medical interventions in which they may remain passive. By enhancing their capacity for reality testing, the supportive psychotherapist can assist patients in coming to see their own stress-reactivity and toward beginning to appreciate their involvement in the pain-stress cycle.

Few patients would deny that their pain is *one* of, if not *the* greatest source of stress in their lives; and this simple acknowledgment is often the beginning of a psychoeducational breakthrough. For many patients, this shift heralds their becoming more sophisticated in their understanding of the physiology and psychology of pain and in their appreciation of the differences between pain and injury, hurt and harm. At that point, many are willing to move ahead by working with a psychotherapist toward developing strategies to make the most of their own strengths and resources for coping with stress and managing pain.

Operant-Behavioral Therapy

Operant-behavioral therapy (OBT), which has its origins in learning theory, refers to the group of interventions focused principally on the observed behavior of the patient. In the operant model of pain, the reinforcing role of social and environmental factors in the development and maintenance of pain through observed pain behaviors is identified, with the behaviors themselves being targeted for intervention. This approach may prove most effective when patients demonstrate little understanding of the relationship between their pain behaviors and the underlying physiologic damage or disease,[28] and it is especially useful in cases in which the subjective experience of pain appears to go well beyond any established organic basis to the point where secondary gain has become an obvious issue and persistent, often dramatic, pain behaviors have emerged.

The goal of OBT is to encourage the development and practice of more adaptive pain management strategies by establishing and reinforcing new "wellness" behaviors, while discouraging or reducing the reinforcement of "illness" or pain behaviors.[7] Thus, increased self-reliance, activity, and socialization are encouraged, whereas verbal complaints, grimacing, social isolation, and overreliance on family and caretakers are discouraged. As a form of psychotherapeutic management, OBT is not limited to the setting of individual or group psychotherapy but is usually most effective, when supported by the entire team of providers, whether in the setting of office visits, physical therapy sessions, telephone contacts, or walk-in encounters.

The basis of OBT suggests that both wellness and pain behaviors can be shaped—developed, increased, reduced, or extinguished—according to the principles of operant conditioning. Reinforcement increases the likelihood that behaviors will occur, whereas punishment or the withdrawal of reinforcement decreases the likelihood of their occurrence. When attention from a provider or family member, for example, is offered solicitously in response to the patient's facial grimacing, there is immediate reinforcement, ensuring that this pain behavior will recur and possibly become habitual. When reinforcement is withdrawn—when the behavior no longer elicits the sought-after attention—it will decrease and possibly extinguish.

Similarly, when the patient experiences an exacerbation of pain, following an increase in activity, the exacerbation itself can serve to punish any motivation toward self-reliance and the development of wellness behaviors. Finding reinforcements that can modulate or offset the negative consequences of increased activity can encourage the patient to adopt wellness behaviors, even at the cost of some discomfort. Again, because what occurs at the clinic or psychotherapist's office is a comparatively small sampling of behavior, encouraging the patient's consistency of motivation—through supportive interventions and his or her family's participation in family meetings—will result in the most successful outcome. In severe or poorly tractable cases—in which it is apparent that setting limits and assisting the patient in the development of more adaptive responses on an outpatient basis is failing—an inpatient pain program, in which the highest level of operant control is possible, may become necessary.

Whether outpatient or inpatient, individual or group, informal or structured, a variety of OBT techniques can be adapted to the patient's particular situation, including (1) pacing and graduated activity, (2) scheduling and tapering of pain medications, and (3) social reinforcement.[7] Because these techniques of operant conditioning are common to the interventions of a broad range of behavioral and psychotherapeutic approaches to the management of pain, they can be employed as a milieu therapy or as an adjunct to supportive and cognitive-behavioral interventions. On the minutest of levels, no physician or nurse or psychotherapist can sit with a patient for long, without reinforcing some responses and discouraging others with as small an intervention as a facial expression, gesture, or well or poorly chosen word.[38]

Cognitive-Behavioral Therapy

Whereas OBT may be considered a core behavioral therapy, basic to all programs of pain management, cognitive-behavioral therapy (CBT) has more specific psychotherapeutic goals and is usually undertaken in the formal setting of individual or group psychotherapy, whether outpatient or inpatient. CBT is directed toward changing patients' maladaptive responses to chronic pain by examining and posing alternatives to the thoughts, attitudes, and beliefs underlying them, as well as by encouraging the acquisition of new coping skills and techniques to take their place. CBT usually includes a range of behavioral components, most notably, relaxation training and keeping a pain diary; however, the emphasis is placed on modifying emotional and behavioral responses, those that tend to affect the patient's level of functioning adversely, by challenging and restructuring their cognitive underpinnings.

The focus of CBT, therefore, is on the development of self-control and self-regulation.[28] The work of treatment is often undertaken in a threefold stepwise progression, including (1) a psychoeducational phase, (2) a skills-building phase, and (3) an application phase,[7] with each phase roughly corresponding to a new milestone in self-regulation and a new stage in the patient's readiness for change.[25] In CBT, the goal is the establishment of a higher level of functioning, which the patient is now motivated to sustain and has developed the skills to maintain. In the process, the patient becomes more resilient to the comorbid development of anxiety and depression, increasing his or her perception of pain as a controllable or manageable experience.

The first or psychoeducational phase of CBT is designed to enlist the patient's efforts as an active participant in his or her own recovery and rehabilitation. It is here that what is often referred to as the *mind-body* model of understanding pain is introduced to the patient. Concepts, such as stress-reactivity and the pain-stress cycle, are presented in such a way as to assist the patient in the identification of those thoughts, attitudes, and beliefs that tend to make his or her pain less tractable and his or her suffering, more severe. These self-defeating cognitions typically develop under the influence of anxiety, misinformation, secondary gain, and poorly resolved intrapsychic conflicts and often lead to depression and feelings of worthlessness, hopelessness, and helplessness. When a patient believes, "I'll never be able to work or provide for my family or have a normal life with this pain," despair cannot be far behind. Yet most patients come to treatment with a personalized array of such poorly examined and unchallenged cognitions.

The second or skills-building phase of CBT is designed to develop cognitive strategies enabling the patient to recognize the negative impact of his or her self-defeating cognitions and replace them with self-affirming statements, emphasizing control and adaptive coping. When a patient believes, "I have faced many problems, and I can handle this one, too," or, "I may not be able to do everything I want, but I can do much more than I previously thought," the motivation for rejecting pain behaviors, nurturing wellness behaviors, and raising the level of activity and social interaction becomes apparent. The cognitive restructuring techniques employed in CBT not only help patients to recognize those thoughts, attitudes, and beliefs about their pain that make them feel stuck, but also encourage the systematic substitution of more stable and positive ones that are likely to facilitate treatment across all modalities, from medications and procedures to physical and complementary therapies.

Part of the skills-building phase may also be devoted to the acquisition of other supportive coping strategies, such as stress management, anger management, assertiveness training, relaxation training, and pacing. Most of these techniques are employed in the service of identifying and modifying the patient's response to those environmental, interpersonal, and intrapsychic triggers that increase autonomic arousal and musculoskeletal tension and adversely affect the subjective experience of pain. Relaxation training, in particular, offers a broad range of behavioral techniques designed to quiet the autonomic nervous system and relieve musculoskeletal rigidity and tension. Various forms of meditation, autogenic training, guided imagery and visualization, self-hypnosis, as well as yoga and even tai chi, have been used successfully in pain management programs, with the National Institutes of Health favorably reviewing the recent empirical data in support of the efficacy of relaxation techniques in the treatment of chronic pain.[39]

Biofeedback is another psychoeducational and training device that allows the patient to monitor his or her ongoing progress at developing an effective regimen of relaxation techniques. During a biofeedback session, the patient is connected by surface (skin) electrodes or receptors to an electronic or computerized instrument designed to measure, amplify, and *feed back* physiologic information to the patient and psychotherapist or technician.[40,41] The latter, in turn, assists the patient to refine and increase the efficacy of one or more relaxation techniques in order to counteract the effects of dysponesis—maladaptive compensatory bracing in response to pain—and autonomic overarousal.[42]

By monitoring the level of musculoskeletal tension, through surface electromyographic leads, and the level of autonomic activity, through measures of heart rate, blood pressure, blood-volume pulse wave amplitude, skin temperature, oxygen saturation, and electrodermagraphic response, patients can see firsthand the extent to which they are having success at gaining control through the practice of regular and disciplined relaxation over processes that they previously felt were unmanageable. There is sufficient and still growing evidence to suggest that biofeedback monitoring in conjunction with behavioral therapy is an effective treatment in a number of chronic pain conditions, including migraine headache, tension-type headache, disorders of intestinal motility, musculoskeletal pain, including low back pain, and Raynaud's disease.[40,43]

There is also growing interest in its application as a psychoeducational tool applied to nociceptive desensitization in patients who have become so highly sensitized to pain and other noxious sensations that their pain perception appears to have an augmented affective component or heightened emotional intensity.[44] In this category, we find patients who are suffering from what may represent limbically augmented pain syndromes (the LAPS hypothesis) characterized by pain that is frequently out of proportion to clinical findings and associated with neurovegetative problems and disturbances of mood.[45] This group includes patients who are suffering from fibromyalgia, chronic fatigue syndrome, certain types of visceral and headache pain, chronic regional pain syndromes, and phantom pain; and biofeedback training has been shown, in some cases, to be useful by assisting these individuals to countercondition sensations of pain with sensations of relaxation, warmth, and well-being.

Biofeedback can help patients to move toward the third or application phase of CBT in which their newly acquired collection of cognitive skills, behavioral techniques, and coping strategies develops into a more enduring and adaptive approach to pain management. Cognitive-behavioral therapy concludes, then, as patients learn to apply their skills and maintain their new outlook in progressively more challenging situations.[7] In this way, it becomes, not merely a collection of tools or techniques, but a template for successfully adjusting to the ongoing intrusion of chronic pain. Patients who have successfully completed courses of CBT often refer to it as though they have undergone a change in lifestyle in which relaxation exercises and pacing have become as second nature as eating breakfast and brushing one's teeth.

Complementary Techniques

Two additional techniques or therapeutic approaches are often undertaken in the attempt to enhance pain management, whether applied on their own or combined with other individual psychotherapies in an eclectic treatment. These are hypnosis and, of more recent origin, eye movement desensitization and reprocessing (EMDR). Whether hypnosis can play an effective first-line role in the management of chronic pain remains controversial.[46] As a technique for inducing genuine analgesia, it is applied far more often in the management of acute and surgical pain, and many practitioners see its principal worth in addressing chronic pain as simply that of evoking the relaxation response. For those patients who cannot master meditative techniques or comfortably employ progressive muscle relaxation, self-hypnosis can become an essential skill in the management of musculoskeletal tension and autonomic overarousal. In the case of those patients with chronic pain who have used hypnosis—whether hypnotherapy with a practitioner or self-hypnosis—to achieve analgesic relief from exacerbations or flare-ups or who use it regularly for time-limited relief or respite, additional study is needed to discern the generalizability and applicability of the technique.

EMDR is a comparatively new addition to the panoply of psychotherapeutic approaches to the management of pain, but its role in facilitating the cognitive processing of physical and emotional trauma associated with the origin of chronic pain is already promising. EMDR was developed as a precise technique, which, like hypnosis, requires specialized training for the practitioner.[47] Although compatible with psychodynamic and cognitive-behavioral approaches, its techniques are directed toward the evocation of the patient's capacity for rapid information processing to facilitate the processing of traumatic or dysfunctional thoughts and feelings.

The goal of this approach is to disengage affective memories that may be linked to pain through remembered or associated experience but not to the specific situation giving rise to pain in the present. By detaching or releasing these affective memories, EMDR restores the affective dimension of pain to a level more consonant with the actual situation giving rise to the pain. In effect, like the goal of psychodynamic psychotherapy, the result of EMDR is to separate past from present trauma, allowing the patient to process what were heretofore overwhelming emotions, focus on his or her present dilemma, and move forward in his or her recovery and rehabilitation. The possible applications of EMDR to limbically augmented pain syndromes are obvious and compelling; but, as with hypnosis, additional study is needed to discern the generalizability and criteria for applying the technique in cases of chronic pain.

GROUP PSYCHOTHERAPY

The formal practice of conducting group psychotherapy with medically ill patients is nearly a century old.[48] In the first recorded groups of this nature, the leaders—usually medical personnel—instructed patients on the medical aspect of their illness and encouraged them to present weekly reports to the group regarding their medical and spiritual progress.[49] The goal of these groups was to help patients cope more adaptively with their illnesses by addressing issues of self-confidence, self-esteem, and physical well-being[50]; and what began with tuberculosis sufferers was soon extended to groups for patients with other illnesses, including asthma, cancer, irritable bowel syndrome, skin disorders, and chronic pain.

Participation in groups offers a variety of advantages for patients with chronic pain. Group psychotherapy tends to be more affordable than individual treatment for both patients and health insurance carriers, and there is increasing evidence that participation in a group reduces the number of visits and telephone calls to physicians, further relieving strain on the medical care system.[51] Far more importantly, however, the effectiveness of group psychotherapy in the reduction of the psychological and physical distress accompanying chronic medical illness is well documented,[50,52] and patients with a broad range of medical illnesses demonstrate improved compliance, decreased physical symptoms, decreased symptoms of anxiety and depression, and increased self-esteem.[53,54]

In the treatment of patients with chronic pain, three approaches have emerged as dominant: support groups, psychodynamic groups, and structured cognitive-behavioral or behavioral medicine groups.[55] There is considerable evidence to suggest that groups with a strong CBT or behavioral medicine component are the most effective,[7,50] but, despite their differences in theory of approach and intervention, all three models share a range of common goals for treatment. Group psychotherapy can offer patients with chronic pain (1) validation of their experience, (2) increased self-esteem, (3) decreased social isolation, (4) opportunities to express frustration appropriately and practice assertiveness, (5) enhanced reality testing through opportunities to compare experiences with others, (6) a sense of satisfaction from helping others, (7) education about the pain-stress cycle and other psychosocial and medical factors involved in chronic pain, (8) the acquisition of a new set of coping skills, (9) encouragement for the development of more adaptive strategies for stress and pain management, and (10) reduction in symptoms.

Support Groups

The most popular and numerous groups for patients with chronic pain are support groups, which are frequently led by patients themselves and are often affiliated with patient- and volunteer-staffed organizations, as opposed to medical clinics, hospitals, or professional personnel. Many of the virtual support groups, electronic bulletin boards, and chat rooms of the various on-line services may be included in this category. Their emphasis is on providing social and emotional support for their members, as well as a forum for sharing medical information, but they often lack the specific goals of acquiring new coping skills and developing more adaptive stress and pain management strategies. In certain situations, they can also promulgate the spread of misinformation and lend uncritical endorsement to maladaptive strategies for pain management.

Although support groups can be effective for many patients who would otherwise have little opportunity to compare their experiences with others and seek validation, the cohesiveness and continuity of these groups may suffer from a lack of direction or supervision. A number of factors can spark disagreements between members and lead to fragmentation of the group, including erratic attendance by some members; differences in need, level of functioning, and interpersonal skills; dominance of the discussion by stronger personalities; and differences in perceived goals. Having an assigned lay leader or even a skilled professional leader may not rule out all of these pitfalls, but it will likely ensure greater cohesion and longevity of purpose and direction.

Psychodynamic Groups

Less structured than cognitive-behavioral groups, psychodynamic group psychotherapy in the setting of chronic pain has as its goal the creation of an interpersonal laboratory in which communications among the members can be examined within the dynamics of the group.[56] By observing, analyzing, and interpreting how each member relates to the group, the group's leader—always a professional mental health specialist—can assist each member, as well as enlist each member's help in assisting the others, to come to a better understanding of how chronic pain is affecting his or her relationships, social and occupational functioning, outlook on the world, and self-esteem. As with individual psychodynamic psychotherapy, the goal is to make the unconscious basis of conflicts and maladative defensive strategies more accessible to each member by examining the interpersonal impact that each member has on the group.

The psychotherapist in the psychodynamic group uses interventions designed to foster connections between the members and facilitate the give and take of the members' reactions to one another. The use of maladaptive defenses or the adoption by one of the members of self-defeating or interpersonally destructive choices are examples of behaviors that are typically challenged by the psychotherapist and other group members. To consolidate these insights and therapeutic gains, the psychotherapist often will articulate the themes and shared struggles of the group in an effort to move the members toward (1) a more realistic appreciation of their situations and the impact of their communications on others, (2) a greater reliance on their own natural resources and strengths, and (3) the acquisition of new behaviors and patterns of communication, reflecting more adaptive strategies for coping and more functional and health-affirming choices.

Behavioral Medicine Groups

*Behavioral medicin*e and *mind-body medicin*e are terms often used to describe a model of care that addresses the effects of stress on a disease or symptom, as well as the stress of chronic illness on the individual patient. Treatment according to this model addresses the biologic, psychological, and social issues, not just the biomedical ones, with the mode of intervention being CBT. In effect, behavioral medicine groups are highly structured, time-limited CBT groups, directed toward specific populations of medical patients, such as patients with chronic pain. The varieties of intervention can include any or all of the techniques one would find in individual CBT, including relaxation training—meditation, autogenic training, hypnosis, self-hypnosis, guided imagery and visualization, and even yoga or tai chi—cognitive therapy, pacing activities, and keeping a pain diary.

Behavioral medicine has traditionally involved a multidisciplinary effort that recognized and supported the synergy created by bringing together professionals in *both* mind *and* body to focus their expertise on the treatment of medical problems, such as cardiovascular disease, cancer, and chronic pain. Such collaboration has produced considerable research in the clinical efficacy of these combined treatments and in the cost-effectiveness of offering them to patients.[57] Behavioral medicine distinguishes itself from psychiatry and psychology by attending principally to the physical symptoms of patients and their effects on stress, coping, and emotions, as well as the effects of stress, coping, and emotions on the experience of physical symptoms. If psychopathology proves to be a determining factor in a particular patient's expression of physical symptoms, then that patient is referred to psychiatric providers; however, many depressed, anxious, and even personality disordered patients with chronic pain nevertheless benefit from participation in behavioral medicine groups, along with their psychiatric care.

Applications of Behavioral Medicine Groups to Chronic Pain In October 1995, the National Institutes of Health (NIH) convened a Technology Assessment Conference to consider the integration of behavioral and relaxation approaches into the treatment of chronic pain and insomnia.[39] The consensus panel concluded that there were sufficient data to recommend the inclusion of cognitive-behavioral therapies in the treatment of chronic pain. In a review of the relevant research, the panel cited a range of findings—including that all six of six factors identified in the correlation of treatment failures of low back pain are psychosocial—and recommended the integration of relaxation techniques with conventional medical procedures as a *necessary* step in the successful treatment of chronic pain.

Cognitive-behavioral skills can benefit the majority of patients experiencing chronic pain, because the emphasis is on the pain-stress cycle—both the stressful effects of pain and the effects of stress on pain. Groups can, therefore, be composed of patients with different diagnoses or etiologies of pain if there are not sufficient members for a single diagnostic group. Mixing diagnoses, furthermore, may actually have advantages, because patients come to realize that the experience of pain has universal features, qualities, and consequences. This realization frequently leads, in turn, to the inevitable comparisons patients make between their circumstances, often accompanied by the observation, "Things could be worse!" One of the principal advantages of group over individual psychotherapy is the power of the experience of validation that comes from sharing a common crisis in one's life with others who have similar experiences. That experience of psychosocial support has been shown repeatedly to have a significant positive influence on patients' coping and the course and outcome of disease.[58]

A further advantage is that the format of the behavioral medicine group can be adapted to small or large numbers of patients, depending on whether the model is largely psychoeducational or more psychotherapeutic. Psychoeducational models can accommodate groups of up to 25 or 30 patients, whereas psychotherapy groups are generally limited to 6 to 10. The format of behavioral medicine groups is flexible enough, in most cases, to adjust to the needs of the setting, the credentials of the providers or leaders, and the mechanism of reimbursement. Some models even incorporate the use of patients who have previously "graduated" from the group—or who have received special training—as assistant facilitators or, with ongoing professional supervision, even as lay providers, conducting groups largely on their own.[59]

Goals and General Format of Behavioral Medicine Groups Behavioral medicine groups are applied to the problem of chronic pain with three specific goals: to assist patients with (1) mastering skills for both stress and pain management, (2) mobilizing those skills routinely but especially during periods of increased stress and pain, and (3) developing self-efficacy—the belief and attitude that engaging in certain behaviors will reach a desired outcome. Encouraging patients to set and discuss the goals they hope to achieve in the group can help them to identify unrealistic expectations and engage them in taking the first steps toward the development of self-efficacy.

Ideally, the recommendation to participate in a cognitive-behavioral group is part of a coordinated multidisciplinary treatment plan, formulated after a comprehensive evaluation of the patient. There have been many attempts to predict the attributes associated with the successful completion of behavioral medicine groups, but only a few trends—and multifactorial ones, at that—have been identified.[60] In general, patients who are psychologically or cognitively impaired or who exhibit disruptive behaviors or who are nonambulatory are at greatest risk for failing to enter treatment or for attrition from a group they have begun, whereas patients who

TABLE 14-1 **Format of a Schedule of Sessions in a Behavioral Medicine Group**

Session	Description
Session 1: Understanding Pain	Psychoeducation on the pathophysiology of pain, presentation of a rationale for acute and chronic pain therapies, and review of the program's content *Members may invite a guest to this initial session.*
Session 2: Mind/Body Connection	Instruction on relaxation techniques and breathing exercises *Pain puts stress on the body, and many people in pain experience multiple symptoms of stress, as well as pain. Relaxation techniques assuage the harmful effects of prolonged stress on the body and mind. Techniques specific to pain management are introduced during succeeding sessions.*
Session 3: Body/Mind Connection	Instruction on exercise, pleasurable activities, pacing, and body awareness *Patients with chronic pain make two frequent errors: (1) they cut off awareness of body sensations and become "numb" to signals that might allow them to pace themselves adequately, and (2) they stop "moving" so that deconditioning contributes to dysfunction.*
Session 4: Body/Mind Connection and Nutrition	Review of patients' observations on pacing and exercise and instruction in the role of nutrition in chronic pain *Good nutrition promotes good health and may assist in the management of pain.*
Session 5: Power of the Mind	Introduction to basic cognitive therapy strategies: (1) identification of negative automatic thoughts and the cognitive distortions behind them, and (2) reframing them into more realistic thoughts and attitudes *Many patients with chronic pain find their coping skills challenged to the point of being overwhelmed. Cognitive restructuring offers them greater flexibility and a way out of their anxiety, anger, and depression.*
Session 6: Adopting Healthy Attitudes	Instruction in the uses of empathy and humor, as well as the adoption of "stress-hardy" attitudes *Patients' negative thoughts come from old cognitive-behavioral "tapes" applied inappropriately to new situations. Through the adoption of healthy attitudes, they need not suffer twice—with pain* and *negative emotional responses.*
Session 7: Effective Communication I	Review and role play of effective communication skills *People frequently do not say what they mean, with the result that conflicts emerge that were often never intended. Patients are encouraged to understand what their intentions are, when they see their health care providers, and to make their internal conflicts, expectations, and assumptions more consciously accessible.*
Session 8: Effective Communication II	Instruction on making statements match intent and review of the three styles of communication: passive, aggressive, and assertive *Once patients know what they want and begin to repair their self-esteem from the damaging effects of chronic pain, adopting an appropriate style of communication can support their new attitudes and help them to resolve previous conflicts.*
Session 9: Effective Problem-Solving	Instruction in problem-solving as an aid to setting goals *Many people are ineffective at setting goals, especially when an emotional "hook" is in conflict with the goal. The goal of losing weight, for example, may be in conflict with the feeling that food is the only means of comforting oneself. Patients in pain have difficulty accomplishing goals, because the wish to be able to do what they used to do gets in the way. Learning to separate goals from hooks is the first step toward problem-solving more adaptively and effectively.*
Session 10: The End of the Beginning	Review of all the new coping skills acquired and how to use them during exacerbations of pain *The final discussion focuses on relapse prevention and how patients can consolidate and maintain their new, more adaptive strategies for stress and pain management.*

*Caudill MA. Managing Pain Before it Manages You (Revised edition). New York, NY: Guilford Press; 2002.

demonstrate high motivation and a collaborative approach to their own medical care tend to have a high rate of completion.

Group leaders or providers may come from a variety of disciplines, including physicians, psychologists, social workers, nurses, and physical therapists, but essential criteria for their success tend to be that they (1) enjoy working with the chronic pain population, (2) have training in group therapy and group dynamics, and (3) recognize the strong influence of learned helplessness on patient compliance. A setting with pleasant surroundings and comfortable chairs, as well as mats for exercising and lying down, is most conducive to learning, when in pain; and a schedule of weekly meetings that last 1½ to 2 hours does not overtax most patients' capacity for attention and endurance, even if reduced by the presence of pain. Most behavioral medicine groups run for 8 to 10 weeks, which appears to cover the critical period necessary for the three phases of successful CBT: (1) psychoeducation, (2) skills-building, and (3) application and maintenance.[7]

There is considerable latitude in the content of sessions, in the order of presentation, and in the forms of presentation. In most sessions, the time will be divided into several components, with periods allocated for (1) presentation of new instruction; (2) supervised practice of developing skills, such as relaxation techniques; (3) presentation and discussion of homework, for example, pain diaries and checklists of daily relaxation exercises; and (4) stretching and mild exercise or yoga. There are many curricula, designed specifically for behavioral medicine groups with chronic pain patients, available in commercially published workbooks.[61,62] A brief description of the content proposed by one of these workbooks for ten sessions of a group for patients with chronic pain is presented in Table 14-1.[61]

Research has demonstrated that patients with chronic pain who participate in multidisciplinary programs with behavioral medicine groups feel less anxious, less depressed, and less pain, while simultaneously experiencing greater control, increased socialization, and a heightened sense of self-efficacy.[63,64] Patients exposed to CBT programs also appear to rely on the medical system more appropriately, reducing the number of clinic visits and telephone contacts made out of frustration and fear.[51,59,65,66] One patient summarized her experience of her participation in a behavioral medicine group, capturing the essence of the therapeutic goals, when she said, "I know it's going to be a good day, because *I know how to make it a good day.*"[61]

SUMMARY

The goal of psychotherapeutic management of chronic pain is not merely the reduction of pain but the restoration of functioning. The patient with chronic pain will always face limitations, but assisting him or her toward more successful adjustment and more adaptive strategies for coping is the role of psychotherapy in the multidisciplinary approach to pain. Successful psychotherapeutic management involves not only a multidisciplinary approach, but also an interdisciplinary effort in which the interventions of each member of the team of providers can be seen as having a psychotherapeutic impact on the patient, as well as a complementary effect on the interventions of the other providers. Assessing the degree to which any patient is stress-reactive and addressing his or her own unique expression of the pain-stress cycle may involve the application of one or more types of individual or group psychotherapy. An eclectic approach tends to offer the greatest versatility, but cognitive-behavioral therapies, whether individual or group, have demonstrated the greatest efficacy with the chronic pain population.

REFERENCES

1. International Association for the Study of Pain (IASP) Task Force on Taxonomy (Merskey H, Bogduk N, eds.). *Classification of Chronic Pain: Descriptions of Chronic Pain Syndromes and Definitions of Pain Terms.* 2nd ed. Seattle, Wash: IASP Press; 1994.
2. Turk DC, Flor H. Chronic pain: A biobehavioral perspective. In: Gatchel RJ, Turk DC, eds. *Psychosocial Factors in Pain: Critical Perspectives.* New York, NY: Guilford Press; 1999;18–34.
3. Jacobson L, Mariano AJ, Chabal C, et al. Beyond the needle: Expanding the role of anesthesiologists in the management of chronic non-malignant pain. *Anesthesiology* 1997;87:1210–1218.
4. American Medical Association. Pain. In: Cocchiarella L, Andersson GB, eds. *Guides to the Evaluation of Permanent Impairment.* 5th ed. Chicago, Ill: AMA; 2000;565–592.
5. Turk DC. Biopsychosocial perspective on chronic pain. In: Gatchel RJ, Turk DC, eds. *Psychological Approaches to Pain Management: A Practitioner's Handbook.* New York, NY: Guilford Press; 1996;3–32.
6. Ashburn MA, Staats PS. Management of chronic pain. *Lancet* 1999; 353:1865–1869.
7. Compas BE, Haaga DAF, Keefe FJ, et al. Sampling of empirically supported psychological treatments from health psychology: Smoking, chronic pain, cancer, bulimia nervosa. *J Consult Clin Psychol* 1998;66: 89–112.
8. Fordyce WE. *Back Pain in the Workplace: Management of Disability in Nonspecific Conditions: A Report of the Task Force on Pain in the Workplace of the International Association for the Study of Pain.* Seattle, Wash: IASP Press; 1995.
9. Kent J. The treatment of chronic benign pain syndrome in capitated health care. *Managed Care Q* 1996;4:77–83.
10. Weiner R. Chronic pain and stress. In: Margoles MS, Weiner R, eds. *Chronic Pain: Assessment, Diagnosis, and Management.* Boca Raton, Fla: CRC Press; 1999;203–208.
11. Eisendrath SJ. Psychiatric aspects of chronic pain. *Neurology* 1995; 45(suppl):26—34.
12. Gallagher RM. Treatment planning in pain medicine. *Med Clin North Am* 1999;83:823–849.
13. Melzack R. Pain and stress: A new perspective. In: Gatchel RJ, Turk DC, eds. *Psychosocial Factors in Pain: Critical Perspectives.* New York, NY: Guilford Press; 1999;89–106.
14. Lautenbacher S, Krieg J-S. Pain perception in psychiatric disorders: A review of the literature. *J Psychiatr Res* 1994;28:109–122.
15. Banks SM, Kerns RD. Explaining high rates of depression in chronic pain: A diathesis-stress framework. *Psychol Bull* 1996;119:95–110.
16. Kaplan HI, Sadock BJ. *Kaplan and Sadock's Synopsis of Psychiatry: Behavioral Sciences/Clinical Psychiatry.* 8th ed. Baltimore, Md: Williams & Wilkins; 1998.
17. Fishbain DS, Cutler R, Rosomoff HL, et al. Chronic pain-associated depression: Antecedent or consequence of chronic pain? A review. *Clin J Pain* 1997;13:116–37.
18. Von Korff M, Simon G. The relationship between pain and depression. *Br J Psychiatr* 1996;168(suppl):101–108.
19. Ekselius L, Eriksson M, von Knorring L, et al. Comorbidity of personality disorders and major depression in patients with somatoform pain disorders or medical illnesses with long-standing work disability. *Scand J Rehabil Med* 1997;29:91–96.
20. Eimer BN, Freeman A. *Pain Management Psychotherapy: A Practical Guide.* New York, NY: John Wiley & Sons; 1998.
21. Weisberg JN. Personality and personality disorders in chronic pain. *Curr Rev Pain* 2000;4:60–70.
22. Lumley MA, Asselin LA, Norman S. Alexithymia in chronic pain patients. *Compr Psychiatry* 1997;38:160–165.

23. Klapow JC, Slater MA, Patterson TL, et al. Psychosocial factors discriminate multidimensional clinical groups of chronic low back pain patients. *Pain* 1995;62:349–355.
24. American Psychiatric Association. *Diagnostic and Statistical Manual of Mental Disorders.* 4th ed. Washington, DC: APA; 1994.
25. Prochaska JO, Norcross JC, DiClemente CC. *Changing for Good.* New York, NY: William Morrow; 1994.
26. Reid WH, Balis GU, Sutton BJ. *The Treatment of Psychiatric Disorders.* 3rd ed. Bristol, Pa: Brunner/Mazel; 1997.
27. Gatchel RJ, Turk DC. Interdisciplinary treatment of chronic pain patients. In: Gatchel RJ, Turk DC, eds. *Psychosocial Factors in Pain: Critical Perspectives.* New York, NY: Guilford Press; 1999;435–444.
28. Grzesiak RC, Ury GM, Dworkin RH. Psychodynamic psychotherapy and chronic pain patients. In: Gatchel RJ, Turk DC, eds. *Psychological Approaches to Pain Management: A Practitioner's Handbook.* New York, NY: Guilford Press; 1996;148–178.
29. Linton SJ, Larden M, Gillow A-M. Sexual abuse and chronic musculoskeletal pain: Prevalence and psychological factors. *Clin J Pain* 1996; 12:215–221.
30. Goldberg RT. Childhood abuse, depression, and chronic pain. *Clin J Pain* 1994;10:277–281.
31. Glod CA. Long-term consequences of childhood physical and sexual abuse. *Arch Psychiatr Nurs* 1993;7:163–173.
32. Amundson GJG, Norton GR, Alderdings MD, et al. Posttraumatic-stress disorder and work-related injury. *J Anxiety Disord* 1998;12:57–69.
33. Hickling EJ, Blanchard EB, Silverman DJ, et al. Motor vehicle accidents, headaches, and posttraumatic stress disorder: Assessment findings in a consecutive series. *Headache* 1992;32:147–151.
34. Fishbain DA. Secondary gain concept: Definition problems and its abuse in medical practice. *APS J* 1994;3:264–273.
35. Margoles MS. Chronic pain is a family problem. In: Margoles MS, Weiner R, eds. *Chronic Pain: Assessment, Diagnosis, and Management.* Boca Raton, Fla: CRC Press; 1999;65–81.
36. Fishbain DA, Rosomoff HL, Cutler RB, et al. Secondary gain concept: A review of the scientific evidence. *Clin J Pain* 1995;11:6–21.
37. Rockland LH. *Supportive Therapy: A Psychodynamic Approach.* New York, NY: Basic Books; 1989.
38. Birk L. Cognitive behavior therapy and systemic behavioral psychotherapy. In: Nicholi AM Jr, ed. *The Harvard Guide to Psychiatry.* 3rd ed. Cambridge, Mass: Belknap Press of Harvard University; 1999;497–524.
39. NIH Assessment Panel. Integration of behavioral and relaxation approaches into the treatment of chronic pain and insomnia. *JAMA* 1996;276:313–318.
40. Shellenberger R, Amar P, Schneider C, et al. *Clinical Efficacy and Cost Effectiveness of Biofeedback Therapy: Guidelines for Third Party Reimbursement.* 2nd ed. Wheat Ridge, Colo: Association for Applied Psychophysiology and Biofeedback; 1994.
41. AAPB Web site Public Information Area. *What Is Biofeedback?* Available at: http://www.aapb.org/public/AAPBpbiofeedback.html. Accessed February 2, 2001.
42. Devine DA. Psychological and behavioral management approaches to chronic pain. In: Margoles MA, Weiner R, eds. *Chronic Pain: Assessment, Diagnosis, and Management.* Boca Raton, Fla: CRC Press; 1999; 195–202.
43. AAPB Web site Public Information Area. *What Kind of Health Problems Can Biofeedback Help?* Available at: http://www.aapb.org/public/AAPBpbiofeedback.html. Accessed February 2, 2001.
44. Danforth DA. Biofeedback. In: Warfield CA, Fausett HJ, eds. *Manual of Pain Management.* 2nd ed. Philadelphia, Pa: Lippincott Williams & Wilkins; 2002;334–339.
45. Rome H, Rome J. Limbically augmented pain syndrome (LAPS): Kindling, corticolimbic sensitization, and convergence of affective and sensory symptoms in chronic pain disorders. *Pain Med* 2000;1:7–23.
46. Schoenberger NE. Research on hypnosis as an adjunct to cognitive-behavioral psychotherapy. *Int J Clin Exp Hypn* 2000;48:154–169.
47. Shapiro F. *Eye Movement Desensitization and Reprocessing.* New York, NY: Guilford Press; 1995.
48. Lonergan EC. *Group Intervention: How to Begin and Maintain Groups in Medical and Psychiatric Settings.* New York, NY: Jason Aronson; 1982.
49. Stern MJ. Group therapy with medically ill patients. In: Alonso A, Swiller HI, eds. *Group Therapy in Clinical Practice.* Washington, DC: American Psychiatric Press; 1993;185–199.
50. Spira J. Understanding and developing psychotherapy groups for medically ill patients. In: Spira J, ed. *Group Therapy for Medically Ill Patients.* New York, NY: Guilford Press; 1997;3–51.
51. Hellman CJ, Budd M, Borysenko J, et al. A study of the effectiveness of two group behavioral medicine interventions for patients with psychosomatic complaints. *Behav Med* 1990;16:165–173.
52. Locke SE, Chan PP, Morley DS, et al. Behavioural medicine group interventions for high-utilising somatising patients. *Dis Manage Health Outcomes* 1999;6:387–404.
53. Goodman B. Group therapy for medically ill patients. In: Halperin DA, ed. *Group Psychodynamics: New Paradigms and New Perspectives.* Chicago, Ill: Year Book Medical; 1989;107–124.
54. Compton A. Emotional distress in chronic medical illness: Treatment with time-limited group therapy. *Mil Med* 1992;157:533–535.
55. Keefe FJ, Beaupre PM, Gil K. Group therapy for patients with chronic pain. In: Gatchel RJ, Turk DC, eds. *Psychological Approaches to Pain Management: A Practitioner's Handbook.* New York, NY: Guilford Press; 1996;259–282.
56. Levine JB, Irving KK, Brooks JD, et al. Group therapy and the somatoform patient: An integration. *Psychotherapy* 1993;30:625–634.
57. Friedman R, Sobel D, Myers P, et al. Behavioral medicine, clinical health psychology, and cost offset. *Health Psychol* 1995;14:509–518.
58. Hafen B, Frandsaen K, Karen K, et al. *The Health Effects of Attitudes, Emotions and Relationships.* Provo, Utah: EMS Associates; 1992.
59. Lorig KR, Mazonson PD, Holman HR. Evidence suggesting that health education for self-management in patients with chronic arthritis has sustained health benefits while reducing health-care costs. *Arthritis Rheum* 1993;36:439–446.
60. Turk DC, Rudy TE. Neglected factors in chronic pain treatment outcome studies—referral patterns, failure to enter treatment, and attrition. *Pain* 1990;43:7–25.
61. Caudill MA. *Managing Pain Before It Manages You.* Revised edition. New York, NY: Guilford Press; 2002.
62. Jamison RN. *Learning to Master Your Chronic Pain.* Sarasota, Fla: Professional Resource Press; 1996.
63. Keefe FJ, Caldwell DS. Cognitive behavioral control of arthritis pain. *Med Clin North Am* 1977;81:277–290.
64. Flor H, Fydrich T, Turk DC. Efficacy of multidisciplinary pain treatment centers: A meta-analytic review. *Pain* 1992;49:221–230.
65. Caudill MA, Schnable R, Zuttermeister P, et al. Decreased clinic use by chronic pain patients: Response to behavioral medicine intervention. *Clin J Pain* 1991;7:305–310.
66. Young LD, Bradley LA, Turner RA. Decreases in health care resource utilization in patients with rheumatoid arthritis following a cognitive behavioral intervention. *Biofeedback Self-Regulation* 1995;20:259–268.

CHAPTER 15 CONSULTING ON THE DIFFICULT PATIENT IN PAIN

Scott M. Fishman

Treating pain in a difficult patient may raise the challenge and lower the expectations from any analgesic intervention. In this section, the term *difficult* is applied to patients with behaviors, rather than symptoms, that are beyond the norm and that undermine treatment. Discussion of other difficult symptom presentations is beyond the scope of this chapter. Difficult patients who are in pain often are in conflict about whether or not they want care, want the care they are offered, or want pain. Groves has said, "Such patients simultaneously demand and reject care." These patients may also simultaneously obtain and undermine treatment or flatter and frustrate their clinicians. In mild cases, they may strike a cord of uneasiness in their caregivers. In severe cases, caregivers may experience strong emotions such as fear and hate.

Some clinicians find it difficult to acknowledge or discuss patients who strike a negative chord in them. Often, this is because of the intrinsic conflict such patients raise with caregivers. Many clinicians would simply rather not dislike any patients. Disliking a patient is counter to what caregivers consciously strive to achieve—helping in every way. So, even discussing a difficult patient can make some clinicians feel uncomfortable, as if the patient is either being mistreated or ridiculed. Certainly, this may occur with certain individual clinicians in some situations. On the other hand, some patients clearly are difficult, have long histories of inciting strong negative reactions and difficult interactions with many health care providers, and place clinicians in untenable situations in which they ultimately feel bad. Not recognizing this phenomenon is a disservice to the patient. But it is also of paramount importance to recognize that most patients who make you suffer as a clinician are probably suffering much more. Patients with dysfunctional patterns of interactions with physicians usually have similar, if not worse, problems throughout the rest of their lives. Thus, the clinician's discomfort is often just a small reflection of the patient's much greater torment.

Although there is no easy formula for what to do in these difficult interactions, the common mistake is to miss opportunities in which commonsense adjustments can ameliorate problems and prevent escalation. Unfortunately, such difficult cases bring with them frustration and, often, even more severe emotional responses, which taken together diminish the clinician's ability to bring common sense to bear. In such situations, it is critical to recognize dysfunctional patterns of patient and staff interactions as well as monitor one's own internal reactions. By doing so, one can then apply greater awareness, deliberation, planning, patience, and caution to a difficult situation rather than acting from impulse or instinct. This perspective may make the clinician the only member of the treatment team able to change the tide of acrimony and reestablish effective treatment. What follows here is not new and is extensively taken from the work of James E. Groves, as well as Adler, Buie, and Maltsberger, who have published the seminal writings on this subject (see the Bibliography at the end of this chapter). Readers who are interested in furthering their understanding of the difficult patient will be well rewarded by reviewing these works.

It is a first-order task of any clinician caring for patients with complex biopsychosocial problems to expect some emotional response, which all clinicians have to their patients. Some clinicians hide their reactions better than others, whether to others or themselves. The clinician who is unaware of his or her reactions to patients may be more likely to act on these emotions in a counterproductive and potentially harmful manner. Conscious awareness of one's feelings offers the opportunity to recognize these reactions and perhaps use this understanding to respond to difficult patients with more empathy and less animosity.

The difficult patient becomes known to a clinician in one of two ways, either directly or indirectly. Some are directly frustrating and inspire strong negative feelings. Others are noticed indirectly by virtue of the struggle that ensues among the caregivers of the difficult patient. If clinicians honestly pay attention to their reactions to patients, they will notice a constant and wide variety of positive and negative feelings. They may then come to understand some of the motivating forces behind the various ways in which they work with patients and may begin to recognize patterns. Because pain management is often performed in a team treatment setting, the same can be said for the clinician's interactions with the treatment team.

The treatment team can be viewed as a single entity: a system that can be either united or divided. Treatment teams may be harmonious or acrimonious. When there is an unusual amount of conflict or negative feelings among caregivers without an obvious medical controversy, the initial instinct may be to wonder how the individuals on the team can be causing these problems. However, the teams' struggle may be, at least in part, a result of information about the patient. If this scenario is not considered, then a potentially informative piece of the patient care puzzle may be missed. Thus, when the treatment team is both divided and acrimonious, a consultant should avoid the natural temptation to seek blame among the various and potentially divided clinicians. Instead, the team should be viewed as a single unit, contrasted only with the patient. The usual tendency to ally with the patient is a pitfall that may need to be resisted, because the patient's best interest is only served if the treatment team is functional. Because a congruent team best serves the patient, the consultant's alliance must be with the team as a whole. Once seen in this manner, the problematic system may reveal itself.

The difficult patient can elicit intense feelings, ranging from extremely good to extremely bad. Such intense feelings toward a patient should serve as a "red flag" of caution. Being unaware of overly positive feelings toward a patient may lead a clinician to resist addressing issues that may be either unpleasant or otherwise unappealing, yet appropriate. Overly negative feelings may signal conscious or unconscious anger and hostility and can lead to avoidance or inappropriate confrontation. Such strong reactions, particularly when disparately held by members of a treatment team, can bring about chaos. Difficult patients may be extremely independent or dependent, entitled or submissive, engaging or seemingly impossible to connect with, or idealizing or devaluing of their caregivers. Caregivers may be as struck by rage from the patient as from themselves. On the other hand, the only clue for the clinician may be an unusual lack of either concern for, investment in, or connection with the patient. In the most severe form, these patients can become enraged, violent, impulsive, and both physically and emotionally threatening. Although complaints or demands may seem to be endless, there is often another process at work. Sometimes, this process is marked by particular treatment team members being cast in an extremely positive or negative light. Team members may feel like either adored insiders or thankless scapegoats. Their designation by the patient as either all good or all bad may precipitously change from one extreme to the other. This process is termed *splitting* and is a hallmark feature of some difficult patients.

Management in these difficult situations calls on the clinician's greatest tolerance and skill. Understanding why some patients behave in such a difficult manner may serve to de-escalate frustration and help with imparting rational treatment. Often, these patients are extremely frightened and have very low self-esteem. Viewing the world in terms of extremes is often related to past experiences in which they were, in some way, injured or abandoned. As a result, the individual loses the ability to synthesize experiences that are simultaneously good and bad. Much of the struggle with the difficult patient may be a result of the patient's perception of previous and ongoing abandonment. Such individuals often have lives that are marked by persistent feelings of emptiness, with labile moods and unstable personal relationships. It is not uncommon for such patients to present with a counter-intuitive external layer of grandiosity. Some patients may appear to have an almost carefree impassivity that contrasts with marked emotional fragility and the tendency to become easily shamed and enraged. This perspective can now temper the clinician's view of the defense mechanisms resulting from the patient's perceived frightened, if not victimized, position. These defenses—such as splitting, valuing and devaluing, denial and entitlement—may be the only methods the patient has to prevent what he or she perceives as impending doom.

It is all too easy, reflexively and intuitively, to view the overly demanding patient as emotionally secure. However, these patients often have extremely low self-esteem and feel an ever-present, looming risk of imminent shame and humiliation. Entitlement is the external and very thin veneer under which self-loathing and vulnerability hide. Thus, challenging this entitled position serves only to heighten the risk of shame and humiliation and intensifies the need for a demanding and entitled posture. The extreme fragility of these patients underscores the need to avoid challenging their sense of entitlement. While working with such patients, it is best to counter excessive demands with frequent and varied reminders that the patient deserves and will receive the best and most thoughtful care.

Initial management of the difficult patient requires recognizing the dysfunctional system and following some principles, described next. When working with the difficult patient, the role of the consultant is fundamentally different than that of the primary clinician; the primary clinician maintains the continuous therapeutic relationship, which can become stressed by constant demands, whereas the consultant is liberated from such longitudinal constraints. The primary clinician must maintain both an alliance with the difficult patient as well as boundaries within which good health care can proceed and harm can be avoided. Often, it is necessary to use consultants, who can offer an objective perspective, free of the long-term consequences of confronting mixed messages and inconsistent behaviors. In difficult situations, deferring to the consultant may be the primary clinician's only means of minimizing the long-term effects of instituting necessary treatment, setting limits, or avoiding danger.

Patients who consistently encounter turbulent medical experiences may feel most comforted when their physicians are at odds. Some patients, consciously or unconsciously, may feel that a staff that is fighting among itself at least cares, whereas a harmonious team may be disinterested and may even do them harm. These patients may gravitate to a system that casts clinicians as either all good or all bad. Because it is usually insidious and fraught with pitfalls, encountering a case that involves the defense of splitting can be a struggle if not a frightening experience. The clinician who rushes into such a case with disdain for prior management and offers alternatives that inspire the patients effusive gratitude may soon be on the receiving end of disdain. The goal is to avoid this cycle of love and hate and work in a manner that offers solutions that encourage team involvement and minimize fragmentation, all without disrupting the relationship of the primary team with the patient.

Similar cycles and patterns are not limited to patients but are possible for the treatment team, as well. At any point in a case, the treatment team may defer to the consultant for relief. The team may need to overidealize the consultant for the purpose of having him or her assume the role of rescuer. Alternatively, the team may devalue the consultant as they transfer to him or her the burdensome scapegoat role. They may seek company in hating the patient or take an equally righteous but opposite position of defending the patient against the consultant and all other "evil." The latter serves to relieve the guilt of past conflicts or treatment failures.

Because the pain management clinician rarely works in isolation from other care providers, the consultant must offer strategies that preserve self-esteem for both the patient and staff. There is almost never long-term gain to be had by assigning blame, or embarrassing or humiliating the patient or the staff. It is important to appreciate both the patient's sense of enormous vulnerability and the team's sense of hopelessness. The consultant should avoid being part of an atmosphere of anger or resentment toward the patient or the team. As previously noted, the team has primary responsibility for the care of the patient. The consultant who promotes the effectiveness of the primary team best serves the patient. In particularly difficult cases of hospitalized patients, where other practitioners are involved at a greater level of primary care, it is best to interact directly with the patient only as necessary to collect primary information. Otherwise, the consultant should rely on the hospital chart, existing records, and collateral sources to fill in the story. The consultant should intervene directly with the treatment team and guide them in navigating patient interactions, offering options with honor.

The consultant must evaluate both the patient and the team. Self-defeating behavior of the patient and staff should be identified and addressed. Arguing with the patient or with the staff should be avoided; although it may feel good to the frustrated clinician, it will undermine the search for constructive solutions. Sometimes, the consulting clinician may encounter secrets or information that have been revealed selectively to some but not all members of the team. In such situations, one must be wary of important facts that may have become distorted. In the long run, all parties will ultimately feel better when the facts are all true, clear, and consistent.

In the case of difficult patients who are hospitalized or those with treatment providers who can be convened, the consultant can use frequent brief team meetings to interact and ally with key representatives of the treatment team. It is necessary to honestly describe the patient's behavior and needs as well as the pitfalls of managing such impossible demands and contradicting needs. The team may need to hear that it is understandable that there are strong negative feelings toward the patient, which may become displaced onto others. Staff should be reassured that such reactions are normal and linked to their very noble but now frustrated commitment to help others. The consultant should emphasize strengths, such as good rapport, humor, faith, or previous experiences with difficult cases that have been resolved. The team should be offered the chance to vent, and their torment and hopelessness acknowledged.

The consultant should appreciate that the staff may be too frustrated to take its usual rational and understanding position with the current patient. In explaining the complexity of the current interactions, the consultant should be clear that the present brief encounter is probably not going to allow him or her to completely comprehend the complex dynamics of the case, which are probably rooted in events that occurred long ago. The medical or surgical team should be reminded that it is not their primary job to resolve long-standing psychological patterns, issues, or pathology. Their duty is to diagnose and treat the current medical problem. If possible, the consultant can introduce lightheartedness and humor into the team atmosphere, which may have become clouded by emotions of hopelessness and anger. It may help to remember the words of James Groves: *"humor is the mother of empathy."*

Limit setting is a prominent feature of managing the difficult patient in pain. Often, the amount and route of administration of opioids are areas of contention. In such cases, individualized plans must be developed; however, using contracts and strictly holding to rational pharmacotherapy will help with many problems. It is important to remember that the patient has the disease. Nonetheless, he or she may be frightened, impulsive, and very perceptive. Limits must not be confused with punishment or seen as an opportunity for revenge. Management must be offered in a professional and kind manner, without malice or blaming. As previously discussed, confrontation may be self-defeating; however, certain unacceptable or counterproductive behaviors must be addressed and limited. For any suggestion of violent behavior, threats, or imminent harm, patients must be advised of the consequences, including the use of physical restraint. Acts or threats of violence or self-injury must be met with an immediate and clear response that protects the patient and others. In these situations, formal psychiatric assistance is usually necessary.

Finally, the consultant to the difficult patient in pain must help unify the team and implement a rational plan. Unification occurs through communication. When the patient is hospitalized, it may still be impossible to meet with the entire team, so there should be a mechanism for disseminating the plan through caregivers from shift to shift. The patient will be comforted and less agitated by shift changes if staff frequently update the patient with consistent information. The rational plan should have contingencies for various outcomes. The primary team should then present the agreed-on plan, with its contingencies, to the patient and form a contract to follow through on the plan. In the most severe cases, a written agreement offers the patient the opportunity to review and consider the information over time and forms a document that can be recalled if necessary.

Managing the difficult patient in pain can be challenging but also rewarding. It is too often the case that such patients frustrate both their clinicians and themselves. Appreciating the underlying problems and following some basic principles may help deescalate conflict and support or reestablish effective medical care.

BIBLIOGRAPHY

Adler G, Buie DH. The misuses of confrontation with borderline patients. *Int J Psychoan Psychother* 1972;1:109–120.

Gallop R, Lancee W, Shugar G. Residents' and nurses' perceptions of difficult-to-treat short-stay patients. *Hosp Comm Psychiatry* 1993;44: 352–357.

Groves JE. Management of the borderline patient on a medical or surgical ward: The psychiatric consultant's role. *Int J Psychiatry Med* 1975; 6:337–348.

Groves JE. Taking care of the hateful patient. *N Engl J Med* 1978;298: 883–887.

Guziec J, Lazarus A, Harding JJ. Case of a 29-year-old nurse with factitious disorder. The utility of psychiatric intervention on a general medical floor. *Gen Hosp Psychiatry* 1994;16:47–53.

Hahn SR, Thompson KS, Wills TA, Stern V, Budner NS. The difficult doctor-patient relationship: Somatization, personality and psychopathology. *J Clin Epidemiol* 1994;47:647–657.

Maltsberger T, Buie M. Countertransference hate in the treatment of suicidal patients. *Arch Gen Psych* 1974;30:625.

Sansone RA, Sansone LA. Borderline personality disorder. Interpersonal and behavioral problems that sabotage treatment success. *Postgrad Med* 1995;97:169–171, 175–176, 179.

Sharpe M, Mayou R, Seagroatt V, et al. Why do doctors find some patients difficult to help? *QJM* 1994;87:187–193.

Smith S. Dealing with the difficult patient. *Postgrad Med* 1995;71:653–657.

CHAPTER 16 INPATIENT MODEL OF A CHRONIC PAIN MANAGEMENT PROGRAM

Richard T. Goldberg

Chronic pain has been defined by Turk[1,2] as a function of a complex interaction among demographic, physical, psychological, social, and economic factors, including age, sex, education, medical status, pain severity, alcohol and substance abuse, beliefs about pain, increased used of medications and of health care services, and a generalized adoption of the sick role. Because chronic pain is multifactorial in nature, the use of any one modality, pharmacologic treatment, alternative medicine, or psychologic approach is bound to fail. Pain management in an inpatient center provides a model of interdisciplinary treatment consisting of medical care, medication management, physical reconditioning, training in body mechanics, meditation, relaxation, biofeedback psychology, and milieu therapy. Patients who are referred to an inpatient chronic pain program commonly experience functional disabilities, social dysfunction, narcotic and alcohol dependency, child abuse history, vocational impairment, dependency on the public welfare system and the workmen's compensation system, and significant psychiatric disorders that are both antecedent to and consequent from chronic pain. Therefore, the objectives, treatment procedures, outcome measures, and long-term success of inpatient chronic pain management are distinct from treatment of acute pain, malignant pain, and postoperative pain.

OBJECTIVES

The objectives of pain management are manifold. The first objective is to assist the patient in developing coping mechanisms for chronic pain. Patients who have been referred to inpatient programs have failed to adapt to their pain despite numerous treatments that have been given in the community. Upon evaluation, these patients report a history of numerous visits to emergency departments, pain blocks, narcotics, and other standard medical procedures that have failed to provide them with pain relief. The clinician must convince the patient that all standard medical treatments have been offered and given. The task of the patient is to learn coping mechanisms in order that pain no longer is prepotent in their lives.

The second objective is to develop the maximum potential of the patient for normal living, which includes physical, social, psychological-spiritual, and vocational rehabilitation. For too many years, pain management was separated from rehabilitation. When pain management is conducted in isolation from other rehabilitation programs, it focuses on the narrow problems of narcotic addiction and depression. Pain patients, however, have potential for return to work, school, homemaking, and volunteer activities in the community. By keeping the objective on rehabilitation, the focus is changed from a narrow goal of reducing drug dependency to a broader goal of preparation for or return to normal living in the community.[3]

The third objective is to provide functional restoration for patients who have been deconditioned over several months and years. Functional restoration includes physical function, such as walking, stair climbing, standing, balancing, sitting, and endurance in performance of strenuous activities at work or at home. Although few studies have documented the improvement in physical function in pain management centers, Harding and associates[4] showed significant improvement in measures such as a 10-minute walking test and a 20-minute speed walk. One month following treatment, patients showed that they had maintained their gains and had improved in several measures.

The fourth objective is to assist patients to reduce their dependency on narcotic and non-narcotic analgesic medications for the management of chronic pain. Although it may seem surprising to list narcotic taper as fourth on the list of objectives, in view of the fact that this is probably the primary reason for physicians to make a referral to a pain management program (a fact that is documented in my own experience at Spaulding Rehabilitation Hospital in Boston), narcotic taper must be interpreted in the context of pain management as a whole. To reduce dependency on narcotics without concurrently improving the patient's coping, functional, and social capacities is to miss the point of the patient's stay in an inpatient program. Narcotic taper may be accomplished in a drug detoxification program without teaching the patient coping strategies for pain. Moreover, a few, selected patients may require continued opioid therapy, such as methadone for heroin addiction.

The fifth objective is to integrate pain management with rehabilitation as a whole. For too long, pain management has operated in isolation from other rehabilitation programs. The treatment of pain was not accepted as an authentic rehabilitation concern until John Bonica established the first comprehensive pain center at the University of Washington in Seattle.[5] Since then more than 100 pain management centers have sprung up in the United States. Rehabilitation involves the development of the maximal potential for normal living: physically, psychologically, socially, and vocationally. The objectives of pain rehabilitation must focus on the development of potential and, in the cases of acquired disability, the restoration of function. The ultimate objective of pain management must be the integration of the pain patient in the normal activities of family and community.

ASSESSMENT AND TREATMENT

The provision of interdisciplinary procedures in a therapeutic environment enables a chronic pain patient with medical and social pathologies to gain stability and to learn better coping mechanisms. The idea of therapeutic environment and milieu therapy originates in the mental health movement with the studies of Maxwell Jones in England, Morris Schwartz and Milton Greenblatt in the United States.[6–8] These early investigators found that provision of a safe environment in which there can be normal interactions of daily life was therapy for seriously disturbed patients. The role of the physician was important, but was seen in the context of many other specialists who interact with the patient on a daily basis. In the first experiment at Belmont Hospital, England, physicians, nurses, and untrained aides interacted with patients in everyday situations in ways to correct inappropriate behaviors. Patients who entered the hospital with the hope of a cure or of reinforcing their neuroses were quickly disabused of their fantasies. They were expected to express themselves freely but also to assimilate with the culture of the unit. In the United States, the therapeutic community movement quickly spread to the alteration of the custodial psychiatric hospital to community care.

When applied to patients with chronic, nonmalignant pain a therapeutic environment provides the milieu in which treatment can be obtained. The pain unit addresses the physical, psychological, and social impairments caused by chronic pain. The consequences of chronic pain are interpreted as functional and behavioral, not medical. When patients are evaluated for a chronic pain program, they are told that it is assumed that all medical diagnostic tests have been completed. A cure for their pain is not likely in the immediate future. Medications, nerve blocks, and surgery have been tried and found wanting. Narcotics have led to dependency. Moreover, the main problem facing chronic pain patients is not pain sensation but pain behavior, which results in social dysfunction. To alter pain behavior under controlled conditions, a new type of treatment is needed.

Fordyce and associates at the University of Washington applied the principles of operant conditioning to the management of chronic pain.[9–11] Based on the work of B.F. Skinner at Harvard University,[12] the principle is that human behavior is purposive, influenced by consequences, reinforced by positive rewards, malleable, and capable of being altered by a structured series of cues, tasks, environmental conditions, and human experiences. Within the context of a pain program, pain behaviors, such as grimacing, groaning, limping, massaging, and guarding, may be altered through a strategy of both positive and negative reinforcements. Positive reinforcement of any effort or structured activity, such as physical or occupational therapy, is helpful in encouraging well behaviors. Conversely, positive reinforcement of pain behaviors, such as grimacing, limping, not participating in the pain program, or asking for unscheduled pain medication, leads to negative consequences and persistent disability. Avoidance of activity that is associated with pain behaviors is another common consequence. Negative reinforcement takes place when a patient avoids activity or guards against persistent activity, which is consequently reduced. As an example, the spouse of a pain patient who participates in a role reversal may carry out tasks formerly performed by the patient. Negative reinforcement needs to be replaced by positive reinforcement of structured activities that help the patient to build a repertoire of skills.

A behavioral management approach to pain is not appropriate for all chronic pain patients. Very strict criteria for selection and admission to an inpatient pain program must be met. There are several risk factors that should be considered before admission. A patient who is disruptive, is a malingerer, or has a severe somatization disorder is a poor candidate for a pain program. Malingering is present in 1% or 2% of referred patients. Patients with conversion disorder tend to have unsuccessful outcomes. Even when given the opportunity to make improvement in function, they tend to hold onto their somatic symptoms. They also pose a risk to the hospital because of the likelihood of creating a malpractice suit. They may fall out of a wheelchair or lose their balance or cause some self-destructive act to validate their pain. Although it is true that all chronic pain patients have a somatoform component, patients with conversion disorder convert the energy of their inner psychological conflicts into their bodily symptoms without any organic reason for their pain. Classic symptoms of hysterical blindness and deafness are not usually seen in pain clinics. More common disorders such as psychogenic gait disorders or paralyzed limbs without any pathophysiologic mechanism can be found. In one unusual case, the author evaluated a patient who had been diagnosed with stiff-man syndrome, a disorder of which there are not more than 100 examples in the world. The disorder is characterized by continuous spasms and stiffness in the limbs and the trunk, with few periods of remission. However, it was observed that the patient, a man in his early thirties, could enter a period of remission by meditation and relaxation therapy. The resolution of symptoms suggested a diagnosis of conversion disorder.

Patients who have a history of chronic alcoholism or chronic drug addiction prior to chronic pain are less likely to become successful candidates for a pain program. Alcohol and drug addiction are signs of family pathologies that need to be treated either before or concurrent with inpatient pain programs. Because the symptoms are similar in primary and secondary drug addiction, it is important to obtain a complete history of addiction when first evaluating the patient. When a patient presents with long-term addiction, referral to a substance abuse program to cope with the dangers of addiction may be required. In contrast, the judicious use of opioids for the treatment of pain in the absence of an addiction history has moved further into the mainstream. The goal is always the improvement of function and life activities.

A childhood history of physical, sexual, and verbal abuse is often associated with chronic pain. Several studies[13–15] suggest that traumatic events in childhood may be related not only to chronic pain but also to alcoholism, drug dependence, childhood illness, and other major family upheavals. In a recent study,[16] a history of child abuse was found in 55% of 91 patients with chronic pain. These patients were classified into four pain groups: 64% of patients with fibromyalgia, 62% of patients with myofascial pain, 50% with facial pain, and 48% with other chronic pain, consisting of low back pain, had a history of abuse. A logistic regression was conducted to predict membership in the fibromyalgia, myofascial, and facial pain group. The low back pain group was the reference group.

A woman is 11.77 times more likely than a man to be a member of the fibromyalgia, facial, or myofascial group. A person with an alcoholic parent or grandparent is 4.37 times more likely to be a member of the first three groups. Sleep disorder was a negative predictor of membership in the first three groups. The study showed a significant link between history of child abuse and history of alcoholism in the family.

Abuse takes place more frequently in homes where the parent or grandparent is enraged with alcohol. An alcoholic father may strike his son or daughter or may sexually molest his daughter. Sleep disorder was common to all four pain groups, not only to the fibromyalgia group. The tumultuous early family environment of patients with chronic pain may explain, in part, their vulnerability to illness and accident and their difficulty in coping with pain later in life.

Other psychological risk factors include negative pain beliefs.[17] The belief that pain is a punishment for past wrongdoing may influence a patient's cooperation and progress in pain management. Negative pain beliefs may be religious and cultural in origin. In evaluating patients from countries other than the United States, it is important to determine a patient's attitudes toward pain. When pain is perceived as a consequence of some immoral act, or an act of omission, then a patient should be referred for psychotherapy.

Patients who are survivors of the Holocaust or who are children of survivors may express their psychic pain through somatic pain. The stories of the survivors are characterized by dissociation.[18] One patient told me that she survived the concentration camp by remembering her home in Berlin and pretending that she was not really in the camp. Her experiences are similar to those who have suffered childhood sexual abuse.

Some studies suggest that patients with chronic pain selectively attend to pain-related information.[19] Asmundson and colleagues[20] showed that chronic pain patients with low anxiety sensitivity shifted their attention away from stimuli related to pain, whereas patients with high anxiety sensitivity responded selectively to pain cues. Their findings suggest that fear of pain may have implications for coping strategies. Shifting attention away from pain cues may be related to overexertion, potential reinjury, and continued pain. However, there were no differences in selective attention to pain cues between a chronic pain group receiving services in a pain program and health controls recruited from the staff at the pain center.

Positive predictors of success in an inpatient pain management program include age, education, adaptive coping, motivation to work, and an optimistic rehabilitation outlook.[21] Motivation to work or to return to a former life activity, such as school or homemaking, is a major predictor of success. In a study of 21 patients who completed an inpatient pain program and who were followed for 3 months postdischarge, motivation to work predicted for three measures of outcome: reduced depression, lower total pain score on the McGill Pain Questionnaire, and the number of pain words counted on the McGill.[22] An inpatient pain management program should provide a full-time vocational rehabilitation counselor to arouse a patient's aspirations.

A standard multidisciplinary assessment takes place after a patient is admitted into a program. An assessment may consist of standardized measures, such as the Sickness Impact Profile, a 136-item general functional status measure of sickness-related behavior, or the Short-Form Health Survey (SF-36), 36 items that measure physical function, role function, pain, mental health, and health perception.[23] A measure of depression, such as the Beck Depression Inventory II or the Hamilton Scale, is helpful in obtaining a baseline. The intercorrelation between chronic pain and depression is significantly positive, as has been established in numerous studies.[24–26] A measure of pain, such as the McGill Pain Questionnaire or the Multidimensional Pain Inventory, may be useful in establishing a baseline for pain sensation. These commonly used measures are subjective and suffer from unreliability. Moreover, they measure pain perception, and are not objective indices of pain. Another measure of pain that does not suffer from the limitations of verbal description is the visual analog scale, a measure of pain severity and intensity, in which the patient is asked to draw a mark on a straight line representing the extremes of no pain and unbearable pain.[27]

None of the standard measures is useful in measuring functional changes from admission to discharge. Harding and associates[28] designed a battery of measures for assessment of physical functioning of patients with chronic pain. The battery consisted of a 10-minute walk test, a 20-minute speed walk, a 2-minute stair-climbing test, a 30-second balance on one leg, sit-ups, arm endurance, grip strength measured by dynamometer, and peak flow measured by airmed mini-Wright peak flow meter. Three hundred forty-one patients were tested before and after pain management. Patients showed significant improvement in stand-ups and arm endurance at 1 month follow-up. Other functional assessment measures have been developed by Granger.[29] The limitation of both measures is that patients with chronic pain but without significant physical handicaps cannot be assessed by physical measures.

Treatment Procedures

Patients are expected to participate in all activities even when they are feeling sick. If they cannot contribute to the discussion, then they sit in the room and are counted present. They attend groups that focus on different aspects of chronic pain, such as medications, substance use, work, biofeedback, cognitive behavioral approaches, meditation, relaxation, and community. Medication for pain is given at scheduled intervals. Patients are discouraged from asking for breakthrough pain medication on an as-needed basis. Narcotic taper begins within 1 or 2 days after admission and continues for 7 days or until the patient is ready for total withdrawal.

Socialization with staff and other patients is an important aspect of treatment. Television is not permitted in patients' rooms to discourage them from isolating themselves. Inappropriate angry outbursts, sexual behavior, use of obscene words, and other antisocial behavior may be cause for immediate discharge. Deep-seated issues are treated in brief sessions with the psychiatrist. When deep issues cannot be contained within the confines of a pain program, a patient may be transferred to a psychiatric unit. However, the majority of patients are capable of completing a pain program.

Outcome Studies

Very few studies of inpatient pain management programs can stand up to methodologic rigor. Randomized groups, matched case controls, prevention of experimenter bias, specific outcome criteria, estimate of program costs, and comparison with other treatments or with outpatient pain programs have rarely been used. Inpatient pain management takes place in a therapeutic milieu in which multiple disciplines are used to bring about outcomes. The measurement of outcomes must be congruent with the specific treatments employed.

Many interdisciplinary programs incorporate cognitive behavioral techniques, physical reconditioning, stress management, and socialization in a group setting. Outcome measures are reduction of opioid dependency, functional restoration, improvement of mood, and return to work. Studies have attempted to predict these outcomes. Independent measures used to predict outcome include medical conditions,[30–31] depression,[32] pain beliefs,[17] and disability.[33]

In a meta-analysis of 109 studies that assessed outcomes of nonmedical treatments for chronic pain,[34] Malone and Strube found 48 studies that provided sufficient information to aggregate comparable findings. The average sample size was 52.9. The average age was 34.5, and the chronicity of pain was 9.4 years. The percentage of patients improved was calculated for each type of treatment and for no treatment condition. Improvement in the no treatment condition reached 77%. Relaxation training showed a 95% improvement; biofeedback showed 84%; autogenic training showed 68%. The success of relaxation training and biofeedback suggested that these approaches reduce the depression and fear associated with pain, although they do not alter pain intensity, duration, or frequency.

In a meta-analysis of 300 studies of interdisciplinary pain programs, Flor and colleagues[35] found only 65 studies that qualified for systematic comparison. Although the general findings drawn from the meta-analysis tended to support the conclusion that pain programs helped to reduce health care costs by improving function and by returning pain patients to former social and work activities, the authors stated that caution needed to be exercised in making scientific inferences from studies that were inadequately designed.

A comparison of inpatient versus outpatient pain management programs in London, England, randomly assigned patients to three groups: a 4-week inpatient program, an eight half-day outpatient program, and a waiting control group. Mixed pain patients (n = 121) with a mean age of 50 and a mean chronicity of 8.1 years were included in the study. Outcomes showed no significant change in the waiting control group. Both inpatient and outpatient groups showed significant improvement in physical performance and in psychological function, and both had a significant decrease in dependency on medication use. Inpatients, however, made greater gains in the program, maintained gains better at 1 year follow-up, and used fewer health services than outpatients.[36]

In a follow-up of patients 13 years after treatment in a pain management center, Maruta and colleagues[37] contacted 201 patients, which represented 90% of known survivors. Survival rates were identical to those expected in the U.S. population. Questionnaires on health status were returned by 176 patients. Sixty-eight percent of patients reported worse-than-average or an abnormal level of bodily pain, and increased morbidity in physical health and physical and social functioning. Employment questionnaires also were returned by 174 patients. Of those in the working-age group, 65 and younger, 32% were employed full time, 42% were limited in their homemaking activity, and 25% retired early because of pain.

Cost-effectiveness is another major factor for comparison between inpatient and outpatient programs. One study using cognitive behavioral techniques for managing pain showed a 36% reduction in outpatient clinic visits in the first year of an outpatient pain program, with a projected net savings of $12,000 for the first year and $23,000 for the second year.[38] Cicala and Wright[39] showed that the costs of an outpatient pain program were significantly lower than those of a hospital program. However, the return-to-work rates did not differ significantly between the two programs.

The issue of cost-effectiveness is complex, as noted by Grabois[40] in a paper presented for the interest group on pain at the meeting of the American Congress of Rehabilitation Medicine in October 1996. Measures of cost-effectiveness must include return to work or some form of gainful employment, decreased use of narcotics, decreased use of emergency department care, decreased use of medical care by comparison of the costs of care 1 year prior to pain treatment with the costs 1 year after pain treatment, the number of patients requiring rehospitalization for pain, and the number of patients requiring additional surgery for pain.

The amount of savings gained by intervention in pain programs ranges from $9 million to $184 million. There is no accurate estimate of savings beyond individual studies. An estimated $8.8 billion was spent on claims for low back pain alone.[41]

There are several problems in evaluating the effectiveness of pain management programs. Despite the best effort to control for all of the demographic, medical, and psychosocial factors, randomization does not account for the differences between groups. The screening, selection, and approval of patients for inpatient pain programs yields an often skewed sample of patients who are either self-selected or who are selected by referral agents for inpatient pain management. The result is that patients seen in pain clinics differ systematically from pain patients seen in the community by primary care physicians.[42] Patients referred to pain clinics have more severe disability, for a longer duration, and have more work-related accidents. For example, at Spaulding Rehabilitation Hospital one third of patients screened for the pain program are either deferred entrance or rejected because they are not motivated to complete the program, not willing to taper from narcotics, too psychiatrically compromised by depression or more rarely a thought disorder, or they have such severe personality disorders that they would pose a threat of disturbance to others in the inpatient pain unit. Some patients may be better candidates for an outpatient pain program, in which they can be further evaluated to determine their appropriateness for an inpatient program. Outpatient programs may also be used to evaluate for compliance. The best predictors for success in an inpatient program are motivation, realistic assessment of assets and limitations, and an optimistic outlook toward the future.

REFERENCES

1. Turk DC. Biopsychosocial perspective on chronic pain. In: Gatchel RJ, Turk DC, eds. *Psychological Approaches to Pain Management*. New York, NY: Guilford Press; 1996:3–32.
2. Turk DC. The role of demographic and psychosocial factors in transition from acute to chronic pain. In Jensen TS, Turner JA, Wiesenfeld-Hallin Z, eds. *Proceedings of the 8th World Congress of Pain*. Seattle, Wash: IASP Press; 1997:185–213.
3. Goldberg RT. Pain management in today's rehabilitation climate. *Rehabil Outlook* 1997;2:4–12.
4. Harding VR, Williams AC, Richardson PH, et al. The development of a battery of measures for assessing physical functioning of chronic pain patients. *Pain* 1994;58:367–375.
5. Liebeskind JC, Meldrum ML. John J. Bonica: World champion of pain. In Jensen TS, Turner JA, Wiesenfeld-Hallin Z, eds. *Proceedings of the 8th World Congress of Pain*. Seattle, Wash: IASP Press; 1997:19–32.
6. Jones M. The Therapeutic Community. New York, NY: Basic Books: 1953.
7. Schwartz MS, Schwartz CG. *Social Approaches to Mental Patient Care*. New York, NY: Columbia University Press; 1964.
8. Greenblatt M, York RH, Brown EL. From custodial to therapeutic patient care in mental hospitals. New York, NY: Russell Sage Foundation; 1955.
9. Fordyce WE, Fowler R, De Lateur B. An application of behavioral modification technique to a problem of chronic pain. *Behav Res Ther* 1968;6:105–107.
10. Fordyce WE. An operation conditioning method for managing chronic pain. *Postgrad Med* 1973;53:123–138.
11. Fordyce WE. *Behavioral Methods for Chronic Pain and Illness*. St. Louis, Mo: CV Mosby; 1976.
12. Skinner BF. *Science and Human Behavior*. New York, NY: Macmillan; 1953.
13. Rapkin AJ, Kames LD, Darke LL, et al. History of physical and sexual abuse in women with chronic pelvic pain. *Obstet Gynecol* 1990; 76:92–96.
14. Goldberg RT. Childhood abuse, depression, and chronic pain. *Clin J Pain* 1994;10:277–281.
15. Taylor ML, Trotter DR, Cauka ME. The prevalence of sexual abuse in women with fibromyalgia. *Arthritis Rheum* 1995;38:229–234.
16. Goldberg RT, Pachas W, Keith D. Relationship between traumatic events in childhood and chronic pain. *Disability Rehabil* 1999;21:23–30.

17. Williams DA, Keefe FJ. Pain beliefs and the use of cognitive behavioral coping strategies. *Pain* 1991;46:185–190.
18. Langer LL. *Holocaust Testimonies: The Ruins of Memory*. New Haven, Conn: Yale University Press; 1991.
19. Pearce J, Morley S. An experimental investigation of the construct validity of the McGill Pain Questionnaire. *Pain* 1989;39:115–121.
20. Asmundson GJ, Kuperos J, Norton GR. Do patients with chronic pain selectively attend to pain related information? *Pain* 1997;72:27–32.
21. Goldberg RT, Maciewicz RJ. Prediction of pain rehabilitation outcomes by motivation measures. *Disability Rehabil* 1994;16:21–25.
22. Melzack R. The McGill Pain Questionnaire: Major properties and scoring methods. *Pain* 1975;1:277–299.
23. Bergner M, Bobbitt RA, Carter WB, Gilson BS. The Sickness Impact Profile: Development and final revision of a health status measure. *Health Care* 1981;19:787–805.
24. Romano JM, Turner JA. Chronic pain and depression: does the evidence support a relationship? *Psychological Bulletin* 1985;97:18–34.
25. Kleinke CL. How chronic pain patients cope with depression: Relation to treatment outcome in a multidisciplinary pain clinic. *Rehabilitation Psychology* 1991;36:207–218.
26. Kerns R, Turk D, Rudy T. The West Haven Yale Multidimensional Pain Inventory. *Pain* 1985;23:345–356.
27. McCormack H, Horne D, Sheather S. Clinical applications of visual analogue scales: A critical review. *Psychological Medicine* 1988;18: 1007–1019.
28. Harding VR, Williams AC, Richardson PH, et al. The development of a battery of measures for assessing physical functioning of chronic pain patients. *Pain* 1994;58:367–375.
29. Granger CV, Wright BD. Looking ahead to the use of functional assessment in ambulatory physiatric and primary care. *Phys Med Rehabil Clin North Am* 1993;4:3:595–605.
30. Lebovitz AH. Chronic pain: The multidisciplinary approach. Int *Anesthesiol Clin* 1991;29:1–7.
31. Rowlington JC, Hamill RJ. Treatment of low back pain. *Int Anesthesiol Clin* 1991;29:57–68.
32. Banks SM, Kerns RD. Exploring high rates of depression in chronic pain: A diathesis-stress framework. *Psychol Bull* 1996;119:95–110.
33. Dworkin RH. Which individuals with acute pain are most likely to develop a chronic pain syndrome? *Pain Forum* 1997;6:127–136.
34. Malone MD, Strube MJ. Meta-analysis of non-medical treatments for chronic pain. *Pain* 1988;34:231–244.
35. Flor H, Fydrich T, Turk DC. Efficacy of multidisciplinary pain treatment centers: A meta-analytic review. *Pain* 1992;49:221–230.
36. Williams ACdeC, Richardson PH, Nicholas CE, et al. Inpatient vs. outpatient pain management: Results of a randomised controlled trial. *Pain* 1996;66:13–22.
37. Maruta T, Malinchoc M, Offord K, Colligan R. Status of patients with chronic pain 13 years after treatment in a pain management center. *Pain* 1998;74:199–204.
38. Caudill M, Schnable R, Zuttermeister P, et al. Decreased clinic use by chronic pain patients: Response to behavioral medicine interventions. *Clin J Pain* 1991;7:305–310.
39. Cicala RS, Wright H. Outpatient treatment of patients with chronic pain: An analysis of cost savings. *Clin J Pain* 1989;5:223–226.
40. Grabois M. Survival and adaptive strategies for pain treatment in a managed care environment. Paper presented at: the American Congress of Rehabilitation Medicine; October 13, 1996; Chicago, Illinois.
41. Fordyce WE, ed. *Back Pain in the Workplace. Task Force on Pain in the Workplace. International Association for the Study of Pain.* Seattle, Wash: IASP Press; 1995:5–9.
42. Crombie IK, Davies HT. Selection bias in pain research. *Pain* 1998;74: 1–3.

PART IV

PAIN BY ANATOMIC LOCATION

CHAPTER 17 EPIDEMIOLOGY OF HEADACHES

Sandra W. Hamelsky, Walter F. Stewart, and Richard B. Lipton

Headache is a common pain symptom that inflicts a substantial burden on individual sufferers and on society. Headache has many causes; a range of headache diagnoses was defined by the International Headache Society (IHS) in 1988.[1] The IHS distinguishes two broad groups of headache disorders: primary headache disorders and secondary headache disorders. Secondary headache disorders result from an underlying condition, such as a sinus infection or brain tumor. In primary headache disorders, the headache disorder is the fundamental problem. The two most common types of primary headache disorders are episodic tension-type headache (ETTH) and migraine.

The epidemiology of headache varies by headache type and demographics. ETTH, the most common headache type, affects slightly more women than men.[2–7] Between the ages of 18 and 65, about 36% of men and 42% of women suffer from ETTH.[8] In contrast, migraine occurs approximately three times more often in women than in men: approximately 18% of women and 6% of men between 12 and 80 years of age suffer from migraine.[9,10]

ETTH exerts a modest impact on the individual; however, the aggregate societal impact is high because the disorder is so prevalent. Although migraine is less common, individual attacks are considerably more painful and disabling and often result in lost work time. Because the societal impact of both ETTH and migraine is significant, this chapter focuses on the epidemiology of the two disorders. This chapter does not cover secondary headaches because the epidemiology of the underlying condition is an important determinant of the epidemiology of the related headaches. This chapter begins with a review of the diagnostic criteria for migraine and tension-type headache, followed by a review of migraine epidemiology, including incidence, prevalence, and public health impact. We close with a review of the epidemiology of tension-type headache.

DIAGNOSTIC CRITERIA

Migraine is characterized by various combinations of neurologic, gastrointestinal, and autonomic changes that occur during different phases of the migraine attack. Although the IHS defines seven subtypes of migraine (IHS, 1.0), by far, the two most important are migraine without aura (IHS, 1.1) and migraine with aura (IHS, 1.2). The IHS definitions for migraine with and without aura are found in Tables 17-1 and 17-2. Migraine is both a diagnosis of inclusion, because specific diagnostic features are required, and a diagnosis of exclusion, because secondary headache disorders have to be eliminated based on the history, physical examination, or laboratory studies.

The features of the migraine attack can be divided into four phases: premonitory phase, aura, headache phase, and resolution phase. None of these phases is obligatory for diagnosis, and most people with migraine do not have all four phases. The premonitory phase (prodrome) occurs in approximately 60% of migraine sufferers, with equal frequency in both migraine with and without aura.[11] It usually begins hours to days before headache onset. Symptoms that may occur during the prodrome include depression, hyperactivity, yawning, food cravings, and thirst.[11]

In migraine with aura, various focal neurologic symptoms precede or accompany the attack. The aura usually develops over a period of 5 to 20 minutes, and typically lasts less than 1 hour. It is most often characterized by visual phenomena but may also involve other secondary features, motor, language, or brainstem disturbances. The aura is usually, but not always, followed by a headache. Approximately 20% to 25% of individuals have migraine with aura, but even in these individuals, most attacks are migraine without aura.[12]

The third phase is the headache phase. The headache of migraine is typically unilateral, pulsating, of moderate to severe intensity, and aggravated by routine physical activity. Other features, including photophobia, phonophobia, nausea, and vomiting, also occur during the headache phase.

During the final resolution phase the pain and accompanying symptoms subside. Although some migraine sufferers feel euphoric and energetic, others feel lethargic and tired.

The clinical diagnosis of tension-type headache (TTH) is also based on a characteristic symptom profile and the exclusion of secondary headache. Unlike migraine, there is no prodrome or aura in TTH. The headache is usually bilateral, dull, nonpulsating, and of mild to moderate intensity. Although associated features are not required for diagnosis, various symptoms are compatible with the diagnosis.

The diagnostic category TTH (IHS, 2.0) includes two main subtypes, ETTH (2.1) and chronic tension-type headache (CTTH) (2.2). The primary difference between these disorders is the frequency with which the headaches occur. Tension-type headaches that occur less than 15 days per month are classified as ETTH, while those that occur more than 15 days per month are classified as CTTH. In addition, for ETTH nausea is not permitted but either photophobia or phonophobia is permitted. For CTTH, any one of nausea, photophobia, or phonophobia is permitted. The diagnostic criteria for ETTH and CTTH are presented in Tables 17-3 and 17-4.

MIGRAINE EPIDEMIOLOGY AND DISEASE BURDEN

Incidence

Incidence is defined as the rate of onset of new cases of disease in a defined population. Estimating the incidence of migraine is challenging because the disease affects individuals of all ages, and the incidence rate varies substantially by age. To accurately describe incidence requires a large cohort study of individuals ranging in

TABLE 17-1 **International Headache Society (IHS) Diagnostic Criteria for Migraine Without Aura**

1.1 Migraine without aura

Description: Idiopathic, recurring headache disorder manifesting in attacks lasting 4–72 hours. Typical characteristics of headache are unilateral location, pulsating quality, moderate or severe intensity, aggravation by routine physical activity, and association with nausea, photophobia, and phonophobia.

Diagnostic criteria:

A. At least 5 attacks fulfilling B–D

B. Headache attacks lasting 4–72 hours (untreated or unsuccessfully treated)

C. Headache has at least two of the following characteristics:
 1. Unilateral location
 2. Pulsating quality
 3. Moderate or severe intensity inhibits or prohibits daily activities
 4. Aggravation by walking stairs or similar routine physical activity

D. During headache at least one of the following:
 1. Nausea and/or vomiting
 2. Photophobia and phonophobia

E. At least one of the following:
 1. History, physical, and neurologic examinations do not suggest symptomatic headache
 2. History and/or physical, and/or neurologic examinations do suggest such disorder, but it is ruled out by appropriate investigations
 3. Such disorder is present, but migraine attacks do not occur for the first time in close temporal relation to one another

Cephalgia 1988;8:1–96, by permission of Scandinavian University Press.

age from 4 to 60 years. There have been few studies of migraine incidence.

Breslau and colleagues[13] conducted a prospective study to estimate the incidence of migraine. The investigators interviewed 1,007 members of a health maintenance organization who were between the ages of 21 and 30 years. Approximately 98% (972/1,007) of the participants completed a follow-up interview 3.5 and 5.5 years later. The at-risk population was composed of 848 participants who did not meet the criteria for migraine at baseline. The 5.5-year cumulative incidence was 8.4% (71/848; female, 60; male, 11), or a rate of 17.0 per 1,000 person years (24.0, female, 6.0, male).

Two population-based studies estimated the incidence of migraine using the reported age of migraine onset. Stewart and colleagues[14] conducted telephone interviews among 10,169 residents of Washington County, Maryland, who were between the ages of 12 and 29 years. In this study, 392 male and 1,018 female interviewees were identified as migraine sufferers. As shown in Figure 17-1, in both males and females, the incidence rate of migraine with aura peaks 3 to 5 years earlier than migraine without aura. In addition, the onset of migraine in females occurs at a later age than in males. An important strength of this study is that it adjusted for telescoping. Telescoping is the tendency to report the occurrence of past events at times closer to the present.[15] Thus, studies estimating the age-specific incidence of migraine based on recall would likely be biased toward older ages of headache onset.[15,16] To minimize the effect of telescoping, Stewart and colleagues[14] estimated the age-specific incidence rates, adjusted for the time interval between the reported age of onset and the age at interview. However, because of the limited age range of the participants, the generalizability of the results is limited.

The second population-based study, conducted by Rasmussen,[17] reported that the age-adjusted annual incidence of migraine was 3.7 per 1,000 person years (females, 5.8; males, 1.6). Neither age-specific incidence nor incidence by migraine subtypes was reported.

One study, conducted in Olmstead County, Minnesota, used linked medical records to estimate the incidence of migraine.[18] Of the 6,400 patient records reviewed, 629 fulfilled the criteria for migraine. The overall age-adjusted incidence rate was 1.37 per 1,000 person years for males and 2.94 per 1,000 person years for females. The incidence rates in this study are lower than those reported in the aforementioned studies, probably because only individuals who consulted a health care provider for headache were included.

TABLE 17-2 **International Headache Society (IHS) Diagnostic Criteria for Migraine With Aura**

1.2 Migraine with Aura

Description: Idiopathic, recurring disorder manifesting with attacks of neurologic symptoms unequivocally localizable to cerebral cortex or brainstem, usually gradually developed over 5–20 minutes and usually lasting less than 60 minutes. Headache, nausea, and/or photophobia usually follow neurologic aura symptoms directly or after a free interval of less than an hour. The headache usually lasts 4–72 hours, but may be completely absent.

Diagnostic criteria:

A. At least 2 attacks fulfilling B

B. At least 3 of the following 4 characteristics:
 1. One or more fully reversible aura symptoms including focal cerebral cortical and/or brain stem dysfunction.
 2. At least one aura symptom develops gradually over more than 4 minutes or, 2 or more symptoms occur in succession.
 3. No aura symptom lasts more than 60 minutes. If more than one aura symptom is present, accepted duration is proportionally increased.
 4. Headache follows aura with a free interval of less than 60 minutes. (It may also begin before or simultaneously with aura).

C. At least one of the following:
 1. History, physical, and neurologic examinations do not suggest symptomatic headache.
 2. History and/or physical and/or neurologic examinations do suggest such disorder, but it is ruled out by appropriate investigations.
 3. Such disorder is present, but migraine attacks do not occur for the first time in close temporal relation to the disorder.

Cephalgia 1988;8:1–96, by permission of Scandinavian University Press.

TABLE 17-3 **International Headache Study (IHS) Diagnostic Criteria for Episodic Tension-type Headache**

2.1 Episodic tension-type headache

Description: Recurrent episodes of headache lasting minutes to days. The pain is typically pressing/tightening in quality, of mild or moderate intensity, bilateral in location and does not worsen with routine physical activity. Nausea is absent, but photophobia or phonophobia may be present.

Diagnostic criteria:

A. At least 10 previous headache episodes fulfilling criteria B–D listed below. Number of days with such headache <180/year (<15/month).

B. Headache lasting from 30 minutes to 7 days.

C. At least 2 of the following pain characteristics:
   1. Pressing/tightening (nonpulsating) quality.
   2. Mild or moderate intensity (may inhibit, but does not prohibit activities).
   3. Bilateral location.
   4. No aggravation by walking stairs or similar routine physical activity.

D. Both of the following:
   1. No nausea or vomiting (anorexia may occur).
   2. Photophobia and phonophobia are absent, or one but not the other is present.

E. At least one of the following:
   1. History, physical, and neurologic examinations do not suggest symptomatic headache.
   2. History and/or physical and/or neurologic examinations do suggest such disorder, but it is ruled out by appropriate investigations
   3. Such disorder is present, but tension-type headache does not occur for the first time in close temporal relation to the disorder.

Cephalgia 1988;8:1–96, by permission of Scandinavian University Press.

Prevalence

In contrast to the limited number of studies of migraine incidence, there have been many studies of the prevalence of migraine. Prevalence is defined as the proportion of a given population that has migraine over a defined period of time. Lifetime prevalence refers to the proportion of individuals who have ever had the disease. Period prevalence refers to the proportion of individuals who have experienced at least one attack within a defined interval, usually within 1 year of the survey. Prevalence is a function of both the incidence and duration of a disease.

Migraine prevalence estimates have varied widely, largely because of differences in case definitions. Because migraine prevalence varies by age, gender, race, geography, and socioeconomic status, prevalence estimates from different studies also vary because of demographic differences among the populations studied.[19,20] Table 17-5 presents the age- and gender-specific migraine prevalence estimates from population-based studies that used the IHS criteria.[19] Two meta-analyses of published population-based studies that help explain the variation in prevalence will be reviewed in this section.[19,20]

The meta-analysis by Stewart and associates[20] included 24 studies published prior to 1994, only 5 of which used the IHS diagnostic criteria. Over 65% of the variation in prevalence estimates among studies was explained by only a few factors. Case definition accounted for the largest portion of variation in prevalence (36.1%) between studies. Gender (14.5%) and age (age 2.9%; age^2 13.5%) also accounted for a substantial part of the variation. Migraine was more prevalent among females than males, peaking between 35 and 55 years of age in both genders. Factors such as the source of the population, the response rate, and whether diagnoses were confirmed by a clinical examination did not account for a significant portion of the variation among studies.

A second, more recent, meta-analysis included 18 population-based studies all using the IHS criteria.[19] Because this study required the use of the IHS criteria for inclusion and stratified by gender, two major explanations from the first study were eliminated. In this second meta-analysis, migraine was again more

TABLE 17-4 **International Headache Society (IHS) Diagnostic Criteria for Chronic Tension-type Headache**

2.2 Chronic tension-type headache

Description: Headache present for at least 15 days a month during at least 6 months. The headache is usually pressing/tightening in quality, mild or moderate in severity, bilateral, and does not worsen with routine physical activity. Nausea, photophobia, or phonophobia may occur.

Diagnostic criteria:

A. Average headache frequency 15 days/month (180 days/year) for 6 months fulfilling criteria B–D listed below.

B. At least 2 of the following pain characteristics:
   1. Pressing/tightening quality.
   2. Mild or moderate intensity (may inhibit, but does not prohibit activities).
   3. Bilateral location.
   4. No aggravation by walking stairs or similar routine physical activity.

C. Both of the following:
   1. No vomiting.
   2. No more than one of the following: Nausea, photophobia or phonophobia.

D. At least one of the following:
   1. History, physical, and neurologic examinations do not suggest symptomatic headache.
   2. History and/or physical and/or neurologic examinations do suggest such disorder, but it is ruled out by appropriate investigations.
   3. Such disorder is present, but tension-type headache does not occur for the first time in close temporal relation to the disorder.

Cephalgia 1988;8:1–96, by permission of Scandinavian University Press.

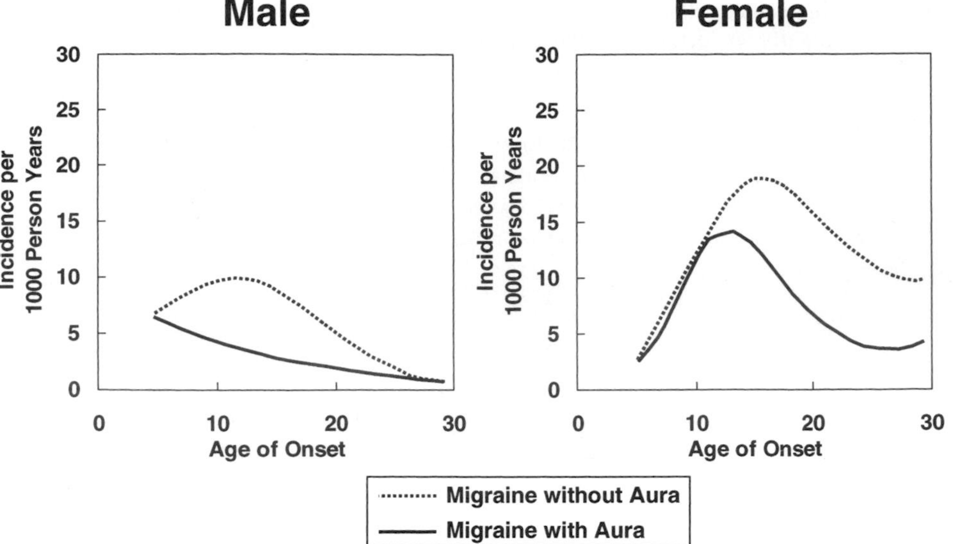

Figure 17-1 Sex- and age-specific incidence of migraine headache with and without aura among 10,131 survey respondents aged 12 to 29 years: Washington County, Maryland, 1987. (Stewart WF, Linet MS, Celentano DD, Van Nutta M, Ziegler D. Age- and sex-specific incidence rates of migraine with and without visual aura. *Am J Epidemiol* 1991;134:1111–1120.)

prevalent among females than males, and peaked during the third and fourth decade of life in both genders. Among females, age and geographic location of the study population accounted for 74% of the variation in migraine prevalence. These two variables accounted for a slightly lower proportion, 58%, of the variation among males. Specifically, prevalence was highest in North America, South America, and Western Europe, intermediate in Africa, and lowest in Asia, as discussed later. Once again, variation in migraine prevalence was not explained by methodologic factors such as sampling method, response method, response rate, and recall period.

After standardizing the definition of migraine across studies, a substantial proportion of the variation in migraine prevalence is explained by remarkably few factors. However, some of the variation remains unexplained. Socioeconomic status, cultural differences in symptom reporting, or other unmeasured factors may account for part of the residual variation in migraine prevalence.[19,20]

Prevalence by Age and Gender Migraine prevalence varies by age and gender. Most studies find that migraine prevalence is higher among females than males. As depicted in Figure 17-2, the prevalence of migraine is higher among females than males and varies considerably with age, with a peak between 35 to 45 years.

Prevalence by Race and Geographic Region Migraine prevalence appears to vary by race and geographic region, two factors that are associated with each other. Stewart and colleagues[32] conducted a population-based study to compare the prevalence of migraine among whites, African Americans, and Asian Americans in the United States. Both before and after adjusting for sociodemographic covariates, other than race, they found the lowest prevalence in Asian Americans (female, 9.2%; male, 4.2%), and the highest prevalence among whites (female, 20.4%; male, 8.6%). Similarly, the meta-analysis[19] found the lowest prevalence in Asia and Africa, and considerably higher prevalence in Europe, Central and South America, and North America.

The international variation in migraine prevalence may be explained in several ways. The variation may be caused by regional differences in genetic susceptibility. This hypothesis is supported by the evidence of lower migraine prevalence in Africa and Asia, as well as among African Americans and Asian Americans in the United States.[32] However, because the prevalence of migraine in Asia is considerably lower than the prevalence among Asian Americans in the United States, it suggests that a role for environmental or cultural factors is likely. A limitation in evaluating the role of genetic and environmental factors in race differences is that the exact same methods have not been used in studies conducted in different countries and race groups.

Prevalence by Socioeconomic Status In the past, migraine was thought to be a disease of the affluent. However, population-based studies conducted in North America indicate that, in the community, migraine prevalence is inversely related to household income or education.[9,10,32,35] That is, as income or education increases, migraine prevalence declines. Prior beliefs regarding the apparent direct relationship between migraine prevalence and income may be explained by patterns of health care utilization. Migraine may appear to be a disease of high income in the physician's office, because medical diagnosis of migraine is more common among high-income groups.[36] The contrasting finding of the National Health Interview Survey (NHIS)[37] supports the inverse association and the role of access to care shaping physicians' perceptions about this condition. In the NHIS study, prevalence was lower in the low-income compared with the middle-income group, and was highest in the high-income group. Because the NHIS relied on self-reported medical diagnosis, the higher prevalence among the high-income group is likely to be the result of an increased likelihood of diagnosis of migraine as income rises. Interestingly, studies outside the United States have generally not reported the inverse relationship between migraine prevalence and income.[21,30,38,39] It is unclear what accounts for the international variation in these findings.

Public Health Significance

Migraine is a disabling disorder that exerts an impact on both the individual and society. The individual impact of migraine is measured by quantifying the frequency and severity of attacks, as well as through quality-of-life studies. The societal impact is measured in economic terms, which include direct costs, such as health care utilization, as well as indirect costs resulting from lost productivity at work.

TABLE 17-5 **Gender- and Age-specific Migraine Prevalence as Reported in Population-based Studies of Migraine That Used International Headache Society (IHS) Diagnostic Criteria[19]***

Author	Age Range	Female	Male	Author	Age Range	Female	Male
Abu-Arefeh[21]	5–15	11.5	9.7	O'Brien[30]	18–24	18.3	10.9
Alders[22†]	5–15	4.4	2.6	O'Brien	25–34	23.0	9.1
Alders	16–25	11.3	8.1	O'Brien	35–44	33.3	8.7
Alders	26–35	11.5	6.7	O'Brien	45–54	32.3	5.9
Alders	36–45	20.3	17.7	O'Brien	55–64	28.7	5.4
Alders	46–55	22.7	7.7	O'Brien	65–74	11.7	1.9
Alders	56–65	6.7	0.0	Rasmussen[2]	45–54	12.0	6.0
Alders	66–87	5.3	0.0	Rasmussen	55–64	19.0	7.0
Arregui[23]	0–9	0.0	0.8	Sakai[31†]	15–19	11.5	2.0
Arregui	10–19	3.7	1.5	Sakai	20–29	13.0	7.0
Arregui	20–29	8.8	0.0	Sakai	30–39	20.0	6.0
Arregui	30–39	8.5	0.0	Sakai	40–49	18.0	2.5
Arregui	40–49	18.0	2.3	Sakai	50–59	11.0	3.0
Arregui	50–59	8.1	3.1	Sakai	60–69	9.0	0.5
Arregui	60–69	4.0	0.0	Sakai	70–79	3.0	0.0
Arregui	0–9	4.8	0.7	Stewart[32‡]	18–25	22.7	10.0
Arregui	10–19	20.1	8.1	Stewart	26–30	22.1	11.5
Arregui	20–29	16.8	5.0	Stewart	31–35	19.0	8.2
Arregui	30–39	22.1	10.0	Stewart	36–40	21.2	9.8
Arregui	40–49	21.5	16.1	Stewart	41–45	21.0	9.1
Arregui	50–59	38.1	12.0	Stewart	46–55	20.9	6.5
Arregui	60–69	15.4	0.0	Stewart	56–65	9.8	3.2
Barea[4]	10–18	10.2	9.6	Stewart[9‡]	12–19	8.1	4.3
Breslau[24]	21–30	12.9	3.4	Stewart	20–29	19.8	7.1
Cruz[25]	0–9	1.4	1.5	Stewart	30–39	28.7	8.9
Cruz	10–19	8.2	8.4	Stewart	40–49	24.4	7.4
Cruz	20–29	9.7	6.2	Stewart	50–59	18.7	6.0
Cruz	30–39	10.1	5.8	Stewart	60–69	10.5	3.4
Cruz	40–49	13.0	6.6	Stewart	70–85	6.6	2.5
Cruz	50–59	10.3	7.1	Tekle-Haimanot[33]	20–29	4.8	1.1
Cruz	60–69	8.1	6.5	Tekle-Haimanot	30–39	5.6	4.3
Franceschi[26]	65–84	2.0	0.0	Tekle-Haimanot	40–49	3.8	1.4
Henry[27‡]	15–24	6.0	2.0	Tekle-Haimanot	50–59	3.4	1.6
Henry	25–34	12.0	3.9	Tekle-Haimanot	60–69	1.9	0.6
Henry	35–49	12.0	2.4	Tekle-Haimanot	70–79	0.6	0.6
Henry	50–64	6.7	2.2	Tekle-Haimanot	80–89	0.0	0.0
Henry	65–75	2.8	0.9	Thomson[34†]	17–29	15.5	13.4
Launer[28]	20–24	17.0	3.0	Thomson	30–49	14.1	10.7
Launer	25–29	24.1	3.8	Thomson	50–70	12.1	5.3
Launer	30–34	21.4	4.4	Wong[3]	15–24	0.8	0.4
Launer	35–39	33.2	8.8	Wong	25–34	2.6	0.9
Launer	40–44	27.5	6.5	Wong	35–44	2.7	1.0
Launer	45–49	27.4	8.3	Wong	45–54	1.4	0.2
Launer	50–54	24.0	15.7	Wong	55–64	0.6	0.4
Launer	≥55	20.4	5.6	Wong	65–74	0.4	0.2
Linet[29‡]	12–17	10.2	5.4				
Linet	18–23	13.1	5.2				
Linet	24–29	18.8	5.4				

*This table was modified slightly from the original publication.

†Data were estimated from published information.

‡Data were obtained from the author.

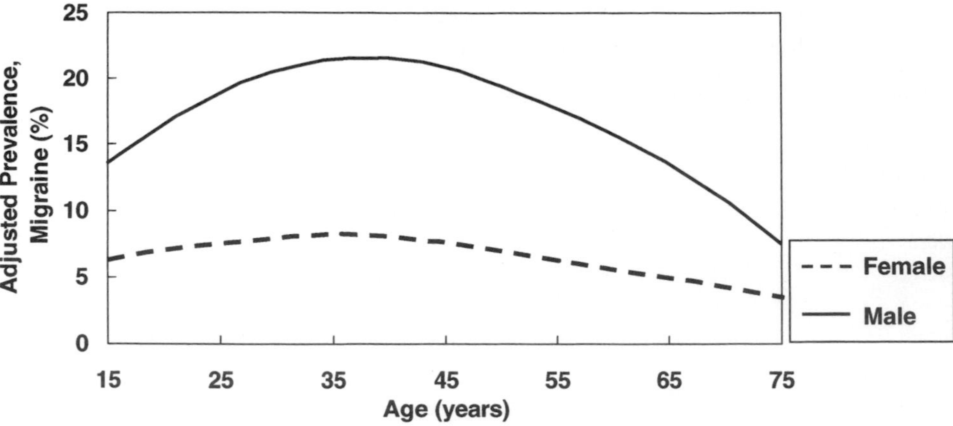

Figure 17-2 Gender- and age-specific estimates of migraine prevalence (North America) based on 18 population studies that used International Headache Society (IHS) diagnostic criteria. (Scher A, Stewart W, Lipton R. Migraine and headache: A meta-analytic approach. In: Crombie I, ed. *Epidemiology of Pain.* Seattle, Wash: IASP Press; 1999:159–170.)

Individual Impact: Frequency and Severity of Attacks The individual impact of migraine is measured by the level of pain intensity, the presence and severity of associated symptoms (nausea, vomiting, photophobia, phonophobia), and the frequency and duration of attacks. The individual impact of migraine has been evaluated in several studies.[9,10,32,40] Most recently, Stewart and colleagues[32] reported the migraine characteristics of 1,748 migraine sufferers residing in Baltimore County, Maryland. In this study, approximately 40% of subjects (female, 38.9%; male, 46.0%) reported severe pain, while an additional 40% reported very severe pain (female, 43.3%; male, 31.8%). The remainder of subjects reported pain that ranged from mild to moderate.

The overwhelming majority of migraine sufferers reported photophobia (overall, 81.9%; female, 83.5%; male, 76.5%) and phonophobia (overall, 77.9%; female, 79.3%; male, 72.9%). More than half (58.8%) of migraine participants reported nausea that accompanies their migraine headache more than half the time (female, 62.1%; male, 47.3%), while only a small proportion reported vomiting.

The majority of subjects reported one to two migraine attacks per month. The duration of an untreated attack varies considerably by gender. Among females, approximately 71% of attacks last longer than 24 hours. In contrast, 48% of males reported attacks that last longer than 24 hours.

The results reported by Stewart and colleagues[32] were comparable to those reported in previous studies.[9,10,40]

Quality-of-Life Studies Measures of quality of life provide a broad-based assessment of the specific and global impact of a condition such as migraine. However, most studies of the impact of migraine have been conducted in clinic-based samples. As such, the quality-of-life impact is likely to be overestimated by these studies. Nonetheless, using the generic health-related quality-of-life (HRQoL) instrument from the Medical Outcomes Study,[41] these studies demonstrate that migraine sufferers have lower quality of life than control subjects in the United States population.[42,43] One study[43] found that individuals with migraine have quality-of-life scores similar to those of patients with osteoarthritis, hypertension, or diabetes. However, quality-of-life as measured in clinic-based samples may differ from that of migraine sufferers in the community. In addition, many studies conducted using clinic-based samples lack a contemporaneous control group. The lack of a control group can lead to an overestimation of treatment benefits because of regression toward the mean.

At least three population-based studies of quality of life in migraine cases versus controls have been conducted.[44–46] In these studies, migraine sufferers had substantially lower HRQoL relative to population controls. In addition, quality of life and frequency of attacks were inversely correlated; as the frequency of attacks increased, quality of life decreased.[44] Lower quality-of-life scores were associated with higher levels of headache-related disability.[46]

A recent study published by Lofland and colleagues[47] assessed the outcomes of migraine sufferers enrolled in a mixed-model staff/independent practice association–managed care organization. The study enrolled patients with migraine when they received their first prescription for sumatriptan. After 6 months of sumatriptan therapy, four of the HRQoL dimensions and the physical component summary score of the Short-Form Health Survey (SF-36) showed significant improvement.[41,48] Furthermore, the Migraine-Specific Quality of Life Questionnaire (MSQ),[49] a disease-specific quality-of-life instrument, showed significant improvement at both 3 and 6 months after initiation of sumatriptan therapy. Despite these striking findings, results are limited by the lack of a control group, leading to a possible overestimation of treatment benefits resulting from apparent improvements that can be explained by regression towards the mean.

Societal Impact

Direct Costs Direct costs related to health care include outpatient visits, hospitalization, the use of emergency department services, the cost of prescriptions, and other treatments. For migraine, most of the direct costs were the result of outpatient visits and the cost of prescription medications. Hospitalization[37,50] and the use of emergency department services[50–52] are uncommon among migraine sufferers.

According to the American Migraine Study,[53] 68% of females and 57% of males have ever consulted a physician for migraine. The study also found that certain demographic and headache characteristics are associated with consultation. For example, females and older age groups are more likely to consult a physician for migraine. In addition, higher pain intensity, the number of migraine symptoms, attack duration, and disability were all associated with an increased likelihood of physician consultation.

Migraine sufferers are more likely to consult their physicians for medical care than individuals in the general population who do not have migraine. Clouse and colleagues[50] compared the health care utilization patterns of migraine sufferers and nonmigraine sufferers enrolled in a United Healthcare Corporation–affiliated plan.

A total of 1,336 migraine sufferers were compared with a matched sample (i.e., matched on the basis of age, sex, duration of enrollment, and subscriber/dependent status) of individuals without migraine. During the 18-month study period, migraine sufferers made 22,587 physician visits, of which, 2,616 were for migraine. In contrast, individuals without migraine made a total of 13,072 visits during the same period. Interestingly, a small proportion of the migraine sufferers accounts for the majority of physician visits among migraine sufferers. Although most migraine sufferers reported only one to four visits per year, 7.6% reported more than 12 visits.

Few studies have translated use of medical care into direct monetary estimates. Hu and colleagues[54] estimated the annual treatment costs of migraine in a population-based sample. They found that the annual treatment costs for migraine were over $1 billion, about $100 per migraine sufferer per year. These are likely to be underestimates because the figures were derived from 1994 data. Consultation and medication use have increased substantially over the past 5 years.[55] Clouse and colleagues[50] reported similar, though slightly higher, average claim costs per member per month ($145). The costs reported by Clouse and colleagues differ from those of Hu because they were not separated by diagnosis. Migraine sufferers are likely to have comorbid conditions; thus, the increased costs may reflect the costs resulting from the treatment of migraine as well as other medical conditions.

Indirect Costs The indirect economic impact of migraine is primarily a consequence of lost productivity at work. Because many migraine sufferers continue to work, even while suffering from a migraine attack, it is important to account not only for lost workdays caused by migraine, but also reduced productivity while at work, when estimating indirect costs.

The early studies of migraine-associated disability had limitations. For example, some studies examined selected populations such as clinical trial participants or individuals with a self-reported diagnosis of migraine.[37,56] Other studies employed designs that were limited by uncertainties regarding the accuracy of recall over a period of up to 1 year.[57–59]

Von Korff and colleagues[60] conducted a population-based diary study as one approach to addressing the limitations of previous studies. They estimated the amount of lost work time among migraine sufferers who completed a daily diary for 3 months. During this 3-month period, migraine sufferers missed an average of 1.1 days per month because of headache. Subjects who worked during a migraine attack reported work effectiveness that was reduced by an average of 41%.

Some studies combine lost workdays and reduced effectiveness days into an overall measure, termed lost workday equivalent (LWDE). The LWDE equals actual days of missed work plus days at work with headache, times one, minus percent effectiveness while at work with headache.[57] In the study reported by Stewart and colleagues,[57] subjects experienced an average of three LWDEs during the study period. The majority of the lost workdays and LWDEs were the result of migraine rather than any other headache type.

The missed workday and LWDE estimates reported by Von Korff and colleagues[60] are higher than those reported in other population-based studies.[37,56,57,61] The use of a daily diary may have improved the accuracy of reporting that is inherently limited by asking people to recall events over the past 3 to 12 months.

In the study reported by Von Korff and colleagues,[60] a relatively small percentage of migraine sufferers accounts for the majority of lost work time. In this study, the most disabled 20% of the participants accounted for 77% of the missed workdays; and 40% of subjects accounted for 75% of the total LWDEs. Similarly, Stewart and colleagues[57] found that 51% of females and 38% of males reported six or more LWDEs per year, which accounted for more than 90% of all lost workdays.

The early studies that attempted to quantify the monetary cost of the lost work also had significant limitations. One study was based on self-identified migraine sufferers[37]; thus, it probably underestimated the cost because it excluded those who did not know they suffered from migraine. Another study[56] probably overestimated the cost because it included a population of clinical trial participants who were likely to be more disabled than migraine sufferers in the community.

Using the human capital method, Hu and colleagues[54] estimated the indirect costs of migraine. Human capital studies assume that the economic value of a missed day of work is equivalent to the wages for that day. According to the results of this population-based study, Hu estimated that migraine costs American employers $13 billion per year as a result of absenteeism and reduced effectiveness at work. Approximately 62% of the cost was a result of absenteeism. Importantly, the greatest indirect costs were found among middle-aged individuals (30–49 years). Although this study provided important information, the human capital method values the indirect costs of the disease according to the sufferers' salary. A lost workday is valued by the individual's wages for that day. This is a reasonable approach, but it may be an overestimate if the worker makes up for lost time or coworkers effectively cover for his or her absence. However, if a migraine sufferer makes an error while at work, it may be an underestimate. In addition, the impact of the disease in a laborer or homemaker would be valued at a lower rate than that of a business executive with a high salary. A limitation of all studies reported to date is that reduced productivity while at work when suffering from a migraine is based on self-report. No studies to date have actually quantified reductions in productivity.

TENSION-TYPE HEADACHE EPIDEMIOLOGY AND DISEASE BURDEN

Prevalence

The prevalence of TTH has not been widely studied. Among published studies of TTH that use the 1988 IHS criteria, the 1-year period prevalence ranges between 14.3[5] and 93.0[2] for ETTH, and 0.0[5,33] and 8.1[33] for CTTH (Table 17-6). Variation in prevalence estimates may be due, in part, to differences in study methodology. Lifetime prevalences are higher than 1-year period prevalences. The age distribution of the population studied influences prevalence estimates. Case definition also plays a role. Studies of the epidemiology of TTH use various levels of diagnostic specificity. Although some studies group all TTH (IHS 2.0) subjects together, other studies distinguish between subjects with ETTH, (IHS 2.1), CTTH (IHS 2.2), and headache of the tension-type fulfilling all criteria except one (IHS 2.3). Prevalence estimates may also vary because of differences in the diagnostic sensitivity and specificity of the methods used to collect symptom data. Methods of data collection (e.g., self-administered questionnaires, telephone interviews, and clinical examinations) as well as the quality of data

TABLE 17-6 **Prevalence of Episodic Tension-type Headache (ETTH) and Chronic Tension-type Headache (CTTH) as Reported in 18 Population-based Studies That Used International Headache Society (IHS) Criteria**

Author, Country	Population Type	Response Method	Sample Size	Headache Type	Prevalence Period	Age Range*	Female
Abu-Arefah[21] (United Kingdom)	Community	Mail SAQ; clinical examination	2,165	Unspecified	1 year	5–15	—
Barea[4] (Brazil)	School survey	In-person interview; clinical examination	538	2.1, 2.2, 2.3	1 year	5th–8th grade	76.7
					1 week	5th–8th grade	35.3
					24 hours	5th–8th grade	10.1
Castillo[62] (Spain)	Community	SAQ; clinical examination	1,883	CTTH	1 month	18–89	2.0
Franceschi[26] (Italy)	Community	In-person interview; clinical examination	312	Unspecified	Lifetime	"Elderly"	4.0
					1 year	"Elderly"	4.0
Gobel[38] (Germany)	Community	Mail SAQ	4,061	ETTH	Lifetime	18–35	
						36–55	
						≥56	
						All ages (≥18)	13.0
				CTTH	Lifetime	18–35	
						36–55	
						≥56	
						All ages (≥18)	1.0
Tekle-Haimanot[33] (Ethiopia)	Community	In-person interview	15,000	CTTH	1 year	20–29	0.0
						30–39	0.7
						40–49	4.3
						50–59	8.1
						60–69	3.9
						70–79	0.0
						80–89	1.7
						All ages (20–89)	2.3
Jabbar[63] (Saudi Arabia)	Community	In-person interview	5,891	Unspecified	Lifetime	16–19	
						20–29	
						30–39	
						40–49	
						50–59	
						≥60	
						All ages (≥16)	
Lavados[5] (Chile)	Community	In-person interview	1,385	ETTH	1 year	15–29	30.5
						30–39	34.8
						40–49	33.0
						50–59	32.1
						≥60	23.2
						All ages (≥15)	
				CTTH	1 year	15–29	1.6
						30–39	2.6
						40–49	7.3
						50–59	5.9
						≥60	6.2
						All ages (≥15)	
Merikangas[64] (Switzerland)	Community	In-person interview	379	ETTH + CTTH	1 year	28–29	18.0
				ETTH	1 year	28–29	
				CTTH	1 year	28–29	

(continued)

TABLE 17-6 **Prevalence of Episodic Tension-type Headache (ETTH) and Chronic Tension-type Headache (CTTH) as Reported in 18 Population-based Studies That Used International Headache Society (IHS) Criteria**

Author, Country	Population Type	Response Method	Sample Size	Headache Type	Prevalence Period	Age Range*	Female
Mitsikostas[65] Greece)	Monks	SAQ; clinical examination	449	ETTH	Lifetime	>50	
				CTTH	Lifetime	>50	
Pereira Monteiro[66] (Portugal)	Medical school students	In-person SAQ	491	ETTH + CTTH	Unknown	18–32	
				ETTH			
				CTTH			
Pryse-Phillips[6] (Canada)	Community	Telephone interview	1,573	ETTH + CTTH	Unspecified	15–24	
						25–34	
						25–44	
						45–54	
						55–65	
						>65	
						All ages (≥15)	64.0
Rasmussen[2] (Denmark)	Community	Clinical examination	740	ETTH	1 year	25–34	93.0
						35–44	92.0
						45–54	82.0
						55–64	74.0
						All ages (25–64)	86.0
					Lifetime	All ages (25–64)	88.0
				CTTH	1 year	All ages (25–64)	
Roh[67] (South Korea)	Community	Telephone interview; mail SAQ	2,500	2.1, 2.2, 2.3	1 year	0–9	
						10–19	
						20–29	
						30–39	
						40–49	
						50–59	
						≥60	
						All ages	14.7
Schwartz[8] (USA)	Community	Telephone interview	13,345	ETTH	1 year	18–29	40.8
						30–39	46.9
						40–49	46.5
						50–59	40.6
						60–65	27.1
						All ages (18–65)	
				CTTH	1 year	18–29	2.6
						30–39	2.5
						40–49	2.9
						50–59	4.2
						60–65	2.7
						All ages (18–65)	
Srikiatkhachorn[68] (Thailand)	Old age home	In-person interview	241	ETTH	1 year	61–98	
				CTTH	1 year	61–98	
Wang[7] (China)	Community	In-person interview; clinical examination	1,533	2.1, 2.2, 2.3	1 year	65–69	45.0
						70–74	44.0
						75–79	47.0
						≥80	48.0
						All ages (≥65)	46.0
				ETTH	1 year	All ages (≥65)	
				CTTH	1 year	All ages (≥65)	
				2.3	1 year	All ages (≥65)	

(continued)

TABLE 17-6 **Prevalence of Episodic Tension-type Headache (ETTH) and Chronic Tension-type Headache (CTTH) as Reported in 18 Population-based Studies That Used International Headache Society (IHS) Criteria**

Author, Country	Population Type	Response Method	Sample Size	Headache Type	Prevalence Period	Age Range*	Female
Wong[3] (Hong Kong)	Community	Telephone interview	7,356	2.1, 2.2, 2.3	1 year	15–24	1.82
						25–34	2.96
						35–44	5.78
						45–54	2.33
						55–64	2.11
						≥65	0.73
						All ages (≥15)	

SAQ, self-administered questionnaire.

*In years, unless otherwise specified.

collection may influence levels of diagnostic accuracy. Finally, the source of the study population, community based or clinic based, is likely to cause varying prevalence estimates. A meta-analysis might help explain how much each of these factors contributes to the variation in prevalence among studies. Following is a summary of several TTH studies that used the IHS criteria.

Schwartz and colleagues[8] conducted the only large-scale population survey in the United States describing the epidemiology of ETTH and CTTH, as defined by the IHS criteria. These investigators used data from a telephone survey of 13,345 residents of the Baltimore County, Maryland, area[32] to estimate the 1-year period prevalence of ETTH and CTTH by sex, age, education, and race. They found that the overall prevalence of ETTH in the past year was 38.3%.

Lavados and colleagues[5] interviewed a representative sample of 1,385 adults (<14 years old) in Santiago, Chile, using an in-person interview. Subjects reported details about the type of headache from which they suffered most often. The 1-year prevalence of ETTH was 24.3%. The lower prevalence in this study compared with that of Schwartz and colleagues[8] may be explained by the case definition used by the Lavados group. Cases were only identified if TTH was the most common headache. When Schwartz and colleagues[8] used similar criteria, they found an ETTH prevalence of 25.3% compared with 38.3% after the second headache type was classified.

Rasmussen and colleagues,[2] on the other hand, reported ETTH prevalence estimates that are higher than those of most other studies (see Table 17-5). In this study, potential participants were identified from the Danish National Central Person Registry and invited to a general health examination, with an emphasis on headache. Of the 1,000 potential study subjects, 740 males and females participated in the study. The 1-year period prevalence of ETTH was estimated to be 74.0%. The prevalence of ETTH may be higher in this study because of the way in which the invitation was worded. Because potential subjects were invited to a health examination with an emphasis on headache, individuals who had headaches may have been more likely to participate. Thus, there may have been an overrepresentation of headache sufferers among the participants.

The prevalence of CTTH is markedly lower than that of ETTH. Schwartz and colleagues[8] found that the overall prevalence of CTTH was 2.2%. Tekle-Haimanot,[33] Lavados,[5] and Castillo and their colleagues[62] reported similar estimates of 1.7%, 2.6%, and 2.2%, respectively, among the subjects they studied.

Prevalence by Demographic Features The prevalences of both ETTH and CTTH vary by age, gender, race, and educational level. TTH is slightly more common among females than males. Schwartz and colleagues[8] found that women had a higher prevalence of ETTH than men (men, 36.3; women, 42.0), with an overall prevalence ratio of 1.16 to 1.0. The female preponderance occurred at all age, race, and educational levels. Several other studies also report a higher prevalence of TTH among women,[2–7] with female-to-male gender ratios ranging from 1.25[2] to 1.9.[5]

Similarly, the prevalence of CTTH is also higher among females than males. In the study published by Schwartz and colleagues,[8] the prevalence was 2.8 in women and 1.4 in men, with an overall prevalence ratio of 2.0. Studies reported by Tekle-Haimanot,[33] Lavados,[5] and Castillo and their colleagues[62] also reported higher prevalence among women than men.

Prevalence by Age The prevalence of TTH varies by age. Prevalence peaks in the thirties and forties, with a decline thereafter.[3,5,8] Pryse-Philips and colleagues[6] reported a similar, although slightly earlier, peak prevalence in the 25- to 34-year-old age group. Rasmussen and colleagues,[2] on the other hand, found that the prevalence of TTH decreased with increasing age, and Gobel and colleagues[38] found no difference in prevalence by age. The lack of association reported by Gobel and colleagues may be attributed to the use of very wide age intervals; whereas in most studies age is categorized into 10-year intervals,[2,3,5,6,8] Gobel and colleagues used 20-year age groupings.

Tekle-Haimanot,[33] Lavados,[5] and Schwartz and colleagues[8] all reported an increase in the prevalence of CTTH with increasing age. This may be explained by the hypothesis that in some individuals, ETTH develops into a chronic form over a prolonged period of time.[17,69] Gobel and colleagues[38] did not find any difference in the prevalence of CTTH by age, but again this may be attributed to the use of very wide age intervals.

Prevalence by Geographic Region and Race Some of the observed variation in the prevalence of TTH among studies may be the result of racial or ethnic differences. Each of the reported studies of the epidemiology of TTH using the IHS criteria was conducted in a different country, and based on these results, prevalence appears to be highest in the western hemisphere[5,6,8] and Denmark,[2] and lowest in the Asian countries.[3]

The only published study of TTH using the IHS criteria that reported the prevalence of TTH by race was that of Schwartz and colleagues.[8] In this study, the prevalence of ETTH was significantly higher in whites than in African Americans in both men (40.1% versus 22.8%) and in women (46.8% versus 30.9%). The prevalence of CTTH by race paralleled that observed for ETTH: prevalence was higher in whites than in African Americans in both men (1.6% versus 1.0%) and women (3.0% versus 2.2%).

Prevalence by Socioeconomic Status The evidence regarding the relationship between socioeconomic status and the prevalence of ETTH is mixed. Schwartz and colleagues[8] reported that the prevalence of ETTH increases with increasing educational level, a measure of socioeconomic status. Prevalence peaked among those with a graduate-level education (men, 48.5%; women, 48.9%). Lavados and colleagues[5] found a similar direct correlation between ETTH prevalence and socioeconomic status. Other studies have not found this direct association.[6,38] Gobel and colleagues[38] reported no significant differences by education; however, their study used only two educational categories (i.e., basic and secondary) and, as such, may simply lack the sensitivity to detect patterns observed in other studies that used a greater number of educational or income categories. It is also possible that the influence of socioeconomic status varies by country.

The relationship between socioeconomic status and migraine may differ for CTTH. Schwartz and colleagues[8] and Lavados and colleagues[5] reported that the prevalence of CTTH declines with increasing educational level, especially among women. Gobel and colleagues[38] found no association between CTTH prevalence and educational level. Schwartz and colleagues[8] suggested that the epidemiology of CTTH, with its higher risk in women and strong relationship to socioeconomic status, is intermediate between that of ETTH and migraine and may reflect the progression of both headache types to a chronic form.

Headache Characteristics

Over 90% of subjects with ETTH report mild to moderate headache pain intensity; attacks typically occur three times per month.[2,8,38] Lavados and colleagues[5] found that more than 86% of TTH sufferers report mild to moderate pain that occurs three to four times per month. The headache frequency reported by Lavados and colleagues is slightly higher than those reported by Schwartz,[8] Gobel,[38] and Rasmussen and their colleagues[2] because the Lavados sample included both ETTH and CTTH sufferers.

CTTH, on the other hand, is typically associated with higher pain intensity and more frequent attacks. In one study, 86% of subjects reported moderate or severe pain (moderate, 44%; severe, 42%).[38] Using a 10-point scale, Schwartz and colleagues[8] found significantly higher pain intensity scores among CTTH subjects than ETTH subjects (CTTH, 5.55; ETTH, 4.98; $P < .001$). For CTTH, headache frequency ranges from 15 to 30 headaches per month.[8,38]

Certain clinical characteristics occur more frequently among TTH sufferers, and these characteristics often differ by gender. Lavados and colleagues[5] reported that bilateral pain occurs in the majority of TTH sufferers but occurs with even greater frequency among women than men (men, 87.9%; women, 61.1%; $P < .01$). Throbbing pain occurs approximately equally in 66.4% of men and 56.8% of women; this feature, often viewed as a hallmark of migraine, does not discriminate the two disorders. These investigators also found that many TTH subjects report pain that is exacerbated with movement (men, 69.8%, women, 75.5%; $P = .4$), which is surprising because pain that is exacerbated by movement is normally associated with migraine rather than TTH. Pressing pain, photophobia, and phonophobia were also frequently reported: each of these characteristics occurred significantly more often among women than men. Nausea was not commonly reported by any of the study participants.

Disability

Rasmussen[58] reported the first population-based study to examine work loss data in ETTH. Of the employed participants with ETTH, 12% reported being absent from work at least once during the previous year because of ETTH. Among those who reported lost workdays, the majority (68%) were absent from 1 to 7 days during the previous year, 25% were absent between 8 and 14 days during the year, and only 16% were absent more than 14 days during the previous year.

In their survey of Baltimore County residents,[8] Schwartz and colleagues also measured the impact of headache in the workplace.[59] In this study, reduced ability to function and an inability to function (actual missed work) were measured separately. Of the lost work time associated with headache, 19% of the missed workdays and 22% of the reduced effectiveness days were specifically the result of ETTH.[59]

Schwartz and colleagues[8] also reported that among subjects with ETTH, 8.3% reported missed workdays, while 43.6% reported reduced effectiveness days because of headache. Among those with missed workdays, an average of 8.9 missed workdays were reported, whereas subjects with reduced effectiveness days reported approximately 5.0 reduced effectiveness days per person.

Lavados and colleagues[5] found higher levels of missed work among their sample of TTH sufferers: 25% of males and 38.9% of females reported missed work because of their headaches. They also found that TTH sufferers were likely to miss family and social activities as a result of their headaches. Approximately 27.6% of males and 25.3% of females missed family or social activities because of their headaches.

In the Schwartz[8] study, the proportions of CTTH subjects reporting lost and reduced effectiveness days were similar to those reported by ETTH subjects: 11.8% of CTTH sufferers reported lost workdays, and 46.5% reported reduced effectiveness days. However, in contrast with the ETTH sufferers, CTTH sufferers reported more frequent lost workdays and reduced effectiveness days. Subjects with lost workdays reported an average of 27.4 lost workdays per person, whereas subjects with reduced effectiveness days reported approximately 20.4 reduced effectiveness days per person.

CONCLUSION

Headache is a very common condition: approximately 36% of men and 42% of women suffer from ETTH,[8] while 18% of women and 6% of men suffer from migraine.[9,10] These disorders impose a burden on the individual, his or her family, and society.

Migraine sufferers report frequent and painful attacks that inhibit their ability to carry out their usual activities. In several population-based studies, migraine sufferers reported notable impairments in quality of life.[44–46] In addition, Hu and colleagues[54] estimated that the annual treatment costs for migraine were more than $1 billion, about $100 per migraine sufferer per year. Furthermore, Hu and colleagues reported that migraine costs American employers $13 billion per year because of absenteeism and reduced effectiveness at work.

When compared with migraine, the impact of ETTH is more modest. ETTH is generally less painful and has a smaller impact on daily functioning.[8,59] However, the aggregate societal impact is large because the disorder is highly prevalent. The individual impact of CTTH is greater than that of ETTH, but the disorder is relatively rare, thus the societal impact is relatively small.

There have been many studies of the epidemiology of migraine; however, TTH has been studied less often. Future research should seek to expand understanding of the variation in TTH prevalence among certain subgroups, as well as heighten awareness of the impact of TTH on the individual and society. This information will enhance understanding about the relative impact of both migraine and TTH.

REFERENCES

1. Olesen J. Classification and diagnostic criteria for headache disorders, cranial neuralgias, and facial pain. Classification Committee of the International Headache Society. *Cephalalgia* 1988;8(suppl):1–96.
2. Rasmussen B, Jensen R, Schroll M, Olesen J. Epidemiology of headache in a general population: A prevalence study. *J Clin Epidemiol* 1991;44:1147–1157.
3. Wong T, Wong K, Yu T, Kay R. Prevalence of migraine and other headaches in Hong Kong. *Neuroepidemiology* 1995;14:82–91.
4. Barea L, Tannhauser M, Rotta N. An epidemiologic study of headache among children and adolescents of southern Brazil. *Cephalalagia* 1996; 16:545–549.
5. Lavados P, Tenhamm E. Epidemiology of tension-type headache in Santiago, Chile: A prevalence study. *Cephalalgia* 1998;18:552–558.
6. Pryse-Phillips W, Findlay H, Tugwell P, Edmeads J, Murray T, Nelson R. A Canadian population survey on the clinical, epidemiologic and societal impact of migraine and tension-type headache. *Can J Neurol Sci* 1992;19:333–339.
7. Wang S, Liu H, Fuh J, et al. Prevalence of headaches in a Chinese elderly population in Kinmen: Age and gender effect and cross-cultural comparisons. *Neurology* 1997;49:195–200.
8. Schwartz BS, Stewart WF, Simon D, Lipton RB. Epidemiology of tension-type headache. *JAMA* 1998;279:381–383.
9. Stewart WF, Lipton RB, Celentano DD, Reed ML. Prevalence of migraine headache in the United States: Relation to age, income, race, and other sociodemographic factors. *JAMA* 1992;267:64–69.
10. Lipton RB, Stewart WF. Migraine in the United States: A review of epidemiology and health care use. *Neurology* 1993;43(suppl):S6–S10.
11. Silberstein S, Lipton R, Goadsby P. *Headache in Clinical Practice.* Oxford, England: Isis Medical Media Ltd; 1998.
12. Johannes C, Linet M, Stewart W, Celentano D, Lipton R, Szklo M. Relationship of headache to phase of the menstrual cycle among young women: A daily diary study. *Neurology* 1995;45:1076–1082.
13. Breslau N, Chilcoat H, Andreski P. Further evidence on the link between migraine and neuroticism. *Neurology* 1996;47:663–667.
14. Stewart WF, Linet M, Celentano D, Van N, Ziegler D. Age- and sex-specific incidence rates of migraine with and without visual aura. *Am J Epidemil* 1991;134:1111–1120.
15. Brown N, Rips L, Shevell S. The subjective dates of natural events in very long-term memory. *Cognit Psychol* 1985;17:139–177.
16. Cummings R, Kelsey J, Nevitt M. Methologic issues in the study of frequent and recurrent health problems. *Ann Epidemiol* 1990;1:49–56.
17. Rasmussen B. Epidemiology of headache. *Cephalalgia* 1995;15:45–68.
18. Stang P, Yanagihara T, Swanson J, et al. Incidence of migraine headache: A population-based study in Olmstead County, Minnesota. *Neurology* 1992;42:1657–1662.
19. Scher A, Stewart W, Lipton R. Migraine and headache: A meta-analytic approach. In: Crombie I, ed. *Epidemiology of Pain.* Seattle, Wash: IASP Press; 1999:159–170.
20. Stewart W, Simon D, Schechter A, Lipton R. Population variation in migraine prevalence: A meta-analysis. *J Clin Epidemiol* 1995;48: 269–280.
21. Abu-Arefeh I, Russell G. Prevalence of headache and migraine in schoolchildren. *BMJ* 1994;309:765–769.
22. Alders E, Hentzen A, Tan C. A community-based prevalence study on headache in Malaysia. *Headache* 1996;36:379–384.
23. Arregui A, Cabrera J, Leon-Velarde F, Paredes S, Viscarra D, Arbaiza D. High prevalence of migraine in a high-altitude population. *Neurology* 1991;41:1668–1669.
24. Breslau N, Davis G, Andreski P. Migraine, psychiatric disorders, and suicide attempts: An epidemiologic study of young adults. *Psychiatry Res* 1991;37:11–23.
25. Cruz M, Cruz I, Preux P, Schantz P, Dumas M. Headache and cysticercosis in Ecuador, South America. *Headache* 1995;35:93–97.
26. Franceschi M, Colombo B, Rossi P, Canal N. Headache in a population-based elderly cohort: An ancillary study to the Italian Longitudinal Study of Aging (ILSA). *Headache* 1997;37:79–82.
27. Henry P, Michel P, Brochet B, Dartigues J, Tison S, Salamon R. A nationwide survey of migraine in France: Prevalence and clinical features in adults. *Cephalalgia* 1992;12:229–237.
28. Launer L, Terwindt G, Ferrari M. The prevalence and characteristics of migraine in a population-based cohort. *Neurology* 1999;53:537–542.
29. Linet MS, Stewart WF, Celentano DD, Ziegler D, Sprecher M. An epidemiologic study of headache among adolescents and young adults. *JAMA* 1989;261:2211–2216.
30. O'Brien B, Goeree R, Streiner D. Prevalence of migraine headache in Canada: A population-based survey. *Int J Epidemiol* 1994;23:1020–1026.
31. Sakai F, Igarashi H. Prevalence of migraine in Japan: A nationwide survey. *Cephalalgia* 1997;17:15–22.
32. Stewart WF, Lipton RB, Liberman J. Variation in migraine prevalence by race. *Neurology* 1996;16:231–238.
33. Tekle-Haimanot R, Seraw B, Forsgren L, Ekbom K, Ekstedt J. Migraine, chronic tension-type headache, and cluster headache in an Ethiopian rural community. *Cephalalgia* 1995;15:482–488.
34. Thomson A, White G, West R. The prevalence of bad headaches including migraine in a multiethnic community. *N Z Med J* 1993;106: 477–480.
35. Kryst S, Scherl E. A population-based survey of the social and personal impact of migraine. *Headache* 1994;34:344–350.
36. Lipton R, Stewart W, Celentano D, Reed M. Undiagnosed migraine headaches: A comparison of symptom-based and reported physician diagnosis. *Arch Intern Med* 1992;152:1273–1278.
37. Stang P, Osterhaus J. Impact of migraine in the United States: data from the National Health Interview Survey. *Headache* 1993;33:29–35.
38. Gobel H, Petersen-Braun M, Soyka D. The epidemiology of headache in Germany: A nationwide survey of a representative sample on the basis of the headache classification of the International Headache Society. *Cephalalgia* 1994;14:97–106.
39. Rasmussen B. Migraine and tension-type headache in a general population: Psychosocial factors. *Int J Epidemiol* 1992;21:1138–1143.
40. Stewart W, Schechter A, Lipton R. Migraine heterogeneity: Disability, pain intensity, and attack frequency and duration. *Neurology* 1994; 44(suppl):S24–S39.
41. Tarlov A, Ware J, Greenfield S, Nelson E, Perrin E, Zubkoff M. The Medical Outcomes Study: An application of methods for monitoring the results of medical care. *JAMA* 1989;262:925–930.
42. Solomon G, Skobieranda F, Gragg L. Quality of life and well-being of headache patients: Measurement by the medical outcomes study instrument. *Headache* 1993;33:351–358.
43. Osterhaus J, Townsend R, Gandek B, Ware J. Measuring functional status and well-being of patients with migraine headache. *Headache* 1994;34:337–343.

44. Terwindt G, Launer L, Ferrari M. The impact of migraine on quality of life in the general population: The GEM study. *Neurology* 1998; 50(suppl):A434.
45. Steiner TJ, Lipton RB, Liberman JN, Kolodner KB, Stewart WF. Work and family impact of migraine: A population-based case-control study. *Neurology* 1999;52(suppl):A470–A471.
46. Lipton R, Liberman J, Kolodner K, Dowson A, Sawyer J, Stewart W. Migraine headache disability and quality-of-life: A population-based case-control study. *Headache* 1999;39:365.
47. Lofland JH, Johnson NE, Batenhorst AS, Nash DB. Changes in resource use and outcomes for patients with migraine treated with sumatriptan. *Arch Intern Med* 1999;159:857–863.
48. Lofland J, Johnson N, Nash D, Batenhorst A. Improvements in managed care patients' health-related quality of life after sumatriptan (Imitrex). *Headache* 1998;38:391.
49. Jhingran P, Osterhaus J, Miller D, Lee J, Kirchdoerfer L. Development and validation of the Migraine-Specific Quality of Life Questionnaire. *Headache* 1998;38:295–302.
50. Clouse J, Osterhaus J. Healthcare resource use and costs associated with migraine in a managed healthcare setting. *Ann Pharmacother* 1994;28:659–664.
51. Edmeads J, Findlay H, Tugwell P, Pryse-Phillips W, Nelson R, Murray T. Impact of migraine and tension-type headache on life-style, consulting behavior, and medication use: A Canadian population survey. *Can J Neurol Sci* 1993;20:131–137.
52. Celentano D, Stewart W, Lipton R, Reed M. Medication use and disability among migraineurs: A national probability sample survey. *Headache* 1992;32:223–228.
53. Lipton R, Stewart W, Simon D. Medical consultation for migraine: Results of the American migraine study. *Headache* 1998;38:87–90.
54. Hu X, Markson L, Lipton R, Stewart W, Berger M. Burden of migraine in the United States: Disability and economic costs. *Arch Int Med* 1999; 159:813–818.
55. Lipton R, Stewart W, Kolodner K, Liberman J. Epidemiology and patterns of health care use for migraine in the United States. *Headache* 1999;39:363–364.
56. Osterhaus JT, Gutterman DL, Plachetka JR. Healthcare resource and lost labour costs of migraine headache in the US. *PharmacoEconomics* 1992;1:67–76.
57. Stewart W, Lipton R, Simon D. Work-related disability: Results from the American migraine study. *Cephalalgia* 1996;16:231–238.
58. Rasmussen B, Jensen R, Olesen J. Impact of headache on sickness absence and utilisation of medical services: A Danish population study. *J Epidemiol Community Health* 1992;46:443–446.
59. Schwartz B, Stewart W, Lipton R. Lost workdays and decreased work effectiveness associated with headache in the workplace. *J Occup Environ Med* 1997;39:320–327.
60. Von Korff M, Stewart WF, Simon DS, Lipton RB. Migraine and reduced work performance: A population-based diary study. *Neurology* 1998;50:1741–1745.
61. van Roijen L, Essink-Bot M, Koopmanschap M, Michel B, Rutten F. Societal perspective on the burden of migraine in the Netherlands. *PharmacoEconomics* 1995;7:170–179.
62. Castillo J, Munoz P, Guitera V, Pascual J. Epidemiology of chronic daily headache in the general population. *Headache* 1999;39:190–196.
63. Jabbar MA, Ogunniyi A. Sociodemographic factors and primary headache syndromes in a Saudi community. *Neuroepidemiology* 1997;16: 48–52.
64. Merikangas K, Whitaker A, Angst J. Validation of diagnostic criteria for migraine in the Zurich longitudinal cohort study. *Cephalalgia* 1993;13(suppl):47–53.
65. Mitsikostas D, Thomas A, Gatzonis S, Ilias A, Papageorgiou C. An epidemiological study of headache among the monks of Athos (Greece). *Headache* 1994;34:539–541.
66. Pereira Monteiro J, Matos E, Calheiros J. Headaches in medical school students. *Neuroepidemiology* 1994;13:103–107.
67. Roh J, Kim J, Ahn Y. Epidemiologic and clinical characteristics of migraine and tension-type headache in Korea. *Headache* 1998;38:356–365.
68. Srikiatkhachorn A. Epidemiology of headache in the Thai elderly: A study in the Bangkae home for the aged. *Headache* 1991;31:677–681.
69. Langemark M, Olesen J, Poulsen D, Bech P. Clinical characterization of patients with chronic tension headache. *Headache* 1988;28: 590–596.

CHAPTER 18 HISTORICAL FEATURES IN PRIMARY HEADACHE SYNDROMES

Gerald W. Smetana

Headache is a nearly universal symptom. As an example of the prevalence of headache, a study of 410 patients who had visited a primary care internal medicine practice found that headache was the fourth most common symptom and was exceeded only by fatigue, back pain, and dyspnea.[1] In an early study of over 1 million unselected individuals from the general population, headache was the single most common current symptom and was reported by 39% of men and 56% of women.[2] As physicians, nearly all of us have had personal experience with headache and can understand the headache descriptions that we hear from our patients. Chapter 17 elegantly details the prevalence of this common symptom and of common primary headache syndromes. Primary headaches are those without a pathologic basis.[3–5] These are benign recurring headaches of unknown cause. The most common primary headache syndromes are migraine, tension-type, and cluster headache. Secondary headaches are the result of an underlying pathologic cause.

When faced with the large numbers of patients who seek medical evaluation for headache, clinicians seek to identify the rare patient with a serious headache from the rest whose headache is benign in nature. Two general approaches assist this effort. Firstly, one must learn the warning symptoms and signs that suggest a pathologic cause for headache. Many published reviews have offered such advice.[4,6,7] A complementary approach is to learn to confidently diagnose benign primary headache syndromes through careful history taking and the systematic application of established diagnostic criteria. Primary headaches are clinical diagnoses that are based on history taking alone. With the exception of the occasional persistence of a partial Horner's syndrome among asymptomatic patients with a history of cluster headaches, the physical examination of a patient with primary headaches is normal during headache-free intervals.

The most commonly used criteria are the International Headache Society (IHS) classification and diagnostic criteria for headache disorders, cranial neuralgias, and facial pain.[8] The use of these criteria helps to identify uniform populations of patients for research and epidemiologic studies. The criteria themselves, however, are complicated, not easily committed to memory, and may be unnecessarily restrictive in the daily clinical care of patients.

When evaluating individual patients with headache, clinicians will benefit from understanding which historical features are most useful in establishing or excluding a particular primary headache diagnosis. In this chapter, I review and summarize published clinical series of patients with migraine, tension-type headache, and cluster headache to determine the sensitivity, specificity, and likelihood ratios of individual historical features.

IS THIS AN OLD OR NEW HEADACHE?

Clinicians may initially classify all headaches as either old or new. Old headaches are similar to those that have occurred repeatedly over time. Primary headaches are old headaches. New headaches are either headaches of recent onset or those that represent a change in the character or pattern of an old headache. A new headache may ultimately prove to be the first instance of a primary headache syndrome; however, clinicians cannot reach this conclusion with certainty until a pattern of similar headaches emerges over time.

A change in the intensity or frequency of an old headache is still an old headache. In this case, the physician must establish the precipitant for the increase in the severity of the old headache. A change in the quality, character, or descriptors of the headache, however, is a new headache. As an example, if a patient's headaches are typically unilateral and throbbing, a headache that is bilateral, constant, and progressive is a new headache. Most old headaches are benign, and the longer a headache syndrome has been present, the more likely it is to be benign.

VALUE OF HISTORY TAKING TO MINIMIZE DIAGNOSTIC IMAGING

In a cost-constrained environment, physicians must minimize the unnecessary use of diagnostic imaging in the evaluation of patients with headache. Neuroimaging is, by definition, normal or unhelpful in patients with primary headaches. A carefully obtained history of migraine, tension-type, or cluster headache minimizes the need for such testing. Several studies have confirmed the low yield of diagnostic imaging among patients with clinical diagnoses of primary headache syndromes.

The history and physical examination may identify patients who need no further diagnostic evaluation. A retrospective study evaluated 592 patients with headache and normal neurologic examinations who had been referred for cranial computed tomography (CT) studies.[9] There were no cases of intracranial pathology sufficient to explain headache in this entire group. Mitchell and coworkers studied 350 patients with headache who were referred by their clinicians for head CT studies.[10] Among the 320 patients with normal neurologic examinations, there were only three clinically significant CT abnormalities. Each of these three patients had a headache of recent onset with worrisome atypical features.

In 1994, the American Academy of Neurology reviewed the role of neuroimaging in the evaluation of patients with headache and normal neurologic examinations.[11] The incidence of clinically important pathologic findings among patients with normal neurologic examinations and migraine or unspecified headache was 0.4% and 2.4%, respectively. They recommended no routine imaging for patients with typical migraine who had no recent change in pattern, seizures, or focal neurologic signs. They acknowledged insufficient evidence, but suggested that neuroimaging may be indicated for patients with atypical headache patterns, seizures, or focal neurologic signs or symptoms.

More recently, the US Headache Consortium reviewed the incidence of significant intracranial abnormalities in patients with migraine or tension-type headache and normal neurologic examinations.[12] They found only two abnormal imaging studies among 1,086 patients with migraine and no abnormal studies among 83 patients with tension headache. In contrast, among patients with unspecified types of headaches and normal neurologic examinations, the prevalence of significant intracranial abnormalities on imaging studies varied from 0% to 6.7%. These reports confirm the importance of careful history taking to identify patients for whom the yield of imaging is sufficiently low that clinicians can establish a clinical diagnosis without further study.

In the same review, focal neurologic symptoms, rapidly increasing frequency of headaches, headaches causing awakening from sleep, lack of coordination, subjective numbness or tingling, and headache with Valsalva maneuver each predicted a significantly higher likelihood of intracranial pathology. By definition, clinicians should not make a diagnosis of a primary headache syndrome if the neurologic examination is abnormal. An abnormal neurologic examination confers a positive likelihood ratio of 3.0 (CI 2.3-4.0) for a significant abnormality on neuroimaging.[12]

MIGRAINE

Migraine headaches are common. In a review by Stewart and colleagues of four prevalence studies that used the IHS criteria, overall migraine prevalence was 6% among men and 16% among women.[13] The initial onset of migraine headaches most commonly occurs during between the ages of 10 and 25 years. Migraine headaches occur for the first time after age 40 uncommonly. In one incidence study, for example, 77% of patients with migraine first sought medical attention for migraine before age 40.[14] The new appearance of a migraine-like headache in a person over age 40 should prompt consideration of other possible diagnoses. Hamelsky and colleagues characterize migraine prevalence in more detail in Chapter 17.

In practice, clinicians most commonly entertain the diagnoses of migraine and tension-type headache for patients with longstanding recurring headaches. Although less common than tension-type headache, migraine is more likely to cause sufferers to be disabled by their headaches and to seek medical attention for their symptoms.[15]

Clinical Features

Tables 18-1 and 18-2 list the IHS criteria for the diagnosis of migraine without aura and migraine with aura, respectively. The principal historical features are headaches that are unilateral, throbbing, moderate to severe in intensity, and worse with ordinary physical activity; last from 4 to 72 hours; and are associated with nausea, photophobia, and phonophobia. All of these features are, however, not equally useful to clinicians in establishing a diagnosis of migraine. Table 18-3 summarizes reported clinical series that detailed the frequency of particular clinical features in patients with migraine and tension-type headache. These data were pooled from multiple series published over the past four decades. All studies were classified as to their use of the IHS diagnostic criteria or other criteria. Sensitivity, specificity, and likelihood ratios were calculated for the diagnosis of migraine as compared with tension-type headache. A positive likelihood ratio indicates the increase in the odds of the diagnosis of migraine if the particular feature is present. A negative likelihood ratio indicates the decrease in the odds of the diagnosis of migraine if the feature is absent.

TABLE 18-1 **International Headache Society Criteria for the Diagnosis of Migraine Without Aura**

A. At least 5 attacks fulfilling B–D.

B. Headache attacks lasting 4–72 hours (untreated or unsuccessfully treated)

C. Headache has at least two of the following characteristics:
   1. Unilateral location
   2. Pulsating quality
   3. Moderate or severe intensity that inhibits or prohibits daily activities
   4. Aggravation by walking stairs or similar routine physical activity

D. During headache at least one of the following:
   1. Nausea and/or vomiting
   2. Photophobia and phonophobia

E. At least one of the following:
   1. History, physical, and neurologic examinations do not suggest a secondary or pathologic cause for headache
   2. History and/or physical, and/or neurologic examinations do suggest such disorder, but it is ruled out by appropriate investigations
   3. Such disorder is present, but migraine attacks do not occur for the first time in close temporal relation to the disorder

Adapted from *Cephalalgia* 1988;8(suppl):1–96, by permission of Scandinavian University Press.

Nausea, exacerbation by physical activity, photophobia, and throbbing headache are the most sensitive features for the diagnosis of migraine. Sensitivities are 81%, 81%, 79%, and 73%, respectively. Despite the origin of the word *migraine* from "hemicrania," only 65% of migraines are unilateral, and this is the least

TABLE 18-2 **International Headache Society Criteria for the Diagnosis of Migraine With Aura**

A. At least two migraine attacks with at least 3 of the following 4 characteristics:
   1. One or more fully reversible aura symptoms indicating focal cerebral cortical and/or brainstem dysfunction.
   2. At least one aura symptom develops gradually over more than 4 minutes or, 2 or more symptoms occur in succession.
   3. No aura symptom lasts more than 60 minutes. If more than one aura symptom is present, accepted duration is proportionately increased.
   4. Headache follows aura with a free interval of less than 60 minutes. It may also begin before or simultaneously with aura.

B. No evidence of secondary or pathologic cause for headache as defined in migraine without aura

C. Migraine with typical aura is diagnosed when in addition to the above criteria, all four criteria under A are met, and one or more of the following types of aurae is present:
   1. Homonymous visual disturbance
   2. Unilateral paresthesias and/or numbness
   3. Unilateral weakness
   4. Aphasia or unclassifiable speech difficulty

Adapted from *Cephalalgia* 1988;8(suppl):1–96, by permission of Scandinavian University Press.

TABLE 18-3 **Headache Features in Migraine With or Without Aura Versus Tension-type Headache (TTH)**

			% (total number of patients)			
Clinical Feature*	Study Selection†	References	Sensitivity for Diagnosis of Migraine	Specificity for Diagnosis of Migraine When Compared with TTH	Positive Likelihood Ratio for the Diagnosis of Migraine (CI)‡	Negative Likelihood Ratio for the Diagnosis of Migraine (CI)
Nausea	IHS	16–29	82 (5,531)	96 (1,443)	23.2 (17.7–30.4)	0.19 (0.18–0.20)
	All		81 (7,780)	96 (1,474)	19.2 (15.0–24.5)	0.20 (0.19–0.21)
Photophobia	IHS	16, 19–29	79 (5,182)	87 (1,443)	6.0 (5.2–6.8)	0.24 (0.23–0.26)
	All		79 (6,524)	86 (1,474)	5.8 (5.1–6.6)	0.25 (0.24–0.26)
Phonophobia	IHS	20, 21, 23, 24, 26–29	69 (2,188)			
	All		67 (3,632)	87 (1,443)	5.2 (4.5–5.9)	0.38 (0.36–0.40)
Exacerbation by physical activity	All	20, 22, 23, 26–28, 30	81 (3,032)	78 (1,843)	3.7 (3.4–4.0)	0.24 (0.23–0.26)
Unilateral	IHS	16–18, 20–23, 25–32	66 (5,925)	78 (1,874)	3.1 (2.8–3.3)	0.43 (0.41–0.45)
	All		65 (8,832)	82 (2,874)	3.7 (3.4–3.9)	0.43 (0.41–0.44)
Throbbing or pulsating	IHS	18, 20–23, 25–32	76 (5,925)	77 (1,874)	3.3 (3.1–3.6)	0.32 (0.30–0.33)
	All		73 (7,832)	75 (2,874)	2.9 (2.7–3.1)	0.36 (0.34–0.37)
Duration 4–24 h	All	16, 26, 32, 33	57 (785)	67 (499)	1.7 (1.5–2.0)	0.64 (0.58–0.71)
Duration 24–72 h	All	26, 32, 33	13 (497)	91 (499)	1.4 (1.0–2.0)	0.96 (0.92–1.0)
Duration < 4 h	All	26, 33	26 (628)	51 (499)	0.52 (0.44–0.61)	1.5 (1.3–1.6)

*In descending order of positive likelihood ratios using data from all studies.

†IHS indicates pooled data from only those studies that used the IHS criteria as the reference standard.

‡95% confidence interval (CI).

Adapted with permission from: Smetana GW. The diagnostic value of historical features in primary headache syndromes: A comprehensive review. *Arch Intern Med* 2000;160:2729–2737. Copyright © 2000, American Medical Association.

sensitive of the major clinical criteria. When compared with tension-type headache, the most specific features for migraine are nausea, phonophobia, photophobia, and unilateral headache, with specificities of 96%, 87%, 86%, and 82%, respectively.

The features with the best overall predictive value are nausea, photophobia, phonophobia, and exacerbation by physical activity. The particularly high positive predictive value of nausea results in part from the inclusion of large numbers of patients who were classified according the IHS criteria. The IHS criteria for the diagnosis of tension-type headache require the absence of nausea. However, questionnaire studies that have used less restrictive criteria for the diagnosis of tension-type headache have also found nausea to be highly specific.[34,35] Headache duration is less useful to distinguish between the two diagnoses, with the exception that headaches lasting less than 4 hours are less likely to be migraine.

Authors used many different diagnostic criteria for migraine and tension-type headache in the pre-IHS era. Despite these varied definitions, the likelihood ratios for all pooled studies are not substantially different than those restricted to studies using the IHS criteria. The data suggest that the pre-IHS studies also included fairly uniform populations of patients.

Features of Migraine Aura Among patients with migraine, one third experience migraine with aura. In a study of 4,000 randomly selected 40-year-olds in a Danish population, the lifetime prevalence of migraine without aura was 11.8%; that of migraine with aura was 5.5%.[36] The migraine aura is sufficiently characteristic that a carefully obtained history of an aura substantially increases confidence in the diagnosis of migraine. Both the subjective aura elements and the duration of the aura are important features. Table 18-4 summarizes the sensitivity of various aura features among pooled series of patients having migraine with aura.

Visual auras are most common; 84% of patients having migraine with aura experience a visual aura. Positive visual phenomena occur slightly more frequently than negative visual phenomena. Positive phenomena include zigzags (fortification spectra), stars, or flashes. Many eloquent descriptions of visual auras exist in the medical literature. In an early review of migrainous visual aura, Alvarez described his personal experience of fortification spectra.[42] "Another time I saw a fine zigzag line running up and down and a coarse one running below it, horizontally. Later, the two ran together, end to end, and bowed out to the right. The line resembles a snake fence, or an old-style fortification with projecting angles. In some spells, the line is so brilliant one can see it easily with the eyes open."*

* Reprinted from the *American Journal of Ophthalmology,* vol. 49, Alvarez WC. The migrainous scotoma as studied in 618 persons, pp. 489–504. Copyright 1960, with permission from Elsevier Science.

TABLE 18-4 **Sensitivity of Aura Features Among Patients Having Migraine With Aura**

Feature	References	Sensitivity % (total number of patients)
Any visual aura	22, 30, 37–39	84 (1,477)
Positive visual phenomena		
Any	30, 37, 39	74 (390)
Zigzags (fortification spectra)	38–40	56 (340)
Stars or flashes	38, 39	83 (263)
Negative visual phenomena		
Any	37, 39, 41	56 (383)
Scotoma	38–40	40 (340)
Hemianopsia	39, 40	7 (177)
Disturbance of visual perception	30, 37, 39, 41	20 (490)
Duration of visual aura		
<30 min	37–39	70 (400)
30–60 min	37–39	18 (400)
>60 min	37–39	7 (369)
Visual aura without headache	38, 42	12 (781)
Sensory aura	22, 30, 37, 38,40	20 (1,454)
Aphasia	22, 30, 37, 38	11 (1,377)
Motor aura	22, 37, 38,40	4 (1,325)

Adapted with permission from: Smetana GW. The diagnostic value of historical features in primary headache syndromes: A comprehensive review. *Arch Intern Med* 2000;160:2729–2737. Copyright © 2000, American Medical Association.

Negative visual phenomena include scotoma and hemianopsia. The presence of hemianopsia is one of the features that establishes a diagnosis of migraine with typical aura (previously referred to as complicated migraine). Disturbances of visual perception are least common. In the study of Queiroz and colleagues,[39] these included, in descending order of frequency, foggy vision, looking through heat waves or water, tunnel vision, mosaic vision, micropsia or macropsia, corona phenomena, and complex hallucinations. Lewis Carroll, the author of *Alice in Wonderland,* was known to suffer from migraine with aura; some authors have speculated that Alice's visual distortions in his novel may have paralleled complex visual hallucinations that he experienced during migrainous auras.[43]

The duration of the aura is also characteristic. IHS criteria require that each aura feature last from 4 to 60 minutes. In practice, the most common aura duration is 20 minutes, and 70% of visual auras last less than 30 minutes (see Table 18-4). Auras that last a few seconds or minutes are distinctly uncommon in migraine and should raise the possibility of seizure phenomena.

Nonvisual auras nearly always occur in conjunction with visual auras rather than as isolated events. In one study, only 4% of auras were complex nonvisual auras that occurred in isolation without accompanying visual auras.[37] Among nonvisual auras, sensory auras are most common, followed by aphasia and motor auras. The sensitivities are 20%, 11%, and 4%, respectively. Sensory auras are unilateral, usually begin in the hand, and then progress to the arm, face, and tongue.[38] Aphasic aura symptoms include paraphasia, impaired production of language, and impaired comprehension of language. Motor auras usually occur in conjunction with sensory auras rather than in isolation.

Historical Features of Migraineurs

Individuals with migraine are more likely to have a family history of migraine, and a childhood history of vomiting attacks or motion sickness. Although these factors, by themselves, are insufficient to establish a diagnosis of migraine, they can be useful in the evaluation of an individual patient if the type of primary headache remains uncertain after taking a careful history.

Of these features, the familial tendency is the least controversial. In a recent review of over 2,500 patients with data on family history, 58% of migraineurs had a family history of migraine as compared with 12% of unselected individuals without headache.[44] In a case-control study, Stewart and colleagues reported a relative risk of 1.50 among family members of probands with migraine.[45] A positive family history was more often present among patients with severe migraine and disability. Russell and coworkers noted different family histories among patients having migraine without aura and those having migraine with aura.[46] In their study of 183 patients, migraine without aura was associated with a 2.9 relative risk of family history of migraine without aura, but no increase in risk of migraine with aura. Patients having migraine with aura were twice as likely to have family histories of both migraine with and without aura than expected.

Neither childhood vomiting attacks nor motion sickness are criteria for the diagnosis of migraine in the IHS classification. However, each of these features is more common in patients destined to develop migraine that in those without migraine. Thirty-two percent of patients with migraine report a history of childhood vomiting attacks as compared with only 14% of individuals without headaches.[44] Data for a history of motion sickness are similar. Children who develop disabling headaches by the age of 5 years are 2.8 times more likely to report motion sickness than those without disabling headaches.[47] In addition, children with migraines score significantly higher on a motion sickness susceptibility questionnaire than children without migraines.[48]

TENSION-TYPE HEADACHE

Tension-type headache is considerably more common than migraine. Thirty-six percent of men and 46% of women suffer from episodic tension-type headache (see Chapter 17). Patients with tension-type headache are, however, less likely to seek medical attention than are those with migraine because their headaches are less frequently disabling.

The IHS criteria define tension-type headache largely as a chronic recurring headache with few or no migrainous features (Table 18-5). Tension-type headache is diagnosed based as much on the absence of particular features as the presence of specific historical features. The principal features are headaches that are pressing or tightening, mild or moderate (not severe) in intensity, and bilateral, and are not associated with nausea, photophobia, phonophobia, or aggravation by ordinary physical activity. Table 18-3 summarizes the prevalence of these features (1-specificity) based on pooled data from clinical series. The IHS criteria are restrictive and do not permit the diagnosis of tension-type headache if nausea is present or if both phonophobia and photophobia are present. As such, published series that report the frequency of particular clinical features run the risk of circular reasoning. Few series precede the publication of the IHS criteria so it is difficult to determine if specific clinical features would be equally frequent using less restrictive criteria.

TABLE 18-5 **International Headache Society Criteria for the Diagnosis of Tension-type Headache**

A. Subtypes of tension-type headache
   1. Episodic tension-type headache:
      At least 10 previous headache episodes fulfilling criteria B–D.
      Headaches are present for less than 15 days per month.
   2. Chronic tension-type headache:
      Headache fulfilling criteria B–D with an average frequency of at least 15 days per month for at least 6 months
B. Headache lasting from 30 minutes to 7 days
C. At least two of the following pain characteristics:
   1. Pressing/tightening (nonpulsating) quality
   2. Mild or moderate intensity, which may inhibit but does not prohibit activities
   3. Bilateral location
   4. No aggravation by walking stairs or similar routine activity
D. Both of the following:
   1. No nausea or vomiting (anorexia may occur)
   2. Photophobia and phonophobia are absent, or one but not the other is present
E. No evidence of secondary or pathologic cause for headache as defined in migraine without aura

Adapted from *Cephalalgia* 1988;8(suppl):1–96, by permission of Scandinavian University Press.

Although the IHS criteria allow tension-type headaches to last from 30 minutes to 7 days, Ulrich and colleagues studied 499 patients with tension-type headache and found that 82% of patients reported headache duration of less than 24 hours.[26] Chronic recurring headaches that usually last more than 72 hours are more likely to be tension-type than migraine, but this occurrence is rare. In general, the duration of headache episodes is not useful as a distinguishing feature between the two diagnoses.

The differential diagnosis of tension-type headache includes several secondary causes for headache. Cervicogenic headache, temporomandibular joint (TMJ) dysfunction, and temporal arteritis may occasionally be confused with tension-type headache. Cervicogenic headache is suggested by a predominantly occipital and occasionally frontal location in addition to neck pain. This headache is more commonly daily as opposed to episodic and may occur for the first time in an older individual more than 50 years of age. In contrast, the peak prevalence of tension-type headache is in individuals aged 30 to 39 years,[49] and the first occurrence is most commonly in the teens or twenties.

TMJ dysfunction is suggested by a temporal location of pain, morning headaches, bruxism with excessive dental wear, and jaw pain. These features help to distinguish it from tension-type headache. The headache of temporal arteritis is variable but, similar to that of tension-type headache, is commonly pressing, bilateral, and without migrainous features.[50] The most important factor that distinguishes the headache of temporal arteritis from that of tension-type headache is the later age at onset. Physicians should consider this possibility in any patient with a new-onset headache who is older than 50 years.

CLUSTER HEADACHE

Cluster headache is a distinct syndrome that is easily recognized by clinicians familiar with its historical features. It is the least common primary headache syndrome. The prevalence has not been well studied but was found to be 0.1% in a single report of nearly 10,000 18-year-old men.[51] Given the mean age of onset of this disorder at age 30,[52–54] the actual prevalence is probably higher and may be as high as 0.4% to 1.0% among men.[55] Table 18-6 lists the IHS criteria for the diagnosis of cluster headache. The principal features are headaches that are severe, unilateral, and supraorbital or temporal; last from 15 to 180 minutes; and are associated with autonomic symptoms on the involved side.

Table 18-7 outlines the sensitivity of particular clinical features of cluster headaches and was derived by pooling data from published clinical series. With one exception, all of the large clinical series of patients with cluster headache precede the development of the IHS criteria. The most commonly used criteria for these series were the Ad hoc criteria,[68] which were published in 1962.

Cluster headache is the only primary headache syndrome that is more common in men than in women; the male:female ratio is

TABLE 18-6 **International Headache Society Criteria for the Diagnosis of Cluster Headache**

A. At least 5 attacks fulfilling B–D

B. Severe unilateral orbital, supraorbital, and/or temporal pain lasting 15–180 minutes untreated

C. Headache is associated with at least one of the following signs, which have to be present on the pain-side:
   1. Conjunctival injection
   2. Lacrimation
   3. Nasal congestion
   4. Rhinorrhea
   5. Forehead and facial sweating
   6. Miosis
   7. Ptosis
   8. Eyelid edema

D. Frequency of attacaks: from 1 every other day to 8 per day

E. No evidence of secondary or pathologic cause for headache as defined in migraine without aura

Adapted from *Cephalalgia* 1988;8(suppl):1–96, by permission of Scandinavian University Press.

6:1. In contrast to patients with migraine, a family history of migraine or other primary headache syndrome is no more common among patients with cluster headache than among individuals without headache. The pain is ocular in 80% of patients; the next most common locations are temporal, frontal, and maxillary. The pain is, by definition, strictly unilateral. Interestingly, in individual patients the headache commonly occurs on the same side.[54,64] In the pooled data, 48% of patients experience their headaches exclusively on the right side, 38% exclusively on the left side, and only 14% of patients on both sides over their lifetimes. The onset of the headaches is rapid, and the most common duration of each headache is 30 to 60 minutes. This is an important distinguishing characteristic from migraine headaches, which nearly always last for at least 4 hours.

These headaches are called cluster headaches because of their tendency to cluster over the lifetime of each patient. In between each cluster, patients are completely asymptomatic. In 57% of patients, each cluster lasts from 1 to 2 months, and the most common cluster frequency is 1 to 2 per year. A patient with cluster headache often reports that during a cluster, each headache occurs at the same time of the day. Nocturnal headaches are most common and are reported by 54% of patients.

The character of the pain is variable and is less helpful to clinicians who seek to make a diagnosis of cluster headache. Tradition holds that cluster headaches are piercing or neuralgic. However the pooled data indicate that only 30% of patients describe their headaches in such a fashion; this is identical to the percentage of patients that report their cluster headaches as throbbing. The pain is excruciating and sufficiently distracting that most patients cannot continue their daily routine during an episode. Patients commonly pace the room and appear restless and agitated to observers.[69] This behavior is in contrast to that of patients with migraine, who usually prefer to rest in a dark, quiet room.

Among ipsilateral autonomic symptoms, lacrimation is experienced by 76% of patients. Next most common are rhinorrhea and a partial Horner's syndrome (miosis and ptosis). The partial Horner's syndrome may persist after resolution of the headache. The differential diagnosis of cluster headache includes trigeminal neuralgia. Clinicians may distinguish trigeminal neuralgia from cluster headache by its briefer duration of seconds to several minutes, the absence of autonomic features, and the lack of periodicity.

HEADACHE PRECIPITANTS

Many patients with recurring primary headaches recognize that certain triggers often precipitate their headaches. Clinicians may be tempted to use these triggers as clues to particular headache diagnoses. Table 18-8 summarizes the published experience on the sensitivity of particular headache precipitants among patients with migraine and tension-type headaches. The only triggers that are significantly more frequent among patients with migraine are chocolate, cheese, and any food. Using pooled data from all series, the positive likelihood ratios for these findings are 7.1, 4.9, and 3.6, respectively. Other precipitants that are present in at least 30% of patients with migraine include stress, alcohol, weather change, menses, missing a meal, lack of sleep, and perfume or odors. None of these triggers is significantly more common among patients with migraine than those with tension-type headache. These data, however, are limited by the relatively small numbers of patients with tension-type headache for whom there are reports of trigger frequency.

The finding that menstrual variation of headache is no more common among patients with migraine than with tension-type headache is particularly surprising but is based on observations of only 221 women with tension-type headache. Most clinicians find this clinical feature to be useful in suggesting a diagnosis of migraine. Migraines occur most commonly in the several days before the onset of menses.[24,79]

Caffeine withdrawal may precipitate headaches both in patients with and in those without a history of primary headaches, but they occur more commonly in patients with a background of primary headaches.[80–82] No data suggest that the development of caffeine-withdrawal headaches distinguishes patients with migraine from those with tension-type headache.

A recent study compared the frequency of precipitating factors for 366 patients with IHS-diagnosed migraine with that of 169 nonmigraineurs.[77] Presumably the nonmigraineurs suffered from tension-type headaches, but they were not required to meet the IHS definition for tension-type headache. Fatigue, stress, certain food or drinks, menstruation, and weather were all significantly more common triggers for patients with migraine than for those without migraine. The stronger association of these factors with migraine than in the pooled data of Table 18-8 may reflect a more heterogeneous population of patients in the nonmigraine category that included patients who would not meet the IHS definition for tension-type headache.

The most common triggers for cluster headache are alcohol and stress. These occur in 32% and 30% of patients, respectively (see Table 18-7). These values are similar to those reported for tension-type and migraine headache and are not helpful in differential diagnosis. From a review of these data, one can conclude that the decision not to include headache triggers in the IHS criteria was

TABLE 18-7 **Sensitivity of Clinical Features Among Patients With Cluster Headache**

Clinical Feature	References	Sensitivity % (total number of patients)
Male gender	52–54, 56–61	86 (1,634)
Family history of primary headache	54, 57, 58, 60, 62–65	26 (1,131)
Location of pain		
Ocular	57, 58, 62–64, 66	80 (952)
Temporal	54, 57, 58, 62–64	72 (846)
Frontal	54, 57, 58, 64	69 (768)
Maxillary	54, 57, 63, 64	30 (766)
Laterality of pain		
Right	54, 57, 58, 63, 64	48 (826)
Left	54, 57, 58, 63, 64	38 (826)
Either	54, 57, 58, 63, 64	14 (826)
Duration of headache		
<30 min	58, 63, 64, 66, 67	11 (795)
30–60 min	58, 64, 66, 67	43 (741)
1–2 h	58, 64, 66, 67	32 (741)
2–3 h	58, 63, 64, 66, 67	10 (795)
Cluster duration of 4–8 wk	54, 58, 61, 64, 67	57 (733)
Cluster frequency of 1–2/yr	54, 58, 61, 64, 67	66 (807)
Nocturnal headaches	54, 58, 62, 67	54 (395)
Headache triggers:		
Alcohol	54, 58, 60–63	32 (446)
Stress	54, 60, 62–64	30 (769)
Character of pain		
Throbbing	54, 57, 58, 62	30 (395)
Neuralgic	54, 57, 62	30 (335)
Ipsilateral lacrimation	54, 57, 58, 62–64	76 (503)
Rhinorrhea	54, 57, 58, 62–64	51 (503)
Nausea	54, 57, 58, 61–64	35 (554)
Partial Horner's syndrome	54, 57, 58, 63, 64	37 (453)

Adapted with permission from: Smetana GW. The diagnostic value of historical features in primary headache syndromes: A comprehensive review. *Arch Intern Med* 2000;160:2729–2737.

appropriate. Obtaining a careful history of headache triggers is most useful to guide subsequent advice to patients related to lifestyle changes that may decrease headache frequency. With the exception of chocolate, cheese, and any food, this information does not make a particular headache diagnosis more or less likely.

SUMMARY

Nausea, photophobia, phonophobia, and exacerbation by physical activity confer the highest positive likelihood ratio for the diagnosis of migraine when compared with tension-type headache. Nausea, exacerbation by physical activity, photophobia, and throbbing headache confer the highest negative likelihood ratio, and their absence makes the diagnosis of migraine significantly less likely. Headache duration is not a useful distinguishing feature.

Among the one third of patients with migraine who experience an aura, visual symptoms are most common, occurring in 84% of patients. Positive visual phenomena, including zigzags and stars or flashes, are more common than negative visual phenomena. Sensory, aphasic, and motor auras are each less common and nearly always occur in conjunction with a visual aura, rather than in isolation.

Headache precipitants are helpful when counseling individual patients about nonpharmacologic approaches to headache management. Only chocolate, cheese, and any food significantly increase the odds that a particular headache is migraine. Other com-

TABLE 18-8 **Headache Precipitants in Migraine With or Without Aura Versus Tension-type Headache (TTH)**

			% (total number of patients)			
Precipitant*	**Study Selection†**	**References**	**Sensitivity for Diagnosis of Migraine**	**Specificity for Diagnosis of Migraine When Compared with TTH**	**Positive Likelihood Ratio for the Diagnosis of Migraine (CI)‡**	**Negative Likelihood Ratio for the Diagnosis of Migraine (CI)**
Chocolate	IHS	26, 70–73	22 (69)	95 (384)	4.6 (2.5–8.8)	0.82 (0.73–0.93)
	All		33 (3,252)	95 (384)	7.1 (4.5–11.2)	0.70 (0.68–0.73)
Cheese	All	70–73	38 (3,252)	92 (52)	4.9 (1.9–12.5)	0.68 (0.62–0.73)
Any food	IHS	16, 24, 25, 70, 71, 74–77	24 (1,157)	86 (407)	1.7 (1.3–2.3)	0.88 (0.84–0.93)
	All		49 (5,020)	86 (407)	3.6 (2.8–4.6)	0.59 (0.56–0.62)
Stress	IHS	24–26, 71, 73–75, 77	50 (797)	57 (751)	1.2 (1.0–1.3)	0.88 (0.80–0.97)
	All		60 (2,008)	57 (751)	1.4 (1.3–1.5)	0.70 (0.65–0.76)
Alcohol	IHS	25, 26, 60, 70, 71, 73, 74, 76	30 (778)	77 (622)	1.3 (1.1–1.6)	0.91 (0.85–0.97)
	All		29 (3,710)	77 (678)	1.3 (1.1–1.5)	0.92 (0.88–0.96)
Weather change	IHS	24, 71, 73–75, 77	31 (554)	74 (388)	1.2 (1.0–1.5)	0.93 (0.86–1.0)
	All		35 (1,765)	74 (388)	1.4 (1.1–1.6)	0.87 (0.82–0.94)
Menses	IHS	16, 17, 24, 25, 60, 71–75, 78, 79	44 (374)	56 (165)	1.0 (0.80–1.2)	1.0 (0.86–1.2)
	All		56 (4,008)	54 (221)	1.2 (1.0–1.4)	0.82 (0.72–0.93)
Missing a meal	All	70, 73, 75	62 (2,876)	46 (32)	1.1 (0.89–1.8)	0.83 (0.61–1.1)
Lack of sleep	All	24, 26, 71, 73, 75, 77	31 (1,646)	62 (553)	0.83 (0.73–0.94)	1.1 (1.0–1.2)
Perfume or odors	All	73, 75	32 (563)	44 (52)	0.58 (0.44–0.76)	1.5 (1.1–2.1)

*In descending order of positive likelihood ratios using data from all studies.

†IHS indicates pooled data from only those studies that used the IHS criteria as the reference standard.

‡95% confidence interval (CI).

Adapted with permission from: Smetana GW. The diagnostic value of historical features in primary headache syndromes: A comprehensive review. *Arch Intern Med* 2000;160:2729–2737.

monly reported triggers, including menses, stress, alcohol, missing a meal, fatigue, and weather change, are equally common among patients with tension-type and migraine headache. Alcohol and stress are the most common triggers of cluster headache but are not helpful in establishing this diagnosis.

Cluster headache is a distinct headache syndrome that is easy to distinguish from the other two primary headache syndromes. It is strictly unilateral, periorbital, lasts most commonly less than 2 hours, occurs primarily in men, and is associated with ipsilateral lacrimation, rhinorrhea, ptosis, and miosis. The most common cluster duration is 1 to 2 months, and affected patients have symptom-free intervals that average 6 to 9 months.

The use of the IHS criteria for diagnosing patients with suspected primary headache syndromes ensures homogeneous populations of patients for inclusion in studies. Practicing clinicians, however, may find these criteria too complicated and restrictive. This chapter identifies those clinical features that are most useful to suggest or exclude particular primary headache diagnoses.

REFERENCES

1. Kroenke K, Arrington ME, Mangelsdorff AD. The prevalence of symptoms in medical outpatients and the adequacy of therapy. *Arch Intern Med* 1990;150:1685.
2. Hammond EC. Some preliminary findings on physical complaints from a prospective study of 1,064,004 men and women. *Am J Publ Health* 1964;54:11.
3. Marks DR, Rapoport AM. Practical evaluation and diagnosis of headache. *Semin Neurol* 1997;17:307.
4. Dalessio DJ. Diagnosing the severe headache. *Neurology* 1994; 44(suppl):S6.
5. Solomon GD, Cady RK, Klapper JA, et al. National Headache Foundation: Standards of care for treating headache in primary care practice. *Cleve Clin J Med* 1997;64:373.
6. Couch JR. Headache to worry about. *Med Clin North Am* 1993;77: 141.
7. Dodick D. Headache as a symptom of ominous disease. What are the warning signals? *Postgrad Med* 1997;101:46.
8. Headache Classification Committee of the International Headache Society: Classification and diagnostic criteria for headache disorders, cranial neuralgias and facial pain. *Cephalalgia* 1988;8(suppl):1.
9. Akpek S, Arac M, Atilla S, et al. Cost-effectiveness of computed tomography in the evaluation of patients with headache. *Headache* 1995; 35:228.
10. Mitchell CS, Osborn RE, Grosskreutz SR. Computed tomography in the headache patient: Is routine evaluation really necessary? *Headache* 1993;33:82.
11. Quality Standards Subcommittee of the American Academy of Neurology. Practice parameter: The utility of neuroimaging in the evaluation of headache in patients with normal neurologic examinations (summary statement). *Neurology* 1994;44:1353.

12. Frishberg BM, Rosenberg JH, Matchar DB, et al, US Headache Consortium. Evidence-based guidelines in the primary care setting: Neuroimaging in patients with nonacute headache. American Academy of Neurology; 2000. Available at http://www.aan.com.
13. Stewart WF, Shechter A, Rasmussen BK. Migraine prevalence: A review of population-based studies. *Neurology* 1994;44(suppl):S17.
14. Stang PE, Yanagihara T, Swanson JW, et al. Incidence of migraine headache: A population-based study in Olmsted County, Minnesota. *Neurology* 1992;42:1657.
15. Silberstein SB, Lipton RB. Headache epidemiology: Emphasis on migraine. *Neurol Clin* 1996;14:421.
16. Selby G, Lance JW. Observations on 500 cases of migraine and allied vascular headache. *J Neurol Neurosurg Psychiat* 1960;23:23.
17. Lance JW, Anthony M. Some clinical aspects of migraine. A prospective survey of 500 patients. *Arch Neurol* 1966;15:356.
18. Olesen J. Some clinical features of the acute migraine attack. An analysis of 750 patients. *Headache* 1978;18:268.
19. Manzoni GC, Farina S, Lanfranchi M, et al. Classic migraine—clinical findings in 164 patients. *Eur Neurol* 1985;24:163.
20. Rasmussen BK, Jensen R, Olesen J. A population-based analysis of the diagnostic criteria of the International Headache Society. *Cephalalagia* 1991;11:129.
21. Lipton RB, Stewart WF, Celentano DD, et al. Undiagnosed migraine headaches: A comparison of symptom-based and reported physician diagnoses. *Arch Intern Med* 1992;152:1273.
22. Dahlof C, Riman E. How does the International Headache Society classification perform in a European headache clinic? In: Olesen J, ed. *Headache Classification and Epidemiology.* New York, NY: Raven Press; 1994:77.
23. Wober-Bingol C, Wober C, Karwautz A, et al. Diagnosis of headache in childhood and adolescence: A study in 437 patients. *Cephalalgia* 1995;15:13.
24. Silberstein SB. Migraine symptoms: Results of a survey of self-reported migraineurs. *Headache* 1995;35:387.
25. Rothrock J, Patel M, Lyden P, et al. Demographic and clinical characteristics of patients with episodic migraine versus chronic daily headache. *Cephalalgia* 1996;16:44.
26. Ulrich V, Russell MB, Jensen R, et al. A comparison of tension-type headache in migraineurs and in non-migraineurs: A population-based study. *Pain* 1996;67:501.
27. Wober-Bingol C, Wober C, Karwautz A, et al. Tension-type headache in different age groups at two headache centers. *Pain* 1996;67:53.
28. Lavados PM, Tenhamm E. Epidemiology of migraine headache in Santiago, Chile: A prevalence study. *Cephalalagia* 1997;17:770.
29. Lipton RB, Stewart WF, Simon D. Medical consultation for migraine: Results from the American Migraine Study. *Headache* 1998;38:87.
30. Roh JK, Kim JS, Ahn YO. Epidemiologic and clinical characteristics of migraine and tension-type headache in Korea. *Headache* 1998;38:256.
31. Friedman AP, von Storch TJC, Merritt HH. Migraine and tension headaches. A clinical study of two thousand cases. *Neurology* 1954;4:773.
32. Phanthumchinda K, Sithi-Amorn C. Prevalence and clinical features of migraine: A community survey in Bangkok, Thailand. *Headache* 1989;29:594.
33. Henry P, Michel P, Brochet B, et al. A nationwide survey of migraine in France: Prevalence and clinical features in adults. *Cephalalgia* 1992;12:229.
34. Michel P, Henry P, Letenneur L, et al. Diagnostic screen for assessment of the IHS criteria for migraine by general practitioners. *Cephalalgia* 1993;13(suppl):54.
35. Gervil M, Ulrich V, Olesen J, et al. Screening for migraine in the general population: Validation of a simple questionnaire. *Cephalalgia* 1998;18:342.
36. Russell MB, Rasmussen BK, Thorvaldsen P, et al. Prevalence and sex-ratio of the subtypes of migraine. *Int J Epidemiol* 1995;24:612.
37. Bana DS, Graham JR. Observations on prodromes of classic migraine in a headache clinic population. *Headache* 1986;26:216.
38. Russell MB, Olesen J. A nosographic analysis of the migraine aura in a general population. *Brain* 1996;119:355.
39. Queiroz LP, Rapoport AM, Weeks RE, et al. Characteristics of migraine visual aura. *Headache* 1997;37:137.
40. Gherpelli JLD, Nagae Poetscher LM, Souza AMMH, et al. Migraine in childhood and adolescence: A critical study of the diagnostic criteria and of the influence of age on clinical findings. *Cephalalgia* 1998;18:333.
41. Hachinski VC, Porchawka J, Steele JC. Visual symptoms in the migraine syndrome. *Neurology* 1973;23:570.
42. Alvarez WC. The migrainous scotoma as studied in 618 persons. *Am J Ophthalmol* 1960;49:489.
43. Rolak LA. Literary neurologic syndromes: Alice in Wonderland. *Arch Neurol* 1991;48:649.
44. Smetana GW. The diagnostic value of historical features in primary headache syndromes: A comprehensive review. *Arch Intern Med* 2000;160:2729.
45. Stewart WF, Staffa J, Lipton RB, et al. Familial risk of migraine: A population-based study. *Ann Neurol* 1997;41:166.
46. Russell MB, Hilden J, Sorensen SA, et al. Familial occurrence of migraine without aura and migraine with aura. *Neurology* 1993;43:1369.
47. Aromaa M, Rautava P, Helenius H, et al. Factors if early life as predictors in children at school entry. *Headache* 1998;38:23.
48. Golding JF. Motion sickness susceptibility questionnaire revised and its relationship to other forms of sickness. *Brain Res Bull* 1998;47:207.
49. Schwartz BS, Stewart WF, Simon D, et al. Epidemiology of tension-type headache. *JAMA* 1998;279:381.
50. Reich KA, Giansiracusa DF, Strongwater SL. Neurologic manifestations of giant cell arteritis. *Am J Med* 1990;89:67.
51. Ekbom K, Ahlborg B, Schele R. Prevalence of migraine and cluster headache in Swedish men of 18. *Headache* 1978;18:9.
52. Ekbom K. Clinical aspects of cluster headache. *Headache* 1974;13:176.
53. Kudrow L. Cluster headache: diagnosis and management. *Headache* 1979;19:142.
54. Manzoni GC, Terzano MG, Bono G, et al. Cluster headache—clinical findings in 180 patients. *Cephalalgia* 1983;3:21.
55. Kudrow L. Clinical symptomatology and differential diagnosis of cluster headache. In: Tollison CD, Kunkel RS, eds. *Headache Diagnosis and Treatment.* Baltimore, Md: Williams & Wilkins, 1993:185.
56. Lovshin LL. Clinical caprices of histaminic cephalalgia. *Headache* 1961;1:7.
57. Ekbom K. A clinical comparison of cluster headache and migraine. *Acta Neurol Scand* 1970;46(suppl):1.
58. Lance JW, Anthony M. Migrainous neuralgia or cluster headache? *J Neurol Sci* 1971;13:401.
59. Graham JR. Cluster headache. *Headache* 1972;11:175.
60. Drummond PD. Predisposing, precipitating and relieving factors in different categories of headache. *Headache* 1985;25:16.
61. Riess CM, Becker WJ, Robertson M. Episodic cluster headache in a community: Clinical features and treatment. *Can J Neurol* 1998;25:141.
62. Friedman AF, Midropoulos HE. Cluster headaches. *Neurology* 1958;8:653.
63. Sutherland JM, Eadie MJ. Cluster headache. *Res Clin Stud Headache* 1972;3:92.
64. Kudrow L. *Cluster Headache, Mechanism and Management.* New York, NY: Oxford University Press; 1980.
65. Andersson PG. Migraine in patients with cluster headache. *Cephalalgia* 1985;5:11.
66. Manzoni GC, Terzano MG, Moretti G, et al. Clinical observations on 76 cluster headache cases. *Eur Neurol* 1981;20:88.
67. Ekbom K. Patterns of cluster headache with a note on the relations to angina pectoris and peptic ulcer. *Acta Neurol Scand* 1970;46:225.
68. Ad hoc Committee on Classification of Headache. Classification of headache. *JAMA* 1962;179:717.
69. Sjaastad O. *Cluster Headache Syndrome.* London, England: WB Saunders; 1992.

70. Dalton K. Food intake prior to a migraine attack: Study of 2,313 spontaneous attacks. *Headache* 1975;15:188.
71. Van den Bergh V, Amery WK, Waelkens J. Trigger factors in migraine: A study conducted by the Belgian Migraine Society. *Headache* 1987;27:191.
72. Davies PT, Peatfield RC, Steiner TJ, et al. Some clinical comparisons between common and classical migraine: A questionnaire-based study. *Cephalalgia* 1991;11:223.
73. Scharff L, Turk DC, Marcus DA. Triggers of headache episodes and coping response of headache diagnostic groups. *Headache* 1995;35:397.
74. Rasmussen BK. Migraine and tension-type headache in a general population: Precipitating factors, female hormones, and relation to lifestyle. *Pain* 1993;53:65.
75. Robbins L. Precipitating factors in migraine: A retrospective review of 494 patients. *Headache* 1994;34:214.
76. Peatfield RC. Relationship between food, wine, and beer-precipitated migrainous headaches. *Headache* 1995;35:355.
77. Chabriat H, Danchot J, Michel P, et al. Precipitating factors of headache. A prospective study in a national control-matched survey in migraineurs and nonmigraineurs. *Headache* 1999;39:335.
78. Epstein MT, Hockaday JM, Hockaday TDR. Migraine and reproductive hormones throughout the menstrual cycle. *Lancet* 1975;1:543.
79. Granella F, Sances G, Zanferrari C, et al. Migraine without aura and reproductive life events: A clinical epidemiological study in 1300 women. *Headache* 1993;33:385.
80. Mosek A, Korczyn AD. Yom Kippur headache. *Neurology* 1995;45:1953.
81. Weber JG, Ereth MH, Danielson DR. Perioperative ingestion of caffeine and postoperative headache. *Mayo Clin Proc* 1993;68:842.
82. Silverman K, Evans SM, Strain EC, et al. Withdrawal syndrome after the double-blind cessation of caffeine consumption. *N Engl J Med* 1992;327:1109.

CHAPTER 19 PATHOPHYSIOLOGY OF HEADACHES

F. Michael Cutrer and Amy O'Donnell

Headaches are estimated to affect over 90% of the general population at some time in their lives[1] and may be encountered by physicians in a wide variety of clinical settings. The overwhelming majority of recurrent headaches occur in the context of what are known as *primary headache disorders,* in which no identifiable underlying cause can be found. Some headaches, however, classified as *secondary headache disorders,* are symptomatic of an underlying abnormality that may include anything from transient viral illness, to intracranial tumor, aneurysm, or drug withdrawal (for differential diagnosis of secondary headache disorder, see Cutrer[2]). Prevalence studies indicate that a benign process, such as a mild febrile illness or alcohol withdrawal, usually causes secondary headaches and that the lifetime prevalence of headache resulting from more ominous intracranial structural lesions is less than 2%.[3]

Head pain occurs when nociceptive neurons within the trigeminal, vagus, or glossopharyngeal cranial nerves or within the upper cervical roots become depolarized. Information from procedures involving intracerebral electrode implantation suggests that direct electrical or mechanical activation of areas within the brain involved in pain processing may also cause head pain.[4] The causes of head pain vary widely and include not only direct mechanical, chemical, or inflammatory stimulation of pain-generating structures but also less well-characterized events that occur in primary headache disorders. Once initiated, the transmission and processing of the painful information is likely to be quite similar regardless of the inciting cause. In this chapter, we first review the anatomy involved in generating generic head pain and then discuss current theories of the pathophysiology of the major primary headache disorders, including migraine, cluster headache, and tension-type headache.

ANATOMY OF HEAD PAIN

Under normal physiologic conditions, the brain is largely insensate. This has been demonstrated in neurosurgical procedures in which stimulation of the brain parenchyma in awake patients caused no pain.[5,6] Head pain is mediated by projections from the trigeminal and upper cervical dorsal root ganglia, which innervate the pial, dural, and extracranial blood vessels. In general, these pseudounipolar neurons innervate the vessels on the same side, which can explain the unilateral distribution of pain in certain headache types, but some of the cells project bilaterally to innervate midline vessels. On activation, these unmyelinated C fibers transmit nociceptive information from perivascular terminals through the trigeminal ganglia[7] to project centrally to synapses on second-order neurons within the trigeminal nucleus caudalis. The primary neurotransmitter for the C fibers is glutamate, but the primary afferents also co-store substance P, calcitonin gene–related peptide and neurokinin A, as well as other neurotransmitters and neuromodulators, in their central and peripheral (e.g., meningeal) axons.

Activity in the trigeminal nucleus caudalis can be modulated by projections from rostral trigeminal nuclei,[8] the periaqueductal gray matter, and the nucleus raphe magnus,[9] as well as by descending cortical inhibitory systems.[9,10] From the trigeminal nucleus caudalis, second-order neurons transmit the nociceptive information, projecting to numerous subcortical sites including the more rostral portions of the trigeminal complex,[11] the reticular formation of the brainstem,[12] midbrain and pontine parabrachial nuclei,[13,14] and the cerebellum,[15,16] as well as to the ventrobasal thalamus,[11,16,17,18] the posterior thalamus,[19,20] and the medial thalamus.[21] From the rostral brainstem, nociceptive information is transmitted to other areas of the brain (e.g., limbic areas) involved in the emotional and vegetative responses to pain.[13] From the ventrobasal thalamus, projections are sent to the somatosensory cortex, where discrimination and localization of pain are thought to occur. The medial thalamus projects to frontal cortex, where the affective and motivational responses to pain are thought to be mediated. However, recent evidence from positron emission tomography (PET) studies indicates that the medial thalamus may participate in the transmission of both discriminative and affective components of pain.[22]

PATHOPHYSIOLOGY OF MIGRAINE

Migraine is one of the most common primary headache disorders and is characterized by unilateral, throbbing headaches associated with nausea, vomiting, photophobia, and phonophobia. Prior to the onset of headache, some migraineurs experience transient focal neurologic symptoms, which may include visual disturbances, unilateral numbness, and weakness, as well as language dysfunction. Probably because of these neurologic symptoms as well as the intensity the headache, the research and speculation surrounding the pathophysiology of migraine has been the most intensive of all primary headache disorders. The speculation that has arisen around migraine has greatly influenced the discussion of pathophysiology of other headache syndromes. Traditional theories of migraine pathogenesis fall into two categories: vasogenic and neurogenic.

Vasogenic Theory

In the late 1930s, Dr. Harold Wolff and coworkers observed that (1) extracranial vessels became distended and pulsated during migraine attacks in many patients, implying that dilation of cranial vessels might be important in migraine; (2) stimulation of intracranial vessels in awake patients resulted in an ipsilateral headache; and (3) vasoconstricting substances, such as ergotamine, could abort headaches, whereas vasodilatory substances, such as nitrates, could trigger migraine attacks. Based on these observations, it was theorized that intracranial vasoconstriction was responsible for the aura of migraine and that the subsequent headache resulted from a rebound dilation and distention of cranial vessels and activation of inflamed perivascular sensory neurons.

Neurogenic Theory

The competing neurogenic theory held that migraine is a brain disorder based on an altered cerebral susceptibility to migraine attacks and that the vascular changes occurring during a migraine were the result rather than the cause of the attack. Advocates of the neurogenic theory pointed to the neurologic symptoms, both focal (in the aura) and vegetative (in the prodrome), that often are prominent components of migraine attacks and cannot be explained on the basis of vasoconstriction within a single neurovascular territory. The expanding nature of the visual and sensory symptoms during migraine aura has led to speculation that the phenomenon of spreading depression might underlie the aura.[23] Spreading depression is a wave of neuronal hyperexcitation followed by suppression that is observed to move across areas of contiguous cortex in experimental animals after chemical or mechanical perturbation.[24] The speculation that spreading depression might be important in migraine aura was reawakened when Olesen, Lauritizen, and their colleagues employed intraarterial xenon 133 (^{133}Xe) blood flow techniques to investigate the hemodynamic changes occurring during aura-like symptoms induced during carotid angiography. Olesen and coworkers reported that aura symptoms were accompanied by reductions in cerebral blood flow, usually in posterior regions of the brain.[25,26] Some studies reported a transient increase in blood flow prior to the blood flow reductions as well as an apparent anterior spread of the blood flow decrements, which moved across neurovascular boundaries.[26] The estimated rate of the spread was about 2 to 3 mm per minute,[26] although the accuracy of this rate has been questioned because of the convoluted nature of the human cerebral cortex. The estimated reductions in blood flow observed in these ^{133}Xe blood flow studies ranged from 17%[27] to 35%,[25] well above the threshold (i.e., > 75%) for frank ischemia, and were therefore termed *spreading oligemia*. However, some researchers have speculated that the artifact of Compton scattering might account for both an underestimation of the magnitude of blood flow reduction and the apparent spreading pattern of the blood flow change.[28]

If applied rigidly, neither of these traditional theories completely explains the clinical symptomatology of migraine. It is likely that migraine is not a disease per se but, rather, a syndrome in which acute attacks occur when one or more triggering environmental events interact with a vulnerable nervous system. Why certain individuals possess this vulnerability to migraine attacks is not fully understood but is likely a result of a combination of genetic and acquired factors. There is great variability among the environmental triggers that are potentially capable of inciting a migraine attack. Most migraineurs are aware of several to which they are sensitive. Those triggers most commonly reported include exposure to certain foods or food additives; certain types of physical exertion; alteration of usual sleep patterns; increased personal or professional stress; hormonal fluctuation; unaccustomed fasting; exposure to glaring, flickering lights, or strong smells; and changes in weather patterns or barometric pressure. The triggers for attacks vary widely from one individual to another and may change with time for an individual migraineur. The mechanism by which these provocative factors start the attack are not well understood. Neither the biochemical nature nor the exact site of migraine initiation is known, but recent advances in functional neuroimaging are beginning to yield some clues.

Initiation A recent investigation performed during the first 6 hours of nine spontaneous attacks of migraine without aura using PET has led to speculation that a so-called migraine generator may exist in the proximal brainstem.[29] In this study, a significant increase in regional cerebral blood flow (rCBF) was observed in the anterocaudal cingulate cortex and in visual and auditory associative cortices. In addition, an 11% increase in rCBF was seen in medial brainstem structures over several planes, slightly contralateral to the headache side. Activation in the medial brainstem but not the cingulate and auditory association cortices persisted even after effective treatment of the headache with 6 mg of subcutaneous sumatriptan. Activation within the medial brainstem was not observed during a subsequent study during a headache-free interval nor was it observed in another series after subcutaneous injection of capsaicin in the forehead.[30] Although this pattern of activation in the brainstem takes place in a region important in nociceptive and vascular control (locus ceruleus and dorsal raphe nucleus), the persistence of the increase in rCBF after relief of symptoms has been interpreted to suggest the presence of a migraine generator. In contrast, other information based on molecular genetic investigations of familial hemiplegic migraine has suggested that altered activation thresholds within cortical neurons may be important in the initiation of migraine attacks in some patients.[31]

Aura Approximately 15% of migraineurs experience attacks in which the headache is preceded by focal neurologic symptoms that persist for up to 1 hour. These transient symptoms, usually called the *aura,* can include transient visual disturbance, unilateral numbness or weakness, language disturbance, and dizziness and are characterized by an unexpected onset and a slow expansion of the area affected by the dysfunction, followed by gradual resolution.

Functional neuroimaging in humans during the opening minutes of spontaneous migraine attacks has shown that decreases in relative cerebral blood flow occur in areas of occipital cortex. In one case, the beginning of a migraine attack was fortuitously captured using PET and ^{15}O-labeled water. A bilateral spreading area of decreased blood flow was observed that started in visual associative cortex (Brodmann's areas 18 and 19) within a few minutes after the onset of a bioccipital throbbing headache. The hypoperfusion progressed anteriorly with time across vascular and anatomic boundaries.[32] Although the subject's difficulty in focusing on the visual target during a part of the study has been interpreted as an atypical migraine aura, it is difficult to draw conclusions about more typical auras, because neither scintillations nor a scotoma were reported, and because the subject had previously only had attacks of migraine without aura.

More recent studies using functional magnetic resonance imaging (fMRI) techniques, such as perfusion- and diffusion-weighted imaging, to study patients during spontaneous migraine visual auras have shown that during the visual symptoms there are increases in mean transit time, the amount of time required for a given amount of blood to move through a set volume of brain parenchyma, of 10% to 54% in the occipital cortex contralateral to the reported visual field symptoms. These studies have also shown decreases in both relative cerebral blood flow (15%–53%) and relative cerebral blood volume (6%–33%) in that area.[33] In between attacks, perfusion weighted imaging and T2-weighted anatomic images in all of the subjects studied (eight thus far) were normal. In one subject, in whom multiple perfusion images were obtained during the same aura, the margin of the perfusion defect appeared to be more anterior in the second image than in the first, suggesting a spread reminiscent of Olesen's findings.

Diffusion-weighted imaging was also performed in subjects during acute migraine with visual auras. Diffusion-weighted imaging, based on the mobility of water molecules, reflects the ability of neurons to maintain normal osmotic membrane gradients. Changes in diffusion-weighted imaging can indicate a loss of this very basic cell function and are seen very early in the evolution of ischemic neuronal injury[34] and in the cortex of experimental animals after the induction of spreading depression.[35] Of the subjects for whom diffusion-weighted images were obtained during visual symptoms, none showed any evidence of regional hyperintensity to suggest the loss of the ability to regulate water mobility. No changes in apparent diffusion coefficient were seen even in areas of occipital lobe that had perfusion decrements of up to 52%.[33] Based on earlier studies in human stroke, the absence of measurable diffusion abnormalities suggests that the threshold for ischemia is not crossed during the migraine aura.[34] Negative diffusion data also suggest that the abnormality that underlies migraine aura in humans, although possibly analogous, is not identical to spreading depression as it occurs in experimental animals.

In general, recent information from functional neuroimaging tends to favor a primarily neuronal rather than vascular origin for the symptoms of migraine aura. The apparent spread across vascular territories and the moderate blood flow reductions seen in both PET[32] and fMRI[33,36] investigations of spontaneous migraine aura symptoms are more suggestive of primary neuronal dysfunction than frank ischemia as the basis for the aura. It is interesting to note that the findings from PET and fMRI (neither of which are vulnerable to Compton scattering) are consistent with the earlier observations using ^{133}Xe blood flow techniques. Whether the characteristics of the neuronal dysfunction prove to be consistent with a human analogue of spreading depression remains to be seen.

Headache Several lines of evidence are consistent with functional neuroimaging findings suggesting that dysfunction within the brain is related to the aura and may provoke head pain. For example, vegetative and affective prodromal symptoms, such as alteration of mood, appetite, and fluid balance, may precede the onset of the headache by up to 24 hours. Furthermore, the majority of patients with aura report that the headache is more severe on the side of the brain hemisphere to which the aura symptoms localize. In addition, the possibility that events intrinsic to the cerebral cortex may be capable of activating meningeal nociceptive neurons is suggested by the fact that seizures are followed by headache in many patients and that repeated spreading depressions in experimental animals results in the induction of c-fos immunoreactivity, (a marker of activation) in second-order nociceptive neurons within the trigeminal nucleus caudalis.[37] Once depolarized, perivascular and meningeal C fibers transmit nociceptive information via the trigeminal nerve and upper cervical nerve roots to areas of pain processing within the trigeminal nucleus caudalis in the distal medulla and dorsal horn of the upper cervical segments.

The gradual intensification and prolongation of headache that occurs during migraine may be governed through a series of events that result in peripheral and central sensitization of the trigeminal system. Information from animal studies indicates that once activated, C fibers release neuropeptides (i.e., substance P, neurokinin A, calcitonin gene–related peptide).[38] Similar increases in neuropeptides have been observed during acute migraine attacks in humans.[39] These neuropeptides generate a neurogenic inflammatory response within the meninges consisting of increased plasma leakage from meningeal vessels, vasodilation, and activation of mast cells and endothelial cells.

Once set into motion, this process is thought to act to lower the threshold of the C fibers to further activation and, as a result, prolong and intensify the headache attack. Drugs known to be effective in ending a migraine attack such as dihydroergotamine or sumatriptan, act at serotonin (5-HT$_{1B}$ and 5-HT$_{1D}$) receptor subtypes to cause constriction of vascular smooth muscle and to block the release of neuropeptides that mediate the development of neurogenic inflammation. Recent animal studies confirm a reduction in activation thresholds after stimulation of the meningeal pain system. After chemical stimulation of the meninges, nociceptive neuronal responses and pain-induced changes in blood pressure were evoked by much smaller levels of dural mechanical stimulation and by previously innocuous cutaneous stimulation, indicating the generation of both central sensitization and cutaneous allodynia.[40]

Generation of an Acute Attack Taking into account the information obtained from recent studies, a possible scenario for the generation of an acute attack in some forms of migraine is as follows:

1. Endogenous neurophysiologic events in the neocortex generate the observed neurologic symptoms of aura and promote the release of nociceptive substances (e.g., H^+ and K^+ ions, arachidonic acid metabolites) from the neocortex into the interstitial space.
2. Within the Virchow-Robin spaces, the released substances accumulate to levels sufficient to activate or sensitize trigeminovascular fibers that surround pial vessels supplying the draining neocortex.
3. Substances that discharge or sensitize small, unmyelinated fibers that transmit pain accumulate in proximity to trigeminovascular fibers and may possibly provide the trigger for headache or sensitize perivascular afferents to blood-borne or other as yet unidentified factors. The headache latency (20 to 40 minutes) may reflect the time needed for extracellular levels to reach a threshold for depolarization.
4. Upon activation, the trigeminal nociceptive neurons transmit the nociceptive information through the trigeminal ganglia to synapse on second-order neurons within the trigeminal nucleus caudalis.
5. Numerous projections from the trigeminal nucleus caudalis then transmit the nociceptive information to various brain areas that underlie various aspects of pain (see the earlier discussion of "Anatomy of Head Pain").

In this scenario, the brain acts as a transducer, interfacing with the environment. Triggering events, such as those associated with emotional stress, glaring lights, or interrupted sleep, modulate activity within brain regions physically contiguous to the meningeal vessels innervated by the trigeminal nerve. In susceptible individuals, these events may be sufficient to initiate neurophysiologic events leading to chemical activation of meningeal fibers. The photophobia, nausea, and vomiting are probably not specific to migraine but are related to meningeal irritation, as similar symptoms are seen with infection or when blood enters the subarachnoid space. This proposed cascade provides a pathogenetic framework for further investigation of migraine and is based on currently understood principles of neurobiology and the physiology of pain. However, the details will need revision as new data emerge from experimental studies in humans and animals.

PATHOPHYSIOLOGY OF CLUSTER HEADACHE

In the past, very little was known about the pathophysiology of cluster headaches, but recent observations have given rise to new speculation about their origins. Similar to other vascular headaches (e.g., migraine), cluster headaches are presumed to develop from pathophysiologic events that ultimately activate the trigeminovascular system.

In the complete form of the syndrome, patients with cluster headache manifest pain in the first and second trigeminal divisions, sympathetic activation (sweating of the forehead and face) and dysfunction (Horner's syndrome), and parasympathetic activation (lacrimation and nasal congestion). This constellation of symptoms and signs can best be explained as the consequence of an abnormality at the point at which fibers from the ophthalmic and maxillary trigeminal division converge with projections from the superior cervical and the sphenopalatine ganglia. This plexus is contained within the cavernous sinus, and narrowing of the cavernous carotid artery has been observed in selected cases of cluster headache. Although a subject of some controversy, changes in the drainage pattern of the cavernous sinus have also been reported in patients with the condition.[41] A history of trauma and variations in the anatomical structure of the cavernous sinus may provide additional clues to the pathophysiologic features of cluster headache. Indeed, recent external craniometric measurements in a groups of 25 patients with cluster headache revealed an apparent narrowing of the anterior-middle cranial fossa when compared with age-matched healthy volunteers ($n = 21$) and migraineurs ($n = 20$).[42] Intraorbital lesions and lesions at remote sites in the middle fossa should be investigated in patients with only a partial set of signs and symptoms.

The circadian rhythmicity of this syndrome is another striking clinical feature that has led to speculation that the hypothalamus or a related structure may be involved in the generation of this headache.[43–45] In a recent PET study of nine patients with acute cluster attacks, investigators observed brain activation in areas known to be involved in pain processing, such as the anterior cingulate cortex bilaterally, the contralateral posterior thalamus, and the insular cortex. They also observed activation in the hypothalamic gray matter.[46] This appears to be specific for cluster headache, as it has not been observed in migraine[47] or in head pain induced by capsaicin injection.[48] Once trigeminal pain fibers are activated, many of the processes associated with the prolongation and intensification of the pain in migraine may apply in cluster headache as well (see the earlier discussion of headache under "Pathophysiology of Migraine").

PATHOPHYSIOLOGY OF TENSION-TYPE HEADACHE

It is ironic that the pathophysiology of the most common of the primary headache disorders is the least well understood. Tension-type headache continues to defy a single or simple pathophysiologic explanation, although the importance of muscular and myofascial structures is acknowledged in many, but not all, cases.[49,50] In one of the more widely accepted paradigms, headache pain is viewed as the sum of nociceptive input from vascular structures, similar input from myofascial and muscular sources, and descending supraspinal modulation.[51] The relative importance of these three factors varies among patients and among attacks in the same patient. In tension-type headache, myofascial input may predominate, although, in migraine, cerebrovascular and meningeal nociceptive stimulation may predominate. Peripheral factors are very important in episodic headaches, whereas chronic headaches seem to be strongly influenced by changes in the supraspinal modulation of pain. This view of tension-type headache may explain the frequent overlap with migraine.

CONCLUSION

The details of the pathophysiology of the various primary and secondary headache disorders undoubtedly differ, especially those pertaining to initiation of the attack. However, the basic biologic principles governing the development, modulation, and prolongation of head pain are likely to be the same regardless of the underlying cause of the headache. As our understanding of these principles increases so, too, will the effectiveness and tolerability of acute therapy. Improvements in prophylactic therapy will require a better knowledge of the factors involved in headache initiation.

REFERENCES

1. Rasmussen BK, Jensen R, Schroll M, Olesen J. Epidemiology of headache in a general population: A prevalence study. *J Clin Epidemiol* 1991;44:1147–1157.
2. Cutrer FM. Headache. In: Borsook D, LeBel A, McPeek B, eds. *The Massachusetts General Hospital Handbook of Pain Management.* Boston, Mass: Little, Brown; 1996:270–302.
3. Rasmussen BK, Olesen J. Symptomatic and non-symptomatic headaches in general population. *Neurology* 1992;42:1225–1231.
4. Raskin NH, Hosobuchi Y, Lamb SA. Headache may arise from perturbation of brain. *Headache* 1987;27:416–420.
5. Ray BS, Wolff HG. Experimental studies on headache. Pain-sensitive structures of the head and their significance in headache. *Arch Surg* 1940;41:813–856.
6. Penfield W. A contribution to the mechanism of intracranial pain. *Assoc Res Nerv Ment Dis* 1935;15:399–416.
7. Mayberg MR, Zervas NT, Moskowitz MA. Trigeminal projections to supratentorial pial and dural blood vessels in cats demonstrated by horseradish peroxidase histochemistry. *J Comp Neurol* 1984;223: 46–56.
8. Kruger L, Young RF. Specialized features of the trigeminal nerve and its central connections. In: Samii M, Janetta PJ, eds. *The Cranial Nerves.* Berlin, Germany: Springer-Verlag; 1981:273–301.
9. Sessle BJ, Hu JW, Dubner R, Lucier GE. Functional properties of neurons in trigeminal subnucleus caudalis of the cat, II. Modulation of responses to noxious and non-noxious stimulation by periaqueductal gray, nucleus raphe magnus, cerebral cortex and afferent influences, and effect of naloxone. *J Neurophysiol* 1981;45:193–207.
10. Wise SP, Jones EG. Cells of origin and trigeminal distribution of descending projections of the rat somatic sensory cortex. *J Comp Neurol* 1977;175:129–158.
11. Jacquin MF, Chiaia NL, Haring JH, Rhoades RW. Intersub-nuclear connections within the rat trigeminal brainstem complex. *Somatosen Motor Res* 1990;7:399–420.
12. Renehan WE, Jacquin MF, Mooney RD, Rhoades RW. Structure-func-

tion relationship in rat medullary and cervical dorsal horns. II. Medullary dorsal horn cells. *J Neurophysiol* 1986;55:1187–1201.
13. Bernard JF, Peschanski M, Besson JM. A possible spino-(trigemino)-ponto amygdaloid pathway for pain. *Neurosci Lett* 1989;100:83–88.
14. Hayashi H, Tabata T. Pulpal and cutaneous inputs to somatosensory neurons in the parabrachial area of the cat. *Brain Res* 1990;511: 177–179.
15. Huerta MF, Frankfurter A, Harting JK. Studies of the principal sensory and spinal trigeminal nuclei of the rat: Projections to the superior colliculus, inferior olive, and cerebellum. *J Comp Neurol* 1983;220: 147–167.
16. Mantle St John LA, Tracey DJ. Somatosensory nuclei in the brainstem of the rat: Independent projections to the thalamus and cerebellum. *J Comp Neurol* 1987;255:259–271.
17. Huang L-YM. Origin of thalamically projecting somatosensory relay neurons in the immature rat. *Brain Res* 1989;495:108–114.
18. Kemplay S, Webster KE. A quantitative study of the projections of the gracile, cuneate, and trigeminal nuclei and of the medullary reticular formation to the thalamus in the rat. *Neuroscience* 1989;32:153–167.
19. Peschanski M, Roudier F, Ralston HJ III, Besson JM. Ultrastructural analysis of the terminals of various somatosensory pathways in the ventrobasal complex of the rat thalamus: An electron-microscopic study using wheatgerm agglutinin conjugated to horseradish peroxidase as an axonal tracer. *Somatosens Res* 1985;3:75–87.
20. Shigenaga Y, Nakatani A, Nishimori T, Suemune S, Kuroda R, Matano S. The cells of origin of cat trigeminothalamic projections: Especially in the caudal medulla. *Brain Res* 1983;277:201–222.
21. Craig AD Jr, Burton H. Spinal and medullary lamina I projection to nucleus submedius in medial thalamus: A possible pain center. *J Neurophysiol* 1981;45:443–466.
22. Bushnell MC, Duncan GH. Sensory and affective aspects of pain perception: Is medial thalamus restricted to emotional issues? *Exp Brain Res* 1989;78:415–418.
23. Milner P. Note on a possible correspondence between the scotomas of migraine and spreading depression of Leao. *EEG Clin Neurophysiol* 1958;10:705.
24. Leao AAP. Spreading depression of activity in the cerebral cortex. *J Neurophysiol* 1944;8:379–390.
25. Olesen J, Larsen B, Lauritzen M. Focal hyperemia followed by spreading oligemia and impaired activation of rCBF in classic migraine. *Ann Neurol* 1981;9:344–352.
26. Lauritzen M, Skyhoj Olsen T, Lassen NA, Paulson OB. Changes of regional cerebral blood flow during the course of classical migraine attacks. *Ann Neurol* 1983;13:633–641.
27. Lauritzen M, Olesen J. Regional cerebral blood flow during migraine attacks by xenon-133 inhalation and emission tomography. *Brain* 1984; 107:447–461.
28. Skyhoj Olsen T, Friberg L, Lassen NA. Ischemia may be the primary cause of neurologic deficits in classical migraine. *Arch Neurol* 1987; 44:156–161.
29. Weiller C, May A, Limmroth V, et al. Brain stem activation in spontaneous human migraine attacks. *Nat Med* 1995;1:658–660.
30. May A, Kaube H, Buchel C, et al. Experimental cranial pain elicited by capsaicin: A PET study. *Pain* 1998;74:61–66.
31. Ferrari MD. Migraine. *Lancet* 1998;351:1043–1051.
32. Woods RP, Iacoboni M, Mazziotta JC. Bilateral spreading cerebral hypoperfusion during spontaneous migraine headache. *N Eng J Med* 1994;331:1689–1692.
33. Cutrer FM, Sorenson AG, Weisskoff RM, et al. Perfusion-weighted imaging defects during spontaneous migrainous aura. *Ann Neurol* 1998; 43:25–31.
34. Warach S, Gaa J, Siewert B, Wielopolski P, Edelman RR. Acute human stroke studied by whole brain echo planar diffusion-weighted magnetic resonance imaging. *Ann Neurol* 1995;37:231–241.
35. Hasegawa Y, Latour LL, Sotak C, et al. Spreading waves of reduced diffusion coefficient of water in the rat brain. *Neurology* 1994;44 (suppl):A341.
36. Cao Y, Welch KMA, Aurora SK, et al. Functional MRI (BOLD) of visually-triggered headache in migraine patients [abstract]. 8th Congress of the International Headache Society. *Cephalalgia* 1997;17:254.
37. Moskowitz MA, Nozaki K, Kraig RP. Neocortical spreading depression provokes the expression of c-fos protein-like immunoreactivity within trigeminal nucleus caudalis via trigeminovascular mechanisms. *J Neurosci* 1993;13:1167–1177.
38. Dimitriadou V, Buzzi MG, Theoharides TC, Moskowitz MA. Ultrastructural evidence for neurogenically mediated changes in blood vessels of the rat dura mater and tongue following antidromic trigeminal stimulation. *Neuroscience* 1992;48:187–203.
39. Goadsby PH, Edvinsson L, Ekman R. Vasoactive peptide release in the extracerebral circulation of humans during migraine headache. *Ann Neurol* 1990;28:183–187.
40. Yamamura H, Makick A, Chamberlin NL, Burstein R. Cardiovascular and neuronal responses to head stimulation reflect central sensitization and cutaneous allodynia in a rat model of migraine. *J Neurophysiol* 1999;81:479–493.
41. Hannerz J. Orbital phlebography and signs of inflammation in episodic and chronic cluster headache. *Headache* 1991;31:540–542.
42. Afra J, Cecchini AP, Schoenen J. Craniometric measures in cluster headache patients. *Cephalalgia* 1998;18:143–145.
43. Ekbom K. Patterns of cluster headache with a note on the relations to angina pectoris and peptide ulcer. *Acta Neurol Scand* 1970;46:225–237.
44. Kudrow L. The cyclic relationship of natural illumination to cluster period frequency. *Cephalgia* 1987;7:76–78.
45. Strittmater M, Hamann GF, Grauer M, et al. Altered activity of the sympathetic nervous system and changes in the balance of hypophyseal, pituitary and adrenal hormones in patients with cluster headache. *Neuroreport* 1996;7:1229–1234.
46. May A, Bahra A, Büchel C, Frackowiak RSJ, Goadsby PJ. First direct evidence for hypothalamic activation in cluster headache attacks. *Lancet* 1998;352:275–278.
47. Weiller C, May A, Limmroth V, et al. Brain stem activation in spontaneous human migraine attacks. *Nat Med* 1995;1:658–660.
48. May A, Kaube H, Buchel C, et al. Experimental cranial pain elicited by capsaicin: A PET study. *Pain* 1998;74:61–66.
49. Jensen R, Rasmussen BK, Pedersen B, Olesen J. Cephalic muscle tenderness and pressure pain threshold in headache. *Pain* 1993;52:193–199.
50. Langemark M, Olesen J. Pericranial tenderness in tension headache. *Cephalalgia* 1987;7:249–255.
51. Olesen J. Clinical and pathophysiological observations in migraine and tension-type headache explained by integration of vascular, supraspinal and myofascial inputs. *Pain* 1991;46:125–132.

CHAPTER 20 COMMON HEADACHE SYNDROMES

Harvey J. Blumenthal and Alan M. Rapoport

Headache is one of the most common painful conditions for which patients consult physicians. Surveys indicate that in any given year, more than 90% of American adults will suffer some kind of headache or head pain.[1] Fortunately, very few headaches are caused by serious organic conditions, and most headaches are actually migraine or tension-type headache. The first step in treating a patient with headache is to establish an accurate diagnosis, and for diagnostic purposes headaches are divided into primary and secondary headache disorders. Secondary headaches have an underlying cause, such as infection, eye disease, tumor, aneurysm, meningitis, and so forth. Primary headache disorders are benign and tend to recur. These headaches are caused by conditions for which the true basis has not yet been established, but altered brain serotonin chemistry clearly plays a role (see Chapter 19 for a discussion of the biology of primary headaches). Chapter 17 outlines diagnostic criteria for migraine, tension-type headache, and cluster headache, the three most common headache syndromes. In this chapter, we comment on differential diagnosis, diagnostic testing, and management of patients with these common primary headache disorders.

MIGRAINE

The two most common patterns of migraine are migraine with aura, formerly called *classic migraine*, and migraine without aura, or *common migraine*. Approximately 18% of women and 6% of men in the United States are plagued by migraine, and 15% will experience an aura with some of their migraine attacks.[1]

Clinical Features and Differential Diagnosis

Blau has described five phases of migraine that are not universally present and may variably occur during different attacks in the same individual.[2] The first phase, or prodrome, occurs in 40% to 60% of migraineurs. It consists of altered mood, irritability, depression or euphoria, fatigue, yawning, excessive sleepiness, craving for chocolate, or other vegetative symptoms, all of which suggest origin of these symptoms in the hypothalamus, perhaps as a result of excessive dopamine stimulation. These symptoms usually precede the headache phase of the migraine attack by several hours or even days, and experience teaches the patient or observant family that the migraine attack has begun.

The second phase of migraine is the aura, consisting of either visual or sensory phenomena (the two most common aura symptoms) or motor weakness, incoordination, or dysphasic symptoms, such as word-finding difficulty. The aura symptoms usually precede the headache phase of the migraine attack, but occasionally occur simultaneously. Sometimes, two aura symptoms occur in the attack, usually visual and sensory symptoms that may occur simultaneously or consecutively. The aura symptoms appear gradually over 5 to 20 minutes and usually subside just before the headache begins.

When examining a patient who has recently experienced only one or two such attacks for the first time, the clinician must determine whether these focal neurologic symptoms represent migrainous aura or manifestations of transient ischemic attack (TIA) or even a focal sensory seizure. Passage of time, repeated identical attacks, and diagnostic testing may be required to obtain certainty, but certain features are more typical of migraine aura. Firstly, visual and sensory symptoms of TIA and seizures usually develop more rapidly than the gradual progression of an aura over 5 to 20 minutes. Secondly, migraine aura is characterized by a combination of negative and positive symptoms; the migraineur experiences a visual scotoma or hole in the vision (negative symptoms) *and* dazzling, glimmering, scintillating lights (positive phenomena). TIA, such as amaurosis fugax or hemianopic scotoma, usually manifests as a black or blank negative visual loss.

Sometimes, especially in the elderly, the visual aura occurs repeatedly without any headache. C.M. Fisher described these features as "late life migraine accompaniments."[3] Sometimes these elderly patients experienced more typical migraine in youth, with the migraine subsiding for many years only to recur as migraine aura without headache in later life. In this setting, the clinician may be more secure in the diagnosis. However, these late life migraine accompaniments often develop with no previous history of migraine. Patients with new late-life migraine symptoms must be carefully evaluated to rule out cerebrovascular disease, structural hemispheric disease, or even retinal detachments.

The sensory auras of migraine usually consist of numbness (negative sensory symptoms) *and* positive symptoms of tingling or paresthesia. Again, these sensory symptoms usually progress over 5 to 20 minutes and are followed by the headache phase, which is the third phase of the migraine attack, and usually the most dramatic. It is the headache phase of migraine for which most patients consult physicians.

Chapter 17 outlines the International Headache Society (IHS) system for diagnosing migraine, but it is important to remember that these strict criteria were designed chiefly for purposes of finding a uniform population of migraine patients to be entered into investigational drug trials. The experienced clinician uses the IHS criteria as a guide but is not rigidly bound by them. Furthermore, both migraine and tension-type headache are very common, and when patients report symptoms of both, there may be overlapping features that make it difficult to tell where one ends and the other begins. In fact, the IHS system of classification is being revised and will be more accurate and complete.

Often, the patient does not initially describe the headache characteristics well, and the skillful clinician must take the time to extract important but subtle historical points. For example, some patients spontaneously report only pressure-type occipital pain, but by digging a little deeper, the examiner can help the patient recall that the worst headaches, occurring infrequently, build to an intense throbbing and radiate to one periorbital region. Patients often report that, because they are unsure at the outset whether the headache will build to severe intensity, they fail to take acute-care medication early and, consequently, obtain less effective relief than if they had treated the migraine earlier in the attack.

The headache of migraine is unilateral in 60% of cases and usually alternates sides from one attack to the next.[4] Often, patients state that the headache is always on one side but when pressed recall that rarely, perhaps 10% of the time, the headache occurs on the opposite side. This alternating hemicrania, however infrequent, makes the clinician more secure in the diagnosis of migraine. Some migraineurs report that the headache is bilateral, but worse on one side. The headache usually builds over a period of 30 minutes to several hours but may occur with sudden intensity. Although the pain of migraine is usually moderate to severe, many patients report milder headaches, which they refer to as "sinus headaches" or "regular headaches" and which, in reality, are milder migraine attacks. Similar benign recurring headaches are much more likely to be migraine or tension-type headache than sinusitis. Sometimes radiography is needed to settle the issue, and computed tomographic (CT) scanning of the sinuses is superior to sinus x-rays in diagnosing acute sinusitis. Many patients are test oriented and anxious to know what the x-ray showed. They may fail to appreciate the knowledgeable opinion of an experienced clinician in making a diagnosis based on a thorough history and examination.

To be sure, clinicians must always be aware of so-called migraine mimics—paroxysmal headaches caused by arteriovenous malformations, pheochromocytoma, repeated exposure to carbon monoxide, transient increased spinal fluid pressure resulting from a colloid cyst of the third ventricle, adult-onset of headaches caused by type II Arnold-Chiari malformations, or other structural brain disease. In the elderly, temporal arteritis must always be considered. Primary central nervous system angiitis may manifest as frequent headaches before other symptoms, such as encephalopathy, seizures, or infarctions, occur as a result of the vasculitis.

The following danger signals warn the clinician that a headache may be more serious than a migraine[1]:

1. Headache that is changing or different from previous headaches may herald a brain tumor superimposed on a long-standing primary headache disorder, such as migraine or tension-type headache.
2. Headache with progressive worsening over 24 hours or several days suggests a mass lesion or infectious disease such as meningitis, abscess, subdural or intracerebral hematoma, or vasculitis.
3. Headache precipitated by exertion, bending over, coughing, or sneezing may result from transient blockage of cerebrospinal fluid (CSF) flow or increased intracranial pressure.
4. Sudden onset of headache during exercise or sexual activity can occur with subarachnoid hemorrhage or with benign exertional headache.
5. Vomiting may result from a brain tumor or other mass lesion with increased intracranial pressure.
6. Early morning headache can occur with obstructive sleep apnea and hypertension.
7. Any abnormal physical or neurologic finding must be considered suspect: fever, stiff neck, rash, lymphadenopathy, scalp tenderness, altered sensorium, or focal neurologic signs. Any patient who presents with his or her "first or worst headache" is cause for alarm.

The young, healthy patient with a textbook history of migraine and a normal examination seldom requires diagnostic investigation. If, however, the patient fails to respond as expected to treatment efforts, diagnostic testing may be wise.

Unsuspected granulomatous inflammations, such as sarcoidosis, meningeal malignancy, and cryptococcal, tuberculous, or Lyme meningitis, can be diagnosed only by CSF examination. Elevated opening spinal fluid pressure may confirm the diagnosis of pseudotumor cerebri.

For structural brain lesions, magnetic resonance imaging (MRI) is much more sensitive than CT scanning and is always preferable unless bone windows are desired. CT scanning is more sensitive for demonstrating subarachnoid hemorrhage in the first 24 hours, whereas MRI becomes more sensitive after 48 hours. Unenhanced CT scans made within 24 hours of subarachnoid hemorrhage demonstrate blood in 90% of cases, but in only 70% of cases after 5 days.[5] If a small subarachnoid hemorrhage, a so-called sentinel bleed, is being considered, CSF examination is essential even when results of the CT are normal. The presence of fresh blood or xanthochromia should prompt angiography. Cerebral angiography is also required if primary central nervous system granulomatous angiitis is suspected. Magnetic resonance angiography is sensitive for identifying unruptured aneurysms as small as 3 to 4 mm, and angiography would be definitive.[5]

There is a high familial incidence of aneurysms; unsuspected asymptomatic intracranial aneurysms were found in 9% of 396 persons having a first-degree relative with an aneurysm.[5] A careful family history is, therefore, important if a warning leak is suspected.

CT scanning of the sinuses is more sensitive than sinus x-rays or MRI. Clinicians must not omit dental disease or jaw dysfunction as a cause of head or facial pain, or localized eye disease, such as glaucoma, which can cause unilateral orbital pain. Cervical spine disease or lesions at the foramen magnum may cause suboccipital pain, and plain x-rays or imaging may be considered.

Certain medications, such as nonsteroidal anti-inflammatory drugs (NSAIDs), estrogen, progestins, selective serotonin reuptake inhibitors (SSRIs), or certain calcium channel blockers, may cause headache. Because these drugs are often used to treat headaches, sorting out the diagnosis may be difficult.

Blau's fourth phase of migraine is the headache termination. Sleep, even a brief nap of 1 or 2 hours, is the most common natural method of resolution, but biofeedback and relaxation exercises may also be beneficial. Today, pharmacologic treatment is the most common medical treatment to terminate an acute migraine attack.

The fifth phase of migraine, the postdrome, was reported by 94% of Blau's patients, but these symptoms have not been widely studied. Postdrome symptoms may last about 24 hours and range from feeling drained or exhausted to an unusual sense of elation or euphoria.

Management

The first step in treating the patient with migraine, or any medical condition, is to establish an accurate diagnosis. The diagnosis must be conveyed to the patient who, very often, is fearful of a tumor or aneurysm, or may erroneously believe he or she has a chronic sinus or psychiatric condition. Many of these patients have been discouraged in the past by physicians who have ignored their complaints of headache. Headache is a common complaint, and many busy physicians are reluctant to take the time required to obtain an adequate headache history, or they may view headache as being a result of nervousness or stress. The busy physician may choose to direct the brief office visit at management of hypertension, diabetes, or arthritis. Headache treatment begins with educating patients about the nature of migraine and reassuring them that this is a biologic disorder caused by altered brain biochemistry with secondary vascular changes, and usually a hereditary predisposition. Patients often are relieved that at last they have found a physician who is knowledgeable about headaches and who expresses an interest in helping them. Sometimes it is helpful to have the spouse present and explain to the couple that headaches, and migraine in particular, are often provoked by hormonal changes, certain food triggers, missing meals, irregular sleep patterns, travel, or specific environmental changes. Visual and sensory stimuli, such as bright lights, excessive noise, cigarette smoking, certain perfumes or smells, or other stimuli, may act as migraine triggers. Some medications, both over-the-counter and prescription drugs, can precipitate headache (Table 20-1). There is also an underlying predisposition for people with migraine to have a biochemical comorbidity of depression or anxiety.

In a specialty headache practice, there is usually a nurse or physician's assistant who instructs the patient to keep a headache calendar, watch for repeated food or environmental triggers, and record the amount of medication taken and response to treatment. Having this accurate record enables the physician to alter pharmacologic treatment depending on the response. The power of the written word cannot be overemphasized, and publications are available that describe and explain many of these issues for the migraineur. Information is available free of charge from the American Council for Headache Education (ACHE) (by phone at 1-800-255-ACHE) and the National Headache Foundation (NHF), (1-800-843-2256).

Some headache patients express a desire to be treated without "drugs" or prefer to take "natural" substances, such as herbal or vitamin supplements. Biofeedback training can be beneficial in conjunction with, or without, medication. Biofeedback training teaches relaxation skills as part of overall headache management.

TABLE 20-1 **Selected Medications Reported to Cause Headaches[4]**

Amantadine	L-dopa
Calcium-channel blockers	Monoamine oxidase inhibitors
Caffeine	Nonsteroidal anti-inflammatory drugs
Cimetidine	Nitrates
Corticosteroids	Nicotinic acid
Cyclophosphamide	Phenothiazines
Dipyridamole	Ranitidine
Estrogens	Sympathomimetic agents
Ethanol	Tamoxifen
Hydralazine	Theophyllines (thioxanthines)
Indomethacin	Tetracyclines
Interferon	Trimethoprim

Patients learn to be aware of skeletal muscle status and how to relax general and specific muscle contraction and tension; they learn breathing techniques and how to enhance blood flow to the peripheral vessels, producing hand warming. With practice, patients can alter autonomic nervous function to produce measurable temperature changes in the hands. These exercises may reduce afferent sensory volleys from peripheral muscular pain and modulate sensory impulses ascending through cervical segments into the trigeminal nerve complex in the brainstem.

Cognitive therapy using behavioral modification can help patients deal with the headache condition in a positive way. If the patient spontaneously asks about stress or if he or she recognizes anxiety or depression as significant problems, consultation with a behavioral psychologist may be very helpful.

Physical therapy with heat or cold applications, ultrasound, myofascial release, and massage therapy are beneficial for some patients. Attention to nutrition and observing for food triggers, especially alcohol, are important. Nutrasweet (Equal, aspartame) has been reported to trigger migraine, and one of the authors has observed this in patients who chew gum containing aspartame.[6] Correcting irregular eating and sleep habits may be beneficial.

Some of these measures, such as keeping an accurate headache calendar, practicing biofeedback exercises, and paying attention to diet, have the added benefit of insisting that the patient play an active role in the treatment program. Many patients express a sense of empowerment and satisfaction that they are contributing to management of the headache condition and gaining more control over their lives and the condition.

Pharmacotherapy

Pharmacotherapy of migraine may be divided into three types: (1) treatment with nonspecific analgesics; (2) acute care treatment with drugs that have specific pharmacologic affinity to bind to certain serotonin receptors and alter the neurochemical, inflammatory, and vascular process of migraine; and (3) the daily use of preventive medications.

Common analgesics, such as aspirin, acetaminophen, or NSAIDs (e.g., naproxen sodium), often provide relief to patients with mild migraine headaches, especially if taken early in the attack. A double-blind placebo-controlled study found Excedrin Extra-Strength was significantly superior to placebo in treating mild to moderate migraine headaches.[7] Combination analgesics, such as Midrin, Fioricet, and Fiorinal, also may be beneficial in migraine if taken early. These compounds have the potential to cause analgesic rebound headache (see later discussion) if taken too often, such as more than three times a week, but they can be very helpful and are safe to take for migraine attacks that occur three or four times a month. Analgesic rebound is more likely related to *frequent* dosing of these drugs, rather than to the total number of doses that may be taken safely in a week.

Treatment of acute migraine attacks was revolutionized in the United States in 1993 with the introduction of sumatriptan and, in 1998, by other triptans—zolmitriptan, naratriptan, and rizatriptan. Dihydroergotamine has been available since 1945 as an injection, but was not widely used until 15 years ago; a nasal spray formulation, Migranal NS, was introduced in 1997.

All of these drugs are effective because of their specific pharmacologic affinity to bind to certain serotonin (5-HT) receptors and interrupt the neurochemical, inflammatory, and vascular changes that occur in migraine. There are differences in lipophilicity of some of the triptans, with variable ability to cross the blood-brain barrier, but whether any central action contributes to meaningful migraine relief remains uncertain. The slight molecular differences of each triptan confer different pharmacologic properties, such as bioavailability, time to peak concentration, onset of action, metabolic half-life, and excretion, among others (Table 20-2). Sumatriptan, zolmitriptan, and rizatriptan are metabolized by the enzyme monoamine oxidase-A (MAO-A) and, therefore, these drugs are contraindicated in patients taking MAO inhibitors. Naratriptan and dihydroergotamine are not so contraindicated.

Triptan metabolism may be inhibited by cimetidine, birth control pills, and propranolol, resulting in higher blood levels and, in turn, increasing the risk of adverse effects. All the triptan drugs share similar adverse effect profiles. Most effects are mild and transient; however, the primary concern with this class of drugs, as well as with dihydroergotamine, is that these compounds can cause coronary vasoconstriction. A few serious and life-threatening cardiac events have been reported in patients using triptans, and caution should be exercised in prescribing any of the triptans or dihydroergotamine for patients with cardiac risk factors. *In vitro* studies of isolated human coronary artery segments demonstrate that these drugs are unlikely to cause myocardial ischemia at therapeutic concentrations in healthy subjects[8]; they are safe for young, otherwise healthy patients with migraine. The triptans and dihydroergotamine have improved the lives of people formerly disabled and suffering several times a month from migraine pain. Because of the pharmacologic differences, one triptan may be very helpful to a patient even if treatment with another triptan has failed.

Rescue treatment refers to using potent opioid analgesia or sedation for an acute attack when specific acute care treatment for migraine fails. Markley provides a thorough review of the appropriate use of opioid analgesics and recommends sound guidelines for the use of these drugs.[9] We agree that it is unfair and unethical to deny patients with intractable pain effective analgesia; however, clinicians must also assume the responsibility to monitor the patient's response and use of these drugs. Once again, we emphasize the importance of having the patient keep an accurate headache calendar, recording the number and severity of headaches and number of and response to acute care medications, including opioids.

Preventive medications may be taken daily by migraineurs who suffer frequent attacks (e.g., three or four times a month or more) or by those who become disabled for 48 to 72 hours even once or twice a month. Only the patient can determine if he or she wishes to take daily preventive medication. Some patients express concerns about side effects or habituation, and clinicians must always monitor continuous medication use in young women who might become pregnant, and caution them of potential harm to the fetus. Patients who are reluctant to take daily medication should be reassured that the drug can be discontinued if they experience any adverse reactions or if their migraine symptoms are not reduced after a trial period. We explain that we begin with a low dose, which can gradually be increased, but at least 4 to 6 weeks of treatment should occur before deciding on effectiveness. The most commonly used preventive medications are listed in Table 20-3. The exact mechanism of action of these medications is not always known, but most have in common the pharmacologic affinity to bind to and downregulate the 5-HT_2 family of serotonin receptors.

Choice of preventive medicine should be determined by consideration of the patient's overall medical condition and any comorbid illnesses. For example, a beta blocker would be a good choice if the patient has mild untreated hypertension, has coexisting essential tremor, or is nervous and excitable. On the other hand, beta blockers should be avoided if the patient has asthma or depression or is taking other vasoactive antihypertensive drugs. Tricyclic antidepressants might be especially helpful for patients who have sleep disturbance, depression, or loss of appetite. Divalproex sodium might be the drug of choice for migraine patients who have obsessive-compulsive traits or are bipolar or who have had seizures in the past, but this drug should be avoided if the patient has known liver disease.

CLUSTER HEADACHE

Cluster headache is so distinctive a condition that once the clinician is aware of the characteristic features, there seldom is any difficulty in making the diagnosis. Of all the headache disorders, cluster headache pain is probably the most excruciating and disabling. The reference to *cluster* in the name of this disorder derives from

TABLE 20-2 **Comparison of Triptan Medications**

	Sumatriptan			Zolmitriptan	Naratriptan	Rizatriptan
	Inject 6 mg	Tab 50 mg	NS 20 mg	Tab 2.5 mg	Tab 2.5 mg	Tab 10 mg
Onset (min)	10	60–90	15–45	40–60	3–4 (h)	30–60
Bioavailability (%)	~90	14	?	40	70	45
Effectiveness (%)						
2 h	81	50–63	60–63	65–67	48	71–77
4 h	?	65–78	?	75	65	?
Recurrence (%)	30–40	26–40	32	22–36	17–28	30–47
Adverse events (%)	85_	29_	25–36_	44_	30_	37_
	53 PL	18 PL	16 PL	30 PL	30 PL	23 PL

_, active drug; Inject, injectable; NS, nasal spray; PL, placebo; Tab, tablet.

TABLE 20-3 **Preventive Medication for Migraine**

Beta blockers
Calcium channel blockers
Tricyclics and miscellaneous antidepressants
Monoamine oxidase inhibitors
Nonsteroidal anti-inflammatory drugs
Antoserotonin drugs
Anticonvulsants
? Leukotriene antagonists (experimental)
? Riboflavin and magnesium
Co-enzyme Q-10
Feverfew

two characteristics of the condition: firstly, the number of headache attacks can occur in a bunch up to eight times per day; and secondly, the frequent headache attacks are clustered, or grouped, over a defined period of several weeks or months, followed by long headache-free intervals for months or years. Another hallmark of cluster headache is its periodicity; hence the British term for this condition, *periodic migrainous neuralgia*. These headaches tend to occur on a regular schedule, often at night, awakening the patient from a sound sleep at precisely the same time every night, seldom deviating by even 5 minutes. Furthermore, the attacks usually have a seasonal periodicity, occurring at the same time every year, often in late autumn or springtime. This may be related to long and short photoperiods of available light, which occur around June 21 and December 21.

The onset of cluster headache is almost immediate, with rapidly escalating intensity. There is no throbbing quality, as in migraine, but instead a deep boring or searing pain, which is often described as being "like a red-hot poker" or squeezing of the eyeball. This intense pain is usually deep in the eye, occasionally in the temple. The duration of cluster headache is briefer than that of migraine, lasting from 15 to 180 minutes, most often 45 to 90 minutes. Unlike migraine, nausea, vomiting, and visual symptoms are absent, despite the orbital location. The associated symptoms of cluster headache are very different from those of migraine and are quite characteristic of each patient's attack. These symptoms, caused by autonomic dysfunction, include ipsilateral oculorrhea, nasal congestion, scleral injection, ptosis, miosis, and forehead sweating. Behavior during the acute cluster headache attack is very different from that during migraine; patients in severe pain with cluster headache cannot lie still, are up walking or sitting, rocking back and forth with pain, or may beat their head with their fists or bang their head on the wall. Patients with migraine want to lie still in a dark quiet room, because movement exacerbates the pain.

The location of the headache and these autonomic features point to the trigeminal nerve and sphenopalatine ganglion anatomic location, but the neurovascular or neuropeptide changes which set in motion this painful periodic disorder remain unknown. Abnormalities of the carotid body and lowered oxygen tension may be causally related.

Cluster headache is always unilateral, and every recurrence over many years is usually on the same side. There are rare reports of the opposite side being involved on occasion.

Like migraine, which has a strong familial tendency, cluster headache has a hereditary predisposition, with first-degree relatives having a 14-fold increase compared with the random population. Only 0.07% of the population is affected, compared with 12% for migraine.[4] Cluster headache occurs chiefly in men, 5:1 over women.[1] These men usually have a characteristic physiognomy: they are athletic or mesomorphic, with prominent thick facial features, furrowed brow, and deep nasolabial folds. They often have an orange-peel–like skin and telangiectasias of the nose and cheeks. They are often intense, busy, dynamic people, heavy smokers and heavy drinkers who have an increased incidence of coronary and gastrointestinal problems. During a cluster headache siege, patients quickly learn that alcohol will trigger a headache attack, but between clusters they may drink with impunity.

Ninety percent of cluster headache sufferers have episodic cluster headache (ECH), with the cluster period lasting 4 to 12 weeks. The pain stops spontaneously, only to return in several months or years. Chronic cluster headache (CCH) develops in 10% of sufferers.[10] This condition usually evolves from ECH, as episodic headaches begin to lengthen in duration and appear more frequently until the attacks are continuous (secondary chronic cluster headache). Rarely, CCH appears at the outset (primary chronic cluster headache). CCH is more resistant to treatment that ECH, and patients suffer terribly.

Differential Diagnosis

Cluster headache must be differentiated from tic douloureux (trigeminal neuralgia), chronic and episodic paroxysmal hemicrania, and SUNCT syndrome (short-lasting unilateral neuralgiform headache with conjunctival injection and tearing). There are rare reports of focal structural lesions, such as ateriovenous malformations, pituitary tumors, intracranial aneurysms, vertebral dissection, or temporal fossa meningiomas, mimicking cluster headache.[4] Occasionally, we encounter patients with cluster headache related to trauma or surgery, especially in the fifth cranial nerve distribution; these cases are often resistant to treatment.

In typical cases of cluster headache in which examination is normal, neuroimaging is not necessary unless the patient fails to respond to treatment and the condition continually worsens.

Management

In cluster headache, unlike migraine, nonpharmacologic treatment is seldom effective. There are two approaches to management of cluster headache: treatment of the acute attack and preventive pharmacotherapy.

Approximately 70% of patients with cluster headache obtain prompt relief within a few minutes by breathing 100% oxygen through a nonrebreathing mask at a flow rate of 7 liters per minute for 15 minutes.[4] Kudrow advocates the patient sitting while leaning forward with arms on knees during the oxygen inhalation. The oxygen cylinder is often kept at the bedside, and prompt relief is achieved for nocturnal cluster attacks.

Subcutaneous injection of sumatriptan is remarkably and rapidly effective for 74% of patients; response is usually consistent without tolerance or loss of effectiveness throughout the cluster period.[11] Sumatriptan nasal spray is sometimes effective. There is less experience with use of the newer triptans in treatment of cluster headache. Migranal NS (dihydroergotamine) or ergotamine tablets or suppositories may be helpful if sumatriptan is ineffective. Lidocaine, 4% nose drops, may be effective but is not a first-line acute care treatment.

As noted, patients with cluster headache are usually middle-aged men who are heavily muscled and frequent smokers, so potent vasoconstrictor medications must be given with caution and are contraindicated if there is a suspected history of heart disease or poorly controlled hypertension.

Preventive treatment may reduce the frequency and severity of individual headaches during the cluster attack and will often interrupt the cluster cycle itself. If this is successful, treatment is usually continued for 3 or 4 weeks and then gradually tapered, but it can be resumed if the headaches return.

A brief tapering course of corticosteroids may break the headache cycle, and can be repeated if the cluster recurs. Calcium-channel blockers are frequently effective; verapamil in high doses has been studied the most thoroughly. Lithium carbonate is often helpful, especially for patients with CCH. Blood levels of lithium, electrolytes, and renal function must be monitored in patients receiving lithium therapy, because high doses may be nephrotoxic. Concurrent use of lithium with diuretics or carbamazepine should be avoided. Indomethacin and the ergot derivatives, such as ergotamine tartrate and methysergide, are often effective for both ECH and CCH. Divalproex sodium, acetazolamide, and intranasal capsaicin have been used successfully. Often, combinations of these medications are required and knowledge of potential toxicity and side effects must be communicated to the patient.[1,4,10]

The pain of cluster headache is intense and disabling, and the fact that 90% of patients can be helped makes treatment of this condition especially gratifying. For the 10% of patients who respond poorly to outpatient medical management, inpatient intensive therapy or surgery may be offered; successful procedures include glycerol injection, radiofrequency thermocoagulation of the trigeminal ganglion, gamma knife procedures involving the trigeminal nerve root entry zone, or sphenopalatine ganglionectomy.[4]

TENSION-TYPE HEADACHE

Tension-type headache (TTH) is the most common kind of headache, experienced by almost everyone at some time in his or her lifetime. Most people take an aspirin or acetaminophen and never even think about consulting a physician for these occasional mild headaches. TTH is less intense than migraine and seldom disabling; these are nonthrobbing, pressure or tight bandlike global headaches that do not have associated symptoms such as nausea or light sensitivity. Chapter 17 includes the IHS criteria used to diagnose TTH. When TTH occurs for more than 15 days per month over a period of more than 6 months, it is termed chronic tension-type headache (CTTH), distinguishing it from less frequent episodic tension-type headache (ETTH).

Before publication of the IHS system of headache classification in 1988,[12] TTH was called *tension headache* or *muscle contraction headache*. We commonly see patients whose symptoms begin with suboccipital tightness or nuchal pressure; these mild headaches can often be relieved with simple analgesics or physical therapy. If not treated early, however, this TTH may progress to assume characteristics of migraine, such as throbbing intensity, and radiating to become localized over one orbital region, accompanied by nausea or photophobia. Modern headache investigators increasingly speculate that migraine and TTH may have a common origin resulting from inflammation, altered pain-regulating neuropeptide dysfunction in the brainstem, and changes in cranial blood vessels.[13] In support of this view are recent reports about response of TTH to sumatriptan in patients who also have migraine.[14] Sumatriptan is believed to decrease migraine symptoms because of its pharmacologic specificity for serotonin 1B and 1D receptors. In any case, patients with ETTH seldom consult physicians, and when they do, treatment is usually straightforward, involving reassurance, simple analgesics, biofeedback, anxiolytics, or tricyclics. Most patients respond to over-the-counter medication, but some require prescription medications such as Fiorinal or Midrin. Occasional use of acetaminophen (Tylenol) with codeine, Fiorinal with codeine, or even butorphanol nasal spray (Stadol NS) may afford rapid relief; these drugs can safely be used up to two times a week, but the patient must be cautioned against dose escalation and increased frequency of use, which can lead to analgesic rebound headaches.

More problematic is the patient with CTTH. Confounding this diagnosis is growing criticism that the IHS classification is not comprehensive; revision of the IHS criteria to subdivide CTTH into patients with or without medication overuse has been proposed.[15] Mathew coined the term "transformed migraine" to describe the phenomenon of patients with infrequent migraine in their teens who develop frequent, milder headaches in their twenties and thirties. They often take increasing doses of medications, both prescription and over-the-counter preparations, which usually contain caffeine, barbiturates, aspirin, or acetaminophen.[1,4] People with a predisposition to headaches often develop a pharmacologic tolerance to these drugs, and as the medicine is metabolized, a rebound headache occurs, usually in the early morning, several hours after the last dose. The patient then takes more of the offending medicine, resulting in a vicious cycle in which the drug is perpetuating and worsening the headache condition and the episodic migraine is transformed into a chronic, daily headache. Patients with analgesic rebound headaches are very difficult to treat, and hospitalization is often necessary for detoxification and development of a more rational and effective comprehensive treatment program. These patients usually report taking Tylenol with codeine, Fiorinal, and other prescription drugs but often neglect to mention the 12 to 16 Excedrin, Anacin, aspirin, or Tylenol they take every day, so the clinician must remember to ask specifically about nonprescription medications.

CTTH must be differentiated from other chronic headache conditions with different natural histories and perhaps different underlying mechanisms; these include transformed migraine, hemicrania continua, and new, daily, persistent headaches. Several investigators were unable to satisfactorily classify 35% to 40% of their chronic headache patients according to existing IHS diagnostic criteria.[15]

A relatively new phenomenon is the increasing popularity of alternative, "natural" substances that patients are reluctant to disclose to the physician. Among these are megadoses of herbal sedatives, such as valerian root; St. John's wort (which can potentiate serotonin reuptake inhibitors); ginkgo biloba (which, combined with aspirin or NSAIDs, can cause serious bleeding); and other herbs and vitamin supplements. These products are sold without FDA regulation or approval as food supplements rather than drugs. Some studies suggest the benefits of oral magnesium, vitamins B_2 and B_6, and, possibly, less for patients with TTH.

Management

Needless to say, treatment of patients with chronic headaches is more difficult than that of patients with straightforward, infrequent, and uncomplicated migraine. The patient-physician relationship, described by Rapoport and Sheftell as having mutuality of input and decision making, is essential more than ever in these situations.[1]

For the difficult patient with chronic headaches, behavioral modification is important, and a cornerstone of treatment must include the patient becoming an active participant rather than a passive consumer of medications. Behavioral treatment begins with the patient keeping an accurate headache diary, which records the following characteristics: (1) when the headaches occur—on weekends, after sleeping late, always at the end of a hectic workday, menstrual-related, and so on; (2) potential food and environmental triggers; and 3)medications, doses, and response to treatment.

Pharmacotherapy begins with the patient being able to distinguish TTH from migraine. Early treatment of TTH may afford complete relief. Aspirin, acetaminophen, Excedrin, and NSAIDs are often effective. Patients must be cautioned about possible gastric irritation, and close monitoring of medication is very important. Combinations of over-the-counter and prescription drugs may be preferred. For example, 2 tablets of naproxen sodium plus 2 tablets of Midrin may give satisfactory headache relief. Daily preventive medications, such as cyclobenzaprine or tricyclic antidepressants, may be helpful in conjunction with the nonpharmacologic treatment methods outlined earlier. The tricyclics are especially effective if the patient complains of sleep disturbance or is depressed. If weight gain or excessive daytime drowsiness develops, reducing the dose or replacing tricyclics with SSRIs may be beneficial. Comorbidity of other conditions should always be considered.

Opiates can be helpful for patients with severe TTH but must be used properly, and limitations must be set and followed by patients.

REFERENCES

1. Rapoport AM, Sheftell FD. *Headache Disorders, A Management Guide for Practitioners*. Philadelphia, Pa: WB Saunders; 1996.
2. Blau JN. *Migraine, Clinical and Research Aspects*. Baltimore, Md: Johns Hopkins University Press; 1987.
3. Fisher CM. Late-life migraine accompaniments as a cause of unexplained transient ischemic attacks. *Le Journal Des Sciences Neurologiques* 1980; 7:9–17.
4. Silberstein SD, Lipton RB, Goadsby PJ. *Headache in Clinical Practice*. Oxford, England: Isis Medical Media; 1998.
5. Schieving WI. Intracranial aneurysms. *N Engl J Med* 1997;336:28–40.
6. Blumenthal HJ, Vance DA. Chewing gum headaches. *Headache* 1997; 7:665–666.
7. Lipton RB, Stewart WF, Ryan RE, et al. Efficacy and safety of acetaminophen, aspirin, and caffeine in alleviating migraine headache pain. *Arch Neurol* 1998;55:210–217.
8. VanDenBrink AM, Reekers M, Bax WA, et al. Coronary side-effect potential of current and prospective antimigraine drugs. *Circulation* 1998;98:25–30.
9. Markley HG. Chronic headache: Appropriate use of opiate analgesics. *Neurology* 1994;44(suppl):518–524.
10. Mathew NT. Cluster headache. *Neurology* 1992;42(suppl):32–36.
11. Ekbom K. Treatment of acute cluster headache with sumatriptan. *N Engl J Med* 1991;325:322–326.
12. Headache Classification Committee of the International Headache Society. Classification and diagnostic criteria for headache disorders, cranial neuralgias and facial pain. *Cephalalgia* 1988;8:1–96.
13. Messinger HB, Spierings ELH, Vincent AJP. Overlap of migraine and tension-type headache in the International Headache Society classification. *Cephalalgia* 1991;11:233–237.
14. Cady RK, Gutterman D, Saiers JA, et al. Responsiveness of non-IHS migraine and tension-type headache to sumatriptan. *Cephalalgia* 1997; 17:588–590.
15. Silberstein SD, Lipton RB, Sliwinski M. Classification of daily and near-daily headaches: Field trial of revised IHS criteria. *Neurology* 1996;47:871–875.

CHAPTER 21 REFRACTORY HEADACHES

Elizabeth Loder

BACKGROUND

With appropriate diagnosis and treatment, the majority of headache sufferers can look forward to improved management (although not elimination) of their headaches. There remains, however, a group of patients whose headaches do not improve with treatment as expected. In addition to the pain of inadequately relieved headache, these patients are at risk of developing chronic pain syndrome, a condition characterized by significant disability, medication dependence and overuse, depression, and worsening headache.

Chronic pain syndrome often develops insidiously over time: as a result of the pain and incapacitation of frequent, poorly relieved headaches, patients miss substantial school or work time, and productivity is often reduced even when they are in attendance. Overuse or dependence on medication may result from desperate attempts to remain functional. This leads to secondary problems with rebound headache, altered sleep-wake cycles, or end-organ dysfunction, such as gastrointestinal hemorrhage related to overuse of anti-inflammatory medications, kidney damage from overuse of acetaminophen, sleep disruption related to sedative misuse, and so forth. Sufferers often limit social or leisure activities in order to devote themselves to essential work or school activities, leading to isolation from family or social contacts. Avoidance of physical exertion that may trigger headache not infrequently leads to profound physical deconditioning. In many patients, depression ensues or worsens.

Once underway, this complex downward spiral is difficult, if not impossible, to address using single-discipline treatment or medication. If the disability resulting from chronic disabling headache could be prevented, tremendous suffering would be avoided. This chapter discusses the magnitude of the problem of refractory headache, suggests ways to intercede in patients currently experiencing refractory headache, and considers how early intervention with appropriate, disease-specific measures might prevent the disaster of chronic headache from developing in many patients.

EPIDEMIOLOGY

Data from the American Migraine Study suggest that 5% of American women and 3% of American men suffer from frequent, severe headaches, defined as headache more than 15 days a month.[1] The vast majority can be assumed to have migraine or transformed migraine, with a small number likely experiencing cluster or other less common types of headache. Although tension-type headache in its chronic form can be debilitating, it is far less frequent than migraine among severely disabled patients.

The gender distribution of headache is not equal, with women more likely than men at all postpubertal ages to suffer from headache, and more likely than men to develop severe, disabling forms of the disorder. Epidemiologic data show that women require more bed rest per attack than do men,[2] and are more likely to be moderately or severely disabled as a result of headache. Regardless of gender, the most disabled segment of the headache population accounts for very large percentages of the indirect costs attributed to migraine,[3] suggesting that treatment targeted to this group of severely affected patients is highly cost-effective.[2]

The level of functioning of patients with chronic headache has been found to be worse in many areas than that of patients with conditions such as diabetes or arthritis. Among a group of patients with chronic illnesses, patients with chronic headache functioned at a level comparable to that of patients with congestive heart failure or recent myocardial infarction.[3]

REASONS FOR REFRACTORY HEADACHE

Five factors, acting singly or in concert, can be responsible for a patient whose headaches have been refractory to treatment, and evidence of them should be vigorously sought when patients do not respond as expected to treatment. They are (1) inappropriate expectations of treatment benefit, (2) inaccurate diagnosis, (3) inadequate treatment, (4) psychiatric comorbidity, and (5) severe disease.

TREATMENT EXPECTATIONS

Headache is most appropriately viewed as a chronic illness of long duration, in which the goal is management, not cure. Chronic nonmalignant headache is currently understood as an inherited vulnerability to headache caused by abnormalities in central nervous system neurotransmitter systems. Changes in central pain processing may also play a role.[4] Although progress has been made in understanding the genetic underpinnings of headache, particularly migraine,[5] it is not possible to alter them, and treatment is aimed at trigger avoidance, improving abortive treatment of migraine, implementing prophylactic measures or medication to decrease headache frequency, and improving the ability of patients to cope with headache.

Patients, their families, or even treating clinicians may have an erroneous understanding of the nature of chronic headache and the ability of medical treatment to alter the natural history of the disease. They may expect that treatment will easily eliminate all headaches with a minimum of side effects, and may not be aware of the importance of active patient involvement in treatment. If uncorrected, these beliefs can lead to physician shopping, dissatisfaction, and poor treatment compliance (especially with prophylactic treatments that produce only gradual, incremental improvement and require relatively long use to become effective).

Thorough exploration of the beliefs of all relevant parties may reveal unrealistic ideas and expectations, providing an opportunity for education and reformulation of treatment goals. In general, realistic treatment goals for this group of severely affected patients are to reduce headache frequency (ideally to two or fewer headaches a week); to find abortive treatment that works quickly, consistently, and well; and to involve the patients in lifestyle alterations that improve their ability to cope with headache, such as regular exercise, good sleep habits, and the use of relaxation or other nonpharmacologic pain control methods. When these goals can be accomplished, most patients remain able to participate in work, school, or social activities despite frequent headache.

INACCURATE DIAGNOSIS

Failure of a patient to respond as expected to headache treatment, or a significant change in headache pattern or characteristics, should prompt reconsideration of the diagnosis. An initial inaccurate diagnosis of a primary headache disorder may have been made in a patient who really has a secondary headache, or a secondary cause of headache may have developed in a patient since the original headache diagnosis was made.

In any case, a thorough review of the headache history and repeat physical and neurologic examination, as well as testing, should be considered. Neurologic and physical findings are generally normal in patients with primary headache disorders, but special attention should be devoted to palpation of the pericranial musculature, funduscopic examination, including the presence of venous pulsations, and mental status. It is important to remember that some secondary causes of headache, such as Arnold-Chiari malformations or high-pressure headaches without papilledema, can present in subtle ways. It is always worth carefully reviewing a patient's medications as well, because many frequently used medications can cause or exacerbate headaches.

There is considerable but not complete overlap in treatment options that are helpful for the various primary headache disorders. This incomplete overlap means that even if the diagnosis of a primary headache disorder has been made correctly, incorrect assignment to the various subtypes of primary headache can have treatment implications. For example, a patient with cluster headache who is considered to have migraine (not an infrequent occurrence) is not likely to benefit from treatment with beta blockers or tricyclic antidepressants, because these drugs are not useful in cluster headache. If such a patient has a partial response to sumatriptan (effective in both migraine and cluster headache), used in the erroneous assumption that the headache in question is migraine, the clinician may be reinforced in the inaccurate diagnosis and recognition of the correct diagnosis delayed. Thus, response to a particular treatment modality should not be considered to have clear diagnostic significance.

INADEQUATE TREATMENT

Evaluation of a patient referred for refractory headaches must include a thorough review of previous courses of treatment. A limited number of medications are useful in the management of headache disorders; it is essential that options for treatment not be discarded as unhelpful on the basis of inadequate previous experience. Detailed information about previous treatment is often difficult to obtain. A complete list may require acquisition of previous medical or pharmacy records. On review, it is clear that many patients referred to specialty clinics with a diagnosis of refractory headache have not had the benefit of aggressive, high-dose trials of treatment. Scrupulous review of previous treatment attempts by an expert in the pharmacotherapy of difficult headache disorders can often produce important suggestions for future treatment trials.

Some patients with frequent or severe headaches have been maintained only on abortive agents, or have never been given the opportunity to try the newer, disease-specific abortive agents such as the triptans, perhaps out of exaggerated fears about the safety of the drugs. Not uncommonly patients report that they are "allergic" or have had an adverse reaction, to an important class of therapeutic drugs for headache. If possible, this claim should be investigated. The author has had many patients report so-called allergic reactions to sumatriptan or dihydroergotamine, for example, which on review represented a dystonic reaction to a phenothiazine antinauseant given concomitantly.

Another common problem is that appropriate medication classes have been tried, but the doses used have not been adequate or the medication has not been tried for an adequate length of time. In general, the maximal benefit of most prophylactic agents requires use for 6 to 8 weeks at the highest safe or tolerated dose before maximal benefit can be assessed.[6] Worsening or improvement in headaches observed over a shorter period of time may be the result of the waxing and waning nature of chronic headaches. Noncompliance may also be a factor in apparently ineffective treatment, and drugs with tolerable side effects and once-daily regimens will likely improve treatment outcome in this chronic disorder.[7]

Treatment attempts can be compromised by concomitant overuse of drugs that cause rebound headache. These are usually short-acting, abortive medications such as combination analgesics, ergotamine, or caffeine-containing drugs. Frequent use of triptans has also been suggested as a cause of rebound headaches.[8] Overuse of these classes of medications has been implicated as the single most important factor leading to the transformation of intermittent migraine to chronic daily headache. In many cases, patients are reluctant to disclose the true extent of medication overuse, or do not report overuse of nonprescription medications.

Withdrawal from such offending medications can be difficult, especially on an outpatient basis. Many patients are reluctant to discontinue their reliance on these medications until their headaches are better; unfortunately, the headaches will not improve until they discontinue these medications.[9] Unproductive treatment stalemates can be avoided by educating the patient about the nature of rebound headache, and outlining a realistic withdrawal regimen and interim headache control plan. The use of repetitive intravenous dihydroergotamine[10] or corticosteroids can be very helpful in weaning patients from these drugs. Patients and physicians need to realize that improvement in chronic headache after withdrawal of excess analgesic medication use will be gradual and can take up to 6 months. Hospitalization may be required if patients cannot successfully complete this step of treatment on an outpatient basis.

In still other cases, rational use of co-pharmacy, or combinations of prophylactic medications, has not been attempted. When possible, therapy with a single agent is preferred to minimize the possibility of drug interactions and adverse events. However, as with other chronic illnesses, the combination of two classes of drugs can prove effective. Often-used combinations include sodium valproate and selective serotonin reuptake inhibitors (SSRIs), or beta blockers and tricyclic antidepressants.

Underuse of nonpharmacologic methods of treatment is common, partly because of poor insurance reimbursement for this treatment. Often such treatments are tried late in the course of the disorder, when a sense of treatment failure is established and the disease well established. In this setting, nonpharmacologic treatment is less effective. Findings from randomized controlled trials support the use of biofeedback (which appeared similar in efficacy to preventive pharmacotherapy); relaxation strategies, such as progressive muscle relaxation, breathing exercises, and imagery; and cognitive-behavioral therapy.[11] Given these data, and considering the substantial side-effect penalties of pharmacologic prophylaxis for migraine, it is disappointing that most insurance and managed care organizations still refuse to pay for these therapies.

Sequential treatment is often all that is possible on an outpatient basis, where formidable bureaucratic barriers and time pressures make it difficult to arrange concomitant treatment with several different modalities. Nonetheless, attempts should be made to capitalize on the synergistic improvements possible with a combination of treatments. For example, many patients obtain better relief with the combination of physical therapy, biofeedback, and pharmacologic treatments when these methods are employed simultaneously, rather than singly. In explaining this to patients, it is often helpful to employ the analogy of a car stuck in a snowbank. Several people pushing together are more likely to meet with success than if each tries alone to move the car. Similarly, if single attempts at headache treatment have not proved effective, it does not necessarily follow that they should be abandoned. Rather, consideration should be given to the use of additional treatment modalities.

PSYCHIATRIC COMORBIDITY

Patients with chronic headache are more likely than controls in the general population to suffer from a spectrum of affective disorders, including depression and anxiety. In specialty headache and pain clinics, personality disorders and a history of childhood trauma are also frequently found. Depression and anxiety disorders are comorbid with migraine, and it has been proposed that the predisposition to develop both is based on inherited disturbances in central nervous system serotonergic systems.[12] Patients suffering from migraine with aura may also be at heightened risk for suicide.[13] It is simplistic to view one as causing the other, and equally ingenuous to assume that treatment of one disorder will somehow cure the other. Adequate treatment of depression can render the burden of headache easier to cope with, and improvement in headache can lead to improvements in depression, but both disorders require specific attention and treatment.

There is no evidence of shared etiologic mechanisms for chronic headache and personality disorders; more likely, the overrepresentation of these patients among refractory populations reflects the fact that when a personality disorder exists in a person who also has a severe headache problem, the personality disorder complicates treatment. The presence of a personality disorder may lead to treatment noncompliance, difficulty establishing a working relationship with caregivers, and less effective coping with the social and occupational burdens of headache. All of this fosters the development of maladaptive behaviors and decreases the success of long-term treatment.

Childhood trauma may cause permanent changes in the central nervous system that increase susceptibility to the development of chronic pain.[14,15] Patients may be reluctant to disclose a history of physical or sexual abuse; tactful queries about these topics are an important part of the history of any patient with refractory headache or pain. If a history of such abuse is elicited, it can alert the clinician to be cautious about such "hands-on" treatment options as physical therapy or biofeedback, techniques which may be poorly tolerated by patients with a history of previous abuse.

Psychosocial factors can amplify or reinforce illness behavior in patients with legitimate headache disorders. For example, the secondary gain of increased attention from family, avoidance of unpleasant work or personal responsibilities, or school avoidance can reinforce the behavior of headache. Caregivers may inadvertently increase the patient's sense of dependence on external factors by overreliance or emphasis on the use of pills, procedures, or passive therapies such as massage. Attention to the role these factors are playing in refractory headache cases is important. Very careful consideration should be given before providing a patient with medical sanction to avoid school or work attendance. Although well-intentioned, such allowances often produce isolating behaviors that prove self-perpetuating and difficult to reverse.

Expert psychiatric and psychological evaluation and ongoing support are invaluable in all cases of refractory headache. Mental health professionals who have experience treating patients with chronic pain or headache, or both, should be sought. Patients may resist such referral unless they understand it does not imply that their headaches are not "real." Most recognize that the burden of living with headache can aggravate any tendency to depression and welcome the opportunity to discuss how to cope with chronic illness. Ideally, the referring clinician will work closely with the mental health professional to coordinate treatment. Some antidepressants can exacerbate headache, and the use of sedatives or tranquilizers may be counterproductive as well, by limiting the options for rescue therapy of severe headache episodes.

SEVERE DISEASE

Although significant progress has been made in understanding and treating headache disorders, not all patients have disease that is amenable to medical therapy. For example, subcutaneous sumatriptan injections, the gold standard in acute migraine therapy, work in only 80% of patients under the best circumstances, and even then provide complete, consistent relief across attacks in an even smaller percentage of patients.[16] Contemporary prophylactic drugs are widely recognized as having limited efficacy with a high side-effect burden, and the best provide improvement of headache in only 50% to 60% of patients.[17] This limited response to treatment likely reflects the underlying genetic heterogeneity of migraine, as well as the spectrum of disease severity. And, as with every other medically based illness, some patients have disease that is simply beyond the reach of currently available medical interventions.

Other patients, over a long course of headache, have developed maladaptive behaviors that significantly limit possibilities for improvement. Entrenched patterns of medication use (or overuse), emphasis on short-term treatment at the expense of long-term improvement, altered family dynamics, expectations of treatment failure, and secondary gain are all extremely difficult to reverse once established. The likelihood of meaningful, successful intervention in a long-established severe headache disorder decreases over time, a strong argument for aggressive intervention at the earliest possible stage.

STRATEGIES FOR INTERVENTION

Specialty Programs

For patients whose headaches have proved refractory to good outpatient management, who are experiencing significant life disruption from their headaches, who require withdrawal from large amounts of problematic medications, or who have medical or psychiatric problems that render traditional, single-discipline outpatient treatment unsuccessful, hospitalization or involvement in a multidisciplinary outpatient pain program are important treatment options. Relatively few specialized inpatient units exist, but the most severely affected patients should be offered this option. Multidisciplinary outpatient programs are increasingly available. A list of treatment programs can be obtained from the Commission on the Accreditation of Rehabilitation Facilities or the American Pain Society. Where possible, these programs should provide access to a clinician skilled in the management of headache patients.

In referring a patient for a multidisciplinary pain management approach, it is important to communicate to the patient the change in treatment strategy and philosophy that such a referral represents. Most such programs emphasize improvement in function rather than pain control as the goal of treatment, and it is important that patients accept this change in emphasis. Rather than focusing on further, largely futile, attempts to find medication or other procedures that will "fix" the pain of headache, these programs attempt to minimize the impact of headache on patients' function. They work to reverse physical deconditioning through physical therapy, teach pacing and organizational strategies to minimize the overdo-underdo cycle in which many patients are trapped, and introduce relaxation and behavioral techniques to manage pain. An emphasis on pain and passive treatments is discouraged, and patients are rewarded for increases in functional behavior and taught to take an active role in their own treatment. Medication reduction programs, in addition to withdrawal from problematic medications, are required for many patients. These programs have been shown to produce measurable and persistent improvements in patients' perceived quality of life despite minimal changes in pain scores. Use of health care resources and emergency department usage also declines.

Maintenance Opioids

Treatment of nonmalignant chronic pain, including headache, with maintenance opioid medications has become increasingly common and accepted in the medical community over the past decade. Several studies have reviewed the impact of such use in patients with chronic headache. The evidence to date suggests that a substantial minority (probably in the neighborhood of 25%) of such patients derive long-term benefit from opioid maintenance without the development of unacceptable adverse events or aberrant drug-related behaviors. The risk of addiction in appropriately selected patients is probably quite low.

If elected, opioid maintenance should be guided by the principles applied in other nonmalignant pain states. A written contract is helpful in clarifying treatment goals and expectations, and regular office visits to monitor progress are essential. It should be remembered that most patients do not derive long-term benefit from this treatment, and that in the majority of cases it simply buys some time to consider other treatment options or obtain a measure of respite from relentless headaches. Those are not inconsiderable benefits, however, and with these realistic goals in mind, opioid maintenance should be considered for every patient truly refractory to other headache therapies.

The danger, of course, is that with the increasing popularity of opioid maintenance therapy for a variety of conditions, and with the emphasis on costs of treatment, opioid therapy (which is relatively inexpensive) will be inappropriately tried before more effective and desirable treatments have been exhausted. This is to be discouraged, for several reasons. In addition to the fact that only a minority of patients ultimately derives long-term benefit from maintenance opioids, they are a nonspecific treatment that masks but does nothing to address the underlying pathophysiology of headache. In addition, the subtle but cumulative effects of mental apathy and cognitive impairment that might be acceptable in terminal cancer patients are much less defensible in generally young, otherwise healthy, and potentially productive patients.

SUMMARY OF TREATMENT APPROACH TO REFRACTORY HEADACHE PATIENTS

Several general principles can be kept profitably in mind when treating patients with refractory headaches who have failed to obtain benefit from careful consideration of the previously mentioned factors. The first is that, despite the apparent failure of previous attempts at prophylaxis, most such patients should be maintained on a reasonable prophylactic regimen for headache—not with the expectation that this will produce improvement, but in the hope that it may delay progression of the underlying disorder. Evidence is slowly emerging that some prophylactics may have disease-modifying effects and delay progression to even more severe levels of headache disability.

The temptation for patients to overuse abortive headache medications is often overwhelming, and strict limits must be agreed on with the patient and enforced. In general, in these severe situations, it is appropriate to allow patients to use strong abortive medications, including opioids, sedatives, or parenteral dihydroergotamine or sumatriptan up to 2 or 3 days a week. Although the clinician may not be able to make these patients better, one certain way to make things worse is to allow too-frequent use of acute medications, with the eventual development of dependence, addiction, or end-organ dysfunction or damage.

All patients should be seen regularly in consultation by a mental health professional and routinely evaluated for depression and suicidal ideation. A regular aerobic exercise regimen and good sleep hygiene should be maintained. Overuse of nonspecific sedative and sleep medications is to be carefully avoided, because this can limit options for rescue treatment of severe headaches.

Finally, as with patients who have other severe, incurable illnesses, these patients benefit from a stable, long-term relationship with an interested clinician. Regular office visits should be geared toward review of the patient's medication and coping strategies, with a goal of preventing further harm from the effects of the illness itself, attendant occupational or social disability, or the injudicious use of medication to treat the illness. Regularly scheduled visits afford the clinician an opportunity to review with patients the merits of herbal, surgical, or alternative medical treatments they may be considering. Ensuring continued psychosocial support and reinforcement of the patient's positive behaviors and attempts to cope constructively with disability are invaluable. Such a long-term relationship usually becomes an important and appreciated resource for a person coping with a chronic illness, and should be viewed as an essential part of the pain physician's practice—to comfort always, even when we cannot cure.

REFERENCES

1. Stewart WF, Lipton RB, Celentano DD, Reed ML. Prevalence of migraine headache in the United States: Relation to age, income, race, and other sociodemographic factors. *JAMA* 1992;267:64–69.
2. Hu XH, Markson LE, Lipton RB, Stewart WF, Berger ML. Burden of migraine in the United States. *Arch Intern Med* 1999;159:813–818.
3. Warshaw LJ, Burton WN, Silberstein SD, Lipton RB. Migraine: A problem for employers and managed care plans. *Am J Man Care* 1997;3:1515–1523.
4. Goadsby P. Nonopioid peptides in migraine and cluster headache. In: Olesen J, Edvinsson L, eds. *Headache Pathogenesis: Monoamines, Neuropeptides, Purines, and Nitric Oxide*. Philadelphia, Pa: Lippincott-Raven Publishers; 1997:201–209.
5. Peroutka SJ. Genetic basis of migraine. *Clin Neurosci* 1998;5:34–37.
6. Saper JR, Silberstein S, Gordon CD, et al. *Handbook of Headache Management*. Baltimore, Md: Williams & Wilkins; 1993.
7. Mulleners WM, Whitmarsh TE, Steiner TJ. Noncompliance may render migraine prophylaxis useless, but once-daily regimens are better. *Cephalalgia* 1998;18:52–56.
8. Gaist D, Tsirpoulus L, Sindrup SH, et al. Inappropriate use of sumatriptan: Population based register and interview study. *BMJ* 1998;316: 1352–1353.
9. Mathew NT, Stubits E, Nigam MP. Transformation of episodic migraine into daily headache: Analysis of factors. *Headache* 1982;22:66–68.
10. Raskin NH. Repetitive intravenous dihydroergotamine as therapy for intractable migraine. *Neurology* 1986;36:995–997.
11. Pryse-Phillips WE, Dodick DW, Edmeads JG, et al. Guidelines for the nonpharmacologic management of migraine in clinical practice. *CMAJ* 1998;159:47–54.
12. Merikangas KR, Angst J, et al. Migraine and psychopathology. Results of the Zurich cohort study of young adults. *Arch Gen Psychiatr* 1990; 47:849–853.
13. Breslau N, Davis GC, Andreski P. Migraine, psychiatric disorders and suicide attempts: An epidemiological study of young adults. *Psychiatry Res* 1991;37:11–23.
14. Domino JV, Haber JD. Prior physical and sexual abuse in women with chronic headache: Clinical correlates. *Headache* 1987;27:310–314.
15. Springs FE, Friedrich WN. Health risk behaviors and medical sequelae of childhood sexual abuse. *Mayo Clin Proc* 1992;67:527–532.
16. Goadsby PJ. A triptan too far? *J Neurol Neurosurg Psychiatry* 1998; 64:143–147.
17. Welch KMA. Drug therapy of migraine. *N Engl J Med* 1993;329: 1476–1483.

CHAPTER 22 CHRONIC DAILY HEADACHE

Egilius L.H. Spierings

Chronic daily headache relates to the daily or almost-daily occurrence of headache. However, not all daily or almost-daily headaches fall under this denominator, as is the case with the daily or almost-daily headaches of (chronic) cluster headache and paroxysmal hemicrania, as well as those of hypnic headache or nocturnal migraine. These conditions can be referred to as *paroxysmal* daily headaches in which the headaches occur in well-defined attack patterns. In cluster headache, the attack pattern is that of headaches occurring once or twice a day and lasting 1 to 2 hours, whereas in paroxysmal hemicrania, it is that of headaches occurring 5 to 15 times per day and lasting 10 to 30 minutes. In hypnic headache or nocturnal migraine, the headaches occur once a day, waking the patient from sleep at night, usually between 4 and 6 AM, and lasting for a variable amount of time, also depending on the efficacy of treatment.

Of the *non*paroxysmal daily headaches, hemicrania continua is a condition that does not fall under the denominator of chronic daily headache, either. However, it is discussed in this chapter because it is very difficult, if not impossible, to distinguish from chronic daily headache on the basis of presentation alone. It differs from chronic daily headache in having a somewhat more consistent and less variable intensity of the pain and in an absolute response to preventive treatment with indomethacin.

Chronic daily headache is not the same as chronic tension-type headache, as defined by the International Headache Society (IHS).[1] The IHS defines chronic tension-type headache as headaches with an average frequency of 15 days per month (180 days per year) or more for at least 6 months. In addition, the headaches must have at least two of the following features: pressing quality, mild or moderate intensity, bilateral location, and no aggravation by routine physical activity. Both of the following have to apply: no vomiting and no more than one of the following symptoms: nausea, photophobia, or phonophobia. Finally, the following conditions must be met: the history as well as the physical and neurologic examination do not suggest the presence of another cause of headache; if the presence of such a cause is suggested, it is ruled out by appropriate investigations or, if such a cause is present, the headaches did not occur for the first time in close temporal relation to occurrence of the disorder.

Although it is stated in the IHS classification that sometimes migraine gradually transforms into chronic tension-type headache, in my opinion, that is incorrect. Migraine may, however, transform into chronic daily headache, as discussed later. The confusion stems from the fact that the IHS identifies chronic daily headache as a synonym for chronic tension-type headache, which is incorrect. Chronic daily headache is, rather, a replacement for the old term, *mixed* or *combined headache*. In the practice of medicine, the group of patients with this condition is also the majority of those with the diagnosis of chronic daily headache. In the general population, such patients may comprise only half of the sufferers, with the other half made up of those with chronic tension-type headache.

PREVALENCE

With regard to the prevalence of *daily* headache in the general population, the only reliable information comes from a study conducted in the Netherlands in 1975–1976.[2] The study was conducted in two districts of Zoetermeer, a middle-size town near Leiden, and involved a random sample of 15,563 subjects. The sample size was 4,522 (29% of the population), and the response rate was 77%, generating 2,198 subjects who were 20 years of age or older. The respondents were asked to fill out a questionnaire that included the following question: "How often do you have headache?" One of the answer options was "daily". In the study, 6% of the respondents aged 20 years or older (4% of the men, 8% of the women) acknowledged the daily occurrence of headache. The highest prevalence was found in the age groups 20 to 24 years (8%) and older than 64 years (8%), and the lowest prevalence in the age group 35 to 54 years (5%).

The prevalence of frequent headache, that is, headaches occurring at least 180 days per year, in the general population is known from two more recent studies.[3,4] One of the studies was conducted in Baltimore County, Maryland. It involved 13,343 randomly selected subjects 18 to 65 years of age, comprising 77% of the total of 17,237 eligible subjects. Of the respondents, 40% were men and 60%, women, and their median age was 38 years. The 1-year prevalence of frequent headache was 4%: 3% in men and 5% in women. Using the IHS criteria for chronic tension-type headache and Silberstein's modified criteria for transformed migraine,[5] the investigators found a prevalence of 2.2% for chronic tension-type headache, 1.3% for frequent headache with migrainous features, and 0.6% for other frequent headaches. They found the prevalence of frequent headache to be highest in the age group 41 to 55 years and lowest in the age group 56 to 65 years.

The other study was conducted in Camargo, Spain. The study involved 1,883 subjects older than 14 years of age, which was 84% of the randomly selected sample of 2,252. Of the respondents, 47% were men and 53% were women. Participants who indicated that they had headaches 10 days per month or more were requested to keep a headache diary for 1 month. On the basis of the diary, the prevalence of frequent headache, that is, headaches occurring 15 days per month or more, was determined to be 4.7%: 1.0% in men and 8.7% in women. The mean age of the subjects with frequent headache was 50 years; the mean age at onset of the frequent headaches was 38 years. Using the criteria presented earlier, the prevalence of chronic tension-type headache was determined to be 2.2% and that of transformed migraine, 2.4%. Overuse of abortive medications was found to be the case in (only) 19% of the patients with chronic tension-type headache and in 31% of those with transformed migraine.

With regard to frequent headache, Langemark and colleagues[6] studied the clinical features of 148 patients with chronic tension headache. The patients had to have at least 10 days with headache

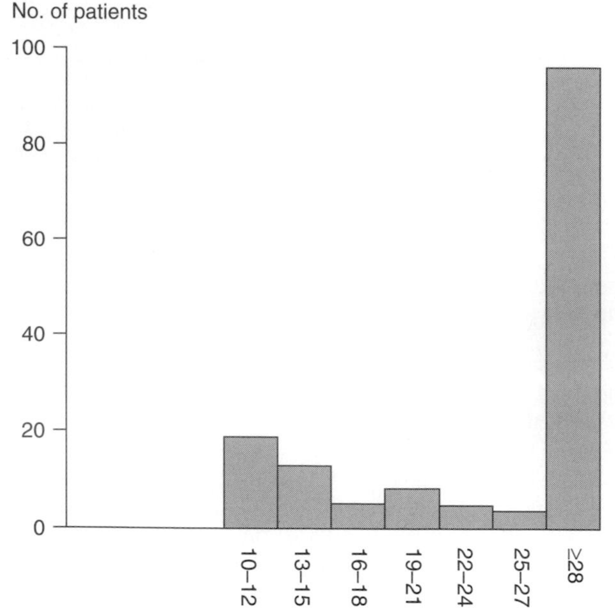

Figure 22-1 Distribution of patients according to the number of headache days per month. (Reproduced from Langemark M, Olesen J, Loldrup D, Bech P. Clinical characterization of patients with chronic tension headache. *Headache* 1988;28:590–596.)

per month and no more than one migraine attack. Ninety-three percent of them turned out to have at least 28 days with headache per month; that is, daily headaches (Figure 22-1). With regard to headache dynamics, this suggests that once headaches have increased to a frequency of 2 or 3 days per week, they rapidly progress to daily or almost-daily occurrence. The implication of this observation for the diagnostic criteria of chronic daily headache is that there is no need for an arbitrary number such as 15 (or 180). The diagnostic criterion for the condition with regard to frequency of headache could simply be "daily or near/almost daily," and the same simplification could be made for chronic tension-type headache. Everything that falls short of this frequency criterion would be episodic; that is, episodic tension-type headache or (episodic) migraine. This observation also means that the prevalence of frequent headache can be equated with that of daily headache.

On the basis of the preceding epidemiologic studies, and taking the study by Langemark and colleagues into account, it can safely be stated that the prevalence of daily headache in the general population is approximately 5%. About half of these headaches are accounted for by chronic tension-type headache as defined by the IHS. With regard to age and gender characteristics of chronic daily headache, women are affected two times more often than are men, but age does not seem to have much of an effect on the prevalence of the condition.

The prevalence of chronic tension-type headache in the general population, as defined by the IHS, was also separately determined in Denmark.[7] The study included 740 (76%) of 975 randomly selected subjects out of a total population of 325,621. The subjects were interviewed clinically, generating a prevalence number for chronic tension-type headache of 3%: 2% in men and 5% in women. It can, therefore, be safely stated that the prevalence of IHS-defined chronic tension-type headache in the general population is 2% to 3%, which accounts for about half of daily headaches.

PRESENTATION

In a study of chronic daily headache that my colleagues and I conducted,[8–10] we defined the condition as headaches occurring at least 5 days per week for a period of 1 year or longer. We excluded only the patients with paroxysmal daily headaches, that is, cluster headache and paroxysmal hemicrania, in order to capture as much of the presentation, development, and outcome of chronic daily headache as possible. The study was conducted in 258 patients from my private headache practice, 19% men and 81% women, with an average age at consultation of 42 years. The distribution of the age of (any) headache onset for the men and women separately is shown in Figure 22-2. Seventy-seven percent of the patients (69% of the men and 79% of the women) experienced the onset of headache before the age of 30 years. The onset of headache occurred in the second decade of life in 36% of the women, compared with 24% of the men. The peak of headache onset in the second decade in women is consistent with the importance of the menstrual cycle in headache occurrence.

With regard to diurnal pattern, the daily headaches were present on awakening or occurred in the course of the morning in 79% of the patients, occurred in the afternoon or evening in 6%, and had a variable time of onset in 15% (Figure 22-3). In 25% of patients, the headaches were worst on awakening or in the course of the morn-

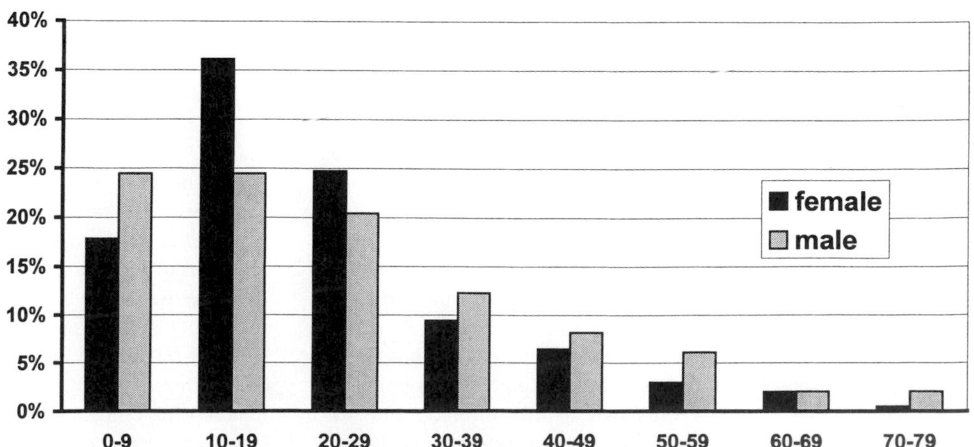

Figure 22-2 Distribution of the age of (any) headache onset per gender (n = 251). (Reproduced from Spierings ELH, Schroevers M, Honkoop PC, Sorbi M. Presentation of chronic daily headache: A clinical study. *Headache* 1998;38:191–196.)

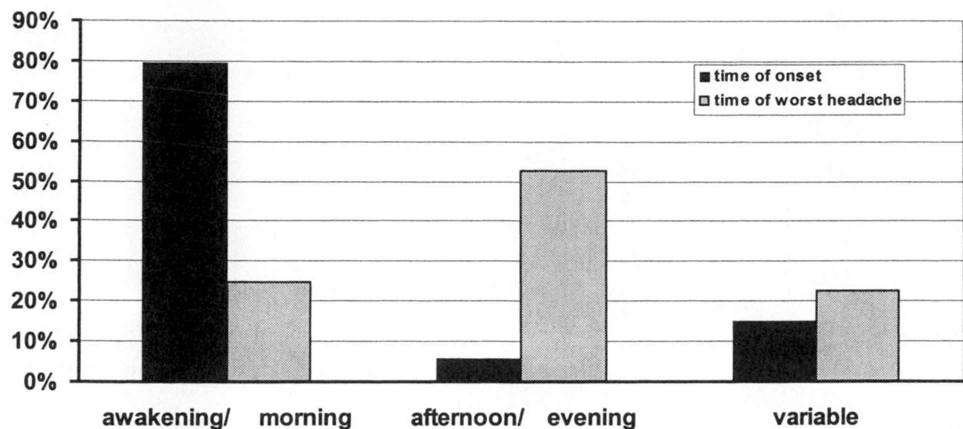

Figure 22-3 Diurnal pattern of the daily headaches (n = 214). (Reproduced from Spierings ELH, Schroevers M, Honkoop PC, Sorbi M. Presentation of chronic daily headache: A clinical study. *Headache* 1998; 38:191–196.)

ing; in 53%, they were worst in the afternoon or evening, and in 22%, they were worst at a variable time of the day. The results agree with my clinical observation that daily headaches come in two distinct diurnal patterns. In the most common pattern, the headaches gradually increase in intensity as the day progresses, becoming worst in the afternoon or evening. According to the results of the study, this is the pattern in more than half of the patients with chronic daily headache. In the less common pattern, which I have referred to as *reversed diurnal pattern*, the headaches are worst on awakening in the morning and gradually improve as the day progresses. This was the case in one quarter of the patients, while in the remaining quarter, the diurnal course of the headaches was variable.

The reversed diurnal pattern is, in my experience, particularly associated with the overuse of analgesics or vasoconstrictors, or both, for headache. Overuse in this context is defined as medication intake that is detrimental rather than beneficial to headache. In the reversed diurnal pattern, the severe headaches on awakening in the morning are caused by the withdrawal of medication overnight, and the gradual improvement during the day results from the resumption of medication intake. This scenario also is associated with the most frequent nighttime awakenings with headache. In the study, nocturnal awakening by headache occurred at least once a week in 36% of the patients. Of those patients who were awakened by headache at least once a week, 48% experienced the worst headache on awakening or in the course of the morning, compared with 22% of the patients who were awakened by headache less than once a week.

Ninety-four percent of the patients experienced severe headaches in addition to the daily headaches. The distribution of the frequency of the severe headaches in days per month is shown in Figure 22-4. Twenty-six percent of the patients experienced severe headaches more than 15 days per month. Otherwise, they experienced severe headaches mostly 10 days per month or less (63%). The results suggest that the majority of the patients with chronic daily headache who seek specialty care for their headaches do *not* have chronic tension-type headache. Instead, they have chronic tension-type headache combined with migraine or, as I prefer to call it, tension-type vascular headache.

In the development of chronic daily headache, medication intake is considered to play an important role, in particular the intake of analgesics and vasoconstrictors. A widely used vasoconstrictor for the abortive treatment of headache is caffeine, which is contained in beverages, especially coffee, but also in prescription and nonprescription medications. We determined the caffeine intake in our patients with chronic daily headache by looking at their coffee and medication intake. A cup of coffee was considered to contain 100 mg of caffeine. We found that 43% of the patients used less than 100 mg of caffeine per day, 35% used between 100 and 300 mg, and 22% used more than 300 mg. The average caffeine intake was 170 mg per day, which is approximately the equivalent of two cups of coffee.

With regard to analgesic use, we considered only the non-opioid medications, because opioids were hardly used by the patients for the treatment of their headaches. Also, of the barbiturate-containing

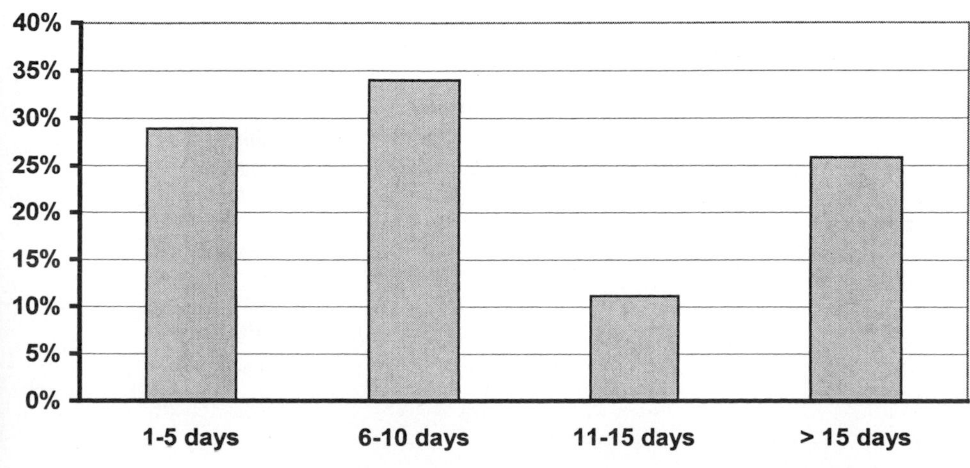

Figure 22-4 Frequency of the severe headaches in days per month (n = 197). (Reproduced from Spierings ELH, Schroevers M, Honkoop PC, Sorbi M. Presentation of chronic daily headache: A clinical study. *Headache* 1998;38:191–196.)

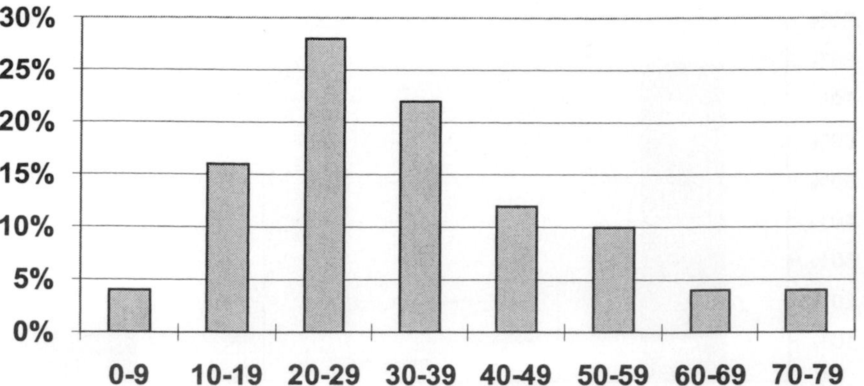

Figure 22-5 Distribution of the age of (daily) headache onset in the patients with primary chronic daily headache (n = 50). (Reproduced from Spierings ELH, Schroevers M, Honkoop PC, Sorbi M. Development of chronic daily headache: A clinical study. *Headache* 1998;38:529–533).

medications, we did not take into account the barbiturate component because it is not strictly an analgesic. With these limitations, we found that 26% of the patients used less than 500 mg of aspirin-equivalents per day and 48% less than 1,500 mg. The average analgesic intake was 1,860 mg of aspirin-equivalents per day.

DEVELOPMENT

Of the 230 patients in the study with known onset of daily headaches, 22% experienced daily headaches from the onset. This could be called *primary* chronic daily headache, in the same way that we speak of primary and secondary chronic cluster headache. The remaining 78% initially experienced intermittent headaches, that is, had *secondary* chronic daily headache. The distribution of the age of onset of the (daily) headaches in the patients with daily headaches from the onset, or primary chronic daily headache, is shown in Figure 22-5. Sixty-six percent of the patients experienced onset of daily headaches between the ages of 10 and 39 years.

Of the patients with daily headaches but who initially had intermittent headaches, that is, of those with secondary chronic daily headache, 19% experienced an abrupt onset of daily headaches and 81%, a gradual onset. The distribution of the age of onset of daily headaches in the patients with abrupt-onset secondary chronic daily headache was similar to that of the patients with primary chronic daily headache shown in Figure 22-5.

The circumstances related to the onset of daily headaches in the patients with primary chronic daily headache and in those with abrupt-onset secondary chronic daily headache are shown in Table 22-1. The table also shows the circumstances of daily headache onset for the two groups combined, as there was no difference in distribution of the circumstances between the two groups. The most common circumstance of daily headache onset in the two groups combined was head, neck, or back injury, caused by a motor vehicle accident in 61%. This was followed by flulike illness or sinusitis and medical illness or surgical procedure as causes of daily headache onset. Examples of medical illness associated with the (abrupt) onset of chronic daily headache are colitis, fibromyalgia, vertigo, encephalitis, and meningitis.

There were also no differences between the patients with primary chronic daily headache and those with abrupt-onset secondary chronic daily headache with regard to the following features: gender distribution, time of daily headache occurrence, worst headache time daily, nocturnal headache awakening, laterality of the daily headaches, occurrence and frequency of severe headaches, laterality of the severe headaches, and parental occurrence of headache. The only difference between the two groups was the association of the daily *and* severe headaches with nausea. Nausea was more common in the patients with abrupt-onset secondary chronic daily headache than in those with primary chronic daily headache. The difference probably results from the fact that 57% of the patients in the abrupt-onset group had a prior history of severe headaches, which tend to be associated with gastrointestinal symptoms.

The distribution of the age of onset of the daily headaches in the patients with gradual-onset secondary chronic daily headache is shown in Figure 22-6 (solid line). Seventy-eight percent of the patients experienced the onset of daily headaches between the ages of 20 and 49 years. The distribution of the age of onset of the ini-

TABLE 22-1 **Circumstances of (Abrupt) Onset of Daily Headaches**

	Primary Chronic Daily Headache (n = 51)	Abrupt-onset Secondary Chronic Daily Headache (n = 34)	Combined Group (n = 85)
Head, neck, or back injury	25%	29%	27%
Flulike illness or sinusitis	12%	18%	14%
Medical illness or surgical procedure	14%	15%	14%
Miscellaneous	18%	12%	15%
No apparent reason	31%	26%	30%

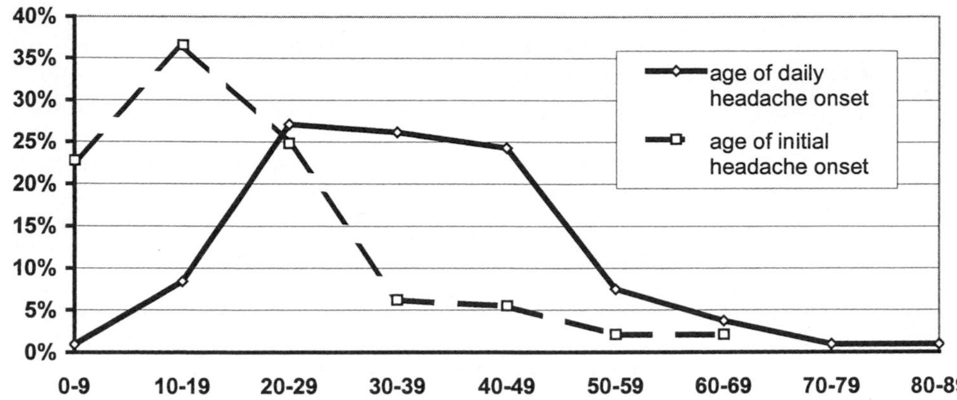

Figure 22-6 Distribution of the age of initial and daily headache onset in the patients with gradual-onset secondary chronic daily headache (n = 106 and 145, respectively). (Reproduced from Spierings ELH, Schroevers M, Honkoop PC, Sorbi M. Development of chronic daily headache: A clinical study. Headache 1998; 38: 529-533.)

tial, intermittent headaches in these patients is also shown in Figure 22-6 (interrupted line). The average duration of the transition of the headaches from intermittent to daily was 11 years, which is reflected in the figure by the separation of the two distributions by approximately a decade.

With regard to parental occurrence, headache in the father or mother, or both, was more common in the patients with gradual-onset secondary chronic daily headache than in the combined group of those with primary chronic daily headache and abrupt-onset secondary chronic daily headache (69% versus 45%). This finding is interesting because conditions that develop abruptly generally have lesser genetic involvement than do those that develop gradually. On the basis of the information gathered on parental headache occurrence, this also seems to be the case in chronic daily headache.

With regard to the intensity of the initial headaches, in the 145 patients with gradual-onset secondary chronic daily headache, the headaches were mild in 33% and severe in 67% (Table 22-2). The mild headaches were associated with nausea in 25% and vomiting in 0% compared with the severe headaches, which were associated with nausea in 84% and vomiting in 72%. With regard to the frequency of the initial headaches, there was no difference between the mild and severe headaches. The mild headaches occurred less than twice per week in 88% and the severe headaches in 91%.

The features of the daily headaches that these patients ultimately developed were the same, whether the initial headaches were mild or severe in intensity. They were the same with regard to age of onset of the (initial) headaches, gender distribution, diurnal headache pattern, nocturnal headache awakening, associated symptoms

TABLE 22-2 **Features of the Initial Headaches in the Patients with Gradual-onset Secondary Chronic Daily Headache**

	Mild	Severe
Headache intensity (n = 112)	33%	67%
Associated symptoms	(n = 12)	(n = 61)
Nausea	25%	84%
Vomiting	0	72%
Headache frequency	(n = 25)	(n = 60)
≤4/mo	60%	73%
5–9/mo	28%	18%
10–19/mo	8%	7%
≥20/mo	4%	2%

and laterality of the daily headaches, occurrence of severe headaches, and the frequency, associated symptoms, and laterality of the severe headaches.

From a classification perspective, does it make sense to distinguish between primary and secondary chronic daily headache as we did and, within the latter group, between abrupt- and gradual onset? Judging from the age of onset of the daily headaches, gender distribution, headache presentation, circumstances of headache onset, and parental headache occurrence, there does not seem to be a reason for the distinction between primary chronic daily headache and secondary chronic daily headache with *abrupt* onset. The two groups probably should be considered as having the same chronic daily headache condition, which could be referred to as *abrupt-onset chronic daily headache*, representing 37% of our study group. However, this group should probably be distinguished from the group having chronic daily headache with *gradual* onset because of the very different development of the headaches and the difference in parental headache occurrence. The latter group could be referred to as *gradual-onset chronic daily headache,* and future studies are needed to determine whether this distinction is meaningful in terms of predicting treatment or outcome, or both.

HEADACHE CONTINUUM

The above mentioned findings with regard to the development of chronic daily headache support the proposed headache continuum, shown schematically in Figure 22-7.[11] The headache continuum includes episodic and chronic tension-type headache, migraine, and tension-type vascular headache. Tension-type headache and migraine are the two most common headache conditions. Episodic tension-type headache is experienced almost universally, whereas migraine affects 10% to 15% of the population. The major distinction between the two, in my opinion, is the intensity of the headaches. Headache intensity is traditionally divided into three categories—mild, moderate, and severe—depending on the extent to which the headache affects the ability to function. A mild headache does not affect the ability to function, a moderate headache affects the ability to function but does not necessitate bed rest, and a severe headache is incapacitating and requires bed rest. Tension-type headaches are mild or moderate in intensity, whereas migraine headaches are moderate or severe.

Related to the (peripheral) mechanisms involved in causing the pain, the migraine headache is localized whereas the tension-type headache is more diffuse in location. The migraine headache is localized not only to one side of the head but, within the side of the

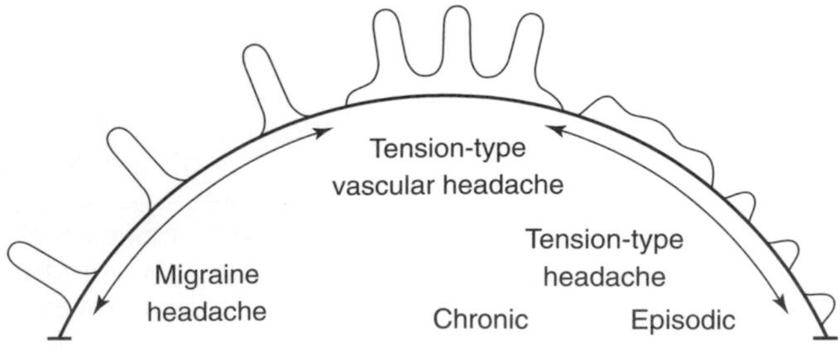

Figure 22-7 The continuum of headache syndromes, which includes episodic and chronic tension-type headache, migraine, and tension-type vascular headache.

head, to areas such as the temple or eye. The pain tends to be throbbing or sharp, steady in nature, whereas the pain of tension-type headache is dull and steady. Also related to the mechanisms involved in causing the pain, the migraine headache is affected by movement and activity, which is not the case with tension-type headache. The migraine headache often develops during the night and is present on awakening in the morning or wakes the patient from sleep at night, usually between 4 AM and 6 AM. Episodic tension-type headache, on the other hand, generally develops during the day, often in the late afternoon, between 4 PM and 6 PM. The episodic tension-type headache lasts a couple of hours, whereas the migraine headache lasts from part of a day to several days. Related to the low intensity of the pain, tension-type headache has few, if any, symptoms associated with it, and when symptoms are present, they are mild in intensity. Migraine headache, on the other hand, has intense associated symptoms related to the high intensity of the pain. Almost universally present in migraine are photophobia and phonophobia; however, nausea also is common and with the most intense migraine headaches, vomiting occurs as well.

There is ongoing debate with regard to the mechanisms involved in causing the pain of tension-type headache and migraine. It is my belief that peripheral mechanisms are important in both headache conditions, although the present thinking is oriented more toward central mechanisms. In tension-type headache, the peripheral mechanism is that of sustained contraction of the craniocervical muscles and in migraine, that of *extra*cranial arterial vasodilation. The arterial vasodilation in migraine activates a secondary mechanism, known as neurogenic inflammation. Stretching of the nerve fibers involved in pain transmission (Aδ and C) surrounding the blood vessels causes the neurogenic inflammation. The stretching causes the nerve fibers to depolarize, which, on the one hand, generates the action potentials that are transmitted to the central nervous system. On the other hand, it causes the release of inflammatory chemicals into the peripheral tissues, such as substance P and calcitonin gene-related peptide. The inflammatory chemicals act to further dilate the arteries and also cause a lowering of the pain threshold locally in the peripheral tissues. Thus, a vicious cycle is created in which vasodilation causes inflammation, which, in turn, accentuates the vasodilation and renders it extremely painful.

When headaches occur regularly, they lead, through an involuntary reflex mechanism, to progressive tightening of the craniocervical muscles. The greater intensity of the pain makes this effect more pronounced in migraine than in tension-type headache. Hence, muscular symptoms are more prominent in migraine patients than in those with tension-type headache. Contributing factors to the process of tightening of the craniocervical muscles are treatment of tension-type headaches with analgesics (as opposed to efforts to relax the muscles) and lack of effective abortive treatment in migraine.

In tension-type headache, the progressive increase in tightness of the craniocervical muscles leads, over time, to an increase in frequency of the headaches. It also leads to a progressive earlier occurrence of the headaches during the day. Ultimately, a daily or almost-daily headache condition develops in which the headaches are present on awakening or begin shortly after arising. As long as the headaches remain mild or moderate in intensity, the condition can be referred to as chronic tension-type headache. However, once the headaches have taken up all available time, they tend to increase in intensity to create "migraine headaches." The condition is then referred to as migraine with chronic tension-type headache. However, a better term would be *tension-type vascular headache,* emphasizing the existence of one single headache condition, rather than suggesting the presence of two separate conditions.

When the regular occurrence of migraine headaches leads to a progressive increase in tightness of the craniocervical muscles, a gradual increase in frequency of the headaches occurs as well as a progressive interposition of the migraine headaches with tension-type headaches. The increase in frequency of the migraine headaches stems from the fact that the muscle tightness itself becomes a trigger of migraine headaches. As the muscles become tighter, they begin to interfere mechanically with their own circulation, creating a stimulus for dilation of the feeding arteries to occur. One such feeding artery is the frontal branch of the superficial temporal artery, which overlies the powerful temporalis muscle. This artery is also involved preferentially in the process of migrainous vasodilation, causing the throbbing or sharp, steady pain in the temple so characteristic of migraine. Ultimately, the migraine and tension-type headaches merge into a condition of daily or almost-daily headaches with frequent migraine headaches. A condition is, thus, created that is identical to what has previously been described as migraine with chronic tension-type headache or tension-type vascular headache. However, the difference is that, in this case, the condition developed out of migraine, whereas the condition described earlier developed out of episodic tension-type headache.

OUTCOME

Of the 145 patients in our study with gradual-onset (secondary) chronic daily headache, we were able to contact 91 (63%) for follow-up telephone interviews. Seven patients refused to participate in the follow-up interview, and 11 no longer remembered the nature of their initial headaches. One patient was excluded from the analysis because of the absence of headaches at the time of contact, and three patients because of missing data. The remaining 69 patients (77%) were able to provide adequate information to classify their initial and present headaches as tension-type headache or migraine according to IHS criteria.

Twenty-three of the 69 patients (33%) still had daily headaches, whereas the remaining 46 (67%) again experienced intermittent headaches. Of the latter 46 patients, the initial headaches were classified as migraine in 39 (85%) and as tension-type headache in 7 (15%). Their present headaches were classified as migraine in 34 (74%) and as tension-type in 12 (26%). Thus, over time a shift had occurred from migraine to tension-type headache, accomplishing an improvement of the intermittent headaches for the group as a whole.

However, the question that we wanted to address was not whether the patients with intermittent headaches had improved in comparison with their initial headaches but whether patients with gradual-onset chronic daily headache revert back to their initial headache condition once the headaches become intermittent again. In the study, of the 39 patients whose initial headaches were classified as migraine, 30 (77%) also had migraine at follow-up and 9 (23%) tension-type headache. Of the 7 patients whose initial headaches were classified as tension-type headache, 3 (43%) had tension-type headache at follow-up and 4 (57%), migraine. Therefore, it seems that after experiencing daily headaches, migraine patients as a rule revert back to migraine, although some find their headaches improved to the extent that they are now classified as episodic tension-type headache. However, the situation is different for those patients who initially had episodic tension-type headache. They seem to be worse after having experienced daily headaches, with some patients experiencing headaches that have features and associated symptoms categorized as migraine according to the IHS classification.

TREATMENT

The first step in the treatment of chronic daily headache is the accurate establishment of the use of analgesics and vasoconstrictors, both prescription and nonprescription. It is important to establish their use in terms of the number of tablets or capsules taken per day and the number of days of use per week or month. Patients tend to be notoriously vague about the intake of medications they use "as needed only". They also often have to be reminded specifically to include nonprescription medications in their tally. Once the exact intake of analgesics and vasoconstrictors has been established, the clinician must determine whether overuse has occurred. As previously mentioned, overuse is defined as medication intake that is detrimental rather than beneficial to headache. It is use that promotes the occurrence of headache long term rather than providing headache relief. Analgesics and vasoconstrictors promote headache when they are taken for headache at time intervals shorter than their duration of action This dosing schedule allows them to accumulate in the system, with a return of headache when their effect wears off, a phenomenon known as rebound.

Rebound headache generally occurs when analgesics or vasoconstrictors are taken more often than 2 days per week on the average. This is particularly true for caffeine-containing medications because of the prolonged vasoconstrictor effect of caffeine, which can last for up to 60 hours. A higher frequency of intake of analgesics or vasoconstrictors can be permitted for simple analgesics and the shorter-acting triptans, such as sumatriptan. A lower frequency of intake should be considered with the longer-acting ergots, ergotamine and dihydroergotamine. However, it must be kept in mind that the rebound threshold has not been determined for any medication or group of medications. Furthermore, the diagnosis of rebound headache can only be made retrospectively, after withdrawal from analgesics and vasoconstrictors has been accomplished and improvement of headaches has occurred. A *suspicion* of rebound headache can be based not only on the frequency of medication intake, but also on increased medication usage over time with decreasing efficacy (Figure 22-8). The decreasing efficacy is often attributed to the development of tolerance but, in my opinion, it is more likely a manifestation of worsening of the headaches and an indication that use has become overuse.

If it is suspected that medication overuse and rebound headache are present, this situation needs to be addressed next. However, it can only be addressed after the patient has been given insight into the situation. With regard to vasoconstrictors, reference can be made to the vascular mechanism of headache. The vascular mechanism is antagonized by the vasoconstrictors, resulting in rebound vasodilation and headache recurrence when the vasoconstrictor effect wears off. Analgesics address only the pain of the headache and not the underlying mechanisms. Consequently—and as with symptomatic treatment in general—the underlying mechanisms deteriorate, resulting in worsening of headaches.

The withdrawal of analgesics or vasoconstrictors is generally best accomplished abruptly. However, whether that is possible also depends on the kind and quantity of the medications taken. When specific quantities of barbiturate-containing or opioid medications are involved, withdrawal may require hospitalization for close monitoring of withdrawal symptoms and intravenous administration of medications. The withdrawal of a significant amount of barbiturate-containing medication also requires a barbiturate taper to prevent seizure. The withdrawal of a significant amount of opioid medication requires expertise in addiction medicine and may have to be carried out in a detoxification center. Otherwise, it can often be accomplished on an outpatient basis, and several protocols have been developed to assist the patient with the withdrawal.

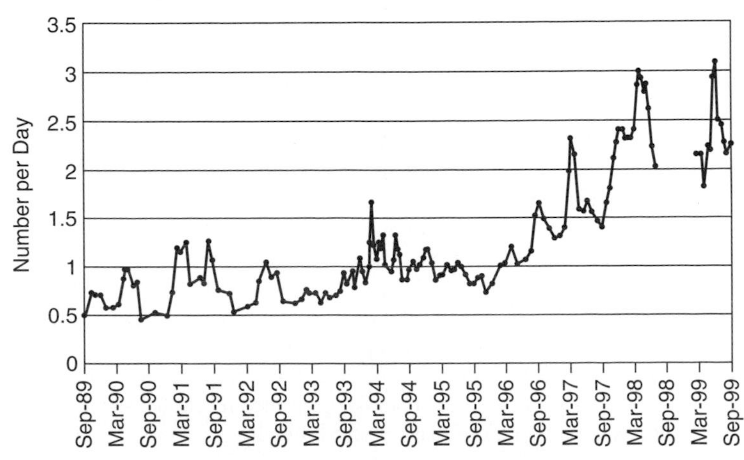

Figure 22-8 Example of increase in the intake of an analgesic for headache, as shown by the number of tablets per day over a period of 10 years.

A recent protocol employs sumatriptan for withdrawal headache after abrupt discontinuation of the rebound-causing medications.[12] Sumatriptan is given in a dose of 25 mg orally, three times per day for 10 days or until the patient is headache-free for 24 hours. Thereafter, it is used only on an as-needed basis for the abortive treatment of moderate or severe headache. Of the 35 sequentially selected patients to be enrolled in a study using this particular protocol, 9 left the clinic and 26 were actually treated. They had suffered from daily headaches for an average of 8.2 years. Of the 26 patients treated, 58% no longer experienced daily headaches after 1 month, and 69% had reverted back to intermittent headaches after 6 months.

An outpatient protocol that I have used successfully for the past 15 years to withdraw patients with daily headaches from daily or almost-daily use of abortive medications uses a short course of prednisone. Depending on the kind and quantity of the medications from which the patient has to be withdrawn, I give the prednisone for 3 or 6 days. The 3-day schedule consists of 15 mg prednisone four times per day for 1 day, 10 mg four times per day for 1 day, and 5 mg four times per day for 1 day; the days are doubled in the 6-day schedule. If the patient exhibits prominent muscular symptoms, that is, complains of tight or sore neck and shoulder muscles, I add diazepam to the schedule in a dose of 1 to 5 mg four times per day to help to relax the muscles.

I have used a similar schedule for patients admitted to the hospital when outpatient withdrawal was unsuccessful because of inability of the patient to tolerate the withdrawal headache or its association with severe nausea or vomiting. Under these circumstances, I add metoclopramide as an antinausea medication, given intravenously in a dose of 10 mg four times per day. It is important to start the metoclopramide immediately, that is, before the patient becomes sick, because once vomiting has developed, it is difficult to control even with intravenous administration of the medication. Instead of prednisone orally, dexamethasone can be given intravenously, in a dose of 4 mg four times per day, for several consecutive days. Diazepam can then be given every 6 hours, but only as needed for severe headache, and can also be given intravenously. An alternative to diazepam intravenously is lorazepam intramuscularly in a dose of 1 or 2 mg as needed every 6 hours.

An alternative to the preceding inpatient protocol with metoclopramide, dexamethasone, and diazepam or lorazepam is a regimen using metoclopramide and dihydroergotamine. In this protocol, both medications are given intravenously on a regular, generally 8-hour, schedule with the metoclopramide administered *before* the dihydroergotamine. This sequence is important to prevent the occurrence of nausea or vomiting as a result of the intravenous administration of dihydroergotamine. The dose of metoclopramide is usually 10 mg, and that of dihydroergotamine is gradually increased from 0.25 to 1 mg, depending on the ability of the patient to tolerate the medication, especially in terms of its gastrointestinal side effects. A long-term follow-up study of 50 consecutive patients with chronic daily headache treated with an intravenous dihydroergotamine protocol showed 44% to have good or excellent results after 3 months and 59%, after 2 years.[13]

After withdrawal from analgesics and vasoconstrictors, headaches may improve for up to 3 months. Often, preventive pharmacologic treatment is initiated immediately after the withdrawal but generally I do not do that. An exception is when the patient has problems sleeping at night, for which I will prescribe amitriptyline, doxepin, or trazodone. These are sedating tricyclic or tetracyclic antidepressants, of which the first two have also been shown to be effective in the preventive treatment of chronic tension headache. However, I do recommend patients to immediately begin nonpharmacologic treatments, such as using a heating pad daily on the neck and shoulders, to help decrease the muscle tightness that many patients have developed over time. At a later stage, I may prescribe more formal physical therapy, consisting of massage, ultrasound, stretching exercises, and so forth, or use trigger point injections to further relax the muscles.

For the daily headaches, I allow patients to use muscle relaxants, such as metaxalone or carisoprodol. For the severe headaches, promethazine, 50-mg suppositories, can be helpful as long as it is judged better for the patient not to use analgesics or vasoconstrictors. Once the headaches have become intermittent, I focus with my abortive treatment on the severe headaches, for which I try to find effective treatment, relying as much as possible on specific antimigraine medications. I define effective treatment as treatment that provides *full* relief of headache and associated symptoms within 2 hours of initiation. It is important for this treatment to be *consistently* effective as well, which would allow the patient to wait until the headache is severe before initiating it. This is the only way that patients can be prevented from falling back, over time, into the pattern of frequent intake of analgesics or vasoconstrictors.

With regard to preventive pharmacologic treatment, a particularly useful combination in those patients with frequent and severe headaches is that of a tricyclic and a beta blocker. The tricyclics that I prefer to use are amitriptyline, doxepin, and imipramine. I prescribe the first two when sedation is needed to help the patient fall asleep or sleep through the night. If sleep is not an issue, I prefer imipramine because it has fewer side effects, in particular a reduced likelihood of increased appetite and weight gain.

With regard to the beta blockers, six medications have been shown in randomized, double-blind, placebo-controlled studies to be effective in migraine prevention. These beta blockers are atenolol, bisoprolol, metoprolol, nadolol, propranolol, and timolol. In the patients with chronic daily headache, they are often effective in decreasing the intensity of headaches, whereas the tricyclics tend to have more of an effect on headache frequency. The calcium-entry blockers, in particular verapamil, I have found helpful if after analgesic or vasoconstrictor withdrawal, the headaches continue to awaken the patient regularly from sleep at night.

Kudrow determined the effect of analgesic withdrawal and preventive treatment with amitriptyline in 200 patients with chronic muscle-contraction headache who used analgesics daily, as documented by 1-month pretrial records.[14] Patients were randomly divided into two groups and four subgroups. Half of the patients were prescribed amitriptyline (25 mg per day for 1 week and 50 mg per day thereafter). In each group, half of the patients were allowed to continue taking analgesics without restriction, while the other half were instructed to discontinue these medications. The percentage of headache improvement observed in the four groups is shown in Table 22-3. Analgesic withdrawal, by itself, resulted in a 43% improvement in headache as determined 1 month after initiation of treatment. The addition of amitriptyline to the analgesic withdrawal increased the headache improvement to 72%.

Our study suggests that with the previously outlined treatment approach, two thirds of patients who have daily headaches can be improved to intermittent headaches. Preventive treatment in these patients may reduce the symptoms of the intermittent headaches somewhat, as suggested by the shift from migraine to tension-type headache observed in our study, when the present headaches were compared with those that occurred initially.

TABLE 22-3 **Headache Improvement 1 Month After Initiation of Treatment in 200 Patients With Chronic Muscle-contraction Headache Who Used Analgesics Daily**

Treatment Protocol	Improvement
Treated with amitriptyline	
Analgesics continued (n = 50)	30%
Analgesics continued (n = 50)	72%
Not treated with amitriptyline	
Analgesics continued (n = 50)	18%
Analgesics withdrawn (n = 50)	43%

What should be done with the patients who continue to have frequent and severe headaches, despite being taken off analgesics and vasoconstrictors and despite efforts at preventive treatment? This situation may be an indication for the use of long-acting opioids to relieve the pain sufficiently to allow these patients to function in their personal and professional lives. The long-acting opioids that I have used in such patients are fentanyl patch, oxycodone, and morphine sulfate. I have found these medications to be effective for a shorter period than manufacturers indicate and, therefore, use the fentanyl patch every 2, rather than 3, days and long-acting oxycodone every 6 or 8, rather than 12, hours. I gradually increase the dose of the medication until *satisfactory* pain control is achieved and the patient has returned to a relatively normal level of functioning. I prefer the use of long-acting to short-acting opioids because of the reduced likelihood that patients will develop tolerance and addiction. For some reason, rebound headache does not seem to develop with the long-acting opioids, although it is a routine consequence of short-acting analgesics, including opioids. The development of tolerance *and* rebound headache increases the use of opioid analgesics over time and makes it very difficult, if not impossible, to accomplish adequate pain control.

HEMICRANIA CONTINUA

As far as its presentation is concerned, hemicrania continua can be looked on as a form of chronic daily headache. It is a nonparoxysmal daily headache, present continuously throughout the day, and limited to one side of the head. However, it is different from chronic daily headache in its treatment. Hemicrania continua is treated with indomethacin to which it has an absolute response, similar to paroxysmal hemicrania.[15] The different treatment suggests a different etiology, which would preclude the condition from being grouped together with chronic daily headache.

It has been suggested that there is a form of hemicrania continua resistant to preventive treatment with indomethacin. Resistance to treatment with indomethacin, however, by definition means that it is *not* hemicrania continua. This does not mean that there are not numerous patients, who have continuous unilateral headaches with fixed lateralization that do not respond preventively to indomethacin. These patients have chronic daily headache and should be treated accordingly. The key to look for in the history is a response to aspirin, which seems to predict the responsiveness of the headaches to indomethacin. This is also the feature that ultimately led to the identification of both paroxysmal hemicrania and hemicrania continua as indomethacin-responsive headache syndromes.

REFERENCES

1. Headache Classification Committee of the International Headache Society. Classification and diagnostic criteria for headache disorders, cranial neuralgias and facial pain. *Cephalalgia* 1988;8(suppl 7):1–96.
2. Instituut Epidemiologie. *Epidemiologisch Preventief Onderzoek Zoetermeer (EPOZ): Tweede en Derde Voortgangsverslag*. Rotterdam, The Netherlands; Erasmus University; 1976.
3. Scher AI, Stewart WF, Liberman J, Lipton RB. Prevalence of frequent headache in a population sample. *Headache* 1998;38:497–506.
4. Castillo J, Muñoz P, Guitera V, Pascual J. Epidemiology of chronic daily headache in the general population. *Headache* 1999;39:190–196.
5. Silberstein SD, Lipton RB, Solomon S, Mathew NT. Classification of daily and near-daily headaches: Proposed revisions of the IHS criteria. *Headache* 1994;34:1–7.
6. Langemark M, Olesen J, Loldrup D, Bech P. Clinical characterization of patients with chronic tension headache. *Headache* 1988;28:590–596.
7. Rasmussen BK, Jensen R, Schroll M, Olesen J. Epidemiology of headache in a general population—a prevalence study. *J Clin Epidemiol* 1991;44:1147–1157.
8. Spierings ELH, Schroevers M, Honkoop PC, Sorbi M. Presentation of chronic daily headache: A clinical study. *Headache* 1998;38:191–196.
9. Spierings ELH, Schroevers M, Honkoop PC, Sorbi M. Development of chronic daily headache: A clinical study. *Headache* 1998;38:529–533.
10. Spierings ELH, Ranke AH, Schroevers M, Honkoop PC. Chronic daily headache: A time perspective. *Headache* 2000;40:306–310.
11. Spierings ELH. Headache continuum: Concept and supporting evidence from recent study of chronic daily headache. *Clin J Pain* 2001; 17:337–340.
12. Drucker P, Tepper S. Daily sumatriptan for detoxification from rebound. *Headache* 1998;38:687–690.
13. Silberstein SD, Silberstein JR. Chronic daily headache: Long-term prognosis following inpatient treatment with repetitive iv DHE. *Headache* 1992;32:439–445.
14. Kudrow L. Paradoxical effects of frequent analgesic use. *Adv Neurol* 1982;33:335–341.
15. Sjaastad O, Spierings ELH. 'Hemicrania continua': Another headache absolutely responsive to indomethacin. *Cephalalgia* 1984;4:65–70.

CHAPTER 23 BOTULINUM TOXINS FOR THE TREATMENT OF HEADACHES

Atif B. Malik and Zahid H. Bajwa

Since the 1980s, botulinum toxins (BTX) have been used for many putative conditions that cause pain. The U.S. Food and Drug Administration (FDA) has not yet approved their use for any specific pain disorders, although two forms of BTX (A and B) have been approved by the FDA for other medical conditions associated with pain and discomfort. However, BTX continues to be used successfully by a range of specialists to address pain control.

Although there are many case reports and open-label studies on the effectiveness of BTX in treating painful conditions, a dearth of double-blind, placebo-controlled, randomized clinical trials exist that directly addresses its use for pain management. Some double-blind, placebo-controlled, randomized clinical studies show that botulinum toxin type A (BTX-A) injections are effective in treating various headache disorders (Table 23-1). However, there are no published clinical trials showing its effectiveness in cluster headaches.

All of the data presented in this chapter, and most of the published experience in headache management is from BTX-A studies, but botulinum toxin type B (BTX-B) also may be effective, given the similarity of the two serotypes.

HEADACHE DEFINITIONS

Headache is one of the most common types of pain disorder, responsible for more than 10 million physician visits annually in the United States. Although the terminology of various types of headaches may be confusing, we limit our discussion here to primary headaches, for which BTX data is available to make preliminary recommendations until more information is available from ongoing large, multi-center, double-blind, randomized, placebo-controlled trials.

Migraine is a neurologic disorder that features recurrent attacks of headache, most often occurring unilaterally. It accompanies various combinations of symptoms, such as nausea, vomiting, and sensitivity to light, sound, and other stimuli. Migraine attacks can occur at any time of day or night. Episodes may last from several hours to days, 4 to 72 hours by International Headache Society (IHS) criteria, and are often disabling. Even routine activity or slight head movement can exacerbate the pain. Pain can migrate from one part of the head to another and may radiate down the neck or shoulder. The majority of patients also experience scalp tenderness during or after an attack.

Tension-type headache has two subcategories: episodic and chronic. The episodic tension-type headache (ETTH) is defined by the IHS[13] as headache frequency of greater than 10 lifetime attacks, but fewer than 15 attacks per month; With an average attack duration of 30 minutes to 7 days; and at least two features that may include mild to moderate pain intensity, pressing, tightening, a bandlike sensation bilaterally, nonpulsatile quality, and no exercise-induced exacerbation.

The IHS chronic tension-type headache (CTTH) criteria are identical to those for ETTH except that the attack frequency is 15 or more attacks per month for at least 6 months. CTTH definition permits one migraine-associated symptom of nausea, photophobia, or phonophobia, in contrast to that of ETTH. Patients who have two different headaches that both meet criteria for ETTH are defined as having CTTH if the sum of the attack frequencies for the two headaches is 15 or more attacks per month.

Chronic daily headache has not been satisfactorily characterized by the IHS but Silberstein and colleagues[14] have proposed that this condition represents a group of disorders that includes CTTH, transformed migraine, new daily persistent headache, and hemicrania continua. Chronic daily headaches usually evolve over a period of months or years but can be of sudden onset. The chronic daily headache spectrum may include transformed migraines that occur more than 4 hours per day, and 15 days per month. There is usually a slow increase in tension-type headache and a concomitant decrease in migraine features. Chronic daily headaches often are associated with analgesic abuse or overuse in many patients.

HISTORY OF BOTULINUM TOXIN

The existence of BTX has been known for centuries, but its positive effects have only recently been realized. Justinus Kerner, a German physician and poet (1786–1862),coined the term "sausage poison," later called "botulism" for the Latin form botulus, which means sausage. Professor Emile Pierre van Ermengem, of Ellezelles, Belgium, identified the bacterium *Bacillus botulinus* in 1885 that was later renamed Clostridium botulinum. In 1944, Edward Schantz cultured C. botulinum and isolated the neurotoxin. In 1949, Burgen and associates discovered that BTX blocks neuromuscular transmission. Dr. Vernon Brooks, in the 1950s, discovered that BTX-A could be injected into hyperactive muscle causing temporary "paralysis" by blocking the release of acetylcholine at the motor nerve ending.

In 1973, Alan B. Scott, MD, of Smith-Kettlewell Eye Research Institute, used BTX-A in monkey experiments, and, in 1980, he was the first to use BTX-A to treat strabismus in humans. In 1988, Allergan acquired the rights to distribute Scott's BTX-A product, Oculinum, and the responsibilities to conduct clinical trials of the drug's effectiveness for other indications, including cervical dystonia. In 1989, the FDA approved Oculinum (renamed Botox in the United States and Dysport in Europe) as an orphan drug to treat strabismus and blepharospasm associated with dystonia, including benign essential blepharospasm or eighth cranial nerve disorder (hemifacial spasms) in patients 12 years of age and older. BTX-A received FDA approval in 2000 for cervical dystonia, and in 2002 for improvement in the appearance of glabellar lines. The newest form of the botulinum toxin, BTX-B, was studied recently, and several products currently are available commercially (MyoBloc in

TABLE 23-1 **Summary of Results from Clinical Trials**

Type/Subtype	Authors/year	Study Type	N	Results
Migraine headache	Silberstein, 2000[1]	Double-blind vehicle-controlled	123	Effective prophylaxis
	Binder, 2000[2]	Open-label	77	Effective with acute attacks and prophylaxis
	Binder, 1998[3]	Retrospective review	96	Effective
Tension-type headache				
ETTH or CTTH	Rollnik, 2002[4]	Double-blind, placebo-controlled	21	No difference with Dysport
CTTH	Relja and Korsic, 1999[5]	Double-blind, placebo-controlled	16	Effective
CTTH and migraines	Smuts, 1999[6]	Double-blind, placebo-controlled	37	Effective
ETTH or CTTH	Schulte-Mattler et al., 1999[7]	Open-label	9	Effective in 8 of 9 patients
CTTH	Wheeler, 1998[8]	Open-label	4	Effective in 4 patients
CTTH	Relja, 1997[9]	Open-label	10	Effective in all 10 patients
—	Zwart et al, 1994[10]	Open-label	6	Unilateral temporal injection not effective
Chronic daily headache				
Secondary to whiplash injury	Klapper and Klapper, 1999[11]	Case studies	5	Effective in 4 of 5 patients
	Freund and Schwartz, 2000[12]	Randomized, double-blind, placebo-controlled	26	Effective in 11 of 14 patients

CTTH, chronic tension-type headache; ETTH, episodic tension-type headache.

the United States; NeuroBloc in Europe). BTX-B (MyoBloc) was approved by the FDA in 2000 for treatment of cervical dystonia to reduce the severity of abnormal head position and neck pain. Clinicians are also using BTX-B when patients become immunologically resistant to serotype A.

BIOCHEMISTRY AND MECHANISM OF ACTION

The BTX molecule is produced by C. botulinum, which is a gram-positive anaerobic bacterium. BTX can be divided into seven neurotoxins (labeled as types A, B, C [C1, C2], D, E, F, and G) that are antigenically and serologically distinct but structurally similar. BTX-A, -B, -E, and, -F (rarely) can cause the clinical syndrome of "botulism," which may occur following ingestion of contaminated food, from colonization of the infant gastrointestinal tract, or from an infected wound. BTX-C and -D cause toxicity only in animals.

BTX is synthesized as a single chain (150 kDa) and cleaved to form a dichain molecule with a disulfide bridge. The light chain (~50 kDa) acts as a zinc (Zn^{2+}) endopeptidase similar to tetanus toxin with proteolytic activity located at the N-terminal end. The heavy chain (~100 kDa) provides cholinergic specificity and binding to the presynaptic receptors. This promotes light chain translocation across the endosomal membrane.

BTX acts by binding presynaptically on the cholinergic nerve terminals, thus decreasing the release of acetylcholine and causing a neuromuscular blocking effect. This effect is temporary, and recovery occurs through proximal axonal sprouting and muscle reinnervation by the formation of new neuromuscular junctions. BTX-A and -E cleave synaptosome-associated protein (SNAP-25), a presynaptic membrane protein required for fusion of neurotransmitter-containing vesicles. BTX-B, -D, and -F cleave a vesicle-associated membrane protein (VAMP), also known as synaptobrevin. BTX-C acts by cleaving syntaxin, a target membrane protein.

CLINICAL EVIDENCE OF BOTULINUM TOXIN AS AN ANTI-HEADACHE AGENT

Clinicians began using BTX with the prospect of reducing pericranial muscular tension and contractions that are thought to contribute to headaches. BTX may reduce muscle spindle activity, and this, in turn, may decrease the sensory feedback. BTX may also directly affect sensory nerves by possibly inhibiting the neuropeptide-containing fibers. Although large multi-center, double-blind, randomized data are lacking, the evidence so far shows that BTX is an effective anti-headache medication when certain criteria are met.

Although there are numerous case studies focusing on use of BTX-A for treating migraines,[1,3] chronic daily headaches with migraine features,[11] and chronic tension-type headache,[4–6,8,9,15] there is no uniformity with the injection techniques or dosages. The studies use two general injection paradigms for treating headaches. In the fixed-site paradigm (Fig. 23-1), BTX is injected in sites that are predetermined and the same for everyone in the study. In the follow-the-pain paradigm, BTX is injected into or around the tender points that are reported by the patients and confirmed on physical examination.

Recent double-blind, placebo-controlled studies have shown consistency and homogeny with injection technique and dosage, allowing better comparative data analysis. An upcoming wave of

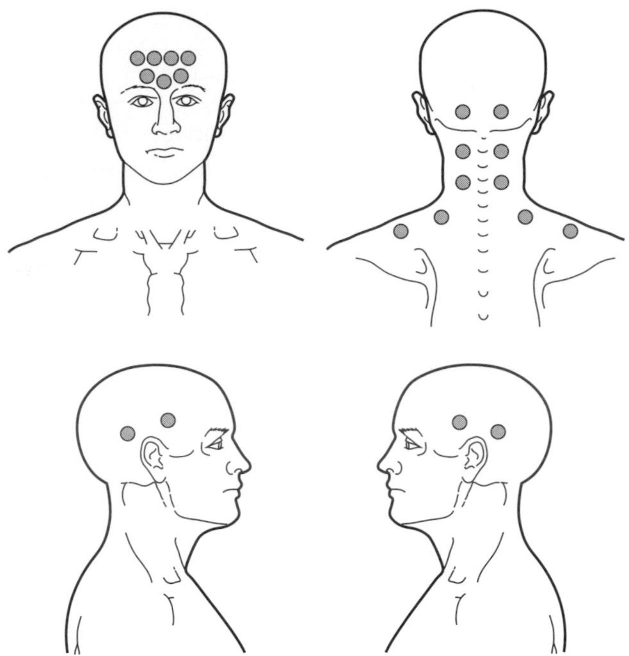

Figure 23-1 This is the protocol we have devised and used successfully for patients with chronic daily headache with migrainous features.

large multi-center, double-blind, randomized placebo-controlled trials will further clarify the role of BTX in the prophylactic treatment of a variety of headache disorders.

Migraine Studies

Silberstein and colleagues, in 2000,[1] reported a double-blind, placebo-controlled study in which 123 patients were randomly assigned into three groups, as follows: placebo (n = 42), BTX-A, 25 units (n = 42), and BTX-A, 75 units (n = 40). Patients who had two to eight moderate to severe, IHS-defined migraine attacks per months were enrolled. BTX-A injection sites were fixed-site and included frontalis, glabellar, and bilateral temporalis muscles. BTX-A decreased the frequency of moderate to severe migraines per month but failed to reach statistical significance. This study also showed a decrease in the number of days of acute medication usage. All treatment-related adverse events were transient, and more commonly associated with the 75-unit dose.

Binder, also in 2000,[2] reported an open-label study that included 77 patients with migraine. Results confirmed the efficacy of BTX-A in reducing the number and severity of acute attacks per month.

In 1998, Binder and colleagues[3] performed a retrospective review of 96 patients who had chronic migraines but were treated with BTX-A for their movement disorder or were seen in the cosmetic surgery clinics. This study evaluated patients who received BTX-A injections into glabellar, temporalis, and occipitalis regions. The mean total dosage of BTX-A was 26 ± 14 units. This study reported that 51% of the 96 patients had complete elimination of their headaches, while 28% of the subjects had more than 50% reduction in the frequency or severity of their headaches. The remaining 21% of the 96 patients either had less than 50% response in headache frequency and severity, or were lost to follow-up. The duration of benefit in the complete responders group was 3.6 ± 2.4 months. The partial responders group (≥ 50% decrease in headache frequency or severity) was 2.9 ± 1.6 months. Adverse effects reported were ecchymosis and transient, local pain at the injection site.

Tension-type Headaches

The first reported study, by Zwart and colleagues in 1994,[10] showed no effect in six patients with tension-type headache, not using the IHS criteria. This study was carried out using the follow-the-pain paradigm, with BTX-A injected unilaterally into the temporal muscle.

Since then, Rollnik and colleagues,[4] in 2000, conducted a double-blind placebo-controlled study involving 21 patients with CTTH or ETTH. The injection sites were specified as follows: "pericranial muscles around the head (2 injections into the fronto-occipital muscle and 3 into the temporal muscles bilaterally)." This study used BTX-A (Dysport) from Ipsen. The total dose used was 200 units. These investigators found no significant difference ($P >$ .5) between the BTX-A and saline-treated groups. The study evaluated the pain intensity (visual analog scale), clinical global impression, headache frequency, and consumption of analgesics. Both groups tended to improve on several measures; however, the pain intensity (P = .051) and clinical global impression (probability not given) at 4 weeks. The authors of this study suggest that given that Dysport is freeze dried and susceptible to breakdown, in contrast to the Botox (an American BTX-A) that is vacuum dried, a higher dose of Dysport may be needed to obtain a successful outcome.

Smuts and colleagues,[6] in 1999, reported a double-blind, placebo-controlled study in which 37 patients with CTTH were randomized into one of two groups: placebo (n = 15) or BTX-A (n = 22). Of the 37 patients, 38% also had history of migraines. The BTX-A injection sites were fixed and included 100 units into bilateral trapezius, splenius capitis, and temporalis muscles. At 3 months, 59% of the patients in the BTX-A group had ≥ 25% improvement in their headache severity score and number of headache-free days, whereas only 13% of the placebo had the same response.

Schulte-Mattler and colleagues,[7] also in 1999, in an open-label prospective study, injected nine patients who had ETTH and CTTH with BTX-A. They reported that eight of the nine patients showed improvement of their headache symptoms.

Wheeler,[8] in 1998, reported four case studies of patients with CTTH for whom previous multiple therapies had been unsuccessful. BTX-A was injected in a follow-the-pain paradigm, using variable doses (20 units to 100 units) at the tender sites. All four patients had subjective pain relief.

Relja,[9] in 1997, did a preliminary open-label study in which 10 patients with CTTH were injected with 15 to 35 units of BTX-A in up to six sites based on local tenderness. All of the patients were refractory to previous pain medications, and all reported elimination or reduction in severity and duration of headaches at 2 weeks.

Relja and Korsic,[5] in 1999, enrolled 16 CTTH patients in a double-blind, placebo-controlled, crossover study. The 35 to 80 units of BTX-A or placebo were injected in up to six sites into bilateral frontalis, trapezius, or sternocleidomastoid muscles based on local tenderness. The patients were followed 1, 2, 4, and 8 weeks post-injection. BTX-A significantly decreased tenderness scores, as recorded in patient diaries, and also decreased severity and duration of attacks (probability values not listed). Adverse events included local pain at the injection site, which occurred in some patients (number not specified) following BTX-A and saline.

Chronic Daily Headaches

Klapper and Klapper,[11] in 1999, reported five case studies of patients who had chronic daily headache with migrainous features. All five received 75 units of BTX-A at 11 fixed injection sites into the frontalis, glabellar, and temporalis muscles. Three of the five patients showed more than 75% subjective improvement. One patient had no response, and one showed only 35% subjective improvement.

Freund and Schwartz,[12] in 2000, reported a double-blind, placebo-controlled study in which 26 patients (n = 14 BTX-A, n = 12 placebo) with daily headaches secondary to cervical whiplash injuries were randomly assigned to one of two groups. The inclusion criteria included neck pain with musculoskeletal signs for more than 6 months. All of the patients were 2 years post-injury and had failed conservative therapy. BTX-A injection involved fixed doses of 100 units and the follow-the-pain paradigm. After 4 weeks, 11 of 14 patients showed a significant decrease in pain, and there was significant improvement in neck pain and range of motion. No adverse effects were reported.

CONCLUSION

Current data suggest that BTX is potentially effective as an agent for treating severe headaches. It has been successfully used to treat not only myofascial pain syndrome but also headaches, although in the United States this use is off-label at the present time. BTX appears to work primarily at the neuromuscular junction by binding presynaptically to the cholinergic nerve terminals, causing a neuromuscular blocking effect. Researchers are also evaluating its effect on substance P and other neurotransmitters involved in pain transmission. It may have a potential direct effect on pain perception.

Although, large multi-center data are yet to be published, based on the current available data on the use of BTX for headaches, we suggest the following guidelines:

1. BTX should be considered in treating migraines that are moderate to severe, resistant to conventional treatments, or cause more than 4 days of disability per month.
2. BTX injections may be efficacious in treating chronic severe tension-type headaches causing missed work or school.
3. BTX may potentially be the most efficacious agent in patients with chronic daily headaches.
4. BTX may be effective in patients with cervicogenic headaches and cervicothoracic myofascial pain syndromes associated with frequent headaches.

All of the headache studies carried out thus far have shown that BTX is a safe drug. The adverse effects are limited to localized pain at the injection site, muscle weakness, and flulike symptoms. There is a possibility of developing immunity to BTX-A, in which case this form of the toxin could be replaced with BTX-B. Current data suggest that headaches can be treated using a relatively low dose, thus further decreasing the potential for developing antibodies. BTX-A doses closer to 100 units show more favorable results in reducing headache frequency and intensity. Data also suggest that the fixed-injection paradigm may be more effective, and it appears to be gaining popularity among headache specialists.

REFERENCES

1. Silberstein S, Mathew N, Saper J. Botulinum toxin type A as a migraine preventive treatment. For the BOTOX Migraine Clinical Research Group. *Headache* 2000;40:445–450.
2. Binder WJ, Brin MF, Blitzer A, et al. Botulinum toxin type A (BOTOX) for treatment of migraine headaches: An open-label study. *Otolaryngol Head Neck Surg* 2000;123:669–676.
3. Binder WJ, Blitzer A, Brin MF. Treatment of hyperfunctional lines of the face with botulinum toxin A. *Dermatol Surg* 1998;123:1198–1205.
4. Rollnik JD, Tanneberger O, Schubert M. Treatment of tension-type headache with botulinum toxin type A: A double-blind, placebo-controlled study. *Headache* 2000;40:300–305.
5. Relja MA, Korsic M. Treatment of tension-type headache by injections of botulinum toxin type A: double-blind placebo-controlled study. *Neurology* 1999;52:A203. (Abstract)
6. Smuts JA, et al. Prophylactic treatment of chronic tension-type headache using botulinum toxin type A. *Europ J Neurol* 1999;6:S99–S102.
7. Schulte-Mattler WJ, Wieser T, Zierz S. Treatment of tension-type headache with botulinum toxin: A pilot study. *Eur J Med Res* 1999;4: 183–186.
8. Wheeler AH. Botulinum toxin A, adjunctive therapy for refractory headaches associated with pericranial muscle tension. *Headache* 1998; 38:468–471.
9. Relja M. Treatment of tension-type headache by local injection of botulinum toxin. *Europ J Neurol* 1997;4:S71–73.
10. Zwart JA, Bovim G, Sand T. Tension headache: botulinum toxin paralysis of temporal muscles. *Headache* 1994;34:458–462.
11. Klapper J, Klapper JA. Use of botulinum toxin in chronic daily headaches associated with migraine. *Headache* 1999;10:141–143.
12. Freund BJ, Schwartz M. Treatment of whiplash associated with neck pain with botulinum toxin-A: A pilot study. *J Rheumatol* 2000;27: 481–484.
13. Headache Classification Committee of the International Headache Society. Classification and diagnostic criteria for headache disorders, cranial neuralgias, and facial pain. *Cephalalgia* 1988;8(suppl):1–96.
14. Silberstein SD, Lipton RB, Solomon S, Mathew NT. Classification of daily and near-daily headaches: Proposed revisions to the HIS criteria. *Headache* 1994;34:1–7.
15. Freund BJ, Schwartz M. Treatment of chronic cervical-associated headache with botulinum toxin A: A pilot study. *Headache* 2000;40: 231–236.

BIBLIOGRAPHY

Barwood S, Baillieu C, Boyd R. Analgesic effects of botulinum toxin A: A randomized, placebo-controlled clinical trial. *Dev Med Child Neurol* 2000;42:116–121.

Blasi J, Chapman ER, Link E. Botulinum neurotoxin A selectively cleaves the synaptic protein SNAP-25. *Nature* 1993;365:160–163.

Brin MF. Botulinum toxin: Chemistry, pharmacology, toxicity, and immunology. *Muscle Nerve Suppl* 1997;6:S146–S168.

Cheshire WP, Abashian SW, Mann JD. Botulinum toxin in the treatment of myofascial pain syndrome. *Pain* 1994;59:65–69.

Coffield JA, Considine RV, Simpson LL. The site and mechanism of action of botulinum neurotoxin. In: Jankovic J, Hallet M, eds. Therapy With Botulinum Toxin. New York, NY: Marcel Dekker Inc; 1994:3–13.

DasGupta BR. Structures of botulinum neurotoxin, its functional domains, and perspectives on the crystalline type A toxin. In: Jankovic J, Hallet M, eds. Therapy With Botulinum Toxin. New York, NY: Marcel Dekker Inc; 1994:15–39.

de Paiva A, Meunier FA, Molgo J. Functional repair of motor endplates after botulinum neurotoxin type A poisoning: Biphasic switch of synaptic activity between nerve sprouts and their parent terminals. *Proc Natl Acad Sci U S A* 1999;96:3200–3205.

Erbguth FJ, Naumann M. Historical aspects of botulinum toxin: Justinus Kerner (1786–1862) and the "sausage poison". *Neurology* 1999;53: 1850–1853.

Foster L, Clapp L, Erickson M. Botulinum toxin A and chronic low back pain: A randomized, double-blind study. *Neurology* 2001;56:1290–1293.

Hyman N, Barnes M, Bhakta B. Botulinum toxin (Dysport) treatment of hip adductor spasticity in multiple sclerosis: A prospective, randomised, double blind, placebo controlled, dose ranging study. *J Neurol Neurosurg Psychiatry* 2000;68:707–712.

Jankovic J. Blepharospasm and oromandibular-laryngeal-cervical dystonia: A controlled trial of botulinum A toxin therapy. *Adv Neurol* 1988; 50:583–591.

Jankovic J, Brin MF. Botulinum toxin: Historical perspective and potential new indications. *Muscle Nerve Suppl* 1997;6:S129–S145.

Kedlaya D, Reynolds LW, Strum SR. Effective treatment of cervical dystonia with botulinum toxin: Review. *J Back Musculoskeletal Rehab* 1999;13:3–10.

Keen M, Blitzer A, Aviv J. Botulinum toxin A for hyperkinetic facial lines: Results of a double-blind, placebo-controlled study. *Plast Reconstr Surg* 1994;94:94–99.

Lew MF, Adornato BT, Duane DD. Botulinum toxin type B: A double-blind, placebo-controlled, safety and efficacy study in cervical dystonia. *Neurology* 1997;49:701–707.

Pearce LB, Borodic GE, Johnson EA. The median paralysis unit: A more pharmacologically relevant unit of biologic activity for botulinum toxin. *Toxicon* 1995;33:217–227.

Porta M. A comparative trial of botulinum toxin type A and methylprednisolone for the treatment of myofascial pain syndrome and pain from chronic muscle spasm. *Pain* 2000;85:101–105.

Porta M. A comparative trial of botulinum toxin type A and methylprednisolone for the treatment of tension-type headache. *Curr Rev Pain* 2000;4:31–35.

Purkiss J, Welch M, Doward S. Capsaicin-stimulated release of substance P from cultured dorsal root ganglion neurons: Involvement of two distinct mechanisms. *Biochem Pharmacol* 2000;59:1403–1406.

Rasmussen BK, Jensen R, Schroll M, Olesen J. Epidemiology of headache in the general population: A prevalence study. *J Clin Epidemiol* 1991; 44:1147–1157.

Rollnik JD, Dengler R. Botulinum toxin (DYSPORT) in tension-type headaches. *Headache* 2001;41:985–989.

Schantz EJ. Historical perspective. In: Jankovic J, Hallet M, eds. Therapy With Botulinum Toxin. New York, NY: Marcel Dekker Inc; 1994:xxiii–xxvi.

Schantz EJ, Johnson EA. Preparation and characterization of botulinum toxin type A for human treatment. In: Jankovic J, Hallet M, eds. Therapy With Botulinum Toxin. New York, NY: Marcel Dekker Inc; 1994:41.

Simpson LL. The origin, structure, and pharmacological activity of botulinum toxin. *Pharmacol Rev* 1981;33:155–188.

Scott AB. Botulinum toxin injection of eye muscles to correct strabismus. *Trans Am Ophthalmol Soc* 1981;79:734–770.

Wheeler AH, Goolkasian P, Gretz SS. A randomized, double-blind, prospective pilot study of botulinum toxin injection for refractory, unilateral, cervicothoracic, paraspinal, myofascial pain syndrome. *Spine* 1998;23: 1662–1666; discussion 1667.

CHAPTER 24

HEADACHES ASSOCIATED WITH ORGANIC PATHOLOGY

Jeremy Goodwin and Zahid H. Bajwa

The vast majority of headaches are of the tension, migraine, and cluster types, which are classified as *primary* headaches and are discussed in Chapter 18. Unfortunately, many patients develop refractory headaches, which usually consist of one or more primary headache disorders complicated by analgesic medication overuse, poor coping patterns, or failure to identify triggers. In such cases, an interdisciplinary management approach is needed.

Of particular concern to patients and clinicians are the *secondary* headaches, also known as organic headaches, accounting for fewer than 10% of all recorded headaches.[1] By definition, they are symptomatic of underlying disease, structural pathology, or pain-inducing processes different from those traditionally ascribed to the primary headaches. Organic headaches may be secondary to elevated cerebrospinal fluid (CSF) pressure, known as benign intracranial hypertension or pseudotumor cerebri; to bleeding from congenital aneurysms or arteriovenous malformations (AVMs); to ischemic or hemorrhagic stroke; as well as to pain caused by mass lesions or mass effect, such as tumors, hematomas, AVMs, and trauma, or infectious processes such as meningitis, encephalitis, and cerebral abscesses. The clinical importance of organic headaches—despite their relatively low prevalence compared with primary headaches—illustrates important principles of diagnosis and treatment useful to the clinician prior to obtaining specialist consultation.

This chapter focuses on the clinical signs, symptoms, and diagnostic workup of selected categories of secondary headaches. Cerebral tumors, stroke, subarachnoid hemorrhage, and vascular anomalies, spinal headache (i.e., spontaneous CSF leaks or those caused by lumbar puncture or epidural misplacement), and infection with the human immunodeficiency virus (HIV) are some of the vehicles used to discuss common clinical scenarios and approaches to decision making. The information that follows is based on both the published literature and our clinical experience as neurologists and headache and pain specialists.

Special emphasis is placed on the importance of maintaining patient comfort, dignity, and self-esteem. This approach is crucial to the success of therapy, even if success is not always defined as "cure," and is especially important in cases of terminal disease or those in which the primary diagnosis or headache symptom is disrupting patient and family dynamics.

DIAGNOSING HEADACHES AS PRIMARY OR SECONDARY

Differentiating secondary from primary headaches can be difficult. The quality of pain may be indistinguishable from that of migraine, tension-type, or other primary headaches. In such cases, the International Headache Society (IHS) states that the *temporal* relationship between the headache and underlying pathology should be the deciding factor.[2] Preexisting headaches *aggravated* by an organic process are still considered primary. If the onset of headache occurs in close proximity to the underlying structural problem, it is considered secondary. Sometimes the question is merely academic or impossible to answer. For example, how does one classify long-standing, stereotypic, but side-locked migraines when a magnetic resonance imaging (MRI) scan of the head, obtained to evaluate the cause of new-onset seizures, reveals the presence of an AVM ipsilateral to the headache, and in a position to cause pain? Are the headaches then primary or secondary? Perhaps the more important question concerns the risk of hemorrhage and neurologic deficits if the malformed blood vessels are left alone, removed, or otherwise treated.

The topic is complex, with potentially far-reaching consequences if errors in the workup are made. The important point for the evaluating clinician is to know *when and what to look for* when suspecting an underlying cause of headache, *and how to evaluate it within the financial limits of today's medical environment or within the constraints of the patient's medical condition.* This requires knowledge of headache presentation, the limits of clinical dogma, awareness of new or less commonly used tests, and a familiarity with imaging and other diagnostic studies, not to mention a compassionate bedside manner.

THE PSYCHOLOGY AND ETHICS OF HEADACHE EVALUATION

Patients (and parents) often seek consultation for their headaches in hope of reassurance that they (or their children) do not have an underlying disease of which pain is but one symptom. They also want to understand *why* they are experiencing headaches. This need to understand is of fundamental importance to many patients and their families, a point often missed by clinicians. In our experience, also supported by literature, patients' need to understand their disease may surpass their need for reassurance that pain medicine will be made available or even that the pain can be relieved.[3] This point is surprising only if one assumes that most patients do not think much about the details of their condition or care. Failure to appreciate this concept may lead to poor communication, mutual loss of respect, and frustration on both sides, which can certainly wind up the level of pain or the frequency of headaches, unnecessarily increasing the patient's suffering.

Pain and headache may either impact or be impacted by patient coping skills, expectation of outcome, or feelings of helplessness and hopelessness.[4] Clinicians need to incorporate the psychology of health and disease in their approach and not merely focus on the more tangible medical signs and symptoms. Patients are people, not diseases; and their fear of brain tumors, for example, often goes unstated. It is beneficial to broach the subject *regardless of whether or not the pattern of headache raises such concern in the clinician's mind.* It is surprising how frequently patients breathe a sigh of relief when they find out *why* their headache is likely to be caused by a tumor. Even when a tumor *is* diagnosed, the patients' anxiety and fear of the unknown can be lowered when they are given an understanding of the mechanism of pain appropriate to their level of interest, as well as knowledge of what to expect over time. This approach minimizes the likelihood of depression caused by the feeling of hopelessness and helplessness that accompanies escalating and misunderstood refractory or frequently recurrent pain.

Diagnostic headache evaluations can be a double-edged sword, especially with regard to ethical considerations. Treatment of structural pathology may prove preventative of serious problems such as stroke, seizures, or even death, and may minimize or eliminate the headaches. However, many identifiable structural anomalies may or may not be amenable to or even appropriately subjected to invasive intervention. *Importantly, there may be no relationship between the pain and the anomaly found.* Risk versus benefit must therefore be carefully considered before embarking on the "latest and the greatest" diagnostics.

Tests alone may carry physical, emotional, and financial risk, leading to significant ramifications for the patient as well as for the family. Contrary to the opinion of many clinicians, *patient refusal to consider invasive treatment is not, per se, reason for psychiatric consultation.* Such refusal certainly merits a gentle, affirming, and understanding discussion though, perhaps over several sessions, in order for the patient to process the information at his or her own speed. Informed consent or refusal is not always accomplished by a 5-minute distillation of the medical "facts" and the dual signing of a piece of paper.

ARTERIOVENOUS MALFORMATION AND HEADACHE

Occasionally, stereotypic-sounding migraine headaches with aura, especially if side-locked (always starting on the same side or in the same place), may turn out to be secondary to underlying structural pathology, sometimes with an associated risk of bleeding and stroke. A good example is an AVM in which veins connect directly to arteries without the usual intervening arterioles.[5,6] Finding an AVM in a family member with migraine may prompt evaluations in relatives known to experience similar headaches, but who have not yet undergone a formal workup. Should all related family members with headache be similarly evaluated? What about those without headache? Whether or not such evaluations are warranted is a matter of controversy and depends on the pathology in question, the philosophy of the clinician, and the individual patient's resources and wishes. In general, focal seizures, vascular bruits, equivocal computed tomographic (CT) scans, and episodes of hemorrhage increase the likelihood that studies will reveal a clinically important headache-related lesion.

Do AVMs cause headache? Some researchers consider them more likely than aneurysms to cause migraine-type symptoms. Even here, though, some investigators postulate AVMs and migraine to be but co-morbid conditions, with the main contribution of the AVM being that of potential cerebral ischemia or severely diminished blood flow leading to temporary or permanent neurologic sequelae. This process may affect the *nature* of the aura but is unlikely to be *causative* of pain, the aura being an independent process added to by the embarrassment of blood flow caused by the AVM. In animal models, and to some extent in humans, a slowly spreading electrical depression of cortical neuronal function appears to correlate with the migraine aura more so than simple blood flow changes. Although a brief leading wave of small vessel hyperperfusion followed by a more prolonged state of hypoperfusion or oligemia may be associated with cortical neuronal depression, actual ischemia (more severe) is not usually observed during the aura.[7] The pathophysiology of migraine remains controversial and is discussed in more detail in Chapter 19.

Finding an abnormality such as an AVM may have unexpected social and behavioral ramifications. It may, for example, place a "red flag" in the person's medical record that could interfere with his or her ability to procure a change in or an upgrade of a health insurance plan. Furthermore, it could lead to patient hypervigilance over somatic sensations, causing anxiety and, therefore, more frequent headaches. The situation is analogous to MRI-discovered disc bulges in those with spinal pain. Such findings are common but may bear no causal relationship to the back pain (although admittedly some disc bulges are associated with internal tears that may, indeed, be the source of spinal pain). Patients may have trouble understanding the logic of the clinician's recommendation that no invasive treatment is advised, so careful explanation is usually necessary. This takes the time that many clinicians feel they do not have. However, not taking the time to fully educate the patient may lead to more clinic phone calls and worsening of headaches due to stress. The patient may eventually find someone willing to operate. Paradoxically, for the "worried well" patients, ordering a head scan, even if likely to be unremarkable, may actually prove cost effective because of the value of reassurance. But the clinician should be aware that an unrelated anomaly might be found, initiating the problematic cascade of events mentioned earlier.

What, then, is the appropriate course of action when a structural lesion is found?

Weighing the relative pros and cons of neurosurgical intervention in a headache-prone but otherwise asymptomatic individual with, for example, a scan-discovered cavernous angioma, requires expert advice and involves a number of variables. If the anomaly has not bled, surgical advice might be to operate only if the headaches become worse or if positive or negative neurologic signs develop, such as seizures or paresis, respectively.[8] An AVM may or may not mandate a more aggressive approach than a cavernous angioma. Much of this decision is made between the consultant specialist (in such cases, a neurosurgeon) and the patient. The primary care clinicians should remain involved, however, because they usually get to know the particular patients better, and can help the specialist and patient to communicate, adding their own perspective, as appropriate.

Sometimes the motivation for further workup is to protect the clinician's legal coverage; for example, when clinician and patient expectations do not coincide. It is important to be honest about this consideration, but separating social from purely medical decision-making may prove difficult. We suggest integrating these points into an informed-consent approach so that the decision to undergo certain tests is a mutual agreement between patient and clinician with careful and detailed documentation. Where appropriate, evaluation by a psychologist specializing in chronic pain can prove extremely helpful in trying to decide between options.

RAMIFICATIONS OF BEING DIAGNOSED WITH A TERMINAL ILLNESS

Many patients, when diagnosed with headaches caused by an inoperable brain tumor or complications from acquired immunodeficiency syndrome (AIDS) or metastatic cancer, feel as concerned (or more so) for those whom they will leave behind as they do for themselves. Spouses and partners diagnosed with a terminal disease may feel that they are abandoning their loved ones in the same way that parents' worry about not being around for their children when they will be needed most. The person *not* diagnosed with the problem may feel guilty about his or her relative health. These fears often go unexpressed and may need to be addressed by caregivers to help patients, friends and family come to terms with these issues. Discussion, clarification, and resolution might also facilitate financial planning, a common concern of dying patients.[9]

Some patients fear severe pain worse than death. Anxiety, depression, and suicidal ideation are common when pain is poorly controlled.[10] However, impending death in those diagnosed with a terminal disease may evoke angst and fear for reasons other than pain and may bring to consciousness spiritual concerns (not necessarily religious) that can interfere with mood and sleep. These feelings and concerns may indirectly worsen pain and suffering and increase the severity and frequency of coincident *primary* headaches.

WHEN SHOULD A HEAD SCAN BE OBTAINED?

In general, a head scan is obtained to rule in or out organic pathology that might account for the headache disorder. As will be evident in the sections that follow, there are times when MRI, magnetic resonance angiography (MRA), magnetic resonance venography (MRV), or CT scanning is clearly the method of choice. As an introduction to the topic, some general principles might prove useful. They are discussed in greater detail elsewhere.[11–15]

CT scanning is less expensive than MRI, is usually more readily available, and takes about one third of the time to perform. This is useful in trauma patients and in those who are delirious or have a hard time lying still. It may also be the imaging modality of choice (with thin cuts and bone windows) when calvarial tumors or skull base pathology is suspected.[16] Except for the superiority of CT in early imaging of hemorrhage, and the clarity with which it reveals bone fractures (MRI being better for bone *marrow* changes), the resolution of MRI is much higher overall.

MRI is not affected by the bone-reflection X-ray artifact that interferes with CT resolution at the bone-soft tissue interface; therefore, it visualizes the brain-stem and posterior fossa much better. Furthermore, MRI reveals subdural hematomas better than CT when blood is in the isodense phase with bone. MRI shows meningeal inflammation well, whereas CT scanning does not. This distinction is helpful when the patient refuses lumbar puncture to assess for meningitis, or when it is inadvisable to perform a lumbar puncture (i.e., when a tumor in the cranium potentially raises the pressure of the cranial contents, putting the patient at risk for a herniation through the foramen magnum in the skull base). It must be noted, however, that lumbar punctures have been reported to cause meningeal enhancement. *A gadolinium-enhanced MRI best precedes the lumbar puncture in these cases and also replaces the need for pre–lumbar puncture CT scanning.*

If the headaches are nonprogressive, and stereotypic, without any sign of raised intracranial pressure or progressive neurologic dysfunction, and the neurologic examination is normal, then imaging is likely to be normal and probably not indicated.[17] *A "nonfocal" neurologic examination, however, cannot rule out a midline lesion for which there may be no lateralizing signs.* Examples include medulloblastomas, cerebellar astrocytomas, craniopharyngiomas, ependymomas, and tumors or cysts of the pineal region.[18]

MRI can visualize AVMs, internal carotid dissection, sinusitis (without having to order special CT views through the sinuses), venous sinus thrombosis, and some aneurysms (although MRA or MRV may do so even better). MRA to a large degree obviates the need for more invasive cerebral angiography and can also be used to investigate the neck vessels in cases where stroke or transient ischemic attacks are of concern. MRA reliably detects aneurysms 5 mm in size or larger. It may even resolve them to 3 mm, but not as reliably as angiography. MRV is particularly useful for ruling in or out thrombosis of the venous sinuses. This is important in the differential workup of benign intracranial hypertension, especially in a potentially hypercoagulable person who has cancer or is pregnant.

When it is necessary to see aneurysms that are smaller than 5 mm, or when the tendency of MRA to overestimate vessel stenosis influences treatment decision making, traditional *cerebral angiography is still the gold standard.* The latter may also more accurately depict the feeding vessels of AVMs. The risks of modern cerebral angiography are really quite low in appropriately selected patients.

MRI is particularly useful for localizing obstruction of CSF pathways and for evaluating Arnold-Chiari malformations and lesions of the skull base. It also depicts white matter lesions associated with multiple sclerosis and small vessel disease, the differentiation between which may depend on age, presence or absence of small vessel disease, and experience of the radiologist and clinician.

Adding iodine contrast to CT or gadolinium to MRI markedly enhances the sensitivity of these scans to a variety of lesions. *There is no cross-allergenicity between these agents, and gadolinium is safer than CT contrast in patients with compromised kidney function.*

Pregnancy, the presence of metal implants, and the types of lesions under investigation (and their expected location) affects the choice of scanning. It is probably best to clarify for the radiologist what is in need of being ruled in or out so that the most appropriate technology can be employed (the radiologist usually being the most up to date on evolving technology).

Situations That Raise Concerns About Organic Pathology of Headache[19]

- Progressive headaches over days or weeks, and increasing in intensity
- New-onset headaches
- New-onset headaches with exertion, coughing, lifting, or orgasm
- Changes in level of consciousness, stiff neck, or papilledema
- Unexplained fever
- Radical increase or change in previously established headache pattern

- New-onset headaches in an immunocompromised patient or one diagnosed with cancers known to metastasize to the brain

Reasons to Obtain Head Scans in Adults With Headache[20]

- *Scenarios noted in the immediately preceding section; in addition:*
- Persistence of headache-associated neurologic deficits
- Neurologic deficits found on examination and referenced to the brain
- Electroencephalographic (EEG) evidence of a focal brain lesion
- A partial or generalized seizure history
- Orbital bruits, especially with eye(s) that protrude, are painful, or reddened
- Side-locked headaches or headaches of unvarying location, or new-onset migraine with aura
- Patient anxiety regarding the potential presence of a structural lesion (if not already ruled out by a scan)
- In cancer patients, depression, personality change, or unusual sensitivity to opioids, with or without headache, should prompt the clinician to order a head scan even if patients have already had one
- Presence of ventriculoperitoneal shunt
- Nocturnal or early AM emesis or headaches that are worse after lying down for hours

Reasons to Obtain Head Scans in Children With Headache[12]

When the headache history is less than 6 months or the child is under the age of 7 years, imaging should be done routinely. Otherwise:

- *Reasons stated above for adult headaches* (substituting the anxious "patient" for "parents")
- Behavioral changes are noted
- Motor or learning skills fail to advance or begin to deteriorate
- Head circumference is considerably out of proportion to height
- Physical growth is not maintained
- Pain is not relieved by simple analgesics
- Diagnosis of neurocutaneous syndromes (neurofibromatosis or tuberous sclerosis)

HEADACHE ASSOCIATED WITH BRAIN TUMORS

The percentage of tumors that cause headache is now estimated to be lower than previously thought. This is because brain imaging for various complaints has become more common, and so-called silent tumors are increasingly being found. But it is important to be aware that tumor-related symptoms and signs are not limited to headache and seizures. For example, sudden loss of consciousness associated with positional changes, stroke, drop attacks, early morning nausea and vomiting with intense headache, or headache exacerbation with the Valsalva maneuver (abdominal straining) may be caused by a third ventricle colloid cyst or a pedunculated tumor blocking CSF flow. This should be evident on imaging studies. Personality changes may also be the first sign of a metastatic or primary tumor.

Headache is overestimated as a symptom of brain tumors, the location and type of which do not correlate well with location or type of tumor.[1,21,22] Headache is a common symptom of tumors, but tumors are a rare cause of headache. Less than 1% of patients presenting to headache clinics, have a brain tumor.[23] The incidence is approximately ten times less when only *chronic* headache is concerned. This is true at least in those who undergo head imaging despite a normal neurologic examination.[24] However, as previously noted, concern over the *potential* presence of a tumor may be the patient's primary motivation for clinical evaluation. Headache as the lone symptom of a brain tumor occurs about 8% of the time.[25] The overall percentage of patients with a tumor-caused headache in neurosurgery clinics may be higher because of referral bias (the mass having often been diagnosed previously and elsewhere by brain scan).

What factors are predictive of pain? The *site* and *rate of tumor growth* may be more predictive of pain than size alone.[1] Infratentorial and posterior fossa tumors tend to present as headache more often than do supratentorial ones,[1,24] especially if CSF obstruction is involved. Sixty percent of childhood brain tumors are infratentorial as compared with 15% to 20% of adult masses. This may explain why children are more likely to present with tumor-associated headaches than are adults. Migraine with aura—*even when successfully controlled with antimigraine medication*—may be tumorous in origin.[26] Furthermore, slow-growing tumors are far more likely to present with *seizures* than with headache.[27,28] And, according to autopsy studies of patients with cancer metastases or primary intracranial tumors, leptomeningeal involvement occurs only 1% to 8% of the time, yet 33% to 76% of such patients experience headache.[29] Other regions within the brain or cranium that are less sensitive to pain are unlikely to result in pain unless expansion raises intracranial pressure or causes a midline shift.

Whether a tumor is primary or secondary may affect the clinical presentation. Although some literature suggests that metastatic tumors are more likely to cause headaches than are primary ones,[30] other studies have found the incidence to be roughly equal.[31] Multiple sites simply make the pain less localized. Thirty percent of the time, metastatic brain tumors are the first sign of cancer anywhere in the body, but only about half of them are traced back to the primary site before death (most commonly the lung).[31] In general, breast, lung, and melanoma cancers are most likely to invade the brain whereas prostate cancer metastasizes to the skull, pelvis, and vertebrae.

Tumors compressing brain tissue from outside tend to induce seizures and neurologic deficits before they cause headache. Whatever the tissue type of origin, when headache occurs, metastatic or primary tumors present as tension-type headache far more often than migraine (77% versus 9%; with 14% mixed).[22] Migraine-like symptoms occur quite often as a result of intraventricular tumors.[32] Anti-migraine medications may occasionally alleviate the pain, and this is reason to not rely too much on the description of headache alone or response to medication as a means of reassuring patients that they do not need an MRI scan to rule out a structural cause of pain. Although most tumor-caused headaches are bilateral, there is some correlation between the most painful side and the site of the tumor. In cases involving considerable swelling and mass effect, however, false localizing signs and symptoms are common. Interestingly, raised intracranial pressure—long assumed to be a pain generator—does not seem to be the cause of pain per se.[33] It is more likely caused by displacement of or traction on pain-sensitive structures within the cranium.[29]

TREATMENT

Most of the following medications are prescribed in the usual adult and pediatric doses. Aspirin and simple analgesics may help with mild pain. Aspirin, however, and most nonsteroidal anti-inflammatory drugs (NSAIDs) should be halted if surgical intervention is likely. Aspirin irreversibly inhibits platelet function and increases the likelihood of bleeding. NSAIDs reversibly inhibit platelet function, but can still increase bleeding time. Using non–platelet-affecting modified aspirin analgesics, such as Trilisate or salsalate, or the new cyclooxygenase-2 (COX-2) selective NSAIDs, seems a reasonable alternative, but there are few data available about this approach.

When edema is present, dexamethasone, 4 mg p.o. b.i.d. to q.i.d., can be helpful for pain, seizures, or neurologic deficits, but this drug can also interfere with the diagnosis of lymphoma because it is a component of lymphoma chemotherapy. Use of the drug can cause the mass to temporarily disappear, resulting in a falsely negative scan. If lymphoma is suspected, steroids should generally be discontinued until the diagnosis is clear. Steroids can also mask a serious anticonvulsant allergy, and patients with terminal diseases at some point may not benefit from continued usage.[34] Although clinicians in neurosurgical practice typically use dexamethasone on a q.i.d. schedule, others feel that a b.i.d. dose is just as effective. To titrate, some advise doubling the dose each time, because improvement in symptoms is dose dependent in some patients.

Opioids, surgery, and radiation may all help to attenuate pain, but other avenues might be tried early on. Tricyclic antidepressants (TCAs) may also decrease the pain but tend to lower the seizure threshold. The same goes for tramadol and bupropion. Selective serotonin reuptake inhibitors (SSRIs), such as fluoxetine, paroxetine, sertraline, or citalopram tend to be less likely to cause seizures, but may also be less effective in terms of pain or headache control. And, although polypharmacy definitely has a role in pain management—often outperforming high doses of single agents—tramadol mixed with TCAs, SSRIs, and opioids can lower the seizure threshold even at relatively moderate doses and can cause seizures even in those who are not predisposed.[35] One must mix agents with caution.

Antiepilepsy medications, such as phenytoin, carbamazepine, divalproex/VPA, gabapentin, oxcarbazepine, and topiramate, used sometimes in combination with phenobarbital, may prove useful at moderate to high doses for tumor-caused headaches using the usual doses for seizures, or exceeding them if clinically well tolerated and demonstrably more efficacious. Of these, only gabapentin and topiramate require no blood work or blood-level checking. Gabapentin, especially, interacts well with most medications and can safely be used in excess of the Food and Drug Administration (FDA)-recommended maximum dose of 1,200 mg p.o. t.i.d. If needed and tolerated, up to 2,000 mg p.o. t.i.d. can be used with safety.[36] One of us (JG) tend to use gabapentin b.i.d. for symptoms of pain and headache alone, using a t.i.d. schedule if seizures are present or if more than 4,000 mg/day is needed (failure of absorption occurs at single doses above 2,000 mg). Topiramate, starting at 25,mg p.o. q.d. to b.i.d., increasing by this amount weekly, soon accelerating to 50-mg weekly incremental jumps (if tolerated) until reaching 150 to –200 mg p.o. b.i.d., is worth trying as there is increasing evidence of its efficacy for the prophylactic treatment of headaches.

Clonazepam is a benzodiazepine that may help diminish the chronic tension-type headache associated with some tumors. It is also an antiepileptic, anxiolytic, and hypnotic that may shorten sleep latency, diminish nocturnal myoclonus (periodic leg movements of sleep) and attenuate restless legs syndrome. It may also reduce myoclonus associated with high-dose opioid use. Whether or not it interferes with deep stages of sleep for long is controversial. A common dose would be 0.5 to 2 mg p.o. q.h.s. or b.i.d. Because clonazepam has a long half-life, it need not be given more frequently than b.i.d., it is often best given 2 hrs before h.s.

Tumor-caused headaches that are migrainous in quality occasionally respond to antimigraine medications. The importance of this response is that migraine as a diagnosis is not ruled *in* by a therapeutic response to antimigraine medications and, conversely, the presence of a tumor is not ruled *out*. Several causes of headache may respond to antimigraine medications, including cluster headache, analgesic rebound headache, and so-called spinal headaches. *In cases of severe anxiety, especially resulting from fear of terminal disease ("dread" in psychiatric parlance), low-dose perphenazine, 2 to 4 mg p.o. b.i.d., may prove more useful than high-dose benzodiazepines in bringing about a sense of calm.* This is about one twentieth to one tenth of the dose used in the management of psychosis. The classes of medications mentioned earlier can be safely used together if the clinician is skilled and experienced in rational polypharmacy.

And what about postoperative pain? NSAIDs are very helpful and can be opioid sparing. The two classes act synergistically to relieve pain. One published regimen for pharmacotherapy following surgery consists of mixing methadone, NSAIDs with or without acetaminophen, hydroxyzine, and a tricyclic antidepressant.[37] Many variations on this theme are possible and reasonable and should be tailored to the patient's reliability, financial means, age, and general health.

BEHAVIORAL INTERVENTION AND ACUPUNCTURE IN SECONDARY HEADACHES

Other headache treatments used alone or in concert with medication play an important role in patient care. It should be borne in mind that relaxation exercises are helpful in terms of coping with mild to moderate pain and bringing it under control, not only in children but in adults as well. In general, 8- to 12-year-olds respond well to hypnosis, but published evidence of efficacy is clearer in the case of primary headaches than it is for secondary cephalalgia.

Suffering from pain and headache varies less between individuals than the wide variety of pain mechanisms might suggest. Support groups and cognitive-behavioral and psychoeducational classes are useful for those suffering from long-standing or life-disrupting pain or recently defined terminal illness, no matter the diagnosis. Children and adolescents have unique social needs and will likely have difficulty relating to others too far out of their age group. This is important when selecting individuals for group therapy.

Mental imagery, deep and slow (diaphragmatic) breathing, meditation, and biofeedback are all useful adjuncts to pain control and are most effective when suited to the patient's personality. We have found, as have others, that acupuncture is helpful in the management of primary headaches,[38] but we do not have enough experience with its use in the management of secondary headaches to comment on its efficacy in the latter case. There is some evidence that it helps in the management of anxiety. However, the range of skills, experience, and depth of training of the acupuncturist has a significant impact on efficacy. It is well to remember that the same must be said regarding allopathic medicine and surgery. There are many who have "certification" but lack in-depth training, making it difficult for the nonpractitioner of acupuncture to evaluate their skills. Unfortunately, and in my experience, when the pain becomes increasingly intense and ever present, adjunctive measures and medications of all types may prove ineffective irrespective of the level of skill of the practitioner, allopathic or otherwise. Only very high doses of opioids, radiation treatment, surgery, or a combination of all three, are likely to help, but often at great cost. Sometimes the only relief from pain seems to come with loss of consciousness.

HEADACHES ASSOCIATED WITH STROKE

The IHS suggests that headaches be considered secondary to a stroke if the pain begins within 48 hours of the development of central nervous system signs and symptoms. The mechanism of headache in such cases is unclear. Data on pain associated with vascular pathologies vary greatly. In general, headache is most likely to occur in the case of large vessel occlusive stroke, least likely as a result of lacunar infarcts, and intermediate in the case of embolism.[39] Hemorrhage may be painful, otherwise symptomatic, or silent. Here, as with tumor-associated headache, the value of lateralization, intensity, and quality of pain is of dubious value and the literature conflicting. Study results depend on methods of patient sampling, type of questionnaire used, and subtype of stroke studied. Not all data are intuitively obvious. In cases of headache associated with *unilateral* stroke of the internal carotid artery territory, about two thirds of patients experience *bilateral* head or neck pain. And regardless of the side(s) affected, the headache often radiates frontally, as it may even if the stroke involves the posterior circulation (vertebrobasilar system). Bleeding into the occipital lobe may refer pain to the ipsilateral eye, whereas temporal lobe pain is often referred anterior to the ipsilateral ear. Pain in the temples may refer from hemorrhage into the parietal lobes, and frontal pain is most likely to originate in the frontal lobe.[40] As stated earlier, there are no clearly useful stereotypic patterns of stroke-caused headache, but it is worth noting that *there exist documented cases of intracerebral hemorrhage being associated with migraine symptoms, remarkable only for an unusually protracted and prolonged course*. As with tumor headaches that sound migrainous, *the danger of misdiagnosis is lessened with the use of appropriate imaging studies.*

SUBARACHNOID HEMORRHAGE-INDUCED HEADACHE

In subarachnoid hemorrhage (SAH), where bleeding occurs within the cerebrospinal fluid, blood pressure and intracranial pressure must be controlled to minimize further blood vessel leakage. Sometimes lowering the blood pressure eases the headache, but this result is more likely to occur with headaches caused primarily by the high blood pressure itself. In SAH, much of the pain comes from meningeal irritation. Several causes for SAH are reported but discussion of all of these is beyond the scope of this chapter. SAH occurs most commonly as a result of head injury, followed by spontaneous rupture of an aneurysm or AVM, and less commonly by hemorrhagic cavernous angiomas and tumors. Surgical excision of cavernous angiomas (a common fortuitous finding on head scan) is recommended only if bleeding has occurred or if their placement is likely to irritate pain-sensitive structures, thereby explaining the headaches. *Hemosiderin staining of surrounding brain tissue, denoting an old site of bleeding, can be discerned by MRI but not by CT, whereas fresh blood is best assessed by CT.* Interestingly, the risk of bleeding depends on the type of vascular anomaly and, according to some studies, on race. An aneurysm is 5 to 25 times more likely to bleed than is a cavernous angioma, but this may not be so in the Asian population for reasons that are unclear.[41] Because of the high prevalence of cerebral aneurysms in persons diagnosed with hypertension, some investigators consider hypertension to be a risk factor for aneurysm formation.[42] The risk of aneurysms bleeding as a result of hypertension is less clear.[43] Approximately one quarter of patients found to have an aneurysm have at least two or three of them.[44] The relationship of this finding to the likelihood of bleeding probably depends on a number of anatomic and physiologic factors. AVMs also have a higher lifetime likelihood of bleeding than do cavernous angiomas, and surgical removal of an AVM or other types of intervention should be considered if the patient is young and if the AVM is accessible. The chance of hemorrhage is approximately 3% per year.

Are there any warning signs or symptoms of the pending hemorrhage of an aneurysm? Sentinel ("thunderclap") headaches may precede SAH by several months, although the association is somewhat controversial. In a recent prospective study of about 100 patients presenting with severe sudden-onset headache, almost two thirds were found to have SAH, two thirds of which were caused by aneurysms.[45] The issue of sentinel headaches, their typical workup, and when to proceed to angiography even if the CT scan and CSF studies are normal, is discussed by Raskin,[46] based on his own extensive experience and that of others.[47–51] Unfortunately, many patients are misdiagnosed or inadequately evaluated and die as a result. In such cases, warning headaches were often dismissed as sinusitis, or tension-type or migraine headaches.[45,52] Exertional factors may also prove important in up to one third of cases. If a hemorrhage occurs, the initially unilateral headache associated with hemorrhage rapidly generalizes and often spreads to the occiput and neck. The neck may become stiff through irritation of the meninges (meningismus). Photophobia, sonophobia, loss of consciousness, seizures, or a combination of these findings, may occur. Such headaches are usually different than any other previously experienced and are classically described by the patient as "the worst ever." *If lumbosacral roots are irritated by blood in the CSF, the patient may even report symptoms of sciatica.*

SAH is a medical emergency requiring both neurologic and neurosurgical consultation. If SAH is strongly suspected and a CT scan is negative, lumbar puncture reduces the false-negative rate of CT scanning from 5% to 10% to under 1%. Xanthochromia (yellowing of the CSF as a result of hemolyzed blood) appears within 4 to 12 hours and lasts 12 to 40 days.[53]

Treatment and assessment techniques of SAH and other vascular disorders are discussed elsewhere,[53] but with regard to pain management, oral or intravenous opioid pain medication may be necessary to decrease the pain, with some clinicians choosing codeine and others stronger opioids. The need for careful attention to changes in mental status in the acute stage may make the latter approach a bit risky unless the clinician is skilled in the dosage of opioids, conduction of the neurologic examination, and pain assessment. A very calm, darkened, and quiet intensive care–level environment (no slamming of doors) will minimize dangerous reactive fluctuations in blood pressure. Some sedation, using phenobarbital or midazolam, both of which prevent or minimize the likelihood of seizures, is often advised. Frequent neurologic assessment is also necessary.

If the workup remains negative, the treatment is usually bed rest for 4 to 6 weeks, with slow or gradual resumption of normal activities. Some clinicians use intravenous calcium channel blockers, followed by oral dosing, in hope of minimizing the risk of delayed vasospasm, but there is reason to doubt that the mechanism of action of calcium channel blockers in the periphery is mirrored in the central nervous system.[54] Pain modulation, for example, may occur via the effects of calcium channel blockers on the serotonin system.

ISCHEMIC STROKE AND HEADACHE

Reports on headache patterns in stroke and transient ischemic attacks vary widely in their conclusions. This has much to do with populations and type of pathology studied as well as variation in study design. It is well to ask about headache, however, because it loosely correlates with the type of circulation involved (anterior versus posterior), and may precede a cerebral vascular accident by days or weeks, serving as a warning of impending problems.[55]

One multi-center prospective study of more than 3,000 patients with a variety of stroke presentations could conclude only generally that deep, small vessel hypertension and anterior circulation–related infarcts were less likely to cause headaches than were posterior circulation and cortically based infarcts. Patients with headache were statistically more likely to have ischemic heart disease, but the duration of pain or ischemic symptoms, and patient sex, were unrelated factors.[56] Other researchers have found headache more likely to occur in females[57] or in males.[58]

In ischemic stroke without bleeding, the reflex leading to a rise in blood pressure is necessary to maintain or restore cerebral perfusion through areas of swelling (although sometimes reperfusion precipitates bleeding). Most neurologists try to maintain systemic systolic blood pressure between 115 and 180 mm Hg. Careful judgment (and some luck) is needed. *For stroke, short-acting nitro-paste is a better choice of antihypertensive medication than the longer acting calcium channel blockers.* J.G. has seen a stroke dramatically worsen with the use of nifedipine, presumably from loss of cerebral perfusion as a result of a profound drop in systemic blood pressure. Nitro-paste can instantly be removed and very quickly metabolized should a drop in blood pressure correlate with re-occurrence or progression of symptoms.

Besides the antihypertensive class of medication, other agents used to diminish pain—such as the "strong" opioids—may also decrease blood pressure, extending the area of ischemia and infarction. Furthermore, in opioid-naive patients, even moderate doses of such analgesics may suppress the rate of respiration if mentation is already depressed. Pain, on the other hand, stimulates respiratory drive. Again, skill in assessment and medication titration is required to treat pain safely in this setting. In general, weaker oral opioids, such as hydrocodone, or lower doses of intravenous opioids might be used more safely. Previous use (tolerance) of opioids may affect the dose needed to gain an effect. High doses or stronger opioids may be required in patients with a high degree of pharmacologic tolerance. Vasoconstrictors for headache relief in ischemic stroke are obviously contraindicated. And the potential complication of analgesic rebound headaches must always be kept in mind if analgesics are used for too long a period of time. It is advisable to reassess the patient periodically to determine the continuing need for regularly taken medication, preventative or abortive.

INTRACEREBRAL HEMORRHAGE, SUBDURAL HEMATOMAS, AND EPIDURAL HEMATOMAS

The data regarding intracerebral hemorrhage (bleeding into the brain tissue itself) is likewise contradictory. Taking stroke as a whole, data range from little to no correlation[57] to fairly well-defined criteria.[59] The latter study found vomiting, younger age, and the presence of headache to be of value in looking for SAH, whereas the absence of headache, older age, and lower systolic pressures were indicative of probable ischemic stroke. *Higher systolic blood pressure in conjunction with headache was somewhat predictive of an intracerebral hemorrhage or hematoma.* Headache is commonly known to follow or to occur in conjunction with a stroke, but it can also precede the event by days or weeks depending, in part, on the mechanism or type of stroke.[60]

In the case of *subdural* hemorrhage, where the headache is unilateral, it is usually ipsilateral to pathology. The hematoma may require surgical intervention. The frequency of headache ranges from 11% to 53% to 81%, depending on whether it is an acute, a subacute, or a chronic condition.[61] When the cause of pain is an *epidural* hemorrhage, focal neurologic signs may accompany the pain as may changes in the level of consciousness (with or without the overemphasized "lucid interval"), making powerful and centrally active painkillers useable only when frequent neurologic evaluations are possible. Otherwise simple analgesics—non–platelet affecting—are used to minimize pain.

TREATING ACUTE HEADACHE WITH OPIOIDS—MANAGING COMPLICATIONS

Fortunately, most cases of stroke-related headache are self-limited. Furthermore, neurologic deficits or changes in mental status often rapidly supersede the headache. Of course, where intracerebral hemorrhage or SAH is concerned, surgical intervention may prove necessary to preserve normal function or to minimize the chance of recurrence.

The type of stroke dictates the direction of treatment. This is the major reason that a CT scan of the head is obtained as early as possible. It differentiates hemorrhagic from ischemic stroke. Unless huge, an ischemic stroke may not appear on CT for up to 24 hours. However, hemorrhage is visible immediately. The amount and location of blood within brain parenchyma or within the subarachnoid space affects the differential diagnosis, prognosis, and direction of evaluation and treatment. Whether anticoagulation is advised in the face of progressive signs and symptoms, as well as which analgesics are best used for severe headache control, depends on the presence or absence of hemorrhage, its location, symptoms and signs, and the amount of bleeding. Consultation with a neurologist is advised.

As yet, few data are available on the use of COX-2 selective inhibitor (COX-1 sparing) NSAIDs for headache management, but these drugs do *not* increase bleeding times, and their use seems reasonable if the pain is not self-limited and if other painkillers are contraindicated. If the pain is intense, as long as the clinician keeps a close eye on the patient's mentation, it is probably safe to carefully titrate short-acting and low-dose opioids for acute pain relief as long as naloxone is on hand. *If sudden deterioration occurs, however, it may be difficult to separate drug-induced sedation from event progression; for this reason many clinicians advise against sedating agents.* If used, especially in the patient who has been using opioids long-term and is physically dependent on them, naloxone can induce a stressful withdrawal syndrome leading to tachycardia, dysrhythmias, noncardiogenic edema, and a rapid increase in blood pressure. In cases of SAH or intracerebral bleeding, the latter may prove devastating.

To minimize complications in using naloxone, we recommend the following approach:

- Dilute a 0.4-mg vial of naloxone in a 10-mL syringe of normal saline, and give it intravenously at a rate of 1 to 2 mL every 1 to 2 minutes, to reverse narcotization without loss of analgesia or induction of withdrawal.
- In patients who have been using opioids for some time (daily for more than 1 to 3 weeks, depending on the route, frequency, and dose) the half-life of naloxone may be shorter than the opioid used so that repeat doses may be needed every 30 to 45 minutes until the situation is stabilized.
- If blood oxygen saturation or the respiratory rate drop ominously, the whole 0.4 mg (or more) dose is rapidly given as a single intravenous bolus.

HEADACHES CAUSED BY LOW CEREBROSPINAL FLUID PRESSURE

It is not only *elevated* CSF pressure that is associated with headache. Headache may result from *low* CSF pressure as well, presumably from traction on pain-sensitive meningeal and intracranial structures. In cases where radioisotope studies show no leak (the radioactive isotope passing directly into the bladder), but with the CSF pressure remaining below 60 mm H_20, the condition is said to be *spontaneous*. If a leak is found following an invasive procedure or if a disease process is considered causative, the condition is said to be *symptomatic*. Although headache-related low CSF pressures may occur above 60 mm H_20, to as high as 90 mm H_20, manometric studies usually reveal pressure readings between 0 and 40 mm H_20.[62]

Leakage or decreased production of CSF is associated with a number of conditions. They include torn dural sleeves around nerve roots, spinal arachnoid cyst rupture, bony erosion by tumors, complications from or incorrect choice of pressure valves in ventricular shunting, procedure-induced dural tears, trauma to the head and neck, as well as sudden physical or even sexual exertion. Systemic illnesses such as uremia, meningoencephalitis, diabetic ketoacidosis, and severe dehydration can also cause low CSF pressures.

SPINAL HEADACHES

Diagnosis

Spinal headaches are not difficult to diagnose. The IHS criteria use 7 days as the window of time following a procedure during which one may attribute a causal relationship. Spinal headaches usually follow an invasive procedure and become intense and generalized within 15 minutes of assuming the upright position. They significantly diminish or resolve within 30 minutes of lying down, but some patients experience an onset and offset within 20 to 30 seconds. Nonspecific associated symptoms of nausea, tinnitus, or lightheadedness may occur. The postural component may become less pronounced if the condition becomes chronic. Cranial nerve VI, being the longest such nerve, is the most likely to be affected by processes causing cranial nerve neuropathy, which manifests as palsy (inability to move the eye laterally).[63] If the duration exceeds 14 days, then the clinician should consider CSF fistula headache (a similar problem that occurs secondary to trauma, neurosurgery, or erosive lesions). As far as diagnostic tests are concerned, manometric assessment by lumbar puncture, radionucleotide CSF flow studies, and pledgets in nasal passages to catch leakage from the cribriform plate and paranasal sinuses are all useful. CT-myelography may pick up dural tears that would otherwise be missed, and MRI of the brain may reveal dural enhancement secondary to vascular engorgement. The latter finding may also occur with infection or inflammation of the meninges and is, therefore, not diagnostic. More sophisticated uses of MRI are coming into vogue. These include specially timed and T2-weighted proton-density studies of the spinal canal or skull base. It is advisable to order the tests with which the radiologists performing the diagnostic testing are most familiar.

Most clinicians focus on postural symptoms as the hallmark of low CSF pressure. However, *postural or exertional factors may be noted in conditions other than that of low CSF pressure*. Obstructions to ventricular CSF flow, Arnold-Chiari malformation type 1, subdural hematomas, cerebral venous thrombosis, and sinus disease can all lead to positional and postural headache. Reactive brain edema (causing slit ventricles) may displace brain tissue downward, accounting for Arnold-Chiari type 1 findings.

Spinal headaches occur most commonly following dural puncture via spinal tap (10% to 30% of the time), and less often following misplaced epidural catheter placement or epidural steroid injections into the intrathecal space. Females and younger patients seem the most likely to develop headaches following lumbar puncture,[64] although prepubertal children rarely, if ever, get them.[65] Larger gauge needles, the angle of the needle-tip bevel (which should be parallel to the length of the body or spine so that it parts rather than cuts dural fibers), the type of bevel itself, and the number of punctures seem to correlate most clearly with this problem; but although these associated factors seem reasonable, their link with spinal headache has not been rigorously proven. It is becoming widely accepted, however, that *positioning of the patient after the procedure has no bearing on the outcome and neither does the length of time of such positioning;* some clinicians even advocate early mobilization.[66,67] J.G. never uses larger than 20-gauge needles (smaller ones making it difficult to obtain 20 to 30 mL of fluid when needed), and I do not have my patients lie prone for more than 15 minutes after a procedure.

Treatment

Caffeine sodium benzoate, 500 mg i.v. t.i.d., may ameliorate the headache; oral caffeine preparations are less effective. We add 500 mg of caffeine to intravenous lactated Ringer's solution or to normal saline (watching for palpitations and insomnia). Simply increasing fluid intake alone rarely helps unless the patient is severely volume depleted or dehydrated. Even theophylline, 282 mg t.i.d., has been used. But none of these approaches is very effective compared with the epidural blood patch. Blood patches can be very effective and should probably be used earlier and more often than they are currently (neurologists and surgeons tending to wait longer than anesthesiologists). Injection of 10 to 20 mL of autologous blood just below the original puncture site is the quickest and most effective way to alleviate the problem, but occasionally the pain worsens. The injection can be repeated if necessary. Fever, coagulopathies, local infection, and the presence of an implanted intrathecal pump (opioids or baclofen, etc.) are contraindications to this procedure. In the latter case, the clinician risks nicking the catheter.

The mechanism of pain relief by blood patch is unknown and controversial; it may involve compression of the dural sac or the formation of a gelatinous tamponade among other mechanisms. Simple analgesics, abdominal binders, and support hose have all been used, at least adjunctively, to hasten relief of headache. Because most spinal headaches spontaneously resolve within 4 to 7 days (53% versus 72%, respectively), some clinicians feel it is worth trying rest and caffeine first. But many patients do not have the time for this less invasive approach. We tend to use blood patches if no improvement is seen with conservative measures in 48 hours. If all of the preceding treatments are unsuccessful, radioisotope studies are used to locate the leak before more invasive intervention is considered.

HEADACHE IN THE HIV-POSITIVE PATIENT

Many HIV-positive patients have, as a cause of headache, relatively benign primary headaches. In outpatients with AIDS, a cause for nonemergent headaches is found only about 50% of the time.[68] Primary pathology has been detected in even fewer cases, about 17%.[69] Headache as a presenting symptom of AIDS occurred in 55% of patients studied in a University of California AIDS clinic,[70] but others have found the number to vary between 12.5% and 27.9%.[71] Among hospitalized patients, however, serious pathology may be found more than 80% of the time.[71,72] Migraine and tension-type headaches alone are common. Analgesic rebound phenomena is a frequent cause of chronic daily headache, and this population, in particular, is likely to overuse prescribed and over-the-counter medications for the pains and anxiety with which they are faced.

Patients may use pain medication primarily to ameliorate anxiety-exacerbated pain, and there may be little insight into this use on the part of the clinician or the patient. Psychological assessment by a *mental health professional who specializes in pain* may prove enlightening and very constructive. Psychosocial stressors must be addressed to avoid the scenario of inadvertent misuse of pain medications, and to effect better headache control. Behavioral training as a means to education and mind-body awareness is crucial to the success of pain and headache management and may cut down the tendency of patients and clinicians to overuse the medical system. Periodic refresher courses may be necessary to reinforce and to maintain gains made.

Etiology

Frequent headaches may be explained by causes other than primary headaches, stress, or overuse of pain medication. Headache resulting from aseptic meningitis, possibly a function of HIV infection itself, is not uncommon. CSF studies may prove of limited value in these cases because the pleocytosis found is nonspecific and seen also in those with asymptomatic HIV infection. Substance abuse is also common and must be considered in the differential diagnosis of frequent headaches. Caffeine and other drug withdrawal syndromes may include headache as a symptom. Amphetamine, crank, crack, and cocaine cause vasculitis, vasospasm, headache, and stroke. Opioids may release histamine, causing head pain. Anti-HIV medications frequently cause headache.

The preceding etiologic factors notwithstanding, secondary headaches occur in the HIV-positive population quite often regardless of the presence or absence of a previous headache disorder. Referral bias skews the reported incidence, but the percentage of headaches considered secondary to serious and potentially fatal complications (such as cryptococcal meningitis) might be quite high. Cryptococcal meningitis is the most common cause of secondary headaches in adults with AIDS, although far less so in children as is true with other opportunistic diseases.[71,73] In patients with AIDS, several disease processes may be occurring simultaneously. *Metabolic, nutritional, psychiatric, and neurocognitive factors may, alone or together, influence the clinical presentation, making diagnosis and management a challenge.*

The likelihood of headaches being secondary in type depends on the stage of HIV infection. The differential diagnosis also varies according to the CD4 count. A CD4 count less than 500 dramatically raises the risk of opportunistic infection or meningitis. These etiologies should be considered if mentation is altered, the patient has a stiff neck (meningismus), or there are localizing neurologic signs such as a cranial neuropathy.

Among patients diagnosed with cryptococcal meningitis and who are HIV-positive, 45% have no history of a previous AIDS-defining illness. Intravenous drug users are especially likely to present with this illness. The headaches may be frontotemporal and accompanied by papilledema, nausea, vomiting, and meningismus. Neuroimaging results are frequently negative, although gadolinium-enhanced MRI may light up infected and inflamed meninges, as with any meningitis, and Virchow-Robin spaces around blood vessels may appear dilated on MRI. A positive serum antigen test, is a reasonable screen for patients not wishing to undergo a lumbar puncture when suspicion is low, or in those for whom lumbar puncture is contraindicated.

Tuberculosis and lymphomas can also affect the meninges, producing headache and neurologic deficits; in these cases, MRI and lumbar puncture are standard elements of the workup. Microbiologic blood studies and polymerase chain reaction (PCR) studies for tuberculin and cryptococcal antigens should be performed routinely, as mentioned in the discussion that follows.

Intracerebral infections also can cause headache. Headache associated with toxoplasmosis may be unilateral, bilateral, or holocephalic and often is accompanied by hemiparesis, language dysfunction, or personality change. The presence of a choreiform movement disorder makes the likelihood of toxoplasmosis very high. Lymphomas may be meningeal or intracerebral, and clinical presentation depends on the location. Differentiation between lymphomas and toxoplasmosis depends on one or more of the following: imaging findings, response to treatment, and brain biopsy.

Typically, serial scans are used to monitor response to medical treatment for 10 to 14 days before biopsies are performed. It is important to follow the lesions to resolution, because more than one type of mass may be present. Use of steroids should be minimized unless there is sufficient swelling to cause brain herniation. As mentioned earlier, steroid-affected lymphomas may diminish on scans only to reappear later. Furthermore, immunosuppression by steroids, in addition to the suppression caused by HIV alone, may put the patient at higher risk for superinfections or interfere with the success of antibiotic and antiviral therapy.

Diagnosing Brain and Meningeal Pathology Associated With HIV Infection

Obtaining a gadolinium-enhanced MRI scan may prove useful, even if the results are negative, because of the likelihood that another scan will be needed later in the course of treatment. Having a baseline scan with which to compare any new scans may significantly clarify equivocal findings. Lumbar puncture, when needed, should include routine microbiologic studies of the CSF including the PCR test for *Mycobacterium tuberculosis*. Both blood and CSF should be evaluated for cryptococcal infection.

A thorough history and physical examination, including but not limited to a detailed neurologic examination, usually is necessary. On occasion, an EEG may prove helpful in differentiating migraine from epilepsy and moderate to severe dementia from depression (pseudodementia). Moderate to severe dementia should show up on an EEG as generalized or regional slowing. The EEG of a depressed person with severe psychomotor slowing and a paucity of verbal output (mimicking some forms of dementia) should be normal unless a concurrent problem exists. Three normal sleep-deprived EEGs have much greater reliability in terms of ruling out a seizure disorder than does a single sleep-deprived or non–sleep-deprived test. Sleep deprivation helps to reveal a seizure disorder by making the brain tired and irritable, increasing the chance of the patient falling asleep. Sharp waves and other signs of epileptiform activity occur most often during the transition from wakefulness to sleep and visa versa. MRI may further evaluate areas of general or focal slowing and other types of abnormal EEG activity. In this way, physiologic and anatomic findings can be correlated.

Treating AIDS pathology–related headaches is a matter of managing the underlying condition and using analgesics judiciously but with attention to alterations in mental status. An excellent and practical overview of this topic, and related ones involving neurologic manifestations of AIDS, is available elsewhere.[74]

REFERENCES

1. Pfund Z, Szapary L, et al. Headache in intracranial tumors. *Cephalalgia* 1999;19:787–790.
2. Headache Classification Committee of the International Headache Society. Classification and diagnostic criteria for headache disorders, cranial neuralgias, and facial pain. *Cephalalgia* 1988;8(suppl):1–96.
3. Packard RC. What does the headache patient want? *Headache* 1979; 19:370–374.
4. Breitbart W, Passik S, Rosenfeld B, et al. Pain intensity and its relationship to functional interference in patients with AIDS. Poster presented at: American Pain Society 13th Annual Scientific Meeting; November 1994; Miami, Fla.
5. Bruyn GW. Intracranial arteriovenous malformation and migraine. 1984;4:191–207.
6. Kowacs PA, Werneck LC. Atenolol prophylaxis in migraine secondary to an arteriovenous malformation. *Headache* 1996;36:625–627.
7. Lance JW, Goadsby PJ. Vascular disorders. In: Lance JW, Goadsby PJ, eds. *Mechanisms and Management of Headache*. 6th ed. Oxford, England: Butterworth-Heinemann; 1998:240.
8. Burchiel KJ. Personal communication, Oregon Health Sciences University, Department of Neurosurgery, 1998.
9. Dunlop R. Delivering palliative care in different settings. In: Dunlop R, eds. *Cancer: Palliative Care (Focus on Cancer)*. New York, NY: Springer; 1998.
10. Breitbart W. Psychiatric management of cancer pain. *Cancer* 1995;76: 2181–2185.
11. Lance JW, Goadsby PJ. The investigation and general management of headache. In: Lance JW, Goadsby PJ, eds. *Mechanism and Management of Headache*. 6th ed. Oxford, England: Butterworth-Heinemann; 1998:291–298.
12. Hockeday JM, Barlow CF. Headache in children. In: Olesen J, Tfelt-Hansen P, Welch KMA, eds. *The Headaches*. Philadelphia, Pa: Raven Press; 1993:795–808.
13. Osborn AE. *Diagnostic Radiology*. St Louis, MO: Mosby-Year Book; 1994:chapters 7, 9–12, 15, 16.
14. Hansman ML, et al. Neuroimaging of acquired immunodeficiency syndrome. In: Berger JR, Levy RM, eds. *AIDS and the Nervous System*. 2nd ed. Philadelphia, Pa: Lippincott-Raven; 1997:297–381.
15. Saper JR. Headache: Urgent considerations in diagnosis and treatment. In: Weiner WJ, Shulman LM, eds. *Emergent and Urgent Neurology*. 2nd ed. Philadelphia: Lippincott Williams & Wilkins; 1999:293–297.
16. Panullo SC, Reich JB, et al. MRI changes in intracranial hypotension. *Neurology* 1993;43:919–926.
17. Report of the Quality of Standards Subcommittee of the American Academy of Neurology. Practice parameter: The utility of neuroimaging in the evaluation of headache in patients with normal neurologic examinations (summary statement). *Neurology* 1994;44:1353–1354.
18. Lewis DW. Case 8: The "MYTH" [of the non focal exam]: Part 3 of The Differential Diagnosis of Pediatric Headache. In: *Education Program Syllabus of the 51st Meeting of the American Academy of Neurology*. vol 9: Headache/Pain section 2AC.008. Toronto, Canada. 1999: 29–32.
19. Robbins LD. *Management of Headache and Headache Medications*. Germany: Springer-Verlag; 1994:5.
20. Selby G. Investigating migraine: When, why, and how. In: Blau JN, ed. *Migraine. Clinical and Research Aspects*. Baltimore, Md: Johns Hopkins University Press; 1987:77–90.
21. Vick NA. Real world neuro-oncology. In: *Education Program Syllabus of the 50th Annual Meeting of the American Academy of Neurology*. Part 6AC.001-6. 1998.
22. Forsyth PA, Posner JB. Headaches in patients with brain tumors: A study of 111 patients. *Ann Neurol* 1992;32:289.
23. Sotaniemi KA, et al. Clinical and CT correlates in the diagnosis of intracranial tumors. *J Neurol Neurosurg Psychiatry* 1991;54:645–647.
24. Evans RW. Diagnostic testing for the evaluation of headaches. *Neurol Clin* 1996;14:1–26.
25. Vasquez-Barquero A, Ibanez FJ, et al. Isolated headache as the presenting clinical manifestation of intracranial tumors: A prospective study. *Cephalalgia* 1994;14:270–272.

26. Pepin EP. Cerebral metastases presenting as migraine with aura [letter to the editor]. *Lancet* 1990;336:127–128.
27. Daumas-Duport C, et al. Dysembryoplastic neuroepithelial: A surgically curable tumor of young patients with intractable partial seizures. *Neurosurgery* 1988;23:545–556.
28. Piepmeier JM. Observations on the current treatment of low-grade astrocytic tumors of the cerebral hemispheres. *J Neurosurg* 1987;67: 177–181.
29. Forsyth PA, Posner JB. In: Olesen J, Tfelt-Hansen P, Welch KMA, eds. *The Headaches*. Philadelphia, Pa: Raven Press; 1993:706.
30. Iversen HK, et al. Brain tumor headache related to tumor size, histology and location. *Cephalalgia* 1987;7(suppl):394–395.
31. Heros DO. Neuro-oncology. In: Weiner WJ, Shulman LM, eds. *Emergent and Urgent Neurology*. 2nd ed. Philadelphia, Pa: Lippincott Williams & Wilkins; 1999:352.
32. Debryne J, Crevits L, Van de Eecken H. Migraine-like headaches in intraventricular tumors. *Clin Neurol Neurosurg* 1982;84:51–57.
33. Schumacher GA, Wolff HG. Experimental studies on headache. *Arch Neurol Psychiatry* 1941;45:199–214.
34. Vick NA. Real world neuro-oncology. In: *Education Program Syllabus of the 50th Annual Meeting of the American Academy of Neurology*. Part 6AC.001-6. 1998.
35. *Physician's Desk Reference (PDR)*. 57th ed. Merck; 2003.
36. Leppik IE. *Contemporary Diagnosis and Management of the Patient with Epilepsy*. 3rd ed. HHC; 1997:96.
37. Caroll EN, Fine E, et al. A four drug pain regimen for head and neck cancers. *Laryngoscope* 1994;104:694–700.
38. Melchart D, Linde K, et al. Acupuncture for recurrent headaches: A systematic review of randomized controlled trials. *Cephalalgia* 1999; 19:779–786.
39. Gorelick PB. Ischemic stroke and intracranial hematoma. In: Olesen J, Tfelt-Hansen P, Welch KMA, eds. *The Headaches*. Philadelphia, Pa: Raven Press; 1993:639–640.
40. Ropper AH, Davis KR. Lobar cerebral hemorrhages: Acute clinical syndromes in 26 cases. *Ann Neurol* 1980;8:141–147.
41. Lance JW, Goadsby PJ. Vascular disorders. In: Lance JW, Goadsby PJ, eds. *Mechanism and Management of Headache*. 6th ed. Oxford, England: Butterworth-Heinemann; 1998:238.
42. Ostergaard JR. Headache as a warning symptom of impending aneurysmal subarachnoid hemorrhage. *Cephalalgia* 1991;11:53–55.
43. Munoz C, Diez-Tejedor E, et al. Cluster headache associated with middle cerebral artery arteriovenous malformation. *Cephalalgia* 1996;16: 202–205.
44. Rinkel GJE, van Gijn J, Wijdicks EFM. Subarachnoid hemorrhage without detectable aneurysm: A review of the causes. *Stroke* 1993;24: 1403–1409.
45. Tolias CM, Choskey MS. Will increased awareness among physicians of the significance of sudden agonizing headache affect the outcome of subarachnoid hemorrhage? *Stroke* 1996;27:807–812.
46. Raskin NH. Paroxysmal head pains. In: *Education Program Syllabus of the 51st meeting of the American Academy of Neurology*. vol 9: Headache/Pain section 5PC.001. Toronto, Canada. 1999:31–35.
47. Day JW, Raskin NH. Thunderclap headache: Symptom of unruptured cerebral aneurysm. *Lancet* 1986;2:1247.
48. Widjdiks EFM, et al. Long-term follow-up of 71 patients with thunderclap headache mimicking subarachnoid hemorrhage. *Lancet* 1988; 2:67.
49. Linn FHH, et al. Prospective study of sentinel headache in aneurysmal subarachnoid hemorrhage. *Lancet* 1994;344:590.
50. Slivka A, et al. Clinical and angiographic features of thunderclap headache. *Headache* 1995;35:1.
51. Hughes RL. Identification and treatment of cerebral aneurysms after sentinel headache. *Neurology* 1992;42:1118.
52. Kassel NF, Kongable GL, et al. Delay in referral of patients with ruptured aneurysms to neurosurgical attention. *Stroke* 1985;16:587–590.
53. Kelley RE. Cerebral vascular disorders. In: Weiner WJ, Shulman LM, eds. *Emergent and Urgent Neurology*. 2nd ed. Philadelphia, Pa: Lippincott Williams & Wilkins; 1999:43–51.
54. Toda N, Tfelt-Hansen P. Calcium antagonists in migraine prophylaxis. In: Olesen J, Tfelt-Hansen P, Welch KMA, eds. *The Headaches*. 2nd ed. Philadelphia, Pa: Lippincott Williams & Wilkins; 2000:477–482.
55. Vestergaard K, Andersen G, et al. Headache in stroke. *Stroke* 1993; 24:1621–1624.
56. Koudstaal PJ, et al, for the Dutch TIA Study Group. Headache in transient or permanent cerebral ischemia. *Stroke* 1991;22:754–759.
57. Portenoy RK, Abissi CJ, Lipton RB. Headache in cerebrovascular disease. *Stroke* 1984;15:1009–1012.
58. Kumral E, Bogoudslavsky J, et al. Headache at stroke onset: The Lausanne Stroke Registry. *J Neurol Neurosurg Psychiatry* 1995;58: 490–492.
59. Gorelick PB, Hier DB, et al. Headache in acute cerebrovascular disease. *Neurology* 1986;36:1445–1450.
60. Vestergaard K, Andersen G, et al. Headache in stroke. *Stroke* 1993;24: 1621–1624.
61. Mckissock W. Subdural haematoma. A review of 389 cases. *Lancet* 1960;1:1365–1370.
62. Saper JR. CSF hypotension and headache: How low is low? In: *Education Program Syllabus of the American Academy of Neurology 51st Annual Meeting*. Toronto, Canada. 1999:5PC.001-45.
63. Wang LP, Schmidt JF. Central nervous system side effects after lumbar puncture: A review of the possible pathogenesis of the syndrome of post puncture headache and associated symptoms. *Dan Med Bull* 1997;44:79–81.
64. Vilming ST, Schrader H, et al. The significance of age, sex, and cerebrospinal fluid pressure in post-lumbar-puncture headache. *Cephalalgia* 1989;9:99–106.
65. Wee LH, Lam F, Cranston AJ. The incidence of post dural puncture headache in children. *Anesthesia* 1996;51:1164–1166.
66. Spriggs DA, Burn DJ, et al. Is bed rest useful after diagnostic lumbar puncture? *Post Grad Med J* 1992;68:581–583.
67. Vilming ST, Schrader H, et al. Post-lumbar-puncture headache: The significance of body posture. A controlled study of 300 patients. *Cephalalgia* 1988;8:75–78.
68. Berger JR, Pall L, Stein N. Headache and human immunodeficiency virus infection: A case control study. *Eur Neurol* 1996;36:229-233.
69. Trenkwalder C, et al. Headache in HIV-infected patients [abstract]. *Int Conf AIDS* 1991;7:215.
70. Levy RM, Bredesen DE. Central nervous system dysfunction in acquired immunodeficiency syndrome. In: Rosenblum ML, Levy RM, Bredesen DE, eds. *AIDS and The Nervous System*. New York, NY: Raven Press; 1988:29–63.
71. Goldstein J. Headache and acquired immunodeficiency syndrome. *Neurol Clin* 1990;8:947–960.
72. Goldstein J. Headache in AIDS. In: Rose FC, ed. *New Advances in Headache Research*. London, England: Smith Gordon and Co; 1988:31–38.
73. Pizzo PA, et al. Acquired immune deficiency syndrome in children: Current problems and therapeutic considerations. *Am J Med* 1988;85: 195–202.
74. Berger JR. Infections of the central nervous system: The neurologic emergencies of acquired immunodeficiency syndrome. In: Weiner WJ, Shulman LM, eds. *Emergent and Urgent Neurology*. 2nd ed. Philadelphia, Pa: Lippincott Williams &Wilkins; 1999:201–222.

CHAPTER 25 FACIAL PAIN

Thomas N. Ward and Morris Levin

The diagnosis and management of patients with facial pain can be daunting even to experienced physicians. The causes are myriad, ranging from the mundane (sinus and dental disease) to the exotic (short-lasting unilateral neuralgiform headache with conjunctival injection and tearing, or SUNCT). Misdiagnosis and mismanagement are common. The goal of this chapter is to discuss some of the more important causes of facial pain, and to guide proper identification and treatment.

Simply because pain is felt in the face does not imply that it necessarily originates in facial structures. As elsewhere in the body, pain may be local in origin, or referred. The role of the trigeminovascular system and the spinal trigeminal nucleus as a point of anatomic and physiologic convergence is discussed in Chapter 19. Suffice it to say that the location of the pain may not be so important diagnostically as other features.

The approach to the evaluation of facial pain requires careful attention to detail. In the history, it is essential to obtain an accurate description of the nature of the pain, or pains, what may have incited it, and what currently provokes and ameliorates it. Are there associated phenomena, such as autonomic changes? Past medical history, including trauma and surgical or dental procedures may provide essential clues. Is there associated depression or any other psychiatric problem? What therapies have been tried, and with what outcomes?

After obtaining a detailed history, a thorough examination is necessary. In addition to the general physical examination, a thorough neurologic examination is essential. The examiner looks for signs of raised intracranial pressure (papilledema, diminished up gaze, sixth cranial nerve palsies) and cranial nerve dysfunction (particularly oculosympathetic paresis). The head and neck require careful attention. Are there trigger points? Is there dental or sinus pathology? Auscultation for bruits and palpation of the carotid artery are sometimes informative maneuvers.

Lastly, the results of prior diagnostic studies are reviewed, noting the timing of the studies. Were the appropriate studies performed? If the situation has changed, perhaps a study should be repeated. Sometimes a diagnosis may become apparent only after serial clinical examinations or diagnostic studies, or both.

After a careful history, examination, and review of the data, a tentative diagnosis may be rendered. Often further consultation is required. Treatment is offered based on the tentative diagnosis and may, in itself, sometimes be diagnostic. The thoughtful physician should always be willing to reconsider the diagnosis.

Facial pain clearly represents a diagnostic challenge. With attention to the fundamental approach outlined in the preceding paragraphs, the vast majority of patients may achieve a satisfying outcome.

NEURALGIAS

Neuralgias are paroxysmal pain in the distribution of a particular nerve. The pain is typically maximal at onset and lancinating, and may be described as "electric shocks" or "jabbing." There may be a single sharp pain, or repetitive pains in succession. The pain may be so brief as to last but an instant, or for several seconds. There is usually a refractory period after the severe pain, during which pain does not occur. Some neuralgic conditions have trigger zones (areas that, when stimulated, provoke an attack) or other triggers. Careful history taking often reveals other pain occurring as well, such as continuous aching, burning, or throbbing. Inquiry must be made about all the sensations that occur, because some patients mention only the severe exacerbations. Response to treatment may provide a clue to diagnosis, but can also be misleading. "Diagnostic blocks" in the setting of facial pain do not necessarily define the site from which the pain arises because of overlap of cranial nerves V, IX, and X (which converge on the spinal trigeminal nucleus and the tractus solitarius).

The best-known facial neuralgia is trigeminal neuralgia, which is discussed in detail in this chapter and, in many ways, serves as a model for understanding other neuralgias causing facial pain.

Trigeminal Neuralgia

Trigeminal neuralgia is a severe, (usually) unilateral facial pain, characterized by lancinating pains in the distribution of one or more divisions of the trigeminal nerve. Although onset may occur in the second and third decades, the majority of cases begin in middle and old age. With an annual incidence rate of 4 to 5 per 100,000, it is one of the most frequently seen neuralgias in the elderly.[1] The pain may be so excruciating that facial muscle spasms can be seen, hence the older term, tic douloureux.

The facial pain tends to occur in paroxysms and is maximal at or near onset. The severe exacerbations tend to last from one to several seconds, but may occur in volleys. There may also be a coexisting continual deep or dull pain. Patients may or may not, therefore, have pain-free periods.

Trigeminal neuralgia most often involves the second and third divisions of the trigeminal nerve (V_2 and V_3), but can include or be limited to the first division, as well. Trigger zones may be present. Often, lightly touching these areas will trigger a paroxysm, and patients tend to protect these areas. Other triggers may include chewing, talking, brushing teeth, cold air, or smiling and grimacing. A refractory period of several minutes typically follows an episode, during which a paroxysm cannot be provoked. In occasional patients, the pain may be bilateral, but not on both sides simultaneously.

This condition may be idiopathic (primary), or symptomatic (secondary). Idiopathic implies no known underlying condition, but in point of fact most idiopathic cases are the result of vascular compression of the trigeminal nerve near its entry into the pons. Symptomatic causes include multiple sclerosis, tumors, and basilar artery aneurysm or ectasia.[2–4]

Unlike some other facial pain conditions, trigeminal neuralgia typically does not awaken patients at night. Some patients have a history of so-called pretrigeminal neuralgia, which is said to be dull, continuous, aching pain in the jaw, evolving eventually into trigeminal neuralgia. This brief, milder pain is sometimes suspected to have a dental origin, and dental procedures are performed. Because trigeminal neuralgia is sometimes precipitated by dental procedures (e.g., dental extraction), confusion about etiology has resulted.[5]

The pathophysiology of trigeminal neuralgia is not fully elucidated. Demyelinative lesions of trigeminal fibers appear to set up ectopic impulses and ephapses. This alteration of afferent input may disinhibit pain pathways in the spinal trigeminal nucleus. Evidence for a role of central pain mechanisms includes the presence of refractory periods after a triggered episode, trains of painful sensations after a single stimulus, and some latency from the time of stimulation to the onset of pain.[6]

Clinically, certain features of the history help in making the diagnosis. Paroxysms of pain in the distribution of the trigeminal nerve, especially if trigger points are present, are typical. The examination may reveal these trigger zones, which often are near the midline. If sensory loss is present, a mass lesion is more likely. In younger patients (20 to 40 years old) with trigeminal neuralgia, multiple sclerosis should be considered. A demyelinative lesion in the pons would explain bilateral symptoms.

Once the diagnosis is suspected on clinical grounds, a careful search for ipsilateral dental pathology should be undertaken (oral surgery consultation should be considered). Magnetic resonance imaging (MRI) and magnetic resonance angiography (MRA) should be performed to look for evidence of demyelinating lesions, a mass lesion in the cerebellopontine angle, or an ectatic blood vessel (rarely seen with MRA). The differential diagnosis includes SUNCT, cluster-tic syndrome, jabs and jolts syndrome, and other neuralgias, all of which are discussed later in this chapter.

Trigeminal neuralgia is usually successfully treated with medication (Table 25-1). Carbamazepine is felt to be the most effective medication. Baclofen, phenytoin, valproate, pimozide, and clonazepam have utility as well, alone or in various combinations.[7] Misoprostol, a prostaglandin E analogue, has been reported as effective in trigeminal neuralgia caused by multiple sclerosis.[8] Gabapentin and lamotrigine have also been reported to be useful, although there is less clinical experience with these agents.[9,10]

Neuroleptic medications, including chlorpromazine and perphenazine, have been used successfully in intractable cases, and novel neuroleptics such as olanzapine and quetiapine are being tried as well. Tizanidine has been used in selected cases. Topiramate has been suggested, because other anticonvulsant medication has been effective.

We have found carbamazepine to be the most useful of all the available drugs. If doses are started low, especially in the elderly (e.g., 50 mg b.i.d.) and advanced gradually, the drug is highly efficacious with few side effects, and few patients develop tolerance. If pain control is insufficient, baclofen may be added. If the patient is desperate for immediate pain relief, intravenous infusion of phenytoin or fosphenytoin (250 to 500 mg at no more than 50 mg/min, monitoring pulse and blood pressure) may be rapidly effective, although many patients quickly develop tolerance to the drug. Nonetheless, intravenous phenytoin may afford immediate temporary relief while oral carbamazepine therapy is begun. This maneuver may also enable the physician to better examine the patient with a sensitive face.[11] Details of the use of these medications may be found elsewhere in this book (see Chaps. 62, 63, and 64).

TABLE 25-1 **Medications for Trigeminal Neuralgia**

Acute
Phenytoin or fosphenytoin intravenously
Chronic*
Carbamazepine
Oxcarbazepine
Baclofen
Valproate
Clonazepam
Pimozide
Gabapentin
Lamotrigine
Topiramate
Perphenazine
Olanzapine
Tizanidine

*See Chapters 48, 49, and 52 for details on the use these agents.

Rarely, there are spontaneous permanent remissions of trigeminal neuralgia. More often, the illness tends to wax and wane in terms of severity and frequency of exacerbations. Therefore, in patients achieving good relief of pain with medications, periodic attempts to gradually withdraw these drugs are warranted.

For patients refractory to therapy with drugs, various surgical procedures may have efficacy. Janetta has popularized microvascular decompression, the dissection away from the trigeminal nerve of various vascular structures, often an ectatic superior cerebellar artery.[12] Long-term outcome is good (over 80% pain-free), but this procedure does involve an intracranial approach with a small morbidity and mortality rate. Other procedures directed against the trigeminal nerve include percutaneous radiofrequency rhizotomy, glycerol rhizolysis, and balloon compression. Complications include anesthesia dolorosa (a central pain disorder resulting from hypersensitization of the second-order spinal trigeminal nucleus neuron) and keratitis, as well as facial weakness caused by injury of the facial nerve. More recently, excellent results with minimal morbidity have been reported with gamma knife therapy.[13] For patients unable or unwilling to tolerate more aggressive surgical procedures, peripheral nerve root avulsion may provide relief. Although often temporarily effective, nerves often regenerate and pain recurs.

Tenser has noted that after surgery for trigeminal neuralgia, herpes simplex virus reactivation occurs in 17% to 94% of patients. The speculation is that altered function of cranial nerve V (CNV) underlies the beneficial response to the various surgical manipulations (injury to the trigeminal root ganglion).[14]

In summary, patients suffering from trigeminal neuralgia deserve a careful evaluation, especially to exclude symptomatic causes such as multiple sclerosis or a cerebellopontine angle mass. Ipsilateral dental pathology should be sought. Pain relief can usually be achieved through aggressive pharmacologic therapy, surgery or both.

Cluster-tic Syndrome

It has been reported that the pains of trigeminal neuralgia and cluster headache may coexist.[15] In the cluster-tic syndrome, there are three types of pain. One component of the pain resembles trigeminal neuralgia—paroxysmal, extremely brief, and severe. The second component is more similar to cluster headache, although of variable length, with autonomic phenomena (lacrimation, rhinorrhea). The third type of pain is a mixture of the first two. This pain may be provoked by trigger points or moving the neck.

Cluster-tic syndrome usually afflicts patients between 20 and 70 years old. It may exist in chronic or episodic forms (remissions and recurrences). Medical therapy is usually unsuccessful, although when surgery (microvascular decompression or trigeminal rhizotomy) relieves the neuralgia, the cluster-like pain may be lessened and become more responsive to therapy.

The differential diagnosis includes SUNCT, which is discussed later in this chapter. Secondary (symptomatic) SUNCT has been reported as a result of arteriovenous malformation in the cerebellopontine angle, and secondary cluster-tic syndrome has been seen associated with an ectatic basilar artery running deep into the cerebellopontine cistern.[16,17] We feel it is possible that so-called cluster-tic syndrome and SUNCT may actually be the same condition.

Glossopharyngeal Neuralgia

Glossopharyngeal neuralgia is defined as paroxysmal pain in areas supplied by cranial nerves IX and X (CN IX, X). There are numerous analogies to trigeminal neuralgia, with which it occasionally coexists.

This entity is much less common than trigeminal neuralgia. Age of onset ranges from childhood to old age, although middle age is most frequent. This condition usually occurs as paroxysmal, severe, unilateral pain involving the ear, larynx, tonsil, or tongue. It is almost never bilateral. Triggers include chewing, swallowing, coughing, speaking, yawning, certain tastes, and touching the neck or external auditory canal (rarely the pre- or postauricular areas).[18]

The pain typically radiates upward from the oropharynx toward the ear. The duration of the severe paroxysms is seconds to minutes, but there may also be a low-grade, constant, dull background pain. Up to several dozen attacks may occur each day, some of which awaken the patient from sleep. Some episodes are associated with strenuous coughing or hoarseness.

Similar to trigeminal neuralgia, glossopharyngeal neuralgia may occur in a pattern of bouts lasting weeks to months, alternating with longer periods of remission. Severe attacks may be associated with bradycardia and asystole, resulting in syncope.[19] Presumably, in these cases, input from CN IX into the tractus solitarius has an effect on the dorsal motor nucleus of X.

Also, similar to trigeminal neuralgia, there are idiopathic and secondary (symptomatic) forms. Presumably, in the idiopathic form, peripheral demyelinization results in brainstem discharges. *Alternatively,* vascular compression of CN IX and X may occur at the nerve root entry zone by the vertebral artery or posterior inferior cerebellar artery. Symptomatic causes include cerebellopontine angle tumor, brainstem demyelinative lesions, peritonsillar abscess, carotid aneurysm, and Eagle's syndrome (in which CN IX is compressed laterally against an ossified stylohyoid ligament).[20]

The evaluation of a patient suspected of suffering from glossopharyngeal neuralgia incudes a careful history, especially inquiring about the presence of trigger factors and nocturnal awakening. All aspects of an attack need to be recorded. MRI and MRA are appropriate, because approximately 25% of cases of glossopharyngeal neuralgia result from secondary causes, such as brainstem mass lesions. Plain skull films might reveal an ossified stylohyoid ligament in Eagle's syndrome.

Medical therapy of glossopharyngeal neuralgia is essentially the same as for trigeminal neuralgia (see Table 25-1). Additionally, the application of local anesthetics to the oropharynx may be both diagnostic and therapeutic. Injection of local anesthetic into the region of the stylohyoid ligament can be diagnostic if Eagle's syndrome is strongly considered. Patients failing drug therapy may be candidates for surgical treatment. Procedures include intracranial sectioning of CN IX along with the upper three to four rootlets of CN X at the jugular foramen, or vascular decompression.[20]

The differential diagnosis of glossopharyngeal neuralgia includes so-called geniculate neuralgia (nervus intermedius neuralgia of Hunt), which is discussed later in this chapter. The obvious overlap of clinical features between the two conditions fosters suspicions that they may actually be variations of the same condition.

Superior Laryngeal Neuralgia

The superior laryngeal nerve is a branch of CN X that runs adjacent to the carotid bifurcation and supplies the cricothyroid muscle of the larynx. A lesion of this nerve produces a weak, hoarse voice. The nerve may be involved by local disease of the carotid or injured by carotid endarterectomy.[21]

Clinically, the patient suffers paroxysmal pain that radiates from the throat to the ear or eye, similar to the pain of glossopharyngeal neuralgia. There is generally hoarseness. The episodes last seconds to minutes, and may occur spontaneously, or be triggered by coughing, swallowing, or speaking. During severe paroxysms, the patient temporarily may be rendered mute.

On examination, hoarseness of speech, and a trigger point superolateral to the thyroid cartilage may be noted. The differential diagnosis includes glossopharyngeal neuralgia, geniculate neuralgia, and carotidynia (all discussed elsewhere in this chapter). Local blockade of the nerve is diagnostic. Some patients respond to carbamazepine and possibly other drugs used for neuralgias. Neurectomy may be curative.[21]

Postherpetic Neuralgia

Acute herpes zoster (shingles) often causes facial pain, especially affecting V_1. The varicella zoster virus persists in sensory nerve ganglia, and may cause a painful rash. Postherpetic neuralgia is variably defined as pain that persists (anywhere from 1 to 6 months) after the rash has healed. Although treatment of acute zoster with acyclovir, valacyclovir, famciclovir, steroids, pain medications, and even sympathetic nerve blocks may shorten the duration and alleviate the immediate pain, none has been clearly proven to prevent the occurrence of postherpetic neuralgia. Age is the major risk factor. Patients younger than 40 years of age rarely develop postherpetic neuralgia, whereas more than 75% of patients older than age 70 years are afflicted.[22] Lesser risk factors include diabetes mellitus, V_1 involvement, and other immunologic compromise.

Clinically, there is usually scarring and pigmentary changes in the affected dermatome. The pain is constant and variably aching, burning, lancinating, or itchy. The mechanism of the pain is likely deafferentation pain. Pathologically, there are degenerative changes in the involved axons, dorsal ganglion, and even the dorsal horn of the spinal cord. Patients complain of allodynia (pain with non-noxious stimulus) in the affected area.[23]

Because this condition preferentially affects the elderly, treatment can be difficult. Unlike trigeminal neuralgia, anticonvulsants are usually ineffective. Amitriptyline is the single most useful agent, although the anticholinergic side effects may be troublesome. Beginning with a low dose (e.g., 10 mg) and slowly escalating toward 75 mg at bedtime may improve tolerance. If side effects are troublesome, either nortriptyline or doxepin, which have fewer anticholinergic side effects, may be substituted (both are available in liquid form, allowing very gradual dose titration if necessary). Approximately 60% of patients obtain significant relief with these agents.[24,25]

Many other agents have been anecdotally reported to benefit patients with postherpetic neuralgia. These include controlled-release oxycodone, capsaicin cream, topical lidocaine gel, EMLA cream, and gabapentin. With persistence, pain relief can usually be achieved. Fortunately, for most patients, the pain eventually spontaneously remits, for the majority in less than 3 years.

Other Neuralgias

Numerous neuralgias have been described as causes of facial pain. However, some share many features with other conditions, and it is likely that some of these conditions simply share several names. Of these, Raeder's paratrigeminal syndrome is the best recognized.

Raeder's syndrome consists of constant, unilateral, burning facial pain with hypesthesia or dysesthesia, or both, in the distribution of the trigeminal nerve, most often V_1, plus oculosympathetic paresis (ptosis and miosis). This syndrome may be caused by carotid artery dissection. It may also occur with trauma, mass or lesion of the middle cranial fossa, syphilis, and sinusitis. In the absence of these underlying conditions, it is generally a self-limited process, remitting in weeks to months.[26]

Sphenopalatine neuralgia (with numerous other synonyms, including greater superficial petrosal neuralgia) is described as unilateral, episodic, perinasal facial pain with nasal congestion.[27] Most of these cases closely resemble cluster headache, and the existence of this neuralgia as a separate diagnostic entity is questionable.

The same may be said for geniculate neuralgia (or nervus intermedius neuralgia of Hunt). This condition has been described as lancinating pains deep in the ear with a trigger zone in the external auditory canal.[28] The existence of geniculate neuralgia as a separate entity also has been called into question. The similarities with the better-accepted diagnosis—glossopharyngeal neuralgia—are obvious.

CAROTID ARTERY PAIN

The carotid artery, like most arteries of its caliber, is sensitive to pain. Distention or inflammation of nociceptive fibers in its walls tends to produce pain, which can seem localized to the neck or, quite commonly, be referred to a number of areas including the jaw, face and periorbital regions, and sinus areas.

Carotidynia

Carotidynia is pain that appears to emanate from the carotid artery. Raskin has described two types: acute and chronic recurrent carotidynia.[29]

The acute form seems to be a self-limited problem. The patient suffers from unilateral or, less often, bilateral pain that may be provoked by swallowing, coughing, or moving the neck. The pain may be pounding, sharp, or dull. The duration is from a few days to (rarely) several months. Corticosteroids have been advocated for relief. The differential diagnosis includes giant cell arteritis and carotid dissection. The evaluation of such complaints should include an erythrocyte sedimentation rate (ESR) and MRI or MRA to evaluate the anatomy of the carotid arteries.

Chronic recurrent carotidynia is felt to be a manifestation of migraine. This condition, like migraine, seems to be more common in women. Pain occurs in the jaw, cheek, or periorbitally. The frequency of attacks is quite variable. Pain may be dull and continuous, or sharp, or throbbing. An association with dental extraction has been speculated. Drugs effective in the prophylaxis of migraine are effective in this condition. Examples include propranolol, methysergide, and amitriptyline. It should be noted that if one examines a migraineur during an attack, the carotid artery is usually found to be tender.

Carotid Artery Dissection

Arterial dissection is caused by penetration of blood into the arterial wall with resultant narrowing of the vascular lumen, sometimes even leading to complete occlusion. Carotid artery dissection may be spontaneous (no discernible inciting event), posttraumatic, or the result of underlying disease of the vessel (such as fibromuscular dysplasia, Marfan's syndrome, cystic medial necrosis).

Carotid dissection is a frequently recognized cause of stroke in the young, especially in migraineurs.[30] Clinically, patients complain of neck pain radiating to the cheek or periorbitally. The pain may be dull, sharp, or throbbing. Uncommonly, the headache is bilateral. Focal ischemic symptoms (transient ischemic attack or stroke) may ensue as a result of loss of blood flow or embolization from the tip of the clot. There may be an ipsilateral oculosympathetic paresis (ptosis, miosis) resulting from involvement of the internal carotid plexus. Bruits may be appreciated, either subjective or objective, or both.[31] MRI and MRA may, in some cases, be as sensitive as angiography for the detection of this lesion.[32] Carotid ultrasound and transcranial Doppler, although less effective for initial detection, are excellent noninvasive methods for studying the resolution of the dissection, which may occur over weeks to months.[33] Treatment may involve antiplatelet agents, heparin, or warfarin. An urgent neurologic consultation is indicated.

POSTTRAUMATIC FACIAL PAIN

Facial pain may occur after trauma. Although bullet wounds and other head injuries may trigger pain, surgery is also a cause. Facial pain may occur after maxillofacial surgery, orbital enucleations, sinus procedures, and dental procedures. Dental procedures may trigger a variety of syndromes, including neuralgia and facial migraine.

In all cases of posttraumatic facial pain, a careful search should be made for underlying pathology, especially dental. Some patients manifest constant burning pain, occasionally with tingling and intermittent stabbing. With trophic changes, edema, and redness, reflex sympathetic dystrophy (complex regional pain syndrome, type 1) should be suspected.[34] In patients who complain of significant burning pain, sympathetic blockade of the stellate ganglion may be effective, even without obvious complex regional pain syndrome.

Treatment of posttraumatic facial pain can be challenging. Brief lancinating pains may respond to agents used in treatment of neuralgias (see Table 25-1). Amitriptyline may reduce pain and lessen associated depression. Other agents useful for treating migraine headaches have been employed empirically for symptomatic benefit. Fortunately, posttraumatic facial pain is a self-limited condition, generally resolving spontaneously within several years.

In some cases, direct trauma to superficial facial nerves, such as the supraorbital and supratrochlear nerves, can lead to persistent lancinating or, less typically, aching pain. Neuroma formation is a postulated mechanism, and local nerve block with lidocaine or bupivacaine can be both diagnostic and therapeutic. We have found percussion tenderness over the nerve in question to be particularly helpful in predicting response to local nerve block.

SINUS DISEASE

Acute sinusitis, maxillary sinusitis being the most common, may cause facial pain. The pain may be felt in the cheeks, upper teeth, or bifrontally. The discomfort may be dull and continuous, throbbing, or sharp. The differential diagnosis includes migraine, which is often misdiagnosed as "sinus headaches."

To make a diagnosis of acute sinusitis as a cause of facial pain, positive findings should be present. On examination, there is tenderness to percussion, often with a purulent nasal discharge, and fever. Laboratory evaluation may show an elevated ESR and white blood count. Sinus imaging (x-rays or computed tomography scan) should be abnormal. Without these findings, alternate diagnoses should be sought. Sphenoid sinusitis can be less obvious, and referred pain can include periorbital and maxillary regions.

The acute condition often responds to decongestants and simple analgesics. More severe, progressive cases require antibiotics. Refractory cases are candidates for ENT consultation for surgery. Chronic sinusitis is rarely a cause of headaches and facial pain.

DENTAL PAIN

Oromandibular conditions as a cause of pain are discussed in detail in Chapter 26. Dental pains are an extremely common cause of facial pain. Specific inquiry regarding prior dental procedures should be made of all patients. Trigeminal neuralgia has been associated with ipsilateral dental pathology. The presence of provocative factors, such as chewing, or the effect of hot or cold liquids may provide useful clues. The teeth and temporomandibular joints should be carefully evaluated in cases of facial pain. Temporomandibular joint syndrome (limitation of jaw movement, crepitus in the joint, and pain with use) may cause pain in the temple, jaw, and neck. Dental or oral surgical consultation may be extremely useful.

Before declaring a diagnosis of dental or sinus disease as the etiology of facial pain, positive evidence must be sought. Many patients with primary headache syndromes have been subjected to numerous dental or surgical procedures, because of where their pain was located, not because of truly local disease.

ATYPICAL FACIAL PAIN

The International Headache Society (IHS) definition of atypical facial pain is "persistent facial pain that does not have the characteristics of the cranial neuralgias classified above and is not associated with physical signs or a demonstrable organic cause."[35] Patients, usually women, present with unremitting facial pain, usually unilateral at onset, sometimes spreading bilaterally. The neurologic examination is, by definition, normal.

Raskin has justly pointed out that a better designation for this entity is "facial pain of unknown cause."[36] In some cases, serious underlying pathology may not declare itself initially. For example, nasopharyngeal carcinoma and other cancers have eventually been implicated in some cases. Only when a neurologic deficit appears (e.g., cranial nerve palsies) may the real diagnosis become evident. Lung cancer has been another reported cause (due to referred pain presumably via CN X).[37] Occult dental pathology, such as infected cavities of maxillary and mandibular bones at the sites of previous extractions, is another consideration. Dental evaluation with injection of anesthetic followed, when effective, by curettage and antibiotics has cured some sufferers.[38]

Many cases have been labeled psychogenic. This may be appropriate if there is evidence for somatization disorder, conversion disorder, or somatic delusions, but probably "psychogenic" is an overused label. Certainly, many patients have concomitant depression, which should be addressed.

All patients presenting with idiopathic facial pain require a careful history and examination. Dental consultation to rule out occult pathology is important. An MRI scan of the head, with attention to the base of the brain is indicated. A chest x-ray, perhaps with a chest CT scan, may help rule out lung cancer, especially in smokers. Serial examinations may be required as the clinician looks for an occult process to declare itself.

The treatment of idiopathic facial pain is extremely challenging. Burning pain may respond to stellate ganglion blocks. Heterocyclic antidepressants may lessen pain as well as help coexistent depression. Behavioral medicine measures, such as biofeedback and cognitive behavioral therapy, may be tried.

(Clearly, "idiopathic facial pain" is a more appropriate designation than "psychogenic" or "atypical." A multidisciplinary approach to both diagnosis and treatment yields the best results.)

OTHER FACIAL PAIN

Primary (Facial) Headache

It should be remembered that migraine, cluster headache, and other so-called headaches (such as chronic paroxysmal hemicrania) may present mainly in the face. Many patients diagnosed with "sinus headaches" are, in fact, migraineurs. Careful attention to details of the history and examination should clarify the diagnosis. Patient reports revealing a family history, trigger factors, or the presence of an aura point toward migraine as the etiology.

Likewise, cluster headache and other short-lasting headaches may present with pain mainly in the face rather than peri- or retro-orbitally. The clarification of the duration of the episodes, plus associated autonomic features (ptosis, rhinorrhea, lacrimation) is diagnostically helpful.

Jabs and Jolts

This head pain syndrome has many names; the IHS terms it *idiopathic stabbing headache*. Other authors refer to it as ice-pick headache. This is a primary headache syndrome with paroxysmal pain lasting up to 10 seconds, but usually less than 2 seconds. Like trigeminal neuralgia, it may occur in volleys.[39] Pain is generally multifocal and can involve the face as well as the head, with the orbital region most commonly affected. The frequency of these sudden brief pains is quite variable, from rare isolated jolts, to 50 or more per day.

These pains may occur as a separate, primary head pain condition or in association with other disorders, including migraine, giant cell arteritis, cluster headache, chronic paroxysmal hemicrania, or even tension-type headache. The differential diagnosis of jabs and jolts syndrome includes SUNCT (see following section), and trigeminal neuralgia. Jabs and jolts syndrome usually responds to treatment with indomethacin. Trigeminal neuralgia often has trigger points and responds much more readily to carbamazepine or other appropriate therapies (see Table 25-1).

SUNCT

Short-lasting unilateral neuralgiform headache with conjunctival injection and tearing (SUNCT) is a rare syndrome. The brief pain (usually 15 to 120 seconds in duration) is typically near the eye, but may occur in the temple or face. Multiple (up to 100) episodes occur daily, sometimes with other autonomic associations (ptosis, rhinorrhea).

The pain is almost always unilateral, and far more common in men. Neck movements trigger the pain in some patients. There are primary and secondary (symptomatic) forms. Secondary causes of SUNCT include cerebellopontine angle arteriovenous malformation.[40] Clinical similarities with trigeminal neuralgia and cluster-tic syndrome are apparent. Because secondary trigeminal neuralgia and SUNCT can be caused by cerebellopontine angle arteriovenous malformations, it may be that microvascular decompression could alleviate other SUNCT cases. MRI is indicated in the evaluation of SUNCT. To date, there is no known effective therapy of primary SUNCT.

SUMMARY

Patients presenting with facial pain often represent a diagnostic and therapeutic challenge. The number of pain-sensitive structures in the face is impressive, and many different entities share similar presenting symptoms. However, close attention to the fundamentals of thorough history taking and examination maximize diagnostic accuracy, the foundation upon which rational treatment rests.

REFERENCES

1. Kateric S, Williams DB, Beard CM, et al. Epidemiology and clinical features of idiopathic trigeminal neuralgia and glossopharyngeal neuralgia: Similarities and differences. *Neuroepidemiology* 1991;10:276–281.
2. Gass A, Kitchen N, MacManus DG, et al. Trigeminal neuralgia in patients with multiple sclerosis: Lesion localization with magnetic resonance imaging. *Neurology* 1997;49:1142–1144.
3. Cheng TM, Cascino TL, Onofrio BM. Comprehensive study of diagnosis and treatment of trigeminal neuralgia secondary tumors. *Neurology* 1993;43:2298–2302.
4. Linskey ME, Jho HD, Janetta PJ. Microvascular decompression for trigeminal neuralgia caused by vertebrobasilar compression. *J Neurosurg* 1994;81:1–9.
5. Fromm GH, Graff-Radford SB, Terrence CF, et al. Pre-trigeminal neuralgia. *Neurology* 1990;40:1493–1495.
6. Fromm GH, Terrence CF, Maroon JC. Trigeminal neuralgia. Current concepts regarding etiology and pathogenesis. *Arch Neurol* 1984;41:1204–1207.
7. Lance JW. *Mechanism and Management of Headache*. Oxford, England: Butterworth-Heinemann; 1993:260.
8. Reder AT, Arnason BG. Trigeminal neuralgia in multiple sclerosis relieved by a prostaglandin E analogue. *Neurology* 1995;45:1097–1100.
9. Khan OA. Gabapentin relieves trigeminal neuralgia in multiple sclerosis patients. *Neurology* 1998;51:611–614.
10. Lunardi G, Leandri M, Albano C, et al. Clinical effectiveness of lamotrigine and plasma levels in essential and symptomatic tri-geminal neuralgia. *Neurology* 1997;48:1714–1717.
11. Raskin NH. *Headache.* 2nd ed. New York, NY: Churchill Livingstone; 1988:343–344.
12. Janetta PJ. Microsurgical management of trigeminal neuralgia. *Arch Neurol* 1985;42:800.
13. Young RF, Vermeulen SS, Grimm P, et al. Gamma knife radio surgery for treatment of trigeminal neuralgia: Idiopathic and tumor related. *Neurology* 1997;48:603–614.
14. Tenser RB. Trigeminal neuralgia: Mechanisms of treatment. *Neurology* 1998;51:17–19.
15. Watson P, Evans R. Cluster-tic syndrome. *Headache* 1985;25:123–126.
16. Bussone G, Leone M, Volta GD, et al. Short-lasting unilateral neuralgiform headache attacks with tearing and conjunctival injection: The first symptomatic case. *Cephalalgia* 1991;11:123–127.
17. Ochoa JJ, Alberca R, Canadillar F, et al. Cluster-tic syndrome and basilar artery ectasia: A case report. *Headache* 1993;33:512–513.
18. Bohm E, Strang RR. Glossopharyngeal neuralgia. *Brain* 1962;85:371–388.
19. Rushton JG, Stevens JC, Miller RH. Glossopharyngeal (vasoglossopharyngeal) neuralgia. *Arch Neurol* 1981;38:201–205.
20. Bryun GW. Glossopharyngeal neuralgia. In: Vinken PJ, Gruyn GW, Klawans HL, eds. *Handbook of Clinical Neurology.* Amsterdam, Holland: Elsevier; 1985:459–473.
21. Bruyn GW. Superior laryngeal neuralgia. *Cephalalgia* 1983;3:235–240.
22. Kost RG, Straus SE. Postherpetic neuralgia-pathogenesis, treatment, and prevention. *N Engl J Med* 1996;335:32–42.
23. Nurmikko T. Clinical features and pathophysiologic mechanisms of postherpetic neuralgia. *Neurology* 1995;45(suppl):554–555.
24. Watson CP. The treatment of postherpetic neuralgia. *Neurology* 1995;45(suppl):558–560.
25. Watson, CPN, Vernick L, Chipman M, et al. Nortriptyline versus amitriptyline in postherpetic neuralgia. *Neurology* 1998;51:1166–1171.
26. Mokri B. Raeder's paratrigeminal syndrome. Original concept and subsequent deviations. *Arch Neurol* 1982;39:395–399.
27. Bruyn G. Sphenopalatine neuralgia (Slyder). In: Vinken PJ, Bruyn GW, Klawanus HC, Rose FC, eds. *Handbook of Clinical Neurology.* Amsterdam, Holland: Elsevier; 1986:475–482.
28. Bruyn GW: Nervus intermedius neuralgia (Hunt). *Cephalalgia* 1984;4:71–78.
29. Raskin NH. *Headache.* 2nd ed. New York, NY: Churchill Livingstone; 1988:353–357.
30. Ganesan V, Kirkham FJ. Carotid dissection causing stroke in a child with migraine. *BMJ* 1997;314:291–292.
31. Mokri B, Sundt TM, Houser W, et al. Spontaneous dissection of the cervical internal carotid artery. *Ann Neurol* 1986;19:126–138.
32. Nguyen BL, Grant-Zawadzki M, Verghese P, et al. Magnetic resonance angiography of cervicocranial dissection. *Stroke* 1993;24:126–131.
33. Sturzenegger M, Mattle HP, Rivoir A, et al. Ultrasound findings in carotid artery dissection: Analysis of 43 patients. *Neurology* 1995;45:691–698.
34. Jaeger B, Singer E, Kroening R. Reflex sympathetic dystrophy of the face. Report of two cases and a review of the literature. *Arch Neurol* 1986;43:693–695.
35. Headache Classification Committee of the International Headache Society. Classification and diagnostic criteria for headache disorders, cranial neuralgia and facial pain. *Cephalalgia* 1988:8(suppl):71–72.
36. Raskin NH. *Headache.* 2nd ed. New York, NY: Churchill Livingstone; 1998:366–367.
37. Copobianco DJ. Facial pain as a symptom of nonmetastatic lung cancer. *Headache* 1995;35:581–585.
38. Ratner EJ, Person P, Kleinman DJ, et al. Jawbone cavities and trigeminal and atypical facial neuralgias. *Oral Surg* 1979;48:3–20.
39. Pareja JA, Ruiz J, de Isla C, et al. Idiopathic stabbing headache (jabs and jolts syndrome). *Cephalalgia* 1996;16:93–96.
40. Pareja JA, Sjaastad O. SUNCT syndrome. A clinical review. *Headache* 1997;37:195–202.

CHAPTER 26 OROFACIAL PAIN

David A. Keith

Pain in the oral and facial structures is a common symptom. Although in most cases, the cause can be determined readily, the anatomy of the area is so complex that the diagnosis may be difficult.

Pain originating in the mouth and face is mediated mainly by the fifth (trigeminal) cranial nerve. This nerve has three branches: ophthalmic, maxillary, and mandibular. In addition, the facial (nervus intermedius root), glossopharyngeal, vagus, and cervical nerves also innervate parts of this region. These nerves have a tortuous anatomic course and distribution and do not follow an orderly pattern. All pain fibers from this region (with the exception of those from the cervical nerves) travel to the spinal nucleus of cranial nerve V. From there, they are connected to higher centers.[1–4]

The emotional significance of pain in this region may be heightened for several reasons. The mouth and face are highly innervated by sensory fibers. This area is represented on the sensory homunculus as much larger than its actual size. The trigeminal nervous system develops early, and reflex suckling activity has been observed in utero. Furthermore, in most western civilizations, the face is one of the few parts of the body exposed to view. It is through the face that humans communicate and express their feelings toward fellow human beings.

PAIN HISTORY

It is imperative that a thorough history be obtained before the patient is examined or special tests are ordered. In most cases, the diagnosis may be made with this information alone.

It also is important to obtain the patient's description of the pain. Primary neuralgias frequently are described as sharp and lancinating, vascular headaches as throbbing, and muscle pain as a continuous, dull ache. The intensity of the pain should be measured against the patient's own experience of pain, need for medication, and effect on lifestyle, for example, sleep, work, and social activities. The origin of the pain should be ascertained by asking the patient to indicate this with one finger. Its distribution pattern should be traced accurately in terms of the local anatomy. The patient should be urged to remember the events surrounding the original onset of the pain, even though this may have occurred several years previously.

Any other instances of similar pain should be determined, although the patient may not associate these with the current problem. The time relationship of the pain should be clarified in terms of duration, frequency of attacks, and possible remissions. In many instances, aggravating factors (e.g., lying down, chewing, the sight or smell of food, alcohol, or stress) and relieving factors (e.g., heat and cold) are important clues. The effect of past treatment should be elucidated carefully (which medications helped, whether surgery altered the nature of the pain, whether endodontic treatment or extractions affected the pain). Finally, the presence or absence of associated factors, such as swelling, flushing, tearing, and nasal congestion, must be ascertained. The patient may not be able to answer all questions during the first interview. Additional information may be required from relatives and friends to obtain a general picture of the pain and its effect on and perception by the patient. This information usually leads the clinician to a diagnosis.

A complete physical examination and appropriate tests, including blood and urine analyses, radiographs, and, where indicated, referral to other specialists or more sophisticated tests—for example, magnetic resonance imaging (MRI) or computed tomography (CT) scan—will help to confirm the clinical diagnosis and exclude other underlying conditions.

CLASSIFICATION OF ORAL AND FACIAL PAIN

There are various classifications of oral and facial pain, but none[5–13] are entirely satisfactory. The International Headache Society classification and diagnostic criteria for headache disorders, cranial neuralgias, and facial pain[14] is valuable, and the amplification in the area of orofacial pain and temporomandibular disorders provided by Okeson[2] help to improve understanding of these conditions. From a clinical point of view, pain in the mouth or face may be divided into the following groups:

I. Pain caused by local disease
   A. Teeth and jaws
   B. Temporomandibular joint and muscles of mastication
   C. Salivary glands
   D. Nose and paranasal sinuses
   E. Blood vessels
II. Pain arising from nerve trunks and central pathways
   A. Group A: no abnormal central nervous system signs (e.g., idiopathic paroxysmal trigeminal and glossopharyngeal neuralgia)
   B. Group B: abnormal central nervous system signs (e.g., nerve involved by pressure, infiltration, or degenerative disease at an intra- or extracranial location)
III. Pain arising from outside the face (e.g., ears, eyes, heart, cervical spine)
IV. Chronic atypical facial and oral pain

CHARACTERISTIC FEATURES OF ORAL AND FACIAL PAIN

Pain Caused by Local Disease

This category includes the greatest number of oral and facial pains encountered in clinical practice. By means of a careful history and appropriate tests, the etiology can be determined.

Teeth and Jaws Pain arising from the teeth, supporting structures, and jaws usually is diagnosed accurately by the patient. Hypersensitivity of a tooth as a result of an exposed root surface or a recent deep restoration is described as sharp, usually transient, and well localized. It is aggravated by hot, cold, or sweet foods. A cracked tooth also may cause transient sharp pain on biting. This may be difficult to identify and lead to an erroneous diagnosis. If the pulp is involved in an inflammatory reaction resulting from dental caries, the pain is spontaneous, severe, and less well localized. Heat aggravates and cold relieves the pain; it may persist for minutes or hours. In time, the pain stops, indicating complete necrosis of the pulpal tissue. This may progress to a periapical abscess in which signs of infection are present, and the tooth is tender to bite on and to percussion. Endodontic treatment will save the tooth and eliminate the infection.

The infection, however, may progress to cellulitis and abscess formation. Incision and drainage can usually be accomplished under local anesthesia, but occasionally, a general anesthetic is required. In the most extreme situation, Ludwig's angina may develop. The infection spreads to the sublingual, submental, submandibular, and pterygomandibular spaces bilaterally and then through the retropharyngeal, pretracheal, and carotid sheath to the mediastinum. In these cases, the airway may be compromised severely. These infections were invariably fatal before antibiotics were discovered. Even today with aggressive antibiotic therapy, surgical drainage, and supportive care, fatalities can occur.

A particularly painful condition occasionally arises after tooth extraction, usually of a mandibular molar. This is termed *localized osteitis* (frequently called *dry socket*). The pain is severe and constant, starting 2 to 3 days after the extraction and lasting for 10 to 14 days thereafter. The socket should be irrigated and dressed on a regular basis until granulation occurs. Osteomyelitis of the jaw (usually the mandible) is rare today, but it may present as an intense deep-seated pain, accompanied by appropriate physical and radiographic signs. The chronic sclerotic variety is more insidious and less readily diagnosed. Treatment is surgical debridement with vigorous antibiotic therapy. Osteoradionecrosis is a relentless, extremely painful condition characterized by postirradiation bone necrosis, predominantly of the mandible, with exposure of the bone into the mouth or externally. In most cases, the condition can be controlled only by radical surgical excision of the affected bone. Hyperbaric oxygen may plan an adjunctive role and can markedly reduce the pain.

Referred pain occasionally is encountered. The patient complains of pain in the mandible, but a maxillary tooth is found to be the cause or vice versa. More common is the complaint of earache accompanying an unidentifiable toothache. Referred pain to the ear indicates mandibular tooth disease. The perception of the anatomic site apparently is mistaken within the branches of the trigeminal nerve.

Temporomandibular Joint Disorders and Diseases Masticatory pain can arise from the muscles of mastication or the temporomandibular joint itself.[15–19] Although these sites are a common cause of facial pain, a thorough history and examination must be done to exclude other potentially more serious diagnoses.

Masticatory system disorders have been classified in many different ways. Because of the difficulty encountered in establishing a precise cause, these disorders often are defined on the basis of symptoms and signs. However, broad categories of masticatory problems include masticatory muscle spasm, internal derangement of the temporomandibular joint, chronic hypomobility, trauma, degenerative joint disease, growth disorders, infections, tumors, and congenital abnormalities.

It is imperative to take a detailed history and perform a thorough clinical examination. In addition, the patient's family, social, and medical history should be ascertained. Clinical examination should include (1) palpation of the muscles of mastication (temporalis, masseter, and medial and lateral pterygoid), (2) observation and measurement of mandibular motion (opening, closing, lateral excursion, and protrusion), (3) palpation or auscultation of joint noises, (4) examination of the dentition and occlusion, and (5) brief neurologic examination of the trigeminal system.

Masticatory muscle spasm (temporomandibular joint or myofascial pain dysfunction) is the most common of all masticatory system disorders. Epidemiologic studies from many countries show that signs and symptoms of such disorders are widespread, and that 28% to 88% of people have detectable clinical signs of dysfunction. Fewer individuals (12%–19%) are aware of symptoms. A smaller group (5% or more) may require treatment.

It is generally agreed that patients with temporomandibular joint dysfunction exhibit one or more of the following signs: (1) decreased range of mandibular motion, (2) impaired function (e.g., deviation, sounds, or sticking), and (3) pain on palpation of the masticatory muscles or joint. One or more of the following symptoms also may occur: (1) temporomandibular joint sounds, (2) fatigue or stiffness of the jaws, (3) pain in the face or jaws, (4) pain on opening the mouth wide, and (5) locking. Radiographic studies of the temporomandibular joint show no evidence of disease.

The cause of this clinical complex is multifactorial. Among the causes most commonly cited are functional, psychological, and structural factors. It is important to understand that, for a particular patient, a single clear etiologic factor rarely is apparent. More often, several possible factors are identified. Likewise, treatment goals should be formulated that address the several likely causes.

Most patients respond to simple noninvasive treatment plans, and these should always be initiated before invasive therapy is contemplated. These measures should include, but are not necessarily limited to the following.

1. *Reassurance.* It is important that patients realize they are not alone with their symptoms, that the symptoms are essentially self-limiting, and that no disease exists. The role of muscle spasm and its benign nature should be explained carefully.

2. *Rest.* Although it is not prudent to immobilize the mandible, patients should be instructed to have a mechanically soft diet for 2 weeks and avoid yawning and laughing with the mouth open. Such habits as chewing gum, biting fingernails, and posturing the jaws should be discouraged.

3. *Heat.* The application of heat to the sides of the face by heating pad, hot towel, or hot water bottle will be comforting and help to relieve muscle spasms. More vigorous treatment can be achieved with ultrasound or short-wave diathermy heat treatments. These are available in physical therapy departments.

4. *Medications.* Nonsteroidal anti-inflammatory analgesics are valuable in the acute stage. The drugs ibuprofen, naproxen, and indomethocin at a low dose for 2 weeks are used most widely. Anxiolytic agents, such as the benzodiazepines, also are used commonly. Several regimens exist, and doses should be individualized. The usual regimen consists of diazepam, 2.5 to 10 mg, two to four times daily, with an increased bedtime dose as necessary to ensure restful sleep. It is important that this treatment be limited to approximately 2 weeks because there is a potential for dependency. Narcotic analgesics should be avoided.

Antidepressants have a long history of effectiveness in the treatment of chronic pain. In view of the strong association between temporomandibular joint dysfunction and psychological factors, their use often is justified especially when this disorder is a part of a more global complex of muscle pains and other signs and symptoms of depression are evident. The tricyclic antidepressants are used most widely. A bedtime-only schedule of 25 to 100 mg of amitriptyline or doxopin often can relieve the symptoms in 1 or 2 weeks. Treatment is maintained for 2 to 4 months; then it is tapered to a low maintenance dose or discontinued. The effect of other antidepressants has not been well studied. There are case reports indicating that some of the selective serotonin reuptake inhibitors may, in fact, potentiate bruxism.

5. *Occlusal therapy*. There are many interocclusal appliances, and their multiplicity suggests that the optimal design has not been found. These devices usually are made of processed acrylic and serve the following functions: (1) improving the function of the temporomandibular joint, (2) improving the function of the masticatory motor system and reducing abnormal muscle function, and (3) protecting teeth from attrition and abnormal occlusal loading. In essence, a full-arch occlusal stabilizing appliance (Fig. 26-1) is the type that has been most effective. Partial-coverage appliances tend to produce significant and irreversible changes in the dentition. An appropriate appliance is effective in most patients (70%–90%). They are most successful in reducing masticatory muscle pain and controlling attrition and adverse tooth loading.

There have been numerous claims that occlusal interferences of various types are the chief cause of masticatory muscle pain and that their elimination by occlusal adjustments will result in improvement. Because masticatory dysfunction is a multifactorial problem, this is unlikely to be true. The negative influence of malocclusion, loss of teeth, and occlusal interferences on masticatory dysfunction is not well supported. On general principles, however, occlusal disharmony (including premature contacts) should be eliminated and missing teeth replaced. The long-term efficacy of repositioning adult nongrowing jaws with occlusal splints or functional appliances has not been proved satisfactorily.

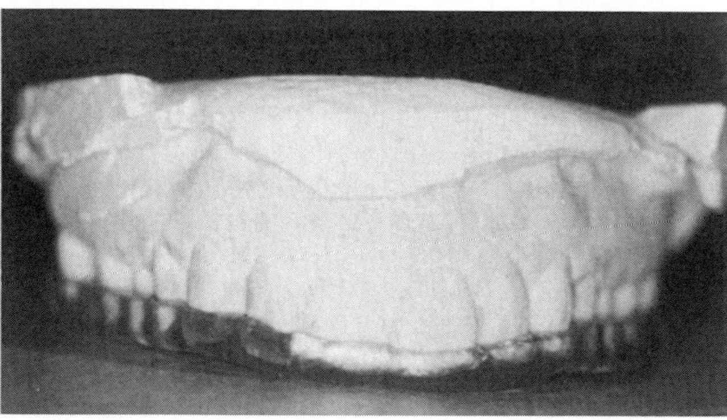

Figure 26-1 Full-arch occlusal stabilizing appliance. (Reproduced with permission from Guralnick WC, Keith DA. Osteoarthritis of the temporomandibular joint. In: Moskowitz RW, et al, eds. *Osteoarthritis. Diagnosis and Management.* Philadelphia, Pa: Saunders; 1984;523–530.)

6. *Behavioral modification*. Bearing in mind the psychological effect in this disorder, attempts to lower patient stress are important. Relaxation techniques, conditioning, and biofeedback all have been advantageous. The most important factor is undoubtedly the therapeutic interaction of the practitioner with the patient.

Internal derangement is another cause of masticatory system disorders. Temporomandibular joint arthrography was developed in the 1940s by Norgaard,[20] but it was not until much later that the potential contribution of internal derangement of the meniscus to the spectrum of temporomandibular joint disorders was recognized.[21] The meniscus can, either temporarily or permanently, be displaced and cause symptoms of sticking, clicking, locking, and pain.

The main categories of internal derangement are, firstly, anterior displacement with reduction. This occurs when the meniscus is displaced in the closed-mouth position and reduces, with a click, to a normal relationship at some time during opening. In these circumstances, the patient complains of the click and a variable amount of pain. On opening, the jaw deviates toward the affected side until the click occurs, and then returns to the midline. Preventing the mouth from closing fully by using a splint, tongue blades, or dental-mirror handle eliminates the click. An MRI study will show a displaced meniscus that is reduced on opening. This clinical situation may include an intermittent locking and may progress to the second category, anterior displacement without reduction (closed lock). Patients again have a variable amount of pain or, if muscle spasm has been relieved adequately, may be pain free. They feel, however, that something in the joint is stopping it from opening. There is usually a history of clicking with intermittent locking. Opening may be limited to 25 to 30 mm, with restriction of motion to the contralateral side. An MRI study shows displacement without reduction (closed lock) and also may demonstrate perforation and degenerative changes. In such cases, the signs and symptoms of degenerative joint disease also may be present.

Initial treatment for internal derangements consists of the noninvasive therapies used for temporomandibular joint disorders (as discussed previously). In patients with anterior displacement with reduction (intermittent locking), these strategies often are successful. In patients with a closed lock, especially those in whom the condition is long standing, these treatments may reduce muscle spasm and pain and restore some motion, but the underlying displacement will remain. When noninvasive treatment has been attempted for several months and the patient remains restricted, arthroscopy or arthrocentesis should be considered.

Chronic hypomobility is a rare but important cause of masticatory system disorders. Ankylosis is the persistent inability to open the jaws. It may result from pathologic involvement of the joint structures (true ankylosis) or limitation produced by extraarticular causes (false ankylosis). Infection and trauma (including previous surgery) are the prime causes of true ankylosis. The findings are severe limitation of opening, possibly with mandibular retrognathism if mandibular growth has been restricted. Radiographs show destruction of the joint surfaces, loss of joint space, and, in extreme cases, ossification across the joint. False ankylosis may be caused by various disorders that can be categorized as myogenic (e.g., masticatory muscle contracture), neurogenic (tetanus), psychogenic (conversion reaction), bone impingement (enlarged coronoid process), fibrous adhesions (occurring after temporomandibular joint surgery, temporal flap, or trauma), and tumors.

Many of these patients require surgery. In those with true ankylosis, even under general anesthesia, it will not be possible to open their mouths. A careful, awake, fiber optic–assisted intubation is required. The key to successful therapy is to identify the cause of the ankylosis and treat it as aggressively as possible. It should be recognized, however, that true ankylosis with fibrosis and calcification can be extremely recalcitrant to treatment.

Trauma is another cause of masticatory system disorders. A blow to the jaw can sprain the temporomandibular joint, cause a joint effusion, or fracture the neck of the mandibular condyle. In an acute sprain, the joint is painful, and there is severe limitation of motion caused by muscle spasm. Heat, rest, and nonsteroidal anti-inflammatory medications resolve the acute symptoms, but other forms of treatment may be required to alleviate residual muscle spasm and pain. In the case of a joint effusion, in addition to pain and limitation, patients are unable to close their teeth together on that side. In a more severe injury, a hemarthrosis may develop, with damage to the meniscus. Active physical therapy is required to restore range of motion and prevent the development of ankylosis. A fracture of the neck of the condyle is a common maxillofacial injury, and, if undisplaced, requires analgesics and a soft diet for a few days. In the unilateral displacement or dislocated variety, the patient has a premature bite on the affected side and deviation to that side on opening. Intermaxillary fixation for 10 days may be required with active physical therapy thereafter to restore function. The patient with bilateral fractures has an anterior open bite and posterior displacement of the mandible, and more aggressive treatment is required to restore the bite and function. Depending on the position of the displaced fragment, it may interfere with mandibular motion.

Degenerative joint disease (osteoarthritis, osteoarthrosis) of the temporomandibular joint is a further cause of masticatory system disorders and may result from several different insults to the joint structure that exceed its capacity to remodel and repair. These insults may be traumatic (acute or chronic), chemical, infectious, or metabolic. The patient complains of pain on jaw movement and limitation of movement, with deviation to the affected side. There may be acute tenderness over the joint itself. Joint sounds are described as grating, grinding, or crunching (but not clicking or popping). Initially, radiographs may be normal, but marked degenerative and remodeling changes are seen later, possibly at a time when the symptoms have subsided. The natural course of the disease suggests that the pain and limitation will disappear after several months.

The features of degenerative temporomandibular joint disease are different from those of most other joints in the body. There is a strong predeliction for women to be affected. A significant number of patients are in their third or fourth decades of life. Few have generalized osteoarthritis.

Most patients can be kept comfortable until remission using the noninvasive techniques outlined earlier. Some require injections of corticosteroids into the joint. This treatment generally is reserved for older patients and is limited to two or three injections. In those who are refractory to these techniques, surgery may be indicated to remove loose fragments of bone (so-called joint mice) and to reshape the condyle. Attention should also be directed toward the meniscus because its displacement may be a primary reason for the degenerative changes.

Rheumatoid arthritis also can afflict the temporomandibular joint, and reports of its incidence range widely. In young patients, an association with micrognathia may be found. In advanced cases, ankylosis may be the presenting complaint. Radiographic findings show joint destruction, possibly involving both the condyle and the articular eminence. Other stigmata of the disease are evident, and if medical management is ineffective, alternative treatment of the degenerative joint disease or ankylosis may be necessary.

Postnatal growth abnormalities also can cause masticatory system disorders. Studies of facial growth show the major contribution made by the mandibular condyle to the adaptive growth of the mandible in the functional soft tissue matrix. Several conditions may reduce growth, including hypothyroidism, hypopituitarism, and nutritional deficiency, such as vitamin D deficiency. In gigantism, all skeletal structures are enlarged; in acromegaly, a marked prognathism is produced. Several local conditions, such as trauma, infection, rheumatoid arthritis, exposure to radiation, and scarring from burns or surgery, are other causes of reduced growth.

Temporomandibular joint infections are uncommon today. When seen, the preauricular area is swollen, hot, and tender. Patients have difficulty opening and closing their mouths. Radiographs may show increased joint space, bony destruction, and sclerosis in the chronic stage. Treatment includes drainage, debridement, and appropriate antibiotic therapy.

Temporomandibular joint tumors are rare, but several varieties of primary and metastatic tumors have been reported. The most common are benign cartilaginous or bony tumors. These may cause limitation of motion or malocclusion, but they are not always painful.

Congenital abnormalities constitute the final cause of masticatory system disorders. Complex coordinated growth of the facial structures is necessary to achieve normal form and function. On occasion, the developmental process is altered, and malformations occur. It is beyond the scope of this chapter to review all the possible anomalies encountered in clinical practice, but many abnormalities of the temporomandibular joint occur in conjunction with recognized syndromes, for example, lateral facial dysplasia or Treacher Collins syndrome. A full clinical and radiologic workup is necessary to evaluate the defect fully. Treatment usually is undertaken by a multidisciplinary team.

Salivary Glands The parotid and submandibular salivary glands occasionally are the site of infection or disease. In the more common condition of submandibular sialolithiasis, Wharton's duct becomes blocked by a stone or nonopaque "sludge." Characteristically, the gland swells, and pain is felt by the patient at the sight, smell, or thought of food. The swelling and pain may decrease after the meal, but they recur at the next meal. If the stone is in the duct, a sialolithotomy often can be done to relieve the problem. Surgical excision of the submandibular gland is frequently necessary, because the gland structure is damaged considerably by repeated infections. A gustatory neuralgia has been desribed after trauma or surgery in the parotid region.

Nose and Paranasal Sinuses Experimental stimulation of various areas in the nose and paranasal sinuses refers pain to well-defined regions of the mouth, face, and cranium. Therefore, in any diagnosis of pain, rhinologic causes should be sought. The most common diagnostic dilemma is differentiating maxillary toothache from maxillary sinusitis, especially because periapical infection from a maxillary premolar or molar occasionally may cause sinusitis.

Blood Vessels The many names ascribed to facial migrainous neuralgias have confused clinicians, as shown by the considerable length of time between onset of symptoms and appropriate diagnosis and treatment of this condition. The Subcommittee on Taxonomy of the International Association for the Study of Pain has provided a provisional summary description for pain of vascular origin.[22]

Cluster headache (see Chap. 25) usually is unilateral in the ocular, frontal, and temporal areas, but it also may be situated in the infraorbital region and maxilla. The condition afflicts men predominantly and usually starts between 18 and 40 years of age. Attacks are grouped in bouts of several weeks to months, with pain-free intervals of several months' duration. Bouts often last from 4 to 8 weeks, with one to three attacks every 24-hour period and a maximum of eight attacks daily. The pain is excruciating. It is described as constant, stabbing, burning, and throbbing. Associated features include ipsilateral ptosis and miosis, tearing, rhinorrhea, and blocked nose. Treatment includes ergot preparations, prednisone, and methysergide. Chronic cluster headache is similar to cluster headache, but it is rarer. The diagnosis requires at least two or more attacks per week over a period of more than a year. Treatment is the same as that for cluster headache, but lithium carbonate tends to work better in patients with chronic cluster headache.

Chronic paroxysmal hemicrania (see Chap. 25) involves the ocular, frontal, and temporal areas and, occasionally, the occipital, infraorbital, aural, mastoid, and nuchal areas (invariably on the same side). It occurs predominantly in women. Patients have attacks every day, usually for 15 to 30 minutes in a 24-hour period. Characteristically, the attacks fluctuate in frequency and severity. Attacks may last 5 to 45 minutes at their maximum, and are excruciating. Ipsilateral conjunctival injection, lacrimation, nasal stuffiness, and rhinorrhea occur in most patients. Attacks occur at regular intervals through the day and night, and patients may be awakened by a nocturnal attack. Indomethacin provides immediate and absolute relief. Although these vascular pains usually are situated in the cranium, they can occur in the infraorbital region of the maxilla and lead to confusion with sinus or dental disease. Such patients frequently undergo extensive dental treatment before the correct diagnosis is made.

Temporal giant cell arteritis (see Chap. 25) afflicts patients older than 60 years of age. There is a dull persistent pain in the temple after chewing. The temporal artery is nonpulsatile, tortuous, and tender. Referral to an ophthalmologist is essential to exclude ophthalmic artery involvement and the possibility of permanent blindness. Corticosteroids ameliorate this condition.

Pain Arising from Nerve Trunks and Central Pathways

Group A: No Abnormal Central Nervous System Signs Facial neuralgias include the primary idiopathic neuralgias. These have been recognized for many centuries and are among the most severe pains felt by humans. The features of trigeminal neuralgia are well described.[23] Characteristically, there is a trigger zone in the area of the nasolabial fold or upper or lower lip. When stimulated by washing, shaving, talking, or any slight movement, pain occurs that is severe, lancinating, and lasts only a few seconds. There is no objective sensory loss. An untreated patient initially may present in an unkempt state, drooling from the mouth, and unwilling to move or touch the trigger area. Injection of a local anesthetic into the area abolishes the trigger for the duration of the anesthesia. Remission for months or years commonly occurs.

Although this description is classic and usually well recognized, patients who have undergone various treatments in the past may give different descriptions that may confuse the diagnosis. Furthermore, several less typical features may be reported, such as continuous or long-lasting aching or burning between paroxysms and spontaneous changes in sensation.

Although no cause has been found, some patients describe a previous traumatic event. Pathologic examination of resected nerve tissue has shown evidence of hypomyelination or demyelination in the region of the trigeminal ganglion. Some neurosurgeons believe that impingement of blood vessels on the nerve in the region of the ganglion is the cause of this disease. It is important to recognize that, in some patients, especially those younger than 40 years of age, symptoms of trigeminal neuralgia may indicate an underlying disease, such as multiple sclerosis or a space-occupying lesion at the cerebellopontine angle.[24]

A similar condition, glossopharyngeal neuralgia, has the same characteristics except that the trigger zones are in the tonsil, lateral pharyngeal wall, or base of the tongue. This condition should not be confused with Eagle's syndrome,[25] in which an elongated styloid process may impinge on the soft tissue of the throat during neck movement or swallowing, or Trotter's syndrome,[26] in which a tumor of the nasopharynx may cause pain in the lower jaw, tongue, and side of the head. In these cases, however, other signs such as deafness (from occlusion of the eustachian tube) and asymmetry in mobility of the soft palate (from tumor invasion of the levator palati muscle) should be sought.

Treatment of the primary neuralgias initially is medical.[27] Carbamazepine, baclofen, or neurontin are effective in many cases. Some patients, however, are allergic to these medications or develop bone marrow depression as an adverse effect. Traditionally, peripheral neurectomy of the maxillary or mandibular division of cranial nerve V or phenol or alcohol blocks have been used to denervate the area permanently. With the introduction of the radiofrequency lesion, the pain fibers specifically supplying the trigger zone may be destroyed selectively without necessarily interfering with sensory function. This is a relatively benign procedure with excellent long-term results. Other neurosurgeons prefer intracranial surgery, in which vascular structures are dissected off the trigeminal ganglion; good results can be obtained despite the greater risks of this major surgical intervention.[28,29] Glycerol injection and other surgical procedures also have been used successfully (see Chap. 35). Gamma knife treatment has recently been suggested as an alternative approach.

Another group A disorder is postherpetic neuralgia[30,31] (see Chap. 40). A significant number of patients (approximately 25%) develop chronic pain after acute herpes zoster, and its incidence increases with age. Although the mechanism is poorly understood, it appears that the initial acute inflammation results in fibrosis of the nerve sheath and dorsal root ganglion, with loss of large myelinated axons.

Herpes zoster also may occur in the distribution of the trigeminal nerve. The first division, especially, is affected, and the possibility of corneal ulceration and scarring should be remembered. The pain is described as a constant burning sensation, with a stabbing component. Hyper- or hypesthesia may be present.

Treatment is not entirely satisfactory. Various medications may reduce the pain of acute herpes zoster, such as topical idoxuridine, oral amantadine, intramuscular interferon, intravenous acyclovir, and intravenous vidarabine. Steroids also have been advocated, and sympathetic block can be useful.

In chronic postherpetic neuralgia, few approaches provide significant relief. Anticonvulsants, antidepressants, and antipsychotic agents all have been used. Occasionally, neurosurgical procedures are indicated.

Group B: Abnormal Central Nervous System Signs The cause in these syndromes may be extracranial or intracranial. This includes trauma, osteomyelitis, Paget disease, primary or metastatic tumors[32] or space-occupying lesions at the cerebellopontine angle[24] and the middle cranial fossa, disseminated sclerosis, cerebrovascular disease, syphilis, and syringobulbia.

Pain Arising From Outside the Face

Pain perceived in the face may be a result of irritation of pain receptors in tissues that are related embryologically to the segmental innervation of the face. This pain may originate in the eyes, ears, heart, or cervical spine. Common ocular causes of pain[33] include refractive error, convergence insufficiency, extraocular muscle imbalance, trauma (e.g., abrasion, contact lens damage, or foreign body), otitis, angle-closure glaucoma, and so-called dry eye syndrome. Common causes of ear pain are outlined in Table 26-1.

Coronary artery disease classically is described as left substernal pain referred to the arm and side of the neck that is brought on by physical exertion, emotional upset, or ingestion of food. It is relieved rapidly by rest or sublingual nitroglycerine. On occasion, the pain sweeps up the neck and into the angle of the jaw. If the pain occurs in the jaw without other related symptoms, the diagnosis may be missed. The dorsal root of cervical nerve III supplies the skin overlying the angle of the mandible. A cervical strain injury, cervical osteoarthritis, or spondylitis may irritate these nerves and cause pain in their distribution. Pressure on the occipital nerve (cervical nerve II) can cause occipital neuralgia with a sharp lancinating quality that shoots forward over the head. Local anesthetic and steroid injections may be necessary.

TABLE 26-1 **Common Causes of Ear Pain**

Types	Examples
Intrinsic	
Infection	Acute otitis media
	Acute otitis externa
	Malignant otitis externa
	Infected cyst of ear canal
Trauma	Barotrauma
	Foreign body
	Direct trauma
Tumor	Carcinoma of the ear
Extrinsic	
Infection	Pharyngitis or tonsillitis
	Sinusitis
	Any cause of cervical adenopathy
	Ramsay Hunt syndrome
Tumor	Carcinoma of the oropharynx, nasopharynx, hypopharynx, or larynx
Other	Temporomandibular joint syndrome
	Dental problems
	Glossopharyngeal neuralgia
	Atypical facial neuralgias

Chronic Atypical Facial and Oral Pain[34–37]

Many patients have intractable facial pain that may be termed *atypical facial pain.* In these patients, the pain is a multifactorial problem characterized by equivocal physical findings, diffuse descriptions, and ill-defined psychiatric symptoms. In addition, malingerers, drug abusers, and patients with Munchausen syndrome may be encountered.

In an effort to diagnose and treat patients with chronic joint pain, a chronic facial pain group (consisting of an oral and maxillofacial surgeon, psychopharmacologist, neurologist, and neurosurgeon), which interviewed and examined patients at the same time. The pain was classified using the McGill-Melzack scale,[38] the International Association for the Study of Pain axes, the *Diagnostic and Statistical Manual, Third Edition, Revised* psychiatric classification, and the International Classification of Disease. In a study[39] of 107 patients, 88 were women, and 19, men (mean age, 44.6 years; range, 17–87 years). These patients had experienced pain for a mean of 7.8 years (range, 0.5–46 years) and had consulted a mean of 5.8 physicians. They typically described their pain as continuous and fluctuating in intensity. All patients had used some medications (mean, 5.7); 58% had used narcotic analgesics, and 34% had used antidepressant medications.

Fifty-one percent of these patients had undergone some previous surgical intervention, and 14% had undergone temporomandibular joint surgery (15 patients and 23 operations). Forty percent of the patients had been treated with physical therapy, and 33% of the patients had used occlusal splints of one type or another. In addition to the facial pain (42% bilateral, 30% left, and 28% right), 58% of the patients had cranial pain, 36% had neck pain, and 46% had pain in other areas.

Most of these patients had more than one diagnosis. According to the classification systems, 65% of the patients had definable psychiatric problems, chiefly depression (38%); 36% had symptoms attributable to the masticatory system (temporomandibular joint and muscles); 29% had neuralgias of the trigeminal nerve; and 15% had pain of vascular origin. The rest were classified as atypical facial pain of unknown or mixed cause.

A variant of atypical facial pain is phantom-tooth pain or atypical odontalgia[40] in which pain is reported in a tooth or its supporting structures. Fillings, endodontic treatment, extractions, and bone currettage often are performed without relief. The same sequence is followed in a neighboring tooth until a whole region of the mouth is rendered edentulous.

Burning mouth and burning tongue (glossodynia) is a troublesome condition with several different causes.[41] On first presentation, a complete oral examination should be performed and a comprehensive history taken. Laboratory tests are necessary to exclude diabetes mellitus, pernicious anemia, and vitamin B_{12} and folate deficiency. Other causes include xerostomia, geographic tongue, median rhomboid glossitis, trauma, candidiasis, and psychogenic factors. In all cases of atypical pain, a thorough physical and radiographic examination is necessary, and a psychiatric workup is indicated. Evidence now exists that burning mouth syndrome may be a neuropathy of thermal sensitivity.

As indicated, depression frequently is associated with chronic pain, either as a premorbid or reactive condition. In either instance, the patient will benefit greatly from treatment. Antidepressant medications have a long history of effectiveness and safety. They can reduce anxiety, reverse both mood and vegetative signs and symptoms of depression, and improve sleep patterns. The tricyclic antidepressants (amitriptyline and doxepin) are used most widely, and a bedtime-only schedule of 25 to 100 mg often achieves improvement in 1 to 2 weeks.[42] The treatment can be continued for several months and then tapered to a low maintenance dose. Monoamine oxidase inhibitors and lithium salts also may be prescibed on occasion.

Anxiety sometimes is associated with chronic facial pain, and it may or may not be associated with a specific major life change, for example, illness, death, or acute stress. A careful history usually uncovers many symptoms, including tachycardia, dizzy spells, headaches, unsteadiness, paresthesias, breathing difficulties, trembling, excessive perspiration, a choking sensation, or hyperventilation. Relaxation techniques (such as meditation, hypnotherapy, behavior therapy, and biofeedback) are useful, and the minor tranquilizers (chlordiazepoxide and diazepam) are prescried widely.[43]

Other psychiatric conditions also may present with pain; for example, hysteria, schizophrenia, and hypochondriasis. Even when these diagnoses have been excluded, there remain many patients with various emotional problems that may contribute to or cause pain. Hackett[44] developed the Madison scale to descnbe the characteristics that correlate with the psychogenicity of pain and are helpful in evaluating such patients.

Treatment for patients with chronic facial pain depends on its cause and may consist of multiple concurrent approaches.[45,46] A multidisciplinary approach has been found to be helpful in the diagnosis and treatment of these patients, but it is evident that, despite the best efforts of physicians and the use of sophisticated imaging techniques and tests, the needs of many of these patients are not met. They continue to seek medical consultations and undergo surgical intervention with no relief of their pain. A pain management program may ultimately be helpful for these individuals.

REFERENCES

1. Wyke B. The neurology of facial pain. *Br J Hosp Med* October 1968: 46–65.
2. Okeson JP. *Bell's Orofacial Pains.* 5th ed. Chicago, Ill: Quintessence; 1995.
3. Sessle BJ. The neurobiology of facial and dental pain: Present knowledge, future directions. *J Dent Res* 1987;66:962–981.
4. Hayashi H, Sumino R, Sessle BJ. Functional organization of trigeminal subnucleus interpolaris: Nociceptive and innocuous afferent inputs. Projections to thalamus, cerebellum, and spinal cord, and descending modulation from periaqueductal gray. *J Neurophysiol* 1984;51:890–905.
5. Bell WE. *Orofacial Pains: Classification, Diagnosis, Management.* 3rd ed. Chicago, Ill: Yearbook Medical Publishers; 1985.
6. Guernsey LH. Facial pain. In: Irby W, ed. *Current Advances in Oral Surgery.* 2nd ed. St Louis, Mo: Mosby; 1977.
7. Gregg J. Neurological disorders of the maxillofacial region. In: Kruger GO, ed. *Textbook of Oral Surgery*. 4th ed. St Louis, Mo: Mosby; 1974: 620–660.
8. Young RR. Basic principles underlying craniofacial pain. In: Shaw JH, Sweeney EA, Cappuccino CC, et al, eds. *Textbook of Oral Biology.* Philadelphia, Pa: Saunders; 1978.
9. Alling CC III, Mahan PK. *Facial Pain.* 2nd ed. Philadelphia, Pa: Lea & Febiger; 1977.
10. Mumford JM. *Orofacial Pain—Aetiology, Diagnosis and Treatment.* 3rd ed. Edinburgh, Scotland: Churchill Livingstone; 1982.
11. Sharar Y. Orofacial pain. In: Wall PD, Melzack R, eds. *Textbook of Pain.* Edinburgh, Scotland: Churchill Livingstone; 1984:338–349.
12. Loeser JD. Tic douloureux and atypical facial pain. In: Wall PD, Melzack R, eds. *Textbook of Pain.* Edinburgh, Scotland: Churchill Livingstone; 1984.
13. Pertes RA, Heir GM. Chronic orofacial pain. A practical approach to differential diagnosis. *Dent Clin North Am* 1991;35:123–140.
14. International Headache Society. Classification and diagnostic criteria for headache disorders, cranial neuralgias and facial pain. *Cephalgia* 1988;8(suppl):1–96.
15. Laskin DM, Greenfield W, Gale E, et al. *The President's Conference on the Examination, Diagnosis and Management of Temporomandibular Joint Disorders.* Chicago, Ill: American Dental Association; 1989.
16. Sarnat BG, Laskin DM. *The Temporomandibular Joint: A Biological Basis for Clinical Practice.* 3rd ed. Springfield, Ill: Charles C Thomas; 1979.
17. Dworkin SF, Huggins KH, LeResche L, et al. Epidemiology of signs and symptoms in temporomandibular disorders: Clinical signs in cases and controls. *J Am Dent Assoc* 1990;120:273–281.
18. Fricton J. Recent advances in temporomandibular disorders and orofacial pain. *J Am Dent Assoc* 1991;122:24–33.
19. LeResche L, Dworkin SF, Sommers E, et al. An epidemiologic evaluation of two diagnostic classification schemes for temporomandibular disorders. *J Prosthet Dent* 1991;65:131–137.
20. Norgaard F. *Temporomandibular Arthrography.* Copenhagen, Denmark: Munksgaard; 1947 [Thesis].
21. Helms CA, Katzberg RW, Dolwick MF. Internal derangement of the temporomandibular joint. San Francisco, Calif: Radiology Research and Education Foundation; 1983.
22. Merskey H. Development of a universal language of pain syndromes. *Adv Pain Res Ther* 1983;5:37–52.
23. Sweet WH. The treatment of trigeminal neuralgias (tic douloureux). *N Eng J Med* 1986;315:174–177.
24. Nguyen M, Maciewicz R, Bouckoms A, et al. Facial pain symptoms in patients with cerebellopontine angle tumors. A report of 44 cases or cerebellopontine angle meningioma and a review of the literature. *Clin J Pain* 1986;2:3–9.
25. Eagle WW. Elongates styloid provess. Further observations and a new syndrome. *Arch Otolaryngol Head Neck Surg* 1948;47:630.
26. Trotter W. On clinically obscure malignant tumours of the nasopharyngeal wall. *Br Med J* 1911;2:1057–1059.
27. Scrivani SJ, Keith DA, Mathews ES, et al. Percutaneous stereotactic differential radiofrequency thermal rhizotomy for the treatment of trigeminal neuralgia. *J Oral Maxillofac Surg* 1999;57:104–111.
28. Janetta PJ. Trigeminal neuralgia: Treatment of microvascular decompression. In: Wilkins RH, Rengachary SS, eds. *Neurosurgery 3.* New York, NY: McGraw-Hill; 1985:2357–2363.
29. Zakrzewska JM. Surgical management of trigeminal neuralgia. *Br Dent J* 1991;170:61–62.
30. Hope-Simpson RE. Postherpetic neuralgia. *J R Coll Gen Pract* 1975; 25:571–575.
31. Taub A. Relief of post herpetic neuralgia with psychotropic drugs. *J Neurosurg* 1973;39:235.
32. Marbach JJ. Current concepts in the management of pain in the head and neck cancer patient. *Dent Clin North Am* 1990;34:251–263.
33. Hitching R. Eye pain. In: Wall PD, Melzack R, eds. *Textbook of Pain.* Edinburgh, Scotland: Churchill Livingstone; 1984:331–337.
34. Feinman C, Harris M. Psychogenic facial pain, l: The clinical presentation; II: Management and prognosis. *Br Dent J* 1984;156:165–168, 205–208.
35. Feinman C, Harris M, Cowley R. Psychogenic facial pain: Presentation and treatment. *Br Med J* 1984;288:436–438.
36. Friction JR. Behavioral and psychosocial factors in chronic craniofacial pain. *Anesth Prog* 1985;32:7–12.

37. Marbach JJ, Lipton JA. Aspects of illness behavior in patients with facial pain. *J Am Dent Assoc* 1978;96:630–638.
38. Melzack R. The McGill Pain Questionnaire: Major properties and scoring methods. *Pain* 1975;1:275–279.
39. Keith DA. Chronic facial pain: A review of 107 patients. Paper presented at the Ninth International Conference on Oral and Maxillofacial Surgery; May 1986; Vancouver, Canada.
40. Marbach JJ, Hulbrock J, Hohn C, et al. Incidence of phantom tooth pain. An atypical facial neuralgia. *Oral Surg* 1982;53:190–193.
41. Zegarellio DJ. Burning mouth. An analysis of 57 patients. *Oral Surg* 1984;58:34–38.
42. Brown RS, Bottomly WK. Utilization and mechanism of action of tricyclic antidepressants in the treatment of chronic facial pain: A review of the literature. *Anesth Prog* 1990;37:223–229.
43. Keefe FJ, Beckman JC. Behavioral assessment of chronic orofacial pain. *Anesth Prog* 1990;37:7681.
44. Hackett TP. The pain patient: Evaluation and treatment. In: Hackett TP, Cassem NH, eds. *Handbook of General Hospital Psychiatry.* St Louis, Mo: Mosby; 1978:41–63.
45. Hutchison I, Nally F. Management of orofacial pain. *Practitioner* 1991;235:72–77.
46. McDonald JS, Pensak ML, Phero JC. Thoughts on the management of chronic facial, head, and neck pain. *Am J Otol* 1990;11:378–382.

CHAPTER 27 NECK PAIN

Mark E. Romanoff, Richard L. Gilbert, and Carol A. Warfield

Neck pain is a common complaint. The prevalance is approximately 75% to 80% in the U. S. population. The neck is composed of many pain-sensitive tissues in a small area, including tendons, ligaments, muscle insertions, vertabrae, zygopophyseal joints, nerve roots, nerves, and plexi. The cervical spine is mobile and situated between an immobile thorax and a relatively weighty head; therefore, it is subject to varying degrees of trauma with body movement. Neck pain ranges from minor self-limited aches to severe pain associated with signs and symptoms of nerve root impingement. Patients with minor neck pain may not consult a physician. Those who see a primary care physician often can be helped by conservative management. A patient with severe chronic symptoms may be best served in a comprehensive pain management clinic. Treatment options can range from the conservative (transcutaneous electrical nerve stimulation [TENS] unit, physical therapy and stretching) to the interventional (facet joint injection and cervical nerve root block). In all cases, a knowledge of the anatomy and the etiology of neck pain is required for definitive treatment.

DIAGNOSIS

Ideally, the cause of a patient's neck pain is determined by a careful history, physical examination, appropriate radiologic and laboratory tests, and diagnostic nerve blocks.[1] It is vital to be aware of the more serious disorders that can cause neck pain and that require urgent referral to a specialist. Table 27-1 lists many causes of neck pain.

History

Some of the more salient aspects of the history that the clinician should focus on include:

1. Precipitating and associated events (trauma, infection, emotional stress, use of medications)
2. Duration (acute, subacute, chronic)
3. Character of pain (sharp, dull, burning, throbbing)
4. Point of origin (and, if present, extent of radicular pain)
5. Aggravating and alleviating factors
6. Areas of maximal pain
7. Associated neurologic symptoms (weakness, numbness, clumsiness, bowel or bladder inccontinence, other long tract signs)
8. Associated medical symptoms (dyspnea, fever, chest tightness, weight loss)
9. Previous treatment
10. Other medical and surgical history
11. Pending litigation or worker's compensation

Acute trauma requires careful neurologic and radiologic investigation. A history of significant or progressive upper extremity weakness or long tract signs indicates neurologic compromise and requires a neurosurgical or orthopedic referral. The presence of meningeal signs in the appropriate setting requires further evaluation and, perhaps, hospitalization. The patient's emotional state and psychosocial factors may aggravate and perpetuate chronic neck pain.

Physical Examination[8]

Inspection should begin by watching the unaware patient as he or she enters the examination room and during history taking. The patient's normal posture and attitude of the head and neck may reveal an underlying disorder. The neck region should be inspected for normal characteristics and disease, including masses, muscular asymmetries, scars, discolorations, and cutaneous lesions. Palpation of the anterior neck can be accomplished best on a patient in the supine position. The bony structures, including the hyoid bone, thyroid cartilage, cricoid cartilage, and first cricoid ring, should be examined for normal contour and motion. The thyroid gland should be assessed for enlargement, tenderness, nodules, and bruits. The carotid artery is examined for bruits, tenderness, and tumor. Abnormal lymphadenopathy may indicate infection or malignancy. Cervical adenitis also may cause torticollis. Parotiditis must be excluded. The sternocleidomastoid muscle should be palpated for trigger points (myofascial pain or disease), hypertrophy, and size discrepancy (torticollis, tenderness and swelling, or hematoma). The supraclavicular fossa must be assessed for masses (tumor, subclavian artery aneurysm, or pathologic lymphadenopathy) and fullness (superior vena cava syndrome).

The posterior bony palpation can be performed best with the examiner's hands cupped underneath the neck of the supine patient, because tense muscles inhibit assessment of the bony prominences. Palpation of the occiput may reveal tenderness of the greater occipital nerves. The mastoid process and superior nuchal line are examined. Each cervical vertebral spinous process is palpated, beginning with C2, and tenderness, irregularity, malalignment, and step-offs are investigated. The facet joints can be assessed by moving each hand laterally about 2 cm from the spinous process. Facet tenderness and increased pain with neck extension and rotation can be observed in facet joint syndrome or osteoarthritis. Soft tissues of the posterior neck can be examined with the patient sitting in front of the examiner. The trapezius muscle is palpated for spasm, trigger points, and tenderness. If there is no evidence of an unstable cervical spine, full range of motion and cervical muscle strength should be tested. The presence of atrophy or hypertrophy and the reproduction of pain symptoms are assessed. The upper extremities and hands are observed for signs of atrophy, color change, edema, and differences in skin temperature (complex regional pain syndrome). Maneuvering the upper extremities to elicit compression syndromes is done.

The neurologic examination is critical in evaluating the patient with neck pain because radicular symptoms and neurologic deficits localize the area of disease (Table 27-2 and Fig. 27-1).

TABLE 27-1 **Classification of Neck Pain**

Neck Pain Without Stiffness

Enhanced by Swallowing

- Carotid artery (carotidynia[2], carotid body tumor, inflamed thyroglossal duct)
- Esophagus (inflamed diverticulum, peptic esophagitis, radiation esophagitis)
- Mediastinum (spontaneous pneumomediastinum)[3]
- Pharynx (pharyngitis or Ludwig's angina)
- Salivary gland (mumps, suppurative parotiditis)
- Thyroid gland (acute suppurative thyroiditis, subacute thyroiditis with pain radiating to ear, hemorrhage, thyroid cystadenoma)
- Tongue (ulcers, neoplasm)
- Tonsils (tonsillitis, neoplasm)

Neck pain enhanced by chewing

- Mandible (fracture, osteomyelitis, periodontitis)
- Salivary gland (mumps, suppurative parotiditis)
- Temporomandibular joint (associated with myofascial pain syndrome in neck)

Neck pain enhanced by head movement

- Cervical spine (whiplash, acute or subacute fracture, dislocation, ligamentous damage, herniated inververtebral disk, rheumatoid neck[4], facet joint syndrome[5], occipital neuralgia with C1 to C2 arthrosis syndrome[6])
- Nuchal muscles or trapezius muscles (viral myalgia, myofascial pain syndrome)
- Sternocleidomastoid (torticollis, hematoma, myofascial pain)

Neck pain enhanced by shoulder movement

- Cervical rib
- Costoclavicular syndrome
- Scalenus anticus syndrome
- Pectoralis minor syndrome

Neck pain not enhanced by movement

- Branchial cleft remnant (inflamed pharyngeal cyst)
- Lymph node, acute (adenitis) or chronic (Hodgkin's disease, scrofula, gummas, actinomycosis, carcinomatous metastasis)
- Nervous system (cervical herpes zoster, postherpetic neuralgia, spinal cord neoplasm, Arnold-Chiari malformation, syringomyelia, epidural abscess or hematoma, poliomyelitis)
- Salivary gland (calculus in duct)
- Skin and subcutaneous tissue (furuncle, carbuncle, erysipelas)
- Soft tissue calcium deposit at first and second cervical vertebrae[7]
- Spinal vertebrae (primary metastatic neoplasm, infectious osteomyelitis, tuberculosis, herniated intervertebral disk)
- Subclavian artery (aneurysm)

Referred neck pain

- Angina
- Bronchus (bronchial tumor)
- Pain from sixth cervical dermatomal band
- Pancoast's (superior sulcus lung) tumor

Stiff Neck, Neck Pain, and Limitation of Motion

- Acquired (spasmodic torticollis)

Acute infections

- Epidural abscess
- Fibrositis (transient stiff neck)
- Reflex spasms (meningitis or adenitis from acute pharyngitis)
- Torticollis

Acute traumatic

- Epidural hematoma
- Cervical spina strain
- Dislocations
- Facet dislocation
- Fractures
- Herniated disk (herniated nucleus pulposus)
- Ligamentous (strain whiplash, rupture)
- Subluxation

Chronic infection

- Infectious arthritis
- Intramuscular gummas
- Tuberculous spondylitis

Chronic posttraumatic

- Contracture from burns
- Nerve injury
- Untreated acute injuries

Congenital (congenital torticollis)

Degenerative

- Cervical spondylosis with fibrositis
- Fibromyalgia, myofascial pain syndrome

Inflammatory bone lesions

- Calcific tendinitis of the longus colli
- Subluxation of atlas

Other useful tests of the cervical spine include[8]:

1. The distraction test. In this test, manual and in-line traction performed by the examiner simulates effective traction on the cervical spine and can relieve pain from nerve root compression and facet joint irritation.
2. The compression test. The examiner presses down on the seated patient's head to reproduce the nerve impinged by the neural foramina or facet joints.
3. The Valsalva test. This test can increase intrathecal pressure, exacerbating nerve root impingement by a tumor or disk in the cervical canal.

TABLE 27-2 **Motor and Reflex Distribution of Cervical Roots**

Disk	Reflex	Muscles
C4, C5, and root C5	Biceps	Deltoid or biceps
C5, C6, and root C6	Brachioradialis	Wrist extensors or biceps
C6, C7, and root C7	Triceps	Wrist flexor, finger extensory, or triceps
C7, TI, and root C8	—	Finger flexors or hand intrinsic muscles
TI, T2, and root TI	—	Hand intrinsic muscles

4. Tests for the compression syndromes. These include the anterior scalene syndrome test (the Adson test)[8] and tests for costoclavicular syndrome and pectoralis minor syndrome. When the history and physical examination warrant, x-rays and additional laboratory studies may be indicated.

NEUROANATOMY AND FUNCTIONAL ANATOMY[9]

There are eight cervical nerves. Each exits above the cervical vertebrae except C8, which exits below the C7 cervical vertebra. The spinal nerves divide into anterior and posterior primary rami, after giving off a meningeal branch that supplies the local vertebral structures. The posterior primary ramus of C1 is entirely motor and runs over the posterior arch of the atlas to the suboccipital triangle, where it supplies the capital movers and neck extensors. The C2 posterior ramus emerges between the axis and the atlas and divides, forming the greater occipital nerve. It is joined by the branches of C3 and supplies cutaneous sensation to the occipital regions. The lateral branch is motor and supplies the posterior cervical muscles. The medial branch of C3 supplies the skin of the lower occiput. The posterior rami of C4 through C8 supply the posterior cervical muscles. The medial branches of C4 and C5 supply the overlying skin. The anterior primary rami of the cervical spinal nerves supply the motor and sensory innervation to the front and side of the neck.

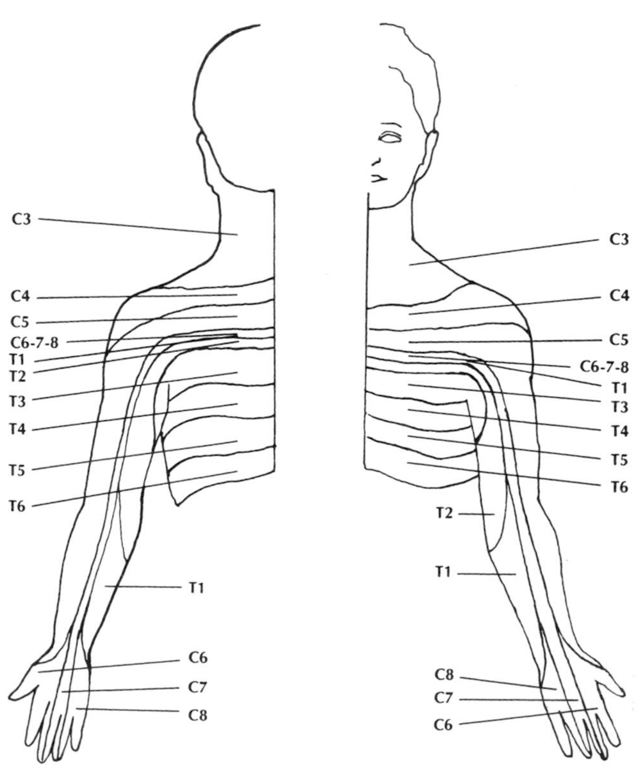

Figure 27-1 Dermatomes of the chest and upper extremities.

The cervical plexus is composed of the anterior divisions of C1 through C4. It supplies the following nerves:

1. The superficial cutaneous branches: lesser occipital nerve (C2), greater auricular nerve (C2 and C3), anterior cutaneous nerve (C2 and C3), and supraclavicular nerve (C3 and C4
2. Deep branches that innervate the anterior vertebral muscles (recti capitus, longus capitus, scalenus medius, and branches of the levator scapular) and contribute to the sternomastoid (C2 and C3) and trapezius (C3 and C4)
3. The phrenic nerve (C3, C4, and C5)
4. The communicating branches to the vagus and sympathetic chain

The brachial plexus is formed by the anterior primary rami of C5 through T1 and provides motor and sensory innervation to the upper extremity. The plexus runs from roots, trunks, divisions, cords, and branches. The pattern of radicular symptoms, including motor, sensory, and reflex deficits, localizes discogenic nerve root compression. Table 27-2 and Figure 27-1 summarize the neuroanatomy of the brachial plexus.

Various pain-sensitive tissues are present in the neck; the musculoskeletal anatomy is considered here. The cervical disk, including the nucleus pulposus and the vertebral body, excluding the periosteum, are considered to be insensitive to pain. The posterior longitudinal ligament is pain sensitive and subjected to pressure from a herniated disk. The anterior ligament also is pain sensitive. The nerve root is a site of pain production from its origin to the aural sleeve and throughout its course in the cervical area. Ischemia secondary to stretching may be the mechanism of pain production. The facet joint is a source of pain; this can be elicited by extension and rotation toward the involved side. Cervical muscular pain may be caused by sustained contracture with resultant ischemia, myofascial pain syndrome, tearing or traction of muscles from the periosteum, and a muscular hematoma.

The healing of torn ligaments and joint capsules may result in hyperplasia, fibrosis, and scarring, with resultant nerve root irritation and compression and characteristic radiculopathy along the distribution of the involved nerve root.[9] Skeletal fractures with degenerative changes may occur. Articular cartilage injury from acute deforming forces, although initially painless because cartilage has no nerve supply, later results in joint wear and tear. Trauma to the sympathetic chain and fascial structures of the neck can result in a complex regional pain syndrome with abnormal sympathetic response.

CERVICAL TRAUMA: SOFT TISSUE INJURIES OF THE NECK

Neck pain from a traumatic origin includes many injuries ranging from self-limited acute cervical strain to cervical fracture with paralysis. This section considers soft tissue injuries without accompanying spinal cord injury.

The anatomic characteristics of the cervical spine predispose it to injury by direct and indirect forces. The neck is situated between the inflexible thoracic spine and the head, a relatively heavy structure that it must support. Reports indicate that 85% of neck disorders result from acute or repetitive neck injuries or chronic stresses and strain.[9]

Minor trauma resulting in acute cervical pain often is secondary to musculoskeletal injury and most frequently is self-limited using conservative treatment. One study[10] examined patients with acute cervical pain without neurologic symptoms in their arms. All patients were encouraged to rest. Most patients improved markedly after 1 week. By 6 weeks, 95% of the patients in all groups were pain free. The patients were divided into three treatment groups: (1) neck collar and analgesics; (2) neck collar, analgesics, and TENS three times a week; and (3) neck collar, analgesics, and physical therapy. There were no differences in outcome between groups except that the TENS group showed improved cervical mobility earlier than the other groups.

Whiplash Syndrome

Neck injuries often result from automobile accidents. One study[11] showed that 60% of patients who were injured in a car accident and presented to a hospital had neck pain. After 1 year, 26% of this group had persistent neck pain. The term *whiplash* describes the resultant injury caused by an abrupt hyperextension of the neck from an indirect force.

When forward flexion of the neck is produced by acceleration or deceleration, the forward flexion of the head is limited by the chin touching the chest.[10] Lateral flexion movement stops when the ear hits the shoulder. These movements are within the physiologic range of motion of the cervical spine. No strain is placed on the intervertebral joints. By contrast, backward extension of the head stops when the occiput hits the posterior thorax. This is beyond the physiologic range of motion. In a rear-end collision, the body is propelled in a linear horizontal direction.[12] The head abruptly moves backward, necessitating acute hyperextension of the cervical spine. This is followed by a recoil of the head with severe cervical neck flexion and, finally, a return to the neutral position. The opposite sequence occurs in head-on collisions. One author feels that cervical facet joint abnormalities are responsible for many of the symptoms seen in whiplash patients.[11] (See the discussion of cervical facet joint syndrome later in this chapter.)

Symptom Complex It is important to note that symptoms may not occur for 12 to 24 hours after a whiplash injury because muscular hemorrhage and edema may need to evolve prior to inciting a nociceptive response. The cervical flexor muscles, specifically the sternocleidomastoid, the scalene muscles, and the longus colli undergo an acute stretch reflex.[13] Some fibers are torn. One study[12] reported characteristic symptoms of patients after a motor vehicle accident. This author followed 146 walk-in patients for 5 years after motor vehicle accidents that caused soft tissue neck injury without fractures or dislocations. Seventy percent of these accidents were rear-end collisions. Loss of consciousness occurred in 10% of patients. Almost all patients complained of neck pain and stiffness. Two thirds of patients had headaches, and one third had shoulder or intrascapular pain. Ten percent had arm and hand pain or arm and hand numbness. Only 3% had a focal neurologic deficit.

Characteristically, the pain is localized to the neck and later may radiate from the neck to the shoulders, arms, or back of the head. Persistent suboccipital pain does not necessarily involve a local lesion at the atlantoaxial region but may be referred pain from a damaged cervical segment.[14] Although pain and numbness radiating down the arm is a prognostic indicator of chronicity of symptoms, it does not necessarily indicate nerve root pressure but may be referred pain.[15] Nonneurogenic radiation of pain and numbness may be caused by chronic irritation of the musculoligamentous joint and intervertebral disk rather than by organic nerve pressure. These radicular symptoms are non-neurogenic; therefore, they follow no specific nerve pathway. They are not well defined by the patient in contradistinction to the well-defined dermatomal pattern of neurogenic symptoms. Subjective numbness in the ulnar distribution may represent anterior scalenus spasm and entrapment of the brachial plexus; this scenario is amenable to injection of the muscle with a local anesthetic and corticosteroid. Although reportedly rare in a whiplash injury, tearing of the longitudinal ligament and intervertebral disk herniation may occur and cause discogenic pain. Radicular type symptoms (across the back, shoulders, and into the arms) may be caused by damage to the posterior scapular muscles.[16] Neurogenic pain is characterized by a clearly defined pattern of sensory, motor, and reflex findings.

Severe hyperextension injury may stretch the esophagus, with resulting edema or retropharyngeal hematoma, and may cause dysphagia. Bilateral vocal cord paralysis inducing hoarseness has been reported after severe flexion-extension injuries.[12] Damage to the cervical sympathetic chain may occur, resulting in symptoms of nausea, dizziness, Horner's syndrome, and tinnitus. Vertebral artery spasm may be responsible for some of these symptoms.[14] The long-term complications of trauma to the sympathetic chain include complex regional pain syndrome. However, it has been found that temporomandibular joint abnormalities are not associated with whiplash syndromes.[17]

Injury to the brain itself from abrupt flexion and extension can cause concussion and cerebral contusion, with symptoms of loss of consciousness, dizziness, and headache. One study found that up to one third of patients with cervical spine or spinal cord injury following trauma had significant head injuries. These included skull fractures, subarachnoid hemorrhages, and intracranial hematomas.[14]

Psychosomatic reactions may occur after soft tissue neck injuries. Factors involved include the chronicity of symptoms, associated emotional reaction to the accident, and secondary gain. One study[15] evaluated the effects of pending litigation on patients with persistent symptoms after a motor vehicle accident. If litigation claims were settled within 6 months, 83% were symptom free at 5 years. However, if litigation settlement did not occur until 18 months after the accident, then follow-up at 5 years revealed that only 38% were symptom free. Two other studies have found persistent symptoms in 12% to 45% of patients after litigation settlements.[14,18] In many cases, patients are not "cured by a verdict," as is commonly thought.

Diagnosis In the patient with neck trauma, a plain-film x-ray study may be useful. In the less severely injured patient, who is conscious, with radiculopathy, but without a neurologic deficit, x-ray studies should include: (1) anteroposterior (AP) view of the atlantoaxial articulation (open mouth), (2) AP view of the lower cervical spine, (3) lateral view, and (4) each oblique view.[19] These should be obtained and examined before additional studies. After excluding an unstable cervical spine, lateral flexion-extension views have been suggested for those with flexion-extension injuries, such as whiplash. Some authors suggest obtaining a pillar view, especially if there is a suspicion of an articular mass. X-rays should be assessed not only for bony damage, but also for soft tissue injury.

Persistent symptoms and neurologic findings may warrant additional investigations, including computed tomograpy (CT) or magnetic resonance imaging (MRI), to exclude nerve root involvement.. These scans can evaluate soft tissue structures as well as disks, facet joints, spinal cord, and nerve roots. Myelography or electromyography may be necessary to confirm suspected spinal cord or nerve root pathology.

Treatment The initial treatment is conservative. Most authors recommend a soft cervical collar, nonsteroidal anti-inflammatory agents (NSAIDs), analgesics, and limited bed rest with gradual increase in activity for the first 1 to 2 weeks. Some suggest physical therapy, such as Greenfield isometric neck exercises, heat, and traction, if the symptoms respond.[14] TENS has been found to be useful for acute cervical strain; it hastens pain relief and the return of range of motion.[15]

One study found that patients who were treated with early mobilization during the first 2 weeks following the injury had significantly better outcomes in pain, neck stiffness, and central nervous system (CNS) functioning after 6 months than patients who were given time off from work and used a soft neck collar during the first 2 weeks.[20]

Despite improvement in most patients' symptoms, a substantial number of patients with whiplash have chronic symptoms. Forty-three percent of patients assessed 5 years after an automobile accident reported persistent symptoms.[15] Prognostic indicators for chronic symptoms included: (1) numbness and pain in the upper extremity, (2) use of a cervical collar for more than 12 weeks, (3) requirement of home traction, and (4) physical therapy restarted more than once. Although a sharp reversal of the cervical curve on x-ray after the injury predicted degenerative changes, it was not associated with persistent symptoms.

If conservative treatment is not effective, then escalation of care is necessary. Tricyclic antidepressants (TCAs), muscle relaxants, analgesics, and injection therapy are often required for pain relief. Table 27-3 summarizes common interventional approaches to neck pain.

Neck Pain of Myofascial Origin

One of the most common and frequently overlooked causes of neck pain is the myofascial pain syndrome. This syndrome is characterized by pain or autonomic phenomena, or both, referred from active trigger points. A myofascial trigger point is a hyperirritable locus that is palpable as an exquisitely tender taut band or knot in a skeletal muscle. Active trigger points are tender, prevent full lengthening of the muscle, weaken the muscle, and can mediate a local twitch response if stimulated adequately. Digital compression causes a characteristic reproducible pattern of referred pain and autonomic phenomena (sweating, vasoconstriction, and pilomotor activity) that is remote from the location of the trigger point.[21] The pain pattern may not be limited to a specific dermatome or peripheral nerve segment. Many times this pattern may superficially mimic other pathology (i.e., herniated nucleus pulposus, radiculopathy) and therefore the diagnosis of myofascial pain syndrome is not entertained.

On a cellular level, the myofascial trigger point seems to originate after an acute muscle stress or strain, causing tissue damage and impairment of calcium regulation. A state of localized sustained muscle contraction is initiated, with increased metabolites and decreased blood flow to the area. Multiple afferent fibers of varying types emanating from the trigger point to the spinal cord are stimulated and initiate the characteristic referred pain or autonomic phenomena.[21]

A myofascial pain syndrome may coexist with other cervical disorders. These other pathologic conditions must be evaluated and treated as well. Myofascial pain is often abrupt in onset, and patients may remember a specific precipitating event, often traumatic, for example, a whiplash injury. However, the pain may be more gradual in onset from a chronically overused muscle. Myofascial pain may develop after, or be worsened by, psychogenic stress, viral illness, visceral disease, exposure to cold or damp weather, and strenuous exercise or prolonged tensing of the involved muscle.[16] The patient often describes pain that is steady, deep, and aching in quality. Although the pain may follow a dermatomal myotomal pat-

TABLE 27-3 **Interventional Treatment**

Diagnosis	Treatment
Complex regional pain syndrome	Stellate ganglion block
Greater occipital neuralgia	Greater occipital nerve block
Traumatic torticollis	Spinal accessory nerve block, trigger point injection
Myofascial pain syndrome	Trigger point injection, cervical epidural steroid injection
Suprascapular shoulder pain	Suprascapular nerve block
Radicular symptoms (degenerative disk disease, herniated nucleus pulposus)	Nerve root block, cervical epidural steroid injection

TABLE 27-4 **Cervical Myofascial Trigger Points**

Muscle	Area of Referred Pain
Trapezius	Neck, shoulder, or temporal region
Splenius capitis or cervicis	Head, occiput, shoulder, or neck (there may be blurred vision)
Posterior neck muscles (semispinalis *capitis*, cervicis, or multifidi)	Suboccipital area, neck, or shoulders
Levator scapulae	Angle of neck or along vertebral border of scapula
Scalene muscles (anterior, medial)	Chest, upper central border of scapula, or along arm
Infraspinatus	Posterior neck, suboccipital area, deltoid, deep in shoulder joint, or front and lateral aspects of arm and forearm

Adapted from Travell JG, Simons DG. *Myofascial Pain and Dysfunction. The Trigger Point Manual.* vol 1. Baltimore, Md: Williams & Wilkins; 1983.

tern, it does not follow a characteristic nerve root pattern nor is there usually dysesthesia or paresthesia, which often is present with nerve root irritation.

Diagnosis In neck pain of myofascial origin, the muscles of the shoulder and neck are often tense with spasm. Palpation of a taut bandlike trigger point that reproduces the patient's pain pattern is pathognomonic for a myofascial pain syndrome. There may be associated weakness but not atrophy of the involved muscles.[16] Loss of full range of motion of the muscle is also seen. Trigger points commonly responsible for pain referred to the cervical area are located in several muscles (Table 27-4). Many patients exhibit a sleep disturbance.

Nerve entrapment by myofascial taut bands has been described. Brachial plexus entrapment by the scalene muscles or the pectoralis minor can occur. Greater occipital nerve entrapment by the semispinalis capitus inferior also may occur.[16] (See the discussion of suboccipital neuralgia later in this chapter.)

Management NSAIDs are useful as adjuvant therapy for decreasing musculoskeletal inflammation in patients with myofascial pain syndrome. Low-dose TCAs are important as well. They increase CNS serotonin levels, which may decrease pain and treat the associated sleep disturbance. Higher doses can help alleviate depression.

Treatment of the myofascial pain syndrome and eradication of acute myofascial trigger points may be achieved by passive stretching and trigger point injections. The involved muscles can be sprayed with vapocoolant coupled with passive stretching of the muscle. A stream of vapocoolant is sprayed in parallel sweeps in the direction of the referred pain over the skin of the involved muscle. The muscle then is stretched passively and slowly to the normal full muscle length in an effort to inactivate the trigger point.

Trigger point injections can be used as well. It is important to identify the trigger point accurately at its point of maximal intensity and inject directly into the taut band with a 22-gauge needle. Needling of the trigger point should reproduce the patient's referred pain pattern. Bupivacaine, 0.25%, or lidocaine, 1%, are usually used. These local anesthetics sometimes are mixed with corticosteroids (triamcinolone or solumedrol, 10–40 mg). Hot packs are applied after injection and stretching. These injections can be quite painful and can have significant side effects. Injections in proximity to the thorax may cause a pneumothorax, great vessels may be lacerated, and nerve chains can be anesthetized. Monitoring for complications is warranted. So-called dry needling can be performed if the use of local anesthetic is contraindicated (e.g., in pregnancy, allergy).

Myofascial pain syndromes of the neck that are resistant to this conservative treatment may be treated with cervical epidural steroid injections, spinal accessory nerve blocks (if the trapezius or sternocleidomastoid muscles are involved; see Fig. 27-2), or specific peripheral nerve blocks (suprascapular nerve, greater occipital nerve).

Because many conditions of daily living contribute to the formation and exacerbation of myofascial trigger points, therapy must incorporate a multifaceted approach. Biofeedback and relaxation techniques are useful in diminishing the psychogenic stress that can cause and exacerbate pain from myofascial trigger points. Driving, typing, heavy shoulder bags, exposure to cold drafts, and improper sleeping positions are a few conditions that contribute to and exacerbate myofascial trigger points and result in cervical pain. Practices and activities that lead to prolonged overutilization, strain, or tensing of the shoulder and neck muscles should be avoided. In addition, a formal physical therapy program often is beneficial. A program that encompasses stretch-and-spray techniques, strengthening exercises, and use of moist heat, ultrasound, and electrical stimulation is useful.[22] The patient also can institute a program of passive stretching while taking a hot shower or with application of moist hot packs.

Torticollis

Torticollis is a severe state of neck muscle contracture. Most commonly the sternocleidomastoid and trapezius muscles are involved. Other muscles that may be associated are the so-called cervical strap muscles. The contracture is sometimes spasmodic but usually is tonic. It is almost always unilateral: the head often is twisted painfully to one side, with the chin directed to the opposite side because of contraction of the sternocleidomastoid. Torticollis results from disease or injury to the CNS or the musculoskeletal tissues of the neck.[23] It may be congenital or acquired (Table 27-5). Long-standing torticollis can produce permanent contracture of the cervical muscles, fibrotic changes in the tissue, and degeneration of the cervical spine. There may be variable degrees of pain associated with the course of the disease.[23]

TABLE 27-5 **Causes of Torticollis**

Congenital Torticollis	Acquired Torticollis
Muscular and postural torticollis	**Traumatic**
Muscle trauma	Fracture
Tumor	Subluxation of the odontoid, C1, C2, or C3
Inflammation	Atlantoaxial instability
C1 to C2 articulations	Trauma to the clavicle, scapula, or cervical ligaments
Atlantoaxial dislocation	Neck muscle injuries
Anomalies of the cervical vertebrae	**Infectious**
Klippel-Feil syndrome	Cervical abscess
Absence of cervical muscles	Osteomyelitis
Neurogenic	Fascitis
Arnold-Chiari malformations	Nasopharyngeal torticollis associated with upper respiratory tract infection
Spina bifida	Cervical adenitis: viral, bacterial, tubercular
Hydrocephalus	**Postinfectious**
Syringomyelia	Influenza
Syringobulbia	Diphtheria
Colloid cyst	Scarlet fever[4]
	Neoplastic
	Bone: multiple myeloma, metastasis
	Muscle: rhabdomyosarcoma
	Lymphatic: lymphoma
	Vascular
	Scar formation
	Vascular abnormalities
	Anterior scalenus syndrome
	Pharmacologic
	Phenothiazines (dystonic reactions)
	Neurologic
	Syringomyelia
	Dystonic syndrome
	Posterior fossae disease: acoustic neuroma
	Herniated cervical disk
	Hydrocephalus
	Postencephalitis
	Spasmodic torticollis

Diagnosis Evaluation of the patient with torticollis should include the history (e.g., trauma, drugs, familial tendencies, and infection), physical findings (including careful neurologic examination and evaluation of the cervical spine), and x-ray findings (including cervical spine films of the odontoid and AP, lateral, and oblique views of the neck). This information enables the clinician to classify torticollis as acquired or congenital, of traumatic origin, or involving musculoskeletal or neurologic structures. When torticollis is associated with a neurologic deficit, additional radiographic investigations are warranted, including CT or MRI scan with and without contrast or myelography.[23]

Treatment Pharmacologic therapy of spasmodic torticollis has been somewhat effective. Therapies manipulating the dopaminergic, cholinergic, adrenergic, and serotonergic systems, and the use of γ-aminobutyric acid (GABA) agonists have had varying degrees of success. Anticholinergics have been recommended for mild symptoms of torticollis, including trihexyphenidyl (2–4 mg/day) or benztropine (1–3 mg/day).[24] Diazepam (5–15 mg/day) or amantadine (100–300 mg/day) have been used for patients with mild to moderate symptoms. Moderate to severe symptoms can be treated with haloperidol (1–8 mg/day). Psychological approaches, such as psychotherapy, hypnosis, behavior modification, and biofeedback also have been advocated.

The spinal accessory nerve innervates the sternocleidomastoid and trapezius muscles. A spinal accessory nerve block can relax the trapezius and sternocleidomastoid muscles in torticollis (Fig. 27-2). Alternatively, local anesthetic may be injected diffusely into

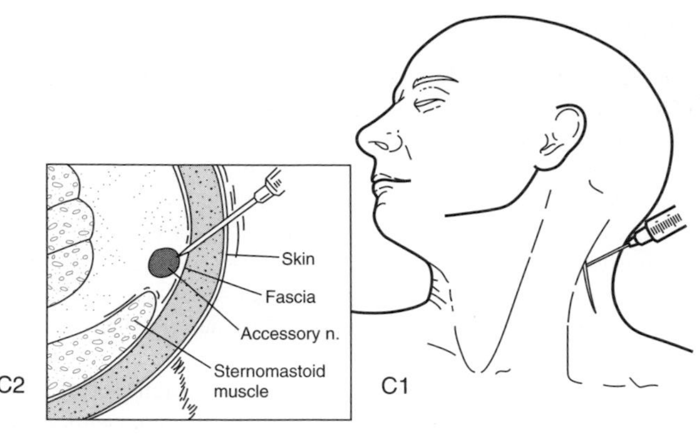

Figure 27-2 Diagram of a spinal accessory nerve block. (Used by permission. Romanoff ME. Somatic nerve blocks of the head and neck. In: Raj P, ed. *Practical Management of Pain.* 3rd ed. 2000).

the muscle belly similar to a trigger point injection. When other neck muscles are involved, a superficial or deep cervical plexus block is required to relieve the spasm (Figs. 27-3 and 27-4). If blocking the cervical plexus and accessory nerves improve the symptoms, repeated blocks are performed, coupled with physical therapy to strengthen opposing muscles. Neurolytic trigger point injections into the offending muscle with phenol may be considered if repeated nerve blocks give only temporary relief of the spasm. Experience over the past decade has shown injection of botulinum toxin complex A (Botox 100–200 units) to be effective.[25]

Cervical spinal cord stimulation may limit symptoms in refractory cases and is a less invasive approach compared with surgery. Surgical options for severe refractory cases include cervical rhizotomy, selective excision of the hyperkinetic cervical muscles, and stereotactic ablative and neuroaugmentative procedures. These surgical approaches have had varied degrees of success.[23] Surgical management of the underlying condition (Arnold-Chiari malformation, syringomyelia, colloid cysts, etc.) may be considered in patients with neurogenic torticollis if medical management and other conservative measures have not provided symptomatic relief.

CERVICAL SPONDYLOSIS

Disk degeneration and cervical spondylosis are common causes of neck pain. Approximately 50% of the population older than age 50 years and 75% of those older than 65 years of age have radiologic evidence of cervical spondylosis.[26] Many of them have associated symptoms.

Pathophysiologic Findings

As a consequence of aging the vascular supply to the disk is diminished resulting in disk degeneration. The anulus dehydrates, leading to approximation of the vertebrae. These changes, which can lead to disk bulging, glycoprotein leakage, inflammation, and fibrosis, may be related to phospholipase A_2 activity.[27] Ultimately this process can result in calcification and osteophyte formation. The resultatnt bone formation can lead to narrowing of the spinal canal, with subsequent cord compression or narrowing of the intervertebral foramina, resulting in nerve root compression. In addition, the ligaments and facet joints hypertrophy.[26,28]

The nerve roots most often involved in spondyloradiculopathy are C5 and C6 because of the increased mobility, angulation, and degeneration that can occur in the midcervical region.[28] Presenting symptoms in patients with radiographic evidence of cervical spondylosis are summarized in Table 27-6.[29]

Neck Pain

Neck pain from a cervical root is caused by acute intermittent nerve irritation, generally as a result of nerve impingement in a narrowed

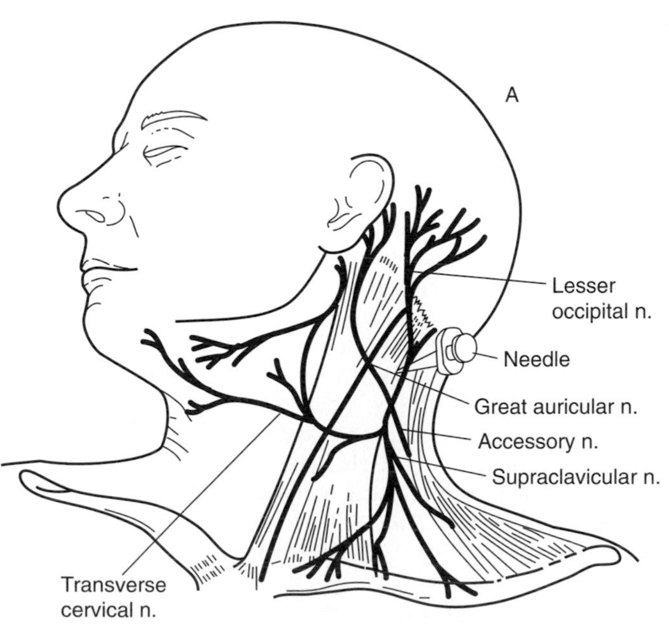

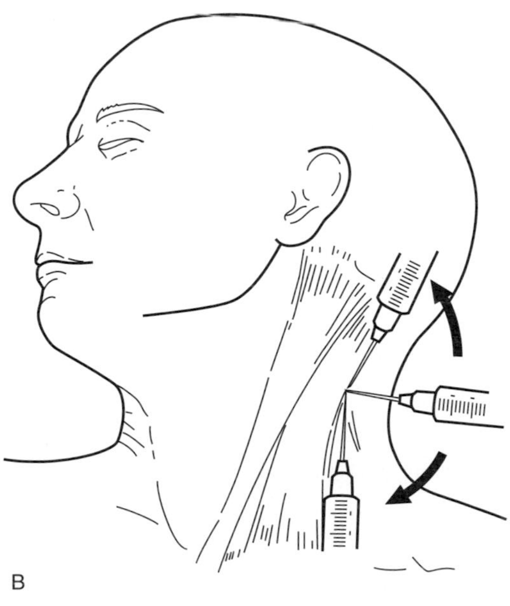

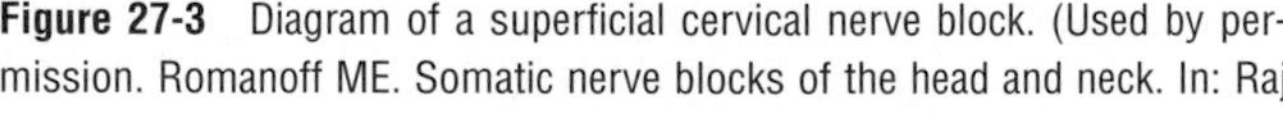
Figure 27-3 Diagram of a superficial cervical nerve block. (Used by permission. Romanoff ME. Somatic nerve blocks of the head and neck. In: Raj P, ed. *Practical Management of Pain.* 3rd ed. 2000).

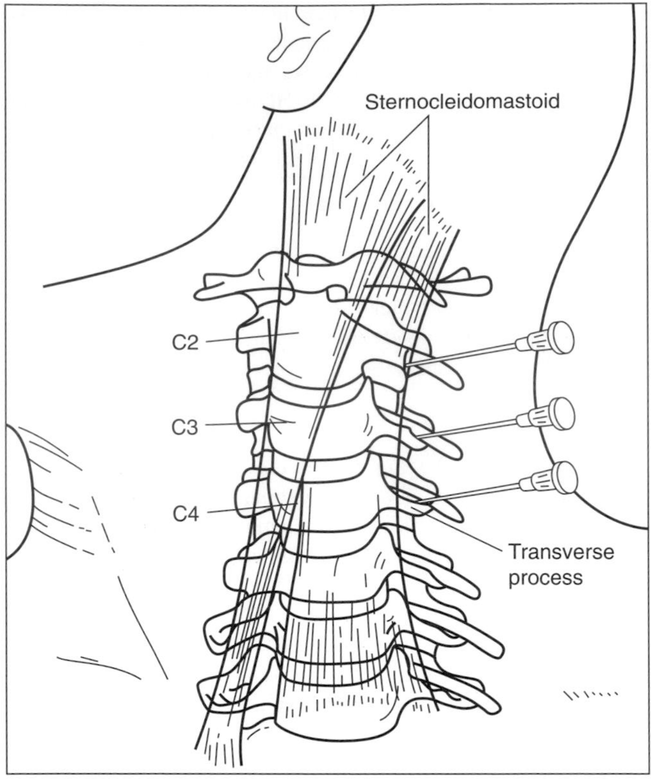

Figure 27-4 Diagram of multiple cervical nerve root blocks or deep cervical plexus block. (Used by permission. Romanoff ME. Somatic nerve blocks of the head and neck. In: Raj P, ed. *Practical Management of Pain.* 3rd ed. 2000).

intervertebral foremen. The pain may occur insidiously, as in cervical spondylosis, but can be precipitated or exacerbated by minor trauma. Alternatively, more acute severe neck pain may occur with a herniated cervical intervertebral disk in the setting of a degenerated spondylitic spine. The neck pain often is poorly localized, worsens with movement, and is associated with muscular spasm.[26] Ill-defined intrascapular pain with muscle spasm and tenderness as a result of anterior disk disease rather than nerve root irritation has been described.[28] This pain can occur months before evidence of root entrapment is seen. Cervical spine x-rays and a CT or MRI scan of the neck are helpful in excluding other causes of neck pain, including primary osteomyelitis, tuberculous osteitis, malignancy, and retropharyngeal abscess.[26] Bone scans also are helpful in the evaluation of infectious causes of neck pain.

TABLE 27-6 **Symptoms of Cervical Spondylosis**

Symptoms	Incidence
Headache, brachial radiculopathy	30%
Vertigo, myelopathy, neck pain	15%
Vertebral-basilar insufficiency	5%
Loss of consciousness	
"Drop attacks"	

Brachial Radiculopathy

The symptom of brachial plexus nerve root impingement at the level of the intervertebral foremen usually is shooting or burning pain, originating in the posterior neck, with radiation across the shoulder and down the outer arm to the elbow or hand.[26] Persistent nerve root impingement leads to a characteristic sensory loss (hypesthesia or anesthesia), motor loss (weakness or atrophy), and diminished reflexes. Radicular pain is sometimes the only presenting symptom. Patients may not recognize the associated mild tricep weakness because of compensation. They may first become aware of this weakness during the neurologic examination.

An acute protruded disk is associated with more severe pain, occurring acutely after trauma or violent movement, with symptoms radiating down the arm. Neurologic deficits soon appear. Other conditions that may produce symptoms similar to brachial radiculopathy include myofascial pain syndrome, apical lung tumors (Pancoast), and shoulder disorders (including capsulitis, rotator cuff injuries, bursitis, and thoracic outlet compression of the brachial plexus nerves or subclavian artery).

Suboccipital Neuralgia

Headache may result from occipital neuralgia. The greater occipital nerve arises from the posterior primary ramus of C2 and C3 and supplies the skin overlying the occiput and scalp. The splenius capitis inferior syndrome is a form of greater occipital neuralgia secondary to a myofascial pain syndrome involving that muscle. Chronic spasm may cause inflammation or direct compression of the nerve. Typically, the pain begins in the upper neck or occipital region and radiates to the ipsilateral forehead or temple. Paroxysmal pain may become continuous. Atlanto-occipital disorders must be excluded radiographically. One author suggests that in children, suboccipital neuralgia must be investigated by a pediatric neurologist or neurosurgeon.[26]

Diagnosis The diagnosis can be made in two ways. Palpation of the greater occipital nerve should reproduce the patient's symptoms. However, if the symptoms are suspicious for greater occipital involvement, and palpation does not completely reproduce the pain, then a diagnostic block may be indicated to rule in or out the possibility of a greater occipital neuralgia.

Treatment Conservative treatment may include the following measures: NSAIDs, TCAs, muscle relaxants, physical therapy, massage therapy, trigger point injections, or greater occipital nerve blocks. These blocks are usually performed using bupivacaine 0.25% (2–5 mL) with or without a corticosteroid. If good results occur, repeating the blocks at 2- to 4-week intervals may produce dramatic results. Resistant cases can be treated by neuroablative procedures. A neurolytic greater occipital nerve block with phenol can be performed. Alternatively, radiofrequency thermocoagulation or cryoablation of the greater occipital nerve can be performed. The effects of both are limited in duration to 3 to 6 months. Neuritis is a complication of all procedures; skin irritation and skin sloughing has occured only with phenol. Surgical treatment includes greater occipital neurectomy or a C2-to-C3 rhizotomy. Postoperative neuritis appears to be more common after surgery than with neuroablative percutaneous procedures.

Cervical Myelopathy

Cervical myelopathy can be a result of compression of the spinal cord by ligaments or protruded disks, trauma, radiation therapy, or compromise of the blood supply. If compression originates anteriorly by an osteophyte or a central disk protrusion, a predominately motor deficit is seen. However, posterior compression from a hypertrophied ligament causes dorsal column dysfunction and sensory loss. The limited mobility of the spinal cord in the cervical area associated with cervical spondylosis magnifies the effect of movement because it contributes to spinal cord compression. Spinal cord compression often is painless, although in the early stages the patient may complain of foot numbness and an unsteady gait.[26] It is essential to perform a thorough neurologic examination to identify lower motor deficits of the upper extremities and associated long tract signs affecting the lower extremities.

Other disorders that may mimic cervical spondylitic myelopathy include dorsal column loss from subacute combined degenerative disease (e.g., vitamin B_{12} deficiency), multiple sclerosis (although often other evidence of CNS plaques and deficits are present), motor neuron disease (e.g., amyotrophic lateral sclerosis), and syringomyelia.[26] Other causes of cord compression (including spinal cord tumors, metastatic disease, infectious processes, and Arnold-Chiari syndrome) can be excluded by more specific radiographic investigations.

Patients with neck pain and cervical radicular symptoms should undergo cervical spine x-rays, including AP, lateral, flexion-extension, atlanto-occipital, and oblique views. A cervical CT or MRI scan may demonstrate significant disk herniation and nerve root impingement. Many elderly patients have some degree of spondylosis and degenerative disk disease, and these findings are not necessarily the cause of the symptoms. One study evaluated the MRI findings in asymptomatic patients.[30] This study revealed that the prevalence of degenerative disc disease was approximately equal to the patient's age in years. That is, a 65-year-old patient has a 65% chance of having degenerative disc disease. The prevalence of a bulging disk was approximately one half of this percentage, and the finding of spinal stenosis was approximately one third.

A chest x-ray is warranted to exclude apical thoracic disease. Progressive neurologic deficit or signs of cord compression are indications for the patient to undergo spinal myelography, MRI or CT scanning, or evaluation by an orthopedist or neurosurgeon.

Treatment A patient with neck pain or cervical radicular symptoms of less than 2 to 4 weeks' duration and with a normal neurologic examination and insignificant radiographic abnormalities may be treated conservatively. Treatment includes a soft collar for up to 2 weeks, NSAIDs, analgesics, and possibly traction. Cervical traction appears to aggravate symptoms in approximately 10% of patients.[31] Any myofascial pain syndrome is treated as mentioned previously.

For symptoms greater than 4 weeks in duration, conservative management includes cervical isometric exercises to increase cervical muscle strength.[26,32] In addition,TENS, TCAs, anticonvulsants (gabapentin, clonazepam), muscle relaxants (baclofen, tizanidine), and local heat or ice can be used.

Cervical epidural corticosteroid injections (CES) for chronic neck pain and cervical radicular symptoms have been reported to be effective. Multiple studies have reported significant improvement in symptoms and pain in patients treated with CES.[32–34] Indications for injection included spondylosis, spinal stenosis, degenerative disk disease with symptoms, cervical arthritis, radiculopathy, cervical disk syndrome, and myofascial pain syndrome. There were no major complications noted in these studies. In addition, one of the authors (CW) published a study of patients with complaints of severe neck and arm pain and numbness in a radicular distribution for at least 3 months with negative CT and myelographic studies. Conservative therapy, including rest, cervical collars, traction, and NSAIDs was ineffective in these patients. Treatment with CES gave more than 65% of patients substantial improvement in their pain, and 36% of patients with abnormal neurologic signs prior to treatment had improvement in these signs. No complications were reported in this study.[35] There have been case reports of intrinsic cervical cord damage after CES injections in sedated patients.[36] It may be prudent to perform these injections with a responsive patient, so any spinal cord irritation can be detected prior to injection.

Cervical nerve root blocks are also effective treatment for radicular symptoms. A patient's history and physical examination may indicate abnormalities in a specific nerve root. These often can be confirmed by CT or MRI studies. Typical findings include a herniated nucleus pulposus, an osteophyte, or epidural scar tissue compressing a cervical nerve root. If conservative treatment has been ineffective, then a cervical nerve root block may improve pain and function. Often, a neurosurgeon or orthopedic surgeon requests a diagnostic nerve root block to determine, prior to attempting any surgical procedure, whether a specific cervical nerve root is the generator of the patient's symptoms.

Surgery usually is reserved for progressive neurologic deficits or signs of cord compression. Minor neurologic deficits that do not seem to interfere with function can be managed nonsurgically. Neurologic deficits that interfere with important functions should be managed surgically.[26,32] Surgery performed for pain, alone, was a controversial approach used 10 to 20 years ago. It is discouraged by most authors because surgical procedures have an extremely low rate of success when performed on patients who do not have radiographic pathology corresponding to their symptoms. The resulting scar tissue, postoperative pain, and rehabilitation often worsens a bad situation.

COMPRESSION SYNDROMES

Compression of the neurovascular bundle in the area of the cervical thoracic dorsal outlet can produce symptoms that mimic the neck pain and extremity dysesthesia and numbness found in cervical radiculopathy. The brachial plexus is formed by the anterior primary rami of C5, C6, C7, C8, and T1. These roots emerge from the intervertebral foramina and become sandwiched between the scalenus anticus and medius. At this point, the roots unite to form three trunks: an upper trunk (C5 and C6), a middle trunk (C7), and a lower trunk (C8 to T1). The three trunks are grouped closely and emerge laterally and between the scalenus, across the posterior triangle of the neck, and across the first rib. At the lateral portion of the first rib and posterior to the clavicle, each trunk separates into an anterior and posterior division. These six divisions descend into the axilla.

In the apex of the axilla, the divisions join to form three cords. Grouped around the axillary artery are (1) the lateral cord, composed of the anterior division of the upper (CS to C6) and middle

TABLE 27-7 **Common Compression Syndromes**

Syndrome	Site of Compression
Anterior scalene syndrome	Triangle formed by scalenus anticus and medius, and first rib
Costoclavicular syndrome	Clavicle and first rib
Pectoralis minor or hyperabduction syndrome	Pectoralis minor and rib cage

(C7) trunk; (2) the medial cord, a continuation of the anterior division of the lower trunk (C8 to T1); and (3) the posterior cord, the posterior division of all three trunks (upper, middle, and lower). Behind the pectoralis minor, the cords orient around the axillary artery according to their names. They continue and form the peripheral nerves and branches of the upper extremity. The lateral and medial cords comprise the median nerve, the medial cord gives rise to the ulnar nerve, and the posterior cord becomes the radial nerve.

The subclavian artery arches over the first rib and joins the brachial plexus immediately behind where the anterior scalenus inserts into the first rib. The subclavian vein runs over the first rib, but usually it is anterior to the anterior scalenus muscle.[28,37]

The most common compression syndromes are described in Table 27-7.

Anterior Scalene Syndrome

Neurovascular entrapment at the level of the anterior scalene may involve the nerve and artery and possibly the vein or lymphatic vessels. Hand edema and finger stiffness may be present because the subclavian vein is compressed between the first rib and clavicle secondary to a taut anterior scalene.[28] Most often, brachial plexus compression occurs with symptoms of numbness, tingling, and hypesthesia in the arms and hands, chiefly in the ulnar distribution. The pain is often dull and aching in quality and may include the neck, shoulders, arm, or hand. Symptoms may occur during the early morning, awakening the patient from sleep, or after prolonged activity using the hands.

These patients may have mild hypesthesia to light touch and pinprick, although other findings often are absent. The Addson test (tensing the scalenus and elevating the first rib) reproduces the patient's symptoms. This test is performed with the examiner abducting and extending the involved arm while monitoring the radial pulse. The patient faces the involved side, extends the neck, and takes a deep breath. Reproduction of the symptoms and obliteration of the pulse constitute a positive result. Normal subjects may have obliteration of the radial pulse with this maneuver, but they do not have the characteristic symptoms. Spasm of the anterior scalene muscle (myofascial syndrome) generally is believed to be the most likely cause. It may result from cervical nerve root irritation from cervical spondylosis or facet syndrome; trauma or stress and strain of the scalene muscles also may be causes. Uncommonly, the presence of a cervical rib with an associated, attached fibrous band may predispose to neurovascular entrapment.[28] However, most patients with cervical ribs have no symptoms, most patients with symptoms have no cervical ribs, and removal of the rib often does *not* afford relief; therefore, surgery rarely is indicated.

Treatment involves conservative measures, including a soft collar and strengthening, stretching, and posture exercises to decrease the cervical lordosis and increase shoulder girdle strength. The anterior scalene muscle and associated trigger points may be injected with a local anesthetic with or without corticosteroid to diminish spasms and relax trigger points.

Costoclavicular Syndrome[28]

As previously described, the neurovascular bundle courses between the first rib and the clavicle. Its compression leads to costoclavicular syndrome. Poor posture, fatigue, and trauma may predispose patients to this syndrome. Pain, paresthesia, and numbness in the arms and hands occur chiefly at night or in the early morning. The diagnosis is made by eliciting symptoms and obliterating the radial pulse by bringing the shoulders back and down (chest elevation and shoulder retraction).

Treatment involves increasing neck flexibility and improving posture by using strengthening exercises for the shoulder girdle. Poor posture secondary to psychogenic factors should be addressed.

Pectoralis Minor Syndrome (Hyperabduction Syndrome)

As previously noted, the neurovascular bundle may be compressed between the pectoralis minor and the rib cage. The symptoms are similar to those of costoclavicular syndrome, except that entrapment often may involve the ulnar and medial distribution.[28] The symptoms usually are transient and without objective physical findings. They frequently occur at night or in the early morning. The diagnosis is made by reproducing the symptoms and obliterating the radial pulse by placing the arms in abduction over the head, while externally rotated and rotated backward. This position stretches the pectoralis minor and compresses the underlying neurovascular bundle.

In addition, hyperirritability and tautness of the pectoralis minor (myofascial syndrome), causing shortening of the muscle, may be responsible for this syndrome. A slumped posture may contribute. Treatment includes improvement in posture and injection and stretching of the pectoralis minor trigger points.

The compression syndromes should be suspected in the patient who has cervical pain and associated extremity symptoms, which may be reproduced by appropriate positioning of the arms and neck. However, it is necessary to exclude other causes, including cervical disk disease, degenerative joint disease, cervical facet joint arthropathy, carpal tunnel syndrome,[4] pericapsulitis,[28] and shoulder-hand syndrome or chronic regional pain syndrome.[28] Disorders of the apical thorax, including Pancoast's tumor, subclavian artery aneurysm, or other supraclavicular fossa or axillary disease, also may mimic compression syndromes.

CERVICAL FACET JOINT SYNDROME

Cervical facet joint, or zygapophyseal, syndrome can cause both local and radicular symptoms that often are indistinguishable from cervical disk disease.[38] Often, cervical facet and disk disorders, leading to cervical pain, occur together.

Each posterior facet joint has a dual nerve supply, with one branch arising from the posterior primary ramus at the same level and the other from the posterior primary ramus from above. Therefore, to block the C4-to-C5 facet joint, for example, the nerves from C4 and C5 must be blocked. Acute facet joint irritation may occur from local trauma or excessive movement. More commonly, facet joint irritation arises from chronic changes of facet joint thickening and hypertrophy initiated by disk degeneration and spondylosis, trauma, or excessive load-bearing stress.[39]

Upper cervical facet joint irritation and lower cervical facet joint arthropathy with muscle spasm may be responsible for symptoms of upper neck pain, with radiation to the occipital region and ipsilateral frontal area. Occipital and vascular headaches may also coexist with facet arthopathy.[5] Radiographic findings (x-rays of the cervical spine, CT, MRI) may reveal degenerative changes of the facet joint (hypertrophy and thickening).

Low cervical pain characterized by neck pain with radicular symptoms to the shoulder and arms may be caused by discogenic nerve root irritation. However, concomitant or secondary facet joint irritation often contributes to this pain syndrome. It is important to remember that facet joint disease may produce radicular symptoms, as well, *without* nerve root involvement.

Diagnosis

Extension and rotation of the neck stresses the facet joints and exacerbates symptoms. Facet joint tenderness may be seen with palpation 3 to 4 cm laterally from the midline. Radiographic studies, if available, will identify the area of pathology. As discussed previously with degenerative disc disease, many patients have a CT- or MRI-documented abnormality involving the cervical spine. In many cases, these are incidental findings. Interventional treatment should be attempted only if the patient's symptom complex and the pathology seen radiographically are concordant. This point needs to be emphasized as the procedures described in this chapter may have significant morbidity. Physical exam can help differentiate the syndromes along with radiographic results.

Treatment

The initial therapy is conservative. Similar to facet syndrome in the lumbar region, patients often respond to NSAIDs,TCAs, physical therapy, TENS, and exercises to strengthen the cervical musculature. Facet joint injections have been beneficial in many patients. These injections usually are performed with 2 to 5 mL of bupivacaine, 0.25% to 0.5%, along with a corticosteroid (depomedrol, 20–40 mg). One study evaluated facet joint injections in patients not responding to conservative therapy. Disk disease was excluded by plane x-rays, and nerve root compression was excluded by electromyographic studies.[40] The facet joint level was selected by the localization of the symptoms from the history or palpation on physical examination, and by the site of the referred pain. More than 60% of patients had pain relief for up to 13 months following treatment. Improvement was more likely if the typical pain was reproduced on distention of the facet joint during the injection.

If facet joint injections with local anesthetic and corticosteroids provide only temporary relief, then the nerve supply to the joint should be addressed. Blockade of the facet joint innervation may be achieved by blocking the posterior primary ramus that supplies the facet joint and the posterior primary ramus above the involved facet joint. The inferior posterior primary ramus also may innervate the joint in some patients. The nerves originate from the cervical root and then curve around the superior facet to innervate the joints. These rami are often referred to as the median branch nerves. Local anesthetic, alone, is injected in these areas. If the injection significantly relieves the symptoms, then permanent blockade can be accomplished with radiofrequency thermocoagulation, cryoablation, or phenol injection.

One study[5] described percutaneous facet denervation in patients with a cervical syndrome emanating from the facet joint that did not respond to conservative therapy, and who were not surgical candidates. A preliminary block of the posterior primary ramus (median branch nerve) was done to evaluate the contribution of the facet joint to the cervical pain. If this alleviated the pain, then a percutaneous facet denervation, using a 12-gauge thermal electrode (60s and 80°C) was performed. Improvement in pain symptoms of 70% to 100% occurred in 40% of patients for up to 18 months. Complications included localized neck pain, which occurred in 20% of patients and lasted 3 to 12 weeks.

There remains controversy about the efficacy of facet joint injections for the treatment of facet joint disease.[41] Surgical treatment includes cervical fusion with iliac crest bone graft or instrumentation.

SUMMARY

The causes of neck pain are many and varied. They may be self-limited, requiring little intervention, or life-threatening, requiring immediate invasive action. A knowledge of the anatomy of the neck is invaluable to the clinician who diagnoses and treats painful cervical conditions. Although the neck may be the source of the patient's pathology, symptoms may involve the neck, head, shoulder, or upper extremities. A thorough history and physical examination, along with carefully chosen ancillary studies (radiographs, CT, MRI, electromyography, nerve conduction velocities, bone scan) often can identifiy the source of the patient's symptoms. Armed with this information, the clinician can provide treatment that is more timely, effective, and rewarding.

REFERENCES

1. Pawl RP. Chronic neck syndromes. *Compr Ther* 1990;16:43–51.
2. Roseman DM. Carotidynia: A distinct syndrome. *Arch Otolaryngol* 1967;85:81–84.
3. Rose VP, Veach JS, Tehranzdeh J. Spontaneous pseudomediastinum as a cause of neck pain, dysphagia, and chest pain. *Arch Intern Med* 1984; 144:392–393.
4. March JS. Rheumatoid neck. *Br J Hosp Med* 1985;33:96–100.
5. Sluijter ME, Koetsveld-Baart CC. Interruption of pain pathways in the treatment of the cervical syndrome. *Anaesthesia* 1980;35:302–307.
6. Ehni G, Benner B. Occipital neuralgia and the C1-2 arthrosis syndrome. *J Neurosurg* 1984;61:961–965.
7. Bernstein SA. Acute cervical pain associated with soft tissue calcium deposition anterior to the interspace of the first and second cervical vertebrae. *J Bone Joint Surg* 1975;57:426–428.
8. Hoppenfeld S. Physical examination of the cervical spine and temporomandibular joint. In: Hoppenfeld S, ed. *Physical Examination of the Spine and Extremities*. New York, NY: Appleton-Century-Crofts; 1976:106–127.
9. Ellis H, Feldman S. *Anatomy for the Anaesthetist*. Boston, Mass: Blackwell Scientific Publications; 1983:164–170.
10. MacNab I. The whiplash syndrome in symposium on disease of the intervertebral disk. *Orthop Clin North Am* 1971;2:389–403.
11. Bogduk N, Lord SM. Cervical spine disorders. *Curr Opin Rheumatol* 1998;10:110–115.

12. Hohl M. Soft tissue injuries of the neck in automobile accidents. *J Bone Joint Surg Am* 1974;56:1675–1681.
13. Silverman JL, Rodrigues AA, Agre JC. Quantitative cervical flexor strength in healthy subjects and in subjects with mechanical neck pain. *Arch Phys Med Rehabil* 1991;72:679–681.
14. Iida H, Tachibana S, Kitahara T, et al. Association of head trauma with cervical spine injury, spinal cord injury, or both. *J Trauma* 1999;46:450–452.
15. Nordemar R, Thorner C. Treatment of acute cervical pain—comparative group study. *Pain* 1981;10:93–101.
16. Cloward R. Acute cervical spine injuries. *Clin Symp* 1980;32:4.
17. McKay DC, Christensen LV. Whiplash injuries of the temporomandibular joint in motor vehicle accidents: Speculations and facts. *J Oral Rehabil* 1998;25:731–746.
18. Gotten N. Survey of 100 cases of whiplash injury after settlement of litigation. *JAMA* 1956;162:865.
19. Harris JH Jr. Radiographic evaluation of spinal trauma. *Orthop Clin North Am* 1986;17:75–86.
20. Borchgrevink GE, Kaasa A, McDonagh D, et al. Acute treatment of whiplash neck sprain injuries. A randomized trial of treatment during the first 14 days after a car accident. *Spine* 1998;23:25–31.
21. Travell JG, Simons DG. *Myofascial Pain and Dysfunction. The Trigger Point Manual*. vol 1. Baltimore, Md: Williams & Wilkins; 1983.
22. Foley-Nolan D, Barry C, Coughlan RJ, O'Conner P, Roden D. Pulsed high frequency (27MJz) electromagnetic therapy for persistent neck pain. A double blind, placebo-controlled study of 20 patients. *Orthopedics* 1990;13:445–451.
23. Maxwell R. Surgical management of torticollis. *Postgrad Med* 1984;75:147–155.
24. Lee C. Spasmodic torticollis and other idiopathic torsion dystonias. Medical management. *Postgrad Med* 1984;7:139.
25. Jedynak CP, de Saint Victor JF. Treatment of spasmodic torticollis by local injections of botulinum toxin. *Rev Neurol (Paris)* 1990;146:440–443.
26. Jeffries RV. Cervical spondylosis in persistent pain. In: Lipton S, ed. *Modern Methods of Treatment*. 2nd ed. New York, NY: Grune & Stratton; 1980:115.
27. Lee HM, Weinstein JN, Meller ST, et al. The role of steroids and their effects on phospholipase A2. An animal model of radiculopathy. *Spine* 1998;23:1191–1196.
28. Cailliet R. *Neck and Arm Pain*. Philadelphia, Pa: FA Davis Co; 1981.
29. Brain L. Some unsolved problems of cervical spondylosis. *Br Med J* 1963;1:771–777.
30. Matsumoto M, Fujimura Y, Suzuki N, et al. MRI of cervical intervertebral discs in asymptomatic subjects. *J Bone Joint Surg Br* 1998;80:19–24.
31. Swezey RL, Swezey AM, Warner K. Efficacy of home cervical traction therapy. Am *J Physical Med Rehabil* 1999;78:30–32.
32. Rothman R. The acute cervical disc. *Clin Orthop* 1975;109:59–68.
33. Rowlingson JC. Epidural analgesic technique in the management of cervical pain. *Anesth Analg* 1986;65:938–942.
34. Pawl RP, Anderson W, Shulman M. The effect of epidural steroids in the cervical and lumbar region on surgical intervention for discogenic spondylosis. In: Fields HL, ed. *Advances in Pain Research and Therapy*. 9th ed. New York, NY: Raven Press; 1985:791–798.
35. Warfield C, Biber M, Crews D, Nath DGK. Epidural steroid injection as a treatment for cervical radiculitis. *Clin J Pain* 1987;3:13–15.
36. Hodges SD, Castleberg RL, Miller T, et al. Cervical epidural steroid injection with intrinsic spinal cord damage. Two case reports. *Spine* 1998;23:2137–2142; discussion 2141–2142.
37. Ellis H, Feldman S. *Anatomy for the Anaesthetist*. Boston, Mass: Blackwell Scientific Publications; 1983:325, fig. 194.
38. Aprill C, Dwyer A, Bogduk N. Cervical zygapophyseal joint pain patterns, II: A clinical evaluation. *Spine* 1990;15:458–461.
39. Boas R. Facet joint injections. In: Stanton-Hick M, Boas R, eds. *Chronic Low Back Pain*. New York, NY: Raven Press; 1982.
40. Dory MA. Arthrography of the cervical facet joints. *Radiology* 1983;149:379–382.
41. Carette S, Marcoux S, Truchon R, et al. Controlled trial of corticosteroid injections into facet joints for chronic low back pain *N Eng J Med* 1991:325:1002.

CHAPTER 28 LOW BACK PAIN

Steven P. Cohen, John Rowlingson, and Salahadin Abdi

EPIDEMIOLOGY

In modern society, one would be hard-pressed to overestimate the impact of low back pain (LBP). The costs of this problem, in both human suffering and dollars, are staggering. Although figures vary widely, the lifetime prevalence of LBP is usually quoted as ranging from 60% to 85%, with an annual rate of about 5%. In one recent study, the point prevalence of LBP was estimated to be 30%.

LBP is the number one cause of worker absenteeism in the United States and most other countries in the industrialized world. In the United Kingdom, it is responsible for 12.5% of all sick days. A 1985 study estimated that 14% of the entire population of the United States misses at least 1 workday per year because of LBP. This figure is highest among people involved in manual labor, with low job satisfaction and poor workplace social support. About 2% of workers each year submit claims for disability from LBP, making it the leading cause of expenditures for workers' compensation.

The chance of someone with LBP returning to work full-time after any significant absence declines exponentially over time. For example, after 6 months of disability, the chance of someone with LBP returning to work full-time is about 50%. After 1 year, this figure plummets to below 20%. After 2 years of missed work, less than 3% of disability patients will ever work regular jobs again. The economic cost of this epidemic is estimated by some experts to exceed $100 billion per year, not to mention the physical, emotional, and psychological tolls it exacts.

Where does all this back pain come from, and who are the people most at risk? Overall, the ratio between men and women is about equal, although younger patients with LBP tend to be disproportionately male, and women report more LBP after the age of 60. For both sexes, the incidence increases with age. Postacchini and colleagues suggested that genetics may play a role in certain types of LBP. In patients with discogenic LBP and those who had undergone surgery for a herniated disk, 35% and 37%, respectively, had at least one first-degree relative with a history of discogenic pain, versus 12% in the control group. In these same two groups, 5% and 10% of patients, respectively, also had at least one family member who had undergone disk surgery, compared to only 1% of patients without complaints of LBP.

Many studies have shown an association between LBP and poor general health. Obesity (and possibly excessive height as well), smoking, low levels of physical activity, and poor strength and flexibility all predispose people to LBP. Interestingly, jobs involving heavy physical labor, and participation in certain sports such as wrestling and gymnastics, have likewise been associated with back pain. Studies have also demonstrated an increased number of sick days taken for other disorders in workers with LBP, and an association between LBP and chronic illness.

ACUTE VERSUS CHRONIC LOW BACK PAIN

Any discussion of LBP must begin with definitions. Chronic LBP is usually defined as LBP that persists longer than 7 to 12 weeks, although some experts define it as LBP that lasts longer than the expected period of healing. As with any form of acute pain, acute LBP represents a nociceptive response to injury. Nociceptors pervade all structures in the spine, so that injury to any of these will be perceived as pain. These structures include the annulus fibrosis, facet joints, paraspinous muscles, periosteum of the vertebral bodies, nerve roots and dorsal root ganglia, ligaments (particularly the anterior and posterior longitudinal ligaments), sacroiliac joints, meninges, and muscle-tendon complexes.

HISTORY

A comprehensive medical history is an indispensable part of the evaluation of any patient presenting with LBP. Although most patients referred to pain specialists present with chronic LBP from nonemergent, progressive medical conditions, a thorough history will rule out causes requiring immediate intervention.

A history of unexplained weight loss and malaise accompanied by back pain that is worse at night requires diagnostic studies to rule out malignancy. New onset of radicular symptoms associated with a rash in a dermatomal distribution may indicate herpes radiculitis. Unexplained fever, chills, night sweats, and a history of intravenous drug abuse or spinal procedures may herald an infection of the meninges or vertebral column. Cauda equina syndrome is a surgical emergency that may be caused by an epidural abscess, hematoma, spinal tumor, or herniated disk. Symptoms include severe back pain with radiculopathy, saddle distribution sensory loss, diminished anal sphincter tone, and urinary retention or incontinence. A history of recent trauma may indicate injury to the facet joints, sacroiliac joints, intervertebral disks, or fracture of the vertebral column. Large quantities of alcohol, caffeine, and smoking may accelerate the development of osteoporosis and predispose patients to spinal fractures. Finally, a ruptured abdominal aortic or iliac artery aneurysm can manifest as severe LBP. Risk factors include diastolic hypertension, chronic obstructive pulmonary disease, male gender, previous vascular procedures, and anticoagulant therapy. A ruptured abdominal aneurysm is a surgical emergency.

Following the general medical history, the physician should focus the interview on the primary complaint. The precipitating event often provides a key clue to the source of LBP. For example, an acute herniated nucleus pulposus (HNP) often causes a person to feel a "pop" in the back, followed shortly thereafter by pain shooting into the foot. The duration and frequency of pain can be important indicators of etiology, as in the case of patients with spondyloarthropathies, who frequently complain of aching LBP of long duration. Conversely, spinal tumors generally cause continuous pain that increases in intensity over time. The location and referral patterns of back pain must be ascertained in a thorough pain history. Pain radiating from the back to the lower limb, or localized exclusively to the lower leg, is strongly suggestive of nerve root irritation. A detailed history that delineates exacerbating and relieving factors can be extremely helpful in distinguishing the myriad sources of LBP. When a herniated disk irritates a nerve root, patients frequently complain of leg pain at rest. When spinal stenosis is responsible, maneuvers that reduce the size of the spinal canal, such as coughing or leaning backward, aggravate the pain. As a general rule, mechanical disorders such as degenerative disk disease and spinal stenosis result in pain that is increased with activity. When inflammatory arthropathies are responsible, pain and function are usually worse in the morning. Regardless of the suspected etiology, accompanying features such as paresthesias, dysethesias, numbness, and changes in bowel and bladder function should always be elicited.

The quality and characterization of pain are integral parts of a good medical interview. Adjectives such as "lancinating" and "shooting" are frequently used to describe pain of neuropathic origin, such as radiculopathy. Words such as "aching" or "pressing" tend to be reserved for nociceptive sources, such as disk disease and facet arthropathy. Finally, the intensity of pain and assessment of disability are essential in determining the effect pain has on a patient's function and quality of life. Clearly, one's perception of pain, the limitations it imposes on one's lifestyle and issues involving secondary gain can have a profound impact on treatment. Several studies have shown that patients with pending litigation tend to have worse outcomes than those who are not entangled with the legal system.

Along similar lines, we inquire about symptoms of depression in all our pain patients. Previous studies have demonstrated an extremely high rate of major depression in patients with chronic pain, with figures ranging from 10% to 85%. In addition to pain management interventions, all patients with significant depressive symptoms are referred to the psychiatry service.

PHYSICAL EXAMINATION OF THE LUMBAR SPINE

Examination of the lumbar spine begins with inspection. To start, the patient is disrobed and examined standing. The spine is viewed posteriorly, laterally, and anteriorly to check alignment. The back is then examined for any superficial abnormalities, such as redness (which may indicate infection or burns from heating pads), unusual skin markings (which can herald underlying bony or neurologic abnormalities), masses (lipomas may denote spina bifida), skin tags (neurofibromatosis), and skin discoloration (bony pathology). Posture should be viewed from multiple angles, because abnormalities can indicate pathology. Absent lumbar lordosis can be a manifestation of severe paraspinal muscle spasm, whereas an exaggerated lumbar lordosis can indicate weakened abdominal musculature. Unilateral muscle spasm can result in scoliosis. In addition to the low back, a complete examination of the lumbar spine must include inspection of the anterior abdominal wall, inguinal area, buttocks, and sciatic region.

Spinal motion is assessed during forward and lateral flexion, extension, and rotation. The normal range of motion for forward flexion is 40 to 60 degrees; for lateral bending, 15 to 20 degrees; for extension, 20 to 35 degrees; and for axial rotation, 3 to 18 degrees. Squatting tests not only lower extremity muscle strength, but joint function as well. Antalgic gait may be the result of back or leg pain. Other ambulatory abnormalities, such as steppage gait, back-knee gait, or flatfoot gait, can indicate weakness in the lower extremities. Patients with numbness in the soles of their feet may broaden their gait to gain stability.

Manual examination of the lumbar spine includes both bony and soft tissue palpation. Among the three layers of paraspinal muscles, only the most superficial layer, the sacrospinalis system, is palpable. On physical examination, it is not possible to distinguish between the three different muscles that comprise the sacrospinalis system. Posteriorly, the spinous processes are covered by ligaments, not muscles, and are thus easily palpated. Prominent gaps between spinous processes may signify spina bifida. A palpable "step-off" between processes may indicate spondylolisthesis. This is a common finding in patients with spondylolysis. Although vertebral tenderness is a sensitive sign for spinal pathology, it cannot reliably discriminate mechanical from medical disorders. To fully examine the coccyx, a rectal examination must be performed.

Neurologic dysfunction caused by abnormalities in the lumbosacral spine is usually manifested as altered sensation, reflexes, or muscle strength in the lower extremites. Lesions involving the T12 and L1 may manifest as weakness in the iliopsoas muscle, along with decreased sensation in the groin region. The L1 nerve root also innervates a small oblique band in the upper, anterior thigh. Patients with T12 and L1 dyfunction of the nerve roots may have diminished superficial abdominal and cremasteric reflexes. Nerve roots L2 through L4 are responsible for hip flexion and adduction (L2–3), and extension at the knee (L3–4). The sensory innervation of these roots includes branches to the back (L2–3), buttock, anterior thigh, and medial aspect of the lower leg and foot (L3–4). The patellar reflex is mediated through nerves originating from L2 through L4, with the L4 nerve root being the major contributor. The L5 nerve root covers the lateral part of the lower leg and the dorsum of the foot, to include the first two toes. To test the L5 nerve root, have the patient dorsiflex the foot or extend the great toe, or both. The associated reflex for this level is the tibialis posterior. The S1 root provides innervation to the sole, heel, and lateral edge of the foot. Muscle testing for S1 involves plantar flexion of the foot and flexion of the knee. The Achilles tendon reflex, mediated through the gastrocnemius muscle, tests the integrity of S1. The S2 nerve root provides sensation to the posterior and medial parts of the leg; its motor component enables flexion of the toes and plantar flexion of the feet. S3 provides sensation to the medial portion of the buttocks, while S4 and S5 nerves innervate the perirectal area. The coccygeal nerve is the sole innervation for the coccyx. There are no muscle tests to evaluate the nerve roots below S2, because there are no motor fibers from these levels. The bulbocavernous reflex is associated with the S3–4 nerve roots, whereas the anal reflex is mediated by S5 and C1. The addendum at the end of this chapter lists special tests used to diagnose specific causes of low back pain; see also Table 28-1.

Radiologic Imaging

With the advent of new procedures, neuromaging has taken on a greater role in recent years for the diagnosis of LBP. Conventional

TABLE 28-1 **Level of Disc Herniation As Differentiated by History and Physical Examination**

L2–3 Disc (L3 nerve root)

Pain: low back, upper buttock to anterior thigh, anterior knee, medial lower leg

Numbness: anterior thigh, knee (may be absent)

Weakness: hip flexion, hip adduction, knee extension

Atrophy: iliopsoas, quadriceps femoris, sartorius, hip adductors

Associated reflex: patellar

L3–4 Disc (L4 nerve root)

Pain: low back, hip, thigh, anterior leg, inner leg to medial portion of foot

Numbness: anteromedial thigh, medial aspect of lower leg (may be absent)

Weakness: knee extension, sometimes dorsiflexion of foot

Atrophy: quadriceps femoris, tibialis anterior, gluteus medius, gluteus minimus, tensor fasciae latae

Associated reflex: patellar, gluteal

L4–5 Disc (L5 nerve root)

Pain: low back, buttock, hip, posterolateral thigh, lateral aspect of lower leg, dorsum of foot, first 2 toes

Numbness: lateral leg, dorsum of foot, first 2 toes

Weakness: dorsiflexion of foot and great toe, difficulty walking on heels, possible foot drop

Atrophy: hamstrings, tibialis posterior, extensor hallucis longus, extensor digitorum brevis, sometimes gluteals

Associated reflex: tibialis posterior, gluteal

L5–S1 Disc (S1 nerve root)

Pain: sacroiliac joint, hip, buttock, posterolateral thigh and leg, lateral edge of foot, heel, sole

Numbness: calf, lateral border of foot, heel, sole, sometimes fourth and fifth toes

Weakness: gastrocnemius, soleus, gluteus maximus, hamstrings, peroneus

Associated reflex: ankle jerk, hamstring

radiographs are frequently used during an initial evaluation of LBP, especially in patients with known musculoskeletal disease, or when a fracture is suspected. Disorders likely to be picked up on plain x-rays include spondylolisthesis, pars interarticularis defects, scoliosis, ankylosing spondylitis, Scheuermann's disease, spinal stenosis, and osteoporosis. However, because of the low yield with radiographs, their utility in patients with LBP is controversial.

Magnetic resonance imaging (MRI) is the diagnostic test of choice for evaluating patients with radiculopathy. Other disorders in which MRI is the preferred imaging tool include syringomyelia, intramedullary tumors of the spinal cord, spinal cord infarction, traumatic injury, and multiple sclerosis. In a study by Jensen et al. published in the *New England Journal of Medicine*, only 36% of individuals without LBP were found to have normal intervertebral disks on MRI scans of their lumbar spine.

The strength of computed tomography (CT) in evaluating patients with LBP lies not in its resolution, but its ability to define spatial relationships between anatomic structures. As such, CT is helpful in patients with spinal stenosis, spinal infections, primary metastatic tumors of the spine, and spinal cord injuries. Because CT provides better images of bone than does MRI, it is preferred for patients with suspected bony abnormalities. Frequently, CT is used in conjunction with myelograms for the evaluation of radiculopathy, and following discography to better delineate disk disease.

Radionuclide bone scanning is the procedure of choice for detecting a variety of bone disorders. Bone scanning is the primary modality used to diagnose and follow skeletal metastases. Whereas osteomyelitis may not be detectable radiographically for more than a week after onset, a bone scan usually shows areas of enhancement within hours of onset. Other indications for bone scanning include occult vertebral fractures, bone disease associated with metabolic disorders, and spondyloarthropathies.

ETIOLOGY

LBP is a symptom, not a disease. The incidence of LBP disability has tended to increase over the years, but the overall prevalence has remained remarkably steady. In spite of the wide variety of disorders that may present with LBP, in the large majority of cases no definitive diagnosis is ever given. Fortunately, most cases (80%–90%) resolve within 6 weeks with or without treatment. Table 28-2 lists the most common causes of chronic LBP by diagnosis.

Infections of the Lumbosacral Spine

Infectious causes of LBP include vertebral osteomyelitis, epidural abscess, and discitis. Vertebral osteomyelitis accounts for between 2% and 4% of all cases of osteomyelitis, with males being affected more than females, and the elderly more than young people. In descending order, the most common sources of infection are the genitourinary system, skin, respiratory tract, and spine surgery. Risk factors include intravenous drug abuse, immune suppression, and rectosigmoid disease. Although vertebral osteomyelitis may sometimes begin abruptly, more often the presentation is insidious. Back pain typically is described as sharp, persistent, and exacerbated with movement. Fever may be minimal or absent. On physical examination, there is usually marked tenderness over the affected vertebra, guarding, and paraspinal muscle spasm. Treatment involves antibiotics and immobilization.

Because of its poor blood supply, most cases of discitis either are iatrogenic or occur secondary to direct spread from an infected vertebra. Classically, patients report the onset of intense, spasmodic pain appearing 1 to 2 weeks after spine instrumentation. Fever is usually absent. In patients without previous surgery, the diagnosis may takes months or even years to make. Pain from discitis may be referred into the groin, flanks, hips, abdomen, or lower extremities. It usually is exacerbated by movement and relieved by rest. In one study, 3 of 13 patients with discitis had neurologic deficits at diagnosis. Physical examination of the spine reveals localized tenderness and restricted range of motion. Treatment is supportive, with antibiotics and pain medication being the mainstays of therapy. Although the treatment course is usually prolonged, surgical debridement is rarely necessary. Some studies have shown discitis to be associated with an increased incidence of chronic LBP.

Epidural abscesses account for approximately 1 in 10,000 hospital admissions. Predisposing factors include intravenous drug abuse, cirrhosis, and alcoholism, with men being affected at a greater rate than women. Although severe back pain that follows

TABLE 28-2 **Final Diagnosis in 2,374 Chronic Low Back Pain Patients Participating in the National Low Back Pain Study**

Diagnosis	Percentage
Herniated disc	36.7
Myofascial pain	19.6
Spinal stenosis	14.0
Lumbar spondylosis	12.2
Osteoarthritis root compression	8.7
Unknown etiology	8.5
Spondylolisthesis	7.3
Discogenic pain	6.1
Facet arthropathy	4.8
Lumbar instability	3.6
Spondylolysis	3.1
Scoliosis	3.1
Pain with psychiatric component	2.2
Compression fracture	1.9
Epidural fibrosis	1.3
Epineural fibrosis	0.8
Arachnoiditis	0.6
Spina bifida	0.5
Other diagnoses	5.1

Adapted from Long DM, BenDebba M, Torgerson WS, et al. Persistent back pain and sciatica in the United States: Patient characteristics. *J Spinal Disord* 1996;9:40–58.

a spinal procedure should arouse suspicion, spinal instrumentation is usually not the cause of an epidural abscess. In a review of 39 cases of spinal epidural abscess over 27 years at Massachusetts General Hospital, only one was secondary to epidural placement.

The four cardinal signs of an epidural abscess are back pain, tenderness, leukocytosis, and fever. Interestingly, back pain is not universal. If left untreated, symptoms progress over a period of days or even months. Generally, the order of progression proceeds from localized back pain to radicular pain, weakness, incontinence, and paralysis. An epidural abscess is a surgical emergency. In one study, whereas patients diagnosed within 36 hours of the onset of symptoms had minimal residual weakness, no recovery was observed in patients paralyzed longer than 48 hours. Other infections that can result in back pain include herpes zoster, Lyme disease, and infectious sacroiliitis.

Vertebral Fractures and Spondylolysis

As the life expectancy of the U.S. population has continued to increase, so too has the incidence of spinal fractures. There are two main reasons for this: increasing disability with age, and a higher incidence of osteoporosis. In clinical practice, only 30% of vertebral fractures come to the attention of physicians, primarily because lack of severe back pain in many patients does not trigger obtaining radiologic studies. However, the prevalence of radiographically demonstrated vertebral deformities rises from 5% of individuals between the ages of 50–54, to 50% in women over 80 years. The most common locations for vertebral fractures are at the thoracolumbar junction, the mid-thoracic spine (T7–8), and the lumbar vertebral column. The prevalence of spinal fractures is highest in white women, owing the their increased incidence of osteoporosis. Aside from the increased propensity for vertebral fractures, some experts believe osteoporosis in and of itself can cause spinal pain. Aside from the increased propensity for vertebral fractures, some experts believe osteoporosis in and of itself can cause spinal pain.

The patient with a vertebral fracture typically presents with acute pain overlying the fracture site. For sacral fractures, pain may radiate into the buttocks or leg. The precise incidence of neurologic deficit depends on the extent, type and location of injury, but is usually cited as being greater than 30%. One way of distinguishing patients with spinal fractures from those with other types of fractures is the fact that more than half of all patients with severe vertebral fractures go on to develop chronic pain. Physical examination of the patient with a vertebral fracture(s) usually reveals marked tenderness on palpation. In patients with lumbar fractures who develop radiculopathy, straight leg raising tests may be positive.

Exercise programs for elderly patients suffering from spinal fractures have been shown to increase bone density, decrease the use of analgesics, and improve quality of life. Since patients with vertebral fractures are at increased risk to develop hip and other fractures, walking programs, fall-prevention courses and even Tai Chi may be beneficial. In most patients with isolated spinal fractures, non-steroidal anti-inflammatory drugs and/or short-acting opiods are sufficient for pain relief. In those with constant pain, sustained release opioids may be necessary. For patients whose main symptoms are consistent with radiculopathy, an epidural steroid injection(s) or trial with neuropathic pain medications may be a worthwhile endeavor. Two treatments that have been shown to both reduce subsequent fractures and provide analgesia for fracture patients are bisphosphonates and salmon calcitonin. In patients with focal pain and limited spinal fractures who do not respond to conservative measures, vertebroplasty, which involves the injection of an actylic polymer into a partially collapsed vertebra, or kyphoplasty should be considered. Finally, surgical intervention may be necessary in patients with unrelenting pain, spinal instability, or worsening neurologic deficit. Physical examination reveals marked tenderness on palpation. In most patients, analgesics and bed rest are sufficient treatment. In those who do not respond to conservative measures, vertebroplasty or surgery may be indicated.

One interesting type of vertebral fracture is spondylolysis, also known as pars interarticularis. For the white adult population, the incidence of spondylolysis has been reported to range between 3% and 6%. There is general agreement that most pars defects occur during childhood, with the large majority of cases being asymptomatic. Risk factors for pars fractures include spondylolisthesis, involvement in sports, and genetics. In active adolescents, spondylolysis can be a significant cause of LBP.

Patients with pars interarticularis usually present with focal LBP, although radiation into the buttock or thigh can occur. This pain may be increased during activities that require extension or rotation of the spine. On physical examination, many patients are noted to have a hyperlordotic posture with tight hamstrings. Diagnosis can be confirmed with plain radiographs, CT, or MRI.

The treatment of patients with symptomatic spondylolysis includes analgesics, bracing, cessation of sports, hamstring stretching, and strengthening of the abdominal muscles. In patients who require further pain management, pars injections may be helpful. In some cases, surgery may be necessary.

Metastatic Spinal Tumors

Bone is the third most common location of tumor metastases after the lungs and liver. In patients with metastatic cancer, tumor invades bone in 60% to 84% of cases, with the vertebral column and pelvis being the most frequently affected sites. In one study, 39% of all skeletal metastases were to the spine. The pain associated with spinal metastases develops slowly over weeks or months, gradually becoming more intense. Frequently, it can be localized to the involved vertebral bodies. Patients typically characterize it as a dull but constant pain. Aggravating factors may include weight bearing, activity, and nighttime, when the patient is trying to sleep. Besides back pain, other signs of spinal metastases include fever, chills, weight loss, and generalized fatigue. Pain treatment includes nonsteroidal anti-inflammatory drugs (NSAIDs), neuropathic pain medications, opioids, orthotics, and activity modification. In patients with neurologic deficits, surgical decompression may be necessary. As an adjunct to conventional modalities, chemotherapy, hormone treatment, corticosteroids, bisphosphonates, salmon calcitonin, radioisotopes, and radiotherapy can be helpful.

Spinal Stenosis

Technically, the term *spinal stenosis* can refer to central canal narrowing, lateral recess stenosis, or foraminal narrowing. The typical presentation of someone with spinal stenosis is an elderly person with axial low back and leg pain brought on by walking, especially down stairs or hills. Frequently, this pain is bilateral and radiates into the ankles. In contrast to patients with vascular claudication, whose symptoms take longer to resolve, those with spinal stenosis find that cessation of walking usually brings immediate relief. Because lumbar extension narrows the spinal canal, patients are often seen bending forward to obtain relief. Numbness and weakness may be present, with sensory complaints usually following a stocking-like distribution.

In contrast to patients with central spinal stenosis, those with lateral recess stenosis or foraminal narrowing tend to have dermatomal symptoms that relate to the irritation of an exiting nerve root(s). Symptoms may be sensory, motor, or both. Sensory complaints are more common than motor dysfunction because of the more peripheral location of sensory fibers in the cauda equina.

The most common causes of spinal stenosis are broad-based disk bulges, facet or ligamentum flavum hypertrophy, and osteophytes. In addition, foraminal narrowing can occur secondary to spondylolisthesis or loss of disk height. The diagnosis of spinal stenosis is usually made by MRI or CT scan.

Most patients with spinal stenosis have only mild to moderate limitation of function and can be treated conservatively. Some noninvasive therapies include lifestyle modification, exercise programs, and pharmacologic treatment with NSAIDs, neuropathic medications, and opioids. In a review of published studies evaluating bed rest for acute LBP and sciatica, Hagen and colleagues found that compared with advice to stay active, bed rest at best has no effect, and at worst may have harmful effects. For the acute exacerbation of radicular symptoms, translaminar epidural corticosteroid injections often provide good pain relief. In patients with foraminal narrowing, the transforaminal approach enables the clinician to deposit corticosteroids directly into the area of pathology. For patients with severe symptoms that are unresponsive to conservative treatment, surgical decompression may be required (Table 28-3).

TABLE 28-3 **Candidates for Epidural Steroid Injections**

Patients with acute radicular pain and corresponding signs or symptoms
Patients with symptoms caused by herniated disc who have not improved with conservative therapy
Patients with cancer in whom tumor infiltration of nerve root(s) may be causing radicular symptoms
Motivated patients with acute exacerbation of discogenic pain or pain from spinal stenosis
Patients with chronic LBP who suffer acute exacerbation, with manifestation of radicular-like symptoms
Patients with epidural fibrosis (epidural lysis of adhesions)

Herniated Disc

A herniated disc, defined as the herniation of the nucleus pulposus (HNP) through the annulus fibrosis, is the most common cause of LBP, accounting for more than one third of cases. Statistically, herniated discs are more likely to occur in the morning, when the disk height is greatest and the compressive forces are increased. In more than 95% of cases, either the L4-5 or L5-S1 disc is affected. There also may be a genetic predisposition for disc herniation. The most common age for disc rupture is during the third and fourth decades of life.

Although the classic picture of an HNP is LBP accompanied by radicular symptoms, in reality less than half of all patients with disc herniations develop true sciatica. Sometimes, radicular pain develops years after an HNP. Clinically, patients may complain of a sharp, lancinating pain radiating down the leg in a dermatomal distribution. Maneuvers associated with an elevation of intrathecal pressure, such as coughing, sneezing, or prolonged sitting, usually aggravate this pain. On physical examination, sensory loss, muscle weakness, or diminished reflexes in the distribution of the affected nerve root may be present. The straight-leg raising test, although highly sensitive, is relatively nonspecific. Conversely, the crossed straight-leg raising test is very specific but poorly sensitive. In severe cases, bowel, bladder, or sexual disturbances may be present. The diagnosis of HNP is generally made by CT, MRI, or myelography. Electromyographic (EMG) findings can be helpful in patients with nerve root impingement.

In most cases, nonoperative treatment is sufficient for pain arising from a herniated disc. Conservative measures that may provide symptomatic relief include controlled exercise therapy, NSAIDs, and, in patients with radicular symptoms, neuropathic medications. Although spinal manipulation and traction may be beneficial in patients with acute axial LBP, there is scant evidence for their routine use in patients with radicular pain. In patients with the acute onset or exacerbation of sciatica, epidural corticosteroid injections can provide pain relief.

Over the past few years, numerous percutaneous techniques have been developed to excise portions of herniated discs without performing an open surgical procedure. Chemonucleolysis by injection of chymopapain into the nucleus pulposus was first described more than 30 years ago, and remains popular in Europe. In clinical studies, this technique has been consistently found to provide better relief than conservative treatment, but less certain results than discectomy. Newer, percutaneous techniques include laser discectomy, arthroscopic microdiscectomy, endoscopic discectomy and nucleoplasty. However, none of these treatments directly removes the portion of nuclear material that has extruded through an annular defect. This may explain their inferior results when compared with conventional surgery. In patients who do not respond to conservative treatments, lumbar discectomy can provide relief in approximately 75% of cases (Table 28-4).

Sacroiliac Joint Pain

The sacroiliac joint is a large (average surface area is 17.5 cm^2 in adults), auricular-shaped, diarthrodial joint connecting the sacral spine to the iliac bones. The function of the sacroiliac joint is to dissipate the load of the upper trunk as it is transmitted to the lower extremities. As a cause of chronic LBP, sacroiliac joint dysfunction is estimated to affect between 15% and 30% of patients. Typically, patients describe a history of pain after falling, lifting and turning, or bracing themselves with their legs during a motor vehicle accident. Mechanistically, the typical injury pattern has been described as "an axial load coupled with abrupt rotation." Patients may describe an aching, usually unilateral, low back or buttock pain that radiates into the groin or thigh area. Prolonged sitting, standing, or bending exacerbates pain. One disorder that is associated with a high incidence of sacroiliac joint pathology is ankylosing spondylitis. Pregnancy, because of the increased axial load, exaggerated lordotic posture, and hormonal-induced ligamentous flexibility, may also precipitate sacroiliac joint pain. Although infection and tumor can cause sacroiliac joint pain, these etiologies are rare.

On physical examination, the most common finding in patients with sacroiliac joint pain is tenderness overlying the joints. Patients with sacroiliac joint arthropathy have also been described as having a higher incidence of leg length discrepancy, pelvic obliquity, and scoliosis. Numerous physical tests have been described as tools to aid in the diagnosis of sacroiliac joint pain, with two of the most common being Patrick's test and Gaenslen's test. However, a study by Dreyfuss and colleagues found that there are no historical or physical examination features that can reliably be used to diagnosis sacroiliac joint pathology. Radiologic studies, such as CT and bone scans, have similarly been shown to be unreliable. As such, the only way to make a definitive diagnosis of sacroiliac joint pain is with diagnostic joint injections, which should be performed with radiologic guidance.

Treatment of sacroiliac joint pain can be a formative task for pain physicians. Pharmacotherapy with medications such as NSAIDs and tricyclic antidepressants can provide relief in some patients, although the benefits are limited. In patients with leg length discrepancies, shoe inserts can result in relief of symptoms by equalizing the pressure across the pelvis. Spinal manipulation has been used for years to provide relief to patients with sacroiliac joint pain, although research is limited. EMG studies have demonstrated muscular abnormalities in patients with sacroiliac joint dysfunction, which have formed the basis for exercise treatment. Two studies have provided preliminary evidence that prolotherapy can be helpful in patients with degenerative joint disease, although none specifically addressed sacroiliac joint pain. For acute pain, noninvasive modalities such as transcutaneous electrical nerve stimulation (TENS), heat and ice packs have been advocated. Perhaps the mainstay of treatment for sacroiliac pain is sacroiliac joint injections with corticosteroids and local anesthetic, which should always be accompanied by physical therapy. Personally, the authors have found that radiofrequency denervation of the L4 and L5 dorsal rami, and lateral branches of S1 to S3, which innervate the sacroiliac joint, can provide long-term relief in patients who respond to diagnostic nerve blocks.

Diskogenic Pain

Pain originating from the intervertebral discs is estimated to affect approximately 39% of patients with chronic LBP. The rationale behind discogenic pain is that as internal disc disruption destroys annular lamellae, the remaining lamellae can no longer bear the load that occurs during normal activities. As the stress on the disc in-

TABLE 28-4 **Prognostic Factors of Positive Outcome With Nonoperative Care for Lumbar Disc Herniation**

Favorable Factors	Unfavorable Factors
Absence of crossed straight-leg raising (SLR)	Positive crossed SLR
Absence of leg pain during spinal extension	Reproduction of leg pain during spinal extension
Large extrusion or sequestration	Subligamentous contained lumbar disc herniation
$>$ 50% reduction in leg pain within first 6 weeks of onset	$<$ 50% reduction in leg pain within 6 weeks of onset
Positive response to corticosteroids	Poor response to corticosteroids
Limited psychosocial issues	Overbearing psychosocial issues
Self-employed	Receiving workers' compensation
Educational level $>$ 12 years	Educational level $<$ 12 years
Good fitness level	Poor fitness level
Absence of spinal stenosis	Presence of spinal stenosis
Progressive return of neurologic deficit within first 12 weeks	Progressive neurologic deficit and cauda equina syndrome

Adapted from Saal JA. Natural history of nonoperative treatment of lumbar disc herniation. *Spine* 1996;21:2S–9S.

creases, the mechanical threshold required to produce nociception is surpassed. The disc may then become chemically sensitized.

Patients with discogenic pain generally complain of the gradual onset of aching LBP that can extend into the buttock, hip, groin, or even a lower limb. This pain is frequently characterized as being exacerbated by prolonged sitting or bending forward, although a study by Schwarzer and colleagues found no clinical features that could reliably distinguish patients with diskogenic pain from those with other sources of LBP. Physical examination reveals an absence of focal neurologic deficits. As sole therapy, the pain relief that accompanies sacroiliac joint corticosteroid injection tends to be short-lived. In patients who respond to diagnostic blocks with local anesthetic, radiofequency denervation of the L4 and L5 dorsal rami and S1–3 lateral branches which innervate the sacroiliac joint, has been shown to provide long-term pain relief. A post-diskography CT scan can provide additional information regarding anatomic abnormalities.

Treatment of diskogenic pain usually begins with conservative therapy, including NSAIDs, weight loss, and physical therapy. In patients with one- or two-level disc disease, intradiskal electrothermal therapy (IDET) has been shown in uncontrolled studies to provide moderate pain relief. Although MRI and CT scans can indicate degenerative disc disease, the diagnois of discogenic pain is best made by provocative discography. False-positive discography is most likely to occur in patients with abnormal psychometric testing, multiple somatic complaints, and previous back surgery. In addition to enhancing sensitivity, obtaining a post-discography CT scan can provide additional information regarding anatomic abnormalities. In patients who have failed or who are not candidates for invasive therapy, opioids may be of benefit.

Facet Arthropathy

First described by Goldthwait in 1911, pain arising from the lumbar zygapophysial (LZ; facet) joints is frequently quoted to affect 15% to 40% of LBP sufferers, although estimates range from as low as 8% to as high as 94%. The LZ joints are paired, true synovial joints that connect adjacent vertebrae posterolaterally. The function of the LZ joints is to limit rotation and assist the intervertebral disk in resisting compressive forces during lordotic postures, so that maximal stress on the LZ joints occurs during lumbar extension and rotation. The load borne by these joints varies between 3% and 25% of the axial load, increasing during disc space narrowing and facet arthritis. During prolonged standing in a lordotic posture, 16% of the axial load is assumed by the facet joints. In patients with lumbar spondylosis, 70% of the compressive load can be transmitted to the joints. Some of the etiologies for facet arthropathy include microtrauma, capsular tears, synovial inflammation and impingement, chondromalacia, microhemorrhage, and meniscoid entrapment. When facet pain is caused by osteoarthritis, morning stiffness may be present. Some studies have found the incidence of facet joint disorders to be more common in women than in men.

Patients with lumbar facet disease typically present with the gradual onset of deep, achy LBP that may be referred into the groin, hip, buttock, or thigh. On physical examination, pain may be aggravated by maneuvers that increase the load borne by the LZ joints, such as hyperextension and rotation of the spine. On palpation of the back, tenderness in the paraspinous region(s) can often be elicited. CT or MRI scan may reveal hypertrophy of the facet joints. However, numerous studies have demonstrated that the only way to definitively identify the LZ joints as pain generators is to perform diagnostic local anesthetic injections under fluoroscopic guidance into either the facet joints themselves or the medial branches that innervate them. For each facet joint, innervation is derived from the medial branch of the primary dorsal ramus at the level of the joint and one level above it. In those patients who obtain significant pain relief from diagnostic nerve blocks, radiofrequency denervation has been demonstrated to provide long-term relief. Some authors have advocated confirmatory blocks before radiofrequency neurotomy.

Myofascial Pain

Myofascial pain is a common cause of LBP, with one study finding its prevalence to be almost 20%, second only to herniated discs. In addition, some studies have found LBP to be associated with elevated levels of paraspinal muscle tension. Myofascial LBP often presents as a deep, achy pain that is aggravated by activity and position changes. It may be localized to the low back, or radiate into the buttock, sacrum, thigh, abdominal wall, or even calf, depending on the affected muscle(s). Pain-induced weakness or paresthesias, or both, may be present but are nondermatomal in distribution. On physical examination, a tender, taut band of muscle may be noted (trigger point) that when palpated results in a characteristic referral pattern. Deep, traverse "snapping" palpation or needle insertion often elicits the characteristic local twitch response.

The treatment of myofascial LBP is conservative. Some of the therapies used for myofascial pain include ischemic compression massage, the so-called spray-and-stretch technique, iontophoresis, and physical therapy. A large, randomized controlled trial compared osteopathic manipulation with conventional noninvasive therapy in patients with axial LBP of less than 6 months' duration. The osteopathic treatment group required less pain medication than the conventional treatment group, but had similar outcomes. When trigger points are identified, trigger point injections using local anesthetic can be helpful. A recent, randomized, double-blind study in patients with chronic LBP found injections with botulinum toxin A to be an effective treatment. When myofascial pain is associated with other pathology of the lumbar spine as is often the case, these problems need to be treated as well.

Piriformis Syndrome

The piriformis is a flat, pyramidal muscle extending from the anterior sacrum, greater sciatic foramen, and sacrotuberous ligament to the greater trochanter of the femur. The major function of the piriformis is to abduct and externally rotate the femur. The possibility that sciatic symptoms may stem from the piriformis muscle dates back to 1928, when Yeoman examined the relationship of the sacroiliac joint, sciatic nerve, and piriformis muscle. Although six anatomic variations between the sciatic nerve and piriformis muscle have been described, in the large majority of cases the sciatic nerve passes anterior to the muscle. Any process that causes the piriformis to spasm or contract inappropriately, or less frequently, results in muscle hypertrophy and sciatic nerve impingement, can lead to piriformis syndrome.

The typical presentation of piriformis syndrome is buttock pain or sciatica, or both, exacerbated by activities that necessitate hip adduction and internal rotation, such as cross-country skiing or prolonged sitting. Pain that accompanies bowel movements may be present and, for women, dyspareunia. Physical examination may reveal tenderness in the buttock extending from the lateral border of the sciatic foramen to the greater trochanter. Both pelvic and rectal examinations may reproduce the pain pattern. Pain is also elicited during resistance to hip flexion, adduction, and internal rotation (Freiberg's sign). The neurologic examination is usually nonfocal, with most patients having a negative straight-leg raising test. Although CT, MRI, and electrodiagnostic studies may be helpful, by themselves these tests are insufficient to make the diagnosis.

For most patients with piriformis syndrome, conservative treatment is sufficient. This includes physical therapy and correction of leg length discrepancies, pelvic obliquity, abnormalities in gait or posture mechanics, and associated back or leg problems. Medications such as NSAIDs and muscle relaxants can sometimes be helpful. Other treatments that have been advocated include transrectal massage, vapocoolant spray coupled with soft-tissue stretching maneuvers, and TENS therapy. When conservative treatment fails, injection of the piriformis with local anesthetic and corticosteroids can relieve muscle spasm and pain. This treatment should be done using either a nerve stimulator to locate the sciatic nerve or fluoroscopy with contrast. In instances in which relief is short-term, piriformis injections can be repeated with botulinum toxin. In rare instances, surgical sectioning of the piriformis muscle may be necessary.

One disorder that is easily mistaken for piriformis syndrome is ischiogluteal bursitis. Patients with ischiogluteal bursitis usually complain of severe pain in the center of the buttock, which is worse with sitting or walking. This pain may radiate into the thigh, but rarely extends below the knee. Tests involving motion at the hip joint, such as straight-leg raising and Patrick's tests, are often positive. Pressure applied on the lateral rectal wall during a digital rectal examination can elicit excruciating pain. Conservative treatment includes NSAIDs and soft pillows or so-called doughnuts for sitting. For patients with severe pain, bursa injections performed with corticosteroids and local anesthetic are indicated.

Failed Back Surgery Syndrome

The definition of failed back surgery syndrome (FBSS) is the persistence or development of low back or leg pain following surgery on the lumbosacral spine. Two statistics highlight the magnitude of so-called failed back syndrome as a pain problem in the United States. First, approximately 300,000 lumbosacral spine procedures are performed each year in the United States as a treatment for chronic LBP. Secondly, depending on the definition of failure, the incidence of FBSS can be as high as 60%.

The reasons why patients continue to have pain following spine surgery can be broadly categorized as follows: (1) poor patient selection (e.g., patients with a somatoform disorder or who are malingering); (2) surgery was not indicated in the first place or the patient underwent the wrong procedure (e.g., a patient with discogenic pain who underwent a laminectomy); (3) clear indication for surgery, but the procedure did not correct the original problem; (4) complication from surgery (e.g., discitis, pseudomeningocele, or a pars defect); (5) recurrent disc herniation; (6) secondary instability or degenerative changes occurring as a consequence of surgery (e.g., discogenic pain or sacroiliac joint pain developing at the level immediate below a spinal fusion, spondylolisthesis following laminectomy, or pain that develops over the site of a donor graft); (7) persistent or established neural injury (e.g., arachnoiditis or epidural scarring); and (8) an intercurrent diagnosis, such as cancer.

The workup of patients with FBSS begins with a detailed history and physical examination. Of particular importance is determining whether the patient's pain is of the same character and quality as before the surgery, or represents a new symptom that has arisen. For instance, a new pain complaint might indicate a surgical complication. Equally crucial is determining whether or not, and for how long, the patient experienced a pain-free interval. The three most common scenarios are as follows:

1. No relief or the worsening of pain shortly after surgery. This category includes a retained disc fragment, failure to remove the offending disc, and certain iatrogenic infections.
2. Initial relief followed shortly thereafter by pain, numbness, or weakness. Examples of this group of disorders are arachnoiditis, epidural fibrosis, and battered-root syndrome with perineural scarring.
3. Excellent relief after the surgery followed by development of pain months or years later. This group includes a recurrent disc at the same or different level, pseudoarthrosis, and lumbar instability.

Overall, the most frequent causes of pain in patients with FBSS syndrome are recurrent disc herniation, spinal stenosis, epidural scarring, and arachnoiditis (Table 28-5). Table 28.5 lists the most frequent diagnoses conferred at one pain management center in patients with failed back surgery syndrome.

After obtaining a detailed history, the physician should arrive at a reasonable differential diagnosis. At this point, diagnostic studies are usually necessary. If a recurrent herniated disc or spinal

TABLE 28-5 **Pain Center Diagnosis in 78 Patients With Failed Back Surgery Syndrome**

Diagnosis	Number of Cases
Normal	16
Minor spondylitic/expected postoperative changes	16
Epidural fibrosis	11
Arachnoiditis	10
Traumatic neuritis	5
Severe spondylosis	4
Spinal stenosis	4
Cancer	3
Musculoskeletal abnormality only	2
Compression fracture	1
Traumatic meningocele	1
Lateral foraminal stenosis	1
Tarsal tunnel syndrome	1
Fractured hip	1
Scoliosis	1
Disc herniation	1

Adapted from Long DM, Filtzer DL, BenDebba M, Hendler NH. Clinical features of the failed-back syndrome. *J Neurosurg* 1988;69:61–71.

stenosis is suspected, an MRI scan is indicated. Because scar tissue is relatively vascular, a gadolinium-enhanced MRI or CT scan is usually necessary to detect epidural fibrosis. This diagnosis can be confirmed with epidural mapping by the injection of contrast media through the caudal canal. In patients with epidural fibrosis, a filling defect is present. When arachnoiditis is suspected, myelography is the diagnostic imaging study of choice. Additional accuracy can be obtained when a myelogram is followed by CT. For osteomyelitis, bone scanning is the preferred test.

The treatment of FBSS is aimed at the underlying cause. Depending on the diagnosis, nerve blocks, including epidural corticosteroid injections, sacroiliac joint blocks, and facet blocks, can sometimes be of benefit. In patients with radicular symptoms, neuropathic pain medications may provide relief. Some clinicians report good results with epidural lysis of adhesions (i.e. Racz procedure) in FBSS patients with epidural fibrosis, although in our experience the analgesia conferred by this procedure tends to be short-lived. Causes of FBSS that may amenable to surgery include a recurrent disk herniation, postlaminectomy instability, recurrent spinal stenosis, nonunion, and a host of surgical complications. However, in a study by North and colleagues that followed 102 patients who underwent repeat back surgery, only 34% had a successful outcome. In patients who do not respond to nerve blocks, repeat surgery, or other medications, opioids are indicated. Finally, spinal cord stimulation may be of benefit for patients with FBSS who have intractable pain, especially those for whom leg pain is the predominant complaint.

Rare Causes

In addition to the usual causes of LBP, the astute clinician must also consider the unusual. Because of their effects on the musculoskeletal system, a host of different metabolic and endocrine disorders can result in LBP, including hyperthyroidism, hyperparathyroidism, and Cushing's disease. For similar reasons, virtually any rheumatologic disorder can present as LBP. Visceral pain emanating from internal organs can be referred to the back secondary to convergence in the spinal cord. These sources of visceral pain include genitourinary organs, the kidneys, gallbladder, bowel, and liver. Vascular disease can manifest as LBP, which if not detected, can be catastrophic. Not only is the spine the site of metastatic tumors, but primary tumors may originate there as well. In some patients, hematologic disorders such as mastocytosis and hemoglobinopathies can lead to low back pain, as can diseases such as sarcoidosis, Paget's disease and infectious endocarditis. Finally, psychiatric and functional disorders can manifest as chronic back pain, which can be extremely difficult to treat.

BIBLIOGRAPHY

Andersson GBJ. Epidemiological features of chronic low-back pain. *Lancet* 1999;354:581–585.

Andersson GBJ, Lucente T, Davis AM, et al. A comparison of osteopathic spinal manipulation with standard care for patients with low back pain. *N Engl J Med* 1999;341:1426–1431.

Baker AS, Ojemann RG, Swartz MN, Richardson EP Jr. Spinal epidural abscess. *N Engl J Med* 1975;293:463–468.

Bloomfield DJ. Should bisphosphonates be part of the standard therapy of patients with multiple myeloma or bone metastases from other cancers? An evidence-based review. *J Clin Oncol* 1998;16:1218–1225.

Borenstein DG, Wiesel SW, Boden SD. *Low Back Pain: Medical Diagnosis and Comprehensive Management.* 2nd ed. Philadelphia, PA: WB Saunders; 1995.

Cohen SP, Dawson T, Abdi S. Lateral branch blocks as a treatment for sacroiliac joint pain: A pilot study. *Reg Anesth Pain Med* 2003;28:113–119.

Dreyer SJ, Dreyfuss PH. Low back pain and the zygapophysial (facet) joints. *Arch Phys Med Rehabil* 1996;77:290–300.

Dreyfuss P, Michaelsen M, Pauza K, et al. The value of medical history and physical examination in diagnosing sacroiliac joint pain. *Spine* 1996;21:2594–2602.

Dreyfuss P, Schwarzer AC, Lau P, Bogduk N. Specificity of lumbar medial branch and L5 dorsal ramus blocks. *Spine* 1997;22:895–902.

Eismont FJ, Montero C. Infections of the spine. In: Davidoff RA, ed. *Handbook of the Spinal Cord.* New York, NY: Marcel Dekker; 1987:411–449.

Foster L, Clapp L, Erickson M, Jabbari B. Botulinum toxin A and chronic low back pain: A randomized, double-blind study. *Neurology* 2001;56: 1290–1293.

Goldberg MS, Scott SC, Mayo NE. A review of the association between cigarette smoking and the development of nonspecific back pain and related outcomes. *Spine* 2000;25:995–1014.

Goldthwait JE. The lumbosacral articulation: an explanation of many cases of lumbago, sciatica and paraplegia. *Boston Med Surg J* 1911;164: 365–372.

Hagen KB, Hilde G, Jamtvedt G, Winnem MF. The Cochrane review of bed rest for acute low back pain and sciatica. *Spine* 2000;25:2932–2939.

Hoppenfeld S. *Physical Examination of the Spine and Extremities.* Norwalk, CT: Appleton-Century-Crofts; 1976.

Jensen MC, Brant-Zawadzki MN, Obuchowski N, et al. Magnetic resonance imaging of the lumbar spine in people without back pain. *N Engl J Med* 1994;331:69–73.

Kraft GH. A physiological approach to the evaluation of lumbosacral spinal stenosis. *Phys Med Rehabil Clin N Am* 1998;9:381–389.

Laslett M, Williams M. The reliability of selected pain provocation tests for sacroiliac joint pathology. *Spine* 1994;19:1243–1249.

Leboeuf-Yde C. Body weight and low back pain. A systematic literature review of 56 journal articles reporting on 65 epidemiologic studies. *Spine* 2000;25:226–237.

Long DM, BenDebba M, Torgerson WS, et al. Persistent back pain and sciatica in the United States: Patient characteristics. *J Spinal Disord* 1996; 9:40–58.

Long DM, Filtzer DL, BenDebba M, Hendler NH. Clinical features of the failed-back syndrome. *J Neurosurg* 1988;69:61–71.

Mayer HM, Wiechert K, Korge A, Qose I. Minimally invasive total disc replacement: surgical technique and preliminary clinical results. *Eur Spine J* 2002:11 Suppl 2:S124–130.

Mercadante S. Malignant bone pain. *Pain* 1997;69:1–18.

North RB, Campbell JN, James CS, et al. Failed back surgery syndrome: 5-year follow-up in 102 patients undergoing repeated operation. *Neurosurgery* 1991;28:685–690.

North RB, Kidd DH, Piantadosi S. Spinal cord stimulation versus reoperation for failed back surgery syndrome: a prospective, randomized study design. *Acta Neurochir Suppl* (Wien) 1995;64:106–108.

Onofrio BM. Intervertebral discitis: Incidence, diagnosis, and management. *Clin Neurosurg* 1980;27:481–516.

Papaioannou A, Watts NB, Kendler DL, et al. Diagnosis and management of vertebral fractures in elderly adults. *Am J Med* 2002;113:220–228.

Parziale JR, Hudgins TH, Fishman LM. The piriformis syndrome. *Am J Orthop* 1996;25:819–823.

Postacchini F, Lami R, Pugliese O. Familial predisposition to discogenic low-back pain. An epidemiologic and immunogenic study. *Spine* 1988; 13:1403–1406.

Saal JA. Natural history of nonoperative treatment of lumbar disc herniation. *Spine* 1996;21:2S–9S.

Schwarzer AC, Aprill CN, Derby R, et al. The prevalence and clinical features of internal disc disruption in patients with chronic low back pain. *Spine* 1995;20:1878–1883.

Sinaki M, Mokri B. Low back pain and disorders of the lumbar spine. In: Braddom RL, ed. *Physical Medicine and Rehabilitation.* 2nd ed. Philadelphia, PA: WB Saunders; 2000;853–893.

Standaert CJ, Herring SA, Halpern B, King O. Spondylolysis. *Phys Med Rehabil Clin N Am* 2000;11:785–803.

Stevens CS, Dubois RW, Larequi-Lauber T. Efficacy of lumbar discectomy and percutaneous treatments for lumbar disc herniation. *Soz Praventivmed* 1997;42:367–379.

Thomas E, Silman AJ, Croft PR, et al. Predicting who develops chronic low back pain in primary care: A prospective study. *BMJ* 1999;318: 1662–1667.

Yeoman W. The relation of arthritis of the sacroiliac joint to sciatica. *Lancet* 1928;2:1119–1122.

Zeidman SM, Long DM. Failed back surgery syndrome. In: Menezes AH, Sonntag VKH, eds. *Principles of Spinal Surgery.* vol 1. New York, NY: McGraw-Hill; 1996;657–679.

ADDENDUM: SPECIAL TESTS FOR LOW BACK PAIN

TESTS FOR RADICULOPATHY

Bow String Sign The patient is seated with the body bent forward and knee flexed to 70 degrees, a position that lengthens the course of the sciatic nerve. The examiner then applies pressure on the sciatic nerve by pressing the fingers into the popliteal fossa. An increase in leg pain signifies a radiculopathy.

Brudzinski's Test With the patient supine, the head is passively flexed to the chest. Reproduction of the patient's leg pain signifies nerve root irritation.

Kernig's Test The patient lies supine with the hip flexed 90 degrees. The patient is then asked to extend the knee. Back pain may be a sign of nerve root irritation.

Lasegue's Test The patient lies supine with the hip flexed 90 degrees. The patient is then asked to slowly extend his knee. A positive test occurs with the elicitation of sciatic pain.

Milgram's Test The patient, lying supine, is asked to elevate both extended legs approximately 2 inches off the examining table. If the patient can hold this position for 30 seconds without pain, it aids the examiner in eliminating intrathecal pathology as a cause of pain. If the patient experiences pain during this maneuver or cannot hold the position, intrathecal pathology, such as a herniated disk, must not be ruled out.

Naffziger's Test The examiner gently compresses the patient's jugular veins for about 10 seconds until the face begins to flush. The patient is then asked to cough, causing an increase in intrathecal pressure. Pain may indicate intrathecal pathology.

Stoop Test The patient is asked to walk briskly for several minutes. When back, posterior thigh, and leg pain appear, the patient sits and flexes forward. Disappearance of the pain suggest neurogenic claudication. During this time, reflexes may be diminished.

Straight-leg Raising Test With the patient lying supine, the affected leg is raised with the knee fully extended. A positive test reproduces the patient's radicular pain at between 30 and 70 degrees of elevation. Straight-leg raising is designed to stretch the affected nerve roots and dura and is especially useful for detecting radiculopathy involving the L4, L5, and S1 nerve roots. A variant of this test is the bilateral straight leg raising test, whereby the patient is asked to raise both legs simultaneously. Movement between 0 and 70 degrees tests the integrity of the sacroiliac joint. Movement above a 70-degree angle places stress on structures of the lumbar spine.

Valsalva's Test The patient is asked to bear down, as during a bowel movement or coughing, thus increasing intrathecal pressure. A positive test suggests intrathecal pathology.

Well Straight-leg Raising Test (Fajersztajn's Test) When the straight-leg raising test is performed on the asymptomatic leg, pain may be reproduced on the affected side. A positive test may indicate a large disk herniation.

TESTS FOR SACROILIAC JOINT DYSFUNCTION

Cranial Shear Test With the patient prone and the pelvis immobilized through the hip, pressure is applied to the coccygeal end of the sacrum. This test may be positive in patients with sacroiliac joint pain.

Extension Test The patient is placed in the prone position, with one hand of the examiner on the thigh of the affected side and other hand over the opposite iliac crest. Downward pressure is exerted on the iliac crest, while pulling slightly on the anterior thigh, to elicit sacroiliac joint pain.

Flamingo Test The patient is asked to stand on the involved leg and hop. Pain in the sacroiliac region is indicative of sacroiliac joint dysfunction.

Gaenslen's Test The patient lies supine on the examining table with both knees drawn to the chest. The patient is then asked to shift over to the edge of the table, so that the leg being tested hovers over the edge. The examiner presses down on the affected side, hyperextending the hip. A positive Gaenslen's test is generally considered a sign of sacroiliac joint pain but may indicate hip pathology as well.

Gillet's Test While the patient stands with the feet approximately 12 inches apart, the examiner sits behind the patient and palpates the S2 spinous process with one thumb and the posterior superior iliac spine with the other. As if taking a large marching step, the patient then flexes the knee and hip of the side being tested. If the posterior superior iliac spine fails to move posteroinferiorly with respect to S2, the test is positive. This test is an indicator of sacroiliac joint dysfunction.

Patrick's Test The patient is positioned supine with the foot of the involved side against the opposite knee. The sacroiliac joint is then stressed by pressing simultaneously against the flexed knee and contralateral anterior superior iliac supine. Although Patrick's test is predominantly used to assess sacroiliac joint dysfunction, pain in the inguinal or hip area may indicate hip pathology as well. Because this test involves *f*lexion, *ab*duction, and *e*xternal *r*otation of the hip, it is also called the FABER test.

Pelvic Compression Test This test compresses the pelvis by the application of lateral pressure to the uppermost iliac crest, directed toward the opposite iliac crest. It is believed to stretch the posterior sacroiliac ligaments and compress the anterior part of the joint.

Pelvic Distraction Test For this test, the examiner applies pressure to both anterior superior iliac spines, directed posteriorly and laterally. This test is alleged to stretch the anterior sacroiliac ligaments.

Pelvic Rock Test The patient lies supine, and the examiner cups both hands around the iliac crests with the thumbs on the anterior superior iliac spine and the palms on the iliac tubercles. The examiner then forcibly compresses the patient's pelvis toward the midline of the body. Complaints of pain may indicate pathology in the sacroiliac joint.

Sacroiliac Shear Test With the patient lying prone, the examiner crosses both hands over the sacrum. The overlying hand delivers a postero-anterior thrust, while the underlying hand is used to detect motion in the joint.

Thigh Thrust Test This test applies a posterior shearing stress to the sacroiliac joint through the femur.

TESTS FOR PIRIFORMIS SYNDROME

Beatty's Maneuver From the lateral decubitus position with the nonpainful side dependent, the patient is asked to abduct the thigh by moving the nonpainful leg off the table. Contraction of the piriformis muscle elicits pain in patients with piriformis syndrome.

Freiberg's Sign Recreation of buttock or leg pain, or both, occurs during internal rotation of the hip. This test may be positive in patients with piriformis syndrome.

Pace Sign An indicator of piriformis syndrome, this test is positive when the patient experiences weakness during resisted abduction and external rotation of the leg.

TESTS FOR MUSCLE PATHOLOGY

Beevor's Sign While the examiner observes the patient's umbilicus, the patient is asked to do a quarter sit-up with the arms crossed over the chest. Normally, the umbilicus should not move. If the umbilicus is drawn up, down, or over to one side (the stronger side), weakness, atrophy, or asymmetry of the anterior abdominal or paraspinal muscles may be present. This sign is frequently positive in patients with meningomyelocele or poliomyelitis.

Sit-up Test Patient's with severe discogenic pain or paraspinal muscle spasm have difficulty sitting up unassisted when flexed at their lumbar spine. They have a tendency to push up with their arms for support.

Tripod Sign As the patient sits with legs dangling and hips flexed 90 degrees, the knees are passively extended. Patients with hamstring muscle tightness will extend the trunk to relieve the pressure.

TESTS FOR MALINGERING OR FUNCTIONAL DISORDER

Hoover's Test This test is helpful when malingering is suspected, and should be performed in conjunction with the straight-leg raising test. A patient who is making a genuine effort to raise the affected leg will automatically put pressure on the calcaneus of his opposite leg in order to gain leverage. By placing one hand under the patient's heel, the examiner can determine whether or not the patient is making a concerted effort.

Kneeling Bench Test While kneeling on a 12-inch bench, the patient is asked to bend forward and touch the floor. The only requisite for this maneuver is flexion at the hips. If the hips are normal and the patient's fingers do not touch the floor, nonorganic pain is suspected.

Voluntary Release Test This test is used to distinguish patients with true organic pathology from those with nonorganic complaints. When attempting a sustained muscle contraction such as flexion at the ankle, patients with nonorganic symptoms sustain the position with jerking and quivering movements, and release the contraction in a similar fashion. In contrast, patients with organic pathology execute these movements smoothly.

Waddell's Signs The following physical signs are used to distinguish patients with organic pathology from those with functional disorders and malingering:

1. Tenderness. The skin is tender to light pinching over a large lumbar area, or deep tenderness is experienced over a wide area and is nonanatomic in distribution.
2. Stimulation tests. The patient complains of low back pain when vertical pressure is exerted on the skull, or reports back pain when the pelvis and torso are rotated in the same plane.
3. Distraction tests. A positive test is elicited in the normal fashion during physical examination. This test is then repeated when the patient is distracted. A positive distraction test finding occurs when pain elicited during a formal examination disappears when the patient is distracted.
4. Discrepancies between symptoms and neuroanatomy. Examples include the patient who exhibits sensory abnormalities in a stocking rather than a dermatomal distribution, or one who demonstrates unexplained motor weakness.
5. Overreaction during the examination. This may take the form of excessive facial expressions, yelling, jumping, or cringing.

TESTS FOR UPPER MOTOR LESIONS

Babinski's Reflex Stimulation is applied to the plantar surface of the foot with a dull object. When the lateral four toes flex and fan and the large toe extends, an upper motor lesion is suspected.

Chaddock Reflex This test is similar to the Babinski's reflex test, except that the lateral aspect of the foot beneath the lateral malleolus is stimulated.

Oppenheim's Test A dull object is run down the anterior portion of the tibia. A positive response is similar to Babinski's reflex.

MISCELLANEOUS TESTS

Femoral Stretch Test With the patient lying prone and the knees flexed, the legs are pushed backward toward the buttock. Pain felt in the anterior thigh may indicate entrapment of the femoral nerve or its nerve roots.

Schober's Test This test measures the flexibility of the lumbar spine. The patient's back is marked twice, once at the level of the sacroiliac dimples, and again 10 cm above this point. As the patient flexes forward, the distance between the two points should increase by at least 4 cm. An abnormal test may indicate spondyloarthropathy.

CHAPTER 29 FACET SYNDROME

Alicja Soczewko Steiner and Daniel P. Gray

More than 60% of people in developed countries will experience spinal pain at some time in their lives. Back pain is the most common complaint of patients referred to pain clinics. The pain is nonspecific in about 85% of the cases, and onset of symptoms is most often between the ages of 35 and 55 years. According to some sources, 15% to 45% of all adults experience lower back pain, and 1 in 20 people present with a new episode annually. Back pain absorbs approximately 40% of the cost of workers' compensation, which was estimated as $24 billion in 1990 and is considerably higher today.

Risk factors for spinal pain include trauma, heavy physical labor, frequent twisting, bending, vibrations, pulling and pushing, and repetitive motion, especially that involving static postures. Psychological features such as anxiety, depression, job dissatisfaction, and stress also can play an important role.

ANATOMIC CONSIDERATIONS

The spine consists of 7 cervical, 12 thoracic, and 5 lumbar vertebrae in addition to sacrum and coccyx. They articulate anteriorly through the disks and posteriorly through the left and right synovial facet joints. Anterior to the ligamentum flavum and covering the facet (apophyseal) joint is a variable amount of vascularized adipose tissue, which directly contacts the dural sleeve of the nerve root. The sleeve is located so close to the facet that it is possible, inadvertently, to inject medication directly into the cerebrospinal fluid. The articular surfaces of the facets are covered by cartilage. Joints are lined by synovium and contain variable amounts of fluid. The fibrous joint capsule forms superior and inferior joint recesses and blends anteromedially with the ligamentum flavum. It is located close to the neural foramen and the nerve root. Enlarged and osteophytic joints can contribute to significant narrowing of the neuroforaminal opening and can cause radicular symptoms.

Computed tomography (CT), magnetic resonance imaging (MRI), and intra-articular contrast medium can be used to demonstrate these anatomic features. The volume of injectate that can be accommodated by the facet joints varies as follows: cervical, 0.5 mL to 1.0 mL; thoracic, 0.4 mL to 0.6 mL; and lumbar, 1.0 mL to 2 mL.

In the upper lumbar spine, approximately 80% of the facet joints are curved and 20% are flat. This situation is reversed in the lower lumbar spine, where approximately 80% of the joints are flat. The upper lumbar facets are oriented more strongly in the sagittal plane, and by the L5 to Sl level, they rotate obliquely. The lumbar facet joints are oriented 45 degrees from the sagittal plane, but because of the curvature of the joints, the posterior part of the joint is close to the sagittal plane. Lumbar facet syndrome has been considered to be a significant source of lower back pain.

The thoracic facet joints are almost parallel to the coronal plane. They extend superiorly and inferiorly from the junctions of the laminae and pedicles and are oriented approximately 20 degrees from the coronal plane. Thoracic facet syndrome is less clearly established as a cause of spinal pain, and further investigation is required into this syndrome.

The anatomy of the cervical facets is significantly different from that of the lumbar ones. The cervical facets extend laterally from the junction of the laminae and pedicles and are oriented in the coronal plane to permit extension, flexion, and lateral bending. The atlanto-occipital and atlanto-axial joints are the C0–1 and C1–2 facet joints. Their structure, function, and innervation are unique. The C2–3 through C5–6 joints are angled 35 degrees from the coronal plane. The C6–7 apophyseal joint is tipped 22 degrees from the coronal plane. All of the cervical facet joints from C2–3 to C7–Tl are angled 110 degrees from the midline posterior sagittal plane, which makes their orientation similar to that of the thoracic facets. The cervical facets play a larger role, physically, in the spinal articular tripod structure and are commonly described as the superior and inferior ends of articular pillars. The vertebral artery, which passes through the transverse foramen of the transverse processes of the C1 to C6 vertebrae, is a landmark of the cervical spine. The prevalence of pain in the cervical spine approaches that of the lumbar spine.

The facet joints appear to function to protect the spine from excessive mobility and distribute axial loading over a broad area. The orientation and shape of the facets are specifically designed to accommodate the stresses and movements expected at each spinal level.

NEUROANATOMY OF THE FACET JOINTS

The nonspecific localization of facet joint pain is explained by profuse overlapping of sensory innervation. The medial branch nerve supplies the lower facet at its own level as well as the upper part of the joint below. Therefore, each of the facet joints receives innervation from a medial branch nerve of two posterior primary rami. These branches also innervate the paraspinal muscles, ligaments, and periosteum, with significant dermatomal sensory overlapping.

In the lumbar region (Fig. 29-1), the medial branch nerve lies in a groove on the base of the superior articular facet and passes between the mammillary and accessory processes. It then runs in a posterior and inferior direction, first sending fibers to innervate the adjacent joint capsule before sending fibers to the next lower level. The course of the L5 medial branch is different, because the transverse process is replaced by the ala of the sacrum. The lumbosacral facet probably has additional innervation from the Sl nerve root branch, which should be blocked to completely anesthetize the L5-S1 zygapophyseal joint. Because of the dual nerve innervation, each joint must be blocked at two segments, both at and

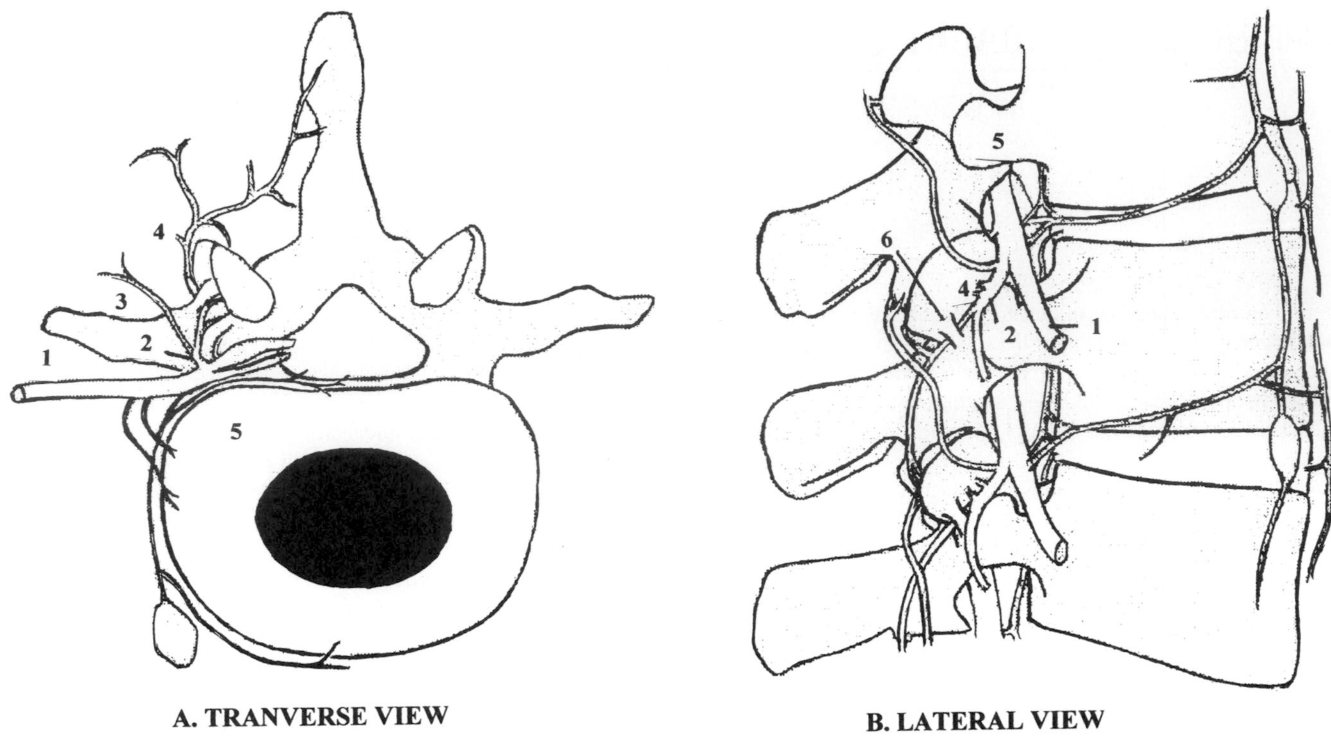

Figure 29-1 Lumbar spine anatomy. **1.** Spinal nerve, **2.** Posterior primary ramus, **3.** Lateral branch, **4.** Medial branch, **5.** Sinu-vertebral nerve (innervation to the disc annulus).

above the level of the involved joint. The lumbosacral facet joint should be blocked at least two if not three levels.

There is evidence of multilevel innervation of the lumbar facet joints, which includes not only the posterior primary rami, but also the sympathetic and parasympathetic ganglia. The sympathetic fibers have been reported to regulate the activity of sensory neurons and may contribute to the experience of lower back pain.

Innervation of the thoracic facets is similar to that of the lumbar spine. Medial branches from two segmental levels innervate each joint. Below the T3 level this pattern is consistent, but the C7 and C8 branches may travel caudally as far as the level of T2 and T3. The exception to this description occurs at the midthoracic level, where the nerves do not reliably make bony contact with the superolateral corner of the transverse process. The T11 branch also has different anatomic features and runs across the lateral surface of the root of the relatively smaller T12 transverse process. At the T12 level, the medial branch localization is analogous to that of the lumbar spine.

The cervical medial branches (Fig. 29-2) mainly supply the facet joints, with minimal innervations of the following posterior neck muscles: multifidus, interspinalis, semispinalis cervicis, and semispinalis capitis. The C3 dorsal branch is the only cervical dorsal ramus below C2 that has a cutaneous distribution. Therefore, if neck pain or headache is caused by cervical facet disease, cervical facet joint blocks can relieve it.

The upper cervical synovial joints—the atlanto-occipital and lateral atlanto-axial joints—are innervated by cervical ventral rami (Fig. 29-3). The only suitable procedure to relieve pain at these joints is an intra-articular injection. The C2-3 facet joint is innervated mainly by the third occipital nerve and sometimes by the C2 dorsal rami (the greater occipital nerve). There are eight cervical nerves and seven cervical vertebrae. The first seven cervical nerve roots exit the spine above the vertebral body, and they are numbered according to the vertebral body below them. The C3–4 through C7–Tl facet joints are supplied by the medial branches at the same level as the joint and from the segmental level above. These nerves branch off from the cervical posterior primary rami and wrap around the waists of the articular pillars (viewed as "centroid" of the articular pillar on the lateral projection). They are attached to the periosteum by fascia and tendons of the semispinalis capitis.

PATHOGENESIS OF FACET SYNDROME

Ghormley was the first to define facet syndrome, describing it as lumbosacral pain with or without sciatic pain and associated with sprain or violent twisting of the facet joint. Since then, much research has been carried out to identify the pathologic processes involved and to find a specific therapeutic approach to this disease.

Neurophysiologic studies have shown that the medial branch nerves transmit nociceptive and proprioceptive signals from the facet joints, which are triggered by inflammatory and mechanical factors. Researchers have identified multiple mechanosensitive somatosensory receptors and neuromodulators of nociception within the facet capsule, including calcitonin gene–related peptide, substance P, and vasoactive intestinal peptide. Chronic inflammation, with consecutive joint hypertrophy, degeneration, and osteophyte formation, may contribute to neuraminal narrowing and compression of the nerve roots. On occasion, this causes referred pain to the extremities, as well as abnormal joint stress with possible subluxation and muscle spasm (Fig. 29-4). Pain originating from the

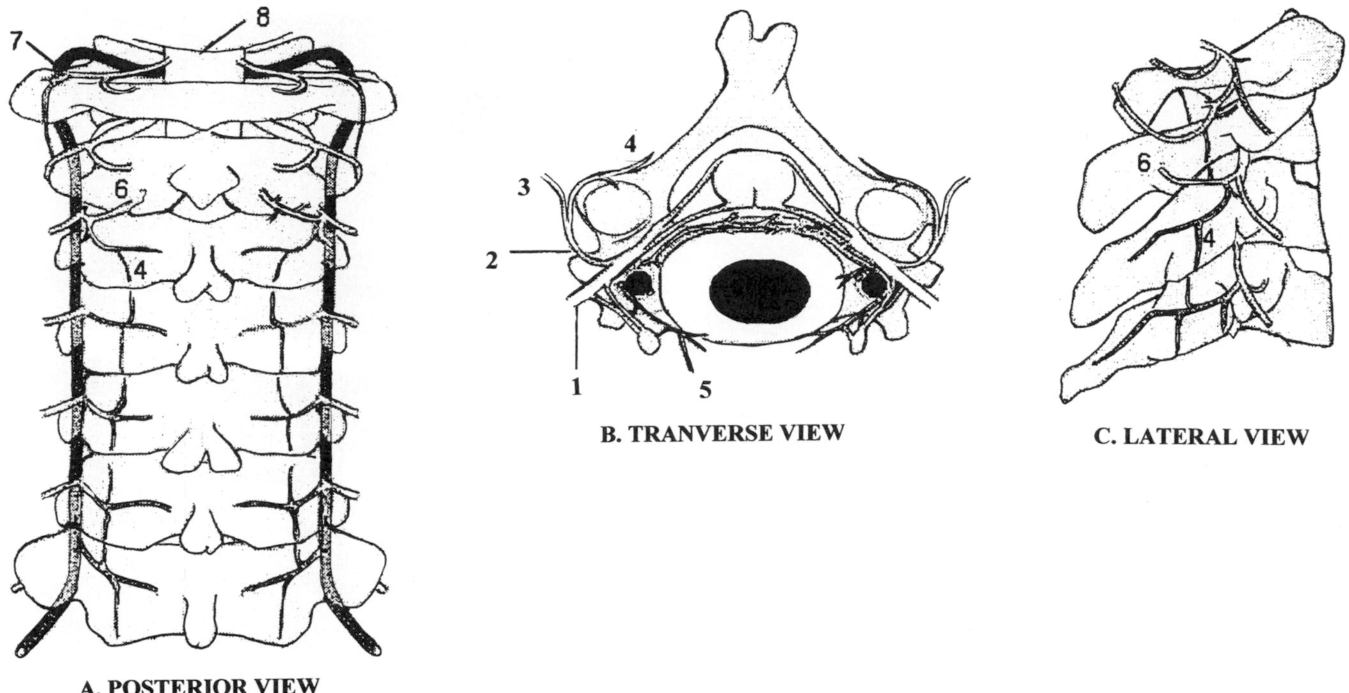

Figure 29-2 Illustration of the cervical zygapophyseal (facet joint) anatomy. **1.** Segmental nerve root, **2.** Posterior primary ramus, **3.** Lateral branch.

apophyseal joints can be attributed to a synovitis, degenerative arthritis, and segmental instability.

The pathophysiology of thoracic and cervical facet syndrome can be explained by the same factors that are exhibited in the lumbar spine. There is also growing evidence that cervical facet syndrome can contribute to the etiology of cervicogenic headaches.

FACET BLOCKING: INDICATIONS AND CONTRAINDICATIONS

The clinical picture of facet joint syndrome is difficult to describe. The diagnosis is one of exclusion based on careful physical examination, medical history, and possible reproduction of pain during facet injections. The classic, unreliable features of the lumbar facet pain include (Fig. 29-5A):

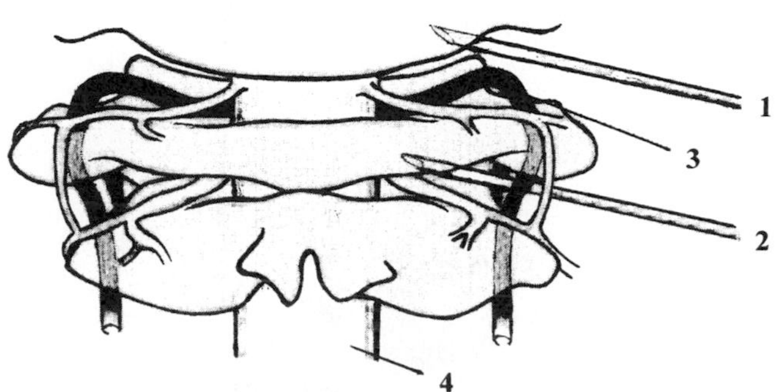

Figure 29-3 Illustration of **1.** Atlanto-occipital joint injection, **2.** Atlanto-axial joint injection, **3.** Vertebral artery, **4.** Spinal cord.

- Pain located in the lower back with occasional (unilateral or bilateral) radiation to the buttock, groin, hip, and lower extremities, usually above level of the knee
- Pain that is dull, deep, and difficult to describe
- No evidence of neurologic deficits
- Paralumbar tenderness with or without muscle spasm
- Onset of symptoms associated with twisting, bending, or rotation
- Deterioration by lateral bending, extension, sitting, and forward flexion in the standing position
- Symptoms improved by walking
- No aggravation on Valsalva's maneuver or during walking
- Evidence of degenerative changes on radiologic studies
- An increased uptake during technetium Tc 99 scanning

The manifestations of thoracic pain syndrome are thought to be similar to those of lumbar pain syndrome, but data are limited on this subject (Fig. 29-5B).

Patients with cervicalgia (Figs. 29-5C and 29-6) can be diagnosed on the basis of the initiating factors. People with prior trauma may have whiplash syndrome and possible cervicogenic headaches. Pathophysiology of this syndrome includes:

- Facet joints sprain with muscle and ligament involvement
- Nerve root irritation
- Muscle spasm
- Occasional periosteal tearing

Patients without a history of trauma may have degenerative disease as a primary diagnosis.

Radiographic facet joint changes are common and nonspecific in adults. Routine lumbar radiographs may be normal or may reveal facet degeneration with or without changes in the discs. Arthrography is an additional study that may provide some limited

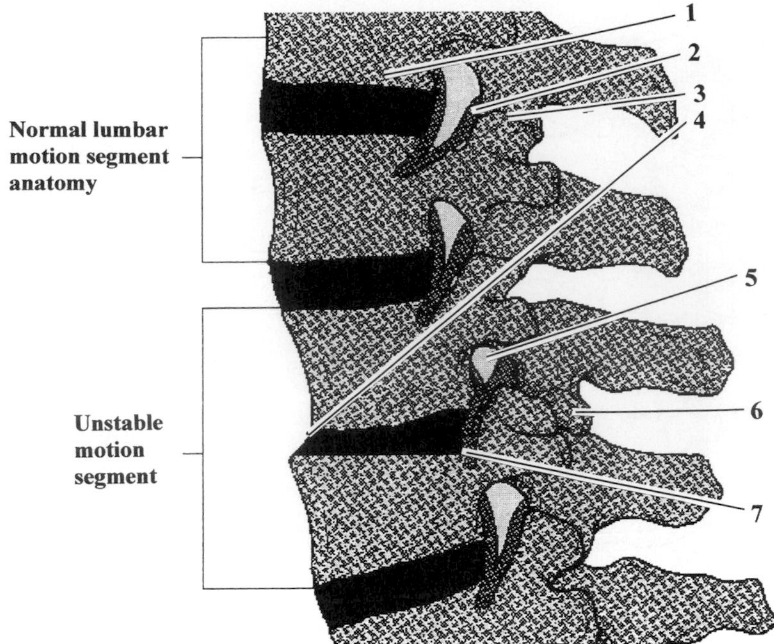

Figure 29-4 Anatomy of normal and degenerative zygopophyseal joints explaining possible mechanisms of facet syndrome. **1.** Vertebrae, **2.** Spinal nerve, **3.** Normal facet joint, **4.** Retrolisthesis, **5.** Narrowing of intervertebral foramen with compression of adjacent nerve root, **6.** Subluxation, **7.** Intervetebral disk narrowing due to degeneration.

data based on the spread of the dye. CT and MRI do not provide specific information, although some studies have suggested that CT and single photon emission computed topography (SPECT) have some value as tools to assess clinically significant facet joint disease. Nevertheless, it seems that a radiographically normal joint is unlikely to be a significant pain generator except in the case of whiplash syndrome.

The clinical criteria for making the diagnosis of facet syndrome are nonspecific. Interventional procedures should be offered to patients without neurologic deficits or other causes for their pain who have exhausted conservative treatment measures (analgesics, bed rest, physical therapy). Interventional techniques consists of:

- Intra-articular or periarticular injections of local anesthetics and corticosteroids
- Medial branch nerve blocks
- Neuroablative facet denervation with radiofrequency and cryotherapy
- Surgical spinal fusion with stabilization of facet joints

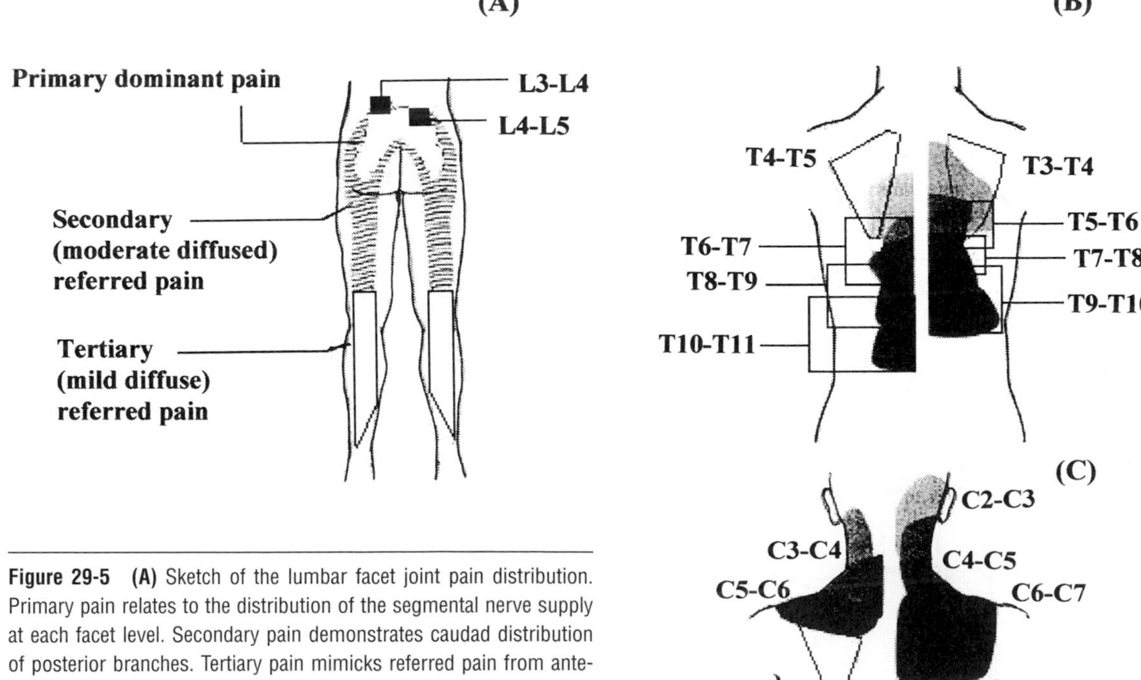

Figure 29-5 **(A)** Sketch of the lumbar facet joint pain distribution. Primary pain relates to the distribution of the segmental nerve supply at each facet level. Secondary pain demonstrates caudad distribution of posterior branches. Tertiary pain mimicks referred pain from anterior division of the segmental nerve. **(B)** Sketch of thoracic facet joint pain distribution. **(C)** Sketch of cervical facet joint pain distribution.

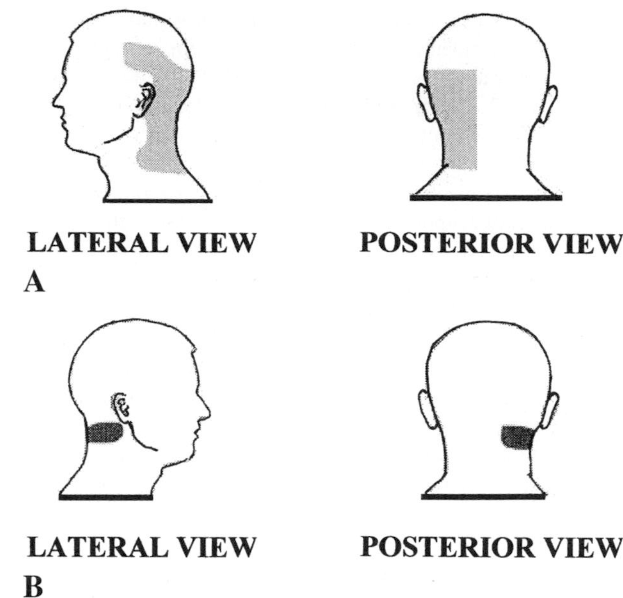

Figure 29-6 **(A)** Atlanto-occipital joint. **(B)** Atlanto-axial (C1-C2) joint.

In the thoracic and cervical spine, the joints to be injected should be selected based on clinical evaluation in conjunction with the presence of radiologic abnormalities analogous to those seen in the lumbar spine.

There are no absolute contraindications to facet injections other than those for any regional block; specifically, coagulopathies and systemic or local infection at the site of the injection. Allergy to contrast media is a relative contraindication, because the procedure can be performed without dye under fluoroscopic guidance or with the use of newer, nonionic contrast agents.

FACET BLOCKING TECHNIQUES

Lumbar Facet Blocks

For this procedure, the patient is placed in the prone position, with the back slightly flexed and the hips supported by pillows. The injection is performed under sterile conditions and with continuous vital sign monitoring. The oblique fluoroscopic view reveals a typical facet joint picture reminiscent of a "Scottie dog." The back of the Scottie dog's head is formed by the inferior articular process, and the front feet are created by the vertebra below. Local anesthetic is injected at the point where an imaginary line from the center of the intensifier intersects the skin on the way toward the facet joint. The clinician advances a 20- or 22-gauge, 10-cm spinal needle, or a thin probe designed for neuroablation, to the desired position under fluoroscopic guidance. A small amount of radiologic dye (0.25 to 0.5 mL) may be injected to visualize placement of the needle tip prior to instilling 1.0 to 1.5 mL of injectate (i.e., 2%–4% lidocaine with 20 mg of triamcinolone or methylprednisolone). The feel of the needle "walking off" the bone into the joint can also confirm the proper position.

Medial branch blocks are performed using a similar technique, but the final needle placement is different. The medial branch is blocked at the junction of the dorsal surface of the transverse process and vertebral body, just caudal to the most medial end of the superior edge of the transverse process. At the lumbosacral level, the posterior primary ramus of L5 is blocked in the groove between the ala of the sacrum and the superior articular process of the sacrum. Blocking a single joint requires that the two medial branch nerves be injected. At the L5-Sl level, the S1 nerve branch should also be blocked. It is located cephalad to the S1 posterior opening in a line between the S1 opening and the L5-Sl facet joint. To make a precise injection, the use of a small volume of local anesthetic (0.5–1.0 mL) is mandatory.

For therapeutic purposes, a less specific periarticular injection can be performed using a larger volume of injectate.

Thoracic Facet Block

There is very limited research into thoracic facet denervation and, at this time, the only recommended injections are either intra-articular or periarticular. This procedure is conducted with the patient in the prone position, using the ribs as the main landmark. The steep angle of the joints requires that the skin entry point overlie the distal pedicle located one or two segments caudally to the intended joint.

Cervical Facet Block

To perform blockade of the C3 through C7 medial branches, the patient is placed in a lateral position with the side to be blocked superior. A 22- or 25-gauge spinal needle is inserted using a posterolateral approach. The target point is the periosteum at the centroid of the projection of the articular pillar as seen on the lateral fluoroscopic image. After a negative aspiration of blood or cerebrospinal fluid, 0.5 mL of local anesthetic is injected very slowly. The medial branch of the C8 nerve crosses the Tl transverse process and runs medially onto the lamina of T1, where it should be blocked.

Intra-articular blockade of cervical facets C3 through C7 is performed using a 22-gauge, 10-cm spinal needle. The needle is inserted one to two levels below the joint to be blocked and is advanced upward and forward into the joint. A maximum of 0.5 to 1.0 mL of injectate (including the dye) should be administered to avoid rupture of the facet joint.

Blockade of the C2-3 facet joint requires location of the third occipital nerve. The target points are located along a vertical line that bisects the articular pillar of C3. Injections should be made immediately above the subchondral plate of the C2 inferior articular process and below the subchondral plate of the C3 superior articular process, as well as at a point between these two. At each of these three sites, 0.5 mL of local anesthetic is injected.

The atlantoaxial joint is usually blocked via a posterolateral approach with the patient in the lateral decubitus position. The patient's head should be slightly flexed and rotated 45 degrees toward the table. The lateral half of the posterior capsule is the final target for a 25-gauge needle. The mastoid process, the occipital prominence, and, located between them, the occipital brim are bony landmarks. With oblique imaging, the C-arm of the fluoroscope and head are moved until the occipital brim is located over the superior, posterior, and lateral aspect of the joint (the destination point). This procedure is complex. The needle is advanced slowly along this path. This position is confirmed regularly with posteroanterior, open mouth, lateral, and oblique views. The final needle placement is visualized using arthrography. Aspiration for blood or cerebrospinal fluid should precede the administration of dye and medication (total volume of 1 mL).

NEUROABLATION OF THE FACET JOINTS

Facet denervation is performed on the medial branch nerves with cryotherapy or, more often, radiofrequency lesioning using the same technique to locate the nerves as for the medial branch blocks. Previous diagnostic blocks determine which facets should be neuroablated. A single lumbar facet denervation requires that two nerves be treated, and three in the case of the L5-Sl facet joint. Two nerves also are denervated for each of the cervical facets, C3-4 to C7-T1. The technique of denervation of these cervical facets is slightly different. The C2-3 facet joint requires three-point lesioning, as in the technique described earlier. Because denervation is obviously a destructive procedure and carries some risk of deafferentation pain and neurologic deficits, there must be clear indications for this treatment. The current criteria for facet denervation are not uniform. The best proposal is to perform the denervation after it has been twice demonstrated that clear pain relief can be achieved using diangostic blocks.

Thoracic medial branch denervation is not recommended because of the lack of a reliable technique for medial branch blocks in this region of the spine.

ADVERSE EFFECTS

Complications secondary to interventions on the facet joints are rare and usually transient. They include:

- Exacerbation of pain
- Failure to relieve pain
- Spinal or epidural anesthesia with or without transient motor and sensory blocks
- Infection and abscess formation
- Chemical meningitis
- Puncture of the vessel, including vertebral artery, with possible local anesthetic toxicity
- Transient ataxia caused by partial blockade of the third occipital nerve and proprioceptive afferents
- Persistent motor or sensory deficits (neuroablative procedures)
- Allergic reactions

EFFICACY OF FACET JOINT BLOCKS

The reported success of facet joint injections and neuroablation varies widely, with positive outcomes cited that range from 16% to 83%. These results were derived mainly from poorly designed studies that were neither randomized nor controlled trials. Accurate clinical diagnosis and careful patient selection are essential to ensure a good outcome. Other causes of low back pain, such as neoplasm, myofascial pain, degenerative disk disease, infection, and spondylolysis, must be excluded.

CONCLUSION

In the assessment of patients with spinal pain, it is essential to rule out serious pathology that requires neurologic or surgical evaluation. Interventions should always be integrated with a well-tailored treatment program that is individually designed for each patient. A one-size–fits-all approach to the problem of spinal pain is neither efficient nor prudent. Facet syndrome remains a diagnosis of exclusion that cannot be confirmed definitively by any specific laboratory, radiologic, or clinical findings. Conservative management should always be offered before scheduling interventional procedures. It is well known that about 80% of people with acute low back pain of a mechanical nature and without a radicular component will recover spontaneously within 6 weeks (with help of simple analgesic and physical therapy), often without any complications or absenteeism from work.

The patient who was screened for other causes of spinal pain and who has a clinical picture of facet pain correlating with radiologic evidence of facet abnormalities usually responds to facet injections. The success rate is significantly reduced in patients with a history of spinal surgery, especially fusion. No one can deny that some of these patients have benefited from the procedure, and there is little to gain and nothing to loose for those who have exhausted other conventional therapies.

The selection of surgical candidates for spinal fusion based on positive facet blocks should be carried out with the knowledge of current diagnostic limitations. These procedures require further extensive studies and well-designed research before clinicians will be able to prove the benefit of such interventions.

BIBLIOGRAPHY

Anderson GBJ. The epidemiology of spinal disorders. In: Frymoyer JW, ed. *The Adult Spine: Principles and Practice.* 2nd ed. New York, NY: Raven Press; 1997:93–141.

Bland JH, Boushey DR. Anatomy and physiology of the cervical spine. *Semin Arthritis Rheum* 1990;20:1–20.

Bogduk N. The innervation of the lumbar spine. *Spine* 1983;8:286–293.

Bogduk N, Anat D. The clinical anatomy of the cervical dorsal rami. *Spine* 1982;7:319–330.

Bogduk N, Marsland A. The cervical zygapophysial joints as a source of the neck pain. *Spine* 1988;13:610–617.

Cavanaugh JM. Lumbar facet pain: Biomechanics, neuroanatomy and neurophysiology. *J Biomech* 1996:29:1117–1129.

Cho J, Park YG, Chung SS. Percutaneous radiofrequency lumbar rhizotomy in mechanical low back pain syndrome. *Stereotact Func Neurosurg* 1997;68;212–217.

Chua WH, Bogduk N. The surgical anatomy of thoracic facet denervation. *Acta Neurochir* 1995;136:140–144.

Deyo RA, Rainville J, Kent DL. What can the history and physical examination tell us about low back pain? *JAMA* 1992;268:760–765.

Dreyfuss P, Michaelsen M, Fletcher D. Atlanto-occipital and lateral atlantoaxial joint pain patterns. *Spine* 1994;19:1125–1131.

Dreyfuss P, Tibiletti C, Dreyer S. Thoracic zygapophyseal joint pain patterns. *Spine* 1994;19:807–811.

Dweyer A, Aprill C, Bogduk N. Cervical zygapophyseal joint pain patterns I. A study in normal volunteers. *Spine* 1990;15:453–457.

Dweyer A, Aprill C, Bogduk N. Cervical zygapophyseal joint pain patterns II. A clinical evaluation. *Spine* 1990;15:458–461.

Falco FJ. Lumbar spine injection procedures in the management of low back pain. *Occup Med* 1998;13:121–149.

Ghormley RK. Low back pain with special reference to the articular facet with presentation of an operative procedure. *JAMA* 1993;101:1773–1777.

Grob D. Surgery in the degenerative cervical spine. *Spine* 1998;23:2674–2683.

Hourigan CL, Bassett JM. Facet syndrome: Clinical signs, symptoms, diagnosis, and treatment. *J Manipulative Physiol Ther* 1989;12:293–297.

Jerosch J, Castro WHM, Liljenqvist U. Percutaneous facet coagulation: Indication, technique, results, and complications. *Neurosurg Clin North Am* 1999;7(1):119–139.

Kaplan M, Dreyfuss P, Halbrook B, et al. The ability of lumbar medial branch blocks to anesthetize the zygapophyseal joint: A physiologic challenge. *Spine* 1998;23:1847–1852.

Lovely TY, Rastogi P. The value of provocative facet blocking as a predictor of success in lumbar spinal fusion. *J Spinal Disord* 1997;10:512–517.

Manchikanti L. Facet joint pain and the role of neural blockade in its management. *Curr Rev Pain* 1999;3:348–358.

Nelemans PJ, deBie RA, DeVet HC, Sturmans AF. Injection therapy for subacute and chronic benign low back pain. *Spine* 2001;26:501–515.

North RB, Han M, Zahurak M, Kidd DH. Radiofrequency lumbar facet denervation: Analysis of prognostic factors. *Pain* 1994;57:77–83.

Savage RA. The relationship between the magnetic resonance imaging appearance of the lumbar spine and low back pain, age, and occupation in males. *Eur Spine J* 1997;6:106–114.

Schwarzer AC, Derby R, Aprill CN, et al. The value of the provocation response in lumbar zygapophyseal joint injections. *Clin J Pain* 1994;10: 309–313.

Tzaan WC, Tasker RR. Percutaneous radiofrequency facet rhizotomy-experience with 118 procedures and reappraisal of its value. *Can J Neurol Sci* 2000;27:125–130.

CHAPTER 30 FAILED BACK SURGERY SYNDROME

Ranjan Dey and Thomas T. Simopoulos

DEFINITION

Failed back surgery syndrome (FBSS) was defined by North and Campbell in 1991 as persistent or recurring low back pain, with or without sciatica, following one or more lumbar spine operations.[1] Van Goethem and colleagues describe it as a syndrome characterized by intractable pain and various degrees of functional incapacitation, following spine surgery.[2] Rowlingson uses the term *failed back surgery syndrome* for patients with chronic debilitating low back pain occurring in a patient after back surgery of a variety of types, such as discectomy, laminectomy, and lumbosacral fusion, that was unsuccessful in relieving the patient's symptoms.[3] Fiume and colleagues consider FBSS to be a severe, long-lasting, disabling, and relatively frequent (5%–10%) complication of lumbosacral spine surgery.[4] Although disability and chronic pain are commonly seen in the lumbosacral region and the lower extremity, similar mechanisms, pathophysiology, diagnostic dilemmas, and management options can be seen and extrapolated to the cervicothoracic region and the upper extremity.

HISTORY

In 1934, Mixter and Barr demonstrated that a herniated disc could cause nerve root encroachment, ultimately producing back pain.[5] In 1951, Barr determined that a patient might have persistent low back pain, sciatica, or both, despite surgical intervention.[6] In 1979, Finneson and Cooper made a statement that, "No matter how severe or intractable the pain, it can always be made worse by surgery."[7] The cause of FBSS has been recognized to be multifactorial over the past decade.

EPIDEMIOLOGY

Population studies indicate that of all patients with acute back and leg pain, only 1% to 2% actually suffer from disc herniation and require surgery.[8] Nearly 300,000 spinal surgeries are performed each year in the United States.[9] Approximately 85% of these procedures involve laminectomy and discectomy and 15% are spinal fusions.[10] The success rate in most surgical series ranged from 80% to 98%.[11–17] Nachemson[17] has pointed out that the success rate drops in a dramatic fashion after the first operation. The success rate drops to about 30% after the second operation, 15% after the third, and 5% after the fourth. The difference in patient populations and evaluation criteria make it difficult to compare the various series published to date. Principally, the results are variable, because of the different procedures being grouped as one.

In a retrospective study by Dvorak and colleagues, 371 post–disc surgery patients were interviewed 4 to 17 years later by neurologists.[18] As many as 70% had residual low back pain; 23% had severe, permanent low back pain; 45% had residual nerve root pain; 35% patients were undertreated; 14% received disability benefits; and 17.2% patients received repeat surgery. Fritch and colleagues conducted a retrospective study on 182 revisions with FBSS from 1965 to 1990, to identify the cause of failure of primary discectomy, the outcome of revisions, and factors that influenced these outcomes.[19] The rate of revision surgery ranged from 5% to 33%. In 80% of patients, the results were satisfactory in short-term evaluation, decreasing to 22% in long-term follow-up (2 to 27 years). Fritch also concluded that laminectomy performed as primary surgery was a major factor leading to a higher rate of revisions. Furthermore, it can be deduced from various studies that a significant percentage of patients who undergo spinal surgery do not achieve what they and their surgeons agree to be a satisfactory result. FBSS is, therefore, a common clinical entity that represents a significant treatment challenge to physicians.

ETIOLOGY

Different authors have classified the various causes of FBSS in multiple ways. Goupille classified it according to the clinical presentation, as follows.[20]

I. No improvement
   a. Faulty technique
   b. Creation of a new source of impingement
   c. Poor patient selection
II. Recurrence after a period of improvement
   a. Recurrent herniation
   b. Other source of impingement
   c. Postoperative "fibrosis"
III. Persistent low back pain
   a. Destabilization
   b. Disc degeneration
   c. Facet joint syndrome
   d. Complications (discitis)

Van Goethem and colleagues subdivided causes of FBSS according to mechanisms, diagnosis, and surgical approach.[2]

I. Mechanical
   a. Recurrent or residual disc herniation
   b. Spinal canal stenosis
   c. Foraminal stenosis
II. Inflammation
   a. Epidural fibrosis
   b. Arachnoiditis
   c. Spondylodiscitis
III. Diagnostic
   Failure to correctly identify the structural source of pain
   a. Conjoined nerve roots
   b. Disc herniation at different level
   c. Peripheral nerve lesion

IV. Surgically induced
  a. Dorsal ramus nerve lesions
  b. Facet joint strain
  c. Sacroiliac joint dysfunction
  d. Erector trunci tendinitis

Poor Patient Selection

Irrespective of the classification, the commonest cause of failed back surgery syndrome is poor patient selection.[1,21] In fact, despite a scoring system for predicting the outcome of lumbar disc excision, the postoperative results have not been very promising.[7,12,17,19] In a multi-center, nationwide, prospective study of the outcome of first-time back surgery, it was determined that over 90% of patients improved when chosen for surgery by expert spinal surgeons. A small group of patients considered to be inappropriate candidates for surgery, as determined by these same experts, had surgery elsewhere. Only 10% improved after an operation performed outside the study, with a resultant worsening of symptoms in a significant portion of these patients.[22]

Waddell, in an assessment of the outcome of low back surgery, stated that it is important to remember that failure of first surgery with residual pain is not an indication for second surgery.[23] He noted that there was a tendency of some surgeons to carry out a decompression procedure with or without discectomy, and then to follow that with fusion when the first procedure failed to relieve pain symptoms. The problem is frequently that the first procedure was ill chosen. In addition, psychological or environmental factors have a major impact on the presentation of low back pain. Indeed, psychological evaluation seems more predictive of the outcome of surgery than the diagnostic studies or surgical findings.

Despite a surgeon's refusal to perform surgery, many patients will "doctor shop"—to pursue a lawsuit, attract sympathy and attention, avoid an unpleasant job or employer, or acquire financial compensation.[24] Thus, inappropriate behavior by the surgeon as well as the patient can lead to FBSS.

Work-related injuries or patients who are sick-listed seem not to benefit from any modalities of treatment.[25] Hansson and Hansson conducted a prospective 2-year cohort study in six countries, including the United States, involving 2,080 subjects who had been sick-listed for more than 90 days. Their objective was to find out the impact of medical interventions, including surgery, in patients with low back pain who are incapacitated at work. The authors concluded that almost none of the frequently practiced medical interventions for patients who are sick-listed because of low back pain had any positive effects on either the recorded health measures or work resumption.

Lastly, some patients have an unrealistic expectation of a complete return to full premorbid function with total absence of pain postoperatively; this expectation can result in some disappointment. It is imperative to explain to the patient that the recovery of damaged nerves is very unpredictable. The expected recovery is variable and may take from months to a year. Clinically, a short duration of symptoms has a much more favorable outcome.

Failure to Correct the Initial Pathology

The failure to decompress the spinal canal, to remove a disc entirely, to decompress a nerve root or roots through foraminotomy, or to miss sequestrated free disc fragments can result in minimal symptomatic improvement. Also, operating at the wrong level or not stabilizing unstable segments can contribute to FBSS. The failures of interventions to correct the primary problem have been confirmed by repeat imaging studies.[26]

Epidural Fibrosis

Epidural fibrosis is one of the major causes of FBSS.[30] The reported incidence of epidural fibrosis ranges from 10% to 75%.[28] The exact pathogenesis of epidural fibrosis is not well established. One possible mechanism accounting for fibrosis following surgery may be related to persistent cotton debris from sponges used during surgery, serving as a fibrogenic stimulus.[29] Metal dust arising from poor-quality surgical tools (e.g., periosteal elevators) has also been identified as one of the potential causative factors leading to the development of epidural fibrosis.[26] The scar tissue that forms at the surgical site does not seem to correlate with the extensiveness of the surgical procedure.[29]

Alternatively, arachnoepiduritis may develop, causing ischemia and atrophy of nerve roots. It has also been shown that there is no correlation between the amount of scar tissue and the severity of symptoms. Although there is no clear evidence that epidural fibrosis can cause symptoms, adhesions may bind the dural sac and nerve root sheaths to the walls of the spinal canal, stretching nerve roots. It seems that postoperative fibrosis is an entity usually associated with a distinctive pattern of pain. The pain-free interval lasts weeks to several months (approximately 6 weeks to 6 months). The pain usually sets in gradually; its distribution is not confined to that of the initially compromised nerve root, but extends to multiple nerve roots. It is commonly described as a burning sensation with occasional lancinations.[20]

Some important nonsurgical causes of epidural fibrosis are annular tear, hematoma, infection, and intrathecal contrast media. Regardless of the cause, the pathology involves collagenous fibers that encapsulate nerve tissues, resulting in lateral spinal stenosis, which could impair arterial tissue perfusion and venous return. This anoxic phenomenon is one explanation for pain at rest. Also, epidural fibrosis causing adhesions may restrict nerve root mobility, leading to increased incidence of lateral herniated disk symptoms with increased tension, decreased blood flow, or additional trauma. Scar tissue is generally found in three components of the epidural space. Dorsal epidural scar tissue is formed by resorption of surgical hematomas and may be involved in pain generation.[29] In the ventral epidural space, dense scar tissue is formed by ventral defects in the disc, which may persist despite surgical treatment and continue to produce chronic low back pain/radiculopathy past the surgical healing phase.[30] The lateral epidural space includes structures like the nerve roots and dorsal root ganglia, called the sleeves that exit the root canals, which are susceptible to lateral disc defects, facet overgrowth, and neuroforaminal stenosis.[31] On the other hand, Pawl investigated post-laminectomy surgical patients with epidural fibrosis and found no clear relationship to pain except in cases with excessive scarring in the first year of surgery.[32]

Recurrent Disc Herniation

Another important cause of repeat symptoms in patients previously operated on for lumbar disc herniation is recurrence of disc herniation at either the same or an adjacent level.[33] In nearly 20% of postoperative patients, there is asymptomatic disc herniation even with impingement of the nerve root. Epidural fibrosis that may coexist with a disc herniation makes it difficult to determine the pain generator.

A herniated disc can cause pain through physical or chemical mechanisms. Pressure-induced changes in nerve fibers are dependent on the degree of force. For instance, an applied pressure of 10 mm Hg decreases the nutrient transport to the nerve roots by 20% to 30%.[34] Compression may also produce edema and lead to formation of intraneural fibrosis. Pressures as high as 200 mm Hg can produce a direct mechanical effect by deformation of nerve fibers, displacement of the nodes of Ranvier, or invagination of the paranodal myelin sheaths.[35] Such high pressure can result in persistent neural injury, especially when compression occurs near the neuronal cell body. Thus, it has been noted that delaying decompression of acute disc herniation for longer than 6 months after the onset is more likely to result in persistent postoperative pain. Moreover, premorbid conditions, including age and coexisting neuropathy, may also influence the recovery of neural function after surgical decompression.[20]

Chemical irritation is another factor responsible for back pain with or without radiculopathy. Degenerative disc disease and tears of the annulus fibrosus may result in the leakage of various chemical irritants. Surgical disc samples from patients with disc herniation have been shown to contain extremely high levels of phospholipase A_2.[36] This enzyme liberates arachidonic, the principal mediator of inflammation and swelling along a nerve root, from cell membranes. In addition it has been theorized that material from the nucleus pulposus might act as a foreign protein and trigger an autoimmune reaction.[34] Obviously, chemically induced irritation can occur in the absence of compression by a disc herniation.

Other Perioperative Surgical Complications

Acute unremitting postoperative pain, tenderness, and neurologic deficits are secondary to hematoma formation. Evacuation of the hematoma produces dramatic pain relief on most occasions. There is an associated low risk of injuries to the spinal cord and nerve roots during surgery. However, more commonly, peripheral nerves, dura, joints, and muscles can be damaged and serve as a source of persistent pain postoperatively.

The failure of fusion can occasionally lead to spinal instability. Pseudoarthrosis in the adjacent joints can occur after a generous laminectomy, or pars fracture. Transition syndrome can result from accelerated degenerative changes at levels adjacent to a spinal fusion.[37] Flat back syndrome follows loss of the normal lordosis. This abnormality is frequently found after extensive fusion or instrumentation. Abnormal posturing is often seen, and a common complication is accelerated degenerative changes causing new pain.

Nonsurgical Causes of Failed Back Surgery Syndrome

Arachnoiditis Inflammatory changes in the nerve roots and the surrounding arachnoid mater secondary to surgical trauma, infection, bleeding, disc disease, or myelography can result in arachnoiditis. Arachnoiditis progresses in three stages. The first stage is radiculitis, characterized by inflammation of the pia-arachnoid mater, with hyperemia and swelling of the nerve roots. There is minimal fibroblast activation, but collagen strands begin to deposit between the nerve roots and pia-arachnoid mater. The second stage is arachnoiditis, characterized by increased fibroblast proliferation and collagen deposition. Although there is less swelling, the nerve roots adhere to each other and to the arachnoid mater. The final stage, adhesive arachnoiditis, marks the end point of the inflammatory process. There is dense collagen deposition and complete encapsulation of the nerve roots, leading to progressive atrophy and stretching.[38] Not all patients with histologic changes develop pain. Neither does a similar degree of trauma consistently give rise to arachnoiditis. The fibrous changes following arachnoiditis may vary from involvement of one nerve root to various parts of the cauda equina.[39]

Clinically, affected individuals present with unremitting pain in the low back and leg, which increases with movement or positions that stretch lumbar nerve roots. There may be patchy neurologic deficits, including bladder dysfunction with variable degrees of motor and sensory changes. Magnetic resonance imaging (MRI) results of patients with lumbar arachnoiditis can be divided into three groups. Group one is characterized by a conglomeration of adherent roots residing centrally within the thecal sac. Group two is distinguished by nerve roots, adherent peripherally to the meninges and giving rise to an "empty-sac" appearance. Group three demonstrates a soft-tissue mass replacing the subarachnoid space.[40]

Spondylodiscitis This condition is seen in less than 0.5% of patients with FBSS. Wound infection immediately after surgery may lead to recurrent or persistent atypical lumbar pain, with or without pain radiating down to the legs, or back muscle spasms. It usually is associated with low-grade fever, leukocytosis, and high erythrocyte sedimentation rate. Aspiration of the disc in the early stages can confirm the diagnosis.[41] MRI findings in the later stages of the disease show central disc enhancement, posterior annulus enhancement, and enhancing edematous bone marrow of both adjacent vertebrae.[2]

Spinal Stenosis Spinal stenosis is one of the most common causes of FBSS.[2] Both central and lateral canal stenosis can coexist. Lateral spinal stenosis is seen commonly as a result of a gradual loss in disc height.[43] The symptoms of pain and neurologic deficit can be episodic and variable, as a result of the somewhat random ischemia of the vascular supply to the spinal nerves. The pain is usually described as deep and aching in the low back area, buttock, and thigh, with radicular pain down the leg, as well. Standing and walking are particularly painful. Most of the pain is dramatically relieved by forward flexion. Walking distance progressively diminishes over time. FBSS occurs if the predominant pain mechanisms are lateral or central canal stenosis.

Facet Joint Arthropathy A previous discectomy, laminectomy, or spinal fusion may cause adjacent facet joints to undergo accelerated degenerative arthritic changes. The pain pattern is mostly axial, seldom radiating below the knee, aggravated by extension and prolonged sitting. Diagnostic block with local anesthetics is one of the easy ways to differentiate facet disease from other causes of low back pain.[2,20]

Pseudomeningocele A pseudomeningocele is a cerebrospinal fluid leakage under pressure, leading to a cerebrospinal fluid–filled cavity. The patient may complain of low back pain. The diagnosis is usually confirmed by MRI, and surgical repair is the recommended treatment.[34] This condition is a rare cause of FBSS.

Tumors A missed diagnosis of spinal cord or cauda equine tumor (e.g., schwannoma or ependymoma) is, rarely, a cause of FBSS.

Central Sensitization Intractable back pain and sciatica may persist despite appropriate surgery to relieve the symptoms caused by a compressed nerve root. Chronic compression of nerve fibers is a source of ectopic discharges. Wall and Devor have shown that normal resting spontaneous discharges in dorsal root ganglia are markedly increased as a result of peripheral neuroma formation.[47,48] Peripheral nerve dysfunction can establish permanent alterations in cell organization and function of the dorsal horn, leading to hypersensitivity. The exaggerated persistence of pain stems from sensitization of the periphery as well as spinal cord mechanisms.

Early surgery is considered as too aggressive, whereas delayed intervention, after central sensitization has taken place, is too late. Hence, there is no clear understanding as to the optimal time for surgery in many cases.

DIAGNOSIS

Diagnosis of FBSS rests mostly on clinical evaluation and imaging studies. Ancillary modes include electromyography, nerve conduction studies, diagnostic blocks, provocative discography, and epiduroscopy. Because the leading cause of FBSS is inappropriate patient selection, a multidisciplinary diagnostic evaluation carried out in a tertiary care center is often warranted. Graham Smith emphasizes the importance of patient selection, particularly after surgery, by admitting patients for 5 days of in-depth assessment.[46] This gives a chance for the different teams, including rehabilitation, to assess the patient's physical, emotional, psychological, and social status in depth. It allows full investigation to make certain that no surgically remediable lesions remain and to determine rehabilitation potential. The role of the psychologist in exploring the patient's attitude to disease and his or her ability to cope with disability is of grave importance in this respect. However, in the current environment of cost containment, a coordinated, multidisciplinary evaluation of patients with disabling, chronic pain is more commonly performed on an outpatient basis.

Clinical History

The medical and surgical history is of paramount importance for evaluating the patient's chronic, disabling low back pain. A thorough review of the patient's self-filed questionnaire and previous medical charts, including previous treatments and imaging studies, can be very helpful in narrowing the differential diagnosis of low back pain. Of foremost importance are the pain characteristics, neurologic symptoms, functional limitations, and comorbid medical and psychological conditions. The outcome of previous treatments will strongly influence the management plan. The identification of an acute neurologic deficit, maladaptive behavioral issues, secondary gain, pending lawsuits, or a history of substance abuse is pivotal in determining treatment options.

Carragee delineated some factors responsible for either favorable or poor outcome influencing surgery.[47] Factors influencing poor outcome are (1) concurrent medical illness, (2) involvement with workers' compensation, and (3) female gender. Factors resulting in favorable outcome are (1) duration of symptoms less than 6 months, (2) absence of litigation, and (3) younger age. Smoking is considered to be a major risk factor for failure of bony union; fusions may be postponed until tobacco abstinence is achieved. Pearce noted some clinical features distinguishing nonlitigants from litigants.[48] Interestingly, when litigation is involved, leg radiation if present is often in the dermatomal distribution of L2 through L4, diffuse, or front of thigh not below the knee (nonanatomic), as opposed to radiation in patients not involved in litigation, which is in the L5-S1 distribution, back and side of buttock, and thigh to foot (anatomic distribution).

Detailed pain assessment is the key factor in the evaluation of patients with low back pain. The type of pain, location, radiation, duration, frequency, severity, association with movement and activity, as well as aggravating and relieving factors are integral to the assessment. Some of the easily distinguishable pain characteristics may help identify the anatomic location. For example pain resulting from spinal stenosis is relieved by forward flexion and aggravated by extension. Axial, deep, low back pain that is worse on extension could be a result of facet arthropathy, spondylolisthesis, or disc pathology. Return of pain within months to years is a result of epidural fibrosis, arachnoiditis, facet joint disease, segmental instability, and recurrent disc herniation.

Physical Examination

As with the clinical history of various pain complaints, review of previous examination findings is crucial in the process of diagnosis. The examination can be divided into components of musculoskeletal, neurologic, functional, and tension signs.

When examining the musculoskeletal system, attention must be given to the curvature of the spine and the limitations on range of motion. For example, pain on repeated lumbar flexion is probably a result of hypermobility problem.[49]

Provocative tests can be secondary to stretch of the spinal cord or sciatic nerve, or tests of increased intrathecal pressure. Tests to stretch the spinal cord or the sciatic nerve are otherwise known as tension tests. The straight-leg raise (SLR) is the most widely used. The pain must typically traverse below the knee to be called positive. The test is only considered provocative between 30 and 60 degrees. It cannot be considered as specific at less than 30 degrees because there has not been enough tension applied to cause movement of the lumbar plexus, which in turn creates movement of the neural structures through the foramina. At greater than 60 degrees, the nerve roots move ventrally and laterally to the pedicle. This causes the test to lose sensitivity.[50] Cross-leg SLR test is considered to be more specific for radicular pain.

Reverse SLR or femoral stretch is specific for L2–3 radiculopathies. With respect to FBSS, the SLR should be interpreted in light of the slump test. The slump test should be performed with proximal and distal initiation. With proximal initiation, allow the patient to sit with legs dangling from the examination table. Then initiate vertical pretension with cervical flexion, thoracic flexion, and lumbar flexion. Follow this by dorsiflexion of the foot and extension of the knee to create slight distal motion and increase tension. A positive result is suggestive of a tension problem, such as a lumbar disc impinging on the nerve root. If the cervical spine is then extended, the tension decreases and there is decreased distal motion. If there is a tension problem, the pain decreases when the tension is diminished. On the other hand, a mobility problem, such as entrapment of the plexus with scar tissue results in increased pain on cervical extension. The results of the slump test should be compared with both distal and proximal initiation, and then with the results of the SLR.[51]

A thorough neurologic examination is compulsory. The "red flag" signs of cauda equina syndrome should be excluded. Any new-onset neurologic sign demands serious consideration. At times, residual neurologic effects, such as foot drop or diminished deep tendon reflexes, may linger despite surgical decompression.[52]

Functional tests, such as the flip-differential SLR test and the Hoover test, must also be performed to identify nonorganic signs.

Waddell designated five cardinal signs of nonorganic low back pain[53]; namely, (1) superficial nonanatomic tenderness, (2) stimulated pain on axial loading, (3) distraction test (otherwise called the flip/differential SLR test), (4) regional or light skin pinch with a wide area of pain or weakness, or both, and sensory loss that is divergent from accepted neuroanatomy, and (5) overreaction with disproportionate verbalization and facial expression. On clinical examination any one of these signs is sufficient to establish an exaggeration of a physiologic state; thus, Waddell's insistence on three factors is not generally necessary. However, one should be cautious in labeling illness behavior, because some functional findings can result from organic problems. For example, patchy, nonanatomic sensory loss is common with arachnoiditis. Allodynia and hyperalgesia secondary to central sensitization can present as "superficial nonanatomic tenderness." Therefore, physical findings should be considered in the context of the whole clinical picture, not in isolation.

Diagnostic Studies

Imaging Studies Interpretation of imaging studies is more difficult in patients with FBSS because they may have superimposed anatomic abnormalities produced by their primary surgery and may have had instrumentation that compromises the quality of certain imaging modalities.[52] Recent advances in diagnostic capabilities have greatly facilitated the possibility of diagnosing the cause of surgical failure. Van Goethem and colleagues, in a review of imaging findings in patients with FBSS, stated that MRI should be the first imaging procedure because many of the most common and important imaging findings in these patients are seen best on MRI.[2] They also commented that it is a misjudgment to first perform computerized tomography (CT). A repeat examination with MRI will usually follow, to differentiate intraspinal soft tissue masses. Furthermore, MRI allows a more accurate assessment of foraminal diameter and visualization of the foraminal contents. In fact, MRI with gadolinium is considered the gold standard modality for consistently diagnosing enhancing scar tissue and recurrent disc herniations or retained disc fragments. The enhancement remains constant regardless of the time since surgery. Scar tissue can have a mass effect and be contiguous with the disc space, demonstrating there remains room for error.[49]

However, Coskun and colleagues, like many others, have found no relationship between the severity of epidural fibrosis and pain following surgery.[27] MRI also avoids the potential morbidity of subarachnoid contrast studies, which have been implicated in the etiology of arachnoiditis. MRI has limitations in defining bony anatomy, which often can be better visualized by plain x-ray and CT. These films are useful for a hypermobility problem. A plain CT may demonstrate the nature of a previous surgery or a pars fracture that was not detected on plain films. CT with myelography has approximately 67% to 100% accuracy in patients with multiple operations to allow the differentiation of scar tissue from disc disease.[54] A detailed review of imaging studies is beyond the preview of this chapter.

Electromyography This method has a reported success rate ranging from 20% to 90% for determining nerve root compression. The specificity is low in patients who have had multiple surgeries because of neurologic changes that are commonly observed postoperatively. At this late stage in patient evaluation, the original lumbar pathology, surgical trauma, or ongoing compression can all yield positive electromyographic results, thereby making a negative study more useful.[55]

Nerve Conduction Studies Nerve conduction studies are useful in correlating clinical symptoms with noncompressed nerve roots (from MRI). Nygaard and colleagues used quantitative sensory testing perioperatively and 12 months after microdiscectomy.[56] They found significant improvement in small, unmyelinated fibers, mostly in the ipsilateral neighboring nerve root, concluding that the observed recovery of function in the adjacent noncompressed nerve roots after successful surgical decompression in monoradiculopathy may result from reduced production of proinflammatory mediators when the disc herniation is removed. Scelsa and colleagues studied the electrophysiologic correlates of weakness in L5-S1 radiculopathy and concluded that low peroneal and tibial compound muscle action potential amplitudes may serve as surrogate measures for segmental weakness of functionally relevant muscles.[55] Electrophysiologic measurements taken in patients with lumbosacral radiculopathy are useful in estimating the degree of physiologic and anatomic injury.

Provocative Diskography Provocative diskography is performed to determine the effect of mechanical loading of individual discs in patients with unremitting, chronic, discogenic low back pain.[57] Elicitation of the patient's characteristic pain is considered a positive sign. Discography is mostly performed as a prelude to either (IDET) intradiscal electrothermal annuloplasty or fusion surgery. Only strongly positive and definite negative results are considered reliable. Manometry is of questionable benefit. It is recommended that an adjacent disc to the clinically correlated level of pain should also be tested as a control. Inappropriate responses most likely suggest illness behavior or a more diffuse pain syndrome.

Epiduroscopy This diagnostic and therapeutic procedure is used for the visualization of fibrosis, neovascularization, granulation tissue, and entrapment of the nerve roots.[58] The epiduroscope is passed through the sacral hiatus to visualize the lumbosacral epidural space. Then a stimulating catheter may be placed for neurophysiologic mapping. It not only is considered the diagnostic method of choice for epidural fibrosis, but also is considered effective in the treatment of radiculitis by mobilization of the adhesions around an entrapped and irritated nerve root (neuroplasty). Corticosteroids in a depot form may be injected, together with local anesthetic. It is not clear whether the therapeutic effects are a result of the accurate placement of medication or the irrigation of the inflammatory mediators.[59]

Diagnostic Blocks Hildebrandt justifies the use of diagnostic nerve blocks, especially in nonspecific spinal pain with poor radiologic correlation.[60] Examples of such blocks include facet joint, sacroiliac joint, and selective nerve roots. In a review, Hildebrandt states that 10% to 15% of axial pain is secondary to a facet joint problem, 15% to 20% is from the sacroiliac joint, and 40% is of discogenic origin. The advantages of blocks are as follows: (1) they allow a peripheral pain pathway to be localized, (2) selectively blocking the specific nerves teases out that faction of the pain generator, and (3) relief of pain after local anesthetic block is attributable solely to block of the target afferent neural pathway. Facet joint pain is commonly associated with other causes of FBSS. Depending on the response to a block, permanent ablative procedures can be considered. Selective nerve root blocks are most often considered when low back pain is associated with monoradiculopathy.

In addition, temporarily abolishing the patient's pain by blocking neuronal activity does not necessarily equate to the primary site of pathology. For instance, a patient with pain and allodynia may experience relief of pain by nerve root block, which temporarily eliminates incoming messages from the painful area. Local anesthetic can spread centrally, as well, giving the impression that a peripheral block is helpful. But if the major pathophysiologic abnormality is within the dorsal horn of the spinal cord, an intervention directed at the primary afferent axons (e.g., foraminotomy or neurectomy) will have limited benefit.[52]

PREVENTIVE MEASURES

As in all disease states, prevention is the most important consideration in reducing the incidence of FBSS. Given the common refractory nature of FBSS, a therapeutic plan must be set up with more realistic patient expectations. It is also important to explain to patients that, as with any other tissues in the body, neural tissue recovery may take months to years to recover. Axonal regeneration can be associated with persistence or worsening of pain. Rarely, patients may have persistence of their radicular pain for months after surgery, with total or near total resolution of pain once reinnervation of the distal target is completed.[52] This recovery-associated pain and paresthesia must be distinguished from FBSS pain. Men who are over 40 years of age, overweight, obese, and heavy smokers (i.e., more than 20 cigarettes/day for more than 20 years) are at increased risk of chronic low back pain.[61,62]

The impact of smoking on the microvascular circulation of peripheral nerves and the vascular network surrounding the intervertebral disks should not be underestimated.[63] Smoking increases the serum proteolytic activity, which increases the intervertebral disk degeneration and also weakens the spinal ligaments, causing spinal instability.[64] Central obesity with associated truncal and lower extremity muscle loss, seen in women over 45 years of age, is considered a risk factor for chronic low back pain.[65] Biologic risk factors, such as osteoarthritis, rheumatoid arthritis, gout, and other collagen diseases, need to be identified. Their impact on surgery, healing, and long-term outcome should be explained to the patient, because it does not alter the progression of the underlying degenerative process. Repeat surgery is more commonly seen in patients with identified biologic risk factors.

Inappropriate or premature patient selection, in this age of advanced diagnostic imaging and other modalities of evaluation, is less likely. Patients with unrealistic expectations must be carefully evaluated prior to any intervention. Unless there is a clear surgical indication, or conservative management has failed, more time should be allowed for surgical decision making, especially with respect to re-exploration. Pearce stated that "there is now good evidence that prolonged, skilled conservative care will sometimes prevent the failed back that so often complicates ill-judged invasive procedures."[48]

Because only 1% to 2% of patients with back pain undergo spinal surgery, the therapeutic approach should begin with conservative management and gradually proceed from less to more invasive options. Goupille emphasized that the decision to perform surgery should be made individually, based on factors such as: (1) clinical correlation of the patients symptomatology with the imaging findings, (2) presence of radicular pain more than axial pain, (3) absence of social or psychological deterrent factors, and (4) patient willingness for surgery.[20] Moreover, it is also important to consider a one-time surgical approach using advanced surgical techniques (e.g., using pedicle screws, plates, interbody cages) to reduce failure of fusion. Pulsed electromagnetic field stimulation has been used for bony bridging in lumbar spinal fusion, to yield a better outcome.[66] Preservation of ligamentum flavum, together with other epidural structures, and limited removal of lamina are important components in preventing epidural fibrosis.[67]

TREATMENT

FBSS is a multifactorial, complex problem that offers a challenging management task for the clinician practicing pain medicine. The literature offers little evidence to substantiate either a conservative or an interventional approach. Many pain centers offer multiple permutations and combinations of pain management strategies to improve quality-of-life measures. As with many complex chronic pain disorders, the primary treatments are frequently combined with physical therapy, occupational therapy, psychotherapy, and mind-body therapy to achieve functional restoration. The minimum criteria defining treatment success is a 50% reduction in pain evaluations. Other important goals include the resumption of employment and activities of daily living, which serve to further assess the response to a therapeutic plan.

Role of Psychologist

Given that the foremost reason for FBSS is poor patient selection, a clinical psychologist can identify confounding behavioral problems that will continue to foster poor responses to interventional and invasive therapies. Psychologists identify how and to what degree depression, anxiety, phobias, maladaptive behaviors, personality disorders, and temperament affect an individual's pain syndrome. The magnitude of any of these psychological conditions can influence the decision to proceed with any additional invasive options. Psychological evaluations are routinely obtained for procedures such as spinal cord stimulation, continuous drug administration systems, and intradiskal therapies. Patients are also assessed to determine appropriateness for psychotherapy, biofeedback, relaxation techniques, psychopharmacology, and mind-body chronic pain programs.

Another key role of the psychologist evaluating chronic pain syndromes is to investigate past or potential future inappropriate use of opioid medications. A past history of substance abuse is thoroughly explored during the evaluation. The psychologist then indicates how closely a patient must be monitored for abuse of opioid medication, if the decision is made to place that individual on chronic narcotic medication. Indeed many patients with FBSS who undergo evaluation have been taking opioids for years. Many of these individuals go on to develop tolerance and dependence but, interestingly, the majority do not develop behavioral signs of addiction.[68]

Role of Physiotherapy

The structural asymmetries, deconditioning, ongoing pain, and attitude of the patient with FBSS represent a formidable rehabilitative challenge. Diminution of the pain behavior that frequently accompanies FBSS is more of a focus for the therapist than actual pain relief.[69] The goals of physical therapy are to improve range of motion, enhance strength, increase activities of daily living, improve ergonomics, and prevent or decrease musculoskeletal injury by increasing physical environment awareness. There is emphasis on daily exercise and stretching routines. In FBSS, there is loss of normal lumbar lordosis, chronic muscle spasm of paravertebral muscles, and tightening and shortening of gluteal, hamstring, and calf muscle groups.[70,71] The rehabilitative process of FBSS is slow and challenging, requiring continuous education and reinforcement.

Pharmacologic Management

A pharmacologic approach remains a cornerstone in any pain management program. Patients who have responded favorably to one surgery in the past are more likely to derive benefit from medical management.[52] But there exists no one medication or class of medications that has demonstrated universal efficacy.

Nonsteroidal Anti-inflammatory Drugs (NSAIDs) NSAIDs remain as the first line of medical treatment against the pain associated with musculoskeletal disorders. Long-term use is much more likely than short-term or sporadic employment to cause adverse effects such as gastrointestinal toxicity, renal dysfunction, platelet inhibition, water and sodium retention, and allergic reactions. Selective inhibition of the cyclooxygenase (COX-2) enzyme may reduce some of the gastrointestinal complications and eliminate platelet dysfunction.[72]

Recently, Mukherjee and colleagues determined that the risk of cardiovascular events is higher with COX-2 inhibitors compared with placebo or traditional NSAIDs, such as naproxen.[73] Regardless of the agent chosen, careful monitoring is necessary. Chronic use of high-dose NSAIDs is common among FBSS patients. Individuals with FBSS may likely have elements of chronic inflammation generating a component of their overall pain and, thus, an NSAID may be of value. COX-2 inhibitors offer an option in patients who do not tolerate or have contraindications to nonspecific NSAIDs.

Systemic Opioids Chronic administration of oral opioids has gained acceptance for the management of long-term nonmalignant pain. Many patients with FBSS are likely to be using pain medications, including narcotic analgesics. The use of chronic opioids does not exclude the possibility of future interventions. In fact, appropriate use of systemic opioids may prevent inappropriate future procedures that can lead to further debilitation. There are some patients who remain stable on chronic opioid therapy over the long term.

In a careful review of the literature, Brown and colleagues formulated recommendations for implementing chronic opioid analgesic therapy (COAT) in patients with chronic low back pain.[74] An analysis of 566 case series reports showed that COAT appears to be safe and effective for many patients suffering from recalcitrant, chronic low back pain. Preexisting substance abuse, personality disorders, certain medical conditions, and occupational factors are identified as relative contraindications. Further work by Jamieson and colleagues in a randomized, prospective, long-term, repeated-dose study that compared either sustained-release morphine or short-acting oxycodone with naproxen found favorable outcomes for mean pain scores, anxiety, depression, and irritability in patients treated with either opioid analgesic in comparison with naproxen.[75] Stable plasma levels of narcotic analgesics improve quality of life, and cause fewer side effects with no cognitive deterioration, when given on a time-rather than pain-contingent basis.[76] Thus, there is now a consensus view that in carefully selected patients with nonmalignant pain, including FBSS, pain and function can be improved with COAT.[77]

There are, however, many patients with FBSS who are refractory to opioids or cease to respond. Incremental dose escalation may lead to copious amounts of narcotics without further benefit. Identification of tolerance, after excluding a new pain disturbance or progression of disease, can be managed by substituting an alternative narcotic or considering additional pain management strategies.[78] The lack of response or intolerable side effects to one narcotic analgesic does not preclude trying several other opioids. Physical dependence is a normal phenomenon in any patient who uses chronic opioids, including patients with FBSS. Many patients choose to avoid using narcotics on a daily basis to avoid addiction or dependence.[79] Actual addiction, or the inappropriate preoccupation with narcotic analgesics induced iatrogenically, has been known to be infrequent since the 1980s.[80] Addiction rates currently estimated in North America indicate that between 3% and 16% of chronic pain patients suffer from an addictive disorder that parallels the life-time prevalence of addictive disease in the general population.[81] Screening patients carefully and instituting vigilant monitoring further reduces the probability of opioid abuse or misuse.[82] Nevertheless, published patient surveys and case reports support the efficacy and long-term safety of opioid analgesics in selected patients with chronic, nonmalignant, and nociceptive more than neuropathic pain.[83]

Adjuvant Analgesic Agents FBSS often has elements of nociceptive pain as well as neuropathic pain, which is commonly refractory to NSAIDs and opioids. Anticonvulsant and tricyclic antidepressant medications have been demonstrated to have efficacy against neuropathic pain syndromes, such as painful diabetic neuropathy and postherpetic neuralgia. These classes of medications have not been formally studied in the context of FBSS; however, they have an accepted role in the treatment of neuropathic pain, and, therefore, enhance analgesia in FBSS.

Other categories of medications include muscle relaxants and α_2 agonists. Muscle relaxants such as carisoprodol, cyclobenzaprine, and metaxalone have been used in patients with persistent muscle spasm with limited success. Two unique agents in the muscle relaxant class are tizanidine (α_2 agonist properties) and baclofen (γ-aminobutyric acid agonist, type B). Baclofen is used as a muscle relaxant, but more appropriately it is an antispastic agent that has shown benefit in patients suffering from neuropathic pain or spasticity. Tizanidine exerts a central α_2 adrenergic agonist effect that has successfully relieved muscle spasm and neuropathic pain.[84] The efficacy of any of these agents in FBSS is uncertain, and clinical experience suggests that as monotherapy, it would be modest.

Epidural Corticosteroid Injections

Despite the lack of randomized, well-controlled studies, the placement of corticosteroids into the epidural space as a treatment for FBSS remains the most common therapeutic modality. The rationale is to reduce any residual inflammation via phospholipase A_2 inhibition. Reduced inflammation and direct C-fiber inhibition by corticosteroids reduces the sensitivity of nociceptors to mechanical stimuli and tensile force.[85] Factors associated with a favorable response to epidural corticosteroids include advanced educational background, lumbar radiculopathy, and pain duration of less than 6 months.[86]

On the other hand, factors that serve to limit the success of epidural corticosteroids are alteration of lumbar anatomy following surgery, limitation in epidural needle placement as a direct result of surgical scarring and altered anatomy, and epidural fibrosis, which interferes with epidural diffusion and penetration to the appropriate targets. A review of 12 randomized controlled trials by Cousins and colleagues found benefit in 6 of the 12 studies.[87] The negative studies essentially found short-term relief. The use of fluoroscopy to improve needle placement and therapeutic response is debated in the literature. But in clinical practice, it has proven invaluable in patients following complex fusions and laminectomy.[88] The incidence of wet tap in patients after laminectomy or fusion can approach 20%, and this is likely reduced through the use of fluoroscopy.[3] Moreover, the injection of radiocontrast into the epidural space confirms placement and spread to the sites of probable pathology.

The use of transforaminal blocks (or nerve root blocks) allows for placement of epidural corticosteroids on the affected nerve root without the necessity of identifying the epidural space. This approach avoids the risk of postdural puncture headache and improves spread of corticosteroid to the affected nerve root by circumventing epidural fibrosis. Devulder and colleagues performed transforaminal blocks for mononeuropathy in 60 patients with FBSS in a randomized, single-blind study.[89] The aim was to compare short- and long-term relief with bupivacaine plus hyaluronidase, and with or without corticosteroid. At 6 months, only 27% of patients had greater than 50% reduction of their initial pain scores, and no benefit was seen from adding corticosteroid to hyaluronidase and bupivacaine. A series of risk factors for failure of this procedure were identified, which include lower level of education, smoking, lack of employment during the initiation of treatment, ongoing litigation, constant nonradicular pain patterns, duration of pain greater than 1 year, pain that is not influenced by activity, pain behavior, and neuropathic features indicative of allodynia and central sensitization. In conclusion, epidural injection of corticosteroids and hyaluronidase appears to be of benefit in selected patient with FBSS. Injection of local anesthetic into the epidural space to silence sympathetic nervous system involvement of nociceptors is without any meaningful long-term efficacy.

Epiduroscopy

The epiduroscope can be used for visualization of epidural fibrosis, neovascularization, granulation tissue, and fibrotic entrapment of nerve roots.[58] Using complete aseptic measures, the scope is introduced at the level of S3. The catheter is fed through the ventral surface until it reaches the L4–5 interspace, which is the usual level of pathology. The catheter can then be maneuvered closer to the sites of epidural scarring. An epidurogram is then performed to detect a so-called filling defect, indicating an area of scarring and possible nerve entrapment. Alternatively, a stimulating catheter may be placed for neurophysiologic mapping. Thereafter, hyaluronidase is injected to hydrolyze excess ground substance in epidural scar tissue, thus allowing diffusion of local anesthetic and corticosteroid to target areas. Racz and colleagues found this technique of epidural neuroplasty effective in 49% of patients with FBSS.[59]

Facet Joint Injections

Degenerative disease of the facet (zygapophyseal) joints is an underappreciated cause of low back pain with radiation to the knee level in FBSS. The clinical examination is, however, unreliable and diagnostic or therapeutic &acet injections can offer more accurate insight. A subjective report of greater than 50% pain relief is regarded as a positive response, in that the pain is derived from the facet joints.

As would be expected, many FBSS patients do not sustain benefit from intra-articular facet injections. The response to medial branch blocks is then evaluated prior to pursuing radiofrequency lesioning of the facet joints. After diagnostic blocks and radiofrequency lesioning, investigators found 50% pain relief in 50% of the patients 3-years follow-up.[90,91]

Facet denervation often alleviates a component of the FBSS, and, therefore, other generators of pain should be considered. A facet problem in FBSS is often accompanied by compensatory muscle spasm. Trigger point injections and physical therapy may be added to offer a more complete rehabilitative approach. Botulinum toxin A has been applied in cases of spasm of the quadratus lumborum, psoas major, piriformis, and paravertebral muscles.[92,93] Chemodenervation is often limited to refractory cases, and its efficacy in FBSS is unknown.

Intradiskal Electrothermal Therapy (IDET)

Patients suffering from FBSS may have internal disruption of a disk as a generator of their pain. The disk may have formerly been operated on, or it may represent new pathology at adjacent levels. The outcomes for IDET procedures on patients with FBSS are unknown. Studies evaluating IDET for patients with diskogenic pain as suggested by history, physical examination, and diskography have generated mixed results.[94–96] Improved patient selection, psychologic testing, and better technique will probably be combined to offer a select group of patients a nonoperative solution to diskogenic pain.

Spinal Cord Stimulation

Neuromodulation has gained increase popularity given the low success rate of ablative procedures. Dorsal root ganglionectomy, whether performed percutaneously with radiofrequency or surgically, has produced only a 15% success rate at 5 years in patients with FBSS.[52] There has been increased recognition of the importance of avoiding deafferentation in a chronic pain syndrome.

Spinal cord stimulation has been used for FBSS since 1967. The pioneering work of Shealy and colleagues has created the basis for interventional pain management for a host of neuropathic pain syndromes.[97] The gate theory of Melzack and Wall and central inhibitory mechanisms evoked by Aβ stimulation are commonly accepted mechanisms of analgesia brought on by spinal cord stimulation.[98]

In the United States, FBSS is the most common indication for spinal cord stimulation. Long-term follow-up studies have shown a success rate of 50% to 75% for FBSS at 5 years.[99] North has demonstrated that spinal cord stimulation is more effective than either dorsal root ganglionectomy or reoperation.[100] Dual lead placement in patients with FBSS allows for more programming options to cover some axial pain, as well as persistent coverage of the extremities even with some lead migration.[100] Indeed, system complications such as lead migration, lead fracture, infection, and battery failure are the most common problems.[101]

Spinal cord stimulation can lower the medical costs of FBSS over time, by reducing office and emergency department visits.[102] Spinal cord stimulation pays for itself within 2.1 years. Medication requirements tend to stabilize or decrease, activities of daily living increase, and some patients are able to return to meaningful employment.[103] Overall, spinal cord stimulation is a viable option for patients who fail to obtain sufficient pain control with less-invasive modalities. Future options may include deep brain stimulation, especially for the nociceptive component of FBSS. Nearly 62% of patients with FBSS derived meaningful analgesia from deep brain stimulation, but only half of these may go on to have sustained benefit over the long term.[104]

Central Neuraxial Infusions

Over the past decade, there has been a significant surge in the use of implantable pump technology for nonmalignant pain, particularly intrathecal opiates for FBSS.[105] Drug administration systems delivering intrathecal narcotics over time can result in tolerance, hyperalgesia, and hormonal disturbances.[106] Despite these problems, long-term intrathecal infusion of opiates can reduce pain scores by 25% to 50% after 2 years of therapy, with improved coping skills in FBSS.[107] Axial pain often respond less favorably than radicular or neuropathic pain to intrathecal infusions. Like spinal cord stimulation, implantable pumps appear to be cost-effective over a period of at least 12 to 22 months.[108] Pump refills and the cost of the technology are far exceeded by frequent emergency department and office visits, as are repeat diagnostic tests, and multiple medication trials.

Reoperation

The rate of success after reoperation varies from 12% to 100%.[1] Reoperation should only be considered if there is a clear anatomic reason for worsening pain and conservative measures have failed. The dogma to reoperate only because alternative methods have failed will simply lead to more morbidity. Epidural fibrosis is always a risk, even in carefully conducted surgery. Reoperation often requires careful evaluation to avoid the enhancement of a syndrome that is already difficult to treat.

CONCLUSION

In all studies of back pain, 10% to 15% of patients account for 80% to 90% of the total health care consumption for spine disorders, and the 2% of patients who undergo spinal surgery are the most expensive group.[109] At least 15% of patients who have spinal surgery develop FBSS. Interestingly, spinal decompression for other reasons, such as tumor, often yields impressive clinical results. The lack of such satisfactory results in nonmalignant pain represents the magnitude of the complexity of back pain in a significant number of patients. In addition to structural abnormalities, psychological factors, social comorbidities, and complex peripheral and central processing of nociceptive information may account for low back pain. The multidimensional nature of this complex clinical problem and the lack of prospective randomized, controlled data have obscured outcome assessment of pharmacologic, surgical, and other interventions in FBSS.

REFERENCES

1. North RB, Campbell JN, James CS, et al. Failed back surgery syndrome: Five years followup in 102 patients undergoing reoperation. *Neurosurgery* 1991;28:685–691.
2. Van Goethem JWM, Parizel PM, Van den Hauwe L, De Schepper AMA. Imaging findings in patients with failed back surgery syndrome. *J Belge Radiol* 1997;80:81–86.
3. Rowlingson J. Epidural steroids in treating failed back surgery syndrome. *Anesth Analg* 1999;88:240–242.
4. Fiume D, Sherkat S, Callovini GM, Parziale G, Gazzeri G. Treatment of failed back surgery syndrome due to lumbo-sacral epidural fibrosis. *Acta Neurochir Suppl (Wien)* 1995;64:116–118.
5. Mixter WJ, Barr JS. Rupture of the intervertebral disc with involvement of the spinal cord. *N Engl J Med* 1934;211:210–215.
6. Barr JS. Low back and sciatic pain. *J Bone Joint Surg Am* 1951;33: 633–649.
7. Finneson BE, CooperVR. A lumbar disc surgery predictive score card. *Spine* 1979;4:141–144.
8. Long DM. Low back pain and sciatica. In: Johnson RT, ed. *Current Therapy in Neurologic Disease*. Philadelphia, Pa: BC Decker; 1985:69–72.
9. Burton CV. Lumbosacral arachnoiditis. *Spine* 1978;3:24–30.
10. Wilkinson HA. Outcome analysis in 654 surgically treated lumbar disc herniations. *Neurosurgery* 1993;32:879.
11. Hakelius A. Prognosis in sciatica: A clinical follow-up of surgical of surgical and non-surgical treatment. *Acta Orthop Scand* 1970; 129(suppl):1–11.
12. Howorth B. Low backache and sciatica: Results of surgical treatment. Part II, Removal of nucleus pulposus and spine fusion. *J Bone Joint Surg Am* 1964;46:1500–1515.
13. Naylor A. The late results of laminectomy for lumbar disc prolapse. A review after ten to twenty-five years. *J Bone Joint Surg Br* 1974; 56:17–29.
14. Salenius P, Laurent LE. Results of operative treatment of lumbar disc herniation. A survey of 886 patients. *Acta Orthop Scand* 1977;48: 630–634.
15. Spangfort EV. Lumbar disc herniation. A computer aided analysis of 2504 operations. *Acta Orthop Scand* 1972;142(suppl):1–95.
16. Abramovitz JN, Neff SR. Lumbar disc surgery: Results of the prospective lumbar discectomy study of the joint section on disorder of the spine and peripheral nerves of the American Association of Neurological Surgeons and the Congress of Neurological Surgeons. *Neurosurgery* 1991;29:301–318.
17. Nachemson AL. Evaluation of results in lumbar spine surgery. *Acta Orthop Scand Suppl* 1993;251:130–133.
18. Dvorak J, Gauchat MH, Valach L. The outcome of surgery for lumbar disc herniation. I. A. 4-17 years of follow-up with emphasis on somatic aspects. *Spine* 1988;13:1418–1422.
19. Fritch EW, Heisel J, Rupp S. The failed back surgery syndrome: Reasons, intraoperative findings, and long term results: A report of 182 operative treatments. *Spine* 1996;21:626–633.
20. Goupille P. Causes of failed back surgery syndrome. *Rev Rhum Engl Ed* 1996;63:235–239.
21. Spengler DM, Freeman C, Westbrook R, Miller JW. Low-back pain following multiple lumbar spine procedures: Failure of initial selection? *Spine* 1980;5:356–360.
22. La Rocca H. Chronic back pain. In: Bonica, J, ed. Management of Pain. 2nd ed. Philadelphia, PA: Lea and Febiger; 1990:549.
23. Waddell G, Reilly S, Torsney B, et al. Assessment of the outcome of low back surgery. *J Bone Joint Surg Br* 1988;70:723–727.
24. Pearce JM. Aspects of failed back syndrome: Role of litigation. *Spinal Cord* 2000;38:63–70.
25. Hansson TH, Hansson EK. The effects of common medical interventions on pain, back function, and work resumption in patients with chronic low back pain: A prospective 2-year cohort study in six countries. *Spine* 2000;25:3055–3056.
26. Burton CV, Kirkaldy-Willis WH, Yong-Hing K, et al. Causes of failure of surgery on the lumbar spine. *Clin Orthop* 1981;157:191–199.
27. Coskun E, Suzer T, Topuz O, Zencir M, Pakdemirli E, Tahata K. Relationship between epidural fibrosis, pain, disability, and psychological factors after lumbar disc surgery. *Eur Spine J* 2000;9:218–223.

28. Gasinski P, Radek M, Jozwiak J, Lyczak P. Peridural fibrosis in lumbar disc surgery—Pathogenesis, clinical problems and prophylactic attempts. *Neurol Neurochir Pol* 2000;34:983–993.
29. Key A, Ford LT. Experimental intervertebral disc lesions. *J Bone Joint Surg Am* 1948;30:621–630.
30. Omnipaque. Package insert. Princeton, NJ: Nycomed; 1996.
31. Imai S, Hukuda S, Maeda T. Dually innervating nociceptive networks in the rat lumbar posterior longitudinal ligaments. *Spine* 1995;19: 2086–2092.
32. Pawl RP. Arachnoiditis and epidural fibrosis: The relationship to chronic pain. *Curr Rev Pain* 1998;2:93–99.
33. Ross JS. Magnetic resonance imaging of the post operative spine. *Semin Musculoskelet Radiol* 2000;4:281–291.
34. Olmarker K, Rydevik B. Pathophysiology of sciatica. *Orthop Clin North Am* 1991;22:223–233.
35. Racz GB, Noe C, Heavner JE. Selective spinal injections for lower back pain. *Curr Rev Pain* 1999;3:333–341.
36. Saal JS, Franson RC, Dobrow R, et al. High levels of inflammatory phospholipase A2 activity in lumbar disc herniations. *Spine* 1990;15: 674.
37. Finnegan WJ, Fenlin JM, Marvel JP, et al. Results of surgical intervention in the symptomatic multiple operated back patient. *J Bone Joint Surg Am* 1979;61:1077–1082.
38. Burton CV. Lumbosacral arachnoiditis. *Spine* 1978;3:24–30.
39. Pawl RP. Arachnoiditis and epidural fibrosis: The relationship to chronic pain. *Curr Rev Pain* 1998;2:93–99.
40. Ross JS, Masaryk TJ, Modic MT, et al. MR imaging of lumbar arachnoiditis. *AJR Am J Roentgenol* 1987;5:1025–1032.
41. Long DM. Overview of failed back syndrome. In: Gildenberg PL, Tasker RR, eds. *Textbook of Stereotactic and Functional Neurosurgery*. New York, NY: McGraw-Hill; 1998:1601–1610.
42. Olmarkar K, Rydevik, B, Nordburg C. Autologous nucleus pulposus induces neurophysiologic and histologic changes in porcine cauda equina nerve roots. *Spine* 1993;11:1425–1432.
43. Carroll SE, Wiesel SW. Neurologic complications and lumbar laminectomy. *Clin Orthop* 1992;284:14–23.
44. Wall PD, Gutnik M. Properties of afferent nerve impulses originating from a neuroma. *Nature* 1974;248:747–743.
45. Wall PD, Devor M. The effect of peripheral nerve injury on dorsal root potentials and on transmission of afferent signals into the spinal cord. *Brain Res* 1981;209:95–111.
46. Graham Smith A. Failed back surgery syndrome. *Florida Orthop J* 1990.
47. Carragee EJ, Kim DH. A prospective analysis of magnetic resonance imaging findings in patients with sciatica and lumbar disc herniation. Correlation of outcomes with disc fragment and canal morphology. *Spine* 1997;22;1650–1660.
48. Pearce JMS. Aspects of failed back syndrome: Role of litigation. *Spinal Cord* 19—;38:63–70.
49. Anderson SR. A rationale for the treatment algorithm of failed back surgery syndrome. *Curr Rev Pain* 2000;4:395–406.
50. Smith AS, Massie JB, Chestnut R, Graffin SR. Straight leg raising. *Spine* 1993;18:990–992.
51. Winkel D, Aufdemkampe G, Matthis O, et al. Surface anatomy of the spine and general aspects of back pain. In: Thersbury G, ed. *Diagnosis and Treatment of the Spine*. Gaithersburg, Md: Aspen; 1996: 168–170.
52. Oaklander AL, North RB. Failed back surgery syndrome: Regional pains. In: Bonica's management of pain. 3rd ed. Lippincott Williams & Wilkins: Philadelphia; 2000:1540–1549.
53. Waddell G, McCulloch JA, Kummel E, Venner RM. Nonorganic physical signs in low back pain. *Spine* 1980;5:117–125.
54. Braun IF, Hoffman JC, Davis PC, et al. Contrast enhancement in CT differentiation between recurrent disc herniation and post operative scar: Prospective study. *AJR Am J Roentgenol* 1985;145:785–790.
55. Scelsa SN, Berger AR, Herskovitz S. Electrophysiologic correlates of weakness in L5/S1 radiculopathy. *Electromyogr Clin Neurophysiol* 2001;41:145–151.
56. Nygaard OP, Kloster R, Solberg T, Mellgren SI. Recovery of function in adjacent nerve roots after surgery for lumbar disc herniation: Use of quantitative sensory testing in the exploration of different populations of nerve fibres. *Spinal Disord* 2000;13:427–431.
57. Bini W, Yeung AT, Caltayud V, Chaaban A, Seferlis T. The role of provocative discography in minimally invasive selective endoscopic discectomy. *Neurochirurgie* 2002;1:27–31; discussion, 32.
58. Saberski LR, Kitahata LM. Direct visualization of the lumbosacral epidural space through the sacral hiatus. *Anesth Analg* 1995;80:839–840.
59. Racz GB, Heavner JE, Raj PP. Percutaneous epidural neuroplasty: Prospective one year follow-up. *Pain Digest* 1999;9:97–102.
60. Hildebrandt J. Relevance of nerve blocks in treating and diagnosing low back pain—is the quality decisive? *Schmerz* 2001;15: 474–483.
61. Kostova V, Koleva M. Back disorder (low back pain, cervicobrachial, and lumbosacral radicular syndrome) and some related risk factor. *J Neurol Sci* 2001;192:17–25.
62. Uematsu Y, Matuzaki H, Iwahashi M. Effect of nicotine on intervertebral disc: An experimental study in rabbits. *Orthop Sci* 2001;6: 177–182.
63. Fogelhom RR, Alho AV. Smoking and intervertebral disc degeneration. *Med Hypotheses* 2001;56:537-539.
64. Toda Y, Segal N, Toda T, Morimoto T, Ogawa R. Lean body mass and body fat distribution in participants with chronic low back pain. *Arch Intern Med* 2000;160:3265–3269.
65. Boden SD, David DO, Dina TS. Abnormal lumbar spine MRI scans in asymptomatic subjects: A prospective investigation. *J Bone Joint Surg Am* 1990;72:403–408.
66. Marks RA. Spinal fusion for discogenic low back pain: Outcomes in patients treated with or without pulsed electromagnetic field stimulation. *Adv Ther* 2000;17:57–67.
67. Aydin Y, Ziyal IM, Duman H, Turkmen CS, Basak M, Sahin Y. Clinical and radiological results of lumbar diskectomy technique with preserving of ligamentum flavum comparing to the standard microdiskectomy technique. *Surg Neurol* 2002;57:5–13.
68. Strumpf M, Linstedt U, Wiebalck A, Zenz M. Treatment of low back pain—significance, principles and danger [in German]. *Schmerz* 2001;15:453–460.
69. Bundschuh CV, Modie MT, Ross JS, et al. Epidural fibrosis and recurrent disc herniation in lumbar spine; assessment with magnetic resonance. *AJNR Am J Neuroradiol* 1988;9:169–178.
70. Manniche C, Lundberg E, Christensen I, Bentzen L, Hasselsoe G. Intensive dynamic back exercises for chronic low back pain. A clinical trial. *Pain* 1991;47:53–63.
71. Holm S, Nachemson A. Variations in the nutrition of the canine intervertebral disc induced by motion. *Spine* 1983;8:866–874.
72. Silverstein FE, Faich G, Goldstein JL, et al. Gastrointestinal toxicity with celecoxib vs nonsteroidal anti-inflammatory drugs for osteoarthritis and rheumatoid arthritis: The CLASS study: A randomized controlled trial. Celecoxib Long term Arthritis Safety Study. *JAMA* 2000;284:1247–1255.
73. Mukherjee D, Nissen SE, Topol EJ. Risk of cardiovascular events associated with selective COX-2 inhibitors. *JAMA* 2001;286:954–959.
74. Brown RL, Fleming MF, Patterson JJ. Chronic opioid analgesic therapy for chronic low back pain. *J Am Board Fam Pract* 1996;9: 191–204.
75. Jamieson RN, Raymond SA, Slawsby EA, Nadeljkovic SS, Katz NP. Opioid therapy for chronic non-cancer back pain. A randomized prospective study. *Spine* 1998;23:2591–2600.
76. Collett BJ. Chronic opioid therapy for non-cancer pain. *Br J Anaesth* 2001;87:133–143.
77. Evans PJD. Opioids for chronic musculoskeletal pain. In: Fields HL, ed. *Opioid Sensitivity of Chronic Noncancer Pain*. Seattle, Wash: IASP Press; 1999:349-365.

78. Quang-Cantagrel ND, Wallace MS, Magnuson SK. Opioid substitution to improve the effectiveness of chronic noncancer pain control: A chart review. *Anesth Analg* 2000;90:933–937.
79. Ytterberg SR, Mahowald ML, Woods SR. Codeine and oxycodone use in patients with chronic rheumatic disease pain. *Arthritis Rheum* 1998;41:1603–1612.
80. Perry S, Heidberg G. Management of pain during debridement: A survey of U.S burn units. *Pain* 1982;13:267–280.
81. Fishbain DA, Rosomoff HL, Rosomoff RS. Drug abuse, dependence and addiction in chronic pain patients. *Clin J Pain* 1992;8:77–85.
82. Savage SR. Addiction in the treatment of pain: Significance recognition and management. *J Pain Symptom Manage* 1993;8:265–277.
83. France RD, Urban BJ, Keefe FJ. Long term use of narcotic analgesics in chronic pain. *Soc Sci Med* 1984;19:1379–1382.
84. Kopf A, Ruf W. Novel drugs for neuropathic pain. *Curr Opin Anaesthesiol* 2000;13:585–590.
85. Johansson A, Hao J, Sjolund B. Local corticosteroid application blocks transmission in normal nociceptive C-fibers. *Acta Anaesthesiol Scand* 1990;34:335.
86. Abram SE, Hoopwood MB. What factors contribute to outcome with lumbar epidural steroids? In: Bond MR, Charlton JE, Woolfe CJ, eds. *Proceedings of the Sixth World Congress on Pain*. Amsterdam, Holland: Elsevier Science Publishers; 1991:495.
87. Cousins MJ, Walker S. Chronic pain management strategies that work. International Anesthesia Research Society; Review course lectures; Cleveland, Ohio: March 2001; 15–25.
88. Anderson VC. Failed back surgery syndrome. *Curr Rev Pain* 2000;4:105–111.
89. Devulder J, Deene P, De Laat M, et al. Nerve root sleeve injections in patients with failed back surgery syndrome: A comparison of three solutions. *Clin J Pain* 1999;15:132–135.
90. Rashbaum RF. Radiofrequency facet denervation: A treatment alternative in refractory low back pain with or without leg pain. *Orthop Clin North Am* 1983;14:569.
91. North RB, Han M, Zahurak M, Kidd DH. Radiofrequency lumbar facet denervation: Analysis of prognostic factors. *Pain* 1994;57:77–83.
92. Raj PP. Botulinum toxin in the treatment of pain associated with musculoskeletal hyperactivity. *Curr Rev Pain* 1997;1:403–416.
93. Foster L, Clapp L, Erickson M, Jabbari B. Botulinum toxin A and chronic low back pain: A randomised double blind study. *Neurology* 2001;56:1290–1293.
94. Saal JA, Saal JS. Intradiscal electrothermal treatment for chronic discogenic low back pain: A prospective outcome study with minimum 1-year follow-up. *Spine* 2000;25:2622–2627.
95. Karasek M, Bogduk N. Twelve-month follow-up of a controlled trial of intradiscal thermal anuloplasty for back pain due to internal disc disruption. *Spine* 2000;25:2601–2607.
96. Barendse GA, van Den Berg SG, Kessels AH, Weber WE, van Kleef M. Randomized controlled trial of percutaneous intradiscal radiofrequency thermocoagulation for chronic discogenic back pain: Lack of effect from a 90-second 70 C lesion. *Spine* 2001;26:287–292.
97. Shealy C, Mortimer J, Reswik J. Electrical inhibitors of pain by stimulation of the dorsal column. Preliminary clinical reports. *Anesth Analg* 1967;46:489–491.
98. Melzack P, Wall P. Pain mechanisms: A new theory. *Science* 1965;150:971–978.
99. Krames E. Mechanisms of action of spinal cord stimulation. *Intervent Pain Manage* 1996;39:407–408.
100. North R, Kidd D, Campbell J, Long D. Dorsal root ganglionectomy for failed back surgery syndrome: A five-year follow-up study. *J Neurosurg* 1994;74:236–242.
101. Deer T. The role of neuromodulation by spinal cord stimulation in chronic pain syndromes; current concepts. *Tech Anesth Pain Manage* 1998;2:161–167.
102. Bell GK, North RB. Cost-effectiveness analysis of spinal cord stimulation in failed back surgery syndrome. *J Pain Symptom Manage* 1997;13:286–295.
103. Devulder J, De Laat M, Van Bastelaere M, Rolly G. Spinal cord stimulation: A valuable treatment for chronic failed back surgery patients. *J Pain Manage* 1997;13:296–301.
104. Levy RM, Lamb S, Adams JE. Treatment of chronic pain by deep brain stimulation: Long term follow-up and review of literature. *Neurosurgery* 1987;21:885–893.
105. Osenbach RK, Harvey S. Neuroaxial infusion in patients with chronic intractable cancer and noncancer pain. *Curr Pain Headache Rep* 2001;5:241–249.
106. Winkelmuller M, Winkelmuller W. Long-term effects of continuous intrathecal opioid treatment in chronic pain of nonmalignant etiology. *J Neurosurg* 1996;85:458–467.
107. Anderson VC, Burchail KJ. A prospective study of long-term intrathecal morphine in the management of chronic nonmalignant pain. *Neurosurgery* 1999;44:289–300.
108. Angel IF, Gould HJ, Carey ME. Intrathecal morphine pump as a treatment option in chronic pain of nonmalignant origin. *Neurosurgery* 1998;49:92–99.
109. Fischgrund JS. Perspective on modern orthopedics: Use of Adcon-L for epidural scar prevention. *J Am Acad Orthop Surg* 2000;8:339–343.

CHAPTER 31

PAIN MANAGEMENT IN RHEUMATOLOGIC DISORDERS

Matthew Lefkovitz, Daniel Ricciardi

"Behind the dazzle of the search for diagnosis and cause, the fundamental concern of rheumatologists and their patients is pain."
CROFT (1996)[1]

Pain resulting from various bone and joint disorders, whether noninflammatory (e.g., degenerative joint disease, osteoarthritis [OA]) or inflammatory (e.g., rheumatoid arthritis [RA]), significantly reduces the quality of life in affected patients. Individuals with chronic pain often become depressed and socially isolated and experience functional decline and disability as well as morbidity and mortality associated with pain. Data on undertreatment of pain in patients with arthritis do not appear to be available. However, as many as 20% of patients with cancer may have inadequate pain relief even when World Health Organization (WHO) guidelines (the analgesic ladder)[2] are used.[3] Pain is frequently underassessed and undertreated in patients with arthritis[4] and in elderly patients. A review of 15 studies of chronic pain in the elderly found a median point prevalence of 15% (range from 2% to 40%) and noted that there were no clearcut differences between estimates based on self-assessment and those made by physicians after clinical examination.[5]

The medications for management of arthritis, especially acetaminophen and nonsteroidal anti-inflammatory drugs (NSAIDs), are not completely satisfactory because of the high incidence of side effects, largely gastrointestinal (GI). As many as 20% of patients experience some toxicity,[6] and 2% to 4% of chronic NSAID users develop upper GI bleeding, a symptomatic ulcer, or intestinal perforation each year, resulting in up to 200,000 hospitalizations and 20,000 deaths in the United States.[7] Long-acting opioid formulations are an underutilized option. In addition, relief of pain may be complicated by age-related changes in organ function, because many patients with arthritis are older adults.

It is important to recognize that the perception of pain caused by arthritis is complex. Trauma or inflammation can result in hypersensitivity at the affected site, which results in alternations of central nervous system processing and amplification of the pain that is perceived.[4] Often there is a discordance between the pain reported and the degree and amount of tissue damage apparent to the examiner. Depression is associated with increased levels of pain and functional impairment. There are advantages to targeting both peripheral and central pain mechanisms. The analgesic and anti-inflammatory action of NSAIDs appears to result from a combination of peripheral and central effects.[4]

The issues in managing pain, including arthritis-related pain, in older individuals has been outlined in clinical practice guidelines.[8,9] Health care providers should aggressively treat the pain with analgesics and nonpharmacologic approaches[10] while evaluating and alleviating the underlying cause of the pain. Monitoring side effects (especially with NSAIDs in older individuals) and using an objective measurement of patient response to pain (e.g., Visual Analog Scale or other validated pain scale) is essential with any analgesic regimen, from acetaminophen, aspirin, or another NSAID to a strong opioid.

Used in addition to analgesics, treatment with various disease-modifying antirheumatic drugs (DMARDs)[11] as well as physical (e.g., exercise, physical therapy) and psychological (e.g., cognitive-behavioral therapy) modalities may be effective in reducing pain and decreasing disability in patients with arthritis.[4] The benefits are modest (15%–20%) reductions in pain that may not be maintained over periods longer than 1 year.[4]

ANALGESICS FOR ARTHRITIS

NSAIDs, Acetaminophen, and Tramadol

NSAIDs are a heterogeneous group of weakly acidic, highly protein-bound drugs that appear to have both peripheral effects, mediated by cyclooxygenase (COX) inhibition (see later discussion), and central effects that may be mediated by prostaglandins or by other mechanisms.[12–16]

GI side effects, often moderate (e.g., dyspepsia, erosions, and ulcers), are frequent in patients; these side effects are sometimes serious (e.g., bleeding, perforation, and gastric outlet obstruction).[17–19] Risk of peptic ulcers associated with NSAID use increases with age; for example, the risk has been estimated to be four- to fivefold higher in patients over 60 years of age and five- to tenfold higher in patients with a history of ulcer disease. Alcohol consumption and smoking result in a modest (twofold or less) increase in ulcer risk.[20,21] A number of large studies have found that adjuvants, such as omeprazole, misoprostol, ranitidine, and other drugs, can reduce but not eliminate the occurrence of gastric or duodenal ulcers.[22]

It is difficult to overstate the importance of GI toxicity associated with NSAID therapy. Patients with arthritis who are taking NSAIDs are much more likely to be hospitalized for GI complications: 2.5% per year for OA and 5.5% per year for RA, which is 2.5 to 5.5 times higher than for the general population.[23] One estimate is that 107,000 patients are hospitalized for NSAID-related GI complications each year and that at least 16,500 deaths occur among patients whose arthritis is treated with NSAIDs.[23]

Aspirin and other NSAIDs may also cause lower GI problems, such as ulcerations, strictures, colitis, or exacerbation of inflammatory bowel disease.[24–26] Aspirin and other NSAIDs, especially diclofenac and sulindac, are also associated with increased risk of hepatotoxicity,[24] but hepatotoxicity of NSAIDs is rare ($<$0.1%) compared with that associated with acetaminophen, especially in alcoholic patients.[27]

NSAIDS, which are weak organic acids, cause gastric damage by a combination of local effects (direct acid damage) and systemic effects related to impaired prostaglandin synthesis (e.g., decreased mucous layer thickness, decreased bicarbonate secretion, and decreased submucosal blood flow).[28] Combination of traditional NSAIDs with misoprostol, a prostaglandin analogue, reduces GI and renal adverse events.[29] Misoprostol reduces both gastric and duodenal ulcers associated with NSAID treatment. Omeprazole and H_2 antagonists (e.g., ranitidine, famotidine) have been shown to reduce NSAID-induced duodenal ulcers. Sucralfate has not been shown to be effective in preventing either type of ulcer.[28,30] Several adjunctive therapies have been considered to reduce GI side effects of NSAIDs, including misoprostol, omeprazole, and various H_2 blockers.

In a 6-month, randomized, double-blind, placebo-controlled trial (Misoprostol Ulcer Complications Outcome Safety Assessment, or MUCOSA), overall complications were reduced by 40% (P = .045) in patients with RA receiving NSAIDs (definite serious GI events occurred in 25 of 4,404 patients treated with misoprostol compared with 42 of 4,439 patients receiving placebo).[31] In this study, there were 242 suspected events reported in 8,843 patients; however, only 95 (about 1%) had definitive or probable upper GI complications (147 patients had alterative causes for GI complications, primarily lower GI bleeding).[28,31–33]

A fixed-dose combination of 50 or 75 mg of diclofenac with 200 μg of misoprostol is available and has been shown to be effective in treating signs and symptoms of both RA and OA and to be well tolerated in most patients.[34,35]

In a 6-month, randomized, double-blind, placebo-controlled trial comparing misoprostol with omeprazole (Omeprazole versus Misoprostol for NSAID-induced Ulcer Management, or OMNIUM), the efficacy in treating ulcers, erosions, and other symptoms of NSAID therapy was similar for the two agents.[36] However, during maintenance treatment more patients remained in remission with omeprazole (61%) than with misoprostol (48%) or placebo (27%). Also, omeprazole was better tolerated than misoprostol.[36]

In a sister study to OMNIUM, the Acid Suppression Trial: Ranitidine versus Omeprazole for NSAID-Associated Ulcer Treatment (ASTRONAUT), omeprazole at 20 or 40 mg/day (89% and 79%, respectively) had a higher success rate against NSAID-associated ulcers than ranitidine at 150 mg twice daily (63%); $P < .001$.[37,38]

In a report of a substudy of the Arthritis, Rheumatism and Ageing Medical Information System (ARAMIS),[39] the authors noted that asymptomatic patients who took antacids or H_2-receptor antagonists (30% of the nearly 2,000 subjects) had a higher risk (OR 2.69; CI 1.36–5.31) of serious GI complications than patients who did not take these agents. A summary of the entire ARAMIS data set estimates the mortality rate for NSAID-related GI complications as much greater than that of cervical cancer, asthma, or malignant melanoma; comparable to that of leukemia; and one third to one half that of diabetes or human immunodeficiency virus (HIV) disease (both about 40,000 deaths per year).[40]

Patients with RA were more willing to accept risks of treatment with NSAIDs than were patients with OA.[41] For example, RA patients would accept mild indigestion or even indigestion requiring an antacid (70% and 60%) more willingly than would patients with OA (45% and 33%); P = .01 and .05, respectively, and were more willing to accept the risk of developing an ulcer or kidney disease.[41] As with opioids, balancing the risk of side effects of NSAIDs with the fact that unrelieved arthritis-related pain results in reduced function and diminished quality of life is important.[4]

Combination of two NSAIDs results in increased toxicity without increased efficacy.[42] Monitoring for GI, renal, and hepatic toxicity is critical, especially in older patients and those with abnormalities in these organs.[42]

The risk of an adverse drug reaction has been estimated to be twice as high in older patients compared with younger patients.[43] In addition, polypharmacy is especially common in older patients; thus, drug interactions are more common. There is a known potential for drug interactions between NSAIDs and certain antihypertensive agents (beta blockers, angiotensin-converting enzyme [ACE] inhibitors, and diuretics), anticonvulsants (phenytoin, valproic acid), hypoglycemics (sulfonylureas), anticoagulants (warfarin), and medications for congestive heart failure (digoxin).[43]

The toxicity of NSAIDs has been ranked using data from a subset of ARAMIS (see earlier discussion), which has been monitoring approximately 17,000 subjects in the United States and Canada.[44] Hospitalizations for GI disorders were monitored in 2,747 patients followed for a total of 9,525 years in five centers. Overall, 107 (87% affecting the upper GI tract) of the 116 hospitalizations for GI disorders occurred while patients were taking NSAIDs. The overall hospitalization rate for GI disorders in patients receiving NSAIDs was 1.6% per year, 5.2 times higher than in the subjects not receiving NSAIDs. Typically GI toxicity accounted for about 67% of the total toxicity, with a few exceptions (e.g., sulindac).[44] The rankings of selected NSAIDs by GI and total toxicity indices deduced from this analysis are listed in Table 31-1. It is important to consider that individual patients often tolerate different NSAIDs to varying degrees based on idiosyncratic factors.

Acetaminophen Acetaminophen has analgesic and antipyretic activity comparable to aspirin, but does not reduce inflammation. Hematologic, renal, and GI toxicities of acetaminophen at standard doses are rare; however, when acetaminophen is used at high doses it can cause serious hepatic (and renal) injury, especially in patients with predisposing factors (e.g., acute alcohol ingestion, especially

TABLE 31-1 **Toxicity Indices From a Subset of Patients in the ARAMIS Study[44]**

Drug	GI Toxicity Index	Total Toxicity Index
Aspirin	1.0	1.77 (Least toxic)
Salsalate	0.87	2.00
Ibuprofen	1.16	2.68
Naproxen	1.78	3.01
Sulindac	1.63	3.92
Piroxicam	2.07	3.97
Tolmetin	2.16	4.13
Fenoprofen	2.48	4.25
Diclofenac	2.27	4.48
Ketoprofen	3.09	4.69
Indomethacin	2.40	5.15
Meclofenamate	4.03	5.94 (Most toxic)

ARAMIS, Arthritis, Rheumatism and Aging Medical Information System; GI, gastrointestinal.

in an individual with chronic alcohol use).[45] Although acetaminophen can relieve mild to moderate pain caused by OA, its efficacy appears to decrease over time, and patients require additional analgesia.[46] In a meta-analysis of randomized controlled trials for OA of the knee, acetaminophen was comparable in efficacy to low-dose naproxin and ibuprofen, 2,400 mg/day.[47] In addition, aspirin and indomethacin were identified as the most toxic NSAIDs.[47]

Aspirin Aspirin use, especially over long periods and especially in elderly individuals, results in GI irritation and GI bleeding, When renal function is compromised, therapy with aspirin can result in accumulation of salicylate and intoxication.

Ibuprofen and other NSAIDs, as appropriate for the patient's individual risk factors for toxicity, are alternatives in patients for whom acetaminophen is not effective. However, for patients whose pain relief is not adequately relieved by agents in this therapeutic class, use of long-acting opioid analgesics should be considered (see later discussion).

COX-2 Inhibitors

The mechanism of action of aspirin and other NSAIDs by inhibition of prostaglandin synthesis was established in 1971.[48–51] The relevant enzyme prostaglandin synthase, also known as cyclooxygenase (COX), catalyzes two different reactions essential for prostaglandin synthesis (Fig. 31-1). COX is inhibited by aspirin and other NSAIDs but not by opioids, acetaminophen, or tramadol.[52] Aspirin irreversibly acetylates a specific serine (530 for COX-1 and 516 for COX-2). The simple competitive inhibition by ibuprofen and naproxen is rapidly reversible, whereas the time-dependent competitive inhibition by indomethacin or diclofenac results from a conformational change and is less easily reversible.[52]

A decade ago it was discovered that COX has two isoforms that share about 75% of their amino acids but have nearly identical enzyme kinetics.[49,50,52–54] The two isoforms vary in their expression and distribution. COX-1, which is the primary target of older NSAIDs,[55] maintains a variety of normal physiologic functions in the GI tract, kidneys, and platelets, whereas COX-2 appears to mediate inflammatory reactions[52] (Table 31-2). When inhibited by aspirin or other NSAIDs, COX-1 is completely inactivated, whereas COX-2 can convert arachidonic acid to the precursor of leukotrienes,[52] which are associated with asthma and anaphylactic shock.

Celecoxib (manufacturer: Searle; trade name: Celebrex, formerly SC-58635),[56–60] the first COX-2 specific inhibitor licensed in the United States, was approved in 1998. In short-term pain studies, celecoxib was effective in relieving pain but did not cause typical side effect associated with NSAIDs (i.e., GI problems, platelet dysfunction, renal insufficiency, or liver toxicity).[46] A new drug application (NDA) for another COX-2 specific inhibitor, rofecoxib (manufacturer: Merck; trade name: Vioxx, formerly MK-0966), has been submitted to the U.S. Food and Drug Administration (FDA).[61]

The potential role of selective COX-2 inhibitors in various diseases, including arthritis, cancer, and Alzheimer's disease has been reviewed.[15,16,53,62,63] However, there are concerns about new adverse effects on normal physiological processes (e.g., ovulation, pregnancy, vascular tone, and renal function) that may emerge over the course of long-term COX-2 inhibition.[53] For example, there has been a report of fulminant liver failure in a patient taking a COX-2 inhibitor.

Two of the newer NSAIDs, nabumetone (a prodrug of the active metabolite 6-MNA) and etodolac, exhibit some preferential inhibition of COX-2.[64] The preference for COX-2 is approximately tenfold for etodolac.[65] Nabumetone and etodolac offer equivalent efficacy profiles but often with markedly reduced GI toxicity compared with older medications.[29] In a head-to-head comparison in treatment of patients with OA, etodolac was as effective as naproxen, and etodolac and nabumetone were equally effective; all drugs had comparable rates of adverse events and drug discontinuation.[66] However, whether this is mediated via COX-2 is not clear for either agent.[67] An NDA for another COX-2 preferential inhibitor, meloxicam,[68–71] has been submitted to the U.S. FDA. These

TABLE 31-2 **Comparison of COX-1 and COX-2**

	COX-1	COX-2
Gene location	Chromosome 9	Chromosome 1
Expression	Constitutive	Constitutively expressed only in brain, induced in inflammation
Range of expression	Can increase 3- to 4-fold	Can increase 10- to 80-fold
Distribution	All tissues	Rapidly induced (1–3 h) during inflammation
Function	Housekeeping	Inflammation
	Platelets	Macrophages
	Stomach	Leukocytes
	Kidney	Fibroblasts
	Endothelium	Endothelium
		Apoptosis
		Tumor cells
Inhibition	Aspirin, NSAIDs	Aspirin, NSAIDs, and specific COX-2 inhibitors
Effect of glucocorticoids	Little or none	Inhibit expression

COX, cyclooxygenase; NSAID, nonsteroidal anti-inflammatory drug.

Adapted from Bjorkman DJ. The effect of aspirin and nonsteroidal anti-inflammatory drugs on prostaglandins. *Am J Med* 1998;105(suppl):10S; and Robinson DR. Regulation of prostaglandin synthesis by antiinflammatory drugs. *J Rheumatol* 1997;24(suppl):32–39.

COX-2 preferential NSAIDs appear to have less GI toxicity than earlier NSAIDs, which typically inhibit both COX-1 and COX-2 at therapeutic concentrations.[72] The advantages of such COX-2 preferential inhibitors are subtle and difficult to verify in clinical trials.[72,73]

Note: Interestingly, several lines of evidence suggest a role for COX-2 in the pathogenesis of malignancy. Increased production of prostaglandin mediated by increased COX-2 expression may be a common mechanism for dysregulation of cell proliferation.[62,74]

NSAIDs and acetaminophen are the mainstays of initial therapy for both RA and for OA.[75] In a survey of 176 primary care physicians using questions about a hypothetical patient,[75] most respondents indicated they would use an NSAID as initial treatment for RA. Ibuprofen (51%) was the most common choice, followed by naproxen (22%) and aspirin (12%).[75] The most common management approach if the initial NSAID was not effective was to change to another NSAID before referring the patient to a rheumatologist after approximately 3 months of treatment. For OA, only one third used acetaminophen (the recommended agent) for initial therapy, and two thirds prescribed an NSAID, most commonly ibuprofen (65%). Typically OA patients received an average of two NSAIDs over the course of 5 months before referral, usually to an orthopedist.[75] If their pain was not controlled by the NSAID or acetaminophen, most patients had to experience uncontrolled pain for several months. As discussed subsequently, the guidelines for treatment of cancer pain note that mild to moderate pain not relieved by NSAIDs or acetaminophen or moderate to severe pain should be treated with more powerful analgesics, including opioids.

These analgesics are underused in patients with pain caused by arthritis. Use of long-acting opioids (sustained-release oral formulations of morphine or oxycodone or transdermal fentanyl), initiated at low doses with an immediate-release opioid (not necessarily the same drug) as a medication for breakthrough pain, is as appropriate in these patients as in cancer patients.

Tramadol is a non-opioid drug with dual analgesic action and analgesic power equivalent to codeine.[76] Tramadol binds weakly to the μ-opioid receptor and also inhibits reuptake of the monoamines norepinephrine and serotonin.[77] The incidence of respiratory depression is low, but side effects such as dizziness and vertigo, nausea, and constipation are common.[77] Because the addictive potential of tramadol is low, it offers an alternative to opioids when a pure analgesic (rather than an NSAID) is desired.[77] Tramadol, however, is not a potent analgesic; 200 to 400 mg/day is equivalent to ibuprofen, 1200 to 2400 mg/day.[78]

Opioids

Adapting the WHO analgesic ladder for cancer pain[8] for arthritis largely involves more extensive trials of NSAIDs before treatment with an opioid. If a weak opioid is inadequate, the recommended approach is to titrate with instant-release morphine, which can subsequently be used as a rescue medication for occasional breakthrough pain, followed by a sustained-release formulation after stable pain control is achieved.[3] In a retrospective study of 644 rheumatology patients, nearly half (45%) had received a prescription for an opioid during the past 3 years. Of these patients, more than half (153) were treated with an opioid for less than 3 consecutive months. Approximately one fourth of all these rheumatology patients received an opioid for pain relief for more than 3 months. Opioids reduced pain severity scores from 8.2 to 3.6 (10-point scale); $P < .001$. Dose escalation occurred in 32 patients and was attributable to worsening disease severity in all but 4 patients (1.4%), who exhibited abuse behaviors.[79] This study indicates that opioid analgesia should not be withheld from patients with pain resulting from arthritis.

For patients likely to require low doses of strong opioids, it is also possible to move from a weak opioid to a long-acting, strong opioid.[3] The opioid analgesics[80] and transdermal fentanyl[81] have been the subject of detailed reviews. One review article discussing chronic pain notes that all opioids have similar side effects (especially constipation, which should be managed preemptively) and raise similar concerns about tolerance and possible addiction. However, unlike NSAIDs which are associated with GI and renal toxicity, chronic opioid use is not associated with organ system toxicity.[82] A reasonable approach to initiation of a strong opioid is to set specific goals that can be measured (e.g., the ability to walk a certain distance or to go to work each day).[82]

Unfortunately, concerns about patient addiction or regulatory oversight cause some physicians to be reluctant to prescribe opioids at all or to prescribe adequate dosages for maintenance and for breakthrough pain.[4] Some patients may resist initiation of opioid analgesics for a variety of reasons, including risk of addiction. However, the risk of drug addiction is extremely low when patients with arthritis are treated for pain. Patients with a history of substance abuse have a higher, but still quite low, risk of addiction when opioids are used appropriately for the relief of pain.[83] Major aberrant drug-related behavior (e.g., prescription forgery, multiple episodes of prescription loss) may be indications to control opioid treatment for pain relief very closely, including providing weekly or even daily supplies. Minor aberrant behaviors (e.g., aggressive complaining about the need for a higher dose, drug hoarding during a period of reduced symptoms, and unsanctioned dose escalation) are less predictive of development of drug addiction.[83]

As with NSAIDs, balancing the risk of side effects of opioids with the fact that unrelieved arthritis-related pain results in reduced function and diminished quality of life is important.[4]

Morphine is the standard against which other strong opioids are compared. Morphine and other pure agonist opioids have no ceiling effect, and greater pain relief can be achieved by higher doses until toxicity (e.g., sedation, impaired cognition, and nausea) occurs. For patients receiving opioids for chronic pain, opioid-related respiratory depression, which is an important side effect in treatment of acute pain, is usually not a serious problem. Patients experiencing toxicity may benefit by substitution of another strong opioid, especially one that is not taken orally, such as transdermal fentanyl.[3]

Opioids are effective against many types of pain, especially nociceptive pain. There is no ceiling effect for the pure agonist opioids, such as morphine, hydromorphone, and fentanyl. Furthermore, opioid therapy has not been associated with major organ toxicity, even in very long-term use. Patient response to opioids varies, and some patients require sequential trials of several different opioids before an effective and well-tolerated regimen is identified.[80]

Opioid dose can be increased until pain is relieved or until side effects limit therapy. Constipation, sedation, and nausea are the most common side effects. Opioid side effects are usually manageable. Many practitioners manage these side effects preemptively. The prevalence of diarrhea is high among patients with HIV disease; thus, constipation is usually not a problem. Antiemetics to control nausea may also cause sedation. Use of caffeine or psychostimulants (dextroamphetamine, methylphenidate, or pemoline) may be helpful. In most cases, pain management with opioids, such as methadone maintenance, is fully compatible with normal function. Instructions to limit driving or other activities are not given unless overt impairment is observed.[84]

Although respiratory depression may occur and can be life threatening, it is rare in patients who have been receiving chronic opioid therapy, even at high doses. Opioid antagonists (e.g., naloxone) should be available for patients initiating opioid therapy.

Weak opioids are often used when stronger opioids are really necessary, which results in inadequate pain relief. A patient with moderate to severe pain should receive a strong opioid initially, with the dose increased until effective pain relief is achieved. Dose titration is limited by the customary formulations combining a weak opioid and aspirin, acetaminophen, or ibuprofen. Codeine is relatively emetogenic and constipating relative to its analgesic potency. Dihydroxycodone and hydrocodone are stronger than codeine but not as strong as oxycodone. Tramadol, a non-opioid with dual analgesic action (modest affinity for the opioid μ receptor and inhibition of uptake of norepinephrine and serotonin) is generally considered equivalent in analgesic power to codeine.[76,78]

Morphine is the prototypical strong opioid and is available in a wide variety of short-acting, immediate-release formulations. Onset of analgesia begins within 30 minutes of oral administration and usually persists for 3 to 4 hours. Maintaining effective levels of morphine with these formulations requires frequent administration, and these formulations are best used to initiate analgesia and to treat breakthrough pain in patients maintained on a long-acting, sustained-release opioid formulation. The usual initial oral dose of morphine for adults and children weighing more than 50 kg (110 lb) is 30 mg every 3 to 4 hours around the clock, which is three times the parenteral dose. Oxycodone, which is 1.5 to 2 times as potent as morphine, should be classed as a strong opioid along with morphine and hydromorphone. The usual initial oral dose of oxycodone is 5 to 10 mg every 3 to 4 hours. Both morphine and oxycodone are available in long-acting formulations.

Hydromorphone is a strong opioid that can be used instead of morphine for patients who do not tolerate morphine or those in whom extremely high doses are needed. The usual initial oral dose of hydromorphone is 7.5 mg every 3 to 4 hours. No sustained-release formulation of hydromorphone is available.

A number of opioid analgesics are not appropriate for chronic pain relief. Meperidine is not suitable for chronic administration because of the accumulation of toxic metabolites associated with CNS excitation and seizures. Agonist-antagonist opioids, such as buprenorphine, butorphanol, and nalbuphine, may interfere with the effects of pure agonist opioids and are not recommended in treatment of chronic pain.

Hydromorphone has been reported to produce excellent analgesia with reduced side effects, but comparative studies with other strong opioids are not available.[3] Oxycodone, which is sometimes considered a weak rather than a strong opioid, has a longer half-life and may have a more favorable side-effect profile than morphine.[3] Oxycodone is now available in both immediate- and sustained-release formulations.

Codeine, hydrocodone, and oxycodone are often formulated with acetaminophen, aspirin, or, recently, ibuprofen. Because the non-opioid component is associated with a ceiling effect, the pain relief available using these agents is limited. These agents, particularly codeine, are often chosen because their addiction potential is presumed to be low. However, codeine, which is very frequently prescribed, is metabolized to morphine and its metabolites, which are responsible for the pain relief from codeine.

Note: The combination of an N-methyl-D-aspartate (NMDA) antagonist with an opioid may have benefits for pain treatment.[85] Good pain relief has been reported with ketamine alone, although the therapeutic window is narrow and adverse effects are common (psychotomimetic syndromes are the most troublesome).[85] Low doses of systemic ketamine reduced the need for opioids for postoperative pain in some studies; however, combined infusion of low doses of ketamine and morphine had no beneficial effects compared with morphine alone in controlling postoperative pain in elderly patients.[85] Clinical studies evaluating the combination of the NMDA antagonist dextromethorphan and opioids are needed. NMDA antagonists, including the investigational agent MK-801, may have a role in treatment of neuropathic pain.[85]

Long-acting Oral Opioids Long-acting morphine, which is indicated for use in patients who will require repeated administration of a strong opioid for more than a few days, is available in two oral formulations, MS Contin and Oramorph. A long-acting formulation of oxycodone, OxyContin, is now available. These formulations are tablets that must be swallowed whole; tablets must not be broken in half, crushed, or chewed. The usual dosing interval is 12 hours. The orally administered, sustained-release morphine results in higher peak levels and lower trough levels than more frequent administration of immediate-release morphine. The release of morphine from these controlled-release tablets is not continuous over the dosing interval.

Patients are typically initially treated with immediate-release morphine and then converted to sustained-release formulations. If opioid-related side effects occur early in the dosing interval, the dose should be reduced. If breakthrough pain occurs near the end of the dosing interval, the dosing interval should be shortened. To avoid acute toxicity from overdosing, the dosing interval should never be longer than every 12 hours.

Transdermal Fentanyl Fentanyl is a potent opioid analgesic whose pharmacologic properties are particularly suitable to transdermal administration.[81] Fentanyl is short acting when administered intravenously, but the transdermal system (Duragesic) provides a long duration and overall smoothing of the plasma concentration curve (reduction in height of peaks and depth of troughs). Most patients change patches every 3 days (72 hours) (Figs. 31-1 and 31-2). A depot of drug concentrates in the viable epidermis under the transdermal fentanyl patch, and this depot is slowly absorbed into the systemic circulation in subdermal tissue through the cutaneous microcirculation in the dermis (Fig. 31-3).

In a randomized, open-label, crossover study comparing 15-day treatment with transdermal fentanyl and sustained-release morphine in patients with cancer, transdermal fentanyl was associated with less constipation and less daytime drowsiness but with greater sleep disturbance and shorter sleep duration than sustained-release morphine.[86] Of the 136 of 202 patients in the study who expressed a preference, 54% preferred transdermal fentanyl and 36%, sustained-release morphine ($P = .037$).[86]

Sustained-release morphine and transdermal fentanyl were compared in a randomized, open-label, crossover study of 202 cancer patients requiring strong opioid analgesia at 38 palliative care centers in the United Kingdom.[86] Patients received one treatment for 15 days followed immediately by the other treatment. Immediate-release morphine was used freely to titrate patients' pain control at the start of the study and at the crossover and for breakthrough pain. Pain relief as recorded by patients was comparable;

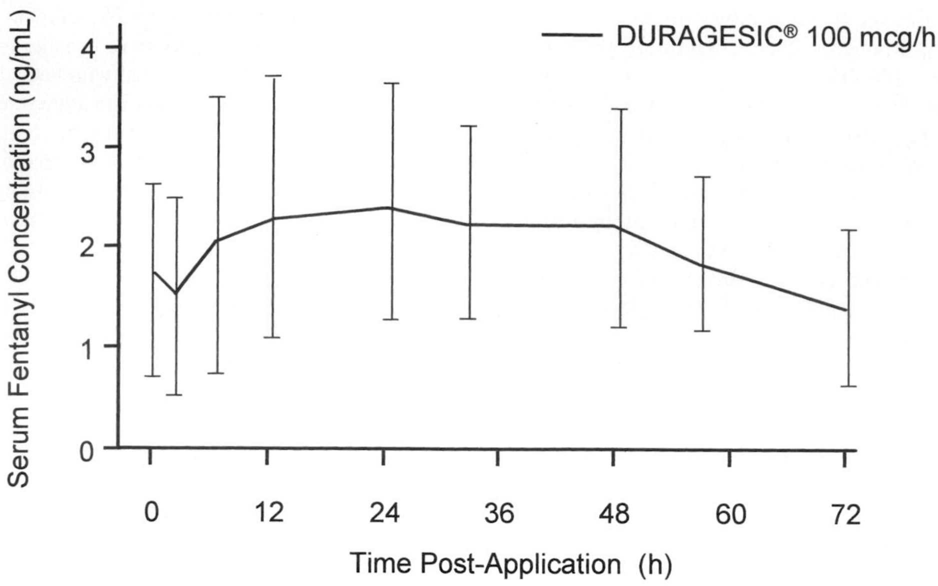

Figure 31-1 Serum fentanyl concentration over three days after application of a single 100 μg/h patch.

however, of those who felt able to express an opinion, transdermal fentanyl was preferred by 54% compared with 36% who preferred sustained-release morphine tablets ($P = .037$).

Fentanyl release may be faster in patients with fever, because there is increased cutaneous circulation; thus, lower dose patches may need to be applied more frequently. Dosing at 2- or 3-day intervals simplifies the pain relief regimen, reducing mediation errors and increasing compliance, especially in patients with cognitive impairment. Patients with reduced body fat may require lower doses of transdermal fentanyl to achieve pain relief.

Because of the slow onset of analgesia, a short-acting opioid prescribed for breakthrough pain should be provided during the first 12 to 24 hours after application of the first transdermal fentanyl patch. The short-acting breakthrough medication can be any strong opioid. The maximum level is typically sustained for 48 hours. After a transdermal patch is removed, plasma fentanyl lev-

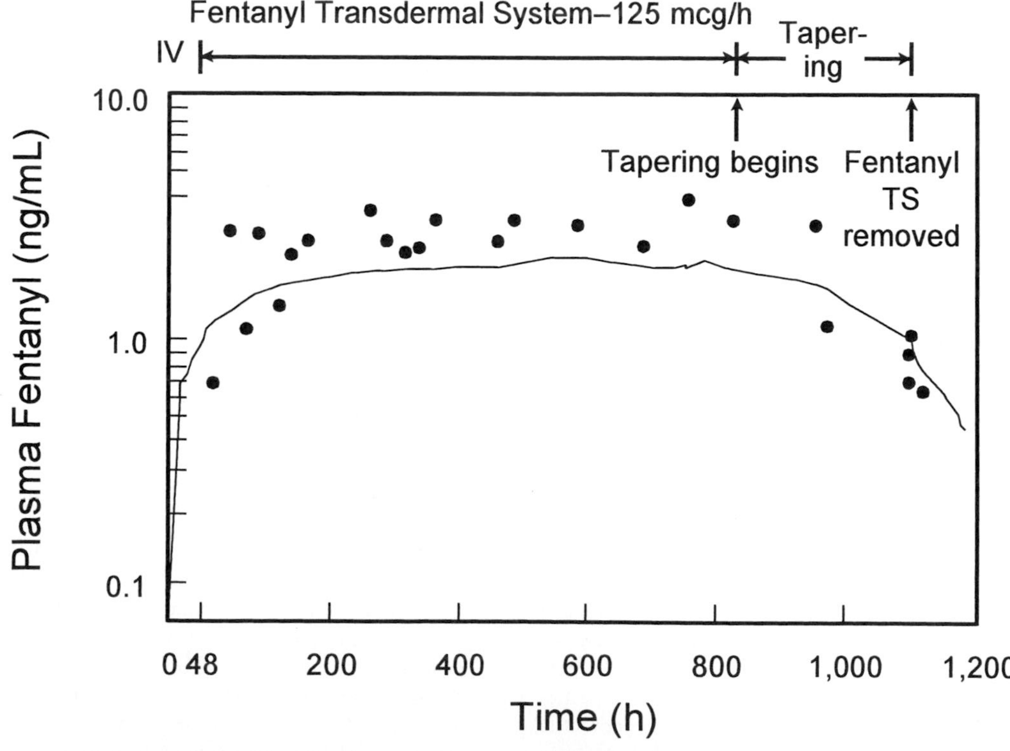

Figure 31-2 Serum fentanyl concentration over 30 days during multiple applications of 125 μg/h patches followed by tapering (From Miser AW, et al. Transdermal fentanyl for pain control in patients with cancer. *Pain* 1989;37:18.)

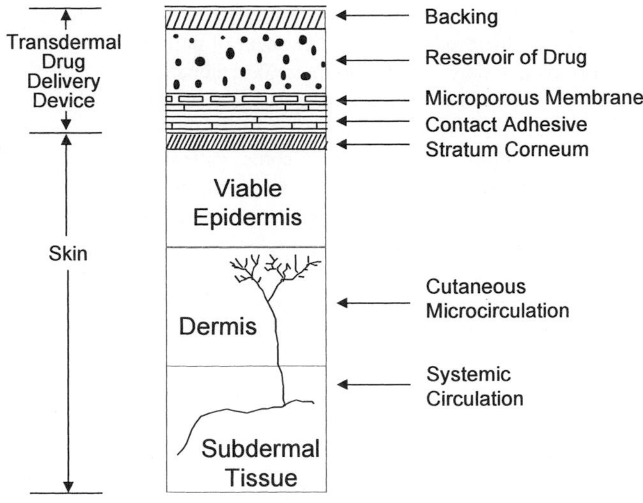

Figure 31-3 Pathway for fentanyl absorption through the layers of the skin (From Varvel JR, et al. Absorption characteristics of transdermally administered fentanyl. *Anesthesiology* 1989;70:928.)

els decline, with a half-life of approximately 17 hours (range: 13–22 hours).

Transdermal administration, which is convenient in most patients, is particularly desirable in patients with GI problems, such as nausea and vomiting or diarrhea, in whom malabsorption of oral medications is likely. Many patients with HIV disease have periods when swallowing is difficult because of opportunistic complications associated with HIV infection. Transdermal fentanyl is particularly useful in such patients, but it is beneficial and effective in all patients with pain. The choice of analgesic and route of administration depend on the pain syndrome, the patient, and the physician's judgment.

The patch must be applied to an area of intact normal skin. Significant dermatologic or allergic reactions are rare, but some patients experience erythema at the site of application.

In opioid-naive patients the initial dose is typically 25 μg/hour, supplemented with a short-acting opioid. Based on use of breakthrough medication, the dose and dosing interval can be adjusted over 1 to 2 weeks to achieve consistent pain relief with minimal use of breakthrough medication.

Potential for Abuse of Long-acting Opioids Although it is possible to abuse almost any psychoactive drug, it is quite uncommon for patients, even those with a history of intravenous drug use, to abuse transdermal fentanyl or other long-acting opioids. The steady blood levels of analgesic provided by these formulations provide effective pain relief but little euphoria, which is associated with the peak levels that occur with frequent dosing of short-acting opioids. Appropriate treatment of moderate to severe pain with opioids, especially long-acting opioids, in my clinical experience rarely results in substance abuse or addiction.

The development of long-acting opioids, including transdermal fentanyl, has simplified treatment of acute pain that requires strong opioids for more than a few days and chronic painful syndromes. In addition, the less-frequent dosing and flatter and lower peak drug levels are associated with less risk of drug abuse. In general, addiction is not a problem in elderly patients treated for arthritis-related pain, especially when the mainstay of treatment is a long-acting oral or transdermal opioid.

ADJUVANT ANALGESICS AND NEUROPATHIC PAIN

Adjuvant analgesics such as antidepressant drugs (both tricyclics and selective serotonin reuptake inhibitors) can benefit patients by relieving clinical depression, which increases sensitivity to pain, and by raising the pain threshold, even in nondepressed individuals. These responses may be the result of increased levels of endorphins.[76]

For patients whose sleep is disturbed by pain, an antidepressant (e.g., amitriptyline or nortriptyline, starting at 10–25 mg and increasing to a maximum of 100–150 mg) given at night may result in improved sleep.[87] In addition, clinical depression is common in patients with RA, especially women. The annual incidence of depression in women with RA was as high at 15% in some prospective studies.[88]

Patients with arthritis may experience neuropathic pain and benefit from treatment with adjuvant analgesics such as tricyclic antidepressants and, for lancinating pain, anticonvulsants. A critical review of controlled trials for treatment of peripheral neuropathic pain supports the analgesic efficacy of tricyclic analgesics and carbamazepine.[89]

Neuropathic pain is generally considered to respond relatively poorly to opioid analgesics. There is a potential for a favorable response in any individual patients; thus, the diagnosis of a neuropathic cause for pain does not justify withholding opioids on the presumption of inefficacy.[84] For example, in a prospective open-label study of transdermal fentanyl for treatment of noncancer neuropathic pain, 35% of patients (17 of 48) reported satisfactory pain relief with acceptable side effects after 12 weeks. For unexplained reasons, neuropathic pain did not recur in 4 of the 17 patients when transdermal fentanyl was discontinued. Of the other 13 patients who had responded to transdermal fentanyl treatment for neuropathic pain, 8 still reported satisfactory pain relief after 2 years of treatment.[90]

The tricyclic antidepressants amitriptyline, nortriptyline, imipramine, or doxepin are frequently used for painful peripheral neuropathy. When they are used as a single nighttime dose, they usually improve sleep with little effect on daytime activities. Two surveys of controlled clinical trials[89,91] found that tricyclic antidepressants were effective analgesics in about half the patients treated. The anticonvulsants carbamazepine, phenytoin, valproic acid, and, more recently, gabapentin have been used successfully for treatment of sharp, shooting (lancinating) pain. In patients whose pain is not controlled with adjuvant analgesic, use of long-acting opioids is a reasonable option. For some patients with debilitating peripheral neuropathy that does not respond to pharmacotherapy, regional anesthetic blockade may be necessary.

OSTEOARTHRITIS

OA, the most common form of arthritis, affects approximately 9% to 12% of the U.S. population, and its incidence increases with age.[87,92] A review of the prevalence of OA noted that in individuals 60 years or older, 17% of the men and 30% of the women had OA based on clinical history.[93] The effect of age is dramatic, with symptomatic OA of the hand occurring in less than 1% of patients younger than 45 years compared with 11.2% of individuals older than 65.[93]

Pain of OA is associated with the presence of radiographic changes and with increased mortality, morbidity, and functional dependence on others. Older age, higher levels of helplessness, and lower levels of education or of income status are associated with increased OA-associated pain.[4] It is important to recognize that NSAIDs are particularly toxic in elderly patients, and, if NSAID therapy is necessary, gastroprotective therapy is prudent in elderly individuals.[94]

Initial treatment of the pain associated with OA, which is primarily caused by degeneration of weight-bearing joints, involves weight loss and exercise. NSAIDs are especially appropriate in the subset of patients who have inflammation secondary to joint degeneration. As discussed later, new COX-2-specific inhibitors may be superior to currently available NSAIDs, which inhibit both COX-1 and COX-2. Some newer NSAIDs, such as nabumetone and etodolac, have some selectivity for COX-2 and less GI toxicity than other NSAIDs.[42]

Acetaminophen alone may provide adequate pain relief for some individuals. Maximal doses of 4 g/day, given in four divided doses for at least 1 week, is an appropriate therapeutic trial for acetaminophen. It is important to consider risks of liver toxicity, especially in patients who drink alcohol or who have liver disease. Acetaminophen, like NSAIDs, has been associated with increased risk of renal failure. Acetaminophen is comparable in efficacy to over-the-counter NSAIDs such as ibuprofen and naproxen.[95] An evidence-based guideline development project[96] in the United Kingdom concludes that acetaminophen (up to 4 g/day) is the preferred initial treatment, with ibuprofen (1.2 g/day) the most appropriate alternative if acetaminophen fails to relieve painful joints. If pain is not relieved, this panel recommends either increasing the dose of ibuprofen to 2.4 mg/day or adding up to 4 g/day of acetaminophen followed by trials of other NSAIDs.[96]

Celecoxib at various doses was compared with placebo in a 2-week trial in patients with painful knee OA. The dropout rate for placebo patients was 14% compared with 1% and 4% for patients receiving celecoxib at 100 or 200 mg twice daily, respectively ($P < .05$).[46]

However, opioids, used in accordance with published clinical guidelines, are appropriate therapy for chronic pain when other analgesics are ineffective.[2,8,9,97] Short-term use of weak opioids, including oxycodone, may be helpful in patients with acute exacerbations of pain.[95] Patients awaiting joint replacement or patients with severe OA who are not candidates for joint replacement may require chronic treatment with a strong opioid,[95] preferably in a long-acting formulation (e.g., sustained-release morphine or oxycodone, transdermal fentanyl).

It is important to recognize that pain resulting from OA varies among individuals and is seldom easily explained by physical or radiographic findings. The perception of pain is a central phenomenon and depends on many factors in addition to those related to the affected joint(s).[98]

Systemic glucocorticoids have no role in routine treatment of OA, although intra-articular injections may relieve painful flares. Such injections, which are most appropriate when only one or a few joints is involved, are typically limited to three or four per joint per year.[42]

Topical capsaicin, which acts locally via inhibition of substance P and can be used with other analgesics, is an option for patients who require additional local pain relief in one or a few joints. The need for administration several times a day and skin reactions, which include burning pain that decreases over time, limit its use.[95,99] According to one review of topical NSAIDs for musculoskeletal conditions,[102] a clear role for this approach in treatment of arthropathies has not yet been defined by long-term studies demonstrating clinical benefit.

Intra-articular injection of hyaluronic acid (weekly for 3 or 5 weeks) is a licensed option for treatment of pain related to OA of the knee, which may be appropriate for certain patients.[95,101,102] One editorial[103] notes that available data (largely relating to the knee) suggest that intra-articular hyaluronic acid injection can provide long-term symptomatic benefit in some patients. However, unequivocal trial-based evidence is lacking, so the procedure should be considered as an alternative in patients who have failed nonpharmacologic and analgesic treatment, for whom NSAID treatment is contraindicated, and who are not candidates for surgery.[103,104]

Note: Glucosamine sulfate with or without concomitant chondroitin sulfate is a popular alternative treatment that may slowly reduce symptoms or NSAID usage.[105] A review of the literature on glucosamine treatment of OA[92] noted that three critically evaluated studies reported a decrease in OA-related symptoms, including decreased pain severity, in patients with OA receiving glucosamine; however, flaws in study design and data analysis prevent the use of these results in modifying current clinical practice.[95] A 6-month randomized, double-blind, placebo-controlled study of oral chondroitin sulfate (800 mg/day) in patients with idiopathic or clinically symptomatic OA of the knee found a statistically significant decrease in pain in the treatment group compared with the placebo group, although the difference in acetaminophen consumption, while trending in the same direction, was not statistically significant.[106]

RHEUMATOID ARTHRITIS

RA, which affects 0.5% to 1% of the population[87,93,107] and is the leading cause of treatable disability in the western world, is underrecognized and undertreated. The American College of Rheumatology (ACR) guidelines initiate treatment of newly diagnosed RA with an NSAID—not acetaminophen, because acetaminophen does not reduce the inflammation associated with RA—with possible use of local or oral corticosteroid.[88,108] Ibuprofen is a good choice because of its low GI toxicity and low cost. For patients with persistent active RA, treatment with DMARDs in consultation with a rheumatologist is indicated. Pain control is an important part of RA management, and successful pain relief leads to improved functional and social integration.[88]

Early identification and institution of treatment with one or more DMARDs before the onset of serious symptoms is desirable and may delay the progression of RA,[108–109] which currently results in disability for about 75% of affected patients.[107] However, the effect of DMARDs on RA-associated pain is incidental, and patients should not be denied adequate analgesia during DMARD treatment. The selection of DMARDs has been reviewed.[11] Chronic, systemic glucocorticoid treatment, although clearly beneficial in controlled circumstances, is controversial owing to adverse events and should be approached using low doses with careful monitoring for anticipated adverse events.[110]

Pain is more commonly associated with RA than with OA. Middle age, lower income status, increased disability, and higher levels of stress and of helplessness are associated with increased RA-associated pain.[4] Although pain in RA is frequently caused by inflammation, in later stages of disease pain may result from secondary OA or from osteoporosis.[4]

Current management of early RA typically focuses on inflammation and frequently does not focus on relieving RA-related pain. Although a pain-free state may not be achievable, a level of pain that allows the patient to cope is reasonable.[4] Clearly, more liberal use of systemic corticosteroids, opioids, and increased doses of NSAIDs and DMARDs may be appropriate in patients with functional limitations resulting from uncontrolled, chronic, RA-associated pain. Rational treatment decisions must involve the patient and physician working together.

Celecoxib was compared with placebo in a 4-week trial in patients with RA. At the end of 1 week, placebo patients reported approximately 20% reduction in pain compared with approximately 70% for patients receiving celecoxib at 200 or 400 mg twice daily ($P < .05$), and these improvements were sustained during the remainder of the study.[46] In this short-term study, celecoxib provided substantial clinical benefit for patients with RA. In addition, even after dosing at 400 mg twice daily for 7 days, celecoxib did not inhibit platelet function, which is mediated by COX-1.[111]

Clearly, short courses of low-dose oral corticosteroids (e.g., prednisolone) are useful for relieving acute exacerbations of RA or as "bridge therapy" before slow-acting DMARDs take effect.[112] Long-term treatment of RA with corticosteroids is often problematic because of adverse effects, even when low doses are used. Meta-analysis of several studies of slow dose corticosteroid has found increased (about 1.5-fold) mortality and hospitalization.[113]

This chapter focuses on treatment of pain in arthritis and does not, therefore, discuss the DMARDs extensively. It is important to note that early use of DMARDs to slow development of RA-associated complications is advocated by some authorities.[114] Also, the introduction of the tumor necrosis factor (TNF)–blocking monoclonal antibody, etanercept, which is indicated for patients with moderate to severe RA with an inadequate response to one or more DMARDs, deserves mention. The role of TNF in the pathogenesis of RA has been reviewed,[107] and the benefits of this expensive parenteral therapy in patients who had failed one to four DMARDs and who were receiving stable doses of corticosteroids (<10 mg/day) or NSAIDs were striking. A randomized, double-blind, placebo-controlled study found that, in addition to benefits on joint swelling and tenderness, pain in treated patients was 4% compared with 56% in patients receiving placebo ($P < .05$).[115]

Drug interactions between methotrexate and various NSAIDs have been reported. One study[116] found that concurrent treatment with aspirin, ibuprofen, naproxen, diclofenac, or indomethacin and methotrexate resulted in increased interpatient variability in methotrexate concentrations; however, there was not a clinically relevant change in its pharmacokinetic parameters.

FUTURE DIRECTIONS

The selective COX-2 inhibitors are anticipated to provide effective therapy for patients with OA and RA without the side effects associated with NSAID therapy. However, the long-term effects of these promising agents when used in clinical practice remain to be established.[46,117,118]

There is increasing evidence that nitric oxide is involved in the pathogenesis of OA.[118,119] The nitric oxide synthase isoforms associated with neural and endothelial tissues are expressed constitutively, whereas a third calcium-independent isoform (iNOS) is induced by following exposure to diverse stimuli such as inflammatory cytokines (e.g., interleukin-1, TNF-α) and inhibited by others (e.g., interleukin-4, interleukin-10, and transforming growth factor-β).[119] The spontaneous production of both prostaglandin E_2 (PGE_2)and nitric oxide in these explants is regulated at the level of transcription and translation. An inhibitor of nitric oxide synthase reduced cellular nitric oxide production by more than 90% but doubled PGE_2 production (a significant increase). Inhibition of PGE_2 production by COX-2 inhibitors (dexamethasone or indomethacin) or addition of exogenous PGE_2 did not significantly affect spontaneous nitric oxide production in this system.[119,120] Although specific drugs targeted to inhibit iNOS and not the constitutive nitric oxide synthase isoforms are not available, many agents currently used to treat rheumatic diseases (e.g., auranofin, glucocorticoids, cyclosporine, methotrexate, tetracycline,[121] and even aspirin[122]) may affect nitric oxide activity.[119] A review article focuses on the role of nitric oxide in the pathophysiology of pain,[123] and another on the potential interactions among isoforms of nitric oxide synthase and COX in various disease states, including OA and RA.[124] In the future, inhibitors of inducible nitric oxide synthase may be developed for a wide variety of conditions associated with inflammation, including OA and RA.[125]

CONCLUSION

The key recommendations adapted from the American Geriatrics Society's clinical practice guidelines for the management of chronic pain in older persons[8] provide a framework for managing pain resulting from OA and RA (Table 31-3). Following published clinical guidelines such as these with clear documentation eliminates concerns some physicians have about involvement of regulatory agencies and malpractice suits if they prescribe opioid analgesics for their patients with arthritis.

In conclusion, patients with pain associated with OA or RA should receive appropriate analgesics at adequate doses (from acet-

TABLE 31-3 **Highlights of the American Geriatrics Society's Clinical Practice Guidelines for Chronic Pain in Elderly Patients[8]**

- Pain should be an important part of each assessment of older patients
  - The underlying cause of pain should be evaluated and alleviated
  - Pain itself should be aggressively treated with appropriate analgesics
- Pain and its response to treatment should be measured objectively using a validated pain scale
- NSAIDs should be used with caution, especially in older patients
- Acetaminophen is the drug of choice in older patients for relieving mild to moderate musculoskeletal pain (Be careful of liver and kidney toxicity)
- Opioids are effective for reliving moderate to severe pain
- Adjuvant analgesics may be appropriate for some patients with neuropathic pain and other chronic pain syndromes
- Nonpharmacologic approaches should be an integral part of care plans for more chronic pain patients
- Referral to a pain specialist or to a multidisciplinary pain management center should be considered when pain management efforts do not meet patient or provider goals
- Regulatory agencies should recognize the need for access to effective opioid analgesics for patients in pain, especially older patients
- Pain management education and practice should be improved at all levels for all health care professionals

NSAIDs, nonsteroidal anti-inflammatory drugs.

aminophen to strong opioids, depending on the circumstances) in addition to treatment for the underlying rheumatic condition using pharmacologic and nonpharmacologic approaches. The goal is not complete relief of pain; this is often not feasible because of the ceiling effect of NSAIDs or side effects. However, patients with painful arthritis deserve pain reduction adequate to improve activities of daily living and quality of life.

REFERENCES

1. Croft P. The epidemiology of pain: The more you have, the more you get. *Ann Rheum Dis* 1996;55:859–860.
2. World Health Organization (WHO). *Cancer Pain Relief and Palliative Care*. WHO Technical Report Series, No. 804.Geneva, Switzerland: WHO; 1990:1–75.
3. Ahmedzai S. Current strategies for pain control. *Ann Oncol* 1997; 8(suppl):S21–S24.
4. Bellamy N, Bradley LA. Workshop on chronic pain, pain control, and patient outcomes in rheumatoid arthritis and osteoarthritis. *Arthritis Rheum* 1996;39:357–362.
5. Verhaak PFM, Kerssens JJ, Dekker J, Sorbi MJ, Bensing JM. Prevalence of chronic benign pain disorder among adults: A review of the literature. *Pain* 1998;77:231–239.
6. Hawker G. Prescribing nonsteroidal antiinflammatory drugs—what's new? *J Rheumatol* 1997;24:243–245.
7. Hamilton GA. Introduction. *Am J Med* 1998;105(suppl):1S.
8. AGS (American Geriatrics Society) Panel on Chronic Pain in Older Persons. Clinical Practice Guidelines: The management of chronic pain in older persons. *J Am Geriatr Soc* 1998;46:635–651.
9. ASA (American Society of Anesthesiologists) Task for on Pain Management, Chronic Pain Section. Practice guidelines for chronic pain management. *Anesthesiology* 1997;86:995–1004.
10. Brandt KD. The importance of nonpharmacologic approaches in management of osteoarthritis. *Am J Med* 1998;105(suppl):39S-44S.
11. Jackson CG, Williams HJ. Disease-modifying antirheumatic drugs: Using their clinical pharmacological effects as a guide to their selection. *Drugs* 1998;56:337–348.
12. Brooks P. Use and benefits of nonsteroidal anti-inflammatory drugs. *Am J Med* 1998;104(suppl):9S–13S.
13. Cashman JN. Mechanisms of action of NSAIDs in analgesia. *Drugs* 1996;52(suppl):13–23.
14. Simon LS. Actions and toxicity of nonsteroidal anti-inflammatory drugs. *Curr Opin Rheumatol* 1996;8:169–175.
15. Simon LS. Biologic effects of nonsteroidal anti-inflammatory drugs. *Curr Opin Rheumatol* 1997;9:178–182.
16. Simon LS. Biology and toxic effects of nonsteroidal anti-inflammatory drugs. *Curr Opin Rheumatol* 1998;10:153–158.
17. Champion DC, Feng PH, Azuma T, et al. NSAID-induced gastrointestinal damage: Epidemiology, risk and prevention, with an evaluation of the role of misoprostol. An Asia-Pacific perspective and consensus. *Drugs* 1997;53:6–19.
18. Cryer B. Gastrointestinal side effects of nonsteroidal anti-inflammatory drugs. *Am J Med* 1998;105(suppl):20S–30S.
19. Griffin MR. Epidemiology of nonsteroidal anti-inflammatory drug-associated gastrointestinal injury. *Am J Med* 1998;104(suppl):23S–29S.
20. Rodríguez LAG. Nonsteroidal antiinflammatory drugs, ulcers and risk: A collaborative meta-analysis. *Semin Arthritis Rheum* 1997;26 (suppl):16–20.
21. Rodríguez LAG. Variability in risk of gastrointestinal complications with different nonsteroidal anti-inflammatory drugs. *Am J Med* 1998; 104(suppl):30S–34S.
22. Hawkey CJ. Progress in prophylaxis against nonsteroidal anti-inflammatory drug-associated ulcers and erosions. *Am J Med* 1998; 104(suppl):67S–74S.
23. Singh G. Recent considerations in nonsteroidal anti-inflammatory drug gastropathy. *Am J Med* 1998;105(suppl):31S–38S.
24. Bjorkman D. Nonsteroidal anti-inflammatory drug-associated toxicity of the liver, lower gastrointestinal tract, and esophagus. *Am J Med* 1998;105(suppl):17S–21S.
25. Wilcox CM, Alexander LN, Cotsonis GA, Clark WS. Non-steroidal antiinflammatory drugs are associated with both upper and lower gastrointestinal bleeding. *Dig Dis Sci* 1997;42:990–997.
26. Wilcox CM, Clark WS. Association of nonsteroidal antiinflammatory drugs with outcome in upper and lower gastrointestinal bleeding. *Dig Dis Sci* 1997;42:985–989.
27. Tolman KG. Hepatotoxicity of non-narcotic analgesics. *Am J Med* 1998;105(suppl):13S–19S.
28. Blower AL. Considerations for nonsteroidal anti-inflammatory drug therapy: safety. *Scand J Rheumatol* 1996;25(suppl):13–24.
29. Benson W, Zizzo A. Newer, safer nonsteroidal anti-inflammatory drugs. Rational NSAID selection for arthritis. *Can Fam Phys* 1998;44: 101–107.
31. Agrawal NM, Aziz K. Prevention of gastrointestinal complications associated with nonsteroidal antiinflammatory drugs. *J Rheumatol* 1998;25(suppl):17–20.
32. Levine JS. Misoprostol and nonsteroidal anti-inflammatory drugs: A tale of effects, outcomes, and costs [editorial]. *Ann Intern Med* 1995; 123:309–310.
33. Silverstein FE, Graham CY, Senior JR, et al. Misoprostol reduces serious gastrointestinal complications in patients with rheumatoid arthritis receiving nonsteroidal anti-inflammatory drugs: A randomized, double-blind, placebo-controlled trial. *Ann Intern Med* 1995;123;241–249.
34. McKenna F. Diclofenac/misoprostol: The European clinical experience. *J Rheumatol* 1998;51:21–30.
35. Shield MJ. Diclofenac/misoprostol: Novel findings and their clinical potential. *J Rheumatol* 1998;25(suppl):31–41.
36. Hawkey CJ, Karrasch JA, Szczepanski L, et al. Omeprazole compared with misoprostol for ulcers associated with nonsteroidal antiinflammatory drugs. *N Engl J Med* 1998;338:727–734.
37. Yeomans ND, Tulassay Z, Juhász L, et al. A comparison of omeprazole with ranitidine for ulcers associated with nonsteroidal antiinflammatory drugs. *N Engl J Med* 1998;338:719–726.
38. Scheiman J, Isenberg J. Agents used in the prevention and treatment of nonsteroidal anti-inflammatory drug-associated symptoms and ulcers. *Am J Med* 1998;105(suppl)32S–38S.
39. Singh G, Ramey DR, Morfeld D, et al. Gastrointestinal tract complications of nonsteroidal anti-inflammatory drug treatment in rheumatoid arthritis. A prospective observational cohort study. *Arch Intern Med* 1996;156:1530–1536.
40. Singh G, Rosen Ramey D. NSAID induced gastrointestinal complications: The ARAMIS perspective 1997. *J Rheumatol* 1998;51(suppl): 8–16.
41. Bagge E, Traub M, Crotty M, Conaghan PG, Oh E, Brooks PM. Are rheumatoid arthritis patients more willing to accept non-steroidal anti-inflammatory drug treatment risks than osteoarthritis patients. *Br J Rheumatol* 1997;36:470–472.
42. Block JA, Schnitzer TJ. Therapeutic approaches to osteoarthritis. *Hosp Pract* 1997;32:159–164.
43. Ruoff G. Management of pain in patients with multiple health problems. *Am J Med* 1998;105(suppl):53S–60S.
44. Fries J. Toward an understanding of NSAID-related adverse events: The contribution of longitudinal data. *Scand J Rheumatol* 1996;25 (suppl):3–8.
45. Makin AJ, Williams R. Acetaminophen-induced hepatotoxicity: Predisposing factors and treatments. *Adv Intern Med* 1997;42:453–483.
46. Lane NE. Pain management in osteoarthritis: the role of COX-2 inhibitors. *J Rheumatol* 1997;24(suppl):20–24.
47. Towheed TE, Hochberg MC. A systematic review of randomized controlled trials of pharmacological therapy in osteoarthritis of the knee, with an emphasis on trial methodology. *J Rheumatol* 1997;26:755–770.

48. Vane JR. Inhibition of prostaglandin synthesis as a mechanism of action for aspirin-like drugs. *Nat New Biol* 1971;231:232–235.
49. Vane JR, Botting RM. Mechanism of action of aspirin-like drugs. *Semin Arthritis Rheum* 1997;26:2–10.
50. Vane JR, Botting RM. Mechanism of action on nonsteroidal anti-inflammatory drugs. *Am J Med* 1998;104(suppl):2S–8S.
51. Vane JR, Bakhle YS, Botting RM. Cyclooxygenases 1 and 2. *Annu Rev Pharmacol Toxicol* 1998;38:97–120.
52. Bjorkman DJ. The effect of aspirin and nonsteroidal anti-inflammatory drugs on prostaglandins. *Am J Med* 1998;105(suppl): 8S–12S.
53. Jouseau J-Y, Terlain B, Abid A, Nédélec E, Netter P. Cyclo-oxygenase isoenzymes: How recent findings affect thinking about nonsteroidal anti-inflammatory drugs. *Drugs* 1997;53:563–582.
54. Smith TJ. Cyclooxygenases as the principal targets for the actions of NSAIDs. *Rheum Dis Clin North Am* 1998;24:501–523.
55. de Brum-Fernandes AJ. New perspectives for nonsteroidal antiinflammatory therapy. *J Rheumatol* 1997;24:246–248.
56. Searle. Draft prescribing information for Celebrex (celecoxib).
57. Anonymous. Celecoxib for arthritis. *Med Lett Drugs Ther* 1999;41: 11–12.
58. Needleman P, Isakson PC. The discovery and function of COX-2. *J Rheumatol* 1997;24(suppl):6–8.
59. Penning TD, Talley JJ, Bertenshaw SR, et al. Synthesis and biological evaluation of the 1,5-diarylpyrazole class of cyclooxygenase-2 inhibitors: Identification of 4-[5-(4-methylphenyl)-3-(trifluoromethyl)-1H-pyrazol-1-yl] benzene sulfonamide (SC-58635,celecoxib). *J Med Chem* 1997;40:1347–1365.
60. Simon LS, Lanza FL, Lipsky PE, et al. Preliminary study of the safety and efficacy of SC-58635, a novel cyclooxygenase 2 inhibitor. *Arthritis Rheum* 1998;41:1591–1602.
61. US Food and Drug Administration. Licensure of Searle's celecoxib 12/31/1998; NDA for Merck's rofecoxib filed 11/23/1998.
62. Dubois RN, Abramson SB, Crofford L, et al. Cyclooxygenase in biology and disease. *FASEB J* 1998;12:1063–1073.
63. Hawkey CJ. Cox-2 inhibitors. *Lancet* 1999;353:307–314.
64. Rothstein R. Safety profiles of leading nonsteroidal anti-inflammatory drugs. *Am J Med* 1998;105(suppl):39S–43S.
65. Dvornik DM. Tissue selective inhibition of prostaglandin biosynthesis by etodolac. *J Rheumatol* 1997;24(suppl):40–47.
66. Schnitzer TJ, Constantine G. Etodolac (Lodine®) in the treatment of osteoarthritis: Recent studies. *J Rheumatol* 1997;24(suppl):23–31.
67. Bolton WW. Scientific rationale for specific inhibition of COX-2. *J Rheumatol* 1998;25(suppl):2–7.
68. Noble S, Balfour JA. Meloxicam. *Drugs* 1996;51:424–430.
69. Barner A. Review of clinical trials and benefit/risk ratio of meloxicam. *Scand J Rheumatol* 1996;25(suppl):29–37.
70. Distel M, Mueller C, Bluhmki E, Fries J. Safety of meloxicam: A global analysis of clinical trials. *Br J Rheumatol* 1996;35(suppl): 68–77.
71. Furst DE. Meloxicam: Selective COX-2 inhibition in clinical practice. *Semin Arthritis Rheum* 1997;26:21–27.
72. Lipsky PE, Abramson SB, Crofford L, Dubois RN, Simon LS, van de Putte LBA. The classification of cyclooxygenase inhibitors. *J Rheumatol* 1998;25:2298–2303.
73. Neustadt DH. Double blind evaluation of the long-term effects of etodolac versus ibuprofen in patients with rheumatoid arthritis. *J Rheumatol* 1997;24(suppl):17–22.
74. Crofford LJ. COX-1 and COX-2 tissue expression: Implications and predictions. *J Rheumatol* 1997;24(suppl):15–19.
75. Spencer-Green G, Spencer-Green E. Nonsteroidal therapy of rheumatoid arthritis and osteoarthritis: How physicians manage treatment failures. *J Rheumatol* 1998;25:2088–2093.
76. Katz WA. The needs of a patient in pain. *Am J Med* 1998;105(suppl): 2S–7S.
77. Katz WA. Pharmacology and clinical experience with tramadol in osteoarthritis. *Drugs* 1996;52(suppl):39–47.
78. Schnitzer TJ. Non-NSAID pharmacologic treatment options for the management of chronic pain. *Am J Med* 1998;105:495.
79. Ytterberg SR, Mahowald ML, Woods SR. Codeine and oxycodone use in patients with chronic rheumatic disease pain. *Arthritis Rheum* 1998;41:1603–1612.
80. Cherney NI. Opioid analgesics: Comparative features and prescribing guidelines. *Drugs* 1996;51:713–737.
81. Jeal W, Benfield P. Transdermal fentanyl: A review of its pharmacologic properties and therapeutic efficacy in pain control. *Drugs* 1997; 53:109–138.
82. Russo CM, Brose WG. Chronic pain. *Annu Rev Med* 1998;49:123–133.
83. Graziotti PJ, Goucke CR. The use of oral opioids in patients with chronic non-cancer pain: Management strategies. *MJA* 1997;167:30–34.
84. Portenoy RK. Opioid therapy for chronic nonmalignant pain: a review of the critical issues. *J Symptom Manage* 1996;11:203.
85. Wiesenfeld-Hallin Z. Combined opioid-NMDA antagonist therapies: What advantages do they offer for the control of pain syndromes? *Drugs* 1998;55:1–4.
86. Ahmedzai S, Brooks D. Transdermal fentanyl versus sustained-release oral morphine in cancer pain: Preference, efficacy, and quality of life. *J Pain Symptom Manage* 1997;13:254–261.
87. Irving GA, Wallace MS. Arthritis. In: *Pain Management for the Practising Physician.* New York, NY: Churchill Livingstone; 1997:91–101.
88. Sewell KL. Rheumatoid arthritis in older adults. *Clin Geriatric Med* 1998;14:475–494.
89. Kingery WS. A critical review of controlled clinical trials for peripheral neuropathic pain and complex regional pain syndromes. *Pain* 1997;73:123–139.
90. Dellemijn PL, van Duijn H, Vannester JAL. Prolonged treatment with transdermal fentanyl in neuropathic pain. *J Pain Symptom Manage* 1998;16:220.
91. McQuay HJ, Tramer M, Nye BA, et al. A systematic review of antidepressants in neuropathic pain. *Pain* 1996;68:217.
92. Barclay TS, Tsourounis C, McCart GM. Glucosamine. *Ann Pharmacother* 1998;32:574–579.
93. Lawrence RC, Helmick CG, Arnett FC, et al. Estimates of the prevalence of arthritis and selected musculoskeletal disorders in the United States. *Arthritis Rheum* 1998;41:778–799.
94. Bird HA. When are NSAIDs appropriate in osteoarthritis. *Drugs Aging* 1998;12:87–95.
95. Creamer P, Flores R, Hochberg MC. Management of osteoarthritis in older adults. *Clin Geriatr Med* 1998;14:435–454.
96. Eccles M, Freemantle N, Mason J. North of England evidence based guideline development project: Summary guideline for non-steroidal anti-inflammatory drugs versus basic analgesia in treating the pain of degenerative arthritis. The North of England Non-Steroidal Anti-Inflammatory Drug Guideline Development Group. *BMJ* 1998;317: 526–530.
97. Jacox A, Carr DB, Payne R, et al. *Management of Cancer Pain: Adults Quick Reference Guide.* No. 9. AHCPR Publication No. 94-0593. Rockville, Md: Agency for Health Care Policy and Research, U.S. Dept Health and Human Services: 1994.
98. Pinals RS. Mechanisms of joint destruction, pain, and disability in osteoarthritis. *Drugs* 1996;52(suppl):14–20.
99. Fusco BM, Giancovazzo M. Peppers and pain: The promise of capsaicin. *Drugs* 1997;53:909–914.
100. Vaile JH, David P. Topical NSAIDs for musculoskeletal conditions. *Drugs* 1998;56:783–799.
101. Wyeth-Ayerst Laboratories. Prescribing information for Synvisc® (hylan G-F 20).
102. Sanofi. Prescribing information for Hyalgan® (sodium hyaluronate).
103. George E. Intra-articular hyaluronan treatment for osteoarthritis. *Ann Rheum Dis* 1998;57:637–640.
104. Marshall KW. Viscosupplementation for osteoarthritis: Current status, unresolved issues, and future directions. *J Rheumatol* 1998;25: 2056–2058.

105. Kelly GS. The role of glucosamine sulfate and chondroitin sulfates in the treatment of degenerative joint disease. *Altern Med Rev* 1998; 3:27–39.
106. Bucsi L, Poor G. Efficacy and tolerability of oral chondroitin sulfate as a symptomatic slow-acting drug for osteoarthritis (SYSADOA) in the treatment of knee osteoarthritis. *Osteoarthritis Cartilage* 1998; 6(suppl):31–36.
107. Camussi G, Luypia E. The future role of anti-tumour necrosis factor (TNF) products in the treatment of rheumatoid arthritis. *Drugs* 1998; 55:613–620.
108. Ad Hoc Committee on Clinical Guidelines. Guidelines for the management of rheumatoid arthritis. *Arthritis Rheum* 1996;39:713–722.
109. van de Putter LBS, van Gestel AM, van Riel PLCM. Early treatment of rheumatoid arthritis: Rationale, evidence, and implications. *Ann Rheum Dis* 1998;57:511–512.
110. Kirwan JR, Russell AS. Systemic glucocorticoid treatment in rheumatoid arthritis—a debate. *Scand J Rheumatol* 1998;27:247–251.
111. Lipsky PE, Isakson PC. Outcome of specific COX-2 inhibition in rheumatoid arthritis. *J Rheumatol* 1997;24(suppl):9–14.
112. Gøtzsche PC, Johansen HK. Meta-analysis of short-term low dose prednisolone versus placebo and non-steroidal anti-inflammatory drugs in rheumatoid arthritis. *BMJ* 1998;316:811–818.
113. Saag KG. Low-dose corticosteroid therapy in rheumatoid arthritis: Balancing the evidence. *Am J Med* 1997;103(suppl):31S–39S.
114. Machold KP, Eberl G, Leeb BF, Nell V, Windisch B, Smolen JS. Early arthritis therapy: Rationale and current approach. *J Rheumatol* 1998; 25(suppl):13–19.
115. Wyeth-Ayerst Laboratories. Prescribing information for Enbrel (etanercept).
116. Iqbal MP, Baig JA, Alic AA, Niazi SK, Mehboobali N, Hussain MA. The effects of non-steroidal anti-inflammatory drugs on the disposition of methotrexate in patients with rheumatoid arthritis. *Biopharm Drug Dispos* 1998;19:163–167.
117. Wallace JL. Nonsteroidal anti-inflammatory drugs and gastroenteropathy: The second hundred years. *Gastroenterology* 1997;112: 1000–1016.
118. Wolfe MM. Future trends in the development of safer nonsteroidal anti-inflammatory drugs. *Am J Med* 1998;105(suppl):44S–52S.
119. Amin AR, Abramson SB. The role of nitric oxide in articular cartilage breakdown in osteoarthritis. *Curr Opin Rheumatol* 1998;10:263–268.
120. Amin AR, Attur M, Patel RN, et al. Superinduction of cyclooxygenase-2 activity in human osteoarthritis-affected cartilage. *J Clin Invest* 1997;99:1231–1237.
121. Amin AR, Attur MG, Thakker GD, et al. A novel mechanism of action of tetracyclines: Effects on nitric oxide synthesis. *Proc Natl Acad Sci U S A* 1996;93:14014–14019.
122. Amin AR, Vyas P, Attur M, et al. The mode of action of aspirin-like drugs: Effect on inducible nitric oxide synthesis. *Proc Natl Acad Sci U S A* 1995;92:7926–7930.
123. Anbar M, Gratt BM. Role of nitric oxide in the physiology of pain. *J Pain Symptom Manage* 1997;14:225–254.
124. Clancy RM, Amin AR, Abramson SB. The role of nitric oxide in inflammation and immunity. *Arthritis Rheum* 1998;41:1141–1151.
125. Nathan C. Perspectives series: Nitric oxide and nitric oxide synthase: What difference does it make? *J Clin Invest* 1997;100:2417–2423.

CHAPTER 32 PAIN IN THE EXTREMITIES

Stephen A. Cohen, Michael J. Stabile, and Carol A. Warfield

Extremity pain can have many causes. This chapter provides a comprehensive differential diagnosis of such pain. The reader should consult the individual chapters dealing with particular pain syndromes to find specific treatment options.

VASCULAR DISORDERS

Acute Arterial Insufficiency (See Chap. 50)

The pain of acute arterial insufficiency is characterized by its sudden onset. Emboli lodge at artery branch points, which are also more likely to be affected by atherosclerosis. Emboli may occlude more than one vessel at a branch point and thereby limit collateral flow. Muscle necrosis and irreversible changes may occur if blood flow is not reestablished within 4 to 6 hours.[1]

The five cardinal features of arterial insufficiency (the five "Ps") consist of pain, pallor, paresthesias, paralysis, and pulselessness. The pain is well localized to an extremity and severe. It may be attenuated by good collateral circulation; that is, occlusion of a brachial artery may not produce as dramatic a clinical picture as occlusion of a common femoral artery or popliteal artery. Nerve endings and muscle tissue are extremely sensitive to hypoxia, and acute obstruction soon leads to anesthesia and paralysis in an affected extremity.[2]

Pulses usually, but not always, are absent distal to the site of obstruction. Therefore, pain and associated signs and symptoms of ischemia in the presence of detectable pulses warrant further investigation.[2] Conversely, pulses may be unusually strong proximal to the site of the occlusion.

Acute ischemia in an extremity also is accompanied by a change in the skin temperature distal to the site of occlusion. The extremity appears pale, and the veins may seem to be empty. Palpation along the course of the artery may reveal tenderness over the site of occlusion. The muscles begin to feel hard and inelastic as the ischemia progresses.[2] Muscular fatigue and weakness are apparent.

Chronic Arterial Insufficiency

Chronic arterial insufficiency can produce a wide variety of painful symptoms. Affected patients can have numbness, coldness, tingling, or total paresis. The degree of insufficiency determines the type of pain in the lower extremity (intermittent claudication or rest pain). Atherosclerosis is the most common cause of chronic lower limb ischemia. Hypertension, diabetes mellitus, hypercholesterolemia, and cigarette smoking increase the incidence and severity of atheroma formation.[3] Thromboangiitis obliterans (Buerger's disease), popliteal artery entrapment, and cystic adventitial disease can also cause lower limb ischemia.

Claudication refers to cramping pain that occurs when blood flow cannot be increased to a muscle mass in response to the increased metabolic demands of exercise. Blood flow is adequate in the extremity at rest. Claudication has several diagnostic features: (1) it is always relieved by rest after exercise, (2) it is produced by a consistent amount of exercise, and (3) it is always experienced in a functional muscle group.[4]

Ischemic rest pain occurs when blood flow in the extremity falls below resting tissue requirements. It is a manifestation of severe chronic arterial insufficiency. Pain can occur in the toes and metatarsal joints and is not confined to functional muscle groups. These patients may experience relief by hanging the affected limb over the side of the bed. The pain is constant and aggravated by limb elevation and exposure to cold.[5] Differentiating between intermittent claudication and ischemic rest pain becomes important because nondiabetic patients with claudication rarely require extremity amputation, although many patients with ischemic rest pain do.[6,7]

Measurement of systolic blood pressure at the ankle facilitates the diagnosis of arterial insufficiency of the lower limbs. The cuff encircles the ankle, and a Doppler probe is placed over the dorsalis pedis or posterior tibial arteries. The ratio of the ankle to arm blood pressure is known as the ankle pressure index. Normally, systolic augmentation occurs, and the ankle pressure should exceed the arm pressure by 10 to 20 mm Hg,[8] which yields an ankle pressure index of 1.10 to 1.20. An index less than 1.0 suggests some degree of arterial insufficiency. Angiographic data correlate with these indices.[9–11] Recently, magnetic resonance angiography has been used to study vascular insufficiency.[12]

Popliteal Artery Entrapment

Popliteal artery entrapment can result in unilateral claudication in even young patients.[13,14] The popliteal artery, instead of coursing downward between the two heads of the gastrocnemius muscle, passes medially to the muscle. Its compression by muscle or fiber spans results in calf and foot claudication. The symptoms of numbness, paresthesias, and cramping associated with exercise may mimic chronic arterial insufficiency. The unilateral nature of the symptoms and the young age of the patient should suggest the diagnosis. Physical examination may reveal either present or absent popliteal and dorsalis pedis pulses, or the latter may disappear with exercise. Palpation may show increased collateral blood flow (palpable geniculate arteries) near the knee. This distinguishes entrapment from chronic arterial insufficiency. Active plantar flexion or passive dorsiflexion may obliterate the pedal pulses and aid the diagnosis. A bruit also may be heard over the popliteal artery.

Arteriography is essential for diagnosis and should be done bilaterally (25% of cases will be bilateral, even in asymptomatic patients).[15] Angiographic confirmation relies on medial deviation of the popliteal artery and segmental occlusion of the popliteal artery.

Adventitial Cystic Disease of the Popliteal Artery

Adventitial cystic disease of the popliteal artery is a rare cause of claudication in young patients.[16] The symptoms are produced by a cyst within the adventitial layer of the popliteal artery, leading to gradual occlusion. These mostly male patients describe a rapid onset of severe claudication. A murmur in the popliteal fossa and the absence of pedal pulses help make the diagnosis. If pedal pulses are present, they can be eliminated by acute knee flexion. The cysts contain mucoproteins and mucopolysaccharides; their exact cause is unclear. Radiographic evidence for the diagnosis includes an "hourglass" appearance using angiography.[16]

Thromboangiitis Obliterans (Buerger's Disease)

Buerger's disease involves the entire neurovascular bundle of the small vessels of the hands and feet. It appears as an intermittent claudication of the arch of the foot and can progress to ischemic digital pain at rest and frank gangrene. Buerger's disease usually affects more than one limb of men younger than 40 who are heavy smokers.[17,18] In contrast to atherosclerosis, Buerger's disease can cause ischemic lesions of the fingers, and recurrent episodes of superficial thrombophlebitis. Angiography shows many small artery occlusions with tapering proximal to the occlusion and the absence of plaques.[19] Its pathologic features include a panangiitis that preserves vessel architecture and infiltration of the vessel walls by giant cells and lymphocytes.

Raynaud's Disease

Raynaud's disease is defined as episodic digital vasospasm precipitated by cold or stress that affects mostly the fingers and hands. It also may affect the feet and toes. The classic attack has three components: (1) initial blanching with relative numbness secondary to arterial vasoconstriction, (2) cyanosis resulting from the desaturation that occurs because of insufficient blood entering the capillaries and small veins, and (3) reactive hyperemia.[20] Usually, neither pallor nor cyanosis predominates. Between 70% and 90% of patients with Raynaud disease are women.[21] The pain, which initially may be mild, becomes more severe and constant as the condition progresses.

The underlying pathophysiology in an attack is digital artery closure.[22] This closure may occur secondary to a vasoconstrictive mechanism (generally in younger women with connective tissue disease) or an obstructive mechanism (usually in older patients with atherosclerosis). The former may be caused by abnormal arterial adrenoreceptors or adrenoreceptor-immune complex interactions. Baseline proximal luminal obstructions are found in the latter group.

Raynaud's phenomenon is associated with various other diseases[23] (Table 32-1) and with occupational hazards, such as operating a chain saw or pneumatic drill. The vibration frequency of these tools (110–140 Hz) presumably causes severe sheer stresses in the arteries of the hands and fingers.[24] Pathologic studies show subintimal fibrosis after long-term exposure to these tools.

The diagnosis is confirmed by the ice-water immersion test. Using a thermistor probe, a baseline digital tip pulp temperature is determined (which must be greater than 32°C, even if external warming must be used). The patient's fingers are submerged in ice water for 30 seconds. Pulp temperature recordings are then made every 5 minutes for up to 45 minutes.[25] A normal patient's digital temperature returns to baseline within 10 minutes. In contrast, patients with Raynaud's syndrome have a prolonged return to baseline temperature.

TABLE 32-1 **Diseases That May Be Associated With Raynaud's Syndrome**

Immunologic and Connective Tissue Disorders
Scleroderma
Mixed connective tissue disease
Systemic lupus erythematosus
Rheumatoid arthritis
Dermatomyositis
Polymyositis
Hepatitis B antigen–induced vasculitis
Drug-induced vasculitis
Sjögren syndrome
Undifferentiated connective tissue disease
Obstructive Arterial Diseases Without Immunologic Disturbance
Arteriosclerosis
Thromboangiitis obliterans
Thoracic outlet syndrome
Occupational Raynaud's Phenomenon
Vibration injury
Direct arterial trauma
Cold injury
Drug-Induced Raynaud's Syndrome Without Arteritis
Ergo
β-Adrenergic blocking drugs
Cytotoxic drugs
Oral contraceptives
Miscellaneous
Vinyl chloride disease
Chronic renal failure
Cold agglutinins
Cryoglobulinemia
Neoplasia
Neurologic disorders
Central nervous system
Peripheral nervous system
Endocrinologic disorder

Other laboratory diagnostic tests include an erythrocyte sedimentation rate, complete blood count, antinuclear antibody, and rheumatoid factor. Hand radiographs are useful for detecting subcutaneous calcinosis typical of scleroderma or CRST syndrome (Calcinosis cutis, Raynaud phenomena, Sclerodactyly, and Telangiectasia).

Thrombophlebitis

Thrombophlebitis of the superficial venous system can occur in either the upper or the lower extremities. The factors responsible for both thrombosis of the superficial venous system and deep vein thrombosis are defined in the Virchow triad: stasis, abnormalities of the vessel wall, and hypercoagulability. Thrombophlebitis may occur after an injury to a limb or secondary to intravenous cannulation. Other causes include varicose veins and carcinoma. Patients may experience pain and redness along the course of a superficial vein, which may feel firm to the touch. Doppler studies show diminished or absent flow through the vein. Treatment is directed toward the underlying disease process and should involve bed rest, elevation of the extremity, and application of moist compresses.

Deep Venous Thrombosis (DVT)

DVT develops commonly near valves in the lower extremity. Initial platelet aggregation elicits fibrin thrombus formation. Both platelets and fibrin contribute to the growing thrombus. In the calf, venous thrombosis usually produces tenderness but minimal swelling. The skin temperature may be increased in the extremity secondary to diversion of blood flow from the deep veins to the superficial veins. Increased tenderness with dorsiflexion (Homan's sign) is notoriously unreliable in the diagnosis of DVT.[26] Femoral vein thrombosis usually results in both calf and popliteal fossa tenderness, and leg swelling. Ileofemoral vein thrombosis is accompanied by sudden severe pain, edema, and discoloration. Patients also may feel tingling, numbness, and weakness. The pain begins in the area of the femoral triangle or in the calf, but rapidly involves the entire leg. This acute venous outflow obstruction can progress to venous gangrene with interference of arterial inflow and limb cyanosis (phlegmasia cerulea dolens).

Conditions that predispose to DVT include obesity, the postpartum state, pelvic surgery, lower extremity fractures, prolonged bed rest, estrogen use, and carcinoma. Detection depends on the following noninvasive laboratory tests.[27–30]

1. *Doppler ultrasonography* recognizes the distorted flow patterns
2. *Impedance plethysmography* quantifies venous obstruction by measuring the rate at which a vein empties when a pneumatic cuff at the thigh is released
3. *Radioactive fibrinogen uptake* tests involve the use of labeled fibrinogen that is taken up by newly formed thrombi. This is the most sensitive test to detect below-the-knee thrombi.

Ascending contrast phlebography also can be used to diagnose DVT, but it is invasive, often painful, and difficult to interpret.

Cellulitis in an extremity, although it does not have a vascular cause, must be differentiated from both superficial and deep venous thrombi. These infections occur after trauma to the skin and subcutaneous tissue. Inflammation is accompanied by edema, hyperemia, and leukocytic infiltration. The hallmarks of infection (swelling, tenderness, heat, and redness) are apparent. Lymphangitis may be evident, with reddish painful streaks and regional node tenderness and enlargement. These patients generally have more systemic symptoms than those with superficial thrombophlebitis. Gram staining of needle aspirates is helpful in diagnosing this disorder and is crucial for further therapy.

Compartment Syndrome

Compartment syndrome is defined as a condition in which increased tissue pressure in a confined space compromises the circulation, resulting in muscle necrosis and neurologic injury. Of the compartment syndromes described (acute, subacute, and chronic Volkmann's contracture), only the acute compartment syndromes are painful. Acute compartment syndromes are seen after tibial fractures, supracondylar fractures, brachial arteriograms, gunshot wounds, circumferential burns, snake bites, reflow after limb reattachment, and crush injuries.

The pathophysiology involves raised tissue pressure leading to altered microcirculation in the compartment.[31–33] Early investigators believed the increased tissue pressure led to arterial spasm and subsequent compromised tissue perfusion. However, newer hypotheses describe increasing tissue pressure that compromises transmural pressure across the walls of the arterioles. At a critical transmural pressure, the vessels close. Small arterioles close at a lower transmural pressure than larger arteries. Hence, tissue ischemia may occur in the presence of palpable pulses. Another hypothesis involves a rise in venous pressure in a compartment in response to the rise in tissue pressure. The venous pressure increase allows blood flow to continue. However, this venous hypertension in the compartment soon disturbs the normal capillary arteriovenous gradient. This, in turn, compromises capillary blood flow and tissue perfusion. Disruption of the Starling gradients leads to decreased extracellular fluid absorption, increased extracellular fluid transudation, and a further increase in compartment tissue pressure.

Acute compartment syndromes usually provoke intense pain, which is well localized to the involved muscle groups. Passive stretching of the involved muscle groups greatly aggravates the pain. For example, passive finger extension in a patient who has flexor forearm compartment syndrome leads to excruciating pain. The second typical finding is induration over the involved muscle groups. Less importantly, patients may have weakness of the involved muscles and paresthesias in the distribution of the involved nerves. Palpable pulses are an unreliable clinical sign (see earlier discussion).

Measuring the tissue pressure in the compartment can aid in the diagnosis. Normal tissue pressure is between 0 and 10 mm Hg. Permanent nerve dysfunction can occur with tissue pressures as low as 30 mm Hg for 6 to 8 hours. The tissue pressure may be measured by the injection method of Whitesides and associates,[34] the wick catheter method of Owen and colleagues,[35] or the continuous infusion method of Matsen and colleagues.[36,37]

Arterial Thrombosis in the Drug Abuser

Extremity pain after drug injection can result from a number of complications[38] (Table 32-2). Intraarterial injection of many agents can result in extremity pain and gangrene. The theoretical mechanisms cited include (1) vasospasm, (2) norepinephrine release, (3) intimal damage, (4) necrotizing arteritis, and (5) particulate embolism. However, the final common pathway is arterial thrombosis. Diluents used in street drugs (lactose, quinine, starch, and talcum powder) compound the vascular insult.[39]

The diagnosis requires eliciting the appropriate history. For example, with an intraarterial injection, patients may describe a so-called *hand trip* that begins with a burning from the point of insertion of the needle to the tip of the fingers.[40,41] This burning is followed immediately by blanching, severe pain, and cyanosis. Addicts also use belts or other vigorous tourniquets for injections; these inadvertently may be left on during the postinjection stupor and further compromise the vascular supply. Pressure necrosis from an abnormal posture after sedation may lead to muscle breakdown and ischemia. Finally, the needle itself, which causes perivascular hematomas, production of an intimal flap, or a false aneurysm, can also lead to thrombosis.[42]

The so-called puffy hand syndrome results from widespread destruction of lymphatic vessels and veins in an extremity used for injections.[43,44] Extremity drainage depends on the deep venous sys-

TABLE 32-2 **Complications of Drug-Induced Vascular Insufficiency**

Infections
Cellulitis
Abscesses
Osteomyelitis
Septic arthritis
Lymphatic Complications
So-called puffy hand
Vascular Complications
Volkmann's ischemic contracture
Crush syndrome
Rhabdomyolysis
Necrotizing angiitis
Direct arterial injury
Thrombosis
Embolism
Mycotic aneurysm
Skin ulcers
Thrombophlebitis
Neurologic Complications
Direct injury to nerve
Polyneuritis
Ischemic neuritis
Acute transverse myelitis

Reprinted with permission from Ritland D, Butterfield W. Extremity complications of drug abuse. *Am J Surg* 1973;126:639.

tem after the superficial lymphatic vessels and veins are destroyed. When perivascular injection or hematomas compromise the deep venous system, swelling and venous hypertension can lead to gangrene. The diagnosis of extremity pain in drug abusers depends on the history and signs of acute ischemia. Identification of the drug used may be helpful. Laboratory tests that may be helpful include Doppler ultrasonography, digital temperature readings, plethysmography, and angiography.

Mycotic Aneurysm[45,46]

Mycotic aneurysms in the extremities can arise through several recognized mechanisms.[47,48]

1. Septic embolization in the arterial lumen, such as occurs with bacterial endocarditis, causes a gradual weakening of the arterial wall, subsequent aneurysm formation, and enlargement of the artery.[49]
2. Local spread from an abscess or area of cellulitis destroys the arterial wall with resulting aneurysm formation.[50]
3. Trauma to an artery and subsequent contamination can cause the formation of a mycotic aneurysm. This commonly occurs after penetrating trauma, radiologic procedures, or inadvertent arterial injection by drug abusers.[51]

Most mycotic aneurysms are arterial, rather than venous, because the high pressure promotes dilation. Aneurysms that result from repeated punctures of arteriovenous dialysis fistulas constitute an exception to this rule. The venous punctures coupled with the high venous pressure seen in these fistulas can cause aneurysm formation.

Patients with a history of rheumatic fever, intravenous drug abuse, immunosuppression, prolonged illness, penetrating trauma, and invasive radiologic procedures may develop mycotic aneurysms. A warm, tender, palpable, pulsatile mass should alert the physician to the diagnosis. A systolic bruit heard over the mass distinguishes aneurysms from arteriovenous fistulas, which have both systolic and diastolic components to their bruits. Signs and symptoms of generalized sepsis also may be present. Occasionally, septic arthritis or petechial skin lesions can develop from emboli originating in the aneurysms. An arteriogram is a useful aid to confirm the diagnosis. Needle aspiration also may be warranted.

Traumatic Aneurysms[52,53]

Traumatic aneurysms are actually false aneurysms produced by arterial penetration. The perivascular hematomas that result may be classified as follows: (1) acute traumatic hematomas, in which through-and-through disruption of the arterial wall leads to a gradual enlarging hematoma contained by surrounding tissue; or (2) chronic traumatic aneurysms, in which the perivascular hematoma is absorbed, and a tissue sac and surrounding fibrosis provide boundaries.

Traumatic aneurysms result from penetrating trauma, invasive radiologic procedures, placement of intra-aortic balloon pumps, vascular procedures, orthopedic reconstructive procedures, and internal fixation of bones.[53]

The interval from initial insult to aneurysm detection is longer than 1 month in more than 50% of cases. Affected patients have a tender pulsatile mass near the course of the artery. As in mycotic aneurysms, a systolic bruit is present. Occasionally, compression by the expanding aneurysm leads to a secondary peripheral neuropathy or venous occlusion. Suspected traumatic aneurysms in the extremity can be evaluated using percutaneous angiography.

NEUROGENIC SYNDROMES

Brachial Plexus Lesions

Several anatomic relationships become important when referring to brachial plexus disorders. The plexus is superficial in the supraclavicular fossa and protected by skin, subcutaneous tissues, and fascia. Also, the brachial plexus is in close proximity to the subclavian artery in the fossa, and both structures lie near the apex of the lung. More distally, the plexus lies close to the first and second parts of the axillary artery, and a thick pad of fat and connective tissue surrounds both. Therefore, many causes can lead to brachial plexus neuropathies (Table 32-3). For example, traction on the upper cervical roots when the shoulder is depressed forcibly and the head turned to the opposite side can lead to neuropathy. Apical lesions of the lung also may depress both the plexus and the vessels that run close to it.

Generally, all lesions of the brachial plexus cause partial or total paralysis of the shoulder. Any lesion involving the T1 root or sympathetic trunk will be accompanied by Horner's syndrome. Sensory deficits will be combined with disturbances of sweating. Most plexus lesions also have long-term complications[54] (Table 32-4).

Plexus lesions can be classified based on anatomic location regardless of their etiology. Superior plexus lesions (Duchenne-Erb)

TABLE 32-3 **Brachial Plexus Neuropathies**[54]

Traumatic
Birth injuries
Stab and gunshot wounds
Motorcycle accidents
Football injuries
Backpack injuries
Electric shock
Laborers carrying heavy loads
Iatrogenic
Axillary artery injuries during cardiac catheterizations
Radiotherapy
Plexus neuropathies from general anesthesia
Vascular
Emboli
Generalized vasculopathies
Heroin injection
Tumors
Primary
Secondary infiltration from lung (Pancoast's tumor)
Metastases (e.g., breast cancer or Hodgkin's disease)
Cryptogenic
Neuralgic amyotrophy
Serum sickness
Anatomic
Thoracic outlet syndrome

result from damage to the fifth and sixth cervical roots. The deltoid, biceps, brachioradialis, and brachialis muscles are affected. There is an inability to abduct and externally rotate the shoulder and an inability to flex the elbow or pronate the forearm. The arm hangs loose, internally rotated, and the palm is visible from behind (so-called porter's-tip position). Sensory loss may be apparent over the deltoid and radial side of the forearm. An isolated middle brachial plexus lesion (C7) is unusual. It is manifested by sensory deficits on the back of the forearm or the radial aspect of the dorsum of the hand. Inferior plexus lesions (C8 to T1) include paralysis of small hand muscles and finger flexors with preservation of finger and wrist extensors. These lesions, therefore, result in hyperextension at the metacarpophalangeal joints and flexion at the interphalangeal joints. Horner's syndrome may be seen. These inferior plexus lesions may result from sudden upward pulling on the shoulder.

TABLE 32-4 **Long-term Complications of Plexus Lesions**

Skin blisters
Ulceration and secondary infection
Joint contractures
Complex regional pain syndrome
Osteoporosis

Lower plexus lesions are divided anatomically into three types. Firstly, posterior cord lesions cause sensory deficits along the distribution of the axillary and radial nerves, weakness of abduction of the arm, and inability to extend the wrist or fingers. Secondly, medial cord lesions cause weakness of the muscles innervated by the ulnar nerve and medial head of the median nerve, thereby leading to severe hand disability. Sensory deficits produce dysfunction of the medial cutaneous nerve of the upper arm and forearm. Isolated medial cord lesions are rare except after radiotherapy. Thirdly, lateral cord lesions involve the lateral part of the median nerve and musculocutaneous nerve, causing weakness of flexion and pronation of the forearm, wrist, and fingers. Sensory loss is limited to the radial aspect of the forearm (Table 32-5).

Because of its superficial position in the supraclavicular fossa, the brachial plexus can be susceptible to traction and exogenous compression. Upper brachial plexus injuries have been reported in laborers who carry heavy loads on their shoulders and U.S. football players. Paralysis from the heavy backpacks carried by soldiers (so-called rucksack paralysis) has been recognized since World War 11.[55–57] The whole plexus (usually on the nondominant side) is affected initially. However, soon only the upper plexus lesions remain, and it is common to see involvement of the nerve to the serratus anterior with winging of the scapula.

Hematomas after anticoagulation or percutaneous axillary artery cannulation may lead to plexus injuries.[58,59] Of special concern to physicians are brachial plexus injuries occurring during general anesthesia. There are three causes. Firstly, shoulder braces may be placed too far medially near the posterior triangle, injuring the plexus before it descends behind the clavicle. Secondly, if the arm is abducted to 90 degrees or more, the head of the humerus descends into the axilla and presses into the plexus as it passes from the supraclavicular area to the axilla. Thirdly, excessive depression of the shoulder girdle with the patient in the Trendelenburg position can stretch the upper roots of the brachial plexus.[60,61]

Vascular insufficiency is a rare cause of brachial plexus injury, but may occur after acute axillary artery occlusions secondary to emboli. Intravenous injection of contaminated heroin can lead to a painless paresis of muscles supplied by the posterior and medial cord.[62] Radiotherapy to the clavicular region or axilla can injure the brachial plexus. Distinguishing radiation injury from direct tumor infiltration can be difficult. Post-radiation intervals shorter than 3 months or longer than 5 years favor metastases. Intense pain, lower plexus lesions, and Horner's syndrome also favor metastases. Skin changes, lymphedema of the extremity, induration over the supraclavicular fossa, and upper plexus lesions favor radiotherapy as the source of the neuropathy. Paresthesias frequently can be elicited by tapping the supraclavicular fossa after radiation-induced lesions[63,64] (Table 32-6).

Inherited Brachial Plexus Neuropathy

A form of recurrent brachial plexus neuropathy can display familial predilection.[65–69] It is similar to neuralgic amyotrophy except for several distinguishing features. In contrast to neuralgic amyotrophy, the familial form of brachial plexus neuropathy is characterized by recurrent episodes over several years separated by intervals of full recovery. Both diseases occur most commonly during the third and fourth decades of life, but in the familial form, affected patients may have their first attacks during the first decade of life. The familial form does not seem to be precipitated as commonly by infections as is neuralgic amyotrophy. However, several

TABLE 32-5 **Physical Findings in Brachial Plexus Injuries**

Vertebral Level	Motor Deficit	Sensory Deficit	Reflex Affected
C5	Shoulder abduction, deltoids, biceps	Radial aspect of arm	Biceps
C6	Wrist extension	Lateral forearm	Brachioradialis
C7	Wrist flexion, finger extension	Middle finger	Triceps
C8	Finger flexion	Medial forearm	—
T1	Finger abduction	Medial aspect of arm	—

Modified from Sola A. Upper extremity pain. In: Melzack R. Wall PD, eds. *Textbook of Pain.* New York, NY: Churchill-Livingstone; 1984:252–262.

authors have reported a dramatic onset of attacks in women several hours after childbirth.[67,70] There may be minor dysmorphic features (e.g., hypotelorism, epicanthic folds, and cleft palate) associated with the familial form of the disease.[67] Finally, there is nerve involvement outside the brachial plexus with such diverse manifestations as Horner's syndrome, Bell's palsy, and lumbosacral weakness in the familial form of the disease.

Pain is the initial manifestation of a familial attack. It is described as sharp and burning, particularly in the shoulder. Movement exacerbates the pain; therefore, affected patients keep their shoulders immobile. Weakness soon follows, and although any muscles controlled by the plexus may be involved, those innervated by the upper trunk of the plexus generally are affected. Sensory dysfunction is not a prominent feature. Affected patients usually have an excellent recovery of strength, but they may accumulate deficits after multiple attacks.[68]

Guillain-Barré Syndrome

Guillain-Barré syndrome occurs worldwide, with an incidence of 1 to 1.5 cases per 100,000 persons annually. There is no age or gender preference; 60% to 70% of cases are preceded by an upper respiratory or gastrointestinal illness 1 to 3 weeks before the onset of the syndrome.[71] An ascending weakness involving both proximal and distal muscles distinguishes Guillain-Barré syndrome. The weakness generally begins in the lower extremities and then can progress to upper extremity, intercostal, and neck muscles. Affected patients also have decreased sensation and possibly transient autonomic dysfunction.

Pain occurs in one third of the cases of Guillain-Barré syndrome as a result of involvement of the posterior roots. There may be tenderness after deep pressure on the muscles. Paresthesias are common. Affected patients also describe a burning, radiating pain.

The clinical diagnosis is aided by examination of cerebrospinal fluid. Normal pressures, increased protein, and acellular fluid are found. Nerve conduction studies show slowing after the paralysis begins.[72] A syndrome identical to Guillain-Barré can occur after infectious mononucleosis.

Fabry's Disease (Angiokeratoma Corporis Diffusum)

Fabry's disease is an X-linked recessive disorder characterized by accumulation of a lipid, ceramide trihexoside, in many organs. Patients are young boys or men with intense burning pain in their feet and lower legs.[73]

The enzymatic defect in Fabry's disease is a deficiency of the enzyme ceramide trihexosidase; the terminal molecule of galactose is missing from this enzyme.[74] Stored glycolipid accumulates in different organ systems. Renal involvement initially is characterized by albuminuria and inability to concentrate urine, which progresses to uremia. Glycolipid accumulates in the endothelial cells of the glomeruli and distal tubular cells. The first manifestations of this disease, angiokeratomas, are found over the perineum, upper thighs, and buttocks. Less commonly, they may be seen on the lip and oral mucosa.[75]

The vascular elements that supply the ganglions of the peripheral nervous system accumulate the lipid. The ganglion cells themselves and the perineural cells may contain the storage material, possibly causing the anhidrosis and pain that are features of this disease.[76]

TABLE 32-6 **Characteristics of Brachial Plexus Injuries Caused by Radiation Versus Tumor[63,64]**

Characteristics	Radiation	Tumor
Site	Upper plexus	Lower plexus
Pain	$< 50\%$	$>75\%$
Lymphedema	Usually present	Usually absent
Time of onset to 1 yr	Between 3 mo and 5 yr	3 mo
Horner's syndrome	Usually absent	Usually present
Skin changes	Usually present	Usually absent

Other systems that accumulate glycolipid include the eye, liver, and reticuloendothelial system. The diagnosis can be confirmed by enzyme assays done on biopsy specimens of small intestinal mucosa.[74] Tissue α-galactosidase activity is decreased in patients with Fabry's disease.

Compression Neuropathies

Compression neuropathies are caused by pressure damage to peripheral nerves. The pressure may be external (a brace or cast), or the nerves may be compressed by adjacent body tissues (tumors, muscle, or synovial thickening). Entrapment neuropathies occur at sites where the nerves normally would be somewhat confined (Table 32-7).

Three degrees of compression neuropathy can be described: neurapraxia, axonotmesis, and neurotmesis. In neurapraxia, functional impairment without axonal structural loss can recover in days to weeks by removing the inciting compressing stimulus. In axonotmesis, wallerian degeneration follows axonal loss and functional restoration may occur only after axonal regeneration, which takes months or years. In neurotmesis, severance of the entire nerve and supporting connective tissue occurs. Such injuries spontaneously regenerate poorly, if at all.

Individual peripheral nerves are more susceptible to compression when already involved by disease states associated with generalized peripheral neuropathies (e.g., diabetes mellitus, renal failure, or alcoholism).[77,78] Affected patients have symptoms of sensory nerve dysfunction. Paresthesias and numbness usually are confined to the cutaneous distribution of the nerve. Pain can occur at rest and is localized, but may be referred to other sites.

Electrophysiologic studies can help localize and assess these neuropathies.[79] Nerve conduction studies may reveal (1) slowing of conduction secondary to focal demyelination, (2) reduced amplitudes of both sensory action potentials and compound muscle potentials secondary to axonal damage, and (3) the presence of a generalized polyneuropathy. Electromyographic studies may show (1) denervation potentials in the muscle secondary to anterior horn cell loss, and (2) motor unit potential variation secondary to reinnervation of the muscle by axons. Computed tomography (CT) scans and radiography may reveal bone or joint abnormalities responsible for compression.[80]

Ulnar Nerve Syndromes

The ulnar nerve derives from the C7, C8, and T1 roots. It courses medially in the upper arm without giving off any branches. At the elbow, it lies behind the medial epicondyle in the ulnar groove. It then descends under a roof formed by the aponeurosis of the flexor carpi ulnaris muscle in the cubital tunnel. Motor branches arise in the cubital tunnel and supply the flexor carpi ulnaris. The nerve then gives off branches to the flexor digitorum profundus of the fourth and fifth digits. The palmar cutaneous branch arises and supplies the hypothenar region. More distally, the dorsal cutaneous branch arises and innervates the medial half of the back of the hand and half of the fourth and fifth digits. The nerve enters the hand superficial to the flexor retinaculum and runs between the hook of the hamate and pisiform bone into Guyon's canal, where it bifurcates and gives rise to a superficial terminal branch and deep motor branch that supplies the hypothenar muscles, third and fourth lumbricales, adductor pollicis, and all the interossei.

Compression Above the Elbow and at the Elbow The elbow is the most common site of ulnar nerve entrapment, particularly in the condylar groove and cubital tunnel. The nerve lies superficially in the groove and is susceptible to compression by leaning on the elbow or improper arm positioning during general anesthesia. Deformities from injuries to the elbow can cause the ulnar nerve to stretch, with a neuropathy appearing long after the actual time of injury (so-called tardy ulnar palsy).[81] The ulnar nerve also may be compressed in the cubital tunnel (so-called idiopathic cubital tunnel syndrome); this may be caused by prolonged flexion tightening of the aponeurosis at the proximal end of the tunnel.[82,83]

Ulnar nerve injuries during anesthesia may result when the patient's arm is adducted along the side of the body and the hand supinated. The patient's elbow may slip out of the restraints, and with the ulnar groove located posteromedially, the edge of the table may compress the nerve. Pronating the forearm will rotate the ulnar groove more posteriorly and laterally and prevent compression

TABLE 32-7 **Common Compression Neuropathies**

Nerve	Site of Entrapment
Anterior interosseous nerve	Between two heads of pronator teres
Median nerve	Carpal tunnel
Ulnar nerve	Condylar groove, cubital tunnel at elbow, palmar fascia–pisiform bone at wrist
Radial nerve (radial tunnel syndrome)	Radial tunnel between superficial and deep heads of supinator
Suprascapular nerve	Spinofenoid notch on upper border of scapula
Lateral femoral cutaneous nerve (meralgia paresthetica)	Inguinal ligament
Obturator nerve	Obturator canal
Deep peroneal nerve (anterior tibial syndrome)	Muscle swelling in anterior compartment
Posterior tibial nerve (tarsal tunnel syndrome)	Tarsal tunnel, medial malleolus–flexor retinaculum
Sural nerve	External pressure over posterior lower calf
Phantom nerve or interdigital nerve (Morton's neuroma)	Adjacent metatarsal heads of third and fourth toes, phantom fascia

Modified from Adams RD, Victor M, eds. *Principles of Neurology.* 3rd ed. New York, NY: McGraw-Hill; 1985:166.

by the table or equipment rail.[84] Patients with entrapment neuropathies at or above the elbows may have pain at the elbow, which may spread to other parts of the arm. Tingling and numbness along the medial portion of the palm and the fourth and fifth digits also occurs. Muscle wasting is prominent in the hypothenar eminence, and affected patients have weakness of the interossei. Severe ulnar neuropathy at the elbow results in a so-called claw-hand deformity. Proximal ulnar entrapment is characterized by weakness of the flexor carpi ulnaris and flexor digitorum profundus muscles; this distinguishes it from more distal entrapments.

Ulnar Nerve Compression in the Wrist or Hand Ulnar nerve compression in the wrist or hand may result in intermittent paresthesias along the volar aspect of the fifth digit and half or all the volar aspect of the ring finger.[85] The sensory branch of the ulnar nerve to the hand courses through Guyon's canal encased by fibrous tissue. Repetitive trauma to the area (e.g., striking a stapler) can lead to compression. Other causes include pressure from a wristwatch band or overuse of the flexor carpi ulnaris. Finally, space-occupying lesions (e.g., ganglions or lipomas), thrombosis of the ulnar artery, or a rapid weight gain may cause nerve compression at the edge of Guyon's canal.

Radial Nerve Syndromes

The radial nerve receives contributions from the C5 to T1 roots. It spirals around the shaft of the humerus in the spiral groove and descends along the lateral aspect of the humerus superficially. It passes distally in front of the lateral epicondyle and divides into the deep motor nerve (posterior interosseous nerve) and superficial radial nerves variably 4 to 5 cm above or below the lateral epicondyle. The deep motor branch (posterior interosseous nerve) passes into the supinator muscle through the arcade of Frohse and finally supplies the extensor muscles of the digits. The superficial radial nerve passes over the supinator and pronator teres muscles along the lateral forearm and supplies sensation to the dorsal aspect of the hand, the thumb, and adjacent fingers.

The radial nerve may be compressed in the axilla secondary to the misuse of crutches. Along with the signs and symptoms described subsequently for more distal radial neuropathies, these patients characteristically have triceps weakness.

Most radial nerve compressions occur between the mid to upper arm and elbow, where the nerve courses laterally around the spiral groove and then passes superficially along the humerus. Improper positioning of the arm during sleep or intoxication (so-called Saturday-night palsy) results in involvement of the extensors of the wrist and fingers and the brachioradialis muscles, with resultant wrist drop and associated variable sensory disturbances.[86] Misuse of tourniquets, external pressure from ether screens and Mayo stands, and failure to pad the dependent arm when a patient is in the lateral decubitus position can produce a radial nerve palsy during anesthesia. Fractures of the shaft of the humerus with callus formation may compress the nerve and cause a neuropathy.

The posterior interosseous nerve (deep motor branch) can be compressed in the radial tunnel between the superficial and deep heads of the supinator. Radial tunnel syndrome is characterized by deep aching pain of the extensor supinator muscles in the dorsal forearm. Affected patients are unable to extend their thumbs and fingers at the metacarpophalangeal joints and cannot deviate their hands in the ulnar direction. Superficial radial nerve compressions can be caused by wearing handcuffs or watchbands or by fractures of the radius. Affected patients feel pain and paresthesias on the dorsum of the thumb and index finger.

Median Nerve Syndromes

The median nerve receives contributions from the C5 to T1 roots. It courses medially in the upper arm where it gives off no branches. The nerve crosses the elbow anteriorly and passes between the two heads of the pronator teres. It then passes deep to the tendon (so-called subliminis bridge) and runs distally between the flexor digitorum profundus muscles and flexor digitorum superficialis muscles. Motor nerves branch off before the median nerve passes between the pronator teres, the muscles responsible for wrist and finger flexion. A purely motor branch, the anterior interosseous nerve, is given off just after the median nerve emerges from the pronator teres. It innervates the flexor digitorum profundus to the second and third digits. The median nerve passes under the flexor retinaculum at the wrist and innervates the first two lumbrical muscles and the adductor pollicis brevis. The digital nerves then provide sensory innervation to the distal palm and palmar surfaces of the first through fourth digits.

Compression in the Carpal Tunnel Compression of the median nerve in the carpal tunnel is the most common compression neuropathy of the upper extremity.[87] Women between the ages of 40 and 60 years are affected predominantly. Any condition that reduces the capacity of the carpal tunnel can precipitate the symptoms.[88] These conditions include (1) fractures, (2) ganglions, (3) xanthomas, and (4) synovial disorders. Systemic conditions predisposing to carpal tunnel syndrome include (1) obesity, (2) pregnancy, (3) hypothyroidism, (4) acromegaly, (5) myeloma, (6) amyloidosis, (7) Raynaud's disease, (8) chronic renal failure, and (9) diabetes mellitus.

Paresthesias and pain occurring during sleep characterize the syndrome. The paresthesias usually are localized to the palmar aspects of the fingers and hands. These patients, however, may complain of wrist and forearm pain. The paresthesias and pain are aggravated by repeated wrist and finger flexion. Affected patients also may feel clumsy and have hand weakness. The symptoms usually begin in the dominant hand, although in more than half of the cases, the disorder is bilateral.[89]

Physical examination reveals decreased sensation over the palmar aspect of the thumb through the ring finger. Atrophy of the thenar muscles can occur as a late sign of median neuropathy. Tinel's sign and Phalen's test help make the diagnosis. Tinel's sign refers to distal paresthesias elicited by percussion of the median nerve either proximal to the flexor retinaculum in the wrist or distally at the base of the palm. Phalen's test is performed by applying a tourniquet to thc arm at 60 mm Hg pressure.[90] The venous congestion will elicit paresthesias in patients with carpal tunnel syndrome. Alternatively, acute flexion of the wrist for 60 seconds will accomplish the same goal.

Median Nerve Compression Proximal to the Carpal Tunnel The median nerve may be compressed proximally, too. For example, compression in the axilla may result from the misuse of crutches. The pronator syndrome, which may appear spontaneously or be caused by excessive forearm pronation (e.g., in tennis players), results from median nerve entrapment between the two heads of the pronator teres.[91] These patients have unlocalized forearm pain combined with numbness in the fingers innervated by the median nerve.[92] Anterior interosseous syndrome is caused by damage to this purely motor branch from fractures or fibrous band compression. Affected patients have proximal forearm pain that increases with exercise.[93]

Diagnostically, these proximal nerve compressions can be distinguished from carpal tunnel syndrome by the characteristic weakness of the flexor digitorum muscles and flexor pollicis longus. These patients are asked to oppose the tip of the thumb to the second digit and are unable to flex both distal phalanges (so-called circle test). Weakness of pronation also is characteristic of proximal median nerve entrapment.[93,94]

Digital Nerve Compression of the Thumb and Fingers

So-called bowler's thumb is caused by constant irritation of the digital nerve at the thumb. Perineural fibrosis and painful nodule formation results. So-called harp player's thumb is caused by strumming musical instruments; painful nodules or hypersensitivity to touch may occur.

Suprascapular Nerve

The suprascapular nerve is a purely motor nerve arising from the upper branch of the brachial plexus. It runs under the trapezius muscle through a notch on the upper border of the scapula and supplies the supraspinatus and infraspinatus muscles.

Damage to the scapula may injure the nerve to produce a syndrome characterized by weakness confined to spinatus muscles without sensory loss. Affected patients have pain after shoulder abduction.[95,96] Tenderness may be elicited by palpating the suprascapular notch. Needle electromyography (EMG) shows denervation of the spinatus muscles.

Femoral Nerve Entrapment Syndrome

The femoral nerve is formed from the posterior branches of L2 to L4 behind the psoas muscle. It then courses around the lateral wall of the psoas muscle into the iliacus compartment located between the psoas and iliacus muscles and covered by the iliacus fascia. It then gives off branches that supply the quadriceps and sensation to the anterior thigh. The nerve terminates as the saphenous nerve, which supplies sensation to the skin on the medial aspect of the leg.

Femoral neuropathy leads to wasting of the quadriceps muscles and sensory disturbances over the anteromedial aspect of the thigh and medial aspect of the lower leg. The patellar reflex also is diminished or absent.

Diabetes is the most common cause of femoral neuropathy.[97] Other causes include injury of the nerve beneath the inguinal ligament as a result of scar tissue or prolonged lithotomy position[98] and compression of the nerve in the iliacus compartment from hematomas secondary to trauma or anticoagulants.[99]

Femoral neuropathy must be differentiated from L3 to L4 radiculopathy. EMG studies can help determine whether motor dysfunction is confined to the femoral nerve distribution. CT scans and radiographs of the lumbosacral spine may help exclude disk disease.

Meralgia Paresthetica or Lateral Femoral Cutaneous Nerve Entrapment (Roth's Disease or Bernhardt's Disease)

The lateral femoral cutaneous nerve, which supplies the anterolateral aspect of the thigh, is a purely sensory nerve formed from the posterior division of the L2 and L3 roots. The nerve emerges along the lateral border of the psoas muscle and courses peripherally around the pelvis between the iliac muscle and its overlying fascia (Fig. 32-1). The nerve then descends under the lateral aspect

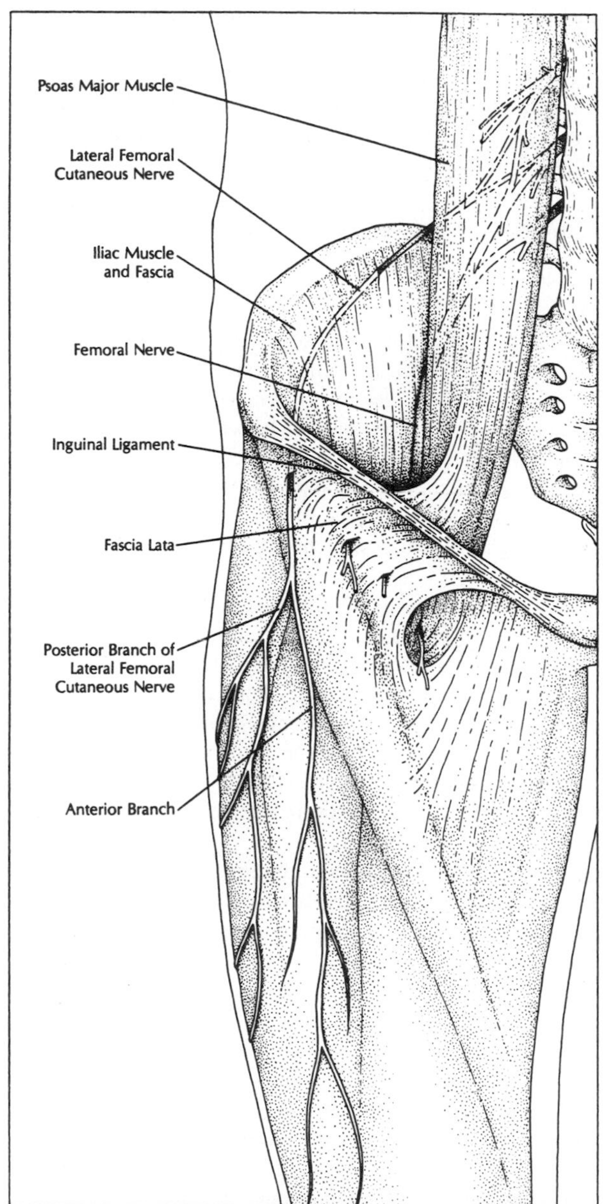

Figure 32-1 Entrapment of lateral femoral cutaneous nerve commonly occurs when nerve passes through inguinal ligament. Entrapment also may occur in fascia of iliac muscle. Tension, mechanical friction, and neural irritation may arise along entire anatomic course, with eventual formation of pseudoganglions and consequent meralgia. (Reproduced with permission from Warfield CA. Meralgia paresthetica: causes and cures. *Hosp Pract Off* 1986;21(2):40c.)

of the inguinal ligament to the anterior-superior iliac spine; finally, it runs beneath the deep fascia and subcutaneous tissue of the upper thigh.[100] The nerve divides into anterior and posterior branches, which supply the anterolateral and posterior aspect of the thigh, respectively. Affected patients have burning pain and dysesthesias along the lateral aspect of the thigh, which are exacerbated by prolonged walking or standing.

The most common site of lateral femoral cutaneous nerve entrapment occurs as the nerve passes from the pelvis into the thigh.[101] Thus, pressure from belts, girdles, and tight pants is cited as a precipitating cause. Also, direct trauma to the area of the anterior-superior iliac spine can lead to increased tension on the nerve. The diagnosis can be confirmed by blocking the nerve with a local anesthetic. A wheal is raised medially and inferiorly to the anterior-superior iliac spine. After the fascia above the inguinal ligament is pierced, 10 to 12 mL of a local anesthetic are injected in a fanlike distribution.

Sciatic Nerve Syndromes

Two distinct nerves, the tibial and common peroneal, comprise the sciatic nerve. The latter arises from the posterior divisions of L4, L5, S1, and S2. The former arises from the anterior divisions of L4 and L5, and S1 to S3. The sciatic nerve leaves the pelvis through the sciatic notch below the piriformis muscle, where it may be compressed by masses. Then it courses between the greater trochanter and ischial tuberosity covered by the gluteus maximus muscle and hamstrings. The fact that the superior and inferior gluteal nerves and posterior cutaneous nerve of the thigh pass with the sciatic nerve through the notch can help to localize sites of sciatic compression.

Aside from penetrating trauma, most injuries to the sciatic nerve occur as a result of fracture dislocations of the hip joint and hip arthroplasty. Deep injections into the buttock may directly injure the nerve or cause muscle fibrosis that compresses the nerve.[102] Masses, such as endometriomas, may compress the nerve at the sciatic notch.[103] In addition to the buttock pain and paresthesias along the back of the leg, a sciatic nerve injury can cause foot drop, impaired hip extension, and decreased sensation over the lateral leg and foot.

Piriformis syndrome is caused by spasm or scarring of the piriformis muscle. Affected patients have symptoms similar to "sciatica," such as buttock pain and burning dysesthesias down the back of the leg.[104,105]

The common peroneal nerve diverges from the tibial nerve in the upper popliteal fossa and passes laterally to the head of the fibula, close to the median margin of the tendon of the biceps femoris. Then it passes superficially to the neck of the fibula. Distal to this, it divides into the superficial peroneal nerve (musculocutaneous nerve) and the deep peroneal nerve. The superficial peroneal nerve courses along the shaft of the fibula with the peroneal muscles that it supplies. Its cutaneous nerve innervates the skin of the lateral and distal portion of the lower leg and the dorsal aspect of the foot. The deep peroneal nerve descends in the anterior compartment of the leg and supplies the tibialis anterior, extensor hallucis longus, and extensor digitorum brevis muscles in the foot.

The common peroneal nerve may be compressed near the neck of the fibula during general anesthesia or coma. Less common causes include prolonged squatting[106] or crossing of the legs.[107] The nerve also may be compressed by ganglions or cysts in the knee joint. Affected patients have foot drop and sensory deficits over the anterolateral aspect of the lower leg and dorsum of the foot (Fig. 32-2).

Anterior tibial syndrome involves compression of the deep peroneal nerve caused by muscle swelling in the anterior compartment of the leg. These patients have exquisite anterior lower leg pain and motor dysfunction. The syndrome may occur after trauma, reperfusion after arterial occlusion, or excessive exercise.

Tibial nerve syndromes involve the tibial nerve, which branches from the sciatic nerve, descends through the popliteal fossa, and passes deep between the heads of the gastrocnemius muscle, which it supplies. The nerve becomes superficial along the medial aspect of the ankle and passes under the flexor retinaculum into the foot. The flexor retinaculum forms the roof of the tarsal tunnel. Distal to this site, the tibial nerve divides into plantar nerves and sensory branches that supply the sole of the heel. The plantar nerve innervates motor and sensory elements of the anterior two thirds of the sole. The sural nerve leaves the tibial nerve in the popliteal fossa and descends in the middle of the calf to supply the skin over the lateral aspect of the ankle.

Compression of the distal part of the tibial nerve or two plantar nerves can cause diffuse foot pain and paresthesias in the sole of the foot. Weakness of foot muscles may be noticed, and physical examination shows plantar nerve sensory abnormalities. Compression or palpation over the medial aspect of the Achilles tendon may elicit pain and paresthesias. This syndrome is called the *tarsal tunnel syndrome,* and it can result from ill-fitting footwear or compression by tendon sheaths.[108,109]

Morton's neuroma (or neuralgia) is caused by compression of the interdigital nerves by adjacent metatarsal heads (generally between the third and fourth toes). The pain radiates from the site of the neuroma into the toes. Initially, the pain occurs while walking, but eventually it becomes continuous.

Sural neuropathy causes paresthesias and pain over the lateral aspect of the ankle and foot. This results from prolonged pressure over the posterior lower calf.[110]

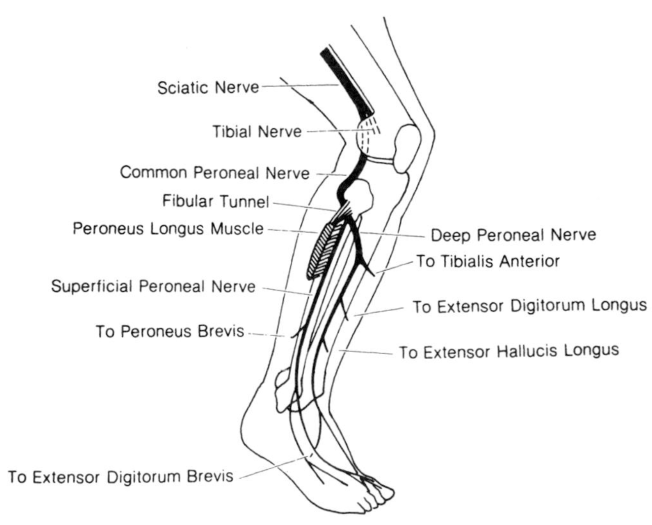

Figure 32-2 Common peroneal nerve (anterolateral aspect of the right leg). Schematic representation of its course, clinically relevant anatomic relations, and major branches. (Reproduced with permission from Dyck PJ, Thomas PK, Lambert EH. Bunge R, eds. *Peripheral Neuropathy.* 2nd ed. Philadelphia: Saunders; 1984:1448.)

Complex Regional Pain Syndrome (See Chap. 39)

In 1994, the International Association for the Study of Pain (IASP) recommended two important changes in the taxonomic classification of pain to reflect more accurately current understanding of the entities. For example, the constellation of signs and symptoms eliciting the diagnosis of reflex sympathetic dystrophy seemed to imply an underlying mechanism, which investigations have so far failed to support. Hence, the terms complex regional pain syndrome (CRPS), types 1 and 2, have replaced reflex sympathetic dystrophy and causalgia, respectively. At one time, clinicians made the diagnosis of CRPS only if a trial of sympathetic blockade ameliorated the pain. Subsequently, it has been discovered that the role of the sympathetic nervous system may vary during the natural course of the chronic pain syndrome. For example, in some patients, early sympatholysis may obliterate the perceived pain, whereas the same intervention later in the course of the disease fails to produce a positive response. Hence, for the same CRPS, a period of sympathetically maintained pain may be followed by a phase of sympathetically independent pain.

Normally, injury stimulates afferent sensory fibers that travel to the dorsal root ganglia and synapse in the posterior horn of the spinal cord. The impulse is relayed as well to sympathetic neurons in the lateral columns, which send efferent impulses through the anterior root. After synapsing in the sympathetic ganglion, these efferent signals can mediate vasoconstriction in the affected extremity. Over time, however, the role of the sympathetic nervous systems becomes less clear.[111]

Pain, swelling, discoloration, and stiffness comprise the four major hallmarks of CRPS. Patients commonly experience constant pain, which has a burning, cramping, or cutting quality. Passive motion of the extremity aggravates the pain. Hyperpathia and tenderness elicited over the joints commonly develop. Swelling often begins at the point of initial trauma and initially feels soft. Eventually it can involve the whole extremity and usually becomes firm. Skin tone changes from red to white as early capillary vasodilation gives way to later vasoconstriction. Stiffness results from the combination of increased swelling and disuse because of the intense pain caused by motion.[112] As the disease progresses, fibrosis of ligamentous structures and adhesion formation further limit joint motion. Forearm and shoulder motion are limited to a much greater extent than elbow motion.

Affected patients also have other signs and symptoms, such as cool skin and positive responses to cold and the ice-water immersion test, and there is decreased skin temperature in the affected extremity. Trophic skin changes may be seen as tight, shiny skin. Later features include atrophy of subcutaneous tissue producing tight, shiny skin and tapering of the pulp area of the fingers (the so-called pencil-pointing sign).

CRPS, type 2 (causalgia), was first described in 1864 among Union soldiers when gunshot wounds to extremities directly injured peripheral nerves. A so-called major form involved proximal nerve injury with resultant pain in the entire extremity.[113,114] Minor causalgia involved injury to distal sensory nerves and is generally confined to one or several fingers.

Hypothyroid Neuropathy

The peripheral nervous system manifestations of myxedema are well described. Affected patients may have either mononeuropathy or polyneuropathy.

The most common mononeuropathy involves compression of the median nerve as it passes through the carpal tunnel at the wrist. With myxedema, the extracellular tissue in the perineurium, endoneurium, and tendons acquires increased amounts of acid mucopolysaccharides. These attract fluid and diminish the available space for nerve in the carpal tunnel.[115]

The extremity pain associated with the polyneuropathy of hypothyroidism has two distinct origins: (1) skeletal muscle, and (2) peripheral nerve. In the first case, affected patients may have edema of the skeletal muscle that is manifested as cramping.[116] Prolonged relaxation and contraction times produce slowed movement. Patients display proximal weakness. The relaxed muscles feel firmer and larger than normal. In the second case, distal extremity pain has a neuropathic origin marked by slowed conduction velocity, decreased tendon reflexes, dysesthesias, and sensory deficits.

A distinct type of muscle cramping has been noticed in patients with both hypo- and hyperthyroidism. These patients experience an undulatory muscular twitching, or so-called myokymia, which may be produced by repetitive discharges from many single motor nerve fibers. The cramping is accompanied by excessive sweating.[117]

Neuropathy in Acromegaly

Patients with acromegaly may have intense pain and tingling in their extremities as a result of hypertrophic neuropathy.[118] In addition, bilateral carpal tunnel syndrome has been reported to be associated with acromegaly.[119] Presumably, the overabundance of growth hormone causes proliferation of the connective tissue and synovium, diminishing the available space in the carpal tunnel. Hypertrophic connective tissue also may compress axons, resulting in sensorimotor disturbances.

Thoracic Outlet Syndrome

Thoracic outlet syndrome results from compression or irritation of the brachial plexus and subclavian vessels as they pass through the costoclavicular space and thoracic outlet.[120,121] Actual compression of the plexus accounts for the symptoms in most patients. Therefore, the disease probably should be viewed as a neuropathy[122] (Fig. 32-3). The syndrome primarily affects young and middle-aged women. The history is essential to separate thoracic outlet syndrome from other causes of upper extremity pain, such as carpal tunnel syndrome and cervical disc disease[123] (Table 32-8). The symptoms may occur spontaneously or after trauma[124] to the shoulder and neck, resulting in chronic muscle spasms.[124,125] The pain initially is unilateral and intermittent, but it increases in severity and frequency with time. It begins over the anterior and posterior shoulder region and radiates down the lateral arm to the hand. The pain also may radiate up the back of the neck to the mastoid and occipital region of the skull and cause severe headaches. Paresthesias accompany the pain, and because the compression typically involves C8 to T1 of the plexus, affected patients localize their numbness and tingling to the ulnar nerve distribution.

A striking feature of the history is that elevating the arm and increased arm activity can initiate or aggravate the symptoms. Muscle cramping, per se, is not a feature of the syndrome. The hands may or may not show increased sensitivity to cold.

Frank arterial occlusion rarely, if ever, accounts for the signs and symptoms of thoracic outlet syndrome. Exertion, which can cause cyanosis and edema of the extremity, may produce subclavian vein thrombosis[126] (the so-called effort thrombotic syndrome

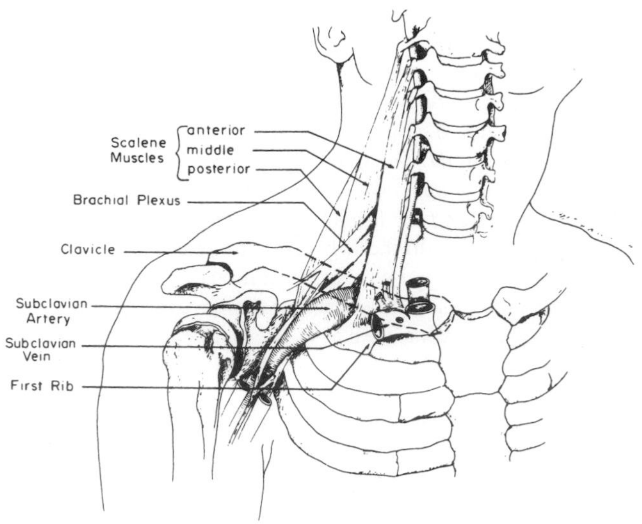

Figure 32-3 Course of the brachial plexus and subclavian artery between the anterior scalene and middle scalene muscles. Dilation of the subclavian artery just distal to the anterior scalene muscle is illustrated. Immediately distal to the anterior and middle scalene muscles is another potential area of constriction, between the clavicle and the first rib. With extension of the neck and turning of the chin to the affected side (Adson maneuver), the tension on the anterior scalene muscle is increased and the subclavian artery compressed, resulting in a supraclavicular bruit and obliteration of the radial pulse. (Reproduced with permission from Adams RD, Victor M. Polymyositis and other acute and subacute myopathic paralyses. In: Adams RD, Victor M, eds. *Principles of Neurology,* 3rd ed. New York: McGraw-Hill; 1965.)

of Paget and Schroetter). The physical examination should include blood pressure measurement in both arms to identify any differences. Muscle atrophy of ulnar-innervated interosseous muscles can be assessed by an interphalangeal card test or by spreading the digits against resistance. Triceps strength may be diminished. Bruits may be heard over the supraclavicular fossa. Moderate pressure over the supraclavicular fossa for 15 seconds may reproduce the symptoms. The reflexes generally are normal. Pinprick sensation may be diminished over the C8 to T1 dermatome.

Several maneuvers that have questionable diagnostic value should be mentioned.[127] Adson's maneuver consists of monitoring the radial pulse while patients take deep breaths, extend their necks, and then turn their chin toward the affected side. A decrease or disappearance of the pulse is a positive test result. A bruit may be heard over the supraclavicular area using this maneuver. The deep breath elevates the first rib, and turning the neck narrows the interscalene triangle. The costoclavicular compressive maneuver consists of monitoring the radial pulse while the patient throws back the shoulders and presses them downward. A positive test result is a decrease or disappearance of the radial pulse with or without a bruit. This maneuver compresses the subclavian artery between the clavicle and the first rib.

By contrast, the elevated-arm stress test described by Roos[125] seems to have some diagnostic value. This test involves a 90-degree abduction and external rotation of the arms. The patient is then instructed to open and close the hands for 3 minutes. A reproduction of symptoms of the thoracic outlet syndrome constitutes a positive test result.

In addition to the history and physical examination, some other tests should be discussed when diagnosing thoracic outlet syndrome. Although thoracic outlet syndrome can be considered an ulnar neuropathy, the actual irritation of the plexus is intermittent and rarely results in neuropathic changes. Hence, nerve conduction studies generally are not useful.[128,129] Also, because the C8 to T1 part of the plexus is both inferior and deep, stimulation would be difficult technically. Only a small minority of patients with thoracic outlet syndrome has disease that involves subclavian arterial compression; therefore, angiograms generally are not indicated. The two exceptions to this rule are when there is (1) a large differential blood pressure between the arms, or (2) interest in excluding a subclavian artery aneurysm. Cervical spine films generally are valuable in patients with thoracic outlet syndrome to exclude any coexisting cervical disc disease.

Cervical Disc Disease (See Chap. 27)

Cervical disc disease is another common cause of neck, shoulder, and arm pain. The root or cord compression may result from ruptured disc material or a degenerative osteophytic lesion. The radiculopathy usually involves, in descending order, C7, C6, C5, and C8. The symptoms may occur after trauma or sudden hyperextension.[130,131]

One common syndrome involving lateral disc lesions between C5 and C6 includes pain felt at the trapezium ridge, tip of the shoulder, radial forearm, and thumb. Affected patients have sensory loss and paresthesias in the same distribution. Unilateral paracervical muscle spasm is present. The patient may experience biceps tenderness in the supraclavicular regions, motor deficit, and loss of deep tendon reflex. The patient has a secondary weakness after forearm flexion.

Another common syndrome is caused by lateral protrusion between the sixth and seventh cervical vertebrae, with involvement of the seventh cervical root. The pain occurs in the shoulder and radiates down the elbow and dorsal forearm to the index and middle fingers. There is tenderness over the third and fourth thoracic spinous processes and the triceps region. The patient has sensory deficits and paresthesias in the second and third fingers. Physical examination shows an absent triceps reflex, with weakness in forearm extension, wrist extension, and hand grip Regardless of the cervical root involved, affected patients relate a history of chronic sharp pain. Events such as coughing or sneezing tend to exaggerate the pain. Most changes in head position (particularly hyperextension) intensify the pain. On examination, turning the head to one side and hyperextending the neck produce neck pain and characteristic radicular paresthesias (Table 32-9).

Neuralgic Amyotrophy

Neuralgic amyotrophy is a syndrome characterized by the acute onset of shoulder pain, which can be severe or aching. Although it frequently affects the shoulder alone, it may also involve the arm, neck, and back. The pain is worse at night and intensifies with movement.[132] The syndrome involves mostly the right side, but almost 25% of cases are bilateral.

Proximal motor weakness in the shoulder and arms, particularly affecting the muscles innervated by the axillary and suprascapular nerves, follows the pain at varying intervals.[133] Complete limb paralysis is rare. Pain relief often occurs after resting the limb with the elbow flexed and the shoulder adducted; however, this may aggravate the weakness. Sensory involvement is not a characteristic feature of this syndrome. The cause remains unknown. However,

TABLE 32-8 **Thoracic Outlet, Carpal Tunnel, and Cervical Disc Syndromes**

	Thoracic Outlet	Carpal Tunnel	Cervical Disc
Symptoms			
Pain	Neck, shoulder and arm (intermittent)	Wrist, volar forearm, fingers 1, 2, and 3 (intermittent)	Neck and shoulder (constant)
Numbness	Ulnar nerve or whole hand or arm asleep	Median nerve, fingers 2, 3, and 4	Radial nerve (dorsal web between fingers 1 and 2)
Awkwardness	All fingers or digits 4 and 5	Fingers 1, 2, and 3	Thumb
Aggravation	Arm elevation	Sustained grasp, pinch	Neck turn or arm stretch
Color	Normal, pallid, cyanotic, or splotchy	Normal, red, or splotchy	Normal or splotchy
Edema	±	±	0
Signs			
Percussion	+ Brachial plexus	+ Tinel volar wrist	+ Neck at disc level
Compression	+ Brachial plexus	+ Phalen (wrist flexion)	+Neck and brachial plexus
Symptoms reproduced	Arm elevation and brachial plexus compression	Wrist flexion	Head turn and tilt, cranial compression
Nerve conduction	± (Unreliable if negative)	± (Unreliable if negative)	
X-rays	Normal, long C7 process, anomalies (venoarteriogram)	Normal, arthritis or old trauma	Degenerative arthritis, narrowed disc myelogram + 85%
Treatment			
Conservative	Shoulder shrug, physical therapy, exercises, avoid arm elevation	Wrist splint, avoid grasp, corticosteroid injection	Cervical traction and collar
Indications for operation	Treatment failure, severe pain, loss of hand function	Return of symptoms, severe pain, loss of function; thenar atrophy	Severe pain unrelieved by treatment
Operation	Resection of first rib and congenital band	Resection of carpal ligament	Discectomy with fusion

Reprinted with permission from Rutherford RD. *Vascular Surgery.* 2nd ed. Philadelphia, Pa: WB Saunders; 1984:710.

a brachial neuritis similar to neuralgic amyotrophy may appear after serum inoculations or infections caused by influenza, typhus, or variola viruses.

The diagnosis depends on obtaining a history consistent with neuralgic amyotrophy. The physical diagnosis is aided by eliciting pain after arm abduction, external rotation at the shoulder, and then extension of the elbow (the so-called flexion-adduction sign described by Waxman).[134] EMG studies show a peripheral plexus lesion with normal spinal roots.[135]

Neuropathy of Serum Sickness

Before the age of antibiotics, bacterial infections often were treated with large volumes of horse or rabbit antisera. The serum sickness that patients developed occasionally was accompanied by neuropathy, usually of the brachial plexus.[136] Heterologous serum rarely is used today, but neuropathies still may occur as a sequela of typhoid or paratyphoid vaccinations or from drugs that form complexes with serum proteins.[137]

The usual clinical features of serum sickness (e.g., lymph node swelling, joint pain, myalgias, and albuminuria) generally are present when the neuropathy appears. There is no relationship between the amount of serum given, the severity of systemic manifestations, and the development of neuropathy.

Pain onset occurs suddenly. It generally starts in the shoulder girdle or upper arm. The pain should be distinguished from more typical myalgic or arthritic types seen during serum sickness in other joints and muscles. Physical examination may reveal tender-

TABLE 32-9 **Most Frequent Clinical Findings With Cervical Disc Disease[131]**

Cervical Root Involved	Clinical Findings		
	Motor Deficit	Sensory Change	Reflex Loss
C5	Deltoid	Proximal shoulder	None
C6	Biceps	Thumb	Biceps
C7	Triceps	Long finger	Triceps
C8	Intrinsic hand muscles	Ring and little fingers	None

ness over the brachial plexus. Weakness involving the shoulder muscles soon follows the onset of pain, and affected patients may be paralyzed totally and have striking atrophy. The reflexes also are decreased or absent, and vasomotor changes may appear. Sensory signs are not prominent, a feature that is found in other brachial neuropathies. The radial nerve is a less common site of involvement.

The pathologic basis of the neuropathy of serum sickness seems to be that immune-complex deposition causes vasculitis and perivascular edema. This, in turn, leads to edema of the nerves. This swelling impinges on the nerves as they exit from the foramina. If the swelling progresses, it may compromise flow further and lead to frank necrosis of the nerves, which explains why severe lancinating pain can be such a prominent feature of this neuropathy.[136,137]

Neuropathy in Connective Tissue Diseases

Peripheral neuropathy may occur in conjunction with various connective tissue diseases. The clinical manifestations and histopathologic findings are similar regardless of the disease. The pathogenic lesion is arteritis involving the small nutrient arteries of the nerves. Thus, it is described as an angiopathic neuropathy that occurs with varying frequencies in rheumatoid arthritis, polyarteritis nodosa, Churg-Strauss vasculitis, systemic lupus erythematosus, and giant cell arteritis.[138]

Patients with rheumatoid arthritis and peripheral neuropathy have certain distinguishing features. Firstly, they usually have had rheumatoid arthritis for an average of 10 years before the onset of neuropathy. Secondly, rheumatoid nodules and destructive joint changes are present. Thirdly, elevated titers of rheumatoid factor are common.[139] Fourthly, these patients have other complications of arteritis (such as nail-bed infarctions, skin ulcers, and Raynaud's phenomenon). Finally, these patients often describe a change in their clinical status involving fever, anorexia, or weight loss. It previously was believed that patients receiving corticosteroids were at risk for an increased incidence of neuropathy. However, these are patients with severe disease, and it is thought currently that corticosteroids may help to check the progression of the arteritis. Thus, rapid tapering of these drugs may exacerbate the arteritis and precipitate the onset of the neuropathy.

The latter usually includes a gradual onset of numbness and tingling confined to the lower extremities. The sensory deficits are symmetric and not accompanied by motor deficits. Patients with rheumatoid arthritis and other connective tissue diseases also may have mononeuritis multiplex or a sudden onset of pain and paresthesias along the course of a peripheral nerve, followed by wrist or foot drop.

Although only a small percentage of patients with rheumatoid arthritis have symptomatic neuropathy, a large percentage have histologic evidence of disease involving the peripheral nerves at autopsy.[139] The range of arterial pathologic changes in the peripheral nerves includes perivascular infiltration with mononuclear cells, fibrinoid necrosis of the media with infiltration of eosinophils and mononuclear cells, intimal proliferation and reduplication of the internal elastic lamina, and hemorrhage around the vessel walls. The damage to nutrient vessels results in both segmental demyelination and wallerian degeneration in the affected nerves.[140]

The diagnosis of rheumatoid arthritis generally is well established before the neuropathy appears. However, patients with neuropathy have an elevated erythrocyte sedimentation rate; mild normochromic, normocytic anemia; and significantly elevated titers of rheumatoid factor.

Polyarteritis nodosa is a multisystem disease characterized by a vasculitis of small and medium-sized muscular arteries, with particular involvement of the kidneys and gastrointestinal tract. Clinical neuropathy is a common manifestation of this disease. The clinical presentation may be similar to that of rheumatoid arthritis. One important distinguishing feature is that the neuropathy of polyarteritis nodosa involves the upper extremities as frequently as the lower extremities. The neuropathy may occur in conjunction with other manifestations of this disease, such as fever, weight loss, renal insufficiency, and skin lesions.[141] Patients with both polyarteritis nodosa and rheumatoid arthritis also may have an accompanying arthritis. The arthritis of polyarteritis nodosa is mild and of short duration. It does not cause the extensive joint destruction and nodule formation seen with rheumatoid arthritis.

The pathologic changes seen in the peripheral nerves involve an arteritis of nutrient arteries that is similar to that described in rheumatoid arthritis. The diagnosis depends on a histologic demonstration of vasculitis in the involved organs. Peripheral neuropathy may be associated with Churg-Strauss vasculitis (eosinophilic granulomatosus). It is considered a variant of polyarteritis nodosa that is characterized by peripheral eosinophilia and a strong association with severe asthma.[142] Both systemic lupus erythematosus and giant cell arteritis (involving the temporal arteries) may include secondary neuropathy.

Porphyric Neuropathy

The porphyrias are a group of metabolic disorders characterized biochemically by an overproduction of porphyrins and porphyrin precursors. Recurrent attacks, which are often precipitated by drugs (such as barbiturates, phenytoin, sulfonamides, and estrogens), are common. The neuropathy and extremity pain is a feature only of one subgroup, the so-called hereditary hepatic porphyrias, which include (1) acute intermittent porphyria, (2) variegate porphyria, and (3) hereditary coproporphyria.[143]

Acute intermittent porphyria, inherited as an autosomal dominant trait, is most common in women of English and Scandinavian origin.[144] Attacks are rare before puberty and are distinguished temporally by three phases: (1) abdominal pain, (2) psychologic disturbances, and (3) polyneuropathy. Abdominal pain initiates the attack. The pain is described as colicky and may be diffuse or confined to one region of the abdominal wall. It often radiates to the back but is not accompanied by abdominal wall guarding or tenderness. Tachycardia is a constant physical sign during attacks.[145] Radiographic studies show distended loops of bowel. Psychologic manifestations follow the acute abdominal attacks. This phase is characterized by restlessness, insomnia, hallucinations, and confusion.[146] Neuropathy is the final phase of the attack. It is symmetric, progressive, and initially involves mostly motor nerves. The upper extremities are affected more than the lower extremities and the proximal, more so than the distal muscles. Tendon reflexes are diminished or absent.[147,148] The extremity pain that occurs can result from various factors. Proximal muscle aching and cramps are common. Paresthesias and dysesthesias also occur in half the cases.

The diagnosis depends on the characteristic history and is confirmed by demonstrations of increased levels of porphobilinogen and δ-aminolevulinic acid in the urine. Variegate porphyria is most common among European descendants in South Africa. The acute attacks are similar to those of acute intermittent porphyria, but in addition, they are accompanied by cutaneous photosensitivity. Hereditary coproporphyria is a rare cause of neuropathy and is distinguished by a predominantly fecal excretion of porphyrins.

Hepatic Neuropathy

Several types of peripheral neuropathy may accompany hepatic dysfunction. These are distinct from alcoholic neuropathy or illnesses that affect both the liver and peripheral nervous system concomitantly.[149] Specifically, the conditions are (1) a painless demyelinating neuropathy that accompanies hepatic dysfunction, regardless of the cause[150,151]; (2) an acute polyneuritis identical to that seen with Guillain-Barré syndrome occurring late in the course of viral hepatitis as jaundice is regressing[152,153]; and (3) a rare but painful neuropathy that occurs with biliary infections.[154]

Patients with biliary cirrhosis and neuropathy have the other common manifestations of this disease: hepatomegaly, pruritus, jaundice, and cutaneous xanthomatosis. Hypersensitivity and paresthesias have been recognized for a long time as a feature of biliary cirrhosis. However, Thomas and Walker[154] also documented the presence of sensory deficits. Xanthomatous involvement of the connective tissue sheaths of the cutaneous nerves is the cause of the painful dysesthesias.

Burning Feet Syndrome

Investigators initially thought that the so-called burning feet syndrome described among prisoners of war after World War II represented a distinct deficiency syndrome. Currently, experts agree that it is merely one manifestation of vitamin B deficiency and can be found in patients with (1) alcoholic neuropathy, (2) beriberi, (3) pellagra, and (4) Strachan's syndrome. The symptom of burning feet, or acrodysesthesia, begins as a persistent burning pain over the metatarsals on the soles of the feet. Various other dysesthesias, tingling, electric shocks, or coldness may accompany this pain. Soon, the entire soles and dorsal surface of the feet are involved symmetrically. The pain worsens at night. Affected patients try a number of methods to relieve the burning: immersing their feet in ice water, constant massage, or walking (despite pain caused by contact). Many authors believed the syndrome had a causalgic basis as a result of findings such as cyanosis and hyperhidrosis. Other features of peripheral neuropathy (e.g., absent reflexes, impairment of sensation, and muscle wasting) may or may not be present. Occasionally, the patient's hands may be involved, too.

Isoniazid- or Hydralazine-induced Neuropathy

The occurrence of isoniazid-induced neuropathy was discovered shortly after the drug was first used to treat tuberculosis. The neuropathy generally involved the motor function, sensation, and reflexes of the lower extremities. The initial symptoms consisted of numbness and tingling, which began in the toes and feet, followed by calf tenderness, and finally continuous burning paresthesias and painful dysesthesias caused by contact stimuli. Increasing severity of symptoms paralleled proximal spread of the neuropathy to the knees. Patients displayed weak toe movements and dorsiflexion and loss of the Achilles reflex.[155] The incidence of the neuropathy varies with the dose of drug administered. It ranges from less than 10% of patients treated with a dose of 4 to 9 mg/kg per day to 40% with doses of 20 mg/kg per day.[156] Vitamin B_6 deficiency causes the neuropathy, which can be prevented by vitamin B_6 supplementation.[157] Isoniazid produces marked excretion of pyridoxine.

Pyridoxine deficiency presumably is the basis for the neuropathy that complicates therapy with hydralazine, which is chemically related to isoniazid.[158]

Pellagra

The first description of pellagra among peasants in northwestern Spain whose diet consisted almost entirely of corn appeared in 1730. The role of sunlight, the seasonal variation (highest in the spring), and the rash that appeared on exposed areas (so-called Casal's collar) were noticed. The first reports of pellagra in the United States were made in the late 1800s, and the disease soon attained epidemic proportions among alcoholic and farming populations. Currently, the disease rarely is seen in the continental United States (except among food faddists). It does occur commonly among poorer vegetarians and the black population of South Africa.

Initially, it was believed that pellagra was caused solely by a niacin-deficient diet. Subsequently, it was shown that (1) administration of tryptophan to humans resulted in increased urinary excretion of niacin metabolites, and (2) the dermal and gastrointestinal manifestations of pellagra responded to large doses of tryptophan. Thus, currently, investigators believe that pellagra is the result of a deficiency of niacin and its amino acid precursor, tryptophan.

Pellagra shows the clinical triad of dermal, gastrointestinal, and neurologic lesions. The skin lesions first appear erythematous, then become brown and hyperkeratotic. They are seen on the face, neck, sternum, and dorsum of the hands and feet. Affected patients have anorexia, diarrhea, weight loss, and dysphagia. The neurologic manifestations consist variously of depression, insomnia, irritability, and signs of spinal cord involvement. The neuropathy, which is identical to that observed with beriberi, is the most common neurologic finding. Affected patients have exquisite tenderness to palpation of the muscles of their calves and feet. Many also feel an intense burning pain in a so-called glove-and-stocking distribution. Diminution or loss of vibratory sensation and deep tendon reflexes occur.

The Syndrome of Amblyopia, Painful Neuropathy, and Orogenital Dermatitis (Strachan's Syndrome)

Strachan (in 1888) and Scott (in 1918) both described a deficiency syndrome among Jamaicans—consisting of amblyopia, painful neuropathy, and orogenital lesions—that was distinct from beriberi and pellagra. These manifestations since have been described among World War II prisoners in Johore and Singapore, in survivors of German concentration camps, and in natives in Trinidad and Senegal. Currently, the syndrome has not been related to a specific vitamin deficiency, although a riboflavin deficiency has been suggested. The few neuropathologic studies performed reveal spinal cord posterior column demyelination, particularly in the cervical region.

Patients with pellagra classically have numbness and tingling in their hands and feet. The dysesthesias consist of severe burning in the soles and palms, which often is worse at night. The numbness extends progressively to the knees or hips, and the patient's gait may be impaired. Often, the symptoms are confined to the lower extremities, or alternatively, they may begin in the fingertips and involve the hands and arms symmetrically. Muscle wasting is progressive, and extremity cramps are common.

Amblyopia is the other constant feature of this syndrome. Visual impairment is accompanied by central and centrocecal scotomas that progress to complete blindness. Ophthalmologic evaluation shows little, except occasionally disc hyperemia is found.

The dermatitis involves the corners of the mouth and eyes, prepuce, anus, and vulva. Deafness and vertigo (so-called camp dizziness) are common features of some outbreaks of the syndrome.

Alcoholic Neuropathy

In a consecutive series of 1,030 alcoholic patients admitted to Boston City Hospital,[159] a 9% incidence of peripheral neuropathy was observed, with a disproportionately higher incidence in women. Nutritional deficiency and the toxic effect of the alcohol, per se, account for the major findings of alcoholic neuropathy. Alcoholic patients not only subsist on a diet of carbohydrates, they also have an impaired capacity to absorb folate and thiamine and to digest fats. Axonal degeneration, with destruction of both myelin and axons, results. The changes are seen predominantly in the longest and largest myelinated fibers. As the neuropathy advances, anterior and posterior nerve root involvement occurs.

Alcoholic neuropathy is a progressive symmetric disorder of the extremities that generally spares both the cranial and truncal nerves. The lower extremities (particularly the feet and ankles) are affected more than the upper extremities; in one study 70% of patients had lower extremity involvement alone. Motor disability and sensory deficits occur concomitantly. These signs can range from mild asymptomatic depression of the Achilles reflex to gross motor deficits (wrist and foot drop). All sensory modalities, both superficial and deep, may be affected with a characteristic distribution (so-called glove and stocking).

The pain that accompanies alcoholic neuropathy typically occurs in several areas. Affected patients have a characteristic tenderness when pressure is applied to the muscles of their feet and calves. The distal lower extremity dysesthesias may have a dull aching quality or a sharp, lancinating, tabes-like pain. These patients also describe a burning feet syndrome that consists of severe paresthesias of the soles aggravated by contact stimuli. Excessive sweating on the volar surfaces of the feet and hands may occur, which presumably is related to postganglionic sympathetic involvement. Other signs, such as stasis edema, glossiness, and pigmentation changes of the skin, and dystrophic changes in the feet, may be present.

Herpes Zoster (See Chap. 40)

Herpes zoster, or shingles, is an infection by the DNA virus varicella-zoster that occurs with an annual incidence of approximately 125 cases per 100,000. Herpes zoster is thought to be a reactivation of the varicella-zoster virus that also causes chickenpox in children, which has remained dormant in the dorsal root ganglia for many years.

When viral antibody titers decline in elderly or immunocompromised patients, the virus may reactivate and begin to replicate. A painful neuralgia results from damage to the sensory ganglia. The virus then spreads peripherally to cutaneous sensory nerve endings, causing vesicular eruptions. Most affected patients are healthy, but the course may be more severe in immunosuppressed patients (Table 32-10).

TABLE 32-10 **Conditions that Place Patients at Increased Risk for Herpes Zoster**

Hodgkin's lymphoma
Lupus erythematosus
Non-Hodgkin's lymphoma
Status post–bone marrow transplantation
Status post–radiochemotherapy
Malignancies
Syphilis
Malaria

Zoster-affected patients usually have pain and dysesthesias along the dermatomal distribution of a single spinal or cranial sensory nerve. The pain at first is usually mild, but it increases in intensity over the succeeding days. Occasionally, patients have accompanying systemic symptoms such as fever, malaise, adenopathy, or headache. After 4 to 5 days, the typical skin lesions appear. Swelling and erythema give way to red papules that progress to clear vesicles, blebs, and pustules that crust over in 2 to 3 weeks. The lesions are unilateral in a dermatomal distribution. The most common dermatomes affected are the thoracic, followed by the cranial, lumbosacral, and cervical. During the acute phase, patients feel continuous dysesthesias that are aggravated by movement or pressure on the skin. As the blebs begin to dry and scale, the intense pain subsides, but many patients still have hyperesthesias and, only gradually, become asymptomatic.

Paresis may accompany the rash, particularly in elderly patients. It follows the appearance of the rash and usually occurs with cervical and lumbosacral eruptions rather than thoracic. Involvement of the facial nerves is common (Ramsay Hunt syndrome). The virus may be recovered from early vesicles, cerebrospinal fluid, and blood. The base of the skin lesions contains multinucleated giant cells and eosinophilic intranuclear inclusions.

Postherpetic neuralgia develop in 10% to 50% of patients with acute herpes zoster; the incidence increases with advancing age. The syndrome consists of pain persisting for 4 to 6 weeks after the skin lesions have disappeared. Such patients generally suffer from a burning pain associated with hyperesthesia.

INTRODUCTION TO PERIPHERAL NEUROPATHIES (SEE CHAP. 37)

Peripheral neuropathies are a common source of extremity pain. Several unique features of the peripheral nervous system make it particularly susceptible to trauma or metabolic derangements. Firstly, it is composed of long axons (1–2 m). Secondly, the spinal roots pass through narrow foramina centrally and many ligaments and tendon sheaths peripherally, making them susceptible to compression. Thirdly, the axons depend on a complex longitudinal network of nutrient arteries that run in the epineurium and perineurium.

The peripheral neuropathies involving smaller afferent fibers are usually painful. Those affecting large-diameter afferent fibers and Schwann cells are generally painless. The pain of a peripheral neuropathy is usually not distinctive, and the diagnosis must, therefore, be based on other criteria.

Regardless of their cause, peripheral neuropathies have several characteristics: (1) paresthesias and dysesthesias, (2) sensory loss, (3) loss or diminution of tendon reflexes, and (4) impaired motor function. Paresthesias and dysesthesias commonly accompany certain types of neuropathies, such as those resulting from diabetes and alcohol. The paresthesias can manifest as tingling, lancinating pain, or numbness. Perversion of sensation may also occur, such as when a tactile stimulus causes a burning or tingling. Commonly, the pain persists after the stimulus is withdrawn. Hyperpathia may be prominent.

TABLE 32-11 **The Diabetic Neuropathies**

Symmetric Polyneuropathies
Sensory polyneuropathy
Acute motor neuropathy
Autonomic neuropathy
Focal and Multifocal Neuropathies
Cranial neuropathy
Limb mononeuropathy
Diabetic amyotrophy

The cause of paresthesias remains poorly understood. One hypothesis suggests that the loss of large touch-pressure fibers no longer inhibits pain-sensing cells in the posterior horn. Another states that ectopic discharges may result from regenerated nociceptive fibers. Some type of sensory loss accompanies most neuropathies. Only one or all sensory modalities (touch-pressure, vibratory, joint position, pain, and temperature) may be affected. Deep tendon reflex loss or diminution characterizes peripheral neuropathy, especially when both sensory and motor involvement exists. The Achilles reflex serves as a particularly sensitive index of polyneuropathy. Tremors and disorders of autonomic function also may be seen with peripheral neuropathies. Useful diagnostic laboratory tests include nerve conduction studies, nerve biopsies, and cerebrospinal fluid examination.[160,161]

Diabetic Neuropathy

Diabetic neuropathy includes a wide range of clinical manifestations. Traditionally, it has been categorized anatomically (Table 32-11). For our purposes, the diabetic neuropathies can be classified into separate pain syndromes: polyneuropathy, mononeuropathy, radiculopathy, and amyotrophy[162,163] (Table 32-12).

Depending on the criteria used to establish the diagnosis, the incidence of diabetic neuropathy varies from 5% to 60% of patients with the disease. Pirart noticed that the neuropathy rarely occurred in the young, and its prevalence increased from 7.5% at the time of discovery of diabetes mellitus to almost 50% after 25 years.[164] Neuropathy may accompany both type 1 and type 2 diabetes mellitus. It also may occur in patients with diabetes after pancreatectomy and hemochromatosis. Several authors have noted the common concurrence of neuropathy, nephropathy, and retinopathy (diabetic triopathy).[165]

Symmetric Sensory Polyneuropathy

A symmetric sensory polyneuropathy is the most frequent form of peripheral nerve disorder in diabetic patients. It may occur acutely after a diabetic coma, as a result of poor serum glucose control, after initiation of therapy, or during periods of emotional stress.[166]

A loss of ankle jerks and vibratory sense in the feet should direct the clinician toward the diagnosis. Symptoms, which consist of tingling, numbness, and burning paresthesias, are generally confined to the lower extremities. A deep aching pain (described by patients as "arising from the bones") that intensifies at night can affect the feet and legs. Symmetric distal sensory impairment occurs in a glove-and-stocking distribution.

Signs and symptoms of diabetic sensory neuropathy display considerable variability. At one extreme, patients show loss of position sense, decreased reflexes, and no pain. At the other end, they manifest cutaneous hyperesthesia, distal burning pain, and autonomic dysfunction but preserved reflexes and large fiber sensory function. Sural nerve biopsies from these patients reveal the involvement of both small myelinated and unmyelinated fibers.[167]

Other less common variants have been described. For example, Archer[168] documented severe distal burning pain without sensory loss or autonomic features that occurred after rapid weight loss in men. The neuropathy subsided after these patients gained weight and had improved diabetic control.

The term *diabetic pseudotabes* refers to a variant that includes symmetric distal loss of cutaneous sensibility, joint position, and vibration, all leading to gait abnormalities and foot ulcers. Autonomic signs and symptoms, including atonic bladder and Argyll Robertson pupils, also may occur.

Neuropathy arthropathy, seen in advanced cases of sensory polyneuropathy, affects mainly the joints of the feet and, less commonly, the ankle. The interphalangeal and metatarsophalangeal joints are affected.[169]

Autonomic dysfunction almost always accompanies the sensory polyneuropathy in diabetes and has a wide range of clinical manifestations (Table 32-13). The disease affects both the longer sensory and autonomic fibers first. Some of the earliest changes involve vascular and sudomotor innervation of the legs. Hence, anhidrosis and an absence of piloerection may be first detected in the feet, but eventually ascend the legs in a symmetric fashion. Peripheral edema of unknown origin also frequently occurs with diabetic neuropathy.[170]

TABLE 32-12 **Features of the Diabetic Neuropathies**

Syndrome	Features
Polyneuropathy	Numbness, painful paresthesias, hyperesthesia, Charcot joints, loss of distal reflexes, edema
Radiculopathy	Lancinating pain in root distribution with segmental sensory and reflex loss
Mononeuropathy	Sudden or gradual loss of cranial nerves (3rd, 4th, 6th, 7th, or 10th) or peripheral nerves (ulnar, median, radial, or femoral)
Amyotrophy	Proximal asymmetric weakness and pain in thighs, or lumbar region with muscle wasting, absence of sensory loss

TABLE 32-13 **Manifestations of Diabetic Autonomic Dysfunction**

Cardiac	Orthostatic hypotension Diminished beat-to-beat variation Peripheral edema
Genitourinary	Neurogenic bladder Retrograde ejaculation Erectile impotence
Gastrointestinal	Nocturnal diarrhea Constipation Decreased gastric motility
Others	Anhidrosis Abnormal pupil reaction

Focal and Multifocal Neuropathies

Diabetes most commonly affects the ulnar, median, radial, femoral, lateral femoral cutaneous, and peroneal nerves. The onset may be abrupt or insidious. These isolated peripheral nerve lesions often occur at sites common for external pressure palsies (e.g., carpal tunnel).

Diabetic Amyotrophy and Proximal Motor Neuropathy

Diabetic amyotrophy connotes a syndrome usually encountered in older patients that consists of asymmetric proximal muscle wasting in the lower limbs. The muscles commonly affected include the iliopsoas, quadriceps, and adductor muscles but not the hamstrings.[171,172] Patients complain of pain, which is generally most severe at night, in the thigh muscles and lumbar region. The patellar reflex may be depressed, but sensation is maintained.

Uremic Neuropathy

Sixty to 70% of patients about to begin dialysis for chronic renal failure display neuropathic features.[173,174] The progression of the neuropathy depends solely on the duration and severity of renal failure. Men seem to have a several-fold higher incidence than women.

The combined motor and sensory dysfunction that occurs with uremic neuropathy invariably occurs in a distal, symmetric distribution.[175] The legs are affected before and more often than the upper extremities. This correlates with histopathologic studies that show a distal axonal degeneration, with shrinkage and nerve fiber loss predominantly involving larger fibers.

The exact cause of the neuropathy is unknown, although the accumulation of toxic substances with molecular weights of 300 to 2000 Daltons (the so-called middle-molecule hypothesis) that are not removed during hemodialysis have been implicated.[176] Two other observations support the middle-molecule hypothesis as the source of neuropathy. One entails the striking remission of neuropathy after successful renal transplantation and the other the fact that peritoneal dialysis, which presumably passes toxic molecules more selectively than hemodialysis, is not associated with neuropathy despite having higher blood levels of urea and creatinine.

Uremic patients can have extremity pain from various causes. Nielsen[177] noticed muscular cramps and the restless-leg syndrome in two thirds of patients in his series. The cramps, which also can occur during acute uremia, probably reflect muscular irritability in the presence of uremic toxins. They are not necessarily associated with any other signs and symptoms of neuropathy (e.g., slowing of conduction velocity). The restless-leg syndrome of Ekbom,[178] characterized by night pain relieved by movement, is associated with clinical neuropathy. Dysesthesias can occur that range from the burning-feet type identical to that seen in alcoholic patients to painful tingling, electric shocks, or constrictive feelings around the ankles and feet. The diagnosis depends on demonstrating a neuropathy with symptomatic uremia and excluding other causes of neuropathy, such as toxins.

Gold Neuropathy

Gold has been used traditionally to treat rheumatoid arthritis. Common side effects of this drug include fever and rashes. The incidence of patients who have peripheral neuropathy after gold therapy is less than 1%. Such patients have painful paresthesias, followed by sudden onset of asymmetric weakness. They may have fever and rashes before the onset of the neuropathy.[179] Controversy exists as to whether the neuropathy results from the direct toxic effect of the drug or from a hypersensitivity reaction.[180]

Perhexiline Neuropathy

Perhexiline maleate was introduced for the treatment of angina in the early 1970s. Peripheral neuropathy was seen in some patients who were treated with doses of 300 to 400 mg/day for 4 months to 1 year. These patients had pain and distal paresthesias, followed by severe distal and proximal muscle weakness. They also had a high incidence of bilateral papilledema, abnormal liver function tests, and weight loss. Perhexiline apparently causes cellular accumulation of abnormal gangliosides, particularly in Schwann cells and liver cells.[181]

Nitrofurantoin Neuropathy

Nitrofurantoin may cause peripheral neuropathy characterized by distal weakness and sensory loss. Pain and paresthesias are the common presenting symptoms.[182] The neuropathy may occur soon after drug therapy begins. It is most commonly seen in patients with impaired renal function who have higher blood levels of the drug.[183]

Disulfiram Neuropathy

Disulfiram therapy for alcohol abuse rarely causes neuropathy.[184] Affected patients generally have taken 1.0 or 1.5 g/day of this drug. They have paresthesias beginning in the lower extremities. The mechanism is unclear; however, carbon disulfide, a by-product of disulfiram, is a known neurotoxin.[185]

Carcinomatous Neuropathy

An association between malignant disease and peripheral neuropathy independent of metastases has been recognized for a long time. In 1948, Denny-Brown[186] described two patients with carcinoma of the lung and sensory neuropathy from degeneration of dorsal root ganglion cells. Studies among different groups of workers revealed an incidence of clinical peripheral neuropathy in the range of 1.7% to 5% of patients with cancer.[187,188] The highest incidence occurs among those with carcinoma of the lung, followed by those with carcinoma of the stomach, colon, and breast.

Most commonly, a combined sensorimotor neuropathy develops, but a pure sensory type also may occur.[188] Painful dysesthesias that begin distally and spread proximally and aching pains characterize the sensory component. Tendon reflexes are depressed, and position and vibratory sense may be impaired. The neuropathy often precedes other symptoms of the neoplasm by a year. Women more commonly display this type of neuropathy. Its course is unaffected by the underlying disease state.

Pathologic changes associated with the sensory neuropathy include severe degeneration of dorsal nerve roots and the posterior columns.[186] Axonal degeneration and segmental demyelination occur with the sensorimotor neuropathy.[189] The etiology of these neuropathies remains unclear.

Vincristine Neuropathy

Casey and associates[190] demonstrated that vincristine, a cancer chemotherapeutic agent, predictably produced a peripheral neuropathy distinct from that caused by the malignancy per se. Affected patients developed finger paresthesias, then painful cramping and weakness in the extensor muscles of their hands and wrists, and commonly lost their ankle reflexes. Symptoms improved somewhat after decreasing or discontinuing the drug. Presumably, the vincristine-induced breakdown of neurotubules and proliferation of neurofilaments in nerve cells plays a role in its neuropathic mechanism.[191]

RHEUMATOLOGIC DISORDERS (SEE CHAP. 31)

Polymyalgia Rheumatica

Polymyalgia rheumatica is a clinical syndrome characterized by morning stiffness in the proximal portion of the extremities or torso.[192] It occurs relatively commonly in persons older than 50; one study documented an annual incidence of 53.7 cases per 100,000 persons and a prevalence of 500 per 100,000.[193] A close relationship exists between polymyalgia rheumatica and giant cell arteritis; polymyalgia rheumatica occurs in 40% to 60% of patients with giant cell arteritis.[194] Hence, some authors suggest that polymyalgia rheumatica may be an expression of an underlying arteritis.

The presence of symptoms in two of the three commonly affected areas (neck, hip, or shoulder) for at least 1 month and evidence of a systemic process, such as an increased erythrocyte sedimentation rate (>40 mm/hour using the Westergren method) confirm the diagnosis.[195] Some definitions also require a rapid response to small doses of corticosteroids. The presence of other diseases, such as rheumatoid arthritis, polymyositis, malignancy, or chronic infection, excludes the diagnosis.

The cause remains unknown. Reports of familial aggregation and the finding that the disease appears almost exclusively in whites suggest a genetic predisposition. Several results suggest a humoral or cellular immune basis. These include (1) the granulomatous histopathologic features of giant cell arteritis, (2) the presence of immunoglobulins and complement deposits adjacent to the elastic lamina in some involved temporal arteries, and (3) the finding that sera from patients with polymyalgia rheumatica contains increased levels of circulating immune complexes during active disease.[196]

These patients are generally in good health before polymyalgia rheumatica develops. Arthralgias and myalgias may occur either slowly or abruptly; they generally begin in one shoulder girdle. However, the disease soon becomes bilateral and eventually involves most of the tendinous attachments, and there is proximal muscle pain with movement (compare the joint pain in rheumatoid arthritis).[197,198] Muscular strength is normal. Synovitis in the knees or sternoclavicular joints may be found. More than half the patients have systemic symptoms such as weight loss or a low-grade fever before the onset of muscle pain.[197,198]

Laboratory findings during the active phase include (1) a markedly elevated erythrocyte sedimentation rate (>100 mm/hour using the Westergren method), (2) a mild-to-moderate normochromic anemia, and (3) an increase in α_2-globulin and fibrinogen.[199] Significant normal laboratory values include serum creatine kinase, muscle biopsies, and EMG studies.

The differential diagnosis of polymyalgia rheumatica includes rheumatoid arthritis, polymyositis, and systemic processes (such as bacterial endocarditis). The absence of swelling and peripheral joint pain should distinguish polymyalgia rheumatica from arthritis. Polymyositis is characterized by muscle weakness, elevated muscle enzyme studies, and abnormal EMG studies.

Psoriatic Arthritis

Psoriatic arthritis is an inflammatory asymmetric polyarthritis found in patients with psoriasis. The cause is unknown, but up to 30% of patients are positive for HLA-B27 antigen.[200] The onset of the arthritis generally follows the psoriasis by months or years. The course of arthritis may or may not parallel that of the skin lesions. The pattern of the arthritis is that of a typical inflammatory arthritis that affects predominantly the upper extremities. The proximal joints of the hands and feet are tender and swollen. The arthritis is limited to several joints and is asymmetric. There are no rheumatoid nodules. Laboratory tests do not show rheumatoid factor. Affected patients may have an increased erythrocyte sedimentation rate and anemia.[200]

The radiologic features of psoriatic arthritis include erosions of the articular surfaces and the so-called pencil-in-cup deformity observed in joints of the fingers and toes. The diagnosis depends on findings consistent with psoriasis and an accompanying inflammatory arthritis without rheumatoid factor or nodules.

Reiter's Syndrome

Reiter's syndrome is an asymmetric inflammatory arthritis coupled with urethritis or cervicitis. Classically, the syndrome also included conjunctivitis. The syndrome has two clinical forms. The postvenereal form occurs predominantly in young men; the postdysenteric form affects both sexes in all age groups. The actual pathogenesis of the disease involves infection of the urogenital tract or gut with one of several organisms in genetically susceptible patients. Sufferers generally have the HLA-B27 alloantigen.[201]

Clinically, the syndrome begins with an asymptomatic serous urethral discharge usually followed by conjunctivitis.[201] Finally, the patient has an acute onset of inflammatory arthritis of the lower extremities. Keratoderma blennorrhagia frequently appear on the palms or soles. Painless mucocutaneous lesions may appear in the mouth, on the palms and soles, or on the glans penis.[201]

Synovial fluid analysis reveals an increased leukocyte count and inflammatory arthritis. The diagnosis, therefore, relies on documenting nonspecific urethritis or cervicitis without rheumatoid factor.

Gout

Gout is a painful disorder of the joints secondary to deposition of crystals of monosodium urate monohydrate. Urate values greater than 7.0 mg/dL in the plasma cause saturation; chronically elevated uric acid leads to gouty attacks. Hyperuricemia, per se, is not synonymous with gout, and most hyperuricemic patients are asymptomatic. Men tend to have higher serum uric acid levels, and more than 95% of cases occur in adult men. Hyperuricemic patients also are prone to acute nephrolithiasis, and approximately 20% of gout sufferers have attacks of renal colic before gouty attacks.[202]

The pathogenesis of an acute gouty attack after years of chronically elevated uric acid levels probably involves crystal deposition and resultant phagocytosis by leukocytes, leading to activation of Hageman factor, coating of crystals with gamma globulins, and complement activation.[202] Lowering the local tissue pH then results in additional precipitation of urate crystals.

Initially, gouty arthritis usually attacks a single joint and is exquisitely painful. Affected patients may describe prior mild attacks (twinges). The distal lower extremities, particularly the great toe (podagra), bear the brunt of the attacks. The following are involved in order of decreasing frequency: instep, ankle, heel, knee, and upper extremities. The attacks may be triggered by trauma, alcohol, surgery, or dietary excesses. Affected patients may have accompanying systemic signs, such as fever, increased erythrocyte sedimentation rate, and leukocytosis. The attacks abate spontaneously and are separated by periods when the patient is completely asymptomatic.[203]

In untreated patients, the hyperuricemia causes deposits of monosodium urate (tophi) in tendons, membranes, and soft tissues. However, these tophi rarely occur before the onset of acute gouty attacks.

Monosodium urate crystals detected using polarized-light microscopy in the leukocytes from synovial aspirates confirms the diagnosis. These crystals appear needle shaped and negatively birefringent. The leukocyte count of the synovial fluid during attacks may vary from 1,000 to 70,000/dL. Extracellular crystals may be found in the synovial fluid during asymptomatic periods. In the absence of microscopic confirmation, the diagnosis can be presumed by the combination of (1) the presence of hyperuricemia, (2) a history typical of gout, and (3) response to colchicine.

Pseudogout

Pseudogout is a crystalline arthritis seen in elderly patients that is characterized by calcium deposits in articular cartilage and caused by release of calcium pyrophosphate crystals into the joint space. There is a definite association with hyperparathyroidism, osteoarthritis, and hemochromatosis. Pseudogout also is seen in metabolic disorders such as Wilson's disease, hypothyroidism, gout, and ochronosis.[204]

Patients with pseudogout have elevated fluid levels of inorganic pyrophosphate. Crystals then form in articular cartilage (chondrocalcinosis). The crystals found in synovial fluid are released from the cartilage, possibly after trauma that disrupts the cartilage or as a result of lowering the Ca^{2+} levels in the synovium. Regardless, the presence of calcium pyrophosphate crystals then causes a classic inflammatory response, and polymorphonuclear leukocytes enter the joint.[204]

The acute arthritic attacks of pseudogout are usually monoarticular. The knee is the most common site. The joint is warm, swollen, and painful. The attacks may be preceded by surgery or trauma.

Showing calcium pyrophosphate dihydrate crystals in the synovial fluid during acute attacks confirms the diagnosis. Under a polarized-light microscope, the crystals appear as positive birefringent blunt rods. They may be intra- or extracellular. Radiologically, these patients have calcium deposits in their articular cartilage.[204]

Osteoarthritis

Osteoarthritis affects predominantly older patients. Articular cartilage absorbs the bulk of joint stress, but over time degenerates. Increased mechanical pressure appears to provoke an elaboration of chondrocytes and synovial fluid. The water and proteoglycan content decreases, and focal cartilage erosions appear. Eventually, joint margins reveal new bone and thickened synovium. The end point of this process is a progressive loss of chondrocytes, development of fissures, osteophyte formation, and replacement of cartilage with bone.[205]

Patients complain of a diffuse, aching pain that usually is limited to one or several joints. Rest relieves the pain, and activity aggravates it. Affected individuals may describe an increase in symptoms with changes in weather. Stiffness generally does not become a major symptom.[206]

Painless Heberden's nodes, which are prominent knobs along the medial and lateral aspect of distal interphalangeal joints, and Bouchard's nodes, which are found on the proximal interphalangeal joints, are a common finding. Occasionally, the joints may appear swollen and warm as a result of the inflammatory synovitis that accompanies an exacerbation of symptoms. The pattern of joint involvement (proximal interphalangeal and distal interphalangeal involvement with sparing of the wrist joint) helps distinguish osteoarthritis from rheumatoid arthritis.[206]

Radiologic findings typical of osteoarthritis include loss of joint space, presence of osteophytes, and subchondral sclerosis. Synovial fluid aspirate shows a low leukocyte count and predominantly mononuclear cells.

Rheumatoid Arthritis

Inflammatory synovitis, which results in eventual cartilage and bone destruction, distinguishes rheumatoid arthritis. The cause remains unknown, but genetics plays a role, as witnessed by its association with HLA-DR4.[207] Women are affected threefold more than men. Symptoms most frequently begin between the ages of 35 and 50 years.

Systemic symptoms, such as fatigue, generalized weakness, and anorexia, generally precede the joint pain of rheumatoid arthritis. The pain affects joints in a symmetric distribution and is aggravated by passive or active motion.[208] Morning stiffness is a universal feature and is an important criterion for the diagnosis. Physical examination reveals synovitis with accompanying swelling, tenderness, and increased warmth in the joints. The pain is secondary to joint swelling, which stretches the joint capsule. The

TABLE 32-14 **American Rheumatism Association Criteria for the Diagnosis of Rheumatoid Arthritis***

1. Morning stiffness
2. Pain on motion or tenderness in at least one joint
3. Swelling (soft tissue thickening or fluid) in at least one joint
4. Swelling of at least one other joint
5. Symmetric joint swelling
6. Subcutaneous nodules
7. Typical radiologic changes
8. Demonstration of rheumatoid factor in serum
9. Poor mucin precipitate from synovial fluid
10. Characteristic histologic changes in synovium
11. Characteristic histologic changes in nodules

*Criteria 1 to 5 must be continuous for at least 6 weeks. Criteria 2 to 6 must be observed by a physician. The presence of seven or more criteria indicates classic disease; five to six criteria indicate definite disease; three to four criteria indicate probable disease.

From Martin JB. *Harrison's Principles of Internal Medicine.* New York, NY: McGraw-Hill; 1987:1950.

wrist joints, proximal interphalangeal joints, and metacarpophalangeal joints usually are involved, but rarely the distal interphalangeal joints. Hand involvement with destruction of cartilage, tendons, and ligaments can cause a number of typical deformities: (1) boutonnäire deformity (which results from flexion deformity of the proximal interphalangeal joints and extension of the distal interphalangeal joints), (2) swan-neck deformity (which results from hyperextension of proximal joint and flexion of distal interphalangeal joints), and (3) radial deviation at the wrist with ulnar deviation at the digits.

Although no specific diagnostic tests exist, the American Rheumatism Association has developed a list of criteria to aid in the diagnosis (Table 32-14). Affected patients may carry the rheumatoid factor (autoantibodies to immunoglobulin G) in their serum. In addition, there may be a normochromic normocytic anemia. Most patients also have increased erythrocyte sedimentation rates. Evaluation of the synovial fluid shows increased leukocytes with polymorphonuclear leukocytes, suggesting an inflammatory process.

MUSCULAR DISORDERS

Most skeletal muscle pain is associated with exercise or trauma.[209] The pain is related temporally to exercise and is of limited duration. Muscle pain is transmitted by the thin myelinated fibers (group III or Aδ) and unmyelinated fibers (group IV or C). These afferent fibers have unencapsulated branching endings throughout the muscle with increasing density in the region of fascia, tendons, and aponeuroses. There are two types of muscle pain receptors: chemoreceptors and mechanoreceptors. The former respond to chemical changes in the environment; the latter are affected by mechanical changes. These receptors can be stimulated by potassium ions, hydrogen ions, histamine, serotonin, or bradykinin.[210–213]

Patients most often describe muscle pain or myalgia as dull or aching in quality. The term *cramp*[214] refers to an acute onset of a painful contraction, and although they can be intensely painful, the quality of pain is described as dull. A muscle *contracture* is similar to a cramp, but of longer duration; it is seen in disorders of muscle metabolism. Muscle *spasms* are reflex contractions of muscles surrounding injured tissues or structures (e.g., abdominal muscle spasm associated with an inflamed appendix). *Myotonia* is tonic spasm of a muscle after voluntary contraction caused by a high-frequency firing of muscle fibers. *Tetany* refers to involuntary cramplike spasms associated with reductions in ionizable calcium or magnesium and attributed to repetitive firing in motor axons. *Dystonia* is an involuntary contraction of muscle that involves both agonist and antagonist activities.

Myalgias can be difficult to distinguish from pain arising from other sites. Pain from the joints is well localized and exacerbated by movement. Patients poorly localize bone pain, but it tends to have a deep, boring quality that generally worsens at night. One must determine whether the muscle pain is accompanied by weakness (failure to achieve strength) or fatigue (failure to maintain strength). As a rule, proximal muscle weakness suggests primary muscle disease; peripheral and localized pain and weakness tend to occur with nerve entrapments. Excessive fatigability is seen in disorders of muscle metabolism, myotonic disorders, and mitochondrial myopathies.

The relationship of diet, alcohol intake, and fasting to muscle pain should be determined. Drinking bouts may precipitate myopathy and myoglobinuria in alcoholic patients. Fasting or prolonged exercise with fasting may precipitate pain and weakness in patients with carnitine palmityl transferase deficiency. A diet lacking in vitamin D may lead to osteomalacic myopathy with bone and muscle pain.

Signs of muscle pain are confined to weakness, fatigability, tenderness, and swelling. Muscle swelling per se is rare, but it may occur in the polymyositis-dermatomyositis complex, acute alcoholic myopathy, phosphofructokinase deficiency, and myophosphorylase.

Useful clinical tests to evaluate muscle pain and disease include (1) presence of myoglobinemia and myoglobinuria, (2) serum creatine kinase levels, (3) erythrocyte sedimentation rate, (4) EMG, (5) quantitation of muscle force generation, (6) exercise testing, (7) ischemic forearm tests, and (8) muscle biopsy.

Myoglobin is a muscle protein involved in oxygen storage. Muscle breakdown or rhabdomyolysis can release myoglobin molecules, which may pass into the urine as a result of their small size (molecular weight 17,500 Daltons) and precipitate oliguric renal failure. Myoglobinemia and myoglobinuria also may arise from various other causes.[215]

Creatine kinase is a muscle enzyme that catalyzes the breakdown and synthesis of phosphoryl creatine. Abnormal increases in serum levels of creatine kinase may indicate muscle damage; however, exercise and intramuscular injections may also cause elevated serum levels.[216] This enzyme is elevated in muscular dystrophies, acute rhabdomyolysis, McArdle's disease, and polymyositis-dermatomyositis complex.

EMG helps distinguish myopathic from neuropathic diseases. Fibrillation and giant action potentials characterize denervation from entrapment; myopathies are associated with brief, small-amplitude motor unit potentials. EMG can also provide information about which nerve roots are involved.

Quantitation[217] of muscle force generation can be done using a hand-held dynamometer or muscle-testing chair. The latter involves electrical activation of the quadriceps with large surface electrodes and provides data concerning muscle fatigability and frequency characteristics. These tools can track the progression of the disease or the distribution of muscle weakness.

Exercise testing uses submaximal effort at approximately 70% of previously determined maximal rate while simultaneously measuring heart rate and blood pressure and levels of blood lactate and pyruvate. Exercise testing can elicit symptoms in patients with muscle disorders, and it is a particularly useful tool in those with suspected metabolic disorders.

The simplicity and advantages of muscle biopsy, particularly in the diagnosis of inflammatory myopathies and mitochondrial myopathies, have been well described. Percutaneous needle biopsy is atraumatic and appears to be as reliable clinically as an open biopsy of muscle.

Muscle Pain and Exercise

Normally, muscle pain with exercise can occur under two situations. Firstly, it can occur with exercise and increase in intensity until the muscle relaxes. When the voluntary contraction stops, the pain disappears immediately. This type of concentric contraction or positive work has a high metabolic cost.[218] The mechanism for this type of ischemic pain appears to be an accumulation of metabolites that occludes blood vessels and stops the blood supply to the muscle. Secondly, vigorous exercise leads to delayed muscle pain. This results from eccentric muscle contractions or negative work where the muscle is lengthened during a contraction.[219] The mechanism of this delayed soreness after eccentric contraction is unknown; however, the muscles show evidence of damage, both biochemically and morphologically.[220]

Cramps are painful involuntary contractions of acute onset that occur more often at night. Stretching of voluntary muscle produces an involuntary contraction that cannot be relaxed. The cramping results from spontaneous firing of groups of anterior horn cells with motor unit contractions. Cramps in the calf muscles generally are considered benign. More generalized cramps, however, may be a sign of muscle disease.[214] Cramps that recur and are confined to one specific muscle group may indicate nerve root entrapment. They also occur with increasing frequency during pregnancy, with electrolyte imbalances, and in patients undergoing hemodialysis. Physical examination during muscle cramping shows a taut, contracted muscle. This can be a distinguishing feature of the cramps caused by intermittent claudication, in which patients have cramplike pain without muscle contraction. The cause of the pain is not understood completely, but it may involve an accumulation of metabolites or a relative ischemia of the muscle. There is a benign form of muscle cramping (idiopathic cramp syndrome) in which no neuromuscular disorder is apparent.

The stiff-person syndrome refers to a progressive form of painful muscle spasm.[221,222] These patients have a boardlike stiffness of their muscles, paroxysms of cramping, and a normal sensory examination. The muscle stiffness resolves during sleep or after the administration of large doses of diazepam. Isaac's syndrome is manifested by excessive sweating, widespread fasciculations, generalized stiffness, and continuous motor unit activity that persists during sleep and anesthesia.[223]

Tetany results from a reduction in ionizable calcium and magnesium. This leads to increased neuromuscular irritability and involuntary, cramplike spasms. The actual level of ionizable calcium needed to produce tetany varies individually and is related to the concentration of other electrolytes in the extracellular fluid. Hyperventilation and ischemia increase the tendency for spasm to occur. The full clinical spectrum of tetany is manifested by perioral and peripheral paresthesias, carpal spasm, pedal spasm, laryngospasm, Chvostek's and Trousseau's signs, and Q-T prolongation on an electrocardiogram. Hypocalcemia causes unstable depolarization of the nerve fiber axons. Thus, there is increased sensitivity of the facial nerve to percussion (Chvostek's sign) and spasm with ischemia (Trousseau's sign).

Drugs also may be a source of muscle pain. Focal myopathy may occur after intramuscular injections from local irritation (e.g., paraldehyde) or after histamine release (opiates).

Painful proximal myopathy with tenderness and weakness can occur after administration of clofibrate, aminocaproic acid, and emetine, particularly after prolonged treatment and elevated serum blood levels. Serum levels of muscle enzymes are elevated, and myoglobinuria may occur. Muscle biopsy reveals multifocal muscle-fiber necrosis. A painful, necrotizing proximal myopathy with an associated peripheral neuropathy has been reported in patients treated with vincristine.[224] Chronic hypokalemia from drug use generally results in painless weakness and hypotonia. However, painful quadriparesis and myoglobinuria have been reported after administration of amphotericin B and chlorthalidone.[224] Finally, some drugs may cause myalgias and cramps from unknown mechanisms. These drugs include lithium carbonate, danazol, isoetharine, cimetidine, and the diuretics metolazone and bumetanide.[224]

The glycogen storage diseases constitute a group of diseases in which an inborn error of glycogen metabolism exists. When the energy supply for muscle contractions is compromised, muscle fatigue and pain may result.

McArdle's disease, or type V, first manifests during adolescence with cramps, weakness, and contractions induced by vigorous exercise. The cramps and pain are relieved by rest, but the contractions may persist for hours. Moderate exercise may be well tolerated. This disorder is caused by a deficiency of the enzyme myophosphorylase. Tarui's disease, or type VII, is a rare enzyme deficiency that begins during early childhood and is characterized by exercise-induced pain without muscle contractions.

Idiopathic Polymyositis and Dermatomyositis

Idiopathic polymyositis and dermatomyositis refer to a category of relatively common diseases that may affect striated muscle only (polymyositis) or skin and muscle (dermatomyositis). They also may occur associated with arthritis, connective tissue diseases, or malignancy. Pain may be a prominent feature.[225]

The cause of polymyositis-dermatomyositis is unknown. Theories include autoimmune processes or a possible viral mechanism.[226] Polymyositis-dermatomyositis may have several different clinical presentations. Polymyositis, confined to striated muscles, begins with an insidious onset over 3 to 6 months of a symmetric weakness of the proximal limb and trunk muscles. In a minority of patients, a febrile illness precedes this subacute muscle weakness. Women outnumber men by 2 to 1, and the age range is generally 30 to 60 years.[226] Rarely, severe muscle weakness occurs acutely with associated myoglobinuria.

Affected patients first notice weakness of the proximal limb muscles when climbing steps, rising from chairs, or combing their hair. The muscle pain that occurs in a minority of patients is of a constant aching quality and follows the same distribution as the weakness.[227]

Physical examination shows a symmetric weakness of the muscles of the hips, shoulders, and thighs. Weakness of the facial and pharyngeal muscles is also common. The muscles are not tender to examination, and atrophy is not a prominent feature.

Dermatomyositis is characterized by skin lesions that may precede, accompany, or follow the muscle involvement. The rash may take one of several forms: localized erythema, maculopapular eruption, or exfoliative dermatitis. The areas most predisposed include the eyelids, the bridge of the nose, and the cheeks. The extensor surfaces of elbows, knees, and knuckles may develop flat plaques known as Gottron's papules.[228] The myositis that accompanies these skin changes is indistinguishable from polymyositis.

Polymyositis or dermatomyositis may occur associated with an underlying neoplasm (group 3) (Table 32-15). The muscle and skin manifestations may antedate the discovery of a carcinoma by 1 to 2 years. This generally occurs with bronchogenic carcinoma.[229] The actual incidence of underlying carcinomas with polymyositis is 2% to 3%; it rises to 15% to 20% with dermatomyositis. Idiopathic polymyositis and dermatomyositis occur less frequently in children than in adults. The childhood form constitutes 8% to 22% of cases in most large series. The clinical features of the disease in children are similar to those in adults; however, children have a high incidence of vasculitis.[230]

Finally, polymyositis or dermatomyositis may occur in collagen vascular disease. Mixed connective tissue diseases also may have an accompanying arthritis that limits joint motion and further diminishes strength.

Laboratory findings common to all the clinical subsets of dermatomyositis-polymyositis include (1) elevated serum levels of skeletal muscle enzymes, particularly creatine kinase (which may be elevated 10–80 times normal); (2) sometimes positive tests for circulating rheumatoid factor and antinuclear antibody; (3) myoglobinuria; (4) EMG studies showing an increase in the insertional activity of the muscle with numerous fibrillation potentials and positive sharp waves at rest[231]; and (5) resultant muscle biopsy consisting of inflammatory infiltrates (lymphocytes and histiocytes) between the muscle fibers and around the small blood vessels in the muscle.[232]

Other Forms of Polymyositis

Trichinosis in humans is contracted by ingesting meat (usually pork) containing the larvae of *Trichinella spiralis.* Once freed from their cysts by gastric digestion, the larvae migrate into the intestinal mucosa, where copulation occurs. The offspring (up to 1,500 per female) enter the circulation and are distributed to muscles throughout the body. After entering the muscle, the larvae grow and become encysted and eventually calcified. The life cycle then ends. The muscles most affected include the eye muscles, diaphragm, deltoid, pectorals, and gastrocnemius.[233]

The clinical severity of the symptoms correlates well with the number of larvae disseminated to the tissues. Patients with less than 10 larvae per gram of muscle are asymptomatic; those with greater than 50 larvae per gram of muscle display gastrointestinal symptoms (e.g., diarrhea and abdominal pain) 1 to 2 days after the infected meat is eaten. This brief period is followed by a stage of muscular invasion that may last up to 6 weeks. Affected patients have muscle pain and tenderness with accompanying weakness. They also may have fever, periorbital edema, conjunctivitis, and a maculopapular rash. Severe cases develop various central nervous system manifestations. Finally, myocarditis may occur, with resultant congestive heart failure and electrocardiographic changes.

Laboratory findings include an eosinophilic leukocytosis (>500 eosinophils/μL) within the first few weeks. Serologic tests may turn positive within the first month and remain positive for years. A definitive diagnosis is made by muscle biopsy. A portion of muscle is excised from the gastrocnemius or deltoid and examined microscopically for the presence of larvae or calcified cysts.[234]

Eosinophilic Myositis

Eosinophilic myositis consists of three separate clinical entities: (1) eosinophilic fasciitis, (2) eosinophilic monomyositis, and (3) eosinophilic polymyositis.[235] The first entity involves tenosynovitis with local pain and stiffness of unknown cause. It progresses from one muscle to another but generally is confined to an extremity. These patients have no systemic manifestations. The muscle, per se, is not involved, and biopsy of fascia and tendon sheaths reveals an inflammatory process with eosinophilic leukocytes.

The second entity includes muscle pain confined to one calf muscle and associated with a tender mass. A muscle biopsy shows an inflammatory necrosis and edema of interstitial tissues. Eosinophilic polymyositis, as described by Layzer and colleagues,[236] is characterized by multiple systemic problems (congestive heart failure, anemia, and pulmonary infiltrates) plus painful proximal muscle weakness. The muscles themselves are swollen and exquisitely tender.[237]

TABLE 32-15 **Classification of the Polymyositis-Dermatomyositis Complex**

Group 1.	Primary idiopathic polymyositis
Group 2.	Primary idiopathic dermatomyositis
Group 3.	Dermatomyositis (or polymyositis) associated with neoplasia
Group 4.	Childhood dermatomyositis (or polymyositis) associated with vasculitis
Group 5.	Polymyositis or dermatomyositis associated with collagen vascular disease (overlap group)

Proposed by Bohan and Peter.[229]

REFERENCES

1. Malan E, Tattoni G. Physio- and anatopathology of acute ischemia of the extremities. *J Cardiovasc Surg (Torino)* 1963;4:2.
2. Perry MO. Acute arterial insufficiency. In: Rutherford RB, ed. *Vascular Surgery*. 2nd ed. Philadelphia, Pa: WB Saunders; 1984.
3. Kempczinski RF. The management of chronic ischemia of the lower extremities. In: Rutherford RB, ed. *Vascular Surgery.* 2nd ed. Philadelphia, Pa: WB Saunders; 1984.
4. Kempczinski RF. Peripheral arterial atheroembolism. In: Miller DC, Roon AJ, eds. *Diagnosis and Management of Peripheral Vascular Disease.* Menlo Park, Calif: Addison-Wesley; 1982.
5. Kempczinski RF. The differential diagnoses of intermittent claudication. *Pract Cardiol* 1981;7:53.
6. Boyd AM. Natural course of atherosclerosis of lower extremities. *Proc R Soc Med* 1962;53:591.
7. Imparato AM, Kim GE, Davidson T, Crowley JG. Intermittent claudication: Its natural course. *Surgery* 1975;78:795.

8. Sumner DS. Measurement of segmental arterial pressure. In: Rutherford RB, ed. *Vascular Surgery.* 2nd ed. Philadelphia, Pa: WB Saunders; 1984.
9. Carter SA. Indirect systolic pressure and pulse waves in arterial occlusive disease of the lower extremities. *Circulation* 1968;37:624.
10. Carter SR. Clinical measurement of systolic pressures in limbs with arterial occlusive disease. *JAMA* 1969;207:1869.
11. Cutajar CL, Marston A, Newcombe JF. Value of cuff occlusion pressures in assessment of peripheral vascular disease. *Br Med J* 1973;2:392.
12. Weiner SD, Reis ED, Kerstein MD. Peripheral arterial disease. Medical management in primary care practice. *Geriatrics* 2001;56:20.
13. Love JW, Whelan TJ. Popliteal artery entrapment syndrome. *Am J Surg* 1965;109:620.
14. Insua JA, Young JR, Humphries AW. Popliteal artery entrapment syndrome. *Arch Surg* 1970;101:771.
15. Ezzet F, Yettra M. Bilateral popliteal artery entrapment: Case report and observations. *J Cardiovasc Surg* 1971;12:71.
16. Bergan JJ. Adventitial cystic disease of the popliteal artery. In: Rutherford RB, ed. *Vascular Surgery.* 2nd ed. Philadelphia, Pa: WB Saunders; 1984.
17. McPherson JR, Juergens JL, Gifford RW Jr. Thromboangiitis obliterans and arteriosclerosis obliterans: Clinical and prognostic differences. *Ann Intern Med* 1963;59:288.
18. Juergens JL. Thromboangiitis obliterans. In: Rutherford RB, ed. *Vascular Surgery.* 2nd ed. Philadelphia, Pa: WB Saunders; 1984.
19. Rivera R. Roentgenographic diagnosis of Buerger's disease. *J Cardiovasc Surg (Torino)* 1973;14:40.
20. Allen EV, Brown GE. Raynaud's disease: A critical review of minimal requisites for diagnosis. *Am J Med Sci* 1932;183:187.
21. VeLayos EE, Robinson H, Porciuncula FV, Masi AT. Clinical correlation analysis of 137 patients with Raynaud's phenomenon. *Am J Med Sci* 1971;262:347.
22. Blunt RJ, Porter JM. Raynaud's syndrome. *Semin Arthritis Rheum* 1981;11:282.
23. Porter JM. Raynaud's syndrome and associated vasospastic conditions of the extremities. In: Rutherford RB, ed. *Vascular Surgery.* 2nd ed. Philadelphia, Pa: WB Saunders; 1984.
24. Taylor W, Pelmar PL. Raynaud's phenomenon of occupational origin: An epidemiological survey. *Acta Chir Scand Suppl* 1976;465:27.
25. Porter JM. Raynaud's syndrome and associated vasospastic conditions of the extremities. In: Rutherford RB, ed. *Vascular Surgery.* 2nd ed. Philadelphia, Pa: WB Saunders; 1984.
26. Bernstein EF. Operative management of acute venous thromboembolism. In: Rutherford RB, ed. *Vascular Surgery.* 2nd ed. Philadelphia, Pa: WB Saunders; 1984.
27. Sumner DS. Hemodynamics and pathophysiology of venous disease. In: Rutherford RB, ed. *Vascular Surgery.* 2nd ed. Philadelphia, Pa: WB Saunders; 1984.
28. Sumner DS. Evaluation of venous circulation with the ultrasonic Doppler velocity detector. In: Rutherford RB, ed. *Vascular Surgery.* 2nd ed. Philadelphia, Pa: WB Saunders; 1984.
29. Wheeler HB. Plethysmographic diagnosis of deep venous thrombosis. In: Rutherford RB, ed. *Vascular Surgery.* 2nd ed. Philadelphia, Pa: WB Saunders; 1984.
30. Baxter BT, Blackburn D, Payne K, Pearce WH, Yao JS. Noninvasive evaluation of the upper extremity. *Surg Clin North Am* 1990;70:87.
31. Rorabeck CH, Clark KM. The pathophysiology of the anterior tibial compartment syndrome: An experimental investigation. *J Trauma* 1978;18:299.
32. Rorabeck CH, Macnab I. The pathophysiology of the anterior tibial compartmental syndrome. *Clin Orthop* 1975;113:52.
33. Sheridan GW, Matsen FA III, Krugmire RB Jr. Further investigations on the pathophysiology of the compartmental syndrome. *Clin Orthop* 1977;123:266.
34. Whitesides TE, Haney TC, Morimoto K, et al. Tissue pressure measurements as a determinant for the need of fasciotomy. *Clin Orthop* 1975;113:43.
35. Owen CA, Mubarak SJ, Hargens AR, et al. Intramuscular pressure with limb compression. Clarification of the pathogenesis of the drug-induced compartment syndrome/crush syndrome. *N Engl J Med* 1979;300:1169.
36. Matsen FA Ill, Winguist RA, Krugmire RB Jr. Diagnosis and management of compartmental syndrome. *J Bone Joint Surg Am* 1980;62A:286.
37. Hargens AR, Mubarak SJ. Laboratory diagnosis of acute compartment syndromes. In: Mubarak SJ, Hargens AR, eds. *Compartment Syndromes and Volkmann's Contracture. Monographs in Clinical Orthopaedics, III.* Philadelphia, Pa: WB Saunders; 1981.
38. Ritland D, Butterfield W. Extremity complications of drug abuse. *Am J Surg* 1973;126:639.
39. Wright CB, Geelhoed G, Hobson R, et al. Acute vascular insufficiency due to drugs of abuse. In: Rutherford RB, ed. *Vascular Surgery.* 2nd ed. Philadelphia, Pa: WB Saunders; 1984.
40. Gay GR. Intra-arterial injection of secobarbital sodium into the brachial artery: Sequelae of a "hand trip." *Anesth Analg (Cleve)* 1971;50:979.
41. Maxwell TM, Olcott C, Blaisdell FW. Vascular complications of drug abuse. *Arch Surg* 1972;105:875.
42. Rich NM, Hobson RW, Fedde CW. Vascular trauma secondary to diagnostic and therapeutic procedures. *Am J Surg* 1973;126:639.
43. Geelhoed GW, Joseph WL. Surgical sequelae of drug abuse. *Surg Gynecol Obstet* 1974;139:749.
44. Neviaser RJ, Butterfield WC, Wieche DR. The puffy hand of drug addiction. *J Bone Joint Surg Am* 1972;54A:629.
45. Anderson CB. Mycotic aneurysms. In: Rutherford RB, ed. *Vascular Surgery.* 2nd ed. Philadelphia, Pa: WB Saunders; 1984.
46. Farooki MA. Aneurysms in the United States and the United Kingdom. *Int Surg* 1973;58:475.
47. Anderson CB, Butcher HR, Ballinger WF. Mycotic aneurysms. *Arch Surg* 1974;109:712.
48. Patel S, Johnston KW. Classification and management of mycotic aneurysms. *Surg Gynecol Obstet* 1977;144:691.
49. Stengel A, Wolferth CC. Mycotic (bacterial) aneurysms of intravascular origin. *Arch Intern Med* 1923;31:527.
50. Yellin AE. Ruptured mycotic aneurysm: A complication of parenteral drug abuse. *Arch Surg* 1977;112:981.
51. Huebl HC, Read RC. Aneurysmal abscess. *Minn Med* 1966;49:11.
52. Rich NM, Hobson RW 11, Collins GJ Jr. Traumatic arteriovenous fistulas and false aneurysms: A review of 558 lesions. *Surgery* 1975;78:817.
53. Rich NM, Hobson RW II, Fedde CW. Vascular trauma secondary to diagnostic and therapeutic procedures. *Am J Surg* 1973;126:639.
54. Mumenthaler M, Narakas A, Gilliatt RW. Brachial plexus disorders. In: Dyck PJ, Thomas PK, Lambert EH, Bunge R, eds. *Peripheral Neuropathy*. 2nd ed. Philadelphia, Pa: WB Saunders; 1984:1383.
55. Ilfeld F, Holder H. Winged scapula. Case occurring in soldier from knapsack. *JAMA* 1942;120:448.
56. Daube JR. Rucksack paralysis. *JAMA* 1969;208:2447.
57. Kraft GH. Rucksack paralysis and brachial neuritis. *JAMA* 1970;211:300.
58. Molnar W, Paul DJ. Complications of axillary arteriotomies. An analysis of 1762 consecutive studies. *Radiology* 1972;104:269.
59. Salam AA. Brachial plexus paralysis: an unusual complication of anticoagulant therapy. *Am Surg* 1972;38:454.
60. Dhumer KG. Nerve injuries following operations: a survey of cases occurring during a six year period. *Anesthesiology* 1950;11:289.
61. Dornette WHL. Compression neuropathies: medical aspects and legal implications. In: Hindman BJ, ed. *International Anesthesiology Clinics*. Vol. 24. Boston, Mass: Little, Brown; 1986.

62. Challenor Y, Richter RW, Brunn B, Pearson J. Nontraumatic plexitis and heroin addiction. *JAMA* 1973;225:958.
63. Kori SH, Foley KM, Posner JB. Brachial plexus lesions in patients with cancer: 100 cases. *Neurology* 1981;31:45.
64. Thomas JE, Colby MY Jr. Radiation-induced or metastatic brachial plexopathy? *JAMA* 1972;22:1392.
65. Geiger LR, Mancall EL, Penn AS, Tucker SH. Familial neuralgic amytrophy. *Brain* 1974;97:87.
66. Dunn HG, Daube JR, Gomey MA. Heredofamilial brachial plexus neuropathy (hereditary neuralgia amyotrophy with brachial predilection) in childhood. *Dev Med Child Neurol* 1978;20:28.
67. Jacob JC, Andermann F, Robb JP. Heredofamilial neuritis with brachial predilection. *Neurology* 1961;11:1025.
68. Windebank AJ. Inherited recurrent focal neuropathies. In: Dyck PJ, Thomas PK, Lambert EH, Bunge R, eds. *Peripheral Neuropathy*. 2nd ed. Philadelphia, Pa: WB Saunders; 1984:1656.
69. Taylor RA. Heredofamilial mononeuritis multiplex with brachial predilection. *Brain* 1960;83:113.
70. Ungley CC. Recurrent polyneuritis in pregnancy and the puerperium affecting three members of a family. *J Neurol Psychopathol* 1933; 14:15.
71. Asbury AK, Amason BGW, Adams RD. The inflammatory lesion in acute idiopathic polyneuritis. *Medicine* 1969;48:173.
72. Adams RD, Victor M. Diseases of peripheral nerve and muscle. In: Adams RD, Victor M, eds. *Principles of Neurology*. 3rd ed. New York, NY: McGraw-Hill; 1986:960.
73. Brady RO. Fabry disease. In: Dyck PJ, Thomas PK, Lambert EH, Bunge R, eds. *Peripheral Neuropathy*. 2nd ed. Philadelphia, Pa: WB Saunders; 1984:1717.
74. Brady RO, Gal AE, Bradley RM, Martensson E, Warshaw AL, Laster L. Enzymatic defect in Fabry's disease: Ceramide trihexosidase deficiency. *N Engl J Med* 1967;276:1163.
75. Imperial R, Helwig EB. Angiokeratoma, a clinical pathological study. *Arch Dermatol* 1967;95:166.
76. Cable WJL, Kolodny EH, Adams RD. Fabry's disease: Clinical demonstration of impaired autonomic function. *Neurology* 1982;32:498.
77. Halter SK, DeLisa JA, Stolov WC, Scardapane D, Sherrard DJ. Carpal tunnel syndrome in chronic renal dialysis patients. *Muscle Nerve* 1980;3:438.
78. Potts G, Shahani BT, Young RR. A study of the coincidence of carpal tunnel syndrome and generalized peripheral neuropathy. *Muscle Nerve* 1980;3:440.
79. Cho DS, Cho MJ. The electrodiagnosis of the carpal tunnel syndrome. *S D J Med* 1989;42:5.
80. Stewart JD, Aguayo AJ. Compression and entrapment neuropathies. In: Dyck PJ, Thomas PK, Lambert EH, Bunge R, eds. *Peripheral Neuropathy.* 2nd ed. Philadelphia, Pa: WB Saunders; 1984:1435.
81. Feindel W, Stratford J. The role of the cubital tunnel in tardy ulnar palsy. *Can J Surg* 1958;1:287.
82. Brown WF, Yates SK, Fergusen GG. Cubital tunnel and ulnar neuropathy. *Ann Neurol* 1980;7:289.
83. Payan J. Cubital tunnel syndrome. *Br Med J* 1979;2:868.
84. Domette WHL. Compression neuropathies: Medical aspects and legal implications. In: Hindman BJ, ed. *International Anesthesiology Clinics.* Vol. 24. Boston, Mass: Little, Brown; 1986.
85. Uriburu IJF, Morchio FJ, Marin JC. Compression syndrome of the deep motor branch of the ulnar nerve (pisohamate hiatus syndrome). *J Bone Surg Am* 1976;58A:145.
86. Trojaborg W. Rate of recovery in motor and sensory fibers of the radial nerve: Clinical and electrophysiological aspects. *J Neurol Neurosurg Psychiatry* 1970;33:625.
87. Spinner RJ, Bachman JW, Amadio PC. The many faces of carpal tunnel syndrome. *Mayo Clin Proc* 1989;64:829.
88. Toranto IR. Aneurysm of the median artery causing recurrent carpal tunnel syndrome and anatomic review. *Plast Reconstr Surg* 1989;84: 510.
89. Gelberman RH, Aronson D, Weisman MH. Carpal tunnel syndrome. *J Bone Joint Surg Am* 1980;62:1181.
90. Stewart JD, Eisen A. Tinel's sign and the carpal tunnel syndrome. *Br Med J* 1978;2:1125.
91. Kopell HP, Thompson WAL. Pronator syndrome. A confined case and its diagnosis. *N Engl J Med* 1958;259:713.
92. Morris HH, Peters BH. Pronator syndrome: Clinical and electrophysiological features in seven cases. *J Neurol Neurosurg Psychiatry* 1976;39:461.
93. O'Brien MD, Upton ARM. Anterior interosseous nerve syndrome. A case report with neurophysiological investigation. *J Neurol Neurosurg Psychiatry* 1972;35:531.
94. Schmidt H, Eiken O. The anterior interosseous nerve syndrome. *Scand J Plast Reconstr Surg* 1971;5:53.
95. Rengachary SS, Neff JP, Singer PA, Brackett CE. Suprascapular entrapment neuropathy: A clinical, anatomical and comparative study. *Neurosurgery* 1979;5:441.
96. Clein LJ. Suprascapular entrapment neuropathy. *J Neurosurg* 1975; 43:337.
97. Bastron JA, Thomas JE. Diabetic polyradiculopathy. *Mayo Clin Proc* 1981;56:725.
98. Hopper CL, Baker JB. Bilateral femoral neuropathy complicating vaginal hysterectomy. *Obstet Gynecol* 1968;32:543.
99. Mukherjee SK. Iliacus haematoma. *J Bone Joint Surg Br* 1971;5313: 729.
100. Warfield CW. Meralgia paresthetica: Causes and cures. *Hosp Pract (Off Ed)* 1986;21:40A.
101. Jefferson D, Eames RA. Subclinical entrapment of the lateral femoral cutaneous nerve: An autopsy study. *Muscle Nerve* 1979;2:145.
102. Rousseau JJ, Reznik M, Le Jenne GN, Franck G. Sciatic nerve entrapment by pentazocine-induced muscle fibrosis. *Arch Neurol* 1979; 36:723.
103. Baker GS, Parsons WR, Welch JS. Endometriosis within the sheath of the sciatic nerve. *J Neurosurg* 1966;25:652.
104. Pace JB, Nagel D. Piriform syndrome. *West J Med* 1976;124:435.
105. Adams JA. The piriformis syndrome-report of four cases and review of the literature. *S Afr J Surg* 1980;18:13.
106. Sandhu HS, Sandhey BS. Occupational compression of the common peroneal nerve at the neck of the fibula. *Aust N A J Surg* 1976;46: 160.
107. Nagler SH, Rangell L. Peroneal palsy caused by crossing the legs. *JAMA* 1947;133:755.
108. Edwards WG, Lincoln CR, Bassett FH, Goldner JL. The tarsal tunnel syndrome. Diagnosis and treatment. *JAMA* 1969;207:716.
109. Lloyd K, Agarwal A. Tarsal tunnel syndrome, a presenting feature of rheumatoid arthritis. *Br Med J* 1970;3:32.
110. Pringle RM, Protheroe K, Mukherjee SK. Entrapment neuropathy of the sural nerve. *J Bone Joint Surg Br* 1974;56:465.
111. Patman RD. Post-traumatic pain syndromes: Recognition and management. In: Rutherford RB, ed. *Vascular Surgery.* 2nd ed. Philadelphia, Pa: WB Saunders; 1984.
112. Lankford LL. Reflex sympathetic dystrophy. In: Evarts CM, ed. *Surgery of the Musculoskeletal System.* New York, NY: Churchill Livingstone; 1983.
113. Mitchell SW, Morehouse GR, Keen W. *Gunshot Wounds and Other Injuries of Nerves.* Philadelphia, Pa: Lippincott; 1864.
114. Lankford LL, Thompson JE. Reflex sympathetic dystrophy, upper and lower extremity: Diagnosis and management. In: *AA OS Instructional Course Lectures.* Vol. 26. St. Louis, Mo: CV Mosby; 1977.
115. Bastron JA. Neuropathy in diseases of the thyroid and pituitary glands. In: Dyck PJ, Thomas PK, Lambert EH, Bunge R, eds. *Peripheral Neuropathy.* 2nd ed. Philadelphia, Pa: WB Saunders; 1984:1834.
116. Hurwitz LJ, McCormick D, Allen IV. Reduced muscle alpha-glucosidase (acid-maltase) activity in hypothyroid myopathy. *Lancet* 1970;1:67.
117. Sheaff HM. Hereditary myokymia: Syndrome or disease entity asso-

ciated with hypoglycemia and disturbed thyroid function. *Arch Neurol Psychiatry* 1952;68:236.
118. Bastron JA. Neuropathy in diseases of the thyroid and pituitary glands. In: Dyck PJ, Thomas PK, Lambert EH, Bunge R, eds. *Peripheral Neuropathy*. 2nd ed. Philadelphia, Pa: WB Saunders; 1984:1841.
119. Oldberg S. The carpal tunnel syndrome and acromegaly. *Acta Soc Med Ups* 1971;76:179.
120. Melliere D, Ben Yahia NE, Etienne G, Becquemin JP, de Labareyre H. Thoracic outlet syndrome caused by tumor of the first rib. *J Vasc Surg* 1991;14:235.
121. Winsor T, Winsor D, Mikail A, Sibley A. Thoracic outlet syndromes—application of microcirculation techniques and clinical review. *Angiology* 1989;40:773.
122. Etheredge S, Wilbur B, Storey RJ. Thoracic outlet syndrome. *Am J Surg* 1979;138:175.
123. Karas SE. Thoracic outlet syndrome. *Clin Sports Med* 1990;9:297.
124. Roos DB. New concepts of thoracic outlet syndrome that explain etiology, symptoms, diagnosis and treatment. *Vasc Surg* 1979;13:313.
125. Roos DB. Congenital anomalies associated with thoracic outlet syndrome—anatomy, symptoms, diagnosis and treatment. *Am J Surg* 1976;132:771.
126. Sanders RJ, Haug C. Subclavian vein obstruction and thoracic outlet syndrome: A review of etiology and management. *Ann Vasc Surg* 1990;4:397.
127. Cuetter AC, Bartoszek DM. The thoracic outlet syndrome: Controversies, overdiagnosis, overtreatment, and recommendations for management. *Muscle Nerve* 1989;12:410.
128. Urschel HC, Razzuk MA. Management of the thoracic outlet syndrome. *N Engl J Med* 1972;286:1140.
129. Cherington M. Ulnar conduction velocity in thoracic outlet syndrome. *N Engl J Med* 1976;294:1185.
130. Brackman R. Cervical spondylotic myelopathy. In: Krayenbuhl, ed. *Advances and Technical Standard in Neurosurgery*. Vol. 6. New York, NY: Springer-Verlag; 1979:137.
131. Bullard DE. Cervical disc lesions. In: Sabiston DC Jr, ed. *Textbook of Surgery: The Biological Basis of Modern Surgical Practice*. 13th ed. Philadelphia, Pa: WB Saunders; 1986:1399.
132. Mumenthaler M, Narakas A, Gilliat RW. Brachial plexus disorders. In: Dyck PJ, Thomas PK, Lambert EH, Bunge R, eds. *Peripheral Neuropathy*. 2nd ed. Philadelphia, Pa: WB Saunders; 1984:1392.
133. Tsairis P, Dyck PJ, Mulder DW. Natural history of brachial plexus neuropathy: Report on 99 patients. *Arch Neurol* 1973;27:109.
134. Waxman SG. The flexion-adduction sign in neuralgia amyotrophy. *Neurology (Minneapolis)* 1979;29:1301.
135. Flaggman PD, Kelly JJ Jr. Brachial plexus neuropathy. An electrophysiologic evaluation. *Arch Neurol* 1980;37:160.
136. Igbal A, Arnason BGW. Neuropathy of serum sickness. In: Dyck PJ, Thomas PK, Lambert EH, Bunge R, eds. *Peripheral Neuropathy*. 2nd ed. Philadelphia, Pa: WB Saunders; 1984:2044.
137. Miller HG, Stanton JB. Neurological sequelae of prophylactic inoculation. *Q J Med* 1954;23:1.
138. Conn DL, Dyck PJ. Angiopathic neuropathy in connective tissue diseases. In: Dyck PJ, Thomas PK, Lambert EH, Bunge R, eds. *Peripheral Neuropathy*. 2nd ed. Philadelphia, Pa: WB Saunders; 1984:2027.
139. Irby R, Adams RA, Toone EC Jr. Peripheral neuritis associated with rheumatoid arthritis. *Arthritis Rheum* 1958;1:44.
140. Dyck PJ, Conn DL, Okazak H. Necrotizing angiopathic neuropathy: Three-dimensional morphology of fiber degeneration related to sites of occluded vessels. *Mayo Clin Proc* 1972;47:461.
141. Lewis DC. Systemic lupus and polyneuropathy. *Arch Intern Med* 1965;116:518.
142. Warrell DA, Godfrey S, Olsen EGJ. Giant-cell arteritis with peripheral neuropathy. *Lancet* 1968;1:1010.
143. Ridley A. Porphyric neuropathy. In: Dyck PJ, Thomas PK, Lambert EH, Bunge R, eds. *Peripheral Neuropathy*. 2nd ed. Philadelphia, Pa: WB Saunders; 1984:1704.
144. Hierons R. Acute intermittent porphyria. *Postgrad Med J* 1967;43:605.
145. Ridley A, Hierons R, Cavanagh JB. Tachycardia and the neuropathy of porphyria. *Lancet* 1968;2:708.
146. Becker DM, Kramer S. The neurological manifestations of porphyria: A review. *Medicine (Baltimore)* 1977;56:411.
147. Ridley A. The neuropathy of acute intermittent porphyria. *Q J Med* 1969;38:307.
148. Mustajaki P, Seppalairen AM. Neuropathy in latent hereditary hepatic porphyria. *Br Med J* 1975;2:310.
149. Asbury AK. Hepatic neuropathy. In: Dyck PJ, Thomas PK, Lambert EH, Bunge R, eds. *Peripheral Neuropathy*. 2nd ed. Philadelphia, Pa: WB Saunders; 1984:1826.
150. Dayan AD, Williams R. Demyelinating peripheral neuropathy and liver diseases. *Lancet* 1967;2:133.
151. Knill-Jones RP, Goodwill CJ, Dayan AS, Williams R. Peripheral neuropathy in chronic liver disease: Clinical electrodiagnostic, and nerve biopsy findings. *J Neurol Neurosurg Psychiatry* 1972;35:22.
152. Phough JC, Ayerle RS. The Guillian-Barre syndrome associated with acute hepatitis. *N Engl J Med* 1953;247:61.
153. Niermeijer P, Gips CH. Guillian-Barre syndrome in acute HBS Ag-positive hepatitis. *Br Med J* 1975;4:732.
154. Thomas PK, Walker JG. Xanthomatous neuropathy in primary biliary cirrhosis. *Brain* 1965;8:1079.
155. Gammon GD, Bunge FW, King G. Neural toxicity in tuberculous patients treated with isoniazid (isonicotinic acid hydrazide). *Arch Neurol Psychiatry* 1953;70:64.
156. Hughes HB, Biehl JP, Jones AP, Schmidt LH. Metabolism of isoniazid in man as related to the occurrence of peripheral neuritis. *Am Rev Tuberc* 1954;70:266.
157. Biehl JP, Vilter RW. The effect of isoniazid on vitamin B6 metabolism and its possible significance in producing isoniazid neuritis. *Proc Soc Exp Biol Med* 1954;85:385.
158. Raskin NH, Fishman RA. Pyridoxine-deficiency neuropathy due to hydralazine. *N Eng J Med* 1965;273:1182.
159. Victor M, Laureno R. Neurologic complications of alcohol abuse: Epidemiologic aspects. *Adv Neurol* 1978;19:603.
160. Thomas PK. Clinical features and differential diagnosis. In: Dyck PJ, Thomas PK, Lambert EH, Bunge R, eds. *Peripheral Neuropathy*. 2nd ed. Philadelphia, Pa: WB Saunders; 1984:1169.
161. Adams RD, Victor M. Diseases of the peripheral nerves. In Adams RD, Victor M, ed. *Principles of Neurology*. 3rd ed. New York, NY: McGraw-Hill; 1985:960.
162. O'Hare JA, Warfield CA. The diabetic neuropathies. *Hosp Pract* 1984;19:41.
163. Ellenberg M. Diabetic neuropathy. In: Ellenberg M, Rifkin H, eds. *Diabetes Mellitus: Theory and Practice*. 3rd ed. New Hyde Park, NY: Medical Examination Pub; 1983:777.
164. Pirart J. Diabetes mellitus and its degenerative complications: A prospective study of 4,400 patients observed between 1947 and 1973. *Diabetes Care* 1978;1:168,252.
165. Root HF, Pate WH, Frehner H. Triopathy of diabetes. Sequence of diabetes, retinopathy and nephropathy in one hundred and fifty-five patients. *Arch Intern Med* 1954;94:931.
166. Ellenberg M. Diabetic neuropathy: A consideration of factors in onset. *Ann Intern Med* 1960;52:1067.
167. Brown MJ, Martin JR, Asbury AK. Painful diabetic neuropathy: A morphometric study. *Arch Neurol* 1976;33:164.
168. Archer A, Watkins PJ, Thomas PK, Sharma AK, Payan J. The natural history of acute painful neuropathy in diabetes mellitus. *J Neurol Neurosurg Psychiatry* 1983;46:491.
169. Sinha S, Municheodappa CS, Koyak GP. Neuroarthropathy (Charcot's joints) in diabetes mellitus. Clinical study of 101 cases. *Medicine (Baltimore)* 1972;51:191.
170. Clarke BF, Ewing DJ, Campbell IW. Diabetic autonomic neuropathy. *Diabetologia* 1979;17:195.

171. Garland H, Taverner D. Diabetic myelopathy. *Br Med J* 1953;1:1045.
172. Garland H. Diabetic amyotrophy. *Br Med J* 1955;2:1287.
173. Robson JS. Uraemic neuropathy. In: Robertson RF, ed. *Symposium: Some Aspects of Neurology.* Edinburgh, Scotland: Royal College of Physicians of Edinburgh; 1968:74.
174. Bolton CF. Letter to the editor. *N Engl Med* 1980;302:755.
175. Asbury AK. Uremic neuropathy. In: Dyck PJ, Thomas PK, Lambert EH, Bunge R, eds. *Peripheral Neuropathy.* 2nd ed. Philadelphia, Pa: WB Saunders; 1984:1811.
176. Scribner BH. Discussion. *Trans Am Soc Artif Intern Organs* 1965; 11:29.
177. Nielsen VK. The peripheral nerve function in chronic renal failure, I: Clinical signs and symptom. *Acta Med Scand* 1971;190:105.
178. Ekbom KA. Restless leg syndrome. *Neurology (Minneapolis)* 1960; 10:868.
179. Hartfall SJ, Garland HG, Goldie W. Gold treatment of arthritis. A review of 900 cases. *Lancet* 1937;2:838.
180. Katrak SM, Pollack M, O'Brien CP, et al. Clinical and morphological features of gold neuropathy. *Brain* 1980;103:671.
181. Wijesekera JC, Critchley EMR, Fahim Y, Lynch PG, Wright JS. Peripheral neuropathy due to perhexiline maleate. *J Neurol Sci* 1980; 46:303.
182. Ellis FG. Acute polyneuritis after nitrofurantoin therapy. *Lancet* 1962;2:1136.
183. Collins H. Polyneuritis associated with nitrofurantoin therapy. *Arch Neurol* 1960;3:656.
184. Moddel G, Bilbao JM, Payae D, Ashby D. Disulfiram neuropathy. *Arch Neurol* 1978;35:658.
185. Rainey JM. Disulfiram toxicity and carbon disulfide poisoning. *Am J Psychiatry* 1977;134:371.
186. Denny-Brown D. Primary sensory neuropathy with muscular changes associated with carcinoma. *J Neurol Neurosurg Psychiatry* 1948;11:73.
187. Lennox B, Prichard S. Association of bronchial carcinoma and peripheral neuritis. *Q J Med* 1950;19:97.
188. Morton DL, Itabashi HH, Grimes DF. Nonmetastatic neurological complications of bronchogenic carcinoma. The carcinomatous neuromyopathies. *J Thorac Cardiovasc Surg* 1967;51:14.
189. Croft PB, Urich H, Wilkinson M. Peripheral neuropathy of sensorimotor type associated with malignant disease. *Brain* 1967;90:31.
190. Cascy EB, Jelliffe AM, Le Quesne PM, Millett YL. Vincristine neuropathy: Clinical and electrophysiological observations. *Brain* 1973; 96:69.
191. Shelanski ML, Wisniewski H. Neurofibrillary degeneration induced by vincristine therapy. *Arch Neurol* 1969;20:199.
192. Hunder GG, Disney TF, Ward LE. Polymyalgia rheumatica. *Mayo Clin Proc* 1969;44:849.
193. Chuang TY, Hunder GG, Ilstrup DM, Jurland LT. Polymyalgia rheumatica. A ten-year epidemiologic and clinical study. *Ann Intern Med* 1982;97:672.
194. Hunder GG, Allen GL. Giant cell arteritis: A review. *Bull Rheum Dis* 1978–1979;29:980.
195. Hunder GG, Disney TF, Ward LE. Polymyalgia rheumatica. *Mayo Clin Proc* 1969;44:849.
196. Papaioannou CC, Gupta RC, Hunder GG, McDuffie FC. Circulating immune complexes in giant cell arteritis/polymyalgia rheumatica. *Arthritis Rheum* 1980;23:1021.
197. Hunder GG, Disney TF, Ward LE. Polymyalgia rheumatica. *Mayo Clin Proc* 1969;44:849.
198. Fernandez-Herlihy L. Polymyalgia rheumatica. *Semin Arthritis Rheum* 1971;1:236.
199. Fauchald P, Rygvold O, Oystese B. Temporal arteritis and polymyalgia rheumatica: Clinical and biopsy findings. *Ann Intern Med* 1972; 77:845.
200. Wright V. Psoriatic arthritis. In: Kelly W, Harris E, Ruddy S, et al, eds. *Textbook of Rheumatology*. Philadelphia, Pa: WB Saunders; 1985:1021.
201. Calin A. Reiter's syndrome. In: Kelly W, Harris E, Ruddy S, et al, eds. *Textbook of Rheumatology*. Philadelphia, Pa: WB Saunders; 1985: 1007.
202. Kelly WN. Gout and related disorders of purine metabolism. In: Kelly W, Harris E, Ruddy S, et al, eds. *Textbook of Rheumatology*. Philadelphia, Pa: WB Saunders; 1985:1359.
203. Kelly W, Harris E, Ruddy S, et al. Gout and related disorders of purine metabolism. In: Kelly W, et al, eds. *Textbook of Rheumatology*. Philadelphia, Pa: WB Saunders; 1985:1359.
204. Howell DS. Diseases due to the deposition of calcium pyrophosphate and hydroxyapatite. In: Kelly W, Harris E, Ruddy S, et al, eds. *Textbook of Rheumatology*. Philadelphia, Pa: WB Saunders; 1985: 1398.
205. Brandt KD. Pathogenesis of osteoarthritis. In: Kelly W, Harris E, Ruddy S, et al, eds. *Textbook of Rheumatology.* Philadelphia, Pa: WB Saunders; 1985:1417.
206. Brandt KD. Osteoarthritis: Clinical patterns and pathology. In: Kelly W, Harris E, Ruddy S, et al, eds. *Textbook of Rheumatology.* Philadelphia, Pa: WB Saunders; 1985:1432.
207. Decker JL, et al. Rheumatoid arthritis: Evolving concepts of pathogenesis and treatment. *Ann Intern Med* 1984;101;810.
208. Harris ED. Rheumatoid arthritis: The clinical spectrum. In: Kelly W, Harris E, Ruddy S, et al, eds. *Textbook of Rheumatology.* Philadelphia, Pa: WB Saunders; 1985:915.
209. Gerr F, Letz R, Landrigan PJ. Upper-extremity musculoskeletal disorders of occupational origin. *Annu Rev Public Health* 1991;12:543.
210. Knighton ES, Dumke PR. *Pain.* Boston, Mass: Little, Brown; 1966.
211. Mense S, Schmidt RF. Muscle pain: Which receptors are responsible for the transmission of noxious stimuli? In: Clifford Rose F, ed. *Physiological Aspects of Clinical Neurology.* Oxford, England: Blackwell Scientific Pub; 1977:265.
212. Kumazawa T, Mizumara K. Thin fibre receptors responding to mechanical chemical and thermal stimulation in the skeletal muscle of the dog. *J Physiol* 1977;273:179.
213. Mense S. Reduction of the bradykinin induced activation of feline Group III and IV muscle receptors by acetylsalicylic acid. *J Physiol* 1982;376:269.
214. Layzer RB, Rowland LP. Cramps. *New Engl J Med* 1971;285:31.
215. Penn AS. Myoglobin and myoglobinuria. In: Vynken PJ, Bruhn GW, eds. *Handbook of Clinical Neurology.* Holland: Elsevier; 1980.
216. Demos MA, Gitlin EL, Kagen LJ. Exercise myoglobinuria and acute exertional rhabdomyolysis. *Arch Int Med* 1974;134:669.
217. Edwards RHT, Wiles CM, Mills KR. Quantitation of human muscle function. In: Dyck P, Thomas PK, Lambert EH, eds. *Peripheral Neuropathy.* Philadelphia, Pa: WB Saunders; 1985.
218. Mills KR, Newham DJ, Edwards RHT. Force, contraction frequency and energy metabolism as determinants of ischemic muscle pain. *Pain* 1982;14:149.
219. Abraham WM. Factors in delayed muscle soreness. *Med Sci Sports* 1977;9:11.
220. Newham DJ, Mills KR, McPhail G, Edwards RHT. Muscle damage following eccentric contractions. *Eur J Clin Invest* 1982;12:29.
221. Moersch FP, Woltman HW. Progressive fluctuating muscular rigidity ("stiff-man syndrome"): Report of a case and some observations in 13 other cases. *Mayo Clinic Proc* 1956;31:421.
222. Valli G, Barbrieri S, Stefano C, et al. Syndromes of abnormal muscular activity: Overlap between continuous muscle fiber activity and the stiff-man syndrome. *J Neurol Neurosurg Psychiatry* 1983;46:241.
223. Isaacs H. A syndrome of continuous muscle fiber activity. *J Neurol Neurosurg Psychiatry* 1961;24:319.
224. Lane RJ, Mastaglia FL. Drug-induced myopathies in man. *Lancet* 1978;2:562.
225. Bohan A, Peter JB. Polymyositis and dermatomyositis. *N Engl J Med* 1975;292:344, 1227.
226. Whitaker JN. Inflammatory myopathy: A review of etiologic and pathogenetic factors. *Muscle Nerve* 1982;5:573.

227. Riddoch J, Morgan-Hughes JA. Prognosis in adult polymyositis. *J Neurol Sci* 1975;26:71.
228. Keil H. The manifestations in the skin and mucous membranes in dermatomyositis with special reference to the differential diagnosis from systemic lupus erythematosus. *Ann Intern Med* 1975;16:828.
229. Bohan A, Peter JB, Bowman RL, Pearson CM. A computer assisted analysis of 153 patients with polymyositis and dermatomyositis. *Medicine* 1977;56:255.
230. Bitnum S, Daeschner CW, Travis LB, Dodge WF, Hopps HC. Dermatomyositis. *J Pediatr* 1964;64:101.
231. Buchthal F, Pinelli P. Muscle action potentials in polymyositis. *Neurology* 1953;3:424.
232. Bohan A, Peter JB, Bowman RL, Pearson CM. A computer assisted analysis of 153 patients with polymyositis and dermatomyositis. *Medicine* 1977;56:255.
233. Gould SE. *Trichinosis in Man and Animals.* Springfield, Ill: Charles C Thomas; 1970.
234. Gross B, Ochoa J. Trichinosis: A clinical report and histochemistry of muscle. *Muscle Nerve* 1979;2:394.
235. Adams RD, Victor M. Polymyositis and other acute and subacute myopathic paralyses. In: Adams RD, Victor M, eds. *Principles of Neurology.* 3rd ed. New York, NY: McGraw-Hill; 1965.
236. Layzer RB, Shearn MA, Satya-Murti S. Eosinophilic polymyositis. *Ann Neurol* 1977;1:65.
237. Stark RJ. Eosinophilic polymyositis. *Arch Neurol* 1979;36:721.

CHAPTER 33 # FOOT PAIN

René Cailliet

Evaluation of the painful foot is simplified because all aspects of the foot that may be designated as the site of pain by the patient are visible, palpable, and reproducible to the examiner. The tissue sites of pain in the foot are the joints, ligaments, tendons, or peripheral nerves. The mechanisms of pain and disability are elucidated by the patient in the history.

ANKLE JOINT INJURIES

The ankle essentially consists of the talotibial joint. The talus fits within the mortise formed by the malleoli of the tibia and the fibula, allowing primarily flexion and extension with limited lateral flexion on rotation. The talus allows no lateral or rotational movement within the mortise when dorsiflexed but allows some lateral motion when fully plantar flexed. It is in the plantar flexed position that the ankle sustains injury to its ligaments when there is excessive lateral rotatory movement upon the fixed foot.

The ankle joint is made stable by its collateral ligaments. The ligaments on the medial side are the deltoid ligaments: anterior talotibial, tibionavicular, calcaneotibial, and posterior talotibial. Those on the lateral side are the anterior talofibular, calcaneofibular, talocalcaneal, and posterior talofibular. All ligaments are named according to the bones they connect and sustain injury when these bones are excessively separated from the sustained injury. The anterior talofibular ligament is the weakest and most frequently injured ligament (Figs. 33-1 and 33-2).

A strain is a force, and a sprain is tissue damage from excessive strain. This damage may involve tearing of individual collagen fibers composing the ligament. The number and degree of sprain depends on the number and extent of the collagen fibers injured.

Symptoms and Clinical Findings

The history reveals the mechanism by which the ligamentous injury occurred. Local pain, tenderness, and swelling are common findings.

Examination reveals the extent of swelling and tenderness. Mere edema implies minor sprain, whereas ecchymosis implies tearing, causing microhemorrhage and more severe injury.

The examination will determine which ligament has been damaged and to what degree. The degree of inversion of the foot compared with the opposite side, using the same technique and moving the feet identically, reveals the degree of ligamentous injury. A complete tear allows excessive motion. A positive drawer sign implicates the posterior or anterior talofibular ligaments.

Diagnosis is basically made by examination, but stress films may reveal talar tilt within the mortise. X-ray studies may also reveal an avulsion fracture when the lateral collateral ligaments have been excessively stressed.

Treatment

Treatment depends on the severity of the injury. Mild sprain (grade I) is an injury that maintains functional integrity with little swelling and tenderness. Moderate sprain (grade II) indicates near-complete ligamentous disruption with moderate swelling and tenderness and functional impairment. Severe sprain (grade III) indicates complete ligamentous disruption. There is tenderness, pain, and marked disability, swelling, and separation of the ankle bones in the foot.

Initial treatment of an acute sprain (grades I and II) involves elevation, ice application, firm wrap, and no weight bearing for at least 24 to 48 hours. This is followed by gradual, active dorsiflexion and extension exercises. Gentle, active inversion and eversion exercises are performed, at first without resistance and then with gradually increased resistance.

Treatment of grade III sprain is more controversial. The decision about whether to use conservative treatment or surgical intervention is determined by the ultimate physical demands on the individual and the expertise of the treating physician.

Rehabilitation treatments are indicated for all grades of sprain, regardless of the definitive treatment, because return of proprioception and strength are mandatory for balance.

OTHER TYPES OF FOOT PAIN

Hind Foot

The hind foot is the weight-bearing part of the foot, containing the talocalcaneus. Pain that occurs predominantly in the calcaneal area is produced by from the Achilles tendon, the bursa behind the tendon, the pad over the plantar area of the calcaneus, and the site of attachment of the plantar fascia on the calcaneus. In the current exercise culture, the jogger's foot includes all painful sites (Fig. 33-3).

Achilles Tendon

The Achilles tendon may be strained or torn, depending on the severity of the injury. Strain implies retained function, with tenderness and possible swelling. Grading is possible, with grade I injury being a sprain, more properly called *peritendinitis,* and grade II being a complete tear. Discomfort is felt on elongation, and tenderness occurs 4 to 8 cm above the site of the tendon's insertion on the os calcis.

Treatment is rest, elevation, local application of ice, and avoidance of any elongation of the tendon for 7 to 10 days. Oral nonsteroidal anti-inflammatory drugs (NSAIDs) are effective. A tear may be treated by casting, with the foot maintained in extreme plantar flexion for many weeks, or by surgical intervention.

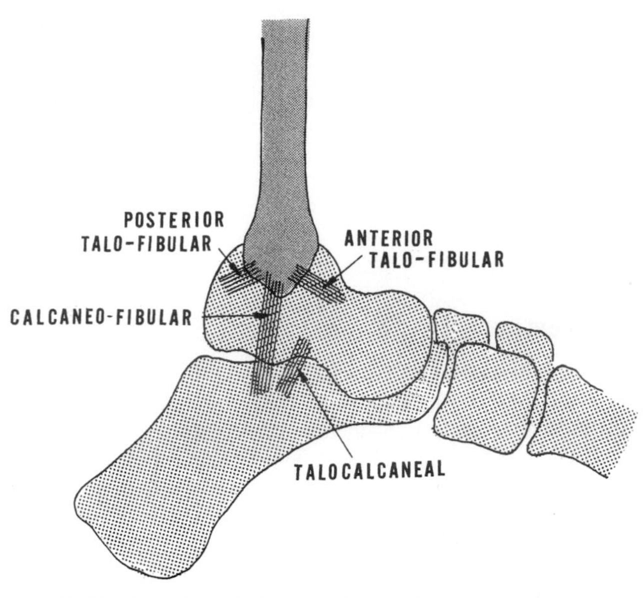

Figure 33-1 Lateral collateral ligaments.

Subtendon Bursitis

An inflamed subtendon bursa reveals tenderness "behind" the tendon on manual palpation. Treatment is generally the same as for tendonitis, but a local injection of analgesic and corticosteroid is usually effective.

Heel Spur (Plantar Fasciitis)

The development of so-called heel spur pain begins with pulling of the plantar fascia at its insertion point on the anterior inferior aspect of the calcaneus. The tendon of the fascia inserts on the periosteum of the calcaneus and, when acutely or chronically strained, causes avulsion of the periosteum from the bone. As the avulsion of the periosteum increases, hemorrhage fills the area. This fluid, containing fibroblasts, ultimately forms a calcific spur. The condition usually occurs in a pronated foot that overstretches the fascia. Hyperextension of the toes further stretches the plantar fascia.

Treatment may include local injection of an analgesic agent and corticosteroid, as well as correction of the pronation.

Talocalcaneal Arthralgia

Movement of the calcaneus on the talus is limited by the talocalcaneal ligaments. Talocalcaneal arthralgia occurs when this articulation is overstretched. This can occur as a result of a severely pronated foot or a severe ankle sprain that moves the calcaneus excessively upon the talus. Pain, which occurs on walking, can be reproduced by immobilizing the talus by placing the foot in extreme dorsiflexion then moving the calcaneus. There usually is tenderness on palpation of the tarsal tunnel, located directly under the lateral (fibular) malleolus, when the foot is markedly inverted and plantar flexed.

Treatment includes local rest, oral NSAIDs, splinting in the acute phase, and then correcting pronation with an appropriate orthosis. Local injection of an analgesic and a corticosteroid into the tarsal tunnel is usually effective.

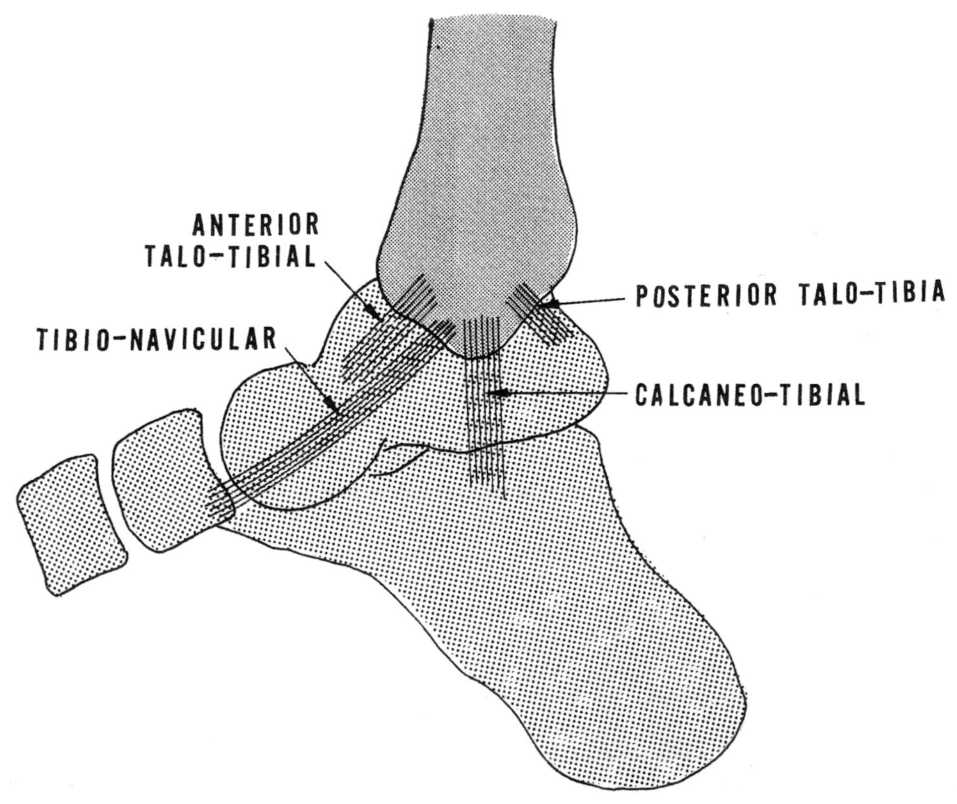

Figure 33-2 Medial (deltoid) collateral ligaments.

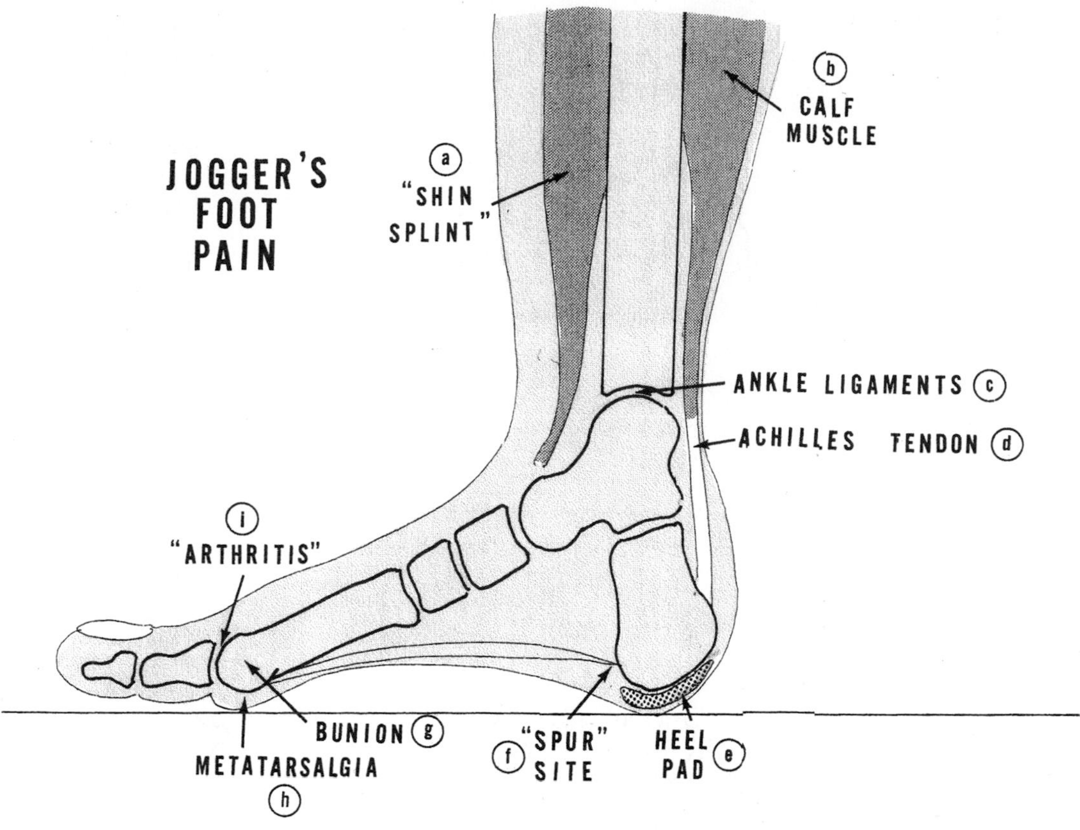

Figure 33-3 Jogger's foot pain. (**A**) so-called shin splint, (**B**) calf muscle, (**C**) ankle ligaments, (**D**) Achilles tendon, (**E**) heel pad, (**F**) "spur" site, (**G**) bunion, (**H**) metatarsalgia, and (**I**) arthritis of metatarsophalangeal joints.

Pronated Foot

The pronated, so-called flat foot causes discomfort and impairment in many people. A pronated foot is often congenital and familial, and may be asymptomatic until the foot is overstressed.

The normal, nonpronated foot has a well-formed longitudinal arch, an adequate transverse arch, and an adequate metatarsal arch. The calcaneus lies directly under the talus in a sagittal line The pronated foot has a depressed longitudinal arch, an everted forefoot, and a depressed metatarsal arch. The heel is in valgus. Gait is usually impaired, with a toe-out pattern (Fig. 33-4).

Patients experience symptoms of aching and fatigue of the foot after walking or prolonged standing. Tenderness is present over the longitudinal arch, anterior heel, and midmetatarsal bones.

Treatment consists of correction of the pronation using an appropriate orthosis, gait correction, and weight loss, if the patient is overweight.

Posterior Tibial Tendonitis

The posterior tibial tendon passes under the medial malleolus and when inflamed can be palpated. When the foot is placed in plantar flexion with active inversion, the tendon is stressed and becomes painful and tender (Fig. 33-5).

Treatment is similar to that for the pronated foot. Local injection of an analgesic agent and a corticosteroid under the sheath containing the tendon also is effective.

Posterior Tibial Neuritis

The posterior tibial nerve passes alongside the posterior tibial tendon and, when inflamed from compression or traction, causes neuritic pain in the dermatomal distribution, branching into the medial and lateral plantar nerves (Fig. 33-6).

Symptoms include tenderness over the nerve at the medial malleolus and paresthesia or burning pain over the medial border of the foot in the plantar surface. Numbness and Tinel's sign can be elicited by the examiner

Metatarsalgia

Metatarsalgia is an ill-defined orthopedic entity of pain—acute, recurrent, or chronic—of any of the metatarsal heads.

The Great Toe Pain in the region of the great toe may result from wearing shoes that cause mechanical pressure on the dorsum or medial aspect of the big toe. The first metatarsal head has no muscles acting upon it, but is supported by a sling.

When the supporting muscles—the extensor hallucis longus and the flexor hallucis longus—slide laterally as a result of structural damage to the great toe, they exert improper pull and add to the

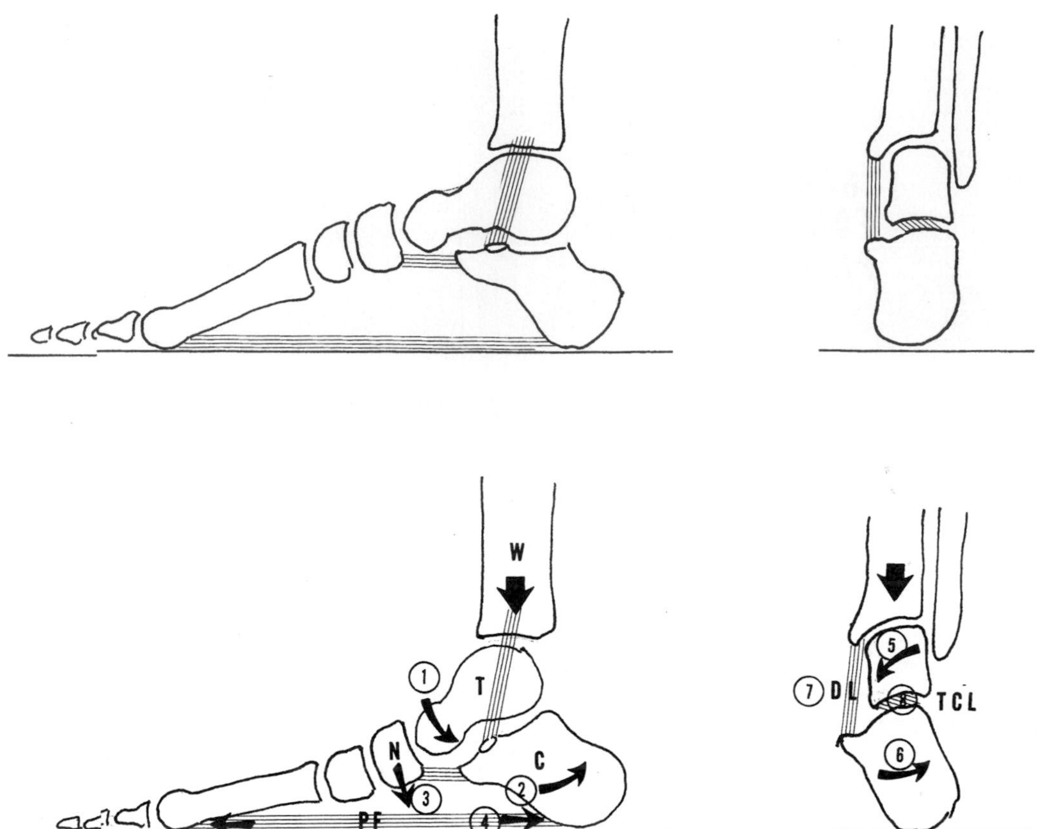

Figure 33-4 Pronated foot. The upper drawing shows the normal foot. The lower drawing shows the components of the pronated foot. W, body weight; T, talus; C, calcaneus; N, navicular; PF, plantar fascia. In pronation, the talus depresses anteriorly (1), and the calcaneus rotates posteriorly (2). The navicular is depressed (3), the plantar fascia is stretched (4), and the talus tilts laterally, (5) as does the calcaneus (6), straining the medial collateral ligaments (7) and the talocalcaneal ligaments (8).

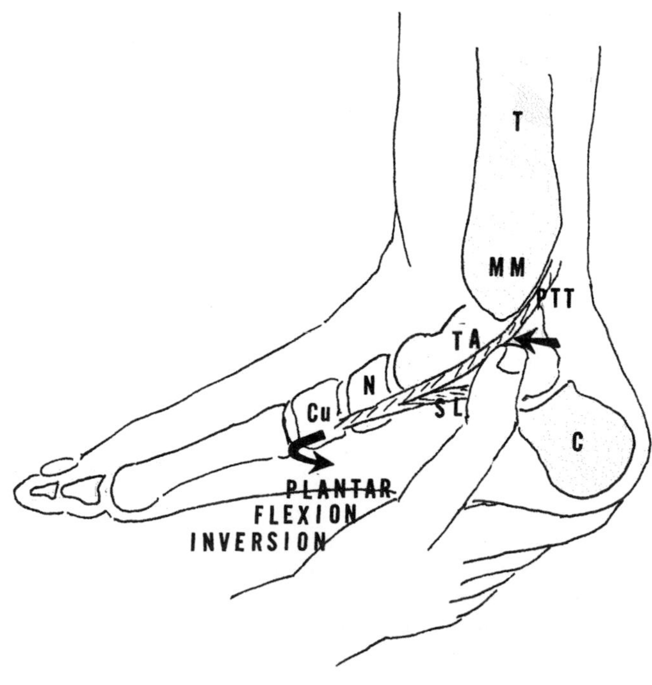

Figure 33-5 Palpation of the posterior tibial tendon. The posterior tibial tendon (PTT) passes under the medial malleolus (MM) of the tibia (T) and over the talus (TA) and navicular (N) to attach on the cuneiforms (Cu). Cis, calcaneus; SL, spring ligament.

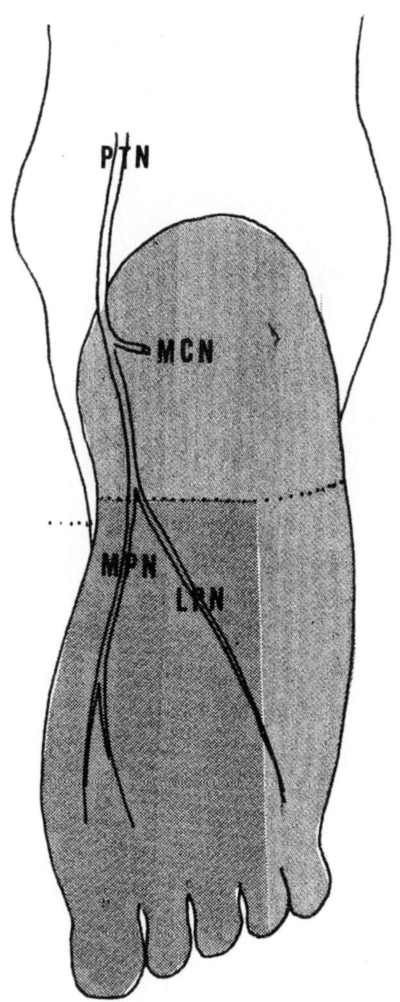

Figure 33-6 Dermatomal distribution of the plantar nerves. The posterior tibial nerve (PTN) divides into the medial calcaneal nerve (MCN), the medial plantar nerve (MPN), and the lateral plantar nerve (LPN). The dermatomal areas are shaded.

deformity. This lateral shift causes malposition of the sesamoid bones, which become painful and tender.

Hallux Valgus In this condition, the great toe deviates laterally to compensate for the internal deviation (varus) of the first metatarsal, which usually is a congenital condition (Fig. 33-7). Standing accentuates the extent of the deformity. In the seated position, the toe is manipulated to determine its stability. Hypermobility is noted in 5% of patients. Crepitation and pain indicate early degenerative changes in the joint cartilage (Fig. 33-8).

Treatment involves ensuring use of an appropriately designed shoe with a wide metatarsal width. Oral NSAIDs, as well as local intra-articular injection of analgesic and corticosteroid, may give temporary relief. Prolonged, intractable pain and impairment are indications for surgical intervention.

Hallux Rigidus Degenerative arthritis of the metatarsophalangeal joint of the great toe results in limitation of passive or active motion of this joint. Initially, the joint range of motion is painfully limited. X-ray studies reveal degenerative changes. The pain diminishes gradually, but motion becomes totally limited.

Treatment consists of modifying the shoe with a rocker bottom and steel-shank insole that prevent dorsiflexion of the toe during gait (Fig. 33-9).

Lesser Metatarsalgia Normally, weight-bearing stress falls on the first (hallux) and the fifth metatarsal heads. With pronation, however, the metatarsal arch is depressed and weight bearing is shifted to the second, third, and fourth phalangeal heads. Pain occurs as a result of weight bearing at these middle toes. Symptoms of pain are felt over the heads of the three middle toes during walking, a feeling that is frequently described as "having a stone in the shoe."

Tenderness is elicited when the heads of the involved toes are compressed digitally by the examiner. Care must be taken to ensure that the pressure is placed on and not between the heads, where the interdigital nerves are located. The foot must also be found to exhibit all the components of pronation.

Treatment consists of preventing the middle metatarsal heads from striking the ground during gait. This can be accomplished by inserting a metatarsal pad in the shoe, under and behind the middle metatarsal heads (Fig. 33-10). Pronation is corrected by an appropriate orthosis, which can be designed to provide the desired metatarsal elevation.

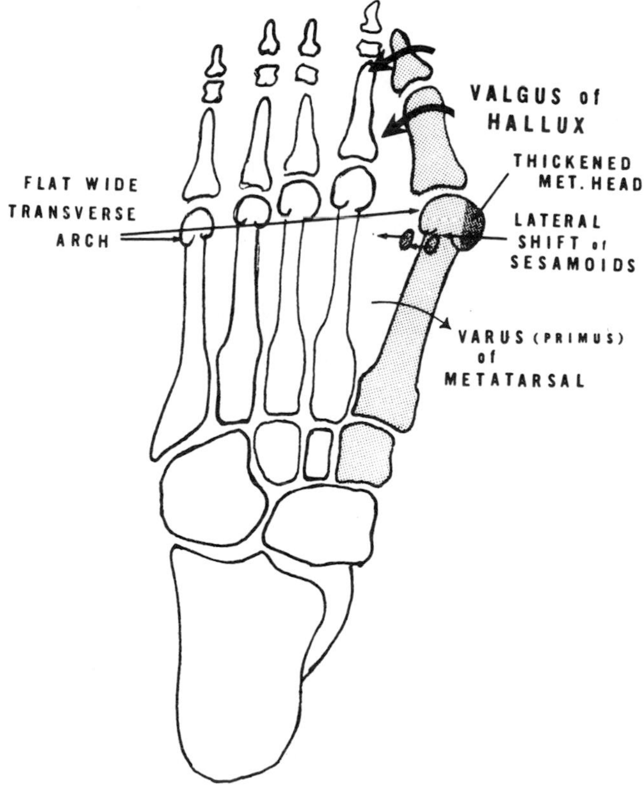

Figure 33-7 Hallux valgus. Lateral deviation of the great toe (valgus) upon a varus first metatarsal exposes the medial aspect of the first metatarsal to external pressure, resulting in hypertrophy and inflammation (darkened area). The flexor tendons migrate laterally.

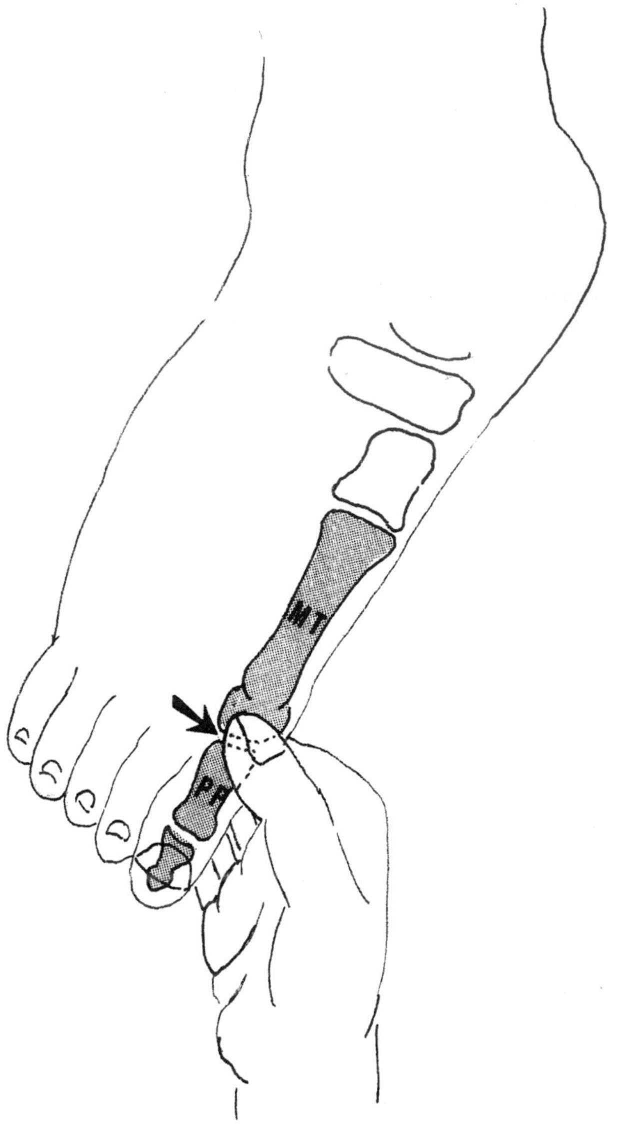

Figure 33-8 Palpation of the first metatarsal phalangeal joint reveals crepitation when the toe is passively or actively flexed and extended. Markedly limited flexibility indicates early hallux rigidus, termed *hallux rigidus limitus*. X-rays reveal the presence and extent of valgus and associated degenerative joint changes.

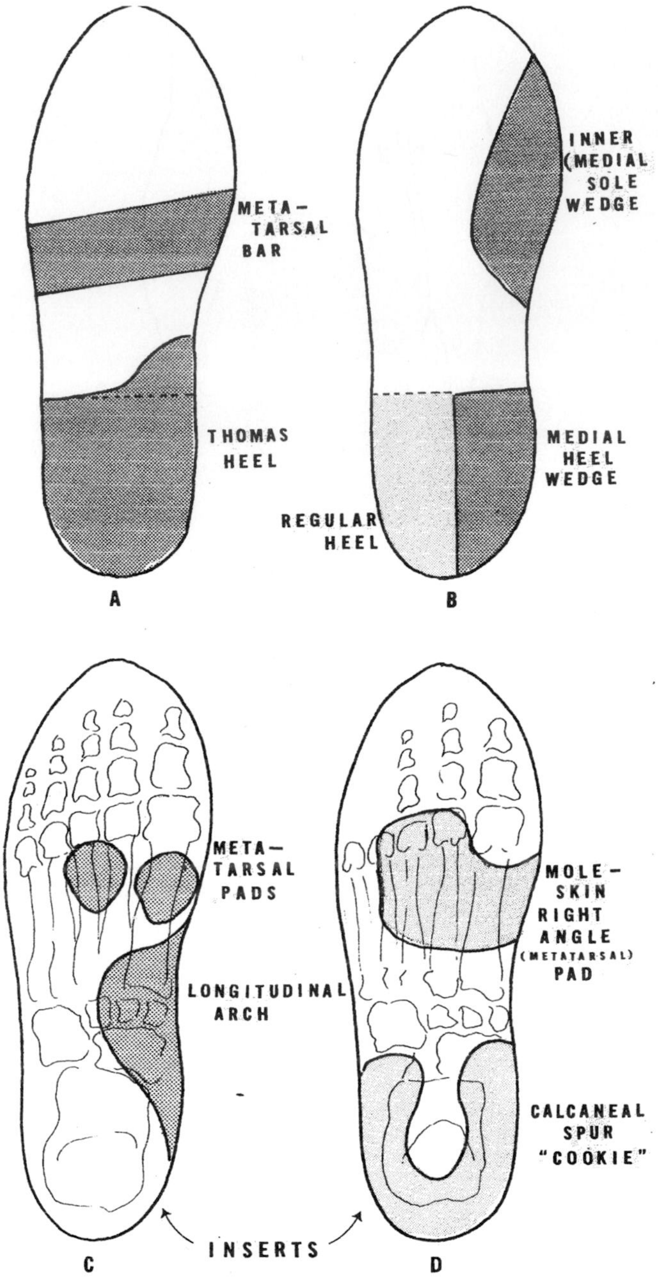

Figure 33-10 Numerous sites for insertion of pads are shown; the placement of metatarsal pads is shown in (**C**).

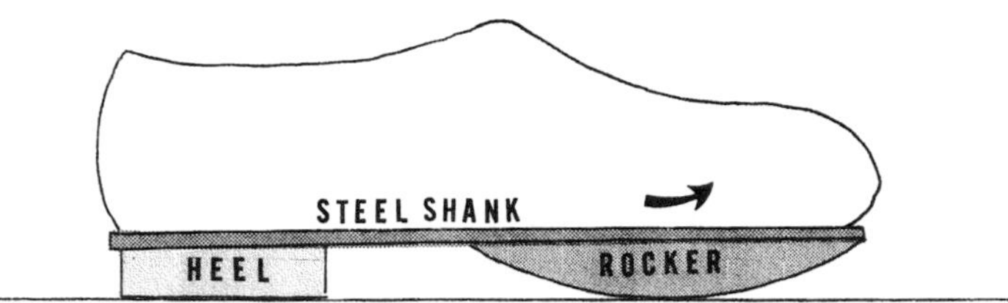

Figure 33-9 Rocker bottom shoe correction for hallux rigidus limitus. The rocker bottom prevents toe dorsiflexion during gait, and the steel shank immobilizes the hallux.

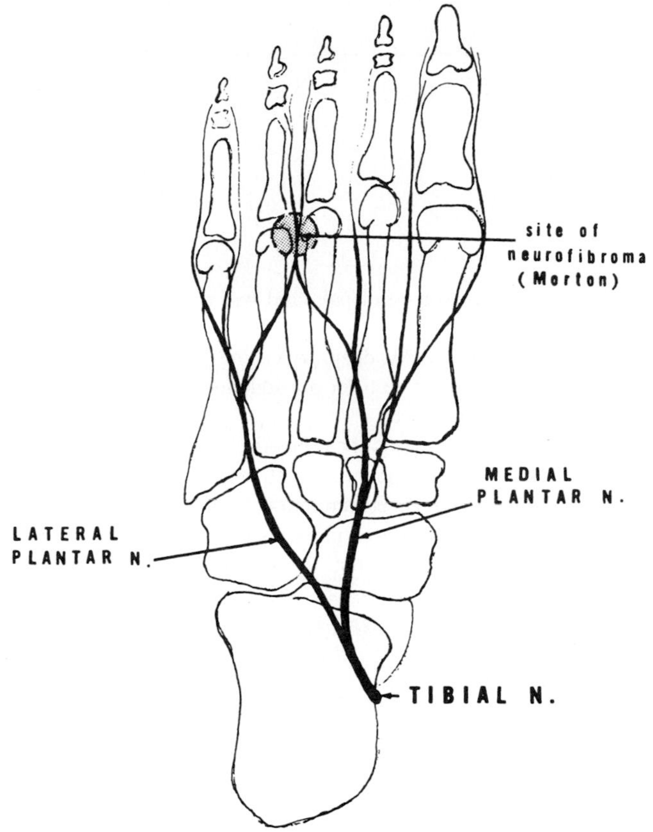

Figure 33-11 The common site of Morton's neuroma is between the third and fourth metatarsal heads at the point where the distal branches of the plantar nerves merge.

Interdigital Neuritis

Neuritis may develop between the metatarsal heads as a result of compression of a nerve between the opposing metatarsal heads. Most often, the distal branches of the lateral and medial plantar nerves are involved, usually between the third and fourth metatarsal heads. The latter condition is termed *Morton's neuroma* (Fig. 33-11).

Morton's neuroma is essentially an interdigital neuritis or a compression neuropathy. Symptoms of "burning" pain occur in the metatarsal area, usually between the third and fourth or the fourth and fifth toes, and are relieved by removing the shoes. The pain can be reproduced on examination by exerting pressure between the implicated toes. Interdigital injection of an anesthetic agent, which relieves the pain, is both diagnostic and therapeutic.

Treatment consists of correction of the foot abnormalities that caused the compression. Corticosteroid and analgesic interdigital injections are effective. When pain is persistent and intractable, surgical intervention is indicated.

Numerous other tissue sites of foot pain exist, but all are revealed by knowledge of functional anatomy and a careful visual and palpable examination.

BIBLIOGRAPHY

Cailliet R. *Foot and Ankle Pain*. 3rd ed. Philadelphia, Pa: FA Davis; 1997.

Gould JS. Metatarsalgia. *Orthop Clin North Am* 1989;20:553–562.

Lassiter TE, Malone TR, Garrett WE. Injury to the lateral ligaments of the ankle. *Orthop Clin North Am* 1989;20:629–640.

Mann R. The great toe. *Orthop Clin North Am* 1989;20:519–533.

Root ML, Oriew WP, Weed JH. Normal and abnormal function of the foot. In: *Clinical Biomechanics*. vol II. Los Angeles, Calif: Clinic Biomech Corp; 1977.

CHAPTER 34 ABDOMINAL PAIN

Alicja Soczewko Steiner

Abdominal pain is one of the most common presenting complaints in the primary care physician's office and often a diagnostic dilemma for surgeons. Despite recent technologic advances, the diagnosis and treatment of chronic, recurrent abdominal pain remain a challenge. Pain is a subjective sensation that patients often find difficult to describe. By contrast with other areas of the body, the abdominal organs have poorly developed sensory systems that also may contribute to the patient's difficulty when trying to describe and localize the pain. In the majority of clinical scenarios, no physical course is apparent and symptoms are transient. The purpose of pain is to protect the organ and the patient from injury. After the source of the pain is found, every effort should be made to control or eliminate it. In chronic pancreatitis or diffuse malignancy, for example, pain control may become as much a challenge as in instances where no underlying cause can be found.

For a patient to perceive pain, the autonomic nervous system must be intact. The anatomy and physiology of pain have been described in detail in previous chapters. Abdominal viscera are relatively insensitive to many stimuli compared with a more sensitive organ such as the epidermis. In addition to the relative paucity of sensory nerve endings, the same group of nerves may innervate several viscera. There are a few well-known nociceptive triggers in the abdominal cavity. These include abnormal distention or contraction of hollow organ walls, ischemia of the visceral musculature, direct action of chemical substances on the mucosa, formation of allogenic mediators, and traction or compression of ligaments, vessels, or mesentery. Pain patterns are not well differentiated as to their location or the cause. Nevertheless, there are some recognizable pain patterns, and a careful history often can lead to the correct diagnosis. The history and physical examination provide diagnosis in two thirds of clinical presentations. Laboratory and radiologic tests are important auxiliary tools for investigative workup. The invasiveness and cost-effectiveness of the proposed tests should always be considered.

There is either a physical (organic) or psychogenic (nonorganic) cause to pain, with one or more elements dominating. Abdominal pain can be classified by the duration of the symptoms, etiology, primary diagnosis, anatomic localization, and its response to treatment. It can be either acute or chronic; chronic pain being arbitrary, based on symptoms persisting for more then 6 months or after the healing process is completed. Some clinicians divide pain into nociceptive (somatic or visceral), neuropathic, psychogenic, or referred.

Visceral pain is transmitted from nociceptors found on the walls of the abdominal viscera via sympathetic (thoracic branches and lumbar splanchnic nerves synapsing in subsidiary plexuses: celiac, splenic, hepatic, aorticorenal, superior mesenteric, adrenal) and parasympathetic (vagus and nervi erigentes S2–4; motor and sensory) pathways. This pain is nonspecific because of wide divergence and relatively small number of afferent fibers innervating a large area with extensive ramification. Patients usually have difficulty localizing the source of pain and will describe it as aching, cramping, or burning that fluctuates in intensity. Visceral pain usually is paroxysmal, colicky, deep, squeezing, and diffuse. Still, today, a theoretical explanation for transduction and transmission of visceral pain is being used.

Centralistic and peripheralistic theories of pain are widely recognized. The centralistic theory is subdivided into the convergence projection and convergence facilitation views. The former states that visceral fibers with nociceptive input converge onto somatosensory spinal neurons, and that the viscerosomatic cells project through nociceptive pathways. The convergence facilitation theory focuses on the fact that visceral activation changes the excitation of multiple spinal units (including pain pathways) without direct activation of spinal neurons. The peripheralistic theory claims that vasoactive substances released into cutaneous and deep tissues lead to hyperalgesia and referred pain from these structures.

Differentiating somatic from referred pain can be accomplished by reviewing the patient's history and selective blocks. Somatic pain tends to be more intense or sharp and is aggravated by movement. It is produced by the stimulation of nociceptors in the parietal peritoneum and intra-abdominal connective tissues. It is usually well localized and described as constant, aching, gnawing, and throbbing. It can be relieved by opiates and peripheral nerve blocks. Referred pain can be explained easily by our knowledge of the segmental distribution of the spinal nerves. The pain can be referred to remote areas of the body if visceral impulses enter the spinal cord at the same level as afferent nerves from another area. These impulses are mistakenly interpreted as pain initiating at the second site. In addition, the pain may spread cranially to adjacent segments. Lower lobe pneumonia may be associated with severe upper abdominal pain and even some associated guarding. This is the most frequently used example of referred pain (Fig. 34-1).

DIAGNOSIS

Examination of the patient with abdominal pain must be done through an organized approach. Description of current and previous disease (including psychiatric treatment) in conjunction with a social and family history will develop a picture of the pain and a presumptive diagnosis. A history of allergies and current medications must be elicited. Knowledge of the pain pattern and character is also important. Following this, the patient should be carefully examined. A useful algorithm is presented in Figures 34-2 and 34-3.)

The patient can differentiate superficial abdominal pain easily. A local process in the abdominal wall usually causes it. Pain over the xiphoid or costal margins that is exacerbated by movement or touch often is attributable to costochondritis, a form of arthritis that usually responds to appropriate therapy with anti-inflammatory agents or intra-articular injections. Sharp, burning pain near a re-

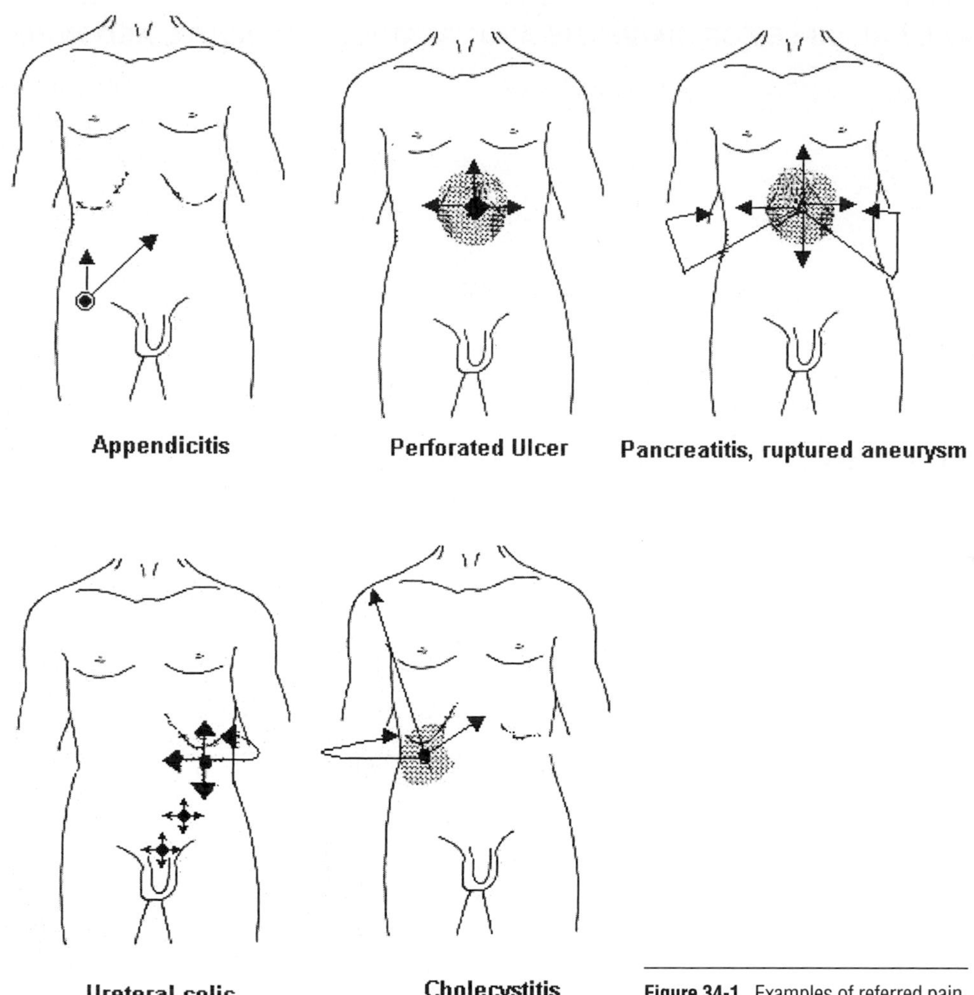

Figure 34-1 Examples of referred pain.

cently healed incision may indicate nerve irritation from surgical transection, entrapment in the healing tissue, or regeneration with neuroma formation. Pain originating in the abdominal wall frequently can be confirmed by Carnett's test and obliterated by blocking the appropriate intercostal or paravertebral nerves. Block of the celiac plexus can be helpful in differentiating abdominal wall or genitourinary pain from intraabdominal visceral pain, because the plexus supplies all abdominal viscera except the rectum, sigmoid, bladder, and reproductive organs.

The more common deep abdominal pain is, by definition, either somatic or visceral (autonomic: sympathetic and parasympathetic). Somatic pain originates in the parietal peritoneum, the root of the mesentery, and is elicited in close proximity to the nociceptive source. It is intense, sharp, precisely localized, associated with external stimuli, and represented at the cortical levels. Severity is related to the intensity of stimulus. Visceral pain is described more often as a poorly localized, vague (can be colicky, cramping, squeezing, dull, aching) pain associated with internal factors. Sometimes the pain can be referred to another part of the body. It can be presented as diffuse midabdominal discomfort. The intensity of the stimulus is as essential as its quality (i.e., cutting or coagulating the bowels is painless, but distention will cause pain). It is a primarily reflex and can be represented at the cord levels. Sometimes severe, visceral pain may generate a secondary physiologic reaction mediated by the autonomic nervous system and manifested by nausea, vomiting, sweating, lightheadedness, and salivation

The pain from the stomach, pancreas, and hepatobiliary tree is referred to the epigastrium. Periumbilical localization occurs from the small bowel and right colon; the rest of the colon and the genitourinary organs cause pain that presents in the epigastrium. The common midline pain location is a result of the bilateral innervation of the abdominal organs from both sides of the spinal cord (Fig. 34-4).

To determine the source of the pain, it is important to assess its intensity, location (Fig. 34-5), and character. It is also important to note its onset, whether acute or insidious, and its temporal profile. The circumstances that intensify or alleviate the pain are significant. Relief with eating or antacids suggests ulcer disease or gastroesophageal reflux. Postprandial pain, depending on its location, character, and timing, could be biliary, ischemic, or associated with a more benign condition, such as lactose intolerance or irritable bowel syndrome. Seasonal patterns frequently are seen in ulcer disease and, occasionally, with regional enteritis. The pain of inflammatory bowel disease and irritable bowel syndrome may be relieved by defecation, whereas heat usually relieves pain of musculoskeletal origin. Posture, sudden movement, coughing, strain-

GENERAL PRINCIPLES OF DIAGNOSIS AND TREATMENT OF ACUTE ABDOMINAL PAIN

HISTORY
DURATION
ONSET
MODE OF PROGRESSION
CHARACTER
-Nature
-Severity
-Periodicity
DIFFERENTIAL DIAGNOSIS

PHYSICAL EXAM
INSPECTION
PALPATION
-Guarding
-Rigidity
-Costal and costovertebral tenderness
PERCUSSION
AUSCULTATION
RECTAL/PELVIC EXAM

CLINICAL TESTING
BLOOD TESTS*
URINALYSIS, STOOL EXAM
ENDOSCOPY, BIOPSY
RADIOGRAPHY, ULTRASOUND
PARACENTESIS
CULDOCENTESIS

ANALGESIA AND RESPIRATORY THERAPY

CONSULTATION

PRIMARY CARE PHYSICIAN
SPECIALIST

HOSPITALIZATION INDICATED
NONSURGICAL TREATMENT
-Conservative measures
-Electrolyte balance
-Pharmacological approach
-Observation
-Further investigational studies**

HOSPITALIZATION NOT INDICATED
Hydration
Analgesia

SURGICAL TREATMENT

ANALGESIC/ANESTHETIC OPTIONS

REGIONAL
NERVE BLOCKS
-Intercostal
-Ilioinguinal
-Splanchnic
-Pudendal
-Intrapleural
WOUND INFILTRATION
NEUROAXIAL BLOCKS
-Epidural
-Intrathecal

PARENTERAL
IM/IV NARCOTICS/NSDAIS
IV PCA
TRANSDERMAL (fentanyl)

ALTERNATIVES
PO ANALGESICS
ACUPUNCTURE
TENS

*Routine baseline screening blood tests
Blood count (CBC)
Electrolytes, creatinine, urea (SMA-7)
Calcium
Glucose
Liver function tests (LFT's)
Erythrocyte sedimentation rate (ESR)
C-reactive protein

**Further investigative studies

GI tract	Gastroduodenoscopy, biopsy (gastroduodenoscopy, colonoscopy, proctosigmoidoscopy, ERCP) Barium swallow test Abdominal x-ray
Pancreas and hepatobiliary system	Ultrasonogram ERCP Choloangiography CT with/without contrast
Abdominal vasculature	Angiogram Radionuclide scan
Genitourinary	Abdominal x-ray Ultrasonogram Cystoscopy, ureteroscopy, hysterescopy

Figure 34-2 How to facilitate diagnosis of acute abdomen.

CLINICAL APPROACH TO CHRONIC ABDOMINAL PAIN

DIAGNOSTIC WORKUP
HISTORY
PHYSICAL EXAM
PSYCHOLOGICAL EVALUATION
LABORATORY RESULTS
RADIOLOGICAL TESTS

INTERDISCIPLINARY DISCUSSION
PRIMARY CARE PHYSICIAN
GASTROENTEROLOGIST
SURGEON
PSYCHOLOGIST/PSYCHIATRIST

MEDICAL THERAPY
PHARMACOLOGICAL (Tx relevant to disease)
ENZYMES REPLACEMENT
DIETARY RESTRICTIONS

SURGICAL OPTIONS
DIAGNOSTIC
-Laparoscopy
-Laparotomy
DEFINITIVE
(e.g. mass resection, pancreatojejunostomy, lysis of adhesions)

ANALGESIC/ANESTHETIC MANAGEMENT
DIAGNOSTIC REGIONAL BLOCKS (local anesthetics)
DEFINITIVE CURATIVE BLOCKS (e.g., neurolitic)
-Celiac
-Splanchnic
-Hypogastric
-Intercostal

Figure 34-3 How to diagnose etiology of chronic abdominal pain.

ing, and sneezing may worsen the pain from peritoneal irritation or of spinal origin. The abdomen is not exempt from psychogenic pain. This may be manifested as a component of irritable bowel syndrome. Although common, psychological pain should and does remain a diagnosis of exclusion.

PHYSIOLOGIC CAUSES OF ABDOMINAL PAIN

Esophagus

Heartburn is the most common symptom referable to the esophagus. It is a burning or hot substernal discomfort that frequently moves up toward the neck, but it may be localized only to the epigastrium. Eating, bending down, lying down after eating, and occasionally vigorous exercise may precipitate it. It is not entirely clear whether heartburn is caused by the chemical irritation of acid or bile, or if secondary muscle spasm plays a role. Occasionally, the pain is described as being a heaviness or tightness in the chest, with secondary restricted respiration and subsequent shortness of breath, simulating myocardial ischemia. The shortness of breath may be caused by an intercostal muscle spasm mediated by spinal reflex arcs.

Usually, the pain from the esophagus is felt at the level of the lesion. In some patients, however, pain caused by a lesion in the lower third of the esophagus is felt in the throat or in the high retrosternal area. The opposite is uncommon. When heartburn is severe, such as that associated with an ulcerating or infiltrating process, esophageal pain can radiate into the back, between the shoulder blades.

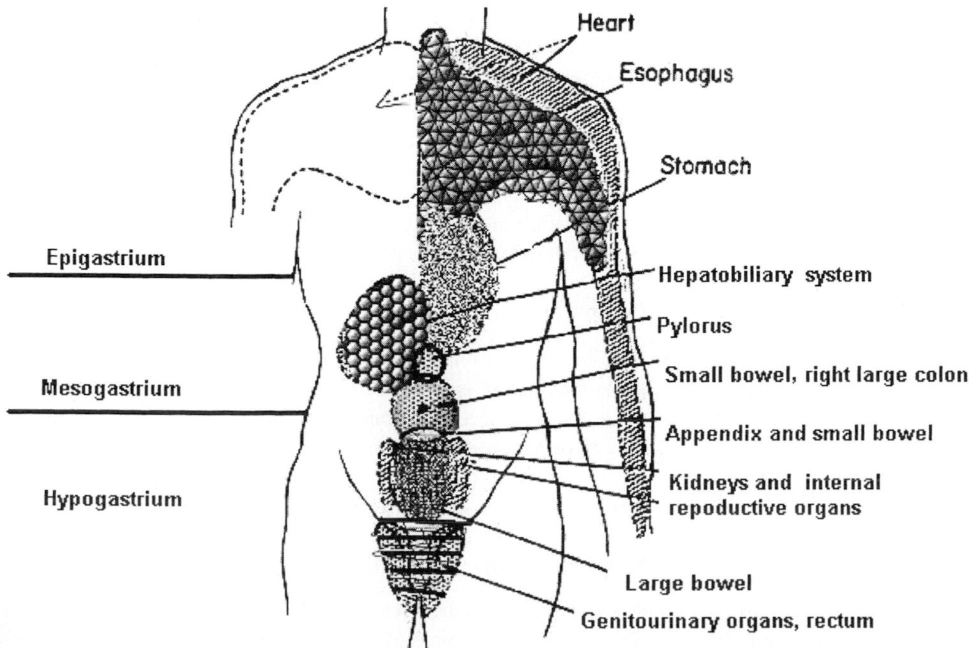

Figure 34-4 Visceral pain sites.

DIFFERENTIAL DIAGNOSIS OF ABDOMINAL PAIN BASED ON LOCALIZATION

EPIGASTRIUM

RIGHT UPPER QUADRANT	LEFT UPPER QUADRANT
Acute cholecystitis Biliary colic Duodenal peptic ulucer disease Liver disease (hepatitis, acute hepatic distention, abscess, carcinoma)	Spleen disease (infarct, rupture, distention) Disease of colon splenic flexure

MESOGASTRIUM

Gastroenteritis
Peptic ulcer disease
Pancreatitis (acute, chronic)
Small intestine and stomach pathology

HYPOGASTRIUM

RIGHT UPPER QUADRANT	LEFT UPPER QUADRANT
Acute and chronic appendicitis Pyogenic sacroiliitis Large and small bowel disease Renal disease (calculus, pyelonephritis) Acute rheumatic fever Ob-Gyn (can be bilateral) (Tubo-ovarian disease, ectopic pregnancy) Mesenteric lymphadenitis	Acute and chronic diverticulitis Pyogenic sacroiliitis Large and small bowel disease Renal disease

Figure 34-5 Differential diagnosis of abdominal pain based on location.

Stomach and Duodenum

The character of pain from ulcer disease varies widely. Typically, it is located in the epigastrium. It may be a sharply localized burning or gnawing pain or just a vague discomfort occurring from ½ to 2 hours after eating. Occasionally, it occurs shortly before meals or on an empty stomach and it may wake the patient up in the early hours of the morning. Food or antacids relieve it. The pain may, at times, be more localized to the right or left upper quadrant. When the pain bores through into the back, it usually indicates a posterior duodenal wall ulcer with secondary irritation of, or penetration into, the pancreas. This pain usually is deep, persistent, poorly localized, and does not respond well to treatment. Unlike heartburn, ulcer pain frequently occurs in clusters; several weeks of daily pain may be followed by variably long pain-free intervals. There may be seasonal variation with the symptoms; that is, they may be worse during the spring and fall.

Pain from gastritis tends to be more persistent and may be more difficult to abolish. The associated nausea and vomiting may be particularly troublesome. As in heartburn, it is not known whether the pain is produced by acid irritation of the nerve endings in the ulcer bed or whether it is secondary to a spasm of antral or duodenal smooth muscle.

Epigastric pain occurring soon after eating, unrelieved by antacids, and with lack of periodicity does not necessarily exclude ulcer disease. Pyloric channel ulcers may present in such a manner, and unless there is associated postprandial vomiting, the diagnosis may not be made until frank gastric outlet obstruction occurs.

Small Intestine

As a rule, pain originating in the small intestine is periumbilical in location and crampy or colicky in nature. Jejunal lesions tend to be associated with pain in the left upper quadrant. Ileal pain tends to localize in the right lower quadrant, and it may result from abnormal bowel motility patterns. A lowered threshold to the pain of bowel distention or contraction also can cause it. A lesion obstructing the lumen of the bowel, such as regional enteritis or a malignant process, may be the precipitating factor.

The pain of irritable bowel syndrome frequently is chronic, and at times, it can be incapacitating. It is unusual, however, for it to wake the patient from sleep. The pain usually is in the lower abdomen, in either the right or left lower quadrants. Its description ranges from burning, sharp, and stabbing to dull. Most commonly, it is intermittent, but it may be constant, with superimposed acute attacks. The pain may remain localized or may migrate with time. Eating usually precipitates it; defecation or fasting tends to relieve it. Nausea, bloating, and dyspepsia frequently occur and may simulate peptic ulcer or biliary tract disease. A change in bowel habits is not a universal finding, but, classically, diarrhea alternates with constipation. Predominant diarrhea or constipation, however, can be part of the syndrome.

Pain from partial small bowel obstruction also occurs after meals. The closer the lesion is to the stomach, the earlier the pain occurs. Moreover, nausea and vomiting are more likely to occur when the lesion is close to the stomach. The pain frequently is described as crampy and comes in waves. Regional enteritis is suggested by localization of the discomfort to the right lower quadrant and associated diarrhea, fever, weight loss, or extraintestinal manifestations, such as arthritis and mouth ulcers. Significant weight loss and cachexia may suggest an underlying lymphoma or metastatic disease to the bowel. It may be several months before complete obstruction occurs. At this time, the diagnosis is more obvious. As in appendicitis, the initial pain may be a nonspecific discomfort, but as the underlying process develops and eventually involves the overlying peritoneum, the pain localizes and approximates the site of the underlying disease.

Postoperative adhesions frequently are blamed for chronic or recurrent abdominal pain. Before exploration is considered, definitive evidence of bowel obstruction using plain abdominal x-rays or angulation and proximal dilation of the bowel using a barium study should be documented.

Colon

Pain from the colon usually is poorly localized to the lower abdomen. However, an adenocarcinoma of the colon or diverticula of the colon with secondary microperforation and abscess formation may have localized symptoms overlying the area of disease. Pain from the rectosigmoid area, in addition to being in the left lower quadrant, may be located in the sacral area.

Pancreas, Liver, and Biliary Tract

Because the pancreas, liver, biliary tract, stomach, and duodenum share some of the same afferent neuropathways, it is easy to understand some of the difficulties involved in the differential diagnosis of chronic epigastric pain. Diseases of the pancreas, and, in particularly, pancreatic cancer, are the most difficult to diagnose. Pain resulting from pancreatic cancer usually signifies infiltration of the retroperitoneal area or celiac axis, or spread to surrounding organs. Some of the pain may be a result of pancreatic duct obstruction and surrounding pancreatitis. Tumors in the head of the pancreas cause pain that is more localized to the epigastrium or right upper quadrant. Those in the tail tend to cause pain in the left upper quadrant. Lesions in the body of the pancreas can cause the pain to radiate into the back. Back pain, alone, also can be a presenting symptom. Because pancreatic cancer is rarely resectable, the physician is able to treat only the symptoms. When the retroperitoneal celiac plexus is involved by the tumor, the anesthesiologist frequently is asked to guide and help manage the pain.

The pain of chronic pancreatitis, which is mainly a result of alcohol abuse, can be constant, debilitating, and frequently lead to drug abuse. The persistent inflammation of the pancreas causes some of the pain, as does the ductal distention secondary to ductal obstruction by creation of strictures. The pain may be dull or sharp, burning, and steady. It commonly radiates into the back. Superimposed, more acute attacks last from days to several weeks. Eating, moving, or lying down may aggravate the pain; sitting up or leaning forward may relieve it. In patients who are not surgical candidates, the anesthesiologist may be asked to intervene. Neurolytic celiac plexus block has been used to treat patients who have not responded to conservative or surgical therapies. It often is used as a last resort, because rendering the abdomen insensitive may allow future abdominal disease to be missed.

Placement of stents during endoscopic retrograde cholangiopancreatography was used initially to decompress a dilated biliary tree. Only recently, this technique has been used to decompress the pancreatic duct. Relief may occur if the dilated biliary (or pancreatic) duct was the cause of the pain. Both benign and malignant lesions are amenable to this technique.

Passing a stone or biliary tree dilation secondary to an obstruction usually causes biliary pain. Contrary to the commonly used term *biliary colic,* the pain tends to have a gradual onset. After it *peaks*, it tends to reach a plateau until again, hours later, it diminishes. An attack can last from several hours to a day or more. The pain characteristically is localized in the right upper quadrant and may radiate to the right shoulder and shoulder blade, but it also is felt commonly in the epigastrium, with radiation into the back. Vomiting occurs in most patients and may provide some relief. After an acute attack, residual soreness may persist for several days. Commonly, these symptoms occur after eating, but they may become constant if the common bile duct is impacted by a stone or infiltrated by a malignant process. Associated dyspepsia is common in approximately one quarter of all patients. It responds to antacids, further confusing its cause. The appearance of complicating cholangitis (with symptoms of fever and jaundice) usually leads quickly to the correct diagnosis.

The liver parenchyma is insensitive to pain, but relatively rapid distention of the liver capsule will initiate well-localized right upper quadrant pain. Acute processes such as viral hepatitis, alcoholic hepatitis, and cardiac decompensation with secondary liver congestion rarely may appear as right upper quadrant pain, but this pain does not evolve into a chronic complaint. Chronic, active hepatitis may follow a course of recurrent attacks of right upper quadrant pain. The pain usually is well localized and accompanied by worsening liver function tests.

Benign focal nodular hyperplasia or adenomas associated with the use of birth control pills may cause recurrent right upper quadrant discomfort or, occasionally, a dramatic crisis of severe abdominal pain and hypotension from a hemorrhage into the capsule or peritoneum. The recurrent warning pains probably are caused by small bleeding episodes into the lesions. Bleeding into or necrosis of malignant lesions in the liver causes similar pain, but this usually is accompanied by fever and jaundice. The pain may be well localized, sharp, and steady. Any movement producing friction between the liver surface and the ribs may exacerbate it. When sought, a bruit over the lesion may he identified in approximately 25% of patients.

Vascular Diseases of the Bowel

Although mainly asymptomatic, occlusive vascular disease may be associated with chronic, recurrent, dull paraumbilical or epigastric pain. The pain of intestinal angina begins approximately 1½ hours after eating and lasts throughout digestion and absorption of the meal. Usually, at least two of the three major splanchnic vessels are affected by significant obstruction from atherosclerotic changes. It is postulated that the collateral supply is insufficient to meet the increased need during digestion, and this state of relative ischemia creates subsequent pain. Classically, this recurrent pain may create a fear of eating and can lead to severe weight loss. When patients with acute ischemia are questioned closely, retrospectively, they often will report postprandial abdominal discomfort preceding the acute event by weeks to months.

Superior mesenteric artery syndrome and celiac compression syndrome frequently are mentioned in the differential diagnosis of chronic abdominal pain, but their validity is controversial. Superior mesenteric artery syndrome is described as occurring in so-called asthenic patients or patients with significant weight loss. The postprandial epigastric pain, vomiting, and distention are believed to be caused by compression of the duodenum by the superior mesenteric artery. The pain of celiac compression syndrome is not necessarily related to meals. The celiac axis frequently has a high take-off and may be compressed by the median arcuate ligament of the diaphragm or by the tissue of the celiac ganglion. Whether bowel ischemia is the cause of the pain or whether the pain originates from the celiac ganglion also is unclear.

Abdominal aortic aneurysm usually presents more acutely, but a slowly expanding or leaking aneurysm may be associated with recurrent, dull midepigastric or back pain over several months. As with pancreatic pain, sitting up or leaning forward occasionally may relieve this pain. The pulsating, sometimes tender, mass can be palpated, and a bruit may be heard.

Peritoneum

The parietal peritoneum is well innervated by the branches of the spinal nerves, and, consequently, the pain perceived is well localized. Such pain frequently is associated with secondary muscle spasm of the overlying abdominal wall. The visceral peritoneum, however, has no pain receptors, and any pain that is generated is poorly defined. A malignant process most often causes chronic pain originating in the peritoneal cavity. Metastatic bowel or ovarian tumors and lymphoma are common. Mesothelioma is the most common primary tumor; teratoma, carcinoid, or sarcoma are much less common. The abdominal discomfort often is compounded by the presence of ascites, which distends the peritoneum further and causes more pain.

In young patients of Mediterranean descent who have chronic recurrent attacks of sudden diffuse or localized peritoneal pain, familial Mediterranean fever should be considered. Abdominal tenderness, fever, and arthritis are common. Despite feeling very ill, the patient recovers in several days and is well until the next attack.

Mesentery and Omentum

Recurrent localized or generalized abdominal pain in an older patient associated with the displacement of the stomach or bowel on x-ray studies should suggest a mesenteric or omental lesion. Fever, weight loss, nausea, vomiting, and a palpable tender mass may be associated with mesenteric panniculitis or retractile mesenteritis. Metastatic tumors to the mesentery are more common than primary lesions. The latter usually are fibromas, myomas, histiocytic or lipomatous tumors. Leiomyomas and leiomyosarcomas tend to involve the omentum.

Genitourinary System

The acute pain of renal colic or pyelonephritis is classic and easy to diagnose. The triad of hematuria, flank pain, and a palpable mass

CLASSIFICATION OF PAIN (PAIN PATTERNS)

INTRAABDOMINAL DISEASE

PARIETAL PERITONEAL DISEASE

GENERALIZED PERITONITIS
- PRIMARY BACTERIAL INFECTION
- SECONDARY BACTERIAL INFECTION (perforated viscera, ruptured abdominal abscess)

LOCALIZED PERITONITIS
- APPENDICITIS, HEPATITIS, PEPTIC ULCER DX, COLITIS, ABSCESS, GASTROENTERITIS, PANCREATITIS, DISTENTION, TRACTION, TORSION OF OMENTUM

ACUTE AND CHRONIC ISCHEMIA

MESENTERIC EMBOLISM, THROMBOSIS, NONORGANIC VENOUS THROMBOSIS
ABDOMINAL ANGINA, CELIAC BAND COMPRESSION
JOGGER'S PAIN (? acute splanchnic ischemia)

RAPID EXTENTION OF SOLID VISCUS OR HOLLOW VISCERA

OBSTRUCTION OF HOLLOW VISCERA

EXTRAABDOMINAL PATHOLOGY

THORACIC ORGAN DISORDERS

LUNG DX (pneumonia, embolism, pneumothorax)
HEART DISEASE (CAD, acute MI, myocarditis)
ESOPHAGUS PATHOLOGY (spasm, rupture, infection, inflammation)

NERUOLOGIC AND MUSCULOSKELETAL DISEASES

DISORDERS OF BRAIN AND BRAIN STEM
SPINE CORD COMPRESSION
THORACIC RADICULOPATHY DUE TO DEGENERATIVE DX OF SPINE/INFECTIOUS PROCESS/TUMORS (E.G. COMPRESSION FRACTURE, DEGENERATIVE DISC DX, HERPES ZOSTER INFECTION AND POSTHERPETIC NEURALGIA)
- MYOFASCIAL PAIN

RIB FRACTURE AND INTERCOSTAL NEURALGIA
COSTOCHONDROITIS AND RIB/COSTAL CARTILAGES DISLOCATION (SLIPPING RIB SYNDROME)
XIPHOIDALGIA
TRAUMATIC HEMATOMA
CICATRICES AND SUBCUTANEOUS NEUROMAS

SYSTEMIC INFECTIOUS AND INFLAMMATORY DISORDERS

TABES DORSALIS
ACUTE RHEUMATIC DISEASE, POLYARTERITIS NODOSA, SLE
HENOCH-SCHONLEIN PURPURA
HERPES ZOSTER
TUBERCULOSIS

DISEASE OF DIAPHRAGM AND PELVIC VISCERA

DIAPHRAGMATIC HERNIA, TUMORS, RUPTURE

GENITOURINARY DISORDERS
- URETERAL AND RENAL COLIC
- PYELONEPHRITIS AND CYSTIS
- RENAL INFARCT OR ABSCESS

GYNECOLOGICAL DISEASE
- ENDOMETRIOSIS
- DYSMENORRHEA
- SALPINGITIS
- ECTOPIC PREGNANCY

METABOLIC DISEASE

ENDOCRINOLOGIC ABNORMALITIES
- *DIABETES MELLITUS, ADDISONIAN CRISIS AND OTHER*

ACUTE INTERMITTENT PORPHYRIA
UREMIA
ACUTE HYPERLIPOPROTEINEMIA
HEREDITARY MEDITERRANEAN FEVER
CARBOHYDRATE MALDIGESTION AND MALABSORPTION
- *HYPOLACTASIA, HYPOSUCRASIA, STAGNANT LOOP SYNDROME*

HEMATOLOGIC DISEASE

SICKLE CELL ANEMIA
ACUTE AND CHRONIC HEMOLYTIC ANEMIA
ACUTE LEUKEMIA

TOXINS AND POISONS AND CERTAIN MEDICATIONS

LEAD AND OTHER HEAVY METAL DIGESTION
SPIDER BITES (E.G. BLACK WIDOW)
OPIATE WITHDRAWAL

PAIN OF PSYCHOLOGIC ORIGIN

SOMATOFORM (PSYCHOPHYSIOLOGIC)
- IRRITABLE BOWEL SYNDROME, PEPTIC ULCER DISEASE, CROHN'S DX, ULCERATIVE DISEASE

HYPOCHONDRIA
HYSTERIA
CONVERSION DX
DELUSIONAL OR HALLUCINATORY PAIN
DEPRESSION AND ANXIETY DX

Figure 34-6 Classification of pain (pain patterns).

suggests renal cell carcinoma, but this triad occurs infrequently. The tumor often is diagnosed from systemic complaints (dull upper abdominal or flank pain may be included). Perinephric abscess, although uncommon, should be considered in a patient with a history of urinary tract infections or pyelonephritis. Typically, dull upper quadrant or flank discomfort is present, accompanied by malaise and low-grade fevers.

Gynecologic problems usually cause acute pain. Depending on the patient's age, chronic lower abdominal pain, usually more localized to one of the lower quadrants, could be a presenting symptom of chronic pelvic inflammatory disease, uterine or ovarian cancer. The pain can be dull, steady, or crampy. The local irritation by the mass or inflammatory process can cause changes in the urine or bowel pattern.

METABOLIC CAUSES OF ABDOMINAL PAIN

Metabolic causes of chronic abdominal pain are rare but should always be sought, particularly when the usual diagnostic avenues have been exhausted. The hepatic porphyrias have many features in common, including their clinical presentation. Abdominal pain is the most prominent symptom. It is thought to result from autonomic neuropathy, which causes disturbances in gastrointestinal motility. Spasm and dilation of the bowel can cause severe pain. The frequent association of fever and leukocytosis mimics an inflammatory process. Although vomiting and constipation frequently are present, the abdomen is soft, without marked tenderness. These attacks may last from days to weeks. Fasting, infections, the menstrual cycle, and drugs whose metabolism involves the hemoproteins of cytochrome P-450 are often the precipitating factors. Such drugs include alcohol, barbiturates, anticonvulsants, estrogens, and contraceptives. Knowledge of so-called safe or probably safe drugs may be useful to the clinician treating the pain. Drugs that are considered safe include morphine and related opiates, which may be required to treat the pain in an acute attack.

In the United States, lead poisoning mainly is encountered in children. Although anemia, peripheral neuritis, and encephalopathy complete the picture, the young patient may have only lead colic, sometimes called *painter's cramps.* Severe, migrating, poorly localized guarding and rigidity of the abdominal wall should raise the suspicion of an acute intraabdominal event that may accompany crampy abdominal pain.

When in a hemolytic crisis, a patient with paroxysmal nocturnal hemoglobinuria may have substernal, lumbar, or abdominal pain, in addition to generalized weakness. The pain may be colicky and last for several days. The abdomen may be tender, with some guarding and even a rebound phenomenon. Venous thrombosis occurs with increased frequency in these patients. It always should be considered if a sudden increase in liver size accompanies these attacks, suggesting thrombosis involving the portal system.

Hyperparathyroidism has been called the syndrome of bones, stones, and groans. Associated peptic ulcer disease or pancreatitis usually causes the abdominal pain.

The lightening-sharp abdominal pain of tabes mainly is associated with syphilis, but it also may occur with diabetes and meningeal tumors. This is a radicular syndrome resulting from damage to the large posterior lumbosacral roots.

The diagnosis of chronic recurrent abdominal pain often can be a challenge to both the therapeutic and diagnostic abilities of the involved physician. Unfortunately, many patients with this type of pain undergo multiple surgical procedures without any significant findings. Good knowledge of the underlying anatomy and pain patterns should make the diagnosis and subsequent treatment easier (Figure 34-6).

PSYCHOSOMATIC CAUSES OF ABDOMINAL PAIN

The abdomen is the third most common site of pain in psychiatric patients. Diagnosis of psychological pain can be made based on exclusion criteria. There are some signs that can be helpful or supportive. Suspicion is raised when location, timing, quality, and distribution of symptoms do not relate to pathophysiologic patterns. There is often marked discrepancy between reported severity of pain and presented behavior. The patient sometimes reports pain in other parts of body and may have a history of many negative diagnostic workups for various complaints. The onset of pain may have an obvious relationship to a stressful event.

TABLE 34-1 **Visceral Pain Pathways and Sites of Nerve Blocks**

Organs	Nervous System Pathways	Sensory Level
Liver, spleen, central part of diaphragm	Phrenic nerve	C3–5, mostly C4
	Sympathetic nerves	T6–11
Gallbladder, peripheral diaphragm	Celiac plexus	T6–12
Pancreas	Celiac plexus	T5–11
Stomach, duodenum	Celiac plexus	T6–9
Jejunum	Celiac plexus	T9–11
Left half of the transverse colon	Mesenteric plexus	T11–12
Descending colon and rectum	Nervi eriggentes	S2–4
Sigmoid colon, kidneys, urethers, testes	Lowest splanchnic nerve	T10–L2
Uterus and cervix	Sympathetic nerves	T6–L2

TREATMENT

Most of this chapter has dealt with the diagnosis of abdominal pain syndromes. When a treatable disorder is identified, appropriate therapy should be instituted. A simplified algorithm was presented at the beginning of this chapter (see Figs. 34-2, 34-3). Unfortunately, in many patients with chronic abdominal pain, a specific diagnosis is not identified despite an extensive workup. In other patients, a condition is diagnosed, but conventional methods fail to treat the disease and pain. Nerve blocks can be helpful in treating acute and chronic abdominal pain (Table 34-1). Nonspecific methods, such as antidepressants, stress reduction techniques, and behavioral approaches, often are useful in treating these difficult problems.

BIBLIOGRAPHY

1. Doherty G, Boey J. The acute abdomen. In: Way L, Doherty G, eds. *Current Surgical Diagnosis and Treatment,* 7th edition. New York: Lange Medical Books/McGraw-Hill; 2003:503–516.
2. Dominitz J, Sekijima J, Watts M. Abdominal pain. In: Kearney DJ, ed. Gastroenterology and Hepatology for the Primary Care Provider. *Principles, Practice, and Guidelines for Referral Current Surgical Diagnosis and Treatment.* University of Washington Division of Gastroenterology, 2000.
3. Gallegos NC, Hobsley M. Abdominal wall pain: An alternative diagnosis. *Br J Surgery* 1990;77:1167.
4. Haubrich WS. Abdominal pain. In: Berk JE, Haubrich WS, eds. *Gastrointestinal Symptoms: Clinical Interpretation.* Philadelphia: BC Decker Inc. 1991:23–58.
5. Haubrich W. Abdominal Pain. In: Haubrich W, Schaffner F, Berk J, eds. *Gastroenterology.* Philadelphia: W.B. Saunders Company, 1995.
6. Kearny D. Approach to the patient with gastrointestinal disorders. In: Friedman S, McQuaid K, Grendell J. *Current Diagnosis and Treatment in Gastroenterology, 2nd edition.* New York: Lange Medical Book/McGraw-Hill, 2003;503–516.
7. Klein KB. Approach to the patient with abdominal pain. In: Yamada T, ed. *Textbook of Gastroenterology, 2nd edition.* Philadelphia: JB Lippincott Co., 1995;750–771.
8. Thompson WG, Creed F, Drossman DA, et al. Functional bowel disease and functional abdominal pain. *Gastroenterology Int* 1992;5:75.
9. Wolf S. Eliciting and interpreting symptoms and signs. In: Haubrich W, Schaffner J. *Gastroneterology.* Philadelphia: WB Saunders Company, 1995.

CHAPTER 35 PELVIC PAIN

Anastasia Kucharski and Jyotsna Nagda

Pelvic pain is a complicated topic and a clinical challenge, because the very definition of this pain can vary. The pelvis has a formal anatomic description; however, *pelvic pain* can refer to pain experienced in the general pelvic cavity or pain that is synonymous with gynecologic pain. In addition, gynecologic pelvic pain, although potentially acute or chronic, can refer to chronic pain with or without an anatomic lesion. Under these circumstances the parameters for describing pelvic pain also fluctuate. In the most general context, pelvic pain can be visceral, somatic, and neuropathic. Causal categories are traumatic, mechanical, and psychological. Organ systems include the genitourinary, gastrointestinal, neurologic, and musculoskeletal. The treatment of pelvic pain encompasses not only discoveries in clinical physiology and pharmacology, but also the social and intellectual assumptions behind the clinical practice.

It is estimated that 9.2 million women in United States have pelvic pain. Ten percent of all gynecologic office visits are for pelvic pain; 44% of all laparoscopies and 10% to 15% of hysterectomies are for chronic pelvic pain; and 30% of women presenting to a pain clinic have already undergone hysterectomy. The male pelvic pain syndrome comprises of 8% of all urologic visits and 1% of all visits to primary care physicians. The economic impact is enormous, with medical costs of $1.2 billion per year and missed work and productivity totalling $15 billion per year.

ANATOMY OF THE PELVIS

Any discussion of pelvic pain requires an appreciation of the spatial relations of the pelvic viscera, along with their vascular supply and innervation. The pelvis has as its walls the bony pelvis and as its floor the pelvic diaphragm. It is lined by a complex vascular structure and traversed by sympathetic and parasympathetic afferent, visceral afferent, and efferent nerves from the lumbar and sacral plexes. The pelvis is divided into a major pelvis and a minor pelvis, separated by the pelvic brim, which also is the boundary between the abdominal and pelvic cavities. The pelvis contains the bladder and the paravesical fossae in front, the rectum and the pararectal fossae in back, and the internal genital organs in the middle.

The bony pelvis includes two hip bones formed from the fusion of the ischium, ilium and pubis, the sacrum, and coccyx. The two innominate bones form the sides of the pelvis. They are joined in front at the symphysis pubis and articulate with the sacrum and coccyx in back.

The pelvic diaphragm, or floor of the pelvis, arises in front from the body of the pubis and continues behind to the coccyx. It includes the levator ani muscles and the coccygeus muscles. The diaphragm holds the lower part of the rectum and supports the bladder, vagina, and prostate by maintaining sufficient intraabdominal pressure. Beneath the diaphragm is the perineum, with the external genitalia.

Although the bony pelvis can be compared to a basin, the pelvic vasculature resembles a woven lining composed of large, thin-walled veins through which the arteries thread their way. The veins are divided into vesicle, uterine and vaginal or prostatic, and rectal venous plexes, which drain into the internal iliac vein and into the inferior mesenteric veins via the superior rectal (hemorrhoidal) vein, eventually reaching the portal vein. The middle rectal vein emerges from the lower part of the side of the rectum, passes to the internal iliac vein, and anastomoses with the superior and inferior rectal veins and with the other plexes of pelvic veins.

The arteries of the pelvis arise from the internal iliac artery, which runs retroperitoneally, is posterior to the ureter, and is divided into anterior and posterior divisions. The anterior division has seven branches, and the posterior division, three. Collateral circulation is abundant.

The major afferent pathways for nociception from the female pelvic organs travel with the sympathetic nerve bundles and have cell bodies in the thoracolumbar distribution. The suprapubic area is innervated by the iliohypogastric nerve (L1, L2). The inguinal area and the base of scrotum or labia are supplied by the ilioinguinal nerve (L1, L2). The skin of the penis is supplied by the two dorsal nerves of the penis, which are branches of pudendal nerves. The skin of the scrotum and perineal skin are supplied by the posterior scrotal nerves (S2, S3, and S4). The skin between the anus and coccyx is innervated by the lower sacral and coccygeal plexus. The lower third of the vagina is supplied by the pudendal nerve. The genital branch of the genitofemoral nerve supplies the lateral side of the scrotum, the vulva, and the cremasteric muscles.

There are sympathetic, parasympathetic, and visceral somatic afferent nerves to the pelvic viscera. The sympathetic nerves cause muscular contraction and vasoconstriction, whereas the parasympathetic nerves relate to relaxation and vasodilation. Most of the autonomic fibers enter the pelvis through the superior hypogastric plexus, which is located bilaterally at the lower third of the fifth vertebral body and the upper third of the first sacral vertebra at the sacral promontory. This plexus is primarily sympathetic and is formed by the confluence of lumbar sympathetic chains and branches of the aortic plexus containing fibers that traverse the celiac and inferior mesenteric plexus (Fig. 35-1). The superior hypogastric plexus divides into the right and the left hypogastric nerves, which descend laterally to the sigmoid colon to reach the inferior hypogastric plexus.

The inferior hypogastric plexus is located against the inside of the pelvis, lateral to the uterovaginal junction and the rectum. It is the major neuronal integrative center in the pelvis. It innervates multiple pelvic organs, including the urinary bladder, proximal urethra, distal ureter, rectum, and internal anal sphincter, as well as genital and reproductive structures via communication through the uterovaginal plexus and the vesical and the inferior rectal plexus. The parasympathetic nerves, which are branches of anterior rami of the S2, S3, and S4 nerve roots, traverse the inferior hypogastric plexus. In contrast to the superior hypogastric plexus, which is

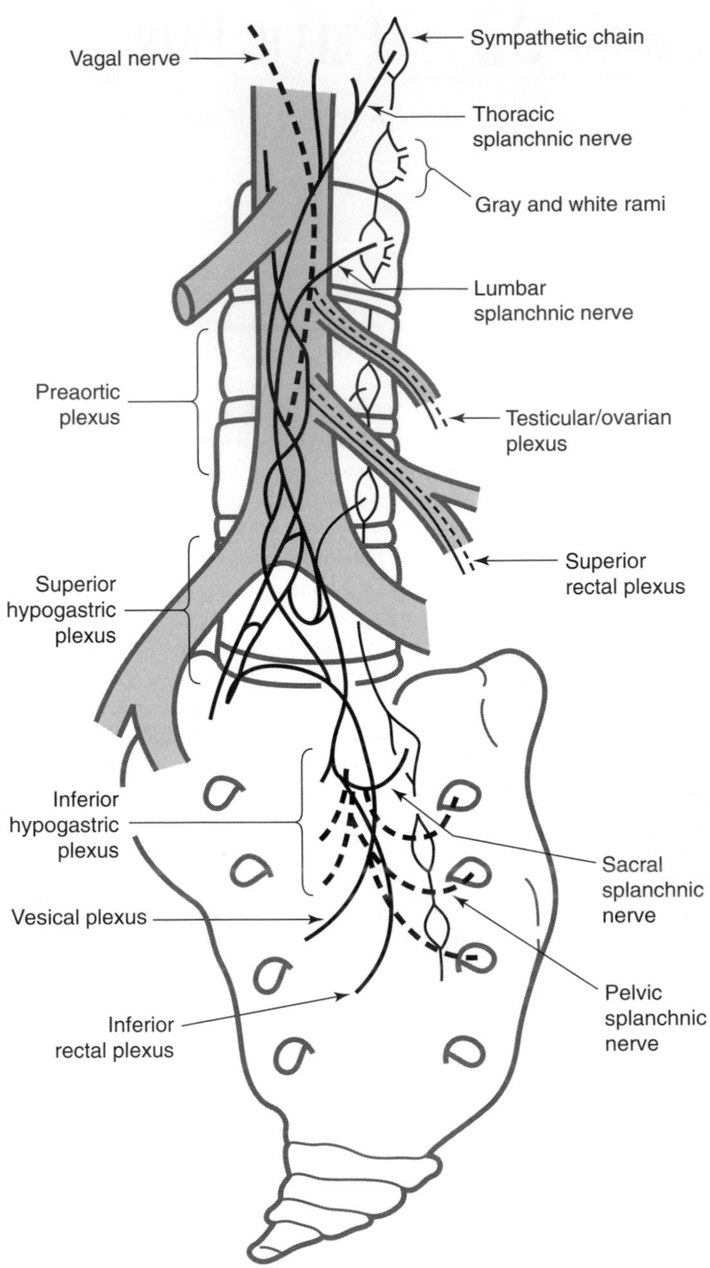

Figure 35-1 Neuroanatomy of visceral pelvic pain. (From Boscher H. Blockade of the superior hypogastric plexus block for pelvic pain. *Pain Practice* 2001;1:165.)

situated predominantly in the longitudinal plane, the inferior hypogastric plexus is oriented more transversely, extending postero-anteriorly and parallel to the pelvic floor. The location and configuration of the inferior hypogastric plexus does not lend itself to surgical or chemical extirpation.

The sensory nerves from the uterus accompany the sympathetic nerves and enter the spinal cord at the T11 and T12 level, and refer pain to the abdomen. The S2, S3, and S4 afferents from the cervix are referred to the lower back and lumbosacral area.[1,2]

The ganglion impar (also known as ganglion of Walther) is a solitary retroperitoneal structure located at the level of the sacrococcygeal junction that marks the termination of the paired paravertebral chains. This structure receives fibers from the lumbar and sacral portions of the sympathetic and parasympathetic nervous system. It provides sympathetic innervation to portions of the perineum, rectum, and genitalia.

GYNECOLOGIC PAIN

Pelvic pain is often considered synonymous with gynecologic pain. Such pain can be acute or chronic. Acute pain is caused by structural disruption or physiologic dysfunction, whereas chronic pain may be the result of persistent pressure on nerves, inflammation of arteries, diseases of the female reproductive organs, and factors not demonstrable by present-day imaging techniques.

Acute Pain

The differential diagnosis of acute pelvic pain includes ectopic pregnancy and complications of pregnancy, ruptured cysts, ovarian and adnexal torsion, uterine fibroids, and pelvic inflammatory diseases. Ninety-eight percent of women with ectopic pregnancy experience unilateral pain, which may be accompanied by light or missed menses. Symptoms of pregnancy, such as nausea and breast tenderness, also may be present.[3]

The pain of ovarian cysts may be dull and aching, localized to the side of the abscess, and accompanied by pelvic tenderness. An ovarian cyst with a twisted pedicle can cause acute pain, which becomes intermittent when the pedicle untwists. Other symptoms include nausea and vomiting, diarrhea or constipation, and leukocytosis.

Symptoms of a palpable mass, delayed menses, and pelvic tenderness also occur with corpus luteum cysts, which can bleed into the peritoneum and mimic pelvic inflammatory disease (PID). PID is defined as a spectrum of upper genital tract inflammatory disorders that may include endometritis, salpingitis, tubo-overian abscess, and pelvic peritonitis. The diagnosis should not be considered conclusive without additional findings, such as a positive cervical culture. The primary pathogens are *Neisseria gonorrhea* and *Chlamydia trachomatis*. Cervical cultures for *Chlamydia* can detect up to 80% of cervical infections; antibody testing, enzyme-linked immunosorbent assay, and DNA probe testing can detect 60% to 90% of infections. Because of this wide range in positive findings, culturing of specimens from the urethra and anus also should be considered. Tubo-ovarian abscess may occur as a complication of PID as well as in postpartum and postoperative patients and in women who use intrauterine devices. The bacteria present in tubo-ovarian access occur in the lower genital tract and may not be the same agents involved in PID.[4]

Chronic Pain

Chronic pain may begin as an acute episode, change into episodic pain, and then persist for 6 months or longer. From a clinical perspective, chronic pelvic pain can be a symptom of a disease or part of a syndrome. Endometriosis and malignancies are examples of primary illnesses, whereas syndromes include dysmenorrhea, premenstrual syndrome, and chronic pelvic pain disorders.

Endometriosis is the presence of ectopic endometrial glands and stroma outside the uterine cavity. Patients with endometriosis may have dysmenorrhea, dyspareunia, back pain, and rectal discomfort in addition to persistent pelvic pain. The symptoms are related to the site of the endometrial implant. However, the intensity of the pain may not correlate with the size of the implant.[5] The incidence is 1% to 2% of the general female population and 15% to 25% in infertile women. Patients may remain asymptomatic until they are being evaluated for infertility. Definitive diagnosis can only be made by laparoscopy, although elevated serum CA-125 levels correlate with severity and reflect the course of the disease. Treatment includes medical and surgical options. The medical treatment for endometriosis includes oral contraceptives, medroxyprogesterone acetate, danazol, and gonadotrophin-releasing analogues. The goals of surgery are to restore normal pelvic anatomy and to resect, coagulate, or vaporize all endometriotic implants.

Adenomyosis is a benign invasion of the wall of the uterus by endometrial tissue. Most patients are 35 to 50 years of age and have had children. Presenting complaints usually dysmenorrhea and menorrhagia.

Uterine *leiomyomas* (fibroids) are painful when they press on or become entangled in other structures, and cause discomfort when they grow. Dyspareunia, dysmenorrhea, and pelvic pressure are frequent symptoms, along with intermenstrual, postmenstrual, and heavy menstrual bleeding. A degenerating leiomyoma may cause only episodic pain at first and then fever, increased pain, and leukocytosis with a left shift later. Leaking purulent material can cause peritonitis. Leiomyomas undergo malignant transformation in 2 to 3 per 100,000 women, but grow slowly. Surgery used in the treatment of women with heavy bleeding, growths of large size, and additional symptoms.[6]

Cervical cancer may cause pelvic pain as it metastasizes. *Ovarian cancer* may be asymptomatic until late stages, when it causes symptoms that are vague and nonspecific. *Endometrial cancer* in 90% of cases presents with vaginal bleeding or discharge. Pelvic pressure or discomfort occurs from uterine enlargement and then spread of the tumor into extrauterine structures. Any tumor that compresses the bladder or rectum can cause pressure, pain, or dyspareunia.[7]

Women with *ovarian remnant syndrome* present with unilateral consent or cyclical pain, as well as postcoital ache, and post-micturition or post-defecation pain. They may have a history of the removal of one or both residual ovaries for pain associated with pelvic adhesions or endometriosis. Although localized abdominal pain is a constant feature of the syndrome, often no mass can be found on pelvic examination. Ultrasound examination is usually diagnostic, revealing a mass that must be distinguished from accessory ovaries, an embrylogic variant of normal development. Treatment is surgical removal of the remnant.[8]

Women with major gynecologic diseases can have pelvic pain in the form of dysmenorrhea. This term is applied to severe cramping in the lower abdomen, lower back, and upper thighs that occurs during menstruation. *Primary dysmenorrhea* is the most prevalent source of chronic episodic pain in premenopausal women. It is caused primarily by prostaglandin release from the endometrium at menses, in particular prostaglandins F_2 alpha and E_2. The cramping pain is often accompanied by nausea, vomiting, headache, diarrhea, and fatigue. *Secondary dysmenorrhea* and *atypical cyclic pain* are caused by underlying intrauterine or extrauterine pathology, such as endometriosis, adenomyosis, and other pathology that alters blood flow, increases pressure, or causes irritation of the pelvic organs.

The treatment of primary dysmenorrhea includes nonsteroidal anti-inflammatory drugs (NSAIDs) and oral contraceptive pills. NSAIDs are effective in up to 80% of cases. Other modes of menstrual hormonal suppression are recommended for patients who obtain no relief with NSAIDs and oral contraceptives. Secondary dysmenorrhea requires a thorough evaluation and then treatment of the underlying cause.

Premenstrual syndrome (PMS) includes mood, behavioral, and physical changes that occur during the luteal phase of most menstrual cycles. Studies suggest that about one third of premenopausal women experience some degree of PMS. As in the treatment of dysmenorrhea, underlying illnesses, such as endometriosis and leiomyomas, should be ruled out. Treatment includes NSAIDs for pain, diuretics such as spironolactone for fluid retention, and antidepressants for dysphoria.

Pelvic congestion syndrome is usually seen in premenopausal women, thus suggesting that there is a hormonal factor involved in the venous dilation.[9] The capacity of pelvic veins to increase 60-fold by the end of pregnancy makes them, in the nonpregnant state, vulnerable to chronic dilation and stasis. Weakened fascial supports during parturition and the vasodilating effects of cyclically fluctuating hormones aggravate the tendency to dilation.[10] The common symptom is a dull, aching pain in the pelvic area that worsens on standing, walking, and lifting and is relieved by lying down. Deep dyspareunia is one of the most consistent symptoms of pelvic congestion syndrome, with an incidence ranging from 71% to 78%. The severity of the pain is determined by the extent of the venous stasis, which leads to hypoxemia and local tissue damage followed by the release of pain-producing substances. The presence of dilated veins in the infundibulopelvic ligament, ovarian hilum, or broad ligament, combined with polycystic changes in the ovary (which may be apparent only on close inspection), is diagnostic of pelvic congestion. Ultrasound and computed tomography (CT) scans are important for revealing polycystic changes in the ovaries and dilated veins in the broad ligament and uterus. Surgical treatment includes hysterectomy and ligation of the ovarian vein. Medical therapy consists of oral contraceptives to suppress ovarian function and intermittent courses of anti-inflammatory agents and antibiotics when inflammation occurs secondary to local infection.[11] Radiologic transcatheter embolization of the ovarian veins has been used with varying success.

Sympathetic pelvic syndrome is a chronic pelvic pain disorder that has been recognized because of developments in the study of chronic pain. It is assumed that visceral illness occurs, with pain transmitted to cutaneous areas. The area of innervation includes the cervix and vagina (with innervation from the pudendal nerves, having derivation from S2 through S4), along with the uterus, fallopian tubes, and ovaries (with innervation from the sympathetic pelvic branches of T10 through T12). Repeated local anesthetic nerve blocks are recommended in addition to the medications used in patients with chronic pain.

Another chronic pelvic pain syndrome is *focal vulvitis*, characterized by burning vulvar pain and superficial dyspareunia. One study found that a majority of patients continued to have symptoms of vulvitis after Woodruff perineoplasty. The authors concluded that surgery was not the best treatment. They noted that these women often had insufficient lubrication or hypertonia of the pelvic floor, or both, during sexual intercourse. Thus, an integrated approach was recommended, including protection of the vulvar skin, relaxation of pelvic muscles, and treatment of psychosexual and relational aspects of the disorder.[12]

These treatment recommendations are similar to those for patients with chronic pain for whom no pathologic findings have been found. Some studies of chronic pelvic pain in women report that 10% to 50% experience pelvic pain without pathology; other studies cite 15% as the percentage of women who have chronic pelvic pain. The studies citing these statistics then tend to look into symptom clusters for this group of patients. The wide incidence range cited suggests there may be some ambiguity in the definition of chronic pain and in the procedures used to evaluate patients with pelvic symptoms.

The initial patient group can be modified after further study and treatment. Nevertheless, there remains a group for whom no physiologic mechanisms have been elucidated.[13,14] These patients have a chronic pelvic pain syndrome that is considered a somatoform disorder similar to irritable bowel syndrome. The prevalence of this syndrome in primary care patients (38%) is comparable to that of asthma and back pain.[15] A syndrome of chronic pelvic pain without obvious pathology (CPPWOP) has also been described, but is unclear in these cases whether pathology has been overlooked or limited to findings for specific diseases,such as endometriosis, thus possibly excluding damage to ligaments and smooth and striated muscle. Patients with CPPWOP have a group of symptoms that includes intermittent pain that can vary with the menstrual cycle and is localized to the low abdomen and back. Dyspareunia may be present. Patients tend to be in their 20s and 30s and have a history of childhood sexual abuse, rape, or incest. Present relationships are marked by abuse, divorce, and prostitution.[16]

Treatment of chronic pelvic pain syndrome or CPPWOP is similar to that of other chronic pelvic pain syndromes and includes NSAIDs and antidepressants. Psychological interventions also have played a role in the treatment of patients with these syndromes. The treatment strategies resemble those for patients with chronic pain with a specific pathology and include methods that help women distract themselves from the pain and encourage them to cope despite the pain.

Women with negative investigations that do not result in an organic diagnosis may then be referred for psychiatric treatment. Despite the apparent presence of anxiety, depression, and possible history of sexual trauma, referral for psychiatric treatment may be resisted. This response is not surprising, given the role psychobiological factors have played in the treatment of women with chronic pelvic pain. Studies of women with chronic pelvic pain syndrome and chronic vulvar pain syndrome have shown a significantly higher incidence of sexual abuse in the two chronic pain groups compared with women who do not have these symptoms. In addition to physical and emotional trauma, there is a significant association between sexual victimization before age 15 years and chronic pelvic pain. Sexual abuse and somatization are highly predictive factors for chronic pain. There also is a higher incidence of depressive symptoms in this group of patients.

The association of sexual abuse, affect and pelvic pain was the basis for psychoanalytic studies of personal development throughout the past century. The first case studies were women with the diagnosis of hysteria, whose symptoms had psychological meaning. The term *hysterus* is Greek for uterus, and the concept of hysteria (derived from a theory of a "wandering" womb as the basis for inexplicable symptoms in women) historically was the basis for treatments that reflected sociocultural values about the status of women. Hysteria is no longer considered a valid diagnosis; it has been replaced by in current practice by the diagnoses of conversion and somatoform disorders, which may affect both men and women. Nevertheless, the legacy of hysteria as a medical condition persists.

Hysterical conversion has been defined as a special type of somatization in which physical symptoms express a psychological conflict (often sexual) that includes affects that were not sufficiently expressed at the time of the incident, and now represented symbolically. In classical psychotherapy, after elucidating the traumatic precipitant, the next step was to clarify how affects were not expressed directly and were converted into physical symptoms. Patients were said to be using the defenses of repression, denial, and somatization to deal with their feelings. Because of social pressure to limit their direct expression of aggression and their vulnerability to sexual abuse, women were more likely to have chronic pain and to express themselves somatically. Eventually, such women came to be identified with their symptoms; the so-called painful woman who resisted the interpretations put forth for her benefit.[17,18]

Even today pelvic pain may be considered psychogenic when there is no explicit organic finding because of the persistence of the triad of affect, sexual abuse, and somatization in clinical and psychometric testing studies. Because not all women with chronic pelvic pain have been abused, an alternative explanation has been sought for pelvic pain that occurs without confirming laparoscopic and imaging findings. The biopsychosocial model attempts to integrate physiologic and psychological causes of pain, suggesting the existence of a mind-body dualism in which psychological factors are secondary to physical symptoms. Keeping in mind that physical symptoms in at least one third of cases have no demonstrable organic findings, this model can lead to clinical situations that are difficult to distinguish from early models of hysteria and thus are subject to patient skepticism. This approach is being replaced by theories of central pain mechanisms focusing on neurotransmitters and neural networks that also express affective and cognitive functions. However, a major deconstruction of the studies for chronic pelvic pain needs to be carried out before the diagnosis of hysteria can be considered obsolete.

MALE PELVIC PAIN

Whereas women with chronic pain have been referred to multidisciplinary treatment centers to treat complex chronic pain, evaluation and treatment for men has included attempts to establish objective criteria for diagnosis of chronic pelvic pain syndrome. *Chronic prostatitis* is a poorly understood form of chronic pelvic pain syndrome in men. The diagnosis is based on symptoms, and no measurable parameter can help in defining the presence of the disease, its severity, or cause. A National Institutes of Health (NIH) classification system showed that 38% of men with chronic prostatis had chronic bacterial prostatitis; with 7% of cases resulting from inflammatory chronic pain syndrome, and 55% from noninflammatory chronic pelvic pain syndrome.[19]

The objectives of current studies include refining and standardizing the evaluation of men with symptoms of chronic prostatitis. Some men have elevated levels of tumor necrosis factor-α and interleukin-1β proinflammatory cytokines. Seminal cytokine levels may provide an objective measure of disease in these patients and suggest specific therapeutic strategies.[20] Patients with prostatitis report more perineal, lower abdominal, testicular, penile, and ejaculatory pain than patients with benign prostatic hypertrophy and sexual dysfunction.

Another attempt at determining objective criteria for chronic pelvic pain syndrome is to look for evidence of T-cell reactivity with normal prostatic proteins in autoimmune prostatitis. In one study, the CD4 T-cell proliferative response to seminal plasma was found to be statistically significant when compared with medium alone in men with a history of chronic prostatitis and chronic pelvic pain syndrome, but it was not statistically significant in normal men. The responses of subjects in the chronic prostate/chronic pelvic pain syndrome group and normal subjects to the recall antigens tetanus toxoid and *Candida* extract were equivalent.[21] In studies using color Doppler ultrasonography, chronic prostatitis was associated with abnormal prostate blood flow in men with and without inflammation in comparison with controls.[22]

In a study of men with pelvic pain, the reported locations of the pain were the prostate or perineal region, or both, in 45.6% of cases, the scrotum or bladder in 38.8% of cases, the penis in 5.8%, the bladder in 5.8%, and the lower abdomen and back in 1.9%.[23] Regardless of the location, most subjects had increased urethral sensitivity, suggesting an apparent association of pelvic floor dysfunction with pelvic pain. Treatment was aimed at modulating the pelvic floor with biofeedback, medication, and sacral anterior root stimulation.[24]

Pelvic floor tension myalgia may contribute to the symptoms in men with chronic pelvic pain syndrome. The presence of detrusor instability, hypersensitivity to filling, or bladder-sphincter pseudodyssynergia on pretreatment urodynamic studies is not predictive of treatment results. Treatment recommendations include a formalized program of neuromuscular reeducation of the pelvic floor muscles plus interval bladder training to improve objective measures of pain, urgency, and frequency in patients with chronic pelvic pain syndrome.[25]

Pelvic varicocele and *seminal vesicle dystrophy* are other causes of pelvic pain. In men, diagnosis of varicocele is based on clinical findings (in contrast with women, in whom instrument evaluation is needed to identify causes such as incontinence of ovarian veins or development of adnexal varicosities). Treatment of male varicocele involves percutaneous sclerotization, surgical excision, or therapeutic embolization.[26]

GASTROINTESTINAL PAIN

One study of women with chronic pelvic pain found that more than 75% had *irritable bowel syndrome*. Of women referred to a gynecologic clinic for dysmenorrhea, dyspareunia, and abdominal pain, half had significantly more symptoms of irritable bowel syndrome than did those referred for symptoms other than pain. Irritable bowel syndrome is a functional bowel disorder of uncertain etiology characterized by a chronic relapsing pattern of abdominal-pelvic pain and bowel dysfunction with constipation or diarrhea, or both. It affects 15% of the population. Symptoms include abdominal pain, bloating, belching, excessive flatus, diarrhea, constipation, passage of mucus, and painful defecation with a sense of incomplete evacuation. Symptoms often are worse during stressful periods and the premenstrual phase of the cycle, and may accompany anxiety and depression.

The pathophysiology of irritable bowel syndrome is multifactorial, involving altered bowel motility, visceral hypersensitivity, and psychosocial factors. Other contributing factors include diet and prior infection. Therapeutic options include increasing dietary fiber to prevent constipation, opioid agents for diarrhea, low-dose antidepressants or infrequent use of antispasmodics for pain, psychotherapy, and hypnotherapy.[27] The diagnosis of irritable bowel syndrome is made by taking a careful history and by use of colonoscopy or barium enema to exclude other conditions.

Inflammatory bowel disease may manifest the same symptoms as irritable bowel syndrome. More than 50% of patients with Crohn's disease and ulcerative colitis present with pain. About 90% of patients with Crohn's disease have a bloody diarrhea, whereas patients with ulcerative colitis have moderate cramping that resolves with defecation. In one study, chronic pelvic pain was reported in 35% of patients with irritable bowel syndrome and in 13.8% of those with inflammatory bowel disease.[28] Women with both irritable bowel syndrome and chronic pelvic pain were more likely to have a lifetime history of dysthymic disorder, current and lifetime panic disorder, somatization disorder, childhood sexual abuse, and hysterectomy than women who had irritable bowel syndrome alone. Logistic regression has shown that the mean number of somatization symptoms was the best predictor of a history of both irritable bowel syndrome and chronic pelvic pain compared with either inflammatory bowel disease or irritable bowel syndrome alone.[29]

UROLOGIC PAIN

Interstitial cystitis is a chronically progressive, severely debilitating, heterogeneous syndrome that affects the urinary bladder and is characterized by urgency frequency and pain. Its etiology is poorly understood; current hypotheses focus on occult or resistant microorganisms, urothelial hyperpermeability from a defective glycosaminoglycan mucus layer, neurogenic or hormonal dysfunction, mast cell activation, and genetic susceptibility as possible causative factors. The diagnosis is made clinically, by cystoscopy with hydrodistention, and sometimes by biopsy when other pathologies have been excluded.[30] This condition is underdiagnosed in women with pelvic pain. Symptoms of urinary frequency and urgency, dysuria, hematuria, and nocturia occur along with the pelvic pain. Patients have often been treated for recurrent urinary tract infections. Urinalysis results may be normal, but microscopic hematuria without white blood cells is sometimes noted. Patients must have at least two of the following symptoms: pain in the suprapubic, perineal, and urethral region; pain on bladder filling that is relieved by emptying; decreased compliance on cystsometrogram; and glomerulations on endoscopy. When these criteria are not met, patients are considered to have *urgency-frequency syndrome*.

Treatment approaches includes use of systemic agents, instillation therapy, and surgical management. Trials of systemic agents, including antihistamines, azathioprine, corticosteroids, heparin, pentosan polysulfate, and tricyclic compounds have shown inconsistent results. Dimethyl sulfoxide (DMSO) has been used for intravesical therapy, with varying response rates. Surgical treatments include urinary diversion procedures and augmentation cystoplasty. Denervation procedures are reserved for patients with severe, intractable disease. Hypogastric plexus block and neuromodulatory procedures have been used with some success.

Infectious cystitis manifests symptoms of suprapubic pain, dysuria, and frequency and urgency, along with pyuria and a positive urine culture. These symptoms respond to antibiotics. In about 25% of women with irritative urinary symptoms and pyuria, *C. trachomatis* is found in the urethra. The *urethral syndrome* occurs when the urinary bacterial count is low, urinalysis is negative, and the *Chlamydia* study is negative. The etiology of this syndrome is unclear, but it may be caused by chronic inflammation of the periurethral glands, or urethral spasticity with periurethral muscle fatigue. Treatment is similar to that of interstitial cystitis and urgency-frequency syndrome, and consists of a combination of medication, biofeedback, and re-education of voiding habits.[31]

MUSCULOSKELETAL AND MYOFASCIAL PAIN

Evolving lumbar disk disease and intradural neoplasms in the upper lumbar area produce symptoms that may be interpreted as pelvic pain. Symptoms consistent with radiculopathy occur late in the course of these diseases. Musculoskeletal pain can be the result of decreased abdominal and pelvic muscle strength, decreased range of motion of the hip, and unequal leg lengths. Trigger points for this pain may be near surgical incisions.

Surgical procedures can lead to serious pain that develops months to years afterward. An example is the Pfannensteil incision, a horizontal incision across the lower pelvis, which can lead to pulling along the pathway of the ilioinguinal and iliohypogastric nerves. The stretching and trauma arising from labor and delivery also can lead to pelvic pain. The pain is from the lower pelvis, although it may be experienced as visceral in origin.[32] Pelvic pain during pregnancy has been associated with symphyseal distention. However, the degree of pain was not proportional to the degree of distention. Studies of pain in pregnancy have attempted to correlate pain with elevated hormones, such as serum concentrations of relaxin and propeptide of type III procollagen measured in early pregnancy.[33,34]

A similar disproportion occurs in *adhesions*, which may be responsible for pelvic pain as sequelae of past infection, chronic active inflammatory state, endometriosis, and postoperative adhesions. Celioscopy is the key diagnostic procedure after history taking and physical examination. There is no systematic relation between the clinical picture and anatomic findings. A diagnosis of chronic pelvic pain is recommended in the absence of any macroscopic, histologic, and bacteriologic lesions.[35]

In laparoscopic studies, about 25% of cases of acute pain and 35% of cases of chronic pain have been attributed to adhesions. The primary sources for the adhesions were in the bowel and omentum. It has been suggested that this pain develops when adhesions fix the pelvic organs in place, hampering their motility. The pain of adhesions can be aggravated by activity. Lysis of adhesions can reduce symptoms of pain, but the duration of relief cannot be predicted. There has been no scientific support for using crystalloids, macromolecular solutions, introperitoneal heparin, corticosteroids, mechanical barriers such as intercede and Gore-Tex, or biodegradable barriers to reduce adhesions.[36]

A study of *laxity in the posterior ligament* support of the uterus suggests that the concurrent pelvic pain is attributable to parasympathetic pain at the T12 to L1 level. The pain may result from gravitational pull on nerves that are not being supported by the lax uterosacral ligaments.[37]

The term *vulvar vestibulitis* refers to pain that occurs during sexual intercourse. The diagnosis is based on the presence of dyspareunia that lasts for at least 6 months and red areas in the vestibulum that are extremely sensitive to touch. The etiology is multifactorial and includes repeated use of antibiotics, local treatment of *Candida* and human papillomavirus infections, use of hormonal contraceptives, frequent use of local substances that may be irritative, lack of arousal, vaginismus, and tense pelvic floor muscles. There is increased intraepithelial innervation and no inflammation. Treatment includes biofeedback, tricyclic antidepressants, psychotherapy, and surgery.[38]

Pudendal nerve entrapment should be considered as a differential diagnosis in patients with anoperineal pain. The idea that pudendal nerve entrapment is the cause of some pelvic pain syndromes has gained momentum in the past 15 years.[39,40] The pudendal nerve navigates along a tortuous path, supplying sensation to virtually the entire pelvic area including the penis, scrotum, perineum, and rectum, as well as motor function to the pelvic floor musculature and urethral sphincter. The two major areas of entrapment include the junction of the sacrotuberous and sacrospinous ligaments, and the pudendal canal of Alcock. Evaluation of this pathology includes reproduction of pain on application of intrarectal digital pressure at the ischial spine. In addition, intrarectal stimulation of the pudendal nerve trunk and a recording response in the bulbospongiosus muscle with distal motor latency longer than 5.0 msec is suggestive of pudendal neuropathy. The pain can be abolished by fluoroscopy or CT-guided local anesthetic and corticosteroid injection at the ischial spine or the canal of Alcock.[41]

Coccygodynia is a common problem, characterized by pain and tenderness at the tip of the spine or in the coccyx. The pain frequently radiates to the perineal, gluteal, and posterior sacral areas; worsens on sitting; and is eased on standing. Treatment consists of massage, local heat, injection of the sacococcygeal joint with local anesthetic and corticosteroid, and, if indicated, psychological therapies. *Tension myalgia* refers to spasm of the involved muscles, which can be the levator ani, the piriformis, or the coccygeus muscle groups. Treatment includes heat and massage, local anesthetic injection of the muscles, and follow-up exercises.[42]

Pelvic joint instability and persistent pelvic pain can occur in instances of precocious puberty and use of oral contraceptives prior to the age of reproduction. Diagnosis is based on a history of early onset of menarche. *Osteoporotic sacral fractures* are associated with pelvic pain.

Sports-related injuries and pain include *pyramidal muscle hematoma*, *osteitis pubis*, and *adductor tendonitis*. Pyramidal hematomas can cause impingement of the sciatic, inferior gluteal, and pudendal nerves when the nerves are compressed between the muscle and the iliac spine. Osteitis pubis, considered to be the most common inflammatory disease of the pubic symphysis, is a self-limiting inflammation secondary to trauma, pelvic surgery, childbirth, or overuse. It occurs more often in men during the third and fourth decades of life, causing pain in the pubic area, one or both groins, and in the lower rectus abdominis muscle. The pain may be exacerbated by exercise or by specific movements, such as running, kicking, or pivoting on one leg, and is relieved with rest. During the physical examination, pain can be elicited by resisted long and flexed adductor contraction. A waddling antalgic gait and symphysis tenderness also can occur. Initial therapy should focus on decreasing inflammation with active rest, ice, NSAIDs, and physical therapy. If necessary, judicious use of local corticosteroids may be attempted.[43]

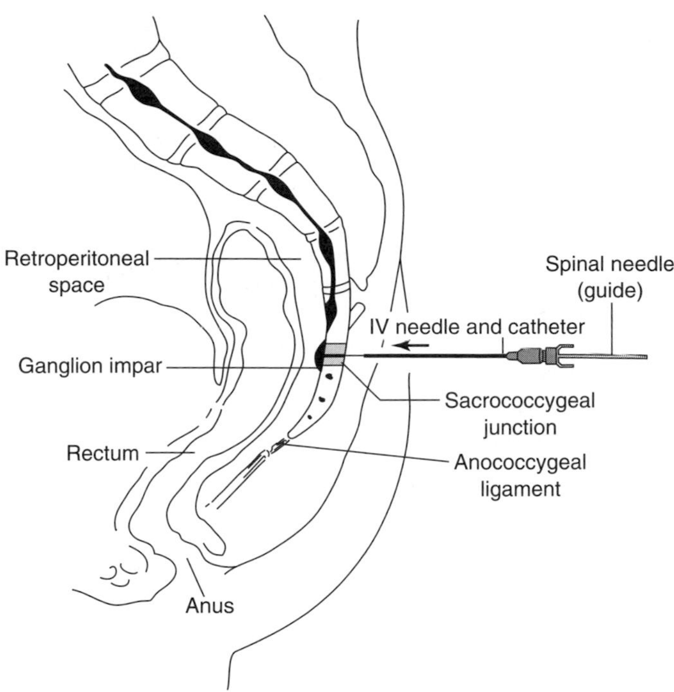

Figure 35-2 A 22-gauge, 7-inch spinal needle (passed through a 10-gauge, 5-inch intravenous needle and angiocath) is percutaneously advanced to the anterior border of the sacrococcygeal disc.

TREATMENT APPROACHES

Medical Therapy

NSAIDs have been studied extensively in the treatment of primary dysmennorrhea and have proven efficacy in various causes of pelvic pain. Combination estrogen-progestin oral contraceptives, danazol, and gonadotropin-releasing hormone agonist are used in a stepwise sequence in the management of pelvic pain secondary to endometriosis. Other adjuvant medications, such as tricyclic antidepressants, have a role in some chronic pelvic pain conditions.

Neural Blockade

Hypogastric Plexus Block This type of block is used to modulate pain that results from a sympathetic mechanism originating in the pelvic viscera. Several techniques have been described for performing hypogastric plexus block. Needle placement with fluoroscopy from the posterior approach, using landmarks and coaxial imaging technique, is commonly used. A transdiskal approach through the L5-S1 disk using fluoroscopy or CT guidance has been reported. An anterior approach under CT guidance may be used in selected cases. Neurolytic hypogastric plexus is quite effective in relieving pelvic pain in patients with gynecologic, colorectal, or genitourinary cancer.[43]

Ganglion Impar Block This block is used to evaluate and manage pain of sympathetic origin that has its root in the perineum, rectum, or genitalia. There are various techniques for performing this block. One technique uses fluoroscopic guidance and an approach via the trans-sacrococcygeal with a straight needle[44] (Fig. 35-2). Another technique involves entering at the level of the anococcygeal ligament with a curved needle[45] (Fig. 35-3). Neu-

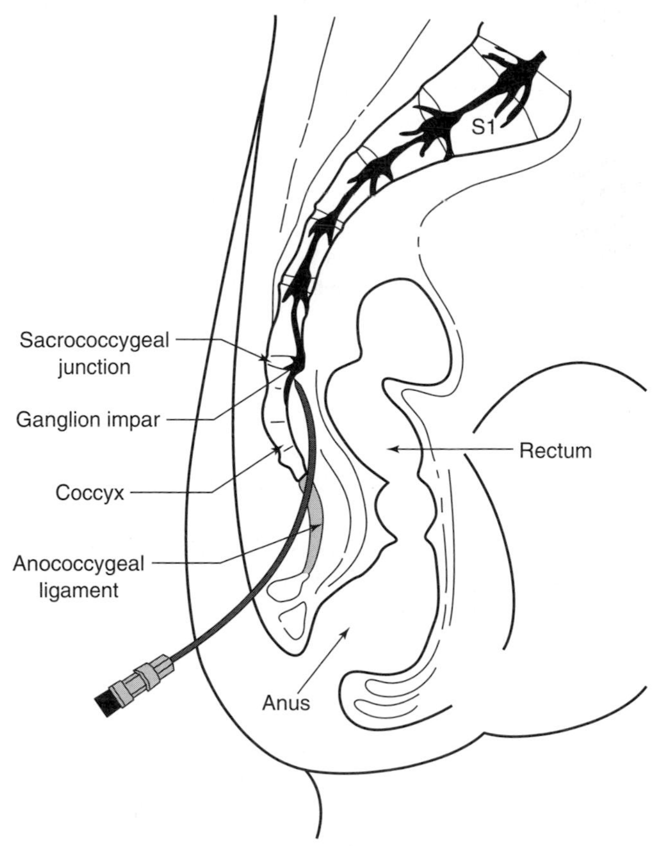

Figure 35-3 Diagrammatic lateral view of the proper placement of curved needle for blockade of the ganglion impar.

rolysis of ganglion impar is used for refractory cases of perineal pain. Neurolysis can be achieved by using chemicals such as phenol or by cryoablation or radiofrequency lesioning.

Pudendal Nerve Blockade Pudendal neuralgia should be considered in the differential diagnosis of long-term anoperineal pain. In women, the block is performed transvaginally with the patient in the lithotomy position. The needle tip must be advanced through the sacrospinous ligament just past the ischial spine. The transperineal approach is used in men, and in women in whom anatomical constraints preclude a transvaginal approach. CT-guided pudendal nerve block has also been reported as a very effective technique in the treatment of pudendal neuralgia.[46]

Neuromodulation

Sacral neuromodulation, which involves insertion of sacral nerve stimulators, has been performed for patients with voiding disorders, including urinary urge continence, urgency-frequency, and nonobstructive urinary retention; for patients with intractable interstitial cystitis; and for those with chronic intractable pelvic pain.[47] This technique is especially beneficial in patients with bladder sphincter dysfunction because it restores balance between the sacral reflexes. Electrical stimulation of the S3 nerve activates the pelvic floor and modulates innervations of the bladder, sphincter, and pelvic floor.

Neuraxial Drug Delivery

Delivery of an analgesic into the epidural or subarachnoid space is used most often in the management of patients with pain secondary to malignancy. Opioids remain the most commonly used drugs for this therapy; however, several other agents, such as local anesthetics and clonidine, can be used in conjunction.

Neuroablation

In patients with unilateral pelvic pain secondary to malignancy cordotomy or rhizotomy can be used in selected patients. The side effects include paresis, ataxia, and bladder dysfunction.

Surgical Therapy

Laparoscopy In a review of 1,524 gynecologic laparoscopies performed for chronic pelvic pain, endometriosis was the most commonly diagnosed disorder (33%), followed by adhesive disease (24%), chronic PID (5%), ovarian cysts (3%), pelvic varicosities (< 1%), leiomyomata (< 1%), and a variety of other diagnoses (4%). No visible pathology was detected in 35% of patients.[12] Resection and ablation of the endometriotic lesions, and lysis of adhesions are the two therapeutic approaches commonly employed laparoscopically.

Nerve Transection Procedures Laparoscopic uterosacral nerve ablation involves the destruction of the uterine nerve fibers that exit the uterus through the uterosacral ligaments. There seems to be little evidence to support the performance of this procedure.[48]

Presacral neurectomy is a procedure designed to interrupt the sympathetic innervation of the uterus at the level of superior hypogastric plexus. It is performed by incising the pelvic peritoneum over the sacrum and then identifying and transecting the sacral nerve plexus. This procedure is more helpful in the management of patients with persistent midline pelvic pain.

Role of Gonadectomy and Hysterectomy Bilateral oophorectomy with or without hysterectomy is the most effective procedure for women who have recurrent symptomatic endometriosis and who have no desire to retain reproductive function.

Multidisciplinary Treatment

Pelvic pain is the end result of disease-initiated stimuli and the interpretation of these stimuli by the central nervous system. It is a complex interaction that involves sensory, psychological, and environmental factors. Hence, applying a multidisciplinary approach, which employs an integrative approach to the psychosocial-mind-body paradigm, is sometimes the most effective strategy in the management of patients with chronic pain states. This approach integrates medical intervention with identification and management of socioenvironmental problems, cognitive behavioral pain strategies, and treatment of concurrent psychological morbidity. Available evidence suggests that outcomes, including pain severity, general health, and functional status and disability, improve more significantly after this approach than after isolated medical or surgical interventions.

Physical Therapy Pelvic floor manual therapy, which involves decreasing the pelvic floor hypertonicity, may ameliorate the symptoms of urgency-frequency syndrome and interstitial cystitis.[49] Other physical therapy modalities, including heat, electrical stimulation, deep ultrasound, and massage, may be used depending on the individual need of the patient.

Psychological Treatment The various psychological modalities of treatment should be selected based on individual need, which can vary dramatically among patients. Behavioral therapy, progressive relaxation training, guided imagery, self-hypnosis, breathing exercises, and biofeedback are some of the techinques employed. Other options that may be more useful in the setting of chronic pelvic pain include group therapy, couples therapy, and sex therapy.

Alternative Medicine Alternative or complementary medicine is receiving greater interest from both patients and health care providers. Yoga, meditation, chiropractic treatment, acupuncture, and magnet therapies are some of the common forms of these modalities used in the treatment of pelvic pain.

CONCLUSION

Pelvic pain remains a diagnostic and therapeutic challenge for the health care provider. It is a source of frustration to both the physician and patient. Physicians have been ill equipped through their training to confront the multifaceted nature of the complaints of patients with chronic pelvic pain. Patients presenting with these pain syndromes are best assessed and treated using a multidisciplinary approach. Close collaboration among gynecologists, urologists, proctologists, neurologists, pain specialist, gastroenterologists, psychiatrists, psychologists, physiatrists, and neurologists is needed. Special emphasis should be placed on preventive strategies, such as screening and treatment of avoidable conditions (e.g., lower genital infection) that can result in PID. Preventive measures also are needed to tackle the growing incidence of childhood and sexual abuse, which play a role in chronic pain syndromes.

REFERENCES

1. Kumazawa T. Sensory innervation of reproductive organs. In: Cervero F, Morrison J, eds. *Visceral Sensation.* New York, NY: Elsevier; 1986: 115–131.
2. McDonald JS. Chronic pelvic pain. In: Copeland LJ, Jarrell JF, eds. *Textbook of Gynecology.* New York, NY: WB Saunders; 2000:741–758.
3. Bjorklund K, Bergstrom S. Is pelvic pain in pregnancy a welfare complaint? *Acta Obstet Gynecol Scand* 2000;79:24–30.
4. Weiner SL. Acute right iliac pain. In: Weiner SL. *Differential Diagnosis of Acute Pain by Body Regions.* New York, NY: McGraw-Hill; 1993:274–276.
5. Vercellini P, Trespidi L, De Giorgi O, Cortesi I, Parazzini F, Crosignani PG. Endometriosis and pelvic pain: Relation to disease stage and localization. *Fertil Steril* 1996;65:299–304.
6. Hillard PA. Benign diseases of the female reproductive tract: Symptoms and signs. In: Berek JS, Adaski EY, Hilard PA, eds. *Novak's Gynecology.* 12th ed. Baltimore, Md: Williams & Wilkins; 1996:331–397.
7. Rigor BM. Pelvic cancer pain. *J Surg Oncol* 2000;75:280–300.
8. Orford VP, Kuhn RJ. Management of ovarian remnant syndrome. *Aust N Z J Obstet Gynaecol* 1996;36:468–471.
9. MacKay HT. Gynecology. In: Tierney LM, McPhee SJ, Papadakis MA, eds. *Current Medical Diagnosis and Treatment.* New York; Lange/McGraw Hill 2003;42:699–733.
10. Foong LC, Gamble J, Sutherland IA, Beard RW. Altered peripheral vascular response of women with and without pelvic pain due to congestion. *Br J Obstet Gynaecol* 2000;107:157–164.
11. Charles G. Congestive pelvic syndromes. *Rev Fr Gynecol Obstet* 1995; 90:84–90.
12. DeJong JM, van Lunsen RH, Robertson EA, Stam LN, Lammes FB. Focal vulvitis: A psychosexual problem for which surgery is not the answer. *J Psychosom Obstet Gynecol* 1995;16:85–91.
13. Howard FM. The role of laparoscopy as a diagnostic tool in chronic pelvic pain. *Ballieres Best Pract Res Clin Obstet Gynecol* 2000; 14:467–494.
14. Zondervan K, Barlow DH. Epidemiology of chronic pelvic pain. *Ballieres Best Pract Res Clin Obstet Gynecol* 2000;14:403–414.
15. Jamieson DJ, Steege JF. The prevalence of dysmenorrhea, dyspareunia, pelvic pain, and irritable bowel syndrome in primary care practices. *Obstet Gynecol* 1996;87:55–58.
16. Badura AS, Reiter RC, Altmaier EM, Rhomberg A, Elas D. Dissociation, somatization, substance abuse and coping in women with chronic pelvic pain. *Obstet Gynecol* 1997;90:405–410.
17. Lipsett DR. The painful woman: Complaints, symptoms and illness. In: Notman MT, Nadelson CC, eds. *The Woman Patient.* Vol. III. New York, NY: Plenum Press; 1982:147–171.
18. Nadelson CC, Notman MK, Miller JB, Zilbach J. Aggression in women: Conceptual issues and clinical implications. In: Notman MT, Nadelson CC, eds. *The Woman Patient.* Vol. III. New York, NY: Plenum Press; 1982:17–29.
19. Strohmaier WL, Bichler KH. Comparison of symptoms, morphological, microbiological and urodynamic findings in patients with chronic prostatitis/pelvic pain syndrome: Is it possible to differentiate separate categories? *Urol Int* 2000;65:112–116.
20. Alexander RB, Ponniah S, Hasday J, Hebel JR. Elevated levels of proinflammatory cytokines in the semen of patients with chronic prostatitis/chronic pelvic pain syndrome. *Urology* 1998;52:744–749.
21. Alexander RB, Brady F, Ponniah S. Autoimmune prostatitis: Evidence of T cell reactivity with normal prostatic proteins. *Urology* 1997;50: 893–899.
22. Cho IR, Keener TS, Nghiem HV, Winter T, Krieger JN. Prostate blood flow characteristics in the chronic prostatitis/pelvic pain syndrome. *J Urol* 2000;163:1130–1133.
23. Krieger JN, Egan KJ, Ross SO, Jacobs R, Berger RE. Chronic pelvic pains represent the most prominent urogenital symptoms of "chronic prostatitis." *Urology* 1996;48:715–721.
24. Zermann DH, Ishigooka M, Doggweiler R, Schmidt RA. Neurological insights into the etiology of genitourinary pain in men. *J Urol* 1999; 161:903–908.
25. Clemens JQ, Nadler RB, Schaeffer AJ, Belani J, Albaugh J, Bushman W. Biofeedback, pelvic floor re-education, and bladder training for male chronic pelvic pain syndrome. *Urology* 2000;56:951–955.
26. Bitker MO, Delcourt A, Yonneau L, Barrow B, Richard F. Seminal vesicle dystrophy as the cause of chronic unilateral pelvic pain in a 20-year-old male. *Prog Urol* 2000;10:461–464.
27. Camilleri M, Heading RC, Thompson WG. Consensus report: Clinical perspectives, mechanisms, diagnosis and management of irritable bowel syndrome. *Alim Pharmacol Ther* 2002;16:1407–1430.
28. Rapkin AJ, Mayer EA. Gastroenterological causes of chronic pelvic pain. *Obstet Gynecol Clin North Am* 1993;20:663–683.
29. Walker EA, Gelfand AN, Gelfand MD, Green C, Katon WJ. Chronic pelvic pain and gynecological symptoms in women with irritable bowel syndrome. *J Psychosom Obstet Gynecol* 1996;17:39–46.
30. Oberpenning F, van Ophoven A, Hertle L. Interstitial cystitis: An update. *Curr Opin Urol* 2002;12:321–332.
31. Yoon SM, Jung JK, Lee SB. Treatment of female urethral syndrome refractory to antibiotics. *Yonsei Med J* 2002;43:644–651.
32. McDonald JS. Chronic pelvic pain. In: Copeland LJ, Jarrell JF, eds. *Textbook of Gynecology.* New York, NY: WB Saunders; 2000: 741–758.
33. Kristiansson P, Svardsudd K, von Schoultz B. Reproductive hormones and aminoterminal propeptide of type III procollagen in serum as early markers of pelvic pain during late pregnancy. *Am J Obstet Gynecol* 1999;180:128–134.
34. Bjorklund K, Bergstrom S, Nordstrom ML, Ulmsten U. Symphyseal distention in relation to serum relaxin levels and pelvic pain in pregnancy. *Acta Obstet Gynecol Scand* 2000;79:269–275.
35. D'Ercole C, Bretelle F, Heckenroth H, Cravello L, Boubli L, Blanc B. Painful pelvic adhesion syndrome. *Rev Fr Gynecol Obstet* 1995;90: 73–76.
36. Saravelos HG, Li TC, Cooke ID. An analysis of the outcome of microsurgical and laparoscopic adhesiolysis for chronic pelvic pain. *Hum Reprod* 1995;10:2895–2901.
37. Petros PP. Severe chronic pelvic pain in women may be caused by ligamental laxity in the posterior fornix of the vagina. *Aust N Z J Obstet Gynecol* 1996;36:351–354.
38. Bohn-Starke N, Rylander F. Vulvar-vestibulitis is a condition with diffuse etiology. *Lakartidningen* 2000;97:483222–483226.
39. Robert R, Prat-Pradal D, Labat JJ, et al. Anatomic basis of chronic perineal pain: Role of the pudendal nerve. *Surg Radiol Anat* 1998; 20(2):93–98.
40. Thoumas D, Leroi AM, Mauillon J, et al. Pudendal neuralgia: CT-guided pudendal nerve block technique. *Abdom Imaging* 1999;24(3):309–312.
41. Roche B, Marti MC. Pelvic pain of proctological origin. *Schweiz Med Wochenschr* 1996;126:316–321.
42. Meyers WC, Foley DP, Garrett WE, Lohnes JH, Mandlebaum BR. Management of severe lower abdominal or inguinal pain in high performacne athletes. *Am J Sports Med* 2000;28:2–8.
43. PlanCarte R, De Leon Casasola OA. Neurolytic superior hypogastric plexus block for chronic pelvic pain associated with cancer. *Regional Anesthesia* 1997;22:562–568.
44. Loev M, Varklet V, Wilsey B, et al. Cryoablation A novel approach to the neurolysis of the ganglion impar. *Anesthesiology* 1998;88:1391–1393.

45. Nebab E, Florence I. An alternative needle geometry for interruption of the ganglion impar. *Anesthesiology* 1997;86:1213–1214.
46. Calvillo O, Skaribas IM, Rockett C. Computed tomography guided pudendal nerve block. A new diagnostic approach to long term anoperineal pain: a report of two cases. *Regional Anesthesia and Pain Medicine* 2000;25:420–423.
47. Siegel S, Paszkiewicz E, Kirkpatrick C, Hinkel B, Oleson K. Sacral nerve stimulation in patients with chronic intractable pelvic pain. *J Urol* 2001;166:1742–1745.
48. Gambone JC, Mittman BS, Munro MG, et al. Consensus statement for the management of chronic pelvic pain and endometriosis: proceedings of an expert-panel consensus process. *Fertility and Sterility* 2002; 78:961–972.
49. Weiss JM. Pelvic floor myofascial trigger points: Manual therapy for interstitial cystitis and the urgency-frequency syndrome. *J Urol* 2001; 166:2226–2231.

BIBLIOGRAPHY

Boescher H. Blockade of the superior hypogastric plexus block for visceral pelvic pain. *Pain Practice* 2001;1:162–170.

Chrousos GP, Gold PW. The concepts of stress and stress system disorders. *JAMA* 1992;267:1244.

Heim C, Ehlert U, Hellhammer DH. The potential role of hypocortisolism in the pathophysiology of stress-related bodily disorders. *Psychoneuroendocrinology* 2000;25:1.

Johnson N, Wilson M, Farquhar C. Surgical pelvic neuroablation for chronic pelvic pain: A systematic review. *Gynaecol Endosc* 2000;9:351–361.

Lampe A, Soder E, Ennemoser A, et al. Chronic pelvic pain and previous sexual abuse. *Obstet Gynecol* 2000;96(6):929–933.

Nader A, Candido KD. Pelvic pain. *Pain Practice* 2001;1:187–196.

Walker EA, Roy-Byrne PP, Katon WJ, Jemelka R. An open trial of nortriptyline in women with chronic pelvic pain. *Int J Psychiatry Med* 1991;21:245–252.

CHAPTER 36 PERINEAL PAIN

Ursula Wesselmann

Chronic, nonmalignant pain syndromes of the perineal area have been well described in the medical literature dating back to the last century. However, the etiology of these focal pain syndromes is poorly understood. The patient who is experiencing pain in the perineal area is often embarrassed, because these areas of the body are considered taboo in our society. These pain syndromes are frequently under-reported and under-recognized.

Patients with these pain syndromes often have seen a variety of specialists in different subspecialties—including urologists, gynecologists, gastroenterologists, proctologists, and internists—and despite an extensive evaluation, no specific etiology has been found in the majority of cases. Not surprisingly, many of these patients are frustrated, because they have suffered from chronic pain for many years, but the disease has not been "given a name" and the pain is not controlled. It is important to recognize that these focal chronic pain syndromes of the perineal area do exist. The etiology of these pain syndromes is not known, and a specific secondary cause can be identified in a minority of patients. Although these patients often are depressed, rarely are these pain syndromes the only manifestation of a psychiatric disease. Currently available treatment strategies are empirical, only. Although complete cures are uncommon, effective treatment modalities exist to lessen the impact of pain and offer reasonable expectations of an improved functional status.

The intent of this chapter is to first give a brief overview of the current knowledge of the neurobiology of the perineal area, and then to review the clinical characteristics and treatment strategies of the different perineal pain syndromes.

NEUROBIOLOGY OF PERINEAL PAIN

The perineum is a highly specialized area of the body, responsible for carrying out a host of basic biologic functions, including defecation, micturition, copulation, and reproduction. The display of these diverse functions relies on precise nervous system control, coordinated with endocrine and other local control mechanisms. Compared with other areas of the body, there has been fairly little research on the neuroanatomy, neurophysiology, and neuropharmacology of the perineum. The complexity of the perineum in carrying out many different specialized functions has largely been considered to account for the slow progress in our understanding of the neurobiology of this area. The fact that these areas of the body often are considered taboo in our society also may account for the scarcity of research on this topic.

A detailed review of the neurobiology of the pelvic floor is provided by Burnett and Wesselmann.[1] Briefly, the innervation of the perineum is served by both components of the autonomic nervous system, the sympathetic and parasympathetic divisions, as well as the somatic nervous systems[2,3] (Figs. 36-1 and 36-2). Sensations from the pelvic floor are mainly conveyed via the sacral afferent parasympathetic system, with a far lesser afferent supply from afferents traveling with the thoracolumbar sympathetics.[4] However, sensations of the testis and epididymis may predominantly involve thoracolumbar afferents.[4] Somatic efferent and afferent innervation to the perineum originates from sacral spinal cord levels S2 to S4. Sacral nerve roots emerge from the spinal cord to form the sacral plexus, from which arises the pudendal nerve.[5] The pudendal nerve also receives postganglionic axons from the caudal sympathetic chain ganglia.[3] The pudendal nerve runs medial to the internal pudendal vessels along the lateral wall of the ischiorectal fossa dorsal to the sacrospinous ligament. First a branch splits off to become the dorsal nerve of the penis (or clitoris), then the remaining pudendal nerve fibers distribute a medial branch to the anal canal, dorsal branches to the urethral sphincter, and dorsolateral branches to the anterior perineal musculature. The posterior perineal musculature is supplied by nerves originating predominantly from sacral level S4. Branches of the S4-5 nerve roots form the coccygeal plexus, distributing fibers to the perineal, perianal, and scrotal (labial) skin.[6]

Neuropeptide release appears to account for perineal sensations.[4] Numerous peptides have been associated with afferent pathways of the pelvic floor, although a preponderance of evidence supports the roles of substance P and calcitonin gene–related-peptide (CGRP) as the primary chemicals released from these sensory neurons.[7]

CLINICAL CHARACTERISTICS AND TREATMENT STRATEGIES

Vulvodynia

Detailed descriptions of hyperesthesia of the vulva can already be found in U.S. and European textbooks of gynecology from the last century.[8,9] Surprisingly, despite these early reports the medical literature did not mention vulvar pain again until the early 1980s, when a new awareness of this chronic pain syndrome developed. In 1984, the International Society for the Study of Vulvar Disease Task Force defined vulvodynia as chronic vulvar discomfort, characterized by the patient's complaint of a burning and sometimes stinging sensation in the vulvar area.[10] Vulvodynia includes several subgroups: vulvar dermatosis, cyclic vulvovaginitis, vulvar vestibulitis, vulvar papillomatosis, and dysesthetic vulvodynia.[11]

The incidence or prevalence of vulvodynia is not known. A recent survey of sexual dysfunction, analyzing data from the National Health and Social Life Survey, reported that 16% of women between the ages of 18 and 59 years living in households throughout the United States experience pain during sex.[12] When these data were analyzed by age group, the highest number of women reporting pain during sex was in the age group of 18 to 29 years. The location and etiology of pain was not analyzed in this study.

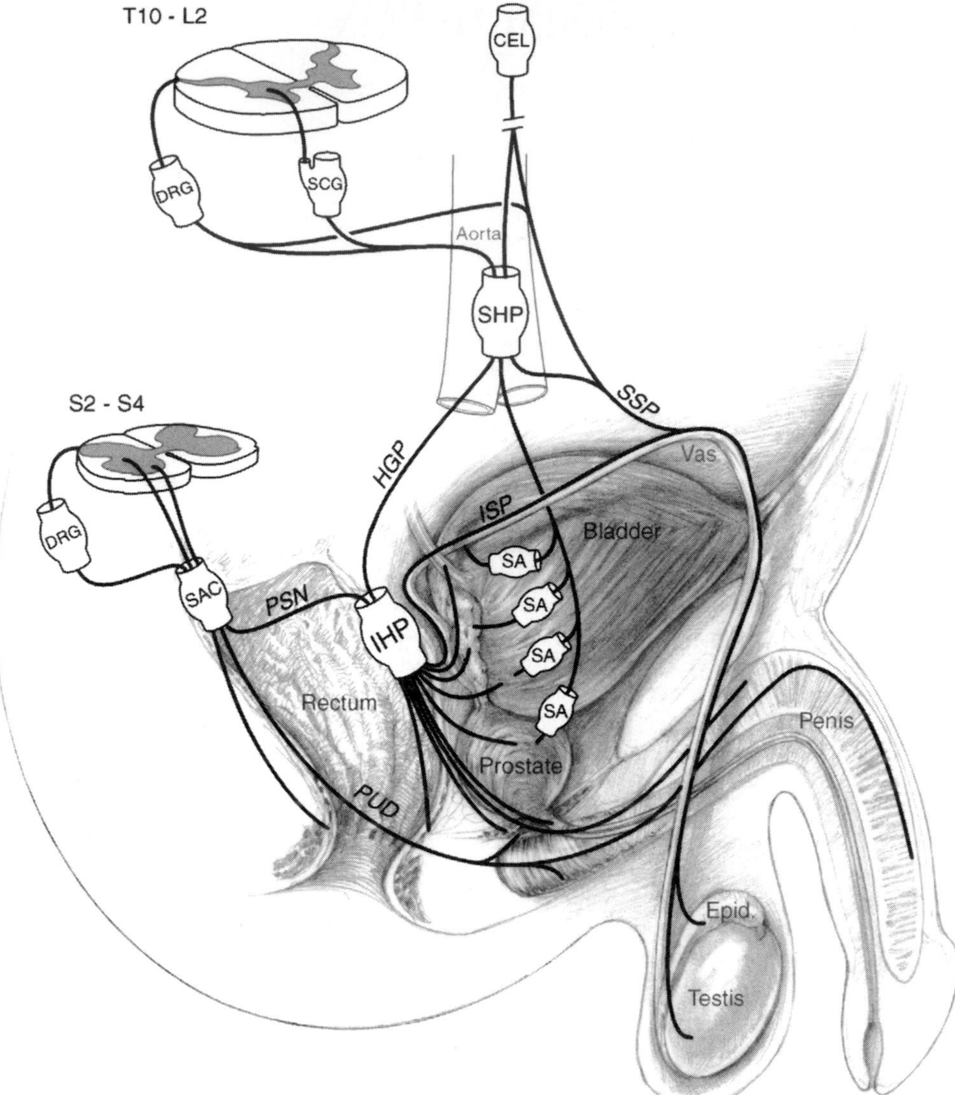

Figure 36-1 Schematic drawing showing the innervation of the pelvic floor in males. Although this diagram attempts to show the innervation in humans, much of the anatomic information is derived from animal data. CEL, celiac plexus; DRG, dorsal root ganglion; HGP, hypogastric plexus; IHP, inferior hypogastric plexus; ISP, inferior spermatic plexus; PSN, pelvic splanchnic nerve; PUD, pudendal nerve; Epid., epididymis; SA, short adrenergic projections; SAC, sacral plexus; SCG, sympathetic chain ganglion; SHP, superior hypogastric plexus; SSP, superior spermatic plexus. (From Wesselmann U, Burnett AL, Heinberg LJ. The urogenital and rectal pain syndromes. *Pain* 1997;73:269–294, with permission.)

Goetsch[13] reported that 15% of all patients seen in her general gynecologic private practice fulfilled the definition of vulvar vestibulitis, a major subgroup of vulvodynia. It is important to point out that these patients had not come for a gynecologic evaluation because of vulvar pain, but for a routine gynecologic checkup. Fifty percent of these patients had always experienced entry dyspareunia and pain with inserting tampons, and most of these, since their teenage years.

It is important to be aware of the different subtypes of vulvodynia, because treatment varies according to diagnosis. The clinical features and treatment strategies for these different subtypes are discussed in the remainder of this section. It is likely that the current classification of different subtypes of vulvodynia will be modified in the future, as physicians learn more about the etiologies of the vulvar pain syndromes. Chronic infections of the vulvar area should be treated before a diagnosis of vulvodynia is made. A number of genital infections have been found to be a frequent cause of chronic vulvar pain,[14] and a thorough evaluation for infections of the vulva and vagina should be carried out by a gynecologist or dermatologist experienced in this area.

Vulvar dermatoses are a frequent cause of chronic vulvar pain. A prospective study[15] of patients presenting with vulvar pain showed that the majority of patients had a corticosteroid-responsive dermatosis. Unlike most other subsets of vulvodynia, vulvar dermatoses are associated with physical signs: redness, blisters, and erosions that can be recognized during a careful physical examination.[16] For the physician who specializes in pain management, these physical signs on examination of the patient should be an indication to evaluate more extensively for an etiology of the pain. The differential diagnosis of these physical signs is complex and may include local as well as systemic disease. Inflammatory dermatoses, chronic contact dermatitis, lichen planus, lichen sclerosus, lichen simplex chronicus, seborrheic dermatitis, psoriasis, herpetic infections, and systemic autoimmune diseases such as Beháet's disease and systemic lupus erythematosus have to be considered.[17] The diagnosis usually needs to be confirmed by vulvar punch biopsy. Vulvar and vaginal redness and erosions also may occur in diabetes mellitus. These patients, however, typically present with vaginal itching and not pain.

Cyclic vulvovaginitis is characterized by episodic "flares" of vulvar pain, often after sexual intercourse (pain is typically worst the next day) or during the luteal phase of the menstrual cycle.[18]

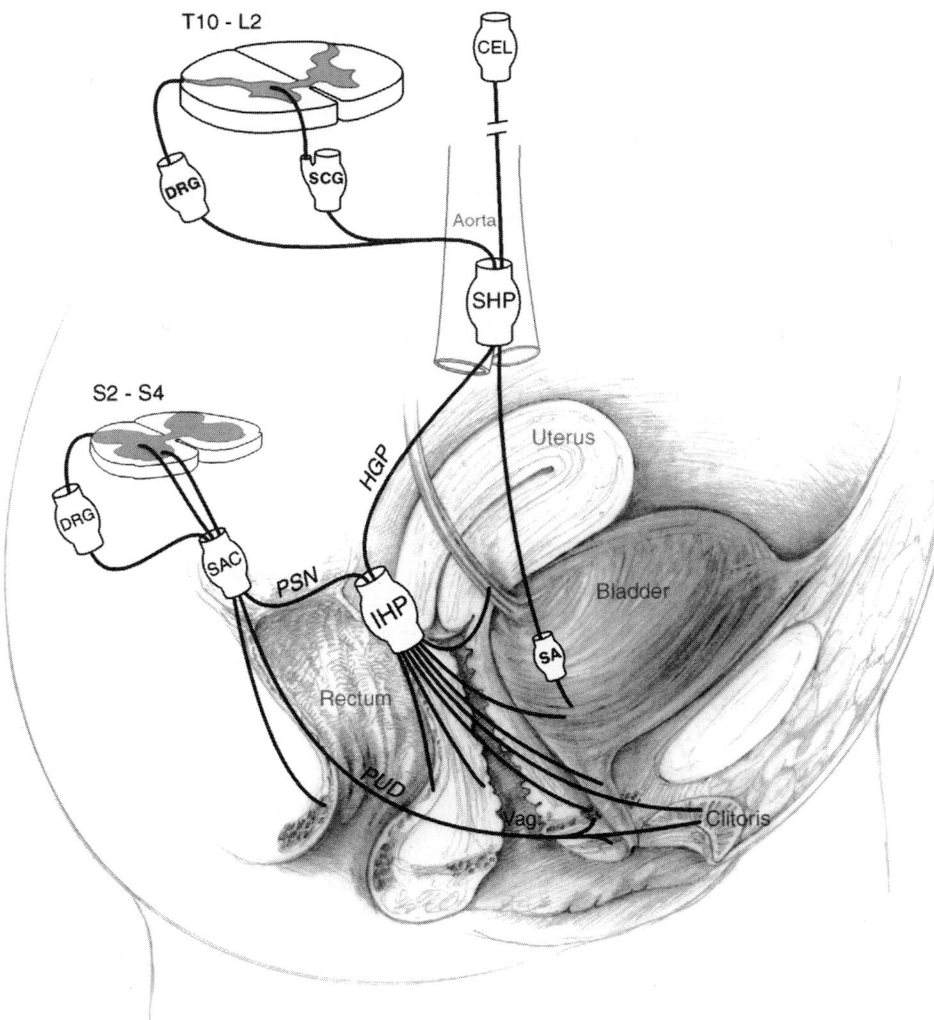

Figure 36-2 Schematic drawing showing the innervation of the pelvic floor in females. Although this diagram attempts to show the innervation in humans, much of the anatomic information is derived from animal data. CEL, celiac plexus; DRG, dorsal root ganglion; HGP, hypogastric plexus; IHP, inferior hypogastric plexus; PSN, pelvic splanchnic nerve; PUD, pudendal nerve; SA, short adrenergic projections; SAC, sacral plexus; SCG, sympathetic chain ganglion; SHP, superior hypogastric plexus; Vag., vagina (From Wesselmann U, Burnett AL, Heinberg LJ. The urogenital and rectal pain syndromes. *Pain* 1997;73: 269–294, with permission.)

Cyclic symptoms have been reported after hormonal changes, such as starting or discontinuing oral contraceptives, or during pregnancy. Cyclic vulvovaginitis might be multifactorial. Several contributing factors have been suggested: hypersensitivity to the Candida antigen,[19] immunoglobulin A deficiency,[20] and cyclic changes in the vaginal environment.[21] Prolonged maintenance therapy with antimycotics, topically or systemically, is usually effective if cultures show the presence of Candida.[16,18]

Vulvar vestibulitis is characterized by a history of entry dyspareunia, pain at the introitus of the vagina when inserting a tampon, and painful sensations when wearing pants, or with bicycle and horseback riding. On examination of the vulva, there is often some vestibular erythema. A typical characteristic of this type of vulvodynia during examination is that touch of the vestibule is very painful.[22] Often, the patient herself can point to a specific spot at the vaginal introitus that is painful to touch. The clinical observation of vestibular erythema associated with dyspareunia was described in 1928 by Kelly[23]: "Exquisitely sensitive deep-red spots in the mucosa of the hymenal ring are a fruitful source of dyspareunia—tender enough at times to make a vaginal examination impossible. Inflamed caruncles with or without these spots often stand guard at the introitus labeled 'noli me tangere'." Earlier studies implicated persistent infection as the cause of vulvar vestibulitis, but histologic and molecular studies have not supported this supposition.[24–28] Interestingly, two recent studies reported vestibular neural hyperplasia,[29,30] which might provide a morphologic and neurologic explanation for the pain in vulvar vestibulitis syndrome.

Approximately half of the patients with clinical symptoms of vulvar vestibulitis eventually experience spontaneous remission.[31] Treatment for vulvar vestibulitis is difficult. Most treatments have been reported as uncontrolled case reports, and no long-term follow-up data have been provided. As a first step in the treatment of vulvar vestibulitis, local irritants and potential allergens should be identified and eliminated. A change to a mild, hypoallergenic laundry detergent should be considered.

The role of urinary oxalate excretion in vulvar vestibulitis is controversial. One initial case report associated vulvar vestibulitis with oxalate crystalluria[32]: the patient experienced pain relief with calcium citrate and a low-oxalate diet. Withdrawal of calcium citrate resulted in reoccurrence of vulvar pain, and reinstitution of calcium citrate alleviated the pain again. A more recent study (published as a commentary, only, without details of the patient population studied) claimed successful pain relief in 75% of patients treated with low-oxalate diet and calcium citrate.[33] However, a controlled study in 130 patients with vulvar pain and 23 volunteers without symptoms showed that urinary oxalates may be nonspecific irritants that aggravate vulvodynia, but that the role of oxalates as instigators is doubtful.[34] Because a low-oxalate diet has no side effects, a trial of this treatment modality is certainly indicated in patients interested in pursuing a dietary approach. Controlled, prospective studies with clearly defined outcome parameters are necessary to further elucidate the role of urinary oxalates in this chronic pain syndrome.

Biofeedback of the pelvic floor musculature has been reported to result in pain improvement in 83% of patients suffering from vulvar vestibulitis.[35] Given that this treatment modality is not associated with any side effects and given the high response rate reported in the literature, a trial of biofeedback is warranted, before considering any more invasive treatment strategies, especially irreversible surgical approaches (see below). Various topical creams or ointments applied to the vulvar vestibule have resulted in pain relief in some patients. A mild hydrocortisone cream or ointment or an estrogen cream applied to the vaginal introitus have been helpful. In mild cases of vulvar vestibulitis, topical lidocaine applied as a 4% solution is often sufficient to make intercourse possible without serious discomfort.[36] Intralesional α interferon injections have been reported to provide substantial or partial improvement in about 50% of patients.[37] Isoprinosine, another agent known to enhance immune function, was found to improve pain in 60% of patients.[38]

Surgical approaches have been suggested with the aim of removing the painful skin area. The most common procedure is perineoplasty. The vulvar vestibule (the hyperalgesic area) is excised, and the vaginal mucosa is then advanced to cover the defect.[39] Risks include general anesthesia, prolonged healing period, intraoperative bleeding, and postoperative disfigurement.[36] A simplified surgical revision under local anesthesia has been suggested in a pilot study,[36] resulting in complete resolution of pain in the majority of patients.

In vulvar papillomatosis, small papillae are seen around the vulvar vestibule. These papillae can be seen in conjunction with lichen simplex chronicus, or with subclinical infection with human papillomavirus. In other cases, this is a normal variant. Colposcopy and biopsy are important to rule out an infection with human papillomavirus. Treatment of the papillomatosis is usually not necessary.[16] If pain persists, symptomatic treatment of the vulvar pain can be considered.

The term essential vulvodynia was originally used to describe chronic vulvar pain for which no secondary cause could be determined.[21] When it was subsequently found that treatment of cutaneous neuralgia was effective in some of these patients, the term essential was replaced by the more appropriate term dysesthetic.[40] Dysesthetic vulvodynia is more common in perimenopausal or postmenopausal women. In contrast to vulvar vestibulitis, in which pain is localized at the vulvar vestibule and evoked by touch, patients with dysesthetic vulvodynia report diffuse, constant hyperalgesia in the vulvar area, often extending throughout the perineum. These women complain less about dyspareunia. Some women present with features of both vulvar vestibulitis and dysesthetic vulvodynia. One article has suggested use of the term vestibulodynia for this symptom complex.[41] It has been hypothesized that the vulvar hyperalgesia in dysesthetic vulvodynia is caused by a neuropathic pain syndrome, possibly of the pudendal nerve.[17] In support of this hypothesis, Sonni and coworkers[42] found that the pain threshold for acid solutions is decreased in women with dysesthetic vulvodynia. Many patients can be helped with medications recommended for other neuropathic pain syndromes.[43] Case reports have demonstrated that low-dose amitriptyline may be effective in women with dysesthetic vulvodynia, especially in elderly women.[40,44] However, no controlled studies have been reported so far, and further clinical research is urgently needed.

Iatrogenic causes have to be considered when evaluating a patient with vulvodynia. Especially as the use of potent topical corticosteroids becomes more widespread, steroid rebound dermatitis in the vaginal area is seen more frequently.[18] Vulvodynia has been recognized as a complication of CO2 laser therapy to the vulva.[17] The literature on the long-term effects of episiotomy on vaginal sensation is sparse. In one older, retrospective study,[45] 16% to 47% of the women interviewed continued to report dyspareunia 1 to 5 years after episiotomy.

In summary, vulvodynia is a recognized disease entity, and an emerging body of literature is reporting on several different etiologic factors, attesting to the multifactorial aspects of this disease. For the treating physician, it is important to realize that many women with vulvodynia are in their reproductive ages and previously had satisfying sexual relationships. In contrast to many other chronic pain syndromes, vulvodynia may only interfere to a moderate extend with the daily activities of a woman, but the disease usually interferes 100% with her sexual life. To confirm the diagnosis of vulvodynia, excluding secondary causes such as dermatitis or gynecologic infections, and to design a treatment plan, a multidisciplinary approach involving collaborations of gynecologists, dermatologists, neurologists, pain specialists, psychologists, and psychiatrists is necessary.

Clitoral Pain

In contrast to the large body of literature that has emerged over the past 15 years on vulvodynia, few reports exist on clitoral pain. In clinical practice, clitoral pain occasionally is seen in women presenting with dysesthetic vulvodynia, if the pain is extending throughout the whole perineum, and the ongoing pain (often a burning, stinging sensation) is usually exacerbated by mechanical stimuli such as tight clothing and sexual contact. Chronic pain is reported as one of the complications of female circumcision. This procedure involves excision of the clitoris and the labia minora, and is still performed on young females in many parts of the world before or as they reach puberty, as an instrument to control female sexuality and maintain cultural pride.[46–48] As mobility is increasing, some of these women have moved to western countries; for example, it is estimated that 2,000 young women living in the Unite Kingdom undergo this ritual per year.[47] Few of these women seem to seek medical attention, and the incidence of chronic clitoral pain in this group is not known.

Urethral Syndrome

Many women present to the urologist, gynecologist, or family physician with painful micturition but no evidence of organic disease, and the urine culture is negative by standard techniques. Gallagher and colleagues[49] in 1965 coined the term urethral syndrome to describe this problem. It has been estimated that urethral syndrome accounts for as many as 5 million office visits a year in the United States.[50] This syndrome is defined as a disease entity characterized by urinary urgency, frequency, dysuria, and, at times, by suprapubic and back pain and urinary hesitancy in the absence of objective urologic findings. Urethral syndrome typically occurs in women during their reproductive years, but it also has been reported in children and in men.[51,52] In contrast to other chronic perineal syndromes involving nonmalignant pain, the rates of spontaneous remission are very high in this patient population.[53,54]

Several different theories have been proposed to explain the etiology of urethral syndrome, most, however, with little supporting evidence. It has been suggested that symptoms are caused by urethral obstruction and thus are surgically treatable.[55,56] It is important to note that there rarely is evidence to support an anatomically obstructive etiology. Although surgical procedures aimed at relieving a urethral obstruction claim excellent results, it must be cautioned that long-term follow-up rarely is provided. These procedures involve some risk of incontinence and are of uncertain and usually temporary efficacy.[57,58] Urinary hesitance, which often is reported by patients with urethral syndrome, might be the result of spasms of the external urethral sphincter, rather than an anatomic obstruction. Several studies reported a staccato or prolonged flow phase during uroflowmetry and increased external sphincter tone detected on urethral pressure profilometry in patients with urethral syndrome.[51] However, these urodynamic findings may also be produced voluntarily in a neurologically intact person, and are, therefore, difficult to interpret.[59] To date, an inflammatory or infectious etiology of the urethral syndrome has not been supported (reviewed in ref. 59), and controlled studies using molecular techniques to assess for infection are necessary to further clarify whether an occult infection is maintaining the chronic pain syndrome.

A thorough diagnostic evaluation is very important, because the symptoms of urethral syndrome are indistinguishable from those caused by urinary infections, tumors, stones, interstitial cystitis, and many other urologic diseases. Urethral syndrome is a diagnosis of exclusion. The urologic evaluation includes urine analysis, culture, and cytology. Radiographic studies, urodynamic studies, and cystoscopy are indicated in selected patients.[59] Systemic diseases affecting the innervation of the urogenital area, including multiple sclerosis, collagen diseases, and diabetes mellitus, have to be included in the differential diagnosis. In female patients a gynecologic examination is necessary to rule out symptoms that may be secondary to a gynecologic cause. As in other chronic pain syndromes, a psychological evaluation should be part of the multidisciplinary evaluation to rule out a psychogenic etiology and to assess for symptoms of depression associated with the chronic pain problem.

Various invasive and medical treatment options have been suggested for patients with urethral syndrome[59]; most are anecdotal clinical reports, and controlled clinical studies are urgently needed to assess which approach might be most successful for this painful disorder. Endoscopic and open surgical procedures have been suggested to eliminate a presumed urethral stenosis. Fulguration, scarification, resection, or cryosurgery has been considered to obliterate cystoscopically apparent urethritis. Bladder instillations with a variety of anti-inflammatory or cauterizing agents and systemic therapy with anticholinergics, α-adrenergic blockers, and muscle relaxants have been advocated. High rates of success were found with skeletal muscle relaxants or electrostimulation combined with biofeedback techniques.[51,58] Realizing the different surgical and nonsurgical treatment options discussed in the literature, a conservative treatment approach has been recommended as the first choice, because this usually is as effective as surgery, less expensive, and, most importantly, less subject to risk.[54,60]

Testicular Pain

Similar to women who suffer from pain syndromes of the reproductive organs, men with chronic testicular pain are usually embarrassed to talk about it, and often wonder if they have a hidden sexual aversion that presents itself as a pain syndrome in the genital region. Many patients cannot recall any precipitating event that led to the onset of the chronic pain syndrome. Secondary causes of chronic testicular pain include infection, tumor, testicular torsion, varicocele, hydrocele, spermatocele, trauma (bicycle accident), and previous surgical interventions.[61,62] The differential diagnosis includes referred pain from the ureter or the hip or lumbar facet joints and entrapment neuropathies of the ilioinguinal or genitofemoral nerve. Chronic testicular pain has been reported as a complication of vasectomy.[63] This chronic genital pain syndrome is usually not associated with erectile or ejaculatory dysfunction.[61]

A careful history, physical examination, and urologic evaluation reveal most secondary causes of chronic testicular pain. In selected patients, a gastroenterologic evaluation might be indicated to rule out referred pain from the lower pelvic organs or herniography to evaluate for an occult hernia. The neurologic evaluation is directed toward the lumbosacral roots, the ilioinguinal, genitofemoral, and pudendal nerves, and the autonomic nerve supply to the testis. In many cases, however, the pain remains unexplained despite a very thorough diagnostic workup. Treatment of chronic testicular pain is directed toward the underlying etiology, if an underlying etiology can be identified. A hydrocele, varicocele, or spermatocele rarely is the cause of chronic testicular pain, but rather is a coincidental finding.[64]

Traditionally, pain management for chronic testicular pain in the urology clinics consisted of a trial of antibiotics and nonsteroidal anti-inflammatory drugs (NSAIDs), with the aim of treating a possible occult inflammatory process. Case reports suggest that medical management, including medications used for other chronic pain syndromes such as low-dose antidepressants, anticonvulsants, membrane-stabilizing agents, and opiates, often are effective for treatment of chronic testicular pain[62,65,66]; however, no placebo-controlled studies have been published yet. Transcutaneous electrical nerve stimulation (TENS) might be helpful.[65] Repeated lumbar sympathetic blocks with local anesthetic and oral sympatholytic drugs have been reported to result in marked pain relief in selected patients in whom a sympathetic component is suspected in the maintenance of chronic testicular pain.[67] In the past, drastic surgical procedures have been recommended for the treatment of chronic testicular pain, such as epididymectomy and orchiectomy. As an alternative to surgical removal of these organs, microsurgical denervation has been suggested.[68]

Prostatitis and Prostatodynia

"Prostatitis" is a diagnosis that is often given to patients presenting with unexplained symptoms or condition that might possibly originate from the prostate gland.[69] In the United States, approximately 25% of men presenting with genitourinary tract problems are diagnosed with prostatitis.[70,71] Drach and colleagues[72] defined four categories of prostatitis: (1) acute bacterial prostatitis, (2) chronic bacterial prostatitis, (3) nonbacterial prostatitis (including nonbacterial infections, allergic and autoimmune prostatitis), and (4) prostatodynia. Prostatodynia is defined as persistent complaints of urinary urgency, dysuria, poor urinary flow, and perineal discomfort and pain, without evidence of bacteria or purulence in the prostatic fluid.[72] In addition to the perineal pain, patients often report that the pain is radiating to the lower back, suprapubic area, and groin. In contrast to patients with chronic testicular pain, patients with prostatodynia often complain about pain with ejaculation. Prostatodynia accounts for approximately 30% of patients presenting with prostatitis, the age range is from 20 to 60 years of age.[73,74]

Physical examination of the prostate is typically normal, without any signs of tenderness. A thorough urologic evaluation is indicated, including urinalysis, urine culture, urine cytology, and urethral cultures.[75] Referred pain from the colon or rectum needs to be ruled out. Prostatodynia is a diagnosis of exclusion, in which it is assumed that the chronic pain syndrome is related to the prostate, but no inflammatory prostatic process can be identified.

The most frequently advocated treatment is antibiotics despite the fact that usually no infectious etiology can be found. The urodynamic abnormalities observed in some patients with prostatodynia suggest that there is increased sympathetic tone. Oral α-adrenergic blockers have been shown to improve the voiding abnormalities as well as pain; however, their use is often limited by side effects, most frequently hypotension.[76] It has been suggested that there is an increase in pelvic floor muscle tone in patients presenting with prostatodynia, and pelvic floor relaxation techniques and muscle-relaxing agents have been reported to result in marked improvement of the symptomatology.[77]

Coccygodynia

Pain localized to the coccyx is a common perineal pain syndrome. The term coccygodynia was first used by Simpson[78] to describe a chronic pain syndrome characterized by tenderness and pain in the area of the coccyx, most severe with sitting. This chronic pain syndrome occurs more frequently in women and among elderly debilitated patients.[79,80] Some patients can remember a history of acute trauma to the coccyx, either a fall in the sitting position or birth trauma. Chronic trauma to the coccyx might result from poor sitting positions in which continued pressure occurs on the coccyx. Although one series related 70% of all cases of coccygodynia to a traumatic etiology,[81] others have suggested that trauma is an unlikely cause of coccygodynia, and instead a rheumatic etiology should be considered.[82]

On physical examination the coccyx is usually tender on palpation. Because pain can be referred to the coccyx from the lumbosacral spine, sacrum, anus, rectum, pelvis, and genitourinary tract, a thorough history is important, including questions regarding a precipitating cause. It is important to evaluate for anal fissures, hemorrhoids, anorectal or gynecologic infections, or rare causes such as space-occupying lesions, including tumors. As in many other perineal pain syndromes, despite a thorough evaluation, no cause can be found in many patients with coccygodynia.

The first step in the treatment of coccygodynia is protection of the painful coccyx from further irritation by sitting in such a position that no pressure occurs on the coccyx.[80] This measure alone often results in significant pain improvement after a few weeks. Physical therapy interventions, including hot sitz bath, pelvic relaxation techniques, and pelvic massage, have been reported to result in pain relief.[77,83] Local infiltrations with local anesthetic of the painful area, coccygeal nerve blocks, and caudal injections with local anesthetic, alone or in combination with corticosteroids, often are helpful.[83,84] Wray and coworkers[84] reported that manipulations of the coccyx under anesthesia resulted in marked pain relief. In these manipulations, the coccyx is repeatedly flexed and extended with the aim of stretching ligaments so that the ordinary ranges of motion were no longer painful. In patients with intractable pain who experience significant temporary pain relief with caudal local anesthetic injections, cryoanalgesia of the posterior rami of the lower sacral nerve roots and the coccygeal nerve should be considered.[85] Surgical removal of the coccyx, the treatment of choice during the nineteenth and early twentieth centuries, is rarely necessary today because conservative measures are usually sufficient.[80,84] In selected patients whose pain is clearly related to the coccyx and in whom conservative measures have failed, coccygectomy is indicated and has a high success rate.[84,86] However, before considering this irreversible surgical procedure, it is important to make use of conservative measures first. Importantly, Wray and coworkers[84] reported a 20% relapse rate in patients who had initial pain relief with conservative measures; however, repeat therapy was usually effective in providing permanent pain relief.

Rectal Pain

Pain in the rectal-anal area can occur as constant pain—proctodynia—or as paroxysms of pain—proctalgia fugax.

Proctodynia is often caused by local disease of the anus or rectum or it can be referred from the urogenital tract or the lumbosacral spine. A comprehensive workup is indicated, because in most cases of proctodynia—in contrast to many of the other perineal pain syndromes—the underlying etiology can be found. Intractable rectal pain has been associated with pudendal neuralgia in 24% of the cases in one study, and has been treated successfully with neuropathic pain medications.[87] A pudendal nerve block with local anesthetic might be helpful to assess the contribution of the pudendal nerve to the chronic pain syndrome. Chronic idiopathic anal pain has been associated with abnormal anorectal manometric profiles, probably resulting from a dysfunction of the striated external anal sphincter. Biofeedback training has been shown to be effective in these cases.[88]

Proctalgia fugax is characterized by sudden attacks of intense pain of short duration in the region of the internal anal sphincter and the anorectal ring. The incidence of proctalgia fugax has been reported to be as high as 14% in the general population, and as high as 33% in patients with gastrointestinal disease.[89,90] Familial forms of proctalgia fugax have been described, and it is important to take a family history. The immediate cause of proctalgia fugax seems to be muscle spasms, but the etiology of this syndrome remains unclear.[91] A consistent phenomenon in all studies seems to be gastrointestinal smooth muscle dysfunction. In the majority of patients with proctalgia fugax, the physical examination is normal, and common anorectal diseases such as hemorrhoids and anal fissures seem to be unrelated to the paroxysmal pain problem, in contrast to patients with constant rectal pain—proctodynia.

Simple and effective remedies have been suggested to end the acute pain attack associated with proctalgia fugax: immediate taking of food or drink, dilation of the anorectum (by digital dilation, attempting a bowel movement or inserting a tap-water enema), hot sitz baths, and firm pressure to the perineum.[92–94] A variety of drugs has been suggested in anecdotal reports: antispasmodics, nitroglycerin, nifedipine, carbamazepine, diltiazem, and salbutamol (reviewed in ref. 43). Eckhardt and colleagues[95] showed in a controlled crossover trial that salbutamol inhalation significantly shortened the duration of the severe pain. Because this is an easy-to-use medication during the acute attack, and given that this is the only controlled study on medications for proctalgia fugax, salbutamol should be the first choice, if a decision is made to use medications to abort pain attacks. It is important to reassure the patient that the symptoms, although quite troublesome (the pain often reaches an intensity of 10/10 on a Visual Analog Scale) are not signs of a life-threatening disease and may improve with time. Psychological assessment is important to rule out a depressive symptomatology contributing to the chronic pain syndrome.

Generalized Perineal Pain

Perineal pain can be localized to a specific area of the perineum, as previously discussed. In some cases, the perineal pain syndrome starts at a specific area and over time extends over the whole perineum. In other cases, perineal pain starts as a diffuse discomfort involving, from the beginning, most of the perineum and gradually increasing in intensity—this is a chronic generalized perineal pain syndrome.

The differential diagnosis is complex: gastrointestinal, proctologic, urologic, gynecologic, and neurologic etiologies have to be excluded. Systemic diseases associated with painful peripheral neuropathies, such as diabetes mellitus and acquired immunodeficiency syndrome (AIDS), have to be considered. French studies have reported a diagnosis of pudendal nerve entrapment in 91% of patients with perineal pain referred to a pain clinic.

Surgical neurolysis-transposition was recommended as the treatment of choice, with best results obtained in patients in whom pudendal nerve entrapment was diagnosed early.[96,97] In patients presenting with perineal pain and sacral meningeal cysts (Tarlov cysts), surgical resection of the cysts has been reported to result in excellent pain relief in the majority of the patients.[98] Perineal pain has been reported in the context of movement disorders. Chronic perineal pain occurred as a complication of neuroleptic drug exposure. Catecholamine depletors resulted in complete resolution of the painful sensations.[99] In addition, chronic perineal pain has been reported in the context of Parkinson's disease, and excellent pain relief was achieved using medications regularly used for Parkinson's disease.[100]

PSYCHOLOGICAL ASPECTS OF CHRONIC PERINEAL PAIN

The literature examining psychological factors in chronic perineal pain has been reviewed in detail.[43] As with other chronic pain syndromes, in the absence of obvious organic pathology, many etiologies regarding a purely psychogenic origin of perineal pain have been entertained. Many of these studies have neglected to examine whether the psychological findings were likely to be preexisting or reactive. It would not be surprising, or necessarily indicative of psychopathology, if a patient with a chronic perineal pain syndrome was depressed. The critical issue is whether this patient was depressed before the chronic pain syndrome started, and whether his or her mood returned to normal after successful therapy for the chronic pain syndrome.

It is important that health care providers treating patients with chronic perineal pain realize that these patients are often embarrassed to talk about their chronic pain syndrome. In addition, they often are afraid of being labeled as not really suffering from a pain syndrome but having a psychosomatic or psychiatric illness, or being hypochondriacs. They also may be afraid that conclusions about their sexual life will be drawn (because the genitalia are either directly affected by the chronic pain syndrome or are close to the painful area), which might further isolate them. The difficulties that many of these patients have in talking about their chronic perineal pain syndrome becomes more obvious if one thinks about two situations in which a patient is in so much pain that he or she cannot come to work: in the first scenario, someone takes a day off from work, telling coworkers that he or she has really bad back pain, in the second scenario, a patient has to take sick leave because of an exacerbation of chronic perineal pain. The patient with perineal pain might invent an excuse, a more legitimate and accepted disease, to prevent any gossip among the coworkers.

Location of pain may be a significant predictor for appraisals of pain and disclosure of pain complaints. Klonoff and colleagues[101] demonstrated that subjects asked to imagine pain in their genitals appraised themselves as more ill than if they were asked to imagine chest, stomach, head, and mouth pain. Further, subjects reported that they would be least likely to disclose genital pain and would be more worried, depressed, and embarrassed by pain in the genitals than in all other areas of the body.

SUMMARY

Although the chronic perineal pain syndromes discussed in this chapter are quite frequent and some were described in detail more than 100 years ago, many of the patients suffering from these pain syndromes do not receive adequate pain management, and some patients do not receive any pain treatment at all. In many cases, the focus is on finding and possibly treating the underlying etiology, and patients go from physician to physician in different subspecialties, hearing after extensive evaluations that nothing abnormal can be found. However, the pain persists, and many patients who have suffered for many years from chronic perineal pain without finding a cure are quite frustrated and angry.

As a first step, it is important to acknowledge that these chronic perineal pain syndromes do exist, and that they are well-described but poorly understood. A thorough workup is mandatory, often including several medial subspecialties. Perineal pain can be a symptom of a malignant or nonmalignant disease, for which specific treatment is available, and the diagnosis of a chronic perineal pain syndrome is a diagnosis of exclusion.

In many patients who present with chronic perineal pain, the workup does not reveal any underlying pathology. In the future, novel treatment strategies might become available, targeted specifically against the pathophysiologic mechanisms of the chronic pain syndromes discussed here. Although these developments are still on the horizon, it is very important to realize what can be done now for patients who suffer from chronic perineal pain. Most currently available treatment options for these pain syndromes are empirical, only. Although these pain syndromes can rarely be cured, some pain relief can be provided to almost all patients using a multidisciplinary approach that includes pain medications (antidepressants, anticonvulsants, membrane-stabilizing agents, and opioids), local treatment regimens, nerve blocks, selected surgical procedures, physical therapy, and psychological support.

REFERENCES

1. Burnett AL, Wesselmann U. Neurobiology of the pelvis and perineum: Principles for a practical approach. *J Pelvic Surg* 1999;5:224–232.
2. De Groat WC, Booth AM, Yoshimura N. Neurophysiology of micturition and its modification in animal models of human disease. In: Maggi CA, ed. *Nervous Control of the Urogenital System*. Chur, Switzerland: Harwood Academic Pub; 1993:227–290.

3. De Groat WC. Neurophysiology of the pelvic organs. In: Rushton DN, ed. *Handbook of Neuro-Urology.* New York, NY: Marcel Dekker; 1994:55–93.
4. JÑnig W, Koltzenburg M. Pain arising from the urogenital tract. In Maggi CA, ed. *Nervous Control of the Urogenital System.* Chur, Switzerland: Harwood Academic Pub; 1993:525–578.
5. Elbadawi A. Functional anatomy of the organs of micturition. *Urol Clin North Am* 1996;23:177–210.
6. Matzel KE, Schmidt RA, Tanagho EA. Neuroanatomy of the striated muscular anal continence mechanism: Implications for the use of neurostimulation. *Dis Colon Rectum* 1990;33:666–673.
7. De Groat WC. Neuropeptides in pelvic afferent pathways. *Experientia* 1987;43:801–812.
8. Thomas TG. *Practical Treatise on the Diseases of Woman.* Philadelphia, Pa: Henry C Lea's Son; 1880:145–147.
9. Pozzi SJ. *Traite de gynecologie clinique et operatoire.* Paris, France: Masson; 1897.
10. McKay M. Burning vulva syndrome. *J Reprod Med* 1984;29:457.
11. McKay M. Vulvodynia. A multifactorial problem. *Arch Dermatol* 1989;125:256–262.
12. Laumann EO, Paik A, Rosen RC. Sexual dysfunction in the United States. Prevalence and Predictors. *JAMA* 1999;281:537–544.
13. Goetsch MF. Vulvar vestibulitis: Prevalence and historic features in a general gynecologic practice population. *Am J Obstet Gynecol* 1991; 164:1609–1616.
14. Mroczkowski TF. Vulvodynia—a dermatovenereologist's perspective. *Int J Dermatol* 1998;37:567–569.
15. Fischer G, Spurrett B, Fisher A. The chronically symptomatic vulva: Aetiology and management. *Brit J Obstet Gynaecol* 1995;102:773–779.
16. Paavonen J. Diagnosis and treatment of vulvodynia. *Ann Med* 1995; 27:175–181.
17. McKay M. Vulvodynia: Diagnostic patterns. *Dermatol Clin* 1992;10: 423–433.
18. McKay M. Vulvodynia. In: Steege JF, Metzger DA, Levy BS, eds. *Chronic Pelvic Pain.* Philadelphia, Pa: WB Saunders; 1998:188–196.
19. Ashman RB, Ott AK. Autoimmunity as a factor in recurrent vaginal candidosis and the minor vestibular gland syndrome. *J Reprod Med* 1989;4:264–266.
20. Scrimin F, Volpe C, Tracanzan G, et al. Vulvodynia and selective IgA deficiency. Case reports. *Brit J Obstet Gynecol* 1991;98:592–593.
21. McKay M. Subsets of vulvodynia. *J Reprod Med* 1988;33:695–698.
22. Marinoff SC, Turner MLC. Vulvar vestibulitis syndrome: An overview. *Am J Obstet Gynecol* 1991;165:1228–1233.
23. Kelly HA. *Gynecology.* New York, NY: Appleton and Co; 1928:236.
24. Chada S, Gianotten WL, Drogendijk AC, et al. Histopathological features of vulvar vestibulitis. *Int J Gynecol Path* 1998;17:7–11.
25. De Deus JM, Focchi J, Stavale JN, et al. Histologic and biomolecular aspects of papillomatosis of the vulvar vestibule in relation to human papillomavirus. *Obstet Gynecol* 1995;86:758–763.
26. Marks TA, Shroyer KR, Markham NE, et al. A clinical, histological, and DNA study of vulvodynia and its association with papillomavirus. *J Soc Gynecol Invest* 1995;2:57–63.
27. Bornstein J, Shapiro S, Goldshmid N, et al. Severe vulvar vestibulitis, relation to HPV infection. *J Reprod Med* 1997;42:514–518.
28. Bornstein J, Shapiro S, Rahat M, et al. Polymerase chain reaction search for viral etiology of vulvar vestibulitis syndrome. *Am J Obstet Gynecol* 1996;175:139–144.
29. Bohm-Starke N, Hilliges M, Falconer C, et al. Increased intraepithelial innervation in women with vulvar vestibulitis syndrome. *Gynecol Obstet Invest* 1998;46:256–260.
30. Westrom LV, Willen R. Vestibular nerve fiber proliferation in vulvar vestibulitis syndrome. *Obstet Gynecol* 1998;91:572–576.
31. Peckham BM, Maki DG, Patterson JJ, et al. Focal vulvitis: A characteristic syndrome and cause of dyspareunia. *Am J Obstet Gynecol* 1986;154:855–864.
32. Solomons CC, Melmed MH, Heitler SM. Calcium citrate for vulvar vestibulitis. *J Reprod Med* 1991;36:879–882.
33. Melmed MH. A low oxalate diet and calcium citrate administration are effective treatment for vulvar pain syndrome (vestibulitis). *J Gynecol Surg* 1996;12:217.
34. Baggish MS, Sze EHM, Johnson R. Urinary oxalate excretion and its role in vulvar pain syndrome. *Am J Obstet Gynecol* 1997;177:507–511.
35. Glazer HI, Rodke G, Swencionis C, et al. Treatment of vulvar vestibulitis syndrome with electromyographic biofeedback of pelvic floor musculature. *J Reprod Med* 1995;40:283–290.
36. Goetsch MF. Simplified surgical revision of the vulvar vestibule for vulvar vestibulitis. *Am J Obstet Gynecol* 1996;174:1701–1707.
37. Marinoff SC, Turner ML, Hirsch RP, et al. Intralesional alpha interferon cost effective therapy for vulvar vestibulitis syndrome. *J Reprod Med* 1993;38:19–24.
38. Petersen CS, Weismann K. Isoprinosine improves symptoms in young females with chronic vulvodynia. *Acta Derm Venereol* 1996;76:404.
39. Woodruff JD, Foster DC. The vulvar vestibule. *Postgrad Obstet Gynecol* 1991;11:1–5.
40. McKay M. Dysesthetic ("essential") vulvodynia, treatment with amitriptyline. *J Reprod Med* 1993;38:9–13.
41. Bornstein J, Zarfati D, Goldshmid N, et al. Vestibulodynia—a subset of vulvar vestibulitis or a novel syndrome. *Am J Obstet Gynecol* 1997; 177:1439–1443.
42. Sonni L, Cattaneo A, De Marco A, et al. Idiopathic vulvodynia: Clinical evaluation of the pain threshold with acetic acid solutions. *J Reprod Med* 1995;40:337–341.
43. Wesselmann U, Burnett AL, Heinberg LJ. The urogenital and rectal pain syndromes. *Pain* 1997;73:269–294.
44. Bornstein J, Isakov D, Fisher M, et al. The burning vulva. *Israel J Obstet Gynecol* 1993;4:23–27.
45. Rageth JC, Buerklen A, Hirsch HA. Spätkomplikationen nach Episiotomie. *Zeitsch Geburt Perinat* 1989;193:233–237.
46. Dirie MA, Lindmark G. The risk of medical complications after female circumcision. *East Afric Med J* 1992;69:479–482.
47. Hanly MG, Ojeda VJ. Epidermic inclusion cysts of the clitoris as a complication of female circumcision and pharaonic infibulation. *Cent Afric J Med* 1995;41:22–24.
48. Briggs LA. Female circumcision in Nigeria—is it not time for government intervention? *Health Care Anal* 1998;6:14–23.
49. Gallagher DJA, Montgomerie JZ, North JDK. Acute infections of the urinary tract and the urethral syndrome in general practice. *BMJ* 1965;1:622–626.
50. Peters-Gee JM. Bladder and urethral syndromes. In: Steege JF, Metzger DA, Levy BS, eds. *Chronic Pelvic Pain.* Philadelphia, Pa: WB Saunders; 1998:197–204.
51. Kaplan WE, Firlit CF, Schoenberg HW. The female urethral syndrome: External sphincter spasm as etiology. *J Urol* 1980;124:48–49.
52. Barbalias GA. Prostatodynia or painful male urethral syndrome? *Urology* 1990;36:146–153.
53. Zufall R. Ineffectiveness of treatment of urethral syndrome in women. *Urology* 1978;12:337–339.
54. Carson CC, Segura JW, Osborne DM. Evaluation and treatment of the female urethral syndrome. *J Urol* 1980;124:609–610.
55. Bergman A, Karram M, Bhatia NN. Urethral syndrome: A comparison of different treatment modalities. *J Rep Med* 1989;34:157–160.
56. Sand PK, Bowen LW, Ostergard DR, et al. Cryosurgery versus dilation and massage for treatment of recurrent urethral syndrome. *J Reprod Med* 1989;34:499–504.
57. Mabry EW, Carson CC, Older RA. Evaluation of women with chronic voiding discomfort. *Urology* 1981;18:244–246.
58. Schmidt RA, Tanagho EA. Urethral syndrome or urinary tract infection? *Urology* 1981;18:424–427.
59. Messinger EM. Urethral syndrome. In: Walsh PC, Retik AB, Stanley TA, Vaughan EDJ, eds. *Campbell's Urology.* 6th ed. Philadelphia, Pa: WB Saunders; 1992:997–1005.

60. Bodner DR. The urethral syndrome. *Urol Clin North Am* 1988;15: 699–704.
61. Davis BE, Noble MJ, Weigel JW, et al. Analysis and management of chronic testicular pain. *J Urol* 1990;143:936–939.
62. Costabile RA, Hahn M, McLeod DG. Chronic orchialgia in the pain prone patient: The clinical perspective. *Am Urol Assoc* 1991;146: 1571–1574.
63. McMahon AJ, Buckley J, Taylor A, et al. Chronic testicular pain following vasectomy. *Br J Urol* 1992;69:188–191.
64. Holland JM, Feldman JL, Gilbert HC. Phantom orchalgia. *J Urol* 1994;152:2291–2293.
65. Hayden LJ. Chronic testicular pain. *Austral Fam Phys* 1993;22: 1357–1365.
66. Wesselmann U, Burnett AL. Treatment of neuropathic testicular pain. *Neurology* 1996;46(suppl):206.
67. Wesselmann U, Burnett AL, Campbell JN. The role of the sympathetic nervous system in chronic visceral pain. *Soc Neurosci Abstr* 1995;21:1157.
68. Levine LA, Matkov TG, Lubenow TR. Microsurgical denervation of the spermatic cord: A surgical alternative in the treatment of chronic orchialgia. *J Urol* 1996;155:1005–1007.
69. Nickel JC. Prostatitis—Myths and realities. *Urology* 1998;51:363–366.
70. Lipsky BA. Urinary tract infections in men. *Ann Int Med* 1989; 110:138.
71. Meares EMJ. Prostatitis and related disorders. In: Walsh PC, Retik AB, Stanley TA, Vaughan EDJ, eds. *Campbell's Urology.* 6th ed. Philadelphia, Pa: WB Saunders; 1992:807–822.
72. Drach GW, Fair WR, Meares EM, et al. Classification of benign diseases associated with prostatic pain: Prostatitis or prostatodynia? *J Urol* 1978;120:266.
73. Brunner H, Weidner W, Schiefer HC. Studies on the role of Ureaplasma urealyticum and Mycoplasma hominis in prostatitis. *J Infect Dis* 1983;126:807–813.
74. Moul JW: Prostatitis: Sorting out the different causes. *Postgrad Med* 1993;94:191–194.
75. de la Rosette JJMCH, Hubregtse MR, Karhaus HFM, et al. Results of a questionnaire among Dutch urologists and general practitioners concerning diagnostics and treatment of patients with prostatitis syndrome. *Eur Urol* 1992;22:14–19.
76. Barbalias GA, Nikiforidis G, Liatsikos EN. Alpha-blockers for the treatment of chronic prostatitis in combination with antibiotics. *J Urol* 1998;159:883–887.
77. Segura JW, Opitz JL, Greene LF. Prostatosis, prostatitis or pelvic floor tension myalgia? *J Urol* 1979;122:168–169.
78. Simpson JY. Coccygodynia and diseases and deformities of the coccyx. *Med Times Gazette* 1859;861:1.
79. Stern FH. Coccygodynia among the geriatric population. *J Am Geriat Soc* 1967;15:100–102.
80. Johnson PH. Coccygodynia. *J Ark Med Soc* 1981;77:421–424.
81. Torok G. Coccygodynia. *J Bone Joint Surg Br* 1974;56B:386–392.
82. Nutz V, Stelzner F. Der Glomustumor als Ursache einer Coccygodynie. *Chirurg* 1985;56:243–246.
83. Bonica JJ. Pelvic and perineal pain caused by other disorders. In: Bonica JJ, ed. *The Management of Pain.* 2nd ed. Philadelphia, Pa: Lea and Febiger; 1990:1384–1385.
84. Wray CC, Easom S, Hoskinson J. Coccydynia: aetiology and treatment. *J Bone Joint Surg Br* 1991;73B:335–338.
85. Evans PJD, Lloyd JW, Jack TM. Cryoanalgesia for intractable perineal pain. *J Royal Soc Med* 1981;74:804–806.
86. Grosso NP, van Dam BE. Total coccygectomy for the relief of coccygodynia: A retrospective review. *J Spinal Disord* 1995;8:328–330.
87. Ger, GH, Wexner SD, Jorge JM. Evaluation and treatment of chronic intractable rectal pain—a frustrating endeavor. *Dis Colon Rectum* 1993;36:139–145.
88. Grimaud JC, Bouvier M, Naudy B. Manometric and radiologic investigations and biofeedback treatment of chronic idiopathic anal pain. *Dis Colon Rectum* 1991;38:690–695.
89. Thompson WG, Heaton KW. Proctalgia fugax. *J Royal Coll Phys (Lond)* 1980;14:247–248.
90. Thompson WG. Proctalgia fugax in patients with the irritable bowel, peptic ulcer, or inflammatory bowel disease. *Am J Gastroenterol* 1984; 79:450–452.
91. Karras JD, Angelo G. Proctalgia fugax. *Am J Surg* 1951;82:616–625.
92. Ewing MR. Proctalgia fugax. *BMJ* 1953;9:1083–1085.
93. Penny RW. The doctor's disease: Proctalgia fugax. *Practitioner* 1970; 204:843–845.
94. Rockefeller R. Digital dilatation for relief of proctalgia fugax. *Am Fam Phys* 1996;54:72.
95. Eckhardt VF, Dodt O, Kanzler G, et al. Treatment of proctalgia fugax with salbutamol inhalations. *Am J Gastroenterol* 1996;91:686–689.
96. Robert R, Brunet C, Faure A, et al. La chirurgie du nerf pudental lors de certaines algies perineales: Evolution et resultats. *Chirurgie* 1993; 119:535–539.
97. Bensignor MF, Labat JJ, Robert R, et al. Diagnostic and therapeutic pudendal nerve blocks for patients with perineal non-malignant pain. Abstract presented at the 8th World Congress on Pain; Vancouver, Canada. 1996:56.
98. Van de Kleft E, Van Vyve M. Sacral meningeal cysts and perineal pain. *Lancet* 1993;341:500–501.
99. Ford B, Greene P, Fahn S. Oral and genital tardive pain syndromes. *Neurology* 1994;44:2115–2119.
100. Ford B, Louis E D, Greene P, et al. Oral and genital pain syndromes in Parkinson's disease. *Mov Disord* 1996;11:421–426.
101. Klonoff E A, Landrine H, Brown M. Appraisal and response to pain may be a function of its bodily location. *J Psychosomatic Res* 1993; 37:661–670.

PART V

PAIN SYNDROMES

CHAPTER 37 POLYNEUROPATHY

Elizabeth M. Raynor and Galit Kleiner-Fisman

Painful polyneuropathy is a debilitating neurologic problem and frequently a challenging therapeutic management issue. Difficulties in managing patients are too often the result of poor understanding of their problem on the part of the treating physician. Many physicians assume that there is no need to work up neuropathy because the final outcome is likely to be an idiopathic, axonal disorder for which there is no effective therapy. In fact, many neuropathies are responsive to immunosuppressive therapies. Although responses to such therapy constitute the minority, they should be vigorously sought before telling patients there is no treatment for their progressive disorder. In many cases, treatment of the polyneuropathy also leads to improved pain control; however, pain is often a primary issue in and of itself and must be treated irrespective of the potential for improvement of the underlying polyneuropathy. In these cases, pain management specialists may work in concert with neurologists to provide a comprehensive treatment approach.

CLINICAL ISSUES IN POLYNEUROPATHY

Introduction

The first step in developing a rational approach to patient management is obtaining a working knowledge of the underlying disorders that fall under the category of neuropathy. Although it is often used loosely to refer to polyneuropathy, the term *neuropathy* is actually not specific and implies any peripheral nerve lesion, focal or diffuse. Classification schemes used widely among peripheral neurologists are based on anatomic and physiologic characteristics of the various disorders affecting peripheral nerves. The use of these classifications is not just an academic exercise but creates a basis for rational decision making in the evaluation and management of patients. The workup and treatment of individual patients with neuropathy must be approached with a basic understanding of the clinical behavior, including the anatomic and pathophysiologic characteristics, of the various neuropathic disorders.

Classification and Clinical Course

The term *polyneuropathy* is used to describe a condition that is fairly symmetric and generalized, as opposed to focal neuropathy (mononeuropathy) or multifocal neuropathy (mononeuropathy multiplex). This chapter focuses on the diffuse disorders, including polyneuropathy and multifocal mononeuropathies. These two groups of disorders may be indistinguishable clinically and are frequently accompanied by severe and disabling pain.

Once a disorder of peripheral nerves is suspected, an attempt should be made to characterize the clinical features based on the time course, anatomic distribution, and physiology. Using this information, a reasonable differential diagnosis can be developed, which will determine appropriate further workup and management. This section further discusses the clinical and physiologic features of the diffuse neuropathies; their diagnostic evaluation is covered in the next section.

Polyneuropathy

Time Course An important clue as to the etiology of a particular polyneuropathy (PN) is its time course. Generally accepted guidelines would classify a neuropathy as acute (< 3 weeks), subacute (weeks to months), or chronic (> 4–6 months). Notably, neuropathies in each of these categories may be associated with debilitating pain. The typical clinic patient presenting with chronic, insidious PN is probably the most easily diagnosed; the more acute neuropathies may be difficult to differentiate from central nervous system disease, particularly spinal cord compression.

Fiber Type and Distribution PN may involve motor, sensory, or autonomic fibers. There is a tendency in some neuropathies for selective involvement of fibers of the same general size distribution. Thus, a neuropathy may involve predominantly large-diameter sensory fibers (mediating vibration and proprioception) in addition to intermediate-sized motor fibers. Conversely, PN may primarily involve small-diameter sensory fibers (mediating pain and temperature) with or without involvement of autonomic fibers. Typically, pain is a prominent feature of these so-called small fiber neuropathies. Certainly, a neuropathy may be generalized in terms of the fiber type involvement (as commonly seen in diabetes); however, careful examination often reveals a predominance of one group of fibers over another.

Pathophysiology A detailed description of the pathophysiologic mechanisms underlying PN in various disorders is beyond the scope of this chapter; instead, we focus on the relevant clinical-pathologic correlates as well as the electrodiagnostic characteristics of the different neuropathies, depending on the primary site of pathologic change.

The two primary sites of pathologic involvement in neuropathy are the axon and the myelin sheath, or Schwann cell; the former being more common in PN. In general, in axonopathies, the longest and larger diameter fibers tend to be involved first, with degeneration originating in distal portions of individual axons and proceeding proximally. This creates a length-dependent pattern, which can be demonstrated both clinically and electrophysiologically. This generalized "dying-back" is theorized to result from metabolic derangement in the cell bodies or diffusely within axons. Axonopathies tend to be quite symmetric in terms of side-to-side involvement, a feature that distinguishes them from the multiple mononeuropathies. These are the most common type of PN; almost all toxic and metabolic insults to the peripheral nervous system result in axonal degeneration.

Less frequently, the axon is largely spared and demyelination is the primary pathologic change. Although myelinopathies may be the result of abnormal Schwann cell development or metabolism, these situations are rare and the most frequent clinical situation is one in which segmental demyelination, or loss of myelin between the nodes of Ranvier, occurs. Segmental demyelination usually is the result of an autoimmune attack on peripheral nerves and nerve roots (as in Guillain-Barré syndrome), with the clinical pattern being somewhat variable; the limbs are involved proximally as well as distally, although usually fairly symmetrically side-to-side.

Etiology and Prognosis Tables 37-1 and 37-2 list the most common causes of PN, based on their physiology (axonal versus demyelinating) and time course.

Although the clinical course of various neuropathies is highly variable, depending on etiology, there are a few generalizable rules regarding prognosis. Any disorder involving significant axonal injury will be less likely to recover than one in which the primary physiology is segmental demyelination. Thus, the differentiation between these two is of practical importance for the clinician. In a disorder characterized purely by the latter, recovery occurs by remyelination and usually occurs over 6 to 8 weeks. In generalized neuropathies, even of primary demyelinating type (e.g., Guillain-Barré syndrome), there is nearly always some accompanying axonal injury and, ultimately, prognosis is dependent on its severity. Thus, recovery may be complete but take months or even years.

In primary axonal neuropathies, the prognosis is dependent on the nature and severity of the axonal injury. For example, in typical mononeuropathy multiplex, in which nerve injury results from ischemic insult, recovery occurs largely through axonal regrowth. Individual regrowth of axons occurs from the proximal nerve stump, at a rate of about 1 inch per month. This form of recovery is very slow and nearly always incomplete. In neuropathies characterized by a dying-back type of physiologic change, there usually is very little regrowth of individual axons. Instead, functional recovery occurs through reinnervation of muscle fibers by nearby healthy axons, a mechanism that probably only limits the severity of the deficit related to axonal loss, rather than allowing any improvement in function.

TABLE 37-1 **Axonal Polyneuropathy—Common Etiologies**

Acute/Subacute	Chronic
Toxins (see acute/subacute)	Toxins (see acute/subacute)
Drugs (see Table 35-6)	Metabolic disorders
Alcohol	(see also acute/subacute)
Lead	Hypothyroidism
Arsenic	Acromegaly
Thallium	Chronic liver disease
Organophosphates	Autoimmune disorder
Pyridoxine (vitamin B_6)	Lupus
Overdose	Rheumatoid arthritis
Acrylamide	Sarcoidosis
	Sjögren's syndrome
Metabolic disorders	
Diabetes	Paraneoplastic (see also acute/subacute)
Uremia	Multiple myeloma
Porphyria	Paraproteinemia
Nutritional/deficiency	Inherited (Charcot-Marie Tooth, type II)
Malabsorption	Lyme disease
Amyloidosis	HIV-related
Paraneoplastic (rare)	
Carcinoma	
Lymphoma	
Guillain-Barré syndrome, axonal form	
Lyme disease	
Cryoglobulinemia	

HIV, human immunodeficiency syndrome.

TABLE 37-2 **Demyelinating Polyneuropathy—Common Etiologies**

Acute/Subacute	Chronic
Guillain-Barré syndrome	Chronic inflammatory demyelinating polyneuropathy (CIDP)
Diphtheria (rare)	
Multifocal motor neuropathy with conduction block (MMNCB)	Metabolic disorders
	Diabetes mellitus
	Uremia
	Hypothyroidism
	Myeloma (osteosclerotic)
	Paraproteinemia
	Cryoglobulinemia
	Hepatitis C
	Inherited (Charcot-Marie Tooth and others)

Mononeuropathy Multiplex

Clinical Course Mononeuropathy multiplex (MM) is a diffuse neuropathic disorder, similar to PN, but it is distinguished by involvement of multiple individual nerves. MM may be impossible to distinguish from PN based on history and examination alone, as the cumulative involvement of multiple nerves can produce a generalized and fairly symmetric picture. A high index of suspicion for MM is important in the appropriate clinical setting. MM is almost invariably the result of ischemic insult to nerves, the most common etiology being small- and medium-vessel vasculitis. MM occurs in the majority of cases of systemic vasculitis and may be its presenting symptom; in rare cases, vasculitis is restricted to the peripheral nervous system (nonsystemic vasculitic neuropathy).[1]

Regardless of etiology, MM typically presents with the acute onset of severe pain and numbness in the involved limb; motor and sensory deficit develop over days. Nerves that are often involved early are those at so-called watershed zones of the vascular tree (e.g., the sciatic nerve in the thigh, the ulnar nerve in the forearm). Progression to other nerves eventually produces a picture suggestive of severe, axonal PN; the progression may be subacute or, rarely, chronic. In all cases, pain remains a prominent feature of the disorder.

TABLE 37-3 **Mononeuropathy Multiplex—Common Etiologies**

Vasculitis
Polyarteritis nodosa
Rheumatoid arthritis
HIV-associated
Diabetes
Sarcoidosis
Lyme disease
Leprosy (rare in United States)

HIV, human immunodeficiency syndrome.

The prognosis is dependent on the underlying etiology of the MM. In vasculitic neuropathy, aggressive treatment of the underlying disease is aimed at preventing further ischemia. Recovery of existing lesions occurs by means of axonal regrowth, at a pace of about 1 inch per month from the site of the injury. An aggressive therapeutic approach to pain is appropriate, particularly early in the course of the disorder, when immunosuppressive therapy has not reached maximum effectiveness. Over time, if the vasculitis can be adequately treated, it may be possible to reduce or withdraw pain therapies.

Etiology Table 37-3 lists the most common etiologies of MM, based on time course.

Diagnostic Evaluation

History and Physical Examination

History The first step in the diagnostic evaluation of any neuropathy is the history and physical examination of the patient. Several important historical points should be reviewed. One should determine the time course of the illness—acute, subacute, or chronic. Next, involvement of nerve fiber types should be ascertained—sensory, motor, and autonomic, with regard to both *positive* and *negative* symptoms. Specific inquiry should be made regarding the presence or absence of pain. Positive symptoms refer to abnormal spontaneous sensory or motor phenomena (e.g., pins and needles, fasciculations), whereas negative symptoms describe a loss of function (e.g., weakness, numbness). Inquiry should be made regarding the symptom distribution and symmetry (i.e., stocking glove versus individual nerve territories), as well as the progression (i.e., slow and insidious versus acute-onset deficits with plateaus). Finally, one should obtain a family history, with an eye to excluding a congenital form of neuropathy.

Characteristic features of neuropathic pain are useful in differentiating it from pain from any other source. It is vital that these symptoms and signs are sought during the history and physical examination as they are often primary evidence for a diagnosis of PN. In some neuropathies, such as those limited to involvement of small fibers, normal laboratory studies are the rule, and diagnosis is based on clinical grounds alone. The presence of positive symptoms is typical of the neuropathic disorders.

Positive symptoms that are typical of PN include (1) *paresthesias*—nonpainful, spontaneous sensory phenomena such as pins and needles or tingling; (2) *dysesthesias*—unpleasant spontaneous or evoked sensory phenomena such as burning; (3) *hyperesthesia*—increased sensitivity to stimuli, often with an unpleasant quality; (4) *allodynia*—pain created by a normally nonpainful stimulus, such as the bedcovers; and (5) *hyperpathia* or *hyperalgesia*—exaggerated pain response created by a normally painful stimulus.

The presence of these symptoms should be sought specifically, in addition to allowing the patient to describe the precise nature of his or her pain. Also, the effect of pain on quality of life and functional status is extremely important. Specific pain measures, such as the Neuropathic Pain Scale,[2] may be used to quantify the patient's pain as well as its effect on the quality of life. Such scales are particularly helpful for patients involved in clinical therapeutic trials and may be used to assess efficacy of treatment regimens outside of experimental trials.

Physical Examination The physical examination should be guided by the patient history. For example, the suggestion of asymmetric onset of symptoms should prompt a careful search for evidence of individual nerve involvement, as opposed to a stocking-glove distribution of sensory loss.

A complete neurologic examination is required. One cannot adequately localize the problem to the peripheral nerve without a careful physical examination to rule out myelopathy, polyradiculopathy, or myopathy, which may mimic or complicate PN. The details of the neurologic examination are not reviewed here, but a few points are worth emphasizing. The goal of the physical examination is to characterize the pattern, symmetry, and distribution of abnormalities and to determine which modalities are involved (motor, sensory, autonomic); the distribution with regard to fiber type should also be demonstrable. The typical pattern to look for is bilaterally symmetric, usually distally predominant. The proximal lower extremities tend to be involved before the distal upper extremities, although this is variable; the anterior thoracic region is often involved in more severe cases. However, there may be proximal predominance, and upper extremities may be involved disproportionately. In MM, the pattern is usually multiple nerve involvement, although it may likely be impossible to differentiate from PN, other than subtle asymmetry in an otherwise stocking-glove distribution. The deep tendon reflexes are part of the overall pattern, as well, and are typically reduced or absent in a distribution consistent with the underlying pathophysiology. For example, patients with distal axonopathies typically have absent ankle jerks, whereas those with chronic demyelinating neuropathies are areflexic.

In patients with painful positive symptoms, there often are correlative signs on the physical examination. Allodynia may be elicited by lightly stroking the involved area (mechanical stimulus) or by testing with a cold instrument (thermal stimulus). Hyperalgesia or hyperpathia may be elicited during pinprick testing. A single, painful stimulus may be reported as a sensory deficit, whereas repeated stimuli in the same area produce an exaggerated pain; this phenomenon is called *summation*.[3] Abnormal sensations may last for several seconds or minutes after discontinuation of the stimulus, a phenomenon called *after sensations*.[3] These examination findings are important, because they are unique to patients with neuropathic pain.

Clinical Neurophysiology

Electrophysiologic Studies The second logical step in the diagnostic evaluation is the electrodiagnostic examination, specifically, nerve conduction studies (NCS) and electromyography (EMG). The utility of these studies is several. Firstly, they usually clarify the diagnosis of PN. Although important, there is a limit to the localizing value of physical examination, even when carefully performed. For example, a detailed physical examination cannot differentiate multiple root involvement from PN or MM in most cases; coexisting neurologic problems may also significantly alter the physical examination. It is important to note that NCS cannot assess the integrity of small-diameter sensory fibers (i.e., those mediating pain and temperature) and so will be normal in patients with pure small-fiber neuropathies. However, these neuropathies are rare, and in those patients with involvement of larger fibers, NCS are more sensitive than physical examination for diagnosing PN.

In addition to establishing a diagnosis with accuracy, electrodiagnostic studies provide several other types of information—the predominant pathophysiology (i.e., axonal or demyelinating), time course and severity of the disorder, and whether motor or sensory fibers, or both, are involved. NCS can differentiate hereditary from acquired forms of PN and is much more sensitive than physical examination for identifying MM. Chapter 9 discusses the use of electrodiagnostic testing in detail. Once the underlying pathophysiology and the time course are understood, the differential diagnostic possibilities are narrowed considerably.

Quantitative Sensory Testing Quantitative sensory testing (QST) is a specialized technique for measuring the intensity of a given stimulus required to elicit specific sensory perceptions.[4] Specifically, QST assesses a sensory detection threshold to various stimuli, including touch-pressure, vibration, heat, and coolness. QST, when properly performed, provides a quantitative, noninvasive means of assessing sensory function. One major advantage is that QST for thermal thresholds allows some quantifiable measure of small-fiber function, which is not possible with routine NCS. Several commercial systems exist for QST. However, a major problem with QST is that it is not widely available for clinical use, and its reliability is highly operator dependent. Notably, its sensitivity in patients with pure small-fiber neuropathies, the group in whom it is potentially of the greatest diagnostic importance, has been reported in several studies to be around 60%.[5,6] Nonetheless, it can be quite helpful in confirming the physical examination findings and substantiating the clinical suspicion of neuropathy. In small-fiber neuropathies, in particular, QST is recommended, as it may provide the only objective means for establishing a diagnosis and can be used to measure efficacy of various therapeutic modalities.[4] QST is typically pursued in the evaluation of PN if the routine NCS are nondiagnostic.

Laboratory Studies The differential diagnostic considerations in any given neuropathy are dependent on the physiologic characteristics and time course of the underlying disorder (see Tables 37-1 through 37-3). Thus, the diagnostic evaluation should proceed initially with electrophysiologic studies, as discussed earlier, and laboratory workup should be guided by the differential diagnostic considerations raised by these findings. The laboratory workup will nearly always include blood studies and occasionally urine studies. Cerebrospinal fluid evaluation is no longer routinely necessary; it is most commonly obtained in fairly acute neuropathies in which Guillain-Barré is suspected.

Table 37-4 outlines the appropriate laboratory workup for PN and MM based on time course and electrophysiology.

TABLE 37-4 **Laboratory Investigation of Diffuse Neuropathies**

Routine Studies

Complete blood count, differential
Liver function studies
Fasting serum glucose
Erythrocyte sedimentation rate, antinuclear antibodies, rheumatoid factor
Lyme titer
Thyroid-stimulating hormone
Vitamin B_{12} level
Serum protein electrophoresis, immunoelectrophoresis, urine protein electrophoresis

Special Studies Based on Physiology

Axonal	Demyelinating	Mononeuropathy Multiplex
Heavy metal screen	HIV titer, if appropriate	HIV titer, if appropriate
Cryoglobulins	Cryoglobulins	Cryoglobulins
HIV titer, if appropriate	Anti-MAG, GM1 antibody	Angiotensin-converting enzyme
dsDNA	CSF evaluation (acute forms)	ANCA
Vitamin levels, if apprpower		Nerve biopsy
Consider CSF evaluation		Consider CSF evaluation
Consider nerve biopsy		

CSF, cerebrospinal fluid; HIV, human immunodeficiency virus.

Biopsy

Nerve and Muscle Nerve biopsy is required in a small proportion of patients with neuropathy, and should be performed only in situations in which the indication is clearly defined. Only rarely is biopsy necessary to establish a diagnosis of PN. Nerve biopsy is most useful in patients with MM, as a means of determining the causative disorder, which is usually inflammatory in nature and has a high morbidity and mortality if untreated. Other disorders appropriately diagnosed by nerve biopsy include sarcoidosis, amyloidosis, and, rarely, leprosy. In the cases of vasculitis and sarcoidosis, a muscle biopsy is usually obtained simultaneously. Nerve biopsy is infrequently performed in cases of progressive PN in which exhaustive workup has failed to reveal an underlying diagnosis. In these cases, the aim of the biopsy is to determine the presence or absence of a potentially treatable disorder.

Skin In recent years, a technique has been developed for quantitative assessment of cutaneous innervation in punch biopsies of the skin. The epidermis contains free nerve endings, which are the terminals of small-caliber, unmyelinated fibers. Using control values obtained from a healthy cohort, investigators have been able to identify abnormal patterns of intraepidermal nerve fiber (IENF) density in patients with small-fiber sensory neuropathies (SFSNs).[5,7] Examination of patients with idiopathic, human immunodeficiency virus (HIV)—associated, and diabetic painful sensory neuropathies indicates a correlation between IENF density and clinical estimates of small-fiber sensory dysfunction.[7] Studies of patients with idiopathic SFSNs suggest that IENF is a more sensitive diagnostic indicator of pure, small-fiber neuropathies than either QST or sural nerve biopsy.[5] Although IENF is still available only in specialized centers, it holds promise as an important tool for routine use in patients with painful sensory neuropathies, whose routine workup may be entirely normal, especially when small-fiber involvement predominates.

NEUROPATHIES WITH PAIN AS A PROMINENT FEATURE

Overview

The painful neuropathies are clinically heterogeneous. Even if one restricts analysis to the diffuse neuropathies, the frequency with which pain will occur in a given setting is impossible to predict based on etiology or physiology. Pain may be present early or late in the clinical course of a given neuropathy. It is important for the clinician to evaluate pain issues in an individual patient with knowledge of the underlying disorder and its clinical course, understanding that the course of the pain may be independent of the disease. To that end, it is worth reviewing the neuropathies most commonly associated with pain.

The most commonly encountered painful PN syndromes occur in the setting of diabetes, HIV, and acquired immunodeficiency syndrome (AIDS) and toxic-metabolic disorders. Aside from these, Guillain-Barré syndrome is probably seen most frequently. These disorders are discussed individually in the following sections. Table 37-5 lists diffuse neuropathies commonly associated with pain as a prominent feature. MM syndromes, although significantly less frequent, are worth noting as they are almost invariably associated with pain. MM is usually the result of ischemic vascular injury, regardless of the underlying etiology (see Table 37-3). Pure SFSNs are classically painful, as well, although they are a rare form of neuropathy.

TABLE 37-5 **Neuropathies With Pain As a Prominent Feature**

Polyneuropathies	Mononeuropathy Multiplex
Toxic	Diabetic syndromes (see section III)
Arsenic	Idiopathic brachial neuritis
Thallium	Idiopathic lumbosacral plexopathy
Drugs	Paraneoplastic
Cisplatinum	Infection
Disulfiram	Lyme
Isoniazid	Cytomegalovirus (HIV-related)
Nitrofurantion	Vasculitis
Thallium	
Vincristine	
Generalized Small-fiber Neuropathies	
Acute pandysautonomia	
Amyloidosis	
Diabetes	
HIV-related	
Idiopathic SFSN	
Sjögren's syndrome	
Metabolic/Nutritional	
Acute alcoholic	
Beriberi (thiamine?)	
Diabetic	
Pellagra (niacin)	
Hereditary	
Fabry disease	
Hereditary sensory neuropathy (dominant or recessive)	
Guillain-Barré syndrome	

HIV, human immunodeficiency virus; SFSN, small-fiber sensory neuropathy.

Diabetic Neuropathies

The diabetic neuropathies are clinically diverse and involve focal, multifocal, and diffuse disorders of varying types. Pain, although not universal, is a characteristic feature of neuropathy in diabetic patients, and the most common cause of painful PN is diabetes. It is worth noting that the majority of diabetic patients suffer from chronic, distal, predominantly sensory PN with involvement of all fiber types; this syndrome is frequently painless for much of its course. However, small sensory fibers may be involved disproportionately or exclusively in diabetes mellitus and, in these syndromes, pain is invariably a feature. Painful diabetic neuropathies include several clinical syndromes, including PN. The acute syndromes include lumbar radiculoplexopathy (i.e., diabetic amyotrophy), acute thoracic radiculopathy, and acute distal sensory PN. Rarely, patients may develop an acute, distal sensory PN shortly after initiation of insulin therapy, this has been termed *insulin neuritis*.

The PN syndromes encountered in diabetics include acute-subacute and chronic forms. Typical, chronic, axonal PN may be associated with pain at any point during its course, usually in proportion to the severity of the overall neuropathy; however, the most important factor appears to be the severity of small-fiber injury, and this may be disproportionate in an otherwise typical axonal PN. Diabetes is the most common etiology underlying pure SFSN, in which small-diameter sensory fibers are almost exclusively involved. These patients typically present with distal lower extremity burning pain as the chief complaint. Clinically, pain and temperature sensation are reduced, with sparing of large-fiber sensory modalities (vibration, proprioception); reflexes are usually intact. Autonomic dysfunction may be prominent in these patients. Nerve biopsies demonstrate a predominant loss of small fibers.[8] The clinical course in these patients is variable, and pain may be a chronic problem.

Acute diabetic PN, although less common, is much more likely to be associated with neuropathic pain. The SFSNs associated with diabetes may be acute; in some of these cases, there may be a mixed pattern of involvement, with large fibers being less affected than small. In rare cases, the onset follows the initiation of insulin therapy (so-called insulin neuritis). A similar picture may be seen following precipitous weight loss in diabetic patients (so-called diabetic cachexia). The relationship to glycemic control is unclear; a similar syndrome has been reported following episodes of ketoacidosis as well as establishment of tight control. These cases appear to be largely self-limited, with slow resolution of symptoms as glycemic control and normal weight are established and appropriately maintained.[8]

HIV/AIDS-related Neuropathies

The neuropathies associated with HIV manifest a wide spectrum of disorders, both clinically and pathophysiologically. The most common HIV-associated neuropathy in which pain is a characteristic feature is distal, primarily sensory, symmetric polyneuropathy (DSPN). Other painful polyneuropathies include those produced by toxins (particularly antiretroviral agents) and Guillain-Barré syndrome. Painful MM occurs in this population but is relatively rare.

DSPN is the most common HIV-related form of neuropathy. A predominantly sensory neuropathy, it has been estimated to affect 10% to 30% of patients with AIDS.[9,10] Although DSPN is a relatively uncommon entity in early HIV infection, electrophysiologic studies have shown that up to one third of patients with AIDS have DSPN.11 As immunologic status worsens, clinical manifestations of DSPN increase in incidence. Clinical features include symmetric numbness; burning paresthesias and dysesthesias in the distal lower extremities, with decreased pinprick, temperature, and vibratory sense in a stocking distribution; and depressed ankle reflexes.

Several of the antiretroviral medications have dose-dependent peripheral nerve toxicities, resulting in a clinical syndrome identical to HIV-associated DSPN. These include the nucleoside analogues didanosine (ddI), zalcitabine (ddC) and the pyrimidine analogue, stavudine (d4T). Didanosine is a now well-known cause of a painful peripheral neuropathy. Early clinical trials found 8 of 37 patients receiving ddI developed a dose-related painful neuropathic syndrome, which resolved within 8 weeks of the removal of the drug.[12] Likewise, ddC and d4T have been clearly shown to cause dose-dependent neurotoxicity, which improves with drug withdrawal.[13–15] Notably, when the offending agent is removed, intensified neuropathic symptoms may persist for several weeks, a phenomenon known as coasting.[13] DSPN is the most important side effect limiting the use of thalidomide in the treatment of painful aphthous ulcers in patients with AIDS.[16] PN is also a well-described complication of therapy with isoniazid, an antituberculous agent used in patients with AIDS.[17] Chemotherapeutic agents such as vincristine and paclitaxel, used in the treatment of Kaposi's sarcoma and lymphoma, also have been associated with DSPN.

Rarely, in early HIV disease, patients may develop MM involving cranial as well as peripheral nerves, which responds either spontaneously or with immunomodulating therapy.[18] In late HIV disease, a more fulminant, progressive MM may develop. In both cases, pain is a prominent feature. Etiologic agents identified include toxoplasmosis, herpes zoster, cryptococcus,[19] cryoglobulinemia,[20] and lymphoma. However, the most prevalent etiologic agent is cytomegalovirus; in these cases, marked improvement in symptoms is expected with ganciclovir or foscarnet therapy.[21] MM in HIV patients also has been associated with vasculitis; in these patients, pain is a presenting symptom and may take months to abate.[22]

Diffuse infiltrative lymphocytosis syndrome (DILS) has been recognized as a rare complication of HIV disease for more than a decade; only recently has it been found to be associated with a characteristic peripheral neuropathy. DILS-associated neuropathy is a painful, symmetric, axonal sensorimotor PN of acute-subacute onset.[23] Immunosuppressive and antiviral therapy are helpful in improving symptoms of the neuropathy.[24]

Otherwise-typical Guillain-Barré syndrome (see later discussion) may occur in patients with early HIV, particularly at the time of seroconversion.[25]

Guillain-Barré Syndrome

Acute inflammatory demyelinating polyradiculoneuropathy, or Guillain-Barré syndrome, is the most common cause of acute-subacute PN. Guillain-Barré syndrome is an immune-mediated PN, which is characterized physiologically by segmental demyelination. The typical clinical picture develops over days to weeks, with limb paresthesias developing in a distal-to-proximal fashion, accompanied by weakness and loss of tendon reflexes in a similar distribution. Weakness may spread to involve craniobulbar and respiratory muscles. A classic laboratory finding is a cerebrospinal fluid protein with relatively few white cells (albuminocytologic dissociation). Electrophysiologic studies reveal evidence of primary demyelination with conduction block. Spontaneous recovery, in variable degrees, occurs over weeks to months. Death from respiratory complications occurs in a small number of patients. Pain has been a relatively underappreciated aspect of the disease but is actually a prominent feature in the majority of cases, as pointed out by Ropper and colleagues.[26]

Patients with Guillain-Barré syndrome describe deep, aching muscular pain involving large muscles of the thighs, buttocks, and back, and, less often, sciatica or painful distal limb paresthesias. Pain is usually worst at night and interferes with sleep. Some patients may respond to simple analgesic agents. There is no published experienced regarding the use of tramadol, a non-narcotic analgesic, in Guillain-Barré syndrome, but its use should be considered before resorting to narcotic analgesic agents. The pain, even dysesthetic limb pain, generally responds poorly to antidepressants and anticonvulsants, therapeutic agents that are considered first-line therapy in chronic PN.[26] The experience to date indicates that narcotics have been the most effective treatment and should be used appropriately to control pain, particularly when it is interfering with sleep. In patients whose respiratory status is so marginal that there is a concern of decompensation with the use of narcotics, intubation should be considered.[26]

Toxic Neuropathies

The largest number of toxic neuropathies is related to the use of pharmaceutical agents in appropriate clinical situations. Environmental and occupational toxins are much less frequently seen. Table 37-6 lists pharmaceutical agents that are commonly associated with neuropathy. The typical clinical scenario is a distal axonopathy that develops after sustained use of the medication, although the time course to onset of symptoms is highly variable. Sensory and motor symptoms and signs develop in a length-dependent fashion, in a time course ranging from weeks to months, or even years, depending on the dose and neurotoxic properties of the drug. Painful paresthesias and dysesthesias are common complaints. Prognosis is variable, but in most cases, significant resolution of clinical signs and symptoms occurs with drug withdrawal; however, recovery is variable and related to the severity of the underlying axonal injury.

TABLE 37-6 **Drugs Commonly Associated With Toxic Neuropathy**

Antiarrhythmics	Antineoplastic Agents
Amiodarone	Cis-platinum
Antibiotics/Antituberculous Agents	Doxorubicin
Chloramphenicol	Misonidazole
Dapsone	Vincristine
Ethambutol	Taxol
Isoniazid (INH)	Antiretroviral Agents
Metronidazole	Didanosine (ddl)
Nitrofurantoin	Stavudine (d4T)
Anticonvulsants	Zalcitabine (ddC)
Phenytoin	Other
Antihypertensives	Gold
Hydralazine	Disulfiram
	Nitrous oxide (chronic abuse)
	Pyridoxine
	Thalidomide

PATHOPHYSIOLOGY: PAIN IN THE NEUROPATHIC DISORDERS

Proposed Mechanisms of Pain in Polyneuropathy

Peripheral Mechanisms

Anatomic and Physiologic Considerations The perception of pain is the result of a complex interplay among cells at multiple levels of the nervous system. When an insult results in damage to a peripheral nerve, the transmission and sensation of pain involves the axon, the dorsal root ganglion, and the central nervous system, as well. In this section, we review theories concerned with the role of the peripheral nervous system in the generation and propagation of pain. These include a number of possible pathophysiologic mechanisms, such as ectopic generation, afferent sensitization and hyperexcitability, amplification of neural pacemakers, and electrical cross-talk. We also focus on the pathophysiology of neuronal damage in common illnesses associated with peripheral neuropathies, including diabetes mellitus and HIV infection.

Neuroma Formation and Ectopic Generation When an axon is injured and disconnected from its cell body, it undergoes wallerian degeneration, or so-called dying-back. Subsequently, nerve regeneration occurs through axonal sprouting and elongation from the proximal terminal. If there is some obstacle to forward progress, the axonal sprouts grow in a disorganized fashion and may form a neuroma, a mass of tangled neuronal tissue.[27] Several studies have found the neuroma to function as the nerve's sensory terminal,[28,29] as well a being a source of ectopic discharge in both myelinated and unmyelinated axons.[27] Thus, axonal injury may result in positive symptoms (e.g., paresthesias), as well as negative symptoms (e.g., numbness).

The function of a sensory axon is to propagate information from the sensory receptors to the central nervous system. In normal nerve, a temporary noxious stimulus results in transient pain, because the axon ceases its firing once the stimulus is removed.[30] The development of ongoing pain and paresthesias following the removal of an external stimulus implies a fundamental change in the properties of the axon. Instead of functioning purely as an impulse conductor, it has become an impulse generator.[27] It has been proposed that this metamorphosis following nerve injury results from the formation of a neuroma that has spontaneous pacemaker activity. The neuroma can depolarize and fire continuously in response to various different types of stimulation and may depolarize in the absence of a stimulus; this phenomenon is termed *ectopic generation.*[27] An electrically active neuroma is demonstrated in Figure 37-1.

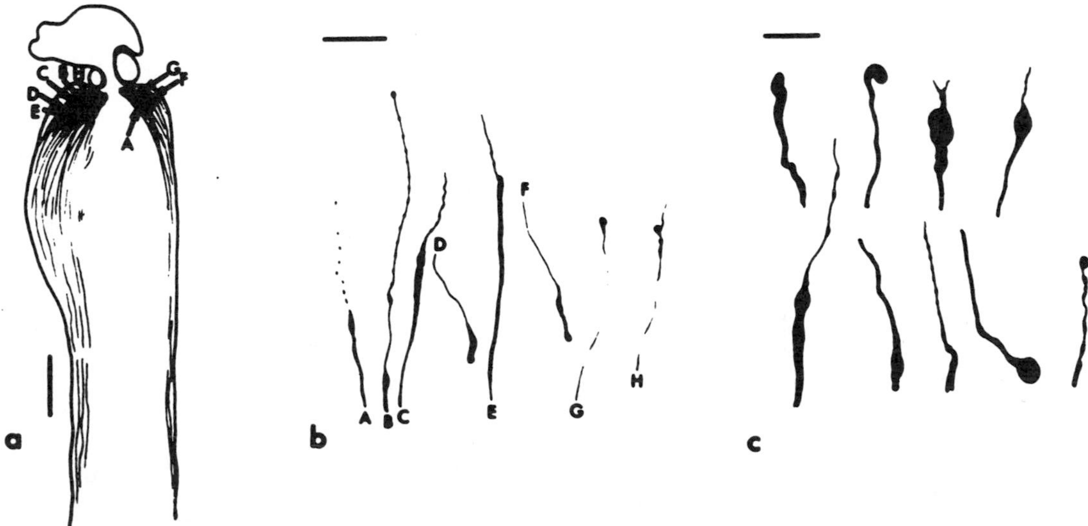

Figure 37-1 (**A**) Structure of an electrically active rat nerve-end neuroma (15 days post-injury). (**B**) End-structure of individual sensory axons (A–H). (**C**) High-magnification of individual end-structures. Such end bulbs are the probable source of spontaneous and evoked ectopic neuroma discharge. (From Fried K, Devor M. End structure of afferent axons injured in the peripheral nervous system. *Somatosens Mot Res* 1988;6:79–99, with permission.)

The development of electrogenetic potential in nerve fibers is one of the key changes that underlie the generation of neuropathic pain. Once an ectopic generator has been established, various stimuli affecting membrane excitability can induce repeated nerve depolarization. Examples of such stimuli include ischemia, mechanical stimuli, and neuroactive substances, including histamines, prostaglandins, and catecholamines.[31]

Unlike peripheral afferents, which develop pacemaker capability as a result of injury, there are a small number of cells in the dorsal root ganglia (DRG) that normally discharge spontaneously. This intrinsic rhythmogenicity is amplified by chronic nerve damage.[32] It has been postulated that enhanced pacemaker activity in the DRG, as well as changes in central pathways, might explain why peripheral nerve blocks may fail to relieve sensory symptoms associated with peripheral nerve lesions.[27] Figure 37-2 demonstrates a prolonged afterdischarge of an afferent axon following mechanical stimulation of the DRG.

Sensitization and Hyperexcitability Several studies have shown that, following injury, intact nerve fiber endings adjacent to injured nerve fibers start to grow and exhibit collateral sprouting. It appears that nociceptive afferent fibers proliferate preferentially. Thus, following nerve injury, an area of denervation may become surrounded by an area that is partially reinnervated but has increased sensitivity to noxious stimuli.[33]

Other changes that take place as a result of nerve injury include axonal membrane remodeling, with an accumulation of voltage-sensitive sodium channels in the end bulb of the axon.[34] These channels are normally in a constant state of turnover, and there is continuous transport of sodium channels downstream.[35] However, if the axon is disrupted, the sodium channels accumulate in the end bulb and render the cell membrane hyperexcitable. Even minor injury, resulting in the loss of myelin without any damage to the axon, triggers the deposition of sodium channels in areas of the axon where they are not usually present.[36]

Amplification Initiation of an action potential by an undamaged neuron is an all-or-none phenomenon, which occurs when a threshold potential is reached. However, the attainment of a certain threshold potential by a damaged neuron can result in *amplification*, or repetitive firing. For example, ectopic neuronal pacemakers that are depolarized to their threshold potentials will fire repetitively, despite a single stimulus. Further increase in intensity of a stimulus can cause a linear, proportional increase in the rate of firing. As ectopic neuronal pacemakers and DRG pacemaker cells have resting membrane potentials near the repetitive-firing threshold potential, even a weak stimulus may initiate repetitive firing, resulting in symptoms of ongoing pain or parasthesiae.[37]

Electrical Cross-Talk Experiments performed in the 1940s by Granit and Skoglund[38] suggest that if the glial insulation between adjacent axons is disrupted, current may flow from severed axons to neighboring fibers. This electrical cross-talk initially subsides following acute injury but may reappear during the process of nerve regeneration and neuroma formation. Because different fiber types lie adjacent to one another (e.g., large, myelinated IA afferent fibers next to nociceptive C fibers), a low-threshold large fiber may be stimulated distally but, because of electrical cross-talk at the site of nerve damage, current might be transferred to a proximal nociceptive afferent.[39]

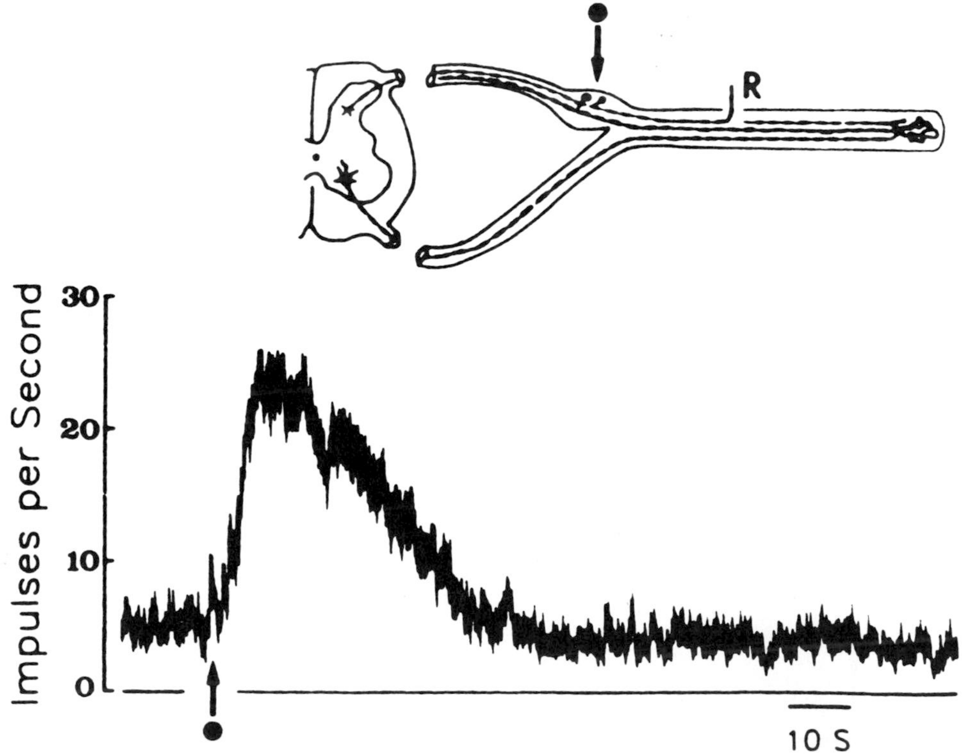

Figure 37-2 Prolonged afterdischarge of an afferent axon following mechanical disturbance of the dorsal root ganglia using a 150-mg von Frey hair (*arrow*). The sciatic nerve had been cut 11 days previously. (From Devor M. The pathophysiology of damaged nerves. In: Wall P, Melzack R, eds. *Textbook of Pain.* Edinburgh, Scotland: Churchill Livingstone, 1994:79–99, with permission.)

Central Mechanisms Individuals with pain syndromes associated with both peripheral and central nervous system lesions may have altered firing in thalamic neurons, changes in the somatotopic organization of the ventrobasal complex of the thalamus, and altered responses to electrical stimulation of the central nervous system.[40] Thus, both the peripheral and central nervous systems play an important pathophysiologic role with respect to pain in peripheral nerve disorders.

Mechanisms of Nerve Injury in Specific Disorders

The two disorders most commonly associated with painful PN are diabetes and HIV/AIDS. Although mechanisms of pain in these specific disorders are not well studied, the pathophysiology of nerve injury in these diseases may shed light on the underlying process that ultimately leads to some of the peripheral mechanisms discussed in the previous section.

Diabetes The diabetic neuropathies are clinically heterogeneous. Pain related to diabetic neuropathies occurs in several clinical syndromes, including DSPN (predominantly involving small fibers), diabetic amyotrophy, truncal radiculopathy, and mononeuritis multiplex.

Several theories have been proposed to explain the pathophysiology of diabetic neuropathies; the most widely accepted are those invoking either metabolic derangement or microangiopathy as primary mechanisms. In spite of intensive study, it remains unclear how metabolic and vascular abnormalities affect the excitability of nerve cell membranes to result in the clinical manifestations of diabetic PN, including pain.

Metabolic Theories It is generally agreed that chronic hyperglycemia plays a key role in complications of diabetes, including neuropathy. In 1993, the Diabetes Control and Complications Trial (DCCT) provided evidence that intensive glycemic control delayed the onset and slowed the progression of the long-term complications of insulin-dependent diabetes mellitus, including neuropathy.[41,42] Additionally, several studies have shown improvement of diabetic PN following pancreatic or pancreatic-renal transplants.[43–45] Two proposed mechanisms for the induction of neuropathy by hyperglycemia are (1) the aldose reductase-sorbitol model, and (2) the glycation model.

In the first model, investigators note that, in the setting of hyperglycemia, glucose is converted to sorbitol by aldose reductase within the nerve. Sorbitol competitively inhibits myoinositol uptake into nerve cells; theoretically, reduced uptake of myoinositol into nerve results in decreased Na^+/K^+-ATPase activity at the nodes of Ranvier. Ultimately, sodium accumulates within the axon, leading to loss of sodium channels and potassium current leak.[46] Loss of sodium channels is, in turn, associated with disruption of the junctional complexes between myelin and axons in the paranodal region. Subsequent paranodal demyelination and axonal shrinkage are the predecessors to clinical neuropathy.

Although attractive, this hypothesis has been challenged based on incomplete metabolic, electrophysiologic, and morphometric evidence.[47,48] Additionally, aldose reductase inhibitors and supplementation with myoinositol have failed to demonstrate therapeutic efficacy in clinical trials of patients with diabetic neuropathy.[49]

According to the glycation model, the presence of excessive glucose in the extracellular matrix results in the formation of so-called advanced glycation end products (AGE). Theoretically, these compounds interfere with several cell functions; DNA and nuclear proteins also may be modified by AGE.[48] In animal studies, diabetic complications have been reduced by the administration of aminoguanidine, an inhibitor of AGE formation.[50,51]

Vascular Theory Another putative mechanism for the development of painful diabetic neuropathy is through microangiopathic changes in the *vasi nervorum*. Theoretically, nerve injury results directly from ischemia, or from ischemia and inflammation associated with immune-mediated vasculitis. Various studies have demonstrated pathologic evidence in nerve biopsy samples for both inflammation and immune complex deposition in vessel walls in patients with various painful forms of diabetic neuropathy.[52,53]

In addition, significant structural changes are seen in blood vessels of patients with diabetes, including basement membrane thickening and deposition of cellular debris. A significant increase in vascular mural area resulting from to deposition of cellular debris is described in diabetes, even in the absence of clinical neuropathy.[54] These microvascular changes appear to precede the development of clinical neuropathy and their severity correlates with duration of diabetes and with the severity of the neuropathy.[55] These pathologic findings, although well described, are of unclear significance in the development of neuropathy in diabetes.

Nitric Oxide Endoneurial blood flow has been shown to be reduced in experimental animal models of diabetes.[56] The pathogenesis of this is unclear; however, it appears that the endothelium-derived relaxing factor nitric oxide (NO) may be involved. Depletion of NO or reduced smooth muscle sensitivity to NO is thought to decrease endothelium-dependent relaxation of smooth muscle, a function that has been found to be reduced in diabetic animal models and humans.[56–58] Alternatively, NO may act indirectly on endoneurial blood by modulating sympathetic tone; depletion of NO may result in nerve ischemia as the result of increased vasoconstriction.[59–61]

The metabolic and vascular mechanisms proposed as underlying diabetic neuropathy may converge with the NO theory.[62] Studies have demonstrated a metabolic competition for NADPH by aldose reductase, the enzyme that converts glucose to sorbitol, and NO synthetase, the enzyme that converts L-arginine to NO. It has been shown that aldose reductase inhibitors improve nerve blood flow and restore endothelium-dependent relaxation to normal.[63,64] Figure 37-3 demonstrates the theoretical mechanism by which this metabolic defect might lead to endoneurial ischemia and abnormalities in nerve conduction.

HIV/AIDS-related Neuropathies The HIV-associated neuropathies manifest a wide spectrum of disorders, both clinically and pathophysiologically. The most common HIV-associated neuropathy in which pain is a characteristic feature is DSPN. Of the HIV-related neuropathies, this one is the best studied with regard to pathophysiology. The leading theories that have undergone rigorous investigation propose either direct HIV infection or immune-mediated nerve injury as the primary mechanisms underlying DSPN.

Several studies have demonstrated perivascular inflammatory infiltrates in peripheral nerves of patients with HIV-associated DSPN, consisting of macrophages and T lymphocytes, suggesting an immune mechanism underlying the disorder.[10,65,66] It appears unlikely that immune complex deposition is involved in the patho-

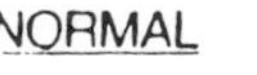

DIABETIC

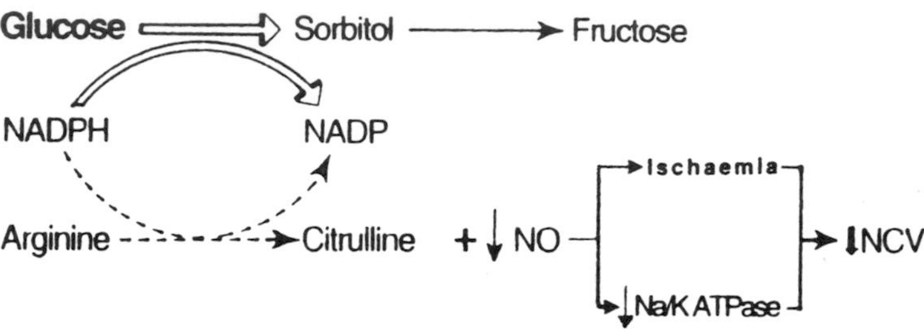

Figure 37-3 Metabolic competition for NADPH by aldose reductase and nitric oxide synthase in normal and diabetic state. AR2, aldose reductase; NO, nitric oxide; NOS, nitric oxide synthase; NCV, nerve conduction velocity; SDH, sorbitol dehydrogenase. (From Stevens MJ, Feldman EL, Greene DA. The aetiology of diabetic neuropathy: The combined roles of metabolic and vascular defects. *Diabet Med* 1995;12:566–579, with permission).

genesis of this neuropathy, based on the absence of electron microscopic evidence for immune globulin or complement deposition in nerves.[65,67] However, HIV could lead to a cell-mediated immune attack on the nerves, with resultant demyelination and axonal degeneration.[65] Evidence of cytokine activation and T cells and macrophages at all levels in the peripheral nervous system suggests that the damage to the peripheral nervous system in AIDS is a multifocal, immunologic process.[10,66]

The isolation of HIV, HIV-like particles and HIV-associated mRNA in peripheral nerves of patients with DSPN led some investigators to postulate that neuropathy resulted from direct invasion of peripheral nerve by the virus.[67,68] Others have suggested direct infection by the virus of lumbosacral dorsal root ganglion cells, with subsequent central-peripheral distal axonal degeneration as a possible mechanism of DSPN.[69] Subsequent pathologic studies have not been able to confirm HIV particles or antigens in peripheral nerves, nerve roots, or DRG cells.[69,70] Furthermore, in the patients in which HIV was isolated from peripheral nerve in the original studies, the diagnosis of DSPN was subsequently revised to other types of neuropathy.

THERAPEUTICS OF PAIN IN POLYNEUROPATHY

Approach to Pain in Polyneuropathy

The pharmacologic approach to patients with PN who suffer from positive symptoms, particularly pain, is the same, regardless of the underlying cause of the neuropathy. To date, most clinical studies looking at pharmacologic efficacy in painful neuropathy have been done in patients with diabetic neuropathies, and only a limited number of studies have used double-blind, controlled methodology. Nonetheless, management of pain in PN is often successful using standard agents, particularly when the appropriate principles are considered. Often, patients fail to achieve pain control because of inadequate dosing rather than inefficacy of a particular agent.

In neuropathy, amelioration of pain may be achieved with the use of agents that block pain transmission centrally or peripherally; the role of agents that act on the sympathetic nervous system is less clear. Certainly, some patients with PN may have an element of sympathetically maintained pain. Often, patients require trials with various agents and dosages before optimal therapeutic effect is achieved. The choice of therapy must be tailored to the individual patient (i.e., with regard to age, medical illnesses, previous medication record, and concomitant medications). Drug dosages must be titrated slowly to achieve relief of pain without intolerable side effects. One of the primary principles of pharmacologic management should be the use of single drug therapy whenever possible.

Several classes of drugs are currently used to treat patients with painful peripheral neuropathies. These include tricyclic antidepressants, anticonvulsants, antiarrhythmics, analgesics, and narcotic agents. For an extensive discussion of pharmacologic therapies for pain, including specific pharmacologic agents, see Part VI (Chaps. 58 to 64). A brief review of the efficacy of the most commonly used agents for painful PN is presented next.

Pharmacologic Agents

Antidepressants Tricyclic antidepressants have been shown to be safe and effective in alleviating the pain of peripheral neuropathy. Commonly used agents include amitriptyline, nortriptyline, imipramine, and desipramine. These agents have been studied in double-blind, randomized controlled trials with results suggesting that each of them reduces pain independent of their effect on depression.[71–74] In one study, 74% of patients who received 75 to 150 mg of amitriptyline attained moderate or greater relief of their pain compared with 41% of patients receiving placebo.[71] Similar results were seen with desipramine.

The tricyclic antidepressants are thought to exert their analgesic effect by inhibiting norepinephrine and serotonin reuptake in the central nervous system. They also affect cholinergic, histaminergic, and adrenergic transmission, resulting in some limiting side effects. These include sedation, orthostasis, cardiac arrhythmia, and urinary retention. Nortriptyline and desipramine, secondary amine tricyclics, tend to have fewer of these adverse effects, which is preferable for many patients, especially the elderly. Side effects may be minimized by slow titration, starting with 10 to 25 mg at night and increasing the dose by 10 to 25 mg once or twice weekly. There is no specific target dose; however the dose usually associated with pain relief is between 50 and 150 mg/day.[75]

Anticonvulsants The classic anticonvulsant agents phenytoin and carbamazepine have been used in treating neuropathic pain since the 1960s. It is postulated that anticonvulsants modulate pain by suppressing neuronal firing.[76] These agents have been examined in controlled trials and found to be efficacious in treating pain associated with diabetic neuropathy. A systematic review of these agents found them to be efficacious in treating some neuropathic pain syndromes, including trigeminal neuralgia and diabetic neuropathy, but noted that the risk of adverse effects was equal to the likelihood of significant benefit.[77] Other agents such as clonazepam and valproate have been used anecdotally without much success in pain relief. Overall, the clinical experience suggests that these older anticonvulsant agents are less beneficial in treatment of pain in PN than tricyclic antidepressants or the newer anticonvulsants.[3]

In 1994, gabapentin was approved for use in the United States as an anticonvulsant. It has subsequently enjoyed broad use, including off-label use in the treatment of neuropathic pain. A recent randomized, controlled trial of gabapentin for treatment of pain in diabetic neuropathy found that patients treated with gabapentin had clinically significant alleviation of daily pain severity and improvement of quality-of-life measures.[78] Patients were started on 900 mg/day and the dose increased by 900 mg/day every week for a total of 4 weeks. Sixty-seven percent of patients achieved the maximum dose of 3,600 mg/day, although patients reported therapeutic effect at doses of 900 to 1800 mg/day. Reported side effects included mild dizziness and somnolence. It was concluded that gabapentin monotherapy was efficacious and safe in treating the pain of diabetic neuropathy.

Antiarrhythmics Studies in animal models have shown that antiarrhythmic agents modulate pain pathways by decreasing spontaneous discharges associated with pain generation in injured nerves.[79] Oral mexiletine has been evaluated in several controlled studies; the general consensus is that mexiletine is safe and effective in treating neuropathic pain.[80–82] The dose found to be efficacious in the studies has been 450 to 675 mg/day. It is recommended that the drug be started at 150 mg/day and titrated upward for effective pain relief. Side effects in the studies were mild and included nausea and dizziness. Electrocardiogram changes were not demonstrable in patients without cardiac disease.

Analgesics

Non-narcotic Agents Another recent addition to the pain therapy armamentarium is tramadol, a centrally acting, synthetic, nonnarcotic analgesic that has been available in the United States since 1995. Its two mechanisms of action are (1) low affinity binding to μ-opioid receptors, and (2) weak inhibition of norepinephrine and serotonin reuptake.[83] A recent double-blind, randomized, placebo-controlled trial of patients with painful diabetic neuropathy found that patients receiving an average dose of 210 mg/day of tramadol had significant pain relief with better physical and social functioning compared with patients receiving placebo.[84] The most frequently occurring side effects were headache, constipation, nausea, and somnolence.

Narcotic Agents Clinicians often prescribe narcotics when other therapies have failed. As with other therapeutic agents, it is recommended that a low dose be begun initially and titrated upward to achieve either effective pain relief or intolerable side effects. Patients should be informed of the risk of tolerance. When prescribing an opiate for painful neuropathies, it is recommended that a long-acting agent, such as extended-release morphine, oxycodone, or methadone, be used.[3]

Topical Agents Capsaicin is an alkaloid found in capsicum peppers. When applied topically, it produces desensitization to noxious stimuli.[85] It has been studied in patients with painful diabetic neuropathies with mixed results. One double-blind comparison of topical capsaicin and oral amitriptyline found topical capsaicin to be equally efficacious as amitriptyline but without any systemic side effects.[86] Another randomized, controlled trial of the drug in painful diabetic neuropathy found it to be of no benefit.[87] Although the literature appeared optimistic originally, clinical experience has been disappointing. Patients find the drug difficult to use because care must be taken not to allow contamination of unaffected body parts. Even in affected body parts, the drug causes significant burning pain on application, which most patients find an intolerable side effect.

Other Agents Dextromethorphan, a low-affinity *N*-methyl-D-aspartate (NMDA) receptor antagonist and dextro isomer of the codeine analogue levorphanol, has been studied in a randomized, double-blind, placebo-controlled crossover trial of patients with a painful diabetic neuropathy and patients with postherpetic neuralgia.[88] In diabetic neuropathy, patients who received dextromethorphan had their pain decrease by an average of 24% relative to patients who received placebo. Dextromethorphan did not alleviate pain for patients with postherpetic neuralgia. The average dose received by the diabetic patients was 381 mg/day. The limiting side effects of treatment with dextromethorphan include ataxia and sedation. Although this study suggests that NMDA receptor antagonists may useful in the treatment of painful neuropathies, the clinical experience has been disappointing.[3]

REFERENCES

1. Dyck PJ, Benstead TJ, Conn DL, et al. Nonsystemic vasculitic neuropathy. *Brain* 1987;110:843–853.
2. Galer BS, Jensen MP. Development and preliminary validation of a pain measure specific to neuropathic pain: The Neuropathic Pain Scale. *Neurology* 1997;48:332–338.
3. Galer B. Painful polyneuropathy. *Neurol Clin* 1998;16:791–812.
4. Peripheral Neuropathy Association. Quantitative sensory testing: A consensus report from the Peripheral Neuropathy Association. *Neurology* 1993;43:1050–1052.
5. Holland NR, Crawford TO, Hauer P, et al. Small-fiber sensory neuropathies: Clinical course and neuropathology of idiopathic cases. *Ann Neurol* 1998;44:47–59.
6. Giuliani M, Tobin K. Small-fiber neuropathy: Evaluation recommendations. *Neurology* 1996;46(suppl):A312.
7. McCarthy BG, Hsieh ST, Stocks A, et al. Cutaneous innervation in sensory neuropathies: Evaluation by skin biopsy. *Neurology* 1995;45:1848–1855.
8. Thomas P, Tomlinson D. Diabetic and hypoglyemic neuropathy. In: Dyck P, Thomas P, Griffin J, et al, eds. *Peripheral Neuropathy.* Philadelphia, Pa: WB Saunders; 1993:1222–1250.

9. Cornblath D, McArthur J. Predominantly sensory neuropathy in patients with AIDS and AIDS-related complex. *Neurology* 1988;38:794–796.
10. Rizzuto N, Cavallaro T, Monaco S, et al. Role of HIV in the pathogenesis of distal symmetrical peripheral neuropathy. *Acta Neuropathol (Berl)* 1995;90:244–250.
11. So Y, Holtzman D, Abrams D, et al. Peripheral neuropathy associated with acquired immunodeficiency syndrome: Prevalence and clinical features from a population based survey. *Arch Neurol* 1988;45:945–948.
12. Lambert J, Seidlin M, Reichman R, et al. 2′,3′-dideoxyinosine (ddI) in patients with the acquired immunodeficiency syndrome or AIDS-related complex. A phase I trial. *N Engl J Med* 1990;322:1333–1340.
13. Berger A, Arezzo J, Schaumburg H, et al. 2′,3′-dideoxycytidine (ddC) toxic neuropathy: A study of 52 patients. *Neurology* 1993;43:358–362.
14. Simpson D, Tagliati M. Nucleoside analogue-associated peripheral neuropathy in human immunodeficiency virus infection. *J Acquir Immune Defic Syndr Hum Retrovirol* 1995;9:153–161.
15. Browne M, Mayer K, Chafee S, et al. 2′,3′-didehydro-3′-deoxythymidine (d4t) in patients with AIDS or AIDS-related complex: A phase I trial. *J Infect Dis* 1993;167:21–29.
16. Ochonisky S, Vernoust J, Bastuji-Garin S, et al. Thalidomide neuropathy incidence and clinicoelectrophysiologic findings in 42 patients. *Arch Dermatol* 1992;130:66–69.
17. Figg W. Peripheral neuropathy in HIV patients after isoniazid therapy initiated. *DICP* 1991;25:100–101.
18. So Y, Olney R. The natural history of mononeuritis multiplex and simplex in patients with HIV infection. *Neurology* 1991;41(suppl 1):375.
19. Engstrom J, Lewis E, McGuire D. Cranial neuropathy and the acquired immunodeficiency syndrome. *Neurology* 1991;41(suppl 1):374.
20. Stricker R, Sanders K, Owen W, et al. Mononeuritis multiplex associated with cryoglobulinemia in HIV infection. *Neurology* 1992;42:2103–2105.
21. Roullet E, Assuerus V, Gozlan J, et al. Cytomegalovirus multifocal neuropathy in AIDS: Analysis of 15 consecutive cases. *Neurology* 1994;44:2174–2182.
22. Said G, Lacroix-Ciaudo C, Fujimura H, et al. The peripheral neuropathy of necrotizing arteritis: A clinicopathological study. *Ann Neurol* 1988;23:461–465.
23. Moulignier A, Authier F, Baudrimont M, et al. Peripheral neuropathy in human immunodeficiency virus–infected patients with the diffuse infiltrative lymphocytosis syndrome. *Ann Neurol* 1997;41:438–445.
24. Price R. Neuropathy complicating diffuse infiltrative lymphocytosis. *Lancet* 1998;352:592–594.
25. Vendrell J, Heredia C, Pujol M, et al. Guillain-Barre syndrome associated with seroconversion for anti-HTLV-III. *Neurology* 1987;37:544.
26. Ropper A, Wijdicks E, Truax B. *Guillain-Barre Syndrome.* Philadelphia, Pa: FA Davis; 1991.
27. Devor M, Rappaport Z. Pain and the pathophysiology of damaged nerve. In: Fields H, ed. *Pain Syndromes in Neurology.* London, England: Butterworth & Co; 1990:42–83.
28. Gouvrin-Lippmann R, Devor M. Ongoing activity in severed nerves: Source and variation with time. *Brain Res* 1978;159:406–410.
29. Blumberg H, Janig W. Discharge pattern of afferent fibers from a neuroma. *Pain* 1984;20:335–353.
30. Ruiz J, Kocsis J, Preson R. *Repetitive Firing Characteristics of Mammalian Myelinated Axons: An Intra-axonal Analysis.* Vol. 7. Bethesda, Md: Society for Neuroscience; 1981.
31. Devor M, White D, Goetzl E, et al. Eicosanoids, but not tachykinins, excite C-fiber endings in rat sciatic nerve-end neuromas. *Neuroreport* 1992;3:21–24.
32. Kajander K, Wakisaka S, Bennet G. Spontaneous discharge originates in the dorsal root ganglion at the onset of a painful peripheral neuropathy in the rat. *Neurosci Lett* 1992;138:225–228.
33. Inbal R, Rousso M, Ashur H, et al. Collateral sprouting and sensory recovery after nerve injury in man. *Pain* 1987;28:141–154.
34. Devor M, Gouvrin-Lippmann R, Angelides K. Na^+ channel immunolocalization in peripheral mammalian axons and changes following nerve injury and neuroma formation. *J Neurosci* 1993;13:1976–1992.
35. Matzner O, Devor M. Na^+ conductance and the threshold for repetitive neuronal firing. *Brain Res* 1992;597:92–98.
36. Devor M. The pathophysiology of damaged nerves. In: Wall P, Melzack R, eds. *Textbook of Pain.* Edinburgh, Scotland: Churchill Livingstone; 1994:79–99.
37. Lisney S, Devor M. Afterdischarge and interactions among fibers in damaged peripheral nerve in the rat. *Brain Res* 1987;415:122–136.
38. Granit R, Skoglund C. Facilitation, inhibition, and depression at the "artificial synapse" formed by the cut end of a mammalian nerve. *J Physiol* 1945;103:435–448.
39. Bernstein J, Pagnarelli D. Long-term axonal opposition in rat sciatic nerve neuroma. *J Neurosurg* 1982;57:682–684.
40. Willner C, Low P. Approaches to neuropathic pain. In: Dyck P, ed. *Peripheral Neuropathy.* Vol 2. Philadelphia, Pa: WB Saunders; 1993:1709–1720.
41. Diabetes Control and Complications Trial and Research Group. The effect of intensive treatment of diabetes on the development and progression of long-term complications in insulin-dependent diabetes mellitus. *N Engl J Med* 1993;329:977–986.
42. Diabetes Control and Complications Trial and Research Group. Effect of intensive diabetes treatment on nerve conduction in the diabetes control and complications trial. *Ann Neurol* 1995;88:869–880.
43. Kennedy W, Navarro X, Goetz F. Effects of pancratic transplantation on diabetic neuropathy. *N Engl J Med* 1990;322:1031–1037.
44. Orloff M, Greenfield G, Gerard B. Reversal of diabetic somatic neuropathy by whole pancreas transplantation. *Surgery* 1990;108:179–190.
45. Navarro X, Sutherland D, Kennedy D. Long-term effects of pancreatic transplantation on diabetic neuropathy. *Ann Neurol* 1997;42:727–736.
46. Greene D, Lattimer S, Sima A. Sorbitol, phosphoinositodes, and sodium-potassium ATPase in the pathogenesis of diabetic complications. *N Engl J Med* 1987;316:599–605.
47. Dyck P, Giannini C. Pathologic alterations in the diabetic neuropathies of humans: A review. *J Neuropathol Exp Neurol* 1996;55:1181–1193.
48. Brownlee M. Glycation products and the pathogenesis of diabetic complications. *Diabetes Care* 1992;15:1835–1845.
49. Krentz A, Honigsberger L, Ellis S. A 12-month randomized controlled study of the aldose reductase inhibitor ponalrestat in patients with chronic sympatomatic diabetic neuropathy. *Diabet Med* 1992;9:463–468.
50. Hammes H, Martin S, Federlin K, et al. Aminoguanidine treatment inhibits the development of experimental diabetic retinopathy. *Proc Natl Acad Sci U S A* 1991;88:11555–11558.
51. Yagihashi S, Kamijo M, Baba M, et al. Effect of aminoguanidine on functional and structural abnormalities in peripheral nerve of STZ-induced diabetic rats. *Diabetes* 1992;41:47–52.
52. Said G, Goulon-Goeau C, Lacroix C, et al. Nerve biopsy findings in different patterns of proximal diabetic neuropathy. *Ann Neurol* 1994;35:559–569.
53. Younger D, Rosoklija G, Hays A, et al. Diabetic peripheral neuropathy: A clinicopathologic and immunohistochemical analysis of sural nerve biopsies. *Muscle Nerve* 1996;19:722–727.
54. Yasuda H, Dyck P. Abnormalities of endoneurial microvessels and sural nerve pathology in diabetic neuropathy. *Neurology* 1987;37:20–28.
55. Giannini C, Dyck P. Basement membrane reduplication and pericyte degeneration precede development of diabetic polyneuropathy and are associated with its severity. *Ann Neurol* 1995;37:498–504.
56. Mayhan WG, Simmons LK, Sharpe GM. Mechanism of impaired responses of cerebral arterioles during diabetes mellitus. *Am J Physiol* 1991;260:H319–H326.
57. Vallance P, Collier J, Moncada S. Effects of endothelium-derived nitric oxide on peripheral arteriolar tone in man [see comments]. *Lancet* 1989;2:997–1000.

58. Calver A, Collier J, Vallance P. Inhibition and stimulation of nitric oxide synthesis in the human forearm arterial bed of patients with insulin-dependent diabetes. *J Clin Invest* 1992;90:2548–2554.
59. Greene DA, Sima AA, Stevens MJ, et al. Complications: Neuropathy, pathogenetic considerations. *Diabetes Care* 1992;15:1902–1925.
60. Bult H, Boeckxstaens GE, Pelckmans PA, et al. Nitric oxide as an inhibitory nonadrenergic non-cholinergic neurotransmitter [see comments]. *Nature* 1990;345:346–347.
61. Cameron NE, Cotter MA, Low PA. Nerve blood flow in early experimental diabetes in rats: Relation to conduction deficits. *Am J Physiol* 1991;261:E1–E8.
62. Stevens MJ, Dananberg J, Feldman EL, et al. The linked roles of nitric oxide, aldose reductase and, (Na^+,K^+)-ATPase in the slowing of nerve conduction in the streptozotocin diabetic rat. *J Clin Invest* 1994; 94:853–859.
63. Yasuda H, Sonobe M, Yamashita M, et al. Effect of prostaglandin E1 analogue TFC 612 on diabetic neuropathy in streptozocin-induced diabetic rats. Comparison with aldose reductase inhibitor ONO 2235. *Diabetes* 1989;38:832–838.
64. Cameron NE, Cotter MA. Impaired contraction and relaxation in aorta from streptozotocin-diabetic rats: Role of polyol pathway. *Diabetologia* 1992;35:1011–1019.
65. de la Monte S, Gabuzda D, Ho D, et al. Peripheral neuropathy in the acquired immunodeficiency syndrome. *Ann Neurol* 1988;23:485–492.
66. Bradley W, Shapshak P, Delgado S, et al. Morphometric analysis of the peripheral neuropathy of AIDS. *Muscle Nerve* 1998;21:1188–1195.
67. Bailey R, Baltch A, Venkatesh R, et al. Sensory motor neuropathy associated with AIDS. *Neurology* 1988;38:886–891.
68. Ho D, Rota T, Schooley R, et al. Isolation of HTLV-III from cerebrospinal fluid and neural tissues of patients with neurologic syndromes related to the acquired immunodeficiency syndrome. *N Engl J Med* 1985;313:1493–1497.
69. Rance N, McArthur J, Cornblath D. Gracile tract degeneration in patients with sensory neuropathy and AIDS. *Neurology* 1988;38:265–271.
70. Grafe M, Wiley C. Spinal cord and peripheral nerve pathology in AIDS: The roles of cytomegalovirus and human immunodeficiency virus. *Ann Neurol* 1989;25:561–566.
71. Max M, Lynch S, Muir J, et al. Effects of desipramine, amitriptyline, and fluoxetine on pain in diabetic neuropathy. *N Engl J Med* 1992; 326:1250–1256.
72. Gomez-Perez F, Rull J, Dies H, et al. Nortriptyline and fluphenazine in the symptomatic treatment of diabetic neuropathy: A double blind cross-over study. *Pain* 1985;23:395–397.
73. Max M, Kishore-Kumar R, Schafer S, et al. Efficacy of desipramine in painful diabetic neuropathy: A placebo-controlled trial. *Pain* 1991; 45:3–9.
74. Kurnsdahl B, Molin J, Froland A, et al. Imipramine treatment of painful diabetic neuropathy. *JAMA* 1984;251:1727–1730.
75. Portenoy R. Painful polyneuropathy. *Neurol Clin* 1989;7:265–288.
76. Maciewicz R, Bouckoms A, Martin J. Drug therapy of neuropathic pain. *Clin J Pain* 1985;1:39–49.
77. McQuay H, Carroll D, Jadad A, et al. Anticonvulsant drugs for management of pain: A systematic review. *Br Med J* 1995;311:1047–1052.
78. Backonja M, Beydoun A, Edwards K, et al. Gabapentin for the symptomatic treatment of painful neuropathy in patients with diabetes mellitus: a randomized controlled trial. *JAMA* 1998;280:1831–1836.
79. Chabal C, Jacobson L, Russell L, et al. Pain response to perineuromal injection of normal saline, epinephrine, and lidocaine in humans. *Pain* 1989;38:333–338.
80. Oskarsson P, Ljunggren J, Lins P. Efficacy and safety of mexiletine in the treatment of painful diabetic neuropathy. The Mexiletine Study Group. *Diabetes Care* 1997;20:1594–1597.
81. Dejgard A, Petersen P, Kastrup J. Mexiletine for treatment of chronic painful diabetic neuropathy. *Lancet* 1988;1:9–11.
82. Stracke H, Meyer U, Schumacher H, et al. Mexiletine in the treatment of diabetic neuropathy. *Diabetes Care* 1992;15:1550–1555.
83. Raffa R, Friderichs E, Reimann W, et al. Opioid and nonopioid components independently contribute to the mechanism of action of tramadol, an 'atypical' opioid analgesic. *J Pharmacol Exp Ther* 1992; 260:275–285.
84. Harati Y, Gooch C, Swenson M, et al. Double-blind randomized trial of tramadol for the treatment of the pain of diabetic neuropathy. *Neurology* 1998;50:1842–1846.
85. Tandan R, Lewis GA, Krusinski PB, et al. Topical capsaicin in painful diabetic neuropathy. Controlled study with long-term follow-up [see comments]. *Diabetes Care* 1992;15:8–14.
86. Biesbroek R, Bril V, Hollander P, et al. A double-blind comparison of topical capsaicin and oral amitryptiline in painful diabetic neuropathy. *Adv Ther* 1995;12:111–120.
87. Chad DA, Aronin N, Lundstrum R, et al. Does capsaicin relieve the pain of diabetic neuropathy? [letter]. *Pain* 1990;42:387–388.
88. Nelson K, Park K, Robinovitz E, et al. High-dose oral dextromethorphan versus placebo in painful diabetic neuropathy and postherpetic neuralgia. *Neurology* 1997;48:1212–1218.

CHAPTER 38 CENTRAL PAIN STATES

Ronald R. Tasker

Central pain, defined as "pain associated with lesions of the central nervous system,"[1] is a type of neuropathic pain whose features are summarized in Table 38-1, as discussed by many authors.[2–9] Central pain of spinal cord origin is essentially a young man's disease, usually resulting from trauma, whereas central pain of brain origin is usually the result of stroke.

One of the amazing things about central pain is that the clinical picture is similar in a patient with a cord lesion so slight it produces no clinically detectable sensory loss to that seen after complete cord transection.[10–13] Furthermore, stroke pain after a lesion so massive that it essentially produces a hemispherectomy is similar to that after a stroke with no persisting sensory loss. Furthermore, only a certain percentage of patients with apparently identical lesions develop central pain.

A chief problem is that the mechanism of this pain is poorly understood, making attempts at treatment difficult to rationalize. It must be remembered that the most common feature is the steady, constant, burning, dysesthetic or aching element for which there is no laboratory model. Patients must serve as models, because only they can tell us what they feel.

CORD CENTRAL PAIN

As has been mentioned, not every patient who suffers cord damage develops central pain; the reported incidence ranges from 6% to 94%.[9,14–24] The etiology is usually trauma. In a personal series of 127 patients,[25] 65% were victims of trauma, 12% suffered from iatrogenic lesions, 9% from inflammatory lesions, 6% from neoplastic lesions, 4% from congenital lesions, 2% from vascular lesions, and 2% from skeletal pathology. The location of lesions in these patients was as follows: cervical, 42%; T1 to T9, 21%; and T10 to L2, 37%. Thirty-two percent of lesions were clinically complete, 64% were incomplete, and 4% of patients had no clinically detectable sensory loss. Etiology and level or completeness of lesion did not correlate with presence, severity, or quality of pain, except as discussed subsequently.

Clinical Features

One of the startling features of cord central pain is the fact that its onset may be delayed after the causative event, sometimes for years. Among patients I have treated, 24% experienced immediate onset of pain; 18% had pain that appeared in the first month; 26%, pain after 1 month but before 6 months; and 18%, pain after 6 but before 12 months. The longer the delay in pain onset, the more likely it is that syrinx is present[26]—a lesion that must be identified and treated to protect the patient from neurologic deterioration. Syrinx decompression is, however, disappointing as a means of pain control, as the experience of Milhorat and colleagues[26] and my own experience[25] have shown. Milhorat and colleagues found that only 19% of their patients were totally relieved of pain soon after surgery, while 41% were partially relieved of pain soon after, and 24% were better after 1 year. It is my impression that, of syrinx-related pain, the neuralgic element running down the arms responds best, and the steady element remains intractable.

Cord central pain often has multiple components. It is important to listen to how the patient describes the pain because, as Boureau and coworkers[27] have shown, these descriptors reflect the pathophysiology on which treatment is based. This chapter offers my views on these matters. If one disregards pain associated with skeletal, soft tissue, and urologic problems, cord central pain falls into a number of categories.[6,15,21,22,26,28–33] In the previously described group of 127 patients, 75% reported pain that was burning, 26%, dysesthetic, 31%, shooting, 44%, evoked (allodynia and hyperpathia), 15%, musculoskeletal-like, and 3%, visceral-like pain, with multiple components often being present. For consideration of treatment, these have been grouped into four main components: (1) steady (burning, dysesthetic, or aching), (2) shooting, (3) evoked and visceral, and (4) musculoskeletal. Although most (96%) patients had steady pain, 2% had shooting pain, and 4%, allodynia or hyperpathia in isolation. Three percent of complete lesions and 2% of incomplete lesions were associated with facial pain.

The clinical correlates were as follows. By definition, evoked pain occurred only in the presence of at least some preserved sensation, often in a band or in radicular distribution at the upper level with a complete lesion, more diffusely in incomplete lesions. Facial pain was always associated with syrinx. Visceral-like pain often mimicked intraabdominal pathology, causing diagnostic dilemmas (especially in incomplete lesions), whereas musculoskeletal-like pain strongly suggested actual nociceptive pain, presenting diagnostic difficulties except when it occurred below a complete level, and often prompting extensive negative investigation and futile treatment. The most important clinical correlate was with neuralgic pain. This correlation was most common with conus–cauda lesions, present in 82% of the patients with complete T10 to L2 lesions and in 64% of those with incomplete T10-L2 lesions. When associated with other pain types, shooting pain was usually the most severe.

Patterns of sensory loss were variable. In a review of 72 patients,[25] 42% experienced complete loss of all modalities; 39% had incomplete loss; 16%, dissociated loss, and 3%, no clinically detectable sensory loss.

Few laboratory studies have examined the possible pathophysiology of cord central pain. Levitt and Levitt[34] found that pain, as evidenced by autotomy in rats, followed anterolateral quadrant cord lesions or hemisection as long as some sensation was preserved in ipsilateral nociceptive pathways. Pain did not result after posterior quadrant section or simultaneous section of ipsilateral, lateral, or anterolateral quadrant accompanied by contralateral section of the anterolateral quadrant or hemisection. These observations are difficult to correlate with clinical experience, however, because in hu-

TABLE 38-1 **Characteristics of Neuropathic and Central Pain**

Results from damage to somatosensory pathways; damage may be slight (with no sensory loss) to massive (with anesthesia)
Pain is idiosyncratic (appears genetically determined in animals) and occurs in distribution of sensory damage
Onset may be delayed
May be reversible (brain central pain)
Has three common components: (1) steady and neuralgic, (2) spontaneous, and (3) evoked
Proximal or distal somatosensory local anesthetic blockade, or both, may temporally relieve it, as may sympathetic blockade, if evoked element is present
Steady pain may be better relieved by intravenous sodium thiopental than by opiate infusion
Steady element is not usually relieved by proximal transection but may respond to chronic stimulation that induces paresthesia in pain area
Evoked and neuralgic elements may be relieved by proximal neural interruption

man patients, pain onset was delayed and pain, once established, was not alleviated by morphine administration or cord transection proximal to the level of the causative lesion nor to lesions made in the same structures that caused pain rostral to the causative lesion.

Functional imaging with single photon emission computed tomography (SPECT) and positron emission tomography (PET) scans[35,36] reveals diminished thalamic perfusion contralateral to pain in various pain syndromes, including cord central pain, the hypoperfusion being normalized by strategies that abolish the pain. The fact that the steady component of cord central pain is not relieved by transection of the cord rostral to the causative lesion or by destructive lesioning of pain pathways in the brain suggests that this pain is being generated centrally at the cortical level. Melzack and Loeser concluded that it is the result of a "pattern generating mechanism."[37]

Treatment

Treatment of cord central pain can be divided into surgical and nonsurgical strategies, there being no prophylactic measures. Prior to directly addressing the pain, attention to issues such as spasticity and spasms, wound healing, skin hygiene, skeletal stabilization, urologic therapy, pulmonary function, nutrition, seating, physiotherapy, and occupational therapy are essential to establish the optimal milieu in which to deal with a difficult problem.

In considering therapy for the central pain itself, whether medical or surgical, the first requirement is to be realistic. Therapy for chronic pain often fails, and if successful is usually only partly so, with a tendency to recurrence over time.[38] Next, the patient's pain must be dissected into its component parts, each to be treated with the relevant strategy, which differs according to the pain syndrome present. Above all, it is necessary to remember that therapy suitable for nociceptive (e.g., cancer) pain is not relevant in neuropathic pain.[2–6,39] In planning a treatment strategy, the physician must consider not only the patient's expectations for outcome, as determined using a Visual Analog Scale, but also related to satisfaction with the treatment, and the resulting lifestyle and work patterns, balancing out the expected gains against the risks.[40]

Medical Therapy Initial therapy should be noninvasive, as indicated in Figure 38-1, an algorithm for the treatment of cord central pain. Drugs that have been found to be ineffective include trazodone,[41] valproate,[42] and mexilitine.[43] Some benefit was found with ketamine and alfentanil,[44] intrathecal baclofen,[45] possibly combined with clonidine,[46] amitriptyline, clonazepam, nonsteroidal anti-inflammatory drugs, 5-hydroxy tryptophane, desipramine,[47] and intrathecal morphine.[48] Probably the use of amitriptyline is the most popular medical therapy.[49,50] According to Watson, there are no controlled studies of the use of anticonvulsants and opioids.[49]

Surgical Treatment Medical therapy may fail, leading the physician to turn to surgical measures in many patients.[5,6,51] The simplest surgical approach should be tried first.

I have been impressed by a number of published reports indicating that the steady and neuralgic components of cord central pain respond differentially to destructive procedures that interrupt pain pathways rostral to the injury site, such as cord transection (cordectomy), cordotomy, and the dorsal root entry zone (DREZ) procedure (Table 38-2). These reports parallel my own experience.[25] And, in my experience, the same is true for allodynia and

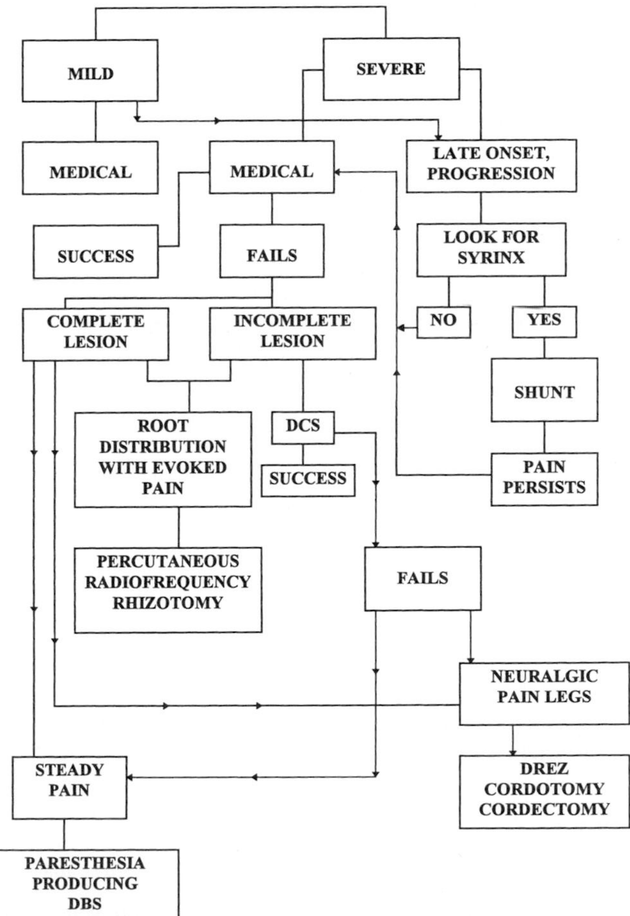

Figure 38-1 Algorithm for the treatment of cord central pain. (Reproduced with permission from Loeser JD, ed. *Bonica's Management of Pain.* 3rd ed. Baltimore, Md: Lippincott Williams and Wilkins; 2001:436.)

TABLE 30-2 **Response of Central Pain of Spinal Cord Origin to Surgery: Percentage of Patients With Any Degree of Relief**

	Type of Pain		
Type of Surgery	**Steady**	**Neuralgic**	**Allodynia and Hyperpathia**
Destructive			
Cordotomy, cordectomy, DREZ procedure	25	83	82
Stimulation to produce paresthesia in area of pain			
DCS, DBS	36	0	16

DBS, deep brain stimulation; DSC, dorsal column stimulation; DREZ, dorsal root entry zone.

hyperpathia. There is no certain explanation of this dichotomy, which is statistically significant, but one interpretation follows. In peripheral neuropathic pain, allodynia is the result of garbled processing in the dorsal horn so that normally non-noxious input is transmitted in the spinothalamic tract.[52,53] How this is produced in cord lesions is unclear, but my own surgical experience suggests that it, too, is dependent on spinothalamic transmission, because it is relieved by destructive surgery that interrupts that tract. The steady pain, on the other hand, may be organized at a cortical level because it is not relieved by cord transection above the lesion site[18,25,54] or by central interruption of pain pathways. This idea is in keeping with the observation that paresthesia-producing stimulation may suppress it. The more exciting aspect of the problem is the response of the neuralgic pain. I equate this with the end-zone pain of Nashold and coworkers[32] and that described by Jefferson,[18] which extends caudally from the level of the cord lesion for several dermatomes[32,55] and is often the most severe component. This is relieved by interrupting spinothalamic transmission.[18,24,25,32,56–59] It is possible such pain may arise from ectopic impulse generation at an injury site,[60,61] conceivably in damaged roots.

Simple Percutaneous Procedures Diagnostic local anesthetic blockade can be treacherous, because it can temporarily relieve neuropathic pain, encouraging surgical interruption at the same site, which nearly always fails.[2–4,7] Repeated local anesthetic blockade, as used therapeutically by Livingston,[7] does not appear to be in current use. Intrathecal injection of hypertonic saline, cold saline, phenol, or alcohol are also probably seldom used today, though alcohol or phenol blocks, which produce similar effects to radiofrequency lesions, may be useful in carefully selected patients. However, such injections tend to be more difficult to localize than radiofrequency lesions and effect unpredictably variable depths of penetration into the target fibers.

Procedures Performed on the Spinal Cord

Percutaneous Radiofrequency Rhizotomy Dorsal rhizotomy is occasionally useful to relieve disabling allodynia or hyperpathia in the distribution of a single, usually brachial, root, usually in a quadriplegic patient. It should be preceded by local anesthetic diagnostic blockade to identify the culprit root and to ensure that no disabling position sense loss will ensue from interruption of that root.

Cordectomy This operation is really transection of the spinal cord above the level of the lesion responsible for the pain. Intuitively, it would be imagined that cordectomy would eliminate cord central pain, but it has proved useful only for the relief of the lancinating and evoked elements. Nashold[32] has reviewed the history of the operation, noting that most published experience is based on small series of patients in whom pain quality was not elaborated. Jefferson, however, reported experience with 19 patients in whom two features determined outcome.[18] If the cord lesion causing the pain was at or above the level of T10, only 25% of patients derived any pain relief after cordectomy, whereas all patients with lower lesions enjoyed some degree of relief. Jefferson also noted that pain was more likely to be relieved if it was episodic and extended to the anterior thighs or knees: 60% of 12 patients undergoing cordectomy enjoyed good relief and 40%, fair relief, of neuralgic pain, and 80% had some relief of evoked pain. However the expectation that cord-injured patients have for eventual restoration of cord function usually makes cordectomy unacceptable, leaving two alternatives: cordotomy and the DREZ procedure.

Cordotomy Originally performed by open, more recently by percutaneous, means, cordotomy is also capable of relieving the neuralgic and evoked but not the steady elements of cord central pain.[14,15,24,25,31,62] Among my own patients, 54% of those undergoing cordotomy enjoyed good relief of neuralgic pain and 32%, fair relief; in addition, 50% had good relief and 25% fair relief of evoked pain.

As mentioned earlier, pain tends to recur gradually after relief by surgical or medical therapy. Cordotomy is no exception, as Rosomoff and colleagues have pointed out in a mixed group of patients.[63] I have found a steady decline over years in the incidence of pain relief after cordotomy accompanied by the recovery of appreciation of pain and temperature sensation below the level of the cordotomy; sometimes repetition of the cordotomy restores pain relief and dissociated sensory loss.[64]

The DREZ Procedure Percutaneous cordotomy carries a small risk of producing ipsilateral arm paresis—a disastrous consequence in a paraplegic patient, and a risk that can be avoided by using the DREZ procedure, instead. The latter is a more massive operation than cordotomy; it requires laminectomy at the level of the cord injury and risks aggravating bladder dysfunction in a continent patient.

The DREZ operation can be performed by cutting the segregated pain fibers as they enter the dorsal horn—with a knife,[56] as Sindou has advocated, or by a series of small radiofrequency lesions, as advocated by Nashold and colleagues. To be successful, the operation must be performed at cord sites that are related somatotopically to the cord central pain. Reported series quote pain relief in 20% to 77% of patients.[32,58,59,65–71] The researchers at Duke University[58,67] and others[71] have emphasized that the procedure preferentially relieves so-called end zone, or root radicular, pain but not diffuse, steady, burning or so-called phantom body pain. End zone pain extends distally from the level of injury into the dermatomes immediately caudal to the level of injury.

Dorsal Column Stimulation For the diffuse steady element of cord central pain, destructive surgery is disappointing. Artificial production of paresthesias in the patient's pain area appears to be the most useful surgical strategy. Although dorsal column stimulation (DCS) is the simplest means of accomplishing this, the technique is seldom successful in cord central pain because of two problems. Firstly, the injury itself or surgery for its emergency treatment may interfere with access to the dorsal columns. Secondly, after major or complete cord lesions, the dorsal columns die back to the dorsal column nuclei, making it impossible to produce paresthesias in the area of pain by stimulating the dorsal columns. In a personal series, of 22 patients with incomplete lesions, 22% enjoyed good relief[25] with DCS; however, none of 11 patients with complete lesions did so. The modality was most useful in patients with incomplete conus–cauda lesions, in which at least some of the pain might have originated in damaged roots. Published results are equally disappointing.[6,25,72–78]

Operations on the Brain

Destructive Procedures In my experience, there is little room for destructive brain operations to treat cord central pain because they add nothing to the benefits achieved from destructive cord lesions and because, like the latter, they are not effective for the relief of the steady pain. In a review of the literature, I found 22% to 36% of patients with central pain were helped by mesencephalic tractotomy[79] or thalamotomy at various sites.[80] Other authors share this pessimistic view,[51,81] although some have suggested a 50% success rate.[5,82,83] The review by Gybels and Sweet[84] suggested that mesencephalic tractotomy relieved 44% of cases of neuropathic pain of all types, including central pain. Although lesions have been made at other sites in the brain in attempts to relieve pain, most of these procedures are of historical interest today.

Deep Brain Stimulation As previously mentioned, DCS is usually technically impossible in cord central pain, which leaves paresthesia-producing deep brain stimulation (DBS) as the only surgical alternative for treating the steady element of cord central pain. There has been controversy as to whether DBS in periventricular-periaqueductal grey matter (PVG/PAG) might be useful in treating neuropathic including central pain. My colleagues and I[85] have shown that when electrodes were inserted in both PVG/PAG and sensory thalamus in patients with neuropathic pain, only electrodes in sensory thalamus were effective. Bendok and Levy,[86] in a literature review, found paresthesia-producing DBS never relieved nociceptive pain but helped 56% of patients with neuropathic pain, whereas PVG/PAG DBS was successful in 59% of patients with nociceptive pain, and in 23% with neuropathic pain. In my experience treating 16 patients with cord central pain, 31% of patients who underwent a trial of DBS and 67% of those permanently implanted achieved useful relief.

BRAIN CENTRAL PAIN

This central pain syndrome results from brain injury, usually stroke. Despite the fact that brain central pain has long been recognized,[87,88] and despite detailed functional imaging and clinical neurophysiologic studies, its mechanism remains obscure and treatment, disappointing. Another example of neuropathic pain, brain central pain shares the characteristics of the group at large.

Clinical Features

Brain central pain can arise from brain lesions of any etiology and severity that interfere with sensory pathways at any level between the foramen magnum and the cerebral cortex. It may occur even after a brain insult that leaves no permanent, clinically detectable sensory loss. Like cord central pain, it has three common components—(1) steady, (2) neuralgic, and (3) evoked (allodynia and hyperpathia)—but whereas in cord central pain the steady and neuralgic components are most common, in brain central pain, steady and evoked pain predominate.

Ninety-one percent of a series of personal cases resulted from vascular lesions: 67% from supratentorial thrombotic stroke, 11% from supratentorial hematoma, and 7% from infratentorial hemorrhage. Although it has been suggested that 1% to 2% of strokes result in pain,[9] Andersen and colleagues[89] found 8% of 207 consecutive patients went on to develop central pain, which was severe in 5%, and 7% developed allodynia. Although Dejerine and Roussy[88] popularized the concept that brain central pain resulted from thalamic lesions, it is now known that this type of pain can arise after lesions anywhere from the medulla to cerebral cortex that affect sensory structures,[90–92] with cortical lesions, especially, involving the second somatosensory area.[93] Various thalamic sites have been incriminated without complete consensus.[94–96]

It is curious that craniocerebral injury and craniotomy rarely result in central pain[97] and that certain common brain lesions, made during neurosurgical operations, virtually never cause central pain (e.g., those in the nonspecific spinoreticulothalamic tract, limbic system, hypothalamus, dorsomedian, center median, intralaminar and reticular nuclei in the thalamus, and lesions in the kinesthetic pathway and the basal ganglia).[4,5,78,98] However, lesions made in the tactile relay nucleus of thalamus cause central pain in from 4% to 18% of patients.[39]

The onset may be immediate, as it was in 29% of 73 personal cases, whereas in 18%, it was delayed up to 1 month, and in 26%, from 1 month to 1 year. Occasionally, onset was delayed for years after the causative event.

If the thalamus is involved in a pain-producing stroke, it is more likely to be on the right side than on the left.[99–101] There are intriguing instances of reversibility of brain central pain, such as after a stroke,[102] removal of a tumor,[103] or resection of cortex,[104,105] but it has not been possible to reverse it consistently by surgical procedures.[4]

In the cases reported by Dejerine and Roussy,[88] dystonia on the same side as the pain was a feature of the syndrome, but only 8.2% of patients I studied[101] had dystonia, always associated with thalamic lesions. And, of course, strokes can produce dystonia without pain. An action tremor of a cerebellar type most commonly associated with brainstem lesions was noted in 6.8% of my cases.

Pathophysiology

Attempts to understand the mechanism of brain central pain have been based on clinical features, imaging, and neurophysiologic studies. Functional imaging has shown thalamic hypoperfusion on the side of the stroke,[35,36] and hyperperfusion in cases with allodynia when allodynia is induced. Canavero and colleagues[106] found reduced perfusion in the parietal lobe in patients with brain central pain and a further reduction occurred after inducing allodynia. These abnormalities disappeared after successful treatment of the pain with injection of propofol. Hirato and coworkers[107] found perfusion was increased in the centrolateral nucleus but reduced in the ventral intermediate nucleus.

The clinical features of strokes associated with central pain have been explored in attempts to define the pathogenesis. Among my own cases, 98.6% of 73 patients complained of steady pain; this pain was described as burning in 64.4%, dysesthetic in 31.6%, and aching in 38.6%. In addition, 64.9% had allodynia or hyperpathia, or both, evoked by single or multiple stimuli; and only 16.4% had intermittent or neuralgic pain. On examination 46.5% of patients showed hemibody deficiencies of all somatosensory modalities; 20.5% showed dissociated sensory loss; 8.2% had loss in all modalities, but especially pain or temperature appreciation; 6.8% had isolated allodynia or hyperpathia, or both; 5.5%, isolated impairment of touch, vibration, or position sense; and 5.5%, no clinically detectable sensory loss. There were no clear correlates between pain and features such as lesion size or location, or degree or quality of sensory loss.[89,101]

Boivie and Leijon[108] concluded that virtually all patients with stroke pain have sensory loss, with diminished appreciation of pain and temperature appearing to be key. However, 1 patient outside their 63-patient study series had no sensory loss, and others have recorded such cases.[5,6,97,101] Vestergaard and coworkers[109] found an increased threshold for pain appreciation in all 11 cases they studied. Neuralgic pain was more common in brainstem lesions in my experience, as in the case reported by Nashold and Wilson.[110] Pain after selective damage to lemniscal pathway such as my colleagues and I have found is very rare, there being apparently only one other reported case.[111] However central pain is a well-known accompaniment of tabes dorsalis, in which the chief destruction of neural tissue occurs in the medial lemniscus.

Based on these clinical data, several authors have suggested that brain central pain is based on central disinhibition resulting from damage to some portion of the spinothalamic tract.[108,112,113] Presumably, subclinical damage could explain pain in cases with no clinically detectable sensory loss, but it is difficult to apply the argument to cases of selective lemniscal loss. Cassinari and Pagni[5] and Bowsher[114] have suggested that pain results from disinhibition caused by selective damage to the neospinothalamic tract that spares spinoreticulothalamic fibers. Craig[115] has suggested that selective loss of thermal sensitivity paths with disinhibition of cold-evoked pain pathways results in brain central pain. Jensen and Lenz[116] hypothesized that pain results from the stroke-deafferentated cells in the reticular nucleus of the thalamus giving rise to a burst in thalamic relay neurons, which projects to the cortex through collaterals from the reticular nucleus.

There is no satisfactory explanation for the idiosyncratic incidence whereby out of a group of patients with similar lesions and similar sensory loss, not all will develop pain.

To study brain central pain, my colleagues and I have taken advantage of thalamic explorations with microelectrodes that were performed to guide DBS implants. Recording examines the receptive fields and the sensory pathway from periphery to thalamus, whereas microstimulation explores the projected fields of the patient's thalamic neurons. We have concluded that neither the presence or pattern of bursting cells nor the somatotopographic reorganization relate to the pain, both features being found in deafferentated patients without pain.

An interesting finding has been the induction of pain by macrostimulation of the medial mesencephalon and thalamus in patients with neuropathic pain of various types, especially stroke pain.[117] These are structures that give no response on stimulation in patients with cancer pain or no pain. This observation suggests that the medial nonspecific polysynaptic pain pathways, such as the spinoreticular, spinomesencephalic, and spinoreticulothalamic, are implicated in neuropathic pain. This suggestion recalls the proposal by Bowsher[114] and Cassinari and Pagni[5] that differential section of the spinothalamic, sparing the spinoreticulothalamic, pathway is somehow related to disinhibition of the latter system, causing pain. In addition, stimulation of these structures in some way enters consciousness and achieves somatotopographic organization.

A second interesting observation is that in patients with stroke pain, stimulation of the tactile relay nucleus of the thalamus often induces pain rather than the usual paresthesias, a feature not seen in other neuropathic pain syndromes.[118–121] My own personal view is that this phenomenon nearly always occurs in patients with allodynia and hyperpathia. This observation suggests that disordered central, presumably cortical, processing of normally non-noxious input results in pain in these patients in a similar manner to that generated at dorsal horn level after peripheral lesions that induce neuropathic pain. An alternative proposition is that the allodynia arises at the dorsal horn as a result of disordered feedback from the cortex. Curiously, just as proximal interruption of spinothalamic tract in cord central pain eliminates allodynia and hyperpathia, so did PVG DBS in 3 of my patients.[122]

The most enlightening observations, however, were made in a patient[123,124] who had suffered a massive thrombotic right-hemisphere stroke that produced spastic left hemiplegia, left homonymous hemianopsia, and left multimodality hemisensory loss with allodynia and hyperpathia (Fig. 38-2). During an unsuccessful attempt to treat the pain with DBS, 14 microelectrode trajectories for recording and microstimulation and 3 macrostimulation trajectories were made in the right hemisphere (on the side of the stroke) between the third ventricle and the right 17 mm lateral sagittal plane. These microelectrodes failed to detect any functioning neurons or any response to stimulation; recording and microstimulation on the opposite hemisphere, performed to implant a PVG DBS electrode, gave typical responses.

These observations led to several conclusions. Firstly, somatosensory function (light touch, position, vibration and kinesthetic sense, appreciation of pain and temperature) is preserved, although diminished, after loss of the contralateral thalamus and cortex; a fact known from studies of patients suffering from infantile hemiplegia or undergoing hemispherectomy. Preserved function on the hemiplegic side is presumably mediated by surviving ipsilateral somatosensory projections both in spinothalamic and medial lemniscal pathways, the diminished appreciation of the sensation presumably corresponding to the relative paucity of ipsilateral, compared with contralateral, fibers. Because of the extent of the patient's stroke, no commissural pathways above midbrain could have survived to explain the findings. Secondly, stroke-induced steady pain, allodynia, and hyperpathia can still occur contralateral to a stroke that eliminates the thalamus and cortex, the clinical picture being identical to that seen after less severe strokes that leave the contralateral hemisphere functioning. This conclusion is in keeping with the fact that central pain has been observed after hemispherectomy.[5,6]

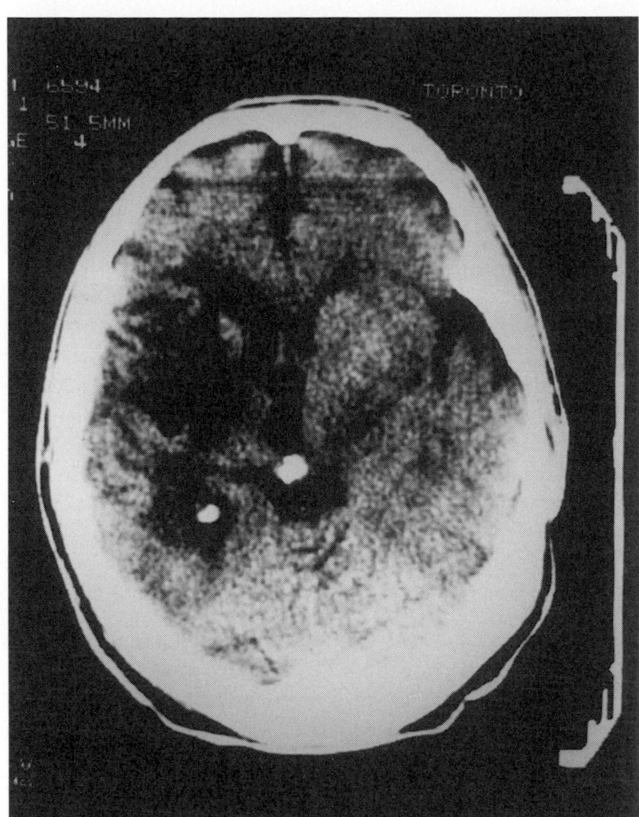

Figure 38-2 Computed tomography scan of head of a patient with brain central pain. (Refer to the accompanying text discussion.)

The following proposal is a preliminary attempt to explain these observations. Firstly, the mechanisms of steady pain and of allodynia and hyperpathia after stroke differ from each other, but it is assumed that the mechanisms are the same regardless of stroke severity, whether causing a tiny infarct in the thalamus or a hemispherectomy. Secondly, stroke pain is signaled by somatosensory cortical mechanisms that are somatotopographically organized, either ipsilateral or contralateral to the pain according to the extent of the stroke. This abnormal pain signaling is driven by mechanisms related to the disconnection, through stroke, of sensory, possibly noxious, receptors from the cortex. This disconnection may be so massive as to result in ipsilateral processing or so slight that the patient demonstrates no enduring, clinically detectable sensory loss.

The most likely pain-driving mechanism resulting after this disconnection is disinhibition of somatotopographically organized somatosensory, possibly nociceptive, pathways. In the previously described patient with a massive stroke that destroyed thalamus and cerebral cortex, the pain-causing disinhibition could act either on the multisynaptic nonsomatotopographically organized structures in the brainstem (e.g., the spinoreticulomesencephalic system) or through a direct descending effect on dorsal horn. This action is possible because all the contralateral specific sensory pathways, including those for temperature and pain, have been eliminated by the stroke, along with the possibility of interplay between specific and nonspecific systems above these levels. There can be no selective damage to the surviving ipsilateral fibers, all of which the stroke left intact. A role for the multisynaptic system would fit with the concepts of other investigators, described earlier,[5,114] and with my own observation of the peculiar pain sensitivity in medial brainstem structures.[117] It is known that spinothalamic fibers project to the nonspecific brainstem and medial thalamic nuclei, and also that in primates, there are ipsilateral projections of spinothalamic tract.[125 p 230]

Thus, I am proposing that steady stroke pain is the result of hyperactivity in brainstem nuclei that mediate the polysynaptic nonsomatotopic portion of the pain pathway induced by disinhibition of those structures by the stroke, with resultant signaling of pain in the paucisynaptic somatotopographically organized system on the side of the brain contralateral to the pain in small strokes and ipsilateral, in massive ones. This explanation might be extended to explain cord central pain or peripheral neuropathic pain if one postulates that the deafferentation in each case is sufficient to result in disinhibition in the same way.

Neuralgic pain is rare after strokes but may be more common after brainstem strokes. The observations of Nashold and Wilson[110] support the concept of ectopic impulse generation at a lesion site, as has been suggested in cord central pain from conus-cauda lesions. In Nashold and Wilson's cases,[110] recordings from the midbrain demonstrated bursts of slow wave activity that correlated with paroxysms of pain. Such pain was relieved by proximal destructive lesions in Nashold's hands.

Treatment

Medical Therapy The same general principles outlined for cord central pain apply to the treatment of brain central pain (Fig. 38-3). Neither medical nor surgical treatment has been very promising. As in other neuropathic pain syndromes, distal local anesthetic blockade can temporarily relieve the pain,[126–128] but offers little permanent therapeutic benefit. This experience has possibly led to the use of intravenous lidocaine perfusion[129,130] and the oral use of mexiletine,[130,131] a drug related to lidocaine. Loh and colleagues[127] have found stellate block and guanethidine infusion useful, but there is little published experience with the technique. There is conflicting information on the use of opioids.[132,133] Other suggested medications include propofol,[134] adrenergically active antidepressants,[131] naloxone,[135] and intrathecal baclofen.[136,137] However, the most frequently employed drugs are amitriptyline and carbamazepine,[49] which were found to be statistically significantly useful in a three-phase, placebo-controlled study.[50]

Surgical Treatment

Peripheral Procedures and Those Performed on the Cord For the most part, surgical strategies for stroke pain must be aimed at the brain. Although cases of relief of stroke pain have been reported after cordotomy,[6] there does not appear to be evidence that this approach is useful. I have found published mention of only two cases of stroke pain relieved by the trigeminal DREZ procedure.[138] DCS is disappointing for the treatment of brain central pain.[6] In my experience, 17% of 12 patients submitted to this simple technique derived ongoing relief. The one promising experience with peripheral procedures, although based on scant evidence, is with chronic trigeminal stimulation.[139] I have used this technique in seven patients with brain central pain in the face, (three with lateral medullary syndrome, one with middle cerebral artery area in-

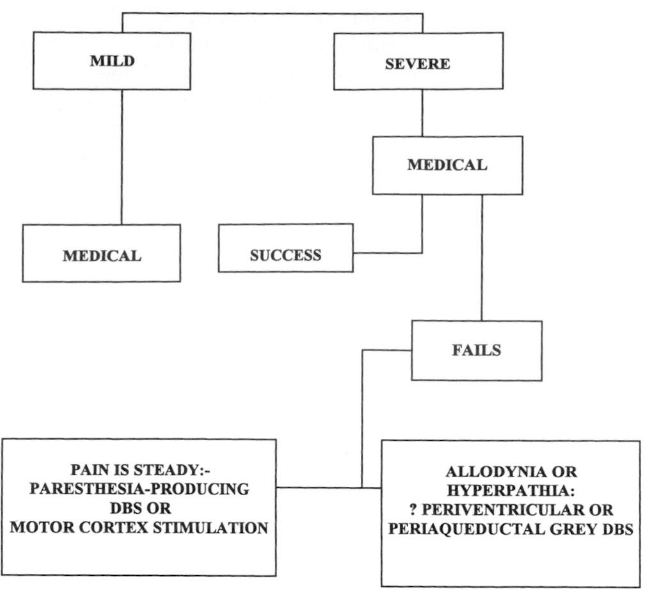

Figure 38-3 Algorithm for the treatment of brain central pain. (Reproduced with permission from Loeser JD, ed. *Bonica's Management of Pain.* 3rd ed. Baltimore, Md: Lippincott Williams and Wilkins; 2001:452.)

farct, one with a massive thalamocortical infarct, one with an infarct from internal carotid artery ligation, and one following medullary trigeminal tractotomy), five of whom (71%) enjoyed more than 50% pain relief after implantation of a permanent device.

Procedures on the Brain In view of the preceding statistics, most procedures for brain central pain have been directed at the brain, particularly mesencephalic tractotomy, medial thalamotomy, and DBS.

Mesencephalic Tractotomy It has always appeared to me from literature reviews that mesencephalic tractotomy carries a low success rate in neuropathic, particularly central, pain, providing 27% to 45% relief of brain central pain. Two recent publications, one by Amano and colleagues in Tokyo[140] and the other by Shieff and Nashold,[141] have reported much more promising outcome data: 64% and 62% relief, respectively, of brain central pain. Both groups of authors stress the inclusion in the mesencephalotomy lesion of the structures medial to the neospinothalamic tract but lateral to the aqueduct in which lies the spinoreticulothalamic system discussed earlier. It is hoped that further data will accumulate to restore general interest in the procedure.

Medial Thalamotomy Medial thalamotomy is the other popular destructive brain procedure used to treat brain central pain. Although different authors have chosen differing targets in the medial thalamus (center median, intralaminar, centrolateral, parafascicular nuclei), all involve the spinoreticulothalamic pathway. Again, my review of the literature has suggested disappointing outcomes after medial thalamotomy for stroke pain, with low initial success rate and frequent recurrence reported.[142–144] A recent article by Jeanmonod and colleagues[145] is much more encouraging, reporting 67% relief. This success may reflect target choice (centrolateral nucleus) and the use of microelectrode guidance. These authors, and Rinaldi and coworkers,[146] have drawn attention to the presence of bursting cells in the medial thalamus and appear to use them to guide the site of their thalamotomy lesion. These authors appear to consider the bursting cells to be deafferentation pain generators, the destruction of which abolishes pain. This is a fascinating proposal; however, my own experience suggests that bursting cells are normal in some brain sites, including the areas under consideration, and that they are markers of deafferentation but not of pain in other sites. Further studies of bursting cells in humans offer many opportunities. In a personal communication with one of my colleagues, Dr. Zelma Kiss of Calgary Alberta, Jeanmonod kindly provided a further update on his work. Of 85 patients with neuropathic, including stroke-induced, pain, 56% enjoyed more than 50% pain relief. Of the various elements of the pain syndromes treated, so-called pain attacks, allodynia, pins and needles, and electrical pain responded best; continuous tearing or compressive deep pain and proprioceptive allodynia were least affected. The other outstanding experience is that of Young and coworkers,[147] who report 60% relief of neuropathic pain in their cases.

Of further interest, Levin and colleagues[148] reported successful treatment of three cases with intrahypophyseal alcohol injection.

Deep Brain Stimulation DBS has frequently been used to treat stroke pain, by stimulating both PVG/PAG and sensory thalamus or medial lemniscus to produce paresthesias in the patient's area of pain. However, in my experience[79] when DBS electrodes were placed for trial stimulation in both PVG and sensory thalamus in the same patient, only the paresthesia-producing electrode proved useful. The experience of Bendok and Levy[86] also leads to the conclusion that DBS is to be preferred for neuropathic, including central, pain. However, DBS in the sensory thalamus, rather than producing pleasant paresthesias, is often too painful to be tolerated by patients who have stroke central pain with allodynia and hyperpathia.[79] In three such patients, PVG DBS alleviated the allodynia and hyperpathia.[122] Published outcome data have suggested a 0% to 80% incidence of useful pain relief with DBS in brain central pain, usually less than 50%. In Levy's reviews,[149,150] 30% to 50% relief was reported, and in Gybels' and Sweet's[84] review, 20%. In my own experience, of 17 cases of brain central pain in whom DBS was attempted, 35% enjoyed significant relief, while 75% of those receiving permanent implants did so.

Motor Cortex Stimulation The remaining therapeutic strategy, motor cortex stimulation, although reported infrequently, appears promising. Tsubokawa and colleagues,[151] who introduced the technique, reported 90% relief after 1 year in their initial experience with 10 patients with brain central pain, and 45% after 2 years' follow-up.[152] Hosobuchi[153] controlled pain in three of six cases. Clearly, in a condition in which therapy has been so disappointing, clinicians will look forward eagerly to further experience with this technique. One of the drawbacks of motor cortex stimulation is the difficulty of accurate electrode localization in patients with massive cortical destruction. Yamamoto and colleagues[154] found that patients had better outcomes if their pain was relieved during a preoperative test injection of thiamytal and ketamine, but not of morphine.

CONCLUSION

Central pain, whether of cord or brain origin, is an astonishing entity whose pathogenesis remains unclear. Yet the condition invites clinical investigative studies to define its neurologic and neuropharmacologic substrate, future understanding of which will, it is hoped, result in more successful therapy, possibly in the form of sophisticated drug infusion techniques. For the present, the relative success in relieving the neuralgic pain down the legs after conus-cauda lesions and the relief of facial pain with trigeminal stimulation must be emphasized.

REFERENCES

1. Merskey H. Classification of chronic pain: Descriptions of chronic pain syndromes and definitions of pain terms. *Pain* 1986;3(suppl): S1–S225.
2. Tasker RR. Deafferentation. In: Wall PD, Melzack R, eds. *Textbook of Pain*. Edinburgh, Scotland: Churchill Livingstone; 1984:119–132.
3. Tasker RR, Organ LW, Hawrylyshyn P. Deafferentation and causalgia. In: Bonica JJ, ed. *Pain*. New York, NY: Raven; 1980:305–329.
4. Tasker RR, Tsuda T, Hawrylyshyn P. Clinical neurophysiological investigation of deafferentation pain. In: Bonica JJ, Lindblom U, Iggo A, eds. *Advances in Pain Research and Therapy*. New York, NY: Raven; 1983:713–738.
5. Cassinari V, Pagni CA. *Central Pain: A Neurosurgical Survey*. Cambridge, Mass: Harvard University Press; 1969.
6. Pagni CA. Central pain due to spinal cord and brain stem damage. In: Wall PD, Melzack R, eds. *Textbook of Pain*. Edinburgh, Scotland: Churchill Livingstone; 1984:481–495.
7. Livingston WK. *Pain Mechanisms: A Physiologic Interpretation of Causalgia and Its Related States*. 2nd ed. New York, NY: Plenum; 1976.
8. Melzack R. Central pain syndromes and theories of pain. In: Casey KL, ed. *Pain and Central Nervous System Disease: The Central Pain Syndromes*. New York, NY: Raven; 1991:59–64.
9. Casey KL. Pain and central nervous system disease: A summary and overview. In: Casey KL, ed. *Pain and Central Nervous System Disease: The Central Pain Syndromes*. New York, NY: Raven; 1991:1–11.
10. Bors E. Phantom limbs of patients with spinal cord injury. *AMA Arch Neurol Psychol* 1951;66:610–631.
11. Berger M, Gerstenbrad F. Phantom illusions in spinal cord injuries. In: Siegfried J, Zimmermann M, eds. *Phantom and Stump Pain*. Berlin, Germany: Springer-Verlag; 1981:66–73.
12. Wall PD. On the origin of pain associated with amputation. In: Siegfried J, Zimmermann M, eds. *Phantom and Stump Pain*. Berlin, Germany: Springer-Verlag; 1981:2–14.
13. Carlen PL, Wall PD, Nodvorna H, Steinbach T. Phantom limbs and related phenomena in recent traumatic amputations. *Neurology* 1978; 28:211–217.
14. Porter RW, Hohmann GW, Bors E, et al. Cordotomy for pain following cauda equina injury. *Arch Surg* 1966;92:765–770.
15. White JC, Sweet WH. *Pain and the Neurosurgeon: A Forty-Year Experience*. Springfield, Ill: Charles C Thomas; 1969:435–477.
16. Mariano AJ. Chronic pain and spinal cord injury. *Clin J Pain* 1992; 8:87–92.
17. Nepomuceno C, Fine PR, Richards JS, et al. Pain in patients with spinal injury. *Arch Phys Med Rehabil* 1979;60:605–609.
18. Jefferson A. Cordectomy for intractable pain. In: Lipton S, Miles J, eds. *Persistent Pain*. Vol 4. New York, NY: Grune & Stratton; 1983: 115–112.
19. Burke DC. Pain in paraplegia. *Paraplegia* 1973;10:297–313.
20. Yezierski RP. Pain following spinal cord injury: The clinical problem and experimental studies. *Pain* 1996;68:185–194.
21. Rose M, Robinson JE, Ellis P, Cole JD. Pain following spinal cord injury: Results from a postal survey [letter]. *Pain* 1988;34:101–102.
22. Richards JS, Meredith RL, Nepomuceno C, et al. Psychological aspects of chronic pain in spinal cord injury. *Pain* 1980;8:355–366.
23. Richardson RR, Meyer PR, Cerullo LJ. Neurostimulation in the modulation of intractable paraplegic and traumatic neuroma pains. *Pain* 1980;8:75–84.
24. Botterell EH, Callaghan JC, Jousse AT. Pain in paraplegia: Clinical management and surgical treatment. *Proc R Soc Med* 1954;47:281–288.
25. Tasker RR, De Carvalho GTC, Dolan EJ. Intractable pain of spinal cord origin: Clinical features and implications for surgery. *J Neurosurg* 1992;77:373–378.
26. Milhorat TH, Kotzen RM, Mu HTM, et al. Dysesthetic pain in patients with syringomyelia. *Neurosurgery* 1996;38:940–947.
27. Boureau F, Doubrère JF, Luu M. Study of verbal description in neuropathic pain. *Pain* 1990;42:145–152.
28. Pollock LJ, Brown M, Boshes B, et al. Pain below the level of injury of the spinal cord. *Arch Neurol Psychiatr* 1951;65:319–322.
29. Waisbrod H, Hansen D, Gerbershagen HU. Chronic pain in paraplegics. *Neurosurgery* 1984;15:933–934.
30. Beriü A, Dimitrijevic MR, Lindblom J. Central dysesthesia syndrome in spinal cord injury. *Pain* 1988;34:109–116.
31. Davis L, Martin J. Studies upon spinal cord injuries: II The nature and treatment of pain. *J Neurosurg* 1947;4:483–491.
32. Nashold BS Jr. Paraplegia and pain. In: Nashold BS Jr, Ovelmen-Levitt J, eds. *Deafferentation Pain Syndromes: Pathophysiology and Treatment*. New York, NY: Raven; 1991:301–319.
33. Siddall PJ, Taylor DA, Cousins MJ. Classification of pain following spinal cord injury. *Spinal Cord* 1997;35:69–75.
34. Levitt M, Levitt JH. The deafferentation syndrome in monkeys: Dysesthesias of spinal origin. *Pain* 1981;10:129–147.
35. Pagni CA, Canavero S. Functional thalamic depression in a case of reversible central pain due to a spinal intramedullary cyst. *J Neurosurg* 1995;83:163–165.
36. Cesaro P, Defer G, Moretti JL, Dagos JD. Central pain and thalamic activation. *Pain* 1990;(suppl 5):S433.
37. Melzack R, Loeser JD. Phantom body pain in paraplegics: Evidence for a central "pattern generating mechanism" for pain. *Pain* 1978;4: 195–210.
38. Tasker RR. The recurrence of pain after neurosurgical procedures. *Qual Life Res* 1994;3(suppl 1):S43–S49.
39. Tasker RR. Pain resulting from central nervous system pathology (central pain). In: Bonica JJ, ed. *The Management of Pain*. 2nd ed. Philadelphia, Pa: Lea & Febiger; 1990:264–283.
40. Tasker RR, Gybels J. Central neurosurgery. In: Wall PD, Melzack R, eds. *Textbook of Pain*. 4th ed. Churchill Livingston: Edinburgh; 1999:1307–1339.
41. Davidoff G, Guarricini M, Roth E, et al. Trazodone hydrochloride in the treatment of dysesthetic pain in traumatic myelopathy: A randomized, double-blind, placebo-controlled study. *Pain* 1987;29: 151–161.
42. Drewes AM, Andreasen A, Paulsen LH. Valproate for treatment of chronic central pain after spinal cord injury. A double-blind crossover study. *Paraplegia* 1994;32:565–569.
43. Chiou-Tan FY, Tuel SM, Johnson JC, Priebe MM, Hirsh DD, Strayer JR. Effect of mexiletine on spinal cord injury dysesthetic pain. *Am J Phys Med Rehabil* 1996;75:84–87.
44. Eide PK, Stubhaug A, Stenehjem AE. Central dysesthesia pain after traumatic spinal cord injury is dependent on N-methyl-D-aspartate receptor activation. *Neurosurgery* 1995;37:1080–1085.
45. Kawabatake H, Iseki H, Ueda A, Takakura K. A new approach to the control of central deafferentation pain—spinal intrathecal baclofen. *Acta Neurochir* 1995;64(suppl):136–138.
46. Middleton JW, Siddale PJ, Walker S, Molloy AR, Rutkowski SB. Intrathecal clonidine and baclofen in the management of spasticity and neurogenic pain following spinal cord injury: A case study. *Arch Phys Med Rehabil* 1996;77:824–826.
47. Leijon G, Boivie J. Pharmacological treatment of central pain. In: Casey KL, ed. *Pain and Central Nervous System Disease: The Central Pain Syndrome*. New York, NY: Raven; 1991:257–266.
48. Fenollosa P, Pallares J, Cervera J, et al. Chronic pain in the spinal cord injured: Statistical approach and pharmacological treatment. *Paraplegia* 1993;31:722–729.

49. Watson CPN. Nonsurgical considerations in neuropathic pain. In: Gildenberg PL, Tasker RR, eds. *Textbook of Stereotactic and Functional Neurosurgery*. New York, NY: McGraw-Hill; 1998:1637–1643.
50. Leijon O, Boivie J. Central post-stroke pain—a controlled trial of amitriptyline and carbamazepine. *Pain* 1989;36:27–36.
51. Meglio M. Evaluation and management of central and peripheral deafferentation pains. In: Gildenberg PL, Tasker RR, eds. *Textbook of Stereotactic and Functional Neurosurgery*. New York, NY: McGraw-Hill; 1998:1631–1635.
52. Woolf CJ. Evidence for a central component of post-injury pain hypersensitivity. *Nature* 1983;306:686–688.
53. Woolf CJ. Central mechanisms of acute pain. *Pain* 1990;(suppl 5): S218.
54. Tasker RR, Tsuda T, Hawrylyshyn P. Clinical neurophysiological investigation of deafferentation pain. In: Bonica JJ, Lindblom U, Iggo A, eds. *Advances in Pain Research and Therapy*. New York, NY: Raven; 1983:713–738.
55. Friedman AH, Bullitt E. Dorsal root entry zone lesions in the treatment of pain following brachial plexus avulsion, spinal cord injury and herpes zoster. *Appl Neurophysiol* 1988;51:164–169.
56. Sindou M, Fischer G, Goutelle A, Mansuy L. La radicellotomie postérieure sélective: Premiers résultats dans la chirurgie de la douleur. *Neurochirurgie* 1974;20:397–408.
57. Nashold BS Jr, Ostdahl RH. Dorsal root entry zone lesions for pain relief. *J Neurosurg* 1979;51:59–69.
58. Nashold BS Jr, Bullitt E. Dorsal root entry zone lesions to control central pain in paraplegics. *J Neurosurg* 1981;55:414–419.
59. Nashold BS Jr, Ostadahl RH, Bullitt E, et al. Dorsal root entry zone lesions: A new neurosurgical therapy for deafferentation pain. In: Bonica JJ, Lindblom U, Iggo A, eds. *Advances in Pain Research and Therapy*. Vol 5. New York, NY: Raven; 1983:739–750.
60. Raymond SA, Rocco AG. Ephaptic coupling of large fibres as a clue to mechanism in chronic neuropathic allodynia following damage to dorsal roots. *Pain* 1990;(suppl 5):S276.
61. Nordin M, Nystrom B, Wallin U, Hagbarth KE. Ectopic sensory discharges and paresthesiae in patients with disorders of peripheral nerves, dorsal roots and dorsal columns. *Pain* 1984;20:231–245.
62. White JC. Anterolateral chordotomy: Its effectiveness in relieving pain of non-malignant disease. *Neurochirurgia* 1963;6:83–102.
63. Rosomoff HL, Papo I, Loeser JD, et al. Neurosurgical operations on the spinal cord. In Bonica JJ, ed. *The Management of Pain*. 2nd ed. Philadelphia, Pa: Lea & Febiger; 1990:2067–2081.
64. Tasker, RR. Percutaneous cordotomy. In: Schmidek HH, Sweet WH, eds. *Operative Neurosurgical Techniques, Indications, Methods, and Results*. 3rd ed. Philadelphia, Pa: WB Saunders; 1995:1595–1611.
65. Richter HP, Seitz K. Dorsal root entry zone lesions for the control of deafferentation pain: Experience in ten patients. *Neurosurgery* 1984; 15:913–916.
66. Sweet WH, Poletti CE. Operations in the brain stem and spinal canal, with an appendix on open cordotomy. In: Wall PD, Melzack R, eds. *Textbook of Pain*. Edinburgh, Scotland: Churchill Livingstone; 1984: 615–631.
67. Friedman AH, Nashold JRB, Nashold BS Jr. DREZ lesions for treatment of pain. In: North RB, Levy RM, eds. *Neurosurgical Management of Pain*. New York, NY: Springer-Verlag; 1997:176–190.
68. Young RF. Clinical experience with radiofrequency and laser DREZ lesions. *J Neurosurg* 1990;72:715–720.
69. Powers SK. Laser-induced DREZ lesions. *J Neurosurg* 1984;60:871.
70. Wiegand H, Winkelmüller W. Bejhandlung des Deafferentierungsschmerzes durch Hochfrequenzläsion der Hinterwurzeteintrittszone. *Dtsch Med Wochenschr* 1985;110:216–220.
71. Sampson JH, Cashman RG, Nashold BS Jr, Friedman AH. Dorsal root entry zone lesions for intractable pain after trauma to the conus medullaris and cauda equina. *J Neurosurg* 1995;82:28–34.
72. Sweet WH, Wepsic JG. Stimulation of the posterior columns of the spinal cord for pain control: Indications, technique, and results. *Clin Neurosurg* 1974;21:278–310.
73. Lazorthes Y, Verdie JC, Arbus L. Stimulation analgésique médullaire amtérieure et postérieure par technique d'implantation percutanée. *Acta Neurochir (Wien)* 1978;40:253–276.
74. Urban BJ, Nashold BS. Percutaneous epidural stimulation of the spinal cord for relief of pain. *J Neurosurg* 1978;48:323–328.
75. Richardson RR, Meyer PR, Cerullo LJ. Neurostimulation in the modulation of intractable paraplegic and traumatic neuroma pains. *Pain* 1980;8:75–84.
76. Cioni B, Meglio M, Plentimalli L, Visocchi M. Spinal cord stimulation in the treatment of paraplegic pain. *J Neurosurg* 1995;82:35–59.
77. Lazorthes Y, Siegfried J, Verdie JC, Casaux J. Chronic spinal cord stimulation in the treatment of neurogenic pain. Cooperative and retrospective study on 20 years of follow-up. *Neurochirurgie* 1995;41: 73–86.
78. Nashold BS Jr. Central pain: Its origins and treatment. *Clin Neurosurg* 1974;20:311–322.
79. Tasker RR. Stereotaxic surgery. In: Wall PD, Melzack R, eds. *Textbook of Pain*. Edinburgh, Scotland: Churchill Livingstone; 1984; 639–655.
80. Tasker RR. Thalamic procedures. In: Schaltenbrand G, Walker AE, eds. *Stereotaxy of the Human Brain: Anatomical, Physiological and Clinical Applications*. Stuttgart; 1982:484–497.
81. Pagni CA. Place of stereotactic technique in surgery for pain. In: Bonica JJ, ed. *Advances in Neurology*. Vol 4. New York, NY: Raven; 1974:699–706.
82. Nashold BS Jr. Brain stem stereotaxic procedures. In: Schaltenbrand G, Walker AE, eds. *Stereotaxy of the Human Brain: Anatomical, Physiological and Clinical Applications*. Stuttgart; 1982:475–483.
83. Davis RA, Stokes JW. Neurosurgical attempts to relieve thalamic pain. *Surg Gynecol Obstet* 1966;123:371–384.
84. Gybels JM, Sweet WH. *Neurosurgical Treatment of Persistent Pain: Physiological and Pathological Mechanisms of Human Pain*. Basel, Switzerland: Karger; 1989.
85. Tasker RR, Vilela Filho O. Deep brain stimulation for the control of intractable pain. In: Youmans JR, ed. *Neurological Surgery*. 4th ed. Philadelphia, Pa: WB Saunders; 1996;3512–3527.
86. Bendok B, Levy RM. Brain stimulation for persistent pain management. In: Gildenberg PL, Tasker RR, eds. *Textbook of Stereotactic and Functional Neurosurgery*. New York, NY: McGraw-Hill: 1998: 1539–1546.
87. Riddoch G. The clinical features of central pain. *Lancet* 1938;1093–1098, 1150–1156, 1205–1209.
88. Dejerine J, Roussy G. La syndrome thalamique. *Rev Neurol (Paris)* 1906;14:521–532.
89. Andersen G, Vestergaard K, Ingeman-Nielsen, Jensen TS. Incidence of central post-stroke pain. *Pain* 1995;61:187–193.
90. Biemond A. The conduction of pain above the level of the thalamus opticus. *Arch Neurol Psychiatr* 1956;75:231–244.
91. Agnew DC, Shetter AG, Segall HD, Flom RA. Thalamic pain. In: Bonica JJ, Lindblom U, Iggo A, eds. *Advances in Pain Research and Therapy*. Vol 5. New York, NY: Raven; 1983:941–946.
92. Bowsher D, Lahuerta J, Brock L. Twelve cases of central pain, only three with thalamic lesions. *Pain* 1984;2(suppl):S83.
93. Schmahmann JD, Leifer D. Parietal pseudothalamic pain syndrome: Clinical features and anatomic correlates. *Arch Neurol* 1992;1032–1037.
94. Bogousslavsky J, Regli F, Uske A. Thalamic infarcts: Clinical syndromes, etiology and prognosis. *Neurology* 1988;38:837–848.
95. Walker AE. The anatomical basis of the thalamic syndrome. *J Belge Neurol Psychiatr* 1938;38:69–95.
96. De Ajuraguerra J. *La douleur dans les affections du système nerveux central*. Paris, France: Doin; 1937.
97. Marshall J. Sensory disturbances in cortical wounds with special reference to pain. *J Neurol Neurosurg Psychiatry* 1951;14:187–204.
98. Tasker RR, Sequeira J, Hawrylyshyn P. Whatever happened to VIM thalamotomy for parkinsonism? *Appl Neurophysiol* 1983;46:68–83.

99. Kameyama M. Vascular lesions of the thalamus on the dominant and nondominant side. *Appl Neurophysiol* 1976–1977;39:171–177.
100. Nasreddine ZS, Saver JL. Pain after thalamic stroke: Right diencephalic predominance and clinical features in 180 patients. *Neurology* 1997;48:1196–1199.
101. Tasker RR, De Carvalho G. Pain in thalamic stroke. In: Proceedings of Stroke Rehabilitation: A conference and workshop on pain and ethical and social issues. Stroke Rehabilitation XIII Annual Scientific Meeting of the Inter-Urban Stroke Academic Association; May 4–5, 1990; Toronto, Ontario.
102. Soria ED, Fine EJ. Disappearance of thalamic pain after parietal subcortical stroke. *Pain* 1991;44:285–288.
103. Portagas C, Avdelidis D, Singounas E, Missir O, Sessopos A. Episodic pain associated with a tumor on the parietal operculum: A case report and literature review. *Pain* 1997;72:201–208.
104. Hamby WB. Reversible central pain. *Arch Neurol* 1961;5:82–86.
105. Erickson TC, Blackwenn WJ, Woolsey CN. Observations on the postcentral gyrus in relation to pain. *Trans Am Neurol Assoc* 1952:57–59.
106. Canavero S, Pagni CA, Castellano G, et al. The role of cortex in central pain syndromes: preliminary results of a long-term technetium-99 hexamethylpropylene amineoxime single photon emission computed tomography study. *Neurosurgery* 1993;32:185–191.
107. Hirato M, Watanabe K, Takahashi A, et al. Pathophysiology of central (thalamic) pain: Combined change of sensory thalamus with cerebral cortex around central sulcus. *Stereotact Funct Neurosurg* 1993; 62:300–303.
108. Boivie J, Leijon G. Clinical findings in patients with central poststroke pain. In: Casey KL, ed. *Pain and Central Nervous System Disease*. New York, NY: Raven; 1991:65–75.
109. Vestergaard K, Nielsen J, Andersen G, et al. Sensory abnormalities in consecutive, unselected patients with central post-stroke pain. *Pain* 1995;61:177–186.
110. Nashold BS Jr, Wilson WP. Central pain. Observations in man with chronic implanted electrodes in the midbrain tegmentum. *Confin Neurol* 1966;27:30–44.
111. Garcin R. La douleur dans les affections organiques du système nerveux central. *Rev Neurol (Paris)* 1937;68:105–153.
112. Leijon G. *Central Post-stroke Pain: Clinical Characteristics, Mechanism and Treatment*. Linkoping University Medical Dissertations, Sweden, No 281, 1988.
113. Boivie J, Leijon G, Johansson I. Central post-stroke pain: A study of the mechanisms through analyses of the sensory abnormalities. *Pain* 1985;37:173–185.
114. Bowsher D. The problems of central pain. *Verh Dtsch Ges Inn Med* 1980;86:1535–1537.
115. Craig A. A new version of the thalamic disinhibition hypothesis of central plain. *Pain Forum* 1998;7:1–14.
116. Jensen TS, Lenz FA. Central post-stroke pain: A challenge for the scientist and the clinician [guest editorial]. *Pain* 1995;61:161–164.
117. Tasker RR, Organ LW, Hawrylyshyn PA. *The Thalamus and Midbrain of Man: a Physiological Atlas using Electrical Stimulation*. Springfield, Ill: Charles C Thomas; 1982:154–172.
118. Davis KD, Kiss ZHT, Tasker RR, Dostrovsky JO. Thalamic stimulation-evoked sensations in chronic pain patients and in nonpain (movement disorder) patients. *J Neurophysiol* 1996;75:1026–1034.
119. Davis KD, Dostrovsky JO, Tasker RR, et al. Increased incidence of pain evoked by thalamic stimulation in post-stroke pain patients. *Soc Neurosci Abstr* 1993;19:1572.
120. Lenz FA, Tasker RR, Dostrovsky JO, et al. Abnormal single-unit activity and responses to stimulation in the presumed ventrocaudal nucleus of patients with central pain. In: Dubner R, Gebhart GF, Bond MR, eds. *Proceedings of the V World Congress on Pain*. Amsterdam, Holland: Elsevier; 1988:158–164.
121. Gorecki J, Hirayama T, Dostrovsky JO, et al. Thalamic stimulation and recording in patients with deafferentation and central pain. *Stereotact Funct Neurosurg* 1987;52:219–226.
122. Parrent A, Lozano A, Tasker RR, Dostrovsky J. Periventricular gray stimulation suppresses allodynia and hyperpathia in man [abstract]. *Stereotactc Funct Neurosurg* 1992;59:82.
123. Parrent AG, Lozano AM, Dostrovsky JO, Tasker RR. Central pain in the absence of functional sensory thalamus. *Stereotact Funct Neurosurg* 1992;59:9–14.
124. Parrent AG, Tasker RR. Can the ipsilateral hemisphere mediate pain in man? [abstract] *Acta Neurochir* 1992;117:89.
125. Willis WW. *The Pain System. The Neural Basis of Nociceptive Transmission in the Mammalian Nervous System*. Karger, Switzerland: Basel; 1985:130.
126. Crisologo PA, Neal B, Brown R, McDanal J, Kissin I. Lidocaine-induced spinal block can relieve central poststroke pain: Role of the block in chronic pain diagnosis. *Anaesthesiology* 1991;74:184–185.
127. Loh L, Nathan PW, Schott GD. Pain due to lesions of central nervous system removed by sympathetic block. *Br Med J* 1981;282:1026–1028.
128. Kibler RF, Nathan PW. Relief of pain and paresthesiae by nerve block distal to a lesion. *J Neurosurg* 1960;23:91–98.
129. Galer BS, Miller KV, Rowbotham MC. Response to intravenous lidocaine infusion differs based on clinical diagnosis and site of nervous system injury. *Neurology* 1993;43:1233–1235.
130. Edmondson EA, Simpson RK Jr, Stubler DK, Beric A. Systemic lidocaine therapy for poststroke pain. *South Med J* 1993;86:1093–1096.
131. Bowsher D. The management of central post-stroke pain. *Postgrad Med J* 1995;71:598–604.
132. Dehen H, Willer JC, Cambier J. Pain in thalamic syndrome. In: Bonica JJ, Lindblom U, Iggo A, eds. *Advances in Pain Research and Therapy*. Vol 5. New York, NY: Raven; 1993:935–940.
133. Strumpf M. Zenz M. Opioid therapy of central pain conditions—long-term therapy? An expanded indication for opioid drugs. *Fortschr Med* 1994;112:227–228.
134. Canavero S, Bonicalzi V, Pagni CA, et al. Propofol analgesia in central pain: Preliminary clinical observations. *J Neurol* 1995;242: 561–567.
135. Budd K. The use of the opiate antagonist, naloxone, in the treatment of intractable pain. *Neuropeptides* 1985;5:419–422.
136. Taira T, Tanikawa T, Kawamura H, Iseki H, Takakura K. Spinal intrathecal baclofen suppresses central pain after a stroke. *J Neurol Neurosurg Psychiatry* 1994;57:381–382.
137. Taira T, Kawamura H, Tanikawa T, et al. A new approach to the control of central deafferentation pain—spinal intrathecal baclofen. *Acta Neurochir* 1995;64(suppl):136–138.
138. Sampson JH, Nashold BS Jr. Facial pain due to vascular lesions of the brain stem relieved by dorsal root entry zone lesions in the nucleus caudalis. Report of two cases. *J Neurosurg* 1992;77:473–475.
139. Taub E, Munz M, Tasker RR. Chronic electrical stimulation of the gasserian ganglion for the relief of pain in a series of 34 patients. *J Neurosurg* 1997;86:197–202.
140. Amano K, Kawamura H, Tanikawa T, et al. Long term follow up study of rostral mesencephalic reticulotomy for pain relief: report of 34 cases. *Appl Neurophysiol* 1986;49:105–111.
141. Shieff C, Nashold BS. Stereotactic mesencephalic tractotomy for thalamic pain. *Neurol Res* 1987;99:101–104.
142. Pagni CA. The treatment of central deafferentation pain syndrome. In: Nashold BS Jr, Ovelmen-Levitt J, eds. *Deafferentation Pain Syndromes*. New York, NY: Raven; 1991;275–283.
143. Namba S, Nakao Y, Matsumoto T, et al. Electrical stimulation of the posterior limb of the internal capsule for the treatment of thalamic pain. *Appl Neurophysiol* 1984;47:137–148.
144. Niizuma H, et al. Follow-up results of centromedian thalamotomy for central pain. *Appl Neurophysiol* 1982;45:324–325.
145. Jeanmonod D, Magnin M, Morel M. Thalamus and neurogenic pain: Physiological, anatomical and clinical data. *Neuroreport* 1993;4:475–478.
146. Rinaldi PC, Young RF, Albe-Fessard D, Chodakiewitz J. Spontaneous neuronal hyperactivity in the medial and intralaminar thalamic nuclei of patients with deafferentation pain. *J Neurosurg* 1991;74:415–521.

147. Young RF, Jacques DS, Rand RW, Copcutt BC, Vermeulen SS, Posewitz AE. Technique of stereotactic medial thalamotomy with the Leksell gamma knife for treatment of chronic pain. *Neurol Res* 1995;17:59–65.
148. Levin AB, Remirez LF, Katz J. The use of stereotaxic chemical hypophysectomy in the treatment of thalamic pain syndrome. *J Neurosurg* 1983;59:1002–1006.
149. Levy RM, Lamb S, Adams JE. Deep brain stimulation for chronic pain: Long-term follow-up in 145 patients from 1972–1984. *Pain* 1984;(suppl 2):S115.
150. Levy RM, Lamb S, Adams JE. Treatment of chronic pain by deep brain stimulation: Long-term follow-up and review of the literature. *Neurosurgery* 1987;21:885–893.
151. Tsubokawa T, Katayama Y, Yamamoto T, et al. Motor cortex stimulation for control of thalamic pain. *Pain* 1990;(suppl 5):491.
152. Tsubokawa T, Katayama Y, Yamamoto T, et al. Chronic motor cortex stimulation for the treatment of central pain. *Acta Neurochir* 1991; 52(suppl):137–139.
153. Hosobuchi Y. Motor cortical stimulation for control of central deafferentation pain. In: Devinsky O, Beriü A, Dogali M, eds. *Electrical and Magnetic Stimulation of the Brain and Spinal Cord.* New York, NY: Raven; 1993:215–217.
154. Yamamoto T, Katayama Y, Hirayama T, Tsubokawa T. Pharmacological classification of central post-stroke pain: Comparison with the results of chronic motor cortex stimulation therapy. *Pain* 1997; 72:5–12.

CHAPTER 39 COMPLEX REGIONAL PAIN SYNDROME

Michael Stanton-Hicks

Ever since Claude Bernard implicated the sympathetic nervous system in sensation, its role in nociception has been the subject of debate.[1] No one would argue with the fact that the sympathetic nervous system is intimately involved with the preservation of homeostasis and noxious challenges in humans, although the manner in which it influences the sensation of pain has, until recently, escaped explanation.[2] Anatomically, the sympathetic nervous system constitutes a highly complex arrangement of preganglionic and postganglionic neurons that subserve specific and diverse functions of target organs, including enteric neurons, smooth muscle, syncytial muscle, and striated muscle.[3] Physiologically, the sympathetic nervous system is associated in some way with both systemic and specific local reactions, which are expressed by supratentorial and confrontational aspects that are represented in the periaquaductal gray matter of the midbrain (e.g., non-opioid analgesia).[4,5] In contrast, rest and quiescence are represented in the ventrolateral periaquaductal gray matter, being associated with endogenous opioid analgesia.

The stress response described by Selye,[6] "fight or flight," involves both spinal levels of integration, with hypothalamo-mesencephalic centers, but is associated with adrenocortical and hypothalamo-hypophyseal responses designed to protect the organism under normal biologic conditions. A secondary set of responses to sympathetic activity that can be considered pathophysiologic and occur with or without obvious nerve injury are those changes in blood flow, sudomotor and muscle activity, with subsequent trophic changes and abnormal sensation long after the noxious event.[7,8] Sensory changes include allodynia, hypoalgesia, hyperalgesia, hyperesthesia, and hyperpathia. Why, and in what manner, the sympathetic nervous system is involved in these changes that occur in a small but readily identifiable group of patients is still unclear. However, recent research has clarified some of the previous misconceptions with regard to levels of sympathetic activity, involvement of the central nervous system, and the possibility of preexisting immunologic factors. Interestingly, similarities in the characteristics of complex regional pain syndrome (CRPS) are seen in other chronic pain states, such as irritable bowel syndrome, interstitial cystitis, nonulcer dyspepsia, and certain cases of angina pectoris.

During the Civil War, Weir Mitchell[9] drew attention to the exaggerated response to nerve injury that was distinct from the neurogenic inflammation that is associated with most nerve injuries. These patients typically suffered from a penetrating injury in the vicinity of a major nerve, in most cases without disruption, and typically caused by a musket shot. Mitchell called this *causalgia* because of the bizarre swelling, heat (*causa*), and pain (*algia*), which were out of all proportion to the signs and symptoms of most nerve injuries. Leriche,[10] a French surgeon, also described similar syndromes in the lower extremities for which he developed the surgical procedure of stripping the sympathetic nervous plexus from the large vessels in the lower extremities. Sudeck, in a series of articles, provided similar descriptions with detailed observations of the bony and trophic changes following injury that came to be described in German-speaking countries as "morbus Sudeck" or "Sudeck's atrophy."[11]

Perhaps Livingston, more than any other individual, would influence contemporary thinking with regard to these CRPSs. Livingston[12] proposed the concept of a vicious circle that involved the spinal cord at the level of sensory interneurons, which are maintained in a state of abnormal repetitive firing from the periphery (Fig. 39-1). In other words, Livingston proposed that a linkage existed between afferent nociception, and the efferent responses generated by spinal neurons in some manner contributed to an exaggeration of the nociceptive signals in the local injured tissue. This so-called sympathosomatic coupling suggested the genesis of a reflex mechanism that was fundamental to these disorders.

Obviously influenced by Livingston's thinking, Evans[13] coined the term *reflex sympathetic dystrophy,* in a single stroke implying a mechanism that had not yet been scientifically validated. It is interesting to note that Lewis,[14] also a contemporary, made the suggestion that secretory dysfunction might be responsible for the dystrophic changes and atrophy that are seen in integumentary structures, although he did not specifically imply that there was a disturbance of autonomic function. He suggested that the nocifensor nerves actually became irritated in causalgic states, thereby potentiating the clinical process.

Experiments by Walker and Nulsen,[15] who were interested in autonomic physiology, determined that stimulation of the sympathetic trunk in patients who had undergone a thoracic sympathectomy for causalgia elicited burning and tingling paresthesias in the affected extremity. Twenty years later, these observations were confirmed by White and Sweet,[16] who contended that a *sympathetically dependent* mechanism is responsible for the disturbance that is seen in patients with causalgia and reflex sympathetic dystrophy. Other clinical observations that support a role of the sympathetic nervous system in pain are the relief that frequently attends interruption of the paravertebral ganglia with local anesthetics, chemical or physical modalities, and surgery; as well as intravenous regional application of guanethidine, bretylium, and systemic intravenous phentolamine.[17–20]

With regard to intravenous regional sympatholysis, placebo-controlled, double-blind studies have supported the use of this modality and method of inducing analgesia.[21] Observations by Jänig and McLachlan,[22] Blumberg and Jänig,[23] Häbler and colleagues,[24] Jänig and Koltzenburg,[25] and Price and colleagues[26] provide evidence in favor of a role for the sympathetic nervous system in the generation of pain in such patients. Likewise, Torebjörk and coworkers[27] have demonstrated that α-adrenoceptor agonists that are applied by injection or iontophoresis in a previously affected extremity rekindle symptoms in patients who had been in remission for periods exceeding 15 years. Similar responses have been elicited by injection of epinephrine into a chronic neuroma.

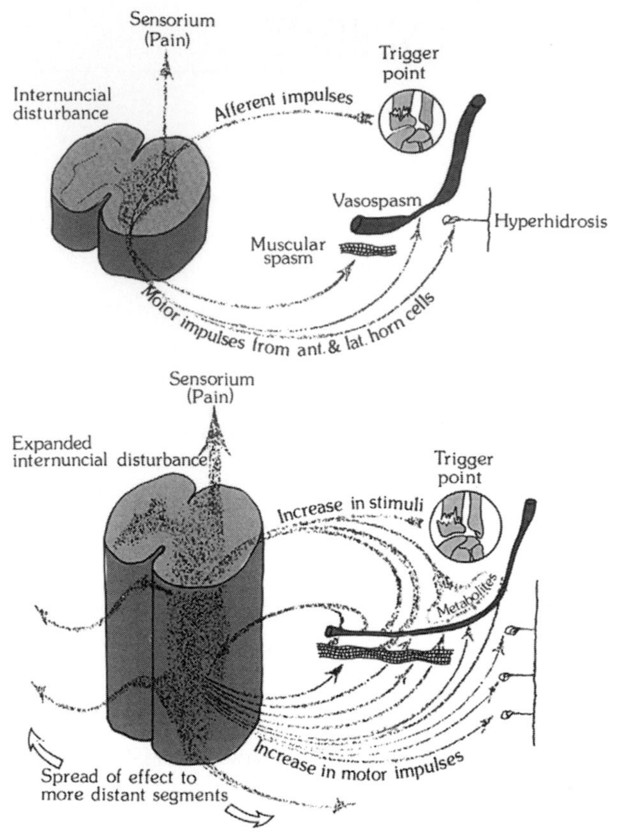

Figure 39-1 Figure illustrates the concept of a vicious circle involving the spinal cord both at the level of the sensory disturbance and the temporal and spatial expansion that was proposed by Livingston[12] in 1943.

In 1986, Roberts[28] introduced the concept of sympathetically maintained pain (SMP), which he postulated accompanies CRPS at some point in the natural history of the condition. His suggestion that low-threshold mechanoreceptors types I and II (Aβ fibers) are induced by postganglionic sympathetic activity that, in turn, induces chronic firing in wide-dynamic-range (WDR) multi-receptive neurons, (lamina 5, dorsal horn), thereby maintain the status quo (Fig. 39-2). The hypothesis is supported by animal experiments that demonstrate an activation of mechanoreceptors by sympathetic postganglionic sympathetic efferents. Although there is a qualitative difference from the proposal by Livingston[12] some 40 years earlier, there are striking parallels between the two hypotheses. Indeed, Torebjörk and Hallin[29] were unable to demonstrate any lowering of nociceptor mechanical threshold nor the relief of pain by C-fiber block, but did demonstrate analgesia by pressure (differential) ischemic block induced by tourniquet in patients who exhibited hyperalgesia following nerve injury (i.e., hyperalgesia was in this instance mediated by large, myelinated afferents).

Campbell and coworkers[30] and Raja and coworkers[31] believe that the genesis of SMP results from an expression of additional α_1-adrenoreceptors on primary afferent nociceptors that, in turn, are stimulated by postganglionic sympathetic efferents (i.e., physiologic and not a result of sympathetic dysfunction). This theory would imply a peripheral and not central cause for the clinical syndrome.

In fact, the studies already referred to by Torebjörk, using microneurography in the 1970s, and an analysis of catecholamine levels in affected extremities have never reflected any increase in sympathetic activity. To the contrary, in many cases sympathetic activity in patients with CRPS was actually found to be less than normal.[32] However, studies by McLachlan[33] in rats have demonstrated adrenergic sprouting at dorsal root ganglia within 2 weeks following complete sciatic nerve transection, suggesting functional adrenergic change in response to injury. These investigators were able to demonstrate evoked activity in primary sensory neurons that were blocked by α-receptor antagonists when the postganglionic sympathetic fibers were stimulated. Using the Chung model[34] of neuropathic pain (chronic constriction injury), they found accelerated sympathetic sprouting at the dorsal root ganglion of segmental nerves within 4 days of this injury. They noted a reduction in mechanosensory threshold that preceded changes in the thermal threshold. These authors felt that the more rapid manifestation of changes in the sympathetic nervous system could be attributed to the influence of nerve growth factor expressed by the damaged axon. Drummond, et al had produced evidence that an increased density of alpha-1 adrenoceptors are found in the epidermis of hyperalgesic skin of patients with CRPS.[35]

All of the foregoing observations do not support the previously held opinion that sympathetic hyperactivity is necessary to explain the clinical features of CRPS. In fact, an alternate theory, and one whose origins go back to Sudeck, suggests that local inflammatory mediators with changes in vascular hydrostatic pressure resulting from dorsal root reflexes may amplify inflammatory responses and pain in the periphery. Wall,[36] in a recent editorial, has drawn attention to the current understanding of neuropathic pain mechanisms and relationship, if it exists and in what manner, by which the sympathetic nervous system might be involved. Two recent important communications underscore a possible central origin for the expression of CRPS, whether of clinical nerve injury or tissue damage. Sieweke and colleagues[37] showed that hyperalgesia in association with SMP is mechanical (brush evoked) whereas thermal hyperalgesia is not present. This finding, together with the ineffectiveness of acetylsalicylic acid in treatment, strongly supports a major central component that contributes to pain, at least in the early stages of CRPS. The second study, by Schürmann and colleagues[38] using laser Doppler flowmetry, found that a loss of the normal sympathetic control of the microcirculation in an ipsilateral extremity of patients with CRPS was also a systemic-wide phenomenon; a finding that strongly supports a central foundation for CRPS. In fact, this study corroborates earlier observations by Schwartzman and McClellen.[39] Although predisposing psychological characteristics have not found support in numerous studies, there has been some suggestion that patients who developed CRPS may acquire an excessive preoccupation with or hypervigilence about their disease.[40] In this regard positron emission tomographic studies reveal extensive cortical and subcortical activity in several neuropathic pain states.[41] Rommel determined that in 24 patients with CRPS-1 were found to have hemisensory and motor impairment suggestive of supratentotial areas of central processing.[42] Likewise, it has not been possible to distinguish between the protective response behavior that occurs in association with these diseases as being merely a response to the excessive pain or an abnormal psychological response that is seen only in patients with these syndromes.[43]

DEVELOPMENT OF A NEW TAXONOMY

The foundations for a new taxonomy had their origins in a meeting that was held in 1988 at Schloss-Rettershof, Germany[44] A consensus statement describing reflex sympathetic dystrophy in the

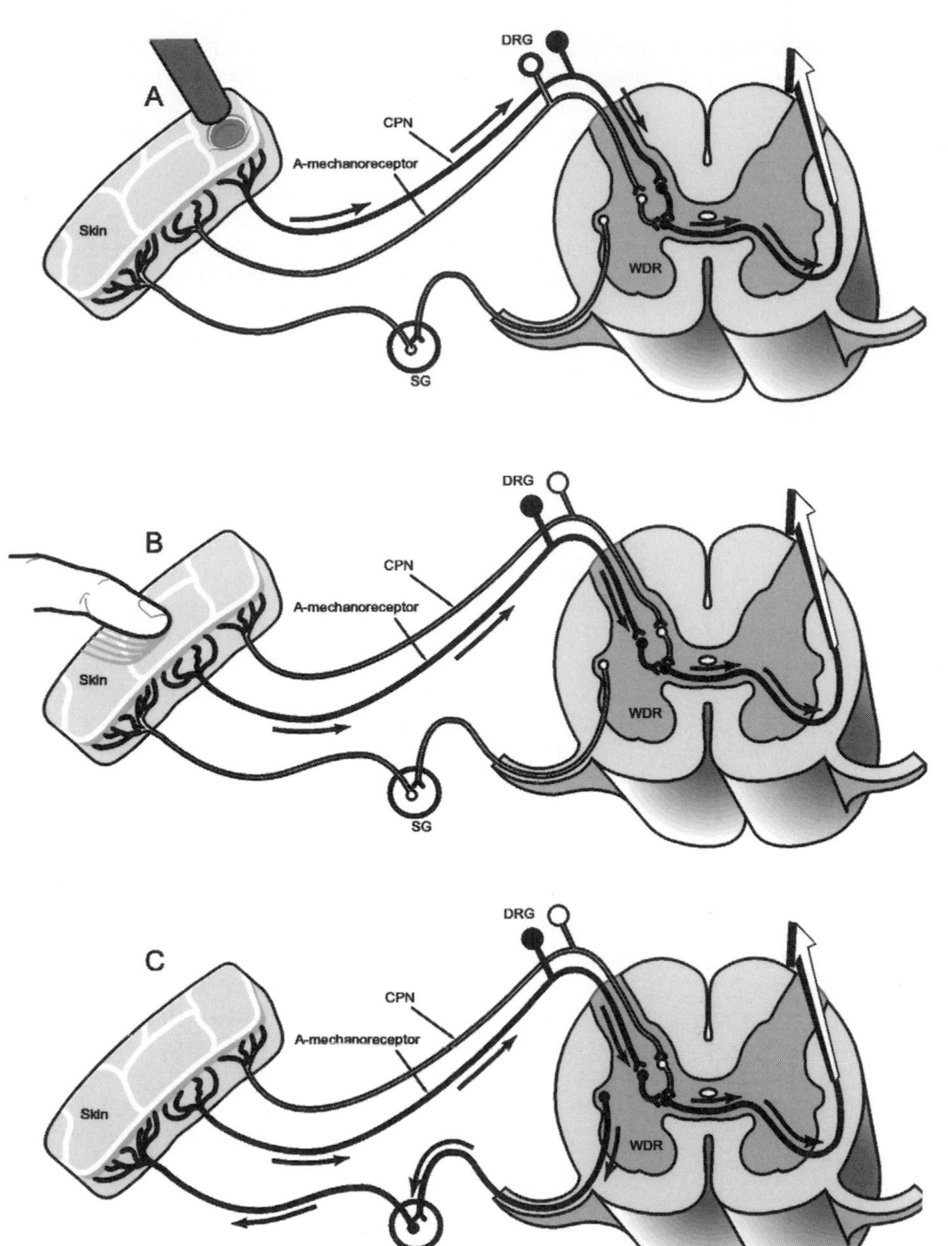

Figure 39-2 This figure illustrates the hypothesis of Roberts,[28] introduced in 1986, to explain the phenomenon of sympathetically maintained pain. (**A**) Initiation of C-nociceptor response to injury with excitation of the wide-dynamic-range (WDR) neurons and spinothalamic transmission. (**B**) WDR neurons now become sensitized to activity in large-diameter A-mechanoreceptors, which respond to light touch (allodynia). (**C**) Increased WDR response to A-mechanoreceptor activity resulting from sympathetic efferent action at the nociceptor. *Note:* This last phase represents sympathetically maintained pain and requires no further cutaneous stimulation. DRG, dorsal root ganglion; SG, sympathetic ganglion; CPN, C-polymodal nociceptor.

following terms was presented at a meeting of the Special Interest Group (SIG), Pain and the Sympathetic Nervous System of the International Association for the Study of Pain (IASP) at the Sixth World Congress on Pain in Adelaide, Australia, in 1990. This statement read: "Reflex Sympathetic Dystrophy is a descriptive term meaning a complex disorder or group of disorders that may develop as a consequence of trauma affecting the limbs, with or without an obvious nerve lesion. RSD may also develop after visceral disease, central nervous system lesions, or rarely without an obvious antecedent event. RSD consists of pain and sensory abnormalities, abnormal blood flow, decreased or increased sweating, abnormalities of the motor system, and changes in the structure of both superficial and deep tissues (trophic changes). It is not necessary that all components be present. The name 'Reflex Sympathetic Dystrophy' is used in a descriptive sense and does not imply any specific underlying mechanisms."[45] As would be expected, making a change in concepts that had been introduced to characterize certain aspects of reflex sympathetic dystrophy and causalgia such as SMP and sympathetically independent pain tended to complicate rather than improve the level of understanding, at least by those practitioners of whichever discipline who are faced with the diagnosis and treatment of these syndromes.

In November 1993, under the auspices of the SIG, Pain and the Sympathetic Nervous System, another closed workshop convened in association with the annual scientific meeting of the American Pain Society in Orlando, resulted in the development of a strict set of clinical descriptors to characterize features of these medical entities in order to distinguish them from other diseases, the mechanism for which, or their pathophysiology, is well known. These recommendations were made to the Committee on Taxonomy of Chronic Pain Conditions of the International Association for the Study of Pain and formed the basis for the term *complex regional pain syndromes* that was published in the second edition of the *Classification of Chronic Pain: Description of Chronic Pain Syn-*

dromes and Definition of Pain Terms, published by the IASP Press in 1994.[46,47]

Requirements for a New Taxonomy

1. Any new taxonomy for reflex sympathetic dystrophy should suggest areas of basic research and development of animal models that identify how the sympathetic nervous system is involved, and should promote clinical investigation or corroborate hypotheses born out of the basic research.
2. A new taxonomy should improve the differential diagnosis from other medical entities that have features similar but not identical to those found in reflex sympathetic dystrophy.
3. A new taxonomy should suggest tests in support of a diagnosis of reflex sympathetic dystrophy.

New Taxonomy

The term *complex regional pain syndrome* was chosen to replace the former terminology of reflex sympathetic dystrophy and causalgia.[47] Acknowledging that at the time no mechanism was available to explain the clinical features of these disorders, and using a linguistic convention adopted by the Subcommittee on Taxonomy for inclusion in the classification of chronic pain, the term allows for the later inclusion of a variety of painful conditions that may occur after injury. These conditions are manifested regionally, mostly in an extremity, predominantly distal; and with findings that exceed in magnitude and duration the expected course following such an inciting event. The taxonomy also acknowledges that in some cases these disorders may occur on the trunk or face, and spread to other body areas. Frequently, there is impairment of motor function, which is evident as tremor, dystonia, or muscle weakness. Because a temporal sequence is variable, the terms *complex* and *regional* were used to distinguish this from other syndromes. The taxonomy emphasizes that the clinical features tend to commence in the distal part of an extremity, and tend to extend proximally, involving the musculature of the shoulder or pelvic girdles, respectively; but in a small percentage of cases the syndrome may emanate proximally.

The order of classifying these conditions was changed, with the term *CRPS type I (RSD)* being the generic disease and *CRPS type II (causalgia)* being applied to conditions in which there is obvious nerve injury. The previous listing in the first edition of the IASP classification was historical in deference to the description by Mitchell.[9] Causalgia is well described by both Richards[48] and Bonica[49] and requires no elaboration here.

The terminology for CRPS types I and II acknowledges that both spontaneous and touch-evoked (allodynia or hyperalgesia) pain may be concurrent in the affected region. Pain of either nature is regarded as a cardinal symptom in these medical disorders, although in rare cases, pain in association with all other clinical features that satisfy the diagnosis may be absent.

In patients who do not fulfill the criteria for a diagnosis of CRPS type I or II, allowance was made in the taxonomy for a third type of CRPS, not otherwise specified (NOS). With this instrument, the taxonomy encourages the clinician to identify specific types or subgroups of CRPS types I and II. For example, one patient group may meet all the criteria specified for CRPS type I but uniformly have in addition another specific symptom or clinical finding. The temporal course of their disease process follows a uniformly different course or their response differs from that of the main type I group, in which case the classification could be changed to include this as a specific subgroup within the main CRPS type I group. Bonica[50] introduced the concept of staging, which he felt was important to the description of these diseases, but experience has questioned the utility of this in diagnosis or treatment and, as a consequence, it was eliminated from the taxonomy. It was agreed that experience with the new taxonomy may suggest a reappraisal and inclusion of staging in the future.

Although the epidemiology of CRPS has not been systematically studied, recent publications in relation to Colles fracture[38] and statistics from Sweden (T. Gordh, 1998, personal communication) suggests a prevalence of about 10%. Also, a clinical study by Mailis and Wade[51] concerning the development of CRPS types I and II in white women suggest genetically similar profiles, whereas Devor and Raber[52] and Bhatia and colleagues,[53] in two separate studies that demonstrated the predisposition for neuropathic pain behavior in genetically selected laboratory animals, provide support for this concept.

Motor symptoms and signs frequently are reported in patients with CRPS types I and II. During preparation of the new taxonomy, a lack of scientific evidence in support of this being a specific movement disorder resulted in the exclusion of these findings from the standard clinical criteria, although they are mentioned in the draft criteria of the taxonomy. Likewise, the response to sympathetic blockade is also removed from the taxonomy of CRPS types I and II but receives attention in the discussion of sympathetically maintained pain and other neuralgias.

Specific exclusion criteria for the definition of CRPS types I and II were necessary to prevent the inclusion of other clinical entities and syndromes in which the findings are consistent with a particular injury but resemble those of CRPS types I and II. One example might be a patient who met the criteria for causalgia but whose signs and symptoms lay outside of the territory of the injured nerve. If the clinical findings were to occur within the regional territory of that nerve, however, they would then satisfy inclusion criteria under this definition. Another exception might be a patient in whom the clinical findings are localized to the trunk or face but not associated with a particular injured nerve. Although these entities might be classified as a subset within the main definition, like the primary classification, they must have signs and symptoms that are completely disproportionate in both nature and severity to the injury.

Signs of vasomotor instability may not be present at the time of clinical examination. However, a patient history of swelling, sweating, color, and temperature changes would, of necessity, satisfy the diagnostic criteria for CRPS.

Sympathetically Maintained Pain

SMP is defined as *pain that is maintained by sympathetic efferent innervation or by circulating catecholamines.*[46] A positive response to sympatholysis (sympathetic block) historically was necessary before a diagnosis of CRPS could be made. Given the current ignorance of the manner in which the sympathetic nervous system is involved in the pathophysiology of these conditions and the contradictory literature in this regard, it has been necessary to abandon the convention that only following a positive response to sympatholysis can a diagnosis of CRPS be supported. The concept of sympathetically independent pain was introduced to explain those cases in which sympatholysis (either pharmacologic or nerve blockade) provides no pain relief. This concept[4] is illustrated in Figure 39-3.

In this figure, a symbolic patient (A) may be seen at one time in the course of his or her disease in which most of the patient's pain is sympathetically maintained (i.e., it responds to sympatholysis) but temporarily becomes less responsive to blockade and ultimately is composed mostly of sympathetically independent pain.

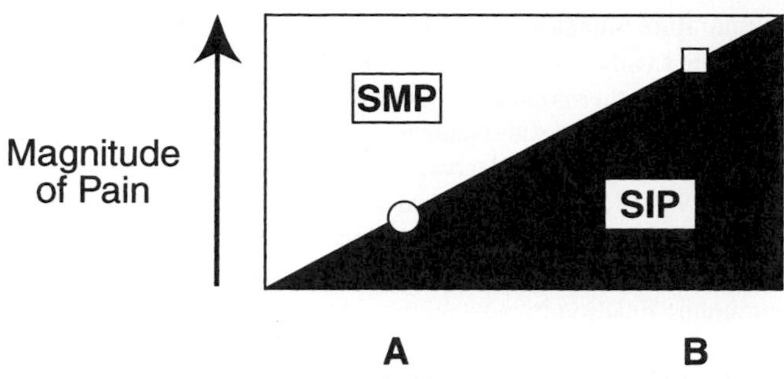

Figure 39-3 This figure illustrates the relative contribution of sympathetically maintained pain (SMP) to the overall pain. A symbolic patient *A* would demonstrate maximum response to sympatholysis (i.e., demonstrating a large component of SMP), whereas patient *B* would have almost no response to sympathetic block, therefore exhibiting sympathetically independent pain. It should be noted that points *A* and *B* may also represent the same patients at different times in the course of their disease.

Similarly, (A) and (B) may be two separate patients who, at the time of their physical examination, exhibit these distinguishing characteristics of pain by their response to sympathetic blockade. This example illustrates the poor diagnostic specificity when sympathetic blockade is used for this purpose and is the reason for which a positive response to sympathetic block is no longer regarded as being necessary for a diagnosis of CRPS to be sustained.

However, the response to sympatholysis may contribute to other clinical signs and symptoms that support the diagnostic criteria for CRPS. This and other tests, including temperature measurement, sudomotor function, skin blood flow, and skin resistance, have been developed to assess sympathetic activity.[54–56] The hypothesis for SMP already discussed may be as important to treatment as it is to diagnosis. The sensitization of C-polymodal nociceptors and sensitization of WDR neurons in laminar-5 fibers of the dorsal horn may, as a response to sympatholysis, subside but can only be regarded as a contributory phenomenon or symptom in CRPS or, for that matter, in many other conditions (Fig. 39-4).

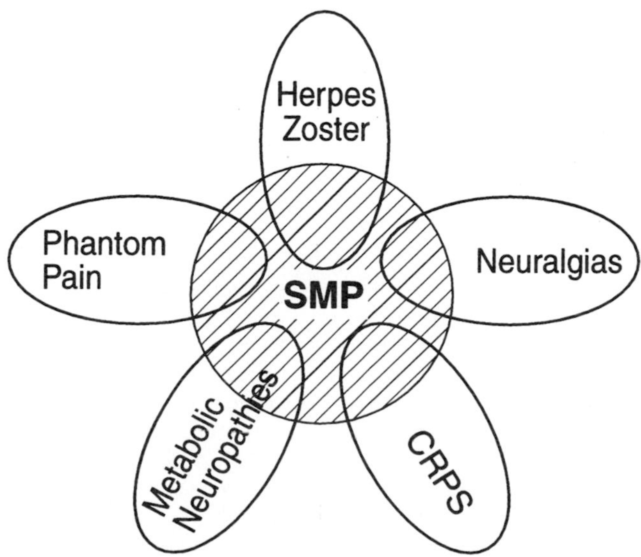

Figure 39-4 Wen diagram showing the conceptual relationship of sympathetically maintained pain to medical conditions other than complex regional pain syndrome. The figure in no way implies any quantitative relationship.

Musculoskeletal Disorders and Pain Dysfunction Syndromes

Those medical entities that do not satisfy specific diagnostic criteria for a specific condition are described in the International Classification of Diseases (ICD-9) as NOS codes. The diagnostic criteria for CRPS types I and II use a similar device. As an example, pain in a limb without the other characteristics of CRPS is defined as limb pain, NOS type III. The IASP classification of chronic limb pain conditions provides a code for such instances: X1.19 pain in the limbs, NOS: upper limb (S) 2XX. XXZ, and lower limb (S) 6XX. XXZ. Pain in the hand (musculoskeletal disorder) that does not meet the criteria for CRPS might be diagnosed as pain dysfunction syndrome (a nonstandard classification)[57] (see the discussion of differential diagnosis later in this chapter). Several medical conditions that have been described using nonstandard terminology, including cumulative trauma disorder, repetitive strain injury, overuse syndrome, and tennis elbow,[58–61] are included under the umbrella term *pain dysfunction syndrome*. The International Coding Diseases Manual classification of such conditions is musculoskeletal disorders, which includes a large number of diseases and syndromes such as carpal tunnel syndrome. Many of these conditions that are associated with mechanical hyperalgesia, pain that is out of the ordinary, temperature changes, and myofascial pain syndrome might be considered as CRPS type III. However, the differential diagnosis, depending on tenderness and hyperalgesia that is found specifically over a particular muscle group or epicondylar region, would favor occupational overuse, bursitis, a nerve entrapment, or tennis elbow, for example. Often a long antecedent history of fibromyalgia with hyper-responsiveness, associated headache, fatigue, sleeplessness, depression, and other subjective symptoms may occur in conjunction with CRPS or these musculoskeletal entities.[61]

It also should not be forgotten that the specialty of the physician may influence the primary or secondary diagnosis, particularly its differential, if sufficiently stringent criteria do not satisfy a diagnosis of CRPS.

Differential Diagnosis

Many medical entities have characteristics that are similar to the clinical features of CRPS. Although many of these conditions are frequently found in the distal part of an extremity, they must be distinguished from other musculoskeletal and neuropathic pain conditions. As already discussed, their clinical presentation may suggest SMP; however, its interpretation, at least early in the course of the disease, must be circumspect. Pain relief after sympatholysis is not specific for reflex sympathetic dystrophy (see Fig. 38-3) but may merely reflect an altered response to physiologic sympathetic activity.

Patients with myofascial dysfunction, a frequent accompaniment, may present with regional temperature differences and mechanical hyperalgesia yet still not satisfy all of the criteria for a diagnosis of CRPS. The broad group of musculoskeletal disorders that have been described as pain dysfunction syndromes may have some clinical signs and symptoms but are insufficient in number or character to satisfy a diagnosis of CRPS. Table 39-1 is a list of conditions that should be considered in the diagnosis of CRPS.

Motor dysfunction, although not an inclusion criterion of CRPS, is found sufficiently frequently for its mention in the classification. In fact, recent papers have all identified motor dysfunction as an independent and almost invariable finding.[62–64] Dystonia, limita-

TABLE 39-1 **Conditions to Be Considered in the Differential Diagnosis of Complex Regional Pain Syndrome**

Musculoskeletal disorders
Pain dysfunction syndrome
Cumulative trauma disorder
Repetitive strain injury
Overuse syndrome
Tennis elbow
Shoulder-hand syndrome
Nonspecific thoracic outlet syndrome
Fibromyalgia
Posttraumatic vasoconstriction
Undetected fracture
Peripheral vascular disease

tion of movement, and weakness must be carefully distinguished from a lack of voluntary effort or dystrophic changes in joint components.

The differential diagnosis of CRPS II can be distinguished from a nerve injury in which neurogenic inflammation is associated with pain and by symptoms that are out of proportion, as described in the new taxonomy. The additional criteria are edema, skin temperature, color changes, and sudomotor changes that also are out of proportion to those that would be found in association with a painful nerve injury. Although one or more of these signs and symptoms may dominate, all should be found at some time during the course of the disease. The pain, including allodynia and hyperalgesia, without vasomotor changes by itself would not satisfy the criteria for CRPS. Only rarely do patients present with all or most of the clinical features of CRPS, but without pain. Although the temporal course and response to treatment modalities may be identical with that of CRPS, the taxonomy requires that such patients should remain outside the CRPS umbrella.

A few patients with CRPS types I and II may have premorbid psychological or psychiatric disturbances, the occurrence of which does not exclude their primary diagnosis. Likewise, malingering and factitious disease are well-recognized clinical entities that are separate from a diagnosis of CRPS but must be included in the differential diagnosis. Conversion disorders and somatization, well recognized in association with chronic pain, have their own specific criteria and may occur independently or in association with CRPS types I and II.[65] Occasionally, the diagnosis of these conditions is difficult and may only be determined after medical treatment is instituted. In the final analysis, pain that is neuropathic and out of proportion to that occurring as a symptom of many other medical conditions is required for a diagnosis of CRPS. SMP is neuropathic pain that is associated with many conditions; for example, postherpetic neuralgia, diabetic neuropathy, and most cases of CRPS types I and II early in the course of the disease.

Diagnostic Tests

Although no diagnostic tests specifically support a diagnosis of CRPS, a number of measurements and laboratory tests may contribute to the clinical diagnosis.

Temperature Measurement Temperature change that is reflective of changes in the cutaneous blood flow[66] may be measured by thermometry, telethermometry, passive infrared methods, or thermography. For these measurements to have any relevance, they should also be taken on corresponding sites or areas of the contralateral extremity. At least 1.5°C is required for the difference to be significant. Thermography in conjunction with cold physiologic stress testing of an unaffected independent extremity is a useful test of autonomic function in the ipsilateral extremity. This test should be undertaken only in a thermostable, and preferably comfortable—about 22°C—environment. Either the failure to respond to cold stress or the delay in rewarming, particularly when the contralateral temperature side differences are 1.5°C or greater, does this test indicate dysfunction of the autonomic nervous system.

Caution is necessary when interpreting temperature changes as has been demonstrated by Wasner, et al.[32] When whole-body temperature changes were induced, three distinct vascular patterns were identified, namely inhibition of cutaneous sympathetic vasoconstrictor neurons as characterized by a warmer affected limb early in the disease. In chronic CRPS, sympathetic vasoconstrictor neurons are still inhibited, but secondary changes in neurovascular transmission caused the skin changes to remain cold, and an intermediate change characterizes the dynamic vascular abnormalities that depend on the specific activity of sympathetic vasoconstrictor neurons at the time. These authors noted that the maximal difference in skin temperature during induced thermoregulatory changes is a reliable means of distinguishing CRPS from other extremity pain syndromes.[67]

Peripheral Blood Flow This measurement may be made by laser Doppler flowmetry. As already mentioned, Schürmann and colleagues have clearly demonstrated that this test is an early predictor of sympathetic dysfunction and, therefore, supportive of a diagnosis of CRPS.[38,39]

Quantitative Sweat Testing The quantitative sudomotor axon reflex test (QSART) is another clinical laboratory test that focuses on abnormalities of evoked sweat production. Taken together with the resting sweat output (RSO) and alteration in vasomotor activity, QSART provides a good laboratory correlation with the clinical features of CRPS.[66,68]

Quantitative Sensory Testing This test is a useful evaluation of vibratory, thermal, and cold responses that, although not specific for CRPS, may contribute to the clinical picture and support a differential diagnosis of CRPS.[69]

Sympathetic Skin Response This response may be used to identify increased conductance when comparing the ipsilateral with the contralateral extremity.[55]

Bone Scan Three-phase bone scintigraphy with technetium diphosphonate usually demonstrates a reduction in flow during the early phase of CRPS but increased periarticular uptake during the third phase. Sensitivity is approximately 60%, and specificity of 86% has been claimed, but many reports describe 30% false-positive and 30% false-negative responses.[70]

Muscle Strength and Joint Testing The measurement of muscle strength depends on patient cooperation, psychological factors, and pain. Nevertheless, grip strength with thumb adduction and opposition, along with pinch testing and goniometry, may be important measurements both as baseline and as prognostic indicators. Joint mobility, including range of motion (ROM), although subjective, may be obtained most reliably by a therapist who works frequently with orthopedic patients.

Psychological Tests The most useful instruments for psychological testing are the Beck Depression Inventory and the McGill Pain Questionnaire.

TREATMENT

Physical Therapeutic Algorithm

If early diagnosis is crucial to the institution of an appropriate treatment plan, incorporating a graduated and stepwise approach to treatment using modalities that experience has shown to be most effective is a natural corollary.

Until a mechanism for CRPS is established, functional restoration using physiotherapeutic methods is regarded as essential to providing a remission in most cases. Three requirements are necessary if physical therapy is to be successful.

1. Pain control
2. "Turning off" the disturbance
3. Development of patient rapport and confidence in the requirements of a treatment program

Depending on the complexity or fulminant nature of the disease in a particular patient, it may be necessary to increase the proposed time for each step in the physical therapeutic algorithm.[71] This point is arbitrary and serves two purposes: (1) to prevent the patient who, because of symptoms, may no longer progress with a particular treatment modality, and (2) to reassess the disease process and introduce measures of symptom control that will permit exercise therapy to continue.

Initially, it is important to gain rapport with the patient so that he or she will develop confidence in the planned investment of effort and time using the various therapeutic modalities that will be necessary, in most cases, to achieve a remission. Once each patient buys into this approach, the business of motivation, mobilization, and desensitization are introduced. It is important at each step to rapidly achieve increments of symptomatic improvement using non-narcotic or narcotic analgesics,[72] while at the same time addressing the disturbances of sleep, anxiety, depression, and motor dysfunction.[73,74] Some patients with recent onset of CRPS may respond well with a reduction in pain to anticonvulsants or antiarrhythmic medications.[75–79] Unacceptable side effects, together with the length of time (3 to 4 weeks) to realize any efficacy, may preclude their use. Further deterioration in functional integrity, failure to improve, or an increase in symptoms should trigger the use of a therapeutic and prognostic sympathetic block.

Figure 39-5 is an updated clinical pathway illustrating the main domains of rehabilitation, pain management and psychological treatment that are fundamental to regaining function and, ultimately, a remission of CRPS.[67,120] The new clinical pathway (guideline) emphasizes an intra-disciplinary, time-contingent guidance that incorporates the recently published treatment options. These are addressed simultaneously and will vary according to the patient's response to treatment. Important to the use of this clinical guideline is the recommendation to use whichever treatment

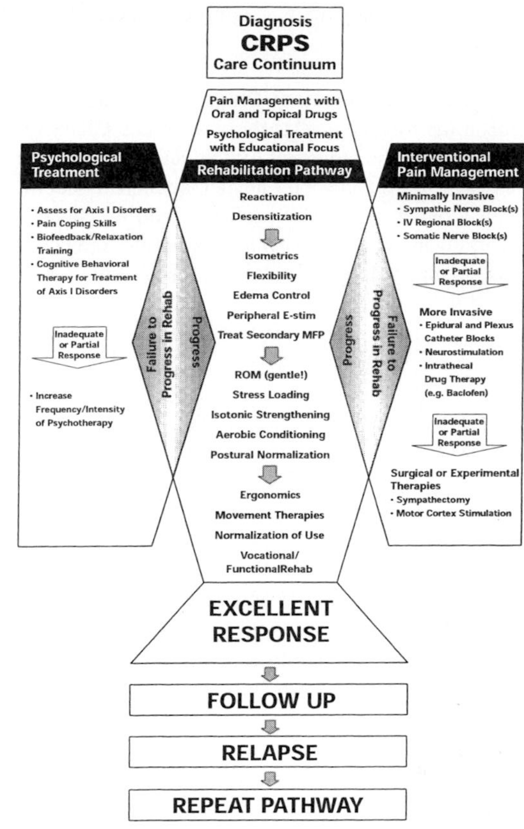

Figure 39-5 Revised therapeutic pathway with emphasis on the therapeutic modalities that are used in response to the patients clinical progress in the rehabilitation algorithm. Adapted from the 1998 guidelines.[68]

modality, when a patient fails to respond to whatever level of treatment after 12–16 weeks. The clinical pathway focuses on quality of life, as well as function.

A word should be said about joint movement, and particularly ROM, in patients with these syndromes. Orthopedic experience in particular has shown that the use of aggressive or passive ROM, or both, may be deleterious for progress or worse, because mechanoreceptor stimulation in the joint structures can cause a dramatic worsening of both pain and the inflammatory response.[80] This is evident by immediate increase in edema, allodynia or hyperalgesia, and hyperpathia.

The technique of so-called stress loading with isometric exercises and gentle ROM has been found most effective.[80] It may be necessary to use cognitive behavioral methods to assist the patient against pain avoidance, kinesophobia, bracing, and overprotection, all of which may develop in a patient in whom previously *inappropriate* exercise therapy may have been employed.[81–83] Treatment of the nociceptive and neuropathic generators is required using the following pharmacologic, regional anesthetic, and neuromodulation techniques. In fact, a combination or sequence of these modalities may, in some cases, be required to ultimately achieve a return of function.

Pharmacologic Management

The following section summarizes drugs that have been found useful in the treatment of CRPS. Although none is specific for the disease, each has a place in managing an aspect of the clinical presentation.

Nonsteroidal Anti-inflammatory Drugs These agents are most successful in the treatment of early or very late CRPS types I or II. Their use should be tempered by the development of gastrointestinal or renal side effects.[71] If one member is without effect, then others with a better side effect profile should be chosen. It may also be worth using one of the cyclooxygenase-2 (COX-2) agents. Topical use of these drugs has also been suggested. It should be remembered that these agents have a tendency to cause water retention, with edema, a side effect that may interfere with rehabilitation.

Opioids Although opioids are more effective in the treatment of nociceptive pain, they have a place in treatment of pain of a neuropathic nature.[72] If tolerated by the patient, the use of slow-release opioids on a round-the-clock basis is preferable to as-needed dosing. The side effects of one class of opioid do not preclude use of another class. It is important to remember that abrupt discontinuation of opioids may lead to an extreme exacerbation of a patient's symptoms, as well as other signs and symptoms of withdrawal. It should be noted that there is a greater acceptance in the use of opioids for neuropathic pain, such as CRPS.

Anticonvulsants and Antiarrhythmics Agents generally classified as so-called membrane stabilizers include anticonvulsants, local anesthetics, and antiarrythmic agents. Drugs that are the most effective for neuropathic pain are carbamazepine, gabapentin, lamotrigine, phenytoin, and valproic acid.[75–79] Recent studies with gabapentin, a selective voltage-gated Na^{2+} channel blocker, have demonstrated some efficacy in the treatment of CRPS pain. The oral antiarrhythmic lidocaine analogue, mexiletine, may prove quite effective in a small but significant number of patients with CRPS.[78] The drug has been found effective in the treatment of diabetic neuropathy in a dose of 10 mg/kg. An intravenous bolus and infusion of lidocaine can be used to predict the response to oral analogues.[84] In addition, transdermal lidocaine, which has been shown to be quite effective in the treatment of postherpetic neuralgia, can in some patients reduce the touch-evoked allodynia of CRPS.[85] The conotoxin SNX-111 (Ziconitide), infused intrathecally, may be successful in the treatment of long-standing CRPS that has proved refractory to all other treatment.[86]

Tricyclic Antidepressants The serotonin and norepinephrine reuptake blocking agents, amitriptyline, desipramine, maprotiline, have all demonstrated efficacy in the treatment of neuropathic pain syndromes, including CRPS.[87–89] These agents are much more effective than the selective serotonin reuptake inhibitors (SSRIs), suggesting that it is the catecholaminergic aspect of the former three agents that is therapeutic. These agents are also particularly useful in providing sedation and reducing nocturnal symptoms. They should, therefore, be prescribed for use at night.

Adrenergic Drugs The α_1-adrenoceptor blocking agents (terazosin, prazocin, and phenoxybenzamine) may be strikingly effective in patients with SMP.[90] They do, however, have a poor side effect profile—with tachycardia, chest pain, gastric symptoms, and, in some cases, sedation that preclude their use. However more than 30% of patients with SMP respond dramatically to these agents. The α_2 agonist, clonidine, is most effective when introduced by the epidural or intrathecal route of administration.[91] It may be tried topically and, in some cases, it may be dramatically effective when applied to a discrete area of hyperalgesia.[92,93]

Corticosteroids Corticosteroids have been successful in the treatment of early CRPS when the acute inflammatory response may be most pronounced.[94,95] It is during this phase that intraosseous plasma extravasation can be demonstrated scintigraphically by labeled immunoglobulins. It should be noted that corticosteroids are most successful when sympathetic blocks are completely effective in relieving the continuous pain.

Regional Anesthesia

Regional anesthetic techniques have two purposes: firstly, the relief of symptoms otherwise not controlled by pharmacologic means; and secondly, the demonstration of pain that is sympathetically maintained (SMP).[31,66] Traditionally, this approach has been used in the treatment of CRPS involving both the upper or lower extremities. Significantly, when used early in the course of the disease, pain relief that is either partial or complete, depending on the degree of SMP, may be realized. Blocks of the sympathetic nervous system interrupt efferent vasomotor, sudomotor, and visceromotor fibers as well as visceral afferents, somatic afferents, and nociceptor fibers.

For sympatholysis in the upper extremity, the paratracheal technique of stellate ganglion block at the level of C6, with the development of Horner's syndrome (myosis, ptosis, and enopthalmos), has been a standard approach for many years. However, as has been pointed out by many authors, including Bonica, Kuntz, and others, the anatomic position of the stellate ganglion anterior to the costovertebral articulation and neck of the first rib makes it more amenable to block at the lower portion of the C7 vertebral body.[96–98] In addition, the local anesthetic has a greater chance of diffusing on the longus colli muscle to reach the T2 through T4 ganglia, thereby providing a more effective sympathetic blockade to the upper extremity. Signs of a successful sympathetic block include a temperature rise to 35°C, measured at the finger pulp. Supplementary tests of sympathetic function are the sympathetic skin response using a modified electrocardiogram and cold pressor test to demonstrate that this response has been disabled when a noneffected extremity is placed in ice-cold water. Laser Doppler flowmetry is an excellent noninvasive measurement of changes in skin blood flow, the loss of which is clearly evident.

In the same manner, lumbar sympathetic blockade can be realized using a single needle under fluoroscopic guidance at the lower third of the body of L3.[99] The correct anatomic site is clearly demonstrated by the flow of radiocontrast in the gutter formed by the fascia overlying the psoas muscle and its continuation as the periosteum overlying the vertebral bodies of L2 through L4. Verification of effective sympatholysis can be demonstrated by using one of the previously described measurements.

If sympathetic blockade completely eliminates the patient's symptoms, consideration should be given to effecting a prolonged block by neurolysis, using either an agent such as phenol, which may be prepared with radiocontrast material (e.g., Meglumine [Conray 420, Malingkrodt, St. Louis, Mo.]) or radiofrequency lesions.[100] A duration of effect lasting up to 6 months may be achieved by these methods. Demonstration of SMP by sympathetic blockade also should trigger the use of an α-adrenoceptor blocker, such as terazosin. A good pharmacologic response with these agents may preclude further sympathetic blockade, which in any case should be discontinued if the symptomatic relief fails to outlast the duration of local anesthesia.

Mixed conduction block of peripheral nerves or the brachial or lumbar plexus, or in the form of a central neural block, are useful alternatives to the use of sympatholysis. They should be employed only when analgesia by pharmacologic means is insufficient to support exercise therapy. Although intermittent blocks are helpful to initiate therapy, in some cases it is necessary to use continuous conduction analgesia.[101] A catheter implanted in the brachial or lumbosacral plexus allows infusions for 1 to 2 weeks but is subject to technical failure or infection when used for longer periods. The epidural route with a tunneled catheter offers the greatest utility and enables the long-term administration of local anesthetics and adjuncts for many months. This facilitates exercise therapy,[102,103] although technical failure with dislodgment, breakage, and infection, mostly at the skin entry site and less frequently in the deeper tissues, will require removal, treatment, and replacement of the catheter.

A word of caution with regard to implanted catheters is in order. Because these devices may be used for long durations, they should be treated as minor surgical procedures and can only successfully achieve their purpose if placement is made under strict asepsis using fluoroscopic guidance to ensure that the epidural infusion is ipsilateral, or if the contralateral extremity is also involved, that bilateral spread can be assured.

In a few cases, a long-acting local anesthetic such as bupivacaine or ropivacaine may be sufficient to provide analgesia commensurate with exercise therapy. However, it is frequently necessary to add an opiate, such as fentanyl, or other agents, including morphine, hydromorphone, sufentanil, or buprenorphine, to achieve a sufficient level of "working" analgesia. Occasionally, it may be necessary to consider the use of an α_2-adrenoceptor agonist, clonidine, when hyperalgesia or allodynia prevent effective physical therapy. A short, 2- to 5-day hospital admission is required to determine the clinically most effective infusion in each case.

From this account, it should be clear to the reader that where once regional anesthetic techniques such as sympathetic blockade were necessary to support a diagnosis of CRPS, their conventional application is primarily to determine pain that is modified by sympathetic block (SMP) and as a means of supporting exercise therapy and other treatment modalities that will ensure the return of function.

Neuromodulation

Neuromodulation incorporating either spinal cord stimulation or peripheral nerve stimulation aims to change or modify function of the central or peripheral nervous systems. Although neuromodulation has been in use since its introduction by Shealy[104] in 1967, it is the past 10 years that have seen such a dramatic increase in its use for the treatment of neuropathic and vasculopathic pain.[105–108] Although the posterior columns were thought to be the primary target for spinal cord stimulation, stimulation of the descending inhibitory pathways and the dorsal root fibers are now recognized as being equally important for modulating nociception.[109]

Computer modeling of spinal cord stimulation has helped to determine the putative clinical response that could be achieved by electrode geometry and the ratio of dorsal column to dorsal root fibers.[110] The pain in CRPS tends to be more global than dermatomal, and electrodes that have a longitudinal and central disposition tend to have greater spatial selectivity and are likely to be more efficient in providing pain relief to the affected extremity.

If, as has already been mentioned, CRPS is a neurologic disease, it should be amenable to treatment by neurostimulation. Perhaps one of the best indications for either spinal cord or peripheral nerve stimulation is injury to a peripheral nerve. Similarly, CRPS with its altered cutaneous sensibility, tactile allodynia to cold, and mechanical stimuli, is also likely to respond well to spinal cord stimulation. The autonomic effects of spinal cord stimulation, with improvement in both the micro- and macrocirculation in the stimulated region, appear to be a result of preganglionic modification of the autonomic nervous system function.[111]

Although there have only been two prospective studies describing the successful use of neuromodulation in the treatment of pain resulting from CRPS, a number of clinical retrospective case studies support use of the modality.[112,113] Functional restoration is central to the treatment of CRPS, and adequate relief of pain and correction of the autonomic disturbance positions this modality well among other modalities in achieving this end.

Because time is of the essence in the treatment of CRPS, any failure to progress through the therapeutic algorithm, must be regarded as a trigger to introduce regional anesthetic or neuromodulatory methods to support progressive rehabilitation. The temporal introduction of the different treatment modalities must be seen only as a guide, and their order does not constitute priority (see Figure 39-5).

For patients with CRPS of either the upper or lower extremities, a single quadrapolar or octapolar lead is most effective. In cases where bilateral stimulation is required, it may be necessary to employ two electrodes to ensure adequate paresthesias (coverage) in both extremities. For CRPS II, selection of a peripheral nerve stimulator is more likely to provide stable and specific control of symptoms relative to the injured nerve.

All patients considered suitable for neuromodulation must first satisfy behavioral criteria and undergo a structured psychological examination.[71,114] Self-report tests such as the Beck Disability Inventory and McGill Pain Questionnaire are suitable instruments.

It can be concluded that for cases characterized by failure to progress through the physiotherapeutic algorithm or an exacerbation of the patient's symptoms, a trial of spinal cord stimulation may prove to be a most effective tool when other modalities have failed.

Psychological Aspects

Most studies in patients with CRPS have failed to show any correlation with a preexisting psychological disorder.[115,116] However, a significant percentage of these patients develop behavioral abnormalities and require psychological support during treatment. Not uncommonly, 6 months into their disease, patients demonstrate varying degrees of depression manifested by disturbed sleep, anxiety, and despair that their disease is not improving. Measures such as biofeedback, relaxation, temperature control, and reduction in muscle tension are indicated. Group therapy, in which a spouse or family member is present, is sometimes helpful for CRPS patients, as for other patients with chronic pain. Use of a single antidepressant, particularly a tricyclic such as amitriptyline, is preferable to a combination of different antidepressants or the newer SSRIs.

Complex Regional Pain Syndrome in Children

It can be categorically stated that CRPS in children, particularly before puberty, and in adolescence, is a different disease from that in the adult.[117,118] Although the same signs and symptoms constituting the clinical entity are present, the course of the disease and its response to treatment suggest early behavioral and psychological aspects that may require special skills in cognitive management. Because of their dependence on parents, children exhibit more behavioral aspects reflecting problems of enmeshment and bizarre responses to the slightest degree of family dysfunction.[119] In fact, in many cases one sees a parallel in the adult with a conversion disorder.

Usually, children do not require the use of interventions and will respond appropriately to pharmacologic measures and good psychological support.[120] Physical therapy should be presented either as a challenge or as a game, with goals being set to win and overcome the disability. Transcutaneous electrical nerve stimulation often provides sufficient analgesia (in over half the patients) to allow for their participation in physical therapy.[120] It is preferable to avoid invasive therapies; however, a lumbar sympathetic block or an epidural catheter should not be withheld if there is failure to progress in exercise therapy or the disease process has remained refractory to conservative treatment. In rare cases, it may actually be necessary to use a spinal cord, or even peripheral nerve, stimulator, which in either case may be subsequently removed once the disease process is in remission. In principle, at least 60% of children will respond well to physical therapeutic measures and pharmacologic therapy, but almost all require strong support with these, or whichever additional psychological measures are used, to gain confidence in and increase compliance with their therapy.

SUMMARY

CRPS is a disease, the pathophysiology and mechanism of which remain unknown. The disease is complex and generally commences in a particular region of the body, usually the distal aspect of an extremity. Sometimes it occurs in other parts of the body, and it may also spread to other areas. Pain is the *sine qua non* of CRPS but, in rare cases, may actually be minimal or absent. The diagnosis is one of exclusion after having eliminated, in the differential diagnosis, those other conditions for which the pathophysiology is well categorized. The treatment plan should be orderly, and one that uses a structured physiotherapeutic approach facilitated by pharmacologic, interventional, and behavioral components. Time is of the essence, and any delay or failure to progress with exercise therapy after 2 to 3 weeks of treatment should prompt the introduction of modalities that at the time seem most appropriate and more likely to facilitate therapy and achieve a remission. It frequently is necessary to make continuous adjustments in physical therapy commensurate with the clinical response. Such therapy, in each case, must be individualized to be successful.

REFERENCES

1. Bernard C. Influence du grand sympathique sur la sensibilit et sur la calorification. *CR Soc Biol (Paris)* 1851;3:163–164.
2. Hess WR, Brhgger M. Das subcorticale Zentrum der affecktiven Abwehreaktion. *Helv Physiol Acta* 1943;1:33–52.
3. Jänig W. Organization of the lumbar sympathetic outflow to skeletal muscle and skin of the cat hind limb and tail. *Rev Physiol Biochem Pharmacol* 1985;102:119–213.
4. Jänig W. Vegetatives nervensystem. In: Schmidt RF, Thews G, eds. *Physiologie des Menschen.* 26th ed. Heidelberg, Germany: Springer-Verlag; 1995:340–369.
5. Jänig W. The sympathetic nervous system in pain. *Eur J Anesthesiol* 1995;12(suppl 10):53–60.
6. Selye H. *The Stress of Life*. New York, NY: McGraw-Hill; 1957.
7. Jänig W, Schmidt FR, eds. *Reflex Sympathetic Dystrophy: Pathophysiological Mechanisms and Clinical Implications.* Weinheim, Germany: VCH Verlags Gesell Schaft; 1992.
8. Jänig W, Koltzenburg M. What is the interaction between the sympathetic terminal and the primary afferent fiber? In: Basbaum AI, Besson, JM, eds. *Towards a New Pharmacotherapy of Pain.* Chichester, England: Dahlen Workshop Reports, Wiley; 1991:331–352.
9. Mitchell SW. *Injuries of Nerves and Their Consequences.* Philadelphia, Pa: JB Lippincott; 1872.
10. Leriche R. *La Chiurgie del la Douleur.* Paris, France: Masson cie; 1939.
11. Sudeck D. gber die akute entzundliche Knochenatropie. *Arch Klin Chir* 1962:147–156.
12. Livingston WK. *Pain Mechanisms: A Physiological Interpretation of Causalgia and Its Related States.* New York, NY: Plenum; 1976.
13. Evans JA. Reflex sympathetic dystrophy. *Surg Clin North Am* 1946; 26:780–790.
14. Lewis T. *Pain*. London, England: MacMillan; 1942.
15. Walker AE, Nulsen F. Electrical stimulation of the supper thoracic portion of the sympathetic chain in man. *Arch Neurol Psychiatr* 1948; 59:559–560.
16. White JC, Sweet WH. *Pain and the Neurosurgeon.* Springfield, Ill: Charles C Thomas; 1969.
17. Bonica JJ. Causalgia and other reflex sympathetic dystrophies. In Bonica JJ, Lieberskiend JC, Albe-Fessard, DG, eds. *Advances in Pain Research and Therapy.* Vol 3. New York, NY: Raven; 1979:141–166.
18. Casale R, Glynn CJ, Buonocore M. The role of ischemia in the analgesia which follows Bier's block technique. *Pain* 1992;50:169–175.
19. Jadad AR, Carroll D, Glynn CJ, et al. Intravenous regional sympathetic blockade for pain relief in reflex sympathetic dystrophy: A systematic review and a randomized double-blind crossover study. *J Pain Symptom Manage* 1995;10:1313–1320.
20. Ramamurthy S, Hoffman J, The Guanethidine Study Group. Intravenous regional guanethidine in the treatment of reflex sympathetic dystrophy/causalgia: A randomized double-blind study. *Anesth Analg* 1995;81:718–723.
21. Dellemijn PL, Fields HL, Allen RR, et al. The interpretation of pain relief and sensory changes following sympathetic block. *Brain* 1994; 17:1475–1487.
22. Jänig W, McLachlan E. The role of modifications in noradrenergic peripheral pathways after nerve lesions in the generation of pain. In Fields HC, Liebeskind JC, eds. *Pharmacological Approaches to the Treatment of Chronic Pain: New Concepts and Critical Issues, Progress in Pain Research and Management.* Vol 1. Seattle, Wash: IASP Press; 1994:101–129.
23. Blumburg H, Jänig W. Clinical manifestations of reflex sympathetic dystrophy and sympathetically-maintained pain. In: Wall PD, Melzack R, eds. *Textbook of Pain.* 3rd ed. Edinburgh, Scotland: Churchill Livinstone;1994:685–697.
24. Hábler HJ, Jänig W, Koltzenburg M. Activation of unmyelinated efferents and chronically lesioned nerves by adrenalin and excitation of sympathetic efferents in the cat. *Neurosci Lett* 1987;82:35–40.
25. Jänig W, Koltzenburg M. Sympathetic reflex activity in neuroeffector transmission change after chronic nerve lesions. In: Bond MR, Charlton JE, Woolf CJ, eds. *Proceedings of the Sixth World Congress on Pain, Pain Research and Clinical Management.* Vol 4. Amsterdam, Holland: Elsevier; 1991:365–371.
26. Price DD, Long S, Huitt C. Sensory testing of pathophysiological mechanisms of pain in patients with reflex sympathetic dystrophy. *Pain* 1992;49:163–173.
27. Torebjörk HE, Wahren LK, Wallin G, et al. Noradrenalin-evoked pain in neuralgia. *Pain* 1995;63:11–20.
28. Roberts WJ. A hypothesis on the physiological basis for causalgia and related pains. *Pain* 1986;124:297–311.
29. Torebjörk HE, Hallin RG. Microneurographic studies of peripheral pain mechanisms in man. In: Bonica JJ, Lieberskind JC, Alb-Fessard DG, eds. *Advances in Pain Research and Therapy.* Vol 3. New York, NY: Raven; 1979:121–131.

30. Campbell JN, Meyer RA, Raja SN. Is nociceptor activation by alpha-1 adrenoceptors the culprit in sympathetically-maintained pain? *APS J* 1992;1:3–11.
31. Raja SN, Treede RD, Davis KD, et al. Systemic alpha-adrenergic blockade with phentolamine: A diagnostic test for sympathetically-maintained pain. *Anesthesiology* 1991;74:691–698.
32. Wasner G, Heckmann K, Maier C, et al. Vascular abnormalities in acute reflex sympathetic dystrophy (CRPS I)—complete inhibition of sympathetic nerve activity with recovery. *Arch Neurol* 1999;56:613–620.
33. McLachlan EM, Jänig W, Devore M, et al. Peripheral nerve injury triggers noradrenergic sprouting within dorsal root ganglia. *Nature* 1993;363:543—545.
34. Carlton SM, Lekan HA, Kim SH, et al. Behavioral manifestation of an experimental model for peripheral neuropathy produced by spinal nerve ligation in the primate. *Pain* 1994;56:155–166.
35. Drummond PD, Skipworth S, Finch PM. Alpha-1 adrenoceptors in normal and hyperalgesic skin. *Clin Sci* 1996;91:73–77.
36. Wall PD. Inflammatory and neurogenic pain: New molecules, new mechanisms. *Brit J Anesth* 1995;75:123–124.
37. Sieweke N, Birklein F, Riedl B, et al. Patterns in hyperalgesia in complex regional pain syndrome. *Pain* 1999;80:171–177.
38. Schürmann M, Grad LG, Andress HJ, et al. Assessment of peripheral sympathetic nervous function for diagnosing early post-traumatic complex regional pain syndrome type I. *Pain* 1999;88:149–159.
39. Schwartzman RJ, McLellan TL. Reflex sympathetic dystrophy: A review. *Arch Neurol* 1987;44:555–561.
40. Eccleston C, Crombez G, Aldrich S, et al. Attention and somatic awareness in chronic pain. *Pain* 1997;72:209–215.
41. Darbyshire SW, Jones AK, Davani P, et al. Cerebral responses to pain in patients with atypical facial pain, measured by positron emission tomography. *J Neurol Neurosurg Psychiatry* 1994;57:1166–1172.
42. Rommel O, Gehling M, Dertwinkel R, et al. Hemisensory impairment in patients with complex regional pain syndrome. *Pain* 1999;80: 95–101.
43. Vlaeyen JWS, Kole-Snijders AMJ, Boern RGB, et al. Fear of movement/re-injury in chronic low back pain and its relation to behavioral performance. *Pain* 1995;62:363–372.
44. Stanton-Hicks M, Jänig W, Boas RA. *Reflex Sympathetic Dystrophy.* Boston, Mass: Kluwer; 1990.
45. Jänig W, Blumburg H, Boas RA, et al. The reflex sympathetic dystrophy syndrome: Consensus statement and general recommendations for diagnosis and clinical research. In: Bond MR, Charlton JE, Woolf CJ, eds. *Proceedings of the Sixth World Congress on Pain, Pain Research and Clinical Management.* Vol 4. Amsterdam, Holland: Elsevier; 1991:372–375.
46. Stanton-Hicks M, Jänig W, Hassenbusch S, et al. Reflex sympathetic dystrophy: Changing concepts and taxonomy. *Pain* 1995;63:127–133.
47. Merskey H, Bogduk N, eds. *Classification of Chronic Pain: Descriptions of Chronic Pain Syndromes and Definitions of Pain Terms.* 2nd ed. Seattle, Wash: IASP Press; 1994.
48. Richards RL. Causalgia: A centennial review. *Arch Neurol* 1967; 16:339–350.
49. Bonica JJ. Causalgia and other reflex sympathetic dystrophies. In: Bonica JJ, Lieberskiend JC, Albe-Fessard, DG, eds. *Advances in Pain Research and Therapy.* Vol 3. New York, NY: Raven; 1979:141–166.
50. Bonica JJ. *The Management of Pain.* Philadelphia, Pa: Lea & Febiger; 1953.
51. Mailis A, Wade J. Profile of Caucasian women with possible genetic predisposition to reflex sympathetic dystrophy: A pilot study. *Clin J Pain* 1994;10:210–217.
52. Devor M, Raber P. Heritability of symptoms in an experimental model of neuropathic pain. *Pain* 1990;42:51–67.
53. Bhatia KP, Bhatt MH, Masden CD. The causalgia-dystonia syndrome. *Brain* 1993;116:843–851.
54. Low PA, Caskey PE, Tuck RR, et al. Quantitative sudomotor axon reflex test in normal and neuropathic subjects. *Ann Neurol* 1983;14: 573–580.
55. Knezevic W, Bajada S. Peripheral autonomic surface potential: Quantitative technique for recording autonomic neural function in man. *Clin Exper Neurol* 1985;21:201–210.
56. Glynn C, Walsh JA, Basedow RW, et al. A model for investigating the effect of drugs in the peripheral sympathetic nervous system in man. *J Auton Nerv Syst* 1982;5:195–205.
57. McCain GA, Scudds RA. The concept of primary fibromyalgia (fibrositis): Clinical value, relation and significance to other chronic musculoskeletal pain syndromes. *Pain* 1988;33:273–287.
58. Browne CD, Nolan BM, Faithfull DK. Occupational repetition strain injuries: Guideline for diagnosis and management. *Med J Aust* 1984; 140:329–332.
59. Frye HJH. Overuse syndrome in musicians: Prevention and management. *Lancet* 1986;11:728–731.
60. Punett L, Robbins JM, Wegman DH, et al. Soft tissue disorders in the upper limbs of female garment workers. *Scan J Work Environ Health* 1985;11:417–425.
61. Lautenbacher S, Rolman GB, McCain GA. Multi-method assessment of experimental and clinical pain in patients with fibromyalgia. *Pain* 1994;59:45–53.
62. Deuschl G, Blumburg H, Lückling CH. Tremor in reflex sympathetic dystrophy. *Arch Neurol* 1991;48:1247–1258.
63. Schott G. Clinical features of algodystrophy: Is the sympathetic nervous system involved? *Funct Neurol* 1989;4:131–134.
64. Jancovic J, van der Linden C. Dystonia and tremor induced by peripheral trauma: Predisposing factors. *J Neurol Neurosurg Psychiat* 1988;51:1512–1519.
65. American Psychiatric Association. *Diagnostic and Statistical Manual of Mental Disorders: DSM IV-TR.* Washington, DC: American Psychiatric Association; 2000.
66. Stanton-Hicks M, Raj PP, Racz GB. Use of regional anesthetics for diagnosis of reflex sympathetic dystrophy and sympathetically-maintained pain: A critical evaluation. In: Janig W, Stanton-Hicks M, eds. *Reflex Sympathetic Dystrophy: A Reappraisal, Progress in Pain Research and Management.* Vol 6. Seattle, Wash: IASP Press; 1996:217–237.
67. Birklein F, Sittl R, Spitzer A, Klaus D, Neundorfer B, Handwerker HO. Susomotor function in sympathetic reflex dystrophy. *Pain* 1997; 69:49–54.
68. Sandroni P, Low PA, Ferrer T, Opfer-Gehring TL, Willner CL, Wilson PR. Complex Regional Pain Syndrome I (CRPS I): Prospective study and laboratory evaluation *Clin J Pain* 1998;14:282–289.
69. Gracely RH, Price DD, Roberts WJ, et al. Quantitative sensory testing in patients with complex regional pain syndrome (CRPS) I and II. In: Janig W, Stanton-Hicks M, eds. *Reflex Sympathetic Dystrophy: A Reappraisal, Progress in Pain Research and Management.* Vol 6. Seattle, Wash: IASP Press; 1996:151–172.
70. Kozin F, Genant HK, Bekerman C, et al. The reflex sympathetic dystrophy syndrome, II. Roentgenographic and scintigraphic evidence of bilaterality and of periarticular accentuation. *Am J Med* 1976;60:332–338.
71. Stanton-Hicks M, Baron R, Boas R, et al. Complex regional pain syndromes: Guidelines for therapy. *Clin J Pain* 1998;14:155–166.
72. Portenoy RK, Foley KM, Inturrisi CE. The nature of opioid responsiveness and its implications for neuropathic pain: A new hypothesis derived from studies of opioid infusions. *Pain* 1990;43:273–286.
73. Macks MB, Schafer SC, Culnane M, et al. Amitriptyline, but not lorazepam relieves post herpetic neuralgia. *Neurology* 1988;38:1427–1432.
74. Macks MB, Kisore-Kumar R, Schafer SC, et al. Efficacy of desipramine in painful diabetic neuropathy: A placebo-controlled trial. *Pain* 1991;45:69–73.
75. Swerdlow M. Anticonvulsants in the therapy of neuralgia pain. *Pain Clin* 1986;1:9–19.
76. Chaturvedi SK. Phenytoin in reflex sympathetic dystrophy. *Pain* 1989;36:379–380.
77. Mellick GA, Mellick LB. Gabapentin in the management of reflex sympathetic dystrophy. *J Pain Symptom Manage* 1995;10:265–266.

78. Dajgard A, Petersen P, Kastrup J. Mexiletine for treatment of chronic painful diabetic neuropathy. *Lancet* 1988;1:9–11.
79. Kastrup J, Angelo HR, Peterson P, et al. Treatment of chronic painful diabetic neuropathy with intravenous lidocaine infusion. *Br Med J* 1985;292:173.
80. Carlson LK, Watson HK. Treatment of reflex sympathetic dystrophy using the stress-loading program. *J Hand Ther* 1988;1:149–154.
81. Egle UT, Hoffman SO. Psychosomatic aspects of reflex sympathetic dystrophy. In: Stanton-Hicks M, Janig W, Boas RA, eds. *Reflex Sympathetic Dystrophy*. Boston, Mass: Kluwer; 1990:26–36.
82. Geertzen JB, DeBruyn H, DeBruyn-Kofman AT, et al. Reflex sympathetic dystrophy: Early treatment and psychological aspects. *Arch Phys Med Rehabil* 1994;75:442–446.
83. Wilder RT, Wolohan M, Vieyra MA, et al. Reflex sympathetic dystrophy in children. *J Bone Joint Surg* 1992;74:910–919.
84. Boas RA, Covino BG, Shahnarian A. Analgesic responses to lidocaine. *Br J Anaesth* 1982;54:501.
85. Rowbotham MC, Davies PS, Galer BS. Multicenter, double-blind vehicle controlled trial of long-term use of lidocaine patches for postherpetic neuralgia. Paper presented at the 8th World Congress on Pain, IASP; August 17–22, 1996; Vancouver, Canada.
86. Nebe J, Vanegas H, Scaible HG. 1998 Spinal application of ?-conotoxin GIVA, an H-type calcium channel antagonist, attenuates enhancement of dorsal spinal neuronal responses caused by intraarticular injection of mustard oil in the rat. *Exp Brain Res* 1998;120:61–69.
87. Kishore Kumar R, Schafer SC, et al. Efficacy of desipramine in painful diabetic neuropathy: A placebo-controlled trial. *Pain* 1991;45: 69–73.
88. Watson CP, Evans RJ, Reed K, et al. Amitriptyline vs. placebo in postherpetic neuralgia. *Neurology* 1981;32;671–673.
89. Watson CP, Chipman M, Reed K, et al. Amitriptyline in postherpetic neuralgia: A randomized, double-blind crossover trial. *Pain* 1991; 48;29–36.
90. Ghostine SY, Comair YG, Turner DM. Phenoxybenzamine in the treatment of causalgia: Report of 40 cases. *J Neurosurg* 1984;6; 1263–1268.
91. Rauck RI, Eisenach JC, Jackson K, et al. Epidural clonidine treatment for refractory reflex sympathetic dystrophy. *Anesthesiology* 1993;79;1163–1169.
92. Byas-Smith MG, Max MB, Muir J, et al. Transdermal clonidine compared to placebo in painful diabetic neuropathy using a 2-stage enriched enrollment design. *Pain* 1995;60;267–274.
93. Davis KD, Treede RD, Raja SM, et al. Topical application of clonidine relieves hyperalgesia in patients with sympathetically-maintained pain. *Pain* 1991;47:309–317.
94. Christiansen K, Jensen EN, Noer I. The reflex sympathetic dystrophy syndrome: Response to treatment with corticosteroids. *Acta Chir Scand* 1982;148;653–1985.
95. Oyen WJ, Arntz I, Claessens RM, et al. Reflex sympathetic dystrophy of the hand: An excessive inflammatory response. *Pain* 1993;59: 151–157.
96. Kuntz A. *Autonomic Nervous System.* 4th ed. Philadelphia, Pa: Lea & Febiger; 1953.
97. Racz G, Stanton-Hicks M. Radiofrequency (RFA) sympatholysis for CRPS. *Pain Practice* 2002;2:250–256.
98. Moore DC. Anterior (paratracheal) approach for block of the stellate ganglion. In: *Regional Block: A Handbook for Use in the Clinical Practice of Medicine and Surgery.* 4th ed. Springfield, Ill: Charles C Thomas; 1975:123–137.
99. Hatangdi DS, Boas RA. Lumbar sympathectomy: a single needle technique. *Br J Anesth* 1985;57:285–289.
100. Pernak J. Percutaneous radiofrequency thermolumbar sympathectomy. *Pain Clinic* 1995;80:99–106.
101. Raj PP. Continuous epidural infusion and patient-controlled epidural analgesia in the management of pain. In: Waldman S, Winnie A, eds. *Interventional Pain Management.* Philadelphia, Pa: WB Saunders; 1996:333–338.
102. Raj PP, Denson DD. Prolonged analgesia technique with local anesthetics. In: Raj PP, ed. *Practical Management of Pain.* Chicago, Ill: Yearbook Medical Pub; 1986:687–700.
103. DuPen S, Williams A. Management of patients receiving combined epidural morphine and bupivacaine for the treatment of cancer pain. *J Pain Symptom Manage* 1992;7:56–58.
104. Shealey CN, Mortimer JT, Hagfors NR. Dorsal column electroanalgesia. *J Neurosurg* 1970;32:560–564.
105. Meyerson BA, Linderoth B, Lind G. Spinal cord stimulation in chronic neuropathic pain. *Lakartidningen* 1991;88:727–732.
106. Nashold BS Jr, Goldner L, Mullen JB, et al. Long-term pain control by direct peripheral nerve stimulation. *J Bone Joint Surg Am* 1982; 64:1–10.
107. Augusinsson L, Linderoth B, Mannheimer C. Spinal cord stimulation in various ischemic conditions. In: Illis L, ed. *Spinal Cord Dysfunction. Vol 3. Functional Stimulation.* Oxford, England: Oxford Medical Pub; 1992.
108. Hassenbusch SJ, Stanton-Hicks M, Schoppa D, et al. Long-term results of peripheral nerve stimulation for reflex sympathetic dystrophy. *J Neurosurg* 1996;84:415–423.
109. Alo KM, Yland MJ, Redko V, et al. Lumbar and sacral nerve root stimulation (NRS) in the treatment of chronic pain: A novel anatomic approach and neurostimulation technique. *Neuromodulation* 1999;2: 1;23–31.
110. Holsheimer J, Struijk JJ, Tas NR. Effects of electrogeometry and combinational nerve fiber selectivity in spinal cord stimulation. *Med Biol Eng Comput* 1995;33:676–682.
111. Linderoth B. Neurophysiological mechanism involved in vasodilatation and ischemic pain relief by spinal cord stimulation. In: Galley D, Illis SL, Krainick M, Sier J, Staaf M, eds. *First Congress of the International Neuromodulation Society.* Bologna, Italy: Monduzzi Editore; 1993:27–40.
112. Kember MA, Barendse GA, van Kleef M, et al. Spinal cord stimulation in patients with chronic reflex sympathetic dystrophy. *N Engl J Med* 2000;343:618–624.
113. Oakley JC, Weiner RL. Spinal cord stimulation for complex regional pain syndrome. A prospective study in 19 patients. *Neuromodulation* 1999;2:47–50.
114. Burchiel KJ, Anderson VC, Wilson BJ, et al. Prognostic factors of spinal cord stimulation for chronic back and leg pain. *Neurosurgery* 1995;36:1101–1111.
115. Bruehl S, Carlson CR. Predisposing psychologic factors in the development of reflex sympathetic dystrophy: A review of the empirical evidence. *Clin J Pain* 1992;8:287–299.
116. Haddox JD. Psychological aspects of reflex sympathetic dystrophy. In: Stanton-Hicks M, ed. *Pain and the Sympathetic Nervous System.* Boston, Mass: Kluwer; 1990:207–224.
117. Ruggeri SB, Arthreya BH, Doughty R et al. Reflex sympathetic dystrophy in children. *Clin Orthop* 1988;163:225–230.
118. Wilder RT, Berde CB, Wolohan M, et al. Reflex sympathetic dystrophy in children: Clinical characteristics in follow up of 70 patients. *J Bone Surg Am* 1992;74A:910–919.
119. Stanton RP, Malcolm JR, Wersdock KA, et al. Reflex sympathetic dystrophy in children: An orthopedic perspective. *Orthopedics* 1993; 16:773–779.
120. Kessler RW, Saulsbury FT, Miller LT, et al. Reflex sympathetic treatment with transcutaneous nerve stimulation. *Pediatrics* 1988;82:728-732.
121. Stanton-Hicks M, Burton AW, Bruehl SP, Carr DB, Harden RN, et al. An updated interdisciplinary clinical pathway for CRPS: report of an expert panel. *Pain Practice* 2002;2:1–16.

CHAPTER 40 ACUTE HERPES ZOSTER AND POSTHERPETIC NEURALGIA

P. Prithvi Raj

ACUTE HERPES ZOSTER

Acute herpes zoster, commonly called *shingles*, is an acute infectious viral disease that primarily affects the posterior spinal root ganglia of the spinal nerves. A single posterior spinal root ganglion or a small number of adjacent ones may be affected, usually on the same side. The corresponding ganglia of the cranial nerves also may be involved similarly. The causative virus, varicella-zoster, belongs to a DNA group of viruses that is host specific. The same virus produces chickenpox or varicella in children and young people.

Etiology

Herpes zoster most frequently occurs in adults who previously have had chickenpox. It is thought that the virus remains dormant in the dorsal root ganglia until, many years later, it is reactivated and produces herpes zoster. The decrease in immunity that permits the reactivation may be caused by infection or malignancy, or it may occur in the iatrogenically immunosuppressed patient. The impact of stress on varicella-zoster virus has not been well studied, but major depression has been associated with markedly decreased varicella-zoster virus–specific cellular immunity.[1] Patients experiencing stress during a zoster episode are more likely to have more severe pain, increasing their risk of postherpetic neuralgia.[2] Patients with herpes zoster occasionally relate a history of recent contact with the virus exogenously; but it is rare, if ever, that an infection so develops. The incidence of herpes zoster does not increase during seasonal chickenpox epidemics.

It is thought that, after the virus multiplies in the dorsal root ganglion, it is transported along the sensory nerves to the nerve endings, where the lesions are formed. In the immunocompetent patient, the disease is confined to a local distribution because there is a rapid mobilization of defense mechanisms.

Although the posterior root ganglia of the spinal and cranial nerves are involved most commonly, any part of the central nervous system can be affected. For example, the anterior motor horn may be involved, or the patient may have myelitis or encephalomyelitis. In rare cases, only the sympathetic ganglia are affected, resulting in a syndrome resembling reflex sympathetic dystrophy.

The location of the herpes zoster infection may be determined by the site of a primary inflammatory disease, malignancy, or trauma. Patients with neoplasms, especially lymphomas, are more susceptible to herpes zoster. This high incidence may be the result of recent radiation of affected nodes, advanced disease, and possible splenectomy. Other associated diseases include meningitis, spinal cord tumors, anterior poliomyelitis, syringomyelia, tabes dorsalis, intoxication from arsenicals or carbon monoxide, and malignant neoplasms such as breast, lung, or gastrointestinal tumors.

Incidence

Estimates of the incidence of herpes zoster in the U.S. population indicate an approximate 64% increase in the general population over the past 30 years, to approximately 215 cases per 100,000 person years.[3] Men are affected more frequently than women. African Americans 65 years of age or older are significantly less likely to develop zoster than their white counterparts.[4] The incidence of herpes zoster is usually low in immunocompetent children[5] but is a problem in immunosuppressed children, such as transplant recipients.[6] The disease is more common in debilitated patients.

Our knowledge of cellular immune events in herpes zoster is still somewhat scanty. Experimental and clinical studies suggest that symptomatic herpes zoster occurs only when cell-mediated immunity to varicella-zoster is depressed.[1,7,8] There is an inverse correlation between the capacity of the host to mount a specific cellular immune response and the incidence of zoster. Cell-mediated immune responses to zoster have been difficult to evaluate because the response generally is suppressed during the disease and usually takes time to develop. The function of lymphocytes and monocytes is impaired in herpes zoster. As in other herpetic infections, the normal ratio of helper T cells to suppressor T cells is reversed. It has recently been suggested that T-cell recognition of varicella-zoster virus proteins is a likely mechanism involved in the control of reactivation of the virus from latency.[9] The infection is limited by the cell-mediated immune lymphocytic transformation, lymphocyte-monocyte inactivation of the virus, and local host responses of interferon production and polymorphonuclear inflammatory response in the vesicle. Antibody administration also modifies the disease, perhaps by altering membrane antigens and cellular cytotoxicity.

POSTHERPETIC NEURALGIA

Postherpetic neuralgia is a continuation of herpes zoster that generally occurs in older patients. Although spontaneous resolution of herpes zoster may be expected in most patients, a significant number have intractable pain. Postherpetic neuralgia, which persists for months or years after the skin lesions have healed, occurs in approximately 10% of patients older than 40 years of age and 20% to 50% of patients older than 60 years of age. Some young patients may have postherpetic neuralgia for 1 or 2 weeks after the lesions have healed, although hypesthesia or hyperesthesia may persist; however, the probability is extremely low.[5]

This is one of the most difficult problems encountered by physicians. Few other conditions create such agonizing pain and suffering for the patient. Many patients consider suicide as a means of relief from the torturous pain.

DIFFERENTIAL DIAGNOSIS

Acute Herpes Zoster

The diagnosis of herpes zoster usually is difficult to make in the preeruptive stage. After the lesions appear, the clinical features are so typical that the diagnosis is easy. Before eruption, herpes zoster often is mistaken for other pain-causing conditions, such as coronary disease, pleurisy, pleurodynia, cholecystitis, neural disease, appendicitis, peritonitis, and collapsed intervertebral disk. Occasionally, localized herpes simplex may occur. Differentiation between the two herpesvirus conditions can be made by virus isolation procedures in the laboratory.

To confirm the diagnosis of herpes zoster, the virus can be isolated from vesicular, but not usually from pustular or crusting, lesions 7 or 8 days after eruption. Specific antigens also can be found in vesicular fluid and in the crusts of lesions using a simple gel-precipitation technique.

Epithelial cells with eosinophilic intranuclear inclusions and multinucleated giant cells can be identified in material scraped from the base of a vesicular lesion. The leukocyte count is normal in uncomplicated herpes zoster. Mononuclear pleocytosis is present in the cerebrospinal fluid of patients with herpes zoster, particularly those with cranial nerve involvement.

Visceral pain can be differentiated from herpetic pain by a somatic sensory nerve block; this will not relieve visceral pain.

Postherpetic Neuralgia

Postherpetic neuralgia also can be confused with other problems, but the patient usually has a history of a previous unilateral skin eruption, and there may be residual scarring of the skin. Hyperesthesia, dysesthesia, and anesthesia also may be present in the affected areas. Skin eruption may be minimal in some cases, and few or even no scars may be present with postherpetic neuralgia (zoster *sine herpete*). In these patients, the central nervous system was damaged by the original infection, resulting in neuralgia without producing any scars to the skin. A rising zoster antibody titer in the acute stage confirms the infectious agent.

SIGNS AND SYMPTOMS

Acute Herpes Zoster

The development and course of herpes zoster depend on contributions from both the virus and the host. The disease can progress in three stages, with virus and host factors interacting at each stage (Table 40-1).

Acute herpes usually has pain that is localized to the dermatomal distribution of one or more affected posterior root ganglia. The pain may be accompanied by fever and malaise. It usually is mild at first, but it may grow more severe over the succeeding few days. It can be dull, sharp, burning, aching, or shooting. Commonly, paresthesia also is present. Skin lesions usually appear 4 to 5 days later, but they may appear immediately.

At first, there is a local redness and swelling followed by red papules that progress through vesicles, blebs, pustules, and then to the crusting stage over the succeeding 2 to 3 weeks. The lesions characteristically are unilateral, running along the dermatome in a band. In mild cases, the skin lesions may not affect the whole dermatome, but sensory involvement of the whole dermatome usually is present. In severe cases, larger blebs usually cover the entire dermatome and tend to coalesce. The area is likely to be extremely painful; the pain is aggravated by contact or movement.

TABLE 40-1 **Stages of Herpes Zoster**

Stage I	Viral replication Loss of immune surveillance
Stage II	Clinical syndrome (acute herpes zoster) Viral effect on ganglion-nerve-dermatome Antiviral immune response by the body Cytolysis from virus and host inflammatory reaction
Stage III	Sequelae of herpes zoster Central nervous system and visceral spread Antiviral immune response

Reproduced with permission from Raj P. Pain due to herpes zoster. In: Raj P, ed. *Practical Management of Pain.* 2nd ed. Chicago, Ill: Mosby-Year Book; 1992.

The lesions appear in thoracic dermatomes in more than 50% of patients. The next region where they commonly are seen is the trigeminal distribution, with an incidence of 3% to 20%. The ophthalmic division is involved in 75% of these patients. Lumbar and cervical eruptions occur in 10% to 20% of patients, with a sacral distribution being much less common. With advancing age, the incidence of trigeminal (ophthalmic) zoster increases and that of spinal zoster declines. Bilateral zoster occurs in less than 1% of patients. Recurrent zoster has been reported in 1% to 8% of patients; approximately one half of the recurrences are at the site of the previous eruption (Table 40-2).

Occasionally, motor paralysis in the intercostal and abdominal muscles, arms, legs, and muscles innervated by cranial nerves may be associated with herpes zoster. These motor deficits may be reversible over a period of years.

If the trigeminal (gasserian) ganglion is affected, the symptoms usually include pain in the nerve distribution, headache, weakness of the eyelid muscles and, occasionally, an Argyll Robertson pupil. Lesions may appear on the face, cornea, mouth, and tongue. Scarring and anesthesia of the cornea may occur. The first division of the trigeminal nerve most often is affected. If there is involvement of the geniculate ganglion, there may be Bell's palsy, vertigo, disorders of hearing, and lesions of the external ear and canal and the anterior portion of the tongue.

TABLE 40-2 **Site and Incidence of Acute Herpes Zoster**

Site of Herpes Zoster	Incidence (%)
Thoracic	50
Face (ophthalmic)	3–20
Cervical	10–20
Bilateral	<1
Recurrent	1–8
Recurrent at the site of previous herpes zoster	50

Reproduced with permission from Raj P. Pain due to herpes zoster. In: Raj P, ed. *Practical Management of Pain.* 2nd ed. Chicago, Ill: Mosby-Year Book; 1992.

The crusts generally fall off at approximately 5 weeks, leaving irregular pink scars. These scars eventually become hypopigmented and anesthetic. They form characteristic pocks, which usually are surrounded by mottled pigmentation and may last for years. The hyperesthesia and pain usually subside and disappear at approximately the same time the crusts fall off.

Risk factors for severe, persistent pain associated with acute herpes zoster include prodromal symptoms, age greater than 50 years, or moderate or severe pain at presentation.[10] The duration of pain has been shown to correlate with severity of lesions at worst phase and the involved region, with age over 60 years and those with trigeminal involvement most likely to have significantly longer duration of pain.[11]

Postherpetic Neuralgia

In 10% to 50% of patients with herpes zoster, pain and hyperesthesia persist after the lesions are healed. This condition, called *postherpetic neuralgia,* may improve slowly, but after it has been present for 6 months, complete spontaneous cure is unlikely.

The discomfort of postherpetic neuralgia is of two types: pain and dysesthesia. The persistent intractable pain, which is constant and never varies, often is associated with a feeling of heat. It is described variously as burning, shooting, twisting, lancinating, pressing, and gripping. A feeling of tightness also may be present. Relief usually is found during sleep. In chronic postherpetic neuralgia, the patient commonly has hyperpathia, often associated with damage to a peripheral nerve, the spinothalamic tract, or the thalamus. It may be caused by a reduction in the number and proportion of conducting nerve fibers.

Dysthesia often is interpreted as pain. Uncomfortable unpleasant sensations make the patient unable to bear the lightest contact with the skin. Some patients even cut holes in their clothing to minimize the problem. A slight breath of wind can incite a paroxysm of pain. Curiously, most patients can tolerate firm pressure on the affected area but not light pressure. They may wear especially tight clothing or keep their hands pressed over the painful region. Patients may complain about a feeling of worms under the skin or of ants crawling over the skin (formication).

PATHOPHYSIOLOGY

Acute Herpes Zoster

Early lesions of herpes zoster are minute unilocular vesicles involving the epidermis and corium. There is a ballooning degeneration of the involved epithelial cells, and intranuclear inclusion bodies often are present. Huge giant cells with multiple inclusions are found in mature lesions. Necrosis and hemorrhaging into the uppermost portion of the dermis may occur if there is destruction of the germinal layer.

Typical varicella vesicles are formed from serum that collects around the damaged cells. The fluid in the vesicle soon becomes cloudy from polymorphonuclear leukocytes, multinucleated giant cells, degenerated cells, and fibrin. A scab is formed when the fluid is absorbed.

Occasionally, patients develop persistent papules that do not progress to vesicles. No difference has been found in cell-mediated immunity or immunophenotype in lymphocytic infiltrates between the vesicular and papular types of herpes zoster, suggesting that the clinical appearance is dependent on the infected site of virus in the tissue.[12]

The dorsal root ganglion of the affected nerve is hemorrhagic and swollen. There is round cell infiltration and eventually neuronal destruction. Ganglion and satellite cells may have intranuclear inclusions. Maximum degeneration is seen in the posterior nerve root approximately 2 weeks after dermal lesions first appear. Similar changes may be seen in the posterior column and sensory nerves. Rarely, the anterior horn may be involved or a localized meningitis may occur, on both. Eventually, the ganglion may be replaced by scar tissue.

When dermal nerves in 48 cases with cutaneous and mucosal herpesvirus infection were examined retrospectively, all had perineural inflammation consisting of a dense, mixed lymphocyte-polymorphonuclear cell infiltrate. Other abnormalities also were noted, including peripheral nerve twig inflammation and more distant neural involvement, suggesting that nerve twigs may be directly involved in infection.[13]

Postherpetic Neuralgia

Many hypotheses have been postulated to explain the intractable nature of postherpetic neuralgia. Noxious impulses may become established in centrally located, closed, self-perpetuating loops; and progressive facilitation may develop in these synapses. Eventually, pain that is entirely unaffected by surgical section of peripheral pathways occurs spontaneously. Sensitized nociceptors may not return to normal after inflammation subsides; initiation of nociceptor-evoked central hyperexcitability and axonal damage may result in ectopically discharging nociceptor sprouts.[14,15] Patients who develop postherpetic neuralgia usually have areas of cutaneous scarring and sensory loss.[16] In general, possible mechanisms for generating pain and allodynia in peripheral nerve injury usually include: (1) central nervous system mechanisms (loss of large-fiber inhibition; deafferentation hyperactivity of central pain transmission neurons; aberrant connections resulting from reorganization of the central nervous system; central sensitization; summation; secondary hyperalgesia; and allodynia); and (2) peripheral mechanisms (ectopic impulse generation; enhanced adrenergic sensitivity; and inflammation of the nerve trunk).[17] Two different mechanisms are believed to cause postherpetic pain. In most patients it may be related to abnormally hyperactive primary afferent nociceptors. For patients with constant pain in an area with profound sensory loss, pain may result from a change in the functional connectivity and activation state of central nervous system pain transmission neurons produced by deafferentation.[2] There also is a possibility that the infection involves higher pathways in the cord and brain than formerly was believed. For instance, subclinical extension of viral inflammation of acute zoster into the central nervous system has been identified as common; and brainstem and cervical cord lesions attributed to zoster, visualized using magnetic resonance imaging, have been associated with development of postherpetic neuralgia.[18] If this is true, the infection is outside the reach of extradural and intrathecal medication and, possibly, cordotomy.

The gate-control theory might explain some features involved in the occurrence and persistence of postherpetic neuralgia. It is postulated that pain is carried by small unmyelinated nerve fibers to the central nervous system, where the input is modified by pathways in larger myelinated nerve fibers. Nerve impulses are transmitted faster in the large, myelinated nerve fibers than in the small, unmyelinated nerve fibers. In acute herpes zoster, there is a tendency, proportionately, for more of the larger fibers to be damaged and destroyed than the small fibers. The larger fibers also regenerate more slowly than small fibers, and their diameter after regeneration usually is smaller than originally. Hence, there is an increase in the percentage of smaller fibers over large fibers.

According to the gate-control theory, this is the situation in which minimal small-fiber stimulation might produce the sensation of pain because the normal modulation of large nerve-fiber stimulation is no longer present. It is important to notice that older patients have fewer large fibers initially, and they lose more after herpes zoster infection. Therefore, such patients are more likely to feel a greater degree of pain than younger patients and to be more susceptible to the intractable pain of postherpetic neuralgia.

LABORATORY DIAGNOSIS

Because most viral replication occurs early in the disease process, optimal drug treatment depends on an early and accurate diagnosis. The varicella-zoster virus may be recovered from early vesicles and has been recovered from blood, lung, liver, and cerebrospinal fluid, but, only occasionally, from the oropharynx. The virus is cell associated; therefore, scraping the base of the vesicle is more productive than using a fluid overlay. Scrapings also provide cellular material containing multinuclear giant cells. Acidophilic intranuclear inclusions can be seen in the Tzanck smear stained with hematoxylin and eosin, Giemsa, Papanicolaou, or Paragon multiple stain. A pouch biopsy for electron microscopic examination provides even more reliable material; the more reliable material may permit a diagnosis before the vesicular stage develops (Table 40-3).

PREVENTION

A vaccine against herpesvirus is now being tested and has shown good results in certain groups of older adults and immunosuppressed children in terms of decreased incidence and severity of herpes zoster.[6,19,20]

MANAGEMENT

Acute Herpes Zoster

The goals of treatment are early resolution of the acute disease and prevention of postherpetic neuralgia. The earlier the institution of treatment, the less likely is the development of postherpetic neuralgia.[21]

Pain should be treated aggressively, especially in elderly patients and immunosuppressed patients, who are prone to postherpetic neuralgia.[14,15] After postherpetic neuralgia is established, there is no reliable treatment for this syndrome. Unfortunately, no treatment regimen is fully effective; this has led to many different treatments with varying success rates.

TABLE 40-3 **Laboratory Diagnosis of Acute Herpes Zoster**

Techniques	Comment
Virus recovery from Vesicles Blood Lung Liver Cerebrospinal fluid Oropharynx (only occasionally)	Rapid diagnostic tests allow for early diagnosis
Scrapings from the vesicles contain cellular material with multinucleated giant cells	Show acidophilic intranuclear inclusions
Tzanck smear Hematoxylin-eosin stain Giemsa stain Papanicolaou stain Paragon multiple stain	
Punch biopsy for electron microscopy	More reliable and provides diagnosis before vesicular stage develops
Culture tests (in human epitheloids or fibroblasts) Virus specifically identified in culture by intranuclear inclusions after staining and by gel-precipitation techniques	Focal lesion with swollen refractile cells in 3–4 days
Staining of cellular material with direct fluorescent antibody of Tzanck smear	Readily identifies infected cells

Reproduced with permission from Raj P. Pain due to herpes zoster. In: Raj P, ed. *Practical Management of Pain.* 2nd ed. Chicago, Ill: Mosby-Year Book; 1992.

Some physicians do not treat acute herpes zoster because they believe it will resolve spontaneously if left alone. They institute treatment only if postherpetic neuralgia develops. This is a great disservice to the group of patients with intractable pain from postherpetic neuralgia. Treatment during the early stages of acute herpes zoster is the best means of preventing needless pain and suffering.[21,22]

There is no available treatment that is effective in all cases. Success is usually limited with any method. Many methods of management have been tried for acute herpes zoster and postherpetic neuralgia.

Drug Therapy The various drugs used in the treatment of the acute stage of herpes zoster are summarized in Table 40-4.

Antiviral Agents Antiviral agents are now standard therapy for herpes zoster. The varicella-zoster virus, like all viruses, is a parasite that takes over healthy cells and uses their DNA to reproduce itself. It is believed that, if viral DNA synthesis can be slowed or inhibited, then specific host immune systems might have more time to help control the viral infection. Some substances that grossly inhibit DNA synthesis were developed as possible anticancer drugs and have been found to have a more significant antiviral than anticancer activity. Theoretically, these agents could either kill the virus or alter its replication. To be effective, the agents must be given before significant tissue damage occurs. Such agents include acyclovir, cytarabine, vidarabine, idoxuridine, sorivudine, famciclovir, valaciclovir, and brivudine.

Experimental trials using systemic administration of cytarabine in various dose schedules gave conflicting results, ranging from apparent success in early, uncontrolled studies to no benefit or apparent worsening of infection in controlled trials. Controlled studies of vidarabine in the treatment of herpes zoster in immunosuppressed patients have been promising. Therapy was most successful when administered early and to patients younger than 38 years of age or to those with reticuloendothelial malignancy. Cutaneous healing was accelerated, pain was relieved acutely, and the incidence of postherpetic neuralgia was low.

TABLE 40-4 **Drug Therapy for Acute Herpes Zoster**

Antiviral Agents
- Acyclovir
- Cytarabine
- Vidarabine
- Idoxuridine
- Thymidine analogues
- Sorivudine
- Famciclovir
- Valaciclovir
- Brivudine
- Interferon
- Zoster immune globulin
- Adenosine monophosphate

Analgesics
- Anti-inflammatory agents
- Prednisone

Antidepressants and Tranquilizers
- Amitriptyline and fluphenazine
- Dozepin

Other
- Vitamin B_{12}
- B-complex vitamins
- L-tryptophan

Acyclovir masquerades as one of the building blocks of the DNA needed by the herpesvirus to reproduce itself. This stops the chain, and the virus ceases to replicate. Although acyclovir accelerates cutaneous changes in herpes zoster, the intensity and duration of acute herpetic neuralgia appear to be directly related to time of therapy initiation (not later than 6 days after onset).[21] The author of a meta-analysis of 30 clinical trials in immunocompetent patients found five homogeneous, randomized, placebo-controlled trials that showed that oral acyclovir, 800 mg/day within 72 hours of rash onset, may reduce the incidence of residual pain at 6 months by 46%.[22] However, at an estimated cost of from $250 to $300 for 7 days' treatment with oral acyclovir, use of this antiviral agent may not be economically justified in immunocompetent younger patients, especially in developing countries.[23]

Some ophthalmologists have used idoxuridine for treating herpetic lesions of the conjunctiva and cornea. Prompt treatment is necessary, and best results are obtained when the drug is used within 4 or 5 days of the onset of infection. This drug's effects are variable, and it will not prevent postherpetic neuralgia. Varying concentrations of idoxuridine in dimethyl sulfoxide have been used in New Zealand to treat patients with herpes zoster, and it has been shown that pain decreased faster and that fewer vesicles developed after topical applications. Early initiation of treatment is necessary. Similar positive results have been reported from Denmark. Idoxuridine in dimethyl sulfoxide 35% to 40% has been used in Great Britain on herpes zoster skin lesions. Faster healing of lesions and a shorter duration of postherpetic neuralgia have been reported, and late sequelae are uncommon. Success depends on early institution of treatment. The solvent decreases inflammation and edema and has a bacteriostatic action. It is an extremely strong solvent that has not been approved by the Food and Drug Administration for this use.

Thymidine analogues have been found to have some inhibitory effect on certain strains of varicella-zoster virus.

Although acyclovir has been shown to be effective in shortening duration of zoster pain, other newer agents may offer some advantages. Sorivudine has compared favorably with acyclovir in terms of accelerating cutaneous healing[24] and preventing recurrences and new episodes.[25] Valaciclovir may be more efficacious than acyclovir in shortening time to complete resolution of herpes zoster–associated pain[26,27] and appears to offer cost benefits.[28] Famciclovir has been shown to be efficacious in treating herpes zoster.[29–31] It has also been shown to accelerate healing of genital herpes in humans,[32–34] in preventing further outbreaks of genital herpes (unpublished data on file, SmithKline Beecham, 1998, Philadelphia) in humans, and in preventing herpes simplex virus-1 latency in mice.[35–37] Famciclovir may be as or more effective than acyclovir in prevention of latency for genital herpes.[38,39] Intravenous foscarnet is the current treatment of choice for acyclovir-resistant zoster.[40,41]

Interferon, which is produced by the body's immune system, appears to play a role in the control of disease. It seems to work more effectively in tandem with other components of the body's immune system. Large doses, however, can cause adverse effects. It has been reported that interferon production in the vesicle fluid of patients with disseminated herpes zoster is delayed in comparison with that of patients with localized disease. When human leukocyte interferon has been administered, it has been shown to increase circulating interferon. It may, therefore, be used in cases where there might be a risk of herpetic dissemination.

Zoster immune globulin is not effective in altering the clinical course of herpes zoster in immunocompromised adults. It is used currently, however, for the passive protection of susceptible leukemia patients who have been exposed to chickenpox. It also is recommended for use in immunocompromised children at risk for chickenpox.

Adenosine monophosphate given intramuscularly also has been used in the treatment of acute herpes zoster. The exact mechanism by which it provides certain therapeutic benefits is not understood. It may correct underlying biochemical imbalances or defects at the cellular level. Beneficial effects also may occur as a result of the vasodilating effect of the drug and its ability to decrease tissue edema and inflammation.

I believe that the ultimate answer to the problem of herpes zoster and its sequela, postherpetic neuralgia, lies in the field of antiviral therapy. An antiviral agent is needed that will kill the virus safely and reliably before there is neurologic damage. Investigation is still needed to find the most effective antiviral agents against the varicella-zoster virus.

Analgesics Analgesics are an important adjunctive therapy. They may be categorized as nonaddictive, moderately addictive, or strongly addictive agents. Selecting the optimal agent for a specific patient involves consideration of various factors, the most important of which are quality, intensity, duration, and distribution of pain.

Non-narcotic, nonaddictive drugs are used for the control of mild pain. Oral aspirin and acetaminophen are effective drugs with a low incidence of side effects. However, they are not effective in controlling severe pain. Evidence suggests that topical application of acetylsalicyclic acid markedly reduces the spread of infection and produces an analgesic effect.[42,43]

Codeine, propoxyphene, pentazocine, and oxycodone are examples of moderately addicting drugs. The incidence of addiction is relatively low, but dependence may occur with these agents. They are good analgesic agents, but they sometimes produce adverse side effects (such as constipation).

When used properly, the strongly addictive narcotics are effective in the treatment of severe refractory pain, providing relief to varying degrees. In acute herpes zoster, strong medication may be needed to control severe pain. Because the acute stage is short, strongly addictive drugs may be used for a limited period. In such cases, the narcotic is tapered off as treatment decreases the degree of pain. When pain is at a level that can be controlled by non-narcotic drugs, the narcotics should be discontinued. Examples of strongly addictive drugs are morphine, hydromorphone, and meperidine.

Anti-inflammatory Agents The effects of corticosteorid therapy on herpes zoster are still unclear, but reports are encouraging. Results of recent, limited studies suggest that corticosteroids such as prednisone are well tolerated and may significantly reduce the duration of acute neuralgia and improve quality of life; however, they have not been shown to be efficacious in preventing postherpetic neuralgia.[44] Inflammation and scarring are reduced with anti-inflammatory agents. Despite the uncertain effects of corticosteroid therapy on herpes zoster, these drugs have been used extensively to treat this infection.

The role of anti-inflammatory drugs in acute herpes zoster is controversial. If host responses contribute significantly to tissue injury, then attenuation of these responses may be beneficial. Unfortunately, the host defenses that cause tissue injury may be inseparable from those that eliminate or prevent the spread of infection. Currently, dissociation of protective from harmful host responses to the virus has not been demonstrated clearly. However, in the immunocompetent individual, a vigorous antiviral response is altered only very mildly by corticosteroids. Similarly, in the presence of potent antiviral therapy, even in the immunosuppressed patient, a reduction in the inflammatory response eventually may be safe and have a salutary effect. These are important issues for future investigation.

These drugs usually are administered in the first 10 days and continued for as long as 3 weeks. Prednisone is usually the agent of choice. It may be given orally in doses of 60 mg/day the first week, 30 mg/day the second week, and 15 mg/day the third week.

Corticosteroids also have been administered by subcutaneous injection under affected skin, with and without a local anesthetic. Enthusiastic anecdotal reports of large numbers of patients claim 80% to 100% success in treating acute herpes zoster, with a rapid resolution of pain and diminished incidence of postherpetic neuralgia. The experience of others has been less enthusiastic.

Antidepressants and Tranquilizers Major depression has been associated with a marked decline in varicella-zoster virus–specific cellular immunity.[1] Antidepressants have two actions: they can relieve pain, and they can relieve depression. Tricyclic drugs are known to block serotonin reuptake. Therefore, they would be expected to enhance the action of this neurotransmitter at synapses, and such enhancement can produce analgesia in laboratory animals. One of the mechanisms active in central pain states is some defect in the transmission system in the neuraxis; specifically, a deficit in serotonin.

There is a strong consensus among clinical investigators that centrally active antidepressants should be tried in any patient who is not obtaining pain relief, whether or not he or she appears depressed. Tricyclics and anxiolytics frequently are given together because, although depression is not common in acute herpes zoster, many patients experience anxiety along with the severe pain. The most widely used combination is amitriptyline and fluphenazine. Amitriptyline alone has been shown to significantly reduce pain in older patients by more than one half, making a strong argument for its use with an antiviral in this group of patients.[45] In addition to their antidepressant and analgesic properties, tricyclics are also sedatives (for sleep regulation).

Amitriptyline and doxepin may correct the sleep disturbance, frequent awakening, and early morning awakening that are common in severe chronic pain states. Adverse side effects of tricyclic antidepressants include hypotension or hypertension, tachycardia, arrhythmias, drowsiness, confusion, disorientation, dry mouth, blurred vision, increased intraocular pressure, urinary retention, and constipation.

Other Drug Therapies It is thought that the host immune system is incompetent during the acute outbreak. Vitamins, minerals, and improved general nutrition may help improve the immunologic state or replace a missing element.

Nerve Blocks

Local Infiltration In a large group of patients, subcutaneous injections of triamcinolone 0.2% in normal saline have been administered under areas of eruption and sites of pain and itching, with excellent results and reduction of postherpetic neuralgia to a negligible percent. Subcutaneous injections of corticosteroids and local anesthetics offer an effective treatment for acute herpes zoster. The procedure is not associated with any significant complications, the Y technique is simple and inexpensive, and the response to treatment is fairly predictable, as borne out by our own experience.

Somatic Nerve Blocks Because nerve root involvement is suspected in acute herpes zoster, somatic nerve blocks have been used in its treatment. These can include brachial plexus, paravertebral, intercostal, and sciatic blocks. They are of limited value in the acute phase and of no value in the postherpetic stage.

Sympathetic Nerve Blocks As understanding of the pathology of herpes zoster developed, attention was directed toward the sympathetic ganglia. Sympathetic blocks have been used to relieve the vasospasm that was thought to cause the pain and nerve damage. Evidence suggests that sympathetic blockade during the acute phase of herpes zoster can help the immediate pain problem, often dramatically. Of greater value, however, is the possibility that it can prevent the development of postherpetic neuralgia. Although the evidence for this is less compelling, it is probably a worthwhile prophylactic measure that should be used as early as possible.

Trigeminal herpes zoster has been treated with a bupivacaine block of the ipsilateral stellate ganglion.

Sympathetic blocks have been very successful in treating herpes zoster, with just one block often proving to be effective. However, success depends on administration within the first 2 or 3 weeks after onset of the outbreak. The incidence of success decreases thereafter. This therapy also apparently prevents lesions from progressing into the postherpetic syndrome, at least in younger patients.

Epidural Blocks Epidural blocks using local anesthetic have been successful in acute herpes zoster.[46] The duration of the infection is shorter, the lesions dry faster, and the pain is relieved.

Spinal Blocks Spinal blocks usually are not indicated because they are not as specific as epidural blocks. A patient who has had a laminectomy in the affected area would be an exception to this general rule. The use of lumbar plexus blockade has been reported to relieve pain in an elderly patient for whom other approaches were contraindicated.[47]

Neurolytic Blocks Neurolytic blocks are not indicated in acute herpes zoster.

Complications Complications that may result from any nerve block procedure include pain, local hemorrhage, infection, needle soreness, sterile abscess (usually in the immunosuppressed patient), vertigo, and Cushing's syndrome.

Psychological Interventions Because the acute phase of herpes zoster is short, psychological interventions are not mandatory. However, some patients (especially those with severe anxiety and fear) benefit from a support program. Some studies show that interventions such as psychotherapy can also positively affect certain components of the immune response.[48–50] A regimen consisting of psychological support, administration of antiviral agents, and patient education has been described by one author as the ". . . best available option for the management of herpes virus infections."[51]

Other Therapies Usually, transcutaneous electrical nerve stimulation (TENS) is not used in the treatment of acute herpes zoster. However, results of a preliminary, randomized, single-blind study suggest that a new form of electroanalgesia—percutaneous electrical nerve stimulation—may be useful in treating acute herpes zoster lesions.[52] Ice therapy is a counterirritation technique based on the gate-control theory. It sometimes is used alone in the acute stage to cool the area. Acupuncture and hypnosis usually are not used in the treatment of acute herpes zoster because other conventional methods are more appropriate. Surgery and neurosurgery are not indicated. The acute stage is self-limited and does not require such drastic measures. Autohemotherapy has been shown to be effective in eliminating clinical sequelae of herpes zoster, but this alternative method requires further investigation.[53]

Recommended Therapeutic Strategey It is useful to categorize affected patients according to their immune status and age (Table 40-5). This allows the clinician to direct efforts toward all or either antiviral, anti-inflammatory, or antinociceptive effects, based on the probability of success and risk factors involved. These patients can be categorized into four groups: (1) immunocompetent young, (2) immunocompetent older, (3) immunosuppressed young, and (4) immunosuppressed older patients.

TABLE 40-5 **Therapeutic Strategy for Acute Herpes Zoster**

		Treatment		
Type of Patient	**Age (years)**	**Antiviral**	**Anti-inflammatory**	**Pain Relief**
Young immunocompetent	< 50	–	–	Sympathetic block
Older immunocompetent	> 50	–	+	Epidural, somatic, and/or sympathetic block—helpful
Young immunosuppressed	< 50	++ Within 72 h	–	Systemic narcotics
Older immunosuppressed	> 50	+ Within 72 h	±	Nerve blocks + systemic oral analgesics; adjuvant oral analgesics

–, not required; +, useful; ++, necessary.

Reproduced with permission from Raj P. Pain due to herpes zoster. In: Raj P, ed. *Practical Management of Pain.* 2nd ed. Chicago, Ill: Mosby-Year Book; 1992.

Immunocompetent Young Patients Patients in this group have no defined underlying illness, are younger than 50 years of age, and have normal immunologic responsiveness. Although they have acute herpes zoster, their reaction to the infection is brisk, enabling them to confine the rash in the initial unit. Likewise, postherpetic neuralgia does not occur. The acute morbidity is low, and healing is rapid. The rationale for treatment of this group of patients is to relieve their intolerable pain and prevent inflammatory damage of the tissues. Antiviral agents administered during the first 72 hours may be helpful in stopping the replication of the virus and spreading the infection to the peripheral nerves. Anti-inflammatory agents (i.e., corticosteroids administered locally or systematically) are useful in decreasing tissue damage and keeping the inflammatory reaction of the host to a minimum. The obligatory treatment is to decrease the severe pain of neuralgia. This is best done using sympathetic or epidural blocks in the first 3 to 4 weeks after onset of infection. Antidepressant agents also are helpful as adjuvant agents.

Immunocompetent Older Patients The major objective of therapy in this group is to prevent postherpetic neuralgia. Although suffering no underlying disease, the response to varicella-zoster virus in this group may be less vigorous than in young patients, leading to a slower viral clearance and perhaps a higher incidence of spread beyond the initial unit of infection. Nonetheless, nervous system and visceral complications are still infrequent and, by themselves, probably do not warrant the use of potentially toxic therapy at this time. However, both antiviral and anti-inflammatory therapies may be valuable in preventing postherpetic neuralgia. Of these, the latter has been shown prospectively to be effective in this group of patients. It is reasonable on the basis of the current evidence to treat older patients with acute herpes zoster who are immunologically normal with a limited course of corticosteroids (e.g., 60 mg of prednisone or its equivalent daily for 5 days, tapering the dose over the following 2 weeks).

The value of antiviral agents in this group of patients has not been tested carefully, although one trial suggested no effect in the incidence of persistent pain in patients treated with acyclovir despite an effect on acute pain. This issue deserves careful study. A four-treatment-arm study of the individual and combined effects of antivirals and corticosteroids is needed. At this point, antiviral therapy in this group probably is indicated only in an investigative setting. Pain relief should be addressed in these patients. Conventional narcotics should be avoided because these patients are usually older and frail. In addition, there is a high incidence of postherpetic neuralgia. Non-narcotic analgesics in association with nerve blocks (epidural and sympathetic blocks or local intracutaneous infiltration with bupivacaine and corticosteroids) are recommended.

Immunosuppressed Young Patients The principal concern in immunodeficient younger patients is the spread of the virus in and outside the primary ganglion-nerve-dermatome unit. Postherpetic neuralgia is not a major issue. Therapy, therefore, is directed at confining the viral infection. Currently, acyclovir is available, is of proven efficacy, and can be recommended for patients. It seems reasonable to recommend hospitalization for patients in this group who are at greatest risk of developing complications, particularly those with lymphoproliferative disease or early dissemination. It also must be emphasized that, if therapy is given, every effort should be made to start treatment early. When newer agents become available, they will require similar consideration, with their convenience, cost, and toxicity weighted against the magnitude of their potential benefit. It can be predicted, however, that, when other oral drugs are introduced, their efficacy proved, and their toxicity demonstrated to be low, the indications for treatment will expand. The clinical decision to administer these drugs to this group of patients would be an easy one, with virtually all patients in this group routinely receiving such treatment. Pain relief in such patients should be obtained by the techniques that are common for acute pain management.

Immunosuppressed Older Patients In this group of patients, therapeutic objectives include prevention of both viral spread and postherpetic pain. As discussed previously, antiviral therapy may be helpful in both respects. Acyclovir has been effective in reducing infection, and it may reduce postherpetic pain. The latter requires additional confirmation. More importantly, because of the risk of viral dissemination, patients in this group require antiviral treatment. However, the use of corticosteroids to prevent postherpetic neuralgia warrants separate comment. In older immunocompetent patients, corticosteroids appear to cause no special risk and to be therapeutically beneficial; but in the immunosuppressed individual, greater caution is required. These patients are more susceptible to viral spread and central nervous system and visceral complications. Corticosteroids may impair their remaining defenses below a critical level, increasing the risk of these complications. Data from a collaborative study suggest that corticosteroids did not protect against postherpetic pain in this group. This issue must be investigated separately, particularly to consider the effects of combined antiviral and corticosteroid therapy. If potent antiviral coverage were available, corticosteroids might be safe. Pain relief is best provided by nerve blocks.

Postherpetic Neuralgia

Drug Therapy (Table 40-6) A threefold purpose governs the role of drug therapy in the patient with postherpetic neuralgia: (1) to provide analgesia for pain, (2) to reduce depression and anxiety, and (3) to decrease insomnia. Because a considerable degree of depression, anxiety, and insomnia accompany all chronic pain syndromes, hypnotics, tranquilizers, antidepressants, and anticonvulsants frequently have been used as analgesic adjuvants in the management of postherpetic neuralgia. These include the barbiturates, rauwolfia alkaloids, phenothiazine derivatives, benzodiazepines, amphetamines, tricyclic antidepressants, phenytoin, and carbamazepine.

It is important to warn the patient of the potential side effects of any drug. The patient is less likely to stop taking the prescribed medication if he or she knows that certain unpleasant effects are

TABLE 40-6 **Drug Therapy for Postherpetic Neuralgia**

Analgesics
Antidepressants and tranquilizers
Anticonvulsants
Phenytoin
Carbamazepine
Sodium valproate and amitriptyline
Topical capsaicin
Oral antiarrhythmics

expected as a normal occurrence and that they usually are not permanent.

However, it is equally important for the physician to adopt a positive approach regarding the medication. On average, 35% of patients benefit significantly from the placebo effect. This can be used to advantage by describing enthusiastically the desirable effects of each drug which, with time, may be obtained. Patients also are less likely to stop taking their medication before it has had time to provide the desired effect.

Antiviral Agents As a rule, antiviral agents are inappropriate in the treatment of postherpetic neuralgia. An exception may include their use to prevent the possible recurrence of herpes zoster infection in a susceptible patient. For example, the patient with Hodgkin's disease is predisposed to recurrent herpes zoster; antiviral agents may be given before treatment of the primary disease (chemotherapy and radiation therapy) when reactivation of the virus is most likely.

Analgesics These drugs may be required to control the severe intractable pain of postherpetic neuralgia. Narcotics should be used with extreme caution, if at all, because (1) they are addictive; (2) the problem is chronic; (3) these patients usually are not terminally ill; (4) the side effects, such as nausea, loss of appetite, and constipation, usually make these patients miserable; (5) there may be adverse drug interactions with antidepressants and other drugs; and, (6) most importantly, adequate pain relief may be obtained with other drugs. The temporary initial use of narcotics to relieve extreme pain may be necessary, however, until the patient begins to respond to therapy.

Antidepressants and Tranquilizers Antidepressants and tranquilizers frequently are used in conjunction with analgesics. Some patients become depressed as a reaction to their pain. The signs of depression may be so subtle that they easily are missed. As many as 90% of patients may be depressed. Approximately 85% of these patients will respond to antidepressant drugs.

Tricyclic antidepressants are the most commonly used drugs, and they are the most effective single drug class used in the management of postherpetic neuralgia. Antidepressants may act at a higher level than the neurotransmitters, perhaps on pressure molecules in the hypothalamus or pituitary. This could explain why only some depressed patients fit the catecholamine hypothesis (i.e., a deficit of serotonin or norepinephrine is the cause of the problem). Both chronic pain and depression may represent neurotransmitter deficiencies, and the antidepressants may restore these to normal levels. These drugs should be given in appropriate doses, and several should be tried before concluding that there is no response.

Topical application of a local anesthetic plus a tricyclic antidepressant can be effective.[14,15]

Tricyclics and anxiolytics commonly are given together because many patients have anxiety with their depression. This feeling may be caused by anticipation of painful spasms, social obligations that may exacerbate the pain by increasing stress, fear of having a painful episode in public, or fear that the pain may never leave. Many patients who did not obtain relief with tricyclics alone may benefit when a phenothiazine is added. For lasting pain relief, treatment must be continued throughout life. The usual recommended doses are as follows: amitriptyline, 50 to 75 mg/day, and fluphenazine, 1 mg three or four times a day.

As a last resort, immediate relief has been obtained in some hospitalized patients who had not responded to any other therapy with a short course of high-dose chlorprothixene, 50 mg every 6 hours for 5 days. Because this protocol requires hospitalization and is associated with adverse effects, this treatment is recommended only if all other methods fail and if the pain is severe, because pain often returns in a few weeks or months.

Anticonvulsants Anticonvulsants sometimes are useful when other medications have failed. Phenytoin, 100 mg three to four times a day, or carbamazepine, 500 to 1000 mg daily in three to four divided doses, can be used to relieve sharp pain.

Sodium valproate, 200 mg twice a day, and amitriptyline, 10 to 25 mg twice a day, have been successful. If the stabbing component of pain continues, the dose of amitriptyline can be increased. The dull-ache component of the pain is most resistant to therapy. If it persists, the scar can be infiltrated with a local anesthetic and corticosteroids, or TENS, can be started.

Gabapentin has been shown to effectively reduce pain and sleep interference and improve mood and quality of life in patients with postherpetic neuralgia and those with painful neuropathy.[54,55] Maximum dosage administered was 3,600 mg/day.

The side effects of anticonvulsants tend to limit their use. These include bone marrow depression, ataxia, diplopia, nystagmus, abnormal liver function tests, nausea, lymphanadenopathy, confusion, and vertigo.

Topical Capsaicin This drug depletes substance P from sensory nerve endings in the skin and has been used topically for various dermatologic diseases.

Antiarrhythmics Intravenous lidocaine has been advocated for the treatment of many types of chronic neurogenic pain, including postherpetic neuralgia. The oral antiarrhythmics (e.g., mexiletine) have been tried, and reports are encouraging. However, definitive studies on the efficacy of oral antiarrhythmics for the treatment of postherpetic neuralgia are lacking.

Nerve Blocks The pathogenesis of postherpetic pain is unknown. Autopsy studies have shown that the entire sensory pathway, including the brain and sympathetic ganglia, may be involved. There appear to be multiple areas along this pathway that can initiate pain. This provides a rationale for the various methods of treatment and an explanation of treatment failures.

Analgesic blocks can be used as prognostic, therapeutic, and prophylactic tools in managing pain. As prognostic tools, blocks help predicts the effects of prolonged interruption of nerve pathways achieved through injection of neurolytic agents or surgery. By interrupting pain pathways, therapeutic blocks influence the autonomic response to noxious stimulation. They break the cycle of this disease. Patients with severe intractable pain who are not suited to other treatment regimens may be relieved by blocks with neurolytic agents.

Local Infiltration Subcutaneous infiltration of corticosteroids has been used; pain relief was obtained in approximately 64% of patients. A solution of triamcinolone 0.2% in normal saline was injected daily under all areas of pain, burning, or itching until the desired effect was obtained. Maximum benefit was achieved in the first 12 treatments. In a comparison study, subcutaneous infiltration of bupivacaine 0.25% and triamcinolone 0.2% was used, alone or in conjunction with systemic medication and sympathetic blockade. Overall results showed moderate to significant improvement in 70% of patients. A difference in response to treatment was noticed in relation to duration of symptoms; patients with symptoms for less than 1 year responded better (85% success) than patients with symptoms for more than 1 year (55%).

Subcutaneous infiltration of corticosteroids can offer an effective treatment for postherpetic neuralgia. No significant complications have been recorded, the technique is simple and inexpensive, and the response to treatment is fairly predictable. Most importantly, it offers relief for some patients with postherpetic neuralgia of many months' duration.

The total number of such treatments ranges from one to ten (average, four to six injections). In acute herpes zoster, treatments usually are given two or three times weekly and tapered to one per week, if the patient is responding well.

Somatic Nerve Block Nerve root involvement is an obvious characteristic of postherpetic neuralgia, and sensory nerve blocks were used in early attempts to relieve its pain. The results were limited, depending primarily on the duration of the blocks, although there were some reports of success in managing pain in the early stages of the disease. Coincidental spontaneous resolution may have been responsible. Nerve blocks primarily are used in postherpetic neuralgia for diagnosis and prognosis, especially as a prognostic block before neurolytic block. Corticosteroids injected around the dorsal nerve have had unpredictable and limited success.

Sympathetic Nerve Block Sympathetic blocks are sometimes helpful in alleviating pain, although results are sometimes temporary and may only be obtainable in patients with neuralgia of less than 2 months' duration. Sympathetic blocks of the stellate ganglion and trigeminal branch blocks often are used to treat trigeminal zoster.

Epidural Block Epidural corticosteroid administration has been successful in treating various lumbosacral conditions. For instance, epidural nerve blocks often are used to treat zoster in the fifth cervical dermatome.

Neurolytic Block Neurolytic blocks may be considered when other blocks have not given the patient significant relief. They should be performed only after a prognostic block has shown that an effective block of the appropriate can be achieved. Neurolytic agents are used in cases of prolonged destruction of nerves. These blocks include ethyl alcohol 50% in aqueous solution, absolute alcohol 95% in aqueous solution, and phenol 6%. Ethyl alcohol causes a higher incidence of neuritis than phenol. This is primarily a result of incomplete peripheral nerve block after inaccurate needle placement or spillage of the agent on somatic nerve fibers. The duration of effects may vary from days to years, but usually it ranges from 2 to 6 months.

Ammonium compounds also can be used for peripheral nerve block. Pain relief follows selective destruction of unmyelinated C fibers by the ammonium ion. A solution of ammonium sulfate 10% in lidocaine 1% or ammonium chloride 15% is used. The duration of action ranges from 4 to 24 weeks. Neuritis does not occur with either ammonium sulfate or chloride. The most annoying side effect is numbness, which can be as bad as the pain for some patients.

Cryoanalgesia also has been used as a means of producing long-term neural blockade.

Psychosocial Therapy It is especially important in patients with postherpetic neuralgia to treat the whole patient and not just an area of the skin. The emotional stability of the patient almost always is affected, and the stresses involved for the patient and all members of the household require thoughtful management.

Severe depression is seen in more than 50% of these patients and, as previously noted, suicide commonly is considered by those with long-term intractable pain. Counseling by a psychologist or clinical social worker who is experienced in pain management is a valuable adjunct to drug therapy. Training the patient in stress management and relaxation techniques is important. Anxiety and stress can exacerbate and prolong the pain. By practicing these techniques, the patient may be able to control pain to some degree.

In some patients, the pain-tension-anxiety cycle can convert acute pain symptoms into a chronic condition. Often, no matter what is done to treat these patients, the pain is not relieved unless the stress factors also are removed. Basically, two types of persons are susceptible to chronicity: the tense, hard-driving, conscientious perfectionist, and the dependent individual unable to cope with life but burdened with repressed anger and hostility. Reinforcement of the patient's response to pain (such as moaning, grimacing, asking for medication, and remaining in bed) or favorable consequences of the pain(such as attention and expressions of sympathy, perhaps also the occasion to manipulate others) may lead to chronic behavior that, eventually, is independent of the original underlying pathologic condition.

The most important guideline in preventing chronicity is complete honesty. Make patients aware of the relationship between the psyche and pain, and relieve them of the fear of organic disease. After the patient fully accepts the emotional causes of pain, he or she can learn to relieve the pain by controlling anxiety and tension.

Family and friends should be included in counseling sessions. They, too, must cope with the pain a loved one is experiencing. The counselor not only can ease their anxiety but also can teach them how to provide effective emotional support to help the patient endure an extremely difficult period. Concentrating on the special needs of families may require extra effort on the part of the staff, but it should result in a greater number of patients who recover with the physical and emotional well-being of the family intact.

Many patients are elderly and live alone. They are unable to turn to family and friends to provide the assistance they need for routine daily tasks. The counselor should contact appropriate social service agencies to provide transportation and other necessities (such as prepared meals, grocery shopping, housework, and regular contact with the patient to check on his or her well-being).

Other Therapies Because many patients continue to have some residual pain of varying degrees that can be aggravating, they may require management with other techniques. The following techniques are used when all others fail (Table 40-7).

TENS This has been used in an attempt to relieve the intractable pain of postherpetic neuralgia. Although the success rate is low, relief can be sufficient to permit a return to normal activity without analgesic therapy.

Ice and Other Cold Therapies Ice is applied to the skin for 2 to 3 minutes several times a day, starting with the least sensitive area and approaching the most sensitive area. A vibrator then is used in the same manner in conjunction with psychotropic drugs. Ethyl chloride, or other cold sprays, can be used alone as treatment. Fluid

TABLE 40-7 **Other Therapies for Postherpetic Neuralgia**

Transcutaneous electrical nerve stimulation
Cold therapies
Ice
Ethyl chloride
Cryocautery with dry ice
Acupuncture
Hypnosis
Surgery and neurosurgery

is sprayed over the entire painful area, beginning at the upper area and working down. Evaporation cools the area. The procedure is repeated twice at 1-minute intervals until the skin is thoroughly cooled. When beneficial, these treatments will relieve pain for varying lengths of time. When pain returns to near its former intensity, the treatment can be repeated. If the patient responds satisfactorily, the pain is relieved by two or three sets of sprays per day. Good-to-excellent pain relief has been maintained in patients with refractory postherpetic pain using cryocautery with a stick of solid carbon dioxide (dry ice) applied directly to the hyperesthetic sites.

Acupuncture Significant pain relief has been obtained in patients with postherpetic neuralgia treated with acupuncture. Further investigation is underway.

Hypnosis Hypnosis acts at the level of the cerebral cortex. Impulses are sent down from higher centers to close the neurophysiologic gate that controls pain. Pain relief through hyponosis is sometimes complete but, more often, it is not. Hypnotism is reported to be helpful in patients with chronic unbearable pain; this changes to bearable discomfort by breaking up patterns of suffering.

Dimethyl Sulfoxide The treatment value of this agent in postherpetic neuralgia is unknown. It may be tried as a benign last resort. Only a few states have approved this solvent for medical use.

Surgery and Neurosurgery Surgery is the last resort for the treatment of severe intractable postherpetic pain. It is not always successful. More effective management techniques learned in recent years have limited this option further.

Surgery usually attacks the pain pathway in stages at progressively higher divisions. Because it was suspected that the origin of the pain lay in the scar and peripheral receptors, wide excision and skin graftings were tried. This was not found to be effective and rarely is used today.

Rhizotomy of the somatic afferents and sensory root ganglia also has had poor results. Investigators who have had some success recommended that ablation include several segments above and below the affected area. Sympathectomy has not been successful in treating postherpetic neuralgia.

Cordotomy has been used with good results. In most cases, however, the pain returns. Early recurrence has been blamed on failure to ablate all the nerves in the pathway, which resume function after the swelling has decreased. Stereotactic ablation of the conducting paths in the thalamus and mesencephalon and frontal lobotomy have been used. These should be tried only in patients with short life expectancies who have not had success with any other methods.

Because of the finality of surgery and the unpredictable results, many surgeons in recent years have taken advantage of technologic advances in other areas to replace destructive procedures. These include electronic stimulators used to block transmission of nerve impulses. An implantable electrode placed over the dorsal columns of the spinal cord has been tried with some success. Deep brain stimulators, which are patient activated, have been applied to the mesencephalic medial lemniscus to block the pain-conducting systems and stimulate endorphin secretion, the body's natural pain reliever. Good pain relief has been achieved in many patients.

COMPLICATIONS

Acute Herpes Zoster

The most common complications of acute herpes zoster usually appear after eruption of the rash (Table 40-8). They include neuralgia, facial or oculomotor palsy, paralysis of motor nerves, and myelitis. Meningoencephalitis, which has its onset either during or 2 to 4 days after the rash appears, also can be a complication. Postherpetic neuralgia seems to occur more frequently and is more protracted in immunosuppressed patients, especially in those with Hodgkin's disease or other lymphomas.

There is a marked increase in the incidence of infection in immunosuppressed or immunoincompetent patients. The clinical course in these patients is exaggerated. It is acutely disabling in many cases, and it may become life threatening if visceral involvement occurs with dissemination. In the early stages, the infection often spreads segmentally to involve ipsilateral and, less frequently, contralateral dermatomes. It usually is associated with fever and increasing debilitation. Although some of the old lesions are healing, new lesions continue to appear. Many patients have dissemination and visceral involvement that ultimately may be fatal.

Generally, patients in whom the disease remains localized for 4 to 6 days do not experience complications. The greatest morbidity and mortality usually occur with visceral involvement through dissemination, especially in patients older than 40 years of age.

Systemic toxicity, fever, chills, and sometimes secondary bacterial sepsis occur. Varicella pneumonia, which is associated with a high mortality, occurs less frequently.

TABLE 40-8 **Complications of Acute Herpes Zoster**

Neuralgia
Facial or oculomotor palsy
Paralysis of motor nerves
Myelitis
Meningoencephalitis
Postherpetic neuralgia
Systemic toxicity or dissemination
Fevers
Chills
Bacteria sepsis
Varicella pneumonia

Postherpetic Neuralgia

Although physical complications occur with acute herpes zoster, the complications from the postherpetic stage primarily are emotional. Depression is common and may include suicidal tendencies. Destruction of the patient's lifestyle (inability to work, breakup of the family, and restricted mobility that prohibits former social activities) may be the tragic human consequences that affect the patient with long-term pain. Physical function may be impaired beyond that seen during the acute stage because of the longer period of immobility.

PROGNOSIS

There is a close relationship between the duration of neuralgia and therapeutic efficacy; prompt treatment shortens the progressive course of the disease and also decreases its severity. There also appears to be a correlation between the age of the patient and the response to therapy. Patients younger than 60 years of age generally respond better to therapy and, even untreated, have a lower incidence of postherpetic neuralgia than do older patients. In addition, older patients do not respond as well as young patients to therapy and specifically to sympathetic nerve blocks. For unknown reasons, postherpetic neuralgia lesions in the ophthalmic division of the trigeminal nerve are often the most difficult lesions to treat successfully. The psychological makeup of the individual patient is also important. Lastly, one fifth of patients with neoplasms who have had herpes zoster will have this disease at least once again.[2]

REFERENCES

1. Irwin M, Costlow C, Williams H, et al. Cellular immunity to varicella-zoster virus in patients with major depression. *J Infect Dis* 1998;178 (suppl 1):S104–108.
2. Fields HL, Rowbotham MC. Pathophysiology of postherpetic neuralgia. Presented at the Herpes Zoster and Postherpetic Neuralgia Satellite Symposium; August 13 and 14, 1996; Whistler Mountain, British Columbia.
3. Donahue JG, Choo PW, Manson JE, et al. The incidence of herpes zoster. *Arch Intern Med* 1995;155:1605–1609.
4. Schmader K, George LK, Burchett M, et al. Racial and psychosocial risk factors for herpes zoster in the elderly. *J Infect Dis* 1998;178 (suppl 1):S67–70.
5. Petursson G, Gelgason S, Gudmundsson S, et al. Herpes zoster in children and adolescents. *Pediatr Infect Dis J* 1998;17:905–908.
6. Broyer M, Tete MJ, Guest G, et al. Varicella and zoster in children after kidney transplantation: Long-term results of vaccination. *Pediatrics* 1997;99:35–39.
7. Terada K, Tanaka H, Kawano S, et al. Specific cellular immunity in immunocompetent children with herpes zoster. *Acta Paediatr* 1998; 87:692–694.
8. Glaser R, Jones JF, eds. *Herpes Virus Infections.* New York, NY: Marcel Dekker; 1994.
9. Sadzot-Delvaux C, Arvin AM, et al. Varicella-zoster virus IE63, a virion component expressed during latency and acute infection, elicits humoral and cellular immunity. *J Infect Dis* 1998;178(suppl 1):S43–47.
10. Whitley RJ, Shukla S, Crooks RJ. The identification of risk factors associated with persistent pain following herpes zoster. *J Infect Dis* 1998;178(suppl 1):S71–75.
11. Higa K, Mori M, Hirata K, et al. Severity of skin lesions of herpes zoster at the worst phase rather than age and involved region most influences the duration of acute herpetic pain. *Pain* 1997;69:245–253.
12. Yi JY, Kim TY, Shim JH, et al. Histopathological findings, viral DNA distribution and lymphocytic immunophenotypes in vesicular and papular types of herpes zoster. *Acta Derm Venereol* 1997;77:194–197.
13. Worrell JT, Cockerell CJ. Histopathology of peripheral nerves in cutaneous herpesvirus infection. *Am J Dermatopathol* 1997;19:133–137.
14. Bennett GJ. Animal models and their relation to neuropathic pain: Particularly HZ and PHN. Presented at the Herpes Zoster and Postherpetic Neuralgia Satellite Symposium; August 13 and 14, 1996; Whistler Mountain, British Columbia.
15. Bennett GJ. Hypotheses on the pathogenesis of herpes zoster-associated pain. *Ann Neurol* 1994;35:538–541.
16. Nurmikko T, Wells C, Bowsher D. Sensory dysfunction in postherpetic neuralgia. In: Boivie J, Hansson P, Lindblom U, eds. *Touch, Temperature and Pain in Health and Disease: Mechanisms and Assessments.* Vol 3. Seattle, Wash: IASP Press; 1994:133–141.
17. Fields HL, Rowbotham MC. Multiple mechanisms of neuropathic pain: A clinical perspective. In: Gebhart GF, Hammond DL, Jensen TS, eds. *Proceedings of the 7th World Congress on Pain.* Vol 2. Seattle, Wash: IASP Press; 1994:437–454.
18. Haanpaa M, Dastidar P, Weinberg A, et al. CSF and MRI findings in patients with acute herpes zoster. *Neurology* 1998;51:1405–1411.
19. Levin MJ, Barber D, Goldblatt E, et al. Use of a live attenuated varicella vaccine to boost varicella-specific immune responses in seropositive people 55 years of age and older: Duration of booster effect. *J Infect Dis* 1998;178(suppl 1):S109–112.
20. Redman RL, Nader S, Zerboni L, et al. Early reconstitution of immunity and decreased severity of herpes zoster in bone marrow transplant recipients immunized with inactivated varicella vaccine. *J Infect Dis* 1997;176:578–585.
21. Jovanovic J, Cvjetkovic D, Pobor M, et al: Herpes zoster—Treatment with a acyclovir. *Med Pregl* 1997;50:305–308.
22. Jackson JL, Gibbons R, Meyer G, et al. The effect of treating herpes zoster with oral acyclovir in preventing postherpetic neuralgia. A meta-analysis. *Arch Intern Med* 1997;157:909–912.
23. Kubeyinje EP. Cost-benefit of oral acyclovir in the treatment of herpes zoster. *Int J Dermatol* 1997;36:457–459.
24. Gnann JW Jr, Crumpacker CS, Lalezari JP, et al. Sorivudine versus acyclovir for treatment of dermatomal herpes zoster in human immunodeficiency virus–infected patients: Results from a randomized, controlled clinical trial. Collaborative Antiviral Study Group/AIDS Clinical Trials Group, Herpes Zoster Study Group. *Antimicrob Agents Chemother* 1998;42:1139–1145.
25. Bodsworth NJ, Boag F, Burdge D, et al. Evaluation of sorivudine (BV-araU) versus acyclovir in the treatment of acute localized herpes zoster in human immunodeficiency virus–infected adults. The Multinational Sorivudine Study Group. *J Infect Dis* 1997;176:103–111.
26. Wood MJ, Shukla S, Fiddian AP, et al. Treatment of acute herpes zoster: Effect of early (<48 h) versus late (48–72 h) therapy with acyclovir and valaciclovir on prolonged pain. *J Infect Dis* 1998;178(suppl 1): S81–84.
27. Stein GE. Pharmacology of new antiherpes agents: Famciclovir and valacyclovir. *J Am Pharm Assoc* 1997;NS37:157–163.
28. Grant DM, Mauskopf JA, Bell L, et al. Comparison of valaciclovir and acyclovir for the treatment of herpes zoster in immunocompetent patients over 50 years of age: A cost-consequence model. *Pharmacotherapy* 1997;17:333–341.
29. Stott GA. Famciclovir: A new systemic antiviral agent for herpesvirus. *Am Fam Physician* 1997;55:2501–2504.
30. Tyring S, Barbarash RA, Nahlik JE, et al. Famciclovir for the treatment of acute herpes zoster: Effects on acute disease and postherpetic neuralgia. A randomized, double-blind, placebo-controlled trial. *Ann Intern Med* 1995;123:89–96.
31. Degreef H. Famciclovir Herpes Zoster Clinical Study Group. Famciclovir, a new oral drug: Results of the first controlled clinical study demonstrating its efficacy and safety in the treatment of uncomplicated herpes zoster in immune-competent patients. *Int J Antimicrob Agents* 1994;4:241–246.

32. Sacks SL, Martel A, Aoki F, et al. Clinic-initiated treatment of recurrent genital herpes using famciclovir: Results of a Canadian multicenter study. Presented at the Sixth International Congress for Infectious Diseases; 1994; Prague, Czechoslovakia.
33. Sacks SL, Aoki FY, Diaz-Mitoma F, et al. Patient-initiated, twice daily oral famciclovir for early recurrent genital herpes: A randomized, double-blind multicenter trial. *JAMA* 1996;276:44–49.
34. Mertz G, Loveless MO, Levin MJ, et al. Oral famciclovir for suppression of recurrent genital herpes simplex virus infection in women. *Arch Intern Med* 1997;157:343–349.
35. Field JH, Thackray AM. The effects of delayed-onset chemotherapy using famciclovir or valacyclovir in a murine immunosuppression model for HSV-1. *Antiviral Chem Chemother* 1995;6:210–216.
36. Field JH, Tewari D, Sutton D, et al. Comparison of efficacies of famciclovir and valacyclovir against herpes simplex virus type 1 in a murine immunosuppression model. *Antimicrob Agents Chemother* 1995;39:1114–1119.
37. Thackray AM, Field JH. Differential effects of famciclovir and valacyclovir on the pathogenesis of herpes simplex virus in a murine infection model including reactivation from latency. *J Infect Dis* 1996; 173:291–299.
38. Ahmed A, Woolley PD. Comparison of famciclovir and acyclovir in first episodes of genital herpes: Possible effect on latency. Presented at the European Conference on Herpesviruses; 1996; Paris, France.
39. Loveless M, Sacks SL, Harris JRW. Famciclovir in the management of first-episode genital herpes. *Infect Dis Clin Pract* 1997;6(suppl 1): S12–16.
40. Breton G, Fillet AM, Katlama C, et al. Acyclovir-resistant herpes zoster in human immunodeficiency virus–infected patients: Results of foscarnet therapy. *Clin Infect Dis* 1998;27:1525–1527.
41. Wutzler P. Antiviral therapy of herpes simplex and varicella-zoster virus infections. *Intervirology* 1997;40;343–356.
42. Bareggi SR, Priola R, De Bendittis G. Skin and plasma levels of acetylsalicylic acid: A comparison between topical aspirin/diethyl ether mixture and oral aspirin in acute herpes zoster and postherpetic neuralgia. *Dur J Clin Pharmacol* 1998;54:231–235.
43. Primache V, Binda S, De Benedittis G, et al. In vitro activity of acetylsalicylic acid on replication of varicella-zoster virus. *New Microbiol* 1998;21:3997–401.
44. Ernst ME, Santee JA, Klepser TB. Oral corticosteroids for pain associated with herpes zoster. *Ann Pharmacother* 1998;32:1099–1103.
45. Bowsher D. The effects of pre-emptive treatment of postherpetic neuralgia with amitriptyline: A randomized, double-blind, placebo-controlled trial. *J Pain Symptom Manage* 1997;13:327–331.
46. Higa K, Hori K, Harasawa I, et al. High thoracic epidural block relieves acute herpetic pain involving the trigeminal and cervical regions: Comparison with effects for stellate ganglion block. *Reg Anesth Pain Med* 1998;23:25–29.
47. Hadzic A, Vloka JD, Saff GN, et al. The "three-in-one block" for treatment of pain in a patient with acute herpes zoster infection. *Reg Anesth* 1997;22:575–578.
48. Applegate KL, Cacioppo TJ, Keicolt-Glaser JK, et al. The effects of stress on the immune system: Implications for reactivation of latent herpesviruses. Presented at the Herpes Zoster and Postherpetic Neuralgia Satellite Symposium; August 13 and 14, 1996; Whistler Mountain, British Columbia.
49. Lutgendorf S, Antoni MH, Jumar M, et al. Changes in cognitive copying strategies predict EEBV-antibody titre following a stressor disclosure induction. *J Psychosom Res* 1994;38:63–78.
50. Esterling BA, Antoni MH, Fletcher MA, et al. Emotional disclosure through writing or speaking modulates latent Epstein-Barr virus antibody titers. *J Consult Clin Psychol* 1994;62:130–140.
51. Tyring SK. Advances in the treatment of herpesvirus infection: The role of famciclovir. *Clin Ther* 1998;20:661–670.
52. Ahmed HE, Craig WF, White PF, et al. Percutaneous electrical nerve stimulation: An alternative to antiviral drugs for acute herpes zoster. *Anesth Analg* 1998;87:911–914.
53. Olwin JH, Ratajczak HV, House RV. Successful treatment of herpetic infctions by autohemotherapy. *J Altern Complement Med* 1997;3:155–158.
54. Rowbotham M, Harden N, Stacey B, et al. Gabapentin for the treatment of postherpetic neuralgia. A randomized controlled trial. *JAMA* 1998;280:1837–1842.
55. Backonja M, Beycoun A, Edwards KR, et al. Gabapentin for the symptomatic treatment of painful neuropathy in patients with diabetes mellitus. A randomized controlled trial. *JAMA* 1998;280: 1831–1836.

CHAPTER 41 PREEMPTIVE ANALGESIA

Thomas T. Simopoulos

The understanding of postoperative pain has evolved greatly during the past decade. Many laboratory investigations have established that peripheral tissue injury during surgery can trigger a prolonged state of spinal cord excitation. A reduction in neuronal thresholds in the central nervous system (CNS) is thought to amplify pain in postsurgical patients. Preemptive analgesia is an antinociceptive treatment targeted to block CNS hyperexcitability, and thereby leads to a reduced postoperative pain state. Despite numerous investigations, the clinical relevance of such treatment is, at present, an issue of controversy.

HISTORY AND BACKGROUND

The concept of preemptive analgesia was postulated by George Washington Crile during the early 1900s.[1,2] Crile proposed that trauma induced by surgery caused a "shock and exhaustion" to the CNS. He went on to advocate preincisional and intraoperative local anesthetic infiltrations in addition to general anesthesia. In this way, noxious stimuli could be prevented from reaching the brain, thus establishing the "shockless operation." Rekindling of this idea was not to occur until the 1980s.

Wall, based on laboratory data and several clinical studies, postulated in an editorial in 1988 that (1) a reduction in massive small-fiber input into the CNS during surgery would prevent a central sensitization, and (2) analgesia that is present preoperatively has the potential to render prolonged effects, well beyond the known time frame of drug action.[3] Consistent with this proposal was experimental data by Wall and Woolf demonstrating that low doses of opioids, given prior to a painful stimulus, can effectively prevent central sensitization.[4] In contrast, much higher doses of opioids are required to suppress an already sensitized spinal cord. Since the editorial by Wall, a large number of investigations have been carried out; the overall results are to date equivocal. Appreciation for the multiple variables that influence postoperative pain as well as limitations in outcome measures have become more evident.

PATHOPHYSIOLOGY OF POST-INJURY PAIN

Peripheral Sensitization

The establishment of sensitization in the periphery involves the transition of high-threshold nociceptors into ones of low threshold, as induced by the release of various chemicals soon after surgical incision.[5] At the site of damage, a complex array of inflammatory mediators, as outlined in Table 41-1, are mobilized from injured tissue, while others are delivered by the circulation.[6] Small-diameter primary afferent neurons, Aδ and C fibers innervating the region of insult, subsequently enter a state characterized by ongoing discharge, a lowered activation threshold, and excitation elicited by suprathreshold stimulation (hyperalgesia).[7] The center of a surgical wound, which is the primary zone of injury, would be expected to demonstrate static mechanical hyperalgesia.

Immediately surrounding the primary zone is an area of erythema, edema, and hyperalgesia initiated by axon reflexes.[8] Activation of C fibers leads to neurogenic inflammation as a result of antidromic release of neuropeptides (e.g., substance P) from collateral axons.[9] Substance P release degranulates histamine and serotonin, and causes vasodilation to further fuel peripheral sensitization. The skin, muscle, tendons, and other deep somatic structures become sore, achy, and tender. Clinically, patients refrain from movement and deep breathing, and guard their surgical site. With ensuing healing, inflammatory mediators decrease and primary afferent neurons resume their usual high threshold state, emphasizing the normal reversibility of peripheral sensitization.

Central Sensitization

Peripheral sensitization provoked by surgical incision leads to massive and prolonged afferent nociceptor input into the CNS, particularly the spinal cord.[10] C fibers release neuropeptides (substance P, neurokinin A, calcitonin gene–related peptide) and excitatory amino acids (glutamate, aspartate) on second-order neurons (nociceptive-specific and wide dynamic range) in the dorsal horn.[11] Second-order neurons enter a state of increased spontaneous firing, prolonged cell discharge ("windup"), reduced thresholds, and expansion of peripheral receptive fields.[12] This process is central sensitization at the level of the spinal cord, which now abnormally amplifies future incoming impulses (Table 41-2).

Sensitized wide-dynamic-range (WDR) neurons receive input not only from Aδ and C fibers, but also from low-threshold Aβ fibers (mediating light touch). Such convergence results in an innocuous stimulus being perceived as painful (allodynia).[13] Receptive fields are expanded to involve normal-appearing areas surrounding the primary site of tissue injury. Such secondary hyperalgesic zones are characteristically painful to light touch, indicating that large Aβ fibers are transmitting impulses to a spinal cord that is sensitized.[14] Dynamic allodynia is established through the convergence of Aβ and C fibers on hyperexcitable WDR cells. Of note is that peripheral sensitization causes Aδ and C fibers to respond to low-intensity stimuli. Central sensitization alters dorsal horn cell processing such that impulses from large-diameter, low–threshold, mechanoreceptive afferents fibers (Aβ) produce pain. Under physiologic conditions, central sensitization, like peripheral, is reversible.

Cellular and Biochemical Mechanisms of Central Sensitization

The central changes produced by tissue damage and noxious stimulation associated with surgery have been the focus of in-

TABLE 41-1 **Biochemical Mediators That Induce Peripheral Sensitization**

Hydrogen ions	Purines
Noradrenaline	Cytokines
Bradykinin	Serotonin
Potassium ions	Leukotrienes
Histamine	Nerve growth factor
Prostaglandins	Neuropeptides

tense investigation. The molecular physiology underlying central neuroplasticity is understood with a fair degree of confidence, and therefore deserves further discussion. Indeed, the prevention of central sensitization forms the basis of preemptive analgesia.

As indicated previously, neuropeptide and excitatory amino acid release in the dorsal horn initiates central sensitization. Both types of ligands lead to increases in intracellular calcium.[15,16] Neuropeptides bind to neurokinin-G protein–coupled receptors that activate voltage-gated calcium channels to enhance the flux of calcium ion into the dorsal horn cells. Similarly, aspartate interaction with the *N*-methyl-D-aspartate (NMDA) receptor leads to increases in intracellular calcium, which is thought to be the predominant mechanism responsible for persistent abnormal neuronal hypersensitivity following noxious stimulation.[17]

In addition, glutamate interacts with metabotropic receptors to activate phospholipase C (PLC), a common second messenger system.[18] Receptor-triggered activation of PLC results in hydrolysis of polyphosphatidylinositol (a cell membrane phospholipid) into two intracellular messengers, inositol triphosphate (IP_3) and diaylglycerol (DAG). IP_3 stimulates the release of calcium from internal cellular stores, whereas DAG activates protein kinase C (PKC). PKC is enzymatically active only in the presence of calcium. Increased calcium concentrations, together with PKC, result in increased expression of proto-oncogenes, such as c-fos and c-jun.[19] The gene products of c-fos and c-jun regulate the encoding of dynorphin and enkephalin peptides. These peptides are then thought to mediate long-term changes in cellular function.[20,21] Finally, PKC itself can phosphorylate NMDA receptors, leading to sustained alterations in cell membrane conduction[19] (Table 41-3). Cellular memory for pain (long-term potentiation) results in enhanced response to noxious stimulation.

PREVENTION OF CENTRAL SENSITIZATION

NMDA Antagonists

The concept of preemptive analgesia makes ketamine a very suitable candidate for investigation of postoperative pain reduction. Ketamine is a noncompetitive antagonist of the NMDA receptor, thereby reducing associated ion channel conduction.[22] The NMDA receptor, as indicated previously, is thought to be considerably involved in central pain processing and spinal cord neural plasticity. Preclinical models strongly suggest the importance of administering specific NMDA antagonists prior to noxious stimulation to effectively block central sensitization.[23] Clinical trials have shown significant benefit in the management of acute postoperative pain, even when administered after surgical insult.[24] Unlike other, more selective, NMDA antagonists (e.g., MK-801), ketamine does not lead to reduced spinal Fos protein.[25] Mechanistically, the neuropharmacology of ketamine is complex. Ketamine may inhibit sodium and L-type calcium channels, α-amino-hydroxy-5-methyl-4-isoxazole-proprionic acid (AMPA) and kainate receptors, neuronal uptake of norepinephrine, as well as have agonist actions on opioid receptors.[26] In addition, ketamine inhibits the NMDA receptor when the channel is in an open state.[27] This latter point may help explain the clinical findings that ketamine is effective not only in reducing central facilitation after an acute noxious input, but also in chronic painful conditions (e.g., postherpetic neuralgia).[28,29]

Ketamine in clinical investigations has been administered intravenously and epidurally. Unfortunately, ketamine has not consistently been shown to reduce postoperative pain scores or analgesic usage. A preemptive effect would consist of a reduction of secondary hyperalgesia, by diminishing or ablating central sensitization. Prolonged analgesic effects would then be appreciated. Tverskoy and colleagues administered preincisional ketamine intravenously and demonstrated a reduction in wound hyperalgesia, compared with controls, by measuring pain threshold to pressure.[30] Despite profound reductions in wound hyperalgesia after abdominal hysterectomy, there was no significant effect on postoperative pain or opioid consumption. Similar results in kidney donors have been reported later by Stubhaug and coworkers, which have led investigators to question the relevance of central sensitization in postoperative pain.[31]

On the other hand, studies not assessing secondary hyperalgesia have been able to show a moderate reduction in postoperative opioid consumption lasting between 24 and 48 hours, with early administration of low-dose ketamine (0.15 mg/kg).[32–34] Pain

TABLE 41-2 **Terms Indicating Sensitization or Facilitation of the Dorsal Horn**

Term	Description
Central sensitization	Persistent changes in second-order neuron processing due to lower thresholds, which result in amplified peripheral receptive fields
Windup	Increased and prolonged discharge of dorsal horn cells
Central hyperexcitability	Exaggerated and prolonged responsiveness of second-order neurons to normal stimulation
Long-term potentiation	Cellular memory for pain, giving rise to enhanced response to noxious stimulation

TABLE 41-3 **Summary of the Biochemical Basis of Central Sensitization**

Biochemical Mediator	Effect
Excitatory amino acid (e.g., glutamate) and neuropeptides (e.g., substance P)	Neurotransmitters that initiate an increase in intracellular Ca^{2+} of second-order neurons
N-methyl-D-aspartate (NMDA) receptor	Key role in windup, allowing large influx of Ca^{2+} after binding excitatory amino acids
Second messengers (e.g., G proteins and phospho-inositol cascade)	Further enhance the increase in Ca^{2+} and activate protein kinase C
Protein kinase C	Increased expression of proto-oncogenes
Proto-oncogenes (e.g., c-fos, c-jun)	Regulate mRNA encoding of dynorphin and enkephalin peptides
Dynorphin, enkephalin peptides	Enhanced excitability and long-term alterations in cell function

scores, in general, appear to be reduced in patients undergoing abdominal and knee procedures, although not consistently.[32,35] The analgesic effects of ketamine are, therefore, variably expressed in terms of decreases in opioid use, pain scores, and wound hyperalgesia. Interestingly, all of the sustained benefits of ketamine far exceed the plasma half-life of ketamine (distribution half-life of 17 minutes).[36] Plasma levels of greater than 100 ng/mL associated with analgesia would not be expected to be maintained.[37] The extended benefits of ketamine suggest a preemptive effect, yet diminution of secondary hyperalgesia has not correlated with pain reduction. Noncompetitive interaction of ketamine at the NMDA receptor may limit the development of acute opioid tolerance.[38] This can, in turn, offer a partial explanation for the observed decrease in postoperative opioid consumption.

Similarly, epidural ketamine can result in prolongation to first analgesic request, as well as reduction in postoperative analgesic needs in patients after total knee replacement and hysterectomy.[39,40] These beneficial effects appear to be independent of whether ketamine is administered before or after incision.[40] In both studies, however, doses were generous (30–60 mg) and, therefore, may still be adequate to ablate central sensitization even after it has been initiated. Reduction of wound hyperalgesia was not assessed in either study. Clearly, epidural ketamine requires further evaluation. Safe dosing of epidural ketamine in humans is unknown, as is the potential for neurotoxicity. Animal studies thus far have demonstrated the relative safety of neuraxial ketamine, but dose-related neurotoxicity studies have not been performed.[41]

Opioids

Preclinical studies have evaluated both systemically and spinally administered opioids in their ability to prevent central facilitation. Neuraxial opioids are known to yield significant dose-dependent analgesia via modulation at the dorsal horn of the spinal cord. Opioids render analgesia at the level of the spinal cord by two distinct mechanisms: (1) preventing the release of excitatory neurotransmitters from small, primary afferent fibers, and (2) hyperpolarization of second-order neurons.[42] Intraspinal opioids would be reasonable to investigate as agents that may produce preemptive analgesia. Systemically administered opioids are felt to have a more complex mechanism of action that is not fully understood.[43] Supraspinal sites have been implicated in studies evaluating animals with high-spinal transections. Supraspinal opioid targets activate descending inhibitory pathways, which lead to dorsal horn modulation.[44] The impact of this descending inhibition on the release of excitatory neurotransmitter from primary afferent fibers, or the response of dorsal horn cells, is unknown. Although the main mechanism of action of opioids is agreed to be CNS modulation, peripheral opioid receptors may contribute to analgesia. Aside from intraarticular application, opioid interaction with peripheral receptors does not appear to manifest in clinically significant pain reduction[45]; therefore, peripheral sensitization would be at best be modestly affected by systemically or neuraxially administered opioids.

At the present time, both spinally and systemically administered opioids have given inconsistent results in preemptive trials. Post-injury facilitation of dorsal horn cells using subcutaneous formalin has been shown to be routinely blocked by intrathecal μ agonists. Interestingly, Yamamoto and Yaksh demonstrated that central facilitation (phase II of the formalin test) may be suppressed, even if intrathecal morphine is given after noxious stimulation (phase I of the formalin test, corresponding to acute C fiber–evoked activity in spinal neurons).[46] Previous studies had stressed the failure of post-injury administration of intrathecal μ agonists to entirely ablate central sensitization.[47] Other animal models, which involve the generation of more intense peripheral inflammation by either deep tissue injury with 5% formalin (e.g., into a knee joint) or a plantar incision of the hind paw, have identified that ongoing input from the periphery may be adequate to sustain central sensitization long after injury.[48,49] Actual incisional pain with associated hyperalgesia may progress during the surgery, and actually peak shortly after. It is, therefore, not so surprising that these latter studies, which inflicted an intense and prolonged inflammatory injury, were unable to document a significant difference in pain behavior between subjects administered intrathecal opioids pre- and post-injury.

Systemic opioids have produced mixed results in experimental animal models. Abram and Olson employed the rat formalin test to show that high doses of morphine or alfentanil, administered systemically, were unable to prevent central sensitization.[50] Even at high intravenous doses, morphine concentrations achieved in the subarachnoid space remained an order of magnitude lower than those achieved by direct subarachnoid injection. In contrast, Lascelles and colleagues, using a model of ovariohysterectomy in rats, were able to prevent surgically induced hyperalgesia by early administration of meperidine.[51] Applying the same rat ovariohysterectomy model, Gonzalez and coworkers reported a preemptive effect with subcutaneous morphine prior to surgical incision.[52] The conflicting experimental results involving preemptive analgesia stem in part from the different animal models studied. It is of critical importance that a model parallel as much as possible the usual human intraoperative and postoperative pain state. Finally, it remains unclear if typical doses of systemically administered opioids are capable of suppressing dorsal horn activity.

Clinical trials have evaluated both systemic and spinal opioids, given preincision and postincision, to determine whether a preemptive effect exists. This in turn, would generate appreciable postoperative pain reduction. Initial trials with systemic opioids appeared to reduce wound hyperalgesia. Richmond and colleagues reported reductions in Visual Analog Scale (VAS) scores and postoperative opioid consumption when pretreating women undergoing abdominal hysterectomy with 10 mg of morphine prior to incision,[53] as well as an associated decrease in secondary hyperalgesia. In a follow-up study, Collis and colleagues reported similar findings in women undergoing abdominal hysterectomy, but found no advantage with increasing the preemptive dose of morphine to 20 mg.[54] Tverskoy and colleagues demonstrated a decline of secondary hyperalgesia in women after abdominal hysterectomy with early administration of fentanyl, but without significant impact on VAS or opioid use.[30] Griffin and coworkers demonstrated less morphine consumption in posthysterectomy patients at 48 and 72 hours with preincisional high-dose alfentanil (70 μg/kg),[55] but VAS pain scores did not differ significantly between preincisional and post-incisional groups. Several other investigators, using the hysterectomy model, have not shown a difference with presurgical versus postsurgical administration of systemic opioids.[56–59] Given the experimental uncertainty of systemic opioids to affect central sensitization in animal models, it should be expected that human studies would generate inconsistent results. Moreover, recent data suggest that tolerance can develop rapidly in both rats and humans.[60–62] Large preincisional doses of opioids may potentially increase the dose requirements of analgesics postoperatively, because of acute opioid tolerance.

Studies of epidural opioids, alone or in combination with epidural or systemic ketamine, have demonstrated consistent differences between preincisional and post-incisional groups. Clinical studies evaluating the value of epidural opioids in thoracotomy, lumbar laminectomy, and prostatectomy have shown a significant reduction in postoperative pain scores, as well as analgesic consumption, in preemptive groups compared with controls.[63–65] Unfortunately, assessment of secondary hyperalgesia was not performed. Interestingly, Gottschalk and colleagues found that preemptive epidural fentanyl for radical prostatectomy can decrease postoperative pain at 9.5 weeks and increase function after hospital discharge.[65]

Enhanced blockade of dorsal horn cell excitation offered by ketamine, when added to epidural opioids, has consistently been shown to decrease postoperative pain and analgesic requirements. Ketamine may also reduce acute opioid tolerance, as already noted; therefore, reduced postoperative opioid consumption is probably a less valid measure of preemptive analgesia. The degree of diminution of secondary wound hyperalgesia was not evaluated using this combination of analgesics. Choe and coworkers showed that epidural ketamine (60 mg) plus morphine (2 mg) for upper abdominal surgery, given preincisionally, provided longer analgesia than post-incisional treatment.[66] Similarly, Wong and colleagues found that administration of preincisional epidural ketamine and morphine for total knee replacement, performed under epidural lidocaine anesthesia, was more effective than post-incisional adminstration.[39] More recently, in a randomized, double-blind study, Aida and colleagues concluded that a combination of epidural morphine (0.06 mg/kg followed by infusion 0.02 mg/kg per hour) and intravenous ketamine (1 mg/kg) was more definitive in reducing VAS scores and morphine consumption than either agent alone for patients undergoing gastrectomy.[67] There appears to be reasonable support for using preincisional epidural opioids to decrease postoperative pain and opioid consumption. These effects can be boosted by ketamine given prior to surgical trauma. This clinical impression would be consistent with laboratory work described earlier. Unfortunately, although the results of these studies suggest that reduction of dorsal horn activity decreases postoperative pain, they do not attempt to directly correlate a decrease of secondary wound hyperalgesia with a decline in postoperative pain, and thus the need for decreased analgesic administration.

Nonsteroidal Anti-inflammatory Drugs (NSAIDs)

NSAIDs have both peripheral and central effects. Indeed, C fiber–evoked activity in dorsal horn cells may be reduced by intrathecal NSAIDs.[68] Furthermore, case reports have shown that although NSAIDs were ineffective as systemic therapy, intense and prolonged relief was achieved when these drugs were given epidurally.[69] Cyclooxygenase inhibition in second-order neurons results in decreased excitation of the dorsal horn.[70] However, the predominant mechanism of parenteral or oral NSAIDs is thought to be peripheral reduction in prostaglandin synthesis.[1] Subsequently, inflammation is reduced, followed by pain. Thus, drugs that significantly modify peripheral sensitization would be inappropriate when the goal is to establish the role of blocking central facilitation on postoperative pain.[65]

Local Anesthetics

Local anesthetics prevent impulse generation and propagation by blocking initiation of an action potential.[71] The predominant mechanism is "plugging" of transmembrane sodium channels that allow for the intracytoplasmic increase in the concentration of sodium ions. Thus, local anesthetics allow a clinically reliable method for preventing afferent input into the spinal cord during noxious stimulation. In both preemptive preclinical and clinical studies, neuraxial, local infiltration, and peripheral nerve blockade by these agents have been evaluated. Direct infiltration of local anesthetics into the wound can abolish the axon reflex, thereby reducing the spread of inflammation.[72] Central or peripheral nerve blockade is less likely to interfere with peripheral sensitization and can more appropriately be used to assess the value of preemptive analgesia.

Laboratory investigations modeling the inflammatory generating nature of surgery have not demonstrated a clear advantage of preadministration versus postadministration use of local anesthetic. Brennan and colleagues characterized a rat model of surgical pain, with an incision on the plantar aspect of the hindpaw.[73] Skin, fascia, and muscle were cut, yielding mechanical hyperalgesia with an expected duration. Preincisional treatment with intrathecal bupivacaine did not differ from post-incisional treatment using measures of hyperalgesia in this model.[48] Yashpal and coworkers provided further insight to the declining value of preemptive intrathecal lidocaine as peripheral sensitization (induced by escalating doses of formalin injection) becomes more intense and sustained.[74] They speculated that peripheral inflammation must fall below a certain level to allow preemptive treatment to become appreciated. Kissin and colleagues demonstrated that paw hyperalgesia induced by carrageenan injection in rats can be prevented by administration of a nerve block, either pre- or post-injury.[75] Long-lasting, effective peripheral nerve blockade (tonicaine, 16-hour duration), administered 5 hours after injury, reversed secondary hyperalgesia almost entirely. Trials comparing prenerve block versus post-nerve block by local anesthetics run a high probability of not showing a significant difference.

As would be expected, human trials have generated varied results depending on the duration of analgesia provided. For example, analgesic requirements for patients undergoing abdominal hysterectomy did not differ whether they received spinal bupivacaine before or after surgery.[76] Comparable results were obtained when evaluating preincisional and postincisional epidural bupivacaine in a similar population posthysterectomy.[77] There was no apparent difference between preincisional and postincision caudal block on postoperative analgesic consumption for patients undergoing hypospadias repair, herniorrhaphy, orchidopexy, and circumcision in multiple investigations.[78–81] In all of these studies, secondary hyperalgesia was not assessed between groups. Central sensitization was probably reestablished once the block (spinal or caudal) wore off, given that there is adequate tissue injury during these procedures. Dahl and colleagues examined the difference between extradural analgesia with bupivacaine and morphine initiated before and after colonic surgery and total knee arthroplasty.[82,83] Following either surgery, a continuous infusion of bupivacaine-morphine was administered for 48 hours in the knee arthroplasty group and for 72 hours in the post-colectomy patients. There was no significant difference in request for additional analgesics or VAS pain scores for either group of patients. The results of these trials parallel the results of Kissin and colleagues' laboratory findings, discussed earlier, whereby central sensitization can be reversed by late neural blockade, and prevented from returning by intense postoperative analgesia. Ilioinguinal and iliohypogastric nerve blocks together with spinal anesthesia in patients post-inguinal hernia repair provided better pain control up to 48 hours after the surgery than did spinal anesthesia alone.[84] This study illustrates the importance of ongoing afferent blockade while peripheral sensitization declines. The authors then appreciated a prolonged analgesic effect.

In contrast to laboratory investigations, Carr and colleagues were able to show that individuals receiving interscalene block with 0.5% levobupivacaine prior to shoulder surgery, rather than after, had a lower incidence of requests for analgesic medication as well as lower pain scores for the first 8 hours after surgery.[85] Use of opioids and VAS scores approximated each other by 24 hours post–shoulder surgery. Katz and coworkers demonstrated a more pronounced effect with early administration of 15 mL of 0.5% bupivacaine, given epidurally, in patients undergoing lower abdominal procedures.[86] Postoperative pain was controlled by patient-controlled analgesia. There was an average reduction of morphine consumption by 25% for up to 72 hours post-procedure, as well as McGill Pain Questionnaire ratings, in those receiving preincisional treatment compared with the postincisional group. Likewise, Gottshalk and colleagues, with preemptive use of epidural fentanyl, found comparable results using epidural bupivacaine in the recovery of patients after radical prostatectomy.[65] Here investigators showed not only benefit in the immediate postoperative period, but also increased activity and function long after discharge from the hospital. These later studies hint at the potential benefit of preemptive treatment, but it is difficult to reconcile all the incongruities among the various studies.

THE COMPLEXITY OF DEMONSTRATING PREEMPTIVE ANALGESIA

The overall clinical expectation of preemptive analgesia was that it would reduce subsequent postoperative pain, and this would consistently and easily be measured by VAS or postoperative analgesic consumption, or both. Unfortunately, the effect of preemptive analgesia may not be so apparent. The complexity of clearly demonstrating preemptive analgesia has been evolving in the literature during the past decade. Multiple variables continue to be identified and require adequate control or defining, as pointed out in an editorial by Kissin.[87] It has become evident that high-intensity noxious stimuli are not only present during surgical incision, but persist well into the postoperative period in the form of peripheral sensitization. Neglecting to block immense small-fiber afferent input during the postoperative period may certainly establish central sensitization, even if there was adequate block of peripheral input throughout the surgery and immediately postoperatively.[88] Very painful operations, such as a thoracotomy or total knee arthroplasty, certainly mandate ongoing intense analgesia during the postoperative period, even if very sufficient afferent blockade occurred during the procedure. By the same token, the nature of the surgery must generate enough noxious signals to induce central sensitization so that preemptive analgesia can, in fact, have the opportunity to alter the postoperative pain state.

To prevent central sensitization, one must ensure that the treatment provides adequate disruption of the afferent barrage on dorsal horn cells. Although laboratory studies can determine the appropriate doses of drug necessary to achieve this end, this goal becomes more challenging in the clinical setting. Performing highly noxious surgery under regional anesthesia (e.g., epidural), with ongoing interruption of afferent central input is likely the most practical method of ensuring that central hyperexcitability is avoided.

To complicate matters further, many investigators feel that there have been inadequate controls. Opioids are commonly given to both the control group and preemptive group on induction, as is nitrous oxide for maintenance. The analgesic properties of nitrous oxide may lead to a preemptive effect.[89] Potent inhaled anesthetics are also known to suppress spinal cord sensitization, and the degree of this effect varies among the inhaled agents.[90] Furthermore, early studies investigating preemptive analgesia did not include a control group. There was no comparison of preincisional analgesic treatment with the same therapy instituted postoperatively.

Opioid consumption as a measure of outcome is not without its problems. Multiple confounding factors influence any patient's analgesic usage. Anxiety, depression, perception of the surgical course, and overall care may contribute to opioid use. Kissin further added that pain intensity and analgesic requirements have not been demonstrated to consistently correlate.[87] Despite multiple confounding factors and shortcomings, total opioid consumption delivered via patient-controlled analgesia devices has been most commonly employed to assess preemptive analgesia.

CONCLUSION

Despite a significant number of clinical studies throughout the past decade, the contribution of central sensitization to the overall postoperative pain state remains unclear. To what degree central facilitation amplifies pain after surgery is unknown in humans. Many of the studies did not evaluate secondary wound hyperalgesia, and then attempt to correlate this with improved pain control. The preemptive trials comparing preincisional with postincisional treatment groups are now regarded by many authors to be too simplistic.[88,91] As mentioned earlier, many of the post-injury interventions are adequate to reverse central sensitization. Furthermore, once adequate afferent blockade to the spinal cord is lost, postsurgical inflammatory injury may establish central facilitation. Thus, any preemptive treatment is unlikely to render any benefits. Investigators now agree that the initial postoperative period must be covered.[88]

Even with these shortcomings, several studies have documented modest benefit comparing patients' preincisional interventions with those administered postoperatively. Aggressive control of postoperative pain may manifest more of its beneficial effects not in the immediate postsurgical time frame, but weeks later. Improved functional restoration, marked by more rapid return to the usual activity level and employment postprocedure, may be an outcome of preemptive analgesia. Lastly, reduction of chronic pain following surgery may be another benefit of preventing central sensitization.

REFERENCES

1. Crile GW. The kinetic theory of shock and its prevention through anoci-association. *Lancet* 1913;185:7–16.
2. Katz J. George Washington Crile, anoci-association, and pre-emptive analgesia. *Pain* 1993;53:243–245.
3. Wall PD. The prevention of postoperative pain. *Pain* 1988;33: 289–290.
4. Woolf CJ, Wall PD. A dissociation between the analgesic and antinociceptive effects of morphine. *Neurosci Lett* 1986;64:238.
5. Woolf CJ, Chong M-S. Preemptive analgesia-treating postoperative pain by preventing the establishment of central sensitization. *Anesth Analg* 1993;77:362–789.
6. Levine J, Taiwo Y. Inflammatory pain. In: Wall PD, Melzack R, eds. *Textbook of Pain*. 3rd ed. London, England: Churchill Livingstone; 1994:45–56.
7. Fields HL, Rowbotham M, Baron R. Postherpetic neuralgia: Irritable nociceptors and deafferentation. *Neurobiol Dis* 1998;5:209–227.
8. Chapman LF. Mechanisms of the flare reaction in human skin. *J Invest Dermatol* 1977;69:88–97.
9. Lembeck F. Mediators of vasodilation in the skin. *Br J Dermatol* 1983;109(suppl 25):1–9.
10. Cook AJ, Woolf CJ, Wall PD, McMahon SB. Dynamic receptive field plasticity in the rat spinal cord dorsal horn following C-primary afferent inputs. *Nature* 1987;325:151–153.
11. Nagy I, Maggi CA, Dray A, et al. The role of neurokinin and *N*-methyl-D-aspartate receptors in synaptic transmission from capsaicin sensitive primary afferents in the rat spinal cord in vitro. *Neuroscience* 1993;52: 1029–1037.
12. Coderre TJ, Katz J, Vaccarino AL, Melzack R. Contribution of central neuroplasticity to pathologic pain: Review of clinical and experimental evidence. *Pain* 1993;52:259–285.
13. Woolf CJ, King AK. Dynamic alterations in the cutaneous mechanosensitive receptive field of dorsal horn neurons in the rat spinal cord. *J Neurosci* 1990;10:2717–2726.
14. Simone DA, Sorkin LS, Oh U, et al. Neurogenic hyperalgesia: Central neural correlates in responses of spinothalamic tract neurons. *J Neurophysiol* 1991;66:228–246.
15. MacDermott AB, Mayer ML, Westbrook GL, Smith SJ, Barker JL. NMDA-receptor activation increases cytoplasmic calcium concentration in cultured spinal cord neurons. *Nature* 1986;321:519–522.
16. Womack MD, MacDermott AB, Jessell TM. Sensory transmitters regulate intracellular calcium in dorsal horn neurons. *Nature* 1988;334: 351–353.
17. Woolf CJ, Thompson SWN. The induction and maintenance of central sensitization is dependent on *N*-methyl-D-aspartic acid receptor activation; implications for the treatment of post-injury pain hypersensitivity states. *Pain* 1991;44:293–299.
18. Sugiyama H, Ito I, Hirono C. A new type of glutamate receptor linked to inositol phospholipid metabolism. *Nature* 1987;325:531–533.
19. Naranjo JR, Mellstrom B, Achaval M, Sassone-Corsi P. Molecular pathways of pain: Fos/Jun-mediated activation of a noncanonical AP-1 site in the prodynorphin gene. *Neuron* 1991;6:607–617.
20. Iadorola MJ, Sanders SR, Draisci G. Differential activation of spinal cord dynorphin and enkephalin neurons during hyperalgesia: Evidence using cDNA hybridization. *Brain Res* 1988;455:205–212.
21. Dubner R, Ruda MA. Activity-dependent neuronal plasticity following tissue injury and inflammation. *Trends Neurosci* 1992;15:96–103.
22. Yamamura T, Harada K, Okamura A, Kemmotsu O. Is the site of action of ketamine anesthesia the *N*-methyl-D-aspartate receptor? *Anesthesiology* 1990;72:704–710.
23. Yamamoto T, Yaksh TL. Comparison of the antinociceptive effects of pre- and posttreatment with intrathecal morphine and MK801, and NMDA antagonist, on the formalin test in the rat. *Anesthesiology* 1992; 77:757–763.
24. Schmid RL, Sandler AN, Katz J. Use and efficacy of low-dose ketamine in the management of acute postoperative pain: A review of current techniques and outcome. *Pain* 1999;82:111–125.
25. Gilron I, Quirion R, Coderre TJ. Pre-versus postformalin effects of ketamine or large-dose alfentanil in the rat: Discordance between pain behavior and spinal fos-like immunoreactivity. *Anesth Analg* 1999;89: 128–135.
26. Kohrs R, Durieux ME. Ketamine: Teaching an old drug new tricks. *Anesth Analg* 1998;87:1186–1193.
27. Eide PK, Strubhaug A, Oye I. The NMDA-antagonist ketamine for prevention and treatment of acute and chronic post-operative pain. *Baillieres Clin Anesthesiol* 1995;9:539–540.
28. Eide PK, Stubhaug A, Oye I, Breivik H. Continuous subcutaneous administration of the *N*-methyl-D-aspartic acid (NMDA) receptor antagonist ketamine in the treatment of post-herpetic neuralgia. *Pain* 1995; 61:221–228.
29. Eide PK, Jorum E, Strubhaug A, Bremnes J, Breivik H. Relief of post-herpetic neuralgia with the *N*-methyl-D-aspartic acid receptor antagonist: A double-blind, cross-over comparison with morphine and placebo. *Pain* 1994;58:347–354.
30. Tverskoy M, Oz Y, Isakson A, Finger J, Bradley EL, Kissin I. Preemptive effect of fentanyl and ketamine on postoperative pain and wound hyperalgesia. *Anesth Analg* 1994;78:205–209.
31. Stubhaug A, Breivik H, Eide PK, Kreunen M, Foss A. Mapping of punctate hyperalgesia around a surgical incision demonstrates that ketamine is a powerful suppressor of central sensitization to pain following surgery. *Acta Anaesthesiol Scand* 1997;41:1124–1132.
32. Fu ES, Miguel R, Scharf JE. Preemptive ketamine decreases postoperative narcotic requirements in patients undergoing abdominal surgery. *Anesth Analg* 1997;84:1086–1090.
33. Roytblat L, Korotkoruchko A, Katz J, Glazer M, Greemberg L, Fisher A. Postoperative pain: The effect of low-dose ketamine in addition to general anesthesia. *Anesth Analg* 1993;77:1161–1165.
34. Suzuki M, Tsueda K, Lansing PS, et al. Small-dose ketamine enhances morphine-induced analgesia after outpatient surgery. *Anesth Analg* 1999;89:98–103.
35. Frederic A, Libier M, Oszustowicz T, Lefebvre D, Beal J, Meynadier J. Preoperative small-dose ketamine has no preemptive analgesic effect in patients undergoing total mastectomy. *Anesth Analg* 1999; 89:444–447.

36. Clements JA, Nimmo WS. Pharmacokinetics and analgesic effect of ketamine in man. *Br J Anesth* 1981;53:27–30.
37. Pekoe GM, Smith DJ. The involvement of opiate and monoaminergic neuronal systems in the analgesic effects of ketamine. *Pain* 1982;12: 57–73.
38. Eisenach JC. Preemptive hyperalgesia, not analgesia? *Anesthesiology* 2000;92:465–472.
39. Wong CS, Lu CC, Cherng CH, Ho ST. Preemptive analgesia with ketamine, morphine, and lidocaine prior to total knee replacement. *Can J Anaesth* 1997;44:31–37.
40. Abdel-Ghaffar ME, Abdulatif M, Al-Ghamdi A, Mowafi H, Anwar A. Epidural ketamine reduces post-operative epidural PCA consumption of fentanyl/bupivacaine. *Can J Anaesth* 1998;45:103–109.
41. Yaksh TL. Epidural ketamine: A useful, mechanistically novel adjuvant for epidural morphine? *Reg Anesth* 1996;21:508–513.
42. Dickinson AH. Mechanisms of the analgesic actions of opiates and opioids. *Br Med Bull* 1992;47:690–702.
43. Advokat C, Burton P. Antinociceptive effects of systemic and intrathecal morphine in spinally transected rats. *Eur J Pharmacol* 1987; 139:335–343.
44. Fields HL, Basbaum AI. Brainstem control of spinal pain transmission. *Ann Rev Physiol* 1978;40:217–248.
45. Stein C. The control of pain in peripheral tissue by opioids. *N Engl J Med* 1995;332:1685–1690.
46. Yamamoto T, Yaksh TL. Comparison of the antinociceptive effects of pre- and posttreatment with intrathecal morphine and MK801, an NMDA antagonist, on the formalin test in the rat. *Anesthesiology* 1992;77: 757–763.
47. Dickerson AH, Sullivan AF. Subcutaneous formalin-induced activity of dorsal horn neurones in the rat: Differential response to an intrathecal opiate administered pre or post formalin. *Pain* 1987;30:349–360.
48. Brennan TJ, Umali EF, Zahn PK. Comparison of pre-versus postincision administration of intrathecal bupivacaine and intrathecal morphine in a rat model of postoperative pain. *Anesthesiology* 1997;87: 1518–1528.
49. Yashpal K, Katz J, Coderre TJ. Effects of preemptive or postinjury intrathecal local anesthesia on persistent nociceptive responses in rats. *Anesthesiology* 1996;84:1119–1128.
50. Abram SE, Olson EE. Systemic opioids do not suppress spinal sensitization after subcutaneous formalin in rats. *Anesthesiology* 1994;80: 1114–1119.
51. Lascelles BDX, Waterman AE, Cripps PJ, Livingston A, Henderson G. Central sensitization as a result of surgical pain: Investigation of the pre-emptive value of pethidine for ovariohysterectomy in the rat. *Pain* 1995;62:201–212.
52. Gonzalez MI, Field MJ, Bramwell S, McCleary S, Singh L. Ovariohysterectomy in the rat: A model of surgical pain for evaluation of preemptive analgesia? *Pain* 2000;88:79–88.
53. Richmond CE, Bromley LM, Woolf CJ. Preoperative morphine preempts postoperative pain. *Lancet* 1993;342:73–753.
54. Collis R, Brandner B, Bromley LM, Woolf CJ. Is there any clinical advantage of increasing the pre-emptive dose of morphine or combining pre-incisional with postoperative morphine administration? *Br J Anaesth* 1995;74:396–399.
55. Griffin MJ, Hughes D, Knaggs A, Donnelly MB, Boylan JF. Late-onset preemptive analgesia associated with preincisional large-dose alfentanil. *Anesth Analg* 1997;85:1317–1321.
56. Mansfield M, Meikle R, Miller C. A trial of pre-emptive analgesia: Influence of timing of preoperative alfentanil on postoperative pain and analgesic requirements. *Anaesthesia* 1994;49:1091–1093.
57. Wilson RJT, Leith S, Jackson IJB, Hunter D. Pre-emptive analgesia from intravenous administration of opioids: No effect with alfentanil. *Anaesthesia* 1994;49:591–593.
58. Sarantopoulos C, Fassoulaki A. Sufentanil does not preempt pain after abdominal hysterectomy. *Pain* 1996;65:273–276.
59. Fassoulaki A, Sarantopoulos C, Zotou M, Papoulia D. Preemptive opioid analgesia does not influence pain after hysterectomy. *Can J Anaesth* 1995;42:109–113.
60. Kissin I, Bright CA, Bradley EL. Acute tolerance to continuously infused alfentanil: The role of cholecystokinin and *N*-methyl-D-aspartate-nitric oxide systems. *Anesth Analg* 2000;91:110–116.
61. Vinik HR, Kissin I. Rapid development of tolerance to analgesia during remifentanil infusion in humans. *Anesth Analg* 1998;86:1307–1311.
62. Kissin I, Bright CA, Bradley EL. The effect of ketamine on opioid-induced acute tolerance: Can it explain reduction of opioid consumption with ketamine-opioid analgesic combinations? *Anesth Analg* 2000;91: 1483–1488.
63. Katz J, Kavanagh BP, Sandler AN, et al. Preemptive analgesia: Clinical evidence of neuroplasticity contributing to postoperative pain. *Anesthesiology* 1992:77;439–446.
64. Kundra P, Gurnani A, Bhattacharya A. Preemptive epidural morphine for postoperative pain relief after lumbar laminectomy. *Anesth Analg* 1997;85:135–138.
65. Gottschalk A, Smith DS, Jobes DR, et al. Preemptive epidural analgesia and recovery from radical prostatectomy. *JAMA* 1998;279:1076–1082.
66. Choe H, Choi Y-S, Kim Y-H, et al. Epidural morphine plus ketamine for upper abdominal surgery: Improved analgesia from preincisional versus postincisional administration. *Anesth Analg* 1997;84:560–563.
67. Aida S, Yamakura T, Baba H, Taga K, Fukuda S, Shimoji K. Preemptive analgesia by intravenous low-dose ketamine and epidural morphine in gastrectomy. *Anesthesiology* 2000;92:XX.
68. Malmberg AB, Yaksh TL. Hyperalgesia mediated by spinal glutamate or substance P receptor blockade by spinal cyclooxygenase inhibition. *Science* 1992;257:1276–1279.
69. Lauretti GR, Reis MP, Mattos AL, Gomes JMA, Oliveira AP, Pereira ML. Epidural nonsteroidal antiinflammatory drugs for cancer pain. *Anesth Analg* 1998;86:117–118.
70. Saito Y, Kaneko M, Kirihara Y, et al. Intrathecal prostaglandin E_1 produces a long-lasting allodynic state. *Pain* 1995;63:303–311.
71. de Jong RH. Nerve impulse blockade. In: de Jong RH, ed. *Local Anesthetics*. St Louis, Mo: Mosby; 1994:45–63.
72. Meyer RA, Campbell JN, Raja SN. Peripheral neural mechanisms of nociception. In: Wall PD, Melzak R, Bonica JJ, eds. *Textbook of Pain*. 3rd ed. Edinburgh, Scotland: Churchill Livingstone; 1994:13–44.
73. Brennan TJ, Vandermeulen EP, Gebhart GF. Characterization of a rat model of incisional pain. *Pain* 1996;64:493–501.
74. Yashpal K, Katz J, Coderre TJ. Effects of preemptive or postinjury intrathecal local anesthesia on persistent nociceptive responses in rats. *Anesthesiology* 1996;84:1119–1128.
75. Kissin I, Lee SS, Bradley EL. Effect of prolonged nerve block on inflammatory hyperalgesia in rats: Prevention of late hyperalgesia. *Anesthesiology* 1998;88:224–232.
76. Dakin MJ, Osinubi OYO, Carli F. Preoperative spinal bupivacaine does not reduce postoperative morphine requirement in women undergoing total abdominal hysterectomy. *Reg Anesth* 1996;21:99–102.
77. Pryle BJ, Vanner RG, Enriquez N, Reynolds F. Can pre-emptive lumbar epidural blockade reduce postoperative pain following lower abdominal surgery? *Anaesthesia* 1993;48:120–123.
78. Ho JWS, Khambatta HJ, Pang LM, Siegfried RN, Sun LS. Preemptive analgesia in children. *Reg Anesth* 1997;22:125–130.
79. Holthusen H, Eichwede F, Stevens M, Willnow U, Lipfert P. Preemptive analgesia: Comparison of preoperative with postoperative caudal block on postoperative pain in children. *Br J Anaesth* 1994;73:440–442.
80. Rice LJ, Pudimat MA, Hannallah RS. Timing of caudal block placement in relation to surgery does not affect duration of postoperative analgesia in paediatric ambulatory patients. *Can J Anaesth* 1990;37: 429–431.
81. Gunther JB, Forestner JE, Manley CB. Caudal epidural anesthesia reduces blood loss during hypospadias repair. *J Urol* 1990;144:517–519.
82. Dahl JB, Hansen NC, Hjortso NC, Erichsen CJ, Moiniche S, Kehlet H. Influence of timing on the effect of continuous extradural analgesia with bupivacaine and morphine after major abdominal surgery. *Br J Anaesth* 1992;69:4–8.

83. Dahl JB, Daugaard B, Rasmussen B, Egebo K, Carlsson P, Kehlet H. Immediate and prolonged effect of pre-versus postoperative epidural analgesia with bupivacaine and morphine on pain at rest and during mobilisation after total knee arthroplasty. *Acta Anaesth Scand* 1994; 38:557–561.
84. Bugedo G, Carcamo CS, Mertens RA, Dagnino JA, Munoz HR. Preoperative percutaneous ilioinguinal and iliohypogastric nerve block with 0.5% bupivacaine for post-herniorraphy pain management in adults. *Reg Anesth* 1990;15:130–132.
85. Carr DB, Sternlicht A, Carabuena JM, Wurm WH, Robelen G. Efficacy and safety of pre-emptive levobupivacaine in elective shoulder surgery. *Reg Anesth Pain Med* 2000;25S:20.
86. Katz J, Clairoux M, Kavangh BP, et al. Pre-emptive lumbar anesthesia reduces postoperative pain and patient-controlled morphine consumption after lower abdominal surgery. *Pain* 1994;59:395–403.
87. Kissin I. Preemptive analgesia: Why its effect is not always obvious. *Anesthesiology* 1996;84:1015–1019.
88. Kissin I. Preemptive analgesia. *Anesthesiology* 2000;93:1138–1143.
89. Goto T, Marota JJA, Crosby G. Nitrous oxide induces preemptive analgesia in the rat that is antagonized by halothane. *Anesthesiology* 1994; 80:409–416.
90. O'Connor TC, Abram SE. Inhibition of nociceptive-induced spinal sensitization by anesthetic agents. *Anesthesiology* 1995;82:259–266.
91. Brennan TJ, Taylor BK. Analgesic treatment before incision compared with treatment after incision provides no improvement in postoperative pain relief. *J Pain Symptom Manage* 2000;1:96–98.

CHAPTER 42 ACUTE PAIN MANAGEMENT IN ADULTS

Christine G. Peeters-Asdourian and Vimal K. Akhouri

Pain relief in an acute pain situation, besides having a humane value, has an important bearing in the well-being of an individual. Although it may not be possible to achieve total relief in all situations, a serious effort should be made.

Since the discovery of opioid receptors in 1978, efforts have been made to improve the delivery of analgesic drugs in a more effective way. Thanks to these advances in basic science on the clinical front, the last two decades have witnessed major strides in postoperative analgesia with the creation of acute pain services, the increased use of epidural analgesia, and the introduction of the concept of patient-controlled analgesia.

The tissue damage produced by surgery is similar to that of acute injury. It causes local and systemic noxious stimuli that initiate nociceptive impulses, relays, and reflexes throughout the nervous system. In addition to the disturbances associated with the conscious interpretation of theses impulses, there are autonomic effects generated that may disrupt the healing and recovery process. The deleterious physiologic side effects of acute pain are well recognized. In the patient who is breathing spontaneously, muscle splinting (seen in conjunction with discomfort of chest or abdominal origin) may result in decreased vital capacity, decreased functional residual capacity, and ultimately decreased alveolar ventilation. Atelectasis is a frequent postoperative complication. Discomfort experienced during coughing may result in retention of secretions and subsequent pneumonia. The sympathetic response to pain may cause increased cardiovascular demands. This may be apparent clinically by signs of tachycardia, increased peripheral resistance, and hypertension; these signs are associated with increased cardiac work and myocardial oxygen consumption. The potential for myocardial ischemia and infarction is obvious. Muscle spasm produced by segmental and suprasegmental reflex motor activity may perpetuate pain. In the chest wall and abdomen, pain and muscle spasm may compromise respiratory function. The gastrointestinal tract similarly is affected by increased sympathetic activity. Pain increases intestinal secretions and smooth muscle sphincter tone and decreases intestinal motility. By similar mechanisms, pain may produce urinary retention. Acute injury also has an impact on the endocrine system, causing sodium and water retention and hyperglycemia. Immobility from acute postoperative pain may predispose the patient to deep vein thrombosis and pulmonary embolism as a result of venostasis and platelet aggregation. In a complex intertwined relationship, psychological alterations may occur concomitantly with the physiologic ones.[1]

Numerous guidelines have been published about the management of postoperative pain. First the Agency for Health Care Policy and Research (AHCPR) took the lead in educating caregivers as well as the public. The American Pain Society as well as the American Society of Anesthesia then followed suit, and the Joint Commission on Accreditation of Healthcare Organizations (JCAHO) has published "Standards for Pain Management in Hospital Settings" that were implemented in 2001.[2,3]

PAIN AS THE FIFTH VITAL SIGN

The guidelines from JCAHO incorporate pain measurements in the bedside chart in addition to tracking the patient's temperature, blood pressure, heart rate, and respiratory rate, thus making pain rating the fifth vital sign.

However, a simple numerical assessment of pain on the visual analog scale or verbal rating scale does not differentiate between pain at rest and pain with movement or incident pain, which is usually more challenging to manage.

Also, to effectively adjust the analgesic regimen, one needs to track sedation and other possible adverse effects associated with the administration of analgesics such as nausea and vomiting, respiratory depression, and cognitive impairment.

The importance of good postoperative analgesia and its impact on favorable postsurgical outcomes are undeniable. Pain in the postoperative period may contribute to adverse outcomes including thromboembolic and pulmonary complications.

Many factors influence our perception of postoperative pain. Determinants of the intensity, quality, and duration of postoperative pain include:

- The site, nature, and duration of the operation, including the type of incision and the amount of intraoperative trauma
- The physiologic and psychological makeup of the patient
- The preoperative psychological, physical, and pharmacologic preparation of the patient
- The presence of serious related complications
- The anesthetic management
- The quality of postoperative care. Some of the ineffectiveness of current medical analgesic therapy can be attributed to inadequate understanding by nurses of the pharmacology of narcotics.

Inadequate understanding by physicians of the nature of pain also has been demonstrated. A structured interview of 37 medical inpatients showed that 32% had severe distress despite a narcotic analgesic regimen; an additional 41% declared themselves to be in moderate distress. As part of the study, a questionnaire survey of 102 staff physicians showed an underestimation of effective dose ranges, overestimation of the duration of action, and an exaggerated concern with the addictive potential of meperidine in a therapeutic dosing range. It is thought that the development of addiction in patients with no previous addictive history is rare. Children, perhaps the most dependent group in the hospital population, also bear the burden of postoperative suffering. As a reaction to discomfort, many children withdraw and vegetate. This may be misinterpreted as coping with the pain. Many immature patients fear injection, deny pain, and are unable to realize that a short-term discomfort may grant a longer period of analgesia.[4,5]

In summary, at least three major factors contribute to the inadequacy of traditional analgesic therapy. Foremost is the incomplete comprehension by medical personnel of analgesic pharmacodynamics. This lack of knowledge coupled with overconcern about respiratory depression and addiction liability leads to the administration of inadequate doses. Second, the logistics of administering narcotics often leads to a long lag period between the onset of pain and the administration of pain-relieving drugs. Coupled with the delay in absorption of intramuscularly administered analgesics, this interval may distress the patient greatly. A third barrier to adequate analgesia is a common hospital community attitude that stoicism is a virtue. The suffering patient may sense such an attitude and, rather than attacking this formidable barrier, refrain from requesting appropriate medication.[6]

POSTOPERATIVE PAIN: THE PROBLEM

A surgical incision cuts through a variety of tissues including nerve endings and activates specific nociceptors (pain receptors) as well as free nerve endings. It is associated with the release of inflammatory mediators such as bradykinin, serotonin, and histamine, which contribute to *peripheral sensitization*. Clinically, this phenomenon is manifested by hyperalgesia, which is an amplification of noxious pain signals. These painful signals are transmitted to the dorsal horn of the spinal cord in an amplified fashion and are increased in duration.

The nociceptor information is transmitted to the cord via the A-δ (myelinated) fibers and the C (unmyelinated) fibers. When peripheral sensitization occurs, painful information can also be carried by A-α and A-β fibers. This is manifested by *allodynia*, a pain state where non-noxious stimuli are transformed and expressed as painful. Signals entering the central nervous system from the periphery will be increased in amplitude and duration. This is the phenomenon of "wind up" or central sensitization.[7]

Analgesic techniques, to be effective, will need to counteract these activations of nociceptors at the periphery as well as centrally, thus the need for a multimodal or "balanced" analgesia to ensure patient comfort, to improve early mobilization, and decrease the consequences of the postsurgical stress.

Traditional methods of intermittent on request, intramuscular, or subcutaneous administrations of opioids have failed to provide satisfactory analgesia. Failure to adequately relieve postoperative pain contributes not only to discomfort, but to postoperative morbidity, poor patient outcome, and prolonged hospital stay.

PHYSIOLOGIC RESPONSE TO ACUTE PAIN

Endocrine and Metabolic Response

Any injury provokes a neurohumoral response involving the hypothalamic-pituitary-adrenal axis, activation of sympathetic nervous system, and an increase in glucagon secretion.[1] Surgery leads to a similar reproducible response, which causes hyperglycemia, increased lipolysis, lipid oxidation, accelerated protein breakdown, and nitrogen loss.[2,3]

These responses begin during surgery and may be maintained for days, especially after major abdominal or thoracic surgery. The stress response peaks in the postoperative period.[4] Clinically, this presents as hypertension, tachycardia, arrhythmias, myocardial ischemia, protein catabolism, immune system suppression, and impaired renal excretory function. Suppression of the stress response is possible, though not completely. The intensity of the stress response depends on the site of surgery (extremities versus thoracic or abdominal), pain control modality, (neuraxial versus systemic), medication used (local anesthetic versus opioid), and initiation and maintenance of treatment (intraoperative versus postoperative). Studies have shown that stress response and morbidity in the first 24 hours is less in patients receiving epidural analgesia with local anesthetics with or without opioids.[8,9]

Pulmonary Function

Pulmonary dysfunction is commonly seen after thoracic and upper abdominal surgery and is more important than after extremity or laproscopic surgery. This is a major source of morbidity and mortality in the perioperative period. Primary mechanisms are decreased phrenic nerve activity and diaphragmatic dysfunction, reflex increased spinal arc activity causing increased intercostals, and abdominal muscle tone. Clinically, it is manifested as a decrease in functional residual capacity and a decrease in tidal volume. Existing pulmonary disease or respiratory depression due to opioid analgesics may compound these problems.[10]

Gastrointestinal Motility

A combination of surgery and anesthesia in addition to pain produces a decrease in gastric motility, especially in the colon. The stomach and small intestines recovers within 12 to 24 hours after abdominal surgery, whereas the colon is inhibited for at least 48 to 72 hours. Early enteral feeding is known to decrease the surgical stress response, thus making a difference to the postoperative morbidity.[11]

Possible mechanisms to explain illeus are sympathetic hyperactivity in response to surgical stress and pain, especially after abdominal surgery, and abdominal pain that activates spinal reflex, which inhibits intestinal motility. Use of opioids for pain control would further promote illeus. Epidural opioids also inhibit gastrointestinal motility, but somewhat less than systemic opioids.[12]

Cardiovascular

Uncontrolled pain causes increased sympathetic tone and a resetting of baroreceptors that cause an increase in heart rate and blood pressure. The neural outflow also causes redistribution of blood to and within various organs. This predisposes to myocardial ischemia in the presence of coronary artery disease and may induce arrhythmias. Stress per se is also arrhythmogenic in nonischemic myocardium.[13]

Besides the increase seen in catecholamines and sympathetic neural outflow, there is a reflex decrease in parasympathetic outflow due to pain. This imbalance in the autonomic system alters the baroreceptors settings.[14]

Immune System

There is a large amount of clinical evidence showing suppression of both humoral and cellular mechanisms of the immune system following trauma and surgery. There is a decrease in responsiveness to antigen and mitogen, delayed hypersensitivity, natural killer cell activity, and antibody response.[15] The exact causative mechanism is not known. Increased release of glucocorticoids is seen as one of the reasons, but other stress response hormones may also cause immune modulation.[16]

Coagulation System

Changes in the coagulation system primarily occur from surgery in the form of activation of the coagulation cascade, increased platelet activity, and decreased fibrinolytic activity leading to increased coagulability. Use of epidural analgesia in the perioperative period has been found to produce less platelet activity and improved fibrinolysis, which may be related to the systemic effects of local anesthetic.[17]

Cognitive Dysfunction

Postoperatively, 10% to 50% of patients develop transient cognitive impairment, which is worse on the second day, but they usually recover within a week. Elderly patients may take up to 3 months to recover baseline cognitive function. Exact mechanisms are not clear and there is no conclusive data to suggest a particular choice of anesthetic technique. Delirium occurs in about 10% of patients undergoing noncardiac surgery after age 50. Electrolyte abnormality, sleep apnea, history of alcohol abuse, and benzodiazepines and meperidine intake are risk factors for delirium. Studies have found that high levels of postoperative pain can cause delirium and, vice versa, delirium can impair cognition and cause exacerbation of pain.

Options for pain management in the postoperative period include the following:

1. Systemic analgesics
2. Neuraxial opioids and local anesthetics
3. Regional anesthetic techniques
4. Adjunct treatments, e.g., transcutaneous electrical nerve stimulation (TENS) unit, heat application, and self-hypnosis.

SYSTEMIC ANALGESICS

Opioids

Opioids remain the mainstay of postoperative analgesia and have demonstrated their efficacy in the management of severe pain. The main concerns about the use of opioids remain their side effects: nausea, vomiting, ileus, biliary spasms, respiratory depression, and the potential for abuse, although in the immediate postoperative period this is rarely an issue. Opioids can be administered intramuscularly, subcutaneously, or intravenously.

The administration of opioids by intramuscular injections prescribed on an as-needed basis provide fluctuating opioids levels resulting in sedation and other adverse effects when levels are high and inadequate analgesia when levels are low. A better method of administration of opioids is via a microprocessor-controlled infusion pump or patient-controlled analgesia (PCA).[18]

A preset dose of opioids is delivered to the patient when activating the demand switch, given that a predetermined time has elapsed since the previous dose; this is the "lockout" time. An upper limit per hour or per 4 hours is predetermined and set in the program as an additional safety device. Numerous studies have demonstrated the safety and opioid-sparing effect of PCA (Table 42-1).

Patients taking opioids preoperatively will show some tolerance intraoperatively and postoperatively. One can safely assume that patients taking two tablets of combination analgesics such as Percocet (5 mg oxycodone/tablet) or Vicodin (5 or 7, 5 mg hydrocodone) four times daily will require 1 mg of morphine per hour postoperatively to replace their regular opioids.

Non-Opioid Analgesics

With opioids alone, intramuscularly or intravenously, the analgesia may be marginal and side effects intolerable (nausea, vomiting, sedation), thus the need for synergy, choosing drug classes that will overlap for analgesia but not for side effects. Drug classes that fit these requirements are as follows: cyclooxygenase inhibitors, alpha$_2$ agonists, nitric oxide synthetase inhibitors, NMDA (N-methyl-D-aspartate) receptor blockers, and local anesthetics when delivered by thoracic epidural catheters. This balanced analgesia or delivery of different classes of analgesics will result in effective pain relief by synergistic or additive effect with reduced incidence of side effects.[19]

Nonsteroidal Anti-inflammatory Drugs

Nonsteroidal anti-inflammatory drugs (NSAIDs) produce their effect by inhibiting the prostaglandin synthesis and releasing at the level of cyclooxygenase. These drugs have proven efficacy as the sole analgesic agent for management of mild to moderate pain in minor surgical procedures.

TABLE 42-1 **Patient-Controlled Analgesia (PCA) Suggested Dosing**

	PCA Dose	Lockout Time	1-Hour Limit	Basal Rate†
Morphine 1 mg/mL	0.5–3 mg	5–10 minutes	10–20 minutes	0.5–2 mg/1 h
Hydromorphone 0.2 mg/mL	0.1–0.5 mg	5–10 minutes	1–2 mg	0.1–0.2 mg/h
Fentanyl	25–50 μg	5–10 minutes	250 μg	25–50 μg/h
Meperidine 10 mg/mL	10–20 mg	5–10 minutes	100 mg*	100–200 mg/h

*Toxic metabolite normeperidine may accumulate rapidly if patient is getting more than 1000 mg/day.

†Basal rates should not be used routinely and can be reserved for nighttime when indicated.

TABLE 42-2 **Epidural Catheter Insertion Site**

Cord Segment	Target For	Central Bony Location	Landmark
Upper Thoracic Cord	Thorocotomy	T3	Root of scapular spine
Lower Thoracic Cord	Upper abdominal surgery	T6	Scapular tip
Lumbo Sacral Cord	Lower abdominal surgery	T11–12	12th Rib
	Lower extremity surgery above the knee	L1–L2	12th Rib
	Perineal surgery	L3–L4	Tuffier's line L4–L5
	Lower extremity surgery below the knee	L3–L4 L4–L5	Tuffier's line L4–L5

Ketorolac, the only parenteral NSAID presently available, is a nonspecific inhibitor of both cyclooxygenase isoenzymes (COX-1 and COX-2). The COX-1 isoenzyme is normally found in blood vessels, platelets, the gastrointestinal tract, and the kidney. On the other hand, the COX-2 isoenzyme is induced by inflammation in peripheral tissues. The inhibition of the COX-1 isoenzyme is responsible for the gastric and renal side effects of NSAIDs and for its inhibitory effect on platelet function.[20,21]

One should be cautious when using NSAIDs in the immediate postoperative period, taking into consideration such risk factors as a history of bleeding peptic ulcers, volume depletion (for NSAID-induced acute renal failure), especially in elderly patients, or when the risk of hemorrhage is considerable and the surgical site involves the airway. The usual dose of ketorolac is 15 mg intravenously every 6 hours for 24 to 48 hours. COX-2 inhibitors appear to be safer but parenteral forms of these molecules are not yet available.

Analgesic Adjuvants

Other classes of drugs may enhance the effects of opioids or may have independent analgesic effects. Most of these drugs are not available in parenteral forms and are usually reserved for patients not responding to more routine therapies. The addition of an alpha$_2$ agonist may be beneficial and opioid sparing. Clonidine, dexmedetomidine, and tizanidine are representative of that class but only clonidine is Federal Drug Administration (FDA) approved and may contribute to hypotension in the perioperative period.

Antihyperalgesic drugs, which block the effect of the transmitter release, include nitric oxide synthetase inhibitors and NMDA receptor blockers. There is no available pure nitric oxide synthetase inhibitor. However, there is some evidence that acetaminophen exerts its action by inhibition of nitric oxide production. For this reason, acetaminophen administered around the clock in the immediate postoperative period may be very useful. Proparecetamol, the precursor of acetaminophen, is being clinically investigated in a parenteral form. Otherwise, acetaminophen is available orally (pill form and elixir) and rectally. The only concern may be that acetaminophen, because of its antipyretic properties, will mask febrile states in the immediate postoperative period.

Dextrometorphan is the most readily available NMDA blocker, although it is often in combination with other drugs such as cough suppressants.[22] The clinically useful dose appears to be 30 to 60 mg every 4 to 6 hours. Ketamine in low doses (up to 10 mg per hour intravenously) may also be a useful NMDA blocker for postoperative pain.[23]

NEURAXIAL OPIOIDS AND LOCAL ANESTHETICS

These agents can be provided by the epidural or intrathecal route. Of these, the epidural catheter infusion is the most commonly used method and, recently, a cumulative meta-analysis of various postoperative therapies shows that epidural opioids and epidural local anesthetics with or without opioids decreased the incidence of pulmonary complications as opposed to systemic opioids. Epidural analgesia is also associated with a lower incidence of cardiovascular events and provides a decreased stress response to surgery, earlier ambulation, rapid return of bowel function, shortened hospitalization, reduced costs and, overall, a lower mortality.

Large surveys show that the most effective placement of the epidural catheter for infusion of local anesthetic (bupivacaine or ropivacaine in dilute concentration) with a lipophilic opioid such as fentanyl is the upper thoracic region (T3) for thoracic surgery, the mid-thoracic region (T6) for upper abdominal surgery, and the lower thoracic region (T9) for lower abdominal surgery (Table 42-2).

The amount of opioids needed by the neuraxial route to provide effective analgesia is less than by the systemic route, especially when combined with local anesthetics. This is definitely the case with morphine, and to a lesser degree with fentanyl and hydromorphone, but systemic side effects of opioids may be less frequent.

When using a combination of local anesthetic and opioids, an infusion technique is required. The advantages of the combination are a synergistic effect with lower opioid doses and overall fewer side effects. However, with an infusion technique there is a risk of local anesthetic toxicity, a risk for catheter migration, potential sympathetic block, and orthostatic hypotension (Table 42-3).[24–26]

A large recent study shows an incidence of respiratory depression of 0.07%, nausea and vomiting 22%, and pruritus 22%. An-

TABLE 42-3 **Epidural Local Anesthetic and/or Opioid**

Local Anesthetic		Opioid
Bupivacaine	0.0625%–0.125%	Morphine 25 to 50 mg/mL
Ropivacaine	0.05%–0.2%	Hydromorphone 3 to 13 mg/mL Fetanyl 1 to 10 μg/mL

Usual rate 4 to 16 mL/h.

other equally large study showed an overall rate of complications of 3% associated with the placement of thoracic epidural catheters. The complications included dural perforation (0.7%), unsuccessful catheter placement (1.1%), postoperative radicular type of pain (0.2%), responsive to catheter withdrawal in all cases, and peripheral nerve lesions (0.6%), 0.3% of which were peroneal nerve palsies probably related to surgical positioning and other transient peripheral nerve lesions (0.2%).[27]

Coagulopathy and systemic infection associated with bacteremia are definite contraindications to neuraxial techniques.

Anticoagulation is a relative contraindication. The American Society of Regional Anesthesia recently published a concern statement on neuraxial anesthesia and anticoagulation.[27] For postoperative analgesia, the timing of the epidural catheter removal is important since most case reports of epidural hematomas have been documented on removal of the epidural catheter.

Patients receiving low-dose warfarin therapy during epidural analgesia should have their prothrombin time and internationalized normalized ratio (INR) monitored on a daily basis, and checked before catheter removal, if the initial dose was >36 hours before. Initial studies evaluating the safety of epidural analgesia in association with oral anticoagulation utilizing low-dose warfarin may require more intensive monitoring of the coagulation status.

Neurologic testing of sensory and motor function should be performed routinely on patients on anticoagulation with epidural analgesia and continued for at least 24 hours after.

An INR >3 should prompt the physician to withhold or reduce warfarin dose in patients with indwelling neuraxial catheters.

The use of antiplatelet drugs alone does not create a level of risk that will interfere with the performance of neuraxial blockade. When used in combination with other anticoagulant regimens, there may be an increased chance of hematoma formation.

It is recommended that indwelling catheters be removed prior to initiation of low-molecular-weight heparin thromboprophylaxis. If a continuous technique is selected, the epidural catheter may be left indwelling overnight and removed the following day, with the first dose of low-molecular-weight heparin administered 2 hours after the catheter removal.

For any low-molecular-weight heparin prophylaxis regimen, catheter removal should be delayed for at least 10 to 12 hours after a dose of low-molecular-weight heparin.

A single intrathecal opioid injection can also be used either alone or in combination with epidural infusion and other methods for pain control. However, the pain relief achieved with this method usually is not longer than 12 to 18 hours and the need for monitoring for possible respiratory depression is the same as for epidural opioid administration.[28]

With the use of neuraxial opioids, it is paramount to adequately educate the nursing and support staff to the monitoring and possible side effects of the techniques. Policies and protocols need to be in place to ensure patient safety, and it has been demonstrated that an organized acute pain service provided superior postoperative analgesia care compared to standard delivery of analgesics.

REGIONAL ANESTHESIA TECHNIQUES

Interpleural Analgesia

Interpleural analgesia (IPA) has been well studied for its use in providing postoperative analgesia. IPA may also be utilized for analgesia in trauma victims with multiple rib fractures. The major mechanism of action of IPA is thought to be local anesthetic diffusion through the parietal pleura, which yields multiple segmental intercostals nerve blocks. The efficacy of IPA has been variable and factors, which may be partially related to affecting efficacy include: catheter position; presence of blood/clot; infection; scar adhesions fibrosis; presence of thoracostomy drainage tubes; and abnormal distribution of local anesthetic possibly secondary to altered lung mechanics (e.g., postsurgery).

IPA may be administered via:

1. Surgical placement of a catheter under direct vision
2. Percutaneous insertion of an interpleural catheter
3. Injection through a double-lumen chest tube.

If there is no chest tube on continuous suction present, the catheter may be bloused with 0.4 mL/kg of 0.5% bupivacaine with 1:200,000 epinephrine, followed by a continuous infusion of 0.125 mL/kg/h of 0.25% bupivacaine. If a chest tube on continuous suction is present, the chest tube should be clamped for about 30 minutes following an interpleural bolus (assuming that there is no surgical contraindication for clamping the chest tube for that period of time). Bupivacaine 0.5% with 1:200,000 epinephrine may be bloused interpleurally every 6 hours (or, alternatively, lidocaine or ropivacaine).

There are multiple possible contraindications of interpleural analgesia but the major ones include positive end-expiratory pressure, pleuritis, pleural fibrosis/adhesions, pleural effusion pneumonothorax, bullous emphysema, recent pulmonary infection, local anesthetic allergy, and infection at the insertion site/bleeding diathesis (especially if percutaneous placement is planned). Advantages of IPA include surgical placement under direct vision is less operator-dependent than epidural placement; the catheter can be "transduced" to confirm "interpleural" placement, and it avoids potential epidural hematoma/abcess. Although there are multiple complications of IPA, the major ones include local anesthetic toxicity, pneumothorax, Horner's syndrome, allergic reaction, shoulder pain, bronchopleural fistula, and intrapulmonary injection.[29,30]

Femoral Nerve Analgesia

Femoral nerve analgesia (FNA) is a technique that may be utilized as a potentially useful adjunct to opioids and other acute pain analgesic regimens. FNA has been used for analgesia in patients with femoral shaft fracture and various knee surgeries for postoperative analgesia. FNA is generally administered using 0.25% bupivacaine by continuous infusion 7 to 10 mL per hour. Potential advantages of FNA include decreased quadriceps muscle spasm/splinting and diminished opioid usage. A pitfall of the technique is that it is only effective for the anterior aspects of the knee; the sciatic nerve supplies the posterior aspects of the knee joint.

Many other techniques have been utilized for acute pain management, including continuous intercostal nerve block, continuous thoracic paravertebral block, and continuous brachial plexus catheter techniques.[29,30] Although some of these techniques can be extremely useful (especially in certain circumstances), most continuous catheter techniques remain underutilized, potentially because of fears of complications, unfamiliarity, time constraints, and possibly reimbursement issues.

For both PCA and epidural analgesia, standard orders for monitoring and for medications such as antiemetics (e.g., droperidol), anti-pruritus agents (e.g., diphenlydromine), as well as orders for small titrations greatly facilitate the delivery of postoperative care (See Appendix A).

Nonpharmacologic methods of pain management and stimulation-induced analgesia can be used in the postoperative period with either acupuncture or TENS. With TENS, a small electrical current presumably stimulates the touch pressure and proprioception fiber (A-β) to release endogenous opiates and closes the "gate" of pain transmission at the spinal level. The TENS technique is considered safe but does not reliably provide analgesia in all cases. It is best used for amputations, back surgery, and postcesarian sections. Sterile electrodes are available to be placed close to surgical sites. TENS is contraindicated for patients with demand pacemakers and may interfere with electrocardiogram monitoring.

Behavioral techniques such as relaxation therapy and hypnosis have also been successfully used in the treatment of postoperative pain, but these techniques require postoperative preparation and motivation on the part of the patient to be effective in the immediate postoperative period.

REFERENCES

1. Sinatra RS. Acute pain management and acute pain services. In: Cousins MJ, Bridenbaugh PO, eds. *Neural Blockade in Clinical Anesthesia and Management of Pain.* 2nd ed. Philadelphia, Pa: Lippincott-Raven, 1988:793–836.
2. Acute Pain Management Guidelines Panel. *Acute Pain Management: Operative or Medical Procedures and Trauma. Clinical Practice Guideline.* Rockville, Md: US Dept of Health and Human Services, Agency for Health Care Policy and Research; 1992. AHCPR publication 92-0032.
3. Practice Guidelines for Acute Pain Management in the Perioperative Setting. ASA Task Force on Pain Management. *Anesthesiology* 1995; 82:1071.
4. Cohen FL. Postsurgical pain relief: patient status and nurses' medication choices. *Pain* 1980;9:265.
5. Houck C, Berde C, Anand K. Pediatric pain management. In: Gregory G, ed. *Pediatric Anesthesia* New York, NY: Churchill Livingstone, 1994:743–771.
6. Marks RM, Sachar EJ. Undertreatment of medical inpatients with narcotic analgesics. *Ann Intern Med* 1973:78:173.
7. Woolf CJ, Chong M. Preemptive analgesia – treating postoperative pain by preventing the establishment of central sensitization. *Anesth Analg* 1993;77:362.
8. Kehlet H. Modification responses to surgery by neural blockade. In: Cousins MJ, Bridenbaugh PO, eds. *Neural Blockade in Clinical Anesthesia and Management of Pain.* 2nd ed. Philadelphia, Pa: Lippincott-Raven, 1998:129–175.
9. Basbaum AI. Spinal mechanisms of acute and persistent pain. *Reg Anesth Pain Med* 1999;24:59.
10. Ballantyne JC, Carr DB, deFerranti S, et al. The comparative effects of postoperative analgesic therapies on pulmonary outcome: cumulative meta-analysis of randomized, controlled trials. *Anesth Analg* 1998; 86:598.
11. Bardram L, Funch-Jensen P, Jensen P, et al. Recovery after laparoscopic surgery with epidural analgesia, and early oral nutrition and mobilization. *Lancet* 1995;345:763.
12. Kehlet H. Acute pain control and accelerated postoperative surgical recovery. *Surg Clin North Am.* 1999;79:431–443.
13. Carr DB, Saini, V, Verrier RL. Opioids and cardiovascular function: neuromodulation of ventricular ectopy. In: Inkelburtus HE, Francle G, eds. *Neurocardiology.* New York, NY: Futura, 1980:223.
14. Randall DC. Plasticity of the unconditioned response: evidence linking pain and cardiovascular regulation. *J Cardiovasc Electrophys* 1991; (suppl 2):576.
15. Dantzer R, Kelly KW. Stress and immunity: an integrated view of the relationship between the brain and the immune system. *Life Science* 1998;44:1995.
16. Liebeskind JC. *Pain can kill* [editorial]. *Pain* 1991;44:3.
17. Kehlet H. Multimodal approach to control postoperative pathophysiology and rehabilitation. *Br J Anaesth* 1997;78:606.
18. Ballantyne JC, Carr DB, Chalmers TC, et al. Postoperative patient-controlled analgesia: meta-analyses of initial randomized control trials. *J Clin Anesth* 1993;5:182.
19. Power I, Barratt S. Analgesic agents for the postoperative period. *Surg Clin North Am* 1999;79:275–295.
20. Shen Q, et al. Preoperative rofecoxib 25 mg and 50 mg: effects on postsurgical morphine consumption and effort-dependent pain. *Anesthesiology* 2001; 95:A961.
21. Camu F, Beecher T, Recker DP, Verburg KM. Valdecoxib, a COX-2 specific inhibitor, is an efficacious, opioid-sparing analgesic in patients undergoing hip arthroplasty. *Am J Therap* 2002;9:43.
22. Grace RF, Power I, Umedaly H, et al. Preoperative dextromethorphan reduces intraoperative but not postoperative morphine requirements after laparotomy. *Anesth Analg* 1998;87:1135.
23. Kohrs R, Durieux ME. Ketamine: teaching an old drug new tricks. *Anesth Analg* 1998; 87:1186.
24. Yeager MP, Glass DD, Neff RK, Brinck-Johnsen T. The safety and efficacy of intrathecal opioid analgesia for acute postoperative pain: seven years' experience with 5969 surgical patients at Indiana University Hospital. *Anesth Analg* 1999;88:599.
24. Liu S, Carpenter RL, Neal JM. Epidural anesthesia and analgesia. *Anesthesiology* 1995;76:342.
25. Bylon JF, Katz J, Kavanagh BP, et al. Epidural bupivacaine-morphine analgesia versus patient-controlled analgesia following abdominal aortic surgery. *Anesthesiology* 1998;89:585.
26. Wang, LP, Hauerberg J, Schmidt JF. Incidence of spinal epidural abscess after epidural analgesia. *Anesthesiology* 1999;91:1928–1936.
27. Consensus on anticoagulation and neuraxial anesthesia. American Society of Regional Anesthesia and Pain Medicine. Available at *http://www.asra.com*
28. Ready LB. Acute perioperative pain. In: Miller RD, ed. *Anesthesia.* Philadelphia, Pa: Churchill Livingstone, 2000;2323–2350.
29. Reiestad F, Stromskag KE. Interpleural catheter in management of postoperative pain. *Reg Anesth* 1986;11:89.
30. Sinatra RS. Acute pain management and acute pain services. In: Cousins MJ, Bridenbaugh PO, eds. *Neural Blockade in Clinical Anesthesia and Management of Pain.* 2nd ed. Philadelphia, Pa: Lippincott-Raven, 1998:793–836.

CHAPTER 43 ASSESSMENT AND TREATMENT OF PAIN IN SPORTS INJURIES

Joseph Audette and Walter Frontera

OVERVIEW

As our knowledge increases regarding the health benefits of exercise, more and more people attempt to stay healthy and physically fit with sports-related activities. As a result, sports injuries are no longer confined to a small group of competitive athletes but affect an ever-growing segment of the population. Improper training techniques, over-ambitious routines, and the use of faulty equipment have led to an increase in sports injuries (especially overuse injuries) and resultant pain syndromes. In the pediatric population, younger and younger children engage in highly competitive sports with training schedules that put them at increased risk for injury. Elite athletes, under the pressure of commercial interests and more widely disseminated knowledge about exercise physiology and training methods, are driven to greater extremes in order to gain small but significant advantages over the competition. This has led to overambitious workouts with inadequate rest periods. Many athletes suffer from chronic pain and injury as a result.

This chapter presents a brief review of the essential elements of bone, joint, tendon, ligament, and muscle physiology to lay the foundation for understanding both acute and repetitive stress injuries that are commonly seen in athletics. We then give an overview of treatment strategies for both acute and more chronic pain syndromes.

BASIC PHYSIOLOGY

Bone

Bone is composed of organic proteins, matrix, and cells. The organic component of bone is 90% collagen type I and provides the tensile strength. The mineral phase of bone matrix accounts for 50% of the volume and 65% of the weight of bone and is composed of highly structured hydroxyapatite crystals and amorphous calcium phosphates. Bone cells account for only 3% of bone volume and include osteoblasts, osteoclasts, and osteocytes. Bone remodeling is ongoing throughout life and occurs predominantly at the trabecular part of the skeleton. Wolff's law of adaptation states that mechanical remodeling of bone occurs in response to deforming strain. Both osteoblasts (responsible for erosion of existing bone) and osteoclasts (responsible for repair and remodeling of erosions) are involved. The exact mechanism of how mechanical strain activates osteocytes to initiate remodeling is still unknown, but both chemical messengers (dependent on the prostaglandins PGI_2 and PGE_2, IGF-1, and parathyroid hormone) and piezoelectric effects are believed to be involved.[1]

High levels of physical activity and stress loading in athletes increase bone density. The degree of increase in bone density is proportional to the level of stress loading accomplished in the athletic activity. For example, the bone mineral density (BMD) of the distal femur is found to be highest in world-class weightlifters followed by throwers, runners, soccer players, and then swimmers. This positive effect on BMD from mechanical loading is also observed in young women skaters and may counter the adverse estrogen-deficient effects on bone density seen in woman who are thin and amenorrheic.

Studies on both the elderly and young confirm that strength training at higher loads increases BMD more when compared with endurance training at low weights with high repetitions.[2]

Joints

Diarthrodial or synovial joints are capable of large degrees of motion and, under normal circumstances, tolerate high levels of friction, shear, and wear with little deterioration throughout a normal life span. A typical knee or hip joint may withstand loads up to six times body weight on a repetitive basis for up to a million times a year.[3] Synovial fluid and soft connective tissue are common to all diarthrodial joints. The soft connective tissue includes the articular cartilage, joint capsule, meniscal cartilage, and ligaments. The primary load-bearing structure of the joint is the articular cartilage. Cartilage is primarily made up of type II collagen with up to 150 proteoglycan (PG) monomers linked to a central core of hyaluronic acid (Fig. 43-1). The link between PG and hyaluronic acid is essential for the structural integrity of cartilage. These macromolecules are highly hydrophylic, but, because they are confined in the semirigid collagen matrix, reach only 20% of their theoretical swell volume. The swelling pressure caused by the embedded PG is resisted by the tension that develops in the collagen matrix, and it is this balance of forces that is essential for modulating the compressibility of the structure under various loads.

Immobilization of a joint for prolonged periods causes significant loss of PGs in the cartilage, which in turn causes a loss of resistance to compression. In the recovery process after injury, both joint range of motion and stress loading is necessary to reverse the above changes.

Tendons and Ligaments

Tendons and ligaments are made up of highly organized collagen fibers (predominantly type I) arranged in a linear fashion. Tendons transmit the force generated by muscle actions to bones and generate movement about a joint. Ligaments are capsular if they extend off of the joint capsule, or accessory when extending between bones. In contrast to tendons, ligaments prevent excessive movement and contribute to joint stability. Both tendons and ligaments are made up of collagen fascicles that spiral on each other with successive folds or crimps that permit stretch and buffer elongation. The blood supply to tendons and ligaments is sparse when compared with joints, muscle, and bone. For example, avascular regions are found in the central region of the anterior cruciate ligament of the knee and the supraspinatus tendon of the shoulder.

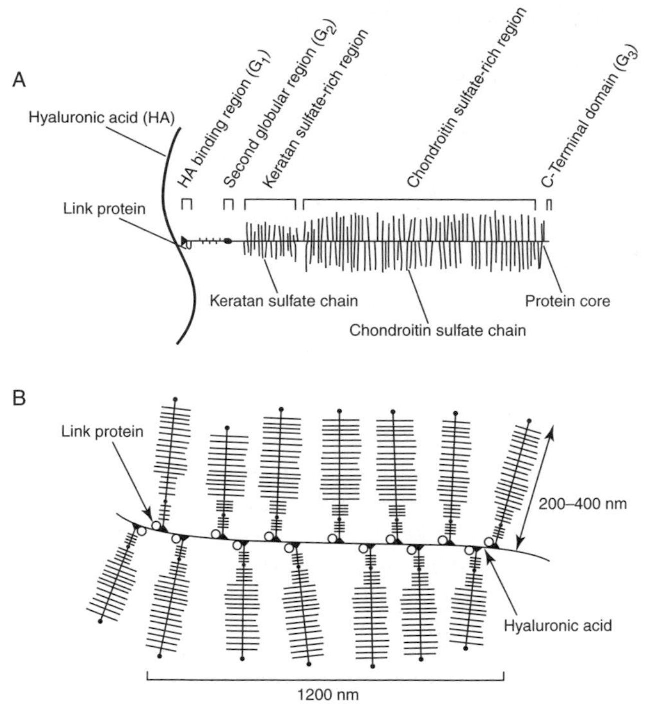

Figure 43-1 **(A)** Schematic depiction of the molecular arrangement of the PG monomer. **(B)** The PG aggregates along a hyaluronate chain. (From Zimmerman JR, et al. In: Downey JA, Myers SJ, et al, eds. *The Physiological Basis of Rehabilitation Medicine.* 2nd ed. Boston, Mass: Butterworth-Heinemann, 1994.)

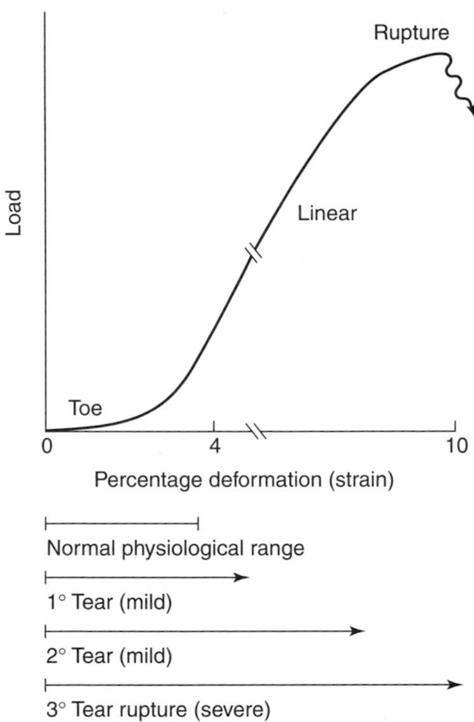

Figure 43-2 Load-deformation (strain) curve for ligaments and tendons. The "toe" region of the curve is within the normal physiologic range. Greater than 4% strain causes tissue damage. (From Oakes BW. Tendon/ligament basic science. In: Harries M, Williams C, et al. *Oxford Textbook of Sports Medicine.* 2nd ed. Oxford, England: Oxford University Press, 1998.)

Tendons are often surrounded by synovial sheaths when there is a significant pulley action present (e.g., the digit flexor tendons of the hand). At the junction with the bone, or enthesis, small synovial bursa are often present to prevent friction (e.g., greater trochanter bursa, retrocalcaneal bursa, and subacromial bursa).

Golgi and Pancinian organs lie at the myotendinous junction and transmit information to the central nervous system about muscle tension and pressure. Tendons demonstrate nonlinear deformation in response to stress. In the first phase, collagen fibers straighten and elastic fibers elongate. The second phase requires much greater force, and is characterized by breaking of collagen cross-links and disruption of smaller collagen fibers. Finally, increased forces will result in tendon rupture and failure occurs when a tendon is stretched 5% to 8% beyond its resting length (Fig. 43-2).

Changes in activity significantly affect tendons and ligaments. Physical training increases the weight and size of tendons and ligaments and increases the cross-links between collagen fibers. Immobilization decreases these cross-links and thus diminishes the tensile strength.

Muscle

Skeletal muscle makes up approximately 40% to 45% of the total body weight. There are two major types of muscle fibers (type I and II), which were originally identified with basic histochemical staining techniques (Fig. 43-3). These staining differences correlate with underlying differences in structural, contractile, and biochemical properties. Subtypes of type I and II have been characterized as well, and Table 43-1 summarizes the differences among fiber types.

The response of muscle to changes in levels of physical activity can be profound. There are two basic forms of muscle actions: static (or isometric), in which there is no joint movement, and dynamic in which there is a change in the length of the muscle and joint movement occurs. Dynamic actions can be further divided into concentric, in which the muscle shortens during the increased load (triceps in a shotput hurl), and eccentric, in which the mus-

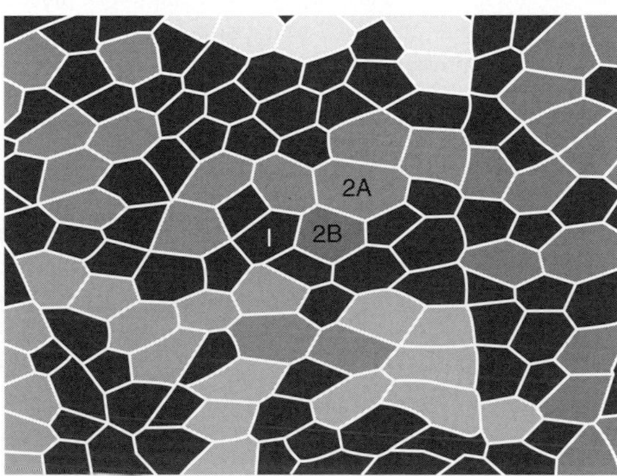

Figure 43-3 Photomicrograph of vastus lateralis from a 21-year-old man stained for ATPase at pH 4.6 showing type I, type IIA, and type IIB fibers. (From Lieberman JS, et al. Skeletal muscle: structure, chemistry, and function. In: Downey JA, Myers SJ, et al, eds. *The Physiological Basis of Rehabilitation Medicine.* 2nd ed. Boston, Mass: Butterworth-Heinemann, 1994: 88.)

TABLE 43-1 **Muscle Fiber Type Classification**

	Type I	Type IIA	Type IIB
Glycogen Content	Low	High	High
Mitochondria	Many	Many	Few
Oxidative Enzymes	High	Intermediate	Low
Contraction Speed	Slow	Fast	Fast
Fatigue Resistance	High	High	Low
Aerobic Capacity	High	Medium	Low
Anaerobic Capacity	Low	Medium	High
Strength	Low	High	High

cle lengthens during the increased load (quadriceps when landing from a jump). Eccentric actions have lower energy requirements but carry an increased risk of muscle damage and tearing due to higher forces.

Increases in muscle mass with resistance training are primarily brought about by type II fiber hypertrophy (with a contribution from type I hypertrophy) rather than by muscle fiber proliferation. It has been found in animal models that repetitive stretching of muscle fibers alone is sufficient to cause massive increases in gene expression of contractile proteins causing muscle hypertrophy. The resistance to fatigue that develops with endurance training results from a number of factors including increases in capillary supply and mitochondrial content (i.e., increase in oxidative capacity) of the muscle fibers and metabolic adaptations favoring fat metabolism and glycogen sparing. It is still a contested question whether transformation of fiber types contributes to the adaptation of muscle to various training stimuli. The predominance of type I fibers in distance runners probably results from genetic influences, environmental factors such as training, and the interaction between the two. Some studies have shown changes in type IIB to type I with high-intensity interval training, but others did not show such changes or have only shown a shift from type IIB to type IIA with endurance training. In disuse atrophy, the reduction of muscle bulk can be profound, with up to 30% reduction in cross-sectional area after 1 month of immobilization. Both type I and II fibers are reduced in size to varying degrees depending on the individual.[4]

Aging alone has been thought to lead to the loss of muscle mass and strength. There is a loss of both cross-sectional area and total number of muscle fibers with age, predominantly affecting type II. This loss in muscle mass coincides with loss of bone density. However, recent studies have supported that many of the changes seen are not inevitable but are the result of decreased activity. The positive training effects seen on muscles in the young also occur in the elderly. Even in the 10th decade of life, an elderly person can make significant increases in muscle mass and strength if given a progressive resistance-training program. Similar positive changes in muscle respiratory capacity seen in the young can occur with endurance training in the elderly.[5]

Finally, the central nervous system also changes with training. This is evidenced by the marked improvement in performance that can occur with training in a specific activity over time, with much less dramatic changes in peripheral muscle strength. For example, during a 12-week period of training that included lifting boxes from the floor to the waist by knee extension, a 200% increase in weight was achieved with only a 15% increase in absolute isometric strength of the quadriceps muscle group. Also, the untrained contralateral limb will show an improvement in performance when the ipsilateral limb is repetitively trained, suggesting that the central mechanism plays a role. These changes are felt to result from neural adaptations including synchronization of motor units in the trained activity with a more advantageous balance of agonist versus antagonist muscle activation.[2]

INJURY IN SPORTS

Injuries in sports can be caused by a sudden overload to structural components of the bones, joints, and soft tissue or from chronic overuse. The forces that various structures must withstand during athletic activity are enormous. For example, a runner weighing 165 pounds will absorb a total of nearly 500,000 pounds of force on each foot during a 1.6-km run. There are various extrinsic and intrinsic factors that influence the type and severity of injury listed in Table 43-2. In the majority of injuries that are not traumatic, there has usually been a sudden change in the training routine that underlies the onset of pain. Typically, either there was a recent initiation of a new sport activity or there was a recent marked increase in training load involving changes in frequency, duration, and intensity.

Bone and Joint

Bone injury can occur with the extremes of repetitive forces seen in athletics and is characterized by the formation of stress fractures. The incidence of stress fractures in athletic populations of men is approximately 2% and of woman from 3.8% to 10%. Up to 49% of woman track runners with fewer than five menstrual periods a year develop stress fractures, suggesting that a hypoestrogenic state increases the risk. In runners, stress fractures account for nearly 25% of all injuries.[6] Stress fractures are seen more commonly in different bones depending on the athletic endeavor[7] (Table 43-3).

The most common joints injured in sports are the shoulder and the knee. The shoulder is the most unstable joint in the body and depends almost exclusively on ligaments and the tendons of the intrinsic muscles to maintain a balance between the extremes of range of motion and stability. As a result, these ligamentous and tendinous structures are commonly injured in sports where this tenuous balance is tested to achieve optimal performance. Both acute and chronic repetitive injuries are seen. Table 43-4 lists some less common shoulder injuries in the athletic population.[8]

TABLE 43-2 **Factors that Influence Injuries in Healthy Athletes**

Extrinsic Factors	Intrinsic Factors
Excessive Loads	Structural Malalignment
Training Errors	Muscle Weakness/Imbalances
Adverse Environment (such as training surface)	Decreased Flexibility
Poor Equipment	Joint Laxity
Sport Rules	Gender/Age

TABLE 43-3 **Stress Fracture Sites**

Fracture Site	Return to Sport	Comments
Lower Extremity		
Femoral Neck	7 to 12 weeks	High incidence of late nonunions and avascular necrosis. Surgical management often necessary.
Femoral Shaft	8 to 14 weeks	Vague thigh or groin pain often only clue.
Tibia	Prolonged	Common in runners, dancers, and jumping sports. Casting may be necessary. Most common stress fracture in LE.
Fibula	6 weeks	Differential includes compartment syndrome and peroneal nerve entrapment.
Tarsal Navicular	16 to 20 weeks	Commonly missed. 6 weeks of casting, followed by semirigid shoe with medical arch necessary.
Metatarsal	4 to 6 weeks	March fracture. 2nd and 3rd rays most common. Rigid shoe recommended to promote healing.
Upper Extremity		
Ribs	6 to 8 weeks	Rare. Seen in rowers, baseball players.
Clavicle	8 weeks	Rare. Found typically with throwing activity.
Scapula	6 to 8 weeks	Rare. Intense weightlifting is common etiology.
Humerus	10 to 16 weeks	Seen in adolescent athletes.
Olecranon	8 to 12 weeks	Seen in throwers and gymnasts.
Ulna	4 to 6 weeks	More common. Seen in a variety of sports.
Radius	12 to 16 weeks	Commonly seen in gymnasts.
Metacarpals	4 weeks	Tennis racquet gripping or ball gripping underlie injuries.

From Brukner P. Stress fractures of the upper limb. Sports Med 1998;26:415.
LE denotes lower extremity.

The knee is typically injured acutely because of sudden forces that overwhelm the supporting ligaments. Often, if the loads are sufficient to disrupt the relatively tough intrinsic ligaments of the knee, the cartilagenous structures such as the menisci will also be torn. Common causes of knee pain in the athlete include meniscal tears, patellofemoral pain syndrome, ligamentous injuries, patellar tendinitis, and osteochondral injury. In the juvenile population apophysitis of the tibia (Osgood-Schlatter's syndrome) is often seen. Table 43-5 lists some less common injuries to the knee in the athletic population.[9]

TABLE 43-4 **Uncommon Causes of Shoulder Injuries in Athletes**

Causes	Comments
Neurovascular	
Suprascapular Nerve Compression	Commonly due to traction or blunt trauma. Seen in volleyball players.
Long Thoracic Nerve Palsy	Scapular winging due to serratus anterior, weakness.
Axillary Nerve Compression	Seen in throwing athletes.
Spinal Accessory Nerve Injury	Trapezius weakness with shoulder sagging following trauma.
Thoracic Outlet Syndrome	Brachial plexus compression. Often seen after clavicle fracture.
Effort Thrombosis	Axillary vein injury commonly with repetitive throwing.
Soft Tissue	
SLAP lesions	Deceleration injury to anterior glenoid labrum transmitted by biceps.
Posterior-Superior Impingement	Injury to posterior-superior labrum in throwing sports.
Tendon Ruptures	Biceps, pectoralis major, subscapularis, coracobrachialis, and serratus.
Snapping Scapula Syndrome	Usually myofascial in origin.

TABLE 43-5 **Less Common Causes of Knee Injuries in Athletes**

Causes	Comments
Neurovascular	
Saphenous Nerve Entrapment	Fascia of sartorius and vastus medialis 10 cm proximal to medial condyle of femur.
Soft Tissue	
Iliotibial Band Syndrome	Pain at site of friction over lateral femoral condyle, common in runners, cyclists.
Popliteus Tendinitis	Commonly seen with downhill walking or running.
Hoffa's Disease	Infrapatellar fat pad syndrome, injured during repetitive extension.
Semimembranosus Tendinitis	Pain at posteromedial corner of knee, more common with runners.
Pes Anserinus Tendinitis	Common insertion of sartorius, gracilis, and semitendinosus.
Tibial Collateral Ligament Bursitis	Deep to medial collateral ligament, pain without locking or instability to valgus stress.

Spine

Just as in the occupational arena, low back pain (LBP) is common in sports. Pain can develop as a result of any of the causes seen in nonathletes. Of particular interest to adolescent athletes is the development of symptomatic spondylolysis with pars interarticularis defects. Spondylolisthesis can occur with bilateral pars defects. Excessive loading of spinal elements during growth in adolescence is felt to be harmful and puts athletes in this age group at greater risk for developing LBP than sedentary controls. The cumulative prevalence of LBP in juveniles is 30% with only 8% having more chronic or recurrent problems.[10] Among adolescent athletes referred for evaluation of LBP, up to 47% have been found to have spondylolysis. Stress loading in extension and rotation is felt to be particularly problematic, and as a result, there is a higher prevalence of spondylolysis in sports such as soccer, tennis, wrestling, gymnastics, football, volleyball, and rugby. The level most frequently involved is L5 (88.6%) with L4 seen less often.[11] Spina bifida occulta has been found to be more prevalent in patients with spondylolysis.

Soft Tissue

Tendons Tendinitis and muscle strains account for 30% to 50% of all sports injuries. A recent review of the literature on the etiology and treatment of tendinitis suggests that there are few well-controlled prospective studies that can guide care.[12] Nevertheless, some basic concepts are generally accepted. The forces that injure a tendon can be either extrinsic to the tendon itself, causing an impingement on the tendon, or intrinsic, related to excessive stretch forces on the tendon during activity. A common example of an extrinsic tendinitis is *shoulder impingement syndrome*, where there is inadequate space between the humeral head and the acromion for free passage of the rotator cuff tendons during overhead activity (throwing and swimming), leading to direct tendon trauma. Intrinsic tendinitis commonly results from repetitive overuse or sudden excessive loading as is seen with weightlifting. Eccentric loading of the tendon applies greater forces and under many circumstances can be more traumatic. This occurs when the muscle tendon complex is lengthening during an action. An example of acute eccentric loading to the patellar tendon occurs when landing from a jump as the knee bends and the quadriceps muscle lengthens to absorb the shock. In addition, a lengthening of the muscle to maximize force generation briefly precedes most concentric actions. This puts the maximum force on the tendon when the tendon is elongated, potentially causing damage.

Ligaments Ligament injuries, or sprains, commonly occur in the knees and ankles of athletes. The etiology of such injuries is almost always the result of a sudden excessive force on the ligament. Examples include a sudden valgus stress to the knee with a football tackle at the knees causing disruption of the medial collateral ligament, or a sudden change in direction on a tennis court or football field with the foot firmly planted, which can lead to anterior cruciate ligament injury. Joint stability may be significantly impaired with serious ligamentous injury and, if improperly treated, can lead to chronic stresses to the joint and supporting muscles and tendons.

Muscles Muscle injuries occur either from an acute excessive load or from excessive chronic use. Myotendinous failure is a function of the force applied and the strength and level of fatigue of the muscle. The myotendinous junction is highly infolded, increasing the contact surface area by 20 times to provide added strength. As a result, tears occur near but not at the true histologic junction. If severe enough, muscle and tendon tears can occur and be associated with hematomas. Muscles that cross two joints or have a higher percentage of type II fibers are more prone to strain patterns. Examples of such muscles include the hamstrings, rectus femoris, and the gastrocnemius.

Eccentric actions put muscles at greater risk for strain and can cause the disruption of contractile elements at the Z lines. Delayed onset muscle soreness is more common after eccentric loading.[13] This condition usually appears 24 to 48 hours after an exercise bout and is associated with high serum levels of intramuscular enzymes such as creatine kinase.

Other causes of muscle pain in sports include muscular contusions by blunt trauma. Myositis ossificans is a complication of muscle contusion characterized by intramuscular calcifications. Exertional rhabdomyolysis can also occur, with or without direct trauma, and is potentially fatal. Complications include compartment syndrome in the affected limb due to excessive muscle swelling and renal failure.[14] Compartment syndrome can also occur in chronic

TABLE 43-6 **Grading of Acute Ligament Injuries**

Injury Grade	Examination Feature	Comments
I	Applied stress meets with distinct endpoint	Minimal swelling, discomfort, and functional loss
II	Soft endpoint with applied stress	More swelling, ecchymosis, and functional loss (i.e., inability to walk)
III	Lack of distinct endpoint	Other structures often involved (i.e., torn cartilage)

situations and results from repetitive injury to a muscle group, leading to swelling and increased pressures in the muscle with exertion (often seen in the lower extremities of runners).

ASSESSMENT PRINCIPLES

History

Historically, it is important to determine if there has been a recent change in duration, intensity, and frequency of the training regimen. Symptoms usually present approximately 2 to 4 weeks after a training regimen change. In addition, other common risk factors for injury include changes in environment or terrain and changes in equipment such as new running shoes or tennis racquets. The exact mechanism of injury (inversion sprains or decelerating injuries) contributes to establishing a diagnosis. Associated disease states should be looked for, including arthritis, circulation problems, and prior history of injuries. Special considerations for female athletes and athletes in the pediatric and elderly age groups are highlighted later in the chapter.

Examination

When examining an athlete, even with a specific, well-localized pain problem, it is important not to focus too narrowly on the problem. Biomechanical factors that underlie an injury can only be determined by viewing the relationship of the various joints involved at least one level above and below the area of pain, both at rest and dynamically in the sports-related activity. Side-to-side comparisons of muscle strength and mass should be made to get a better understanding of muscle imbalances. In sports that involve the asymmetrical use of an extremity (such as tennis), one should expect to find significant differences, but, in many cases, large differences can be problematic. Strength testing of antagonist and agonist muscle groups (such as hamstrings and quads) should also be made in the injured and noninjured side to help with future training recommendations. Finally, grading of the ligamentous sprains and overuse injuries is important to help with clinical decision making regarding immobilization, rehabilitation, and the need for surgical interventions (Tables 43-6 and 43-7). Assessment of problems in the upper or lower extremities should include a thorough examination of the peripheral vascular and nervous system integrity.

Imaging

In most injuries, imaging can be delayed until treatment response is assessed. Of particular concern in an athletic population is the increased prevalence of stress fractures. Stress fractures can be observed under ideal circumstances as little as 3 weeks and at times up to 3 months after injury with conventional radiology. Initial plain films will be negative up to 67% of the time. Classic findings include periosteal new bone formation with sclerosis and radiolucent lines called DBLs (dreaded black lines) that are transverse cortical striations. The three-phase bone scan is the gold standard with virtually 100% sensitivity, but poor specificity. For example, infection and arthritic conditions will also cause positive findings requiring other tests to provide clinical correlation. Changes in bone scan can be seen as early as 48 to 72 hours after the onset of symptoms and can remain positive for 6 months to 2 years after injury. Only 10% to 25% of bone scan positive stress fractures show evidence of fracture on plain films. By using the technetium 99 methylene diphosphonate three-phase technique (angiogram, blood pool, and delayed image phases), other stress injuries can be observed in addition to stress fractures. For example, stress fractures will be positive in all three phases, whereas medial-tibial stress syndrome (shin splints) will only be positive in the third or delayed image phase. In up to 50% of athletes with positive bone scans, asymptomatic sites of uptake will be seen and are felt to be areas of subclinical bone strain (Table 43-8).[15]

Magnetic resonance imaging (MRI) has excellent sensitivity and superior specificity for bone abnormalities. The advantage over CT scanning is in being able to differentiate between stress fractures and bone tumors or infectious processes. Single photon emission computed tomography (SPECT) is more sensitive for the early detection of spondolytic changes in the spine than bone scan or plain films, but may not be effective for detection 3 months after symptomatic onset.

Imaging of muscles in athletes is rarely indicated. If there is concern over severe muscle tears or soft tissue masses, MRI is the technique of choice, although there is a growing literature about the positive sensitivity and specificity of diagnostic ultrasound in soft tissue injury.[16]

TABLE 43-7 **Grading of Overuse Injuries**

Injury Grade	Symptom	Duration
I	Pain only after activity	2 weeks
II	Pain during and after activity with no functional disability otherwise	More than 2 weeks
III	Pain during and after activities with significant functional limitations	Greater than 6 weeks
IV	Constant pain, unable to train or compete	Impending tissue failure

TABLE 43-8 **Classification of Stress Reactions**

Grade	Nomenclature	Exam	Pain with Activity	Bone Scan	Radiograph
0	Normal remodeling	None	–	+	–
I	Mild stress reaction	Pain with activity	+	+	–
II	Moderate stress reaction	Pain with activity Mild tenderness	+	+	+
III	Severe stress reaction	Pain with activity Marked tenderness Palpable mass	+	+	+
IV	Stress fracture	Rest pain Palpable mass	+	+	+

SPECIAL CONSIDERATIONS

Female Athletes

After puberty, significant differences emerge between male and female athletes. Females maintain a higher percentage of body fat, gain less muscle mass, have lower lung capacities, and lower oxygen-carrying capacity than men. In addition there are biomechanical differences that may put female athletes at more risk for injury. For example, woman have a higher incidence of genu valgus, which can lead to patellar tracking disorders and injury.

Perhaps more important than these differences are the effects that excessive training can have on normal endocrine function in the female population. Recognition of problems related to athletic ammenorrhea has improved among trainers and physicians. Up to 28% of women participating in college varsity athletics will be ammenorrheic. The prevalence increases to 57% in cross-country runners and is high in dancers, swimmers, and cyclists. The most significant physiologic consequence of this is the effect on bone density, and as a result, stress fractures are more common in this group. Special attention must be given to the risk factors for *anorexia athletica,* which can in some cases be fatal[17] (Table 43-9).

Elderly Athletes

Acute injuries are common in the elderly participating actively in sports. The safety margin of an exercise routine is much narrower and puts this population at greater risk. Changes in the cardiovascular and neurologic system will inevitably compromise aerobic capacity and coordination of the athletic elderly and should be taken into account when recommending training regimens. Injury rates vary from 14% to 57% in the athletic elderly in different series. Common sites of injuries involve the shoulder or knee and are often due to preexisting orthopedic problems in those joints. In general, lower extremity injuries are most common.[18]

Muscle strains occur frequently and rupture of muscle and tendons is more likely to occur than in younger populations. Acute injuries related to falls are a common scenario seen in this group. Overuse injuries typically involve tendons and muscles rather than bone, and recovery can be extended up to 2 years in some studies. Stress fractures are rare, but it should be noted that the sensitivity of bone scan may decrease to 80% to 95% in patients older than 65 years of age.

Pediatric Athletes

In children and adolescents, the muscles and tendons are stronger than the bone, and thus bone avulsions are seen more frequently than in adults. The growth plates at the apophyses in the pelvis and hips are particularly at risk and are common sites of acute avulsion. In addition, skeletal immaturity puts the pediatric population at greater risk for stress fractures if overambitious training routines are followed.

Exercise performance is limited compared with adults partly because of lower anaerobic capacity. During exertion, children use more oxygen per kilogram of body weight and thus will experience a higher metabolic cost than adults for an equivalent, absolute

TABLE 43-9 **Diagnostic Criteria for Anorexia Athletica**

Symptom	Absolute Criteria	Relative Criteria
Weight loss > 5% of IBW	+	
Absence of medical or other psychological illness	+	
Excessive fear of being obese	+	
Excessive restriction of food intake	+	
Delayed puberty (>age 16)		
Ammenorrhea or other menstrual dysfunction		+
Distorted body image		+
Use of purging methods (vomiting, diuretics, laxatives)		+
Binge eating		+
Compulsive exercise		

IBW denotes ideal body weight.

TABLE 43-10 **Common Sites of Apophysitis in Pediatric Athletes**

Injury Site	Sport Activity	Comments
Medial Epicondyle Little League Elbow	Throwing sports	Due to repetitive valgus stress
Tibial Tubercle Osgood-Schlatter disease	Football, running, soccer, basketball	Affects 10- to 13-year-olds
Inferior Pole Patella Sinding-Larson-Johansson disease (Jumper's Knee)	Basketball, jumping sports, running	Affects 10- to 12-year-old boys
Iliac Bone	Runing, dancing	Affects 16 year olds
Calcaneous Bone Sever's Disease	Soccer, hockey, basketball	Seen with tight calf muscles

exercise level (i.e., walking at a given speed). The response to strength training in children is also different than in adults. In the prepubescent population, the muscle responds to training with central neurogenic adaptations in firing rate and recruitment, but not by muscle fiber hypertrophy, and increases in lean muscle mass. As a result, aggressive strength training with high weights and low repetitions should not be attempted in this population because it increases the risk of tendon and bone trauma without benefit. However, strength training is safe in children if the program is properly designed and supervised by individuals experienced with this age group. In addition, during growth spurts, the apophyses (the site of tendon insertion into the bone) are particularly at risk for injury and training regimens should be reduced[19] (Table 43-10).

TREATMENT PRINCIPLES

Treatment of injured athletes has three primary goals: (1) control pain and inflammation, (2) restore normal pain-free range of motion, and (3) return individuals to prior levels of strength, endurance, and optimal biomechanical coordination for the sport-specific activity. There have been studies suggesting that highly trained athletes may have a decreased sensitivity to noxious stimuli.[20] Athletes as a group tend to be highly motivated and often overaggressive in the implementation of a treatment plan. Recognition of this phenomenon is important to prevent further injury during the recovery phase. One must also take into account that athletes may not have a normal response to pain during training and fail to appropriately limit activity in response to nociceptive input. There is still debate about the etiology of this phenomenon. Whether training produces sustained effects on raising the pain threshold, or whether competitive athletics preselects individuals with high pain thresholds, not enough is currently known to decide. Clearly, the culture of highly competitive athletics is to endorse the notion that without pain there will be no significant gains made in performance. This can engender repetitive injuries and a balance must be struck between encouraging normal soreness of aggressive conditioning and strengthening routine versus pain caused by a repetitive injury associated with the athletic activity.

Acute Injuries

A useful acronym for managing an acute sports-related injury is RICE: rest, ice, compression, and elevation of the injured part. With grade II or III sprains, appropriate immobilization will be necessary. Treatment can be broken up into three phases for grade I and II injuries: acute, subacute, and chronic. Briefly, in the acute phase, ice should be applied to the inflamed structure for 15 to 20 minutes several times a day with range of motion allowed within the limits of pain. Relative rest is preferred rather than complete lack of activity to avoid severe deconditioning. If the injury involves a weight-bearing structure, crutches should be used when active. This phase can last from a few to several weeks, up to 2 to 5 weeks depending on severity. After the acute inflammatory phase of the injury, ice is not necessary and heat can be applied to improve circulation to the area of injury and can ease stretching of the affected area to prevent dense scar tissue formation in the injured tissue. During this phase, atrophy is prevented with isometric or static muscle actions. Functional electrical stimulation (FES) can also be used to maintain muscle mass. In the subacute phase, gradual increases in range of motion and progressive, active strengthening and endurance training of the involved muscles as well as cardiovascular conditioning should be attempted. Finally in the final phase of rehabilitation, sport-specific training should occur. Initially, training should begin at 25% of the preinjury level and then increase by 10% to 20% each session if no symptoms are provoked during the first two thirds of the training session.[21]

Repetitive Injuries

In repetitive or overuse injuries, correction of underlying external and internal risk factors are essential. In addition to a careful analysis and correction of the biomechanical factors that may underlie the injury, changes in training routines will also have to be made. Treatment must be more cautious than in acute traumatic injuries and is often more prolonged, but many of the same principles of treating acute injuries apply. If there is an acute exacerbation of a chronic problem, ice in the first 48 hours can be helpful to reduce inflammation and swelling. Subsequently, heat is likely to be of more benefit. Initially, flexibility training is more important than is strength training. When strength training is introduced, the focus should be directed at muscle imbalances observed during the examination. When the pain has subsided, eccentric exercises for chronic tendinitis have been found to be extremely effective to increase the strength of the involved structure and can help prevent re-injury.[22]

The treatment of stress fractures is somewhat different from that outlined above for chronic soft tissue injuries. There are two phases to the treatment of stress fractures. Phase I involves modified weight bearing (ADLs allowed but not sports) and time to allow the bone to heal. Active treatment includes use of NSAIDs and ice for pain control (ultrasound is contraindicated), with stretching and cross training to maintain aerobic fitness using a method that avoids stress to the affected limb (upper extremity bicycle if lower extremity is injured). Use of casting or immobilization is not necessary unless there are hormonal or other factors that may lead to late nonunion of the fracture. When the athlete has been pain free for 2 to 3 weeks, percussion tenderness is negative, and plain films show bone healing, phase II can begin. Here the focus is on the gradual reintroduction of sport with a focus on better controlling any biomechanical and training factors that may have led to the original injury.

Stress fractures of the spine are in general more difficult to treat than other bones given the difficulty in isolating the structure for rest. The treatment of spondylolysis of the lumbar spine is focused on limiting extension of the spine to promote healing. If there is a normal plain film but positive bone scan or SPECT, many advocate treatment without bracing of the spine. Mean time for fracture healing is about 7 months. Specific spine stabilization exercises have been shown to be superior to rest and general conditioning exercises.[23] When braces are used after failure of more conservative measures, they must immobilize both the thoracolumbar and the lumbosacral segment. Recommendations are to remain immobilized for 23 to 24 hours a day for up to 6 months. Surgery is needed if this approach fails.[10]

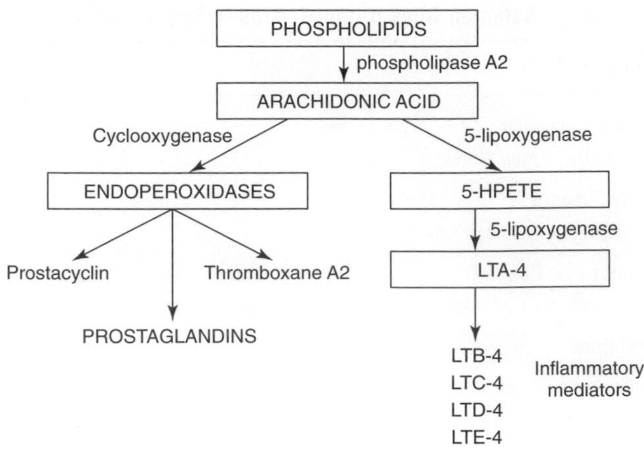

Figure 43-4 The arachidonic acid pathway. (From Stanley KL, et al. Pharmacologic management of pain and inflammation in athletes. *Clin Sports Med* 1998;17:375.)

Medications

The use of medications for controlling pain and inflammation in sports-related injuries is not without controversy. Many injuries seen in sports are associated with swelling and inflammation, and this makes the use of anti-inflammatory medications for pain con-

TABLE 43-11 **Dosage of Currently Available NSAIDs**

Generic Name	Brand Name	Common Unit Dose (mg)	Usual Dosing Frequency
Aspirin		325	Q 2–4 h
Diclofenac	Voltaren	75	BID
Diflunisal	Dolobid	500	BID
Etodolac	Lodine	400	BID
Fenoprofen	Nalfon	600	QID
Flurbiprofen	Ansaid	100	TID
Ibuprofen	Motrin	800	QID
Indomethacin	Indocin	25	TID
Ketoprofen	Orudis	75	TID
Ketorolac	Toradol	10	QID
Meclofenamate	Meclomen	100	TID
Nabumetone	Relafen	500	2 QD
Naproxen	Naprosyn	500	BID
Oxaprozin	Daypro	600	2 QD
Piroxicam	Feldene	20	QD
Salicylsalicylic Acid	Disalcid	750	QID
Sodium Salicylate		650	Q 4 h
Sulindac	Clinoril	200	BID
Tolmetin	Tolectin	400	TID

Modified with permission from Leadbetter WB. Anti-inflammatory therapy in sports injury: the role of nonsteroidal drugs and corticosteroid injection. *Clin Sports Med* 1995;14(2):353.

TABLE 43-12 **Common Sites of Injection in Athletes**

Injection Sites	Needle	Volume (mL)	Comments
Joints			
Ulno-carpal	#25, 1.5 in.	1–3	Steroid volume to anesthetic ratio 1:1
Radiocarpal			
Carpometacarpal			
Elbow	#25, 1.5 in.	2–3	Steroid volume to anesthetic ratio 1:2
Ankle			
Shoulder	#25, 1.5 in.	7–10	Steroid volume to anesthetic ratio 1:6 to 9
Knee			
Sacroiliac Joint			
Bone-Tendon			
Medial/Lateral Epicondyle	#27, 1.25 in.	2–3	Steroid volume to anesthetic ratio 1:1
Plantar Fascia			
Patellar Tendon			
Achilles Tendon			
Pubic Symphysis	#25, 1.5 in.	3–5	Steroid volume to anesthetic ratio 1:2 to 4
Hamstrings			
Adductors			
Tendon Sheaths			
Thumb Extensor	#27, 1.25 in.	1–3	Steroid volume to anesthetic ratio 1:1
Finger Flexors			
Posterior Tibial	#27, 1.25 in.	3–5	Steroid volume to anesthetic ratio 1:2 to 4
Biceps (Long Head)			
Bursae			If aspirating, will need #18–20 needle first.
Prepatellar	#25, 1.5 in.	2–3	Steroid volume to anesthetic ratio 1:1
Pes Anserine			
Olecranon			
Subacromial	#25, 1.5 in.	7–10	Steroid volume to anesthetic ratio 1:6 to 9
Greater Trochanter			
Perineural			
Carpal Tunnel	#27, 1.25 in.	2–5	Steroid volume to anesthetic ratio 2:1
Tarsal Tunnel			
Suprascapular Notch			
Cubital Tunnel			

Use 1% lidocaine or 0.25% bupivicaine with long-acting, insoluble steroids salts such as triamcinalone acetate or betamethasone acetate.

trol an obvious choice. Both nonsteroidal anti-inflammatory medications (NSAIDs) and corticosteroids are known to have suppressive effects on the inflammatory response to injury. Tissue injury causes the release of cell membrane phospholipids, which degrade to arachidonic acid. This in turn leads to a cascade of enzymatic reactions that release pro-inflammatory substances including the prostaglandins, thromboxanes, and leukotrienes (Fig. 43-4). Corticosteroids act early in the cascade to inhibit phospholipase A_2. This limits the production of inflammatory mediators by both the cyclooxygenase and the lipoxygenase pathways and underlies the greater potency of corticosteroids and the adverse effects retarding normal tissue repair. Most NSAIDs inhibit cyclooxygenase (COX-1 and COX-2) nonspecifically, thereby limiting production of both PGE_1 and PGE_2. PGE_1 is a constitutive enzyme involved with normal *housekeeping* activity in the body, including the maintenance of normal renal and gastric function. PGE_2 is an inducible form of the enzyme and is expressed only in inflamed tissue. There has been great interest in the recent marketing of more specific COX-2 inhibitors. It is still unclear whether they will provide any additional safety or benefit when used to control pain and inflammation in sport-related injuries. Both NSAIDs and corticosteroids also have other cellular and noncellular effects on suppressing the response to inflammation.

The controversy with using anti-inflammatory medications revolves around the concern that the inflammatory response to injury is not purely pathologic, and that it is necessary to remove necrotic tissue and disrupted connective tissue from the injured area. Studies of the effects of NSAIDs on tissue repair in an acute muscle strain injury animal model has shown a delay in the degradation of damaged tissue and slowed muscle regeneration. The majority of the evidence also shows that corticosteroids strongly inhibit tendon and ligament healing following injury.

Nevertheless, in a recent review of clinical studies addressing the benefit of short-term use of NSAIDs for sports injuries, modest benefits were seen with slight decreases in pain symptoms, disability, and inflammation. No clinical evidence for delaying healing was found. Generally, short-term use of NSAIDs (3 to 5 days) is recommended to control pain, to assist in the reduction of swelling, and promote early mobilization of the involved structure. Long-term use is not recommended and vastly increases the risk of potentially lethal side effects including gastric and renal compromise. These side effects can be a serious consequence of overuse of these medications in highly trained athletes during the extremes of competition. Anti-inflammatory medications should not be used to mask a persistent pain problem in the athlete because this will promote further injury and does not address the underlying training or biomechanical issues. There has been no well-controlled study to justify the use of steroids in soft tissue injuries. A list of available NSAIDs and dosing frequency can be found in Table 43-11.

Stronger pain medications are generally not encouraged in athletics, and the International Olympic Committee (IOC) bans most of the opioids. Obviously, use of opioid analgesics in an acute traumatic injury may be appropriate, when the pain is severe. However, in the recovery period, strong analgesics should not be used to mask pain while training.

Injection Principles

Appropriate use of injection techniques into joints, tendon sheaths, bursa, muscle trigger points, and other soft tissue structures can be of great benefit both from a diagnostic and therapeutic point of view in the athlete. It is often useful before injecting to have the athlete provoke the pain by performing the activity that induces the discomfort. This can help with localization of the inflamed tissue. If in doubt about the pain generator, it can be useful to inject with local anesthetic alone initially and then try to provoke the pain 10 to 20 minutes later to determine whether the location was accurate before infusing corticosteroid (Table 43-12).

The risk of tendon rupture with repeated steroid injections is real. The maximum load strength of tendons and ligaments after steroid injection has been demonstrated to be reduced in many animal studies. This effect is particularly predominant immediately after injection. Unfortunately, there is a general lack of well-designed clinical studies to guide the safe use of steroids.[24]

A conservative approach would permit only 1 to 2 tendon or tendon sheath injections in 1 year, and some would recommend that no vigorous muscle loading should be performed for at least 2 weeks after injection to avoid complications. Many would advocate, however, never to inject a tendon in an athlete, given the potential for loss in tissue durability. Joints can typically be injected up to 3 times in a year. Bursa can be injected more frequently. With injections into superficial structures such as the epicondyles of the elbow or the pes anserine bursa, avoid depositing the steroid into the skin because this can cause depigmentation. One technique is to pinch the skin and pull away from the deeper structures before inserting the needle to avoid such complications. When injecting into perineural areas such as the carpal tunnel, it is safe to touch the nerve if using a 27-gauge needle and then pull back 1 to 2 mm before injecting. Infection or bleeding can be avoided with proper sterile and hemostatic technique. Other risks of steroid use are summarized in Table 43-13.

TABLE 43-13 **Local and Systemic Complications with Local Injections of Corticosteroids**

Local	Systemic
Subcutaneous Atrophy	Transient hyperglycemia in diabetics
Pigmentation Abnormalities	Vasovagal symptoms with syncope
Tendon/Ligament Rupture	Cognitive affects "steroid psychosis"
Accelerated Joint Destruction	Allergic reactions
Local Sterile Abscess	Systemic infection
Peripheral Nerve Injury	Suppression of pituitary-adrenal axis
Muscle Necrosis/Vascular Injury	Avascular necrosis of hip

CONCLUSIONS

Treating pain syndromes in athletes can often present major challenges. Although the group as a whole is highly motivated, the goals of treatment are often more difficult to attain than in the general population. The athlete does not only want to be pain-free but to be pain-free while performing an extremely stressful activity that requires a high degree of tissue, biomechanical, and psychological integrity. A complex set of intrinsic and extrinsic factors must be taken into account and corrected in order to be successful and prevent chronic re-injury. As a result, a thorough understanding of both the underlying physiology of the structural elements involved as well as the external factors that are often unique to each sport is essential.

REFERENCES

1. Smith EL, Gilligan C. Dose response to mechanical loading. *Bone*. 1996;18(1):45S.
2. Kerr DA, Prince RL, et al. Does high resistance weight training have a greater effect on bone mass than low resistance weight training? *J Bone Miner Res* 1994;9:S152.
3. Zimmerman JR, Mow VC. Physiology of synovial joints and articular cartilage. In: Downey JA, Myers SJ, et al, eds. *The Physiological Basis of Rehabilitation Medicine*. 2nd ed. Boston, Mass: Butterworth-Heinemann, 1994:149.
4. McComas AJ. Human Neuromuscular adaptations that accompany changes in activity. *Med Sci Sports Exerc* 1994;26(12):1498.
5. Kirkendall DT, Garrett WE. The effects of aging and training on the skeletal muscle. *Am J Sports Med* 1998;26(4):598.
6. Fredericson M. Common injuries in runners: diagnosis, rehabilitation, and prevention. *Sports Med* 1996;2:49.
7. Brukner P. Stress fractures of the upper limb. *Sports Med* 1998;26:415.
8. Schulte KR, Warner JJP. Uncommon causes of shoulder pain in the athlete. *Sports Med* 1995;26:505.
9. Safran MR, Fu FH. Uncommon causes of knee pain in the athlete. *Orthop Clin North Am* 1995;26(3):547.
10. Duggleby T, Kumar S. Epidemiology of juvenile low back pain: a review. *Disabil Rehabil* 1997;19(12):505.
11. Micheli LJ, Wood R. Back pain in young athletes. *Arch Pediatr Adolesc Med* 1995;149:15.
12. Almekinders LC, Temple JD. Etiology, diagnosis, and treatment of tendinitis: an analysis of the literature. *Med Sci Sports Exerc* 1998;30(8):1183.
13. Garrett WE. Muscle strain injuries. *Am J Sports Med* 1996;24:S2.

14. Arrington ED, Miller MD. Skeletal muscle injuries. *Sports Med* 1995; 26:411.
15. Monteleon GP. Stress fractures in the athlete. *Orthrop Clin North Am* 1995;26(3):423.
16. El-Khoury GY, Brandser EA, Kathol MH, et al. Imaging of muscle injuries. *Skeletal Radiol* 1996;25(1):3..
17. Beim G, Stone DA. Issues in the female athlete. *Orthop Clin North Am* 1995;26(3):443.
18. Kallinen M, Markku A. Aging, physical activity, and sports injuries. An overview of common sports injuries in the elderly. *Sports Med* 1995;20:41.
19. Cook PC, Leit ME. Issues in the pediatric athlete. *Sports Med* 1995; 26:453.
20. O'Connor PJ, Cook, DB. Exercise and pain: the neurobiology, measurement, and laboratory study of pain in relation to exercise in humans. *Exerc Sport Sci Rev* 1999;27:119.
21. Curwin SL. The aetiology and treatment of tendonitis In: Harries M, Williams C, et al. *Oxford Textbook of Sports Medicine*. 2nd ed. Oxford, England: Oxford University Press, 1998.
22. Renstrom AFH. In: Harries M, Williams C, et al. *Oxford Textbook of Sports Medicine*. 2nd ed. Oxford, England: Oxford University Press, 1998.
23. O'Sullivan PB, et al. Evaluation of specific stabilization exercise in the treatment of chronic low back pain with radiologic diagnosis of spondylolysis or spondylolisthesis. *Spine* 1997;22:2959.
24. Leadbetter WB. Anti-inflammatory therapy in sports injury: the role of nonsteroidal drugs and corticosteroid injection. *Clin Sports Med* 1995; 14(2):353.

CHAPTER 44 CANCER PAIN SYNDROMES

Stuart W. Hough and Ronald M. Kanner

OVERVIEW

Pain in cancer patients has numerous possible causes. The vast majority of pain syndromes are caused by direct tumor involvement of pain-sensitive structures, a smaller number are treatment-related, and fewer than 10% are unrelated to the cancer. Metastatic disease may invade bone, obstruct a hollow viscus, and compress nerve or spinal cord. Radiation treatment may cause fibrosis of nerve or spinal cord. Chemotherapeutic agents may cause peripheral neuropathy, aseptic bone necrosis, and predispose to painful opportunistic infections. Surgical treatment leads to acute postoperative pain, and may cause deafferentation pain if major nerves or nerve plexi are cut. In any given patient, one or more of these factors may be in play, and more than 50% of cancer patients with pain have more than one source of pain.[1]

Primary care physicians and oncologists should be able to recognize and treat most of cancer-related pain. They should be able to initiate treatment for the more common causes with opioids and nonopioid analgesics. More than 70% of patients can be treated effectively with simple analgesics and adjuvant drugs. Effective pain relief, without intolerable side effects, is occasionally difficult to obtain with the use of conventional analgesics. When this occurs, consultation with a specialist in pain management may be necessary.

DIMENSIONS OF THE PROBLEM

Daut and Cleeland found that while 36% of 286 patients with nonmetastatic cancer reported pain, 59% of 381 with metastatic disease did.[2] Cleeland and colleagues found that 67% of 1308 outpatients with metastatic cancer had pain, and 62% of those had severe pain. Thirty-six percent reported disability due to pain, and 42% of those with pain reported inadequate analgesia.[3] Terminal pain, refractory to escalating opioid administration, is a more challenging problem. Depression, uncontrolled pain, the adverse effects of opioids, and fear of pain may precipitate suicidal thoughts or requests for aid in dying.[4,5] Pain also adds to the discomfort experienced by those caring for the dying patient.

The likelihood of pain associated with cancer depends on the type and stage of disease. Foley, in a 1-week survey of 540 patients hospitalized at Memorial Sloan-Kettering Cancer Center, showed that the prevalence of pain requiring analgesic drugs varies by cancer type (Table 44-1).[6] In contrast, among 1308 outpatients with metastatic cancer, Cleeland and colleagues did not find variation in pain prevalence according to cancer type.[3]

THE THREE TYPES OF PAIN

Pain can be divided into three pathophysiologic categories: somatic nociceptive, visceral nociceptive, and neuropathic, on the basis of the inferred mechanisms of pain (See Chapter 3, Pathophysiology of Pain). It is useful to characterize pain in this way, because the approach to treating each type is somewhat different. However, they are not mutually exclusive, and cancer patients, in particular, may have pain with multiple causes. The mechanisms of each type are the subject of considerable ongoing research.

Somatic Nociceptive Pain

This is the typical pain that we all have experienced acutely or chronically: the cutaneous burn and arthritic joint are examples. The painful site is tender and corresponds to the site of tissue damage. Somatic pain is described as constant, and sometimes throbbing or aching. Bone metastases are the most common malignant cause of somatic pain and, in fact, are the most common source of pain in cancer.[7]

Noxious (potentially tissue-damaging) mechanical, thermal, and chemical stimuli trigger nociceptive ischemia, inflammation, and perhaps substances produced by a nearby tumor may sensitize nociceptors to ordinarily non-noxious stimuli. Pain signals are carried by small, myelinated Aδ fibers (mechanical and thermal stimuli) and unmyelinated C fibers (all three stimulus types) to the dorsal horn of the spinal cord. From there, they ascend in the contralateral spinothalamic and spinoreticular tracts to the thalamus and reticular formation, respectively (See Chapter 2, Anatomy and Physiology of Pain). Although most research into nociceptive mechanisms has focused on cutaneous pain, nociceptors exist in most tissues to varying degrees.

Visceral Pain

Pain originating from the viscera is familiar to many of us: abdominal cramps and the pain of passing a renal stone are examples. It may be less constant than somatic pain, occurring in dull, colicky waves. Visceral pain is poorly localized, and often referred to a distant cutaneous site, which may be tender. Unlike somatic pain it is often associated with nausea and diaphoresis. Cancer patients experience primary and referred visceral pain from pancreatic cancer, bowel obstruction, and other causes.

The mechanisms of visceral pain transduction and transmission are not well characterized. Visceral autonomic afferents may by involved.[8] The noxious stimuli required to trigger visceral pain include ischemia, inflammation, torsion, traction, distension, and impaction. In fact, cutting, crushing, and burning may not be felt as painful.[9] Pain referral is poorly understood, but may involve convergent somatic and visceral nociceptive input in the dorsal horn.[10] This hypothesis explains the cutaneous sensation of visceral pain in a dermatome corresponding to the innervation of the affected organ, for example, diaphragmatic irritation felt in the shoulder.

Neuropathic Pain

In everyday life, chronic neuropathic pain is uncommon. However, acute and transient neuropathic pain is felt whenever the "funny bone" is struck, or an extremity "falls asleep" from pressure. Per-

TABLE 44-1 **Prevalence of Pain in Hospitalized Cancer Patients**

Type of Cancer	Patients with Pain (%)
Bone	85
Oral Cavity	80
Male Genitourinary	75
Female Genitourinary	78
Breast	52
Lung	45
Gastrointestinal	40
Lymphoma	20
Leukemia	5

From Foley KM. Pain syndromes in patients with cancer. In: Bonica JJ, Ventafridda B, eds. Advances in Pain Research and Therapy. Vol. 2. New York, NY: Raven Press, 1979:59. Used with permission of Lippincott Williams & Wilkins.

haps the most frequent nonmalignant chronic neuropathic pain is that produced by nerve root compression from a herniated intervertebral disk. Neuropathic pain is often described as prolonged, severe, burning, lancinating, squeezing, and is often associated with focal neurologic deficits. It is usually constant, but may be interrupted by paroxysms of dramatically increased pain. There may be no area of tenderness, or areas of exquisite sensitivity to normally innocuous stimuli (allodynia). Symptoms and signs of autonomic instability may accompany neuropathic pain. The clinical hallmarks of neuropathic pain are spontaneous pains and painful responses to non-noxious stimuli. Neuropathic pain is also characterized by its relative resistance to opioids, making it the most challenging of pain conditions to treat.[11] Cancer patients experience neuropathic pain from a variety of causes. Direct infiltration of neural structures by tumor is the most common, but iatrogenic causes, such as radiation fibrosis and surgical injury, also occur.

Injury to any part of the nervous system, whether central or peripheral, may result in neuropathic pain. A number of theories have been advanced to explain both peripheral and central mechanisms for maintaining the perceived pain. In the periphery, C fibers may become sensitized by direct injury or by ongoing nociception from injured tissues. This sensitization would make them susceptible to stimuli that are not normally perceived as painful, including sympathetic discharges.[12,13] Two other peripheral mechanisms include neuroma formation (in which an injured nerve's attempt to regrow results in an overly sensitive, disordered jumble of fibers), and abnormal foci of sensitivity along the course of a nerve, resulting in ephaptic transmission (cross talk) or ectopic discharges.[14,15]

Regardless of the initial site of neurologic injury, the central nervous system probably plays a significant role in maintaining the pain syndrome. Increased sensitivity to peripheral stimuli can be demonstrated in the dorsal horn of the spinal cord, as can spontaneous activity. This spinal cord hypersensitivity could explain both the spontaneous pain and the allodynia felt in neuropathic pain syndromes.

CANCER PAIN SYNDROMES

Most pain syndromes in patients with advanced cancer are caused by direct tumor invasion of pain-sensitive structures. The specific pain syndrome depends more on the type of structure involved (e.g.,bone pain, visceral pain, mucosal irritation) than on the causative tumor. Similarly, though less commonly, the injury is iatrogenic from diagnostic, surgical, chemotherapeutic, and radiotherapeutic interventions. In many patients, pain has multiple causes. Since increasing pain may signal advancing disease, determining its cause is important.[16] In addition, knowing the cause of pain assists in selecting the most appropriate analgesic approach. The following are several common, recognizable painful conditions that occur in cancer patients. They are grouped according to the type or location of pain.

Bone Pain

Tumor involvement of bone is the most common cause of cancer pain.[7] Any tumor may involve bone, but the most common include metastatic cancer of the breast, lung, prostate, and thyroid, and multiple myeloma.[1] This is purely somatic pain, unless pathologic fracture or tumor extension disrupts nerve. As such, pain is usually described as focal and constant, but may be referred. Typically, patients experience several days or weeks of increasing pain. Acutely increased bone pain may signal fracture or neural impingement. Tumors may activate nociceptors by pressure, ischemia, or secretion of algesic substances (e.g., prostaglandin E2, osteoclast activating factor).[17] Most pain is probably sensed in periosteum and synovium; these are quite sensitive to surgical manipulation. Common sites of bony metastasis are the vertebral column, skull, humerus, ribs, pelvis, and femur.[6]

Diagnosis of bony metastases in known cancer patients may be made by plain x-ray when tumor involves the cortex. A computed tomography (CT) scan further defines the morphology of bone lesions that are seen on x-ray films. When the radiography is normal, radionuclide scintigraphy (bone scan) may identify osteoid formation in the marrow, before cortical destruction has occurred. Even in predominantly osteolytic tumors, some reactive osteoid formation usually occurs, and the bone scan is positive (Table 44-2).[18] A bone scan, however, is often normal in purely lytic tumors, such as multiple myeloma, and in previously irradiated bone. Furthermore, it lacks the anatomic detail of x-ray film. Magnetic resonance imaging (MRI) is more sensitive than x-ray and bone scan, and can identify bony metastases in previously irradiated bone.[6] MRI is not used as the initial diagnostic tool because it is expensive, time-consuming, and often not immediately available.

Other forms of bone pain in cancer are iatrogenic: avascular necrosis of the femoral and humeral heads from steroid treatment, osteoradionecrosis following radiation treatment, and pseudo-

TABLE 44-2 **Primary Bone Response to Some Tumors**

Osteoblastic	Osteolytic
Prostate	Thyroid
Breast	Kidney
Carcinoid	Colorectal
	Breast (may be either)
	Non-Hodgkin's lymphoma
Hodgkin's Disease	Lung
	Multiple myeloma

rheumatism from steroid withdrawal. X-ray films do not confirm avascular necrosis for several weeks or months after the onset of pain, whereas a bone scan is more sensitive.[6] Osteoradionecrosis usually occurs in the mandible, and may develop months or years after irradiation. It must always be distinguished from recurrent tumor, radiation-induced sarcoma, and osteomyelitis.[19] Reinstitution of steroid treatment, followed by slow withdrawal, confirms the diagnosis of pseudorheumatism by relieving the arthralgias and myalgias.[6]

Back Pain

The vertebral column (particularly the thoracic spine) is the most common site of bony metastasis.[20] Although cancer causes less than 1% of back pain in the general population, 98% of known cancer patients who present with back pain have underlying malignancy.[21] Up to one third of cancer patients develop metastases to the spine, with prostate, breast, thyroid, and lung cancers being most common.[20,22] Because back pain in cancer patients usually signifies bone or epidural metastasis, aggressive investigation to define the presence and extent of tumor is necessary. Left untreated, metastases destabilize the axial skeleton and encroach on the spinal cord or cauda equina.

Investigation of back pain should begin with a detailed history and physical examination, attending to the presence of rapid pain progression, referral patterns, and neurologic symptoms and findings. Points that should raise the suspicion of epidural disease include failure of pain to resolve with recumbency, point tenderness of the spine on examination, and, of course, any history of bowel or bladder dysfunction or focal neurologic deficit.

Vertebral disease at certain levels of the spine may initially have a confusing presentation. High cervical spine metastases may produce only posterior headache, which could be mistaken for tension headache. Involvement of C7-T1 causes pain in the interscapular region. Lesions of T12 or L1 may refer pain to the flank, iliac crest, or sacroiliac joint. Sacral destruction may refer pain in a saddle pattern.[1] Radiation myelopathy causes local burning pain, which radiates bilaterally, and progressive neurologic deficits.[23]

Stable back pain in cancer patients, without neurologic symptoms or signs, warrants nonurgent x-ray films of the affected area. Radiographs will detect approximately 70% of vertebral tumors.[21] If plain films are normal, radionuclide bone scan is indicated, because it has a higher sensitivity than radiography for early osteoblastic lesions, fractures, and infection. If x-ray or bone scan is positive or equivocal, MRI should be performed to detect or define the extent of disease, especially that involving soft tissue.[18] If both x-ray and bone scan are normal, CT or MRI of the paraspinal and retroperitoneal areas is warranted to detect a source of referred or extraaxial soft tissue pain.

MRI is always the test of first choice when there is evidence of neural compression, and should be completed urgently if cord compression is suspected. MRI is sensitive for early metastases, easily images the entire spine in one scan (unlike CT), and accurately defines the extent of adjacent soft tissue disease.[18] CT with myelography may be used when MRI is not available.

Even when there is no evidence of neural compression by history or physical examination, radiologic evaluation should not be delayed for more than several days if back pain is positional or progressing. Unstable vertebral fractures may lead to acute cord compression and may require prophylactic stabilization or irradiation.[24]

Some patients with back pain due to epidural malignancy do not have vertebral metastases. Tumor may reach the epidural space by hematogenous spread or by direct extension along nerves, through the intervertebral foramina. MRI should be completed when radiologic evaluation and bone scan are negative if radiculopathy, plexopathy, or myelopathy develops.[22,25] Other patients with back pain in the absence of vertebral disease may have leptomeningeal carcinomatosis (LM). They have signs of neurologic dysfunction at several levels, and usually complain of headache, nausea, and nuchal rigidity, but may also have lumbar radicular pain.[23] Contrast-enhanced MRI of the entire spine and head, followed by lumbar puncture, is appropriate when LM is detected. LM may require treatment with radiation, steroids, or intrathecal chemotherapy.

Loss of motor function, hyper- or hyporeflexia and bowel or bladder disturbances are suggestive of myelopathy. Their presence should prompt immediate intervention, even before diagnostic imaging has been obtained, to prevent permanent neurological impairment (Fig. 44-1). Even in the absence of myelopathy, certain situations require urgent radiologic evaluation. Rapidly progressing pain is highly suspect for tumor, and should be investigated until the extent of disease is known. Increased pain when supine or erect may signal positional cord compression, which will progress to overt myelopathy unless treated. In these situations, MRI of the entire spine should be performed to define the extent of disease and the threat to neural tissue.[26]

Brachial Plexopathy

Brachial plexopathy is a common neurologic complication of cancer.[23] Metastatic brachial plexopathy (MBP) and radiation-induced brachial plexopathy (RBP) are the most likely culprits when shoulder and arm pain are present in the cancer patient. The differential for arm pain includes cervical radiculopathy, osteoarthritis, bursitis of the shoulder, and myofascial pain. Less common cancer-related causes are iatrogenic plexus injury during surgery or central venous catheter placement, chemotherapeutic neurotoxicity, and secondary plexus tumors following radiation.[27]

MBP, also called Pancoast syndrome and thoracic inlet syndrome, presents in 2% to 9% of patients with lung and breast cancer,[28,29] and is also seen in lymphoma, thyroid cancer, and others.[27] Tumor may spread to the plexus from the apex of the lung or from nearby lymph nodes. Differentiating MBP from RBP may be difficult when a patient has received radiation (Table 44-3). MBP typically presents with neuropathic pain in the ipsilateral shoulder or arm, which is rapidly progressive. Although both conditions may eventually involve the entire plexus, selective lower plexus involvement implies MBP, and upper plexus involvement occurs with RBP. The time from cancer diagnosis to presentation (3 to 6 years) is similar for MBP and RBP in patients who have received radiation.[27] Horner's syndrome is much more likely in MBP than RBP, and is highly associated with epidural tumor spread, which occurs in 25% of MBP patients, often without abnormalities on x-ray film, bone scan, or myelogram.[30] MRI is more sensitive than myelography for epidural disease, and should be used in the evaluation of patients with cancer and brachial plexopathy (Fig. 44-1).[25,31]

Olsen and colleagues found that 14% of 128 breast cancer patients receiving surgery and radiation developed RBP. The addition of cytotoxic chemotherapy increased the likelihood of RBP. Forty-seven percent of the RBP patients had pain.[32] The dose of radiation may also affect the incidence of RBP, as does treatment tech-

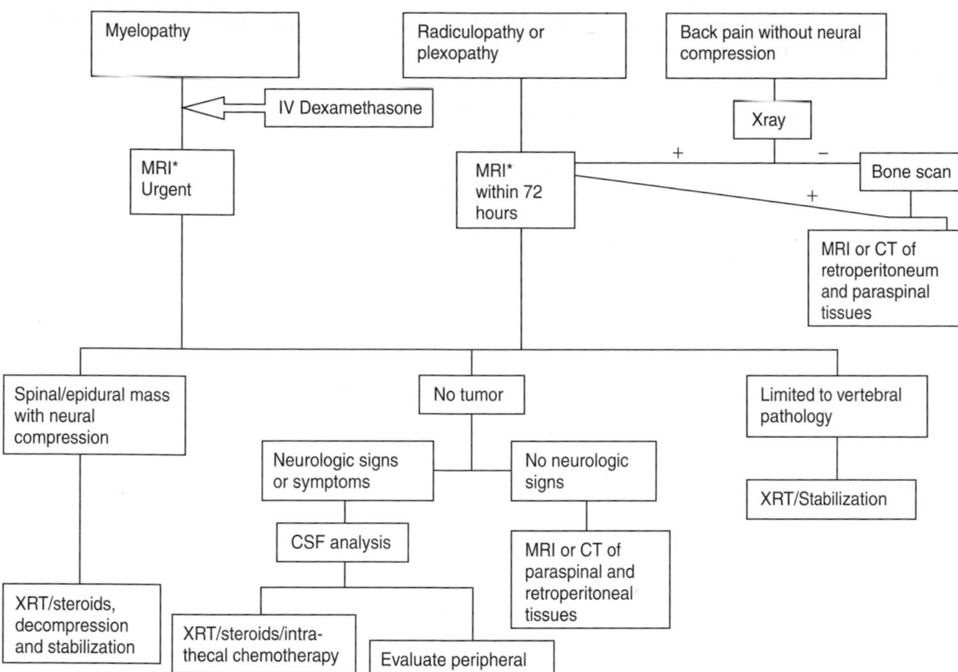

Figure 44-1 Diagnostic approach to back pain in the cancer patient. (*Combined CT and myelogram may be used in place of MRI if MRI is unavailable or contraindicated.)

nique. RBP is associated with progressive fibrous constriction of nerve bundles, thickening of endoneurium, loss of myelin, and obliteration of small blood vessels. Initial symptoms of RBP are paresthesiae, numbness, heaviness, weakness, and swelling. Pain is a presenting symptom in 18%, and becomes a major symptom in 35%. Sensory and motor loss progress gradually, eventually rendering the arm useless. Reversible radiation-induced plexopathy has been reported in conjunction with chemotherapy for breast cancer. This entity presents earlier than RBP, rarely causes pain or weakness, and resolves in time.[33]

MRI is the best imaging modality to differentiate MBP from RBP.[31] If MRI is not available, however, computed tomography should be performed with intravenous contrast. An electromylogram (EMG) of the affected arm and shoulder muscles shows fibrillation potentials and myokymia in RBP, but not in pure MBP. However, patients with brachial plexus tumor may also have some radiation fibrosis, so EMG cannot rule out MBP. Biopsy also may confirm fibrosis or tumor, but cannot rule out either one. When pain presents many years following radiation in a patient who was thought to be free of cancer, MRI and biopsy should be utilized to rule out radiation-induced secondary neoplasm.[1]

Lumbosacral Plexopathy

Pelvic tumors may invade or compress the lumbar and sacral plexuses to produce pain, bowel and bladder dysfunction, and leg weakness. Jaeckle and colleagues studied 85 patients with pelvic tumor and low back or leg pain.[34] The most common primary tu-

TABLE 44-3 **Clinical Presentation of Patients with MPB versus RBP**

	MBP		
Presenting Symptom	**With Prior Radiation (n = 44)**	**Without Prior Radiation (n = 34)**	**RBP (n = 22)**
Pain	33 (75%)	39 (89%)	4 (18%)
Arm Swelling	0 (0%)	0 (0%)	9 (40%)
Dysesthesia	11 (25%)	2 (6%)	12 (55%)
Arm Weakness	0 (0%)	2 (6%)	6 (27%)
Horner's Syndrome	23 (53%)	19 (56%)	3 (14%)
Lymphedema	6 (13%)	5 (15%)	16 (73%)
Upper trunk (C5-6)	0 (0%)	3 (9%)	17 (77%)
Lower (C8-T1)	33 (75%)	23 (68%)	0 (0%)
Whole Plexus	11 (25%)	8 (23%)	5 (23%)

mors were colorectal, uterine, cervical, breast, sarcoma, and lymphoma. Seventy percent presented with pain, and 98% eventually developed pain, which was aching and pressure-like. Pain was local, radicular, or referred, and a combination of local and radicular was common. Two thirds developed weakness, and one half developed sensory symptoms. Twenty-seven percent had bilateral plexopathy. Epidural extension was detected in 35% of patients. Radiation-induced lumbrosacral plexopathy (LP) is rare, and, as in RBP, sensory and motor symptoms commonly precede pain; approximately one half of patients never develop pain. Plexopathy follows radiation by an average of 5 years, but there is a considerable range. Symptoms are usually bilateral, but asymmetric.[35]

Diagnosis of LP starts with a history of unilateral or bilateral pain or weakness in the low back, abdomen, perineum, or leg. Bowel and bladder function may be spared when only the upper plexus is involved. Involvement of the lower lumbosacral plexus (sciatic nerve), occurring in one half of patients resembles sciatica from a herniated intervertebral disk, with a positive straight leg raising test and tenderness in the sciatic notch. Upper plexus involvement, occurring in one third of patients, produces tenderness in the lumbar region.[34] Lower (sacral) plexopathy results in urinary incontinence, sexual impotence, and neuropathic perineal and genital pain. Radiologic evaluation of LP begins with MRI or contrast-enhanced CT of the lumbosacral spine. If these are negative, an extraaxial pain source is sought (see Fig. 44-1). If the history suggests radiation fibrosis of the plexus, EMG to detect fibrillation potentials and myokymic discharges is useful but does not rule out tumor as the cause of LP.[35]

Cervical Plexopathy

Injury to the cervical plexus, whether from tumor or surgery, causes pain in and around the ear or in the anterior neck to the clavicle. The phrenic nerve may also be paralyzed. Horner's syndrome is seen if the superior cervical ganglion is affected. The differential includes disease of the upper cervical spine and the base of the skull.[23] In a patient who has had surgery in the area, Horner's syndrome, phrenic nerve paralysis, and signs of cervical myelopathy or contralateral radiculopathy should suggest recurrent tumor. In such patients, and in those who have not had neck surgery, MRI with contrast is indicated to define the extent of disease.

Headache and Facial Pain

Headache occurs in about 60% of patients presenting with primary brain tumors, and is the presenting symptom in 50% of patients with cerebral metastases (See also Chapter 19, Pathophysiology of Headaches). It is usually of mild or moderate intensity, similar to a tension-type headache. Only 25% of patients have awakening or morning headaches. Cancer patients with new headaches or a change in headache pattern should be investigated for cerebral metastases. Neurologic signs are more common than neurologic symptoms in these patients. Weakness is a presenting symptom in approximately 30%, but a hemiparesis can be found in about 60%.[36] Papilledema is surprisingly uncommon, appearing in only 25%, so its absence should not be taken as reassuring. Investigation of the suspicious headache should include MRI or CT, both with intravenous contrast. MRI is more sensitive, especially for skull base and posterior fossa tumors, and delineates the extent of disease more precisely than CT. Initial management is with corticosteroids, followed by antitumor therapy and/or symptomatic treatment.[37] Brain tumor headache characteristically responds rapidly to the administration of corticosteroids.

Not all headaches in patients with cancer are due to cerebral metastases. Leptomeningeal metastases cause headaches that are commonly associated with radicular or cranial nerve findings. Multiple metastases, posterior fossa metastases, and leptomeningeal carcinomatosis are the most frequent intracranial causes of head pain. Other cancer-related causes include ischemic or hemorrhagic stroke, pseudotumor cerebri from superior vena cava syndrome, and sagittal sinus occlusion by tumor or thrombus.[23] Fever and migraine are the most common noncancer causes of headaches in patients with cancer.

Cancer is a rare cause of facial pain. Extracranial bony or soft tissue metastases may impinge on cranial and upper cervical nerves, causing headache or facial pain. Pain in these cases is usually unilateral, and may be accompanied by focal tenderness. Glossopharyngeal neuralgia may be seen in patients with leptomeningeal metastases, jugular foramen invasion, or more peripheral primary head or neck malignancies. Pain occurs in the pharynx and base of the tongue, and sometimes around the ear. Pain in the trigeminal distribution has been described with middle and posterior fossa tumors, skull base metastases, and with lymphomatous meningitis.[23] Of 2,972 patients with a diagnosis of trigeminal neuralgia at the Mayo Clinic, 10% were found to have tumors, the majority of which were benign.[38] Unilateral facial pain has been described as a presenting symptom of ipsilateral nonmetastatic lung cancer. It is typically severe, around the ear and temple, and resolves with radiation of the tumor. It probably occurs when tumor invades the vagus nerve.[39]

Metastases to the base of the skull produce distinct patterns of head and facial pain.[23,37] Breast, lung, prostate, and nasopharyngeal tumors are common primaries. A tumor in the orbit produces progressive pain in the supraorbital area, proptosis, and external ophthalmoplegia. A parasellar tumor may present with unilateral supraorbital and frontal headache with diplopia. Middle fossa tumors often present with pain and sensory changes in the mandibular and maxillary trigeminal distributions, which may be followed by headache, diplopia, dysarthria, and dysphagia. Tumor invading the jugular foramen affects the glossopharyngeal, vagus, and accessory nerves to cause throat pain, hoarseness, dysphagia, and weakness of the sternocleidomastoid and trapezius muscles. Involvement of the occipital condyle causes occipital pain and neck stiffness with associated hypoglossal nerve paralysis. Metastasis to the clivus presents with vertex headache, worse with neck flexion, and eventual lower cranial nerve dysfunction. Sphenoid sinus tumor may cause bifrontal headache radiating to the temples and retro-orbital areas, sometimes with abducens nerve palsy. Fracture of the odontoid process (dens), pathologic or not, causes posterior headache with increased pain on neck flexion. The resulting cervical spine instability or mass effect from such a tumor may cause spinal cord or brain stem compression.

Peripheral Neuropathies

Peripheral neuropathies in cancer can be divided into mononeuropathies and more symmetric polyneuropathies. Any nerve may be directly affected by tumor, but radicular pain and intercostal entrapment from rib metastasis are the most common.[23]

The most common symmetric polyneuropathies are paraneoplastic syndromes and those resulting from chemotherapy. One paraneoplastic syndrome associated with oat-cell lung cancer, breast, colon, and ovarian cancers is a painful sensory neuropathy. It is characterized clinically by tingling, burning, and lancinating pains in the extremities. Pathologic examination reveals an inflammatory process in the dorsal root ganglia, followed by loss of peripheral myelinated and unmyelinated fibers.[40] This syndrome may be a presenting feature of the cancer. Multiple myeloma is commonly associated with a painful sensorimotor neuropathy that responds to tumor therapy.[23] Ovarian, lung, and breast cancer may also cause sensorimotor neuropathy as they progress.[41, 42] In these cases, segmental demyelination and axonal degeneration are seen histologically.[40]

Chemotherapy often produces a painful peripheral neuropathy with dysesthesias. The vinca alkaloids and cisplatinum are most commonly to blame, and symptoms are dose-related and often irreversible. Burning in the feet and hands and vibratory and proprioceptive deficits are characteristic.[23,43]

ACUTE ZOSTER AND POSTHERPETIC NEURALGIA

Painful varicella-zoster reactivation causes a dermatomal rash and neuropathic pain. It occurs two to three times as frequently in cancer patients as in the general population. Lymphoma and breast cancers cause a disproportionate number of cases. The dermatome involved is likely to correlate with the site of primary tumor in breast, lung, and gynecologic cancer.[44] Advancing age, the severity of the initial rash and pain, and an ophthalmic distribution predispose to the later development of postherpetic neuralgia. Cancer does not appear to increase the likelihood of postherpetic neuralgia when age is accounted for.[45] A thorough review of zoster and related pain is provided in another chapter (See Chapter 40 Acute Herpes Zoster and Postherpetic Neuralgia).

Abdominal and Pelvic Pain

In a review of 5675 patients presenting with acute abdominal pain to a group of five European hospitals, 106 (1.9%) were eventually found to have intraabdominal cancer. The risk of cancer for those over 50 years old was 10%.[46] Abdominal pain from cancer is typically visceral in nature. As such, it is poorly localized and often referred to distant sites, and often accompanied by nausea and vomiting. Diaphragmatic irritation and distension of the hepatic capsule produce ipsilateral shoulder pain, retroperitoneal tumor may cause back pain, and pelvic tumor may cause perineal pain. Viscus or duct blockage and distension, peritoneal inflammation or tension, mesenteric torsion, and vascular or lymphatic obstruction typically produce pain. Pelvic cancer pain occurs primarily in patients with malignancies of the rectum and genitourinary tracts. Extra-abdominal cancers also often metastasize to the sacrum and pelvis.

Abdominal pain not directly caused by intraperitoneal or retroperitoneal malignancy is also common. Radiation-induced enteritis occurs in acute and chronic forms. Acute injury manifests as abdominal or pelvic pain, diarrhea, or tenesmus in up to one half of patients. Chronic injury, occurring in 2% to 5% of patients, presents as stricture, bleeding, perforation, or fistula 6 to 24 months after radiation. Pain may be associated with bowel ischemia, obstruction, or intraabdominal infection in patients with chronic enteritis.[47] Pain may radiate or refer to the abdomen from destructive low thoracic and high lumbar spine disease and nerve root compression. Following abdominal surgery for cancer, adhesions may form and cause painful bowel obstruction.

Pain from pancreatic cancer is of particular interest because of its frequency, severity, and amenability to celiac plexus block. Up to 80% of patients with this disease present with significant pain. With advanced disease, the figure rises to 90%, and probably represents gastric or retroperitoneal invasion. Most tumors are at the head of the gland, and may cause bile duct obstruction early in the disease. Pain from the pancreatic head localizes to the right epigastrium, whereas that from the body is felt in the mid-epigastrium, and tumor in the tail produces pain in the left epigastrium and posterior intercostal space.[48]

Mucositis

In about 70% of patients, chemoradiotherapeutic conditioning for bone marrow or stem cell transplantation causes noninfectious mucositis (stomatitis) by killing cells with high mitotic rates.[49] Several days following conditioning, hemorrhagic degradation and ulceration of the oropharyngeal mucosa begins. While initially causing constant mild or moderate burning discomfort, the condition progresses to preclude talking, eating, or swallowing. Significant pain requiring opioid use persists in one half of patients at 3 weeks after transplant.[50] Mucositis from head and neck radiation usually develops in the second or third week of therapy, affects almost all patients, and is otherwise similar to that from bone marrow conditioning. Normal doses of chemotherapeutic agents also cause mucositis in about 40% of patients.[49] Pain may be more severe or prolonged when mucosal ulcers become superinfected with bacteria or fungus, and when graft-versus-host disease occurs. Reactivation of herpes simplex, cytomegalovirus, or varicella-zoster infections in the immunocompromised cancer patient may present with vesiculo-ulcerative mucositis.

Chronic Postsurgical Pain

Four postsurgical chronic pain syndromes have been identified. They result from injury to nerve or plexus, so the pain is neuropathic in nature.

Mastectomy Burning, aching, and tight constriction of the axilla, medial upper arm, and chest with superimposed lancinations and scar sensitivity are characteristic of postmastectomy pain. Phantom breast pain is also described, and uncomfortable lymphedema of the arm is common. Whereas previously less than 10% of mastectomy patients were said to develop chronic pain,[23] one half of 467 mastectomy patients recently surveyed went on to develop pain, paresthesias, and phantom sensations.[51] Less extensive surgery was more often associated with pain in the ipsilateral arm. In fact, the radiation and chemotherapy that followed less extensive surgery were probably responsible for much of the arm pain. Progressive pain was more common in patients with recurrent disease.

Maunsell and colleagues studied arm symptoms in 223 women who underwent breast surgery with or without axillary dissection.[52] About one half complained of arm pain at 3 months postoperatively, and a similar proportion at 15 months. Patients who had axillary dissection were more likely to have arm pain, although this result did not reach statistical significance. Wallace and colleagues also found that breast reconstruction with implants after mastectomy increases the likelihood of chronic pain from about 30% (mastectomy alone or with simple reconstruction) to 50%.[53] Submuscular implant placement may injure the long thoracic, thoracodorsal, lateral pectoral, and medial pectoral nerves. Capsule formation around the implant may entrap the long thoracic and the two pectoral nerves.

Evaluation of chest and arm pain after mastectomy should focus on the nature of the pain and its location, as well as neurologic examination to define the areas of sensory loss and hypersensitivity. A neuroma is sought in the chest wall and axilla. Autonomic changes and limited shoulder motion may be present in the "frozen shoulder" syndrome. Scapular winging is seen when the long thoracic nerve has been disrupted. Pain that is not typical of postmastectomy pain syndrome should prompt evaluation for infection and tumor recurrence.

Neck Dissection During radical neck dissection, the superficial cervical plexus is dissected out. The result is often neuropathic pain and sensory loss in the anterolateral neck and extending to the shoulder. Division of the accessory nerve and removal of the sternocleidomastoid muscle may also lead to chronic pain via postural changes that affect the shoulder girdle and entrap the upper brachial plexus.[23] Loss of trapezius function leads to drooping of the shoulder, mild scapular winging, inability to abduct the shoulder above 90°, and forward rotation of the scapula, often with sternoclavicular subluxation (Fig. 44-2).[54] Frozen shoulder often develops as a result of weakness and pain.[55]

Ewing and Martin described 100 radical neck dissection patients in 1952.[54] Of 89 with unilateral operations, 42 patients had persistent shoulder pain. In two more recent studies, 76 of 100 radical neck dissection patients had shoulder pain and dysfunction when evaluated at least 6 months after surgery.[57,58] In 31, the pain was severe. The deep cervical plexus innervates enough of the trapezius muscle to maintain shoulder mobility and prevent shoulder-arm pain in some patients.[58] Any patient who has increasing pain following neck dissection should be evaluated for infection and tumor recurrence.

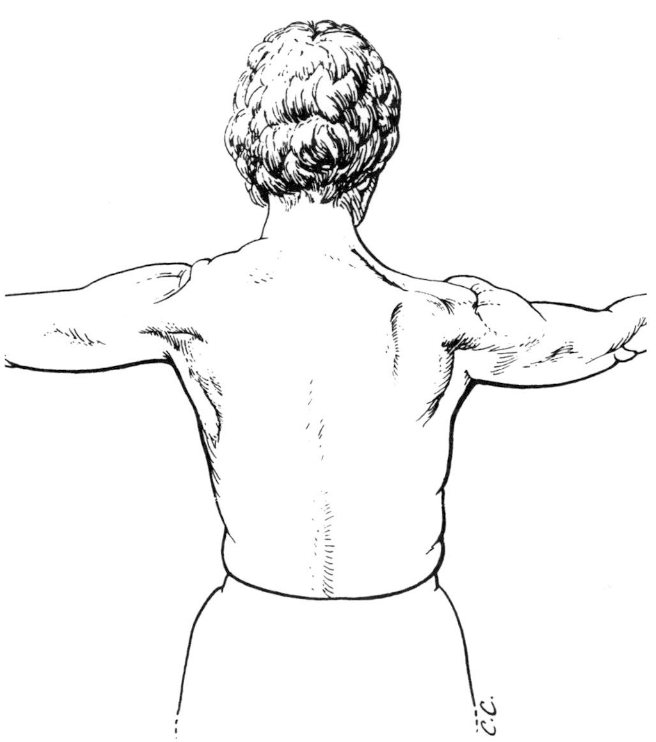

Figure 44-2 Posterior view of musculoskeletal changes seen after radical neck dissection. (From Braddom RL, Buschbacher RM, Dumitru D, et al, eds. *Physical Medicine and Rehabilitation.* Philadelphia, Pa: WB Saunders, 1996. With permission of Baylor College of Medicine, Houston, TX.)

Thoracotomy Chronic chest pain after thoracotomy affects up to 55% of patients followed for more than 1 year.[59] Keller and colleagues reviewed the records of 238 consecutive thoracotomy patients.[60] Post-thoracotomy pain was defined as that requiring regular use of analgesics beyond 3 months from surgery. Eleven percent of patients met this definition, but one half of these used opioid analgesics preoperatively. Chest wall resection and pleurectomy increased the likelihood of chronic pain when compared with pulmonary resection. Importantly, all 20 patients with recurrence of pain after initial control were found to have tumor regrowth. The use of video-assisted thoracic surgery (VATS) for pulmonary resection may decrease the incidence of chronic pain and disability when compared with thoracotomy.[61]

Mechanisms for chronic pain after thoracotomy are several. The intercostal nerves may be injured during rib resection, or compressed with a retractor. Incidental rib fractures may entrap an intercostal nerve during healing. These patients may develop dermatomal chest wall numbness and neuropathic pain complaints, including point tenderness from neuroma formation. Severe rib retraction may also disarticulate the costochondral and costovertebral junctions, resulting in somatic pain and tenderness. Because the latissimus dorsi and serratus anterior muscles are often cut during thoracotomy, ipsilateral shoulder disability is also common. Untreated thoracotomy pain and inadequate rehabilitation may lead to frozen shoulder. Symptomatic myofascial trigger points often develop in chest wall muscles. All patients with increasing or recurrent pain after thoracotomy should be evaluated for tumor and infection.[60]

Amputation Chronic pain following limb amputation is either stump pain or phantom pain or both. Wartan and colleagues surveyed 590 war-related amputees in England to assess the prevalence of chronic pain.[62] Of these, 55% reported phantom pain, and 56% had stump pain. Sherman and colleagues surveyed 5000 American veterans with amputations.[63] Fifty-five percent responded, and 78% of those reported phantom pain. Stump pain is due to local disease, most commonly infection or neuroma formation. Neuroma formation several weeks after amputation produces exquisite stump tenderness and pain that is either constant or elicited by palpation or movement. An ill-fitting prosthesis, recurrent tumor, infection, or ischemia may also cause local pain and tenderness.[64]

Phantom sensation, the sensory experience that the amputated limb is still present, occurs in most amputees. Phantom pain is often described as a paroxysmal burning, crushing, and twisting in the missing part. Phantom pain peaks in the first month after surgery and may fade slowly as it "telescopes" toward the stump.[63] It is more common after more proximal amputations.[65] Patients with extremity pain prior to amputation are more likely to develop immediate postamputation phantom pain,[66] and preemptive analgesia with lumbar epidural blockade may reduce the incidence of phantom pain.[67]

TABLE 44-4 **Prevalence of Psychiatric Disorders and Pain in 215 Cancer Patients**

Psychiatric Diagnoses	Patients, No. (%)	Psychiatric Diagnoses (%)	Patients with Significant Pain, No. (%)
Adjustment Disorders	69 (32)	68	–
Major Affective Disorders	13 (6)	13	–
Organic Mental Disorders	8 (4)	8	–
Personality Disorders	7 (3)	7	–
Anxiety Disorders	4 (2)	4	–
Total with Psychiatric Diagnosis	101 (47)		39 (39)
Total without Psychiatric Diagnosis	114 (53)		21 (19)
Total Patients	215 (100)		60 (28)

From Derogatis LR, Morrow GR, Fetting J, et al. The prevalence of psychiatric disorders among cancer patients. JAMA 1983;249:751. © 1983, American Medical Association. As adapted by Breitbard W. Psychiatric management of cancer pain. Cancer 1989;63:2336. © 1989 American Cancer Society. Reprinted by permission of Wiley-Liss, Inc., a subsidiary of John Wiley & Sons.

Numerous neurophysiologic explanations for phantom pain have been advanced, from changes at the stump to functional cortical changes. Sensory deafferentation in primates and arm amputation in humans causes cortical somatosensory reorganization.[68] This may explain the elicitation of phantom pain by sensory stimulation at other sites. As with the other postsurgical pain syndromes, an unexpected increase in or recurrence of pain should prompt evaluation for infection, ischemia, or tumor recurrence.[64,65]

PSYCHOLOGICAL ASPECTS OF CANCER PAIN

It is important to recognize that the experience of cancer pain is not merely physical. Cancer patients and those close to them suffer emotionally as well as physically. The way in which a patient and his or her family adjust to the experience of pain and dying markedly influences their perception of physical pain. Conversely, uncontrolled pain causes or contributes to anxiety, depression, and delirium in many cancer patients.[69] Derogatis and colleagues evaluated 215 unselected cancer patients for psychiatric disorders. Forty-seven percent had a DSM-defined (*Diagnostic and Statistical Manual of Mental Disorders*) psychiatric disorder (Table 44-4).[70]

Suicide is only slightly more common in cancer patients than the general population, but suicidal ideation is frequent, and strongly associated with mood disturbance. Successful suicide typically occurs in patients with uncontrolled pain. Self-destructive personality traits and delirium also contribute to suicide attempts. The degree to which noncompliance and refusal of life-extending treatment represent suicide is not known.[71]

Fear of opioid addiction and abuse in cancer patients is a factor in the ongoing underuse of these medications for cancer pain. Tolerance (the need for increasing doses to achieve the same effect) and physical dependence (the occurrence of withdrawal symptoms when stopping or reducing opioid dosage) are expected with chronic opioid use. Addiction (a behavioral pattern of compulsive drug procurement and use for nonmedical reasons) is quite rare in cancer pain patients, and may be less common than in those with nonmalignant pain.[72] Given their utility and safety, the sparing use of opioid analgesics in cancer pain is inappropriate.

REFERENCES

1. Portenoy RK. Cancer pain: epidemiology and syndromes. *Cancer* 1989;63:2298.
2. Daut RL, Cleeland CS. The prevalence and severity of pain in cancer. *Cancer* 1982;50:1913.
3. Cleeland CS, Gonin R, Hatfield AK, et al. Pain and its treatment in outpatients with metastatic cancer. *New Engl J Med* 1994;330:592.
4. Coyle N, Adelhardt J, Foley KM, Portenoy RK. Character of terminal illness in the advanced cancer patient: pain and other symptoms during the last four weeks of life. *J Pain Symptom Manage* 1990;5:83.
5. Quill TE. Doctor, I want to die. Will you help me? *JAMA* 1993;270:870.
6. Foley KM. Pain syndromes in patients with cancer. In: Bonica JJ, Ventafridda B,eds. *Advances in Pain Research and Therapy* Vol. 2. New York, NY: Raven Press, 1979:59.
7. Foley KM. The treatment of cancer pain. *New Engl J Med* 1985;13:84.
8. McMahon SB. Mechanisms of cutaneous, deep, and visceral pain. In: Wall PD, Melzack R, eds. *Textbook of Pain* 3rd ed. New York, NY: Churchill Livingstone, 1994:129.
9. Capps JA, Coleman GH. *An Experimental and Clinical Study of Pain in the Pleura, Pericardium, and Peritoneum.* New York, NY: McMillan, 1932.
10. Cervero F, Laird JMA, Pozo MA. Selective changes of receptive field properties of spinal nociceptive neurones induced by noxious visceral stimulation in the cat. *Pain* 1992;51:335.
11. Portenoy RK, Foley KM, Inturrisi CE. The nature of opioid responsiveness and its implications for neuropathic pain: new hypotheses derived from studies of opioid infusions. *Pain* 1990;43:273.
12. Cline MA, Ochoa J, Torebjork HE: Chronic hyperalgesia and skin warming caused by sensitized C nociceptors. *Brain* 1989;112:621.
13. Hu S, Zhu J. Sympathetic facilitation of sustained discharges of polymodal nociceptors. *Pain* 1989;38:85.
14. Devor M. Neuropathic pain and injured nerve: peripheral mechanisms. *Br Med Bull* 1991;47:619.
15. Burchiel KJ. Abnormal impulse generation in focally demyelinated trigeminal roots. *J Neurosurg* 1980;53:674.
16. Gonzales GR, Elliott KJ, Portenoy RK, Foley KM. The impact of a comprehensive evaluation in the management of cancer pain. *Pain* 1991;47:141.

17. Payne R: Cancer pain: anatomy, physiology, and pharmacology. *Cancer* 1989;63(suppl):2266.
18. Tryciecky EW, Gottschalk A, Ludema K. Oncologic imaging: interactions of nuclear medicine with CT and MRI using the bone scan as a model. *Semin Nucl Med* 1997;27:142.
19. Friedman RB. Osteoradionecrosis: causes and prevention. *NCI Monogr* 1990;9:145.
20. Posner JB. Back pain and epidural spinal cord compression. *Med Clin North Am* 1987;71:185.
21. Deyo RA, Diehl AK. Cancer as a cause of back pain: frequency, clinical presentation, and diagnostic strategies. *J Gen Intern Med* 1988; 3:230.
22. Ruff RL, Lanska DJ. Epidural metastases in prospectively evaluated veterans with cancer and back pain. *Cancer* 1989;63:2234.
23. Elliott K, Foley KM. Neurologic pain syndromes in patients with cancer. *Crit Care Clin* 1990;6:393.
24. Hoskin PJ. Radiotherapy in the management of bone pain. *Clin Orthop Rel Res* 1995;312:105.
25. Sarpel S, Sarpel G, Yu E, et al. Early diagnosis of spinal-epidural metastasis by magnetic resonance imaging. *Cancer* 1987;59:1112.
26. Heldmann U, Myschetzky PS, Thomsen HS. Frequency of unexpected multifocal metastasis in patients with acute spinal cord compression. Evaluation by low-field MR imaging in cancer patients. *Acta Radiol* 1997;38:372.
27. Kori SH. Diagnosis and management of brachial plexus lesions in cancer patients. *Oncology* 1995;8:756.
28. Berrino F. Epidemiology of superior pulmonary sulcus syndrome (Pancoast syndrome). In: Bonica JJ, Ventafridda V, Pagni CA,eds., *Advances in Pain Research and Therapy*. Vol.. 4. New York, NY: Raven Press, 1982:15.
29. Ampil FL. Radiotherapy for carcinomatous brachial plexopathy. *Cancer* 1985;56:2185.
30. Kanner RM, Martini N, Foley KM. Epidural spinal cord compression in Pancoast syndrome (superior pulmonary sulcus tumor): clinical presentation and outcome. *Ann Neurol* 1981;10:77.
31. Thayagarajan D, Cascino T, Harms F. Magnetic resonance imaging in brachial plexopathy of cancer. *Neurology* 1995;45:421.
32. Olsen NK, Pfeiffer P, Johannsen L, et al. Radiation-induced brachial plexopathy: neurological follow-up in 161 recurrence-free breast cancer patients. *Int J Radiat Oncol Biol Phys* 1993;26:43.
33. Salner AL, Botnick LE, Herzog AG, et al. Reversible brachial plexopathy following primary radiation therapy for breast cancer. *Cancer Treat Rep* 1981;65:797.
34. Jaeckle KA, Young DF, Foley KM. The natural history of lumbosacral plexopathy in cancer. *Neurology* 1985;35:8.
35. Thomas JE, Cascino TL, Earl JD, et al. Differential diagnosis between radiation and tumor plexopathy of the pelvis. *Neurology* 1985;35:1.
36. Cairncross JG. Neurological emergencies in cancer patients. *Prog Clin Biol Res* 1983;132D:319.
37. Jaeckle KA. Causes and management of headaches in cancer patients. *Oncology (Huntingt)* 1993;7:27.
38. Cheng TMW, Cascino TL, Onofrio BM. Comprehensive study of diagnosis and treatment of trigeminal neuralgia secondary to tumors. *Neurology* 1993;43:2298.
39. Capobianco DJ. Facial pain as a symptom of nonmetastatic lung cancer. *Headache* 1995;35:581.
40. Lamarche J, Vital C. Carcinomatous neuropathy. An ultrastructural study of ten cases. *Ann Pathol* 1987;7:98.
41. Cavaletti G, Bogliun G, Marzorati L, et al. The incidence and course of paraneoplastic neuropathy in women with epithelial ovarian cancer. *J Neurol* 1991;238:371.
42. Peterson K, Forsyth PA, Posner JB. Paraneoplastic sensorimotor neuropathy associated with breast cancer. *J Neurooncol* 1994;21:159.
43. van der Hoop RG, van der Burg MEL, Huinink WWB, van Houwelingen JC. Incidence of neuropathy in 395 patients with ovarian cancer treated with or without cisplatin. *Cancer* 1990;66:1697.
44. Rusthoven JJ, Ahlgren P, Elhakim T, et al. Varicella-zoster infection in adult cancer patients. A population study. *Arch Intern Med* 1988;148: 1561.
45. Choo PW, Galil K, Donahue JG, et al. Risk factors for postherpetic neuralgia. *Arch Intern Med* 1997;157:1217.
46. deDombal FT, Matharu SS, Staniland JR, et al. Presentation of cancer to hospital as 'acute abdominal pain.' *Br J Surg* 1980;67:413.
47. Nussbaum ML, Campana TJ, Weese JL. Radiation-induced intestinal injury. *Clin Plast Surg* 1993;20:573.
48. Alter CL. Palliative and supportive care of patients with pancreatic cancer. *Semin Oncol* 1996;23:229.
49. Berger AM, Bartoshuk LM, Duffy VB, Nadoolman W. Capsaicin for the treatment of oral mucositis pain. *PPO Updates* 1995;9:1.
50. Chapko MK, Syrjala KL, Schilter L, et al. Chemoradiotherapy toxicity during bone marrow transplantation: time course and variation in pain and nausea. *Bone Marrow Transplant*. 1989;4:181.
51. Tasmuth T, von Smitten K, Hietanen P, et al. Pain and other symptoms after different treatment modalities of breast cancer. *Ann Oncol* 1995;6:453.
52. Maunsell E, Brisson J, Deschenes L. Arm problems and psychological distress after surgery for breast cancer. *Can J Surg* 1993;36:315.
53. Wallace MS, Wallace AM, Dobke MK. Pain after breast surgery: a survey of 282 women. *Pain* 1996;66:195.
54. Ewing MR, Martin H. Disability following radical neck dissection. *Cancer* 1952;5:873.
55. Patten C, Hillel AD. The 11th nerve syndrome. Accessory nerve palsy or adhesive capsulitis. *Arch Otolaryngol* 1993;119:215.
56. Garden FH, Gillis TA. Principles of cancer rehabilitation. In: Braddom RL, Buschbacher RM, Dumitru D, et al, eds. *Physical Medicine and Rehabilitation*. Philadelphia, Pa: WB Saunders, 1996:1210.
57. Shone GR, Yardley PJ. An audit into the incidence of handicap after unilateral radical neck dissection. *J Laryngol Otol* 1991;105:760.
58. Krause HR. Shoulder-arm syndrome after radical neck dissection: its relation with the innervation of the trapezius muscle. *Int J Oral Maxillofac Surg* 1992;21:276.
59. Dajczman E, Gordon A, Dreisman H, Wolkove N. Long-term postthoracotomy pain. *Chest* 1991;99:270.
60. Keller SM, Carp NZ, Levy MN, Rosen SM. Chronic post thoracotomy pain. *J Cardiovasc Surg* 1994;35(6 suppl 1):161.
61. Landreneau RJ, Mack MJ, Hazelrigg SR, et al. Prevalence of chronic pain after pulmonary resection by thoracotomy or video-assisted thoracic surgery. *J Thorac Cardiovasc Surg* 1994;107:1079.
62. Wartan SW, Hanann W, Bedley JR, McColl I. Phantom pain and sensation among British war amputees. *Br J Anaesth* 1997;78:652.
63. Sherman RA, Sherman CJ, Parker L. Chronic phantom and stump pain among American veterans: results of a survey. *Pain* 1984;18:83.
64. Weinstein SM. Phantom pain. *Oncology* 1994;8:65.
65. Sugarbaker PH, Weiss CM, Davidson DD, Roth YF. Increasing phantom limb pain as a symptom of cancer recurrence. *Cancer* 1984;54:373.
66. Jensen TS, Krebs B, Nielsen J, et al. Immediate and long-term phantom limb pain in amputees: incidence, clinical characteristics, and relationship to pre-amputation limb pain. *Pain* 1985;21:267.
67. Bach S, Noreng MF, Tjelden NY. Phantom limb pain in amputees during the first 12 months following limb amputation, after preoperative lumbar epidural blockade. *Pain* 1988;33:297.
68. Flor H, Elbert T, Knecht S, et al. Phantom-limb pain as a perceptual correlate of cortical reorganization following arm amputation. *Nature* 1995;375:482.
69. Breitbart W. Psychiatric management of cancer pain. *Cancer* 1989;63: 2336.
70. Derogatis LR, Morrow GR, Fetting J, et al. The prevalence of psychiatric disorders among cancer patients. *JAMA* 1983;249:751.
71. Breitbart W. Cancer pain and suicide. In: Foley KM, ed. *Advances in Pain Research and Therapy*.Vol. 16. New York, NY: Raven Press, 1990: 399.
72. Kanner RM, Foley KM. Patterns of narcotic use in a cancer pain clinic. *Ann NY Acad Sci* 1981;362:161.

CHAPTER 45 MEDICAL MANAGEMENT OF CANCER PAIN

Stuart W. Hough and Russell K. Portenoy

OVERVIEW

Cancer pain is usually caused directly by neoplastic injury to pain-sensitive structures. For this reason, primary antineoplastic therapy, including radiation, chemotherapy, and palliative surgery, should be considered part of an analgesic strategy in some cases. When therapy directed at the tumor is inappropriate, is not feasible, or is ineffective, symptomatic analgesic therapies become the overriding concern. Opioid-based pharmacotherapy is the mainstay approach, but adjunctive anesthetic, surgical, psychiatric, and physical modalities may be essential in some cases (See Chapter 46, Anesthetic Interventions in Cancer Pain). Pharmacologic approaches may be systemic or regional (anesthetic). This chapter addresses only systemic pharmacologic analgesics.

The World Health Organization (WHO) proposed a three-step approach to the selection of drugs for the treatment of cancer pain (Fig. 45-1).[1] The first step, for mild pain, utilizes non-opioid analgesics and adjuvant drugs. Adjuvant drugs can be either nontraditional analgesics (so-called adjuvant analgesics) or drugs added to manage the side effects of the primary analgesics. For more intense pain, an opioid is added. Some opioids are used conventionally for moderate pain and others are used for severe pain. This approach is designed to be simple to understand and useable around the world. Uncontrolled field testing has found the WHO guidelines effective for 70% to 100% of patients with cancer.[2]

PAIN ASSESSMENT

Pain is often underrecognized in cancer patients. Cleeland et al surveyed outpatients with metastatic cancer and physicians from 54 treatment centers.[3] They found that 42% of 597 patients with pain were not receiving adequate analgesia by the WHO guidelines (Fig. 45-1). Insufficient pain relief was particularly common among minorities, women, and the aged. An important barrier to effective pain management was a discrepancy between the patient's and physician's assessments of the extent to which pain was interfering with daily activities. The data underscore the importance of accurate pain assessment in providing adequate cancer pain relief.

The assessment should allow inferences about the pain mechanisms, identification of the pain syndrome (See Chapter 44, Cancer Pain Syndromes), and classification of the relationship between the pain and the disease. The clinician must also assess the functional impact of the pain and psychosocial comorbidities. It is essential to accept the patient's report of pain at face value. Pain should be assessed frequently and systematically, especially when a new pain is reported or a new analgesic treatment is initiated. The location, intensity, and quality of the pain, aggravating and relieving factors, and the patient's emotional and cognitive response to pain should be noted.

Pain Measurement Tools

Although there is no quantitative biochemical or neurophysiologic test for pain, tools have been devised to assess pain intensity [4] (See Chapter 6, Evaluating the Patient with Chronic Pain). Categorical scales, which ask patients to rate pain using adjectives such as "mild" and "excruciating," are simple to use, but assume an understanding of the adjectives. Pain relief may also be rated with a categorical or percentage scale. The verbal numeric scale, rating pain from zero for "no pain" to 10 for "the worst imaginable pain," is easily implemented and recorded during frequent assessments. The use of numbers removes any linguistic misunderstanding of categorical descriptors. Similarly, a 100-mm visual analog scale may be used, with or without intensity descriptors (Fig. 45-2). Although a visual analog pain score may not mean the same thing to different patients, it is reliable on repeated use with the same patient.[5] This permits serial assessments by different clinicians, if necessary, over the course of treatment. Patients must be instructed in the use of these analog scales.

All of these pain scales are unidimensional. They do not reflect the complexity of the pain experience. Nonetheless, they provide a score that can be recorded, as vital signs are[6] This is useful for tracking pain intensity and can prompt intervention when pain exceeds an acceptable level.

When the patient cannot communicate, pain intensity must be evaluated by other means. Next of kin are usually able to verify the existence of pain, but they cannot accurately describe its intensity, location, and treatment.[7] Non-English speakers will need a translator or a pain scale with instructions in their language. Originally designed for use in children, the faces pain scale might also be useful in some cognitively impaired adult patients (Fig. 45-3).[8]

Attention to nonverbal pain manifestations is also important. Autonomic changes may be present, including hypertension, tachycardia, and diaphoresis. Patients with organic brain disease may show agitation or confusion, or they may be apathetic, inactive, or irritable. They may also refuse to eat without explanation, protect the painful part, and show facial grimacing. While these manifestations are not specific for pain, empiric analgesic treatment in such situations, after ruling out more serious acute illness, will often confirm the assessment.

Several multidimensional assessment instruments incorporate pain quality, intensity, location, emotional and functional impact, and effectiveness of coping skills.[9] The best known of these is the McGill Pain Questionnaire (MPQ).[10] The patient chooses among 16 groups of descriptive words to characterize the sensory, affective, and evaluative qualities of his or her pain. Four additional word groups are specific to certain pain conditions. A pain intensity scale, a questionnaire on the use of analgesics and prior pain experience, and a human figure drawing on which the patient indicates his or her pain location are also included in the MPQ. A shorter instrument, the Memorial Pain Assessment Card, is de-

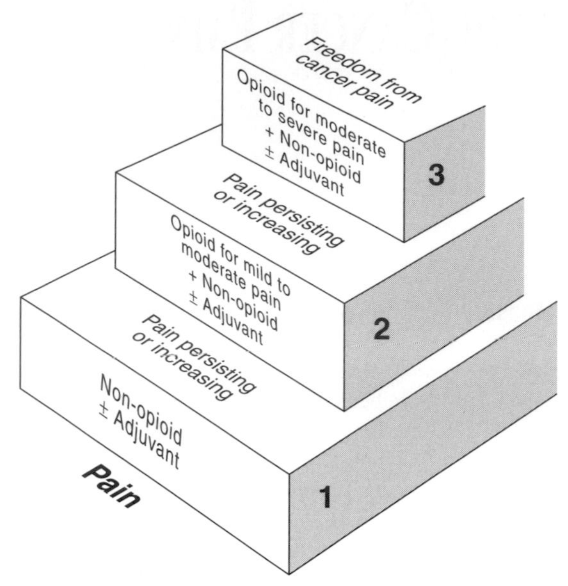

Figure 45-1 The three-step analgesic ladder for cancer pain treatment. (Reproduced by permission of WHO, Cancer Pain Relief. 2nd ed. Geneva, World Health Organization, 1996.)

signed to allow rapid assessment of cancer pain intensity, effectiveness of analgesics, and general psychological distress.[11] It uses three visual analog scales and a set of eight pain intensity descriptors (Fig. 45-4). It appears to correlate with some of the more complicated instruments, yet it can be administered repeatedly without the evaluator's assistance.

NON-OPIOID ANALGESICS

Nonsteroidal anti-inflammatory drugs (NSAIDs) and acetaminophen are routinely used in the treatment of cancer pain (See Chapter 61, NSAIDs). In general, they should be used on an around-the-clock schedule for patients with mild pain before advancing to step 2 of the pain ladder.[1] At that step and beyond, they may be continued in addition to opioids. NSAIDs may be especially effective for bone pain,[12] but they are probably useful in all types of pain, since they provide at least additive analgesia. They can act synergistically with opioids in the spinal cord [13] and allow reduction of opioid dose, lessening the likelihood of opioid side effects. When one NSAID is ineffective or poorly tolerated, another drug should be tried. When the oral route is not available, as in the patient with unremitting nausea, some NSAIDs and acetaminophen may be given rectally. Ketorolac is available for intramuscular and intravenous use in the United States, but is not recommended for prolonged use because of concern about gastrointestinal toxicity (Table 45-1).

NSAID Side Effects

Before initiating NSAID or acetaminophen therapy, the potential for toxicity must be considered (See Chapter 61, NSAIDs).[14] Nonselective NSAIDs inhibit cyclooxygenase 1 and 2 (COX-1 and COX–2), and produce gastroduodenal irritation and ulceration, renal cortical ischemia, hepatotoxicity, and platelet dysfunction. These toxicities are believed to be primarily related to COX-1 inhibition.[15] COX-2 is induced by injury or inflammation, and likely that NSAID analgesia is mainly related to inhibition of this isoenzyme. Certain NSAIDs, including choline magnesium trisalicylate, nabumetone, diclofenac, and etodolac, may be less likely to cause gastrointestinal toxicity because they show relative selectivity for COX-2.[16] Celecoxib and rofecoxib cause less gastrointestinal toxicity than traditional NSAIDs.[17]

NSAID-induced dyspepsia is best managed prophylactically by taking the drugs with food. If this is insufficient, addition of an H_2-receptor blocker, misoprostol, omeprazole, lansoprazole, sucralfate, or an oral antacid may be necessary. NSAID-induced ulcers may be prevented with H_2 blockers (e.g., famotidine 40mg per day, or ranitidine 150 mg twice daily) or misoprostol (200 μg orally three times daily).[18] Yeomans et al showed that omeprazole (20 mg or 40 mg taken orally every day) is somewhat more effective in preventing and healing gastric and duodenal ulcers than ranitidine.[19] The same group also found that omeprazole is better than misoprostol in healing gastric and duodenal ulcers and in preventing their reappearance during NSAID therapy.[20] The risk of ulceration during NSAID therapy increases with age, previous NSAID intolerance, history of peptic ulcer disease, and smoking.[21] In such patients, prophylactic use of an H_2 blocker, proton, pump inhibitor, or misoprostol is warranted.

Most NSAIDs interfere with platelet aggregation. Choline magnesium trisalicylate does not prevent normal platelet aggregation as measured experimentally, and appears to be associated with less occult gastrointestinal bleeding.[22] COX-2 inhibitors have less platelet effects,[17] but the clinical implications of this effect remain to be determined. Despite its short elimination half-life, aspirin irreversibly inhibits platelet aggregation for the lifetime of the platelet (4 to 7 days). The platelet effect of other NSAIDs lasts about 2 days after the drug is discontinued.

Renal effects of NSAIDs include reversible renal insufficiency, interstitial nephritis, and predisposition to acute tubular necrosis in the patient with low renal perfusion. NSAIDs should be prescribed with caution for patients with hypertension, renal insufficiency, or congestive heart failure. Although COX-2 inhibitors might eventually prove less nephrotoxic than conventional NSAIDs, present evidence is insufficient to draw this conclusion.[23]

Other toxicities are also possible: both acetaminophen and NSAIDs may cause hepatic toxicity, even at normally recommended doses.[24] Confusion and inability to concentrate are possible central nervous system (CNS) effects of the NSAIDs. Patients who are allergic to aspirin or to an NSAID may be cross-reactive to other NSAIDs.

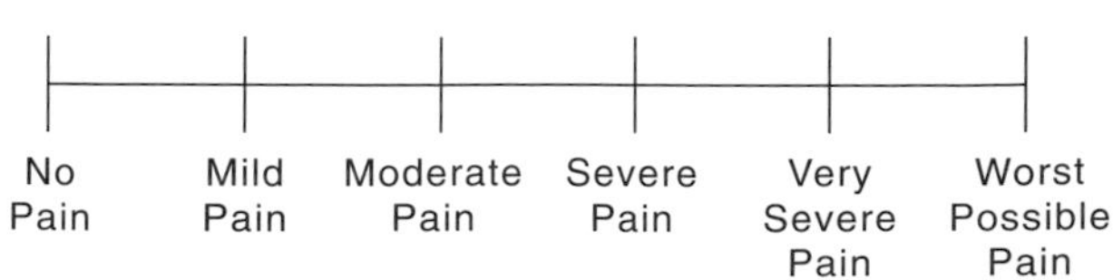

Figure 45-2 A visual analog scale, with intensity descriptors. The patient is asked to mark a point on a 10-centimeter line that represents the level of pain. (Scale to 10 centimeters.)

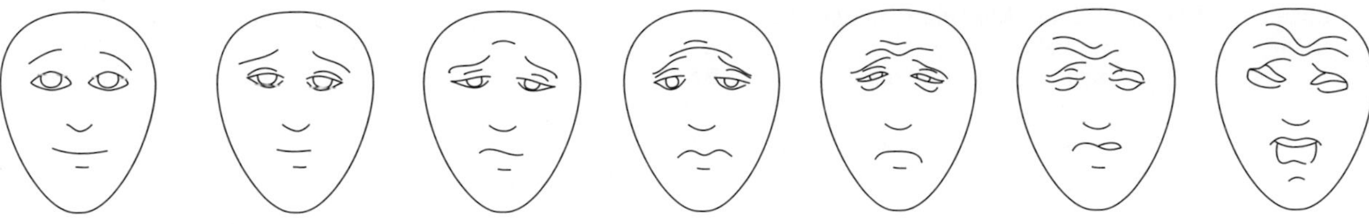

Figure 45-3 The faces pain scale. The patient chooses the face that represents his pain experience. (Reprinted from Bieri D, Reeve RA, Champion GD, et al. The faces pain scale for the self-assessment of the severity of pain experienced by children: development, initial validation, and preliminary investigation for ratio scale properties. Pain. 1990;41:139. Copyright 1990, with permission from Elsevier Science.)

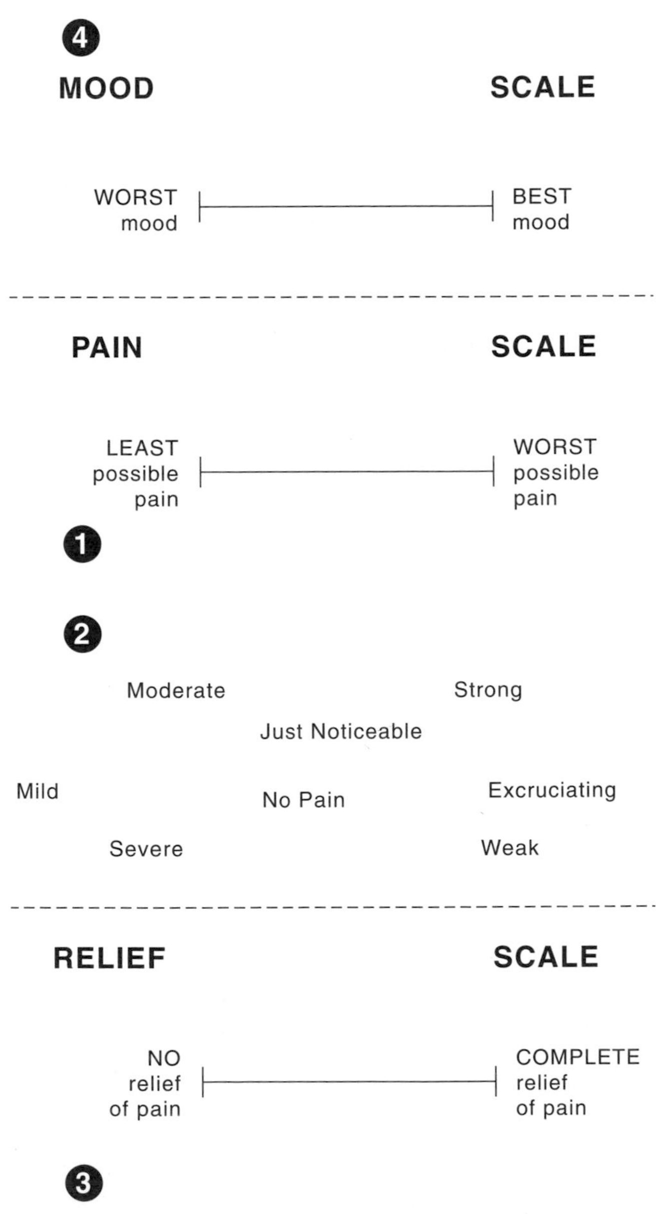

Figure 45-4 The Memorial Pain Assessment Card. (From Fishman B, et al. Cancer. 1987;60:1151. Copyright 1987 American Cancer Society. Reprinted by permission of Wiley-Liss, Inc., a subsidiary of John Wiley & Sons, Inc.)

OPIOIDS

Opioids are indicated for the treatment of cancer pain because of their effectiveness, reliability and safety, and ease of administration (See Chapter 58, Opioid Pharmacology). Although neuropathic pain may be more difficult to treat with opioids, its presence does not preclude a favorable response to opioid-based analgesia.[25]

Steps 2 and 3 of the WHO ladder advocate the addition of opioids for moderate to severe pain, with or without an adjuvant drug.[1] "Weak" and "strong" opioids (for step 2 and step 3, respectively) are not inherently different in their ability to control pain, but are customarily used in amounts appropriate for milder and stronger pain, respectively. The so-called weak opioids (codeine, hydrocodone, dihydrocodone) are commonly prepared in combination with coanalgesics (acetaminophen, aspirin, or an NSAID). The coanalgesic limits dose escalation, necessitating a change to another opioid or preparation as pain increases.

Tolerance, Physical Dependence, and Addiction

Opioids can induce tolerance and physical dependence. Addiction—defined as loss of control over drug use, compulsive use, and use despite harm—is rare in patients with no history of substance abuse.[26] Although demands for opioids and dramatic pain behavior are commonly interpreted as markers of addiction, undertreatment of pain is an alternative explanation (pseudoaddiction).[27]

Although tolerance to opioid analgesia occurs, disease progression is usually to blame for increasing analgesic requirements.[28] Tolerance to adverse effects, such as respiratory depression and somnolence, is favorable and allows dose escalation to analgesic levels. Physical dependence is another pharmacologic effect of opioid drugs, and is defined solely by the development of abstinence after abrupt discontinuation of therapy or administration of an antagonist. Physical dependence is not a clinical problem if abstinence is avoided.

Choosing an Opioid

Comparative clinical trials do not exist to differentiate opioids according to responsiveness. Hence, they are usually chosen on the basis of familiarity by the prescriber. Other factors to consider are the route of administration, cost, convenience, and availability. Individual patients vary greatly in their response to different opioids, supporting the practice of sequential opioid trials (opioid rotation)

TABLE 45-1 **Doses and Routes of Some Nonopioid Analgesics**

Drug	Dose	Frequency	Route	Daily Maximum	Comments
Acetaminophen	500–1000 mg	q4-6h	PO/PR	4000 mg	Liquid available.
Aspirin	500–1000 mg	q4-6h	PO/PR	4000 mg	
Diflusinal	500 mg	q8h	PO	1500 mg	First dose 1000 mg.
Choline Magnesium Trisalicylate	750–1500 mg	q8-12h	PO	3000 mg	Liquid available. Less dyspepsia and platelet dysfunction
Ibuprofen	200–600 mg	q4-6h	PO	2400 mg	
Ketoprofen	25–75 mg	q4-8h	PO	300 mg	
Flurbiprofen	50–100 mg	q4-6h	PO	300 mg	
Naproxen	250 mg	q6-8h	PO	1250 mg	Sustained release available First dose 500 mg.
Indomethacin	25–50 mg	q8-12h	PO/PR	100 mg	Frequent side effects.
Ketorolac	10–30 mg	q6h	PO IV/IM	40 mg 60 mg	Lower dose for repeated use. Limit to 5 days (PO/IV).
Etodolac	200–400 mg	q6-8h	PO	1200 mg	
Diclofenac	25–100 mg	q6-12h	PO	200 mg	
Nabumetone	500–1500 mg	q24h	PO	1500 mg	
Oxaprozin	600–1200 mg	q24h	PO	1200 mg	
Celecoxib	100–200 mg	q12	PO	400 mg	COX-2 inhibitor.
Rofecoxib	12.5–50 mg	q24h	PO	50 mg	COX-2 inhibitor.

to find the most acceptable balance between analgesia and side effects (See Changing opioids and routes of administration later in this Chapter).[29]

The initial opioid should be a short-acting drug when the patient has severe pain and requires rapid dose titration, when the patient has intermittent pain, or when the patient is opioid naïve and there is concern about delayed toxicity from a long-acting preparation. In other cases, a long-acting drug may be the initial opioid. Long-acting opioids include methadone, levorphanol, and extended-release preparations of morphine, oxycodone, and fentanyl.

There are differences among opioids in toxicity. Meperidine should be avoided for cancer pain treatment, especially in patients with renal failure.[30] Its active metabolite, normeperidine, has a long half-life, and causes CNS excitability, including seizures. It accumulates with high doses, prolonged use, and renal dysfunction. Morphine is metabolized to a potent opioid compound, morphine-6-glucuronide. It does not tend to cause problems in patients with normal renal function, but can lead to toxicity in those with renal failure. In these patients, morphine should be used with caution.

Partial opioid receptor agonists (buprenorphine) and mixed agonist-antagonists (pentazocine, dezocine, nalbuphine, and butorphanol) also should be avoided. They may precipitate withdrawal symptoms and pain in patients already physically dependent on opioids. When used alone, increasing amounts provide less incremental analgesia, a phenomenon known as a "ceiling effect." Some of the mixed agonist-antagonists have relatively greater toxicity than the pure mu agonists.[31]

Combination analgesics, which often contain acetaminophen, should be used with caution because of the possibility of acetaminophen toxicity. Daily acetaminophen intake should be limited to 4 g. Alcohol use, coexisting hepatic disease, and starvation (which may be present in debilitated cancer patients) predispose to acetaminophen hepatotoxicity at lower doses.[24]

Methadone and levorphanol have long half-lives and may be considered in place of extended-release preparations for baseline opioid requirements. One advantage of these drugs is that they are absorbed easily by the gut, and may be effective in patients with bowel pathology who are unable to completely absorb the extended-release preparations.[32] These drugs, particularly methadone, may be difficult to titrate, however, because the initial duration of action (4 to 6 hours) is shorter than the half-life, leading to drug accumulation with repeated dosing over 2 to 5 days. Furthermore, methadone pharmacokinetics are highly variable among patients, owing to differences in protein binding, urinary excretion, and induction of metabolism by methadone and other drugs.[32,33] Methadone's half-life is usually about 24 hours, but may be as short as 12 hours, or longer than 150 hours. Therefore, it may be prudent to use these two opioids on an as-needed basis initially, allowing an adjustment for drug accumulation by titrating to the analgesic effect and to the degree of sedation.[34]

Opioid Dosing

The appropriate opioid dose and interval control pain without end-of-dose failure and unacceptable side effects at peak concentration (i.e., without bolus effects). The required dose varies with the severity of pain, the type of pain, preexisting opioid exposure, psychological distress, and other factors.[25] The elderly are more sensitive to opioid-induced analgesia, but may also be more susceptible to side effects.[35] Large doses may be necessary as the disease progresses. Although there is no theoretical limit to the dose, a practical limit is imposed by the occurrence of intolerable side effects, a large injectate volume, numerous pills or suppositories, or excessive skin surface required for fentanyl patches.

When initiating opioid therapy, a short-acting drug may be given as needed every 2 or 3 hours (Table 45-2). After 5 or 6 half-lives (1 day for morphine), the basal daily opioid requirement is determined and a long-acting opioid preparation may be substituted. Alternatively, a long-acting opioid may be used initially when pain is constant and not severe or progressive. Long-acting opioids should be provided regularly to prevent most pain. An additional short-acting opioid (5% to 15% of the basal daily requirement) is made available for breakthrough pain every 1 to 3 hours.[34] If the short-acting opioid is needed more than three times per day, the amount of long-acting opioid is usually increased. It is inconvenient and unnecessary to increase the dosing frequency of long-acting oral preparations when increasing the total daily dose. Dose changes should be in increments of one third to one half of the preceding dose, or according to the patient's usage of breakthrough opioid. If side effects prevent dose escalation, a switch to another opioid should be considered before changing to another route of administration or abandoning opioids.[29]

Cessation or reduction of opioid use may be appropriate when the patient is pain-free following antitumor therapy, or after a successful anesthetic or neuroablative procedure. Based on clinical observation, reduction of the daily dose by 50% every 3 days will usually prevent symptomatic withdrawal. Withdrawal is marked by yawning, nausea, vomiting, abdominal cramps, diarrhea, insomnia, anxiety, irritability, temperature instability, diaphoresis, and salivation.

Route of Administration

The usual route of systemic opioid administration is oral. Peak effect is typically in 20 to 90 minutes, and duration is 3 to 6 hours.[38] Extended-release oral preparations (morphine and oxycodone) are available for maintenance of steady analgesia, with peak effect at 2 to 3 hours, and a duration of 8 to 24 hours.[39,40,41] The clear advantages of oral administration are the numerous drugs available and their ease of use. However, some patients may not be able to use oral medications, including those with oral mucositis, dysphagia, bowel obstruction, and severe nausea.[42]

Fentanyl is the only opioid prepared for transdermal use, which is especially important when the oral route is made unavailable by dysphagia or impaired gastrointestinal function.[43] Transdermal fentanyl might also be selected if patient compliance with oral analgesics has been a problem. The onset of analgesia is 12 to 14 hours from initial patch application, and continues for 16 to 24 hours after removal. A comparative trial against extended-release morphine suggests that transdermal fentanyl is associated with less constipation.[44]

Morphine, oxymorphone, and hydromorphone are manufactured for rectal use. Injectable methadone and sustained-release morphine have also been used rectally.[42,45] A disadvantage of rectal administration is the inter-patient variability in absorption and degree of first-pass metabolism. Partial avoidance of the portal circulation may result in slightly increased bioavailability compared to oral opioids. Whereas morphine suppositories are slowly absorbed,[42] morphine microenema (10 mg in 1mL) has a more rapid onset and longer duration than the same dose given orally.[46] Mucositis or transmucosal lesions, diarrhea, thrombocytopenia, and neutropenia contraindicate the rectal route.

Fentanyl is newly available in an oral transmucosal form (Actiq) for breakthrough pain, but experience is limited. Some pharmacies can compound concentrated solutions of morphine,

TABLE 45-2 **Equivalent and Recommended Opioid Doses and Routes**

	Approximate Equianalgesic Dose		Usual Starting Dose	
Drug	**Oral**	**Parenteral**	**Oral**	**Parenteral**
Morphine[1,3,4]	30 mg q 3–4 h	10 mg q 3–4 h	20–60 mg q 3–4 h	10 mg q 3–4 h
Hydromorphone[4]	7.5 mg q 3–4 h	1.5 mg q 3–4 h	4–8 mg q 3–4 h	1–2 mg q 3–4 h
Methadone	20 mg q 6–8 h	10 mg q 6–8 h	20 mg q 6–8 h	10 mg q 6–8 h
Levorphanol	4 mg q 6–8 h	2 mg q 6–8 h	2–4 mg q 6–8 h	1–2 mg q 6–8 h
Meperidine[2]	300 mg q 2–3 h	100 mg q 3 h	300 mg q 2–3 h	100 mg q 2–3 h
Codeine	200 mg q 3–4 h	130 mg q 4 h	30–60 mg q 3–4 h[5]	60 mg q 2 h[5]
Hydrocodone	30 mg q 3–4 h	N/A	5–10 mg q 3–4 h[5]	N/A
Oxycodone[3]	30 mg q 3–4 h	N/A	5–10 mg q 3–4 h[5]	N/A
Fentanyl	N/A	100 μg/h[6]	N/A	25–50 μg/h[6]

[1]Doses of morphine shown are for chronic use. Larger doses of oral morphine are needed for equivalent acute analgesia.[36]

[2]Meperidine is not recommended for chronic use.

[3]Morphine and oxycodone are available in controlled release forms, which are given two or three times per day. The total daily dose is unchanged.

[4]Available as a rectal suppository. Rectal opioids are roughly equianalgesic to oral opioids.[37]

[5]Doses recommended for codeine, hydrocodone, and oxycodone are for milder pain. Usually used in fixed combinations with acetaminophen or NSAIDs.

[6]Provided as a transdermal patch, which is changed every 2 to 3 days. Fever increases drug uptake.

oxycodone, and hydromorphone (up to 50 mg/mL) for sublingual use. These preparations might be useful for patients with dysphagia or gastrointestinal dysfunction.

Injected opioids may be useful for patients who cannot take opioids by the oral, sublingual, or rectal routes, for those who need rapid dose titration, and for those whose high opioid needs cannot be easily met by other routes. Subcutaneous injection is preferred over intramuscular, as the latter is more painful. Intravenous injection of most opioids provides peak effect in 5 to 15 minutes, with similarly shortened duration of effect. Continuous infusion (subcutaneous or intravenous) or frequent redosing is usually necessary to maintain analgesia with injected opioids. Subcutaneous infusion volume should be limited, especially in cachectic patients, to permit stable absorption.[47] Moulin et al compared subcutaneous to intravenous opioid infusion in 15 patients with cancer pain in a double-blind, randomized, crossover trial.[48] The mean bioavailability was 78% with subcutaneous infusion, but pain scores and the need for breakthrough medication were no different from intravenous infusion.

Patient-controlled analgesia (PCA) may be useful for initiation of parenteral opioid therapy, rapid opioid titration with changing pain intensity, and treatment of incident pain.[49] Since the patient controls the delivery of opioid, individual differences in pain intensity, drug clearance, and effectiveness are less likely to interfere with therapy. In a study of 26 patients with oral mucositis following bone marrow transplantation, psychological dependence was no more likely, total opioid consumption and side effects were less, and analgesia was the same or better with PCA as with nurse-administered opioids.[50] PCA devices are individually programmed for the size of the dose, the minimum time between doses (lockout interval), and the cumulative dose allowed in 1 or 4 hours (several times higher than the anticipated need). Continuous infusion may be programmed in addition to the demand doses to allow sleep and to cover baseline pain. An important safety feature of PCA is that the patient will not request additional medication when overly sedated. Those attending to the patient must not circumvent this safety feature by pressing the demand button.

Recommended PCA settings for morphine, hydromorphone, and fentanyl are shown in Table 45-3. Much larger doses may be needed for the opioid-tolerant patient. To limit the total volume of injectate, hydromorphone may be chosen over fentanyl and morphine because of its potency and solubility. Fentanyl is commercially available only at 50 μg/mL, whereas morphine and hydromorphone can be compounded to 50 mg/mL for injection.

PCA is an efficient means of determining a patient's opioid requirement when initiating or changing opioids. The pump records the amount of drug used, which is then converted to continuous infusion, transdermal fentanyl, or a sustained-release oral preparation. PCA is available for use in the home as well as the hospital. Patients without intravenous access may use subcutaneous PCA.[49]

Changing Opioids and Routes of Administration

Dose-limiting side effects and the loss of the previous route of administration are the usual reasons for changing drugs or routes. Trials of several opioids should be considered before abandoning systemic opioids for treatment of cancer pain, as patients may respond differently to different drugs. Incomplete cross-tolerance between opioids may account for the apparent decrease in required dose when changing analgesic drugs.[29,51] When changing one opioid to another drug or route of administration, conversion is made with the assistance of opioid conversion charts (Table 45-2).

All opioid doses can be expressed as equianalgesic doses. Typically, 10 mg of parenteral morphine is considered the unit dose, and doses of other drugs for oral or parenteral administration are listed in equianalgesic amounts. The conversion tables (Table 45-2) contain approximations based largely on short-term use of smaller opioid doses. When converting large opioid doses, caution dictates dose reduction by one third to one half to account for incomplete cross-tolerance.[29,51] When changing to methadone, a 75% to 90% initial dose reduction is indicated because of the greater potential for drug accumulation and the possibility of unexpectedly high potency.[29] If inadequate analgesia necessitates the conversion, and there are no significant side effects, the new drug may be started closer to the equianalgesic dose.[34] Additional short-acting opioid is made available while titrating the new drug to achieve stable analgesia. When any change in opioid or route is made, frequent assessments are needed to keep pain controlled and to prevent side effects.

ANALGESIC ADJUVANTS

Analgesic adjuvants are rarely adequate analgesics when used alone for cancer pain. They are used especially to relieve neuropathic pain and to provide an opioid-sparing effect, thus lessening opioid-related side effects. Many patients with neuropathic pain, however, can be treated with opioids alone.[25]

Antidepressants

Tricyclic antidepressants (TCAs) were used as analgesics shortly after their introduction.[52,53,54] The mechanism of their analgesic

TABLE 45-3 **Suggested Post-Controlled Analgesia Opioid Programming for the Opioid-Naïve Patient, After a Loading Dose of the Opioid is Given**

Drug	Bolus Dose	Lockout Interval	Hourly Maximum
Morphine 1 mg/mL	0.5–2.5 mg	5–15 minutes	5–15 mg
Hydromorphone 0.25 mg/mL	0.125–0.375 mg	5–15 minutes	1.25–3 mg
Fentanyl 25 or 50 μg/mL	12.5–50 μg	5–10 minutes	100–300 μg

action is not certain, but probably includes enhancement of monoamine concentrations in the dorsal horn,[55] and stimulation of $alpha_2$ receptors[56] (See Chapter 62, Adjuvant Analgesics). They are useful in treating neuropathic pain, and have been proven analgesic in well-designed trials for postherpetic neuralgia, diabetic neuropathy, atypical facial pain, migraine headache, fibrositis, and central poststroke pain.[53,54] There are few controlled trials of TCAs for the treatment of cancer pain, perhaps because cancer pain encompasses so many somatic, visceral, and neuropathic entities (See Chapter 44, Cancer Pain Syndromes). Amitriptyline has been shown effective in a placebo-controlled study of 20 patients with neuropathic postmastectomy pain.[57] The analgesic effect of the TCAs on neuropathic pain seems to be separate from their antidepressant or sedative effects.[57–61]

TCAs are most appropriate for cancer patients with neuropathic pain, which is often described as burning, searing, aching, or dysesthetic, and occurs in the setting of known or probable nerve injury. The choice of drug is empiric; there is no clearly superior drug. A patient having difficulty with sleep may benefit from a more sedating drug, such as amitriptyline, imipramine, or doxepin. Nortriptyline is less sedating, and desipramine has the fewest side effects.[58,62] Trazodone is not an effective analgesic for neuropathic pain, but may be indicated in the cancer pain patient with a sleep disturbance. Probably fewer than half of patients with neuropathic pain achieve greater than 50% pain relief with an antidepressant,[54] and a lack of complete relief should not be interpreted as treatment failure.

Suggested dosing for the TCAs is shown in Table 45-4. Because these drugs are usually sedating, they are best given in the evening. If the initial low dose is not effective, it should be increased every few days until an effect is seen or side effects become intolerable. As with opioids, greater analgesia is seen with higher doses.[59]

Adverse effects with TCAs are common.[54] They are primarily anticholinergic, including sedation, constipation, urinary retention and overflow incontinence, tachycardia, dry mouth, blurred vision, dysphoria, and agitation. Antihistaminergic effects are responsible for sedation and weight gain, and may exacerbate hypotension. $Alpha_1$ and $alpha_2$ blockade contribute to orthostatic hypotension and tachycardia. Most of these side effects are not life-threatening and diminish with time. Dry mouth tends to persist. The side effects are troubling, however, and often prevent the continued use of TCAs. Cardiac conduction abnormalities and seizures are more concerning effects. A history of seizure is a relative contraindication to TCA use.[63] An electrocardiogram should be obtained prior to TCA initiation to rule out bundle branch block and bifascicular block, which are also relative contraindications.[64] Dose adjustment according to drug levels may help to prevent these consequences of antidepressant therapy.[63] When a patient experiences unwanted side effects, it is wise to switch to another TCA, since patient responses are variable and often idiosyncratic. Persistence in treatment is essential, as analgesic response may take 4 weeks to achieve.[53]

Selective serotonin reuptake inhibitors (SSRIs) are newer antidepressants than TCAs. They are usually better tolerated than TCAs, but there is little evidence to support their use in cancer pain. Although SSRIs are commonly used to treat fibromyalgia and migraine headaches, most studies have found them to be less effective in neuropathic pain.[54,61,62] SSRIs should be tried when TCAs are not tolerated or relatively contraindicated.

Anticonvulsants

Carbamazepine has long been used for treatment of trigeminal neuralgia.[65] Several anticonvulsants are now commonly employed to treat lancinating and burning dysesthesias complicating nerve injury (See also Chapter 62, Adjuvant Analgesics). In addition to trigeminal neuralgia, glossopharyngeal neuralgia, tabes dorsalis, diabetic neuropathy, postherpetic neuralgia, postamputation pain, migraines, central pain, and other conditions have been reported to respond to anticonvulsants in case reports, case series, and poorly controlled trials.[66] Two randomized, double-blind, placebo-controlled studies support the use of gabapentin for diabetic neuropathy and postherpetic neuralgia.[67,68]

Swerdlow studied 200 patients with lancinating pain in an open-label, uncontrolled trial of carbamazepine, phenytoin, valproate, and clonazepam.[66] Patients were switched from one drug to another if they failed to obtain relief. Most patients did respond to one of the drugs, but there was no clearly superior medication in general or for any particular condition. McQuay et al conducted a recent systematic review of 20 randomized, controlled anticonvulsant trials.[69] Trigeminal neuralgia responded to carbamazepine, and diabetic neuropathy responded to both carbamazepine and phenytoin. Valproate and carbamazepine were effective for migraine prophylaxis. While there are few prospective, controlled trials of anticonvulsants for patients with cancer pain, individual patients may respond dramatically, and these medications should not be withheld from patients in pain, pending definitive evidence of their efficacy. Yajnik et al compared phenytoin with buprenorphine and the combination in three groups of 25 patients with cancer pain resulting from various causes.[70] A low dose of phenytoin (100 mg twice daily) provided greater than 50% pain relief in most patients, and enhanced the effect of buprenorphine without increasing side effects.

TABLE 45-4 **Doses of Some Tricyclic Antidepressants Used for Pain Management**

Antidepressant	Dose Range	Comments
Amitriptyline	10–150 mg	Sedation and hypotension are common. Effective for insomnia.
Imipramine	10–150 mg	Sedating.
Nortriptyline	10–100 mg	Sedating, but less so than amitriptyline.
Desipramine	10–150 mg	May have an alerting effect. Tachycardia.
Doxepin	10–150 mg	Very sedating.

Gabapentin is receiving considerable attention in pain management, and there is now convincing evidence to support its use in diabetic neuropathy and postherpetic neuralgia.[67,68] It has not been studied in cancer pain, but it is commonly used because of its few side effects and relative absence of drug interactions. It is usually started at 300 mg at bed time, and increased as high as 3600 mg/day in divided doses. Dosage should be reduced in patients with renal failure. Side effects (somnolence, ataxia, and dizziness) are not life-threatening and plasma concentrations are not monitored, making this an easy anticonvulsant to use.[71] Other new anticonvulsants, lamotrigine, tiagabine, oxcarbazepine, and topiramate are also being investigated for analgesic activity.

Carbamazepine is started at 100 mg twice daily, and is escalated until toxicity occurs, pain is relieved, or the safe plasma level is exceeded (12 μg/mL). Bone marrow suppression often manifests as mild leukopenia or thrombocytopenia, and rarely aplastic anemia. If bone marrow suppression is anticipated from radiation, chemotherapy, or tumor replacement, carbamazepine should be avoided. Patients receiving carbamazepine should have their complete blood counts and hepatic transaminases monitored. Reversible hepatotoxicity, resembling viral hepatitis, occurs rarely, and fatal hepatic necrosis is less common.[72] Cutaneous reactions may also occur, and require cessation of the medication. Sedation, vertigo, ataxia, hyponatremia, and nausea are more common effects.[66]

Phenytoin and valproate are available in oral and intravenous forms. A new form of phenytoin, fosphenytoin, may be administered intramuscularly. Treatment with phenytoin begins with an oral loading dose, and maintenance therapy, starting at 100 mg three times daily, is adjusted to control pain with a plasma concentration of less than 20 μg/mL. Side effects may include anemia, anorexia, nausea, somnolence, and ataxia. Bone marrow suppression is less likely with phenytoin than carbamazepine. The potential for hepatotoxicity mandates periodic monitoring of liver function tests.[66] Hypersensitivity to phenytoin is rare but potentially fatal, and manifests with rash, fever, and hepatitis. Up to 19% of patients on phenytoin develop cutaneous reactions, usually without hypersensitivity.[73] Oral valproate therapy usually starts at 125 mg twice daily. The most common side effects are nausea and epigastric pain,which are reduced by taking it with food and with enteric-coated tablets. Hepatotoxicity is rare.[66]

Clonazepam is available for oral or parenteral use, and is started at 0.25 to 0.5 mg daily. It is the most sedating anticonvulsant, and may be useful for patients with anxiety and insomnia. The dose is increased as needed. Plasma concentrations are not measured and the principal toxicity is sedation.

Systemic Local Anesthetics

Systemic local anesthetics are often used to treat neuropathic pain (See also Chapter 62, Adjuvant Analgesics). Intravenous lidocaine (5 mg/kg over 30 minutes) has been found effective for postherpetic neuralgia (PHN) and diabetic neuropathy.[74,75] Painful peripheral neuropathies may also respond to oral mexilitine (10 mg/kg/day).[76,77] Systemic local anesthetics have not been studied for cancer pain.

Topical Analgesics

Topical local anesthetics are often used in the treatment of mucocutaneous pain states. Topical lidocaine and benzocaine provide temporary relief of pain from oral mucositis. This is necessary to allow the patient to eat and for oral hygiene. Likewise, Rowbotham et al showed that topical application of 5% lidocaine gel relieves the pain of PHN for up to 24 hours in a blinded, placebo and site-controlled trial.[78] The effect is greatest when lidocaine is applied in the painful dermatome. A lidocaine patch was recently approved in the United States for treatment of PHN.

Capsaicin is the compound in chili peppers that makes them taste hot. When it is applied to the skin or a mucus membrane, it produces a burning sensation as a result of C fiber activation. Repeated application causes desensitization.[79] Although it is promoted for relief of arthritis pain, topical capsaicin has been found useful for some types of neuropathic pain.[79,80] Postmastectomy pain, diabetic neuropathy, and postherpetic neuralgia may respond. Studies have been complicated by difficulty in blinding because only the active preparation causes a burning sensation. Capsaicin is available over the counter in 0.25% and 0.75% concentrations in a cream vehicle and a roll-on. The cream should be used four to five times daily. Unfortunately, many patients do not persist in applying the cream after the first few treatments because of the uncomfortable burning.[80]

Corticosteroids

Corticosteroids are used as coanalgesics when inflammation or the mass effect of vasogenic edema causes pain.[81] They reduce inflammation by inhibiting phospholipase activity, and thus prostaglandin synthesis. In addition, they may reduce axonal sprouting and neurokinin concentration in sensory fibers near injured tissue.[82] Regenerating axons in neuromas discharge spontaneously or with minimal tactile stimulation because of high sodium channel expression[83]; locally injected corticosteroids reduce neuroma discharge in animal models, and appear to be effective in humans as well. Acute neural compression, intracranial hypertension, bony and soft tissue infiltration, and visceral distention cause pain that may respond to steroids.

Corticosteroid therapy for cancer pain usually includes dexamethasone, 4 to 8 mg, methylprednisolone, 8 to 40 mg, or prednisone 10 to 50 mg. Multiple daily doses are not needed, except for hydrocortisone.[81] High initial doses are continued until a response is seen, then tapered to the minimum effective dose. Concurrent use of phenytoin, carbamazepine, or phenobarbital induces hepatic metabolism of corticosteroids, increasing the required dose. Dexamethasone may be given in very high doses (40 to 100 mg intravenously) for the initial treatment of spinal cord compression and for selected patients with other causes of crescendo pain.

Corticosteroids have numerous toxicities when taken chronically.[81] These include fluid retention and electrolyte disturbances, hypertension, proximal myopathy, osteoporosis and aseptic necrosis, insomnia, psychosis, gastritis, hyperglycemia, and impaired cellular immunity. These adverse effects may be undesirable in cancer patients who are expected to survive for more than several months. Mood elevation, antiemesis, and appetite stimulation are often desirable side effects of corticosteroids, but they may diminish with prolonged use.[81]

Sedatives and Tranquilizers

Most benzodiazepines and barbiturates have no significant primary analgesic effect, but may reduce anxiety associated with uncontrolled pain and cancer. Clonazepam, when used for lancinating neuropathic pain and myoclonus, may be an effective coanalgesic (See Sections entitled Anticonvulsants, and Myoclonus and Hyperalgesia). Benzodiazepines may also be effective for reducing muscle spasm, which may accompany pain and spinal cord injury, and have a coanalgesic role in these conditions. Lorazepam has been used to prevent nausea associated with chemotherapy.

Phenothiazines have been used commonly in conjunction with opioids for acute pain management. Although they have a tranquilizing effect, only methotrimeprazine, which is no longer marketed, is analgesic when used alone.[84] Extrapyramidal side effects, sedation, and hypotension make chronic phenothiazine use impractical for cancer pain treatment. They are more often indicated in the treatment of nausea and anxiety.

Most antihistamines are mild analgesics. The mechanism of analgesic activity is unknown. Hydroxyzine (50 to 100 mg intramuscularly) is commonly used in conjunction with opioids for acute pain. It is also effective in cancer pain.[85] These drugs are most useful for their sedative, muscle relaxing, and antiemetic properties, though opioids are more effective analgesics.

Calcitonin and Bisphosphonates

Pain from osteolytic metastases may be caused by bony destruction alone or by neural or soft tissue compression by pathologic fracture. Bisphosphonates and calcitonin are noncytotoxic agents that inhibit osteoclast activity. They are often used for the management of hypercalcemia of malignancy.[86] They have also been found to reduce bone pain from metastases, and may induce healing of lytic lesions.[87] Calcitonin also inhibits malignant osteolysis, and reduces bone pain in patients with advanced, progressive disease.[88]

Calcitonin has also been investigated for the treatment of neuropathic pain. The mechanism of analgesia is uncertain, but binding of calcitonin in the hypothalamus and limbic system, areas rich in serotonin, may have a role. A double-blind crossover study of intravenous salmon calcitonin (200 μg) in 21 patients with acute phantom limb pain showed a decrease in pain intensity and frequency with calcitonin.[89]

Alpha$_2$ Agonists

Clonidine, an alpha$_2$ receptor agonist, may contribute to analgesia by stimulating presynaptic or postsynaptic receptors in the superficial dorsal horn, decreasing sympathetic outflow, and enhancing noradrenergic inhibitory fibers from the brain stem.[90] These mechanisms may make clonidine a useful analgesic adjuvant for opioids, especially in the setting of neuropathic pain.[91,92] Max et al found a single dose of oral clonidine (200 μg) superior to placebo, ibuprofen (800 mg), and codeine (120 mg) in the treatment of postherpetic neuralgia.[90] The epidural route appears to be more effective than the systemic route for clonidine.[92] Side effects associated with clonidine include orthostatic hypotension, sedation, dry mouth, and constipation. Clonidine does not appear to aggravate opioid-induced respiratory depression, however.

Tizanidine is a newer alpha$_2$ agonist that has been used to treat pain associated with muscle spasm,[93,94] and neuropathic pain.[95] Because it causes less hemodynamic disturbance than clonidine, it may be more useful in treating debilitated patients. Animal studies suggest that tizanidine is also effective when administered intrathecally.[96] Tizanidine, like clonidine, produces sedation.

MANAGEMENT OF ANALGESIC SIDE EFFECTS

Many of the analgesics described produce dose-limiting side effects. Unfortunately, patients and their families are often asked to accept a compromise between pain and these other symptoms. As the use of opioids and other analgesics becomes more widespread for cancer pain, control of side effects is receiving increased attention.

Nausea and Vomiting

Opioids have three emetogenic mechanisms: a direct effect on the chemoreceptor trigger zone, an enhancing effect on vestibular sensitivity, and a slowing effect on gastric emptying. Although nausea is common with opioids, tolerance to this effect occurs quickly. Treatment is therefore given as needed.[34] When evaluating opioid-induced nausea, refractory constipation and impaction of stool must be considered and treated first. If nausea follows meals or is accompanied by postprandial vomiting, metoclopramide is an appropriate choice. If it occurs with movement, meclizine may be more effective. In the absence of these associations, a phenothiazine, butyrophenone, antihistamine, or serotonin antagonist is appropriate (Table 45-5). If these are ineffective, a corticosteroid[81] or benzodiazepine may also be useful.

Constipation

Opioids bind to specific receptors in the gastrointestinal tract and central nervous system to produce constipation by direct and anticholinergic effects.[97] Increased gastrointestinal transit time causes excessive water and electrolyte reabsorption from the feces. Decreased biliary and pancreatic secretion further dehydrates the stool. Tricyclic antidepressants, clonidine, dehydration, surgical procedures, and bowel obstruction by tumor contribute to constipation as well. Elderly patients are particularly susceptible to constipation and impaction of stool.[98]

Opioid-induced constipation is so common that cathartic and stool-softening medications should be routinely initiated with around-the-clock opioid orders in predisposed patients, such as the elderly. The coadministration of docusate (100 mg taken orally

TABLE 45-5 **Some Antiemetics**

Drug	Dose	Route
Metoclopramide	10 mg QID	PO/IV
Cisapride	10–20 mg BID	PO
Meclizine	12.5–25 mg QID	PO
Proclorperazine	25 mg BID	PR
	10 mg QID	PO/IV/IM
Promethazine	12.5–25 mg BID-QID	IM/IV
Droperidol	0.625 ng QID	IV
Hydroxyzine	10–50 mg QID	PO
	50–100 mg	IM
Ondansetron	4–32 mg in one to four divided doses	PO/IV

twice daily) and senna (2 to 6 tablets twice daily) is appropriate for most patients. Adequate hydration, physical activity, and regular toileting are also helpful. If constipation develops or persists with this regimen, then an osmotic laxative, such as lactulose (15 to 30 mL) or magnesium citrate (200 mL), is added after ruling out fecal impaction. Bisacodyl suppository or sodium phosphate/biphosphate enema is used for patients who are too nauseated to take oral cathartics. Disimpaction may be facilitated with mineral oil or saline enemas. Refractory constipation may respond to oral naloxone (1 to 12 mg), which acts at enteric opioid receptors. Because naloxone is only about 3% bioavailable, systemic opioid withdrawal and recrudescence of pain may be avoided with low doses. Oral naloxone should be avoided in patients with bowel obstruction.[99,100] Methylnaltrexone, a peripherally acting opioid antagonist, shows promise as a treatment for opioid-induced constipation.[101]

Sedation

Somnolence and mental clouding are common complaints when opioids are initiated or escalated. Some patients continue to have these problems, especially when certain coanalgesics (antidepressants, anticonvulsants, benzodiazepines, antihistamines, and phenothiazines) are being used. After ruling out primary central nervous system abnormalities and metabolic derangement, unnecessary sedative medications should be gradually eliminated. If symptoms persist, and analgesia is adequate, the opioid dose may be reduced or the opioid drug may be changed. If analgesia is unsatisfactory, coanalgesics may be initiated or increased to achieve an opioid-sparing effect. An anesthetic or neuroablative procedure may be necessary if the patient finds sedation particularly troubling.[34]

Psychostimulants, such as caffeine (100 to 200 mg orally per day), dextroamphetamine (2.5 to 10 mg orally twice daily), and methylphenidate (5 to 10 mg orally twice daily), are commonly used to offset the sedative effects of opioids.[102] Bruera et al studied the cognitive effects of methylphenidate versus placebo in a double-blind, crossover trial involving 20 patients with cancer pain who were receiving continuous infusions of opioids.[103] Cognitive function was improved by methylphenidate, and most patients preferred it to placebo. Amphetamines, like antidepressants, have mood elevating and analgesic properties as well.[102]

Respiratory Depression

Respiratory depression occurs with sedation when opioids are given systemically, and tolerance to this effect occurs quickly. All opioids affect the medullary respiratory center directly. No pure opioid agonist is less likely to cause respiratory depression than any other when given at an equianalgesic dose. For most patients, mild respiratory depression (respiratory rate of 8 to 12 per minute) is well tolerated. For those with limited ventilatory or respiratory reserve, it may be problematic. If a low respiratory rate and moderate sedation occur after the expected peak of opioid activity, it is best to withhold further opioids until the respiratory rate rises or pain returns. If necessary, ventilatory support and a small dose of dilute naloxone (20 to 80 μg intravenously) may be given and repeated as necessary. Because naloxone's effects are shorter than those of most opioids, continued close monitoring for recurrence of respiratory depression is necessary.[34]

Myoclonus and Hyperalgesia

Myoclonus, uncontrollable spasms of certain muscle groups, and hyperalgesia, excessive sensitivity to mildly noxious stimuli, are sometimes seen at very high doses of opioids. Their occurrence, separately or together, may limit the ability of opioids to control pain at the end of life.[104] The mechanisms of these conditions are not certain, but may include the inhibition of non-opioid CNS inhibitory systems,[105] and the potentiation of glutamate activity at NMDA receptors.[106] Morphine-3-glucuronide accumulates with chronic morphine administration, and also may play a role in these hyperexcitability conditions by stimulating non-opioid receptors in the CNS.[107] A change to another opioid and the addition of coanalgesics and adjuvants may allow a reduction in the opioid dose, relieving either condition.[51] Clonazepam (0.5 to 2 mg orally three times daily), and perhaps other anticonvulsants, may also be used to suppress myoclonus.[51,108] Finally, an anesthetic or neuroablative procedure may be indicated for the rare patient with a more favorable prognosis.

REFERENCES

1. World Health Organization. *Cancer pain relief.* 2nd ed. Geneva, Switzerland: World Health Organization, 1996.
2. Jadad AR, Browman GP. The WHO analgesic ladder for cancer pain management. Stepping up the quality of its evaluation. *JAMA* 1995; 274:1870.
3. Cleeland CS, Gonin R, Hatfield AK, et al. Pain and its treatment in outpatients with metastatic cancer. *New Engl J Med* 1994;330:592.
4. Cleeland CS. Pain assessment in cancer. In: Osoba D. *Effect of Cancer on Quality of Life.* Boca Raton, Fla: CRC Press, 1991.
5. Revill SI, Robinson JO, Rosen M, Hogg MIJ. The reliability of a linear analogue for evaluating pain. *Anaesthesia* 1976;31:1191.
6. McCaffery M, Pasero CL. Pain ratings: the fifth vital sign. *Am J Nurs* 1997;97(Feb):15.
7. O'Brien J, Francis A. The use of next-of-kin to estimate pain in cancer patients. *Pain* 1988;35:171.
8. Bieri D, Reeve RA, Champion GD, et al. The faces pain scale for the self-assessment of the severity of pain experienced by children: development, initial validation, and preliminary investigation for ratio scale properties. *Pain* 1990;41:139.
9. Bruera E, Watanabe S. New developments in the assessment of pain in cancer patients. *Support Care Cancer* 1994;2:312.
10. Melzack R. The McGill pain questionnaire: major properties and scoring methods. *Pain* 1995;1:277.
11. Fishman B, Pasternak S, Wallenstein SL, et al. The Memorial Pain Assessment Card: a valid instrument for the evaluation of cancer pain. *Cancer* 1987;60:1151.
12. Stambaugh JE, Drew J. The combination of ibuprofen and oxycodone/acetaminophen in the management of chronic cancer pain. *Clin Pharmacol Ther* 1989;44:665.
13. McCormack K. Non-steroidal anti-inflammatory drugs and spinal nociceptive processing. *Pain* 1994;59:9.
14. Amadio P, Cummings DM, Amadio PB. NSAIDs revisited: selection, monitoring, and safe use. *Postgrad Med* 1997;101:257.
15. Siebert K, Zhang Y, et al. Distribution of COX-1 and COX-2 in normal and inflamed tissues. *Adv Exper Med Biol* 1997;400A:167.
16. Cryer G, Feldman M. Cyclooxygenase-1 and cyclooxygenase-2 selectivity of widely used nonsteroidal anti-inflammatory drugs. *Am J Med* 1998;104:413.
17. Bombardier C. An evidence-based evaluation of the gastrointestinal safety coxibs. *Am J Cardiol* 2002;89:30–90.
18. Dajani EZ, Agrawal NM. Prevention and treatment of ulcers induced by nonsteroidal anti-inflammatory drugs: an update. *J Physiol Pharmacol* 1995;46:3.

19. Yeomans JD, Tulassay Z, Juhasz L, et al. A comparison of omeprazole with ranitidine for ulcers associated with nonsteroidal antiinflammatory drugs. *New Engl J Med* 1998;338:719.
20. Hawkey CJ, Karrasch JA, Szczepanski L, et al. Omeprazole compared with misoprostol for ulcers associated with nonsteroidal antiinflammatory drugs. *New Engl J Med* 1998;338:727.
21. Robinson M, Mills RJ, Euler AR. Ranitidine prevents duodenal ulcers associated with nonsteroidal anti-inflammatory drug therapy. *Aliment Pharmacol Ther* 1991;5:143.
22. Stuart JJ, Pisko EJ. Choline magnesium trisalicylate does not impair platelet aggregation. *Pharm Therapeutica* 1981;2:547.
23. Ahmad SR, Kortepeter C, Brinker A, Chen M, Beitz J. Renal failure associated with the use of celecoxib and rofecoxib. *Drug Saf* 2002; 25:537–544.
24. Schiodt FV, Rochling FA, Casey DL, et al. Acetaminophen toxicity in an urban county hospital. *New Engl J Med* 1997;337:1112.
25. Portenoy RK, Foley KM, Inturrisi CE. The nature of opioid responsiveness and its implications for neuropathic pain: new hypotheses derived from studies of opioid infusions. *Pain* 1990;43:273.
26. Kanner RM, Foley KM. Patterns of narcotic drug use in a cancer pain clinic. *Ann NY Acad Sci* 1981;362:161.
27. Weissman DE, Haddox JD. Opioid pseudoaddiction—an iatrogenic syndrome. *Pain* 1989;36:363.
28. Gonzales GR, Elliott KJ, Portenoy RK, et al. The impact of a comprehensive evaluation in the management of cancer pain. *Pain* 1991; 47:141.
29. Galer BS, Coyle N, Pasternak BW, Portenoy RK. Individual variability in the response to different opioids: report of five cases. *Pain* 1992;49:87.
30. Chan GL, Matzke GR. Effects of renal insufficiency on the pharmacokinetics and pharmacodynamics of opioid analgesics. *Drug Intell Clin Pharm* 1987;21:773.
31. Houde RW. Analgesic effectiveness of narcotic agonist-antagonists. *Br J Clin Pharmacol* 1979;7:2975.
32. Fainsinger R, Schoeller T, Bruera E. Methadone in the management of cancer pain: a review. *Pain* 1993;52:137.
33. Plummer JL, Gourlay GK, Cherry DA, Cousins MJ. Estimation of methadone clearance: applications in the management of cancer pain. *Pain* 1988;33:313.
34. Cherny NI, Portenoy RK. The management of cancer pain. *CA Cancer J Clin* 1994;44:262.
35. Kaiko RF, Wallenstein SK, Rogers AG, et al. Narcotics in the elderly. *Med Clin North Am* 1982;66:1079.
36. Kaiko RF. Commentary: equianalgesic dose ration of intramuscular/oral morphine, 1:6 versus 1:3. In: Foley KM, Inturrisi CE,eds. *Advances in Pain Research and Therapy*. Vol. 8. New York, NY: Raven Press, 1986: 87.
37. Ellison NM, Lewis GO. Plasma concentrations following single doses of morphine sulfate in oral solution and rectal suppository. *Clin Pharmacol* 1984;3:614.
38. Sawe J, Dahlstrom B, Rane A. Steady-state kinetics and analgesic effect of oral morphine in cancer patients. *Eur J Clin Pharmacol* 1983; 24:537.
39. Shepard K. Review of a controlled-release morphine preparation. In: Foley KM, Bonica JJ, Ventafridda V,eds. *Advances in Pain Research and Therapy*. New York, NY: Raven Press, 1990:191.
40. Broomhead A, Kerr R, Tester W, et al. Comparison of a once-a-day sustained-release morphine formulation with standard oral morphine for cancer pain. *J Pain Symptom Manage* 1997;14:63.
41. Kaiko RF, Benziger DP, Fitzmartin RD, et al. Pharmacokinetic-pharmacodynamic relationships of controlled-release oxycodone. *Clin Pharmacol Ther* 1996;59:52.
42. Ripamonti C, Zecca E, Brunelli C, et al. Rectal methadone in cancer patients with pain. A preliminary clinical and pharmacokinetic study. *Ann Oncol* 1995;6:841.
43. Grond S, Zech D, Lehmann KA, et al. Trandermal fentanyl in the long-term treatment of cancer pain: a prospective study of 50 patients with advanced cancer of the gastrointestinal tract or the head and neck region. *Pain* 1997;69:191.
44. Ahmedzai S, Brooks D. Transdermal fentanyl versus sustained-release oral morphine in cancer pain: preference, efficacy, and quality of life. The TTS-Fentanyl Cooperative Trial Group. *J Pain Symptom Manage* 1997;13:254.
45. Campbell WI. Rectal controlled-release morphine: plasma levels of morphine and its metabolites following the rectal administration of MST Continus 100mg. *J Clin Pharm Ther* 1996;21:65.
46. DeConno F, Ripamonti C, Saita L, et al. Role of rectal route in treating cancer pain: a randomized crossover clinical trial of oral versus rectal morphine administration in opioid-naïve cancer patients with pain. *J Clin Oncol* 1995;13:1004.
47. Bruera E, Brenneis C, Michaud M, et al. Continuous SC infusion of narcotics using a portable disposable device in patients with advanced cancer. *Cancer Treat Rep* 1987;71:635.
48. Moulin DE, Kreft JH, Murray-Parsons NM, et al. Comparison of continuous subcutaneous and intravenous hydromorphone infusions for management of cancer pain. *Lancet* 1991;337:465.
49. Ripamonti C, Bruera E. Current status of patient-controlled analgesia in cancer patients. *Oncology* 1997;11:373.
50. Chapman CR, Hill HF. Prolonged morphine self-administration and addiction liability: evaluation of two theories in a bone marrow transplant unit. *Cancer* 1989;63:1636.
51. MacDonald N, Der L, Allan S, Champion P. Opioid hyperexcitability: the application of alternate opioid therapy. *Pain* 1993;53:353.
52. Paoli F, Darcourt G, Corsa P. Note preliminaire sur l'action de l'imipramine dans les etats douloureux. *Rev Neurol* [Paris] 1960;2: 503.
53. Magni G. The use of antidepressants in the treatment of chronic pain. A review of the current evidence. *Drugs* 1991;42:730.
54. McQuay HJ, Tramer M, Nye BA, et al. A systematic review of antidepressants in neuropathic pain. *Pain* 1996;68:217.
55. Spiegel K, Kalb R, Pasternak GW. Analgesic activity of tricyclic antidepressants. *Ann Neurol* 1983;13:462.
56. Yaksh TL. Pharmacology of spinal adrenergic systems which modulate spinal nociceptive processing. *Pharmacol Biochem Behav* 1985; 22:845.
57. Eija K, Tiina T, Pertti NJ. Amitriptyline effectively relieves neuropathic pain following treatment of breast cancer. *Pain* 1996; 64:293.
58. Kishmore-Kumar R, Schafer SC, Lawlor BA, et al. Desipramine relieves postherpetic neuralgia. *Clin Pharmacol Ther* 1990;47:305.
59. Max MB, Schafer SC, Culnane M, et al. Amitriptyline, but not lorazepam, relieves postherpetic neuralgia. *Neurology* 1988;38:1427.
60. Max MB, Culnane M, Schafer SC, et al. Amitriptyline relieves diabetic neuropathy pain in patients with normal or depressed mood. *Neurology* 1987;37:589.
61. Watson CPN, Evans RJ. A comparative trial of amitriptyline and zimelidine in postherpetic neuralgia. *Pain* 1985;23:387.
62. Max MB, Lynch SA, Muir J, et al. Effects of desipramine, amitriptyline, and fluoxetine on pain in diabetic neuropathy. *New Engl J Med* 1992;326:1250.
63. Preskorn SH, Fast GA: Tricyclic antidepressant-induced seizures and plasma drug concentration. *J Clin Psychiatry* 1992;53:5.
64. Dietch JT, Fine M. The effect of nortriptyline in elderly patients with cardiac conduction disease. *J Clin Psychiatry* 1990;51:2.
65. Blom S. Tic douleureux treatment with new anticonvulsant. *Arch Neurol* 1963;9:285.
66. Swerdlow M. Anticonvulsant drugs and chronic pain. *Clin Neuropharmacol* 1984;7:51.
67. Backonja M, Beydoun A, Edwards KR, et al. Gabapentin for the symptomatic treatment of painful neuropathy in patients with diabetes mellitus: a randomized controlled trial. *JAMA* 1998;280:1831.
68. Rowbotham M, Harden N, Stacey B, et al. Gabapentin for the treatment of postherpetic neuralgia: a randomized controlled trial. *JAMA* 1998;280:1837.

69. McQuay H, Carroll D, Jadad AR, et al. Anticonvulsant drugs for management of pain: a systematic review. *BMJ* 1995;311:1047.
70. Yajnik S, Singh GP, Singh G, Kumar M. Phenytoin as a coanalgesic in cancer pain. *J Pain Symptom Manage* 1992;7:209.
71. Ramsay RE. Clinical efficacy and safety of gabapentin. *Neurology* 1994;44(suppl 5):S23.
72. Horowitz S, Patwardham R, Marcus E. Hepatotoxic reactions associated with carbamazepine therapy. *Epilepsia* 1988;29:149.
73. Conger LA, Grabski WJ. Dilantin hypersensitivity reaction. *Cutis* 1996;57:223.
74. Rowbotham MC, Reisner-Keller LA, Fields HL. Both intravenous lidocaine and morphine reduce the pain of postherpetic neuralgia. *Neurology* 1991;41:1024.
75. Kastrup J, Peterson P, Dejgard A, et al. Treatment of painful diabetic neuropathy with intravenous lidocaine infusion. *Br Med J* 1986;292:173.
76. Chabal C, Jacobson L, Mariano A, et al. The use of oral mexilitine for the treatment of pain after peripheral nerve injury. *Anesthesiology* 1992;76:513.
77. Dejgard A, Petersen P, Kastrup J. Mexilitine for treatment of chronic painful diabetic neuropathy. *Lancet* 1988;29:9.
78. Rowbotham MC, Davies PS, Fields HL. Topical lidocaine gel relieves postherpetic neuralgia. *Ann Neurol* 1995;37:246.
79. Lynn B. Capsaicin: actions on nociceptive C-fibers and therapeutic potential. *Pain* 1990;40:61.
80. Watson CP. Topical capsaicin as an adjuvant analgesic. *J Pain Symptom Manage* 1994;9:425.
81. Twycross R. The risks and benefits of corticosteroids in advanced cancer. *Drug Saf* 1994;11:163.
82. Hong D, Byers MR, Oswald RJ. Dexamethasone treatment reduces sensory neuropeptides and nerve sprouting reactions in injured teeth. *Pain* 1993;263:830.
83. Devor M, Govrin-Lippmann R, Raber P. Corticosteroids suppress ectopic neural discharge originating in experimental neuromas. *Pain* 1985;22:127.
84. McGee JL, Alexander MR. Phenothiazine analgesia—fact or fantasy? *Am J Hosp Pharm* 1979;36:633.
85. Stambaugh JE, Lane C. Analgesic efficacy and pharmacokinetic evaluation of meperidine and hydroxyzine, alone and in combination. *Cancer Invest* 1983;1:111.
86. Kinirons MT. Newer agents for the treatment of malignant hypercalcemia. *Am J Med Sci* 1993;305:403.
87. Bloomfield DJ. Should bisphosphonates be part of the standard therapy of patients with multiple myeloma or bone metastases from other cancers? An evidence-based review. *J Clin Oncol* 1998;16:1218.
88. Blomqvist C, Elomaa I, Porkaa L, et al. Evaluation of salmon calcitonin treatment in bone metastases from breast cancer—a controlled trial. *Bone* 1988;9:45.
89. Jaeger H, Maier C. Calcitonin in phantom limb pain: a double-blind study. *Pain* 1992;48:21.
90. Max MB, Schafer SC, et al. Association of pain relief with drug side effects in post-herpetic neuralgia: a single-dose study of clonidine, codeine, ibuprofen, and placebo. *Clin Pharmacol Ther* 1988;43:363.
91. Ossipov MH, Lopez Y, Bian D, et al. Synergistic antinociceptive interactions of morphine and clonidine in rats with nerve-ligation injury. *Anesthesiology* 1997;86:196.
92. Eisenach JC, DeKock M, Klimscha W. α2-adrenergic agonists for regional anesthesia: a clinical review of clonidine (1984-1995). *Anesthesiology* 1996;85:655.
93. Fogelholm R, Murros K. Tizanidine in chronic tension-type headache: a placebo controlled double-blind cross-over study. *Headache* 1992; 32:509.
94. Berry H, Hutchinson DR. A multicentre placebo-controlled study in general practice to evaluate the efficacy and safety of tizanidine in acute low-back pain. *J Int Med Res* 1988;16:75.
95. Fromm GH, Aumentado D, Terrence CF. A clinical and experimental investigation of the effects of tizanidine in trigeminal neuralgia. *Pain* 1993;53:265.
96. McCarthy RJ, Kroin JS, Lubenow TR, et al. Effect of intrathecal tizanidine on antinociception and blood pressure in the rat. *Pain* 1990; 40:333.
97. Canty SL. Constipation as a side effect of opioids. *Oncol Nurs Forum* 1994;21:739.
98. Portenoy RK. Pain management in the older cancer patient. *Oncology* (Huntington) 1992;6(suppl 2):86.
99. Culpepper-Morgan JA, Inturrisi CE, Portenoy RK, et al. Treatment of opioid-induced constipation with oral naloxone: a pilot study. *Clin Pharmacol Ther* 1992;52:90.
100. Sykes NP. An investigation of the ability of oral naloxone to correct opioid-related constipation in patients with advanced cancer. *Palliat Med* 1996;10:135.
101. Murphy DB, Sutton JA, Prescott LF, Murphy MB. Opioid induced delay in gastric emptying: a peripheral mechanism in man. *Anesthesiology* 1997;87:765.
102. Sjogren P. Psychomotor and cognitive functioning in cancer patients. *Acta Anaesthesiol Scand* 1997;41:159.
103. Bruera E, Miller MJ, Macmillan K, Kuehn N. Neuropsychological effects of methylphenidate in patients receiving a continuous infusion of narcotics for cancer pain. *Pain* 1992;48:163.
104. Truog RD, Berde CB, Mitchell C, Grier HE. Barbiturates in the care of the terminally ill. *New Engl J Med* 1992;327:1678.
105. Dickenson AH. Mechanisms of the analgesic actions of opiates and opioids. *Br Med Bull* 1991;47:690.
106. Chen L, Huang L-Y. Sustained potentiation of NMDA receptor-mediated glutamate responses through activation of protein kinase C by a mu opioid. *Neuron* 1991;7:319.
107. Sjogren P, Jonsson T, Jensen NH, et al. Hyperalgesia and myoclonus in terminal cancer patients treated with continuous intravenous morphine. *Pain* 1993;55:93.
108. Eisele JH, Grigsby EJ, Dea G. Clonazepam treatment of myoclonic contractions associated with high-dose opioids: case report. *Pain* 1992;49:231.

CHAPTER 46 ANESTHETIC INTERVENTIONS IN CANCER PAIN

Stuart W. Hough, Leonidas C. Goudas, and Daniel B. Carr

OVERVIEW

In this chapter we present a broad overview of a variety of approaches including, but not limited to, anesthetic interventions. A roster of excellent clinicians and researchers discuss in prior chapters, in great detail a variety of approaches used in the management of pain in general. These prior approaches are used for the management of pain directly attributable to cancer as well as pain resulting from cancer treatment. We feel that it would be useful to the reader of this textbook — at the expense of some overlap with other chapters — to present a broad overview and synthesis of these approaches with emphasis on the unique attributes of cancer patients. Patients with cancer comprise a traditionally undertreated group. Even when the World Health Organization (WHO) guidelines for cancer pain treatment are followed (See Chapter 45, Medical Management of Cancer Pain), up to 30% of patients report inadequate analgesia.[1,2] In addition, some patients with adequate analgesia may experience intolerable side effects from opioids and other pharmacologic treatments. This chapter first addresses the role of psychological and physical approaches to cancer pain management. Then, a variety of palliative procedures, including anesthetic, radiologic, and neurosurgical interventions, are presented.

PSYCHOLOGICAL APPROACHES

Psychosocial aspects of cancer pain, often underestimated by clinicians who adopt a disease-centered rather than a patient-centered focus, have a profound impact on pain management.[3] Nonpharmacologic methods used in conjunction with analgesics have as their goal to help the patient gain or maintain functionality and restore a sense of psychological control over their pain and their circumstances. These approaches ordinarily have no negative side effects. The perception of pain resides within the brain[4] and is closely influenced by the patient's ever-evolving emotions, behaviors, and attitudes toward pain. As mentioned previously, during the treatment of cancer pain one must be aware of the patient's mood, coping strategies, family support structure, social beliefs, ability to express pain, cognitive level, and expectations regarding pain management.[5] Pain is characterized not only by location, quality, and intensity, but also by affective, cognitive, and behavioral responses.[6] Modifying these responses is part of treating pain. Although pain may diminish when the patient's responses to it are optimized, there may remain issues of self-control, fear of death, dependency, and confusion about the meaning of pain.[7] Adequate pain control is difficult to achieve without addressing these issues. Psychological interventions for cancer pain have continually demonstrated efficacy and are likely to be cost-effective[8] (See Chapters 12 through 16). It is important for health care providers never to conclude that if psychological interventions are of benefit, then the pain was purely psychogenic ("it was all in his head").[9]

Psychotherapy

Depression and adjustment disorder with depressed mood are common among cancer patients.[10] They are often caused by, and usually interfere with, the management of pain.[6,11] Derogatis et al studied 215 patients with newly diagnosed cancer who were not physically disabled or near death.[12] Forty-seven percent were found to have a psychiatric diagnosis by DSM (*Diagnostic and Statistical Manual of Mental Disorders*) criteria; 85% of those had psychiatric diagnoses in which depression, anxiety, or both are a central feature. Thirteen percent (6% of total) had major affective disorders, primarily major depression. Those with a DSM diagnosis were twice as likely to have pain as those without. Bukberg et al found that the prevalence of major depression was 42% among 62 patients with advanced disease.[13] In addition to pain and past history of mood disorders, a number of social, cancer, and treatment-related factors are associated with depression and anxiety.[11,13]

Depression hinders the application of coping skills that patients may otherwise use to deal with pain.[14] Effective treatment of depression is therefore helpful in managing cancer pain. The converse is also true: effective analgesia may resolve an apparent psychiatric disturbance.[6,10] Because cancer patients may appear depressed for a variety of reasons, a psycho-oncologist is often useful in diagnosing depression and in sorting out the precipitating factors.[11]

Short-term crisis-oriented therapy provides patients and families with support, knowledge, and skills to cope with cancer treatment, pain, and death. Patients and families learn to utilize their preexisting coping abilities and to develop new ones for difficult situations, including uncontrolled pain. Peer support groups provide unstructured cognitive and emotional support to patients who often feel isolated by their disease. Pastoral counseling is valuable to some patients suffering with pain and spiritual or existential fears.

Cognitive-Behavioral Techniques

Individuals are equipped with varying capacities to handle pain. Self-assured personality, social support, spiritual belief, and preexisting coping strategies give the patient some control over pain, whereas isolation and a lack of self-efficacy aggravate suffering.[7] Cognitive-behavioral teaching is a short, structured, individualized intervention that provides the patient with tools to control physical and emotional distress.[14,15] By giving the patient some control over pain, self-efficacy is enhanced. The patient cannot control severe pain with cognitive-behavioral techniques alone, but may use them in conjunction with medications to reduce pain intensity and the emotional distress that accompanies and exacerbates pain. Patients with delirium, dementia, severe or acute pain, acute nausea, and depression are less capable or unable to use these techniques.[14]

Patients often inaccurately attribute negative meaning to new pain symptoms, feeding their anxiety and blocking effective responses.[6] Cognitive techniques reshape the patient's perception of symptoms and events so that they will seem predictable and controllable.[14] The simplest way to do this is to forewarn the patient of expected symptoms, and to explain events as they occur.[16] The appropriate use of medications for pain and other symptoms should also be explained. Having the expectation of and the tools to deal with pain, the informed patient is less likely to become anxious when uncomfortable.[7]

More complicated cognitive methods require self-monitoring of mental processes to allow transformation of self-defeating mental reactions into rational coping strategies.[14,15] Reframing and cognitive restructuring are self-administered cognitive therapies. Negative thoughts and images are replaced with positive ones. Patients who become anxious every time pain breaks through their baseline opioid can gain control over their anxiety (and thereby their pain) by realizing that past breakthrough pain experiences have been self-limited and have yielded to additional medication. Self-defeating thoughts may be redirected toward pleasant or neutral ones, or replaced with self-affirmations, prayer, and songs. Distraction is the refocusing of mental energy away from pain and toward other subjects, such as prayer, listening to music, and reading. Several cognitive techniques are often tried before one is found that works well for a patient.[7]

Behavioral techniques modify physical and social responses to pain to eliminate those reactions that interfere with analgesia.[14,15] The most basic behavioral approach is self-monitoring. With it, the patient tracks symptoms and his or her responses to them, including analgesic usage. After reviewing this diary, the patient and clinician optimize medication use and alter dysfunctional behaviors, such as inactivity. Systematic desensitization and graded task assignment aim to prevent situational anxiety and avoidant behavior, such as that accompanying a painful medical procedure.

Some patients can also reduce anticipatory anxiety and pain intensity with behavioral methods designed to induce mental and physical relaxation.[14,15] Four basic easily taught techniques are presented in the Agency for Health Care Policy and Research guideline for cancer pain management.[17] They are focused-breathing, progressive muscle relaxation, meditation, and music-assisted relaxation. When used to treat acute symptoms, behavioral methods must be simple. Pleasant mental imagery may add to the analgesic and calming effects.[18,19]

Relaxation techniques are aimed at helping the patient diminish muscle tension and anxiety, and often employ pleasant imagery to enhance pain control.[9] Relaxation is useful in most age groups and should be taught early in situations where patients are expected to experience escalating pain and anxiety. Cognitive therapy has patients "redefine" or "reframe" their negative perception of bodily sensations including pain into more positive, productive ones. Reframing the patients' perception often assist relaxation training and may help hypnosis to be more effective in controlling a patient's pain. Cognitive therapy is facilitated by simply providing the patient and family with information about pain and the medications employed to treat it. The goal of the distraction technique in cognitive therapy is to divert attention away from pain by the performance of external, enjoyable tasks or by deliberately employing a variety of internal visual images. Distraction has been used successfully in conjunction with cognitive-behavioral therapy and hypnosis.[20] Stress inoculation is a cognitive therapy, which involves preparing the patient to employ behavioral pain control methods (e.g., hypnosis and distraction therapy) during an imagined future painful procedure prior to its occurrence.

Hypnosis promotes suggested changes in behavior, sensations, thoughts, and perceptions. It can be used alone but more often it is used in conjunction with relaxation and cognitive therapy so as to boost the efficacy of these other approaches.[20] The efficacy of hypnosis is related more to the ability and expectations of the patient than to the skill of the hypnotist. Golden et al[21] and Spira and Spiegal[22] outlined specific steps in the application of hypnosis for cancer pain control, beginning with first educating the patient about hypnosis and what to expect prior to starting. Typical hypnotic suggestions include: (1) anesthesia of a painful site, (2) dissociation from one's body that enables one to perform enjoyable imaginary tasks, and (3) substitution of distressing situations by more pleasant ones. The ability of hypnosis to permit patients to tolerate escalating nociception does not appear to be mediated by endogenous opioids, since hypnotic pain control is not reversed by naloxone.[23] Nor are differences in somatosensory-evoked potentials or electroencephalographic patterns apparent during hypnosis.[24] Kiernan et al[25] demonstrated that hypnosis reduced the R-III spinal reflex similar to morphine, indicating that its mechanism of action might involve both spinal cord and higher cortical processing. Hypnosis can benefit the patient by: (1) altering the appreciation of the sensation, (2) altering the affective or emotional response to the sensation, and (3) augmenting segmental analgesia (biasing the "gate") via the descending modulation of spinal processes.

An evidence synthesis on the treatment of cancer-related pain was conducted recently by the New England Medical Center Evidence Practice Center.[26] The topic of cancer-related pain was selected by the Agency for Healthcare Research and Quality in response to a request from the American Pain Society. The report includes a review of published literature on the epidemiology of cancer pain and its relief, and also summarizes predominantly randomized controlled trials so as to gauge the efficacy of major treatments. Of six major questions formulated to address this broad topic, one concerned the relative efficacy of current adjuvant (nonpharmacological/noninvasive) physical or psychological (relaxation, massage, heat and cold, music, and exercise) treatments in the management of cancer-related pain.

Investigators found a small number of studies that incorporated a variety of types of interventions. Studies of education evaluated different interventions applied to patients, medical staff, and the community at large. Also, different types of pain seemed to be addressed, though specifics were not always provided. Only a few randomized studies examined hypnosis in conjunction with cognitive-behavioral techniques, in the context of acute procedure-related pain and oral mucositis pain after bone marrow transplant. They included studies in the pediatric and adult age groups. Hypnosis seems to help with both procedural and mucositis-related pain. Cognitive-behavioral treatments may also be helpful. More studies are needed, with larger numbers and with control groups.

Because various interventions are evaluated, comparisons between studies are not possible. The most consistent finding, however, is that relaxation and imagery are useful in reducing the intensity of incidental pain.[27] In one of the better studies, Syrjala, et al found that a combination of relaxation and imagery (hypnosis) was effective for reducing oral mucositis pain after bone marrow transplantation (BMT) in 67 patients.[19] Unstructured supportive therapy and cognitive-behavioral techniques that excluded guided imagery were not effective for pain. In a follow-up study of 94 BMT patients, Syrjala, et al compared relaxation/imagery to treatment as usual, supportive therapy, and a combination of cognitive-behavioral techniques and relaxation/imagery.[28] Again, the relaxation/imagery group reported less pain, but the addition of cognitive-behavioral techniques did not enhance pain control further. The results of these studies, however, might apply only to predictable, incidental pain, as occurs for several weeks following BMT. When pain is less predictable, and is not expected to resolve in the short term, patients might find these techniques less useful. Alternatively, patients might master the more difficult techniques over time, increasing their usefulness.

PHYSICAL MODALITIES

Various noninvasive physical stimulatory methods exist to diminish pain, but they are often overlooked in cancer pain management.[29] Physical modalities can be applied by the patient, family, and health care providers and include heat, cold, physical therapy, external electrical stimuli (TENS), acupuncture, and immobilization (See also Chapter 79, Physical Medicine and Rehabilitation). Their use is intended to augment, not replace, analgesic drug therapy. Importantly, physical measures should be applied early on to minimize the generalized deconditioning and myofascial pain associated with reduced activity and intervals of immobility associated with cancer and its therapy. These are especially useful as adjuncts for mild to moderate pain, and while awaiting the effect of a breakthrough analgesic. The choice of technique is empirical: different modalities are used until one is found effective.[29] They are never adequate alone to manage moderate or severe cancer pain. Although these analgesic approaches receive support from experts in cancer pain,[17] few have received rigorous attention in clinical trials.

Thermal Therapy

Various superficial and deep heating methods have been applied to control pain, and are popular among cancer pain patients.[29,30] Heat is analgesic in part by increasing blood flow and decreasing joint stiffness. It also may induce a state of mental relaxation.[29] Superficial heating, with hot packs, heating pads, or baths, improves cutaneous blood flow and relaxes muscles and ligaments to a depth of 0.5 cm. Deep heating (diathermy) to 3 to 5 cm involves converting electromagnetic or acoustic energy to heat.[31] Care should be taken to avoid burns, and to avoid heating skin that has been irradiated.[17] Deep heating should be avoided near a tumor, since increased blood flow may stimulate growth.[31]

Cold application, with ice packs, malleable chemical gel packs, and vapocoolant sprays reduces nerve conduction, muscle spasm, inflammation, and edema.[29,31,32] Initial vasoconstriction is followed by vasodilation. Cold may be used in cancer pain when heat has failed to reduce spasm, for acute inflammatory conditions, and over neuromas and myofascial trigger points. Ice massage, in which a small area of skin overlying focally tender tissue is rubbed with a block of ice, produces analgesia after several minutes.[33] Controlled studies of cold-induced analgesia for cancer pain do not exist. Cold should also be avoided in ischemic and irradiated tissues.[17]

Exercise

Exercise is the ideal means of preventing joint stiffness and muscle spasm.[14] Physical rehabilitation is also useful after mastectomy and radical neck dissection to maintain shoulder girdle mobility and perhaps to decrease pain.[34,35] It may also be effective in reducing acute pain.[30] Exercise, however, may not be possible for patients with advanced cancer. Massage, mechanical vibration, and repositioning are useful alternatives to exercise for reducing muscle tension and relieving pain.[29,30,36] Physical therapy, consisting of massage and bandaging, is also effective in reducing painful lymphedema following mastectomy.[37] When acute pain is associated with movement, as after surgery or fracture, temporary immobilization is appropriate. Prolonged immobilization should be avoided.[17]

Electrical Stimulation

Transcutaneous electrical nerve stimulation (TENS) and acupuncture are peripheral stimulatory techniques that appear effective for certain patients. TENS might work by stimulating A-a fibers to "close the gate" to incoming pain signals on C and A-delta fibers.[38] One uncontrolled study of 60 cancer patients found TENS effective in 65% after 2 weeks of treatment, but only 33% after 3 months.[39] Those with trunk or extremity pain responded best to TENS. In our experience and that of others, TENS is especially useful for phantom limb and post-thoracotomy pain syndromes (Fig. 46-1).[19,40]

Acupuncture

Acupuncture might also work by the gate mechanism, or by activating opioidergic, serotonergic, or noradrenergic modulatory systems (See Chapter 78, Acupuncture).[41–43] Our experience with these techniques in cancer pain is limited. The motivated patient, however, seems more likely to respond with a feeling of well-being (especially acupuncture) and a temporary reduction in pain. Since these methods are free of adverse effects, they should not be withheld from interested patients.

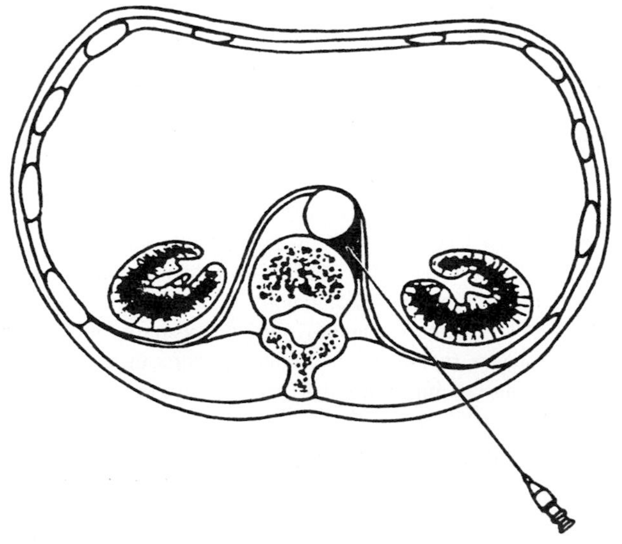

Figure 46-1 Celiac plexus block. Classic retrocrural approach, wherein a neurolytic agent is injected bilaterally behind the crus of the diaphragm, adjacent to the aorta and vena cava (Illustration from Mercadante S, Nicosia F. Celiac plexus block: a reappraisal. Reg Anesth Pain Med 1998;23:37).

INVASIVE, NONPHARMACOLOGIC PALLIATIVE PROCEDURES

About one in ten patients with pain due to cancer continues to experience pain despite maximal application of noninvasive analgesic methods. With few exceptions, noninvasive analgesic approaches should precede invasive forms of palliation such as neurolytic blocks and other anesthetic techniques, neurosurgery, radiation therapy, spinal column stimulation, or neurosurgical division of ascending pathways. Among these exceptions are palliative radiotherapy for pain at the site of a long bone metastasis or an isolated brain metastasis, and celiac block for a patient with pancreatic or other retroperitoneal tumor who presents with pain. These procedures are designed to improve analgesia or minimize analgesic side effects. Most are intended for pain that is localized to a nerve or plexus distribution. Loss of sensory, motor, visceral, and autonomic function must be considered before proceeding to a neurolytic procedure. Because of their complexity, risk, and cost, invasive procedures are reserved for patients with intractable pain despite full application of the WHO guidelines,[1] and those with intolerable side effects from systemic pharmacologic pain treatment. However, it is important not to delay excessively when conventional pharmacologic management appears inadequate. Referral to a multidisciplinary pain clinic might be considered early in the course of cancer pain to optimize current pharmacologic, psychological, and physical management techniques, and to educate the patient, family, and referring physician about pain progression and future management options. Following an anesthetic or neurosurgical procedure, sudden analgesia may prompt discontinuation of opioids. Gradual opioid taper is necessary to avoid uncomfortable withdrawal symptoms. The more common procedures are presented and illustrated here.

ANESTHETIC PROCEDURES

The following techniques have an increasing role in cancer pain management, as patients are surviving longer, even with advanced stages of disease. They are usually used in conjunction with or as an extension of pharmacologic pain management.

Myofascial Injection

Pain from muscle spasm, which may accompany and aggravate any underlying pain condition, is easily treated with local anesthetic injection (See Chapter 49, Fibromyalgia and Myofascial Pain Syndrome).[44] This is especially useful for bedridden patients who cannot employ the physical modalities for muscle spasm that are described above. Muscle injection is sufficiently simple and safe that most physicians should be comfortable performing it. Pain relief from a myofascial injection often lasts for days or weeks.

Neuroma and Intralesional Injection

Painful neuromas are easily treated with local anesthetic injection. A corticosteroid is added to prolong the effect by decreasing spontaneous discharges in the sprouting axons.[45] If frequent injections are needed, the neuroma may be frozen with the cryoprobe (See following section, Cryoanalgesia), or injected with neurolytic solutions.[46] Painful surgical scars, which may accompany post-thoracotomy and postmastectomy syndromes (See Chapter 44, Cancer Pain Syndromes), are also amenable to local anesthetic injection. The absence of a discrete neuroma makes cryoablation and neurolytic injection impractical. One effective analgesic treatment for postherpetic neuralgia is intralesional injection of local anesthetic and steroid (See Chapter 40, Acute Herpes Zoster and Postherpetic Neuralgia).

Somatic Nerve Block

Somatic and neuropathic pain localized to a single nerve, plexus, or dermatome distribution are amenable to local anesthetic block of the nerve. Common examples are pain from herpes zoster, surgery, and neuromas. Although pain relief is often dramatic, the longest lasting local anesthetics wear off within a day. Occasionally, the duration of analgesia outlasts that of sensory or motor block by days or weeks. Kirvela and Antila retrospectively analyzed 281 thoracic paravertebral blocks they performed on 32 patients with post-thoracotomy or postmastectomy pain.[47] Among the post-thoracotomy pain patients, 58% of blocks produced at least 75% relief for at least 1 month. Among postmastectomy patients, 88% of blocks produced at least 75% relief for 1 week to 1 month.

To prolong the effect of local anesthetics, anesthesiologists may insert a catheter for continuous delivery to a nerve or plexus. The brachial plexus and femoral nerve sheath are the usual sites of peripheral catheter placement. Interpleural catheters were once used more frequently, but epidural catheters have largely replaced them (See following section, Intraspinal Anesthesia).[48] Maintenance of peripheral catheters is difficult, as movement may easily displace them. The high daily doses of local anesthetics may lead to serious toxicity. Corticosteroids are often added to local anesthetics to enhance and prolong the nerve-blocking effect, but experimental support for this practice is lacking.[49,50] Several efforts are underway to design longer acting local anesthetics and delayed release delivery systems to allow weeks or months of analgesia.[51]

Somatic Neurolytic Block

Neurolytic blocks are often performed following a successful local anesthetic blocks to extend relief for weeks or months (See Chapters 68 and 73).[52,53] Because neural disruption causes motor, sensory, and autonomic dysfunction, these blocks are reserved for those who cannot get relief by other means. Commonly used chemical neurolytic agents are ethanol 50% to 100%, phenol 6% to 12%, ammonium salts 6%, glycerol 50%, hypertonic saline 10%, and butamben (a butylamino derivative of benzoic acid known for decades but not yet FDA approved). Phenol and ethanol are the most popular agents for chemical neurolysis. Both agents cause extensive damage to the neuron. Subsequent inflammation and fibrosis of the nerve and adjacent tissues may cause secondary neuralgic pain.[52,54] Radiofrequency neurolysis coagulates nerves by heating a small area around the tip of a needle-shaped probe. The size and shape of the lesion are more controlled than with chemical neurolysis, which may decrease the likelihood of damage to adjacent tissues.[55] Neurolytic blocks are not permanent, despite the neural injury they entail. Neural regrowth limits the analgesic effect of these procedures to weeks or months.[52]

Few case series of somatic neurolytic blocks have been published.[53,54,56] Doyle reported on 46 advanced cancer patients treated with phenol intercostal blocks for chest wall pain.[53] All patients responded favorably, for a mean duration of 3 weeks. Ramamurthy et al treated 28 patients with a variety of pain problems with either phenol or cryoneurolysis.[54] Only 28% of patients had at least 40% relief 4 weeks after treatment. These low success rates further restrict the use of peripheral neurolysis to patients in the last few months of life.

Cryoanalgesia

More recently, cryoanalgesia has been used for neurolysis, particularly in the treatment of cancer-related perineal pain.[57] Freezing a nerve or neuroma to −60°C temporarily disrupts myelinated fibers while leaving intact unmyelinated fibers, endoneurium and perineurium.[58,59] The nerve regrows along its intact sheath over several weeks,[58,59] and the neuroma probably regenerates in a similar period. Because the nerve regrows normally, with minimal inflammation or fibrosis, cryolesions are unlikely to be followed by neuroma formation or deafferentation pain.[54,57,58] In their comparison of phenol and cryoneurolysis, Ramamurthy et al found that 6% phenol solution was more effective than cryoneurolysis to −20°C.[54] Zhou et al showed that freezing nerves to −20°C does not affect fiber morphology or function, perhaps explaining these unfavorable results.[58] In our experience, cryoanalgesia lasts for several weeks to months. With both chemical and physical neurolysis, sensory and motor functions may be lost. Prognostic local anesthetic block must therefore precede neurolysis to confirm that analgesia is significant and that the resulting functional deficit is acceptable to the patient.

Sympathetic Block

Local anesthetic and chemical neurolytic blocks are used extensively to treat sympathetically maintained (reflex sympathetic dystrophy), ischemic, and visceral pain.[55,60-,62] Visceral cancer pain, which may be difficult to control within opioids and other analgesics, is especially suited for sympathetic plexus and splanchnic nerve blockade. Visceral afferents travel with the autonomic nervous system, permitting their blockade without resulting in somatosensory or motor dysfunction.[62] Sympathetic blocks are successful and safe enough that they should be offered early in the course of cancer pain, especially if the patient has any difficulty with opioid side effects.[61,63] Neurolytic injections may provide months of visceral pain relief.

Celiac plexus block Pain from tumor involvement of the upper abdominal viscera (pancreas, liver, diaphragm, spleen, stomach, small bowel, kidneys, abdominal aorta, adrenals, mesentery, and proximal colon) is treated with celiac plexus block (Fig. 46-1).[64] The celiac plexus lies anterior to the aorta at the level of the celiac artery, and has contributions from the T5 to T12 preganglionic sympathetic fibers. It contains splanchnic afferents, preganglionic parasympathetic fibers, and postganglionic sympathetic fibers. It is accessed intraoperatively[65] or percutaneously from a bilateral posterior or midline anterior approach. Fluoroscopic or computed tomography (CT) guidance is used to facilitate proper needle placement, avoid organ puncture, and to monitor the spread of neurolytic solutions.

A meta-analysis of 24 papers on celiac plexus block, including only two randomized and controlled studies, found that 90% of suitable cancer patients had partial to complete analgesia 3 months after the procedure.[66] About 20% of patients experienced recurrent pain before death. Repeat celiac block should be offered in these cases.[64] Intraoperative chemical splanchnicectomy (interrupting the preganglionic sympathetic fibers) has been used prophylactically in pancreatic cancer patients at the time of surgical exploration and palliation.[65] When compared to placebo in a randomized trial, prophylactic splanchnicectomy delayed the onset of pain or decreased its intensity.[65] Among patients with pain at the time of surgery, splanchnicectomy provided analgesia and appeared to improve survival. By providing constant, prolonged analgesia and limiting side effects,[63] neurolytic celiac plexus block appears to maintain quality of life for pancreatic cancer patients better than systemic opioid and adjuvant treatment.[61]

Failure of the celiac plexus block to provide analgesia is often due to extension of tumor to the peritoneum or abdominal wall, which are innervated by somatic pain fibers. Hypotension, back pain, and diarrhea are expected outcomes of celiac plexus block.[64,66] The patient compensates for relative hypovolemia, caused by mesenteric vasodilation, over a period of about 2 days. Diarrhea is often a desirable outcome for the patient with opioid-induced constipation, and is also usually limited to 2 days. Less common complications, such as unilateral paresis from somatic neurolysis, paraplegia from subarachnoid neurolysis or anterior cord infarction, pneumothorax, and retroperitoneal bleeding, are rare.[66] In a 5-year retrospective survey, only 4 of 2730 neurolytic celiac plexus blocks resulted in paraplegia or loss of sphincter function.[67]

Superior hypogastric plexus block Pain from the pelvic viscera (rectum and sigmoid colon, bladder and ureters, uterus and adnexa) is often responsive to superior hypogastric plexus block.[68] The superior hypogastric plexus lies in the retroperitoneum and extends from the anterior aspect of L5 to the superior sacrum (Fig. 46-2). Afferent fibers from the pelvic viscera pass through the plexus, which also contains sympathetic postganglionic fibers. As with celiac plexus block, only visceral pain responds to superior hypogastric plexus block. Somatic pain from sacral or muscle involvement, and neuropathic pain from nerve root compression or infiltration do not respond to this block. An initial local anesthetic block is used to predict response to neurolytic phenol block.[68]

The superior hypogastric plexus is accessed intraoperatively[69] or percutaneously via a bilateral posterior approach. Fluoroscopy is used to facilitate needle placement and to confirm appropriate spread of phenol. Plancarte et al studied 227 pelvic cancer pain patients who had poor analgesia or intolerable sedation with opioid management.[68] Seventy-nine percent of patients had a favorable response to local anesthetic test block. Visual analog pain scores decreased from >7 of 10 to <4 of 10 in 72% of the responders. The other 28% experienced more modest pain reductions. Both groups of responders reduced opioid usage after the neurolytic block. Of 18 patients who were enrolled because of excessive sedation, 16 showed improvement after the procedure. There are no placebo-controlled studies of this block, nor studies that comprehensively evaluate other outcomes, such as quality of life, complications, and symptoms other than pain. Because the plexus lies over the sacrum, hypotension, diarrhea, and injury to the aorta or spinal cord are unlikely. Lumbar plexus injury, bladder puncture, and iliac artery puncture with retroperitoneal bleeding or cholesterol plaque embolization might occur. In the Plancarte study, no significant complications occurred.[68]

Other sympathetic blocks Anesthetic blocks are also possible elsewhere along the sympathetic chain. Blockade of the cervicothoracic (stellate), middle, and superior cervical ganglia—stellate ganglion block—affects sympathetic tone and visceral afferent sen-

A

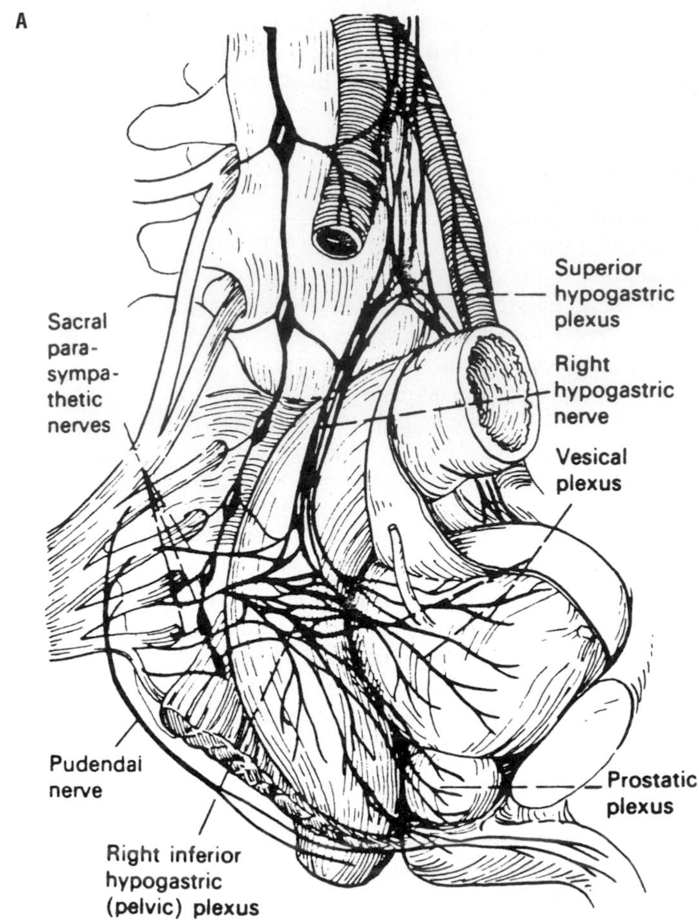

B

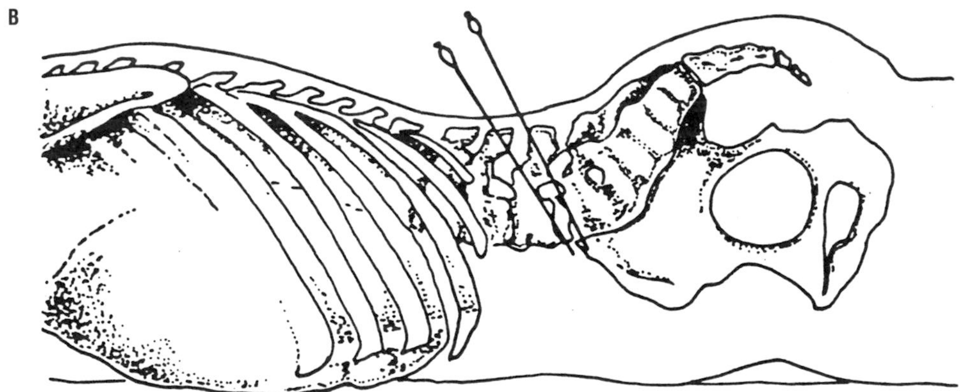

Figure 46-2 Superior hypogastric plexus block. **(A)** Relevant anatomy. **(B)** Needle placement anterior to the L5-S1 interspace (Illustrations from Lee RB et al. Presacral neurectomy for chronic pelvic pain. Obstet Gynecol. 1986;68(4):517–521).

sation of the head, neck, and arms. These ganglia are easily reached anteriorly at the C6 transverse process. Some patients with cancer pain in the head and neck might benefit from stellate ganglion block. The thoracic and lumbar sympathetic ganglia are accessed via a posterior approach with fluoroscopic guidance. Rarely used for cancer pain treatment, these blocks may be useful for phantom pain sensations, postmastectomy pain, and post-thoracotomy pain.[70,71] Sympathetic block is also effective for acute zoster pain[72] (See Chapter 40, Acute Herpes Zoster and Postherpetic Neuralgia). Neurolytic blockade of the sympathetic ganglia is possible with chemical and thermal modalities.[55]

Intraspinal Anesthesia

When cancer pain is located below the T1 level, and systemic opioids are inadequate to provide analgesia without intolerable side effects, neuraxial drug delivery is appropriate. Hogan et al reviewed 1205 oncology service hospitalizations over a period of 3 years.[73] It is not stated how many patients were admitted for pain management, but 16 required epidural morphine after aggressive titration of systemic analgesics. Six of those responded well to morphine alone, and the other 10 obtained relief with the addition of a local anesthetic. Temporary and permanent epidural and spinal catheters are used frequently to deliver opioids, local anesthetics, and clonidine. The main differences between epidural and intrathecal catheters are that lower drug doses are used intrathecally, and analgesia may be confined to fewer dermatomes with epidural delivery. Temporary catheters are always inserted prior to permanent catheter placement, to ensure that the goals of intraspinal analgesia (better analgesia and/or fewer side effects) can be met for the selected patient. After a successful trial of 1 to 5 days, a permanent catheter, with or without an implantable pump, is placed under local anesthesia. Implantable pump systems, which are refilled percutaneously, are often chosen for patients with life expectancies of 3 or more months (Fig. 46-3).[74] Tunneled catheters, resembling venous access devices, require an external pump (Fig. 46-4). They are appropriate for patients with shorter life expectancies.

Initially bleeding and later epidural abscess, meningitis, and pump pocket infection are the most significant possible complications of catheter placement. With proper maintenance, few intraspinal systems become infected over time.[75,76] Cerebral spinal fluid hygroma and pump pocket seroma may occur after pump placement, but are usually self-limited. Catheter migration and blockage occur rarely, especially with continuous infusion.[75] Systemic infection, thrombocytopenia, and coagulation defects must be treated before catheter placement.

By delivering opioids closer to their site of action in the substantia gelatinosa of the dorsal horn, intraspinal catheters allow reduction in the total opioid dose, possibly decreasing side effects. Since most opioid side effects are mediated by the central nervous system, intraspinal is not uniformly superior to systemic opioid delivery.[73,76] Of particular concern, gradual cephalad spread of morphine in the cerebrospinal fluid introduces the possibility of delayed respiratory depression, 12 to 18 hours after injection. When opioids and local anesthetics are delivered together, activity-induced pain and side effects are less than when either drug is used alone.[77,78] Because they are synergistic in the dorsal horn, small amounts of each drug may be used to treat regional pain by delivering the mixture epidurally at the appropriate spinal level. Taking advantage of drug synergy may reduce sensory and motor block, urinary retention, pruritus, nausea, and respiratory depression. During the initial 24 hours of treatment, patients must be monitored hourly for life-threatening complications of respiratory depression, hypotension, and intraspinal hematoma.

There have been no prospective, randomized, controlled studies of intraspinal versus oral opioid treatment for cancer pain. Sjogren and Banning compared pain, sedation, and continuous reaction time (CRT, a measure of cerebral dysfunction) in 14 cancer pain patients during treatment with oral opioid, and then with epidural morphine treatment.[79] There were no statistically significant changes in these measures with the institution of epidural therapy. However, CRT before treatment was slower than in healthy controls, whereas CRT after epidural treatment was not significantly different from controls. Four patients did experience better pain control with less sedation during epidural morphine infusion. Hassenbusch et al studied epidural morphine treatment in 69 terminal patients.[75] Forty-one responded favorably to trial infusion, and had continuous infusion pumps implanted. These patients noted large reductions in pain scores and systemic opioid con-

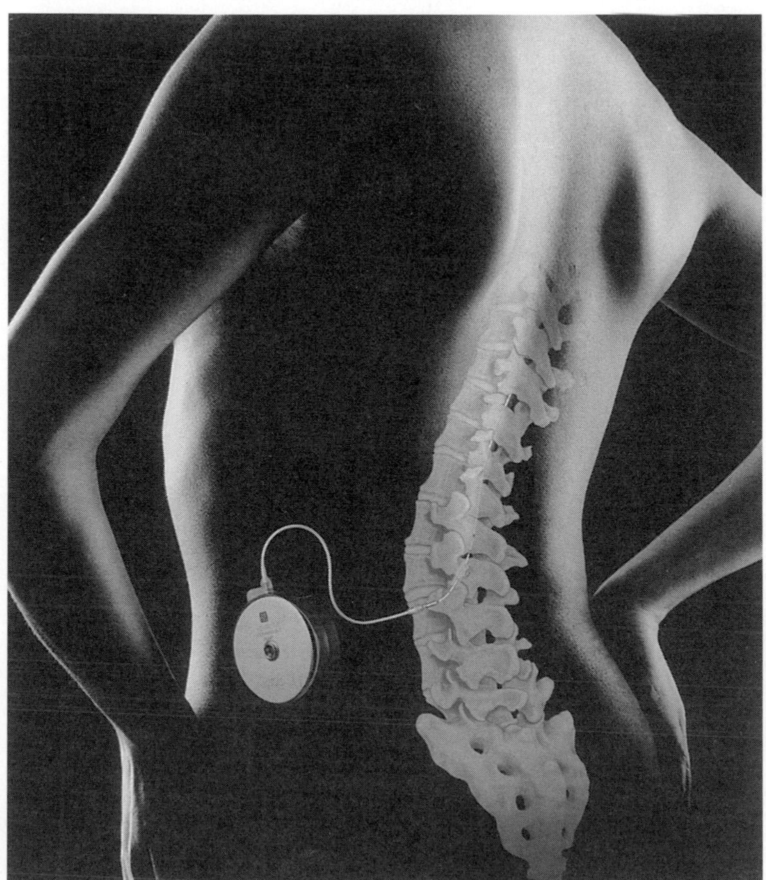

Figure 46-3 SynchroMed® implantable intrathecal delivery system, including pump and catheter. (Used with permission of Medtronic Neurological, Minneapolis, MN).

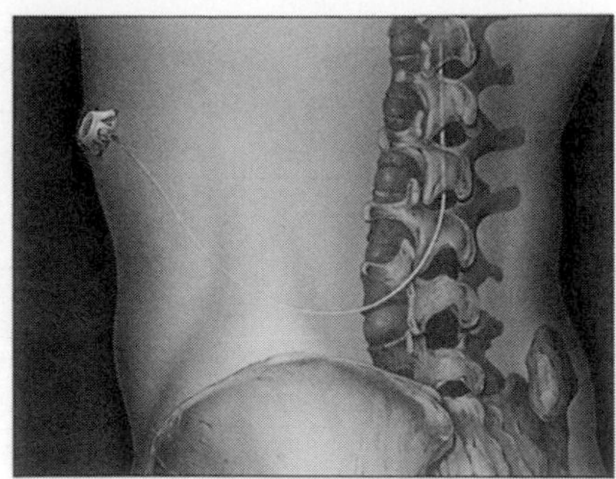

Figure 46-4 Permanent epidural catheter with subcutaneous port. PORT-A-CATH II Epidural Low Profile Implantable Access System. (SIMS Deltec, Inc., St. Paul Minnesota.)

sumption during the first month of treatment, reductions that were sustained over subsequent months. It is not clear, however, whether rapid escalation of systemic opioid treatment might have produced equivalent analgesic results without significant side effects. Intrathecal opioid delivery might produce fewer side effects than epidural delivery by further lowering total drug dose.[80]

Local anesthetics and clonidine may also contribute to intraspinal analgesia without aggravating opioid side effects.[73,78] This synergy may be especially important in treating neuropathic, cutaneous, and intermittent somatic pain.[76] Sjoberg et al treated 53 patients with intractable cancer pain with an intrathecal bupivicaine/morphine combination.[76] All patients had acceptable analgesia and improved sleep until death. Despite large bupivicaine doses, motor block, urinary retention, hypotension, and paresthesias occurred in a minority of patients. Eisenach et al added clonidine or placebo to epidural morphine infusions in 85 patients with cancer pain.[81] Clonidine was an effective analgesic in 56% of patients with neuropathic pain, but did not improve morphine analgesia in others. Hypotension and bradycardia were occasionally problematic with clonidine infusion. Sensory and motor block, respiratory depression, pruritus, nausea, and urinary retention are not seen with intraspinal clonidine treatment.[81]

The best approach to intraspinal analgesia at this time is to select appropriate patients who have fared poorly with the aggressive use of systemic analgesics, and to give them an intraspinal analgesic trial over several days. Patients who experience reduced pain intensity and improved function are likely to do well with a permanent system.

Intrathecal and Epidural Neurolysis

Absolute alcohol (ethanol) and phenol may be used to selectively interrupt dorsal root function when pain is limited to four dermatomes.[82,83] This anesthetic version of the neurosurgical rhizotomy (See section, Dorsal Rhizotomy) is easily accomplished on the awake patient. It lacks the precision of an open rhizotomy, resulting in damage to Lissauer's tract and the posterior columns, in addition to the dorsal roots. This procedure is limited to use for regional somatic pain in the trunk or in a functionless limb. Visceral pain is not affected, and neuropathic pain may not be susceptible inasmuch as it is due to deafferentation and pathologic changes in the spinal cord or brain.

For intrathecal neurolysis, the patient is positioned on his side and a spinal needle is introduced at the appropriate cord level (Fig. 46-5).[82] Small aliquots of the neurolytic agent are injected until analgesia develops in the area of pain. Pelvic and perineal pain are also amenable to intrathecal neurolysis with phenol, wherein the patient is seated and the agent is allowed to pool around the sacral roots.[83] Epidural neurolysis is performed similarly, although the effect cannot be reliably limited to one side.[84] Epidural injection of phenol via the sacral hiatus is useful for treating perineal pain. Bowel, bladder, and sexual dysfunction may result, especially when treating perineal pain.[83] Paresis, from anterior root or cord injury, is possible with any of these procedures, although it is uncommon.[82] In several large studies of intrathecal neurolysis, about three quarters of patients experienced fair to good relief.[82] As with peripheral neurolytic procedures, pain may recur in weeks to months after the procedure.[82,84]

Spinal Cord Stimulation

Spinal cord stimulation (SCS) is used to treat intractable, regional neuropathic pain.[85] A set of electrodes is inserted into the epidural space to deliver electrical stimulation to the appropriate segment of the spinal cord. The electrodes are then connected to an implantable pulse generator, similar to a pacemaker. Primarily used for treatment of pain caused by spine disease, SCS is rarely used for patients with advanced cancer. It may be appropriate, however, for patients with neuropathic pain related to surgery, such as phantom limb pain.[86] The cost of SCS and the need for patient in-

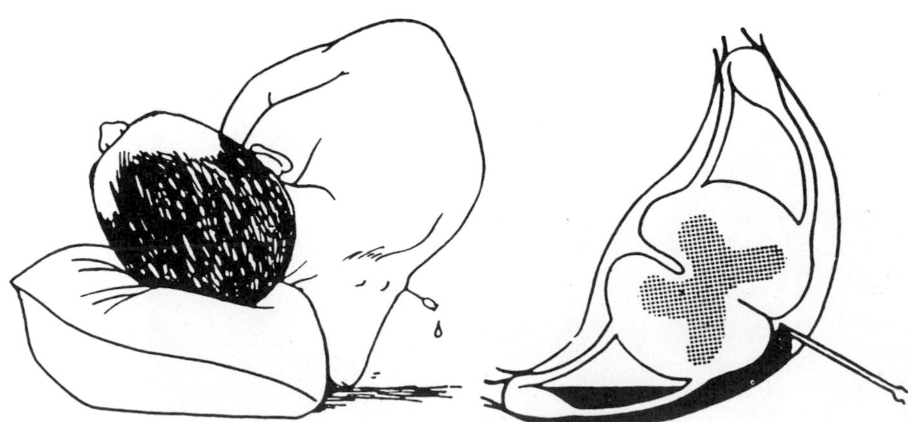

Figure 46-5 Intrathecal neurolysis – patient positioning for phenol injection (From Swerdlow M. Inrathecal neurolysis. *Anaesthesia* 1978;33:733. Used with permission of Blackwell Science.)

volvement in its use makes it unsuitable for debilitated cancer patients near the end of life.

RADIATION THERAPY

Radiation is an adjunct to pharmacologic pain management. Often used in the treatment of primary cancers, it has a prominent role in palliation of pain due to bony metastases.[87] Pain from neural compression and soft tissue metastases may also respond, but liver and kidney do not tolerate radiation. The biological basis of analgesia following radiation is not fully understood, as pain from tumors felt to be radiation-insensitive often responds.[88] Acute radiation toxicity includes mucositis, enteritis, dermatitis, and bone marrow suppression. Radiation causes tissue fibrosis over time, including painful damage to the nervous system.[89]

Palliative external beam radiation is prescribed according to the patient's condition, the site to be treated, the tumor type, and previous exposure to radiation. Re-irradiation of bone is possible within the toxicity limits of surrounding soft tissues. Frequent treatments with low doses allow greater total radiation dose and less late toxicity. For example, metastatic plexopathy is treated with longer radiation courses to decrease the likelihood of late neural fibrosis. Single treatments and short courses, however, may be less acutely toxic and are often just as effective for bone pain.[87,88,90]

Localized radiation of bone metastases is an effective analgesic in 35% to 100% of cases.[90] Tumor type and treatment regimen might not predict response to radiotherapy when pain relief is the measured outcome.[87,90-92] Renal and non-small cell lung carcinomas are less responsive in this regard, but should be treated.[87] In a retrospective study, retreatment of previously responsive bone metastases outside of the spine reduced pain at 48 of 57 sites.[91] Of patients with diffuse metastatic bone pain, 75% to 100% responded to hemibody radiation in a large single dose.[90] Pain relief often follows hemibody radiation within 24 hours, but associated morbidity, including nausea, diarrhea, bone marrow depression, and fatal radiation pneumonitis, is more frequent.

Long bone metastases meeting certain size and location criteria, whether painful or not, are irradiated to prevent pathologic fracture and to promote their healing.[90] Although surgical fixation is indicated to decrease pain and facilitate rehabilitation after pathologic fracture, patients with inoperable fractures and those who are physically debilitated may get pain relief from palliative radiation alone. Irradiation of vertebral metastases might prevent bony collapse and spinal compression, but criteria for prophylactic spinal irradiation are not established. Whereas patients who already have vertebral body collapse and spinal instability are best treated with surgical fixation,[93] palliative radiation alone may be offered to those in whom surgery is too risky. Radiation treatment is initiated urgently for patients with new onset of spinal cord compression.[90] Those with established paraplegia for several days from cord compression will not recover neurologic function, but radiation may still relieve their back pain. Irradiation is also indicated to treat cranial nerve palsies from skull base metastases. Symptoms of pain and neurologic deficit improve in 50% to 78% of patients with skull base irradiation.[90]

Radiopharmaceuticals localize to areas of osteoblastic activity or to specific tumor types.[90] Because of their widespread effects, treatment is similar in principle and effect to hemibody radiation. Moderate myelosuppression from systemic radiopharmaceuticals occurs 4 to 6 weeks after treatment. Iodine 131 is used to treat differentiated thyroid cancer. Phosphorous 32 orthophosphate (P-32) and strontium 89 (Sr-89) are used to treat bone pain from predominantly osteoblastic lesions, such as prostate and some breast and lung metastases. P-32 is taken up in normal and diseased bone, and has been associated with a high incidence of pancytopenia. Sr-89, which behaves like calcium, is more selective for areas of increased osteoblastic activity and is retained at these sites for weeks. Robinson et al measured a 77% response rate to Sr-89 in 375 patients with prostate or breast cancer.[94] Porter et al showed that high doses of Sr-89 improved and prolonged analgesia from external beam radiation in a prospective, randomized, controlled study of 126 prostate cancer patients with bone pain.[95] New pain sites appeared less frequently in patients treated with Sr-89. Thrombocytopenia occurred in 32% of Sr-89 treated patients, but only 7.5% required platelet transfusion, and 10% of Sr-89 treated patients developed leukopenia. Rhenium-186-diphosphonate and samarium-153-EDTMP, not yet approved in the United States, are similar in effect to Sr-89.

PALLIATIVE SURGERY

Even when curative surgery is impossible, certain operations may reduce pain and other symptoms. A few common palliative surgeries are mentioned here.

Pathologic fracture stabilization improves function and decreases pain for well over 80% of patients.[96] With improved survival with advanced cancer, patients may now obtain substantial benefit from aggressive surgical management of long bone, pelvic, and vertebral fractures and impending fractures. Metastatic plexopathy may be treated with en bloc resection of tumor and surrounding structures, together with radiation and chemotherapy.[93] Ninety percent of patients with bowel obstruction have continuous pain.[97] Tumor resection, ostomy placement, and gastrointestinal bypass may permit continued enteral nutrition and relieve obstruction in patients who have not responded to conservative measures.[97] Few patients with pancreatic cancer can be cured, and the vast majority have abdominal pain at the time of death. Nonetheless, aggressive surgical treatment, including tumor resection, biliary bypass, and decompression, is warranted to improve survival and decrease pain.[98] Chronic radiation enteropathy, often associated with crampy abdominal pain, is effectively palliated with proximal jejunostomy, ileostomy, or colostomy. Focal areas of radiation necrosis may be resected or bypassed.[99]

Spinal decompression and stabilization relieves pain from epidural cord compression, and prevents impending paralysis. Extensive vertebral body destruction may leave the spine unstable, and positional changes may be painful.[93,96] Surgical stabilization provides complete pain relief in over 80% of these patients, even if neural compression is absent.[93]

NEUROSURGERY

Several neurosurgical treatments have been designed to interrupt pain pathways and stimulate modulatory systems. Over the last two decades, high-dose opioid treatment has replaced many of these surgeries.[93] But some patients, especially those with localized pain, may find more benefit and less morbidity in neuroablative procedures than in systemic analgesics. Of course, the WHO analgesic ladder should be followed before resorting to a neurosurgical pain procedure.[1] Following a neurosurgical procedure, care must be taken to taper the opioid dose so as to avoid symptomatic withdrawal. The most common procedures are presented here, and the reader is referred to a recent review for details on other procedures.[100]

Intraventricular Opioid Delivery

Morphine may be injected into the cerebral ventricles after placement of an Ommaya reservoir or with a continuous infusion pump. It is appropriate for certain patients with pain from head and neck cancer, but no studies have demonstrated superiority of intraventricular over systemic opioid delivery. The relatively small experience with this technique has shown 50% to 90% good to excellent initial relief.[93,101] As with intrathecal and epidural opioid delivery, respiratory depression and bleeding are potential early complications. Infection is the most concerning late complication.

Cordotomy

A lesion in the anterolateral quadrant of the spinal cord blocks the spinothalamic tract (Fig. 46-6), which carries pain signals from the contralateral body to the thalamus. A percutaneous modification makes this a minimally invasive procedure for an experienced operator.[83] Cordotomy is most useful for patients with unilateral somatic pain below the C5 dermatome, but useless in cases of deafferentation pain.[83] Lumbosacral plexopathy from tumor invasion is ideally suited to cordotomy. High cervical cordotomy may be used for arm pain. Bilateral cordotomy may be used for bilateral or midline pain conditions.[102] Because corticospinal and reticulospinal tracts are also located in the anterolateral quadrant, voluntary and involuntary respiration may be hampered by high cordotomy. Autonomic fiber disruption may interfere with bowel and bladder function in about 2% of patients. Persistent paresis is seen in 2%. These complications are more likely when bilateral lesions are made.[102] While initial success with cordotomy is high (71% to 98%), recurrence of pain is common months to years later.[83,93,100]

Dorsal Rhizotomy and Dorsal Root Entry Zone Lesions

Dorsal rhizotomy is the surgical version of intrathecal neurolysis (See section, Intrathecal and Epidural Neurolysis). Interruption of dorsal roots blocks all regional sensation, including pain. Motor function is impaired if proprioception is blocked, so this procedure is limited to several dermatomes serving the trunk or functionless limbs. Of patients with chest wall pain from tumor invasion, 50% to 80% experience relief with rhizotomy.[93] Sindou's highly selective rhizotomy involves making small incisions in the intermediate posterolateral sulcus of the cord, adjacent to the dorsal root entry sites.[104] Pain sensation may be selectively interrupted without loss of normal sensation or proprioception. As with intrathecal neurolysis, rhizotomy is not effective for purely neuropathic pain. Dorsal root entry zone (DREZ) lesioning destroys Lissauer's tract and the outer laminae of Rexed, preventing the development of deafferentation pain (Fig. 46-7).[105] DREZ is classically used to treat pain from brachial plexus avulsion, but it has also been successfully applied to phantom limb pain, radiation plexopathy, and postherpetic neuralgia.[106108]

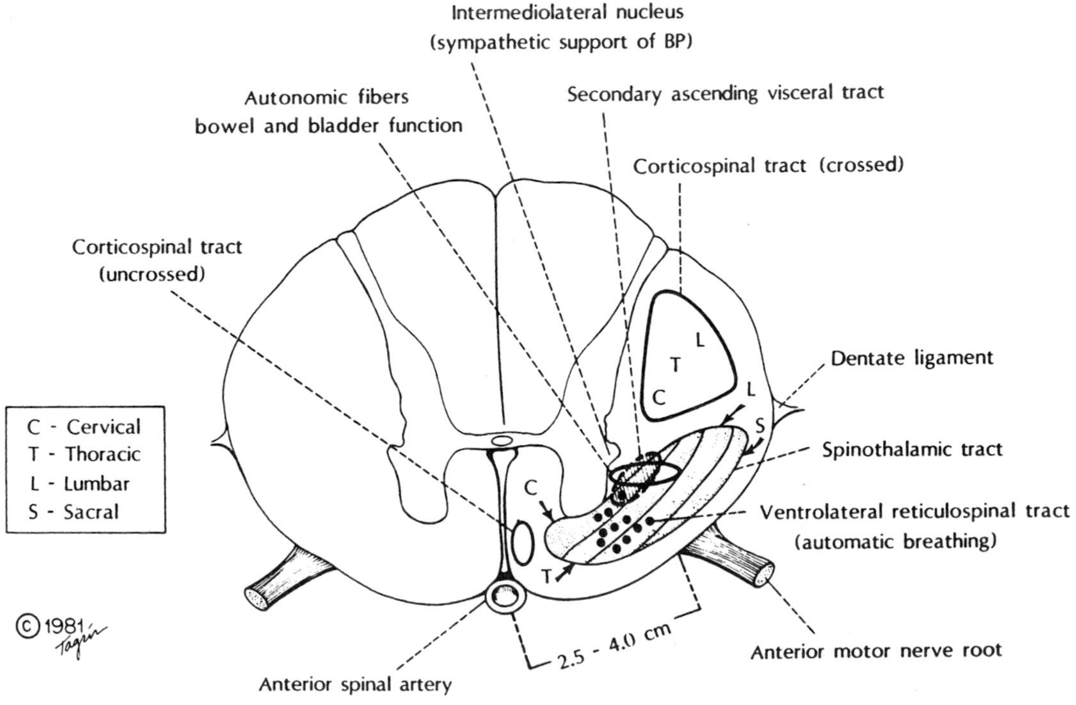

Figure 46-6 Cross section of the spinal cord showing the locations of spinothalamic, autonomic, reticulospinal (automatic breathing) and corticospinal (motor) tracts. Anterolateral cordotomy interrupts the spinothalamic tract, but complications may occur if surrounding fibers are affected. (From Poletti CE. Open cordotomy medullary tractotomy. In: Schmidek HH, Sweet WH, eds. Operative Neurosurgical Techniques: Indications, Methods, Results. New York, NY: Grune and Stratton, 1988.)

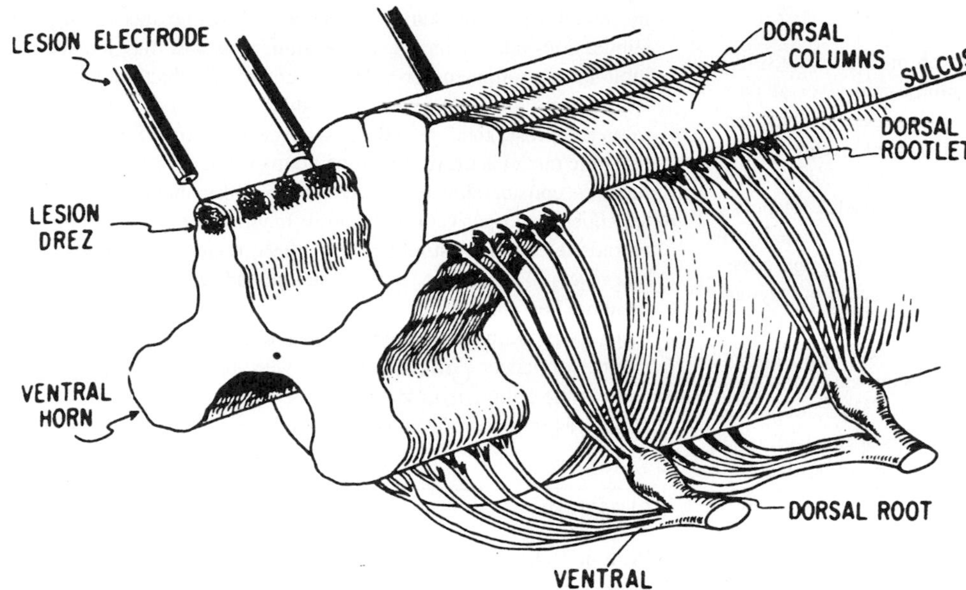

Figure 46-7 Radiofrequency dorsal root entry zone (DREZ) lesions as originally described by Nashold. (From Nashold BS, Ostdahl FH. Dorsal root entry zone for pain relief. *J Neurosurg* 1979;51:59. Used with permission of the American Association of Neurological Surgeons.)

Cranial Rhizotomies

When tumor growth causes somatic or neuralgic orofacial pain, radiation and resection are effective palliative treatments.[109,110] Percutaneous and open rhizotomies of the glossopharyngeal and trigeminal nerves may also be effective in these situations.[111,112] Giorgi and Broggi performed percutaneous rhizotomies on one patient with glossopharyngeal and four patients with combined glossopharyngeal and trigeminal neuralgia due to tumor.[111] Four patients were pain-free and one was improved at the last follow-up, between 4 months and 3 years later. Surgical section, thermal, and chemical ablation have all been used. These procedures may result in prolonged pain relief, but neurologic deficit is expected and recurrent pain is not uncommon.

Hypophysectomy

Widespread pain from metastases may respond well to ablation of the pituitary. Hypophysectomy was introduced in 1953 for treatment of breast and prostate tumors.[113] An unexpected result of these early operations was the rapid onset of analgesia, which frequently was not associated with tumor regression. The analgesic mechanism is still unknown. Over the last 40 years, thousands of palliative hypophysectomies have been performed surgically and by closed chemical and thermoablation, primarily for widespread bone pain. Most hypophysectomy patients achieve partial or total pain relief that lasts weeks to months, and infrequently over 1 year.[114,115] Alcohol instillation via the transsphenoidal route is now the most popular technique (Fig. 46-8).[116] While patients with hormone-sensitive tumors are usually treated in this way, pain from other tumors may also respond.[114,117] Hypophysectomy is appropriate for patients who have diffuse pain, especially above the clavicles, in whom antitumor treatments and conservative analgesic approaches have failed. CSF leakage, infection, coma, and cranial nerve palsies may result. Hypopituitarism is expected, but not uniformly with chemical and thermoablation.

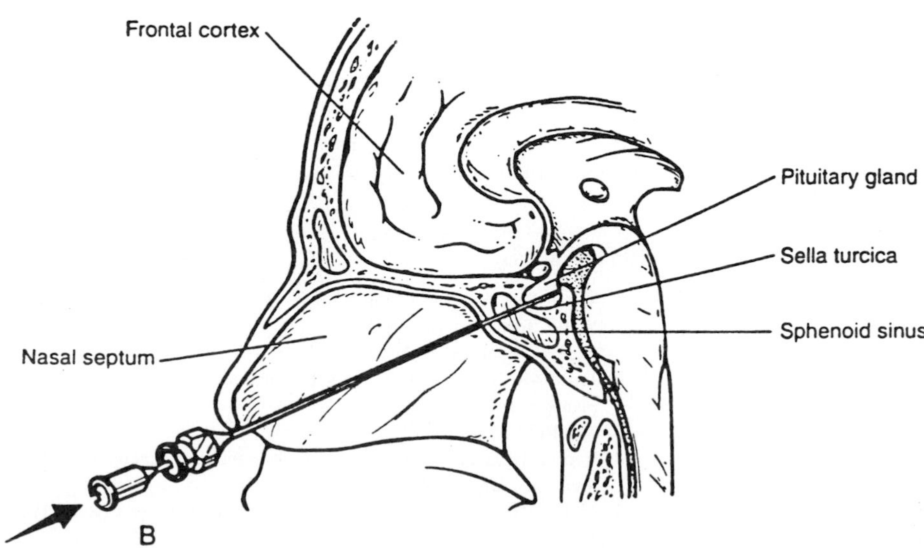

Figure 46-8 Sagittal illustration of needle placement for chemical hypophysectomy. (From Waldman SD, Winnie AP, eds. Interventional Pain Management. Philadelphia, Pa: WB Saunders, 1996:519.)

Midline Myelotomy

Conventional anterolateral cordotomy, which interrupts the spinothalamic tract, is often ineffective for midline and visceral pain. Furthermore, bilateral cordotomy often produces paresthesias, sensory disturbances, and bladder dysfunction. Recent research points to a midline dorsal column pathway for visceral pain.[119] A small dorsal column lesion at the T8 level has proven useful for pelvic visceral pain control in a case report (Fig. 46-9).[120]A related procedure, commissural myelotomy, involves interrupting the crossing spinothalamic pain fibers as well as a hypothetical polysynaptic visceral pathway that runs posterior to the spinal canal (Fig. 46-9).[100] Gildenberg and Hirshberg treated 14 patients with midline pelvic cancer pain. Ten experienced significant relief, and there were no complications or neurologic side effects.[121] Although it is possible that a central pain pathway exists, it now seems likely that the dissection for commissural myelotomy causes some dysfunction of the dorsal column visceral pathway.[120]

Neurostimulation

Unlike neuroablation, neurostimulation is reversible and may be patient-controlled.[93] Motor and sensory functions are generally preserved with stimulatory procedures. Possible mechanisms of stimulation-induced analgesia are numerous, and may include inhibitory neurotransmitter release, sensory conduction blockade, dorsal horn "gate" closure,[4] and others. Spinal cord stimulation, often a neurosurgical procedure, is described above. Stimulation of thalamic nuclei is useful for some neuropathic pain conditions, but requires considerable expertise for lead placement.[122] The periaqueductal and periventricular gray matter contains receptors for opioids. Deep brain stimulation of these regions produces naloxone-reversible analgesia. Since systemic and neuraxial opioid treatment has become more accepted, these procedures have fallen from favor. Deep brain stimulation has been used successfully in a small number of cancer pain patients who were refractory to intraspinal or systemic opioid treatment, but more conservative approaches are at least as effective for most patients.[100,123]

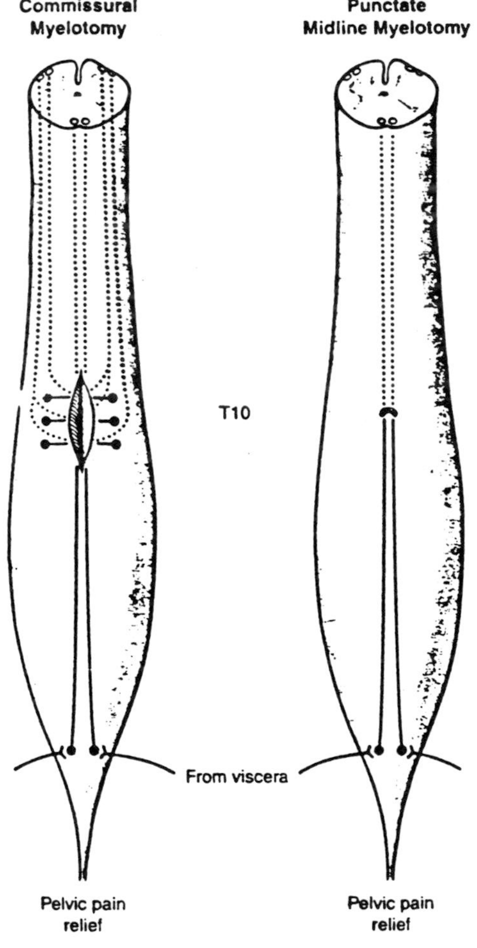

Figure 46-9 Commissural myelotomy interrupts crossing spinothalamic fibers at several levels, and may inadvertently affect the dorsal column visceral pain pathway. Midline myelotomy selectively interrupts the visceral pathway. (From Nauta HJW et al. Surgical interruption of a midline dorsal column visceral pain pathway. *J Neurosurg* 1997;86:538.)

SUMMARY

Profound changes have taken place in the public's and medical professionals' attitudes related to cancer pain. Hopeless resignation has been replaced by widespread acceptance of the importance of routine pain assessment and control, and the institutionalization of this new view in clinical practice guidelines[9,124] and quality assurance processes[125] and standards of the Joint Commission for the Accreditation of Healthcare Organizations.[126] This acceptance of the importance of pain control for optimizing quality of life has had a ripple effect to the benefit of many other patients with pain, such as those experiencing postoperative pain, burn patients, and pediatric patients. As society realizes it must face limits in providing medical care at the end of life, this ripple effect has extended further to intensifying interest in palliative care at the end of life. Indeed, it is now clear that pain medicine will play a substantial role in the 21st century medical practice not only from a humanitarian viewpoint, but also from an economic one. Cancer pain control is still a common cause for hospital admissions that could be averted if proactive planning and continuity of pain management between care settings (home, hospital, hospice) were the rule. The importance of educating patients, families, and health care providers to monitor and manage pain cannot be overemphasized. Patients should be taught to report changes in their pain or any new pain so that these can be assessed and their treatment plan adjusted, or diagnostic studies arranged. Recently, the concept of "disease management" has gained currency as a means to provide optimal, cost-effective care that involves an array of specialists for the patient with an illness episode or a chronic illness. Pain control must now be considered an integral part of the disease management process for all patients with cancer.

REFERENCES

1. World Health Organization. *Cancer Pain Relief and Palliative Care*. WHO Technical Report Series, 804. Geneva, Switzerland: World Health Organization, 1990.
2. Jadad AR, Browman GP. The WHO analgesic ladder for cancer pain management. Stepping up the quality of its evaluation. *JAMA* 1995; 274:1870.
3. Redd WH. Behavioral intervention for cancer treatment side effects. *Acta Oncologica* 1994;33:113.
4. Melzack R. Pain: past, present, and future. *Can J Exp Psychol* 1993; 47:615.

5. McGrath P, McAlpine L. Psychologic perspectives on pediatric pain. *J Pediatr* 1993;122:S20.
6. Ahles TH, Blanchard EB, Ruckdeschel JC. The multidimensional nature of cancer-related pain. *Pain* 1983;17:277.
7. Breitbart W. Psychiatric management of cancer pain. *Cancer* 1989; 63:2336.
8. Friedman R, Sobel D, Myers P, et al. Behavioral medicine clinical health psychology and cost offset. *Health Psychol* 1995;14:509.
9. Jacox A, Carr DB, Payne R, et al. Cancer Pain Guideline Panel: Non-pharmacologic management: physical and psychosocial modalies. In: *Clinical Practice Guideline Number 9: Management of Cancer Pain.* Rockville, Md: US Dept of Health and Human Services, Agency for Health Care Policy and Research; 1994. AHCPR publication 94-0592.
10. Cleeland CS. The impact of pain on the patient with cancer. *Cancer* 1984;54(suppl):2635.
11. Spiegel D. Cancer and depression. *Br J Psychiatry* 1996;168(suppl 30):109.
12. Derogatis LR, Morrow GR, Fetting J, et al. The prevalence of psychiatric disorders among cancer patients. *JAMA* 1983;249:751.
13. Bukberg J, Penman D, Holland J. Depression in hospitalized cancer patients. *Psychosom Med* 1984;46:199.
14. Loscalzo M. Psychological approaches to the management of pain in patients with advanced cancer. *Hematol Oncol Clin North Am* 1996; 10:139.
15. Fishman B, Loscalzo M. Cognitive-behavioral interventions in management of cancer pain: principles and applications. *Med Clin North Am* 1987;71:271.
16. Mishel MH. Perceived uncertainty and stress in illness. *Res Nurs Health* 1984;7:163.
17. Jacox A, Carr DB, Payne R, et al. *Clinical Practice Guideline No. 9: Management of Cancer Pain.* Rockville,Md: US Dept of Health and Human Services, Agency for Health Care Policy and Research; 1994. AHCPR publication 94-0592.
18. Graffam S, Johnson A. A comparison of two relaxation strategies for the relief of pain and its distress. *J Pain Symptom Manage* 1987;2:229.
19. Syrjala KL, Cummings C, Donaldson GW. Hypnosis or cognitive behavioral training for the reduction of pain and nausea during cancer treatment: a controlled clinical trial. *Pain* 1992;48:137.
20. Kirsch I, Lynn SJ. The altered state of hypnosis: changes in the theoretical landscape. *Am Psychologist* 1995;50:846.
21. Golden WL, Gersh WD, Robbins DM. Pain control. In: *Psychological Treatment of Cancer Patients: A Cognitive Behavioral Approach.* New York, NY: MacMillan, 1992:46–47.
22. Spira JL, Spiegel D. Hypnosis and related techniques in pain management. *Hospice J* 1992;8:89.
23. Montgomery G, Kirsch I. Mechanisms of placebo pain reduction: an empirical investigation. *Psychol Sci* 1996;7:174.
24. Meier W, Klucken M, Soyka D, Bromm, B. Hypo- and hyperalgesia: divergent effects on pain ratings and pain-related cerebral potentials. *Pain* 1993;53:175.
25. Kiernan BD, Dane JR, Phillips LH, Price DD. Hypnotic anagelsia reduces RIII nociceptive reflex: further evidence concerning the multifactorial nature of hypnotic analgesia. *Pain* 1995;60:39.
26. Goudas LC, Carr D, Balk E, et al. *Management of Cancer Pain. Evidence Report/Technology Assessment Number 35.* Services, Public Health Service. Rockville, Md: US Depart of Health and Human Services, Agency for Healthcare Research and Quality; 2001. *http://www.ahrq.gov/clinic/canpainsum.htm*
27. Wallace KG. Analysis of recent literature concerning relaxation and imagery interventions for cancer pain. *Cancer Nurs* 1997;20:79.
28. Syrjala KL, Donaldson GW, Davis MW, et al. Relaxation and imagery and cognitive-behavioral training reduce pain during cancer treatment: a controlled clinical trial. *Pain* 1995;63:189.
29. Rhiner M, Ferrell BR, Ferrell BA, Grant MM. A structured non-drug intervention program for cancer pain. *Cancer Pract* 1993;1:137.
30. Barbour LA, McGuire DB, Kirchhoff KT. Nonanalgesic methods of pain control used by cancer outpatients. *Oncol Nurs Forum* 1986; 13:56.
31. Lehmann JF, deLateur BJ. Ultrasound shortwave, microwave, laser, superficial heat, and cold in the treatment of pain. In: Wall PD, Melzack R, eds. *Textbook of Pain.* Edinburgh, Scotland: Churchill Livingstone, 1994:1237.
32. Ernst E, Fialka B. Ice freezes pain? A review of the clinical effectiveness of analgesic cold therapy. *J Pain Symptom Manage* 1994;9:56.
33. Michlovits S. *Thermal Agents in Rehabilitation.* Philadelphia, Pa: F.A. Davis, 1986.
34. Wingate L. Efficacy of physical therapy for patients who have undergone mastectomies. A prospective study. *Phys Ther* 1985; 65:896.
35. Herring D, King AI, Connelly M, et al. New rehabilitation concepts in management of radical neck dissection syndrome. A clinical report. *Phys Ther* 1987;67:1095.
36. Weinrich SP, Weinrich MC. The effect of massage on pain in cancer patients. *Appl Nurs Res* 1990;3:140.
37. Morgan RG, Casley-Smith JR, Mason MR, Casley-Smith JR. Complex physical therapy for the lymphoedematous arm. *J Hand Surg* [Br]. 1992;17:437.
38. Melzack R, Wall PD. Pain mechanisms: a new theory. *Science* 1965; 150:69.
39. Avellanosa AM, West CR. Experience with transcutaneous electrical nerve stimulation for relief of intractable pain in cancer patients. *J Med* 1982;19:46.
40. Sherman RA, Sherman CJ, Parker L. Chronic phantom and stump pain among American veterans: results of a survey. *Pain* 1984;18:83.
41. Sjolund B, Eriksson M. Electro-acupuncture and endogenous morphines. *Lancet* 1976;13:1085.
42. Liu X, Zhu B, Zhang SX. Relationship between electroacupuncture analgesia and descending pain inhibitory mechanism of nucleus raphe magnus. *Pain* 1986;24:383.
43. Tsai HY, Lin JG, Inoki R. Further evidence for possible analgesic mechanism of electroacupuncture: effects on neuropeptides and serotonergic neurons in rat spinal cord. *Jpn J Pharmacol* 1989;49:181.
44. Borg-Stein J, Stein J. Trigger points and tender points: one and the same? Does injection treatment help? *Rheum Dis Clin North Am* 1996; 22:305.
45. Devor M, Giovrin-Lippmann R, Raber P. Corticosteroids suppress ectopic neural discharge originating in experimental neuromas. *Pain* 1985;22:127.
46. Kirvela O, Nieminen S. Treatment of painful neuromas with neurolytic blockade. *Pain* 1990;41:161.
47. Kirvela O, Antila H. Thoracic paravertebral block in chronic postoperative pain. *Reg Anesth* 1994;17:348.
48. Myers DP, Lema MJ, deLeon-Casasola OA, Bacon DR. Interpleural analgesia for the treatment of severe cancer pain in terminally ill patients. *J Pain Symptom Manage* 1993;8:505.
49. Johansson A. Methylprednisolone shortens the effects of bupivicaine on sensory nerve fibers in vivo. *Acta Anaesthesiol Scand* 1996;40:595.
50. McCleane G, Mackle E, Stirling I. The addition of triamcinolone acetonide to bupivicaine has no effect on the quality of analgesia produced by ilioinguinal nerve block. *Anaesthesia* 1994;49:819.
51. Kuzma PJ, Kline MD, Calkins MD, Staats PS. Progress in the development of ultra-long-acting local anesthetics. *Reg Anesth* 1997; 22:543.
52. Ferrer-Brechner T. Neurolytic blocks for cancer pain. *Curr Manage Pain* 1989;3:111.
53. Doyle D. Nerve blocks in advanced cancer. *Practitioner* 1982;226: 539.
54. Ramamurthy S, Walsh NE, Schoenfeld LS, et al. Evaluation of neurolytic blocks using phenol and cryogenic block in the management of chronic pain. *J Pain Symptom Manage* 1989;4:72.
55. Rocco AG. Radiofrequency lumbar sympatholysis. The evolution of a technique for managing sympathetically maintained pain. *Reg Anesth* 1995;20:3.

56. Patt RB, Millard R. A role for peripheral neurolysis in the management of intractable cancer pain. *Pain* 1990;5(suppl):S358.
57. Evans PJ, Lloyd JW, Jack TM. Cryoanalgesia for intractable perineal pain. *J R Soc Med* 1981;74:804.
58. Zhou L, Kambin P, Casey KF, et al. Mechanism research of cryoanalgesia. *Neurol Res* 1995;17:307.
59. Barnard D. The effects of extreme cold on sensory nerves. *Ann R Coll Surg Engl* 1980;62:180.
60. Cross FW, Cotton LT. Chemical lumbar sympathectomy for ischemic rest pain. A randomized, prospective controlled clinical trial. *Am J Surg* 1985;150:341.
61. Kawamata M, Ishitani K, Ishikawa K, et al. Comparison between celiac plexus block and morphine treatment on quality of life in patients with pancreatic cancer pain. *Pain* 1996;64:597.
62. Bonica JJ. Autonomic innervation of the viscera in relation to nerve block. *Anesthesiology* 1968;29:793.
63. Mercadante S. Celiac plexus block versus analgesics in pancreatic cancer pain. *Pain* 1993;52:187.
64. Mercadante S, Nicosia F. Celiac plexus block: a reappraisal. *Reg Anesth Pain Med* 1998;23:37.
65. Lillemoe KD, Cameron JL, Kaufman HS, et al. Chemical splanchnicectomy in patients with unresectable pancreatic cancer. A prospective randomized trial. *Ann Surg* 1993;217:447.
66. Eisenberg E, Carr DB, Chalmers TC. Neurolytic celiac plexus block for treatment of cancer pain: a meta-analysis. *Anesth Analg* 1995;80:290.
67. Davies DD. Incidence of major complications of neurolytic coeliac plexus block. *J R Soc Med* 1993;86:264.
68. Plancarte R, deLeon-Casasola OA, El-Helaly M, et al. Neurolytic superior hypogastric plexus block for chronic pelvic pain associated with cancer. *Reg Anesth* 1997;22:562.
69. Lee RB, Stone K, Magelsen D, et al: Presacral neurectomy for chronic pelvic pain. *Obstet Gynecol* 1986;68(4):517–521.
70. Papay FA, Verghese A, Stanton-Hicks M, Zins J. Complex regional pain syndrome of the breast in a patient after breast reduction. *Ann Plast Surg* 1997;39:347.
71. Wartan SW, Hamann W, Wedley JR, McColl I. Phantom pain and sensation among British veteran amputees. *Br J Anaesth* 1997;78:652.
72. Tenicela R, Lovasik D, Eaglstein W. Treatment of herpes zoster with sympathetic blocks. *Clin J Pain* 1985;1:63.
73. Hogan Q, Haddox JD, Abram S, et al. Epidural opiates and local anesthetics for the management of cancer pain. *Pain* 1991;46:271.
74. Bedder MD, Burchiel K, Larson A. Cost analysis of two implantable narcotic delivery systems. *J Pain Symptom Manage* 1991;6:368.
75. Hassenbusch SJ, Pillay PK, Magdinec M, et al. Constant infusion of morphine for intractable cancer pain using an implanted pump. *J Neurosurg* 1990;73:405.
76. Sjoberg M, Nitescu P, Appelgren, L, Curelaru I. Long-term intrathecal morphine and bupivicaine in patients with refractory cancer pain. *Anesthesiology* 1994;80:284.
77. Penning JP, Yaksh TL. Interaction of intrathecal morphine with bupivicaine and lidocaine in the rat. *Anesthesiology* 1992;77:1186.
78. Dahl JB, Rosenberg J, Hansen BL, et al. Differential analgesic effects of low-dose epidural morphine and morphine-bupivicaine at rest and during mobilization after major abdominal surgery. *Anesth Analg* 1992;74:362.
79. Sjogren P, Banning A. Pain, sedation and reaction time during long-term treatment of cancer patients with oral and epidural opioids. *Pain* 1989;39:5.
80. Onofrio BM, Yaksh TL. Long-term pain relief produced by intrathecal morphine infusion in 53 patients. *J Neurosurg* 1990;72:200.
81. Eisenach JC, DuPen S, Dubois M, et al Epidural clonidine analgesia for intractable cancer pain. *Pain* 1995;61:391.
82. Swerdlow M. Intrathecal neurolysis. *Anaesthesia* 1978;33:733.
83. Ischia S, Luzzani A, Ischia A, et al. Subarachnoid neurolytic block (L5-S1) and unilateral percutaneous cervical cordotomy in the treatment of pain secondary to pelvic malignant disease. *Pain* 1984;20:139.
84. Dobrogowski J, Kus M. Epidural neurolytic block in cancer patients. In: Erdman W, Oyama R, Pernak MJ, eds. *The Pain Clinic I. Proceedings of the First International Symposium*. Utrecht, The Netherlands:VNU Science Press, 1985:51.
85. Bedder MD. Spinal cord stimulation and intractable pain: patient selection. In: Waldman SD, Winnie A, eds. *Interventional Pain Management*. Philadelphia, Pa: WB Saunders, 1996:412.
86. Krainick JU, Thoden U, Riechert T. Pain reduction in amputees by long term spinal cord stimulation: long term follow-up study over 5 years. *J Neurosurg* 1980;52:346.
87. Arcangeli G, Micheli A, Arcangeli G, et al. The responsiveness of bone metastases to radiotherapy: the effect of site, histology and radiation dose on pain relief. *Radiother Oncol* 1989;14:95.
88. Bates T, Yarnold JR, Blitzer P, et al. Bone metastasis consensus statement. *Int J Radiat Oncol Biol Phys* 1992;23:215.
89. Mathes SJ, Alexander J. Radiation injury. *Surg Oncol Clin North Am* 1996;5:809.
90. Hoskin PJ. Radiotherapy in the management of bone pain. *Clin Orth Rel Res* 1995;312:105.
91. Mithal NP, Needham PR, Hoskin PJ. Retreatment with radiotherapy for painful bone metastases. *Int J Radiat Oncol Biol Phys* 1994;29:1011.
92. Rutten EHJM, Crul BJP, van der Toorn PPG, et al. Pain characteristics help to predict the analgesic efficacy of radiotherapy for the treatment of cancer pain. *Pain* 1997;69:131.
93. Sundaresan N, DiGiacinto GV, Hughes JEO. Neurosurgery in the treatment of cancer pain. *Cancer* 1989;63:2365.
94. Robinson RG, Blake GM, et al. Strontium-89: treatment results and kinetics in patients with painful metastatic prostate and breast cancer in bone. *Radiographics* 1989;9:271.
95. Porter AT, McEwan AJB, Powe JE, et al. Results of randomized phase-III trial to evaluate the efficacy of Sr-89 adjuvant to local field external beam irradiation in the management of endocrine resistant metastatic prostatic cancer. *Int J Radiat Oncol Biol Phys* 1992;25:805.
96. Harrington KD. Orthopedic surgical management of skeletal complications of malignancy. *Cancer* 1997;80(suppl):1614.
97. Ripamonti C. Management of bowel obstruction in advanced cancer. *Curr Opin Oncol* 1994;6:351.
98. Lillemoe KD, Barnes SA. Surgical palliation of unresectable pancreatic carcinoma. *Surg Clin North Am* 1995;75:953.
99. Mann WJ. Surgical management of radiation enteropathy. *Surg Clin North Am* 1991;71:977.
100. Hassenbusch SJ. Surgical management of cancer pain. *Neurosurg Clin North Am* 1995;6:127.
101. Dennis GC, DeWitty RL. Long-term intraventricular infusion of morphine for intractable pain in cancer of the head and neck. *Neurosurgery* 1990;26:404.
102. Ischia S, Luzzani A, Ischia A, Maffezzoli G. Bilateral percutaneous cervical cordotomy: immediate and long term results in 36 patients with neoplastic disease. *J Neurol Neurosurg Psychiatry* 1984;47:141.
103. Poletti CE. Open cordotomy medullary tractotomy. In: Schmidek HH, Sweet WH, eds. *Operative Neurosurgical Techniques: Indications, Methods, Results*. New York, NY: Grune and Stratton, 1988:1155.
104. Sindou M, Giontelle A. Selective posterior rhizotomies for the treatment of pain. In: Krayenbul, et al, eds. *Advances and Technical Standards in Neurosurgery*. New York, NY: Springer-Verlag, 1983:147.
105. Nashold BS, Ostdahl FH. Dorsal root entry zone lesions for pain relief. *J Neurosurg* 1979;51:59.
106. Saris SC, Iacono RP, Nashold BS. Dorsal root entry zone lesions for postamputation pain. *J Neurosurg* 1985;62:72.
107. Zeidman SM, Rossitch EJ, Nashold BS. Dorsal root entry zone lesions in the treatment of pain related to radiation-induced brachial plexopathy. *J Spinal Disord* 1993;6:44.

108. Friedman AH, Nashold BS, Ovelman-Levitt J. Dorsal root entry zone lesions for the treatment of post-herpetic neuralgia. *J Neurosurg* 184; 60:1258.
109. Tacconi L, Arulampalam R, Johnston F, Symon L. Adenocarcinoma of Meckel's cave: a case report. *Surg Neurol* 1995;44:553.
110. Mastronardi L, Lunardi P, Osman Farah J, Puzzilli F. Metastatic involvement of the Meckel's cave and trigeminal nerve. A case report. *J Neurooncol* 1997;32:87.
111. Giorgi C, Broggi G. Surgical treatment of glossopharyngeal neuralgia and pain from cancer of the nasopharynx. A 20-year experience. *J Neursurg* 1984;61:952.
112. Cheng TM, Cascino TL, Onofrio BM. Comprehensive study of diagnosis and treatment of trigeminal neuralgia secondary to tumors. *Neurology* 1993;43:2298.
113. Luft R, Olivercrona H. Experiences with hypophysectomy. *J Neurosurg* 1953;10:301.
114. Katz J, Levin AB. Treatment of diffuse metastatic cancer pain by instillation of alcohol into the sella turcica. *Anesthesiology* 1977;46:115.
115. Lipton S, Miles JB, Williams N, Bark-Jones N. Pituitary injections of alcohol for widespread cancer pain. *Pain* 1978;5:73.
116. Levin AB, Katz J, Benson RC, Jones AG. Treatment of pain of diffuse metastatic cancer by stereotactic chemical hypophysectomy: long term results and observations on mechanism of action. *Neurosurgery* 1980;6:258.
117. Tindall GT, Nixon DW, Christy JH, Neill JD. Pain relief in metastatic cancer other than breast and prostate gland following transsphenoidal hypophysectomy. A preliminary report. *J Neurosurg* 1977;47: 659.
118. Waldman SD. Neuroadenolysis of the pituitary: indications and technique. In: Waldman SD, Winnie AP,eds. *Interventional Pain Management.* Philadelphia, Pa: WB Saunders, 1996:519.
119. Al-Chaer ED, Feng Y, Willis WD. Visceral pain: a disturbance in the sensorimotor continuum? *Pain Forum.* 1998;7:117.
120. Nauta HJW, Hewitt E, Westlund KN, Willis WD. Surgical interruption of a midline dorsal column visceral pain pathway. *J Neurosurg* 1997;86:538.
121. Gildenberg PL, Hirshberg RM. Limited myelotomy for the treatment of intractable cancer pain. *J Neurol Neurosurg Psychiatry* 1984;47:94.
122. Turnbull IM, Shulman R, Woodhurst WB. Thalamic stimulation for neuropathic pain. *J Neurosurg* 1980;52:486.
123. Young RF, Brechner T. Electrical stimulation of the brain for relief of intractable pain due to cancer. *Cancer* 1986;57:1266.
124. Carr DB. The WHO concept of cancer pain treatment: a guideline prototype and its context. In: Chrubasik J, Cousins M, Martin B,eds. *Advances in Pain Therapy I.* Berlin, Germany: Springer-Verlag, 1992: 8–17.
125. American Pain Society Quality of Care Committee. Quality Improvement Guidelines for the Treatment of Acute Pain and Cancer Pain. *J Neurosurg* 1995;274:1874–1880.
125. Joint Commission for the Accreditation of Healthcare Organizations. Available at www.jcaho.org

CHAPTER 47 PAIN MANAGEMENT IN END OF LIFE: PALLIATIVE CARE

Lachlan Forrow and Howard S. Smith

"Pain is a more terrible master than Death itself."
DR. ALBERT SCHWEITZER

Basic principles of the diagnosis and management of pain syndromes are similar across all clinical settings. Details of the application of these principles, however, can vary significantly depending on the clinical context. One context that is especially important is the care of patients with incurable, progressive, and ultimately fatal illnesses who are in or approaching the terminal phase. This is sometimes referred to as the context of "palliative care," and that term, while not fully satisfactory,[1] is used throughout most of the discussions in this chapter. The range of pain syndromes that arise in these situations include most of the acute and chronic pain syndromes addressed in detail in other chapters in this text, and their management primarily involves the same diagnostic and therapeutic strategies and skills. Nonetheless, pain management in the "end-of-life" or "palliative care" setting often raises clinical and ethical issues that are at least somewhat different from those in other settings. This chapter focuses primarily on those differences.

PAIN MANAGEMENT AND PALLIATIVE CARE: OVERVIEW

The World Health Organization (WHO) has defined palliative care as: "The active total care of patients whose disease is not responsive to curative treatment. Control of pain, of other symptoms, and of psychological, social and spiritual problems, is paramount. The goal of palliative care is achievement of the best quality of life for patients and their families . . . Palliative care . . . affirms life and regards dying as a normal process . . . neither hastens nor postpones death . . . provides relief from pain and other distressing symptoms . . . and integrates the psychological and the spiritual aspects of care, . . . [including helping] the family cope during the patients illness and in their own bereavement."[2]

A more recent statement developed by the Task Force on Palliative Care of the Last Acts Campaign,[3] formulated by representatives of many leading U.S. professional organizations, states that "palliative care affirms life and regards dying as a natural process that is a profoundly personal experience for the individual and family. The goal of palliative care is to achieve the best possible quality of life through relief of suffering, control of symptoms, and restoration of functional capacity while remaining sensitive to personal, cultural and religious values, beliefs, and practices." The Task Force goes on to specify five "core precepts" of the evolving field of palliative care:

1. Respecting patient goals, preferences, and choices
2. Comprehensive caring of the patient
3. Utilizing the strengths of interdisciplinary resources
4. Acknowledging and addressing needs and concerns of family caregivers
5. Building systems and mechanisms of support for the field.

While it is clear that the field of palliative care encompasses a far broader range of issues than the narrower field of pain management, it is also clear from these definitions that the two fields overlap in important ways. These include a focus on quality of life as the primary goal of care; a recognition that psychological, social, and spiritual aspects of care are often deeply intertwined with strictly biological aspects; and an appreciation of the importance of interdisciplinary teams in effectively addressing these multifaceted issues.

Whether identified as such or not, palliative care has been an important part of medical practice for as long as medicine has existed. Prior to the 20th century, physicians rarely had any truly effective curative options within their therapeutic armentaria. The scientific transformation of medicine in the 20th century changed this dramatically. With the onset of the antibiotic era, many previously life-threatening infectious diseases were suddenly curable. The development of insulin for the treatment of diabetes, later advances in the diagnosis and treatment of coronary disease, major improvements in several forms of cancer therapy, and the revolutionary development of the field of organ transplantation all delayed or definitively eliminated many previously fatal disorders. These historic and justifiably celebrated successes, however, have contributed to increasing difficulty in accepting death as a tolerable outcome of any specific illness, and have even led to questions about whether mortality need be accepted as an inevitable fact of human existence.

As medical and lay cultures increasingly viewed death as a "defeat," tragic repercussions of heroic medical efforts to forestall death became more and more common in the latter part of the 20th century. These were most thoroughly documented in the Study to Understand Prognoses and Preferences for Outcomes and Risks of Treatment (SUPPORT). This study followed 9,105 patients (and their families) hospitalized in the United States who had a diverse range of illnesses with anticipated 50% mortality within 6 months of enrolling in the study. Investigators found that nearly half of these patients spent the last phase of their lives on ventilators in intensive care units, with family members reporting moderate to severe pain for approximately half of patients during the last 3 days of life.[4–6] This study helped catalyze a rapid increase in efforts to improve the experiences of patients and their families during the last phase of life, building from knowledge and experience gained in preceding decades in the United Kingdom, Canada, the United States, and elsewhere through the so-called hospice movement and other palliative care initiatives.[7–12]

MISCONCEPTIONS ABOUT PALLIATIVE CARE

Several common misconceptions about palliative care need to be confronted directly.

Misconception #1: *A palliative care approach should usually be considered only when all curative or life-prolonging efforts have been exhausted.*

A commonly held, but profoundly mistaken, model of the relationship between curative or life-prolonging efforts and palliative care approaches is shown in Figure 47-1.

There are three fundamental flaws with this model. First, during life-prolonging interventions in any illness, but especially for an illness that is potentially fatal, efforts to maximize the quality of each day of life are a mandatory part of all good clinical care. Life prolongation and palliation are not mutually exclusive. Second, achieving some of the most important emotional, psychological, and spiritual goals of first-rate palliative or hospice care can require a significant amount of time. If efforts to achieve those goals are not instituted until the last hours or days of a patient's life, or until a patient is so debilitated that his or her available energy and ability to communicate are severely limited, the likelihood that those goals can be achieved is severely compromised.

The third and final fundamental flaw is embodied in standard hospice reimbursement rules, at least in the United States. In choosing hospice services that focus on maximizing the quality of each day of life, a patient must agree to forgo interventions designed to lengthen life. But if the patient, because of the very effectiveness of those hospice services, comes to find that each day of life has fewer burdens and greater meaning than before, it is natural for the patient to want *more* of those days — that is, at least some interventions designed to lengthen life. In most cases, to receive those services the patient must leave the hospice program. He or she thereby risks losing exactly the services that helped make longer life more appealing.[13–14]

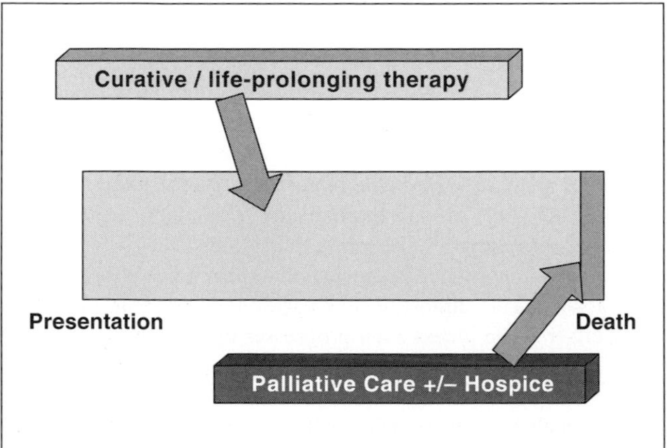

Figure 47-1 Common view of the relationship between curative and life-prolonging therapy and palliative care. (Adapted from the EPEC Project. Educating Physicians on End-of-Life Care. Chicago, Ill: American Medical Association.)

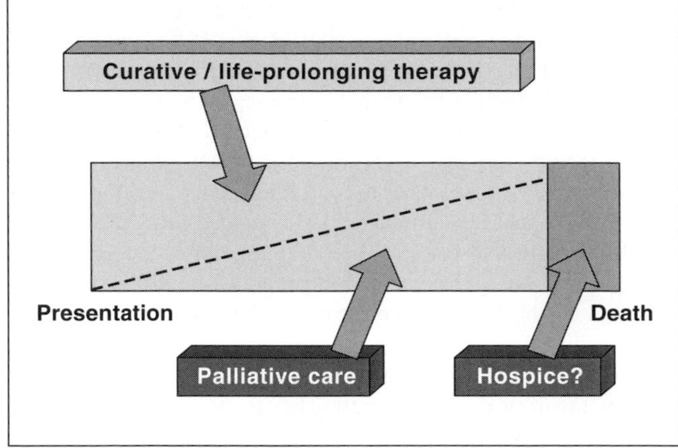

Figure 47-2 Preferred model of the relationship between curative and life-prolonging therapy and palliative care efforts. (Adapted from the EPEC Project. Educating Physicians on End-of-Life Care. Chicago, Ill: American Medical Association.)

Both in the care of individual patients, and in the reform of reimbursement rules and other features of our health care system, physicians and other health care workers must consistently fight against the dichotomization of the clinical world into curative "versus" palliative approaches. Figure 47-2 provides a preferred model for thinking about the relationship between these often coexisting approaches.

Misconception #2: *"Comfort" is the primary goal of good palliative care.*

This is often stated much more strongly, in the form of "Comfort Measures *Only*" orders (or some such variant) that are commonly written in the terminal phases of an illness. But "comfort," or the relief of symptoms generally, is *not* the most important goal of good palliative care. Using the language of the WHO definition of palliative care cited above, "Control of pain, of other symptoms, and of psychological, social and spiritual problems, is paramount." But control of symptoms is not the ultimate goal; it is, more precisely, the *prerequisite* for accomplishing something more fundamental: "The goal of palliative care is achievement of the best quality of life for patients and their families." Exactly what the "best quality of life" involves will vary considerably from individual patient to individual patient, but the latter stage of an ultimately fatal illness can be one of most important and meaningful periods of a person's life.[15–16] For some patients, mental alertness sufficient to allow maximal interactions with loved ones is more important than physical comfort, and an optimal pain regimen would reflect that. For others, being home during the last stage of illness, untethered to a continuous intravenous line, is more important to their quality of life than the potentially more reliable symptom control that might be achieved in a closely observed inpatient setting with continuous intravenous access.

Misconception #3: *Palliative care is "low tech" and "lower cost."*

A predominantly palliative approach to care is characterized by its primary (though not necessarily exclusive) focus on quality of life. This does not imply anything about the modalities (e.g., "high tech" or "low tech") that should be used to optimize quality of life. Numerous palliative interventions may involve highly sophisticated technology. These include bronchoscopic laser treatment of a malignant endobronchial lesion that is interfering with quality of life (i.e., via compromise of ventilation, or recurrent hemoptysis); radiation therapy for pain control; and a variety of interventional radiology-guided approaches to controlling pain or other symptoms for which an anatomical intervention is judged most effective.

The tragedy that occurs when dying patients undergo highly burdensome but ineffective life-prolonging efforts is compounded by the fact that the resources that are consumed in the process are often enormous. Nonetheless, extreme caution must be used in even considering cost reduction as a partial justification for favoring palliative approaches to these patients. This is not only true for obvious ethical reasons, and for the practical reason that if patients or family members believe that cost reduction is a priority of the physician who suggests a palliative approach there will likely be great resistance if not outright hostility and anger at that suggestion. But it is also far from proven that systematically providing palliative care with the same standards of excellence that characterize most life-prolonging ICU efforts would significantly reduce overall costs of medical care during the last year of life.[17-18] Too often, for example, home care near the end of life is touted as not only more consistent with patients' priorities, but also less expensive than inpatient care. To the extent that that is true, it is in part because a transfer to home usually involves a transfer of responsibility for hour-to-hour patient monitoring and for other aspects of care to family members, with very limited in-home support. In the SUPPORT study, many families faced near-bankruptcy as a result of increased costs and lost income during a terminal illness.[19] This transfer in most cases would be more accurately described as *cost-shifting* rather than *cost-saving*. If adequate hours of home health aides, and nursing, social work, pastoral, and medical staff were provided to ensure that patient and family needs during the last weeks or months of life were optimally addressed, the costs to the health care system of home-based palliative care would increase. For involved clinicians, however, the first concern must be to determine what services will best meet a patient's needs, then taking steps to ensure that those services are provided to the maximal extent possible in the context of finite (and sometimes severely constrained) resources. To the extent that a change in the priorities of health care financing (currently heavily tilted toward life-prolonging interventions) would allow improvements in palliative care services, clinicians should be prepared to undertake advocacy roles.[20]

PATIENT-CENTERED GOALS: ETHICAL AND PRACTICAL IMPORTANCE

As already alluded to above, defining clear patient-centered goals of care is a prerequisite to developing optimal diagnostic and therapeutic strategies. In the medical ethics literature, four core values that physicians are obligated to consider are frequently identified: autonomy; beneficence; justice; and non-maleficence. The physician's professional integrity is an additional important value. While cases in which these values are in conflict can pose exceedingly difficult ethical dilemmas, in most cases involving the clinical care of an individual patient the central question that should be posed about *any* proposed intervention is:

Do the expected benefits outweigh the expected burdens from the patient's perspective?

If the answer is yes, the intervention should almost always be instituted, unless an alternative is even more favorable. If the answer is no, the intervention should never be instituted, and if it is already in place, it should be withdrawn. This assessment applies equally to minor interventions such as phlebotomy or a plain radiograph and to much more complex interventions such as surgery or a course of radiation therapy.

There are obviously cases in which the answer to this question is *not* the sole ethical consideration. These include cases where the proposed intervention would violate other important moral values, such as when physician-administered active euthanasia would be considered a "benefit" by the patient. In addition, in some cases costs may be morally relevant, or considerations of "fairness" in allocating limited resources. Nonetheless, in almost all decisions about the care of individual patients, the answer to this question is the overriding consideration in determining the ethically appropriate approach to the patient's care.

The simplicity of this framework should not mask the frequent complexity of its application, which requires as full as possible an understanding of what the individual patient considers a "benefit" or a "burden," as well as an assessment of the probability of those benefits and burdens for each intervention under consideration. In this process, there is a natural division of labor between the respective roles of the patient (or his or her surrogate) and the patient's physician and/or other members of the clinical team, as illustrated in Figure 47-3. The patient (or surrogate) is the appropriate expert and authority about what goals and values are most important in developing a plan of care—that is, what kinds of things would count as important benefits and what others would constitute significant burdens. The physician and/or clinical team is usually the appropriate expert and authority about whether specific benefits are achievable (and burdens avoidable), and about what clinical interventions are most likely to achieve those benefits (and avoid or minimize unwanted burdens).

In developing plans of care, it is therefore vitally important for the clinician to engage the patient (or surrogate) in a careful consideration of the relative priority of a wide range of possible goals of care.

One common error in planning care is that discussions of relative priority for various potentially competing goals of care are limited to comfort versus length of life. As described above, however, comfort is rarely the most important human life goal, but rather the prerequisite to achieving other goals. Table 47-1 lists some of the goals of care that are most commonly expressed by patients confronting an ultimately fatal illness.

It is also important to appreciate that the relative priority of various goals of care almost always varies over the course of an illness, either as the illness itself progresses or as the person changes during the process of living with the illness. The clinician therefore needs to review regularly with the patient not only how well various goals of care are being achieved, but also whether the relative priority of various goals has changed (or whether entirely new goals have been identified).

A second common error in planning care is to confuse the articulation of *goals* of care with the determination of the most appropriate *means* of accomplishing those goals. This is a frequent shortcoming of both written and orally conveyed advance directives, which are often framed in terms of preferences for or against

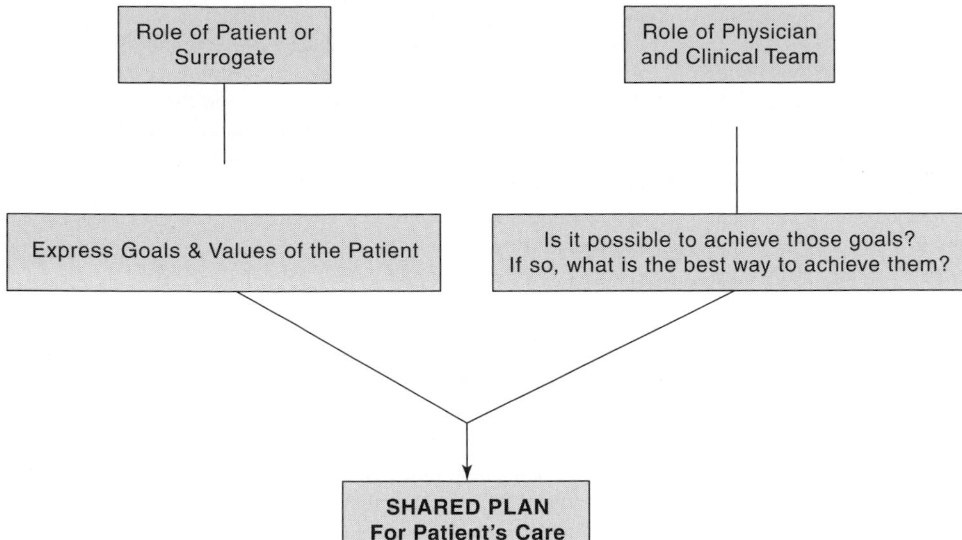

Figure 47-3 Shared decision making.

various clinical interventions (such as mechanical ventilation, CPR, or "feeding tubes"). For example, many patients who express with great confidence some variant of "I would never want to be kept alive by machines" will, on further discussion, quickly agree that "if a limited period of extremely intensive ICU care might restore me to near-normal condition, I would want it." For some patients who have previously adamantly expressed the view that they do not want any further "surgery," the expected benefits of an anatomical pain intervention that includes a relatively minor surgical procedure may far outweigh any likely burdens.[21]

In the opposite direction, patients are frequently asked some variant of "if your heart stops, would you want to be resuscitated?" The common affirmative response leads to a "full code" status that clinical staff may believe is inappropriate. But the desire to be "resuscitated" is an expression of a *goal*, which may not at all reflect a well-informed judgment about whether the expected benefits of administering CPR are likely to outweigh the expected burdens. A discussion that is much more likely to yield a plan of care that optimally serves the patient's most important goals might begin with a conversation about the patient's attitude toward death ("At this point in your illness, is death the enemy?"), as well as what conditions of prolonged life are most hoped for or feared. From an understanding of those, the clinician may offer specific suggestions of the clinical interventions that are most likely to achieve goals that are important to the patient, and most likely to avoid burdens or outcomes to which the patient is particularly averse.

TABLE 47-1 **Goals of Care**

Examples of Possible Goals of Care
Longer Life
Relief of Symptoms
Time at Home
Ability to Travel
Mental Clarity
Physical Mobility
Ability to Interact with Loved Ones
Minimizing Burdens on Loved Ones
Personal/Spiritual Growth
"Dignity" (specific meaning will vary)

PAIN, SUFFERING, AND MEANING IN THE END-OF-LIFE: PALLIATIVE CARE CONTEXT

As discussed at length elsewhere in this text, pain is a complex phenomenon that includes nociceptive, psychological, behavioral, and social components [See Chapter 4]. Pain must also be distinguished from suffering, which is not directly related to the severity of physical symptoms.[22,23] As Cassell suggests, suffering is experienced by *persons,* not bodies, and generally stems from conditions or events that threaten the integrity of the person as a complex psychological and social entity. Absence or loss of affirmative meaning and purpose, absence or loss of control, and absence or loss of hope are major sources of suffering.[24]

In his landmark study *Man's Search for Meaning*, psychiatrist Viktor Frankl analyzed experiences of his fellow concentration camp inmates at Auschwitz, in part to try to understand what distinguished those who survived from those who did not. He quotes Friedrich Nietzsche: "He who has a *why* to live for can put up with almost any *how*."[25] Analogously, for patients confronting serious or even life-threatening illnesses, the *meaning* (or absence thereof) of their continued life is often the strongest determinant of whether symptoms are bearable. A growing number of studies of requests for physician assistance in suicide support this insight: patients who ask for such assistance do not have higher levels of pain or other physical symptoms than those who do not make such requests. Rather, the primary concerns of many (if not most) patients asking for such assistance have more to do with issues of *meaning*, including the loss of a sense of any purpose in continued life, and concerns that the terminal phase of illness will involve a serious loss of personal dignity.

Biomedical efforts to control pain and other symptoms therefore constitute only a limited component of a broader effort to relieve suffering and help a patient find affirmative value in the last phase of life. Nonetheless, a failure to achieve consistent control of pain and other symptoms may make achievement of any other goals quite impossible. It is obvious that uncontrolled severe pain or other symptoms can so dominate a person's consciousness that he or she has no energy or capacity to focus on any affirmative goals or meaningful experiences. Even when pain is recently well controlled, fears that severe pain will recur and not be controllable can interfere with or even overwhelm other psychological processes. In addition, a perceived lack of control over pain often interacts synergistically with other perceptions by the patient that he or she has lost control over important parts of life, fueling a downward spiral of increasing depression and hopelessness. Conversely, the demonstrated controllability of pain not only has the direct benefit of relieving important symptoms; it can also help fuel an upward spiral of increasing optimism and hope.

TOLERANCE, DEPENDENCE, AND ADDICTION IN PALLIATIVE CARE

A comprehensive understanding of these three distinct phenomena is vital in many areas of pain management, and is covered in detail elsewhere in this text. In the palliative care setting, misconceptions about these phenomena, or a lack of attention to their potential importance, can significantly compromise the quality of pain management involving opioids.

Tolerance

Tolerance is characterized by the need to use escalating doses of a drug to maintain the same effect. When the underlying disease process is clearly stable, and when there is no evidence for either addiction or drug "diversion" (See following section, Addiction), the need for increased doses can with reasonable confidence be attributed to this phenomenon. In some cases switching to another opioid, for which a patient may have only partial cross-tolerance, can be useful. In actual practice, however, once a chronically effective dose has been well established in the treatment of a stable disease process, it is unusual for subsequent tolerance to be an important clinical problem.

In the palliative care context, however, the underlying disease process is rarely stable, and when increased doses are needed to achieve the same analgesic effect, the clinician's primary suspicion should always be disease progression. If disease progression is in fact the cause, then further increases in the dose of the current opioid may be effective. These increases may be quite large, as high as 20-fold.[26,27]

Physical Dependence

Physical dependence is characterized by symptoms of withdrawal following abrupt discontinuation of the drug, and can be a severe problem in the context of chronic use of significant doses of opioids. In the palliative care context, clinicians rarely if ever consciously stop chonic opioids abruptly. Nonetheless, serious withdrawal syndromes can become manifest in the terminal phase of illness if the route of administration of chronic opioids is suddenly no longer available – as in the case of a patient taking opioids orally who becomes moribund and unable to swallow. In this situation, it is important to find an alternate route to administer a minimum of the 25% of the previous daily dose of opioid that is generally regarded as required to prevent withdrawal symptoms. (This may not be as necessary in cases of acute renal or hepatic failure, which may alter the pharmacokinetics of the administered opioid and its active metabolites in ways that obviate the need for additional administered drug.)

Addiction

Addiction is characterized by psychological dependence on the involved drug, compulsive use, loss of control, associated loss of interest in other pleasurable activities and, most importantly, continued use in spite of evident harm. It is rare for this to be a problem in pain management in the setting of terminal illness, and it is virtually unheard of in terminally ill patients with no preexisting history of addiction or substance abuse. For patients with such a preexisting history, the risks of addiction must be carefully assessed and proactively addressed in planning any pain management regimen. Concern about these risks, however, must not lead to plans of care that leave a dying patient with inadequate symptom relief. Furthermore, even when there is an apparent pattern of opioid consumption or "lost prescriptions" that suggests the possibility of substance abuse, anectodal experience in the care of terminally ill patients suggests that two alternative explanations (neither with a simple solution) must be considered at least as strongly: another household member may be stealing the patient's medication, or the patient himself or herself may be selling the medication to cover other living expenses.

A much more frequent problem than true addiction is the unwarranted concern of patients (or their loved ones) that they will become addicted if they consume significant opioid doses over time. This concern can become a major obstacle to adequate symptom management and should be explicitly addressed with all patients. This can begin by simply inquiring about whether the patient or involved family members have any concerns about addiction to prescribed medications. Any concerns about addiction should be addressed with appropriate information and reassurance, emphasizing that the physical, psychological, and spiritual problems associated with uncontrolled pain take a far, far greater toll on most patients confronting a life-threatening illness.

OPIOIDS, RESPIRATORY SUPPRESSION, AND HASTENING DEATH

When high (or at least increasing) doses of opioids are required for effective pain control, clinicians are often concerned that in administering these doses they may depress a patient's respiratory drive and thereby hasten death. Even clinicians deeply committed to ensuring comfort at the end of life may exercise such caution in opioid administration that they fail to achieve adequate analgesia.

Although it is true that respiratory suppression can be a primary drug effect of opioids, it is in fact far less common than many physicians believe they "know" from their own clinical experience.[28–30] Tachypnea is a frequent manifestation both of acute pain and of anxiety, and the decreased respiratory rate that almost always follows administration of an opioid in the setting of intense, acute pain is in most cases a secondary result of the drug's primary analgesic and anxiolytic effects. In addition, a large number of anecdotal reports of death occurring shortly after the administration of a high-dose opioid (manifest, obviously, by a cessation of respiration) would be expected even if opioids themselves *never* played a causal role. This is a simple statistical phenomenon. It is not uncommon for patients to receive escalating doses of opioids in the final hours of the dying process, often in bolus dosing and often at increasingly short intervals, to help control terminal dyspnea, pain, or agitation. If a bolus is given hourly during this period, then even if death occurs at a random moment unrelated to the bolus, there is a 10% chance that death will transpire within 6 minutes of the bolus. It is therefore unsurprising that not only many clinicians but also family members have had experiences that suggest to them that the opioid was a direct precipitant of death; it would be far more surprising if this were *not* the case.

Given the widespread belief that administration of opioids in the terminal setting may hasten death, there is a surprising dearth—indeed, a virtual absence—of convincing data that this is a real phenomenon, with the exception of rapid dose escalation in previously opioid-naive patients. Experienced palliative care clinicians are generally adamant that, as long as escalations in opioids are carefully titrated on the basis of appropriate symptoms and signs (usually of pain or dyspnea), concerns that death will thereby be hastened are simply unfounded. Twycross argues that "the use of morphine in the relief of cancer pain carries no greater risk than the use of aspirin *when used correctly*," [italics in the original] and, far from being the cause of death, "the correct use of morphine is more likely to prolong a patient's life . . . because he is more rested and pain-free."[31] Portenoy and Coyle report that "the development of new respiratory symptoms is virtually never a primary drug effect in patients who have been receiving stable doses or who are undergoing dose increases following substantial prior opioid intake."[32] Foley adds that "respiratory depression is not a significant limiting factor in the management of patients with pain because with repeated doses, tolerance develops to this effect."[33]

Nonetheless, even though it is far less commonly a real clinical issue than is generally perceived, the possibility in a specific case that opioid administration may directly hasten death cannot be completely excluded, particularly for a patient who has had limited previous exposure to opioids. Some clinicians (and also some family members) will therefore at least occasionally confront the difficult clinical and ethical challenge of trying simultaneously to fulfill their duty to relieve suffering and their obligation not to knowingly cause a patient's death. The most widely used analytic framework for deciding what to do when a proposed action has two foreseeable effects, one good and one bad, and is known as the "doctrine of double effect."

Doctrine of Double Effect

Historically rooted in Roman Catholic theology dating back to Aquinas, the doctrine of double effect states that when an action (such as administering escalating doses of opioids to relieve pain in the terminal setting) has the possibility of both a "good" effect (relief of pain) and a "bad" effect (hastening death), the action is ethically permissible if *all* of the following conditions are met:[34,35]

1. The action itself must be morally good or at least indifferent (i.e., not intrinsically evil).

Administering effective medication to a suffering patient unquestionably qualifies. Most people would agree that killing the patient with a weapon would not.

2. Only the good effect must be intended, even though the bad effect is foreseeable.

The only morally acceptable goal of the clinician is the relief of the patient's symptoms. It is ***not*** *morally acceptable for the clinician to* ***intend****, as a stated or unstated goal of administering the opioid, to shorten the patient's life.*

3. The good effect must not be achieved as a result of the bad effect.

Relieving suffering ***by*** *causing death (as would be the case if the drug in question were a bolus of intravenous potassium) is not acceptable.*

4. The good effect must outweigh the bad effect.

The benefit to the patient of the relief of suffering must be greater than the harm to the patient of a shortened life. When the administered opioid offers the best available likelihood of relieving suffering, and when the length of time by which the patient's life might be shortened is small (minutes, hours, or perhaps a few days), and when that time would add little or no value to the patient's life (e.g., if the patient is permanently incapable of meaningful interaction), this condition is clearly met. In different circumstances (e.g., administering the drug risks greatly shortening a patient's life that has clear ongoing meaning), an opposite conclusion might be reached.

Both the conceptual framework and the practical application of the doctrine of double effect have been criticized in recent years.[28,36,37] The second condition of the doctrine has been attacked as hopelessly subjective, and as providing a "politically correct" public mask for actions by clinicians who in fact do not consider the hastening of death in some terminal care situations a bad effect at all. Quill, for example, urges abandonment of the doctrine, except perhaps in cases where the involved clinician(s) (or patient or family members) would otherwise find himself or herself ethically unable to respond effectively to accelerating terminal pain or dyspnea.[38] Alternative criteria that he proposes, however, would not clearly exclude administering a lethal bolus of potassium as a definitive comfort measure, which leads even those sympathetic to critiques of the doctrine of double effect to conclude that it still has an important role to play in clinical-ethical reasoning.[39] Although a resolution of this debate is beyond the scope of this chapter, it is not even necessarily true that a clear, unanimously supported, and reassuring (to clinicians, patients, and families) ethical framework is really desirable. Any analytic framework or abstract set of principles that makes profound ethical dilemmas seem easy or uncontroversial risks reducing the sensitivity of those involved to the extraordinary seriousness and complexity of some moral choices. And there are few if any moral challenges more profound than the task of finding a course of action that simultaneously: (1) expresses reverence for an individual human's life as something of incalculable value, and (2) ensures that suffering is relieved when the only reliably effective approach risks causing the person's death. Fortunately, when opioids are properly used, situations such as this are rare, and thus in most cases the difficult ethical dilemma simply does not exist.

OTHER OPIOID-RELATED ISSUES IN THE PALLIATIVE CARE CONTEXT

There are several additional important issues related to the use of opioids in the palliative care context. Details of each of these are covered in other chapters in this text, and only major points will be reviewed here.

Routes of Administration

A wide variety of routes of administration are available, including oral, intravenous, subcutaneous, rectal (morphine, oxymorphone, hydromorphone, or methadone suppositories), sublingual (concentrated morphine elixir or hydromorphone), and transdermal and oral transmucosal (fentanyl citrate). Continuous intravenous infusion with the possibility of frequent additional doses of small boluses, generally administered through a patient-controlled (PCA) system, usually provides both the most consistent blood concentrations as well as the most rapid response to breakthrough pain. The continuous infusion facilitates maintenance of the minimum reliably effective blood concentration, minimizing some of the adverse effects (including sedation and confusion) that can accompany the bolus effects of intermittent dosing. During a phase of life in which final interactions with others can be of the utmost importance, minimizing these adverse effects is particularly important.

Continuous intravenous infusion with self-administered breakthrough bolusing however requires an alert patient and continuous intravenous access. The former may not be the case during the terminal phase of illness, and the latter may not be desired by the patient, particularly in the home setting. To achieve a stable level of the minimum reliably effective blood concentration without intravenous access, slow-release preparations are preferred. For breakthrough dosing, the most rapidly acting available preparation and route should be used. If decreased level of consciousness is not a reason for concern from the patient's perspective, it may be possible to achieve analgesia with maximal convenience by giving higher doses at longer intervals.

As new forms of opioid delivery have become available, cost has become an increasing factor. Transdermal preparations of fentanyl citrate, for example, provide stable blood levels in most patients, but at far greater cost than slow-release forms (either oral or rectal) of morphine or oxycodone. Similarly, oral transmucosal fentanyl citrate has been shown to be highly effective for breakthrough pain in alert patients, but again at far greater cost than other alternatives. Often pharmacy colleagues can be helpful not only in creatively shaping an approach that is well-suited to an individual patient's circumstances, but also in choosing the most cost-effective approach if there is more than one clinically suitable alternative.

Undesirable Effects

As discussed in detail elsewhere (See Chapter 60), optimal use of opioids requires careful attention to identifying and treating their undesirable effects, and to preventing their occurrence whenever possible. Since the beneficial effects of the opioid can sometimes be adequately achieved at a lower dose, that should always be considered first. Opioid rotation can also be helpful.[40] Other alternatives include: using localized routes of administration (e.g., spinal) that do not generate such high circulating drug levels; using nonopioid analgesics, either as adjuvants that allow reduction in the opioid dose or as substitutes; continuing the opioid while adding pharmacologic agents that counteract the undesirable effect(s); and nonpharmacologic approaches (See Chapters 58, 60, 62).

Common opioid effects that will be addressed briefly here include constipation, nausea, vomiting, sedation, and delirium. For all of these except constipation, tolerance may develop and patients should be counseled that even if the undesirable effects are significant with initial doses, a trial of at least a few days may be warranted before deciding that an alternative medication should be used or that the dose of the opioid can be reduced. In the meantime, symptoms should be monitored closely and vigorously treated.

Constipation is a predictable effect of chronic opioid use. In the palliative care setting, where patients frequently have markedly reduced levels of physical activity and other serious comorbidities, it is even more significant, and can become a cause of significant abdominal discomfort. A proactive bowel regimen designed to prevent constipation, with daily monitoring of its effectiveness, is a mandatory component of chronic opioid therapy in this setting. Bulk-forming agents should generally be avoided unless the patient is physically active, since an increase in the volume of stool can pose difficulties for the bed-bound patient.

Nausea and vomiting can be treated with a variety of pharmacologic agents, including trials of compazine, haloperidol, metaclopromide, and ondasteron. If tolerance to these adverse effects does not develop, alternative opioids should be tried.[40] It is important to keep in mind, however, that many palliative care patients are suffering from illnesses or taking other medications which may themselves be the cause of the nausea or vomiting, and the opioid may be only partially to blame, or may even be an entirely innocent bystander.

Delirium is a common problem for patients in the terminal setting, with estimated prevalence rates ranging from 25% to 85%.[41–48] Many of these patients are receiving opioids, but even when administration of the opioid is the precipitating factor, the cause is frequently multifactorial,[49] including the contributing factors indicated in Table 47-2.

Delirium can take both agitated and non-agitated forms,[50] with the latter more frequently unrecognized. When the delirious state is clearly distressing to the patient, its evaluation and treatment should have the same urgency as that of uncontrolled pain. In some cases, however, it is unclear whether or not the delirious patient is suffering from his or her loss of mental clarity, and some near-death experiences that many would categorize as delirious are reported by patients as extremely peaceful, reassuring, and pleasant.[41,51] Nonetheless, even when the patient is not clearly suffering the delirious state interferes with his or her ability to have meaningful interactions with loved ones, and it thus warrants close attention.

Because some forms of delirium do not manifest themselves with obvious behavioral abnormalities, it is important to screen all patients at risk, which includes virtually all patients receiving opioids in the terminal phase of illness. The simplest and most commonly used assessment tool is the Mini-Mental State Exam (MMSE).[52] When evidence of delirium is detected, a comprehensive evaluation of potentially contributing factors is warranted, with efforts to treat the underlying cause(s) whenever the benefits of doing so would outweigh the burdens from the patient's perspective. Although delirium in the terminal care setting may not be reversible in the majority of cases, some authors estimate that up to 33% of cases are.[41,44,46,53,54]

Changing the opioid can be useful.[53] In addition, a variety of pharmacologic agents can be used to treat delirium, and nonpharmacologic approaches can also be useful.[41,55] Haloperidol has generally been considered the drug of choice, and has been shown superior to lorazepam and chlorpromazine in a double-blind, controlled study of the treatment of delirium in hospitalized patients with AIDS.[56] In one small series, all four patients who developed delirium while taking an opioid improved after being switched to an alternative opioid supplemented by haloperidol.[57] An alterna-

TABLE 47-2 **Risk Factors for Delirium in Terminal Illness**

Risk Factors
Impending death
Advanced age
Severity of illness
Limitations on physical mobility
Social isolation
Reduced sensory acuity (vision, hearing)
Underlying neurologic degeneration or injury
Seizures
Brain tumors, abscesses, hemorrhages
Fever or hypothermia
Hypoxia
Severe anemia
Infection
Dehydration
Metabolic imbalances
Low serum albumin
Polypharmacy
Drug withdrawal (e.g., benzodiazepines, alcohol, opiates)
Medications
Opiates (especially meperidine and anileridine)
Anticholinergic agents (e.g., antihistamines)
Corticosteroids
Antiemetics
Psychostimulants
Sedative-hypnotics
Drugs of abuse (including alcohol)

Adapted from Schuster JL. Delirium, confusion, and agitation at the end of life. J Palliat Med 1998;1:177.

tive agent that may be considered is methotrimeprazine.[58] In some cases of agitated delirium, only sedation is effective.[59–62] If benzodiazepines are used for this purpose, close monitoring for a paradoxical increase in agitation (attributed to the disinhibiting effects of benzodiazepines) is warranted.[41]

Sedation is an effect of opioids that can be either desirable or undesirable in the palliative care setting. If the latter, and if dose reduction is not possible without a return of unacceptable symptoms, a psychostimulant such as methylphenidate, caffeine, or amphetamine should be tried unless there is a specific contradindication.[63–65] Modafinil, a relatively new agent, may prove useful for this purpose in the future,[66] since it may be useful ameliorating the sedation of other sedating medications.

Finally, if other efforts to address undesirable side effects have been unsuccessful, careful titration of an extremely low dose of an opioid antagonist (e.g., naloxone via continuous intravenous administration, or repeated parenteral boluses of nalmefene, essentially a long-acting form of naloxone) may be a viable option. There is preliminary evidence to suggest that opioid antagonists, in extremely low doses, may exhibit the potential to increase analgesia, diminish side effects, and diminish tolerance.[67] The use of larger, conventional bolus doses of an opioid antagonist to attempt to reverse opioid side effects is usually ill-advised in the palliative care setting, because of the substantial risk of precipitating recurrent pain or even a withdrawal syndrome.[27,68,69]

OPIOIDS AND RENAL INSUFFICIENCY

In the terminal phase of end of life care, end-organ insufficiency is not uncommon. In renal failure, the opioid of choice is hydromorphone. Hydromorphone is mainly metabolized to hydromorphone-3-glucuronide, which is a reasonable opioid metabolite relative to others, although it may contribute to hyperexcitability in large amounts.[70] Commercial morphine preparations may contain bisulfite (which in large doses may contribute to seizures) or chlorobutanol (which may contribute to somnolence).[71] Morphine is metabolized to morphine-3-glucuronide (M3G) and morphine-6-glucuronide (M6G). M3G is inactive at opioid receptors and M3G and/or normorphine may contibute to hyperexcitability with accumulation of large amounts.[72,73] It is possible that hyperexcitability secondary to high-dose opioids (especially in renal failure) may be mediated via spinal antiglycinergic effects and therefore not responsive to and perhaps even worsened by naloxone administration.[74] M6G is twice as potent as morphine as an analgesic and accumulates in renal dysfunction.[27,75] It may be responsible for the increased and prolonged effects of morphine in renal failure, since the elimination of morphine itself is unimpaired.[76] In clinical practice, an actively dying patient who has been receiving morphine and has now become oliguric or anuric may need little or no additional morphine to maintain adequate analgesia. Because opioid needs in the terminal phase in some patients increase markedly, however, close individual observation and titration of dosing is required.

ADDITIONAL SPECIAL ISSUES IN THE TERMINAL PHASE

The management of other symptoms in the palliative care setting is beyond the scope of this text, and is well covered in other sources.[77,78] A few remaining issues are covered in this section.

Identification and Treatment of the Underlying Etiology of Pain

A cardinal principle of pain management is that an accurate delineation of the pathophysiology of a particular pain syndrome is crucial to the formulation of an optimal plan of management. Although this is more often than not true in the palliative care setting as well, there are clear exceptions, especially in the latter phases of illness. The burdens of diagnostic assessments, including the amount of time spent undergoing them when life expectancy may be measured in days or even hours, may outweigh the sometimes small incremental benefits of more precise pathophysiologic understanding and resulting targeting of analgesic therapies. As always, however, the balancing of burdens and benefits, from the patient's perspective, of attempting more precise definitions of the etiology of a pain syndrome depends on an assessment of the relative priorities of various goals of care. A patient with advanced pancreatic cancer and intractable abdominal or back pain, for whom continued mental clarity or longer life is no longer important, may be appropriately managed simply by increasing opioid dosages to whatever level is needed to ensure comfort. Optimal management of another patient with exactly the same symptoms and identical underlying pathophysiology, who continues to value additional time and interactions with others, may involve a detailed diagnostic evaluation, including extensive imaging studies, to determine whether anatomically based interventions might achieve adequate analgesia without compromising cognitive function.

Symptom Assessment in Patients with Reduced Levels of Consciousness

Assessing the adequacy of analgesia in a patient with a reduced level of consciousness can be exceedingly difficult. If increased alertness is either not an important goal or has become impossible to attain (at least without unacceptable symptoms), then even ambiguous signs of discomfort should usually be treated. At the same time, a patient who is actively dying may groan or grunt in ways that cause clinical staff, and especially family members, to have concern that he or she is in pain. Although it is not possible to know with certainty what an incommunicative patient is experiencing, some clues may be useful. Signs of possible discomfort that are accompanied by increases in respiratory rate or heart rate should be taken more seriously. If physical stimulation of the patient elicits signs of discomfort, either during bathing or by deliberate, gentle administration of a noxious stimulus and increased analgesia may be warranted. Tachypnea by itself may not be a sign of discomfort, especially if it occurs in the setting of metabolic acidosis with respiratory compensation, because even conscious patients in those situations infrequently report a sense of dyspnea. Nonetheless, prolonged respiratory rates over 20/minute can be uncomfortable because of muscle fatigue, and it is reasonable even in the absence of other evidence of discomfort to adjust opioid dosing with a target respiratory rate of 15 to 20/minute.

Nutrition and Hydration

Family members and clinicians often experience considerable anguish about providing adequate nutrition and hydration in the terminal phase of illness, both for clinical and ethical reasons.[79-84] This issue is often miscast as a choice about whether to withhold food or fluids from the patient, which raises concerns about whether the patient is being "starved to death." As in all other clinical decisions, the fundamental question regarding various alternative methods of providing nutrition or hydration is whether the benefits outweigh the burdens from the patient's perspective. Family members should be counseled to let the patient's own expression of interest be their primary guide. If a dying patient shows interest in either food or fluids, they should *never* be withheld unless providing them clearly causes greater suffering than satisfaction to the patient, as can be true in patients for whom oral feeding reproducibly causes significant discomfort because of dysphagia, aspiration, or postprandial abdominal pain. In most cases, however, such patients either do not show an active interest in food or are satisfied with very small amounts of specific foods (such as sweet custards or ice cream) that are reasonably well tolerated. The *forced* administration of nutrients, either parenterally or through a nasogastric or gastrostomy tube, has little or no benefit to most patients in the last days or weeks of life, and the placement or continuation of the required intravenous line or enteral feeding tube can be burdensome. When an enteral feeding tube is used during the terminal phase of illness, it is actually often more useful as a mechanism for administering medications than calories.

Concerns about continuing adequate hydration are often even more seriously misplaced. Relative dehydration can be beneficial during the terminal phase for several reasons. First, with decreased urine output the problem of urinary incontinence, or of discomfort or difficulty in trying to use a bedpan or commode, is reduced. Decreased gastrointestinal secretions may lead to reduced nausea and vomiting, particularly when obstruction is present. More speculatively, pain may be improved by a reduction in tumor edema.

Perhaps most importantly, reduction in oropharyngeal and pulmonary secretions may lead to reduced airway congestion and diminished pooling of secretions the patient is too weak to clear. In one study of 200 patients during the last 48 hours of life, the most common symptom was "noisy and moist breathing," occurring in 56% of patients.[85] Even if this is not a source of discomfort to the patient, the "death rattle" that is familiar to clinicians can be extremely disturbing to family members. In addition to avoiding overhydration (or even consciously aiming at relative dehydration), gentle suctioning may occasionally be needed to remove secretions that have already pooled, and anticholinergic agents such as hyoscine hydrobromide (scopolamine) or atropine are often helpful in reducing additional secretion production.

Terminal Sedation

The vast majority of patients can be helped to die peacefully with carefully targeted symptom management. Nonetheless, a small percentage of patients may continue to suffer (e.g., from pain, agitated delirium, or multifocal myoclonus) in ways that are refractory to all symptom- or pathophysiology-specific modalities. In these cases, the only available mechanism to achieve symptom relief may be complete sedation. This may raise ethical concerns that are analogous to those raised in regard to the possibility that opioid administration may hasten death (See foregoing section, Opioids, Respiratory Suppression, and Hastening Death). While concerns that opioids may contribute to hastening death are often unfounded, there is little question that complete sedation of patients who will not subsequently receive adequate hydration to sustain life can play a causal role in death. Nonetheless, there is a growing clinical, ethical, and legal consensus that when other alternatives are ineffective, terminal sedation is an appropriate therapeutic modality.[86–94] This subject is addressed in more detail in Chapter 86 of this text.

Caring for Families

Although most of this chapter has focused on the needs of patients, the definitions of palliative care with which this chapter began emphasize the needs and concerns of family members as well. In part this is because family members are often centrally involved in providing important aspects of care to the patient, and providing these caregivers with adequate education, counseling, and other support can be crucial to ensuring that their care is effective. In addition, however, the impact of terminal care extends far beyond the death of the patient, through the memories and adaptations of bereaved loved ones. Family members often remember vividly the last days of their loved one's life, especially whether he or she seemed comfortable. These family perceptions of the patient's dying process can profoundly influence not only their own bereavement course, but also how they approach their own deaths. Simple steps on the part of involved clinicians, both during the terminal phase and after the patient's death, can make a significant difference to involved family.[95-99] The effort and skills (or shortcomings therein) that clinicians bring to the care of dying patients and their families thus not only have frequently profound benefits for patients themselves, but also are likely to have positive (or negative) repercussions throughout the lives of surviving loved ones.

REFERENCES

1. Doyle D, Hanks G, MacDonald N. Introduction. In: *Oxford Textbook of Palliative Medicine.* 2nd ed. Oxford, England: Oxford University Press, 1998:3–8.
2. *Cancer Pain Relief and Palliative Care.* Technical Report Series 804. Geneva, Switzerland: World Health Organization, 1990.
3. Task Force on Palliative Care, Last Acts Campaign, Robert Wood Johnson Foundation. Precepts of Palliative Care. *J Palliat Med* 1998;1(2): 109.
4. SUPPORT Principal Investigators. A controlled trial to improve care for seriously ill hospitalized patients: the Study to Understand Prognoses and Preferences for Outcomes and Risks of Treatments (SUPPORT). *JAMA* 1995;274:1591.
5. Desbiens NA, Mueller-Rizner N, Connors AF Jr, et al. The symptom burden of seriously ill hospitalized patients. *J Pain Symptom Manage* 1999;17:248.
6. Lynn J, Teno JM, Phillips RS, et al. For the SUPPORT Investigators. Perceptions by family members of the dying experience of older and seriously ill patients. *Ann Intern Med* 1997;126:97.
7. Institute of Medicine, Committee on Care at the End of Life. *Approaching Death: Improving Care at the End of Life.* Washington, DC: National Academy Press, 1997.
8. Meier DE, Morrison RS, Cassel CK. Improving palliative care. *Ann Intern Med* 1997;127:225.
9. Lynn J, Schuster JL, Kabcenell A. *Improving Care for the End of Life: A Sourcebook for Health Care Managers and Clinicians.* New York, NY: Oxford University Press, 2000.
10. Lynn J, Schall MW, Milne C, et al. Quality improvements in end-of-life care: insights from two collaboratives. *Joint Comm J Qual Improve* 2000;26:254.
11. Cassel CK, Foley KM. *Principles for Care of Patients at the End of Life: An Emerging Consensus among the Specialties of Medicine.* New York, NY: Milbank Memorial Fund, 1999.
12. *The EPEC Project: Educating Physicians on End-of-Life Care.* Chicago, Ill: American Medical Association, 2000.
13. Mahoney JJ. The Medicare hospice benefit—15 years of success. *J Palliat Med* 1998;1(2):139.
14. Walsh D. The Medicare hospice benefit: a critique from palliative medicine. *J Palliat Med* 1998;1(2):147.
15. Byock I. *Dying Well: The Prospect for Growth at the End of Life.* Riverhead Books, New York 1997.
16. Quill TE. *A Midwife through the Dying Process: Stories of Healing and Hard choices at the End of Life.* Baltimore, Md: Johns Hopkins University Press, 1996.
17. Kidder D. Hospice: does it still save Medicare money? *J Palliat Med* 1998;1(2):151.
18. Emanuel EJ. Cost savings at the end of life. What do the data show? *JAMA* 1996;275:1907.
19. Covinsky K, Goldman L, Cook E, et al. The impact of serious illness on patients' families. *JAMA* 1994;272;1839.
20. Forrow L, Arnold RM. Preventive ethics. *J Clin Ethics* 1993;4:287.
21. Forrow L. The green eggs and ham phenomena. *Hastings Cent Rep* 1994;24(6 suppl):S29.
22. Fishman B. The treatment of suffering in patients with cancer pain: cognitive-behavioral approaches. In: Foley K, Bonica J, eds. *Advances in Pain Research and Therapy.* New York, NY: Raven Press: New York, 1990:310–316.
23. Portenoy RK. Pain and quality of life. *Oncology* 1990:4:172.
24. Cassell E. *The Nature of Suffering and the Goals of Medicine.* Oxford University Press, New York, NY 1991.
25. Frankl, VE. *Man's Search for Meaning.* New York, NY: Washington Square Press, 1984.
26. Foley KM. Clinical tolerance to opioids. In: Basbaum AL, Besson JM, eds. *Towards a New Pharmacotherapy of Pain.* Chichester, England: John Wiley & Sons, Inc, 1991:181–204.
27. Foley KM. Pain and symptom control. In: Curtis JR, Rubenfeld GD, eds. *Managing Death in the Intensive Care Unit.* Oxford University Press, New York, NY 2001:103–125.
28. Fohr SA. The double effect of pain medication: separating myth from reality. *J Palliat Med* 1998;1:315.
29. Walsh TD. Opiates and respiratory function in advanced cancer. *Recent Results Cancer Res* 1984;89:115.
30. Grond S, Zech D, Schug SA, et al. Validation of the World Health Association guidelines for cancer pain relief during the last days and hours of life. *J Pain Symptom Manage* 1991;6:411.
31. Twycross RG. Ethical and clinical aspects of pain treatment in cancer patients. *Acta Anaesthesiol Scand Suppl* 1982;74:83.
32. Portenoy RK, Coyle N. Controversies in the long-term management of analgesic therapy in patients with advanced cancer. *J Pain Symptom Manage* 1990;5:307.
33. Foley KM. The relationship of pain and symptom management to patient requests for physician-assisted suicide. *J Pain Symptom Manage* 1991;6:289.
34. Garcia JLA. Double effect. In: Reich WT, ed. *Encyclopedia of Bioethics.* New York, NY: Simon & Schuster, 1995:636–641.
35. Beauchamp TL, Childress JF. *Principles of Biomedical Ethics.* 3rd ed. New York, NY: Oxford University Press, 1989:128.
36. Sulmasy DP. The use and abuse of the principle of double effect. *Clin Pulm Med* 1996;3:86.
37. Quill TE, Dresser R, Brock DW. The rule of double effect. A critique of its role in end-of-life decision-making. *N Engl J Med* 1997;337: 1768.
38. Quill TE. Principle of double effect and end-of-life pain management: Additional myths and a limited role. *J Palliat Med* 1998;1:333.
39. Brody H. Double effect: does it have a proper use in palliative care? *J Palliat Med* 1998;1:329.
40. Ashby MA, Martin P, Jackson KA. Opioid substitution to reduce adverse effects in cancer pain management. *Med J Aust* 1999;170:68.
41. Shuster JL. Delirium, confusion, and agitation at the end of life. *J Palliat Med* 1998;1:177.
42. Massie MJ, Holland J, Glass E. Delirium in terminally ill cancer patients. *Am J Psychiatry* 1983;140:1048.
43. Bruera E, Chadwick S, Weinlick A, MacDonald N. Delirium and severe sedation in patients with terminal cancer. *Cancer Treatment Rep* 1987;71:787.
44. Leipzig RM, Goodman H, Gray G, et al. Reversible, narcotic-associated mental status impairment in patients with metastatic cancer. *Pharmacology* 1987;35:47.
45. Fainsinger R, MacEachern T, Hanson J, et al. Symptom control during the last week of life on a palliative care unit. *J Palliat Care* 1991;7:5.
46. Bruera E, Miller L, McCallion J, et al. Cognitive failure in patients with terminal cancer: a prospective study. *J Pain Symptom Manage* 1992;7:192.
47. Minogawa H, Uchitomi Y, Yamawaki S, Ishitani K. Psychiatric morbidity in terminally ill cancer patients: a prospective study. *Cancer* 1996;78:1131.
48. Conill C, Verger E, Henriquez I, et al. Symptom prevalence in the last week of life. *J Pain Symptom Manage* 1997;14:328.

49. Caraceni A, Martini C, De Conno F, Ventafridda V. Organic brain syndromes and opioid administration for cancer pain. *J Pain Symptom Manage* 1994;9:527.
50. Lipowski ZJ. *Delirium: Acute Confusional States*. New York, NY: Oxford University Press,1990.
51. Callanan M, Kelley P. *Final Gifts: Understanding the Special Awareness, Needs, and Communications of the Dying*. New York, NY: Bantam Books, 1992.
52. Folstein MF, Folstein SE, McHugh PR. Mini-Mental State: a practical method of grading the cognitive state of patients for the clinician. *J Psychiatr Res* 1975;12:189.
53. Maddocks I, Somogyi A, Abbott F, et al. Attenuation of morphine-induced delirium in palliative care by substitution with infusion of oxycodone. *J Pain Symptom Manage* 1996:182.
54. de Stoutz ND, Tapper M, Fainsinger RL. Reversible delirium in terminally ill patients. *J Pain Symptom Manage* 1995;10:249.
55. Breitbart W, Chochinov HM, Passik S. Psychiatric aspects of palliative care. In: Doyle D, Hanks GWC, MacDonald N, eds. *Oxford Textbook of Palliative Medicine*. 2nd ed. Oxford, England: Oxford University Press, 1998:933–954.
56. Breitbart W, Marotta R, Platt MM, et al. A double-blind trial of haloperidol, chlorpromazine, and lorazepam in the treatment of delirium in hospitalized AIDS patients. *Am J Psychiatry* 1996;153:231.
57. Bruera E, Schoeller T, Montejo G. Organic hallucinosis in patients receiving high doses of opiates for cancer pain. *Pain* 1992;48:397.
58. Foley KM. Management of cancer pain. In: DeVita VT, Hellman S, Rosenberg SA, eds. *Cancer Principles and Practice of Oncology*. 3rd ed. Philadelphia, Pa: JB Lippincott, 1997:2807–2841.
59. Mercadante S, De Conno F, Ripamonti C. Propofol in terminal care. *J Pain Symptom Manage* 1995;10:639.
60. Moyle J. The use of propofol in palliative medicine. *J Pain Symptom Manage* 1995;10:643.
61. Truog RD, Berde CB, Mitchell C, Grier HE. Barbituates in the care of the terminally ill. *N Engl J Med* 1992;327:1678.
62. Cherny NI, Portenoy RK. Sedation in the management of refractory symptoms: guidelines for evaluation and treatment. *J Palliat Care* 1994;10:31.
63. Bruera E, Chadwick S, Brenneis C, Hanson J. Methylphenidate associated with narcotics in the treatment of cancer pain. *Cancer Treat Rep* 1987;71:67.
64. Forrest WH, Brown BW, Brown CR, et al. Dextroamphetamine with morphine for treatment of postoperative pain. *N Engl J Med* 1977; 296:712.
65. Laska EM, Sunshine A, Mueller F, et al. Caffeine as an analgesic adjuvant. *JAMA* 1984;251:1711.
66. Teitelman E. Off-label uses of modafinil. *Am J Psychiatry* 2001;158: 1341.
67. Crain SM, Shen KF. Antagonists of excitatory opioid receptor functions enhance morphine's analgesic potency and attenuate opioid tolerance/dependence liability. *Pain* 2000;84:121.
68. Fins JJ. Acts of omission and commission in pain management: the ethics of naloxone use. *J Pain Symptom Manage* 1991;17:1210.
69. Manfredi PL, Ribeiro S, Chandler SW, Payne R. Inappropriate use of naloxone in cancer patients with pain. *J Pain Symptom Manage* 1996; 11:131.
70. Babul N, Darke AC. Putative role of hydromorphone metabolites in myoclonus. *Pain* 1992;51:260.
71. Gregory RE, Grossman S, Sheidler VR. Grand mal seizures associated with high dose intravenous morphine infusions: incidence and possible etiology. *Pain* 1992;51:255.
72. Mcquay HF, Carrol D, Foura CC, et al. Oral morphine in cancer pain: influences on morphine and metabolite concentration. *Clin Pharm Ther* 1990;48:236.
73. Glare PA, Walsh TD, Pippenger CE. Normorphine, a neurotoxic metabolite. *Lancet* 1990;335:725.
74. Hagen N, Swanson R. Strychnine-like multifocal myoclonus and seizures in extremely high-dose opioid administration: treatment strategies. *J Pain Symptom Manage* 1997;14:51.
75. Tiseo P, Thaler HT, Lapin J, et al. Morphine-6-glucurinide concentrations and opioid related side effects—a survey in cancer patients. *Pain* 1995;61:47.
76. Woolner DF, Winter D, Frendin TJ, et al. Renal failure does not impair the metabolism of morphine. *Br J Clin Pharmacol* 1986;22:55.
77. Doyle D, Hanks GWC, MacDonald N. *Oxford Textbook of Palliative Medicine*. 2nd ed. Oxford, England: Oxford University Press, 1998.
78. Wrede-Seaman, L. *Symptom Management Algorithms. A Handbook for Palliative Care*. 2nd ed. Yakima, Wash: Intellicard, 1999 (www.intelli-card.com).
79. Twycross R, Lichter I. The terminal phases. In: Doyle D, Hanks GWC, MacDonald N, eds. *Oxford Textbook of Palliative Medicine*. 2nd ed. Oxford, England: Oxford University Press, 1998:977–992.
80. Winter SM. Terminal nutrition: framing the debate for the withdrawal of nutritional support in terminally ill patients. *Am J Med* 2000;109:723.
81. Lynn J,ed. *By No Extraordinary Means: The Choice to Forgo Life-Sustaining Food and Water*. Bloomington: Indiana University Press, 1989.
82. Dunphy K, Finlay I, Rathbone G, et al. Rehydration in palliative and terminal care: if not—why not? *Palliat Med* 1995;9:221.
83. Micetich KC, Steinecker PH, Thomasma DC. Are intravenous fluids morally required for a dying patient? *Arch Intern Med* 1983;143:975.
84. Fainsinger R, Bruera E. The management of dehydration in terminally ill patients. *J Palliat Care* 1994;10:55.
85. Lichter I, Hunt E. The last 48 hours of life. *J Palliat Care* 1990;6:7.
86. Krakauer EL, Penson RT, et al. Sedation for intractable distress of a dying patient: acute palliative care and the principle of double effect. *Oncologist* 2000;5:53.
87. Quill TE, Byock IR. Responding to intractable terminal suffering: the role of terminal sedation and voluntary refusal of food and fluids. *Ann Intern Med* 2000;132:408.
88. Chater S, Viola R, Paterson J, Jarvis V. Sedation for intractable distress in the dying—a survey of experts. *Palliat Med* 1998;12:255.
89. Hallenbeck JL. Terminal sedation: ethical implications in different situations. *J Palliat Med* 2000;3:313.
90. Mount B. Morphine drips, terminal sedation, and slow euthanasia: definitions and facts, not anecdotes. *J Palliat Care* 1996;12:31.
91. Rousseau P. The ethical validity and clinical experience of palliative sedation. *Mayo Clin Proc* 2000;75:1064.
92. Fainsinger RL, Landman W, Hoskings M, Bruera E. Sedation for uncontrolled symptoms in a South African hospice. *J Pain Symptom Manage* 1998;16:145.
93. Ethics Committee of the National Hospice and Palliative Care Organization. *NHPCO Policy Statement on Total Sedation*, NHPCO Alexandria, VA 2000.
94. Burt RA. The Supreme Court speaks: not assisted suicide but a constitutional right to palliative care. *N Engl J Med* 1997;337:1234.
95. Tilden V, Tolle S, Garland M, Nelson CA. Decisions about life-sustaining treatment. Impact of physicians' behaviors on the family. *Arch Intern Med* 1995;155:633.
96. Schulz R, Beach SR, Lind B, et al. Involvement in caregiving and adjustment to death of a spouse: findings from the caregiver health effects study. *JAMA* 2001;285:3123.
97. Billings JA, Kolton E. Family satisfaction and bereavement care following death in the hospital. *J Palliat Med* 1999;2:33.
98. Casarett D, Kutner JS, Abrahm J, et al. Life after death: a practical approach to grief and bereavement. *Ann Intern Med* 2001;134:208.
99. Prigerson HG, Jacobs SC. Caring for bereaved patients. *JAMA* 2001; 286:1369.

CHAPTER 48 PAIN IN HIV AND AIDS

Matthew Lefkowitz

IMPORTANCE OF PAIN IN HIV DISEASE

In the era of highly active antiretroviral therapy, HIV-infected patients live longer and healthier lives, which makes relief of pain associated with the complications of HIV infection an important factor in improving the quality of life. Relief of acute pain is important not only because pain relief affects the quality of life of caregivers as well as the individual suffering pain, but also because unrelieved pain can become chronic pain, which is much more difficult to manage because a vicious cycle that sustains pain develops.[1,2]

Acute pain may be classified in various ways, but is usually more or less directly related to some pathologic condition, although the intensity of the pain experienced may be out of proportion to the physiologic cause. When unrelieved acute pain has become chronic pain (often called "benign" when it is not associated with malignancy), special management considerations not found in acute pain become important.

A variety of studies have found the prevalence of pain in patients with HIV disease to vary from 40% to 60%, with even higher rates of pain found in inpatient settings and in patients near the end of life.[3–5] Although different risk groups (eg, men who have sex with men, intravenous drug users, women) have different degrees of unrelieved pain, in general pain in HIV-infected individuals is underdiagnosed and undertreated. In one survey, only 7.3% of 110 patients with AIDS who reported "severe" pain received a strong opioid according to treatment guidelines, whereas 11.8% received no analgesic and 39.1% received a nonsteroidal anti-inflammatory drug.[6]

A French study[7] found that doctors underestimated pain severity in more than half (52%) of AIDS patients and that only a fifth (21%) received a strong opioid, whereas 57% received no analgesic treatment. This is somewhat higher than a recent estimate based on a meta-analysis of 15 studies that found a median point prevalence of chronic pain of 15% (range 2% to 40%) in adults.[8]

Many studies show that the intensity of pain in HIV disease is comparable to that experienced by cancer patients. However, a patient with AIDS often experiences several painful syndromes simultaneously. Table 48-1 lists some causes of HIV-related pain.

Painful syndromes may be nociceptive, neuropathic, or idiopathic. Nociceptive (somatic or visceral) pain, which is mediated by pain receptors, accounts for the majority of painful syndromes reported by ambulatory AIDS patients. Nociceptive pain is usually effectively relieved by conventional analgesics. Although non-opioid analgesics may be enough in many situations, a strong opioid may be necessary to effectively manage some severe nociceptive pain syndromes. Neuropathic pain, which is due to damage within the nervous system, may occur in a quarter of patients with HIV disease, who may also be experiencing nociceptive pain. Often neuropathic pain is poorly localized and described as a sensation other than pain, for example, burning, shooting, tingling, itching, or crawling. Adjuvant analgesics, often with conventional analgesics given concurrently, are the treatment of choice for neuropathic pain.

BARRIERS TO EFFECTIVE PAIN RELIEF

Studies have shown that pain is dramatically undertreated in patients with HIV disease and that opioids in particular are underprescribed.[9]

In a recently published study of 199 ambulatory AIDS patients in New York City, pain management was inadequate in 83% (165/199).[9] This sample included a high proportion of women (only 36% were men), of African-Americans and Hispanics (only 27% were white), and drug users (only 15% were homosexuals).[9] Table 48-2 lists the most frequently patient-endorsed barriers to pain management, which focus on potential addiction and, to a lesser extent, on side effects. Effective pain management should address such patient-related barriers as well as those related to clinicians and the health care system.[9]

PRINCIPLES OF PAIN RELIEF

The most well-established principles for pain relief have been developed for the management of pain in patients with cancer[10–12] and, more recently, patients with chronic pain.[13] However, patients with HIV disease are typically younger and less psychologically prepared for the consequences of devastating illness and chronic pain than cancer patients and older patients with chronic pain due to arthritis. In addition, patients with HIV disease are often taking a variety of medications that are metabolized by the cytochrome P450 system and are likely to cause drug interactions. In patients with HIV disease, diarrhea, either associated with various opportunistic infections or with antiretroviral drug therapy, can complicate use of sustained-release oral analgesic formulations. Finally, concomitant drug abuse is common in patients with HIV disease, which presents a significant barrier to effective pain relief. The general principles of pain management are largely derived from experience with pain associated with cancer (Table 48-3).

The WHO three-step analgesic ladder suggests initial treatment with a non-opioid, typically acetaminophen, aspirin, or a nonsteroidal anti-inflammatory drug (NSAID) for mild to moderate pain.[10] These agents are all associated with a "ceiling effect," that is, higher doses do not increase analgesia but do increase toxicity, which is increasingly recognized as quite significant, especially to the gastrointestinal (GI) system.

If the pain persists or increases, the second step is a weak opioid, often in the form of a combination product that includes a weak opioid and acetaminophen, aspirin, or ibuprofen. The pain relief available from weak opioids is limited, especially if they are

TABLE 48-1 **Selected Causes of Pain in Persons with HIV Disease**

Related to HIV/AIDS
- HIV neuropathy or myelopathy
- Opportunistic infections
- Kaposi's sarcoma

Related to medications
- Antiretrovirals (eg, nucleoside-associated neuropathy)
- Procedures (biopsies, bronchoscopy)
- Cancer treatment with radiation, surgery, or chemotherapy

Unrelated to HIV or its treatment (idiopathic)
- Diabetic neuropathy
- Headache
- Intervertebral disc disease

combined with an agent that has a ceiling effect. Because hepatic disease is common in patients with HIV disease, acetaminophen-containing formulations should be avoided because of potential hepatotoxicity.

For moderate to severe pain or for mild to moderate pain that is uncontrolled by a step 1 or step 2 agent, a strong opioid is indicated. For chronic pain, patients should receive adequate doses of a long-acting agent around the clock with a short-acting agent available for breakthrough pain as needed. Long-acting opioid treatments currently available are oral formulations of morphine and oxycodone and transdermal fentanyl. The short-acting agent for breakthrough pain does not have to be the same chemical entity as the long-acting agent. Often, the short-acting opioid is used before instituting treatment with a long-acting opioid. The amount of the rescue medication is used to adjust the dose of the long-acting medication.

The general strategies to control pain in patients with HIV disease are similar to those for cancer pain but also include considerations specific to HIV disease such as the observation that patients often experience several painful syndromes simultaneously (Table 48-4 and Table 48-5).

Since self-report is the primary source of information about pain and pain relief, consistent use of one of the validated intensity/severity rating systems (eg, numerical, visual analog, happy/sad faces) is very helpful. Systematically monitor and record information about side effects and quality of life.

TABLE 48-3 **General Principles of Pharmacotherapy for Pain**

- Choose analgesic based on severity and etiology of pain.
- Around-the-clock (ATC) administration of long-acting opioids such as oral sustained-release formulations of either morphine or oxycodone or transdermal fentanyl is preferred for moderate to severe pain that is chronic or persistent.
- Short-acting analgesics are useful for intermittent pain or for breakthrough pain.
- Adjust the dose of long-acting opioid based on use of breakthrough pain medication.
- Use least invasive modalities, but consider potential effects of diarrhea (a common complication in patients with HIV disease) on absorption of oral medications, especially sustained-released formulations.
- Do not equate opioid tolerance and physical dependence (pharmacologic phenomena) with addictions (a psychosocial phenomenon).
- Recognize and treat analgesic side effects aggressively.

NON-OPIOID ANALGESICS

Nonsteroidal anti-inflammatory drugs (NSAIDs) and acetaminophen are effective for a variety of mild to moderate painful syndromes, especially when the pain is due to inflammation. These

TABLE 48-2 **Barriers to Pain Management Endorsed by AIDS Patients**

Barrier	Any Endorsement (%)	High (%)
People get addicted to pain medication easily.	96.4	74.5
There is a real danger of becoming addicted to pain medication.	95.0	78.4
Pain medication is very addictive.	92.4	74.7
It's a good idea to "save" pain medication for later when you might really need it.	85.4	67.3
Nausea from pain medicine is really distressing.	84.8	64.6
Having pain means that the disease is getting worse.	82.8	54.5
Constipation from pain medicine is really upsetting.	82.2	63.5
I do not like having shots.	80.4	65.8
Drowsiness from pain medicine is really a bother.	79.4	58.3
Confusion from pain medicine is really a bother.	78.9	55.3

From Breitbart W, et al. Patient related barriers to pain management. *Pain.* 1998;76:9.

TABLE 48-4 **General Strategies to Control Pain in Patients with HIV/AIDS**

Diagnose and treat the painful syndrome whenever possible.

Record the pain reported by the patient.

Immediately begin to relieve pain with analgesics.
- Individualize therapy.
- Use adequate doses of appropriately potent analgesics.
- Supplement analgesics with adjuvant analgesics and nonpharmacologic approaches as needed

Document pain relief and change treatment as indicated.

Provide analgesic during diagnosis and treatment of the underlying disease process(es).

drugs, alone or in combination with weak opioids, are limited by a ceiling effect. Although there are many different NSAIDs, toxicity, especially GI toxicity, is common to all of them. NSAIDs can also damage renal function. Acetaminophen, particularly, is associated with liver toxicity. These highly protein-bound drugs can interact with other highly protein-bound medications, including HIV protease inhibitors. Masking fever may delay diagnosis of certain opportunistic infections.

OPIOID ANALGESICS

Opioids are effective against many types of pain, especially nociceptive pain. There is no ceiling effect for the pure agonist opioids such as morphine, hydromorphone, and fentanyl. Also, opioid therapy has not been associated with major organ toxicity even in long-term use. Patient response to opioids varies, and some patients require sequential trials of several different opioids before an effective and well-tolerated regimen is identified.[14]

Opioid dose can be increased until pain is relieved or until side effects limit therapy. Constipation, sedation, and nausea are the most common side effects. Opioid side effects are usually manageable. Many practitioners manage these side effects preemptively. The prevalence of diarrhea is high among patients with HIV disease, so constipation is usually not a problem. Antiemetics to control nausea may also cause sedation. Use of caffeine or psychostimulants (dextroamphetamine, methylphenidate, or pemoline) may be helpful. In most cases, pain management with opioids, such as methadone maintenance, is fully compatible with normal function. Instructions to limit driving or other activities is not given unless overt impairment is observed.[15]

Although respiratory depression may occur and can be life-threatening, it is rare in patients who have been receiving long-term opioid therapy, even at high doses. Opioid antagonists (ie, naloxone) should be available for patients initiating opioid therapy.

Weak opioids are often used when stronger opioids are necessary, which results in inadequate pain relief. A patient with moderate to severe pain should receive a strong opioid initially, with the dose increased until effective pain relief is achieved. Dose titration is limited by the customary formulations, combining a weak opioid and aspirin, acetaminophen, or ibuprofen. Codeine is relatively emetogenic and constipating, relative to its analgesic potency. Dihydroxycodone and hydrocodone are stronger than codeine but not as strong as oxycodone. Tramadol, a nonopioid with dual-analgesic action (modest affinity for the opioid μ-receptor and inhibition of uptake of norepinephrine and serotonin) is generally considered equivalent in analgesic power to codeine.[16,17]

Morphine is the prototypical strong opioid and is available in a wide variety of short-acting,immediate-release formulations. Onset of analgesia begins within 30 minutes of oral administration and usually persists for 3 to 4 hours. Maintaining effective levels of morphine with these formulations requires frequent administration, and these formulations are best used to initiate analgesia and to treat breakthrough pain in patients maintained on a long-acting, sustained-release opioid formulation. The usual initial oral dose of morphine for adults and children weighing more than 50 kg (110 lb) is 30 mg every 3 to 4 hours around the clock, which is three times the parenteral dose. Oxycodone, which is 1.5 to 2 times as potent as morphine, should be classed as a strong opioid along with morphine and hydromorphone. The usual initial oral dose of oxycodone is 5 to 10 mg every 3 to 4 hours. Both morphine and oxycodone are available in long-acting formulations.

Hydromorphone is a strong opioid that can be used instead of morphine for patients who do not tolerate morphine or if extremely high doses are needed. The usual initial oral dose of hydromorphone is 7.5 mg every 3 to 4 hours. No sustained-release formulation of hydromorphone is available.

A number of opioid analgesics are not appropriate for chronic pain relief. Meperidine is not suitable for long-term administration because of the accumulation of toxic metabolites associated with central nervous system excitation and seizures. Combination agonist-antagonist opioids such as buprenorphine, butorphanol, and nalbuphine may interfere with the effects of pure agonist opioids and are not recommended for treatment of chronic pain.

The development of long-acting opioids, including transdermal fentanyl, has simplified treatment of acute pain that requires strong opioids for more than a few days and chronic painful syndromes. In addition, the less frequent dosing and flatter and lower peak drug levels are associated with less risk of drug abuse.

Long-Acting Oral Opioids

Long-acting morphine, which is indicated for use for patients who will require repeated administration of a strong opioid for more than a few days, is available in two oral formulations, MS Contin and

TABLE 48-5 **Special Considerations for Using Opioids in HIV/AIDS**

Unique pharmacologic considerations
- Potential drug interactions, especially in patients taking HIV protease inhibitors
- Malabsorption, due to diarrhea or altered stomach acidity
- Skin lesions

Potentially increased sensitivity to drug side effects.

Polypharmacy

Substance use
- Physician reluctance to prescribe opioids to persons with current or past substance use.
- Patient reluctance to use opioids, especially if in recovery.
- Complications relating to patient's concurrent use of recreational drugs.

Oramorph. A long-acting formulation of oxycodone, OxyContin, is now available. These formulations are tablets that must be swallowed whole; tablets must not be broken in half, crushed, or chewed. The usual dosing interval is 12 hours. The orally administered sustained-release morphine results in higher peak levels and lower trough levels than more frequent administration of immediate-release morphine. The release of morphine from these controlled-release tablets is not continuous over the dosing interval.

Patients are typically initially treated with immediate-release morphine and then converted to sustained-release formulations. If opioid-related side effects occur early in the dosing interval, the dose should be reduced. If breakthrough pain occurs near the end of the dosing interval, the dosing interval should be shortened. To avoid acute toxicity from overdosing, the dosing interval should never be longer than every 12 hours.

Transdermal Fentanyl

Fentanyl is a potent opioid analgesic whose pharmacologic properties are particularly suitable to transdermal administration.[18] Fentanyl is short-acting when administered intravenously, but the transdermal system (Duragesic) provides a long duration and overall smoothing of the plasma concentration curve (reduction in height of peaks and depth of troughs). Most patients change patches every 3 days (72 hours) (Fig. 48-1 and Fig. 48-2).

A depot of drug concentrates in the viable epidermis under the transdermal fentanyl patch, and this depot is slowly introduced into the systemic circulation in the subdermal tissue through the cutaneous microcirculation in the dermis (Fig. 48-3).

In patients with fever, not uncommon in patients with HIV disease, fentanyl release may be faster since there is increased cutaneous circulation. Therefore, lower dose patches may need to be applied more frequently. Dosing at 2- or 3-day intervals simplifies the pain-relief regimen, reducing mediation errors and increasing compliance, especially in patients with cognitive impairment.

Because of the slow onset, analgesia using the short-acting opioid prescribed for breakthrough pain should be provided during the first 12 to 24 hours after application of the first transdermal fentanyl patch. The short-acting breakthough medication can be any strong opioid. The maximum level is typically sustained for 48 hours. After a transdermal patch is removed, plasma fentanyl levels decline with a half-life of approximately 17 hours (range 13 to 22 hours).

Transdermal administration, which is convenient in most patients, is particularly desirable in those patients with GI problems such as nausea, vomiting, or diarrhea, where malabsorption of oral medications is likely. Many patients with HIV have periods during which swallowing is difficult because of opportunistic complications of HIV infection. Transdermal fentanyl is particularly useful in such patients, but it is beneficial and effective in all patients with pain. The choice of analgesic and route of administration depends on the pain syndrome, the patient, and the physician's judgment.

The patch must be applied to an area of intact normal skin. Significant dermatolgoic or allergic reactions are rare, but some patients experience erythema at the site of application.

In opioid-naive patients the initial dose is typically 25 μg/hour, supplemented with a short-acting opioid. Based on use of break-

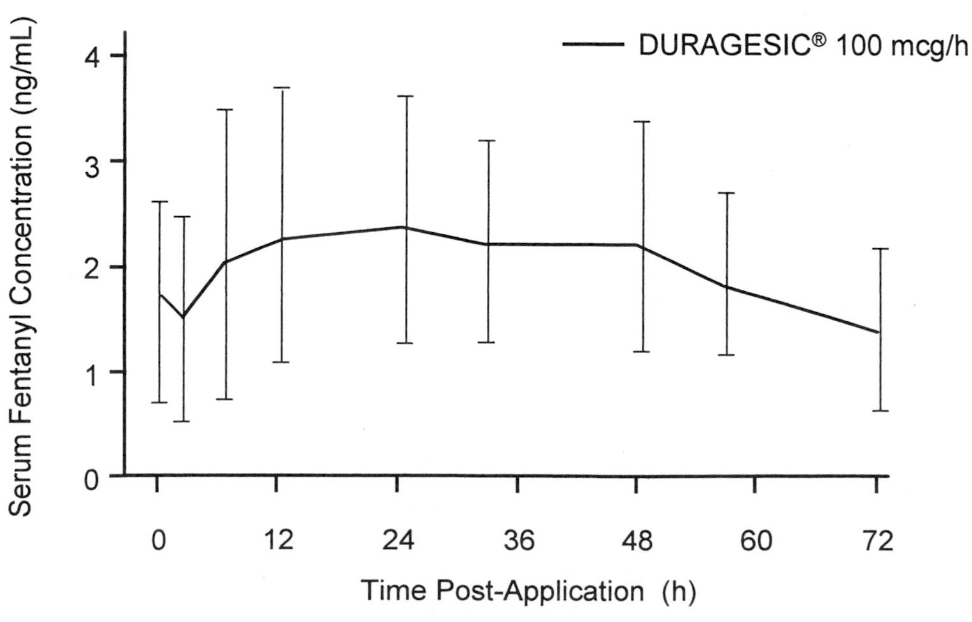

Figure 48-1 Serum fentanyl concentration over 3 days after application of a single 100-μg/hour patch.

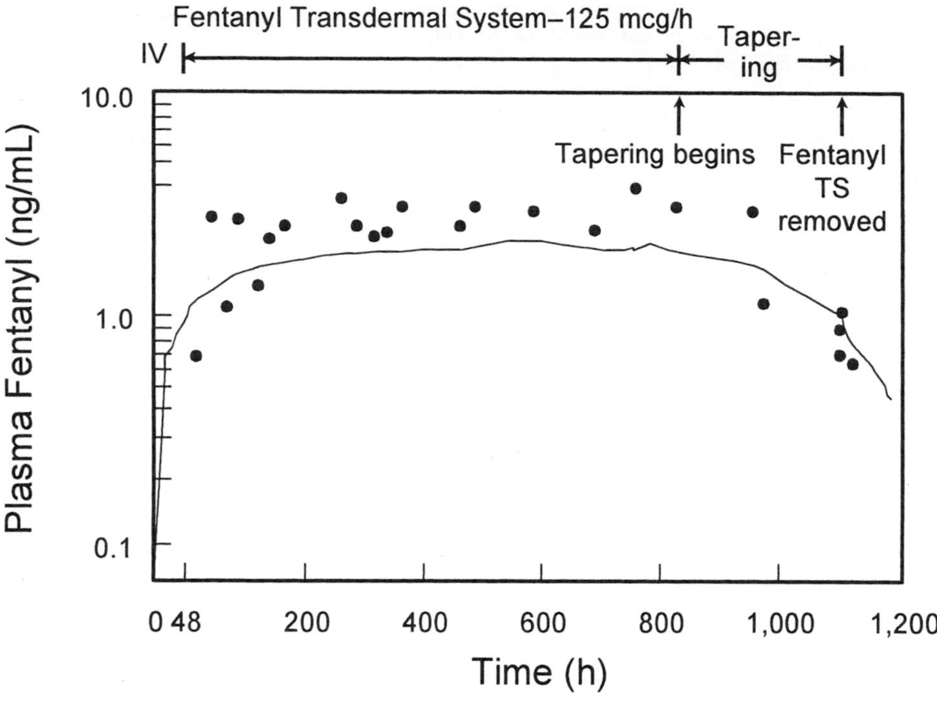

Figure 48-2 Serum fentanyl concentration over 30 days during multiple applications of 125-μg/hour patches followed by tapering. (From Miser AW, et al. Transdermal fentanyl for pain control in patients with cancer. *Pain.* 1989;37:18.)

through medication, the dose and dosing interval can be adjusted over 1 to 2 weeks to achieve consistent pain relief with minimal use of breakthrough medication.

Sustained-release morphine and transdermal fentanyl were compared in a randomized, open-label, crossover study of 202 cancer patients requiring strong opioid analgesia at 38 palliative care centers in the United Kingdom.[21] Patients received one treatment for 15 days, followed immediately by the other treatment. Immediate-release morphine was used freely to titrate patient's pain control at the start of the study, at the crossover, and for breakthrough pain. Pain relief as recorded by patients was comparable; however, of those who felt able to express an opinion, transdermal fentanyl was preferred by 54% compared with 36% who preferred sustained-release morphine tablets, $P = .037$.

Potential for Abuse of Long-Acting Opioids

Although it is possible to abuse almost any psychoactive drug, it is quite uncommon for patients, even those with a history of intravenous drug use, to abuse transdermal fentanyl or other long-acting opioids. The steady blood levels of analgesic provided by these formulations provide effective pain relief but little euphoria, which is associated with the peak levels that occur with frequent dosing of short-acting opioids. Appropriate treatment of moderate to severe pain with opioids, especially long-acting opioids, in my clinical experience rarely results in substance abuse or addiction.

ADJUVANT ANALGESICS

Adjuvant analgesics, that is, agents that are not primarily considered analgesics such as antidepressants and anticonvulsants, may be added to any of the previously described regimens if indicated. The most common complication treated with adjuvant analgesics is peripheral neuropathy, which can arise from a variety of causes (Table 48-6). As a general rule, any medications associated with peripheral neuropathy should be promptly discontinued and alternatives substituted for patients who develop peripheral neuropathy. The incidence of peripheral neuropathy has decreased because, currently, patients are treated typically earlier in the course of the disease with lower doses than in the past. A recent review estimates that approximately 10% of patients receiving stavudine or zalcitabine will discontinue due to peripheral neuropathy with didanosine. The discontinuation rate specifically attributable to peripheral neuropathy is only 1% to 2%.[22]

Progressive polyradiculopathy should be considered when treating patients with CMV infection and they should be treated immediately with anti-CMV drugs.

Neuropathic pain is generally considered to respond relatively poorly to opioid analgesics. There is a potential for a favorable re-

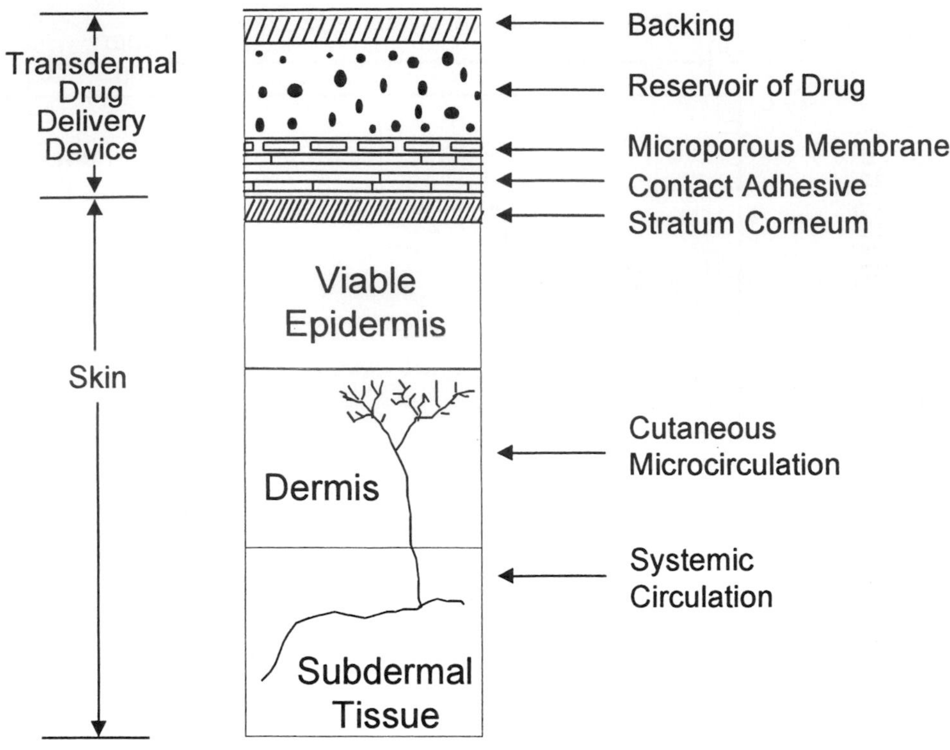

Figure 48-3 Pathway for fentanyl absorption through the layers of the skin. (From Varvel JR, et al. Absorption characteristics of transdermally administered fentanyl. *Anesthesiology*. 1989;70:928.)

sponse in any individual patients, so the diagnosis of a neuropathic cause for pain does not justify withholding opioids on the presumption of inefficacy.[15] For example, in a prospective open-label study of transdermal fentanyl for treatment on noncancer neuropathic pain, 35% (17/48) reported satisfactory pain relief with acceptable side effects after 12 weeks. For unexplained reasons, neuropathic pain did not recur in 4 of the 17 patients when transdermal fentanyl was discontinued. Of the other 13 patients who had responded to transdermal fentanyl treatment for neuropathic pain, 8 still reported satisfactory pain relief after 2 years of treatment.[23]

TABLE 48-6 **Common Causes of Painful Peripheral Neuropathy in Patients with HIV/AIDS**

- Viral infections
  - HIV (usually a distal symmetrical polyneuropathy that is predominantly sensory)
  - CMV (cytomegalovirus)
  - VZV (varicella-zoster virus), also associated with postherpetic neuralgia
- Toxic (medications or alcohol)
  - antiretroviral agents (zalcitabine > stavudine > didanosine)
  - antineoplastic agents (vincristine, vinblastine)
  - anti-TB agents (isoniazid, rifampin, ethionamide)
- Nutritional deficiency
  - Vitamin B_2 (riboflavin)
  - Vitamin B_6 (pyridoxine)
  - Vitamin B_{12} (cobalamin)

The tricyclic antidepressants amitriptyline, nortriptyline, imipramine, or doxepin are frequently used for painful peripheral neuropathy. When they are used as a single nighttime dose, they usually improve sleep with little effect on daytime activities. Two surveys of controlled clinical trials[24,25] found that tricyclic antidepressants were effective analgesics in about one half the patients treated. The anticonvulsants carbamazepine, phenytoin, valproic acid and, more recently, gabapentin have been used successfully for treatment of sharp, shooting (lancinating) pain. In patients whose pain is not controlled with adjuvant analgesic, use of long-acting opioids is a reasonable option. For some patients with debilitating peripheral neuropathy that does not respond to pharmacotherapy, regional anesthetic blockade may be necessary.

DRUG INTERACTIONS

Patients with HIV infection take large amounts of a wide variety of medications to control HIV infection and to treat or prevent opportunistic infections. A comprehensive medication history of

TABLE 48-7 **Cytochrosome p450 3A4: Substrates, Inducers, and Inhibitors**

3A4 Substrate	Alternative(s)
Disopyramide, lidocaine, quinidine	Agent depends on indication
Warfarin	Agent depends on indication
Carbamazepine, ethosuximide	Gabapentin, lamotrigine, valproic acid
Itraconazole, ketoconazole	Fluconazzole
HIV protease inhibitors	Reverse transcriptase inhibitors
Fluoxetine, fluvoxamine, nefazodone, sertraline	Paroxetine, venlafaxine
Dronabinol, ondansetron	Metoclopramide
Astemizole	Cetirizine, clemastine, loratadine
Cisapride	Metoclopramide
Alprazolam, midazolam, triazolam	Temazepam
Calcium channel blockers	Decrease dose by 50%
Oral contraceptives	Other form of birth control
Lovastatin, pravastatin, simvastatin	Gemfibrozil
Alfentanil, fentanyl	Other opioid analgesics
Hydrocodone, oxycodone, methadone	Other analgesics
Etoposide, paclitaxel, tamoxifen, vinblastine, vincristine	Decrease initial dose by 50%
Sildenafil	Yohimbine
3A4 Inducer	**Alternative(s)**
Carbamazepine, ethosuximide, valproic acid, phenobarbital, phenytoin	Gabapentin, lamotrigine, topiramate
Dexamethasone	Agent depends on indication
Troglitazone	Other oral hypoglycemic agents
Efavirenz, nevirapine	Nucleoside reverse transcriptase inhibitors
3A4 Inhibitor	**Alternative(s)**
HIV protease inhibitors	Reverse transcriptase inhibitors
Clarithromycin, erythromycin	Azithromycin, dirithromycin
Cimetidine	Famotidine, nizatidine, ranitidine
Azole antifungal agents	Amphotericin B, terbinafine
Cisapride	Metoclopramide
Omeprazole	Lansoprazole
Fluoxetine, fluvoxamine, nefazodone, sertraline	Paroxetine, venlafaxine
Norfloxacin	Ciprofloxacin, levofloxacin, trovafloxin
Grapefruit juice	Other fruit juices
Zafirlukast	Albuterol, inhaled steroids
Delavirdine	Nucleoside reverse transcriptase inhibitors

Data from: Gelone SP. Clinically significant drug interactions. Hosp Med. 1998;(July):44. And from Deeks SG, Volberding P. Antiretroviral therapy for HIV disease: a review of the clinical pharmacology, safety, efficacy, and resistance patterns of each currently available data. Available at http://hivinsite.ucsf.edu/akb/1997/04arvrx/index.htm.l.

all current drugs, including over-the-counter drugs and herbal medications, and dosage regimens is essential.

The HIV protease inhibitors, which are a component of most highly active antiretroviral regimens,[26] interact with the cytochrome p450 enzyme system, especially the isoenzyme, which is responsible for more than half of the drugs that are metabolized.[27–29] Table 48-7 lists commonly used medications that are substrates of, or interact with, the p450 3A4 isoenzyme.[29–30] Concurrent administration either of an inducer or an inhibitor and a substrate should be approached with caution. Another isoenzyme 2D6 is responsible for metabolism of another 30% of drugs, including codeine and many psychotherapeutic agents.[28,30] These drug interactions may be complex and unpredictable.

Ritonavir is the most potent inhibitor and is associated with the most drug interactions including increased levels (usually measured by total drug exposure or AUC, area under the time-concentration curve) of, for example, saquinavir and rifabutin. Indinavir and nelfinavir are more modest inhibitors of p450, and saquinavir is a weak inhibitor.[27]

Many drugs metabolized by the liver are likely to be affected by concurrent administration of any of the HIV protease inhibitors and there are many drugs not recommended for concurrent use. The prescribing information of the relevant HIV protease inhibitor should be consulted as well as the most recent National Institutes of Health guidelines for antiretroviral therapy.[26] Of particular note, the anticonvulsants phenytoin, phenobarbital, and carbamazepine are enzyme inducers and would be anticipated to reduce levels of HIV protease inhibitors.[32]

Nucleoside analogues have more limited potential for drug interactions compared with other antiretroviral drugs.[32] Zidovudine, like morphine, is glucuronidated to a significant extent, but there is no documented drug interaction between zidovudine and morphine based on this similar metabolic pathway. Interestingly, induction of p450 also induces the glucuronyl transferases that add glucuronide to increase water solubility and facilitate renal excretion.[27]

Of the nonnucleoside reverse transcriptase inhibitors, nevirapine induces cytochrome p450 enzyme and delavirdine inhibits them. Efavirenz is a mixed inducer/inhibitor of cytochrome p450 3A4 isoenzymes, and concentrations of concomitant drugs may be increased or decreased, depending on the specific enzyme pathway involved.[26]

PATIENTS WITH A HISTORY OF PAST OR CURRENT SUBSTANCE USE

Substance abuse is an important risk factor for HIV infection. The prevalence and intensity of pain experienced by substance abusers is not different from that reported in persons who do not use substances. However, substance abusers are more likely to be undertreated for pain. Physicians are usually reluctant to prescribe opioids for patients using other substances, whereas patients in recovery may be reluctant to accept appropriate opioid therapy.

Pain was compared in a sample of AIDS patients that included 270 who reported intravenous drug use as their HIV transmission risk factor and 246 individuals who did not report a history of intravenous drug use (IVDU).[33] Pain was similar in the two groups, whereas pain relief differed between the two groups (Table 48-8). The percentage of IVDUs receiving adequate pain relief was less than half that of non-IVDUs, but pain relief was very poor with 80% to 90% of these patients receiving inadequate pain relief.

TABLE 48-8 **Pain and Pain Relief in AIDS Patients With and Without IV Drug Use History**

	IVDUs	non-IVDUs	*P*
Presence of pain	67%	59%	NS
Number of pains	2.51	2.43	NS
Pain intensity			
at present	3.51	3.68	NS
on average	5.49	5.57	NS
at its worst	7.46	7.24	NS
Adequate pain relief	8.4%	19.7%	.003

From Breitbart W, et al. A comparison of pain report and adequacy of analgesic therapy in ambulatory AIDS patients with and without a history of substance abuse. Pain. 1997;167:30.

IVDUs denotes intravenous drug users; non-IVDUs, non-intravenous drug users; NS, not significant.

Management of such patients can be challenging. A thorough and accurate substance abuse history is essential. Concerns are very different in active users than in patients in recovery (either abstinent or receiving methadone maintenance therapy). Individualization of therapy must include the pattern of past or current substance use. Objective assessment of the cause and probably severity of the pain in a patient with HIV disease and substance abuse is critical, but the patient's report of pain and pain relief is the ultimate guide. The physician must accept and respect the report of pain in spite of the possibility of being misled. Realistic treatment goals and conditions for opioid therapy must be set. Clear limits and predetermined consequences for drug abuse behaviors must be established by a single prescriber who is experienced in recognizing drug abuse behaviors (Table 48-9). Major aberrant behavior may be managed by very frequent weekly or even daily supply of opioid or discontinuation (weaning). Minor aberrant behaviors may be managed by reassessing medication (dose may be too low) and expectations (complete pain relief all the time may not be possible), consider changing to another drug, or reducing time interval between supply of opioid. Minor aberrant behaviors may be evidence of unrelieved pain or patient self-knowledge about what analgesics work and do not work for him or her.

It is critical to distinguish between tolerance and physical dependence, which are pharmacologic properties of opioids, and addiction or drug abuse, which is a complex psychological phenomenon involving drug craving, compulsive use despite physical, psychological, or social harm to the user, and various aberrant drug-related behaviors. Interestingly, in patients receiving opioids for pain relief over long periods, the opioid dose typically stabilizes and dose increases are associated with a worsening physical lesion or a change in psychological status.[15]

In my clinical experience, it is possible to use opioids for pain relief in patients with a history of substance abuse. Short-acting opioids are more problematic than long-acting opioids, which have a much lower abuse potential since the peak levels are much flatter and lower than those with short-acting opioids. Transdermal fentanyl patches replaced every 2 to 3 days are much less subject to abuse than two Percocet tablets taken every 3 to 4 hours.

TABLE 48-9 **Major and Minor Aberrant Drug Behaviors Predictive of Developing Addiction**

Major aberrant behaviors (more predictive)
Selling drugs
Prescription forgery
Seeking prescriptions from other providers
Stealing or borrowing drugs from others
Concurrent use of illicit drugs
Multiple nonsanctioned dose escalations
Multiple episodes of prescription loss
Functional deterioration apparently related to drug use
Minor aberrant behaviors (less predictive)
Aggressive complaining about need for more drug or a more potent drug
Drug hoarding during periods of reduced pain
Requesting specific drugs
Unsanctioned dose escalation

Data from: Portnoy RK. Opioid therapy for chronic nonmalignant pain: a review of the critical issues. J Pain Symptom Manage. 1996;11:203. And from Graziotti PJ. Goucke CR. The use of oral opioids in patients with chronic non-cancer pain: management strategies. MJA 1997;167:30.

CONCLUSION

Chronic pain is underrecognized and undertreated in patients with HIV infection. Patients receiving effective antiretroviral therapy may live for long periods with HIV infection and often experience HIV-related pain. Once the underlying medical complication(s) signaled by pain have been diagnosed and treatment initiated, the pain should be relieved, since unrelieved pain contributes greatly to psychological and functional morbidity in patients living with HIV infection. Although a multidisciplinary approach is optimal and may be necessary, especially in patients with a history of past or current substance use, many of the painful syndromes associated with HIV disease can be readily managed by the primary care practitioner. It is important to give pain a high priority in patients at all stages of HIV disease. Documenting pain and its management, including its efficacy and side effects, clearly in the patient's chart will allow prescription of strong analgesics in appropriate doses to effectively relieve AIDS-related pain and suffering without fear of regulatory action. Table 48-10 outlines an approach to managing pain in patients with HIV disease. Some patients with an AIDS diagnosis receiving multiple-drug antiretroviral therapy and appropriate prophylaxis for opportunistic infections may be able to work if they are not suffering from unrelieved pain. Other patients should receive effective pain relief as part of palliative terminal care.

TABLE 48-10 **An Approach to Managing Pain in Patients with HIV Disease**

- Do a complete physical examination.
- Obtain a thorough history including current and past medications, history of substance use, and, if appropriate, neurologic and psychologic asssssments.
- Localize, characterize, and document the pain(s), considering possible multiple etiologies.
- Treat medical and psychological causes of pain with analgesic and, if necessary, psychotropic medications.
- Document pain therapy and side effects, and pain relief experienced.
- Individualize therapy
  - Consider around-the-clock treatment with long-acting opioids as initial therapy chronic moderate to severe pain and for less severe pain that persists despite treatment.
  - Provide short-acting opioids for breakthrough pain.
- Consult specialists in pain management or substance abuse when necessary.

REFERENCES

1. Markenson JA. Mechanisms of chronic pain. *Am J Med* 1996;101(suppl 1A):6S.
2. Russo CM, Brose WG. Chronic pain. *Annu Rev Med* 19098;49:123.
3. Hewitt DJ, McDonald M, Portenoy RK, et al. Pain syndromes and etiologies in ambulatory AIDS patients. *Pain* 1997;70:117.
4. Breitbart W, McDonald MV, Rosenfeld B, et al. Pain in ambulatory AIDS patients: I. Pain characteristics and medical correlates. *Pain* 1996;68:315.
5. Rosenfeld B, Breitbart W, McDonald MV, et al. Pain in ambulatory AIDS patients. II. Impact of pain on psychological functioning and quality of life. *Pain* 1996;68:323.
6. Breitbart W, Rosenfeld BD, Passik SD, et al. The undertreatment of pain in ambulatory AIDS patients. *Pain* 1996;65:243.
7. Larue F, Fontaine A, Colleau SM. Underestimation and undertreatment of pain in HIV disease: a multicentre study. *BMJ* 1997;314:23.
8. Verhaak PFM, Kerssens JJ, Dekker J, et al. Prevalence of chronic benign pain disorder among adults: a review of the literature. *Pain* 1998; 77:231.
9. Breitbart W, Passik S, McDonald MV, et al. Patient related barriers to pain management. *Pain* 1998;76:9.
10. World Health Organization [WHO]. *Cancer Pain Relief and Palliative Care.* WHO Technical Report Series, 804. Geneva, Switzerland: World Health Organization, 1990:1-75.
11. Jacox A, Carr DB, Payne R, et al. *Management of Cancer Pain: Adults Quick Reference Guide* Number 9. Rockville, Md: US Dept of Health and Human Services, Agency for Health Care Policy and Research; March 1994. AHCPR publication 94-0593.
12. Levy MH. Pharmacologic treatment of cancer pain. *N Engl J Med* 1996; 335:1124.
13. American Society of Anesthesiologists [ASA] Task for on Pain Management, Chronic Pain Section. Practice guidelines for chronic pain management. *Anesthesiology* 1997;86:995.
14. Cherny NI. Opioid analgesics: comparative features and prescribing guidelines. *Drugs* 1996;51:713.
15. Portenoy RK. Opioid therapy for chronic nonmalignant pain: a review of the critical issues. *J Pain Symptom Manage* 1996;11:203.
16. Katz WA. The needs of a patient in pain. *Am J Med* 1998;105(suppl 1B):2S.
17. Schnitzer TJ. Non-NSAID pharmacologic treatment options for the management of chronic pain. *Am J Med* 1998;105(suppl 1B):45S.
18. Jeal W, Benfield P. Transdermal fentanyl: a review of its pharmacologic properties and therapeutic efficacy in pain control. *Drugs* 1997; 53:109.
19. Miser AW, Narang PK, Dothage JA, et al. Transdermal fentanyl for pain control in patients with cancer. *Pain* 1989;37:18.

20. Varvel JR, Shafer SL, Hwang SS, et al. Absorption characteristics of transdermally administered fentanyl. *Anesthesiology* 1989;70:928.
21. Ahmedzai S, Brooks D. Transdermal fentanyl versus sustained-release oral morphine in cancer pain: preference, efficacy, and quality of life. *J Pain Symptom Manage* 1997;13:254.
22. Moyle GJ, Sadler M. Peripheral neuropathy with nucleoside antiretrovirals—risk factors, incidence and management [abstract]. *Drug Saf* 1998;19:481.
23. Dellemijn PLI, van Duijn H, Vannester JAL. Prolonged treatment with transdermal fentanyl in neuropathic pain. *J Pain Symptom Manage* 1998;16:220.
24. Kingery WS. A critical review of controlled clinical trials for peripheral neuropathic pain and complex regional pain syndromes. *Pain* 1997; 73:123.
25. McQuay HJ, Tramèr M, Nye BA, et al. A systematic review of antidepressants in neuropathic pain. *Pain* 1996;68:217.
26. Fauci AS, Bartlett JG, Goosby EP, et al. Guidelines for the use of antiretroviral agents in HIV-infected adults and adolescents [revised 1 December 1998]. Available from the CDC National AIDS Clearinghouse, PO Box 6003, Rockville, MD 20849-6003 (1-800-458-5231 or 1-301-217-0023), or the CDC home page at *http://www.cdc.gov*.
27. Flexner C. Understanding and managing drug interactions. *PRN Notebook.* 1998;3(3):9. See also *http://www.healthcg.com/hiv/treatment/interactions/*.
28. Cupp MJ, Trace TS. Cytochrome P450: new nomenclature and clinical implications. *Am Fam Physician* 1998;57:107.
29. Thummel KE, Wilkinson GR. In vitro and in vivo drug interactions involving human CYP3. *Ann Rev Pharmacol Toxicol* 1998;38:389.
30. Gelone SP. Clinically significant drug interactions. *Hosp Med* 1998; (July):44.
31. Deeks SG, Volberding P. Antiretroviral therapy for HIV disease: a review of the clinical pharmacology, safety, efficacy, and resistance patterns of each currently available drug. Available at: *http://hivinsite.ucsf.edu/akb/1997/04arvrx/index.html.*
32. Barry M, Gibbons S, Back D, Mulcahy F. Protease inhibitors in patients with HIV disease: clinically important pharmacokinetic considerations. *Clin Pharmacokinet* 1997;32:194.
33. Breitbart W, Rosenfeld B, Passik S, Kaim M, Funesti-Esch J, Stein K. A comparison of pain report and adequacy of analgesic therapy in ambulatory AIDS patients with and without a history of substance abuse. *Pain* 1997;72:235.
34. Graziotti PJ, Goucke CR. The use of oral opioids in patients with chronic non-cancer pain: management strategies. *MJA* 1997;167:30.

CHAPTER 49 FIBROMYALGIA AND MYOFASCIAL PAIN

Lance J. Lehmann and Zahid H. Bajwa

Fibromyalgia syndrome (FMS) is one of the most frequent causes of widespread musculoskeletal pain and disability. It is a painful condition predominantly involving muscles and soft tissue rather than joints.[1] Patient's with FMS are commonly seen by rheumatologists and are often referred to pain centers. A multidisciplinary approach to treatment appears to be most beneficial, and may include pharmacologic management, injection therapy, transcutaneous electrical nerve stimulation (TENS), psychological counseling, and behavior modification.

CLINICAL FEATURES

Etiology and Prevalence

The debate continues as to whether fibromyalgia is a distinct syndrome or a composite of various pain syndromes with overlapping features. FMS has been used interchangeably in the past with other painful muscular conditions such as myofascial pain syndrome. Myofascial pain syndrome (MPS) can best be described as a regional muscle pain disorder accompanied by trigger points.[2] A trigger point, as defined by the International Association for the Study of Pain, is characterized as a discrete point of tenderness, palpable in a taut band of muscle.[3] Palpation of a trigger point usually produces a twitch or "jump sign" as well as a regional referred pain pattern. Myofascial trigger points can also be found in ligaments and tendons and are associated with other chronic pain syndromes including fibromyalgia.

Fibromyalgia syndrome encompasses a broader spectrum of clinical features including sleep disturbance, memory loss, migraine headache, irritable bowel, diffuse pain, and morning stiffness.[4] Women are generally affected more often than men, with the prevalence rate of 3.4% for women, 0.5% for men, and 2.0% for both genders overall. Patients between the ages of 20 and 60 years are most often affected by FMS.[5]

Data on myofascial pain suggest that it is a commonly encountered entity. In a study of 172 patients presenting to a university primary care clinic, 54 patients complained of pain, 30% of whom received a diagnosis of myofascial pain. In another study, myofascial pain was the primary diagnosis in 85% of admissions to a chronic pain center.[6] The incidence of trigger points also appears to be higher in women. Myofascial pain has been shown to increase during the second week of the menstrual cycle, suggesting a hormonal influence. Other studies have shown myofascial pain to be less common in sedentary workers, indicating a possible protective effect of daily activity. In terms of anatomic distribution of pain, the neck, shoulder area, and lower back appear to account for most trigger point activity.[7]

Signs and Symptoms

Correctly diagnosing fibromyalgia can be difficult because of the various symptoms previously mentioned, including widespread musculoskeletal pain, muscle stiffness, and weakness. Timely diagnosis is important to ensure patients obtain both psychological support and relief from pain. It is important to distinguish that fibromyalgia is characterized as generalized diffuse musculoskeletal pain involving multiple tender points in the absence of an underlying condition, such as rheumatoid arthritis or hypothyroidism.[8] Well-defined diagnostic criteria have been developed by the American College of Rheumatology, following a multicenter study.[9] These criteria include generalized pain involving three or more anatomic sites for 3 months or longer, exclusion of other conditions that may cause similar pain, and the presence of reproducible tenderness in 11 out of 18 possible fibromyalgia tender points (FTP; areas of tenderness occurring in muscle, muscle -tendon junctions, or fat pads).[10] Fibromyalgic tender points are found in characteristic locations, which are widely distributed and symmetrical but generally do not produce referred pain, and are not usually associated with the taut band of a trigger point.[11]

In contrast to the more widespread and generalized symptoms of FMS, myofascial pain syndrome is a regional painful muscle condition related to a specific trigger point or points and their associated pain referral pattern. Patients with MPS have relatively few systemic complaints when compared with fibromyalgia patients. Trigger points also occur in FMS and were demonstrated in 18% of patients when classically defined to include a taut band of muscle and twitch response, and in 38% when simple trigger point criteria did not include a taut band and muscle twitch.

Pathophysiology and Pathogenesis

The underlying pathophysiology of FMS remains somewhat of a mystery. Current research has identified possible causes of FMS including serotonin deficiency; emotional trauma; abnormal blood flow to muscles; genetic and familial factors; and generalized hypervigalence along with perceptual amplification of pain.[12,13]

The development of a trigger point in FMS or MPS can be acute, such as following a whiplash type injury or following an episode of severe muscle strain. Trigger points can also have an insidious onset with predisposing factors such as chronic repetitive activities or overexertion, poor posture, lack of exercise, and sleep disturbance. A cycle may develop involving adenosine triphosphate and the release of free calcium ions. This in turn activates the actinomyosin contractile mechanism, causing a tense band of muscle to form. Muscle contraction leads to increased metabolic rate with accumulation of metabolites including serotonin, histamine, and prostaglandins. Local muscle acidity stimulates the firing of nocioceptors, causing local and referred pain. Sustained muscle contraction leads to decreased blood flow to the trigger point and a vicious cycle is established.

Tissue biopsies of muscle tender points have shown a "moth-eaten" pattern in the muscle fibers. Various biochemical abnormalities have been reported, including a reduction of adenosine triphosphate, phosphocreatine, and glycogen with increased levels of adenosine monophosphate and creatine. Abnormally low subcutaneous oxygen tension in trigger points may suggest an increase in metabolism.[14] Fibrocystic nodules have also shown an accumulation of water, fat, mucopolysaccarides, platelets, and mast cells. Platelets and mast cells release serotonin and histamine, which stimulate peripheral nerve endings that contribute to a hyperirritable state. Abnormalities have also been detected by muscle biopsy in FMS, but these are generally considered not diagnostic because of an inadequate definition of cases and lack of control data.[15]

Studies evaluating myofascial trigger points using electromyograpic (EMG) techniques have had limited significance owing to lack of adequate controls and conflicting results. Signs of a local twitch response and increased motor activity of trigger points have been noted following needling or firm palpation. Although some EMG recordings have shown increased local activity in myofascial trigger points including fibrillations, sharp waves, and complex repetitive discharges, other studies have not.[16] Therefore, there are no apparent consistent EMG abnormalities to help aid in the diagnosis.

EVALUATION

Diagnostic Criteria

There are similarities regarding fibromyalgia syndrome versus myofascial pain. The hallmark of myofascial pain is the identification of trigger points and their referred pain pattern. Diagnostic criteria for fibromyalgia are specific and include generalized pain involving three or more anatomic sites for 3 months or longer, the presence of reproducible tenderness in 11 of 18 prespecified sites, and the exclusion of other diseases or conditions that may cause similar symptoms. In addition, FMS patients experience fatigue, morning stiffness, sleep disturbance, irritable bowel syndrome, and headaches (Table 49-1).

TABLE 49-1 **Diagnostic Criteria for Fibromyalgia**

Generalized pain in 3 or more sites for 3 months or longer

Exclusion of other conditions that may cause similar symptoms

Reproducible tenderness in 11 out of 18 prespecified sites

Areas (Bilateral)	Site
Occiput	Suboccipital muscle insertion
Cervical	Anterior aspect C5-C7
Trapezius	Midpoint upper border
Supraspinous muscle	Medial border of scapular
Second rib	Upper surface costochondral junction
Lateral epicondyle	2 cm distal to the epicondyle
Gluteal muscles	Upper outer quadrant of buttocks
Greater trochanter	Trochanteric prominence
Knee	Medial fat pad

Physical Examination

Palpation of the affected muscle and applying sustained pressure is one method frequently used in the diagnosis of FMS and MPS. Once stimulated by pressure, the trigger point may produce radiation of pain. The presence of a taut or "ropy" band of muscle is a typical finding. Occasionally, smaller painful nodules may be felt within the fascial structure of tendons and ligaments.

The patient will often direct the examiner's finger to the affected area and report localized or referred pain during palpation of the area. A "jump sign" involves a behavioral reaction where the patient moves away from the pressure being applied, and twitching of the affected muscle group may also be seen. The referred pain patterns are specific and reproducible; however, they do not follow a dermatomal distribution or specific nerve root. Associated signs, usually absent on physical examination, include joint swelling or neurologic deficits.

The sensation of pain in patients with MPS is described as throbbing, dull, burning, and heavy or pressure-like in nature. Most frequently the head, neck, and shoulder regions are involved. Muscle groups include sternocleiodomastoid, trapezius, masseter temporalis, and levator scapulae (Fig. 49-1 and Fig. 49-2). Temperomandibular joint pain, tension headaches, or torticollis may be present. Myofascial pain with trigger points is one of the most common causes of low back pain. The quadratus lumborum muscle group used for posture and trunk stabilization is commonly affected along with gluteus maximus and minimus muscle groups. Pain referral from these areas can be mistaken for sacroiliac joint disease or simulate pain in the distribution of the sciatic nerve.

Noninvasive Tests

Thermography is a noninvasive imaging technique used to detect body surface temperature distribution. Heat is detected and converted into a visual image. Thermal emission is thought to be symmetrical under controlled conditions in a normal individual and should not vary by more than a few tenths of a degree Celsius at the same site on the same side. Thermography has been used extensively in recent years as a research tool and to study the efficacy of various treatments. Observed "hot spots" have corresponded to the location of active and latent trigger points in 61% of cases. These areas are discoid in shape, 5 to 10 cm in diameter, and 0.5 to 10 degrees Celsius higher in temperature than corresponding areas on the opposite site of the body. Hot spots unassociated with pain may represent latent trigger points. Latent trigger points do not cause spontaneous pain at rest or with movement, as opposed to active trigger points. They are, however, painful to palpation and do cause radiation of pain to typical reference areas. Thermographic studies, however, have also demonstrated inconsistencies with both hot and cold spots being found in active trigger points and this questions the diagnostic value of thermography for the documentation of myofascial trigger points.[17]

Pressure algometry is another noninvasive diagnostic tool used to measure the sensitivity of myofascial trigger points and identify sites of abnormal tenderness. It can help assess the outcome of different treatment modalities such as oral medications, trigger point injections, and physiotherapy. Localized tenderness can be quantified by using a handheld pressure threshold meter to estimate a pressure threshold, which is defined as the minimum pressure that induces pain. Pressure tolerance is measured with a similar device and defined as the maximum pressure that can be endured; this

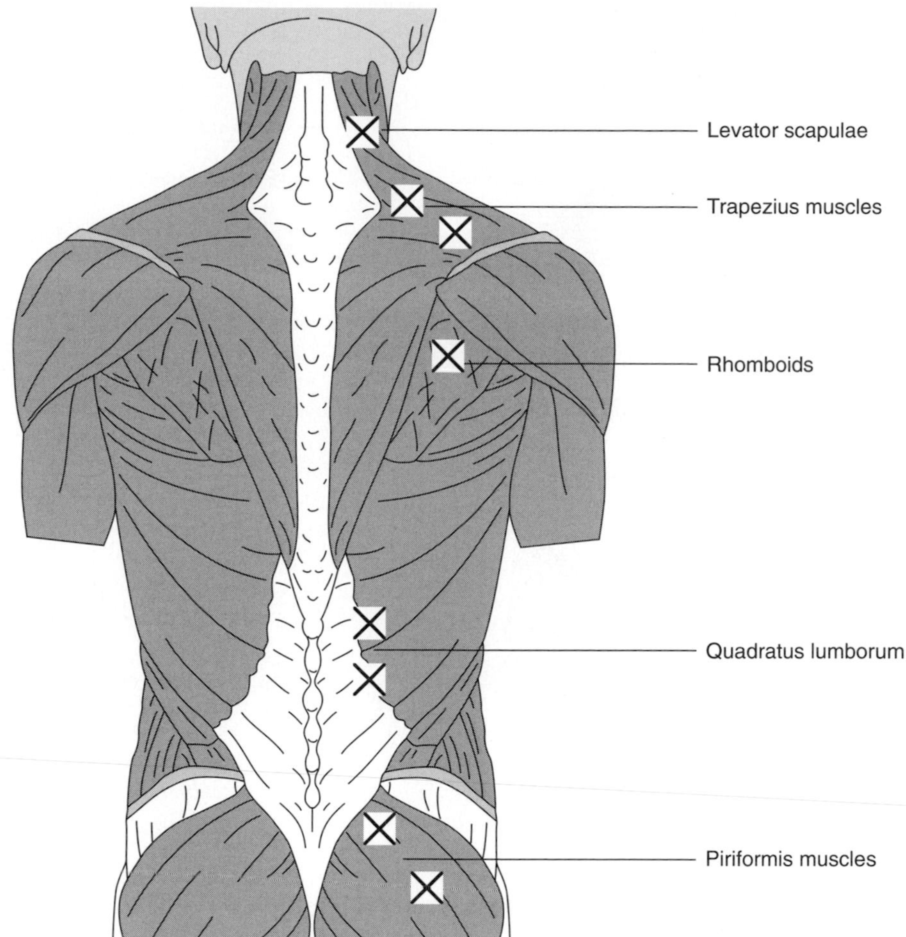

Figure 49-1 Common myofascial trigger points (posterior).

represents sensitivity to painful stimuli. Various studies involving the measurement of trigger points in the head and neck and lower back have demonstrated the reliability of pressure algometer readings in measuring the sensitivity of clinically significant trigger points.[18]

TREATMENT

The treatment of FMS must take into account the chronic nature of the disease, including the physiologic and psychological stresses that contribute to its development and perpetuate the disease process. A multidisciplinary team utilizing anesthesiologists specializing in chronic pain management along with clinical psychologists, physiatrists, physical therapists, and social workers is usually most effective in both reducing the patient's pain and helping to develop coping mechanisms. Treatment options are broad and include trigger point injections, Botox injections, pharmacologic management, electrical stimulation, ultrasound, exercise, and "stretch and spray" techniques.

Injection Therapy

Inactivation of trigger points can be accomplished with injections of local anesthetic with or without steroids, dry needling, stretch and spray techniques, and more recently, Botox injections into affected muscle groups. Proposed mechanisms for the inactivation of trigger points following local infiltration include: mechanical disruption of muscle fibers and/or nerve endings; mechanical disruption of muscle fibers resulting in increased extracellular potassium causing nerve depolarization; interruption of positive feedback mechanisms that perpetuate pain; dilution of nociceptive substances by local anesthetics; or vasodilation effects of local anesthetics that accelerate the removal of various metabolites.

Indications for trigger point injections include tender or taut bands of muscles that produce a jump sign in response to pressure. Twitching of the affected muscle may also be seen. Trigger-point injections are contraindicated during local or systemic infections, bleeding disorders, anticoagulation, allergy to local anesthetics, and acute muscle trauma. Infiltration of trigger points with local anesthetic is widely used to obtain short- and long-term pain relief. This method is preferred over dry needling or the use of saline, which appear to be less effective techniques. Recommended agents include lidocaine 1%, procaine 0.5%, or bupivicaine 0.25 or 0.5%.[19] Steroids are sometimes used in conjunction with local anesthetics to help reduce inflammation at the trigger point. A mixture of 20 to 40 mg is typically mixed with 10 to 12 mL of local anesthetic. Skin depigmentation is the most frequent complication seen following local steroid injection. More serious complications can include tendon atrophy and depression of plasma cortisol levels.

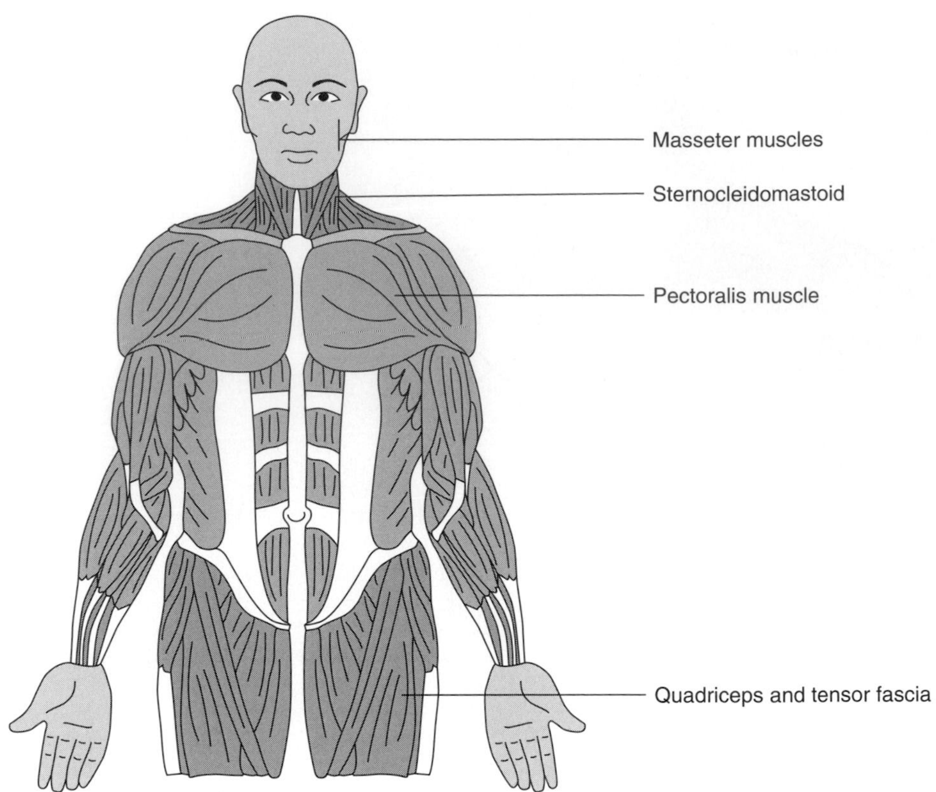

Figure 49-2 Common myofascial trigger points (anterior).

Once the trigger point is identified, the skin is marked and cleansed with either an iodine or alcohol solution. A refrigerated spray such as ethyl chloride can be used before the examiner isolates the trigger point between his or her thumb and index finger. Next, 2 to 4 mL of local anesthetic can be injected in a fanned-out direction in and around the trigger point. When injecting over the scapula or thoracic area, needle depth should remain superficial to avoid causing a possible pneumothorax. Following the injection, the patient's pain should resolve or become markedly diminished, and any prior limited range of motion should resolve. Botulism toxin A appears to be effective when used on myofascial pain affecting cervical paraspinal and shoulder girdle musculature.[20] Its beneficial effect in myofacial pain may occur through the interruption of muscle contraction. The advantage of Botox is its longer lasting effects, on the order of weeks to months.

Dry needling relies on direct stimulation or mechanical disruption of the trigger point. The immediate analgesia produced by needle puncture of the trigger point has been called the *needle effect*. The best analgesic effect is achieved when a fine needle, usually an acupuncture needle, is placed into the most painful spot. The therapeutic effect of this technique has been studied and appears to be mediated by input into the central nervous system.[21] Classic acupuncture has been compared with dry needling and found to be equally effective in terms of pain relief.

Neuro-interruptive Techniques

The stretch and spray technique can be used by itself or as an adjunct to trigger-point injections. The goal is to reduce pain over the trigger point while restoring the muscle to normal length and improving range of motion. Ethyl chloride is usually the agent of choice due to its local anesthetic action and cooling effect. A fine stream of spray is directed toward the tender trigger point as well as the referral pain area using a slow, successive, parallel-sweeping motion. The decreased pain sensation that follows allows the muscles to be passively stretched, thus relieving muscle spasm and any referred pain. The decreased skin temperature is thought to produce transient anesthesia by blocking the spinal stretch reflex and sensation of pain a higher centers.

Transcutaneous electrical nerve stimulation (TENS) is based on the "gate control" theory by Melzack and Wall, first published in 1965.[22] TENS has been extensively studied and shown to be effective for a variety of conditions including trigger points and generalized musculoskeletal discomfort seen in fibromyalgia. The gate control theory states that low-intensity stimulation by TENS selectively activates large diameter nerve fibers that close the "pain gate" located in the dorsal horn of the spinal cord. Other theories attributed to TENS therapeutic effect include release of endogenous opiates, modulation of the autonomic response, and partial block of C fibers.[23] A TENS unit is portable and may consist of 2 to 4 electrodes. These electrodes can be placed directly over the affected muscle group or on the skin overlying a peripheral nerve supplying the affected area. The unit can be applied for several hours at a time, and after it is turned off , the patient may still obtain relief for minutes to hours due to a carry-over effect.

Pharmacologic and Behavioral Management

Several types of medications have been used to treat symptoms commonly associated with FMS. These symptoms include sleep disturbance, depression, anxiety, and musculoskeletal discomfort. Recent studies have shown that patients with fibromyalgia often experience depression and anxiety and report a poorer quality of life associated with their physical condition.[24]

Amitriptyline (Elavil) has been widely used and researched because it both promotes sleep and acts as an antidepressant. Owing to its effect on sleep, clinicians instruct patients to take amitriptyline at night, usually several hours before bedtime. The starting dose is 10 to 20 mg at night; after several weeks the medication can be increased as needed. Side effects include dry mouth and occasional daytime sedation. Newer antidepressants, serotonin reuptake inhibitors, are designed to raise the level of serotonin and include Paxil or Prozac. These medications can interfere with sleep and are often prescribed in the morning. They can be taken by themselves or in combination with amitriptyline at night. Starting dose for Paxil or Prozac is 10 to 20 mg.

Antianxiety agents can also be useful to help with anxiety, muscle spasm, and sleep disturbance. Clonazepam (Klonopin) starting at 0.5 to 1.0 mg at night is effective. Xanax or diazepam can also be used, but may result in prolonged drowziness because of their longer half-lives.

Anti-inflammatory medications can help with musculoskeletal discomfort. The groups of anti-inflammatory medications are too numerous to list, but their use alone or as an adjunct with other medications or treatments may help. Newer agents known as COX-2 inhibitors tout fewer gastrointestinal effects and include Vioxx (rocecoxbid) and Celebrex.

In addition to treating pain, depression, and anxiety, other forms of therapy should emphasize exercise, stretching, and normal sleep patterns. Physical therapy and exercise play an important role in the treatment of FMS and MPS. The goal is to increase blood supply to the affected muscle and overcome any sympathetic activation produced by pain. Modalities of physical therapy that may be helpful include passive and active manipulation of skeletal muscle, deep heat, ultrasound, massage, and TENS. Consultation with a physiatrist will help outline a structured physical therapy program that may also include aquatherapy. Physical therapy is an important part of the patient's overall treatment plan and can be used to measure the patient's progress and results following injection therapy and pharmacologic management.

Finally, the psychological impact of FMS must be addressed. It is not clear whether the patient's psychological state precedes the syndrome or whether it is a result of the physical condition. Relaxation training involving biofeedback, individual psychotherapy, or group sessions emphasizing behavior modification and stress reduction have given patients with FMS significant improvement.[25]

SUMMARY

Fibromyalgia syndrome and myofascial pain syndromes are common yet still poorly understood chronic pain syndromes. Although there is some overlap of symptoms, FMS includes a constellation of symptoms and there are criteria to aid in its diagnosis. The hallmark of myofascial pain syndromes are trigger points demonstrated on physical examination and other means. Undiagnosed patients may feel isolated and misunderstood, further deepening depression and anxiety. They can spend years visiting different specialists and are sometimes mislabeled as drug seeking. Once properly diagnosed, a multidisciplinary approach appears to offer the best outcomes for these difficult to treat patients. As newer treatment options become available and the disease process is further understood, preventive care and behavioral and occupational modifications may significantly reduce or eliminate chronic pain caused by FMS and MPS.

REFERENCES

1. Wallace D. The fibromyalgia syndrome. *Ann Med.* 1997;29: 9.
2. Yunus MB. Fibromyalgia syndrome and myofascial pain syndrome. In: Rachlin ES, (ed). *Myofascial pain and fibromyalgia.*. St. Louis, Mo: CV Mosby, 1994.
3. International Association for the Study of Pain, Subcommittee on Taxonomy. Classification of chronic pain, descriptions of chronic pain syndromes and definitions of pain terms. *Pain* 1986;3(suppl):S81.
4. Tuncer T, Butun B, Arman M, et al. Primary fibromyalgia and allergy. *Clin Rheumatol* 1997;16(1):9.
5. Wolfe F, Ross K, Anderson J, et al. The prevalence and characteristics of fibromyalgia in the general population. *Arthritis Rheumatol* 1995; 38(1):19.
6. Buskilia D, Neumann L, Hazonov I, et al. Familial aggregation in the fibromyalgia syndrome. *Sem Arthritis Rheum* 1996;26:605.7.
7. Yunus MB, Masi AT, Calabro JJ, et al. Primary fibromyalgia: clinical study of 50 patients with matched normal controls. *Semin Arthritis Rheum* 1981;11:151.
8. Campbell SM, Clark S, Tindall EA, et al. Clinical characteristics of fibrositis: a blinded contolled study of symptoms and tender points. *Arthritis Rheum* 1983;26:817.
9. McCain G. A cost effective approach to the diagnosis and treatment of fibromyalgia. *Rheum Dis Clin North Am* 1996;22:323.
10. Wolfe F, Smythe HA, Yunus MB, et al. The American College of Rheumatology 1990 criteria for classification of fibromyalgia: report of the Multicenter Criteria Committee. *Arthritis Rheum* 1990;33:160.
11. Bennett RM. Myofascial pain syndromes and the fibromyalgia syndrome: a comparative analysis. In: Fricton JR, Awad EA, eds. *Advances in Pain Research and Therapy.* New York, NY: Raven Press 1990:43.
12. Aaron L, Bradley L, Alarcon G, et al. Perceived physical and emotional trauma as precipitating events in fibromyalgia. *Arthritis Rheum* 1997;40:453.
13. Nicolodi M, Sicuteri F. Fibromyalgia and migraine, two faces of the same mechanism: serotonin as the common clue for pathogenesis and therapy. *Adv Exp Med Biol* 1996;398:373.
14. Lund N, Bengtsson A, Thorborg P. Muscle tissue oxygen pressure in primary fibromyalgia. *Scand J Rheumatol* 1986;15:165.
15. Yunus MB, Kalylan-Raman UP. Muscle biopsy findings in primary fibromyalgia and other forms of nonarticular rheumatism. *Rheum Dis Clin North Am* 1989;15:115.
16. Durette MR, Rodriguez AA, Agre JC, et al. Needle electromyographic evaluation of patients with myofascial or fibromyalgia pain. *Am J Phys Med Rehabil* 1991;70:154.
17. Swerdlow B, Dieter JNI. An evaluation of the sensitivity and specificity of medical thermography for the documentation of myofascial trigger points. *Pain* 1992;48:205.
18. Reeves JL, Jaeger B, Graff-Radford SB. Reliability of the pressure algometer as a measure of myofascial trigger point sensitivity. *Pain* 1986; 24:313.
19. Hameroff SR, Crago BR, Blitt CD, et al. Comparison of bupivicaine, etidocaine, and saline for trigger point therapy. *Anesth Analg* 1981; 60:752.
20. Cheshire WP, Abashian SW, Mann DJ. Botulism toxin in the treatment of myofascial pain. *Pain* 1994;59:65.
21. Melzack R, Stilwell DM, Fox EJ. Trigger points and acupuncture points for pain: Correlations and implications. *Pain* 1977;3:3.
22. Melzack R, Wall PD. Pain mechanisms: new theory. *Science* 1965;150: 971.
23. Kaada B, Eilsen O. In search of skin vasodilation induced by TENS: serotonin implicated. *Gen Pharmacol* 1983;14:635.
24. Turk D, Okifuji A, Starz T, et al. Effects of type of symptom onset on psychological distress and disability in fibromyalgia syndrome patients. *Pain* 1996;68:423.
25. Minhoto G, Roizenblatt S, Tufik S. The effect of biofeedback in fibromyalgia. *Sleep Res* 1997;26:573.

CHAPTER 50 PERIPHERAL VASCULAR DISEASE

Robert I. Cohen

By late middle age 5% of men and women have developed peripheral arterial disease, and within 5 years one quarter of these will develop pain at rest, ulceration, and gangrene (critical limb ischemia).[1] Physicians practicing in the specialty of pain medicine need to be familiar with the causes and management of pain due to peripheral vascular disease because it has a high prevalence and appropriate management can significantly improve the quality of life for these patients. The pain physician may also be able to significantly improve life expectancy because one half of the patients with symptomatic peripheral vascular disease also have coronary and/or carotid artery disease, and many will not be receiving recommended secondary and tertiary preventive therapy. This chapter outlines the disease conditions and treatments for pain associated with peripheral vascular disease.[2]

Pain similar to that experienced with peripheral vascular disease can be experimentally produced using a sustained tourniquet inflation on an extremity. In experimental studies, as time passes, tissue oxygenation levels fall, metabolic byproducts accumulate, reactive cellular agents are released, nociceptive signals entering the central nervous system increase, and patients report increasing pain intensity. The affective descriptors for this pain may differ and be more difficult to tolerate than pain produced by other experimental modalities. Patients with peripheral vascular disease experience this type of pain but without the ability to restore blood flow by releasing the tourniquet. Effective management of this pain can make a significant difference in quality of life for these patients.

PAIN OF ARTERIAL ORIGIN

Arterial insufficiency is most commonly the result of occlusive diseases with atheroma formation (arteriosclerosis obliterans), but less commonly it occurs in thromboangiitis obliterans (Buerger disease), Raynaud syndrome, diabetic arteritis, and arteritis associated with collagen disease. Other diseases with vascular-related causes such as migraine and cluster headache are discussed elsewhere (Chapter 20).

Atheroma and its Consequences: Arteriosclerosis

The role of lipids was suggested with the early appearance of fatty streaks in young soldiers during emergency surgery and at autopsy in the 1970s. The role of lipids distinguishes arteriosclerosis from other arterial disease. Primary and secondary prevention strategies are available to reduce the incidence and/or aggressively treat the known risk factors of hypercholesterolemia, hypertension, cigarette smoking, and poor control of diabetes. As the disease progresses, plaque formation tends to occur at bifurcations in large- and medium-sized arteries, where turbulence, alteration of laminar flow, and shear stress may provoke an endothelial and/or vascular smooth muscle response. Arteriosclerosis is a dynamic process that involves vascular and inflammatory tissue responses with decreased release of nitric oxide and other protective secretions, increased release of cytokines by inflammatory cells responding to exposed matrix, and release of growth factors from the endothelium, as well as platelet activation. Arteries may initially respond to this process with an increase in size, but this arterial remodeling may not be sustained in the face of ongoing plaque accumulation. Although a full discussion of the process is beyond the scope of this chapter, further understanding of the causes at the gene and cellular level will suggest more effective treatment options.

Progression of Atheromatous Plaques

Although arteriosclerosis is most prominent at bifurcations, the straight femoropopliteal segment is involved in 60% of lower limb disease. Interestingly, the upper limbs are less often involved. Initially, as vessel diameter begins to decrease, flow can be maintained if velocity increases until luminal loss approaches 80 percent (Fig. 50-1). Vessel size also may increase, especially at the arteriolar level, forming a collateral supply. As vessel diameter continues to decrease beyond 70%, the patient may develop symptoms, especially if the process is affecting collateral vessels as well. The initial symptoms usually occur during exercise when the circulation is stressed. Even in patients with severe claudication, blood flow may be near normal at rest. With progression, critical limb ischemia develops with an incidence of 0.5 to 1 per 1000.[3]

Mechanism of Pain from Arterial Disease

Oxygen is the most flow-limited nutrient for muscle and skin. Striated muscle is capable of working anaerobically, with delayed repayment of the oxygen debt. Lactate and pyruvate levels rise as oxygen debt continues. It is assumed that the accumulation of these products of metabolism trigger firing of C-fiber nociceptors, thus triggering the pain cascade.

As oxygen tissue levels fall, hypoxia triggers altered Ca^{2+} signaling in vascular smooth muscle,[4] gene transcription for expression of inflammatory cytokines such as tumor necrosis factor,[5] interleukin-1 and 10[6], and cytokine factors promoting vessel growth, particularly growth of small vessel less than 200 microns in diameter.[9] Endothelial dysfunction is associated with an altered release of mediators such as NO, eicosanoids, endothelium-derived hyperpolarizing factor, endothelin, and angiotensin II.[10] Inflammatory cytokines also affect the coagulation system, for example hypoxia-triggered release of IL-1 can decrease tissue plasminogen activator and stimulate release of plasminogen activator inhibitor-1.[11] Decreased release of NO leads to an increase of endothelial adhesiveness to circulating white blood cells.[12] Inflammatory mediators may both directly and indirectly trigger C-fiber nociceptor barrage into the CNS.

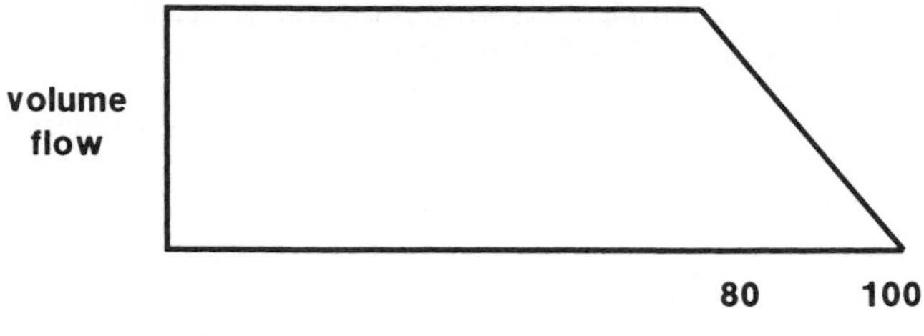

Figure 50-1 Relationship between loss of lumen and volume blood flow.

Clinical Picture of Occlusive Arterial Disease

The patient may complain of claudication and/or rest pain. Claudication is defined as pain in a muscle group (commonly the calf, less often the thigh, instep, or buttock) that occurs while walking and forces the patient to stop. Pain is rapidly relieved by rest, after which walking can be resumed. Walking distance typically decreases as the disease progresses. The diagnosis can often be made with a careful history. Sometimes another disease such as arthritis produces infirmity so the patient cannot exercise. In these cases the diagnosis may be made by examination. In cases of severe coronary disease, the angina linked to very low effort walking may occur before claudication, masking this presentation of the disease. Often the reverse is true, and the presence of claudication may limit the patient's exercise tolerance so that even significant coronary disease may remain quiescent. Because one half of the patients with symptomatic peripheral vascular disease also have coronary artery disease, patients with claudication have only a 50% chance for a 10-year survival rate, with most deaths due to myocardial infarction.[13] For this reason, all patients with claudication should receive preventive treatment to reduce the risk of myocardial infarction and stroke. The differential diagnosis includes venous and neurogenic claudication. The latter is caused by stenosis of the central spinal canal. Spinal stenosis, constricting the cauda equina, can cause pain in the legs during walking. In this case, pain may be worse with trunk extension and better with flexion, so walking downhill (extending the spine) may be more painful than uphill and the peripheral pulses may be good. This diagnosis can be confirmed with computed tomography (CT) or magnetic resonance imaging (MRI) study. If the history is adequate, the site of claudication also may indicate the level of occlusion (Table 50-1). Intermittent claudication is more common in men than in women, in whom it is rare before menopause.

TABLE 50-1 **Relation of Site Claudication to Level of Major Arterial Occlusion**

Site of Claudication	Level of Occlusion
Instep	Popliteal bifurcation or below
Calf	Femoropopliteal
Thigh	Common femoral
Buttock	Aortoiliac

Rest pain (pedal ischemia) consists of pain in the toes or forefoot with or without ulceration or gangrene. The history of ischemic pain is invariably that of pain occurring at night (after a variable recumbent period). This causes the patient to arise and is relieved by dependency of the limb. Patients may volunteer that they prefer to sleep in a chair. As the condition progresses, rest pain becomes more continuous and the condition of the toes deteriorates. Ulceration or gangrene may occur. Spontaneous tissue necrosis may occur in the most peripheral distribution and is likely to affect the toes. It may also occur following trauma, overzealous chiropody, or orthopedic procedures such as operations for bunions and ingrown toenails. Rest pain usually is preceded by claudication, but sometimes it appears in patients who have little or no claudication pain.

Other Relevant History

Arteriosclerosis is a systemic disease, and the history may be positive for myocardial ischemia (infarcts or angina), stroke, hypertension, arrhythmias, and transient ischemic attacks (in the form of focal neurologic deficits resolving within 24 hours). A careful medication history may reveal the extent to which secondary prevention efforts have been successful. The extent of aspirin use and monitoring of cholesterol concentration in a follow-up of patients in the British regional heart study showed that the majority of patients with intermittent claudication who did not have a history of myocardial infarction (MI), angina, or cardiovascular artery disease were not receiving appropriate secondary prevention.[14] Behavioral interventions may be helpful if a history of tobacco use is elicited and psychosocial stressors are present.[15]

PHYSICAL EXAMINATION

The general examination includes blood pressure measurement, cardiac auscultation, and funduscopy. Local examination will reveal ischemic tissue loss and poor capillary circulation. Low input arterial pressure can be enhanced by elevating the legs above the heart for 2 minutes while the patient repeatedly dorsoplantar flexes the ankles; this will produce elevation pallor.

All accessible pulses should be palpated and large vessels (such as the femoral) should be auscultated for presence of a bruit as an indication of proximal stenosis. These data should be charted; an example is shown in Table 50-2.

Investigations

The general assessment of the patient is aided by chest radiography, cardiography, complete blood count, and blood chemistries that include a lipid profile. Echocardiography,[16] testing of coagulation activity including PT, PTT, and INR for patients being treated with coumarin, and, in the future, testing fibrinogen and plasminogen activator inhibitor-1 levels may offer further management options.[17] Noninvasive localization of disease by technology such as combined echocardiography and Doppler (duplex) is preferred for both diagnosis and choosing between surgery and percutaneous transluminal angioplasty (PTA).[18] MRI technology is also capable of providing high-quality noninvasive studies with sensitivity and specificity, comparing favorably with digital subtraction angiography.[19] The standard test remains the ankle-to-arm ratio (ankle-brachial-index [ABI]). Systolic pressure at the ankle is compared

TABLE 50-2 **An Example of a Pulse Chart**

Site	Right	Left
Carotid	+	+
Subclavian	+	+
Radial	+	+
Aorta	[+]	
Femoral	(+)	+
Popliteal	−	+
Dorsalis pedis	−	+
Posterior tibial	−	+
Perforating peroneal	−	−

Note: [ ] indicates aneurysm, ( ) indicates bruit. This patient had an abdominal aortic aneurysm, right iliac stenosis, and right femoropopliteal occlusion.

with systemic arterial pressure measured in the arm. This measure is far more sensitive then pulse oximetry.[20] Observed values are related to clinical state (Table 50-3). When distal vessels are calcified and poorly compressible, the ABI may be unhelpful and values >1.50 may be obtained. Angiography is generally performed prior to reconstructive surgery.

Management of Major Arterial Occlusion

Management of a patient with an ischemic lower limb is summarized in the flow chart seen below:

TABLE 50-3 **Relationship of Severity of Disease to Doppler Ankle-to-Arm Pressure Ratio**

Ankle-to-Arm	Severity of Disease
0.85–1.10	Normal
0.60–0.85	Mild claudication
0.30–0.60	Severe claudication
<0.30	Critical ischemia

Treatment of Claudication

Conservative treatment includes observation and treatment of associated conditions such as diabetes, anemia, or polycythemia. Efforts to assist patients with smoking cessation and to engage in regular exercise have been shown to improve outcome and quality of life.[21] The severity of claudication, response (or lack of response) to medical management, and impact on lifestyle and quality of life must be weighed against the risks of proceeding with a surgical or percutaneous treatment. PTA has high success rates for large vessels with short lesions such as the common iliac, and may be performed as a same-day procedure. Stenting may improve success rates when lesions are more complex or repeat therapy is required. PTA is less effective in smaller vessels, so that, for example, prominent pedal ischemia mandates consideration of vascular surgery if it is technically feasible. Arterial reconstruction may utilize endarterectomy, in situ or reverse venous or synthetic grafting material. The many variations and details are beyond the scope of this

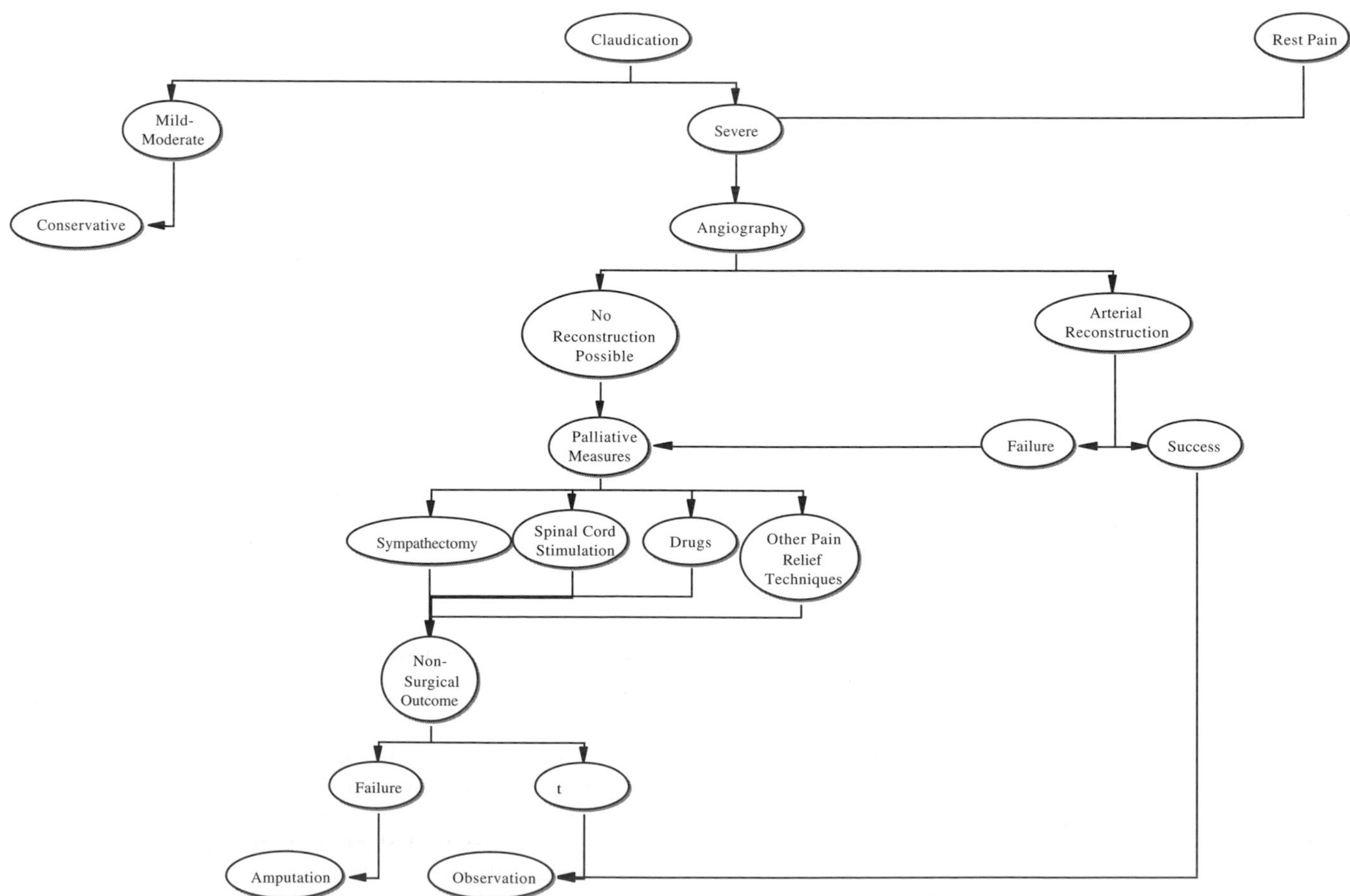

chapter; however the efficacy of bypass surgery for treatment of lower limb ischemia is supported by evidence-based medicine review.[22]

PAIN RELIEF MEASURES

Sympathectomy

Interruption of the lumbar sympathetic chain has a time-honored place in the treatment of peripheral ischemia. Before the advent of arterial reconstruction, it was the only surgical measure that produced pain relief. The indications for sympathectomy have diminished considerably over the last 40 years. Currently, this is a treatment with a limited role.[23,24] Successful reports for the procedure performed by laparoscopy and with chemical sympathectomy continue to appear in the literature.[25,26] Sympathectomy may improve blood flow to the foot and may improve rest pain, heal ulceration, and prevent skin necrosis.

If the affected foot is warmer than the unaffected foot, this suggests that autosympathectomy has occurred (especially in diabetic patients), and that the procedure will not be beneficial. However, there are patients who do not respond despite favorable characteristics. If the popliteal inflow index (Doppler inflow pressure in a popliteal artery versus arm pressure) is ≥ 0.7, a good response can be predicted. It is unlikely that a favorable response will be obtained if the ankle-to-arm ratio is <0.35.[27]

Lumbar sympathectomy can be achieved by injection or surgery. The technique of lumbar sympathetic block is well described in the references.[28] An accurate block of the sympathetic chain at L3 may be adequate and it may not be necessary to use multiple needles (See Appendix A, II). However, the use of radiographic control will make the procedure easier and safer. If repeated blocks with dilute local anesthetic solution produce appreciable circulatory improvement, a neurolytic block with 5 mL aqueous phenol 5% solution can be considered as an alternative to surgical sympathectomy.[29]

Operative sympathectomy may be completed by a relatively atraumatic extraperitoneal approach under general anesthesia in which lumbar ganglia 2, 3, and 4 are excised together with the chain connecting them. Post-sympathectomy neuralgia, an aching pain in the femoral nerve distribution, is a complication that may resolve in 6 to 8 weeks. This is also a complication of chemical sympathectomy if the agent spreads through the prevertebral fascia to the level of the L1 nerve root or through the psoas fascia to reach its major peripheral nerve.

Other Methods of Improving the Peripheral Circulation

Regional Sympathetic Block (See Appendix A, IV) An effective alternative means of producing sympathetic block in a limb is to administer intravenous agents affecting postganglionic neurons to produce noradrenergic block using an intravenous regional anesthesia (IVRA) technique. Before its manufacture was discontinued, guanethidine was used in the last decade with some success in complex regional pain syndrome and peripheral vascular disease.[30,31] By acting on postganglionic neurons, guanethidine first released norepinephrine and then caused noradrenergic block by preventing the reuptake of norepinephrine by the neurons. Other drugs, such as clonidine,[32] phentolamine,[33] bretylium,[34] ketorolac, and corticosteroid, reported effective in management of pain due to complex regional pain syndrome and administered by IVRA technique may also find application in management of pain due to peripheral vascular disease. In the IVRA technique, a tourniquet is placed around the proximal part of the limb and inflated. The limb may be elevated for several minutes to enhance venous drainage prior to inflating the tourniquet. The drug diluted in 50 mL of normal saline may be injected into an indwelling intravenous catheter in the affected leg or arm after tourniquet inflation. Lidocaine can be added to help the patient tolerate the tourniquet. The tourniquet is kept inflated for 15 minutes. This method may be valuable in patients who are receiving anticoagulant therapy in whom paravertebral lumbar sympathetic block could potentially cause significant hemorrhage. IVRA can also be considered in cases in which the effects of operative lumbar sympathectomy are receding.

Spinal Cord Stimulation

Initial reports of the value of large fiber nerve stimulation suggested that patients with pain from peripheral arteriosclerotic disease that had not responded to arterial bypass surgery and/or sympathectomy might respond to stimulation of posterior spinal roots using implanted electrodes. Plethysmographic blood flow and skin temperature were also noted to increase. More recently, it has been suggested that the primary effect may be occurring within the lamina of the dorsal horn of the spinal cord. Pain transmission in this layer is controlled by wide dynamic range neurons. Substance P was one of the first neuropeptides identified as modulating pain transmission, and may be particularly affected by descending traffic modulating pain transmission. It is likely that there are multiple mechanisms involved. The stimulating electrodes may be introduced into the epidural space under direct surgical visualization or by means of a 15-gauge Tuohy needle with the electrodes placed between T 9 and T11.[35] This area of the spinal cord corresponds to lumbar segmental level output. Spinal cord stimulation at this level is associated with increased skin temperature, blood flow, decreased edema, and prolonged pain relief. The stimulating electrodes may be adjusted until stimulation of large fiber afferents produce a tingling paresthesia that overlies the painful region.[36] According to Augustinsson and coworkers,[37] these vasodilating effects of spinal stimulation could be explained by (1) segmental inhibition of vasoconstrictor fibers, (2) antidromic activation of posterior root fibers, and (3) activation of ascending pathways to supraspinal autonomic centers. Interestingly, stimulation over lumbar spines or peripheral nerves was ineffective in these patients.[37,38] The long-term efficacy is reported to be excellent at 70% to 90% when compared with results of 50% to 70% for neuropathic pain.[39,40]

Drug Therapy

The search for a noninvasive treatment of peripheral ischemia has highlighted many drugs that, after a brief popularity, have vanished from our treatment armamentarium. The following discussion of drug therapy approaches includes vasodilators, antithrombotic measures, fibrinolysis, antiplatelet drugs, attempts to modify tissue response to anoxia, prostacyclin, and gene therapy.

Vasodilators Because the regulation of blood flow in the normal foot is affected simply by decreasing or increasing sympathetic tone, alpha-adrenergic blocking agents have been used, including thymoxamine, phentolamine, phenoxybenzamine, and clonidine. Other drugs have a local effect on vascular smooth muscle. These include papaverine and derivatives of nicotinic acid. Priscoline is an alpha-receptor blocker that also has a direct effect.

Systemic use of vasodilators actually may reduce blood flow in the worst affected limb by shunting blood to healthier areas (the vasodilator paradox).[41] A local effect may be obtained by direct intraarterial injection or by retrograde intravenous infusion (Bier technique). Ketanserin, a serotonin$_2$-receptor antagonist, and nifedipine may play a role in therapy,[42] although lowered systemic blood pressure and hence perfusion pressure to the ischemic tissue, and the presence of maximal dilation of local vessels in the ischemic region, suggest vasodilator treatment might not be effective.

Antithrombotic Measures Anticoagulant treatment has not been shown to be helpful in peripheral vascular disease because thrombosis, when it occurs, is only the final episode in the generation of the ischemic limb.

Fibrinolysis Fibrinogen is the substrate for thrombin that converts it to fibrin. Dissolution of fibrin can be achieved using streptokinase, urokinase, and tissue-plasminogen activator. Although it would not affect the atheroma, and restenosis may follow cessation of therapy, it may delay progression and be useful therapy in acute occlusion. Its use should be followed by arteriography to assess the need for reconstruction.

Phosphodiesterase Inhibitors Currently, the only two drugs approved by the FDA for use in intermittent claudication are Cilostazol and pentoxifylline. Both drugs show phosphodiesterase inhibition that can increase the concentration of cyclic AMP, leading to inhibition of platelet aggregation, thromboxane release, and increase in prostacyclin release. Unlike milrinone, which has similar effects on vessels and platelets, Cilostazol does not display significant inotropic effect.[43] Pentoxifylline also affects blood rheology and specifically increases flexibility of red blood cells.

Antiplatelet Therapy Drugs such as aspirin, dipyridamole, ticlopidine, and prostacyclin inhibit release of thromboxane A and prevent platelet aggregation. Because the latter occurs in turbulent flow proximal or distal to atheromatous stenosis or occlusion, such treatment is only of secondary importance in peripheral arterial disease. However, along with lipid-lowering drugs, antiplatelet therapy is the mainstay of secondary prevention to prevent MI and stroke in all patients with peripheral artery disease, even those who do not have signs or symptoms of coronary or carotid disease. Low-dose aspirin, between 81 and 325 mg per day, is the mainstay of preventive treatment for these patients.

Metabolic Agents Naftidrofuryl was marketed first as a vasodilator, but it is purported to influence muscle metabolism beneficially through the Krebs cycle. Although a meta-analysis of seven randomized controlled trials involving 229 patients showed reduction in pain and analgesic consumption, these results were not statistically significant and the drug was withdrawn in the United States for treatment of peripheral arterial disease in 1995.[44] Levocarnitine and propionyl levocarnitine are two drugs that may provide benefit by lessening the acylcarnitine metabolite buildup resulting from an impaired mitochondrial electron transport in ischemic muscle, though propionyl levocarnitine is not yet FDA approved.[45]

Arachidonic Acid Derivatives The term *prostaglandin* was coined by Von Euler,[46] who discovered some of the pharmacologic effects of semen. Endoperoxides derived from cell membrane arachidonic acid are converted to thromboxane A_2 in platelets (vasoconstrictor and platelet aggregator) or to prostacyclin in blood vessel endothelium (vasodilator and inhibitor of platelet aggregation). The balance between these two classes of compounds maintains intravascular hemostasis.

The earliest report of the use of prostacyclin for treating ischemic feet used prostaglandin E_1 by intraarterial infusion; the same team later administered the drug by the intravenous route. In both instances, they reported dramatic relief of rest pain in small patient groups and healing of some ulcers.[47,48] More recently, prostaglandin I_2, also a platelet inhibitor and vasodilator, was administered daily as an intravenous infusion (iloprost), or given orally (beraprost) with encouraging results.[49]

Gene Therapy Gene therapy may be helpful in restoring blood flow to ischemic extremities. A Boston group reported results in a small phase I study. Human DNA coded to make vascular endothelial growth factor (VEGF) was introduced into *Escherichia coli* plasmid, which was grown in culture, purified, and administered by intramuscular injection into ischemic muscles of patients with critical limb ischemia defined as rest pain with nonhealing ischemic ulcers in human volunteers felt to be poor candidates for revascularization surgery. VEGF, secreted by endothelial cells, is the same protein as vascular permeability factor. It has binding sites limited to endothelial cells and so is site-specific. Injection of plasmid VEGF DNA manufactured by *E. coli* produced significant transient edema in the limbs where it was injected. ELISA measured VEGF concentration also increased transiently and was associated in time with increased small blood vessel formation that persisted after VEGF levels returned to baseline, increased ankle-brachial index, healing of ulcers, increased exercise tolerance, and resolved the problem of rest pain. The authors cautiously interpreted their data as supportive for the strategy of intramuscular gene therapy for therapeutic angiogenesis in patients with critical limb ischemia.[50]

PAIN DUE TO PERIPHERAL ARTERIAL DISEASE

Raynaud Phenomenon

This condition differs from all other peripheral arteriopathies because it affects mainly the hands. It was described first by Maurice Raynaud[51] in 1862. Allen and Brown[52] advanced our understanding by separating affected patients into those with and without a known underlying cause.

Raynaud disease (also known as primary Raynaud phenomenon) includes the classic clinical picture of pallor in the distal two-thirds of the fingers (a result of arterial shutdown), cyanosis (from partial relaxation of arterial spasm and deoxygenation of blood), and rubor (reactive hyperemia), all occur in response to cold or emotion. As the condition progresses, the pain becomes more severe and continuous. The condition is more common in women than in men; usually it becomes apparent by the age of 40 years. It occurs much less often in the lower limbs. Raynaud disease describes patients in whom no underlying condition can be found.

Raynaud syndrome (also known as secondary Raynaud phenomenon) comprises those patients with Raynaud phenomenon

TABLE 50-4 **Conditions Associated with Raynaud's Phenomenon**

Immunologic and connective tissue disorders (such as systemic sclerosis, systemic lupus erythematosus, rheumatoid dermatomyositis, hepatitis-B associated vasculitis)
Arterial obstruction (such as thoracic outlet syndrome and Buerger disease)
Vibrating tool disease
Drug induced (such as ergot, β-adrenergic blockers, cytotoxic drugs [vinblastine or bleomycin], or oral contraceptives)
Miscellaneous (such as vinyl chloride disease, cold agglutins, or cryoglobulinemia)

secondary to underlying pathologic disorders (Table 50-4). Interestingly, 10% of patients with primary pulmonary hypertension may exhibit symptoms.[53]

Raynaud syndrome is particularly important because the associated condition may be treatable. In addition, the prognosis is worse, and these patients may develop pathologic changes of ulceration, subungual infection, and pulp loss after digital arterial occlusion (Fig. 50-2). Porter and Rivers[54] reported 383 patients observed in a 10-year period. Of these, 162 had no associated disease and 137 had proven or suspected connective tissue disorder (57 of the latter had systemic sclerosis).

Raynaud Management

General Measures Simple avoidance of cold, either of the body or of the hands, may be all that is required in mild cases. A change of occupation may be necessary if vibrating tools are used. Cessation of smoking has been advocated.

Sympathectomy Because nervous control of digital blood flow occurs simply as a result of increasing or decreasing sympathetic tone, pharmacologic or surgical sympathectomy has been used extensively. Drugs, such as methyldopa, thymoxamine, reserpine, debrisoquine, and phentolamine have been administered orally and intraarterially. Most of the studies are anecdotal, uncontrolled, or rely on subjective assessment. If no effect can be proved when a drug is given intraarterially, it is unlikely that it will work systemically. The pain of Raynaud phenomenon has been controlled by intravenous regional anesthesia (IVRA) sympathetic block with guanethidine (no longer manufactured). Agents used in IVRA to treat other pain syndromes may find application in Raynaud treatment as guanethidine alternatives are investigated (See section, Other Methods of Improving the Peripheral Circulation).

Surgical sympathectomy can be done using an open procedure, but temporary and permanent Horner syndrome may occur. Transaxillary endoscopic coagulation to destroy thoracic ganglia 2 to 5 is another approach.[55] A thoracoscopic approach that is minimally invasive has also been described.[56,57] The immediate effect usually is good, although recurrence is common within 6 to 24 months and this treatment may be less helpful than others.[58] Digital sympathectomy using microvascular techniques has also been reported.[59]

Sympathetic Blockade Where the condition is not severe and particularly if it is seasonal, a stellate ganglion block can be helpful. A paratracheal approach at the C6 level reduces the risk of pneumothorax and intravertebral artery injection. The accuracy may be increased by use of radiographic control and a radiopaque dye that can identify the occurrence of dural cuff injection. A sympathetic block with local anesthetic does not tend to produce a sustained response.

Other Treatments While Ketanserin was initially[60] thought a helpful therapy, recent reviews suggest no significant clinical effect.[61] Temperature biofeedback was recently shown inferior to treatment with calcium antagonist.[62] Nifedipine, or other calcium channel blockers, are highly effective for patients who do not suffer adverse effects. Interestingly, the dihydropyridine calcium channels are closely associated with the endothelin-1 receptor, suggesting endothelin-1, found in higher concentration in Raynaud

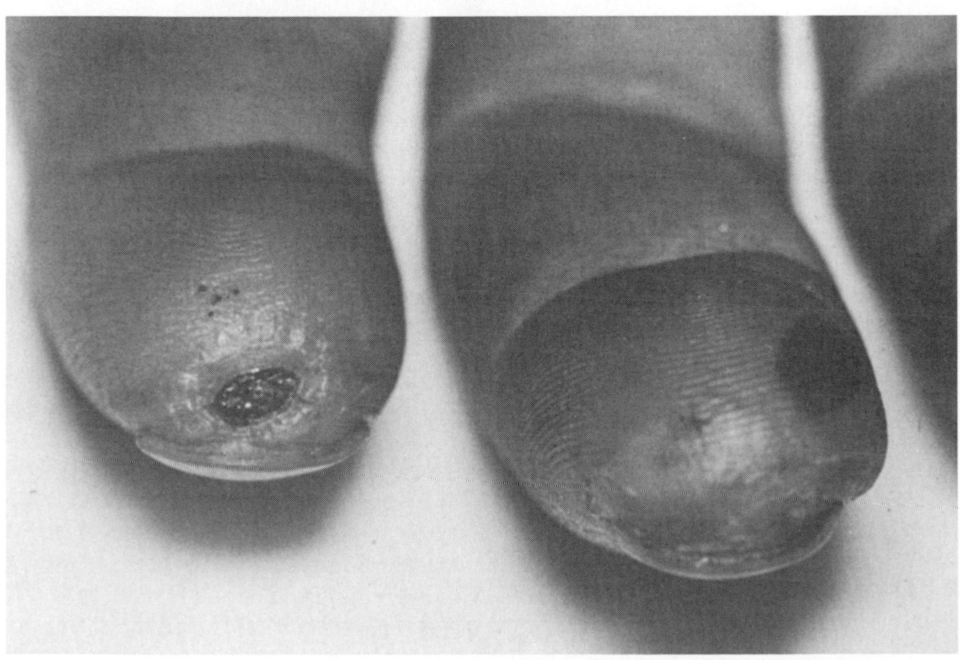

Figure 50-2 Digital ulceration in Raynaud disease.

patient serum, may be a neuron-independent vasoconstrictor.[63] Prostacyclin infusion and administration of a stable oral preparation may be helpful and were previously described. Also as noted above, spinal cord stimulation could be of value.

Buerger Disease

Thromboangiitis obliterans was the name Leo Buerger[64] gave to a specific arterial disease he believed was confined largely to Eastern Europeans. This disease subsequently was shown to be prevalent in Sri Lanka, Korea, and Japan, where it was the most common form of arterial pathology. By the 1970s it was reported that 75% of 1641 cases of femoropopliteal occlusion were caused by this condition.[65] A gradual decrease in the incidence has been reported over the last decade.[66]

Clinical Picture More than 90% of sufferers are men younger than 40 years of age who are smokers. They have instep claudication or painful ischemic changes in the feet. Just less than one half have manifestations in their upper limbs, usually thrombophlebitis or minor ischemic changes. Upper extremity circulation may be assessed with an Allen's test. Have the patient make a fist while occluding radial and ulnar arteries at the wrist. The hand is relaxed and ulnar arterial pressure is released. Failure of the hand to regain color constitutes a positive test. The test is repeated for patency of radial artery. In these patients, foot pulses and, later, popliteal pulses are absent.

Buerger disease is an inflammatory process; the affected artery is surrounded by fibrosis while the normal structure of the vessel wall may be preserved, in contrast to the typical disruption of internal elastic lamina and media in arteriosclerosis and other systemic vasculitides.[67] The pathology is specific with thrombosis in crural arteries and veins. Giant cells are a histologic feature, even in early cases.

Management Universally, it is accepted that for smokers, treatment must begin with smoking cessation. If patients stop smoking, this alone may be sufficient to provide relief.

Local treatment is directed toward debridement and draining infections. Prostaglandin in the form of iloprost may provide benefit, particularly during the period when patients first discontinue smoking.[68] Sympathectomy and spinal cord stimulators also have a place in management of difficult cases. As in arteriosclerosis, gene therapy also may offer some promise.[69]

VENOUS DISEASE

This may be acute (deep venous thrombosis [DVT] or thrombophlebitis) or chronic (DVT with recanalization or gravitational disease). DVT occurs when normal venous flow is disturbed in accordance with the Virchow triad: (1) diminished flow velocity after illness, operation or childbirth; (2) alteration in the characteristics of the contained blood producing increased viscosity, such as polycythemia, abnormal plasma protein fractions, leukemia, or thrombocythemia; and (3) local intimal damage. In most cases more than one factor is responsible. Many cases apparently arise spontaneously in healthy people; however, a search for an underlying condition (such as malignancy or collagen-vascular disease) should be undertaken. Often without initial symptomatology, the disease may present with death due to pulmonary embolism. The focus should be on prevention rather than treatment, particularly for patients at increased risk due to immobility, including patients admitted to the hospital for surgery. For further information, the reader is referred to an excellent discussion of this topic by Geerts and colleagues.[70]

Acute Venous Disease

The clinical diagnosis of DVT is made by the triad of local tenderness, swelling, and color change. Clinical diagnosis alone does not detect the subtler changes, and may overdiagnose the condition. In the presence of atheroma, false-positive and false-negative results comprise 50% of all cases.

When edema is present, it implies that the deep veins are occluded; embolization is less likely, but local sequelae are more likely. The clinical picture is either the white leg (milk leg), which is pale and shows infra-genicular pitting edema, or the blue leg, which involves the entire leg as far proximally as the root of the limb. The former is a result of femoropopliteal obstruction; the latter indicates iliac-caval obstruction. The blue leg causes much dis-

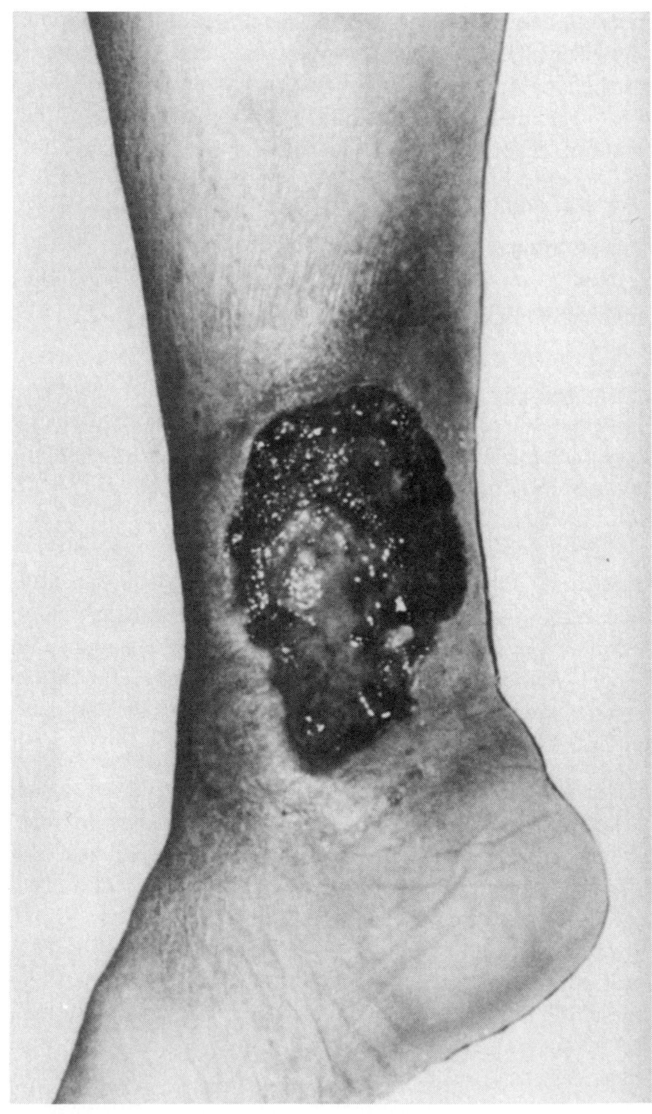

Figure 50-3 Typical venous ulcer.

comfort, and if tissue pressure continues to rise, peripheral gangrene may supervene.

Acute thrombophlebitis is easily recognizable because there is visible swelling and tenderness along the course of a superficial vein. Apart from the underlying conditions already mentioned, the condition may be the harbinger of carcinoma of the pancreas or lung.

Chronic Venous Disease

Occlusion of the major veins is followed by recanalization with valve destruction. This allows transmission of the full force of the column of blood from the right atrium to the heel (+80 to 90 mm Hg). The patient may complain of a resting pain in the calf, which, when associated with walking, is called *venous claudication.*

Gravitational changes are more serious because of their reputation for intractability. These changes include pigmentation, distended intracutaneous veins (in the inframalleolar position, so-called venous flare), edema, liposclerosis, and ulceration (See Fig. 50-3). The pain of a venous ulcer may be excruciating; it usually is worse at night and is unrelated to ulcer size. Investigation of venous disease is directed toward the following:

1. *Proving the diagnosis.* Isotope studies may be helpful in acute DVT. Duplex ultrasonography and impedance plethysmography are useful in establishing the diagnosis. The "gold standard" investigation is venography, which should be universally available. Testing for the D-dimer fibrin degradation product combined with clinical criteria has a high sensitivity and low false-negative results.[71,72]

2. *Demonstrating an underlying cause.* A complete blood count, erythrocyte sedimentation rate, chest x-ray, liver diagnostic tests, urinalysis, renal function tests, serum proteins and immunoglobin level tests, and tests for lupus erythematosus, rheumatoid, and other collagenoses may be required.

Management of Venous Disease

Acute Deep Venous Thrombosis The classic mainstay of treatment used to be a 5000-unit bolus of heparin followed by a continuous intravenous infusion in a dose of 40,000 units in 24 hours. This treatment was designed to prevent the spread of the thrombus and embolization until the clot became adherent and stabilized. In the absence of bleeding complications, therapy was maintained for 5 days, the last 3 days of which overlap with the commencement of oral anticoagulation therapy with coumarin, which was maintained for 3 months. Vitamin K antagonist treatment to maintain an INR of 2.5 is the most frequent secondary treatment for patients with venous thromboembolism. In four studies with 1500 patients, a meta-analysis revealed reduction for risk of recurrent events as long as treatment was maintained. As the risk of recurrent event may decrease over time, this benefit may eventually become outweighed by the risk of hemorrhagic complication that does not decrease over time.[73]

The availability of a low-cost outpatient management option has resulted in shortened hospital stays, with many cases in this country being treated with subcutaneus injections of low-molecular-weight heparin. A meta-analysis of 4754 patients in 14 randomized, prospective, controlled studies showed low-molecular-weight heparin was as effective as unfractionated intravenous heparin in preventing recurrent DVT. The risk of hemorrhage was lower during treatment and mortality at follow-up was also lower for the outpatient treatment protocol.[74]

Acute Thrombophlebitis This usually is a self-limited condition that can be treated by local warm compresses and an anti-inflammatory drug (such as ibuprofen.) If the process involves the saphenous vein in the thigh, it may be necessary to ligate it at the groin to prevent the thrombosis from spreading into the femoral vein.

Chronic Venous Insufficiency The venous hypertension that follows extensive valvular obstruction after DVT includes various stigmata in the gaiter area of the leg, the most disabling of which is ulceration. There are many causes of leg ulceration, and it is important to exclude concomitant arterial disease, diabetes, and rheumatoid disease because these will render standard treatment ineffective. The linchpin of treatment of venous ulcers is effective, graded, dynamic-elastic compression to oppose the harmful effects of venous hypertension. Many topical therapies have been used, including antibiotics, corticosteroids, and enzymes. However, they are all largely ineffective. They also may be expensive and can produce sensitization reactions that may be worse than the original condition.

Pain control with analgesic drugs during the healing phase is important; a decreasing need for analgesia is a good indication of progress toward healing.

SUMMARY

Interestingly, services for patients with pain due to peripheral vascular disease are delivered by a multitude of specialists including vascular surgeons, radiologists, anesthesiologists, rheumatologists, cardiologists, internists, dermatologists, primary care physicians, and podiatrists. The explosion of basic science and clinical research promises improved understanding and additional management options for these severely disabling diseases. Meanwhile, the author encourages the reader, whatever his or her specialty, to take every opportunity to encourage smoking cessation, regular daily exercise, and other preventive measures that produce so much benefit to so many.

REFERENCES

1. Smith FB. Intravenous Naftidrofuryl for critical limb ischemia (Cochrane Review). *The Cochrane Library* 2001 (Issue 2).
2. Swerdlow M, Schraibman IG. Peripheral vascular disease. In: Warfield CA, ed. *Principles and Practice of Pain Management.* New York, NY: McGraw Hill, 1993.
3. European Working Group on Critical Leg Ischemia. Second European consensus document on chronic critical leg ischemia. *Circulation.* 1991;84(suppl IV):IV-1.
4. Sayeed M M. Signaling mechanisms of altered cellular responses in trauma, burn, and sepsis: role of Ca2+. *Arch Surg* 2000;135:1432.
5. Tani T, Fujino M, Hanasawa K, et al. Bacterial translocation and tumor necrosis factor-[alpha] gene expression in experimental hemorrhagic shock. *Crit Care Med* 2000;28:3705.
6. Silvestre J-S, Mallat Z, Duriez M, et al. Antiangiogenic effect of interleukin-10 in ischemia-induced angiogenesis in mice hindlimb. *Circ Res* 2000;87(6):448.
7. Forsythe JA, Jiang BH, Iyer NV, et al. Activation of vascular endothelial growth factor gene transcription by hypoxia-inducible factor 1. *Mol Cell Biol* 1996;16:4604.
8. Akeno N, Czyzyk-Krzeska MF, Gross TS, et al. Hypoxia induces vascular endothelial growth factor gene transcription in human osteoblast-like cells through the hypoxia-inducible factor-2 alpha. *Endocrinology* 2001;142:959.

9. Isner JM. Tissue responses to ischemia: local and remote responses for preserving perfusion of ischemic muscle. *J Clin Invest* 2000;106: 615.
10. Cohen RA. The role of nitric oxide and other endothelium-derived vasoactive substances in vascular disease. *Prog Cardiovasc Dis* 1995; 38:105.
11. Opal S, Thijs L, Cavaillon J-M, et al. Roundtable I: relationships between coagulation and inflammatory processes. *Crit Care Med* 2000;28 (suppl):S81.
12. Kullo IJ, Simari RD, Schwartz RS. Vascular gene transfer: from bench to bedside. *Arterioscler Thromb Vasc Biol* 1999;19:196.
13. Creager MA, Dzau VJ. Vascular disease of the extremities. In: Braunwald E, Fauci AS, Kasper DL, Hauser SL, Longo DL, Jameson JL, eds. *Harrison's Principles of Internal Medicine*. New York, NY: McGraw-Hill, 2001:1036.
14. Vass, A, Leng G, Papacosta O , et al. Secondary prevention may help intermittent claudication. *BMJ* 2001;322:673.
15. DeBenetittis G, Panerai AA, Villamari MA. Effects of hypnotic analgesia and hypnotizability on experimental ischemic pain. *Int J Clin Exp Hypn* 1989;37(1):55.
16. Kapral MK, Silver FL, with the Canadian Task Force on Preventive Health Care. Preventive health care, 1999 update: 2. Echocardiography for the detection of a cardiac source of embolus in patients with stroke. *Can Med Assoc J* 1999;161:989.
17. Philipp CS, Cisar LA, Kim HC, et al. Association of hemostatic factors with peripheral vascular disease. *Am Heart J* 1997;134:978.
18. Kitslaar PJ, Wollersheim H, Zwiers I. Consensus noninvasive diagnosis of peripheral arterial vascular diseases. Central Guidance Organization for Peer Review. *Ned Tijdschr Geneeskd* 1995;139(22):1133.
19. Huber A, Heuck A, Baur A, et al. Dynamic contrast-enhanced MR angiography from the distal aorta to the ankle joint with a step-by-step technique. *AJR Am J Roentgenol* 2000;175:1291.
20. Jawahar D, Rachamalla HR, Rafalowski A, et al. Pulse oximetry in the evaluation of peripheral vascular disease. *Angiology* 1997;48:721.
21. Tan KH, de Cossart L, Edwards PR. Exercise training and peripheral vascular disease. *Br J Surg* 2000;87:553.
22. Leng GC, Davis M, Baker D. Bypass surgery for chronic lower limb ischaemia (Cochrane Review). The Cochrane Library 2001(Issue 2).
23. Belkin M, et al. Peripheral arterial occlusive disease. In: *Sabiston Textbook of Surgery*. 16th ed. Philadelphia, Pa: WB Saunders, 2001:1375.
24. Wronski J. Lumbar sympathectomy performed by means of videoscopy. *Cardiovasc Surg* 1998;6:453.
25. Lee BY, Rangraj MS, Waisbren S. Laparoscopic retroperitoneal lumbar sympathectomy in the treatment of lower extremity reflex sympathetic dystrophy and ischemia. *Contemp Surg* 1998;52:21.
26. Gleim M, Maier C, Melchert U. Lumbar neurolytic sympathetic blockades provide immediate and long-lasting improvement of painless walking distance and muscle metabolism in patients with severe peripheral vascular disease. *J Pain Symptom Manage* 1995;10:98.
27. Yao J, Bergan JJ. Predictability of vascular reactivity relative to sympathetic ablation. *Arch Surg* 1973;107:676.
28. Breivik H, Cousins MJ, Lofstrom JB. Sympathetic neural blockade of the upper and lower extremity. In: Cousins MJ, Bridenbaugh PO, eds. *Neural Blockade in Clinical Anesthesia and Pain Management*. 3rd ed. Philadelphia, Pa: Lippincott-Raven, 1998:411–447.
29. McCollum PT, Spence VA, Marcrae B, Walker WF. Quantitative assessment of the effectiveness of chemical lumbar sympathectomy. *Br J Anaesth* 1985;57:1146.
30. Hannington-Kiff JG. Antisympathetic drugs in limbs. In: Wall PD, Melzack R, eds. *Textbook of Pain*. Edinburgh, Scotland: Churchill Livingstone, 1984:566–577.
31. Stumpflen A, Ahmadi A, Atteneder M, et al. Effects of transvenous regional guanethidine block in the treatment of critical finger ischemia. *Angiology* 2000;51(2):115.
32. Sruben SS, Steinberg RB, Madabhushi L, Rosenthal E. Intravenous regional clonidine in the management of sympathetically maintained pain. *Anesthesiology* 1998;89:527.
33. Malik VK, Inchiosa MA, Mustafa K, et al. Intravenous regional phenoxybenzamine in the treatment of reflex sympathetic dystrophy. *Anesthesiology* 1998;88:823.
34. Hogan QH, Abram SE. Neural blockade for diagnosis and prognosis: a review. *Anesthesiology* 1997;86(1):216.
35. Tesfaye S, Watt J, Benbow SJ, et al. Electrical spinal-cord stimulation for painful diabetic peripheral neuropathy. *Lancet* 1996;348:1698.
36. Stanton-Hicks M, Salamon J. Stimulation of the central and peripheral nervous system for the control of pain. *J Clin Neurophysiol* 1997;14(1):46.
37. Augustinsson LE, Carlson CA, Fall M. Autonomic effects of electrostimulation. *Applied Neurophys* 1982;45:185–189.
38. Naver H, Augustinsson LE, Elam M. The vasodilating effect of spinal dorsal column stimulation is mediated by sympathetic nerves. *Clin Autonom Res* 1992;2:41.
39. Augustinsson LE, Linderoth B, Mannheimer C, Eliasson T. Spinal cord stimulation in cardiovascular disease. *Neurosurg Clin North Am* 1995; 6(1):157.
40. Jivegard LE, Augustinsson LE, Holm J, et al. Effects of spinal cord stimulation (SCS) in patients with inoperable severe lower limb ischaemia: a prospective randomised controlled study. *Eur J Vasc Endovasc Surg* 1995;9(4):421.
41. Gillespie JA. The case against vasodilator drugs in occlusive vascular disease of the legs. *Lancet* 1959;2:955.
42. Tjon JA. Treatment of intermittent claudication with pentoxifylline and cilostazol. *Am J Health Syst Pharm* 2001;58(6):485.
43. Cone J, Wang S, Tandon N, et al. Comparison of the effects of cilostazol and milrinone on intracellular cAMP levels and cellular function in platelets and cardiac cells. *J Cardiovasc Pharmacol* 1999; 34:497.
44. Smith FB, Bradbury AW, Fowkes FGR. Intravenous naftidrofuryl for critical limb ischaemia (Cochrane Review). *The Cochrane Library* 2001 (Issue 2).
45. Hiatt WR. Drug therapy: medical treatment of peripheral arterial disease and claudication. *N Engl J Med* 2001;344:1608.
46. Von Euler US. Uber der spezfishe blutdrucks enkende substanz des menshilichen Prostata-und samen blasensckretes. *Klin Wochenschr* 1935;14:1182.
47. Carlson LA, Erickson I. Femoral artery infusion of prostaglandin E_1 in severe peripheral vascular disease. *Lancet* 1973;1:155.
48. Carlson LA, Erickson I. Intravenous prostaglandin E1 in severe peripheral vascular disease. *Lancet* 1976;2:810.
49. Lievre M, Morand S, Besse B, Fiessinger JN, Boissel JP. Oral beraprost sodium, a prostaglandin I_2analogue, for intermittent claudication: a double-blind, randomized, multicenter controlled trial. *Circulation* 2000;102:426.
50. Baumbartner I. Constitutive expression of phVEGF165 after intramuscular gene transfer promotes collateral vessel development in patients with critical limb ischemia. *Circulation* 1998;97:1114.
51. Raynaud M. De l'asphyxie locale et de la gangrene symmetrique des extremes. Paris, France: Righoux, 1862.
52. Allen EV, Brown GE. Raynaud's disease—a critical review of the minimal requirements for diagnosis. *Ann J Jed Sci* 1932;183.
53. Gaine S. Pulmonary hypertension. *JAMA* 2000;284:3160.
54. Porter JM, Rivers SP. Management of Raynaud's syndrome. In: Bergan JJ, Yao J, eds. *Evaluation and Treatment of Upper and Lower Extremity Circulatory Disorders*. Orlando, Fla: Grune & Stratton, 1984:182.
55. Malone RS, Cameron AEP, Rennie JA. Endoscopic thoracic sympathectomy in the treatmnet of upper limb hyperhydrosis. *Ann R Coll Surg Engl* 1986;68:93.
56. Colt HG. Thoracoscopy: window to the pleural space. *Chest* 1999; 116:1409.
57. Krasna MJ, Jiao X, Sonett J, et al. Thoracoscopic sympathectomy. *Surg Laparosc Endosc Percutan Techniques* 2000;10(5):314.
58. Ho M, Belch JJ. Raynaud's phenomenon: state of the art 1998 [editorial]. *Scand J Rheumatol* 1998;7:319.
59. Yee AM, Hotchkiss RN, Paget SA. Adventitial stripping: a digit sav-

ing procedure in refractory Raynaud's phenomenon. *J Rheumatol* 1998; 25:269.

60. Stranden R, Roald OK, Krohg K. Treatment of Raynaud's phenomenon with the 5-HT_2-receptor antagonist ketanserin. *BMJ* 1982;285:1069.
61. Pope J, et al. Ketanserin for Raynaud's Phenomenon in progressive systemic sclerosis. *The Cochrane Library*. 1999 (Issue 3).
62. Raynaud's Treatment Study Investigators. Comparison of sustained-release nifedipine and temperature biofeedback for treatment of primary Raynaud phenomenon: results from a randomized clinical trial with 1-year follow-up. *Arch Intern Med* 2000;160:1101.
63. Dowd P, Goldsmith P, Bull H, et al. Raynaud's phenomenon. *Lancet* 1995;346:283.
64. Buerger L. Thrombo-angiitis obliterans. A study of the vascular lesions leading to presenile gangrene. *Ann J Med Sci* 1909;136:562.
65. Mishima Y. Curent status of femoropopliteal occlusion in Japan. *J Cardiovasc Surg Suppl* 1970;11(3):97.
66. Matsushita M, Nishikimi N, Sakurai T, et al. Decrease in prevalence of Buerger's disease in Japan. *Surgery* 1998;124:498.
67. Olin JW, Lie JT. Thromboangiitis obliterans (Buerger's disease). In: Loscalzo J, Creager MA, Dzau VJ, eds. *Vascular Medicine*. 2nd ed. Boston, Mass: Little, Brown, 1996:1033–1049.
68. Fiessinger JN, Schafer M. Trial of iloprost versus aspirin treatment for critical limb ischaemia of thromboangiitis obliterans: the TAO Study. *Lancet* 1990;335:555.
69. Isner JM, Baumgartner I, Rauh G, et al. Treatment of thromboangiitis obliterans (Buerger's disease) by intramuscular gene transfer of vascular endothelial growth factor: preliminary clinical results. *J Vasc Surg* 1998;28:964.
70. Geerts WH, Heit JA, Clagett GP, et al. Prevention of venous thromboembolism. *Chest* 2001;119(suppl):132S.
71. Aschwanden M, Labs KH, Jeanneret C, et al. The value of rapid D-dimer testing combined with structured clinical evaluation for the diagnosis of deep vein thrombosis. *J Vasc Surg* 1999;30:929.
72. Wells PS, Anderson DR. Diagnosis of deep-vein thrombosis in the year 2000. *Curr Opin Pulm Med* 2000;6:309.
73. Hutten BA, Prins MH. Duration of treatment with vitamin K antagonists in symptomatic venous thromboembolism (Cochrane review). Cochrane Database Syst Rev (England), 2000, (3) pCD001367.
74. van Den Belt AG, Prins MH, Lensing AW, et al. Fixed dose subcutaneous low molecular weight heparins versus adjusted dose unfractionated heparin for venous thromboembolism. *Cochrane Database Syst Rev.* (England), 2000 (2) pCD001100.

CHAPTER 51 ADVANCES IN THE MANAGEMENT OF ISCHEMIC PAIN

Gisele Girault and Gilbert Fanciullo

Ischemic pain is pain caused by obstruction of the circulation to a body part. Pain management centers have only recently become involved in the care of patients with ischemic diseases such as peripheral vascular disease and angina pectoris because now these centers have something unique to offer. This chapter provides a review of the pathophysiology of ischemic disease, the therapies available and their efficacy, and the role of the pain specialist in the management of patients with peripheral and coronary ischemic disease.

Atherosclerosis obliterans is the principal cause of ischemic pain associated with peripheral vascular disease and coronary artery disease. Ischemic pain in peripheral vascular disease is insidious and gradual in onset. It usually begins with intermittent claudication. Most patients have atherosclerotic changes for 5 to 10 years before they have symptoms. Approximately 25% of patients with intermittent claudication will progress to critical ischemia and pain at rest.

Intermittent claudication is the earliest sign of vascular insufficiency, which is characterized by cramping, tightness, and heaviness that increases with exercise. The pain is relieved with rest and the claudication distance remains fairly constant until further progression of the disease. In the early stages of the disease, collateral circulation develops and may maintain adequate perfusion to the affected limb, but may not provide sufficient blood flow to prevent symptoms, especially during exercise. Over time, both the primary and collateral vessels become stenotic or occluded and critical ischemia develops with pain at rest.

The most common sites of atherosclerosis obliterans are the femoropopliteal arterial segment and the aortoiliac vessels, causing pain in the calves and buttocks, respectively. With progression of the disease, gangrene, ischemic ulcers, and trophic changes can occur in the more distal locations, namely the distal foot and toes. Ischemic ulcers can occur spontaneously; however, trauma is usually the inciting event leading to ulcer formation. The injury is unable to heal due to poor perfusion. Trophic changes, specifically dry scaly skin, loss of hair, and thick nails are also a sign of arterial insufficiency.

Conservative therapy for treatment of intermittent claudication includes smoking cessation and the control of contributing diseases such as hypertension, diabetes, and hyperlipidemia. Protective and prophylactic care of the feet including good hygiene, avoidance of trauma, pressure points, and poorly fitting shoes is imperative to prevent ischemic ulceration and gangrene. Keeping the feet clean, dry and free of infection is also important. In spite of these measures to slow the progression of atherosclerotic occlusive disease, 25% to 50% of patients will require more aggressive treatment

Ischemic pain is described as an achy and crampy sensation that is worse at night and improves when the legs are in a dependent position, which improves blood flow. When rest pain occurs, the degree of vascular insufficiency is severe and these patients are also at increased risk for diffuse atherosclerotic disease of the coronary and cerebral arteries. The differential diagnosis for intermittent claudication is shown in Table 51-1.

Atherosclerotic occlusive disease of the lower extremities can lead to intermittent claudication, ischemic pain at rest, tissue necrosis, and gangrene. In most cases, vascular reconstruction procedures are the treatment of choice. In approximately 10% to 20% of patients, revascularization procedures are not technically feasible or fail secondary to poor outflow. For patients who are not surgical candidates, pain control, tissue salvage, and maintenance of an independent lifestyle are important issues. Unfortunately, limb amputation, which may have a high perioperative mortality, may be the ultimate treatment in some of these patients.

Several noninvasive therapies are in use to treat peripheral vascular disease including antiplatelet, antithrombotic, and fibrinolytic therapies. If a patient has an underlying hereditary predisposition to a hypercoagulable disorder, this should be evaluated and treated first. The most commonly used agents are aspirin, dipyridamole, and sulfinpyrazone. Although aspirin has been shown to be useful in decreasing the incidence of thrombosis in coronary artery disease, the effectiveness of this and other antiplatelet drugs has not been clearly demonstrated for peripheral vascular disease. The fibrinolytic agents urokinase, streptokinase and tissue plasminogen activator have been tested and used extensively for the treatment of acute myocardial infarction. Their efficacy for arterial insufficiency in peripheral vascular disease has not been proven, and may be related to the fact that peripheral vascular disease is not an acute process, but rather a slow and insidious process.

Over recent years, the success and efficacy of percutaneous transluminal angioplasty (PTA) has increased the number of patients treated for occlusive arterial disease who were not surgical candidates because of concomitant disease processes and substantial risk factors associated with surgery. PTA is a minimally invasive procedure that has fewer associated costs, shorter hospital stays, and fewer risks to the patient. The primary concern with PTA of the lower extremities is the long-term patency of the vessel.

Long-term success of iliac artery PTA is dependent on certain predictors as shown in Table 51-2. The early success rate of PTA for the iliac arteries ranges from 90% to 99% patency with a 2-year patency rate of 80% to 95%. Angioplasty for femoropopliteal disease has a 2-year patency rate of 89% and a 4-year rate of 67%. These data indicate that PTA is a valuable and durable alternative to surgical revascularization.

Operative management is still the ultimate therapy if other more conservative efforts fail. Ischemic pain at rest, and not intermittent claudication alone, is the primary indication for surgical intervention. Ischemic rest pain may lead to tissue or limb loss in 20% of patients if untreated. Only 5% of patients with intermittent claudication will require amputation if untreated. In the past, chemical lumbar sympathectomy followed by surgical sympathectomy was widely used for treatment of peripheral vascular disease. Currently, the primary operative interventions are arterial bypass surgery us-

TABLE 51-1 **Differential Diagnosis for Intermittent Claudication**

1. Atherosclerosis obliterans
2. Thromboangiitis obliterans
3. Acute arterial embolism
4. Entrapment syndrome
5. Acute deep venous occlusion
6. Lumbar spinal stenosis
7. Osteoarthritis of the hip and back

ing the saphenous vein or polytetrafluoroethylene grafts and endarterectomy with patch graft.

A large body of evidence now exists supporting the use of epidural spinal cord stimulation (SCS) in the treatment of limb-threatening peripheral vascular disease as well as for intractable angina pectoris. SCS may be a satisfactory alternative to operative revascularization and PTA since the specific anatomy of the arterial stenosis or occlusion is irrelevant. Many patients who were previously not candidates for any type of intervention or who had failed with other therapies may have significant relief of their ischemic symptoms with a SCS device. Since SCS is a minimally invasive procedure and is placed percutaneously under local anesthesia, there are few risks to the patient.

Spinal cord stimulation was first used by Shealy and coworkers in 1967.[1] Early trials were plagued by equipment failures and malfunctions such as lead fracture and electrode movement. Patient selection was also poor since the specific mechanism of analgesia produced by spinal cord stimulation was and still is elusive. SCS was utilized in virtually any patient regardless of the etiology of their pain. The increase in the success rate of spinal cord stimulation over the ensuing years is a result of the combination of improved technology and better patient selection.

In the 1970s Cook et al were using SCS to treat pain in patients with multiple sclerosis and noted that these patients had a significant improvement in lower extremity blood flow and a feeling of warmth in their lower extremities.[2] Further studies showed clinical improvement in pain, microcirculation, and healing of ischemic ulcers in patients with inoperable peripheral vascular disease. Claudication distance, temperature, limb salvage rates, and exercise tolerance were substantially improved. Relief of ischemic pain appears to correlate well with an increase in microcirculatory changes and success rates of 70% to 100% pain relief are common. Macrocirculatory changes do not appear to correlate well with relief of symptoms.

The most common use for spinal cord stimulation in the United States is for back pain with a predominant radicular component. The indications that may have the highest success rates are inoperable angina pectoris, peripheral vascular disease, and complex regional pain syndrome. There is much theory and speculation regarding the physiologic mechanism by which spinal cord stimulation improves symptoms from arterial insufficiency. In general, most researchers concur that relief of ischemic pain is the result of improved microcirculation, since in most studies measurements of macrocirculation were not reliable predictors of long-term success.

Macrocirculatory arterial flow is measured by a variety of noninvasive techniques including segmental pressures, ankle-brachial indices, systolic toe pressures, and duplex scanning. Segmental pressures use a cuff to measure systolic pressures at two different levels of the limb and normally there should be <20 mm Hg difference in any two pressures. The ankle-brachial index, expressed as a percentage, measures the systolic ankle pressure and divides it by the brachial artery systolic pressure. The normal value is 1.0% to 1.2%. The systolic toe pressure should be 80% to 90 % of the brachial artery pressure. Duplex scanning is a combination of ultrasonic imaging of the underlying blood vessel with the capability of estimating velocity changes at different sites and evaluating distal arterial waveform morphology.

The changes that occur during SCS are primarily to the microcirculation or nutritional blood flow. The two techniques used most frequently to measure microcirulatory changes after SCS are transcutaneous oximetry and capillary microscopy. Transcutaneous oximetry measures the oxygen diffusing from the skin ($TcPO_2$). Skin blood flow is determined by the patency of proximal arteries and $TcPO_2$ approaches arterial PO_2 when O_2 delivery is high relative to consumption. $TcPO_2$ will be low when O_2 delivery is low compared with O_2 consumption. Capillary microscopy is used to measure capillary diameter, red blood count (RBC) velocity, peak RBC velocity after a 1-minute occlusion, time-to-peak RBC velocity, and the density of perfused capillaries.

The Fontaine classification of peripheral vascular disease, as shown in Table 51-3, can be used to determine which patients may benefit most from SCS. Studies have shown that patients in the Fontaine class III are the most likely patients to benefit from SCS. Those patients with only intermittent claudication do respond to SCS but not to the same degree as class III patients. Patients that are already experiencing tissue loss may have pain relief from SCS, but the overall limb salvage for the class IV patient is poor.

In a study by Jacobs et al, 20 patients with inoperable ischemic rest pain were evaluated for macro- and microcirculatory changes before and after SCS.[3] These patients had failed other therapies and were not candidates for any further surgical interventions. The macrocirculatory parameters of ankle-brachial index and systolic toe pressure did not change after the SCS procedure. The microcirculatory parameters measured in this study showed dramatic improvements that were statistically significant. Although the diameter of the capillaries did not increase, RBC velocity and peak RBC

TABLE 51-2 **Predictors of Success of Percutaneous Transluminal Angioplasty (PTA)**

1. Site of PTA
2. Indication for PTA (claudication versus limb salvage)
3. Severity of the lesion (stenosis was better than occlusion)
4. Presence of runoff vessels

TABLE 51-3 **Fontaine Classification of Peripheral Vascular Disease**

Class I.	No symptoms
Class II.	Intermittent claudication
Class III.	Rest and night pain without tissue involvement
Class IV.	Grade III plus tissue loss (ulcers, gangrene)

velocity improved within 24 hours of SCS. The long-term limb salvage was 80% at 1 year and 56% at 2 years. The mean hospital stay for patients with SCS implants was 16 days, and for patients with amputations, 91 days.

Positive prognostic factors for success of SCS for peripheral vascular disease in this study included good immediate pain relief after the SCS procedure and for Fontaine class III patients. Patients with existing tissue loss had poorer response to SCS. For patients with gangrene and ischemic ulcers of >3 cm diameter, the limb-saving effect of SCS is minimal. Patients who had no immediate relief of their pain and those who had recurrence of their pain had poorer outcomes and required amputation.

A recent study by Kumar et al included 46 patients with severe limb-threatening ischemia.[4] This study found a significant increase in RBC velocity after 24 hours of SCS. An increase in peak flow velocity of at least 10 cm/second at the level of the common femoral artery was shown to correlate with good long-term success. This study also found that the combination of at least a 75% decrease in pain and an increase of $TcPO_2$ of 10 mm after SCS, when compared with baseline values, were also good predictors of long-term success.

Increases in capillary density, capillary RBC velocity after occlusion, and a decrease in time to peak RBC velocity correlate with a decrease in ischemic pain. Measures of macrocirculation such as ankle-brachial index and systolic toe pressures do not change significantly and do not correlate with long-term success of the SCS procedure.

The actual mechanism of how SCS improves microcirculation is not well understood. There are some theories that postulate that SCS works through inhibition of preganglionic sympathetic activity. This would imply that SCS decreases, or inhibits, the maladaptive responses that occur in the microvasculature distal to an occlusion. Changes in preganglionic autonomic activity is thought to be responsible for the changes seen in ischemic disease. However, if this were the case, then patients who have had either a surgical or chemical sympathectomy would not respond to SCS. In actuality these patients do respond with the microvascular changes previously mentioned. In general, it appears that SCS alters sympathetic outflow, but whether these changes are mediated by a central or peripheral mechanism is unknown. The actual neurohumoral changes that occur with SCS are also poorly understood. There is general agreement that a decrease in ischemic pain correlates well with improved microcirculation after SCS, but is the decreased pain a result of improved circulation or is circulation improved because SCS has relieved pain and lessened the autonomic response to the pain. More research is needed to better understand the underlying mechanisms of SCS.

Angina pectoris is a syndrome that results from an imbalance in myocardial oxygen consumption and myocardial oxygen supply. The disease process can produce severe incapacitating pain, or pressure in the chest, arms, neck, or jaw. Atherosclerotic coronary artery disease is one of the leading causes of morbidity and mortality in westernized countries. The arteries that are most commonly affected by atherosclerosis are the large epicardial arteries; however small vessel disease may also contribute to the overall clinical picture. Atherosclerosis may affect a single vessel and cause a discrete lesion, or it may affect multiple vessels diffusely. There appears to be no correlation between the severity of anginal pain and the severity of atherosclerosis. A single lesion in the left artery descending may produce extreme pain and disability, whereas multiple diffuse lesions affecting several vessels may only produce mild to moderate anginal symptoms or complete absence of symptoms.

Antianginal therapies have focused on decreasing myocardial oxygen consumption while increasing oxygen delivery in an effort to restore the natural balance between supply and demand. The long-term goals of antianginal therapy are to decrease the frequency of anginal attacks, reduce the severity of the attacks, and to prevent the ischemic event from progressing to myocardial damage. Control of anginal symptoms not only preserves the independence and lifestyle of patients, but also improves their long-term prognosis.

Treatment for atherosclerotic coronary artery disease has focused on drug therapy, catheter-based revascularization techniques, surgical revascularization, and more recently, transmyocardial laser revascularization and spinal cord stimulation. The mainstay of pharmacologic treatment has been nitrates, beta-adrenergic blockers, and calcium channel blockers. Beta blockers decrease myocardial oxygen demand and oxygen consumption by decreasing ventricular wall tension, heart rate, and myocardial ionotropic state. Calcium channel blockers work by inhibiting the reuptake of calcium in slow calcium channels, thereby producing vasodilatation. This vasodilatory effect works to increase coronary artery perfusion and oxygen supply. This vasodilation also decreases afterload and increases cardiac output and in effect reduces cardiac work. Nitroglycerin acts as a vasodilator also, and it not only dilates coronary arteries but reduces afterload and preload secondary to its venous pooling effects. Nitrates and the calcium channel blockers both relieve vasospasm, which may contribute to ischemic attacks. These drugs may also be used for patients who have anginal pain but no objective signs of ischemia and normal coronary arteriograms. This syndrome, known as syndrome X, may be the result of small vessel disease and/or coronary vasospasm.

Most patients with atherosclerotic coronary artery disease and anginal pain respond to the medical therapies previously mentioned; however, for those that still have pain and decreased function because of their pain, more aggressive therapies are needed. One new therapy is long-term intermittent urokinase therapy. Urokinase activates circulating and bound plasminogen, which is converted to plasmin. Plasmin degrades fibrin, producing thrombolysis and improving blood rheology. Urokinase may also initiate regression of coronary plaques. The therapy is begun in the hospital with intravenous doses of urokinase three times per week. Once target fibrinogen levels are reached, the patient is discharged to home and the therapy is continued for a total of 12 weeks. Some patients have shown a 70% reduction in anginal attacks with a 20% improvement in exercise tolerance. Patients' symptoms improve for approximately 3 months after the termination of treatment.

More invasive techniques for anginal pain include revascularization procedures such as surgical coronary artery bypass grafting (CABG) and percutaneous transluminal coronary angioplasty (PTCA). The first successful PTCA was performed in 1977, and since then the success rate and the indications for its use have expanded. The current indications for PTCA can be found in Table 51-4. Originally, it was felt that the actual mechanism of PTCA was that the balloon compressed the plaque and caused dilatation or aneurysm formation in the stenosed vessel. Now it is known that the pressure created by the balloon fractures the plaque, and releases the deeper medial and adventitial layers that were previously trapped in the plaque. Once released from the plaque, the vessel wall has improved compliance.

The advantages of PTCA for anginal pain are similar to those for peripheral vascular disease. It is less invasive than surgery, hospital stay is shorter, the procedure can be repeated multiple times, and patients who were not candidates for CABG because of con-

TABLE 51-4 **Indications for Percutaneous Transluminal Coronary Angioplasty**

1. Unstable angina pectoris
2. Acute myocardial infarction
3. Multivessel disease
4. Saphenous vein bypass graft stenosis
5. Acute complete coronary artery occlusion

current diseases may be candidates for a less invasive procedure because the risks are less.

PTCA requires certain anatomical considerations for the procedure to be successful. The lesion should be focal, concentric, proximal, noncalcified, and located on a relatively straight portion of the artery. The long-term restenosis rate is better if the vessel is at least 2.5 mm in diameter, the lesion is at least 50% occlusive, and the occlusion is a focal and not a diffuse stenosis. The complications of PTCA include acute perforation, rupture, total occlusion, dissection, and embolization. The most common complication is acute occlusion at the site of PTCA, which may require emergent CABG. The long-term restenosis rates suggest that approximately 30% of patients will have a return of their symptoms with restenosis in the first 6 months after PTCA. Approximately 70% of patients will have no return of their symptoms at 6 months, and most of these patients will be symptom-free at 5 to 7 years. These success rates refer to single vessel PTCA. Patients with multivessel PTCA have higher long-term restenosis rates and have increased risks associated with PTCA.

The most recent technique in cardiac revascularization is transmyocardial laser revascularization, (TMLR). This technique is based on the fact that myocardial perfusion comes from not only the epicardial arteries but also from ventriculocoronary anastomosis. The technique of artificially creating transmyocardial channels is not new, and was first performed in 1967. The interest in this technique waned because of the advent of CABG and because the channels produced mechanically tended to fibrose and occlude. The development of laser technology has made TMLR a viable technique. The technique uses a carbon dioxide laser to penetrate the myocardium in 50-millisecond discharges. The procedure is done through a thoracotomy incision and can be completed in approximately 2 to 3 hours. The surgeon makes approximately 40 transmyocardial channels that are confirmed using intraoperative transesophageal echocardiography. There is no need for cardiopulmonary bypass to perform the procedure, and the laser portion of the operation may take as little as 15 minutes. The epicardial portion of the 1-mm channel closes almost immediately with compression. The endocardial portion of the channel remains patent. The CO_2 laser vaporizes tissue with minimal thermal damage, which contributes to the long-term success of the treatment. In 1997 the results of an FDA-approved multicenter trial of TMLR showed improvement of symptoms in approximately 79% of patients at 12 months, and approximately 30% of patients were completely symptom-free at 12 months after TMLR. The advantage of this technique over other revascularization procedures is that there are no coronary artery anatomical constraints and patients who were not candidates for CABG or PTCA because of the specific anatomy of their coronary artery lesions may now be candidates for TMLR.

Spinal cord stimulation (SCS), as mentioned earlier, has been used for the treatment of various pain syndromes.[5] Over the past 10 years, SCS has been found to have efficacy in the treatment of intractable angina pectoris in patients refractory to medical therapy who are not candidates for further revascularization procedures. The mechanism by which SCS relieves anginal pain is a subject of much speculation. Various theories suggest that SCS works through a spinothalamic mechanism, which may inhibit neuronal transmission at a segmental level. It is possible that SCS inhibits sympathetic outflow and decreases circulating levels of epinephrine and this in turn reduces cardiac work load and myocardial oxygen consumption. The sympatholytic effect may act directly or indirectly through stimulation of large dorsal column nerve fibers, which inhibit the smaller pain-transmitting fibers. Perhaps the most interesting theory was postulated through the use of positron emission tomography. A recent study evaluating angina patients 6 weeks after SCS showed that patients had no increase in overall myocardial perfusion.[6] There was, however, increased perfusion in previously ischemic regions. This would imply that SCS redistributed microvascular perfusion from non-ischemic areas of the myocardium to ischemic areas.

When SCS was first introduced for anginal pain, it was feared that SCS was merely abolishing nociceptive input and not affecting myocardial oxygen demand or supply. If this were the case, then SCS would obscure or conceal the warning sign of ischemia, namely anginal pain, and not affect the underlying cause of the ischemia. This is not the case and, in fact, SCS seems to work by improving myocardial function through a poorly understood mechanism that decreases myocardial oxygen consumption. Several studies have shown that SCS increases tolerance to pacing, myocardial lactate metabolism, and decreases the duration and magnitude of ST changes during maximal pacing with SCS.[7]

Mannheimer et al looked at the effects of SCS in 20 patients who were on maximal medical therapy and who were not candidates for revascularization procedures.[8] These patients had angina and ST depression during a bicycle ergometry test performed prior to the start of the SCS trial. The investigators used coronary sinus pacing and blood samples to determine the effects of SCS on the parameters of lactate production and coronary sinus blood flow. The investigators evaluated the parameters of coronary sinus blood flow, lactate metabolism, rate pressure product, time to angina, time to ST segment depression, recovery time from angina, and ST segment depression. They measured these parameters before and during the SCS procedure. The results of this study showed that all parameters including tolerance to pacing, time to angina, time to ST segment depression, lactate metabolism, and rate-pressure product improved during SCS. In addition, recovery time from angina and ST segment depression was decreased. Perhaps the most important outcome of this study was that at a maximum pacing rate, all patients experienced anginal pain and ST segment depression comparable to ST segment changes seen in the control. Therefore, SCS not only increases cardiac function, perhaps by decreasing myocardial oxygen consumption, but when there was myocardial ischemia, SCS did not prevent patients from having angina and ST segment depression.

A thorough knowledge of ischemic disease is necessary in order to provide care for these patients. The development of SCS as an option for pain specialists now enables us to render effective and relatively low-risk treatment to these patients that was not previously available. SCS for both peripheral vascular and coronary artery disease is efficacious and has been critically investigated with proven and predictable results and complications.

REFERENCES

1. Shealy CN, Mortimer JT, Resnick, JB. Electrical inhibition of pain by stimulation of the dorsal columns; preliminary clinical report. *Anesth Analg* 1967;46;489.
2. Cook AW, Oygar A, Baggenstos P, et al. Vascular disease of extremities: electrical stimulation of spinal cord and posterior roots. *N Y State J Med* 1976;76;366.
3. Jacobs MJHM, Jorning PJG, Beckers RCY, et al. Foot salvage and improvement of microvascular blood flow as a result of epidural spinal cord electrical stimulation. *J Vasc Surg* 1990;12:354.
4. Kumar K, Toth C, Nath R. Improvement of limb circulation in peripheral vascular disease using epidural spinal cord stimulation: a prospective study. *J Neurosurg* 1997;86:662.
5. Simpson BA. Spinal cord stimulation. *Pain Rev* 1994;1:199.
6. Eliasson T, Augustinsson LE, Mannheimer C. Spinal cord stimulation in severe angina pectoris—presentation of current studies, indications and clinical experience. *Pain* 1996;65:169.
7. Schoebel FC, Frazier OH, Jessurun GAJ, et al. Refractory angina pectoris in end-stage coronary artery disease; evolving therapeutic concepts. *Am Heart J* 1997;134:587.
8. Mannheimer C, Eliasson T, Anderson B, et al. Effects of spinal cord stimulation in angina pectoris induced by pacing and possible mechanisms of actions. *BMJ* 1993;307:477.

CHAPTER 52 SICKLE CELL DISEASE

Natalie Moryl and Richard Payne

INTRODUCTION

Sickle cell disease is one of the most prevalent single gene disorders, affecting over 50,000 Americans. Sickle cell disease is a debilitating condition that is associated with chronic anemia, stroke, splenic and renal dysfunction, susceptibility to bacterial infections, particularly in children, acute chest syndrome, and pain crises. Each year in the US, an average of 75,000 hospitalizations are due to sickle cell disease, costing approximately $475 million. Athough tremendous resources have been invested in looking for a cure and palliative care, the management of acute and chronic pain remains the major intervention, focusing on improving quality of life and decreasing morbidity. In spite of some decrease in mortality in children with sickle cell disease over the last 25 years, median life expectancy for most sickle cell patients remains below age 50 years. Pain, the most frequent symptom experienced by the patients with sickle cell anemia, profoundly impairs patient function at home and work, their social interactions, and their careers. Despite the high prevalence of pain episodes, correlating with morbility and mortality, sickle cell anemia pain remains underestimated and undertreated. There are still multiple misconceptions regarding the use of pain medications, including opioids, tolerance, and addiction.

This review discusses the importance of pain assessment and control in the treatment of patients with sickle cell anemia. The importance of a comprehensive interdisciplinary approach to therapy, including medications, psychological, spiritual and social support, education, as well as availability of the comprehensive support system, is emphasized.

CASE PRESENTATION

The following case illustrates complexity of the management of sickle cell anemia patients.

JF is 21-year-old Hispanic man, admitted to the hospital with severe pain in the legs, shoulders, chest, and abdomen of 2 to 3 days' duration.

History of Present Illness

The patient's condition was diagnosed as hemoglobin SS sickle cell anemia shortly after birth. Severe pain, requiring hospitalizations, has been recurrent for years and most recently has occurred 4 to 5 times a month, lasting from 3 to 4 days to 2 weeks. The patient has developed hemachromatosis, autosplenectomy, hepatomegaly, ascites, left lower leg ulcer, chronic renal failure requiring hemodialysis, and seizures as complications of the disease. At home, pain crises were managed with fentanyl patch 75 mg transdermally every 48 hours, hydromorphone 4 mg orally every 4 to 6 hours as needed, amitriptyline 25 mg orally daily, and diphenhydramine 25 mg orally as needed. When an inpatient, JF was treated with meperidine up to 100 mg intravenously as needed, methadone 10 mg orally every 4 hours, fentanyl patch and hydromorphone intravenously via patient-controlled analgesia (PCA). Clinicians were concerned about his attention-seeking behavior, opioid dependence, preoccupation with his pain, and his withdrawal from social activities. Patient was seen in the Emergency room 3–4 times a month and was frequently admitted to the hospital with pain crises. Opioid analgesics were continued according to the standard protocol at the constant dose in spite of the patient's report of poor pain control and frequent requests to increase the opioid analgesics. At the time of discharge the opioids were changed to oral formulations with significant dose reduction. Patient often reported anxiety, dysphoria and escalation of pain hours after discharge. Continuous pain and agitation after leaving the hospital were managed intermittently by haloperidol, lorazepam, and amiytriptyline.

Physical Examination

The patient was alert, oriented to person, place and time, anxious, and in distress due to pain. Heart rate was 116 beats per minute, blood pressure 110/70 mm Hg, respiratory rate 22/minute, oxygen saturation 97% on room air. His skin was pale. Head, eyes, ears, nose, and throat were unremarkable, except for mild icterus of sclera. Respiratory system: good air entry bilaterally, lungs clear to auscultation. Cardiovascular system: S1, S2 regular, no gallop, and no murmur. Abdomen: distended, moderately tender, no rebound effect, bowel sounds present, present fluid wave liver span 14 cm in midclavicular line, and spleen not palpable. Genitalia: unremarkable. Rectal examination: normal, guaiac test negative for occult blood. Neurologic examination: cranial nerves, motor, sensory examinaton, and reflexes were within normal limits. Routine laboratory studies were done. Of note, hemoglobin 7.9 g/dL, potassium 6.6 mEq/L, BUN 75 mg/dL, creatinine 6.3 mg/dL.

Inpatient Course

In the hospital the patient was treated with Meperidine 75 mg with Hydroxyzine 25 mg every 3 hours, folic acid, hemodialysis, and vitamins. The patient was requesting Meperidene every 2.5 to 3 hours, but was denied earlier than scheduled drug administration. The patient was anxious, angry, or tearful. Behavior was viewed as Opioid dependence and addiction. Placebo was given with good effect. Methadone, Hydromorphone, and Meperidine were given intermittently as needed. Renal failure was progressing, as well as ascites, requiring at this point repeated therapeutic abdominal taps. The patient developed generalized seizure, was transferred to ICU, and started on Phenytoin. Meperidine was continued. In a few days the patient was found unresponsive, and died despite resuscitation.

Case Discussion

"Review of pain management used in this case reveals many common errors: inadequate titration of opioids to pain relief; sudden changes in medications without adjusting the dose for equianalgesic potency; and opioid administration "as-needed" as opposed to around the clock. The use of placebos in this setting should be regarded as unethical and clinical practice guidelines in pain management condemned this practice".[1–3]

Use of Demerol, a traditionally widely used opioid, shown to be associated with serious adverse side effects and should not be used for long term use, especially in patients with seizure disorder and renal insufficiency.

Failure to recognize the nature of pseudo addiction seemed to preclude the appropriate dose escalation. Rapid dose reduction on the day of discharge likely also contributed to pseudo addiction.

Clearly medical staff, social services, and the family shared the common goal of providing adequate and appropriate symptom control, including state of the art pain management for this patient. Failure to achieve this goal demonstrates the need of further education and research, proper utilization of already obtained knowledge, and value of team approach in securing 24 hours a day 7 days a week medical care and social support for patients with sickle cell disease, so far remaining debilitating and in most cases incurable.

Finally, availability and convenience of specialized sickle cell anemia centers for both the pediatric population and adults becomes very important in determining the quality of life and prognosis.

HISTORICAL PROSPECTIVES

Sickle cell disease was first identified in the United States in 1910, when sickle-shaped red blood cells were found in the blood of medical student from Africa.[4] Autosomal dominant inheritance was identified in 1923, and oxygen deprivation of tissues was shown to provoke sickling in 1927.[5] Single amino acid substitution of glutamic acid for valine in the sixth amino acid position of the B chain of hemoglobin was demonstrated to be responsible for physicochemical features of altered hemoglobin.[6] Later studies showed that both altered erythrocytes and endothelial cells express surface molecules that mediate intracellular adhesions, leading to polymerization of deoxygenated hemoglobin S and vaso-occlusion. Advances in basic and clinical research did not significantly change the outcomes for the patients until recently, when antibiotics, hydroxyurea, and bone marrow transplant were introduced. Bone marrow transplant, first performed in 1998, is currently available as a cure only for the selected group of patients.[7–10] Pain management and supportive care have been the cornerstones of the treatment of sickle cell disease since the time of its discovery and still remains the best intervention to reduce morbidity and improve the quality of life for the majority of the patients.

PREVALENCE

Sickle cell disease is widespread in Africa, the Middle East, Mediterranean countries, and India (Department of Health, 1993). Population migration spread it to northern Europe and North America. In some areas of the world, 20% to 40% of the population is homozygous recessive for sickle cell anemia. In the United States, 1 out of 25 black children is a carrier, and 1 out of 500 will develop sickle cell anemia.[11]

PROGNOSIS

The morbidity and mortality of sickle cell anemia result from vaso-occlusion of the microvasculature by sickle cells in multiple organ systems, as well as accelerated hemolysis, anemia, and infection.[12] Early death is associated with acute chest syndrome, renal failure, seizures, persistent leukocytosis, and depressed Hb F levels.[12] The most common cause of death is pulmonary complications, cerebrovascular accidents, causes related to infection, and acute splenic sequestration.

One third of all deaths occurs during vaso-occlusive crisis in the absence of otherwise life-threatening organ failure, whereas only one fifth of all deaths occurred as a result of subacute or chronic organ failure, usually renal or hepatic.[12] Mortality correlates with the frequency of pain crises. Frequency of pain episodes is highly variable: 60% of patients required hospitalization at least once a year, 1% required 6 or more hospital admissions per year.[13]

Only half of adult patients with more than three vaso-occlusive crises per year survive to age 40, whereas patients with fewer than one episode per year will have a 50% chance of survival to age of 55.[12] Median life expectancy for people with homozygous sickle cell anemia is still significantly shortened as compared to the average lifespan: 42 years for men and 48 years for women.[12,14]

MANAGEMENT OF SICKLE CELL DISEASE

Routine management of vaso-occlusive crisis includes hydration, oxygen inhalation, and analgesics. Lately, intravenous hydration and oxygen supplementation have been questioned, as these indices were not found consistently effective in large controlled trials. Corticosteroids remain a controversial modality because these agents were shown to shorten the duration of analgesia requirement, but after discontinuation, led to more episodes of recurrent pain.[15]

Disease-modifying treatment modalities include hydroxyurea, bone marrow transplantation, and gene therapy, most of which are still under investigation and not accessible for most patients. In a randomized, double blind, placebo-controlled study among 299 patients with three or more pain crises a year, hydroxyurea caused a significant reduction in the incidence of both pain crises and acute chest syndrome by increasing Hb F to 20 % and above.[16] Taking hydroxyurea was associated with a 40% reduction in mortality in an observational study with self-selected treatment.[17]

For the most severely affected, bone marrow transplantation and gene therapy are possible options. Bone marrow transplantation was reported to produce good results: cure in young patients with severe sickle cell disease and 90% to 95% survival.[18,19] HLA-matching siblings receive an allogenic bone marrow transplant (BMT) after pretreatment with busulphan cyclophosphamide and antithymocyte globulin. Results of the clinical trials are exciting, but groups are small; children were chosen with clinically advanced disease to justify the risks of bone marrow transplantation. Outcome data of the clinical trials in the United States, Belgium, and France are now available on 136 patients with sickle cell disease who received allogenic HLA-matched BMT.[7,20]

In the United States a multicenter study involved 50 children with severe sickle cell disease. Between 1991 and 1999, children received transplants from HLA-identical siblings after receiving treatment with busulfan, Cyclophosphamide, and antithymocyte globulin conditioning. The actuarial survival was 93% and event-free survival was 82%. Out of 50 patients, 5 patients had graft rejection, 3 died, 2 still exhibited stable-mixed chimerism, and 40 patients had full engraftment. The patients with complete engraftment displayed no symptoms of sickle cell disease after the transplant. Seizures were the most common complications (21% of the patients).

Similar results were obtained in France, where survival and event-free survival were 92% and 75%, respectively.

In Belgium, 50 children received allogenic BMT from HLA-identical siblings or parents after undergoing conditioning with busulfan, Cyclophosphamide, and antithymocyte globulin or total lymphoid irradiation. The outcome was similar to the US study: 96% survival, 86% event-free survival, and 10% graft failure or graft rejection. Of note, in 16 patients who underwent BMT for moderate sickle cell anemia without any significant organ damage or history of long-term transfusions (except for 1 patient) both survival and event-free survival were 100%. No deaths were registered in this group, and the second transplant successfully corrected the only marrow rejection.

Early BMT may offer the obvious advantages. This conclusion correlates with thalassemia studies with much larger numbers of patients. However, sickle cell anemia appears to pose an additional challenge with prognostication: it is impossible to select the individuals with potentially severe sickle cell anemia early on. Accurate predictors of future severity of sickle cell anemia on case-by-case basis are lacking. The role of early transplantation for the reversible complications of sickle cell disease needs to be defined. Thus, the generalization of the results to a larger population is less clear.[21] One of the alternative modalities is plasma exchange.[22]

Gene therapy is under development. Genetic advances enriched pathophysiologic insight and new prospective for the treatment of sickle cell anemia. Gene therapy, however, is far from reality yet.

Even though the genetic mechanisms of sickle cell anemia are well defined, it has been difficult to develop gene therapy because globin gene expression is highly regulated and may be significantly altered after the transfer of the normal adult β-globin gene is completed. Success of gene therapy in sickle cell disease would also depend on the ability to neutralize the effects of already sickled hemoglobin (Hb S, *alpha*$2\beta 2$S).

Using chimeraplasts to replace a single or a few mutant nucleotides constitutes a new technology in gene therapy; however, it failed to correct genetic defects in primary human hematopoietic cells. Stimulation of postnatal overproduction of Hb F is well known approach to the gene therapy of sickle cell disease. It is considered to be a promising therapeutic strategy. Different mouse models for the studying of sickle cell disease have been explored. However, genetic variability of the patient population with sickle cell anemia makes it difficult to determine the level of Hb F needed to alleviate the symptoms of sickle cell anemia in each particular case.

Blood transfusion remains the most common form of disease modification by suppressing Hb S production.[23]

PAIN IN SICKLE CELL DISEASE

According to the International Association for the Study of Pain, pain is "an unpleasant sensory and emotional experience associated with actual or potential tissue damage."[2]

Pain is the reason for up to 90% of hospital admissions in a patient with sickle cell disease.[24] Pain rate is highest in patients between the ages of 19 and 39 year olds. Frequency of pain crises correlates with mortality of inpatients older than 20 years old. Pain was reported to be more severe than pain after major surgery. Typical crisis in an adult lasts for 10.3 days.[24]

Pain can be diffuse or localized. A variety of sites can be involved that determines the complexity of clinical presentation. Pain syndromes encountered in sickle cell anemia[25] are listed in Table 52-1.

In the study of 117 adults the distribution of pain sites is shown in Figure 52-1. Bone pain alone, or in combination with visceral sites of pain, is the most common clinical problem.[26]

Pain in sickle cell can be classified according to the time frame and continuity as chronic, acute, and recurrent pain, and severity and frequency of pain episodes. In general, about 20% of patients have pain only rarely, 60% have one or two episodes each year, and 20% have more than two episodes of pain per month and are considered severely affected.

Traditional classification of pain is based on extensive research of postsurgical and cancer pain (Table 52-2).

Pain of sickle cell disease is different in the way that tissue hypoxia, rather than direct tissue or nerve damage, is a mechanism of such pain.

A number of molecular biological studies regarding ischemic pain as a separate entity have been published. They bring a better understanding of ischemic pain and new treatment modalities. Since 1931 substance P has been considered to be responsible for ischemic pain, accumulating in the ischemic muscle and rapidly disappearing on restoration of blood supply. Since the work of Thomas Lewis it has been known that anoxia and its associated acidification produce the excruciating dull ache of angina. Known inflammatory and pain mediators, such as bradykinin, histamine, serotonin, and acetylcholine, potassium ions, and adenosine, participate in pain conduction disregarding the etiology of pain. Recent studies demonstrated that these mediators show tachyphylaxis of their excitatory action with time, whereas protons produce nonadapting excitation of nociceptors. A proton-gated channel that may be partially responsible for these acid signals has been cloned recently and named ASIC (acid-sensing ion channel).[27] ASIC is expressed in dorsal root ganglia and is also distributed widely throughout the brain. Ischemic muscle pain is thought to be mediated by protons, which could constitute the missing "factor P."[28]

PAIN ASSESSMENT GUIDELINES

1. Pain should become a routinely measurable vital sign, using a simple, preferably universal, scale.
2. Patient self-report should be the primary source of assessment, using behavioral cues in infants.
3. Pain should be frequently reassessed, evaluating and adjusting pain medications as necessary.
4. A comprehensive psychosocial assessment done by interdisciplinary team should be a part of the evaluation, with frequency dependent on the psychosocial conditions and support systems of the patient.
5. Any disparity between the patient's report and clinician's observation should be evaluated professionally, if needed with the help of multidisciplinary team, and until proven otherwise, the patient's self-report should be considered objective.

TABLE 52-1 **Pain Syndromes in Sickle Cell Anemia**

Pain Syndromes	Nature of Pain
Bone Pain	Results from avascular necrosis of bone marrow, which is presumed to cause increased intramedullary pressure as a consequence of the inflammatory response and repair process Osteomyelitis
Priapism	
Abdominal Pain	Splenic sequestration, enlarging spleen, which can cause heart failure and death Splenic infarctions, repetitive, autosplenectomy Mesenteric sickling and bowel ischemia Hepatic sequestration Cholecystitis
Chest Syndrome	One of the most common causes of death in adults, often presents with dyspnea, sickle pain in thoracic cage, hypoxia, and pulmonary consolidations with radiologic changes
Joint Pain	Joint swelling
Renal Papillary Necrosis	Present with renal colic with hematuria Renal failure
Hyphenia and Retinal Detachment	
Ductilities	Caused by avascular necrosis of the marrow, producing painful swelling in the dorsal surfaces of the hands and feet, usually before the age of 5
Skin	Ischemic leg ulceration
Central Nervous System	Ischemic or hemorrhagic stroke

TREATMENT OF PAIN

Pain management in sickle cell anemia follows stepwise ladder approach. It is important to remember that patients and families should be included in the discussion of treatment modalities. Such an approach reduces anxiety, increases compliance and self-efficacy, and puts the patient in charge.[26]

Non-narcotics, narcotics, and adjuvant analgesic drugs are used as a single drug or in combination to achieve pain relief.[29] Mild pain is usually treated at home, and NSAIDs are the first line of drugs.

Narcotic analgesics are usually used in severe pain or if non-narcotic regiment failed. Combinations of narcotic and non-narcotic agents are available; however, NSAIDs limit the amount of the drug that can be administered to the patient. Opioids on the other hand have no "ceiling effect."

Opioids differ in power, side effects, pharmacokinetics, and elimination of the drug and half-life.

Outpatient oral opioid therapy showed good results, improving pain control and reducing the rate of admissions. Sickle cell anemia day hospitals are attractive alternatives to hospital admissions and prolonged emergency room visits.[30] Within 4 years the emergency department admissions in one of the New York sickle cell anemia day hospitals were reduced by 40%. Patients self-referred for pain, screened, and treated in the day hospital required 5 times fewer admissions to the hospital as compared with a similar pa-

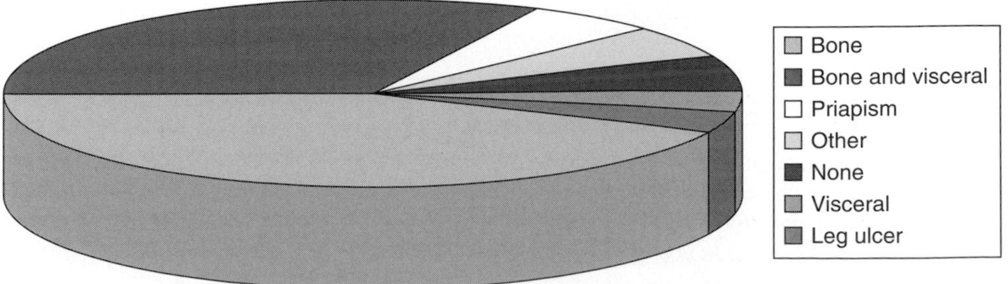

Figure 52-1 Distribution of pain symptoms among 117 adults with sickle cell anemia. (From Payne R. Pain Management in sickle cell anemia. Anesthesiol Clin North Am. 1997;15(2):305.)

TABLE 52-2 **Traditional Pain Classification Based on Cancer Pain**

Type of Pain	Pain Characteristics
Nociceptive	Pain resulting from the activation of nociceptors in somatic or visceral structures by potential tissue-damaging stimuli
Somatic nociceptive	Sharp, aching, throbbing, pressure-like
Visceral nociceptive	Poorly localized, growing or cramping, secondary to hollow viscus involvement, or aching or sharp, secondary to lesion of a capsule or mesentery
Neuropathic	Result of abnormal function of central or peripheral somatosensory systems: dysesthesia, allodynia, hyperalgesia, burning, or stabbing pain
Idiopathic	Not explained by organic pathology or psychological reasons

tient population with sickle-cell-anemia-related pain in the general emergency department. Length of stay for inpatients, followed by the day hospital staff, decreased by 1.5 days, which corresponded to a savings of $1.7 million.[30]

As in cancer pain, constant intravenous infusion appears to have better results as compared with intermittent dosing, and the best results were obtained using patient-controlled analgesia (PCA) via intravenous, which is preferable for most patients. One of the studies showed that inpatient intravenous, rapidly changed to oral morphine given at home, reduced the number of admissions by 44%, the total number of inpatient days decreased by 57%, the length of hospital stay decreased by 23%, and the number of repeat emergency department visits decreased by 67% (Figs. 52-2, 3, and 4). This study used treatment with intramuscular meperidine as a control.[29]

Meperidine given both as boluses and PCA was shown to be associated with seizures.[18,31] Factors increasing likelihood of seizures include renal failure, high meperidine dosage, and coadministration of hepatic enzyme-induced medications and phenothiazine. It is well known that one of the metabolites of meperidine, norperidine, is pharmacologically active, and has central nervous system excitatory properties. In 1992 the Agency for Health Care Policy and Research (AHCPR), a division of the US Department of Health and Human Services, published a clinical practice guideline for acute pain management, which stated that "because of its unique toxicity, meperidine is often contraindicated in patients with impaired renal function." Caution regarding the used of meperidine in patients with sickle cell disease has been reiterated in the most recent clinical practice guidelines.[32] In patients with normal renal function, norperidine has a half-life of 15 to 20 hours; this time is extended greatly in patients with impaired renal function. Norperidine is a cerebral irritant that can cause effects ranging from dysphoria and irritable mood to convulsions. In sickle cell disease with renal insufficiency and frequent necessity of high-dose administration of opioids, all forms of meperidine should be avoided for continuous use. Unfortunately, meperidine still remains the drug that is used frequently in sickle cell anemia.

BARRIERS TO PAIN MANAGEMENT IN SICKLE CELL DISEASE

Common misconceptions about dependence and addiction deserves mentioning.

1. Concern about addiction is still widespread among patients, families, and health care professionals. One should keep in mind, however, the difference between addiction and pseudoaddiction. In the setting of undertreated pain, some patients develop aberrant behavior that may be very similar to addiction.

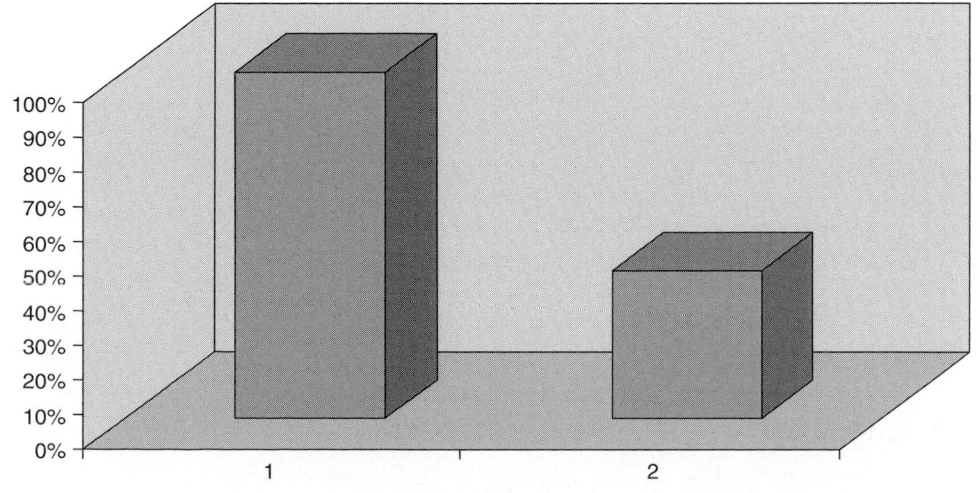

Figure 52-2 Comparison of number of inpatient days for patients in group 1 who were receiving Demerol and those in group 2 receiving intravenous/oral morphine.

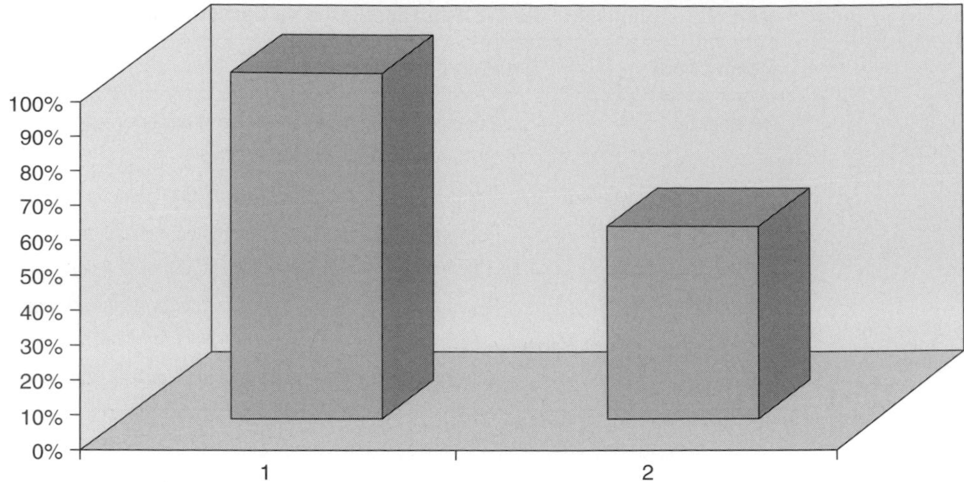

Figure 52-3 Number of admissions for group 1 patients receiving Dermerol and group 2 patients receiving intravenous/oral morphine.

However, when pain is relieved, behavior changes, thus supporting the contention that pain avoidance rather than drug-seeking activities is the major motivation for patient actions. Overestimated risk of adverse side effects and opioid addiction, combined with incomplete assessment of the patients as far as physical, psychological, social, and spiritual dimensions of pain are concerned, and failure to review the effectiveness of the opioid regimen and make appropriate dose adjustment, may lead to inadequate pain control, stimulating pseudoaddictive behavior. Literature data appears reassuring, reporting quite a low rate of addiction.

2. Cross-racial and cross-cultural communication difficulties between the often disabled patient who has both physical and social limitations and the usually highly functioning, often white, physician may reflect some of the societal conflicts.

3. Often needed rehabilitation, social, spiritual, vocational, and other nonpharmacologic interventions may be unavailable or unaffordable, or not covered by the insurance.

4. Clinicians' limited understanding of sickle cell anemia, pain syndrome and its management, leading to disbelief of pain complaints and insufficient analgesics prescriptions, commonly contribute to the challenge of sickle cell management.

SICKLE CELL, QUALITY OF LIFE, AND PALLIATIVE CARE

Palliative care is defined by the World Health Organization (WHO) as the active total care of patients whose disease is not responsive to curative treatment. Symptomatic therapy, including pain control, psychological, and social and spiritual support, is paramount. The goal of palliative care in sickle cell disease is achievement of the best quality of life for patients and their families.[33]

Since sickle cell anemia is a multisystem disorder, it presents with multiple symptoms and syndromes, which include anemia with associated symptoms, pain, and multiorgan dysfunction. The majority of patients depend on supportive care and blood transfusions as the main disease-modifying modality. At this time we are not able to alter the course and the prognosis of the disease for most patients.

Understanding of the pathophysiology of pain, and social and psychological aspects related to it, would augment the experience of using opioids and adjunctive therapy in treatment of acute and chronic pain. A team approach, including providing psychosocial support and psychiatric evaluation, are important because frequent pain episodes and low-family income, common in families with sickle cell disease, correlate with depression.[32] Continuity of care improves the outcome.[35,36] Besides medical and humanistic im-

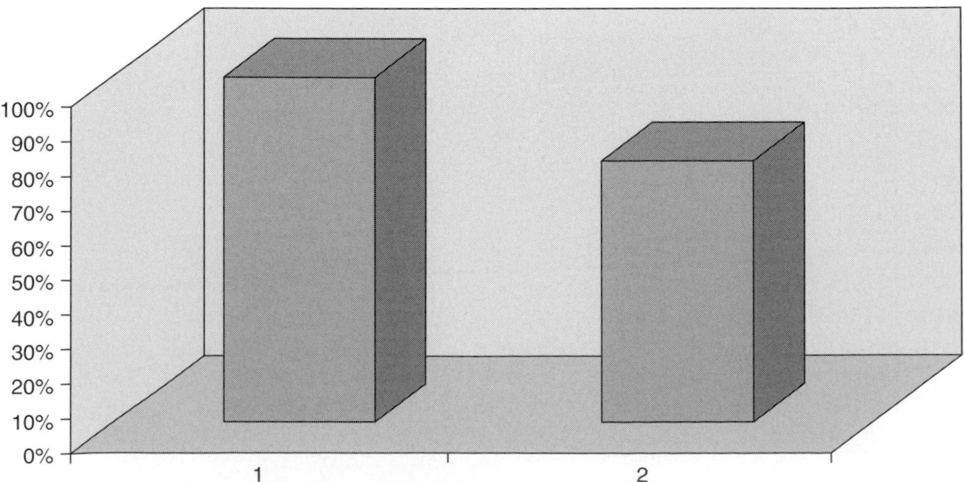

Figure 52-4 Comparison of length of stay of hospital patients for patients in group 1 receiving Dermerol and those in group 2 receiving intravenous/oral morphine.

portance, pain-related disability carries a substantial financial burden on the society. The estimated direct cost per hospitalization is \$6300, or \$475 million per year.[37]

Compared with pain in a patient with cancer pain, where pain starts to affect quality of life only in the end of disease progression, pain in sickle cell disease starts early in childhood and shapes the development of the personality. Pain crises rarely start before the age of 6 months, but after onset, pain has a profound effect on the patient's life, including limitations of physical activity, physical dependence on pain medications, and psychological dependence on the people providing them. Such dependency typically corresponds with immature defense mechanisms, which further put an individual in a dependent position in society.[34] Average life expectancy is shorter in a homozygous patient than the expected 1.5 times. In addition, patients with sickle cell anemia and frequent pain crises and other manifestations of sickle cell disease often achieve less in their professional, social, and personal life. The main objective of care becomes palliative care and functional restoration, including the ability to work.

CONCLUSION

There are three major issues in the treatment of sickle cell anemia with frequent pain crises:

1. Medical: Improved medical knowledge concerning sickle cell disease and the modalities of treatment, including disease-modifying modalities, their availability, as well as pain management, and supportive care, is needed.
2. Social: Concern about addiction, drug-seeking behavior, withdrawal, and tolerance should not overcome concern about providing support and comfort, restoration of function in society, family, and work.
3. Financial: The reduction of pain-related disability that enables patients to return to work and to function in society would relieve a substantial financial burden on society, especially in view of the prevalence of the disease. Adequate pain control reduces hospital stay, doctors' visits, and so forth.

Wide distribution of the disease, marked reduction of lifespan, high morbidity, and adverse effects of chronic and recurrent pain on professional, social, and spiritual life to the extent of social isolation constitute the objective evidence of the need for large, controlled, prospective trials and future research.

REFERENCES

1. Jacox A, Carr DB, Payne R, et al. *Clinical Practice Guideline Number 9. Management of Cancer Pain*. Rockville, M: US Dept of Health and Human Services, Agency for Health Care Policy and Research; 1994.
2. Turk DC, Rudy TE. The robustness of an empirically derived taxonomy of chronic pain patients. *Pain* 1990;43:27.
3. American Society of Pain Management Nurses. *Use of Placebos for Pain Management*. Pensacola, Fla: ASPMN,1998, 2001.
4. Herrick JB. Peculiar elongated and sickle cell shaped corpuscles in a case of severe anemia. *Arch Intern Med* 1910;6:517.
5. Taliaferro WH. The inheritance of sickle-cell anemia in man. *Genetics* 1923;8:594.
6. Conley CL. Sickle-cell anemia: the first molecular disease. In: Wintrobe MM, ed. *Blood, Pure and Eloquent*. New York, NY: McGraw-Hill, 1980:317–319.
7. Walters MC, Storb R, Patience M, et al. Impact of bone marrow transplantation for symptomatic sickle cell disease: an interim report. Multicenter investigation of bone marrow transplantation for sickle cell disease. *Blood* 2000;95:1918.
8. Walters MC, Patience M, Leisenring W,et al. Barriers to bone marrow transplantation for sickle cell anemia. *Biol Blood Marrow Transplant* 1996;2:100.
9. Walters MC. Bone marrow transplantation for sickle cell disease: where do we go from here? *J Pediatr Hematol Oncol* 1999;21:467.
10. Wethers DL. Sickle cell disease in childhood: Part II. Diagnosis and treatment of major complications and recent advances in treatment. *Am Fam Physician* 2000;62:1309.
11. Sickle Cell Disease Guidline Panel. Sickle cell disease screening, diagnosis, management, and counseling in newborns and infants. Clinical Practice Guieline No. 6. AHCPR Pub. No. 93-0562. Rockville, MD: Agency for Health Care Policy and Research, Public Health Service, U.S. Department of Health and Human Services. April 1993.
12. Platt OS, Brambilla DJ, Rosse WF, et al. Mortality in sickle cell disease. Life expectancy and risk factors for early death. *N Engl J Med* 1994;330:1639.
13. Walters MC, Sullivan KM, Bernaudin F, et al. Neurologic complications after allogeneic marrow transplantation for sickle cell anemia. *Blood* 1995;85:879.
14. Wethers DL. Sickle cell disease in childhood: Part I. Laboratory diagnosis, pathophysiology and health maintenance. *Am Fam Physician* 2000;62:1013.
15. Griffin TC, McIntire D, Buchanan GR. High-dose intravenous methylprednisolone therapy for pain in children and adolescents with sickle cell disease. *N Engl J Med* 1994;330:733.
16. Charache S, Terrin ML, Moore RD, et al. Effect of hydroxyurea on the frequency of painful crises in sickle cell anemia. Investigators of the Multicenter Study of Hydroxyurea in Sickle Cell Anemia. *N Engl J Med* 1995;332:1317.
17. Steinberg MH, Barton F, Castro O, et al. Effect of hydroxyurea on mortality and morbidity in adult sickle cell anemia: risks and benefits up to 9 years of treatment. JAMA 2003;1645–1651.
18. Johnson FL, Mentzer WC, Kalinyak KA, et al. Bone marrow transplantation for sickle cell disease. The United States experience. *Am J Pediatr Hematol Oncol* 1994;16:22.
19. Davies SC, Bevan DH. Sickle cell pain crisis. *Lancet* 1996;347:263.
20. Mentzer WC, Kan YW. Prospects for research in hematologic disorders: sickle cell disease and thalassemia. *JAMA* 2001;285:640.
21. Reed W, Vichinsky EP. New considerations in the treatment of sickle cell disease. *Annu Rev Med* 1998;49:461.
22. Geigel EJ, Francis CW. Reversal of multiorgan system dysfunction in sickle cell disease with plasma exchange. *Acta Anaesthesiol Scand* 1997;41:647.
23. Davies SC, Roberts-Harewood M. Blood transfusion in sickle cell disease. *Blood Rev* 1997;11:57.
24. Brozovic M, Davies SC, Brownell AI. Acute admissions of patients with sickle cell disease who live in Britain. *Br Med J* 1987;294:1206.
25. Shapiro BS, Dinges DF, Orne EC, et al. Home management of sickle cell-related pain in children and adolescents: natural history and impact on school attendance. *Pain* 1995;61:139.
26. Payne R. Pain management in sickle cell anemia. *Anesthesiol Clin North Am* 1997;15(2):305.
27. Waldmann R, Bassilana F, de Weille J, et al. Molecular cloning of a non-inactivating proton-gated Na+ channel specific for sensory neurons. *J Biol Chem* 1997;272:20975.
28. Waldmann R, Champigny G, Bassilana F, et al. A proton-gated cation channel involved in acid-sensing. *Nature* 1997;386:173.
29. Brookoff D, Polomano R. Treating sickle cell pain like cancer pain. *Ann Intern Med* 1992;116:364.
30. Benjamin LJ, Swinson GI, Nagel RL. Sickle cell anemia day hospital: an approach for the management of uncomplicated painful crises. *Blood* 2000;95:1130.

31. Kaiko RF, Foley KM, Grabinski PY, et al. Central nervous system excitatory effects of meperidine in cancer patients. *Ann Neurol* 1983;13:180.
32. *Acute and Chronic Pain in Sickle Cell Disease. 2001*. Glenview, Ill: American Pain Society, 2001.
33. Yaster M, Kost-Byerly S, Maxwell LG. The management of pain in sickle cell disease. *Pediatr Clin North Am* 2000;47:699.
34. Gil KM, Carson JW, Sedway JA, et al. Follow-up of coping skills training in adults with sickle cell disease: analysis of daily pain and coping practice diaries. *Health Psychol* 2000;19:85.
35. Anie KA, Green J. Psychological therapies for sickle cell disease and pain (Cochrane review). *CochraneDatabaseSystRev* 2000; CD00 1916, 2000
36. Davis H, Schoendorf KC, Gergen PJ, Moore RM Jr. National trends in the mortality of children with sickle cell disease, 1968 through 1992. *Am J Public Health* 1997;87:1317.
37. Davis H, Moore RM Jr, Gergen PJ. Cost of hospitalizations associated with sickle cell disease in the United States. *Public Health Rep* 1997; 112:40.

CHAPTER 53 ACUTE PAIN MANAGEMENT IN INFANTS AND CHILDREN

Christine D. Greco, Moris M. Aner, and Alyssa LeBel

Pain in children has been historically undertreated. This was in part the result of misguided assumptions, such as children's inability to experience pain because of an immature nervous system and the innocuous effects of untreated pain in children. In addition, limited knowledge of pediatric drug metabolism prevented a clear understanding of how to dose analgesics in children. Over the past two decades, there has been significant progress in the understanding of neuroanatomy, physiology, and pharmacology of analgesics in children, which has led to considerable advancements in pain management. This chapter discusses developmental anatomy and neurochemistry, pain assessment, pharmacologic treatment of pain, and regional techniques in pediatric patients.

DEVELOPMENTAL ANATOMY AND NEUROCHEMISTRY

The late fetus and infant are neurologically sophisticated in their ability to transmit pain signals and respond to stress.[1] Cutaneous sensory nerve terminals are present in the perioral region at 7 weeks' gestation and spread to all body areas by 20 weeks' gestation. Nerve growth factors regulate the extension of peripheral nociceptive fibers into the dorsal spinal cord, with the larger A fibers entering prior to the C fibers at 8 to 12 weeks. At birth, A and C fiber territories overlap in the developing substantia gelatinosa.[2] Therefore, the neonatal response to a nonspecific sensory stimulus is low threshold, nonspecific, and poorly organized. Noxious and non-noxious stimuli produce similar physiologic and behavioral infant responses, complicating an accurate assessment of pain.

In the central nervous system (CNS), the full complement of cortical neurons, approximately 1000 million, are present at 20 weeks' gestation. Pain transmission pathways complete myelination in the spine and brain stem between 22 and 30 weeks' gestation. Myelination extends up to the thalamus by 30 weeks, and to the cortex by 37 weeks or term. Cortical descending inhibition develops post-term.

Excitatory and inhibitory neurotransmitters and neuromodulators are present in the fetus, with the balance favoring excitation. Calcitonin gene-related peptide (CGRP), substance P, and the glutamate-NMDA systems are present at 8 to 10 weeks' gestation. Enkephalin and vasoactive intestinal peptide (VIP) appear at 10 to 14 weeks. Catecholamines are present in late gestation, and serotonin at 6 weeks' postnatal. Of note, the receptors for excitatory neurotransmitters are numerous and widely distributed in the neonate, regressing toward an adult system in the postnatal months. As well, in the developing nervous system, inhibitory chemicals, such as gamma-amino butyric acid (GABA) and glycine, may act as excitatory transmitters. In an experimental murine model, the spinal cord concentration of NMDA receptors, and their ligand-affinity, is greater in neonates than in older animals. NK-1 receptor density is also maximal in late fetal and early postnatal life; however, substance P levels are lower than adult levels at birth.[3]

Regarding stress responses, the functional neuroendocrine pathways between hypothalamus and pituitary are present at 21 weeks' gestation. Corticotrophin-releasing factor (CRF) may stimulate fetal ACTH and β-endorphin from that time, and cortisol and β-endorphin increases have been assayed following intrauterine sampling for exchange transfusion. Norepinephrine is present in paravertebral ganglia and adrenal chromaffin cells at 10 weeks' gestation and is released with intrauterine stress (asphyxia). Epinephrine is present, in smaller amount, after 23 weeks' gestation.[3]

The long-term consequences of untreated pain in the developing organism are not yet defined, but some studies suggest that early pain responses influence later pain behaviors.[4] In one murine model, skin wounds on rat pups caused increased innervation and lowered pain thresholds in the area of injury for 3 months post-injury. In the rats that had recurrent painful stimuli from birth, the changes in the receptive fields of the dorsal horn neurons were persistent.[5] Another study exposed rat pups to repeated hindpaw injections over several days. When compared with control pups and at adult age, the rats that experienced repeated noxious stimuli showed increased responses to painful and nonpainful stimuli relative to their controls. Pathologically, the experimental group showed a loss of nociceptive primary afferents.[6] A third study found that the pain-conditioned behaviors of rats differed according to the timing of the stimulus. Rat pups exposed to early, repetitive noxious stimulation had a decrease in pain threshold compared with control rats. Adult rats given repetitive painful stimuli showed greater stress responses, such as freezing and digging, than controls.[7]

In humans, few empiric studies also show late effects of painful stimuli. One report describes that neonatal males who received a eutetic mixture of topical local anesthetic (Emla Cream; Astra Pharmaceuticals) prior to circumcision had 12% to 25% less facial grimacing and tachycardia than randomized control infants without treatment.[8] An earlier study observed that males circumcised within 2 days of age had longer periods of crying and higher pain ratings than uncircumcised males.[9] Another report compared 18 preterm infants, subject to repeated painful procedures in the neonatal intensive care unit (NICU), with matched full-term infants regarding their somatic complaints at 18 months. Twenty-five percent of mothers of preterm infants with prolonged neonatal intensive care unit stays noted a significantly increased number of somatic complaints in their toddlers as compared with mothers of full-term infants briefly managed in the normal nursery.[10] Alternatively, a recent study of 24 preterm infants compared with matched full-term infants had similar behavioral pain scores when exposed to a finger prick at 4 months of age.[11]

In summary, the neonatal pain transmission system is adequately developed, centrally hyperexcitable, with the necessary components of central sensitization, but generally nonspecific in its response to stimuli. Neonates and infants feel pain, but assessment of this phenomenon remains challenging.[12–14] The long-term effects of neonatal pain are now being investigated.

PAIN ASSESSMENT IN INFANTS AND CHILDREN

Pain assessment is a fundamental and essential part of pain treatment. The ability to reliably assess pain facilitates the diagnosis of painful conditions and helps to evaluate efficacy of pain relief methods. The assessment of pain in infants and children, however, is one of the most difficult challenges faced by health care providers. The subjective nature of pain, cognitive and language limitations, and differences in pain expression and perception account for the difficulty in assessing pain in pediatric patients. As discussed earlier, there is growing evidence to suggest that inadequately treated pain can have both short-term and long-term consequences. For example, it is well established that full-term and preterm infants develop physiologic stress responses to pain and inadequate anesthesia that can result in greater postoperative complications.[1,15,16] Pain is most commonly assessed by asking patients about the quality, location, and severity of their pain. Self-report methods are considered to be the most reliable guides to pain assessment for most patients. However, infants and preverbal children are unable to communicate their experience of pain and must rely on caregivers to interpret signs of pain and distress. Pain assessment methods that combine self-report with other measures, such as behavioral and physiologic responses, may provide more accurate measures of pain. There can be limitations in the use of behavioral and physiologic indices for pain assessment. Distinguishing between pain and distress may be difficult in young children. For example, a young child may cry and exhibit characteristic facial grimacing during an ear examination because of fear and anxiety rather than pain. Physiologic signs may also mislead measures of pain in certain situations. For example, patients who are septic, hypoxic, or receiving vasopressors may have increases in heart rate or blood pressure that reflect other processes not related to pain. Most pain scales have been designed for assessment of acute pain and tend to underestimate pain in children with persistent or chronic pain.

Most pain assessment scales used for infants and preverbal children rely on behavioral observation and physiologic parameters to guide assessment. Observational measures alone may not accurately represent pain intensity since health care workers tend to underestimate pain when compared to a patient or parent report.[17,18] The parent report also tends to underestimate children's pain but to a lesser extent than a report by health care workers.[19] Behavioral parameters typically used are facial grimacing, cry, body movement, and sleep pattern. Facial expression measures appear to be most useful and specific in neonates.[20,21] The typical pain facial expression of eyes tightly closed, furrowed brows, and square mouth is considered to be one of the most consistent signals of pain in infants. Pain cries in infants have been shown to be spectographically different from cries due to hunger or anger and can be recognized by experienced caregivers.[22] Physiologic parameters such as heart rate, oxygen saturation, blood pressure, and palmar sweating provide more objective evidence of pain.

The Premature Infant Pain Profile (PIPP) and CRIES are pain scales used for preterm and full-term infants, respectively, that combine behavioral observations and physiologic criteria to assess pain.[23,24] The PIPP was specifically designed to assess acute pain in preterm infants with consideration to gestational age (Table 53-1). The CRIES is an acronym that refers to Crying, Requires O_2, Increased vital signs, Expression, and Sleepless and consists of five behavioral and physiologic parameters designed to rate postoperative pain in neonates (Table 53-2).

TABLE 53-1 **Premature Infant Pain Profile (PIPP)**

		Premature Infant Pain Profile				
Process	**Indicator**	**0**	**1**	**2**	**3**	**Score**
Chart	Gestational age (at time observed)	≥36 weeks	32–35 weeks	28–31 weeks	<28 weeks	
Observe infant 15 sec		Active/awake	Quiet/awake	Active/sleep	Quiet/sleep	
Observe baseline: Heart Rate: ____ SpO2: ____	Behavioral State	Eyes open Facial movements	Eyes open No facial movements	Eyes closed Facial movements	Eyes closed No facial movements	
Observe infant 30 sec	Heart Rate Max. ________	0 to 4 beats/minute increase	5 to 14 beats/minute increase	15 to 24 beats/minute increase	25 beats/minute or or more increase	
	Oxygen Saturation Min. ________	0% to 2.4% decrease	2.5% to 4.9% decrease	5.0% to 7.4% decrease	7.5% or more decrease	
	Brow Bulge	None 0%–9% of time	Minimum 10%–39% of time	Moderate 70% of 40–69% of time	Maximum time or more	
	Eye Squeeze	None 0%–9% of time	Minimum 10%–39% of time	Moderate 40%–69% of time	Maximum 70% of time or more	
	Eye Squeeze	None 0%–9% of time	Minimum 10%–39% of time	Moderate 40%–69% of time	Maximum 70% of time or more	
Total Score						

TABLE 53-2 **CRIES Neonatal Postoperative Pain Measurement Score**

	CRIES Neonatal Postoperative Pain Measurement Score		
	0	1	2
Crying	No	High pitched	Inconsolable
Requires O_2 for saturation > 95	No	<30%	>30%
Increased vital signs	HR and BP = or < preoperative	HR or BP <20% of preoperative	HR or BP >20% of preoperative
Expression	None	Grimace	Grimace/grunt
Sleepless	No	Wakes at frequent intervals	Constantly awake

HR denotes heart rate; BP, blood pressure.

Children ages 3 to 7 years old become increasingly able to communicate their experience of pain to parents and caregivers. Children in this age group may not understand the abstract concept of pain, but they are able to report "hurt" or "owie" and in general are able to indicate pain intensity. Although self-report measures are most reliable, a variety of factors may alter a child's report of pain.[25] For example, children with inadequately treated persistent pain from cancer or surgery may appear very quiet, still, and withdrawn, giving a false impression of adequate analgesia. Some children may underreport or deny pain for fear of receiving a painful analgesic "shot." Young children are unable to use standard visual analog scales used by older children and adults. Several self-report methods have been developed that are validated and reliable in children as young as 4 years of age.[26,28] The Bieri faces scale is a series of facial expressions depicting degrees of pain and was found to be preferred by most children (Fig. 53-1).[28,29] The Color Continuum Scale is a ruler with numerical anchors where increasing intensity of red signifies more pain (Fig. 53-2).

Children aged 8 years and older generally can use standard "0 to 10" visual analog scales accurately, but many of the scales used in younger children such as the Bieri faces can also be used. Children in this age group may have concerns over loss of control, or may fear painful injections of analgesics that can distort their self-report. Older children and adolescents have the cognitive ability to understand the meaning of pain and tend to use behavioral coping strategies for pain.

Pain assessment in severely cognitively impaired children is particularly challenging for parents and caregivers. As in preverbal children, behavioral observation scales combined with physiologic parameters can be helpful. In some cases when assessment is unclear, therapeutic trials of comfort measures and analgesics can help clarify the situation.

In general, pain assessment is best accomplished by correlating self-report, behavioral, and physiologic measures with the child's overall clinical picture. The choice of pain assessment scale should be individualized and based on a child's age, clinical condition, environment, cognitive abilities, and coping style. Often, explaining and practicing a pain assessment scale to a child during the preoperative visit can help facilitate use after surgery. Table 53-3 summarizes common pain scales used in children and infants.

PHARMACOLOGIC GUIDELINES IN THE NEWBORN AND INFANT

- Neonates have an immature cytochrome P450 hepatic enzyme system, and therefore conjugate opioids and local anesthetics slowly. Delayed toxicity with prolonged infusions is possible.
- Renal function, including glomerular filtration and renal tubular secretion, is decreased in the first few weeks of life (longer for premature infants) compared with adults. The half-life of opioids and, more significantly, their metabolites (MSO4-6-glucuronide) may be increased. Delayed sedation and respiratory depression are limited by increased dosing intervals and decreased doses.
- Neonatal total body water is increased compared with adults. Fat is minimal. Analgesics with high-water solubility have a large volume of distribution.

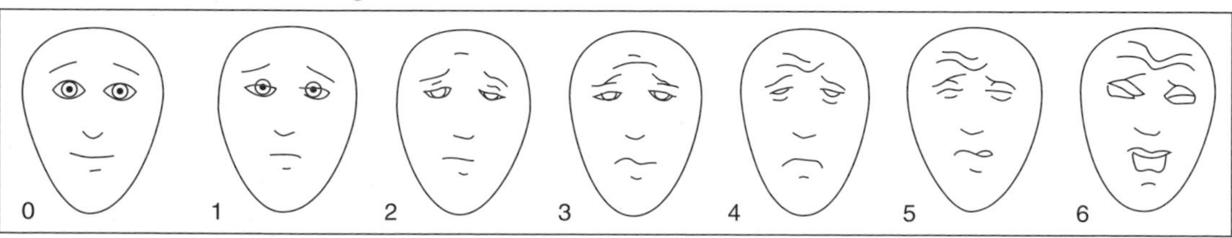

Figure 53-1 Bieri faces scale. From Bieri et al, 1990.

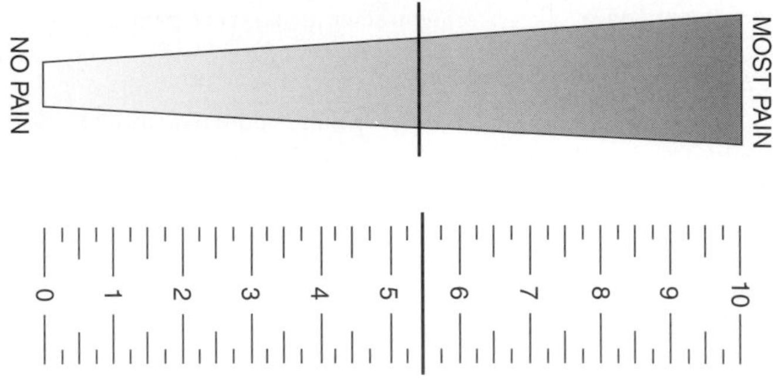

Figure 53-2 Color Continuum Scale.

- Neonates have decreased plasma-protein binding, albumen and α_1 acid glycoprotein, resulting in increased free-drug and greater first-pass toxicity.
- Ventilatory reflexes are immature in the neonate. Infants have a low threshold for hypoventilation secondary to opioids.[30]

PHARMACOLOGIC TREATMENT OPTIONS

Acetaminophen and Nonsteroidal Anti-inflammatory Drugs

Acetaminophen (paracetamol) is the most commonly and widely used analgesic and antipyretic in children. It has no peripheral anti-inflammatory effects and it putatively acts on cyclooxygenase (COX-1 more than COX-2) through CNS mechanisms. Although a weak analgesic, it is a generally safe agent, if proper pediatric doses are administered (Table 53-4). It is a useful adjuvant for acute pain therapy and is often combined, synergistically, with weak opioids. The recommended single doses are 15 to 20 mg/kg, 10 to 15mg/kg with repeated dosing. Toxicity occurs at 90 mg/kg in children and adolescents, 60 mg/kg in infants, and 45 mg/kg in preterm infants. Excess acetominophen is metabolized in the liver to reactive nucleophilic benzoquinones, which bind DNA, leading to parenchymal necrosis. Treatment of overdose must occur within 12 hours of intake in adult patients, with the use of *N*-acetylcysteine or glutathion. Acetaminophen is available in multiple routes of administration—tablets, capsules, suspensions, and suppositories. The rectal dose is 35 to 40 mg/kg every 6 to 8 hours, because of slow absorption and plasma clearance. Rectal absorption peaks at 70 minutes.[31,32]

NSAIDs act peripherally, without significantly crossing the blood-brain barrier, and have a prominent anti-inflammatory effect as well as analgesia and antipyresis. They are generally used for mild to moderate postoperative pain, sickle cell crisis, symptomatic headache, and arthritis. Opioids remain the first choice for moderate to severe pain, such as cancer-related pain, with NSAIDs as adjuvants. Their use is guided as well by their adverse effects, including gastritis, potential gastrointestinal bleeding, and platelet and renal dysfunction. Respiratory depression and dysphoria, often seen with opioid use, are not concerns with these agents.[31–34] In some studies of postoperative pediatric pain, NSAIDs reduce opioid requirements and side effects.[35,36]

The major mechanism of action of nonsteroidal anti-inflammatory drugs (NSAIDs) is through inhibition of prostaglandin synthesis by blockade of constitutive and expressed cyclooxygenase

TABLE 53-3 **Summary of Pain Assessment Scales**

Measure	Features	Age Range	Advantages	Disadvantages
Visual Analog Scale (VAS)	Horizontal 10-cm ruler, markings between "no pain" and "worst pain"	8 years and older	Reliable, well-validated	Not useful for younger children or those with cognitive limitations
Faces Scale (Bieri)	Faces representing different levels of pain intensity	4 years and older	Useful for young children	Choice of facial expressions affects response
Color Analog Scale	Numerical anchors on a ruler where increasing intensity of red signifies more pain	4 years and older	Reliable, useful for young children	Not useful for toddlers or those with cognitive limitations
Behavioral or combined behavioral-physiologic scales (PIPP, CRIES, etc)	Scoring of behavior sometimes combined with physiologic parameters	Many scales are designed for infants and young children	Useful for infants and preverbal children	Underrates persistent pain
Autonomic measures	Measures changes in HR, blood pressure	All ages	Can be useful for patients receiving mechanical ventilation	Autonomic changes may not be related to pain

PIPP denotes Premature Infant Pain Profile; CRIES, Crying, Requires O_2, Increased vital signs, Expression, and Sleepless; HR, heart rate.

From Greco C, Berde B. Pain Management in Children. In: Berhman R, Kliegman R, Jenson H, eds. Nelson Textbook of Pediatrics, 16th Edition. W.B. Saunders Company 2000.

TABLE 53-4 **Pediatric Dosing of NSAIDs**

Drug	Dose
Acetaminophen (PO)	10–15 mg/kg q-4h
Aspirin	10–15 mg/kg q4h
Ibuprofen	4–10 mg/kg q6–8h
Ketorolac (IV)	0.5 mg/kg q6–8h, not for > 5 days

From Berde C, Masek B. Pain in children. In: Wall PD, Melzack R, eds. Textbook of Pain. Edinburgh, Scotland: Churchill Livingstone, 1999.

(COX). The pharmacology of most NSAIDs has been studied in children 2 years old and older, in which population the elimination half-life is similar to adults. In children 3 months to 2.5 years, the volume of distribution and clearance of ibuprofen and ketorolac are increased, suggesting a possible need for higher loading and maintenance dosing in children.[30,31]

Aspirin (acetylsalicylic acid), although used for acute pain and fever for more than 100 years, is contraindicated for fever in pediatric patients because of its association with Reye's syndrome, described 20 years ago. Therefore, acetaminophen and ibuprofen are the primary agents for fever and mild to moderate pain.[30,31] For severe pain, parenteral ketorolac is effective. The oral formulation is similar in stength and efficacy to older NSAIDs. Ketololac has been studied as a single dose in postoperative pediatric patients and is well-tolerated and opioid-sparing. Its' use postoperatively may be limited in tonsillectomy and other procedures associated with significant bleeding. It is generally prescribed every 6 hours over a period of 24 to 48 hours, with frequent reevaluation and a maximum period of 5 days.[37] The newer COX 2 inhibitors, celecoxib and rofecoxeb, are currently being studied in pediatric multicenter pharmacokinetic and postoperative efficacy trials.[38]

Opioids

As in other clinical populations, opioids are also the standard of care for pediatric patients with severe pain. Historically inadequate use is now increasingly replaced by appropriate use, guided by attention to physiologic immaturity, dosing corrected for age and weight, and awareness of potential adverse effects (Table 53-5). In general, as in adults, the use of opioids for the pediatric population is best guided by the adult acute and cancer pain literature. Exceptional patients are premature infants, neonates, and opioid-naïve children requiring high initial bolusing of medication.[30,31]

Pharmacokinetic studies of opioids in children are available for morphine, fentanyl, sufentanil, methadone, and hydromorphone, and in process for such newer oral agents as oxycodone and oxycontin.

In neonates and premature infants, the major concern is respiratory depression, even, at times, with sub-anesthetic dosing. A single large bolus dose in a neonate may result in apnea due to rapid CNS absorption. Adjustment in dosage and dosage interval is necessary in this population. For example, the half-life of parenteral morphine in adults and children is 2 hours, in neonates, 6 to 8 hours, and in premature infants, 10 hours. Pharmacokinetic studies of opioid infusions in neonates suggest the use of lower doses of opioids, monitoring for hypoxemia and hypoventilation, and larger but controlled loading doses because of increased volume of distribution. In healthy infants, 3 months and older, renal clearance of opioids and secondary respiratory suppression is similar to adults.[30,39]

The use of patient-controlled analgesia (PCA) in children has been well studied and is safe and effective, with no increased total opioid administration nor adverse effects. Ages 6 years and older are generally able to comprehend the use of the self-administered bolus dose. Younger children and those with developmental delay may be considered for nurse-administered analgesia (NCA) or continuous infusion. Parent-administered dosing is generally only used in the palliative care setting.[40]

The choice of a specific opioid is based on potency, desired route of administration, and adverse effects. Morphine is the first choice for parenteral boluses and infusions. Children with reactive airway disease may, rarely, be more sensitive to the histaminergic effects of morphine, but generally tolerate this agent well. Rash and pruritis are occasionally present in atopic individuals as well as idiosyncratically. All opioids affect visceral sphincters equally. Meperidine is minimally used secondary to its excitatory effects on the cardiac and central nervous system with repetitive dosing. Hydromorphone is anecdotally preferred in patients with incipient renal failure, putatively due to less accumulation of toxic metabolites compared with morphine (3,6-diglucuronide). Fentanyl is an alternative parenteral opioid, with a short half-life that is useful for painful procedures. It is often a choice in neonates with congenital heart disease because it has little cardiac effect except bradycardia. High doses, and rarely low doses, may produce glottic and

TABLE 53-5 **Initial Opioid Dosing (<50 kg)**

Drug	Oral	Parenteral
Morphine	0.3 mg/kg q3–4h	0.05–0.1 mg/kg q4h, 0.02 mg/kg/h infusion
Hydromorphine	0.04–0.08 mg/kg q3–4h	0.02 mg/kg q2–3h, 0.006 mg/kg/hr infusion
Fentanyl	NA	0.5–1 microgram/kg q1–2h
Methadone	0.2 mg/kg q4–8h	0.1 mg/kg q4–8h
Codeine	0.5–1 mg/kg q3–4h	NA
Oxycodone	0.1–0.2 mg/kg q3–4h	NA

From Berde C, Masek B. Pain in children. In: Wall PD, Melzack R, eds. Textbook of Pain. Edinburgh, Scotland: Churchill Livingstone, 1999.

chest wall rigidity, treated with naloxone and /or neuromuscular blockade. For older patients with chronic pain, fentanyl may be administered rapidly and transmucosally, in a candy matrix, or over 72 hours transdermally via patch placement and subdermal release following deposition. Methadone provides a form of sustained-release administration, with attention to the accumulation of effect, from 3 to 4 hours to 24 hours, with repetitive dosing. It is often used to wean opioids after sustained parenteral infusion. Sufentanil is used primarily as a general anesthetic. Intermittent intramuscular dosing is contraindicated in pediatric patients because of common needle aversion and often incomprehensible pain with injection in this population. As a rough dosing guide, premature infants and neonates require 1/10 the usual adult dosage; 1 month olds, 1/8; 1 year olds, [1/4]; and 7 year olds, [1/2].[30,31,39]

Oral opioid preparations (codeine, oxycodone, morphine elixir, and rapid-release tablets) and opioid / NSAID combination (acetaminophen with codeine, oxycodone with acetaminophen) are often used for the pediatric patients following recovery from acute surgery or trauma for mild to moderate pain.[31] Tramadol is an unusual opioid, recently studied regarding pediatric pharmacokinetics, with morphine-like μ_1-receptor agonism, incompletely antagonized by naloxone, and some additional reuptake blockade of norepinephrine and serotonin.[41,42]

Rectal suppositories of morphine and hydromorphone are available for patients who cannot tolerate oral drugs and who are not neutropenic or immunosuppressed. Neuroaxial opioids, well-tolerated and commonly used in pediatrics, are fentanyl and hydromophone.

Adverse effects of opioids are treated as in adult patients, with the exception of the use of compazine and other dopaminergic agents for nausea and vomiting. These agents may result in frightening dystonic reactions in children. Recommended agents are ondansetron, hydroxyzine, and diphenhydramine.[31]

REGIONAL ANESTHESIA IN CHILDREN

Regional anesthesia techniques are widely used in infants and children for acute postoperative pain management and for diagnosis and treatment of a variety of chronic pain conditions. Because of fear and anxiety of needles and procedures, most children will require general anesthesia for most regional techniques. Some motivated, older children may only require sedation for certain blocks. Regional blockade is typically combined with general anesthesia for most operative procedures. However, patients with neuromuscular diseases requiring muscle biopsy, patients with significant pulmonary disease, or those with a risk for postoperative apnea are often considered for regional techniques without general anesthesia. The regional technique should be explained to the parents and to the child in age-appropriate terms and informed consent should be obtained. Some children become frightened postoperatively with a dense motor or sensory block, and a preoperative discussion about what to expect after surgery can be helpful. Contraindications to the use of regional techniques in children are similar to contraindications for adult patients. These include refusal by patient or parents, infection at the site of needle entry, and clinically significant bleeding disorders.

Pharmacology of Local Anesthetics

The pharmacology of local anesthetics in pediatric patients differs from adult patients. Neonates and infants have delayed hepatic degradation of amide local anesthetics for the first 3 to 6 months of life.[43,44] In addition, infants younger than 3 months old have prolonged elimination half-lives of amide local anesthetics.[43,45] Delayed hepatic degradation and prolonged elimination half-lives may result in higher systemic amide local anesthetic levels with increased risk of toxic effects. Neonates and young infants have reduced serum levels of albumin and α_1-acid glycoproteins involved in protein binding of local anesthetics.[46,47] This may lead to increased levels of free unbound drug and higher risk of systemic toxicity in neonates and young infants.[45,48] Neonates, however, have larger volumes of distribution that may lead to decreases in serum drug levels and may help reduce systemic toxicity.[49]

Ester local anesthetics are metabolized by plasma cholinesterase. Neonates and infants up to 6 months of age have approximately one half the levels of plasma cholinesterase found in adult patients.[50] Therefore, the clearance of ester local anesthetics such as choloroprocaine may be prolonged in infants. However, because of the rapidity with which chloroprocaine is metabolized, even in infants, it is often used for continuous epidural infusions.

Spinal Anesthesia

The use of spinal anesthesia for surgical procedures below the T10 dermatome has been shown to reduce the incidence of postoperative apnea and bradycardia in former preterm infants <55 weeks postconceptual age and full-term infants <44 weeks postconceptual age.[51,52] Short procedures lasting less than 1½ to 2 hours, such as inguinal herniorraphy, circumcision, and hypospadius repair are commonly performed under spinal anesthesia in preterm and full-term infants who may otherwise be at increased risk for postoperative apnea and bradycardia after general anesthesia. Even with the use of spinal anesthesia, patients should continue to be closely monitored for apnea and bradycardia overnight.[53,54]

Hyperbaric tetracaine and bupivacaine are most commonly used for spinal blocks (Table 53-6). In infants, 0.8 to 1 mg/kg of tetracaine provides effective surgical motor block and sensory block to T2-4. Inadequate dosing results in higher failure rates. The level of blockade to T2-4 may lead to motor block of intercostal and abdominal muscles. However, infants are able to maintain adequate tidal volume through diaphragmatic breathing.[55,56] Patients in this age group remain stable with respect to heart rate and blood pressure with this level of blockade.[57]

Spinal block can be performed with the patient positioned in either a sitting or lateral decubitus position (Fig. 53-3). Careful head positioning is required to avoid airway obstruction, particularly in the sitting position.[58] Because the conus medullaris ends at L3 in infants, the dural puncture should be performed at L3 or

TABLE 53-6 **Infant Spinal Anesthetic Solutions***

Local Anesthetic Solution	Dose (mg/kg)	Approximate Duration (min)
Tetracaine 0.5% with 5% dextrose and 20–40 μg epinephrine	0.8–1	90
Bupivacaine 0.75% with 5% dextrose and 20–40 μg epinephrine	0.3–0.5	70–90

*Weight-scaled doses should be diminished after 6-12 months of age.

Adapted from Sethna N, Berde B. Pediatric Regional Anesthesia. In: Gregory G, ed. Pediatric Anesthesia, 4th Edition. Churchill Livingston 2002.

lower. After aseptic skin preparation and draping, the skin is usually infiltrated with local anesthetic. A 25-gauge 1-in. or 22-gauge 1.5-in. spinal needle is slowly inserted. The characteristic loss of resistance felt when puncturing the dura may not be appreciated in infants. The local anesthetic solution should be slowly injected after free flow of CSF is confirmed. Patients may require brief positioning in reverse Trendelenburg if cephalad spread of local anesthetic appears too great. After testing the level of blockade with a light pinprick, the blood pressure cuff and pulse oximetry probe can be moved to the leg to help ensure a still infant during the procedure. A pacifier dipped in glucose solution and a quiet environment may also be helpful. Typically, no sedatives or analgesics are administered, especially with concerns of postoperative apnea.[56]

Caudal Epidural Analgesia

Caudal epidural analgesia is a safe, technically successful, and easily performed block in pediatric patients.[59,60] A "single shot" caudal block is commonly used for outpatient surgical procedures below the T10 dermatome, such as lower extremity orthopedic procedures, herniorraphy, or circumcision. It can be used as continuous catheter infusion for longer and more extensive procedures. Continuous caudal catheter infusions are discussed in the following section on lumbar and thoracic epidural infusions.

Dilute solutions of bupivacaine are frequently used for caudal blocks.[61,62] Doses of 0.75 to 1 mg/kg of 0.25% bupivacaine when combined with general anesthesia provides effective postoperative analgesia, and when placed at the beginning of the procedure, can reduce general anesthetic requirements. This dose is within the recommended maximum safe level of bupivacaine of 2.5 mg/kg.[63,64]

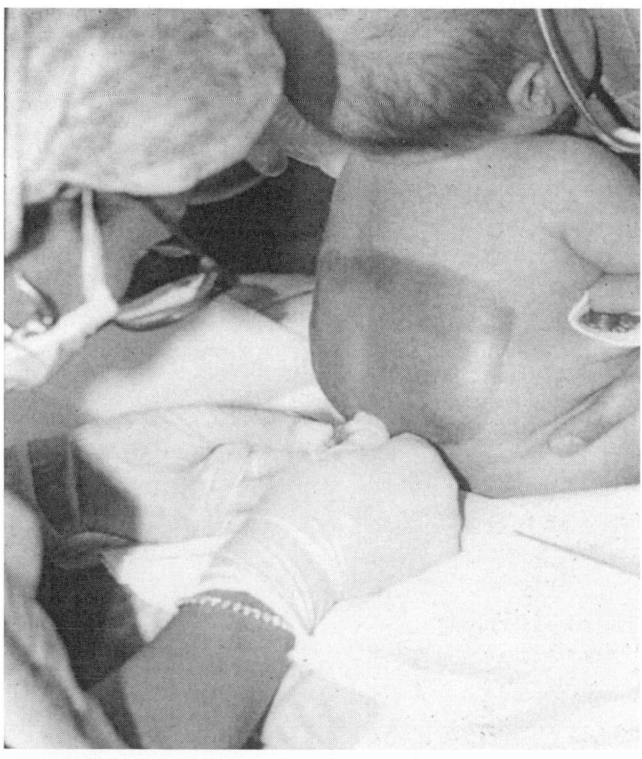

Figure 53-3 Spinal anesthesia in an infant. The head is slightly lifted to avoid airway obstruction.

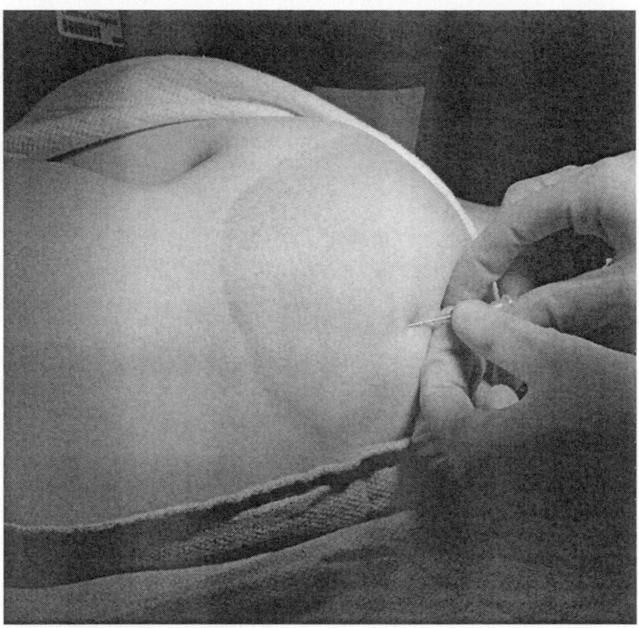

Figure 53-4 Caudal placement in a 4 year old child.

The duration of postoperative pain control varies with caudal epidural analgesia. Some studies estimate the duration of analgesia with caudal blockade with bupivacaine at 5 hours, whereas other studies report that 50% of patients required no analgesics 12 hours after placement of the caudal block.[63,65] The addition of clonidine to the bupivacaine solution may enhance the analgesic effect of the block and prolong duration.[66,68] Although the optimal dose has not been clearly established, we use 1 to 1.5 μg/kg for children older than 1 year of age, up to a maximum dose of 30 μg.

Caudal epidural block is most frequently performed with the patient positioned in a lateral decubitus position. The sacral hiatus is easily palpated between the sacral cornu (Figs. 53-4 and 53-5). Using aseptic technique, the needle is inserted through the sacrococcygeal ligament into the epidural space. Our practice is to use a short-bevel needle. A loss of resistance is typically felt on entering the epidural space. The angle of the needle is lowered and the needle is advanced no further than 2 to 4 mm to avoid intravascular placement. After aspiration for blood and CSF, a test dose of local anesthetic and epinephrine is injected to detect tachycardia or hypertension associated with an intravascular injection.

Lumbar and Thoracic Epidural Analgesia

Lumbar and thoracic epidural analgesia is widely used for infants and children in a variety of surgical procedures, such as lower extremity and pelvic orthopedic surgery, major abdominal surgery, and thoracic procedures. There is evidence to support that epidural analgesia helps with early postoperative extubation and helps to improve postoperative pulmonary function.[69] Because of the need for general anesthesia in performing this technique, children with chronic pain disorders often have continuous epidural catheter infusions rather than repeated epidural injections for treatment of their underlying pain.

Bupivacaine and, in select cases, chloroprocaine are frequently used local anesthetics for continuous epidural infusions in infants

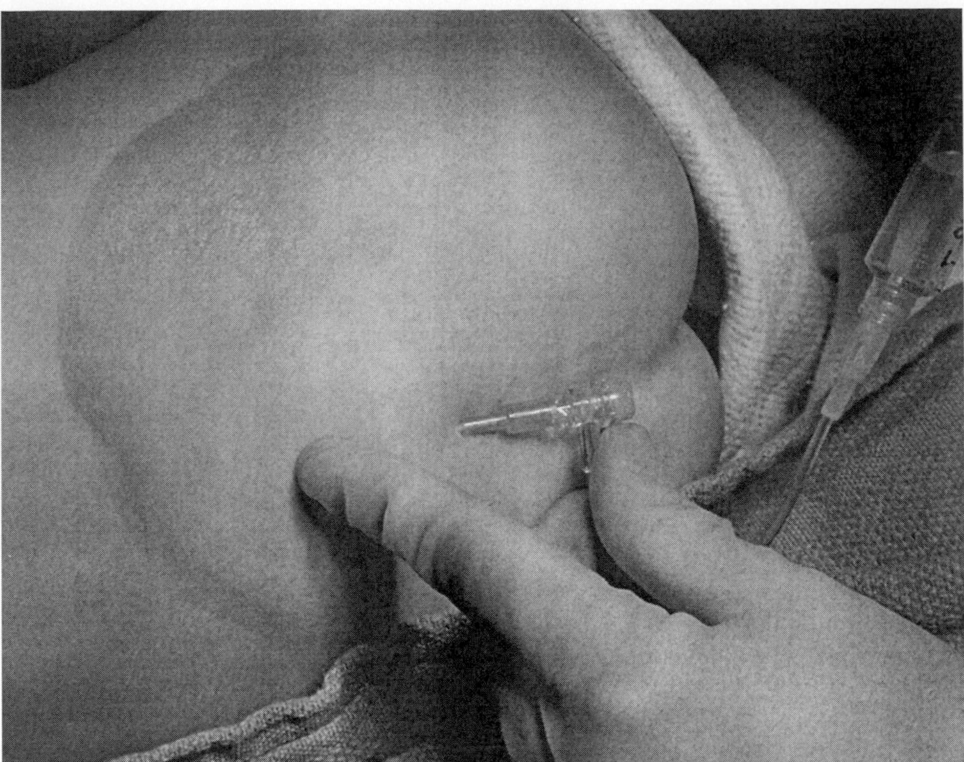

Figure 53-5 Palpation cephalad to the caudal space during injection of local anesthetic can facilitate detection of subcutaneous infiltration.

and children (Table 53-7). Because of age-related differences in hepatic degradation and clearance of amide local anesthetics, it is recommended that epidural bupivacaine infusions should not exceed 0.2 mg/kg/hour in infants younger than 3 months of age and 0.4 mg/kg/hour in children.[43-45,70,71] The addition of opioid and/or clonidine to the bupivacaine solution can provide optimal analgesia while allowing a safe range of bupivacaine infusion rates. We typically use 0.1% bupivacaine combined with fentanyl 2 μg/mL with or without clonidine 0.4 μg/mL, or 0.1% bupivacaine combined with hydromorphone 10 μg/mL. We recommend reduced initial infusion rates when using solutions containing hydromorphone or in cases where the epidural catheter tip is in the thoracic region. Clonidine has less depression of CO_2-response curves in infants compared to fentanyl. Bupivacaine-hydromorphone infusions are rarely used in infants younger than 6 months due to increased risk of respiratory depression. Chloroprocaine 1.5% can be used as a continuous epidural infusion in children younger than 6 months of age, however it can lower the seizure threshold in some patients.

With the patient in a lateral decubitus position, the epidural space is generally located using continuous loss of resistance technique (Fig. 53-6). An 18-gauge 2-in Tuohy needle and a standard 20-gauge catheter are typically used. Loss of resistance to saline rather than air is recommended because of the risk of venous air embolism in infants and small children.[72,73] Because of concerns regarding the risks of direct placement of thoracic epidural catheters in anesthetized children, studies have examined the effectiveness of advancing epidural catheters from the caudal and lumbar regions to a thoracic dermatome.[74–76] Evidence suggests fairly good success rates in caudal to thoracic advancement in infants compared with lumbar to thoracic level. Catheter advancement to the thoracic region should be performed using fluoroscopy, particularly for patients in whom correct catheter placement is crucial, such as for patients with congenital diaphragmatic hernia or for patients requiring palliative care. Our preference is to use styletted 20-gauge catheters with fluroscopic guidance for all thoracic epidural catheters, whether directly placed or advanced from lower levels. Direct thoracic epidural catheters should be placed only in selected patients and by anesthesiologists with considerable expertise in pediatric regional techniques.

Complications associated with epidural techniques in children are similar to adult complications, such as inadvertent intravascular or intrathecal injection of local anesthetics and infection. A neg-

TABLE 53-7 **Representative Pediatric Epidural Infusions***

Solution	Age > 6 months mL/kg/h	Age < 6 months mL/kg/h†
Bupivacaine 0.1% with fentanyl 2 μg/mL	0.1–0.4	0.1–0.2
Bupivacaine 0.1% with fentanyl 2 μg/ml +/− Clonidine 0.4 μg/ml	0.2–0.3	0.1–0.15
†Bupivacaine 0.1% with hydromorphine 10 μg/ml	0.1–0.3	(rarely used)
Chloroprocaine 1.5%	(rarely used)	0.6–0.8

*Adapted from Greco C, Houck C, Berde B. Pediatric Pain Management. In: Gregory G, ed. Pediatric Anesthesia, 4th Edition. Churchill Livingston 2002.

†Cardiorespiratory monitoring required; highly monitored setting for children < 6 months.

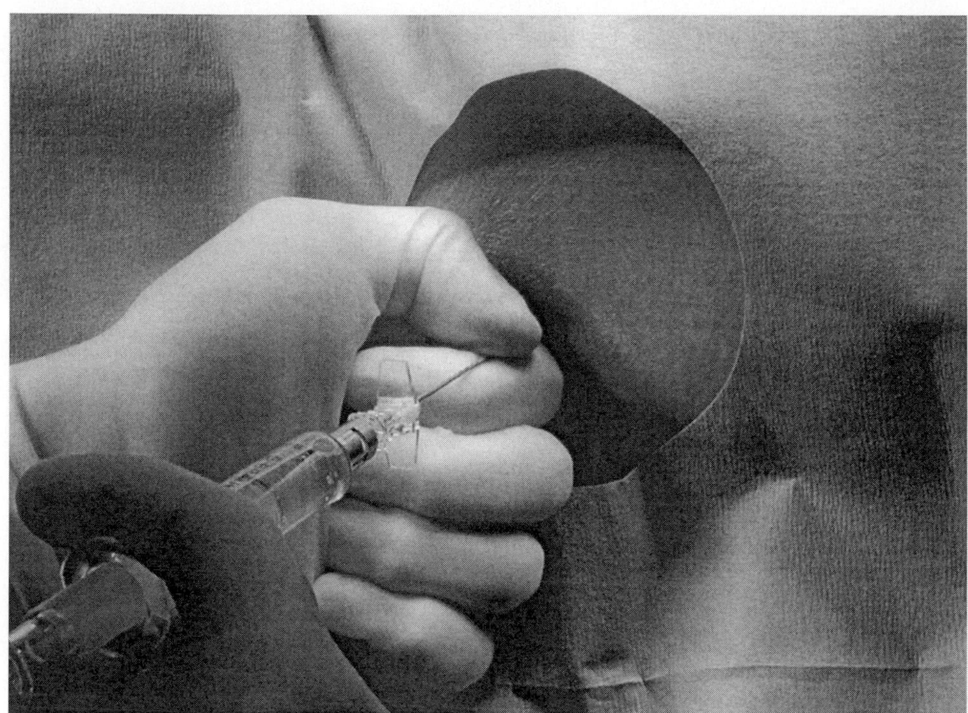

Figure 53-6 Epidural block placement in a 6 year old child.

ative aspiration for blood or CSF helps to reduce the incidence of intravascular or intrathecal injection of local anesthetic.[60] Although a test dose is always recommended, changes in hemodynamic profile as a result of intravascular epinephrine may not be obvious in an anesthetized child.[60,77] A retrospective review of epidural infusions among pediatric patients suggests a very low incidence of infection when used short term for postoperative analgesia.[78]

All patients with continuous epidural infusions require careful nursing observation and regular assessment of level of sedation and pain score and measurement of vital signs. Infants younger than 6 months of age, patients with increased risk for respiratory compromise, or patients receiving epidural hydrophilic opioids require electronic monitoring in addition to close observation.

Axillary Brachial Plexus Block

Axillary brachial plexus blockade is a safe and easily performed block in children undergoing arm or hand surgery, often in conjunction with general anesthesia. The axillary artery is usually readily palpated in children between the coracobrachilis muscle and the pectoralis major.[79] The arm should be flexed and slightly externally rotated. A 22-gauge short-bevel needle is slowly advanced to the perivascular sheath. Proper placement should be confirmed using a nerve stimulator, especially in anesthetized patients. An injection of 0.5 mL/kg of bupivacaine 0.25% provides up to 12 hours of effective postoperative analgesia. Complications with axillary brachial plexus blockade include inadvertent intravascular injection of local anesthetic and direct injury to artery or nerves.[79]

Fascia Iliaca Compartment Block

The fascia iliaca block allows for blockade of the femoral, lateral femoral cutaneous, obturator, and genitofemoral nerves.[80] Proper needle and local anesthetic placement is based on easily identifiable landmarks. The inguinal ligament is identified between the anterior superior iliac spine and the symphysis pubis. A 22-gauge, short-bevel, blunt needle is inserted 0.5 cm caudad to the junction of the lateral one third and medial two thirds of the inguinal ligament (Fig. 53-7). Two distinct "pops" will be appreciated as the blunt needle traverses the fascia lata and the fascia iliaca. There should be a loss of resistance when the iliaca compartment is reached. Aspiration for blood should be checked before and periodically during injection of local anesthetic solution. A solution of 0.8 mL/kg of bupivacaine 0.25% can provide up to 12 hours of postoperative analgesia.[81]

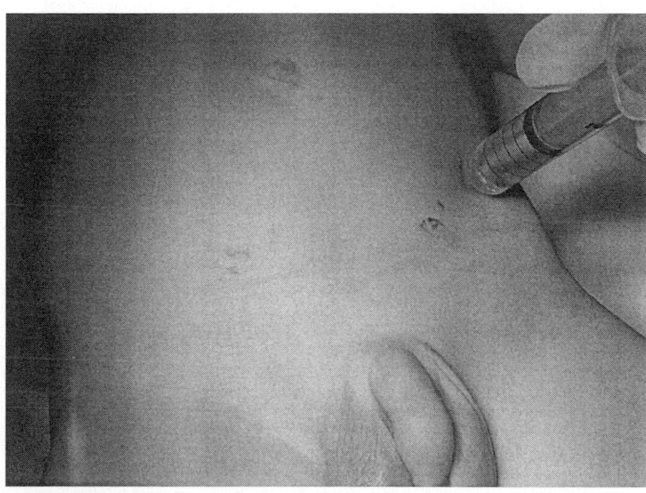

Figure 53-7 Fascia iliaca compartment block.

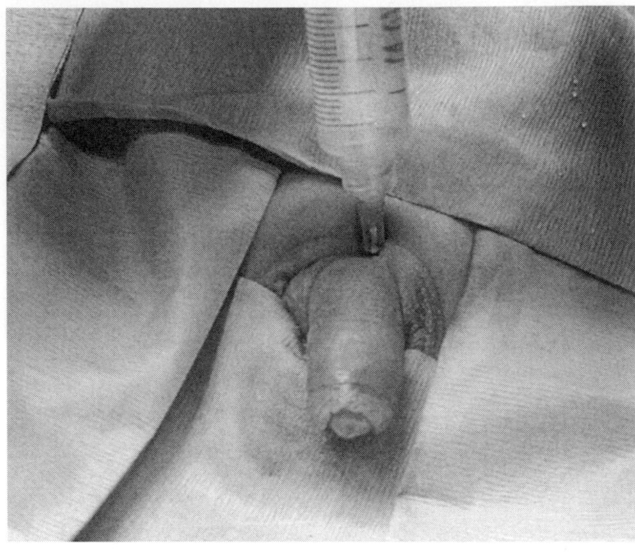

Figure 53-8 Penile block.

Penile Block

The distal part of the penis is innervated by the dorsal penile nerves. These nerves can be reliably blocked in patients undergoing circumcision or distal hypospadius repair.[82,83] Because "single-shot" caudal blocks sometimes cause significant lower extremity weakness and inability to ambulate postoperatively, penile blocks are sometimes preferred to caudal blocks for these types of outpatient procedures.[84,85] The proximal part of the penis and the scrotum are innervated by the genitofemoral and ilioinguinal nerves and are not affected by a penile block.

A penile nerve block is performed by inserting a 25-gauge needles just below the pubic rami, 0.5 to 1 cm on each side of the symphysis pubis (Fig. 53-8).[82] The usual dose of 0.1 mL/kg of 0.25% bupivacaine on each side of the symphysis pubis provides long-lasting analgesia postoperatively. Epinephrine-containing solutions should not be used for penile blocks because of the risk of vasoconstriction of end arteries.

SUMMARY

Over the past 20 years, there have been significant clinical advances in the treatment of acute pain in children. Improved analgesics, better understanding of pediatric pharmacology and neurodevelopment, and increased experience in regional techniques in children have led to these clinical advances. Optimal management of acute pain requires reliable assessment of pain and aggressive management of pain and side effects with consideration to emotional and social factors contributing to pain.

REFERENCES

1. Anand KJS, Hickey PR. Pain and its effects in the human neonate and fetus. *N Engl J Med* 1987;317:1321.
2. Fitzgerald M, Anand KJ. Developmental neuroanatomy and neurophysiology of pain. In: Schecter N, Berde C, eds. *Pain in Infants, Children and Adolescents*. Baltimore, Md: Williams & Wilkins, 1993:11–32.
3. Morton NS. Development of pain perception. In: Morton NS, ed. *Acute Pediatric Pain Management*. Philadelphia, Pa: WB Saunders, 1998: 13–32.
4. Goubet N, Clifton RK, Shah B. Learning about pain in preterm newborns. *J Dev Behav Pediatr* 2001;22:418.
5. Reynolds M, Fitzgerald M. Long-term sensory hyperinnervation following neonatal skin wounds. *J Comp Neurol* 1995;358:487.
6. Reynolds M, et al. Neonatally wounded skin induces NGF-independent sensory neurite outgrowth in vitro. *Brain Res* 1997;102:275.
7. Anand KJ, et al. Long-term behavioral effects of repetitive pain in neonatal rat pups. *Physiol Behav* 1999;66:627.
8. Taddio A, Ilersich AL, Koren G. Effect of neonatal circumcision on pain response during subsequent routine vaccination. *Lancet* 1997;349: 599.
9. Taddio A, Ipp M, et al. Effect of neonatal circumcision on pain responses during vaccination in boys. *Lancet* 1995;345:291.
10. Grunau RV, Whitfield MF, Petrie JH. Pain sensitivity and temperament in extremely low-birth-weight premature toddlers and preterm and full-term controls. *Pain* 1994;58:341.
11. Oberlander TF, Grunau RV, Whitfield MF. Biobehavioral pain responses in former extremely low-birthweight infants at 4 months' corrected age. *Pediatrics* 2000;105:6.
12. Anand KJ, International Evidence-Based Group for Neonatal. Consensus statement for the prevention and management of pain in the newborn. *Arch Pediatr Adoles Med* 2001;155:173.
13. Johnston CC, Stevens BJ. Experience in a neonatal intensive care unit affects pain response. *Pediatrics* 1996;98:925.
14. Fitzgerald M, deLima J. Hyperalgesia and allodynia in infants. In:*Acute and Procedural Pain in Infants and Children*. Seattle, Wash: IASP Press, 2000:1–12.
15. Anand KJS, Hansen DD, Hickey PR. *Hormonal-metabolic* stress responses in neonates undergoing cardiac surgery. *Anesthesiology* 1990; 73:661.
16. Anand KJ, Hickey PR. Halothane-morphine compared with high-dose sufentanil for anesthesia and postoperative analgesia in neonatal cardiac surgery [see comments]. *N Engl J Med* 1992;326:1.
17. Romsing J, et al. Postoperative pain in children. A comparison between ratings of children and nurses[Danish]. *Ugeskrift Laeger* 1997;159:422.
18. Romsing J. Assessment of nurses' judgement for analgesic requirements of postoperative children. *J Clin Pharm Ther* 1996;21:159.
19. Jylli L, Olsson GL. Procedureal pain in a paediatric surgical emergency unit. *Acta Paediatr Scand* 1995;84:1403.
20. Craig KD. The facial display of pain in infants and children. *Pain Res Manage* 1998;10:103.
21. Gilbert CA, et al. Postoperative pain expression in preschool children: validation of the child facial coding system. *Clin J Pain* 1999;15:192.
22. Wasz-Höckert O, et al. *The Infant Cry: A Spectrographic and Auditory Analysis; Clinics in Developmental Medicine*. London, England: Spastics International Medical Publications, 1968.
23. Krechel SW. CRIES: a new neonatal postoperative pain measurement score: initial testing of validity and reliability. *Pediatr Anaesth* 1996; 5:53.
24. Stevens B, et al. Premature Infant Pain Profile: development and initial validation. *Clin J Pain* 1996;12(1):13-22.
25. Beyer JE, McGrath PJ, Berde CB. Discordance between self-report and behavioral pain measures in children aged 3-7 years after surgery. *J Pain Symptom Manage* 1990;5(6):350.
26. Beyer J, et al. The creation, validation, and continuing development of the Oucher: a measure of pain intensity in children. *J Pediatr Nurs* 1992;7:335.
27. Hester NO, Foster R, Kristensen K. Measurement of pain in children: generalizability and validity of the pain ladder and the poker-chip tool. In: Tyler DC, Krane EJ, eds. *Advances in Pain Research and Therapy*. New York, NY: Raven Press, 1990:79–84.
28. Bieri D, et al. The Faces Pain Scale for the self-assessment of the severity of pain experienced by children: development, initial vali-

dation, and preliminary investigation for ratio scale properties. *Pain* 1990;41:139.
29. Keck J, et al. Reliability and validity of the Faces and Word Descriptor Scales to measure procedural pain. *J Pediatr Nurs* 1996;11(6):368.
30. Berde C, Masek B. Pain in children. In: Wall PD, Melzack R, eds. *Textbook of Pain*. 1999, Edinburgh, Scotland: Churchill Livingstone, 1999: 1463–1478.
31. Denman WT, Ballantyne J. Postoperative pain in children. In: Ballantyne J, ed. *The Massachusetts General Hospital Handbook of Pain Management*. Philadelphia, Pa: Lippincott, Williams & Wilkins, 2002: 306–321.
32. Yaster M, et al. *Pediatric Pain Management and Sedation Handbook*. St. Louis, Mo: Mosby-Year Book, 1997.
33. Yaster M, ed. Acute pain in children. *Pediatr Clin North Am* 2000; 47:487.
34. Zwass M, Polaner D, Berde C. Postoperative pain management. In: Cote CJ, et al, eds. *A Practice of Anesthesia for Infants and Children*. Philadelphia, Pa: W B Saunders, 2001.
35. Litalien C, Jacqz-Aigrain E. Risks and benefits of nonsteroidal anti-inflammatory drugs in children: a comparison with paracetamol. *Paediatr Drugs* 2001;3:817.
36. Carney DE, et al. Ketorolac reduces postoperative narcotic requirements. *J Pediatr Surg* 2001;36:76.
37. Chauhan RD, Idom CB, Noe HN. Safety of ketorolac in the pediatric population after ureteroneocystostomy. *J Urol*. 2001;166:1873.
38. Ilowite NT. Current treatment of juvenile rheumatoid arthritis. *Pediatrics* 2002;109:109.
39. Olkkola KT, Hamunen K, Maunuksela EL. Clinical pharmacokinetics and pharmacodynamics of opioid analgesics in infants and children. *Clin Pharmacokinet* 1995;28:385.
40. Doyle E, Harper I, Morton NS. Patient-controlled analgesia with *low* dose background infusions after lower abdominal surgery in children. *Br J Anaesth* 1993;71:818.
41. Murthy BV, et al. Pharmacokinetics of tramadol in children after i.v. or caudal epidural administration. *Br J Anaesth* 2000;84:346.
42. Viitanen H, Annila P. Analgesic efficacy of tramadol 2 mg kg(-1) for paediatric day-case adenoidectomy. *Br J Anaesth* 2001;86:572.
43. Mihaly GW, et al. The pharmacokinetics and metabolism of the anilide local anaesthetics in neonates. I. Lignocaine. *Eur J Clin Pharm* 1978; 13:143.
44. Yaster M, Maxwell LG. Pediatric regional anesthesia. *Anesthesiology* 1989;70:324.
45. Mazoit JX, Denson DD, Samii K. Pharmacokinetics of bupivacaine following caudal anesthesia in infants. *Anesthesiology* 1988;68:387.
46. Lerman J, et al. Effects of age on the serum concentration of alpha 1-acid glycoprotein and the binding of lidocaine in pediatric patients. *Clin Pharmacol Ther* 1989;46:219.
47. Dalens B. Regional anesthesia in children. *Anesth Analg* 1989; 68:654.
48. Mazoit JX, Cao LS, Samii K. Binding of bupivacaine to human serum proteins, isolated albumin and isolated alpha-1-acid glycoprotein. Differences between the two enantiomers are partly due to cooperativity. *J Pharmacol Exp Ther* 1996;276:109.
49. Tucker GT. Pharmacokinetics of local anaesthetics. *Br J Anaesth* 1986; 58:717.
50. Zsigmond E. Plasma cholinesterase activity in newborns and infants. *Can Anaesth Soc J* 1989;18:278.
51. Welborn LG, et al. Postoperative apnea in former preterm infants: prospective comparison of spinal and general anesthesia. *Anesthesiology* 1990;72:838.
52. Krane EJ, Haberkern CM, Jacobson LE. Postoperative apnea, bradycardia, and oxygen desaturation in formerly premature infants: prospective comparison of spinal and general anesthesia. *Anesth Analg* 1995; 80:7.
53. Cote C, Zaslavsky A, Downes J. Postoperative apnea in former preterm infants after inguinal herniorraphy. *Anesthesiology* 1995;82:809.
54. Cox RG, Goresky GV. Life-threatening apnea following spinal anesthesia in former premature infants. *Anesthesiology* 1990;73:345.
55. Pascucci RC, Hershenson MB, Sethna NF, et al. Chestwall motion in infants during spinal anesthesia. *J Appl Physiol* 1990;68:2087–2091.
56. Harnik EV, et al. Spinal anaesthesia in premature infants recovering from respiratory distress syndrome. *Anesthesiology* 1986;64:95.
57. Oberlander TF, et al. Infants tolerate spinal anesthesia with minimal overall autonomic changes: analysis of heart rate variability in former premature infants undergoing hernia repair. *Anesth Analg* 1995;80:20.
58. Gleason CA. Optimal position for a spinal tap in preterm infants. *Pediatrics* 1983;71:31.
59. Dalens B, Hasnaoui A. Caudal anesthesia in pediatric surgery: success rate and adverse effects in 750 consecutive patients. *Anesth Analg* 1989; 68:83.
60. Veyckemans F, van Obbergh LJ, Gouverneur JM. Lessons from 1100 pediatric caudal blocks in a teaching hospital. *Reg Anaesth* 1992;17: 119.
61. Bramwell RGB, et al. Caudal block for postoperative analgesia in children. *Anaesthesia* 1982;37:1024.
62. Broadman LM, et al. Caudal anesthesia in pediatric outpatient surgery: a comparison of three different bupivacaine concentrations. *Anesth Analg* 1987;66:S1.
63. Wolf AR, et al. Bupivacaine for caudal analgesia in infants and children: The optimal effective concentration. *Anesthesiology* 1988; 69:102.
64. Gunter JB, et al. Optimum concentration of bupivacaine for combined caudal-general anesthesia in children. *Anesthesiology* 1991;75:57.
65. Krane EJ, et al. Caudal morphine for postoperative analgesia in children: a comparison with caudal bupivacaine and intravenous morphine. *Anesth Analg* 1987;66:647.
66. Jamali S, et al. Clonidine in pediatric caudal anesthesia. *Anesth Analg* 1994;78:663.
67. Klimscha W, et al. The efficacy and safety of a clonidine/bupivacaine combination in caudal blockade for pediatric hernia repair. *Anesth Analg* 1998;86:54.
68. Constant I, et al. Addition of clonidine or fentanyl to local anaesthetics prolongs the duration of surgical analgesia after single shot caudal block in children. *Br J Anaesth* 1998;80:294.
69. Bosenberg AT, Hadley GP, Wiersma R. Oesophageal atresia: caudothoracic epidural anaesthesia reduces the need for post-operative ventilatory support. *Pediatr Surg Int* 1992;7:289.
70. Maxwell LG, Martin LD, Yaster M. Bupivacaine-induced cardiac toxicity in neonates: successful treatment with intravenous phenytoin. *Anesthesiology* 1994;80:682.
71. Berde CB. Toxicity of local anesthetics in infants and children. *J Pediatr* 1993;122(5 Pt 2):S14.
72. Schwartz N, Eisenkraft JB. Probable venous air embolism during epidural placement in an infant [see comments]. *Anesth Analg* 1993;76: 1136.
73. Sethna NF, Berde CB. Venous air embolism during identification of the epidural space in children [editorial; comment]. *Anesth Analg* 1993; 76:925.
74. Bösenberg AT, et al. Thoracic epidural anesthesia via caudal route in infants. *Anesthesiology* 1988;69:265.
75. Aram L, et al. Tunneled epidural catheters for prolonged analgesia in pediatric patients. *Anesth Analg* 2001;92:1432.
76. Gunter J, Eng C. Thoracic epidural anesthesia via the caudal approach *in* children. *Anesthesiology* 1992;76:935.
77. Fisher QA, Shaffner DH, Yaster M. Detection of intravascular injection of regional anaesthetics in children [see comments]. *Can J Anaesth* 1997;44:592.
78. Strafford MA, Wilder RT, Berde CB. The risk of infection from epidural analgesia in children: a review of 1620 cases. *Anesth Analg* 1995;80: 234.
79. Fisher WJ, Bingham RM, Hall R. Axillary brachial plexus block for perioperative analgesia in 250 children. *Paediatr Anaesth* 1999;9:435.

80. Dalens B, Vanneuville G, Tanguy A. Comparison of the fascia iliaca compartment block with the 3-in-1 block in children. *Anesth Analg* 1989;69:705.
81. Doyle E, Morton NS, McNicol LR. Plasma bupivacaine levels after fascia iliaca compartment block with and without adrenaline. *Paediatr Anaesth* 1997;7:121.
82. Dalens B, Vanneuville G, Dechelotte P. Penile block via the subpubic space in 100 children. *Anesth Analg* 1989;69:41.
83. Lau J. Penile block for pain relief after circumcision in children. A randomized, prospective trial. *Am J Surg* 1984;147:797.
84. Vater M, Wandless J. Caudal or dorsal nerve block? A comparison of two local anaesthetic techniques for postoperative analgesia following day case circumcision. *Acta Anaesthesiol Scand* 1985; 29:175.
85. Yeoman PM, Cooke R, Hain WR. Penile block for circumcision? A comparison with caudal blockade. *Anaesthesia* 1983;38:862.

CHAPTER 54 CHRONIC PAIN IN INFANTS AND CHILDREN

Christine D. Greco and Yuan-Chi Lin

Management of chronic pain is an essential part of pediatric practice that requires an understanding of pediatric illnesses and the psychosocial aspects of chronic pain conditions experienced by children. Many children experience a variety of chronic recurrent pains such as recurrent abdominal pain or headaches. Chronic recurrent pain is more common in children than persistent pain, and is less likely to be associated with underlying organic disease. Chronic pain may become persistent in conditions such as rheumatoid arthritis, malignancies, sickle cell disease, or neuropathic pain syndromes. Because of the complex nature of chronic pain, treatment is often approached from a broad-based medical model that utilizes the expertise of psychologists, neurologists, anesthesiologists, nurses, and other health care providers. This chapter reviews some of the more common types of recurrent and persistent pain among children and summarizes treatment strategies, including pharmacologic as well as nonpharmacologic therapies.

RECURRENT ABDOMINAL PAIN

Recurrent abdominal pain (RAP) is a common problem among school-aged children. Some studies report that as many as 25% of school-aged children will experience recurrent abdominal pain, with the highest prevalence occurring among young girls.[1] Many children with RAP remain functional and maintain normal activities; patients seen at pediatric pain clinics are typically those with more severe patterns of pain and disability. In most cases, there is no clear identifiable cause of RAP in school-aged children.[1,2]

There are certain clinical characteristics that distinguish benign recurrent abdominal pain (RAP) from other types of abdominal pain in children. In general, children with RAP are between the ages of 4 and 16 who experience episodic abdominal pain interspersed with pain-free periods and are otherwise thriving and medically well.[2] Children with RAP frequently describe diffuse periumbilical pain that is poorly localized; it rarely radiates to the back or chest. Pain is often worse at night but rarely awakens the child from sleep. Many children will experience other chronic symptoms such as headaches, nausea, and dizziness.

In the majority of cases, RAP is functional, which refers to the lack of an identifiable biochemical, structural, or other organic cause. The lack of a readily identifiable cause for RAP does not imply psychogenic causes. Most children with RAP are in general medically and psychologically well.[3] A subgroup of patients will have a recognizable underlying disease, such as lactose intolerance, constipation, ureteropelvic junction obstruction, inflammatory bowel disease, or endometriosis.[4–9] For many children, however, an underlying etiology is rarely diagnosed. Some studies have suggested that RAP may be a precursor to irritable bowel syndrome (IBS) in adults, and that some children and adolescents may progress to meet standardized criteria for IBS as adults.[10-12]

The diagnosis of RAP should be based on a thorough history, physical examination, and review of symptoms. A psychosocial history is essential to learn how the child and family cope with pain and to identify school avoidance and reinforcers of pain. A history of fever, weight loss, growth failure, rash, or other symptoms of systemic illness should prompt further investigation of organic causes.[13,14] Occurrence of persistent pain or recurrent abdominal pain in a child younger than 4 years of age is also of concern. A physical examination should include a rectal examination with stool guaiac, evaluation for undescended testes, hernias, and abdominal masses. Findings on history and physical examination that suggest a possible underlying organic disorder should serve as a guide to laboratory and diagnostic testing. In general, extensive routine screening tests such as endoscopies, barium studies, and other radiographic studies are of low yield, particularly when there are no specific clinical suspicions from history or physical examination. In addition to a careful history and physical examination, baseline complete blood count, sedimentation rate, and urinalysis are reasonable screening tests to help rule out occult organic disease. A family history of inflammatory bowel disease in a child with chronic abdominal pain warrants further laboratory and possibly diagnostic testing. In children who experience chronic persistent abdominal pain, rather than the more characteristic episodic pain of RAP, laparoscopy identified treatable conditions in a high percentage of cases.[15,16]

A significant component of treatment is education and reassurance that no serious organic illness appears likely. It should be emphasized that the child's pain is genuine and that clinical reassessments will be ongoing. Treatment is based on improving function and reducing maladaptive pain behaviors through emphasis on cognitive-behavioral therapies.[17–20] Underlying anxiety or depression should be addressed. A return to school and participation in normal family and social activities is essential. Extensive diagnostic testing and referrals to multiple subspecialists may heighten patient and parental anxiety and reinforce a patient's "sick role." Medication trials of tricyclic antidepressants and antispasmodics are sometimes used; however, there is limited data on the efficacy of drug therapy. The routine use of pain medications should be avoided.

Longitudinal studies show that only 30% of children with RAP have resolution of their pain within 5 years and 25% to 50% continue to experience symptoms as adults. Walker and colleagues found that only 1 in 31 children with RAP in a 5-year follow-up were eventually diagnosed with a definable "organic" disease.[21]

HEADACHES

As with many other recurrent pains in childhood, recurrent headaches in children are exceedingly common. As many as 10% of children experience recurrent headaches.[22] The most common types of headaches that occur in children include migraine headaches, tension headaches, and combined migraine-tension headaches. Migraine headaches are more common in boys than girls in young children but become more common in girls after reaching puberty. There is often a strong family history of migraines and almost 60% of adults with vascular headaches experienced symptoms during childhood.[23] Children with migraines typically report an abrupt onset of unilateral or bilateral severe headache pain that is throbbing and often associated with nausea and vomiting. Although some children may experience classic visual or auditory auras of migraines, many experience more subtle premonitory signs such as pallor, irritability, or fatigue.[24] Generally, patients experience relief of the migraine after sleep.[23] Tension headaches are most common among adolescents. Usually, there are no associated auras, nausea, or vomiting. The pain is often described as a squeezing pain located circumferentially around the head. It is not uncommon for tension headaches to occur daily. Children with combined headaches experience chronic tension headaches and episodic acute migraine headaches associated with nausea and vomiting.

Most headaches in children are not associated with serious underlying intracranial pathology or organic disease. A thorough history and physical examination is essential and should include a careful neurologic with funduscopic examination. A careful psychosocial history is helpful in understanding family stressors or maladaptive behaviors that may have a causative role in reinforcing pain behaviors. A history of personality changes, visual disturbances, fever, or headaches associated with neurologic deficits are worrisome signs that mandate neuroimaging. A chronic progressive headache or focal symptoms or signs on neurologic examination also warrant neuroimaging to investigate for structural abnormalities or malignancies.

Treatment for headaches in children without underlying pathology includes pharmacologic therapy, cognitive-behavioral interventions, and lifestyle changes that promote functional and adaptive behavior. Reassurance should be provided that a more worrisome cause for the headaches is unlikely and that re-evaluations will be ongoing. Often, a diary that includes characteristics of the headaches, medications, diet, and stress can help identify aggravating factors.

Combinations of analgesics, anitemetics, and 5-HT serotonin agonists are used for abortive migraine therapy in children. Nonsteroidal anti-inflammatory drugs (NSAIDs) are often used as first-line abortive therapy for migraines, tension headaches, and combined headaches[25] (Table 54-1). Patients should be instructed on proper dosing since excessive use of NSAIDs, acetaminophen, and combination drugs such as Fioricet can cause rebound headaches in some patients[26]. Systematic reviews of NSAIDs among adult patients report little differences in clinical effectiveness. However, parenteral NSAIDs such as ketorolac are often used when patients have persistent vomiting and cannot tolerate oral intake. In a randomized crossover study, ibuprofen was found to be more effective than acetaminophen for interruptive therapy.[25] Ibuprofen in suspension form is commonly used for abortive headache therapy for children who are unable to swallow pills. Recommended pediatric doses are 6 to 10 mg/kg orally. Sumatriptan, a 5-HT agonist, has been shown to be effective for abortive therapy in pediatric patients with severe migraines.[27–29] Chronic opioid use is generally not recommended in the treatment of recurrent or chronic headaches.[30]

Antidepressants, beta blockers, and anticonvulsants are most frequently used for prophylactic migraine therapy. Low-dose tricyclic antidepressants such as amitriptyline or nortriptyline may provide effective migraine prophylaxis. A typical starting dose in children is 0.2 mg/kg administered at bedtime to help promote improved sleep. Doses are titrated on the basis of clinical response and side effects. Trazodone has been shown to be more effective

TABLE 54-1 **Acetaminophen and Nonsteroidal Anti-Inflammatory Drugs (<50 kg)**

Drug	Dosing Guidelines	Comments
Acetaminophen	10–15 mg/kg PO q4h 20–30 mg/kg PR q4h Maximum daily dosing: 90 mg/kg/day (children) 60 mg/kg/day (infants) 30 mg/kg/day (neonates)	No anti-inflammatory effect. No antiplatelet effect. Avoid PR route in patients receiving anti-neoplastic agents. Hepatic failure associated with toxic dosing.
Ibuprofen	4–10 mg/kg PO q6h Maximum daily dosing. 40 mg/kg/day (children)	Anti-inflammatory effects. Gastric and platelet effects.
Naprosyn	5–7 mg/kg PO q8–12 h	Anti-inflammatory effects. Gastric and platelet effects.
Ketorolac	0.25–0.5 mg/kgIV q6h up to a maximum of 5 days	Anti-inflammatory effects. Gastric and platelet effects. Useful for patients unable to tolerate oral dosing.

From Greco C, Berde B. Pain Management in Children. In: Berhman R, Kliegman R, Jenson H, eds. Nelson Textbook of Pediatrics, 16th Edition. W.B. Saunders Company 2000.

than a placebo in crossover trial but should be avoided in teenaged boys because of the potential for priapism.[31] Propranolol is often used in doses of 1 to 2 mg/kg daily; however, controlled studies in pediatric headache management show equivocal results.[32,33] Several studies have shown good clinical results with calcium channel blockers.

Essential in the treatment of chronic headaches in children is cognitive-behavioral therapy. Evidence supports the effectiveness of biobehavioral headache management when compared to pharmacologic agents for certain types of headaches in children.[33,34] Through biofeedback, guided imagery, and progressive muscle relaxation, patients learn to shift their cognitive focus way from pain and decrease their experience of pain. These skills help to reduce stress and anxiety, which can be precipitating factors for many children with headaches. Cognitive-behavioral strategies help patients learn improved coping skills, return to school, recognize maladaptive behaviors, and help reinforce a more functional lifestyle.

CHEST PAIN

Chest pain in children and adolescents is a common presenting symptom to emergency rooms, general pediatric practices, and pediatric pain clinics, accounting for 650,000 physician visits per year.[35] Because chest pain is often an ominous sign among adults, it causes much distress to children and parents. It is, however, uncommonly associated with heart disease in children. Of 67 patients referred to a pediatric cardiology clinic with chest pain, only 6% were found to have underlying cardiac disease.[36] Most common causes in children include costochondritis, idiopathic causes, muscle pain from coughing, and other musculoskeletal causes.[37,38] Other causes in children include slipping rib syndrome and abdominal and gastroesophageal disease.[39]

A thorough medical history and physical examination helps to identify cardiac causes. Selbst and colleagues found that organic causes of chest pain in children were more likely if associated with abnormal findings on physical examination, or if symptoms were present in a younger child.[37] A history of syncope, presyncopal episodes, or a history of palpitations warrants further evaluation. Gastroesophageal reflux or esophageal spasm may cause referred pain to the chest.

In the absence of worrisome findings on history or physical examination, education and reassurance that heart disease is not a likely cause has been shown to be helpful in long-term resolution of symptoms.[36,40] A trial of NSAIDs may be helpful for patients with musculoskeletal causes such as costochondritis. Nonpharmacologic therapies such as transcutaneous electrical nerve stimulation (TENS), heat, progressive muscle relaxation, and physical therapy are helpful for many patients.

PELVIC PAIN

Endometriosis is a common cause of pelvic pain among adolescents, affecting 45% to 70% of adolescents with chronic pelvic pain.[41,42] In general, endometriosis affects women of reproductive age, but young adolescent girls can experience pain from endometriosis prior to beginning menses. Laufer and colleagues studied adolescent patients with chronic pelvic pain not responsive to conservative medical treatment of oral contraceptives and NSAIDs and found that 70% of patients had endometriosis on diagnostic laparoscopy.[41] A variety of other medical conditions such as painful musculoskeletal disorders, constipation, urologic conditions, and irritable bowel syndrome may present as chronic pelvic or abdominal pain.

Many adolescent patients with endometriosis report both cyclic and acyclic pelvic pain. Some patients experience more severe pain at midcycle and with menstruation, but many patients will experience pain throughout the month. There is evidence to suggest that the severity of endometriosis seen on laparoscopy does not necessarily correlate with the severity of pain.[43]

Treatment of chronic pelvic pain and endometriosis can include hormonal suppression of endometriosis, surgical treatment, effective pain control, and minimizing disability. Hormonal therapy with oral contraceptives and gonadotropin-releasing hormone agonists suppress the growth of endometriosis and inhibit progression of disease. Surgical resection of endometriosis has been shown to provide both immediate and long-term relief from chronic pelvic pain due to endometriosis. Long-term follow-up studies in adult patients after laparoscopic resection of endometriosis show symptom improvement in 66% of patients 5 years after surgery.[44]

Chronic pelvic pain in female adolescents can lead to significant disability. Over 90% of adolescent women with chronic pelvic pain referred to the Pain Treatment Services at Children's Hospital, Boston, have endometriosis. A comprehensive approach consisting of biobehavioral therapy, physical therapy, acupuncture, and selected medication trials has been helpful for many patients. As with the treatment of recurrent abdominal pain, emphasis is placed on school attendance, participation in social and family activities, and recognition of maladaptive behaviors. Patients should be thoroughly evaluated for other conditions in addition to endometriosis that may be contributing to pelvic pain such as constipation, irritable bowel symptoms, or urolithiasis. Medication trials of tricyclic antidepressants may be helpful, particularly for patients with sleep disorders, although there is little data on efficacy. Opioids are rarely used for long-term treatment. There is some evidence to suggest that an integrated approach to chronic pelvic pain with attention to organic causes as well as psychosocial factors early in the course of treatment may improve long-term outcome.[45]

NEUROPATHIC PAIN

Neuropathic pain conditions in children are most commonly a result of postsurgical nerve injury, extremity trauma, malignancies, complex regional pain syndromes, and congenital and traumatic amputation. Diabetic peripheral neuropathy and trigeminal neuralgia seen in adult patients are rare in children. Clinical features of neuropathic pain in children include allodynia, hyperpathia, and hyperalgesia to noxious, mechanical, and thermal stimuli. Some children will also experience autonomic dysregulation and motor weakness. Children often have difficulty describing neuropathic pain, and will report pain that is "strange" or "weird."

A thorough history and physical examination, including a careful neurologic examination, is essential when evaluating a child with neuropathic pain. A broad-based evaluation may provide clues to less common causes of neuropathic pain such as underlying cancer, neurodegenerative disorders, or metabolic diseases. Nerve conduction studies are insensitive to abnormalities of C fibers and AÎ fibers, and therefore may be normal in patients with certain neuropathic pain conditions. Quantitative sensory testing (QST), which assesses thermal and vibratory thresholds, may be especially useful in evaluating pediatric patients because it is painless and does not require the use of sedation.[46–48]

The use of medications in the treatment of neuropathic pain in children is based on data extrapolated from adult studies (Table 54-2). Randomized controlled studies of tricyclic antidepressants have shown effectiveness in treating some neuropathic pain conditions in adults, including diabetic neuropathy and postherpetic neuralgia.[49–52] Nortriptyline and amitriptyline are most commonly used in children; desipramine is sometimes a useful alternative if excessive sedation is experienced with other tricyclic antidepressants. Because children metabolize tricyclic antidepressants more efficiently than adults, twice daily dosing is sometimes necessary, although a larger portion of the dose is administered in the evening to help improve sleep disturbances and minimize daytime somnolence. Because of rare case reports of sudden death in children treated with tricyclics attributed to cardiac dysrrhythmias, a thorough cardiac history, physical examination and baseline electrocardiogram is recommended prior to initiating therapy.[53] Other antidepressants such as selective serotonin reuptake inhibitors (SSRIs) are occasionally used in the treatment of neuropathic pain; however, additional studies are needed to determine efficacy. SSRIs can be useful for patients who have neuropathic pain associated with depressed mood or anxiety.

Adult clinical trials have shown effectiveness of anticonvulsants such as carbamazepine, phenytoin, valproic acid, and gabapentin for the treatment of a variety of neuropathic pain conditions.[54–56] Gabapentin has the advantage of a lower side effect profile and fewer severe adverse effects than other anticonvulsants; monitoring of serum levels is not necessary.[57] Most frequent side effects include dizziness and somnolence. Gabapentin may also be effective in the treatment of mood disorders.

There is controversy over the use of opioids in the treatment of neuropathic pain. Some evidence supports that opioids are ineffective in treating neuropathic pain, or that patients experience analgesia only at doses that produce intolerable side effects.[58] Other studies suggest that opioids can provide effective pain relief in patients experiencing neuropathic pain from cancer, limb amputation, and other causes without producing unremitting side effects.[59–60] In general, the use of opioids in selected patients with neuropathic pain not caused by cancer or other terminal illnesses should involve a treatment plan that emphasizes ongoing cognitive-behavioral therapy and maintenance of school and peer activities.

COMPLEX REGIONAL PAIN SYNDROMES

Complex regional pain syndrome type 1 (CRPS 1) is a condition characterized by persistent neuropathic limb pain with cyanosis, coldness, swelling, atrophy, or other signs of neurovascular abnormalities without an associated nerve injury. CRPS 2 refers to this clinical syndrome with a definable nerve injury.

The clinical presentation of CRPS in children differs from that in adults. Most children with CRPS are female with a lower limb affected, which differs from adult presentation of CRPS, where gender differences are not significant and upper and lower extremities are equally effected. CRPS in children occurs most frequently at 10 to 12 years of age and occurs very rarely before the age of 6. In a report by Wilder and colleagues of 70 children with CRPS, all children were able to identify a specific injury prior to developing symptoms, and some patients developed similar symptoms in a second extremity without additional injury.[61] Many pa-

TABLE 54-2 **Commonly Used Non-Opioid Analgesics for Chronic Pain (<50 kg)**

Nortriptyline, amitriptyline	Starting dose 0.1–0.2 mg/kg daily at bedtime; titrate as clinically indicated up to 1.5 mg/kg/day. Some patients require divided dosing, e.g., 25% of dose in daytime.	Useful for neuropathic pain. Screen for rhythm disturbances. Check levels. Side effects include dry mouth, constipation, urinary retention, orthostatic hypotension, palpitations
Gabapentin	5 mg/kg/day PO divided tid Titrate to maximum of 50 mg/kg/day	Useful for neuropathic pain. Reduce dose for renal impairment.
Carbamazepine	Start at 10 mg/kg/day PO, divided bid. Titrate up to maximum of 20 mg/kg/day	Monitor for hematologic and hepatic toxicity. Check levels. Side effects include dizziness, tinnitus, diplopia, urinary retention, Stevens-Johnson syndrome.
Propranolol	1 mg/kg PO bid	Use caution in patients with bronchospastic disease. Screen for rhythm disturbances.

tients experienced eating disorders and were involved in highly competitive sports such as ballet and gymnastics.

Several retrospective pediatric series suggest that conservative treatment with aggressive physical therapy and cognitive-behavioral therapy results in marked improvement of symptoms in children with CPRS.[62–64] In the Wilder study, a noninvasive approach with physical therapy, TENS, and cognitive-behavioral therapy was effective in improving function and reducing pain scores in over 50% of patients.[61] Other studies have emphasized sympathetic blockade.[65] A prospective, randomized, controlled trial by Lee and colleagues[66] showed that a majority of children had clinical improvement with a regimen that emphasized physical therapy and cognitive-behavioral therapy

The approach at the Boston Children's Hospital includes an initial outpatient trial of active physical therapy and cognitive-behavioral therapy. Physical therapy is based on a rehabilitative approach involving desensitization techniques, weight-bearing exercises, and a gradual return to function. Cognitive-behavioral interventions typically include biofeedback training, relaxation techniques, and family and individual counseling. Education of both patients and parents is essential regarding the nonprotective nature of pain with CRPS, and that movement of the affected limb will ultimately diminish pain and dysfunction. Regular school attendance and participation in family and peer activities is emphasized. Often, a home diary that records pain scores and measures of function helps track response to therapy.

Commonly used medications in the treatment of CRPS in children include antidepressants, anticonvulsants, local anesthetic-like drugs, and opioids. There is significant individual variation in response to medication trials. Opioids are used in a selected group of patients. Sympathetic blockade is reserved for patients who do not improve with outpatient therapy and who continue to experience significant pain and limitations of limb mobility. Sympathetic blockade is also used for patients who have severe circulatory impairment with ischemic complications. Typically, sympathetic blockade is performed using continuous catheter techniques combined with an intensive rehabilitative 5- to 7-day hospitalization.

Over the past 15 years, more than 650 children with CRPS have been treated at the Children's Hospital, Boston. Over 85% of patients have experienced pain reduction and good improvement in limb function. Fewer than 5% of patients have received spinal cord stimulation trials or implantations. Fewer than 1% of patients over the past 15 years have received operative or chemical sympathectomies. In all cases, patients underwent sympathectomies to preserve limb circulation rather than for pain control.

AMPUTATION PAIN

Historically, it was assumed that children who have congenital absence of a limb or who have had amputation early in life rarely experience phantom sensations. However, results of several case studies suggest that most children who have limb amputations do experience phantom sensations and pain.[67–69] In a retrospective study of children who had undergone amputation, Krane and Heller found that 100% of patients reported phantom sensations and 75% of patients experienced phantom pain.[67] A study by Melzack and colleagues showed that approximately 20% of patients who had congenital limb absence and 50% of patients who had amputations at an early age experienced phantom limb sensations.[68] There is some evidence to suggest that the children who receive chemotherapy prior to amputation are more likely to experience phantom limb pain than children with amputations who were not exposed to chemotherapy.[70]

Children describe a variety a phantom sensations such as persistent itching, burning, pain, or a perception of the presence of the missing limb. Some patients will experience allodynia and dysesthesia of the stump.

Studies of tricyclic antidepressants, anticonvulsants such as gabapentin and clonazepam, and opioids have shown effectiveness in treating amputation pain; however, there is limited data on the best treatment among adult and pediatric amputees.[61,71,72] Medication trials, biobehavioral techniques, physical rehabilitation, and the early use of a prosthesis have been helpful for many patients.[73] Studies examining whether preoperative neurologic blockade reduces the severity or incidence of phantom pain have shown inconsistent results.[74–76]

SICKLE CELL PAIN

Sickle cell pain ranges from acute vaso-occlusive episodes to chronic, daily pain. Acute painful episodes are characterized by an abrupt and usually unpredictable onset of severe ischemic pain. Vaso-occlusive episodes typically produce pain in extremities, chest, lower back, and abdomen, and may be caused by a variety of factors such as infection, dehydration, hypoxia, and acidosis. Often, there is no obvious cause. Acute episodes of pain account for most hospitalizations and emergency room visits. In a prospective study, Platt and colleagues reported that 5% of patients with sickle cell hemoglobinopathy experienced more than 30% of all painful episodes, and that the patients with the highest rates of painful episodes tended to die earlier than patients with lower rates of painful episodes.[77] Chronic pain may develop as painful episodes become more frequent and severe, resulting in persistent daily pain. Bone infarction or necrosis may result in debilitating chronic pain conditions such as aseptic necrosis of the hip, vertebral compression fractures, and chronic low back pain.

Home management of vaso-occlusive episodes is encouraged through the use of NSAIDs and orally administered opioids (See Chapter 52). Day treatment programs may provide an effective alternative to hospitalizations or emergency room visits for some patients.[78] Hospitalization is necessary for patients who are unable to tolerate oral opioids because of vomiting, or for patients with severe, escalating pain requiring rapid control with intravenous analgesics. Patient-controlled analgesia offers patients the ability to rapidly titrate opioids according to wide fluctuations in pain intensity common in vaso-occlusive episodes (See Chapter 53). A low-dose basal opioid infusion in addition to on-demand doses may provide effective analgesia, particularly during severe episodes of pain; however, there is some evidence showing that this regimen may increase the risk of hypoxemia at night.[79] Continuous epidural analgesia can provide effective analgesia and maintenance of respiratory drive in patients with acute chest syndrome.[80] It has not been established how often to choose epidural analgesia for patients who have frequent painful episodes. Self-report pain scales should be used as much as possible for pain assessment. Close nursing observation and monitoring is necessary, especially for patients at risk for opioid-induced respiratory depression and hypoxemia.

A multidisciplinary approach to sickle cell pain integrates pharmacologic therapy and cognitive-behavioral techniques to provide effective pain control, maintenance of normal functioning, and optimal quality of life. There is often excessive concern among health providers and families about addiction to opioids, which has led to inadequate analgesia in some cases. Education is necessary regarding the use of opioids, home management strategies, and avoidance of precipitating factors of painful episodes. Cognitive-behavioral treatment such as biofeedback, hypnosis, guided imagery, and family therapy can help to improve coping mechanisms and prevent maladaptive behaviors.[81]

CYSTIC FIBROSIS

Patients with cystic fibrosis suffer a variety of recurrent and chronic pains, particularly as lung disease becomes more advanced.[82] Recurrent chest pain is common and may occur from chest wall muscle strain, costochondritis, or spontaneous pneumothorax. Severe coughing may produce painful rib fractures that can significantly compromise respiratory function. Frequent headaches can be caused by sinus disease or by the intense contraction of muscles due to coughing. As respiratory function declines with advanced disease, hypercarbia and hypoxia can contribute to headaches.[82] Other causes of pain in patients with cystic fibrosis include back pain from compression fractures, arthritis pain, and abdominal pain from pancreatitis.[83,84]

Treatment of recurrent and chronic pain of cystic fibrosis should provide optimal analgesia without further impairing respiratory function. Opioids may provide effective pain relief without inducing excessive sedation and respiratory depression in selected patients.[82] Because patients with cystic fibrosis frequently experience constipation with opioid use, laxatives should be used early in the course of treatment. Selective COX-2 inhibitors may help provide analgesia without causing respiratory depression, constipation, and with less risk of hemoptysis than conventional NSAIDs. Continuous thoracic epidural infusions can provide effective analgesia for rib fractures or pneumothoraces, and for postoperative pain control. Intercostal blockade is less preferred than epidural analgesia because of a short duration of effect and the considerable risk of pneumothorax.

COMPLEMENTARY AND ALTERNATIVE MEDICINE

Complementary and alternative medicine (CAM) therapies are increasingly used in pediatric practices and among children with chronic medical illnesses such as cancer and cystic fibrosis.[85] In a survey of pediatric pain clinics in North America, 70% of clinics offered at least one form of CAM therapy, and 30% of clinics offered acupuncture services. In a review of hospitalized patients, children were most likely to use CAM therapy for the treatment of pain, nausea, and insomnia.[86]

Acupuncture is one of the most common CAM therapies and is practiced in a variety of chronic medical conditions including headaches, endometriosis, and nausea. Although children are often reluctant to accept therapy involving needles, even young children report positive experience with acupuncture. One case series reported that 70% of children with chronic pain referred for acupuncture felt that acupuncture treatment helped their symptoms.[87] Acupuncture has a very good safety record; there are very rare reports of adverse events. Additional prospective clinical trials are necessary to determine efficacy in children.

SUMMARY

Central in treatment of pain and distress in children is an in-depth understanding of pediatric diseases and the psychological and social dynamics involved in chronic pain conditions. Analgesics and specialized techniques should be combined with lifestyle changes and nonpharmacologic approaches to provide optimal care. Additional prospective clinical trials are necessary in the understanding and treatment many chronic pain conditions in children.

REFERENCES

1. Apley J, Naish N. Recurrent abdominal pains: a field survey of 1,000 school children. *Arch Dis Child* 1958;33:165.
2. Apley J. *The Child With Abdominal Pains*. London, England: Blackwell, 1975.
3. Astrada CA, et al. Recurrent abdominal pain in children and associated DSM-III diagnoses. *Am J Psychiatry* 1981;138:687.
4. Feldman W, et al. The use of dietary fiber in the management of simple, childhood, idiopathic, recurrent, abdominal pain. Results in a prospective, double-blind, randomized, controlled trial. *Am J Dis Child* 1985;139:1216.
5. Webster RB, DiPalma JA, Gremse DA. Lactose maldigestion and recurrent abdominal pain in children. *Dig Dis Sci* 1995;40:1506.
6. Wewer V, et al. The prevalence and related symptomatology of *Helicobacter pylori* in children with recurrent abdominal pain. *Acta Paediatr* 1998;87:830.
7. Olafsdottir E, et al. Impaired accommodation of the proximal stomach in children with recurrent abdominal pain. *J Pediatr Gastroenterol Nutr* 2000;30:157.
8. Khetan N, et al. Endometriosis: presentation to general surgeons. *Ann Roy Coll Surg Engl* 1999;81:255.
9. Irish MS, et al. The approach to common abdominal diagnosis in infants and children [review]. *Pediatr Clin North Am* 1998;45(4):729.
10. Hyams JS, et al. Characterization of symptoms in children with recurrent abdominal pain: resemblance to irritable bowel syndrome [see comments]. *J Pediatr Gastroenterol Nutr* 1995;20:209.
11. Hyams JS, Hyman PE, Rasquin-Weber A. Childhood recurrent abdominal pain and subsequent adult irritable bowel syndrome [review]. *J Dev Behav Pediatr* 1999;20(5):318.
12. Walker LS, et al. Recurrent abdominal pain: a potential precursor of irritable bowel syndrome in adolescents and young adults. *J Pediatr* 1998;132:1010.
13. Stein M.T, et al. Challenging case: chronic disease—developmental and behavioral implications. *Pediatrics* 2001;107(4).
14. Boyle JT. Recurrent abdominal pain: an update. *Pediatr Rev* 1997; 18(9):310.
15. Stylianos S, et al. Laparoscopy for diagnosis and treatment of recurrent abdominal pain in children. *J Pediatr Surg* 1996;31:1158.
16. Stringel G, et al. Laparoscopy in the management of children with chronic recurrent abdominal pain. *JSLS: Soc Laparoendosc Surg* 1999; 3:215.
17. Gold N, et al. Well-adjusted children: an alternate view of children with inflammatory bowel disease and functional gastrointestinal complaints. *Inflamm Bowel Dis* 2000;6:1.
18. Compas BE, Thomsen AH. Coping and responses to stress among children with recurrent abdominal pain [review]. *J Dev Behav Pediatr* 1999;20:323.
19. Fritz GK, Fritsch S, Hagino O. Somatoform disorders in children and adolescents: a review of the past 10 years [review]. *J Am Acad Child Adolesc Psychiatry* 1997;36:1329.
20. Sanders M, et al. The treatment of recurrent abdominal pain in children: A controlled comparison of cognitive-behavioral family interventions and standard pediatric care. *J Consult Clin Psychol* 1994; 62:306.

21. Walker L, et al. Long term health outcomes in patients with recurrent abdominal pain. *J Pediatr Psychol* 1995;20:233.
22. Bille B. Migraine and tension-type headache in children and adolescents. *Cephalalgia* 1996;16(2):78.
23. Rothner AD. Headaches in children and adolescents [review]. *Child Adolesc Psychiatr Clin North Am* 1999;8(4):727.
24. Barlow CF. Migraine in childhood. *Res Clin Study Headache* 1977; 5:34.
25. Hamalainen ML, et al. Ibuprofen or acetaminophen for the acute treatment of migraine in children: a double-blind, randomized, placebo-controlled, crossover study. *Neurology* 1997;48:103.
26. Symon DN. Twelve cases of analgesic headache. *Arch Dis Child* 1998; 78:555.
27. Linder S. Subcutaneous sumatriptan in the clinical setting: the first 50 consecutive patients with acute migraine in a pediatric neurology office practice. *Headache* 1996;36(7):419.
28. Ueberall MA, Wenzel D. Intranasal sumatriptan for the acute treatment of migraine in children. *Neurology* 1999;52:1507.
29. Hamalainen M, Hoppu K, Santavuori P. Sumatriptan for migraine attacks in children: a randomized placebo-controlled study. Do children with migraine respond to oral sumatriptan differently from adults? *Neurology* 1997;48:1100.
30. Ziegler DK. Opioids in headache treatment. Is there a role? [review]. *Neurol Clin* 1997;15:199.
31. Battistella P, et al. A placebo-controlled crossover trial using trazodone in pediatric migraine. *Headache* 1993;33:36.
32. Lutschg J, Vassella F. The treatment of juvenile migraine using flunarizine or propranolol. *Schweiz Med Wochensch* 1990;120:1731.
33. Olness K, MacDonald J, Uden D. Comparison of self-hypnosis and propranolol in the treatment of juvenile classic migraine. *Pediatrics* 1987;79:593.
34. Sartory G, et al. A comparison of psychological and pharmacological treatment of pediatric migraine. *Behav Res Ther* 1998;36:1155.
35. Ezzati T. *Ambulatory care utilization patterns of children and young adults: National Ambulatory Medical Care Survey United States, January-December 1975.* Hyattsville, Md: National Center for Health Statistics; 1978. Vital and Health Statistics, series 13.
36. Fyfe DA, Moodie DS. Chest pain in pediatric patients presenting to a cardiac clinic. *Clin Pediatr* 1984;23(6):321.
37. Selbst SM. Consultation with the specialist. Chest pain in children. *PediatrRev* 1997;18(5):169.
38. Selbst SM, Ruddy R, Clark BJ. Chest pain in children. Follow-up of patients previously reported. *Clin Pediatr* 1990;29(7):374.
39.. Mooney DP, Shorter NA. Slipping rib syndrome in childhood. *J Pediatr Surg* 1997;32:1081.
40. Lababidi Z, Wankum J. Pediatric idiopathic chest pain. *Mo Med* 1983; 80(6):306.
41. Laufer MR, et al. Prevalence of endometriosis in adolescent with chronic pelvic pain not responding to conventional therapy. *J Pediatr Adolesc Gynecol* 1997;10:199.
42. Laufer MR, Goldstein DP. *Pelvic pain, dysmenorrhea, and premenstrual syndrome.* In: Emans SJ, Laufer MR, Goldstein DP, eds. *Pediatric and Adolescent Gynecology* Boston, Mass: Little, Brown, 1998: 363–410.
43. Fedele L, et al. Stage and localization of pelvic endometriosis and pain. *Fertil Steril* 1990;53:155.
44. Vancaillie T, Schenken RS. Endoscopic surgery. In: Schenken RS, ed. *Endometriosis:Contemporary Concepts in Clinical Management.* Philadelphia, Pa: JB Lippincott, 1989:249–266.
45. Peters A, et al. A randomized clinical trial to compare two different approaches in women with chronic pelvic pain. *Obstet Gynecol* 1991; 77:740.
46. Meier PM, et al. Quantitative assessment of cutaneous thermal and vibration sensation and thermal pain detection thresholds in healthy children and adolescents. *Muscle Nerve* 2001;24:1339.
47. Yarnitsky D, et al. Heat pain thresholds: normative data and repeatability. *Pain* 1995;60:329.
48. Zaslansky R, Yarnitsky D. Clinical applications of quantitative sensory testing (QST) [review]. *J Neurol Sci* 1998;153:215.
49. Max MB, et al. Amitriptyline relieves diabetic neuropathy pain in patients with normal or depressed mood. *Neurology* 1987;37:589.
50. Bowsher D. The effects of pre-emptive treatment of postherpetic neuralgia with amitriptyline: a randomized, double-blind, placebo-controlled trial. *J Pain Symptom Manage* 1997;13:327.
51. McQuay HJ, et al. A systematic review of antidepressants in neuropathic pain. *Pain* 1996;68:217.
52. Sindrup SH, Jensen TS. Efficacy of pharmacological treatments of neuropathic pain: an update and effect related to mechanism of drug action. *Pain* 1999;83:389.
53. Varley CK. Sudden death related to selected tricyclic antidepressants in children: epidemiology, mechanisms and clinical implications. *Paediatr Drugs* 2001;3:613.
54. Ross EL. The evolving role of antiepileptic drugs in treating neuropathic pain. *Neurology* 2000;55(5 suppl 1):S41;discussion S54.
55. Backonja MM. Anticonvulsants (antineuropathics) for neuropathic pain syndromes. *Clin J Pain* 2000;6(2 suppl):S67.
56. Mellick GA, Mellick LB. Reflex sympathetic dystrophy treated with gabapentin. *Arch Phys MedRehab* 1997;78:98.
57. Portenoy RK. Current pharmacotherapy of chronic pain. *J Pain Symptom Manage* 2000;19(1 suppl):S16.
58. Arnér S, Meyerson BA. Lack of analgesic effect of opioids on neuropathic and idiopathic forms of pain [see comments]. *Pain* 1988; 33:11.
59. Portenoy RK, Foley KM, Inturrisi CE. The nature of opioid responsiveness and its implications for neuropathic pain: new hypotheses derived from studies of opioid infusions. Pain 1990;43:273.
60. Huse E, et al. The effect of opioids on phantom limb pain and cortical reorganization. *Pain* 2001;90:47–55.
61. Wilder RT, et al. Reflex sympathetic dystrophy in children. Clinical characteristics and follow-up of seventy patients. *J Bone Joint Surg [Am]* 1992;74A:910.
62. Bernstein BH, et al. Reflex neurovascular dystrophy in childhood. *J Pediatr* 1978;93:211.
63. Sherry DD, et al. Short- and long-term outcomes of children with complex regional pain syndrome type I treated with exercise therapy. *Clin J Pain* 1999;15:218.
64. Stanton RP, et al. Reflex sympathetic dystrophy in children: an orthopedic perspective. *Orthopedics* 1993;16:773.
65. Kesler RW, et al. Reflex sympathetic dystrophy in children: treatment with transcutaneous electric nerve stimulation. *Pediatrics* 1988; 82:728.
66. Lee B, Scharff L, et al. Physical therapy and cognitive-behavioral treatment for complex regional pain syndromes. *J Pediatr* 2002;14:135–140.
67. Krane EJ, Heller LB. The prevalence of phantom sensation and pain in pediatric amputees. *J Pain Symptom Manage* 1995;10:21.
68. Melzack R, et al. Phantom limbs in people with congenital limb deficiency or amputation in early childhood. *Brain* 1997;120(pt 9):1603.
69. Wilkins KL, et al. Phantom limb sensations and phantom limb pain in child *and* adolescent amputees. Pain 1998;78:7.
70. Smith J, Thompson JM. Phantom limb pain and chemotherapy in pediatric amputees. *Mayo Clin Proc.* 1995;70:357.
71. Panerai AE, et al. A randomized, within-patient, cross-over, placebo-controlled trial on the efficacy and tolerability of the tricyclic antidepressants chlorimipramine and nortriptyline in central pain. *Acta Neurol Scand* 1990;82:34.
72. Rusy LM, Troshynski TJ, Weisman SJ. Gabapentin in phantom limb pain management in children and young adults: report of seven cases. *J Pain Symptom Manage* 2001;21:78.
73. Lotze M, et al. Does use of a myoelectric prosthesis prevent cortical reorganization and phantom limb pain? *Nat Neurosci* 1999;2:501.
74. Bach S, Noreng JF, Tjellden NU. Phantom limb pain in amputees during the first 12 months following limb amputation after preoperative lumbar epidural blockade. *Pain* 1988;33:297.

75. Nikolajsen L, et al. Randomised trial of epidural bupivacaine and morphine in prevention of stump and phantom pain in lower-limb amputation [see comments]. *Lancet* 1997;350:1353.
76. Nikolajsen L, Ilkjaer S, Jensen TS. Effect of preoperative extradural bupivacaine and morphine on stump sensation in lower limb amputees. *Br J Anaesth* 1998;81:348.
77. Platt OS, et al. Pain in sickle cell disease. Rates and risk factors [see comments]. *N Engl J Med.* 1991;325:11.
78. Benjamin LJ, . Swinson GI, Nagel RL. Sickle cell anemia day hospital: an approach for the management of uncomplicated painful crises. *Blood* 2000;95:1130.
79. Shapiro BS, Cohen DE, . Howe CJ. Patient-controlled analgesia for *sickle*-cell-related pain. *J Pain Symptom Manage* 1993;8:22.
80.. Yaster M, et al. Epidural analgesia in the management of severe vaso-occlusive sickle cell crisis. *Pediatrics* 1994;93:310.
81. Gil KM, et al. Follow-up of coping skills training in adults with sickle cell disease: analysis of daily pain and coping practice diaries. *Health Psychol* 2000;19(1):85.
82. Ravilly S, et al. Chronic pain in cystic fibrosis. *Pediatrics* 1996;98(4 pt 1):741.
83. Schidlow DV, et al. Arthritis in cystic fibrosis. *Arch Dis Child* 1984; 59:377.
84. Littlewood JM. Abdominal pain in cystic fibrosis [review]. *J Roy Soc Med* 1995;88(suppl 25):9.
85. Eisenberg DM, et al. Trends in alternative medicine use in the United States, 1990–1997: results of a follow-up national survey [see comments]. *JAMA* 1998;280:1569.
86. Kemper KJ, Wornham WL. Consultations for holistic pediatric services for inpatients and outpatient oncology patients at a children's hospital. *Arch Pediatr Adolesc Med* 2001;155:449.
87. Kemper KJ, et al. On pins and needles? Pediatric pain patients' experience *with* acupuncture. *Pediatrics* 2000;105(4 pt 2):941.

CHAPTER 55

CANCER PAIN AND PALLIATIVE CARE IN CHILDREN

Christine D. Greco and Charles B. Berde

The prognosis of cancer in children has improved dramatically over the past 40 years. Unlike many adult cancers, pediatric malignancies are often responsive to initial aggressive induction chemotherapy. The most common childhood cancer, acute lymphoblastic leukemia (ALL), was an almost uniformly fatal disease in the early 1950s. Long-term survival rates in children with ALL now exceed 70%. Children with cancer, however, frequently experience a variety of acute and chronic pains, which can be a result of cancer treatment or of the tumor itself.[1] The treatment of cancer pain in children should involve a multidimensional approach that relies not only on medications for pain and symptom management, but also on cognitive-behavioral interventions and other nonpharmacologic therapies. This approach provides optimal pain control and addresses patients' complex emotional needs related to grief and sense of loss.

TREATMENT-RELATED PAIN

In contrast to adults, children with cancer more frequently experience pain related to aspects of cancer treatment. This is in part because of higher rates of remission in children after initial chemotherapy induction and improved long-term survival rates in childhood cancers.[1,2]

Procedures such as bone marrow biopsies and aspirates, lumbar punctures, and central venous line insertions are common sources of distress and pain in children with cancer. Other sources of pain related to the treatment of cancer include painful mucositis, amputation pain, and painful neuropathies from surgery and chemotherapeutic agents.

Every attempt should be made to minimize distress, fear, and pain in children undergoing brief needle procedures and other more invasive procedures, since initial traumatic experiences with procedures tend to make subsequent procedures more distressing. In general, treatment of procedure-related pain should consist of the individualized use of combinations of cognitive-behavioral interventions, local anesthesia, conscious sedation, and general anesthesia.

There is ample evidence to support the use of cognitive-behavioral strategies in managing procedure-related pain in children with cancer. Through guided imagery, progressive muscle relaxation, and hypnosis, patients can direct their focus away from pain and the procedure and help reduce their experience of pain, fear, and discomfort. Young children or those with developmental deficiencies, however, may not have the cognitive abilities to use these techniques. Explaining the procedure in age-appropriate terms often helps to gain the child's trust and confidence.

The use of local anesthetics and conscious sedation combined with cognitive-behavioral techniques can make procedures less terrifying for children. Applying EMLA (eutectic mixture of lidocaine and prilocaine) to the skin overlying intravenous catheter-insertion sites or lumbar puncture sites can reliably decrease the pain from needle insertion into the skin. This can allow less painful infiltration of local anesthetics deep to the dermis. For more invasive procedures or for children who experience significant distress with brief needle procedures, conscious sedation or general anesthesia should be used. Conscious sedation refers to a level of sedation where a child is comfortable but is able to maintain airway reflexes and spontaneous ventilation. Conscious sedation is often performed by pediatric subspecialists and is widely used for bone marrow aspirates or biopsies, lumbar punctures, or central venous line removals (Table 55-1). A pediatric anesthesiologist is consulted for more invasive procedures or for children with certain risks of conscious sedation, such as airway anomalies, obstructive sleep apnea, or significant gastroesophageal reflux disease.

Centers caring for children with cancer often have a two-tiered approach where certain procedures are performed under conscious sedation by pediatric subspecialists, such as oncologists and radiologists. Sedation protocols guide the choice of sedative used, dosing, monitoring, and indications for when involvement of a pediatric anesthesiologist is required. For young infants, or for patients with certain cardiac, neurologic, or airway diseases that increase risk, sedation or general anesthesia by pediatric anesthesiologists is recommended.

Mucositis refers to painful mucosal inflammation and necrosis due to chemotherapy or radiation therapy. Although it is a self-limiting condition in most cases, it causes significant pain and distress in children. Mucositis associated with bone marrow transplantation can be especially prolonged and painful. Topical therapies such as diphenhydramine, viscous lidocaine, antacids, and sucralfate are sometimes used to provide symptomatic relief; however, there is little evidence to support efficacy. Patient-controlled analgesia (PCA) is frequently used in addition to topical agents. Some children, however, continue to experience significant pain despite aggressive opioid dosing. PCA permits dose titration and treatment of acute exacerbations associated with mouth or perineal care. Some studies have shown lower pain scores, fewer side effects, and lower opioid use in treating mucositis with PCA compared with staff-controlled analgesia.[3]

Vincristine is an antineoplastic agent that can be associated with peripheral neuropathies such as sensory deficits, gastrointestinal dismotility, and paresthesias. Some children treated with vincristine experience burning neuropathic pain of the lower extremities. Additional studies are needed to determine the best treatment strategy; however, opioids, tricyclic antidepressants, and anticonvulsants are often used. In most patients, symptoms will gradually improve but may recur with repeated use of vincristine.

TUMOR-RELATED PAIN

A majority of children experience tumor-related pain at initial diagnosis. A survey by Miser and colleagues showed that 62% of

TABLE 55-1 **Drugs Used for Conscious Sedation in Children**

Midazolam	0.05 mg/kg IV every 5–10 min titrated to clinical effect up to 3–5 doses 0.1–0.2 mg/kg IM (maximum dose 10 mg) 0.3–0.6 mg/kg PO (maximum dose 20 mg)	Good anxiolytic. Can be reversed with flumazenil. Use caution when combining with opioids.
Fentanyl	0.5 μg/kg IV titrated every 5 min up to 3–5 doses	May cause chest wall rigidity. Increased risk of respiratory depression when combined with other sedatives.
Pentobarbital	1 mg/kg IV titrated every 10 min up to 3 doses 2–4 mg/kg IM 4–6 mg/kg PO	Provides no analgesia. Often used for radiologic procedures.
Ketamine	0.2–0.5 mg/kg IV titrated every 10 min up to 3 doses 1–2 mg/kg IM	Causes increased secretions, which may increase risk of laryngospasm. Should be administered by physicians with airway expertise.

Physicians with airway expertise and airway equipment should be readily available. Close observation and monitoring of patients is necessary.

From Greco C, Berde B. Pain Management in Children. In: Berhman R, Kliegman R, Jenson H, eds. Nelson Textbook of Pediatrics, 16th Edition. W.B. Saunders Company 2000.

children reported pain prior to receiving an initial diagnosis of cancer.[4] Other studies show that 25% of outpatient pediatric patients with cancer report experiencing daily pain.[5] Tumors can produce different types of pain through stretch or involvement of bone, viscera, nerves, and other tissues. Leukemias can produce constant, aching bone pain through the proliferation of malignant cells in marrow causing compression of the marrow space. Bone pain can also result from metastasis of solid tumors to localized areas of bone. The involvement of lymphoma, leukemia, and neuroblastoma in solid viscera such as spleen and liver can cause abdominal pain by distension and capsular stretch. Tumors can spread to plexuses, peripheral nerves, or the epidural space causing lancinating and sometimes refractory neuropathic pain. Children with brain tumors and increased intracranial pressure often present with headaches and in some cases focal neurologic signs or seizures. Spinal cord tumors or the extension of tumors into the intrathecal space typically cause back or neck pain.[6]

The assessment of pain in children with cancer can be challenging. Some children with inadequately treated cancer pain may withdraw from their environment and may falsely appear comfortable to care providers. Many pain assessment scales were developed to assess acute pain and frequently under-rate pain when used to assess persistent cancer pain. Physiologic signs such as blood pressure and heart rate may habituate with persistent pain. Gauvain-Piquard and colleagues designed an observational pain scale specifically for young children with cancer that includes depression and anxiety-like descriptors often reported by these patients.[7]

Cancer pain is often best treated using a multidisciplinary approach that combines the aggressive use of pharmacologic agents, psychosocial support, cognitive and behavioral therapy, and nerve blocks when indicated. The World Health Organization (WHO) has proposed an "analgesic ladder" to help guide physicians in treating cancer pain. A study of children with terminal malignancies showed that over 90% of patients had effective pain relief when managed according to standard escalations based on the WHO guidelines.[8] According to this treatment guide, non-opioid analgesics such as acetaminophen or nonsteroidal anti-inflammatory drugs (NSAIDs) are recommended as a first-line therapy. Selective COX-2-inhibitors may be used for children with platelet dysfunction or for children who experience gastric side effects with NSAIDs. Weak opioids, such as low-dose oxycodone or codeine, are often combined with acetaminophen as a "second step" in managing mild pain. Recommended oral dosing of codeine is 0.5 to 1 mg/kg every 4 hours. Patients tend to experience more nausea and other side effects with higher doses of codeine compared with other opioids. In addition, some patients lack sufficient enzyme activity to o-demethylate codeine to morphine, causing a marked reduction in analgesic effect.[9] Dosing of acetaminophen and opioid combination preparations is usually limited by the maximum recommended acetaminophen dose. Weak opioids have a "ceiling effect," where escalation of dose typically causes increased side effects without improving analgesic effect.

With progression of cancer pain, μ-opioid agonists are the cornerstone of treatment (Table 55-2). Oral dosing of opioids is preferable where possible. Regular scheduled dosing of opioids should be used for patients who have continued pain in order to avoid breakthrough pain. Morphine is the most widely used opioid for treating cancer pain in children. Younger infants have an increased risk of hypoventilation with opioids because of both pharmacokinetic factors, such as diminished hepatic conjugation, and pharmcodynamic factors, such as immature ventilatory reflex response to hypoxemia and hypercapnia. A typical starting dose for immediate release morphine in opioid-naïve patients is 0.3 mg/kg orally every 4 hours. Sustained-release preparations of morphine and oxycodone are frequently used and are effective alternatives to frequent dosing of short-acting agents. A significant number of children are unable to swallow pills, which limits the use of sustained-acting preparations in these patients.

TABLE 55-2 **Recommended Initial Opioid Dosing Guidelines***

Drug	Starting IV or SC Dose <50 kg	Starting IV or SC Dose ≥50 kg	Ratio of Parenteral to Oral Dose	Starting PO Dose <50 kg	Starting PO Dose ≥50 kg
Morphine	Bolus: 0.1 mg/kg every 2–4 h Infusion: 0.03 mg/kg/h	Bolus: 5–8 mg every 2–4 h Infusion: 1.5 mg/hr	1:3 chronic use 1:6 single dose	Immediate release: 0.3 mg/kg every 3–4 h Sustained release: 10–15 mg every 8–12 h	Immediate release: 15–20 mg every 3–4 h Sustained release: 30–45 mg every 8–12 h
Codeine	N/A	N/A	1:2	0.5–1 mg/kg every 3–4 h	30–60 mg every 3–4 h
Oxycodone	N/A	N/A	N/A	0.1–0.2 mg/kg every 3–4 h	5–10 mg every 3–4 h
Methadone†	0.1 mg/kg every 4–8 h	5–8 mg every 4–8 h	1:2	0.1–0.2 mg/kg every 4–8 h	5–10 mg every 4–8 h
Hydromorphone	Bolus: 0.02 mg/kg every 2–4 h Infusion: 0.006 mg/kg/h	Bolus: 1 mg every 2–4 h Infusion: 0.3 mg/h	1:4	0.04–0.08 mg/kg every 3–4 h	2–4 mg every 3–4 h
Fentanyl	Bolus: 0.5–1 μg/kg every 1–2 h Infusion: 0.5–2 μg/kg/h	Bolus: 25–50 μg every 1–2 h Infusion: 25–100 μg/h	N/A	N/A	N/A

*For infants younger than 6 months of age, initial dose should be reduced to approximately 25% of the above weight-scaled doses.

†Methadone requires careful vigilance because of potential for drug accumulation.

Adapted from Berde C, Sethna N. Analgesics for the Treatment of Pain in Children. N Engl J Med, Vol 347: 1094–1098, 2002.

Methadone has a prolonged duration of action due to slow hepatic metabolism. The elimination half-life of methadone is approximately 19 hours and the oral bioavailability ranges from 60% to 90%. Elixir preparations are therefore useful for children with continued pain but who are unable to swallow pills. Intermittent intravenous dosing can provide sustained analgesia without the need for a continuous infusion pump or PCA device.[10] Because of the prolonged effect and a slow but variable clearance, the dose-response to methadone can be variable.

Methadone dosing is also complicated by the fact that it is actually a combination drug: the l-isomer is a μ-opioid and the d-isomer of methadone is an antagonist at the *N*-methyl-D-aspartate (NMDA) subgroup of glutamate receptors.[11] NMDA receptor antagonists have been shown to prevent tolerance to opioids. The result of this is that methadone shows incomplete cross-tolerance, meaning that its relative potency for both analgesia and respiratory depression compared with other opioids is much greater in opioid-tolerant patients than in opioid-naïve patients.[12,13] Because of incomplete cross-tolerance and variable dose-response, frequent assessment and careful titration of methadone is recommended to avoid oversedation and hypoventilation. Once adequate analgesia is achieved, the dose of methadone should be reduced or the dosing interval extended to avoid drug accumulation.

Hydromorphone is similar to morphine in onset of action and duration; it is frequently used as an alternative when patients experience dose-limiting side effects with morphine. In a double-blind, randomized, crossover trial comparing morphine with hydromorphone in PCA for children with mucositis, hydromorphone was well-tolerated and had an approximate potency ratio of 6:1 relative to morphine.

Meperidine is most commonly used for rigors following the administration of amphotericin or blood products. The major active metabolite of meperidine, normeperidine, can cause dysphoria, CNS excitation, and seizures, which limits the utility of meperidine in the management of pain in children.

Fentanyl is approximately 50 to 100 times as potent as morphine. It is frequently used for brief needle procedures because of its rapid onset and short duration of action due to rapid redistribution. However, with continuous infusions or multiple dosing, the clinical duration of action becomes significantly more prolonged. Fentanyl is commonly used in PCA for children who have excessive side effects from morphine.

Mixed μ-agonists/antagonists and agonists with activity at kappa receptors, including buprenorphine, butorphanol, and nalbuphine, have limited use in the treatment of cancer pain when compared to μ-agonists. Some of these agents may exhibit a ceiling effect with escalated doses, can cause dysphoria, and can precipitate withdrawal in opioid-tolerant patients. Buprenorphine provides prolonged analgesia and may be a useful agent in countries with limited access to μ-agonists.

ROUTES OF OPIOID ADMINISTRATION

The optimal route of analgesic administration varies in children with cancer. Oral administration of opioids is usually most convenient and relatively easy; however, some children are either unwilling to swallow pills or are unable to tolerate oral drugs due to painful swallowing from mucositis, vomiting, or lethargy associated with terminal disease. Oral analgesics are generally not effective for rapidly escalating pain. In these cases, other routes of administration such as intravenous, subcutaneous, or transdermal are indicated.

Intravenous administration allows for rapid titration in the setting of moderate to severe fluctuating pain. Many children with cancer have indwelling venous catheters, which can be convenient for opioid administration. PCA is widely used in children to manage cancer pain and is useful for both inpatients and outpatients. Nurse-controlled analgesia (NCA) is used for infants or toddlers or those who are unable to push the PCA button. In a palliative care setting, parents often participate in PCA dosing. The use of parent-controlled analgesia in the non-palliative care setting is more controversial.[14] If parent-controlled analgesia is to be considered in a non-palliative care setting, we would advocate formal programs for parent education and standardized protocols for respiratory depression. Morphine is the most commonly used drug in PCA; however, hydromorphone and fentanyl are frequently used alternatives. The addition of a basal infusion appears to provide more consistent analgesia and can promote restful sleep when used at night.

Subcutaneous opioid infusions can be used for children who have limited intravenous access.[15,16] Typically, a 22- or 24-gauge catheter or butterfly needle is inserted in the subcutaneous tissue of the chest or abdomen, with the site changed every 3 to 7 days as needed. Concentrated solutions of morphine or hydromorphone are most commonly used. PCA, NCA, continuous infusions, and intermittent boluses can be administered through subcutaneous catheters.

Transdermal fentanyl patches can provide continuous opioid delivery without the need for intravenous access or PCA devices. Since steady state is reached in approximately 12 to 24 hours after initial patch application, titration by other routes is usually necessary during this time. Transdermal fentanyl patches are not useful for patients who have fluctuating pain intensity. The lowest dose available in the United States is 25 μg per hour, which may be excessive for some children, particularly for opioid-naïve patients.

MANAGEMENT OF OPIOID SIDE EFFECTS

The successful use of opioids in the treatment of cancer pain requires aggressive management of side effects (Table 55-3). Unremitting nausea, vomiting, and pruritus can be as distressing as pain to some children. Constipation should be anticipated, and can be prevented and treated through the early use of stimulant laxatives. 5HT-3 antagonists, antihistamines, and phenothiazines can be effective for opioid-induced nausea in children. Pruritus can be treated with antihistamines or by switching to a different opioid. Sedation can be troublesome to patients as well as parents. The daytime use of dextroamphetamine or methylphenidate can provide additional analgesia and can allow patients to be more alert and interactive during the day. A trial of a different opioid should be considered when managing opioid-induced side effects since some patients experience fewer side effects with one opioid versus another. In general, tolerance to nausea, sedation, and pruritus develops within 1 to 2 weeks after initial opioid dosing. A recent

TABLE 55-3 **Management of Common Opioid Side Effects**

Side Effect	Comments	Drug Dosage
Nausea	Exclude other processes (e.g., bowel obstruction) Consider switching to different opioid Antiemetics	Metoclopramide 0.1–0.2 mg/kg PO/IV q6h Ondansetron 10–30 kg: 1 mg IV q6h >30 kg: 2 mg IV q6h Prochlorperazine 10–40 mg: 2.5 mg PR 1–3 times/day Adult: 2.5–10 mg IV/IM q12h 25 mg PR q12h
Pruritus	Exclude other causes (e.g., drug allergy) Consider switching to different opioid Antipruritic	Diphenhydramine 0.5–1 mg/kg PO/IV q6h Nalbuphine 10–20 μg/kg/dose IV q6h Hydroxyzine Child: 0.5–1 mg/kg PO q6h Adult: 25–75 mg/dose PO/IM q6h
Sedation	Add nonsedating analgesic (e.g., ketorolac) and reduce opioid dose Consider switching to different opioid	Methylphenidate 0.05–0.2 mg/kg PO bid (morning and midday dosing) Dextroamphetamine
Constipation	Regular use of stimulant and stool softener laxatives	Ducosate Child: 10–40 mg PO daily Adults: 50–200 mg PO daily Dulcolax Child: 5 mg PO/PR daily Adult: 10 mg PO/PR daily

retrospective study of parents' recollections following care of children with terminal malignancy suggested that non-painful symptoms, including sedation, fatigue, dysphoria, and sleep disturbances were as important as sources of suffering as pain itself.[17] Increased attention should be directed toward improving methods for management of these symptoms.

ADJUVANT MEDICATIONS

Children with cancer can experience neuropathic pain from tumor invasion of nerves, chemotherapeutic agents, postsurgical trauma, and radiation. Neuropathic pain can range from mild symptoms to severe, lancinating pain that can be refractory to opioids and other medications (See Chapter 54). There is a subgroup of patients with neuropathic pain for whom opioids do provide effective analgesia. In other cases, however, doses of opioids that improve pain also cause intolerable side effects. Tricyclic antidepressants (TCAs) are frequently used in children to treat neuropathic pain, although additional studies are needed to determine efficacy in children. Nortriptyline and amitriptyline are most commonly used. Typically, a bedtime dose is started and titrated according to clinical response and side effects. Plasma levels can help guide titration. A baseline electrocardiogram should be obtained to screen for rhythm disturbances prior to initiating TCAs. Intravenous administration of amitriptyline has been used for patients who cannot tolerate oral routes.[18] Selective serotonin reuptake inhibitors (SSRIs) are considered less effective for treating neuropathic pain; however, they are associated with fewer side effects than TCAs. Some children do experience good analgesic effect with SSRIs and they may be especially helpful for patients with pain and depressed mood. SSRIs have shown some efficacy for patients with depression-related fatigue or those with fibromyalgia.

Anticonvulsants such as gabapentin, valproate, phenytoin, and carbamazepine have all been used for the treatment of neuropathic pain, and are considered to be particularly effective for lancinating, paroxysmal pains. Gabapentin is usually well-tolerated, and unlike other anticonvulsants, monitoring of serum blood levels is not needed.

Corticosteroids are used as adjuvant anlagesics for selected types of cancer pain such as headaches due to increased intracranial pressure, spinal cord compression, and metastatic bone pain.[19] Dexamethasone effectively penetrates cerebral spinal fluid and is most frequently used for pain relief from brain tumors and spinal cord compression. Prolonged used of corticosteroids can result in immunosuppression, mood and behavior disturbances, and fractures.

REGIONAL TECHNIQUES FOR CANCER PAIN MANAGEMENT IN CHILDREN

Despite aggressive opioid dose escalation, some children with cancer experience intractable pain, particularly as the disease becomes widely metastatic. Regional blockade and neurodestructive procedures may be helpful for selected patients with refractory neuropathic pain, unremitting bone pain, severe chest or abdominal pain, and tumor involvement of the spine.[20–22] The use of pharmacologic, nonpharmacologic, and adjuvant therapies should be optimized when considering interventional approaches.

For pain that is largely below the umbilicus, we have found the most success by placing subarachnoid catheters. The subarachnoid route provides great flexibility in escalating local anesthetic dosing without producing toxic plasma levels. We prefer placement of thoracic epidural catheters for pain in upper abdominal and higher dermatomes. Epidural tumor involvement may result in technical difficulty in placing epidural catheters and may interfere with adequate spread of local anesthetics. Most children will require general anesthesia or deep sedation. Fluoroscopic guidance and the use of contrast solution help to ensure proper catheter placement and determine spread of local anesthetics. Tunneling of the catheters facilitates skin care and helps prevent dislodgement. We generally tunnel catheters at initial placement, rather than the two-step process of a temporary catheter followed by an implanted catheter commonly used for adult patients.

The choice of neuraxial solution should be individualized and based on the nature and site of pain, location of catheter tip, and side effects with consideration to a child's other symptoms, such as excessive sedation or air hunger. In our experience, almost invariably, local anesthetics applied in an appropriate dermatomal location are key to providing improved analgesia; neuraxial opioids alone rarely provide sufficient improvement in therapeutic index relative to systemic opioids. If neuraxial opioids produce persistent pruritus, nausea, ileus, or urinary retention, then clonidine may be useful since it provides synergistic analgesia with neuraxial local anesthetics and does not typically produce these particular side effects. In home care of children with subarachnoid or epidural infusions, it is essential that families have the resources to manage issues related to the catheters, pumps, infusions, and any side effects that may occur.

Neurolytic blockade is less commonly used in children with cancer pain; however, it can provide excellent analgesia for some children in terminal stages of their disease. Celiac plexus blockade can provide dramatic pain relief for children with upper abdominal pain due to tumor involvement of viscera.[23,24]

NEURODEGENERATIVE DISEASES

There are a variety of neurologic and neuromuscular diseases in children that can be associated with chronic pain, physical and cognitive impairments, and a shortened life-span. Although there is a wide spectrum of clinical expression, many children with these disorders will require long-term symptom management, palliative care, and end of life care. For example, children with Duchenne's muscular dystrophy and spinal muscle atrophy have intact cognition, but have varying degrees of motor impairment. Some children will experience slowly progressive muscle weakness while others suffer from profound motor devastation, cardiomyopathy, and early death. Tay-Sachs disease causes severe cognitive and motor impairments and death early in life.

A variety of factors make symptom management and palliative care challenging in these patients. Many of these conditions have a variable prognosis and unpredictable clinical course, making long-term care decisions difficult. Cognitive and motor impairments can make diagnosing causes for pain, agitation, and distress quite difficult. Some children will have persistent screaming and agitation without a clearly identifiable cause, which can be extremely distressing to parents and caregivers. Common causes of pain are usually excluded first, such as hip dislocations and gastrointestinal reflux. Therapeutic trials of opioids and sedatives are often used, but many children continue to have unremitting agitation. Baclofen and anticonvulsants trials are also used with varying success.

Improved methods of assisted ventilation have enabled children with myopathies to have an enhanced quality of life and an improved lifespan. Some children require nasal or mask positive pressure devices only at night, without the need for a tracheostomy. However, as motor weakness progresses, many children will eventually require more invasive mechanical ventilation. The decision to provide ventilatory support for patients with advanced neuromuscular disease is invariably difficult and must take into account individual variation. If the decision is made to forego assisted ventilation, then opioids and anxiolytics may have a role in the treatment of terminal air hunger.

CYSTIC FIBROSIS

Cystic fibrosis is a multisystem disorder that affects the pancreas, lung, liver, sinuses, and sweat glands. The associated chronic obstructive lung disease however causes the most pain and suffering. There has been considerable advancement in the life-expectancy of patients with cystic fibrosis. Lung transplantation and heart-lung transplantation offer hope of improved quality of life, although this is limited by a shortage of organ donors and a significant early mortality due to infection and acute rejection.

Patients with cystic fibrosis suffer from a variety of pain and distressing symptoms. A study by Ravilly and colleagues reported that many patients with advanced disease experience daily pains including headaches and chest pain.[25,26] Chronic hypoxemia and hypercarbia and frequent strain of head and neck muscles from violent coughing contribute to chronic daily headaches. In addition, chronic sinusitis can also exacerbate headaches.

Chest pain is a common symptom and can be caused by intercostal muscle strain from coughing and an increased work of breathing. Some patients experience severe chest pain from pneumothoraces, or fracture ribs from violent coughing episodes.

Patients with cystic fibrosis die from progressive respiratory failure. In the final stages of life, patients experience a spectrum of distressing symptoms. Fatigue, air hunger, severe dyspnea, headache, and chest pain are predominant symptoms in children with advanced lung disease. A majority of patients experience daily headaches and chest pain in the final 6 months of life. Opioids can provide relief; however they may exacerbate headaches by increasing hypercarbia. Benzodiazepines may help reduce anxiety associated with dyspnea in some patients. Sleep is often disturbed due to air hunger and anxiety and may be improved through the use of tricyclic antidepressants at bedtime. Tetracyclics, such as trazodone, may be useful if anticholinergic effects of tricyclic antidepressants are bothersome.

Terminal care in patients with advanced disease varies. Prior to the possibility of lung transplantation, patients in our institution died on an in-patient adolescent unit. With the hope of transplantation, many patients in our institution now die in the intensive care unit waiting a transplant.[26] Many of our patients fear suffocation and intractable pain and choose to be in a hospital setting for end-of-life care rather than home care. Other centers report higher patient preference for end-of-life care at home.[27]

TERMINAL CARE

Home care, hospices, or hospital-based programs are chosen by patients and families for end-of-life care. The choice is an individual one involving a variety of factors, including the level of care required, the degree of support for families and caregivers, and the connection to pediatric subspecialists. Home care can provide a secure and comfortable environment for children, free from the anxiety associated with hospital care. Optimal care requires careful individual planning for availability of supplies and medications, often with ongoing support from nurses, physicians, and pharmacists. Some children and families develop close connections to subspecialists and other health care providers at tertiary care institutions through the course of their illness and prefer to remain in this environment in the terminal stages of disease.

Although free-standing hospices are commonly used in adult palliative care, they are used relatively less often for children. More commonly, the choice is between home care, comfort-oriented care at their tertiary pediatric center, or comfort-oriented care at a local community hospital. Where pediatric hospices have been established, they often combine some care of children with advanced cancer, care of infants and children with advanced HIV disease who lack family support, and respite care or end-of-life care for children with neurodegenerative disorders.

Children with cancer, neurodegenerative conditions, and other life-threatening diseases require individualized treatment plans for symptom management through the use of pharmacologic agents, regional techniques, and psychological support. Consideration for quality of life is necessary in all stages of disease. For terminal stages, optimal care should emphasize patient comfort in an emotionally and spiritually supportive environment, which may include home, hospital, or hospice care.

REFERENCES

1. Miser A, et al. The prevalence of pain in a pediatric and young adult cancer population. *Pain* 1987;29:73.
2. Elliot S, et al. Epidemiologic features of pain in pediatric cancer patients: a co-operative community-based study. *Clin J Pain* 1991;7:263.
3. Zucker TP, et al. Patient-controlled versus staff-controlled analgesia with pethidine after allogeneic bone marrow transplantation. *Pain* 1998; 75:305.
4. Miser A, et al. Pain as a presenting symptom in children and young adults with newly diagnosed malignancy. *Pain* 1987;29:85.
5. Elliott SC, et al. Epidemiologic features of pain in pediatric cancer patients. A cooperative community-based study. North Central Cancer Treatment and Mayo Clinic. *Clin J Pain* 1991;7:263.
6. Hahn Y, McLone D. Pain in children with spinal chord tumors. *Child's Brain* 1984;11:36.
7. Gauvain-Piquard A, et al. Pain in children aged 2–6 years: a new observational rating scale elaborated in a pediatric oncology unit—preliminary report. *Pain* 1987;31:177.
8. Collins J, et al. Control of severe pain in children with terminal malignancy. *J Pediatr* 1995;126:653.
9. Caraco Y, Sheller J, Wood AJ. Impact of ethnic origin and quinidine coadministration on codeine's disposition and pharmacodynamic effects. *J Pharmacol Exp Ther* 1999;290:413.
10. Berde C, et al. A comparison of morphine and methadone for prevention of postoperative pain in 3 to 7 year old children. *J Pediatr* 1991; 119:136.
11. Davis AM, Inturrisi CE. d-Methadone blocks morphine tolerance and N-methyl-D-aspartate-induced hyperalgesia. *J Pharmacol Exp Ther* 1999;289:1048.
12. Ripamonti C, et al. Equianalgesic dose/ratio between methadone and other opioid agonists in cancer pain: comparison of two clinical experiences. *Ann Oncol* 1998;9:79.

13. Ripamonti C, et al. Switching from morphine to oral methadone in treating cancer pain: what is the equianalgesic dose ratio? [see comments]. *J Clin Oncol* 1998;16:3216.
14. Monitto CL, et al. The safety and efficacy of parent-/nurse-controlled analgesia in patients less than six years of age. *Anesth Analg* 2000;91:573.
15. Grimshaw D, et al. Subcutaneous midazolam, diamorphine and hyoscine infusion in palliative care of a child with neurodegenerative disease. *Child Care Health Dev* 1995;21(6):377.
16. Miser AW, et al. Continuous subcutaneous infusion of morphine in children with cancer. *Am J Dis Child* 1983;137:383.
17. Wolfe J, et al. Symptoms and suffering at the end of life in children with cancer. *N Engl J Med.* 2000;342:326.
18. Collins JJ, et al. Intravenous amitriptyline in pediatrics. *J Pain Symptom Manage* 1995;10:471.
19. Watanabe, H, Bruera E. Corticosteroids as adjuvant analgesics. *J Pain Symptom Manage* 1994;9:442.
20. Collins JJ, et al. Regional anesthesia for pain associated with terminal *pediatric* malignancy. *Pain* 1996;65:63.
21. Eisenach JC, et al. Epidural clonidine analgesia for intractable cancer pain. The Epidural Clonidine Study Group. *Pain* 1995;61:391.
22. Plancarte R, et al. Superior hypogastric plexus block for pelvic cancer pain. *Anesthesiology* 1990;73:236.
23. Berde CB, et al. Celiac plexus blockade for a 3-year-old boy with hepatoblastoma and refractory pain. *Pediatrics* 1990;86:779.
24. Staats P, Kost-Byerly S. Celiac plexus blockade in a 7-year-old child with neuroblastoma. *J Pain Symptom Manage* 1995;10:321.
25. Ravilly S, et al. Chronic pain in cystic fibrosis. *Pediatrics* 1996;98(4 pt 1):741.
26. Robinson WM, et al. End-of-life care in cystic fibrosis. *Pediatrics* 1997;100:205.
27. Westwood A. Terminal care in cystic fibrosis: hospital vs home? *Pediatrics* 1998;102:436.

CHAPTER 56 ABDOMINAL AND PELVIC PAIN IN CHILDREN AND ADOLESCENTS

Christine D. Greco

RECURRENT ABDOMINAL PAIN

Recurrent abdominal pain (RAP) refers to a condition described by Apley[1] of paroxysmal abdominal pain in children between the ages of 4 and 16 years. These children are otherwise healthy, but the abdominal pain persists for more than 3 months and affects normal activity.[2] RAP is very common, occurring in approximately 10% to 20 % of school-aged children.[3]

RAP has certain characteristic features that help to distinguish it from other sources of chronic abdominal pain in children and adolescents. Typically, patients experience episodes of pain interspersed with pain-free periods. Fewer than 10% of patients report continuous pain. Males and females are equally affected in early childhood; however RAP is more common in females in early adolescence at a ratio of 5:3.[4] Children frequently describe periumbilical pain that is diffuse in location, and many children will have difficulty describing their pain. Rarely does the pain of RAP radiate to the back or chest. Children often report that their pain worsens at night and that they have difficulty falling asleep. Pain that wakes a child from sleep is not characteristic of RAP and should warrant further investigation. Approximately 50% to 70% of children will experience headaches, nausea, or dizziness during the episodes, which can be of variable severity.[5] There is often a family history of migraines, irritable bowel disease, or ulcer disease.

Most cases of RAP are described as functional, which refers to a lack of readily identifiable specific biochemical, structural, infectious, or other organic abnormality. This lack of ability to diagnose a specific physiologic disorder may be a result of limitations in our understanding of RAP or of limitations in ways to test for a physiologic abnormality. Functional RAP does not imply psychogenic causes. Most children with RAP are, in general, medically and psychologically well. A subgroup of patients will have lactose intolerance, ureteropelvic junction obstruction, inflammatory bowel disease, endometriosis, or gastroesophageal reflux. In most cases of functional RAP, an underlying organic cause is rarely eventually diagnosed.[6] A 5-year follow-up study by Walker et al[7] reported that only 1 in 31 patients with RAP eventually received a diagnosis of a specific organic disorder. Other longitudinal studies show that only 30% of children with RAP have resolution of their pain within 5 years, and 25% to 50% continue to have symptoms as adults.[4,8,9]

There can be varying degrees of disability associated with RAP; however, most children with RAP are able to function well despite their symptoms. Children seen at pediatric pain clinics represent a subpopulation with more severe disability. At least 28% of children with RAP miss more than 1 out of 10 days of school. School absenteeism in children and adolescents is a sign of significant functional disability and is analogous to workman disability in adults. Patients with RAP can develop altered peer and family relationships, which may further reinforce a patient's maladaptive behavior. In a study by Gaber et al,[10] mothers of children with RAP reported more child somatic and depressive symptoms than did their children.

A number of studies in the past 6 years have investigated the possibility of a specific underlying organic disorder in RAP. Roma et al[11] performed 396 upper endoscopies in children with RAP and found a remarkably high incidence of gastric inflammation (85%) and *Helicobacter pylori* infection (28%). A limitation of this study was that not all patients had classic symptoms of RAP as described by Apley. A systematic review of six prospective, controlled studies by MacArthur[12] found that current evidence suggests no association between *H. pylori* infection and RAP in children with symptoms based on Apley's criteria. On the basis of these findings, MacArthur concluded that routine endoscopies are not indicated in children with RAP without symptoms of esophageal or gastric pathology.

Webster and colleagues[13] evaluated 137 children with RAP by screening history and physical examination, blood chemistry tests, and breath hydrogen testing. They found lactose intolerance in 24% of patients. The study reported that symptoms of lactose intolerance such as abdominal pain, bloating, diarrhea, and constipation were similar in children with and without lactose maldigestion, and that clinical evaluation alone could not reliably predict which children were lactose intolerant. Children with positive breath testing had improvement in clinical symptoms with a lactose-restricted diet, suggesting that a trial of a lactose-restricted diet may be appropriate in children with RAP.

Gastrointestinal motility studies in children using manometry and measurements of intestinal transit have suggested increased intestinal muscle contraction and delayed transit time in children with RAP. There is controversy in the interpretation of motility tests in children. Olafsdottir et al[14] used ultrasonography to measure proximal and distal gastric volumes following test meals in children with and without RAP. Children with RAP had smaller cross-sectional areas in the proximal stomach with more pain and sensation of bloating. They concluded that differences in gastric volumes following a test meal were related to impaired relaxation of the proximal stomach, which may support the view of altered motility in these patients.

Some studies have suggested that RAP in children and adolescents may be a precursor to irritable bowel syndrome (IBS) in adults. Hyams et al[15] studied 171 patients with RAP and found that 117 patients had IBS that met the standardized criteria for IBS in adults. Walker and coworkers[16] reported on a 5-year follow-up study of children and adolescents with RAP to determine the likelihood of progression to adult-type IBS symptoms. They found that female patients with RAP were more likely than a control group to meet criteria for IBS in adults, and that patients with RAP who had IBS symptoms experienced greater functional disability, higher levels of depression, and more clinic visits. A potential relationship between RAP and IBS may have therapeutic implications as new 5HT3 inhibitors, such as alosetron, are used for treatment in adult patients with IBS.[17,18]

The diagnosis of RAP should be based on a careful history and thorough physical examination that will point the clinician to a presumed diagnosis or to focused diagnostic tests. A physical examination should include a rectal examination and stool guaiac and an evaluation for undescended testes, hernias, abdominal fullness, or masses. Findings on history and physical examination that suggest the possibility of an underlying organic disorder should serve as guide to laboratory and other diagnostic tests. In general, extensive routine screening tests are of low yield, especially in patients with an otherwise normal history and physical examination. Screening radiographic studies and endoscopies have particularly low yield without specific clinical suspicions.[19] A study by Wever et al[20] examined children with RAP by ultrasonography and found an abnormality in 7% of patients. However, other studies examining the use of ultrasound in children with RAP have shown that abnormalities found on ultrasound could have been predicted by history and physical examination and focused laboratory testing. Extensive testing may increase patient and parental anxiety and even reinforce a patient's sick role. In addition to a history and physical examination, baseline complete blood count and urinalysis help rule out occult organic disease such as inflammatory bowel disease and ureteropelvic junction obstruction. In making the diagnosis of RAP, patients should have the characteristic features with respect to age, chronicity, location of pain, and absence of concerning findings on history and physical examination. Any evidence of systemic illness on either history or physical examination such as fever, rash, weight loss, joint pain, or failure to follow growth curve should prompt further investigation of organic causes.[21] Occurrence of persistent or recurrent abdominal pain in a child younger than 4 years should also prompt further workup. A family history of inflammatory bowel disease in a child with chronic abdominal pain warrants further laboratory testing, such as sedimentation rate, and possibly further diagnostic testing, such endoscopy and/or colonoscopy.[21]

Once an organic disorder has been excluded, a significant component of treatment is education and reassurance of patient and parents that a serious illness is not the cause of symptoms. It should be emphasized that the pain is genuine; patients are not "faking it" or malingering. A functional approach with emphasis on cognitive-behavioral treatment is used in our clinic.[22,23] Treatment is directed at reducing maladaptive and pain-reinforcing behaviors in patients and their families and improving coping skills. Underlying anxiety or depression is addressed. Return to school and participation in normal activities is essential. Often a plan to return to school is coordinated with the school and the psychologist, particularly in patients who have developed signs of school avoidance. Extensive diagnostic tests, referrals to subspecialists, and multiple medication trials may heighten anxiety in patients and parents and may reinforce pain behaviors. A trial period of a lactose-restricted diet and lactose supplementation may be helpful. Fiber supplementation was successful in reducing pain episodes in one study of children with RAP; however, excessive fiber supplementation may be associated with increased symptoms. Tricyclic antidepressants are often used in conjunction with biofeedback, self-hypnosis, and other behavioral-cognitive therapy. There are limited data on the efficacy of drug therapy, such as tricyclic antidepressants, antispasmodics, and anticonvulsants, in the treatment of RAP. Tricyclic antidepressants may be helpful in patients with sleep disorders; however, higher doses may worsen symptoms in patients who have constipation.

CHRONIC PELVIC PAIN

Pelvic pain is one of the most frequent presenting symptoms of adolescent women. Typically, chronic pelvic pain (CPP) affects women during their reproductive years but can occur in young adolescents prior to menstruation. Usually, patients have experienced at least 3 months of constant or intermittent pelvic pain and have seen a variety of physicians without significant relief in their symptoms. Patients often experience moderate to severe pain, significant school absenteesim, and have tried a number of analgesics.

In most cases, there is a gynecologic cause for CPP in adolescent women. The more common gynecologic diagnoses among adolescents with CPP are endometriosis and pelvic adhesions.[24] However, a subgroup of patients will have gastrointestinal, urologic, and musculoskeletal disorders that present as pelvic pain. In a review of 282 patients undergoing diagnostic laparoscopy for chronic pelvic pain, Emans et al found that 45% of patients had endometriosis, 13% had postoperative adhesions, and 25% had no identifiable pathology.[24] The authors reported that patients 16 years of age and older were 2 to 3 more times likely to have endometriosis on diagnostic laparoscopy than patients between 11 and 15 years of age; however, the incidence of no identifiable pathology was similar for all age groups. Laufer et al found that on laparoscopy in patients with CPP who did not respond to conservative management with oral contraceptives and nonsteroidal anti-inflammatory drugs (NSAIDs), 70 % of patients had endometriosis and almost 24% of patients had adhesions.[25] In addition to pelvic pain, 34% of patients with endometriosis also experienced gastrointestinal symptoms and 12.5% experienced urologic symptoms.

Endometriosis is the growth of endometrial tissue outside the uterus associated with inflammatory reactions, scarring, and fibrosis. Most endometrial implants contain estrogen, progesterone, and androgen receptors and are regulated by steroid hormones. In general, estrogen stimulates the growth of endometrial implants, and androgens induce their atrophy. The cause of pain associated with endometriosis is unclear but is probably related to the release of prostaglandins, peritoneal inflammation, and scar formation. It occurs in approximately 15% of all menstruating women ranging in age range from 10.5 to 76 years.[26] Endometriosis accounts for 45% of CPP in adolescents, compared with 30% in adult women, and 70% of adolescents with CPP who fail conventional therapy.[24,25] Unlike adult women who primarily experience cyclic pain, adolescent women with endometriosis report both cyclic and acyclic pain.[25]

Over 90% of female adolescents with CPP referred to our clinic have endometriosis. This represents a subpopulation of patients who, despite aggressive surgical and medical therapy, continue to have significant pain and disability. Resistance to medical therapy may be explained in part by insufficient estrogen and progesterone receptors in endometrial implants. Treatment of endometriosis and CPP consists of a combination of medical and surgical management. Once a presumed diagnosis of endometriosis is made, patients begin a trial of NSAIDs and oral contraceptives. Hormonal therapy attempts to create a hypoestrogenic state and atrophy of endometrial tissue, and has been reported to be 90% effective in either reducing or resolving pain in patients with endometriosis. For continued or severe pain, pelviscopy can confirm the diagnosis of endometriosis through biopsy and tissue diagnosis and permits laser ablation of the endometriosis. There is no obvious correlation between the severity of pain and dysfunction and the extent of disease found on laparoscopy. A trial of GnRH agonists such as Lupron usually follows surgical therapy.

Our clinic uses a multimodality treatment plan consisting of biobehavioral therapy, physical therapy, and selected medication trials. Patients should be evaluated for other conditions in addition to endometriosis that might be contributing to their CPP, such as constipation, irritable bowel symptoms, urolithiasis, or psychosocial stresses. The pain associated with CPP may be multifactorial. A prospective, randomized trial by Peters et al compared the outcome of patients with pelvic pain who were evaluated for organic and psychosocial causes of pain at the initial visit with patients with pelvic pain who were evaluated for psychosocial causes of pain only after organic causes were ruled out.[27] The patients in the group that had organic and psychosocial causes of pelvic pain had better response to therapy and had improved long-term outcome. As in the treatment of RAP, a functional approach is emphasized with return to school, participation in social and family activities, and recognition of reinforcers of maladaptive behaviors. Pelvic pain support groups, TENS unit, and acupuncture have been helpful in many of our patients. COX-2 inhibitors may be effective for patients who experience gastrointestinal distress with other NSAIDs. Medication trials of tricyclic antidepressants and anticonvulsants may be indicated, although there are little data on efficacy. Opioids are rarely used for long-term treatment.

REFERENCES

1. Apley J, Naish N. Recurrent abdominal pain: A field survey of 1000 school children. *Arch Dis Child* 1958;33:165.
2. Barr RG. Recurrent abdominal pain syndrome. In: Levine MD, Carey WB, Crocker AC, et al, eds. *Developmental-Behavioral Pediatrics*. Philadelphia, Pa: WB Saunders, 1983:521–528.
3. Rappaport LA, Leichter AM. Recurrent abdominal pain. In: Schechter NL, Berde CB, Yaster M, eds. *Pain in Infants, Children, and Adolescents*. Baltimore, Md: Williams & Wilkins, 1993:561–569.
4. Hodges K, Burbach DJ. Recurrent abdominal pain. In: Bush JP, Harkins SW, eds. *Children in Pain: Clinical and Research Issues from a Developmental Perspective*. New York, NY: Springer-Verlag, 1991:251–273.
5. Boyle TJ. Recurrent abdominal pain: an update. *Pediatr Rev* 1997; 18(9):310.
6. Bury RG. A study of 111 children with recurrent abdominal pain. *Aust Paediatr* 1987;23:117.
7. Walker LS, Garber J, Van Slyke DA, Greene JW. Long term health outcomes in patients with recurrent abdominal pain. *J Pediatr Psychol* 1995;20:233.
8. Magni G, Perri M, Donzelli F. Recurrent abdominal pain in children: A long term follow-up. *Eur J Pediatr* 1987;146:72.
9. Pearl RH, Irish MS, Caty MG, Glick PL. Pediatric surgery for the primary care pediatrician, part II: The approach to common abdominal diagnoses in infants and children. *Pediatr Clin North Am* 1998;45(6): 1287.
10. Garber J, Van Slyke DA, Walker LS. Concordance between mothers' and children's reports of somatic and emotional symptoms in patients with recurrent abdominal pain or emotional disorders. *Abnorm Child Psychol* 1998;26(5):381.
11. Roma E, Panayiotou J, Kafritsa Y, et al. Upper gastrointestinal disease, *Helicobacter pylori* and recurrent abdominal pain. *Acta Paediatr* 1999; 88:598.
12. MacArthur C. *Helicobacter pylori* infection and childhood recurrent abdominal pain: lack of evidence for a cause and effect relationship. *Can J Gastroenterol* 1999;13:607.
13. Webster RB, DiPalma JA, Gremse DA. Lactose maldigestion and recurrent abdominal pain in children. *Dig Dis Sci* 1995;40:1506.
14. Olafsdottir E, Gilja OH, Aslaksen A, et al. Impaired accommodation of proximal stomach in children with recurrent abdominal pain. *J Pediatr Gastroenterol Nutr* 2000;30:157.
15. Hyams JS, Treem WR, Justinich CJ, et al. Characterization of symptoms in children with recurrent abdominal pain: resemblance to irritable bowel syndrome. *J Pediatr Gastroenterol Nutr* 1995;20:214.
16. Walker LS, Guite JW, Duke M, et al. Recurrent abdominal pain: a potential precursor of irritable bowel syndrome in adolescents and young adults. *J Pediatr* 1998;132:1010.
17. Bardhan KD, Bodemar G, Geldof H, et al. A double-blind, randomized, placebo-controlled dose-ranging study to evaluate the efficacy of alosetron in the treatment of irritable bowel syndrome. *Aliment Pharm Ther* 2000;14:23.
18. Camilleri M, Northcutt AR, Kong S, et al. Efficacy and safety of alosetron in women with irritable bowel syndrome; a randomized, placebo-controlled trial. *Lancet* 2000;355:1035.
19. Stylianos S, Stein JE, Flanigan LM, et al. Laparoscopy for diagnosis and treatment of recurrent abdominal pain children. *J Pediatr Surg* 1996;31:1158.
20. Wever V, Strandberg C, Paerregaard A, Krasilnikoff PA. Abdominal ultrasonography in diagnostic work-up in children with recurrent abdominal pain. *Eur J Pediatr* 1997;156:787.
21. Levine MD, Rappaport LA. Recurrent abdominal pain in school children: the loneliness of the long distance physician. *Pediatr Clin North Am* 1984;31:969.
22. Blanchard EB, Schwarz SP, Suls JM, et al. Two controlled evaluations of multicomponent psychological treatment of irritable bowel syndrome. *Behav Res Ther* 1992;30:175.
23. Scharff L. Recurrent abdominal pain in children: a review of psychological factors and treatment. *Clin Psychol Rev* 1997;17:145.
24. Emans SJH, Laufer MR, Goldstein DP, eds. *Pediatric and Adolescent Gynecology*. 4th ed. Philadelphia, Pa: Lippincott-Raven, 1998.
25. Laufer MR, Goitein L, Bush M, et al. Prevalence of endometriosis in adolescent women with chronic pelvic pain not responding to conventional therapy. *J Pediatr Adolesc Gynecol* 1997;10:199.
26. Barbieri RL. Etiology and epidemiology of endometriosis. *Am J Obstet Gynecol* 1990;162:565.
27. Peters AAW, van Dorst E, Jellis B, et al. A randomized clinical trial to compare two different approaches in women with chronic pelvic pain. *Obstet Gynecol* 1991;77:740.

CHAPTER 57 PAIN IN THE ELDERLY

Aida Won

INTRODUCTION

Pain is one of the most common complaints among older people. Conditions such as gout, diabetic neuropathy, herpes zoster, peripheral vascular disease, and cancer are more common with increasing age. The most common complaints are musculoskeletal-related problems such as low back and joint pain. In community dwelling elderly, the prevalence of pain has been estimated between 25% and 50%,[1] with the prevalence of pain complaints being twice as great in those older than age 60 than in those younger than 60 years old.[2] The prevalence of pain in nursing homes is even higher, ranging between 45% and 80%.[3-5] In fact, 25% of nursing home residents with nonmalignant pain experience pain on a daily basis,[6] and up to 40% of nursing home patients with cancer have pain on a daily basis.[7] Unfortunately, the older patient is also at risk for undertreatment of pain. A significant number of elderly people with daily pain do not receive any or enough analgesics. This may be the result of inadequate pain assessment, societal misconceptions about pain in the elderly, as well as the fear of side effects of medications.[6,7]

The management of pain is already quite challenging. However, the management of pain in the older patient often presents additional challenges. These include underreporting of symptoms, multiple medical problems, medication side effects, problems with assessment, problems with communication, mobility and safety issues, as well as consideration of the potential for medical, cognitive, and functional decline.

PAIN ASSESSMENT IN THE ELDERLY

History and Physical Examination

The medical evaluation should begin with a thorough history and physical examination. Because the prevalence of musculoskeletal and neurologic conditions increase with age, special attention should be given to these aspects of the history and physical examination. If the cognitive status of the patient is in question, speak with the primary caregiver to obtain a more reliable history. Always ask about falls and occult trauma in the older population. We should also remember that immobility, contractures, and muscle strain can also be potential sources of musculoskeletal pain. Range-of-motion maneuvers and functional evaluation may reproduce pain and assist in functional assessment. A neurologic examination should also be performed, looking for signs of autonomic, sensory, and motor deficits in order to rule out neuropathic conditions. In addition to establishing a diagnosis, a baseline description of their pain should be made, including intensity, frequency, duration, character of the pain, as well as precipitating and relieving factors. Because many older persons may not refer to their discomfort as pain, but rather use other descriptors such as "ache" and "hurt," we should try to use their language when eliciting a pain history. Documentation of the location of all sites of pain will enable health care professionals target their assessments and determine the functional implications of the pain. It is also helpful to review previous experiences with analgesics, or other therapies. Problems and procedures for the assessment of pain are discussed in the following sections.

Problems with Adequate Assessment

Pain symptoms are frequently underreported in older patients. One study found that 56% of day-to-day health symptoms of older persons (e.g., pain, fatigue, depression) were not reported to health professionals. Some reasons given included responses such as, "the symptoms were no big deal"; "nothing can be done about it"; and "don't want to bother people."[8] Other explanations may include the belief that pain is a natural part of aging, as well as the fear of certain medications or treatment. Thus, decreased reporting of pain by older individuals may have a lot to do with the attitudes and behavior of older people, family, and health professionals. Furthermore, there are special problems in obtaining an accurate history and pain assessment in this population because of cognitive impairment, depression, and reduced vision and hearing that may require modifications in the assessment techniques. However, in cognitively intact community dwelling elders with chronic low back pain, self-reported pain is associated with more pain behaviors (e.g., guarding, shifting weight, slower movements), particularly when observed with testing of activities of daily living (ADL) functions. Therefore observation of pain behaviors, especially during performance of ADL activities, may also be another important method for assessing pain in the elderly.[9]

The presence of dementia compounds the problem of underreporting of pain symptoms. Cognitive impairment is associated with decreased reporting of pain.[6,10,11] Even persons with mild cognitive impairment who are usually able to understand others or make themselves understood, but have difficulties with short-term memory and new situations, appear to have fewer pain complaints than their cognitively intact peers.[6] For this population, we suggest asking about pain symptoms more frequently and regularly, as well as monitoring for pain behaviors more closely.

Patients with mild to moderate dementia have difficulty communicating and may not be able to quantify or describe their pain experience with great detail. However, they can still communicate basic needs in a qualitative way. Because persons with dementia may have difficulty with abstract or complex sentences, as a general rule, always try to speak clearly and keep sentences short, simple, and concrete. Questions should not be open-ended, or require a response to more than two or three choices. Eliciting yes or no responses may be easiest. For example, instead of asking, "What makes your pain worse?" ask "Does your knee hurt more when you walk?" If the patient does not seem to understand you, do not simply repeat the question in a louder or slower voice. Change the sentence and use simpler and different words to explain yourself.

Documenting Pain

A variety of pain assessment tools have been developed in an attempt to document and follow pain symptoms over time. Unidimensional scales, which measure only one element of the pain experience, such as intensity, are used more frequently. Commonly used scales to measure pain intensity include the visual analog scale (VAS), the numerical rating scale (NRS), and the verbal descriptive scale (VDS). The VAS is a 10-cm line, the ends of which are anchored with descriptors of the extremes of pain intensity, ranging from no pain to worst possible pain. Patients indicate the point on the line that best represents their current level of pain. Similarly, the NRS asks patients to quantify the intensity of their pain on a scale of 0 to 10, with 10 being the worst possible pain. The verbal descriptive scale (VDS) asks patients to select adjectives that best describe their pain intensity, ranging from no pain to excruciating (Fig. 57-1).

Although many scales have been found to be reliable, valid, and sensitive to change in younger subjects, visual impairment, manual dexterity, and cognitive impairment may make it difficult for many elders to complete certain scales. Herr and Mobily tested five pain assessment tools in a sample of senior citizens, average age 75, who responded to an advertisement at senior citizen centers and local newspapers.[12] The largest percentage of subjects perceived the VDS to be the easiest to complete (40%) and also best at describing pain (40.7%). The VAS, whether horizontal or vertical in orientation, was rated lowest in both ease of completion and describing pain. Similarly, among nursing home residents with a mean age of 85 years, and moderate dementia (average Mini-Mental State Examination score of 12 out of 30), the VDS was also the easiest to complete, with a 65% completion rate. Only 44% could complete the NRS, and 59% could complete the VAS. Although they were able to answer appropriately to qualitative yes/no questions about the presence of pain during the interview, 17% could not complete any of the quantitative scales. They also found,

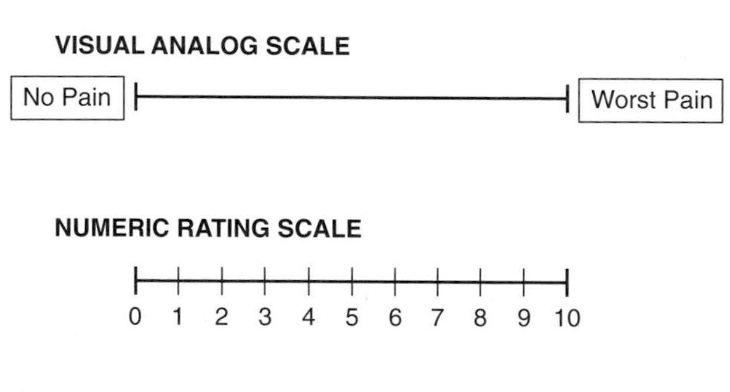

Figure 57-1 Commonly used pain assessment tools for the measurement of pain intensity.

however, that 83% could complete at least one of the five pain assessment tools presented. Therefore, in addition to the use of large print and hearing aids, repeated questioning and the use of different tools may also help elicit responses.[13]

More comprehensive approaches to pain assessment with multidimensional measures also exist. For example, the McGill Pain Questionnaire (MPQ) asks for information on spatial, temporal, affective, as well as sensory qualities of pain. Although comprehensive, the questionnaire was designed and tested in the younger population. It is quite lengthy, requires basic reading and comprehension abilities, and has a large number of choices that might be difficult and overwhelming for individuals with visual and cognitive impairment. Melzack has also created a simplified version known as the SF-MPQ, which was found to be usable in older individuals. It includes descriptors representing sensory and affective components of pain. It also has measures to evaluate pain intensity such as the VAS and VDS.[14]

We must remember that persons with short-term memory impairment may not be able to give an accurate assessment of how their pain compared with last week, or even a few hours ago. We can only rely on the current status of pain. We need to ask caregivers to monitor and record pain symptoms, behaviors, and circumstances every few hours. Therefore, repeated questioning and the use of pain diaries or flow sheets is critical for the documentation and communication of the patient's pain experiences, as it enables the clinician to adjust treatment and determine the overall effectiveness of the pain management program.

For severely demented patients, a structured observation of pain-related behavior is another approach to assessment. Patients with severe dementia or aphasia may communicate pain through behaviors such as crying, calling out, moaning, or guarding of the painful area. Although we cannot know with certainty if the behavior observed is indicative of pain, studies in nursing home residents with mild dementia provide some clues. The most common behaviors identified by these nursing home residents when they experienced pain included using an object for support, shift weight when seated, protect part of body that hurts, move extremely slowly, limp, lie down, and brace self when seated. Negative vocalizations included asking for pain medication, asking someone to do something to help pain, sigh/moan, patient asking himself, "why me?" talk about the pain, tell others to go away, talk more than usual, and scream. Facial expressions included sad, irritable, grimace, angry, and clenched teeth.[15] The family and other caregivers are also important sources of information that can also tell about the likely meaning of such behaviors. They may be able to tell if there are changes in the resident's routine, such as things they are now refusing to do, that may be clues to the source of discomfort.

Others have tried to develop a discomfort scale for patients with advanced Alzheimer's disease. Discomfort was evaluated by rating observations such as noisy breathing, negative vocalization, facial expressions (e.g., content, sad, frightened, frown), or body language (e.g., relaxed, tense, fidgeting).[16] Although the correct use of this assessment tool requires significant training, it is useful. While we await the further development of pain assessment tools for the cognitively impaired, we can instruct the caregiver to look for any of the behavioral responses to pain previously mentioned (Table 57-1). Because severely demented persons cannot tell what is bothering them, a careful medical evaluation and physical examination should be performed if significant changes in behaviors are observed. A careful physical examination may reveal areas of pain, inflammation, or guarding. If it is still unclear whether the person has pain or not, one could consider a trial of an analgesic such as acetaminophen with close follow-up for any changes in behavior. Careful documentation of observations in a pain diary will be helpful.

MULTIDISCIPLINARY EVALUATION

A comprehensive evaluation is extremely important in assessing the older person with pain. With increasing age, problems such as deconditioning, falls, polypharmacy, cognitive dysfunction, and malnutrition become increasingly common. Unfortunately, these conditions can also be potentially worsened by the presence of pain. Patients themselves report that pain has a significant impact on their lives. Ferrell interviewed a sample of 65 nursing home residents and asked them how pain affected their lives. Fifty-four percent reported impaired recreational activities, 53% stated that their ambulation was impaired, 45% claimed sleep disturbances, 32% felt depressed, 26% felt anxious, and 14% had a reduced appetite.[3] This was corroborated by another study looking at resident assessments by nursing staff. Residents with pain were found to have a poorer functional status, more likely to have mood disturbances, and less likely to be involved in activities.[6] This underscores the importance of performing a comprehensive evaluation of the older person with pain. The periodic documentation of changes in function, mood, time involved in activities, caloric intake, and sleep patterns are just as important as the documentation of pain symptoms and behaviors.

TABLE 57-1 **Pain Behaviors**

Facial Expressions
- Sad
- Grimace
- Clench teeth
- Angry
- Wrinkled forehead

Vocal Behaviors
- Ask for pain medication/something to help pain
- Asking "Why me?"
- Telling others to "Go away"
- Sigh
- Moan
- Scream
- Cry
- Call out

Body Movements
- Guarding
- Change in gait
- Shifting weight
- Moving slowly
- Limping
- Increased periods of rest/lying down
- Decreased social interactions
- Sudden change in daily activities

Other
- Sudden onset of confusion
- Irritable

TABLE 57-2 **The Get Up and Go Test for Gait Assessment***

Have the patient sit in a straight-backed high-seat chair

Instructions for patient
- Get up (without use of armrests, if possible)
- Stand still momentarily
- Walk forward 10 feet (3 m)
- Turn around and walk back to chair
- Turn and be seated

Factors to note
- Sitting balance
- Transfers from sitting to standing
- Pace and stability of walking
- Ability to turn without staggering
- Time it takes to complete full sequence (should be less than 20 seconds)

*From Fleming KC, Evans JM, et al: Practical functional assessment of elderly persons: a primary care approach. Mayo Clin. Proc. 1995;70:891.

Assessment of function is important so that mobility and independence can be maximized. Information should be gathered from the history provided by the patient and caregivers. A variety of geriatric assessment tools should be used to evaluate functional status. For example, the "get up and go test" is a timed measure of the patient's ability to rise from an armchair, walk 10 feet, turn around, walk back, and sit down again (Table 57-2). Patients are considered independent for basic transfers if they are able to complete this sequence of maneuvers in less than 20 seconds.[17] Other tests are more comprehensive such as the Katz ADL scale. This scale evaluates activities of daily living such as bathing, dressing, toileting, transferring, continence, and feeding. This is done by asking whether the patient can accomplish these tasks by themselves, if they need some help, or if someone else does it for them (Fig. 57-2).[18] The Lawton IADL scale is similar, and inquires about instrumental activities of daily living such as the ability to use the telephone, transportation, shop, prepare meals, do housework, laundry, take their own medications, and manage their own money (Fig. 57-3).[19] If functional impairment is a concern, the care plan should include physical and occupational therapies. Such therapies can provide assistive devices to help reduce pain and improve safety, as well as teach exercises to improve walking, transfers, balance, and strength. Physical therapies also provide a variety of nonpharmacologic pain management techniques such as heat, ultrasound, and transcutaneous electrical nerve stimulation (TENS). If safety is a concern, a home visit by a visiting nurse may be necessary to assess the home environment to minimize risks of falls and injuries.

Because depression and anxiety are strongly associated with pain in the elderly,[20] a psychological assessment should also be part of the evaluation. A commonly used screening instrument for depression in the geriatric population is the Yesavage Geriatric Depression Scale (GDS).[21] The questions are short and simple, and require only yes or no responses.

Psychosocial factors may also contribute to the perception of pain. Older patients experience many losses in their lives, which

For each area of functioning, check the description that applies. (The word "assistance" means supervision, direction or personal assistance.

1. **Bathing (either sponge bath, tub bath, or shower)**
   - ❑ No assistance
   - ❑ Some assistance in bathing only one part of the body (e.g. back or leg)
   - ❑ Receives assistance in bathing more than one part of the body
2. **Dressing**
   - ❑ No assistance (includes getting clothes and dressing self without help)
   - ❑ Some assistance (dresses without assistance, but need help with tying shoes)
   - ❑ Receives assistance in getting clothes, getting dressed, or stays partly or completely undressed
3. **Toileting**
   - ❑ No assistance (goes to "toilet room" for bowel or bladder elimination, cleans self, and arranges clothes); may manage bedpan or commode, and empty in the morning on own)
   - ❑ Some assistance (with going to the "toilet room", cleansing self, or arranging clothes, or use of bedpan or commode)
   - ❑ Doesn't go to "toilet room", and dependent with cleansing and dressing afterwards
4. **Transfers**
   - ❑ No assistance (able to move in and out of bed or chair without help; may use cane or walker)
   - ❑ Some assistance (needs help or supervision to get in and out of bed or chair)
   - ❑ Total dependence on transfers, or doesn't get out of bed
5. **Continence**
   - ❑ Has full self-control of urination and bowel movements
   - ❑ Has occasional "accidents"
   - ❑ Supervision helps keep continence; catheter used; person often incontinent
6. **Feeding**
   - ❑ No assistance
   - ❑ Some assistance (feeds self but gets help in pre-cutting meat/food)
   - ❑ Completely unable to feed self (needs others to be fed partly or completely by mouth, tubes or IV fluids)

*Adapted with permission (pending) from Katz S, Ford AB, Moskowitz RW, et al. Studies of illness in the aged. The index of ADL: A standardized measure of biological and psychosocial function. JAMA 1963;185:915.

Figure 57-2 Evaluation of activities of daily living (ADL). (Adapted, with permission, from Katz S, Ford AB, Moskowitz RW, et al. Studies of illness in the aged. The index of ADL: a standardized measure of biological and psychosocial function. JAMA. 1963;185:915.)

may result in fear, anxiety, loneliness, and depression. These can affect their perception of pain and other somatic complaints. Once medical factors are addressed, involvement of a mental health professional and social worker is often useful in order to evaluate the social support networks, identify dysfunctional relationships, and determine why the person is unhappy or anxious. Sometimes these feelings are the result of interpersonal conflicts and misunderstandings with family, friends, or caregivers that can be identified and corrected. Sometimes all that is needed is reassurance, encouragement, or more social support, while others may require medication to help with their anxiety or depression. Social work staff can also be helpful in working with the family or living situation, as caregiver stress is also common. Sometimes a more struc-

1. **Use of telephone**
   - ❑ No assistance (looks up and dials numbers, etc.)
   - ❑ Some assistance (answers the phone, dials a few well-known numbers)
   - ❑ Completely unable to use the telephone
2. **Travel**
   - ❑ No assistance (travels independently to places out of walking distance without help)
   - ❑ Some assistance (goes places accompanied or assisted by others)
   - ❑ Completely unable to travel unless special arrangements are made
3. **Shopping**
   - ❑ No assistance
   - ❑ Some assistance (buys only small items independently; needs to be accompanied on any shopping trips)
   - ❑ Completely unable to shop
4. **Food preparation**
   - ❑ No assistance (plans and prepares meals without help)
   - ❑ Some assistance (heats and serves prepared meals)
   - ❑ Completely unable to prepare meals
5. **Housework**
   - ❑ No assistance (maintains house alone with occasional help)
   - ❑ Some assistance (can perform light daily tasks such as dishwashing but may or may not be able to maintain acceptable cleanliness)
   - ❑ Completely unable to do any housework
6. **Laundry**
   - ❑ No assistance
   - ❑ Some assistance (able to launder small items such as socks and stockings)
   - ❑ Completely unable to do any laundry
7. **Medications**
   - ❑ No assistance (able to take right doses at the right time)
   - ❑ Some assistance (takes own medicine if prepared in advance; may need reminders)
   - ❑ Completely unable to take own medicine
8. **Finances**
   - ❑ No assistance (keeps budget, writes checks, pays bills, goes to bank)
   - ❑ Some assistance (able to do day-to-day purchases, but needs help with banking)
   - ❑ Completely unable to handle money

*Republished with permission of the Gerontological Society of America, 1030 15th Street, NW, Suite 250, Washington, DC 20005. *Assessment of older people: Self-maintaining and Instrumental Activities of Daily Living* (Table 2), M.P. Lawton, E.M. Brody, *The Gerontologist,* 1969; Vol. 9. Reproduced by permission of the publisher via Copyright Clearance Center, Inc.

Figure 57-3 Evaluation of instrumental activities of daily living (IADL). (From Lawton, Brody EM. Assessment of older people: self-maintaining and instrumental activities of daily living. Gerontologist. 1969;9. Republished with permission of the Gerontological Society of America.)

tured environment (e.g., senior center, adult day health care) can reduce the risk for loneliness, depression, and anxiety. The family and other caregivers can also be enlisted to provide and reinforce nonpharmacologic and behavioral techniques that can augment medical intervention.

PAIN MANAGEMENT IN THE ELDERLY

Guiding Principles

Many older patients experience pain daily, yet they receive inadequate analgesia. Although many older people have a higher incidence of side effects, this is not a good excuse for undertreatment. Analgesics can still be used, but should be used more wisely and cautiously. The following guiding principles and caveats have been extracted from the American Geriatrics Society Clinical Practice Guidelines, and may help maximize treatment efficacy and minimize adverse effects in the elderly.[22] These principles are summarized in Table 57-3.

Principle 1: A Little Goes a Long Way Hepatic and renal function is often reduced as a normal part of aging. This results in a higher peak plasma level, as well as a longer half-life of many drugs. For example, peak plasma levels of oxycodone are 15% greater in elderly than in younger patients. Persons with a creatinine clearance <60 may have peak plasma levels that are 20% to 50% higher. Thus elderly patients may achieve pain relief from smaller doses of analgesics than those required by younger patients. Therefore, if the pain is mild to moderate, an opioid-naïve elderly person may have a good response with a half tablet to one tablet of oxycodone or hydrocodone. Although the patient may ultimately need higher doses for adequate pain relief, the old adage "start low and go slow" accurately reflects the need for gradual and careful titration. Extra caution should be taken when converting to long-acting forms of analgesics because of the problem of drug accumulation.

TABLE 57-3 **Guiding Principles for Analgesic Use in the Elderly**

A LITTLE GOES A LONG WAY
Start with low doses (one half to one third of usual adult dose)
Increase slowly
Be careful with long-acting forms
USE STANDING DOSES
Avoid relying on prn doses
Premedicate for predictable pain
BE COMPULSIVE ABOUT ASSESSING PAIN AND SIDE EFFECTS
Encourage use of pain assessment flow sheets
Reassess and adjust analgesics within hours/days
Anticipate and monitor side effects closely
INVOLVE THE CAREGIVERS
Caregivers are the gatekeepers of medicines
Caregivers watch for efficacy and side effects
Education and clear written instructions improve cooperation and compliance

Principle 2: Use Standing Doses Medications written as *pro re nata* (prn) often assume that the patient knows when to take or ask for analgesics, which is not often the case, particularly in those with cognitive impairment. This often results in unnecessary suffering. If the pain is experienced at predictable times in the routine of their day, or if there are known triggers, it is better to use standing doses of analgesics to prevent pain. For example, if the person experiences pain mostly during the morning routine of getting up, but are more sedentary most of the day, the standing dose should be taken an hour before arising. If the pain is steady and continuous, analgesics should be used around the clock.

Principle 3: Be Compulsive about Assessing Pain and Side Effects Reassessment of pain relief and side effects should be performed within hours to days, especially during initiation, titration, or after any change in analgesic medications. Adjustments may include changing the drug, dose, or timing of the medication. The assessment of side effects should be performed at the same time. Because we are working with a frailer population in whom drug accumulation occurs easily, adverse effects are more common and more devastating (e.g., confusion, falls), the importance in assessing side effects cannot be emphasized enough, especially when converting to a long-acting form of the drug.

Principle 4: Involve the Caregivers Finally, it is important to include the primary caregivers in the treatment plans because not only are they the gatekeepers of medicines, they also watch for efficacy and side effects. We should give clear written instructions about assessment and materials that explain potential side effects of medications. Without their full understanding and cooperation, it is not uncommon for bad experiences to cause the patient or their family to fear the drug, and lead to noncompliance and needless suffering later on.

Analgesic Drugs in the Elderly

This section provides descriptions of examples of drugs to avoid, as well as those with favorable side-effect profiles for the elderly.

Acetaminophen is the drug of first choice for mild to moderate pain in the elderly. Acetaminophen can be used safely in the elderly up to 4000 mg a day, and must be used cautiously in persons with liver failure. However, there are no gastrointestinal (GI), renal, bleeding, or cognitive side effects compared with nonsteroidal anti-inflammatory drugs (NSAIDs). Acetaminophen has been demonstrated to be equally efficacious in treating osteoarthritis pain as ibuprofen, both at analgesic and anti-inflammatory doses.[23]

Unfortunately, NSAIDs are not as safe as acetaminophen. Common side effects include GI bleeding, renal impairment, constipation, dizziness, and confusion in the elderly. Among NSAIDs, the nonacetylated salicylate preparations such as salsalate and trisalicylate are preferred because they seem to cause less GI erosion and platelet dysfunction.[24–36] Renal toxicity of NSAIDs also should be considered. Since elderly people are more dependent on prostaglandins to maintain renal blood flow, the prostaglandin-inhibiting effects of NSAIDs may reduce glomerular filtration rate and lead to significant azotemia. This adverse effect occurs most frequently among patients taking diuretics or with a history of congestive heart failure. Because creatinine clearance decreases with age, an otherwise healthy 85-year-old person most likely has a calculated creatinine clearance of <40. However, if one still decides to use NSAIDs, we recommend that it be given at half the dose, at half the frequency, and with GI prophylaxis. Patients at high risk of gastrointestinal toxicity include persons older than 60 years old, those with a prior history of ulcers or GI bleeding, or those taking corticosteroids or anticoagulation. Misoprostol (Cytotec) is recommended to prevent both gastric and duodenal ulcers caused by NSAIDs at doses starting at 100 to 200 μg twice daily. Proton pump inhibitors (Prilosec, Prevacid) are also effective, and are less likely to cause diarrhea. H_2-blockers, sucralfate, or antacids are not effective in preventing gastric ulcers caused by NSAIDs.[27]

There is a new class of anti-inflammatory drugs known as Cox-2 inhibitors. These are reportedly less likely to cause significant bleeding and ulcers than other NSAIDs. Furthermore, they do not seem to affect platelet aggregation or interact with warfarin. However, they can cause similar kidney effects including fluid retention and edema, and some remaining Cox-1 inhibitory activity may place the gastric mucosa at risk for bleeding. Although promising, lower doses should be used until more experience is accumulated in frail elderly populations.[28,29]

Drugs used to treat moderate to severe pain include preparations of acetaminophen or aspirin, which are combined with opioids such as codeine (e.g., Tylenol #3), oxycodone (e.g., Percocet), hydrocodone (e.g., Vicodin), or propoxyphene (e.g., Darvon). These combinations augment the efficacy of the opioid. However, there are some preparations we prefer not to use in the elderly, as they often cause more toxicity compared with other preparations. For example, codeine seems to cause more nausea and constipation.[30,31] Propoxyphene is not recommended for use in the elderly since it is no better than aspirin or acetaminophen, and has the potential for development of dependency, renal injury, as well as considerable toxicity. The use of propoxyphene can be dangerous because it interacts with antidepressants, anticonvulsants, and warfarin-like drugs to raise serum levels of these agents. Furthermore, there is also a problem of toxic metabolite accumulation. Its metabolite, norpropoxyphene, has a half-life of 30 to 36 hours and can cause PR and QRS prolongation.[32] Drugs with mixed agonist-antagonist receptor activity such as pentazocine (e.g., Talwin) and butorphanol (Stadol) should never be used, as these frequently cause delirium and agitation in older persons.[33]

Caution should be used with tramadol (Ultram) as well. Although it is not technically an opioid, it has an efficacy similar to codeine. Its mechanism of action is on opioids, norepinephrine and serotonin receptors.[34] Until there is more experience in the older population, caution should be used with higher doses, and should be avoided in persons with seizure risks and those already taking selective serotonin reuptake inhibitors or tricyclic antidepressants.

Of all the opioids used for the treatment of moderate to severe pain, morphine, oxycodone, and hydromorphone are preferred. Demerol should never be used in the elderly, because it is associated with an increased risk of delirium and seizure activity, and has a long-acting and toxic metabolite, normeperidine.[35,36] Furthermore, Demerol often gets used with Vistaril to combat the problem of nausea. However, the anticholinergic activity of these drugs increases the risk of delirium.

The use of long-acting forms of opioids, such as MS Contin, OxyContin, should only be considered when the pain is stable and the opioid requirement is consistent for at least 48 to 72 hours. Because drug accumulation commonly occurs in elderly people, as a rule of thumb, one should use about 75% of the calculated 24-hour requirement when switching to the long-acting form, and cover the difference with a short-acting medication. The caveat should also be applied when switching to different opioid classes because cross-tolerance is incomplete.

Similarly, the fentanyl patch (Duragesic) should be used cautiously in the elderly. When the same doses were given to both elderly and young subjects, the serum concentrations were over two times higher in the older population.[37] Although reduced amounts of subcutaneous fat may decrease the absorption of fentanyl, low protein stores associated with poor nutrition results in higher levels of free drug in the circulation. The combination of increased drug levels and decreased clearance results in more potent opioid effects in the elderly. The use of a 25-μg patch is dangerous in an elderly opioid-naïve patient and increases the risk of delirium, sedation, falls and aspiration. We advise switching to the 25-μg patch only when the morphine requirement is calculated to be consistently about 80 to 90 mg/day over the previous 48 to 72 hours.

Anticipate and Treat Side Effects

Because side effects from opioid use occur more frequently in the elderly, we need to anticipate, monitor, and treat side effects efficiently. All efforts to use the minimum effective dose should be taken. This may include the consideration of more invasive procedures (e.g., hip or knee surgery, steroid injections, or viscosupplementation), if the patient is determined to be a suitable candidate.

Constipation with opioid use is almost always inevitable in the elderly. Tolerance does not occur; therefore prophylactic use of both stool softeners and peristaltic agents is recommended. Ambulation and physical exercise also helps constipation.

Nausea is also common; however, tolerance may develop in 5 to 7 days. So for those who have trouble with nausea, smaller doses of opioids should be used initially. Patients should also be evaluated and treated for other causes of nausea (e.g., gastritis, CNS swelling, chemotherapy). If necessary, the smallest doses of metochlopramide (Reglan 5-mg tablet), prochloperazine (Compazine 5-mg tablet), or promethazine (Phenergan 12.5-mg tablet) should be used sparingly. These agents, however, are not encouraged because they have anticholinergic activity. Dehydration occurs easily in the elderly; therefore fluid intake should be monitored carefully.

Sedation is also common, but like nausea, tolerance develops after a few days. However, this could be compounded by other medications that could be adding to the sedative effects of the opioid. Because of the increased risk for automobile accidents, falls, and other accidents, patients should be evaluated for safety, and efforts toward reducing or discontinuing other sedating medications should be undertaken. If this is not possible, we recommend changing the dosing schedule to minimize administering sedating medications during the daytime. Addition of adjuvant medications may also help minimize opioid requirements. If the person does not have severe or unstable cardiac disease, one could consider a trial of Ritalin at low doses (e.g., 5 to 10 mg once or twice a day).

Delirium is more common among patients with underlying dementia. Other causes of delirium should be considered, such as medications, infections, and concurrent illnesses. Anticholinergic drugs that may be contributing to the problem should be stopped if possible. Some of the most anticholinergic drugs include diphenhydramine (Benadryl), amitriptyline (Elavil), doxepin (Sinequan), cyclobenzaprine (Flexeril), dicyclomine (Bentyl), hyoscyamine (Levsin), and trimethobenzamide (Tigan).[38] Otherwise, one should use the minimum effective opioid dose, try adding an adjuvant, or consider switching to a different opioid.

Adjuvant Therapy

Neuropathic pain is opioid-resistant. Because larger doses of opioids are needed to achieve relief, the person is often better off using adjuvants such as antidepressants or anticonvulsants. There are a few antidepressants that should be avoided. Although amitripyline has been found to be very effective for neuropathic pain, it is also the most highly sedative and anticholinergic of all the tricyclic antidepressants. Doxepin and imipramine are both moderately sedating and anticholinergic. Use of secondary amines such as desipramine and nortriptyline are recommended because not only do they have the lowest incidence of sedation and anticholinergic side effects, they are effective as well. Max et al demonstrated that desipramine and amitriptyline were equally efficacious in treating diabetic neuropathy.[39] In the elderly, these drugs should be started at one half to one third of the usual adult starting dose.

Anticonvulsants such as carbamazepine and valproate are both widely used and have well-established efficacy in the treatment of neuropathic pain. But two other agents might be considered early on because of their very low toxicity: clonazepam, a benzodiazepine, and gabapentin. The only major drawbacks of clonazepam are sedation and ataxia. Gabapentin is a newer anticonvulsant, which has been shown to be effective for peripheral neuropathic pain due to diabetes and postherpetic neuralgia. This drug is preferred in the elderly for several reasons: Gabapentin does not have significant interactions with commonly prescribed medications; it has few side effects; and there is no need to monitor levels. It can also be used in conjunction with low-dose tricyclic antidepressants to augment efficacy. Because it can cause dizziness, drowsiness, and ataxia, we recommend starting with doses as low as 100 mg once or twice a day, and titrating up slowly.[40,41]

Borg Exercise Intensity Scale*

6	
7	**Very very light**
8	
9	**Very light**
10	
11	**Fairly light**
12	
13	**Somewhat hard**
14	
15	**Hard**
16	
17	**Very Hard**
18	
19	**Very very hard**
20	

Base Exercise Prescriptions**

	Endurance Training	**Resistance Training**
Frequency	3–5 days/week	2–3 days/week
Intensity	40–75% max HR or **"somewhat hard"** on Borg Intensity Scale	60–80% max force production, or **"Hard"** to **"Very hard"** on Borg Intensity Scale
Duration	20–30 min/session	2–3 sets of 8–12 repetitions, 6 seconds/ repetition
Examples	Walking, stairs, cycling, swimming, dancing	Weight lifting, elastic bands, isometrics, gravity exercises

Borg Exercise Intensity Scale*

*Source: Fiatarone MA. Fit For Your Life™ Pocket Exercise Reference Guide 1998, Exercise Intensity Scale adapted from Borg G, Linderholme H. Exercise performance and perceived exertion in patients with coronary insufficiency, arterial hypertension and vasoregulatory asthenia. Acta Med Scand 1970;187:17–26.

Guidelines for Exercise Prescriptions**

**Source: Fiatarone MA. Fit For Your Life™ Exercise Program Training Manual, page 3.13, used with permission.

Figure 57-4 Exercise in the elderly: Borg Exercise Intensity Scale. (From Fiatarone MA. Fit for Your Life Pocket Exercise Reference Guide, 1998. Exercise Intensity Scale adapted from Borg G, Linderholme H. Exercise performance and perceived exertion in patients with coronary insufficiency, arterial hypertension and vasoregulatory asthenia. *Act Med Scand.* 1970;187:17.) and Guidelines for Exercise Prescriptions (From Fiatarone MA. Fit for Your Life Exercise Program Training Manual, p. 3.13).

Other adjuvants include steroids for pain from spinal cord compression, soft tissue infiltration, acute nerve compression, or brain tumors. Steroids also help nausea, anorexia, and lethargy. For bony pain from compression fractures, calcitonin nasal spray is a useful adjuvant. It can be used as a nasal spray at 200 IU every day, or given as a subcutaneous injection at 100 IU every day.[42] Topical preparations include capsaicin cream. Because it depletes substance P from nerve endings, capsaicin enhances pain control when added to systemic treatment for osteoarthritis, rheumatoid arthritis, diabetic neuropathy, or postherpetic neuralgia.[43–46] It also appears to be beneficial for other painful cutaneous disorders such as cluster headache, postmastectomy pain, amputation stump pain, and skin tumors.[47] Unfortunately, capsaicin is often limited in use because of the initial burning it causes or the need for frequent application.

Nondrug Pain Management

Nondrug approaches are an important part of the pain management strategy in the elderly for several reasons: Nondrug strategies augment the efficacy of medications; have few adverse effects; give the patient and family a sense of participation and control; and addresses problems of functional decline, mood, and social isolation. An effective program must begin with patient and family education. The clinician should dispel misconceptions that pain, physical disability, and social isolation are normal parts of aging. There should be discussions with the patient, family, and other caregivers concerning the cause of the pain, pain assessment, medication use and side effects, goals of treatment, and use of self-help techniques such as heat, cold, massage, relaxation, and distraction.

Multidisciplinary pain clinics are an important resource in helping patients deal with the functional and psychosocial sequelae of chronic pain, instead of merely focusing on finding a magic cure. Treatments often include physical and occupational therapies, biofeedback, relaxation techniques, psychological support, and cognitive-behavioral therapy (e.g., education about coping mechanisms, stress management, communication skills). Although such programs often result in significant improvement in pain, reduction of health care utilization and less medication use,[48] few elderly are actually enrolled in multidisciplinary pain clinics.[49] One misconception is that older people may be less willing to participate in multidisciplinary treatment. However, studies have demonstrated that when elderly patients were offered participation in multidisciplinary pain clinics, they were as equally likely to accept participation as the younger population. Furthermore, cooperation with treatment, including the psychiatric components, was good, with dropout rates similar to the younger population.[50] We need to find ways of adapting our programs to include those of similar ages and shared experiences.

Although persons with cognitive impairment may not be able to participate in some of the more cognitive therapies, there are strategies that can be used even among persons with dementia. Exercise is one of the most important interventions. Although many older people assume that exercise is an activity for younger persons, exercise in older persons has been shown to have many benefits, including reduction of pain symptoms and amelioration of depression. In a study of community dwelling persons older than 60 years old with self-reports of pain, physical disability, and radiographic evidence of osteoarthritis, enrollment in an exercise program was clearly better than education in relieving pain. Both aerobic and resistance exercises resulted in modest improvements in physical disability, pain, and objective measures such as improved time to climb or descend stairs, and greater walking distances in a timed 6-minute walk.[51] Not only does exercise reduce contractures, weakness, fatigue, recurrent falls, and help with problems such as insomnia and constipation, it also can improve appetite, reduce depression, and improve self-esteem. Furthermore, exercise has the benefit of slowing bone loss in women with postmenopausal osteoporosis.[52] Emphasis on attainable goals rather than on pain symptoms during exercise results in improved mood, less fatigue, increased capacity in most functional tasks, and less perception of pain.[53] Understandably, the exercise program should be adapted to each person's ability and safety. Compliance is improved if low-tech, inexpensive, and simple exercises are emphasized, group socialization is provided, and personal exercise equipment is available such as stationary cycles and free weights. Guidelines for exercise prescriptions are shown in Figure 57-4.

Physical modalities should be employed in the treatment of musculoskeletal or soft tissue pain. Examples include use of heat, cold, and manipulation and massage. Because heat and ice can be self-applied, they give patients some control over their symptoms and treatments. However, precautions must be taken to avoid thermal burns.

Another effective behavioral intervention for those with cognitive impairment is distraction. Examples of distraction techniques include music, conversation, and activity involvement. Ensuring adequate nutrition and sleep will also help make the pain more bearable, and perhaps actually less intense as a sensory experience.

CONCLUSION

We must remember that success is relative. Goals are often different in the older population. The goal of care in the elderly is usually not return to work or prolongation of life, but maximization of quality of life. This might include goals such as being able to walk 100 feet independently, being able to play bingo or bridge every day, or being able to attend religious services on a regular basis. Although improvements may not necessarily be as dramatic as in the younger population, minimal improvements in pain, mood, functional capacity, or activity involvement may lead to large gains in quality of life.

REFERENCES

1. Ferrell BA. Pain management in elderly people. *J Am Geriatr Soc* 1991; 39:64.
2. Crook J, Rideout E, Browne G. The prevalence of pain complaints in a general population. *Pain* 1984;18:299.
3. Ferrell BA, Ferrell BR, Osterweil D. Pain in the nursing home. *J Am Geriatr Soc* 1990;38:409.
4. Lau-Ting C, Phoon WO. Aches and pains among Singapore elderly. *Singapore Med J* 1988;29:164.
5. Roy R, Michael T. A survey of chronic pain in an elderly population. *Can Fam Physician* 1986;32:513.
6. Won A, Lapane K, Gambassi G, et al. Correlates and management of nonmalignant pain in the nursing home. *J Am Geriatr Soc* 1999;47:1.
7. Bernabei R, Gambassi G, Lapane K, et al. Management of pain in elderly patients with cancer. SAGE Study Group. Systematic assessment of geriatric drug use via epidemiology. *JAMA* 1998;279:1877.
8. Brody EM, Kleban MH. Physical and mental health symptoms of older people: who do they tell? *J Am Geriatr Soc* 1981;29:442.
9. Weiner D, Pieper C, McConnell E, et al. Pain measurement in elders with chronic low back pain: traditional and alternative approaches. *Pain* 1996;67:461.
10. Sengstaken EA, King SA. The problems of pain and its detection among geriatric nursing home residents. *J Am Geriatr Soc* 1993;41: 541.

11. Brody EM, Kleban MH. Day-to-day mental and physical health symptoms of older people: a report on health logs. *Gerontologist* 1983;23:75.
12. Herr KA, Mobily PR. Comparison of selected pain assessment tools for use with the elderly. *Appl Nurs Res* 1993;6:39.
13. Ferrell BA, Ferrell BR, Rivera L. Pain in cognitively impaired nursing home patients. *J Pain Symptom Manage* 1995;10:591.
14. Gagliese L, Melzack R. Chronic pain in elderly people. *Pain* 1997;70:3.
15. Weiner D, Peterson B, Keefe F. Chronic pain-associated behaviors in the nursing home: resident versus caregiver perceptions. *Pain* 1999; 80:577.
16. Hurley AC, Volicer BJ, Hanrahan PA, et al. Assessment of discomfort in advanced Alzheimer patients. *Res Nurs Health* 1992;15:369.
17. Fleming KC, Evans JM, Weber DC, et al. Practical functional assessment of elderly persons: a primary-care approach. *Mayo Clin Proc* 1995;70:890.
18. Katz S, Ford A, Moskowitz RW, et al. Studies on illness in the aged. The index of ADL: a standardized measure of biological and psychosocial function. *JAMA* 1963;185:914.
19. Lawton MP, Brody EM. Assessment of older people: self-maintaining and instrumental activities of daily living. *Gerontologist* 1969;9:179.
20. Casten RJ, Parmelee PA, Kleban MH, et al. The relationships among anxiety, depression, and pain in a geriatric institutionalized sample. *Pain* 1995;61:271.
21. Yesavage JA. Depression in the elderly. How to recognize masked symptoms and choose appropriate therapy. *Postgrad Med* 1992;91(1):255.
22. AGS Panel on Chronic Pain in Older Persons. The management of chronic pain in older persons. *J Am Geriatr Soc* 1998;46:635.
23. Bradley JD, Brandt KD, Katz BP, et al. Comparison of an anti-inflammatory dose of ibuprofen, an analgesic dose of ibuprofen, and acetaminophen in the treatment of patients with osteoarthritis of the knee. *N Engl J Med* 1991;325:87.
24. Fries J. Toward an understanding of NSAID-related adverse events: the contribution of longitudinal data. *Scand J Rheumatol Suppl* 1996;102:3.
25. Cryer B, Goldschmiedt M, Redfern JS, et al. Comparison of salsalate and aspirin on mucosal injury and gastroduodenal mucosal prostaglandins. *Gastroenterology* 1990;99:1616.
26. Danesh BJ, Nelson LM, Russell RI, et al. Replacing the acetyl linkage in aspirin with choline and magnesium moieties reduces the occurrence of gastric mucosal injury. *Aliment Pharmacol Ther* 1987;1:51.
27. Scheiman J, Isenberg J. Agents used in the prevention and treatment of nonsteroidal anti-inflammatory drug-associated symptoms and ulcers. *Am J Med* 1998;105:32S.
28. Wallace JL, Bak A, McKnight W, et al. Cyclooxygenase 1 contributes to inflammatory responses in rats and mice: implications for gastrointestinal toxicity. *Gastroenterology* 1998;115:101.
29. Cryer B, Feldman M. Cyclooxygenase-1 and cyclooxygenase-2 selectivity of widely used nonsteroidal anti-inflammatory drugs. *Am J Med* 1998;104:413.
30. Kjaersgaard-Andersen P, Nafei A, Skov O, et al. Codeine plus paracetamol versus paracetamol in longer-term treatment of chronic pain due to osteoarthritis of the hip. A randomised, double-blind, multi-centre study. *Pain* 1990;43:309.
31. Turturro MA, Paris PM, Yealy DM, et al. Hydrocodone versus codeine in acute musculoskeletal pain. *Ann Emerg Med* 1991;20:1100.
32. Beaver WT.: Impact of non-narcotic oral analgesics on pain management. *Am J Med* 1988;84:3.
33. Hanks GW. The clinical usefulness of agonist-antagonistic opioid analgesics in chronic pain. *Drug Alcohol Depend* 1987;20:339.
34. Moore PA, Crout RJ, Jackson DL, et al. Tramadol hydrochloride: analgesic efficacy compared with codeine, aspirin with codeine, and placebo after dental extraction. *J Clin Pharmacol* 1998;38:554.
35. Kaiko RF, Foley KM, Grabinski PY, et al. Central nervous system excitatory effects of meperidine in cancer patients. *Ann Neurol* 1983;13: 180.
36. Foley KM, Inturrisi CE. Analgesic drug therapy in cancer pain: principles and practice. *Med Clin North Am* 1987;71:207.
37. Holdsworth MT, Forman WB, Killilea TA, et al. Transdermal fentanyl disposition in elderly subjects. *Gerontology* 1994;40:32.
38. Beers MH. Explicit criteria for determining potentially inappropriate medication use by the elderly. An update. *Arch Intern Med* 1997;157: 1531.
39. Max MB, Lynch SA, Muir J, et al. Effects of desipramine, amitriptyline, and fluoxetine on pain in diabetic neuropathy. *N Engl J Med* 1992;326:1250.
40. Backonja M, Beydoun A, Edwards KR, et al. Gabapentin for the symptomatic treatment of painful neuropathy in patients with diabetes mellitus: a randomized controlled trial. *JAMA* 1998;280:1831.
41. Rowbotham M, Harden N, Stacey B, et al. Gabapentin for the treatment of postherpetic neuralgia: a randomized controlled trial. *JAMA* 1998;280:1837.
42. Maksymowych WP. Managing acute osteoporotic vertebral fractures with calcitonin. *Can Fam Physician* 1998;44:2160.
43. Deal CL, Schnitzer TJ, Lipstein E, et al. Treatment of arthritis with topical capsaicin: a double-blind trial. *Clin Ther* 1991;13:383.
44. Towheed TE, Hochberg MC. A systematic review of randomized controlled trials of pharmacological therapy in osteoarthritis of the knee, with an emphasis on trial methodology. *Semin Arthritis Rheum* 1997; 26:755.
45. Tandan R, Lewis GA, Badger GB, et al. Topical capsaicin in painful diabetic neuropathy. Effect on sensory function. *Diabetes Care* 1992; 15:15.
46. Rains C, Bryson HM. Topical capsaicin. A review of its pharmacological properties and therapeutic potential in post-herpetic neuralgia, diabetic neuropathy and osteoarthritis. *Drugs Aging* 1995;7:317.
47. Hautkappe M, Roizen MF, Toledano A, et al. Review of the effectiveness of capsaicin for painful cutaneous disorders and neural dysfunction. *Clin J Pain* 1998;14:97.
48. Middaugh SJ, Levin RB, Kee WG, et al. Chronic pain: its treatment in geriatric and younger patients. *Arch Phys Med Rehabil* 1988;69: 1021.
49. Sorkin B, Turk D. Pain management in the elderly. In: Roy R, ed. *Chronic Pain in Old Age*. Toronto: University of Toronto Press, 1995: 56–80.
50. Sorkin BA, Rudy TE, Hanlon RB, et al. Chronic pain in old and young patients: differences appear less important than similarities. *J Gerontol* 1990;45:64.
51. Ettinger WH, Jr., Burns R, Messier SP, et al. A randomized trial comparing aerobic exercise and resistance exercise with a health education program in older adults with knee osteoarthritis. The Fitness Arthritis and Seniors Trial (FAST) *JAMA* 1997;277:25.
52. Preisinger E, Alacamlioglu Y, Pils K, et al. Exercise therapy for osteoporosis: results of a randomised controlled trial. *Br J Sports Med* 1996;30:209.
53. Stenstrom CH. Home exercise in rheumatoid arthritis functional class II: goal setting versus pain attention. *J Rheumatol* 1994;21: 627.

PART VI

Pain Therapies

CHAPTER 58 OPIOID PHARMACOTHERAPY

Arthur G. Lipman and Kenneth C. Jackson II

Among the remedies which it has pleased almighty God to give to man to relieve his sufferings, none is so universal and efficacious as opium.
SIR THOMAS SYDENHAM, 1680

Opium is a heterogeneous drug derived from the milky exudate of the opium poppy, *Papaver somniferum*. The word *opium* is derived from the Greek word for juice. This natural product, which contains over 20 different alkaloids, has been used to control human discomfort for over five millennia. Opium was used clinically in the early days of European medicine, but it fell into disfavor because of toxic outcomes from nonstandardized drugs that were not used with necessary care. Paracelsus repopularized the use of opium in the 16th century, and by the second half of that century, clinical use of opium was understood and adopted by physicians throughout the continent.

The French pharmacist Jean-François Derosne isolated a crystalline precipitate from opium in 1803, but that material was a mixture of morphine and narcotine. It was not until 3 years later that the German pharmacist Friedrich Wilhelm Sertürner isolated the alkaloid morphine from opium. He named this powerful drug after Morpheus, the Greek god of dreams. Other opium alkaloids including papaverine and codeine were soon isolated, and within a few decades, the purified alkaloids began to replace crude opium in clinical practice.

Narcotic—a term derived from the Greek word meaning benumbing—was originally used to describe opium derivatives. Today, narcotic has become a legal term that includes a broad range of sedating and potentially abused drugs, many of which are not at all related to opium. Because the word *narcotic* has such negative connotations, clinicians should *not* use it when talking with patients. Opioid is the preferred term in both clinical and scientific dialogue. Opioids are literally opium-like substances. In the recent past, opioid was used primarily to describe endogenous opium-like substances, and the term *opiate* was used to describe drugs that are opium derivatives. The differences between exogenous opioids, such as morphine, and endogenous opioids, such as β-endorphin, do not justify differing terminology. Opioid accurately describes both types of compounds and is generally considered the preferred term today.

It is not logical that the human body should contain specific receptors for alkaloids derived from a plant. The presence of endogenous opioids was postulated to explain the presence of opioid receptors before the endogenous substances were isolated. Three distinct families of endogenous human opioid peptides, the endorphins, enkephalins, and dynorphins, have been isolated. These peptides are found within the central nervous system (CNS), adrenal medulla, nerve plexi, gastric exocrine glands, and intestines. These peptides appear to have multiple roles including modulation of pain, neurohumoral transmission, and neurohormonal effects.

OPIOID USES

Opioids remain the most effective analgesics available. They are clinically useful in treating diarrhea and gastrointestinal hypermotility because activation of opioid receptors in the intestines slows peristalsis. Opioids decrease respiratory activity that can be useful in anesthetized patients and to help manage air hunger, especially at end of life. They also have an impact on psychological state by lessening anxiety and excitation, and induce a feeling of well-being.

Much of the opioid pharmacology learned by health care professional students is based on studies conducted in lower animals or isolated tissues. Rarely do such studies suggest or consider the profound cognitive effects of pain and analgesia that greatly influence outcomes of opioid therapy in humans. Serious opioid misunderstanding among health care providers results from failure to recognize the great differences between potential acute opioid toxicity and that seen with long-term therapy. Incorrect assumptions and beliefs about opioid toxicity, addiction potential, and tolerance to analgesic effects have led to poor use of these effective drugs in many clinical settings. This has lead to widespread *opiophobia,* which has been defined as the irrational and undocumented fear that appropriate use of opioids causes addiction.[1]

OPIOID AVAILABILITY AND USE

In the middle of the 19th century, many of the patent medicines sold as panaceas or cure-alls contained opioids. Steadily increasing federal and state control of opioids in the United States began with the passage of the Harrison Narcotic Act in 1914. The federal Bureau of Narcotics was created in the 20th century to address use of potentially abused drugs. In recent decades, political and law enforcement demands, rather than scientific or clinical findings, have defined the control system for opioid use in the United States. Creation of the Drug Enforcement Administration (DEA) by the Controlled Substance Act of 1970 assured that control of opioids and other controlled substances would be driven by a law enforcement, not a patient care focus. Numerous initiatives, both within and outside of the government, have worked to emphasize that opioids are important—and frequently underused—clinical drugs. These include the 1979 Report to the White House of the federal Interagency Committee on New Therapies for Pain and Discomfort,[2] the 1985 report of the federal Interagency Committee on Pain and Analgesia,[3] and the 1986 National Institutes of Health Consensus Development Conference Report entitled "The Integrated Approach to the Management of Pain."[4]

When Congress created the Agency for Health Care Policy and Research (AHCPR) of the Public Health Service in 1989, the agency was explicitly charged to develop clinical practice guidelines for areas of health care that were delivered inconsistently. Pain was selected as the first topic to be addressed. This is reflective of the serious concerns that the American public and public health professionals had about the ways in which pain management often was provided. Two federal clinical practice guidelines resulted. *Acute Pain Management* was published in 1992.[5] *Cancer Pain Management* was published in 1994.[6] The full text for both these guidelines is available in a searchable format on the World Wide Web at *www.ahrq.gov*. These scientifically based references document serious misconceptions about use and underuse of opioids in the management of both acute and chronic malignant pain.

The use of opioids in chronic nonmalignant pain was considered controversial by many clinicians well into the 1990s. This controversy existed despite numerous published studies that documented the safety and efficacy of opioids in the management of a variety of chronic nonmalignant pain states, that is, neuropathic, myofascial, arthritic, and osteoporosis pain.[7]

In 1997, the American Academy of Pain Medicine and the American Pain Society published a joint consensus statement entitled, "The Use of Opioids for the Treatment of Chronic Pain."[8] A year later, the Federation of State Medical Boards of the United States published "Model Guidelines for the Use of Controlled Substances in the Treatment of Pain."[9] These two authoritative publications clearly document that opioids have a place in the management of many patients' chronic nonmalignant pain.

Most physicians are far more willing to use opioid analgesics in patients with cancer than noncancer pain. The fact that opioids are seriously underused was underscored by a study of opioid prescribing for cancer pain patients that was published in the *Journal of the American Medical Association* in 1998.[10] Researchers evaluated the records of 13,625 cancer patients discharged from hospitals to Medicare or Medicaid certified nursing homes during the 4-year period 1992 to 1995 in five states. A total of 4003 patients reported and had multiple factors independently associated with daily pain. Only 26% of these patients received morphine or another opioid considered to be on level 3 of the World Health Organization (WHO) analgesic ladder [11] (Fig. 58-1). Only 32 % of the patients received a step 2 analgesic, and 26% received only acetaminophen or a nonsteroidal anti-inflammatory drug (NSAID) for analgesia.

The WHO analgesic ladder that was developed to guide analgesic therapy for cancer patients in developing countries has been shown to be applicable in most pain management in most societies (WHO 1986). This approach describes three levels of analgesia. It suggests that pharmacologic management of mild to moderate pain should include a NSAID or acetaminophen unless there is a contraindication as a first step. When pain persists or increases, add an opioid for the second step. The third step consists of increasing the opioid dose to treat persistent moderate to severe pain. This is not a stepped approach in which prior steps must be tried before initiating more aggressive therapy. Analgesia should be started at the level appropriate for the patient's pain. For cancer pain, a fourth step including palliative radiation and chemotherapy, nerve blocks, and various other modalities exists in developed countries

Morphine remains the standard for opioid comparisons. Most equianalgesic dose tables use parenteral morphine 10 mg every 4 hours as the standard for comparison. Equianalgesic doses are listed in Table 58-1. No such table will always apply for all patients due to great interpatient variances in response to opioids. The tables do provide an approximation of equally effective doses, but patients must often be re-titrated to response when the opioids they are taking are changed. It is important to differentiate among the pure mu (μ)-opioid receptor agonists, mixed agonist-antagonists (which are kappa (κ)-opioid receptor agonists and either antagonistic or neutral at μ receptors), and partial agonists. There is no proven difference in analgesic activity among the pure μ agonists. Greater potency does not imply higher activity. Potency differences simply mean that different amounts of drug must be used to obtain the same activity. However, pharmacokinetic differences can be clinically important. Pharmacokinetic parameters to consider include the peak serum level (C_{max}), time to peak serum level (T_{max}), and elimination half-life ($T_{1/2}$). Oral-to-parenteral dose ratios also vary among opioids. And differences in metabolism (biotransformation) may sometimes make one opioid preferable to another, especially in a patient with impaired metabolism or elimination. Opioids may be long acting due to inherent pharmacologic factors, for example, methadone, levorphanol, or pharmaceutical formulation. Each type has advantages and disadvantages.

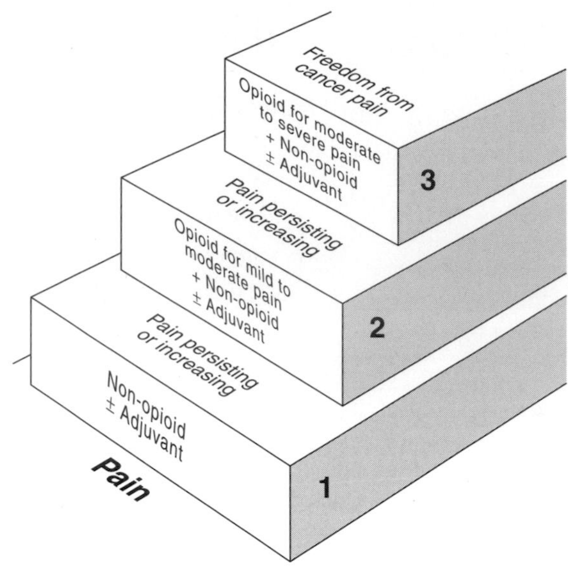

Figure 58-1 World Health Organization analgesic ladder: a progression of analgesics and doses to be used to manage pain of varying intensities.

CURRENTLY AVAILABLE OPIOIDS

Opioids can be administered by a number of routes, including oral, parenteral, rectal, sublingual, transdermal, and transmucosal. Currently, three general types of opioids are available for clinical use. These include μ agonists, mixed agonist/antagonists (i.e., κ agonists), and partial μ agonists. As discussed later, κ agonists and partial μ agonists exhibit a dose ceiling effect that limits their clinical utility (See section, Opioid Mechanism of Action). The reader is referred to Table 58-2 for a list of commercially available μ-agonist opioids.

The μ agonists can be placed into three categories on the basis of their pharmacokinetic parameters (See section, Pharmacokinetics): short-acting, long-acting, and ultrashort-acting. The prototype

TABLE 58-1 **Dosing Comparison for Some Common Opioids**

Drug	Approximate Equianalgesic Oral Dose (mg)	Approximate Equianalgesic IM Dose (mg)	Approximate Time to Onset PO-parenteral (minutes)	Dosing Interval (hours)
Morphine	30 Regular schedule 60 PRN dosing	10	20 15	4–6
Methadone	20	10	30 20	6–8
Levorphanol	4	2	30 20	6–8
Hydromorphone	4–6	1.5–2	20 15	4
Meperidine	150–250*	75–100	15 10	2.5–3.5
Codeine	130**	75	20 15	4–6
Buprenorphine	not available	0.3–0.4*	— 25	6–8
Butorphanol	not available	2*	— 20	3–4
Nalbuphine	not available	10*	— 20	3–6
Pentazocine	150*	60*	20 15	3–6
Oxycodone	10 mg is clinically equivalent to 10–20 mg of oral morphine. The maximum safe daily dose of oxycodone 5 mg/acetaminophen 325 mg is 12 tablets (~4 g of acetaminophen) due to potential for hepatotoxicity. Plain oxycodone can be titrated to higher doses much like morphine. OxyContin labeling recommends a dose ratio of oxycodone to morphine of 1:2. A ratio of 3:4 may be more accurate			
Fentanyl, transdermal	a 50 mcg/hr patch provides similar analgesia to 10 mg of oral morphine on a regular q 4 hour schedule which is equal to 30 mg of sustained acting morphine administered q 12 h. Patients with fever, e.g. tumor fever, may get only about 48 hours of analgesia from a patch; fever or exogenous heat, e.g., heat lamps, electric blankets, may accelerate drug release. The patch requires a mean of 17 hours to reach peak blood levels and effects remain for 12-24 hours after removing a patch. Therefore, patches cannot be used effectively to titrate doses.			

*Meperidine is *not* recommended for pain management > 2 days due to adverse effects from metabolite.

*Agonist-antagonist analgesics are not recommended when pain may increase due to dose ceiling effect

**Codeine doses >65 mg are usually not appropriate due to diminishing incremental analgesia with increasing doses but continually increasing constipation side effect.

Published tables vary in suggested equianalgesic doses. Clinical response is the criterion that must be applied for each patient. There is not complete cross tolerance among these drugs, in patients whose pain is well controlled it is usually necessary to use 10–20% less than equianalgesic doses when changing drugs and then re-titrate to response. If pain is not well controlled, use equianalgesic or 10–20% higher than equianalgesic doses of the new opioid drug and re-titrate to response.

opioid, morphine, represents the most commonly utilized type of opioid. Morphine and other opioids with short half-lives require frequent administration to maintain analgesia. Immediate-release morphine products provide about 4 hours of pain relief, and need to be dosed accordingly. Controlled-release formulations (MS Contin, Oramorph-SR, Kadian, Avinza, and OxyContin orally and Duragesic transdermally) provide alternatives to frequent opioid administration. Medications with longer half-lives, for example, methadone and levorphanol, yield analgesia for 6 to 12 hours. These medications are more expensive than controlled-release products.

The fentanyl series of μ agonists are highly lipophilic, which allows them to be utilized differently from the other μ agonists. They have rapid onset of action, which facilitates use as a preoperative adjunct. The high lipophilicity facilitates transdermal and subcutaneous administration. When administered through or under the skin, these medications depot in subcutaneous fat. Medication is released from the fat slowly. Conversely, when these medications are administered transmucosally or sublingually, they are rapidly absorbed due to the lack of the buccal and sublingual fat. Rapid absorption following transmucosal and sublingual administration makes these drugs useful in managing breakthrough pain.

OPIOID MECHANISM OF ACTION

Opioid receptors are found in the central nervous system and gastrointestinal tract and, to a lesser degree, in peripheral tissues. Opioid drugs manifest analgesic effects primarily by binding to and activating (agonizing) opioid receptors in the central nervous system (CNS). The interaction of exogenous opioids, for example, morphine and opioid receptors, mimics the interaction seen when endogenous opioid peptides (dynorphins, endorphins, enkephalins) bind with these same receptors.[12]

The three generally recognized classes of opioid receptors are the mu (μ), delta (δ), and kappa (κ) receptors.[13–15] Sigma (σ) and epsilon (ϵ) receptors were formerly classified as opioid receptors because opioids can bind to them. However, neither is currently considered to be an opioid receptor per se, because activation does not necessarily result in analgesia and neither of these receptor types is opioid-specific.[16]

TABLE 58-2 **Commercially Available Opioids**

Generic (Proprietary) Name	Dosage Forms Available	Comments
Mu Agonists		
Alfentanil (Alfenta)	Injectable: 500 μg/mL	
Codeine (others) Also available in combinations	Injectable: 50 μg/mL Tablets: 15, 30, and 60 mg	
Fentanyl (Sublimaze, Duragesic, Fentanyl Oralet, Actiq, others)	Injectable: 50 μg/mL Transdermal patch:25,50,75,100 μg/hr(Duragesic) Transmucosal: 100,200,300,400 μg (Fentanyl Oralet) Transmucosal: 200,400,600,800,1200,1600 μg (Actiq)	
Hydromorphone (Dilaudid, others)	Injectable: 1, 2, 3, 4, 10 mg/mL Tablets: 1, 2, 3, 4, 8 mg Oral liquid: 5 mg/5mL Suppositories: 3 mg	
Levorphanol (Levo-Dromoran)	Injectable: 2 mg/mL Tablets: 2 mg	
Meperidine (Demerol, others)	Injectable: 10,25,50,75, 100 mg/mL Tablets: 50, 100 mg Oral liquid: 50 mg/mL	Meperidine with Phenergan (Mepergan Fortis) Capsules: 50 mg with 25 mg promethazine
Methadone (Dolophine, others)	Injectable: 10 mg/mL Tablets: 5, 10 mg Dispersable tablets: 40 mg Oral liquid: 5 mg/5mL, 10 mg/5mL, 10 mg/10mL Oral concentrate: 10 mg/mL	
Morphine (MSIR, MS Contin, Oramorph SR, Kadian, others)	Injectable: 0.5, 1, 2, 3, 4, 5, 8, 10, 15, 25, 50 mg/mL Tablets: 15, 30 mg Soluble tablets: 10, 15, 30 mg Controlled release tablets: 15, 30, 60, 100, 200 mg (MS Contin) Oral liquid: 10 mg/5mL, 10 mg/2.5mL, 20 mg/5mL, 20 mg/mL, 100 mg/5mL Suppositories: 5, 10, 20, and 30 mg	
Oxycodone (Roxicodone, OxyContin, others)	Tablets: 5 mg Controlled-release tablets: 10, 20, 40 mg(OxyContin) Oral liquid: 5mg/5mL Oral concentrate: 20 mg/mL	Available in combination with aspirin (Percodan) and acetaminophen (Percocet, Roxicet, others)
Oxymorphone (Numorphan)	Injectable: 1, 1.5 mg/mL Suppository: 5 mg	
Propoxyphene (Darvon, Darvon-N, others)	Tablets (as HCl): 32 and 65 mg Tablets (as napsylate): 100 mg	Available in combination with acetaminophen (Darvocet N-100)
Sufentanil (Sufenta, others)	Injectable (as Citrate): 50 μg/mL	Solution contains no preservatives
Partial Mu Agonist		
Buprenorphine (Buprenex)	Injectable: 0.3 mg/mL	
Mixed Agonist-Antagonists		
Butorphanol (Stadol, Stadol NS)	Injectable: 1, 2 mg/mL Nasal Spray: 10 mg/mL	
Dezocine (Dalgan)	Injectable: 5, 10, 15 mg/mL	
Nalbuphine (Nubain, various)	Injectable: 10, 20 mg/mL	
Pentazocine (Talwin NX, Talwin)	Injectable: 30 mg/mL Tablet: 50 mg (with 0.5 mg naloxone)	Also in combination with aspirin (Talwin Compound) and acetaminophen (Talacen)

Opioid receptors are composed of glycoproteins found in cellular membranes. These receptors are coupled to G proteins that modulate potassium and calcium ion conduction[17] (Fig. 58-2). When opioid agonists occupy either μ- or δ-opioid receptors, they open a potassium ion channel that permits an increase in potassium conductance. The hyperpolarization inhibits neuronal activity. In contrast, κ-receptor activation inhibits calcium entry via a calcium ion channel. Activation of the opioid receptors decreases transmission of signals from the primary peripheral afferent nerves to higher CNS centers, as well as the processing of the pain stimulus.[18]

Activation of the opioid receptors leads to analgesia as well as adverse effects. All three opioid receptor types have known subtypes (Table 58-3). Two μ subtypes have been best elucidated. Activation of μ_1 leads to supraspinal analgesia, whereas μ_2 activation is commonly thought to be responsible for the adverse sequelae of opioid administration. Activation of κ and δ receptors leads to spinal analgesia. However, κ_3 receptors are thought to mediate supraspinal analgesia.[19] Activation of δ receptors may actually potentiate μ-receptor-induced analgesia. Clinical implications of the δ- and κ-receptor subtypes have not been fully developed at this time.

Recently, the role of peripheral opioid receptors has been described. It is now thought that μ and κ receptors found in peripheral tissues can effect inflammation and exert antihyperalgesic activity.[15] Opioids administered topically or by intraarticular injection have been used to treat pain in soft tissue and joints.[20–22] The clinical significance of the peripheral effects of opioids is currently under debate.[18]

TABLE 58-3 **Opioid Receptors, Subtypes, and Physiologic Effects**

Receptor	Subtypes	Effects
Mu	Mu 1	Supraspinal analgesia
	Mu 2	Physical dependence
		Euphoria
		Sedation
		Respiratory depression
		Constipation
		Orthostatic hypotension
		Arteriolar/venous vessel dilation
Delta	Delta 1, 2	Spinal analgesia
		Euphoria
		Potentiates mu receptor analgesia
Kappa	Kappa 1, 2, 3	Spinal analgesia
		Sedation
		Miosis
		Supraspinal analgesia (K3)

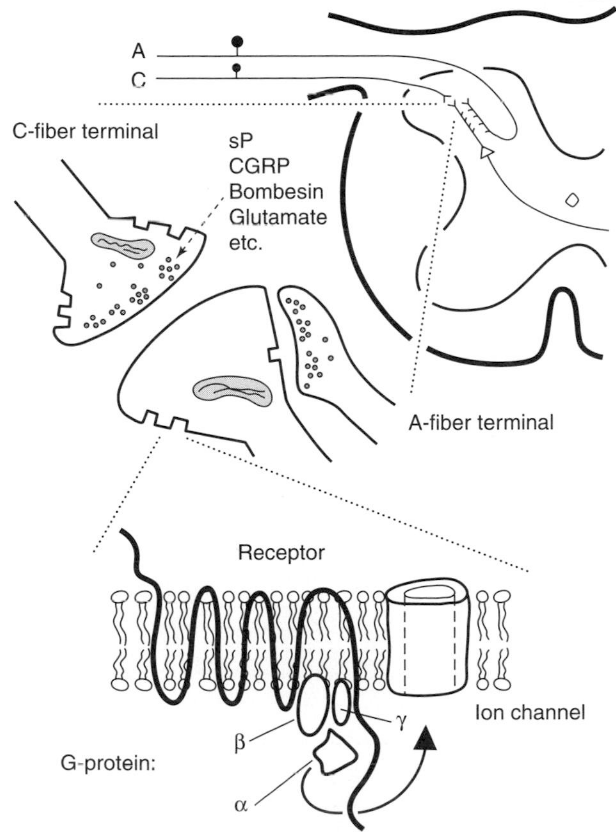

Figure 58-2 Illustration of synapse Aδ and C fibers with second-order neurons in the dorsal horn of the spinal cord and proposed opioid receptor demonstrating the G protein subunits and close approximation to an ion channel. (Adapted with permission from Sabbe and Yaksh.[17])

The lock-and-key receptor theory best describes the interaction of receptors and opioids[23] (Fig. 58-3). Opioids can be full or partial agonists. Partial agonists occupy part of an opioid receptor, resulting in a lesser degree of analgesia than a full agonist. Antagonists can prevent opioid agonists from occupying opioid receptors. Clinically useful antagonists bind to the receptors rapidly and have a higher affinity for the receptors than agonists. Any agonist with a higher affinity for the receptor than one that is already on the receptor may displace the drug with lower affinity. If the second agent (agent with higher affinity) provides less activity than the drug administered previously, withdrawal may occur. Antagonism due to direct receptor binding is competitive, whereas agents that bind near opioid receptors can produce noncompetitive antagonism. Mixed agonist-antagonist opioids are agonists at κ receptors and block μ receptors.

The presence of a dose ceiling effect limits the usefulness of κ agonists and partial agonists as well as codeine as a result of different types of dose ceiling effects. A true dose ceiling is due to lack of additional efficacy after the dose exceeds a predetermined level while incurring additional adverse effects. Both mixed agonist-antagonist opioids (butorphanol, nalbuphine, pentazocine) and the partial agonist (buprenorphine) have true dose ceilings. Therefore, these drugs should not be administered at doses that exceed those listed in the FDA-approved labeling. These analgesics can displace pure μ agonists from μ-receptor sites, resulting in withdrawal. The second type of dose ceiling, which occurs with codeine, is due to unacceptable side effects, that is, nausea and constipation.[24] The oral dose of codeine administered every 4 hours normally should not exceed 65 to 100 mg. Higher doses produce far more incremental side effects than incremental analgesia. Pure μ-opioid agonists (e.g., morphine) do not exhibit a true dose ceiling effect; however, they can present a functional ceiling that varies broadly among patients. For most patients, the functional ceiling

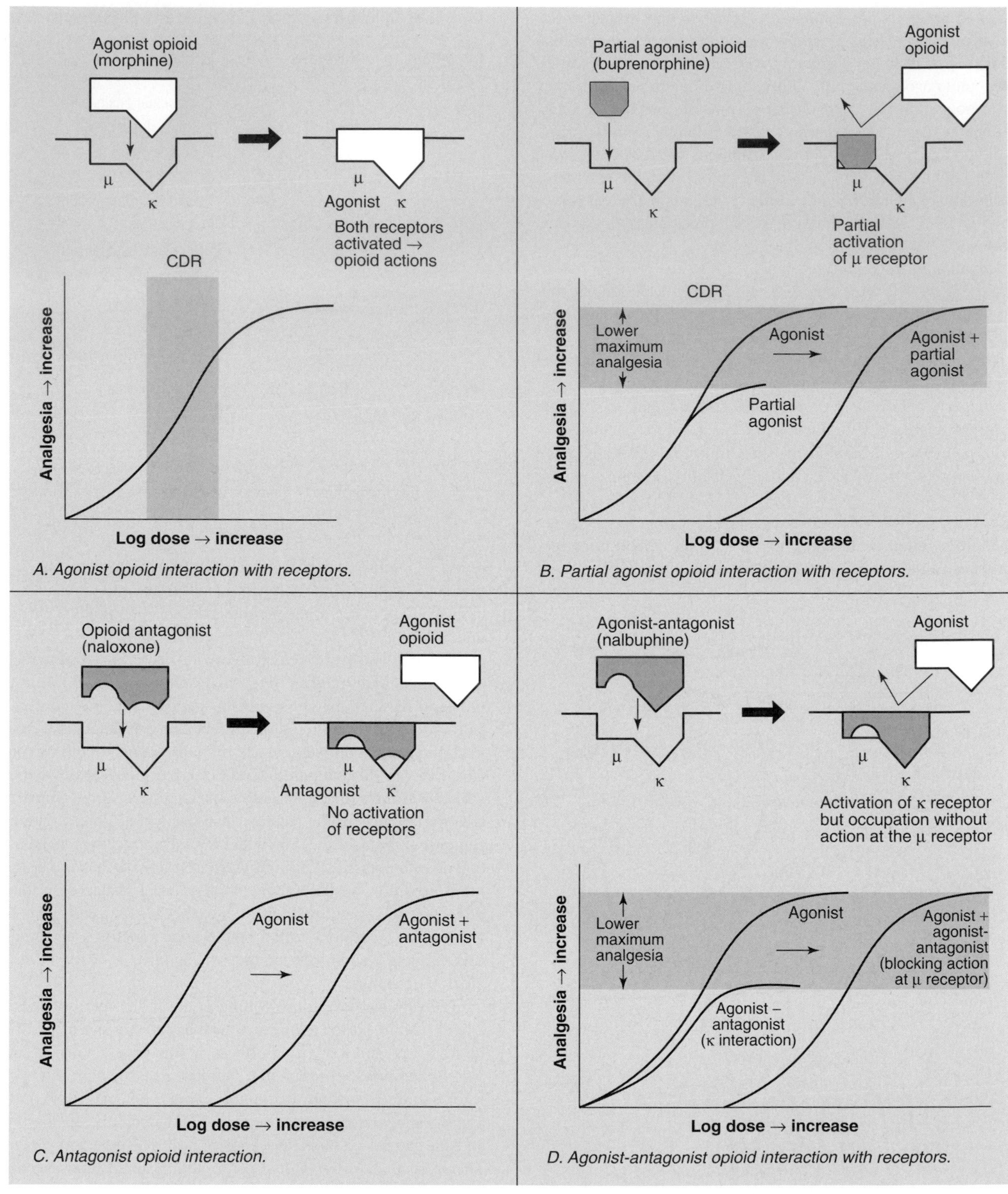

Figure 58-3 Receptor interactions of opioids. The various opioid-receptor interactions are illustrated, both in terms of a key-lock diagram with two receptor sites, mu (μ) and kappa (κ), and a representative dose-response (DR) curve of analgesic effects. (**A**) The agonist opioid such as morphine may stimulate both the μ and κ receptors. The steep portion of the DR curve is in the clinical dose range (CDR) = unlimited analgesia. (**B**) Partial agonists such as buprenorphine combine with the μ receptor, but they have only limited activity. The DR curve is flatter, with a lower maximum effect. The partial agonist will shift the DR curve for an agonist to the right. (**C**) The opioid antagonist, naloxone, can occupy both μ and κ receptors, but it has no intrinsic activity. The antagonist will shift the DR curve for an agonist to the right. (**D**) The agonist-antagonist opioids, ie, nalbuphine, may have mixed effects at the μ and κ receptor. Analgesia occurs because of interaction with κ receptor while blockade with no activity occurs at the μ receptor. This naloxone-like effect would shift the DR curve for a μ-agonist to the right. (Adapted with permission.[23])

is higher than doses needed clinically. The dose or serum concentration at which this functional ceiling occurs cannot be predicted a priori. Therefore, the dose of these drugs should be titrated upward until either analgesia or unacceptable side effects occur (See section, Dosing).

PHARMACOKINETICS

Pharmacokinetic factors impact the effectiveness of any given route of administration. Commonly, four phases of pharmacokinetics are considered: absorption, distribution, metabolism, and elimination. The availability of pharmaceutically formulated controlled-release dosage forms adds another dimension for consideration.

Absorption

Morphine and other opioids are readily absorbed from the GI tract following oral or rectal administration. Oral administration is convenient, simple, and inexpensive. It does not reinforce the sick role, nor does it signal advancing disease as nearly as much as parenteral administration does for many patients. Oral opioids are subject to hepatic first-pass metabolism because orally administered drugs must pass through the liver before reaching the systemic circulation. When that occurs, larger doses of drug are needed than with parenteral routes. Most immediate-release oral opioid formulations have an onset of analgesia of about 20 to 40 minutes for most patients, with peak analgesia occurring about 45 to 60 minutes post-administration. Oral morphine is reported to require 30 to 45 minutes to reach a peak plasma level, whereas oxycodone levels may take 60 to 90 minutes to peak after oral administration.[25] Delayed peak serum concentrations would seem to make oral opioids less than ideal for managing breakthrough pain.[25] Experience, however, has shown that not to be the case; oral opioids usually can effectively manage breakthrough pain. Morphine and oxycodone are available in controlled-release formulations that provide extended pain relief without the need for doses every 4 hours. Methadone and levorphanol are options for long-acting pain management due to the inherently long half-lives of these medications.

Most opioids can be administered rectally when the oral route is not feasible. Rectal administration avoids the hepatic first-pass effect if the dosage form is administered correctly. Three sets of veins are responsible for rectal blood return: the superior, middle, and inferior rectal veins. The rectal superior vein is responsible for the upper portion of the rectum (approximately 15 to 20 cm high) and returns blood to the portal vein that leads to immediate hepatic metabolism. The middle and inferior rectal veins return blood to the inferior vena cava. Drug administration into the lower rectal vault allows for larger amounts of the parent drug to reach the systemic circulation without being affected by the first-pass effect.[26,27] Hydromorphone, morphine, and oxymorphone are commercially available as rectal suppositories. Controlled-release morphine tablets have been used rectally with good results at essentially the same doses as are used orally.[28]

Lipophilicity favors absorption across biological surfaces including the skin and oral mucosa. The more lipophilic opioids (e.g., fentanyl) pass across these surfaces easier and faster than the more hydrophilic opioids (e.g., morphine). Transdermal fentanyl patches permit simple and convenient administration of drug to patients unable to take opioids orally or rectally. The analgesic releases from the gel matrix patch into subcutaneous fat that serves as an *in vivo* drug reservoir from which the drug is released slowly over 2 to 3 days. After patch application, se slowly. The average time to relative steady-state serum le following transdermal fentanyl administration ranges form 15 to 20 hours.[29] Once the patch is removed, the drug continues to move into the serum from the subcutaneous fat depot. Serum fentanyl levels decrease slowly; effects may continue for 12 to 24 hours after patch removal. These pharmacokinetic factors make transdermal fentanyl a poor option for patients with rapidly changing opioid requirements.

Oral transmucosal fentanyl has been commercially available for several years as a lozenge on a handle for both preoperative and preprocedural pain management. Another oral lozenge on a handle dosage form was more recently approved for managing breakthrough cancer pain. Initially, about 25% of the transmucosal dose is readily absorbed across the buccal mucosa. Because some of the medication trickles down the throat and is absorbed from the GI tract, an additional 25% (one third of the remaining 75%) is available systemically after metabolism. Systemic bioavailability is generally considered to be about 50% of an administered dose. Onset of analgesia occurs in 5 to 10 minutes, with a peak effect in 20 to 40 minutes. Other opioids, including morphine and methadone, have been administered as concentrated aqueous sublingual or buccal solutions. Larger doses often are required for morphine and other hydrophilic compounds when they are administered across the oral mucosa. Table 58-4 lists bioavailability variables and data for sublingual opioid administration.

Intravenous opioids provide 100% bioavailability by definition. Subcutaneous opioid infusion provides similar drug levels to those achieved with intravenous infusion.[30] Subcutaneous and intramuscular injections provide similar pharmacokinetics as well. Time to peak effect for intramuscular and subcutaneous administration is delayed due to the need for absorption, but these two routes provide similar levels at similar times. As with transdermal delivery, the more lipophilic compounds (e.g., fentanyl) act more rapidly after injection. Absorption of opioids from the intramuscular route is a rate-limiting step, for which lipophilicity is a major factor. Intramuscular injections are not recommended due to the pain and possible tissue damage they can inflict. Additionally, absorption from intramuscular injections can be erratic.

Distribution

Opioid distribution is a function of plasma protein binding and lipophilicity. Morphine is 30% to 35% bound to plasma proteins and does not appear to be influenced greatly by displacement, a

TBALE 58-4 **Sublingual Opioid Bioavailability**

Drug	% Absorbed
Morphine	22%
Methadone	34%
Fentanyl	51%
Buprenorphine	55%

1 mL sublingual; held for 10 minutes at pH 6.5.

Adapted from Weinberg D, Inturrisi C, Reidenberg B, et al. Sublingual absorption of selected opioid analgesics. *Clin Pharmacol Ther* 1988;44:335.

pharmacodynamic factor. Morphine does not remain in tissues for an extended time. Fentanyl is both highly protein bound (80% to 85%) and quite lipophilic. The free fraction of fentanyl increases in acidosis. Fentanyl also distributes to fat tissue throughout the body from which it redistributes slowly into the systemic circulation.

Metabolism (Biotransformation) and Elimination (Excretion)

Opioids that are not readily eliminated by the kidneys in the parent form are metabolized to form more water-soluble metabolites. The liver metabolizes opioids by numerous processes, including dealkylation, glucoronidation, hydrolysis, and oxidation. Opioids are also metabolized to a minor extent in other body compartments, for example, central nervous system, kidneys, lungs, and placenta. The metabolic fate of a number of pain medications impacts the selection of an appropriate therapeutic regimen (Table 58-5). Some metabolites can cause untoward neurotoxicity,[31] and may displace the more active parent compound from opioid-receptor sites. Many patients are at risk from the toxicities of metabolite accumulation, especially patients with impaired renal function (which includes most elderly individuals) and those receiving high-dose or long-term opioid therapy.

Accumulation of normeperidine, a metabolite of meperidine, causes neurotoxicity, especially in elderly patients and in those with poor renal function. Use of meperidine should be limited to 1 to 2 days for acute pain, and should be avoided in the management of chronic pain.

In man, morphine-3-glucuronide (M3G) and morphine-6-glucuronide (M6G) are the two major morphine metabolites.[32] As much as 50% of the parent drug may be renally excreted as M3G, whereas M6G accounts for about 5%.[33] Both compounds are water-soluble glucuronides that depend on renal elimination for clearance. M3G appears to be antinociceptive and has been associated with hyperalgesia and neurotoxicities including myoclonus.[31,34] M6G possesses analgesic properties, and may be significantly more potent than morphine. Accumulation of both metabolites, as a function of poor renal status, predisposes patients to toxicity as well as poor pain control.

Normorphine, a desmethyl metabolite of morphine, may contribute to the toxic effects seen with high-dose or long-term morphine use. However, reports of normorphine accumulation indicate that M6G and M3G were also elevated.[35] Therefore, whether normorphine accumulation contributes to toxicity remains unclear. It is unclear how often metabolites of other opioids may be problematic in renally impaired patients. Some authors have suggested that caution is advisable with hydromorphone due to metabolites, including the 3 and 6 glucuronides, and with fentanyl, which has a desmethyl metabolite.[31] Oxycodone has only an active analgesic metabolite, hydromorphone, which may make oxycodone safer for some elderly and renally impaired patients.

The kidney accounts for about 90% of the excretion of an opioid (parent drug and metabolites) through the urine. Fecal elimination is a minor pathway and accounts for less than 10% of opioid excretion.

DOSING

Pure μ-opioid agonists do not differ pharmacodynamically, but they do differ in their pharmacokinetic properties. All except codeine normally provide the same level of analgesia when dosed appropriately. For several reasons including genetic polymorphism, some patients respond better to some opioids than others. Clinical trial is the only way to determine a preferred alternative if a patient does not respond as expected to the initial choice. Pharmacokinetic properties and controlled-release formulations play major roles in the drugs' fate in the organism.

As long as a noxious nociceptive stimulus that responds to opioids is present, these drugs should be used on a regular schedule or time-contingent basis. Undertreated acute pain can lead to chronic pain syndromes. Untreated or undertreated pain causes repeated stimulation of the CNS. Repeated stimulation of the afferent nociceptive neurons can sensitize both those neurons, producing the phenomenon known as physiologic windup, and cells in the dorsal horn of the spinal cord resulting in neuronal plasticity.[36] Such sensitization can induce neurologic changes that last long after the initial insult has healed. Neuronal plasticity, or changes in the CNS, may lead to hyperalgesia. Windup is the progressive increase in the frequency of elicited action potentials seen in neurons as a result of a slowly repeated stimulus of C fibers.[37] Long-term potentiation (LTP) is brief high-frequency stimuli that increase the efficiency of synaptic transmission.[38] These processes lead to hyperalgesia as a consequence of central excitability. The use of around-the-clock opioids often breaks the cycle of pain, and can decrease or eliminate the centrally mediated processes that complicate pain control. Thus it may take less drug to prevent the recurrence of pain than would be required to treat recurring pain.

Morphine and the other pure opioid agonists can provide analgesia in most acute and chronic malignant pain patients and many chronic nonmalignant pain patients. There is no *a priori* maximum dose for any pure μ agonists. Patients require individual titration of medication regimens. Morphine dose requirements for comfort following similar noxious stimuli may vary 50- to 100-fold among chronic malignant pain patients,[39] and 10- to 20-fold among acute pain patients.[40]

In addition to the regularly scheduled opioid doses, supplemental doses should be available for management of breakthrough pain. Breakthrough pain can be defined as transitory increases in pain greater than moderate intensity, occurring in addition to baseline pain of moderate or less intensity.[41] Breakthrough pain regimens should be based on the background (time-contingent) dose, not on fixed doses. Sufficient rescue doses of the opioid should be available to the patient as immediate-release dosage forms to provide comfort when breakthrough pain occurs. Incidental pain often occurs predictably when a patient ambulates, gets tired, or undergoes medical procedures. In such cases, an additional dose of an oral, immediate-release dosage form should be administered to provide effective levels about a half-hour before the anticipated pain increase. For unpredictable breakthrough pain, a typical rescue dose order is one half of the every 4-hour scheduled dose (1/6 of the every 12-hour scheduled controlled-release dose) permitted every 2 hours as needed. When a patient with chronic pain requires more than two to three rescue doses for more than 2 to 3 days in succession, an increase in the time-contingent dose should be considered.

When escalation of an opioid dose is warranted, it is important to increase the dose as a percentage of the current regimen, not a set number of milligrams. Increases of 50% should be made as soon as steady-state serum levels are achieved (5 half-lives, which is equal to about 10 hours for morphine) after 5 days of scheduled opioid therapy. An increase from 30 mg every 4 hours to 45 mg

TABLE 58-5 **Opioid Metabolites***

Parent Drug (% excreted unchanged)	Analgesic Duration (hours)	Metabolites (% if known)	Metabolite Half-lives (hours)	Metabolite Elimination Route	Comment
Morphine (~7.2% - iv) (~3.7% - po)	4–6				Elimination of morphine is not affected by renal failure, however, Vd may be smaller ,resulting in increased plasma concentrations; enterohepatic circulation of morphine and glucuronides occur
		Morphine-3-glucuronide (57–74)	2.8–4	Renal	Half life is 41–141 hours in renal failure; 5-20 times more potent than morphine in causing hyperalgesia, EEG spiking, agitation, seizures in animals; possibly by a non-opioid receptor mechanism
		Morphine-6-glucuronide (4.7–12)	Duration cf action 2 times longer than parent	Renal	Half life is 89–136 hours in renal failure; may be responsible for narcosis in patients with renal failure; by IT administration is 100 times more potent than morphine; accumulates with chronic dosing
		Morphine-3-ethereal sulfate (5–10)			
		Normorphine (3.5)			May have toxic effects (myoclonus, allodynia)
		morphine-N-oxide			
Codeine 11.1%	4–6				
		Codeine-6-glucuronide			Primary elimination pathway; profound narcosis has occurred in chronic renal failure
		Norcodeine		Renal	Equipotent to codeine in analgesic activity
		Morphine (10)			May account for analgesic activity of codeine
Fentanyl (<10)	1–2				May be extensively liver metabolized
		Norfentanyl		Renal, hepatic	Metabolized to despropionyl fentanyl May cause neurotoxic side effects Structurally similar to normeperidine
		4-*N*-anilinopiperidine			
Hydromorphone (5.6%)					Clearance dependent on hepatic blood flow
		Hydromorphone-3-glucuronide			Shown to accumulate in renal failure in one patient
		Hydromorphone-6-glucuronide		Renal	Formed from intermediate metabolites, dihydroisomorphine and dihydromorphine
		Nor-metabolites			Significance not known

(continued)

TABLE 58-5 **Opioid Metabolites***

Parent Drug (% excreted unchanged)	Analgesic Duration (hours)	Metabolites (% if known)	Metabolite Half-lives (hours)	Metabolite Elimination Route	Comment
Levorphanol	6–8	Levorphanol glucuronide		Renal	Liver metabolized by glucuronide conjugation
Meperidine 5% (uncontrolled urine pH)	2.5–3.5				Bioavailability increases from 50% to 80% in cirrhosis Half-life of meperidine and normeperidine prolonged in cirrhosis Urinary pH effects elimination of unchanged meperidine in urine 25% in acidic urine vs. 1%–2% in alkaline urine
		Normeperidine (5–30)	15–30	Renal, hepatic	Half-life prolonged significantly in renal failure (>30hrs); twice as potent in CNS stimulatory effects as meperidine; half the analgesic effect of meperidine; urinary excretion pH dependent: uncontrolled pH $f_e = 0.05–0.06$, acidic urine $f_e = 0.30$, alkaline urine $f_e < 0.031$
		Meperidinic acid			Inactive metabolite
Methadone 21% (acidic urine increases the fraction of elimination [f_e])	4–6 initially; 6–12 after steady state (1–2 days)				In one anephric patient, 98% of methadone was found in feces as metabolite, suggesting a shift in metabolism from renal to fecal urinary excretion of methadone and metabolites is dose dependent and is the major route of elimination in doses >55 mg/day; 10–45% of methadone is eliminated in feces as metabolites
		1,5-demethyl-2-ethyl-3,3-iphenyl-1-pyrroline		Renal, biliary	Unpredictable half-life with chronic dosing long-term analgesia is 10 times that of morphine; major metabolite $f_e = 0.30$
		2-ethyl-5-methyl-3,3-diphenyl-1-pyrroline		Renal, biliary	Minor metabolite
		Methadone-*N*-oxide			Minor metabolite
Oxycodone	3–6				Renally excreted, primarily as metabolites
		Noroxymorphone			
		Oxymorphone		Hepatic, renal	Active metabolite; renally excreted as oxymorphone-glucuronide
		Noroxycodone			
Propoxyphene 1.5%	4–6				May depress cardiac conduction secondary to anesthetic properties; half-life not altered in renal failure
		Norproproxyphene (25)	22.9–36.6	Renal	Local anesthetic properties; cardiac conduction abnormalities can result with accumulation (not reversed by naloxone); not hemodiazlyzable

Buprenorphine	6–8			One source says it is almost completely metabolized in the liver, but another source says the majority is excreted unchanged in feces Undergoes enterohepatic circulation with metabolites
		Glucuronidation products	Renal	
		Norbuprenorphine	Renal	May have weak analgesic properties. Primary route of elimination is renal; hepatic, biliary, and fecal routes also involved
Butorphanol 5%	3–4			Extensively liver metabolized; $Cl_{Cr} < 30$ mL/min half-life increased from 5.75 hrs to 10.5 hours in single-dose, intranasal administration
		Norbutorphanol	Biliary	No analgesic activity
		Hydroxybutorphanol	Renal	Analgesic activity; major metabolite; 60–80% renally excreted
Nalbuphine 7%	3–6			Hepatic metabolism; metabolites and parent compound excreted in urine and feces Major route of elimination is biliary secretion
Pentazocine 4.9%	3–6			(l) isomer responsible for analgesic activity; large interpatient variability in metabolism and oral bioavailability Bioavailability in cirrhotic patients increased to 60–70%
		Alcoholic and carboxylic acid metabolites	Renal	Inactive metabolites
		Pentazocine glucuronide	Renal	Inactive metabolite

*Developed in collaboration with the Drug Information Service, Department of Pharmacy Services, University Hospitals and Clinics, University of Utah Health Sciences Center.

Data from: References 79–87.

every 4 hours would be appropriate. If the inadequate dose is 300 mg every 12 hours, the increase should be to 450 mg every 12 hours.

Clinicians should carefully evaluate complaints of increased pain or diminished analgesic effect in patients whose analgesia was adequate before simply increasing the opioid dose. Clinical tolerance to opioid analgesia in itself is uncommon once comfort has been achieved and maintained for a few days. Ineffective analgesia is almost always a result of factors that increase pain or compromise analgesic efficacy. These factors include progressive disease, new disease, increased or excessive activity, poor compliance, change in medication formulation or brand, drug interactions, and opioid addiction or diversion.[42]

Medications with long half-lives, such as methadone and levorphanol, can be useful for managing chronic pain syndromes. Typically these drugs afford analgesia for 8 hours or longer once steady-state serum levels are achieved. Methadone may be required every 4 hours during the first day of analgesic therapy, but can usually be administered every 8 to 12 hours in about 4 days. This longer duration is useful for providing time-contingent opioid therapy to patients with chronic pain who often become noncompliant with every 4-hour opioids after they have a few days of relative comfort. Because of the the long and variable half-life of methadone, clinicians should exercise caution. Patients may achieve adequate analgesia initially, but with continued use they may become toxic due to accumulation of methadone and its metabolites (Fig. 58-4). Methadone has little usefulness in acute pain due to its extended half-life.

ROUTES OF ADMINISTRATION

Currently available μ agonists can be given orally, rectally, parenterally, transdermally, and transmucosally. The mixed agonist-antagonists are available in parenteral dosage forms. Pentazocine also is available in an oral tablet and butorphanol in a nasal spray. For the majority of patients taking time-contingent opioids, oral dosage forms are preferred agents. The oral route is easy to use,

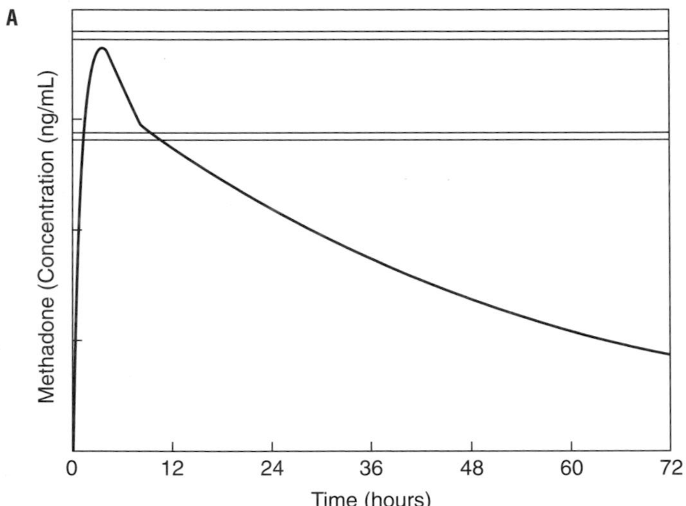

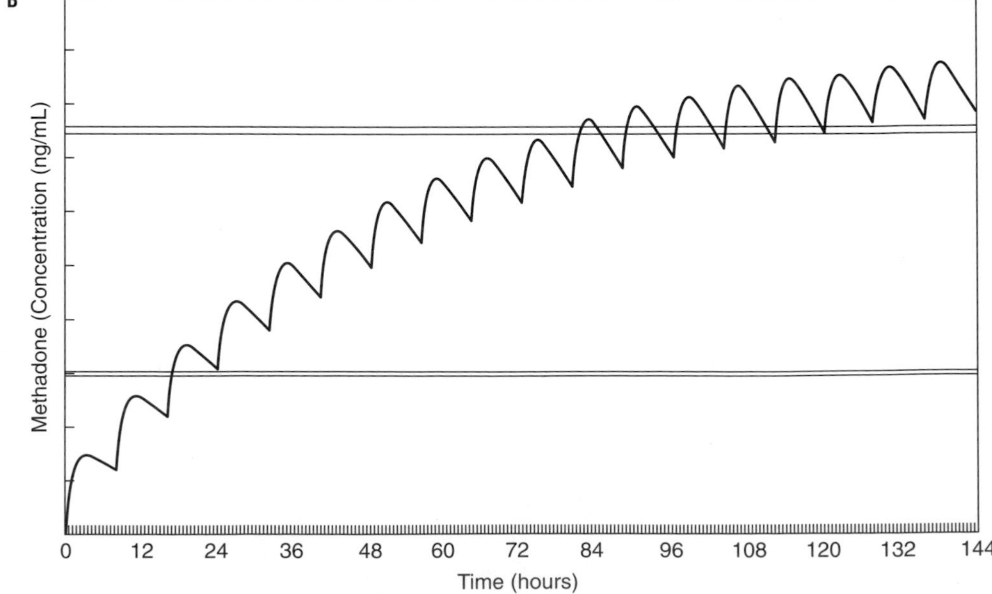

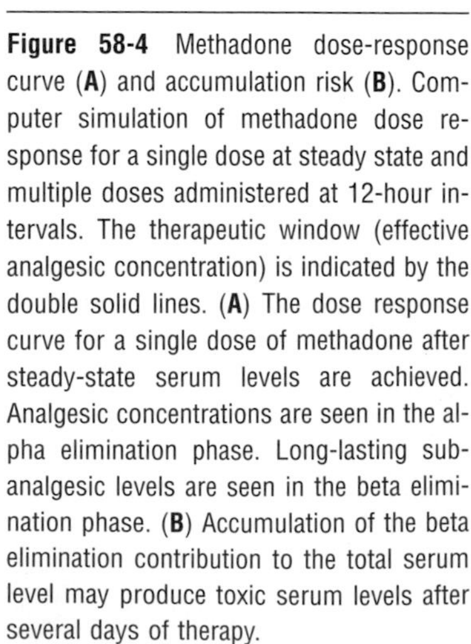
Figure 58-4 Methadone dose-response curve (**A**) and accumulation risk (**B**). Computer simulation of methadone dose response for a single dose at steady state and multiple doses administered at 12-hour intervals. The therapeutic window (effective analgesic concentration) is indicated by the double solid lines. (**A**) The dose response curve for a single dose of methadone after steady-state serum levels are achieved. Analgesic concentrations are seen in the alpha elimination phase. Long-lasting subanalgesic levels are seen in the beta elimination phase. (**B**) Accumulation of the beta elimination contribution to the total serum level may produce toxic serum levels after several days of therapy.

relatively inexpensive, does not signal increasing disease to the patient or family, and is effective. Incomplete bioavailability is not a concern since this limitation is easily overcome by increasing the dose. The only advantage of parenteral over oral administration for a patient able to take a drug orally is delivery of drug to sites of action more quickly. The time difference to analgesic onset and peak levels between oral administration and intramuscular or subcutaneous injections is often negligible. With appropriate scheduling, each dose of opioid can be administered sufficiently in advance of the prior dose to prevent recurrence of pain.

Patients and clinicians often hold false beliefs regarding potency and routes of administration, that is, parenteral versus oral. While intravenous administration affords quicker onset, it does not increase potency. The psychological advantage of oral administration should not be minimized. Fear of loss of control—epitomized by the need to depend on others to administer analgesics—is a major cause of depression among chronic and terminally ill pain patients.

Patients unable to tolerate oral administration often do well on administration, especially in short-term and terminal care. Hydromorphone, morphine, and oxymorphone are commercially available in rectal suppositories. Controlled-release oral morphine tablets have been used effectively via the rectal route[27] (Table 58-6). Mucosal irritation may occur in fewer patients with rectally administered oral controlled-release morphine tablets than with commercial morphine suppositories.[28] No local side effects were noted in a report of controlled-release oral morphine administered rectally.[43]

It is important to insert suppositories and tablets just above the anal sphincter to minimize first-pass metabolism. The inferior and middle rectal veins do not drain into the portal circulation as do the superior rectal veins. Administration higher into the rectal vault could induce a partial first-pass effect, which would lessen the effectiveness of the dose.[27] As with any rectal dosage administration, patients receiving opioids by this route should lie quietly on their sides for about 15 minutes after administration to aid absorption and minimize risk of rectal expulsion of the dose. Rectal administration of oral liquids may be an option in some patients; however, limitations on acceptable rectal fluid volumes and aesthetics may limit this option.

TABLE 58-6 **Rectal Opioid Times to Peak and Duration of Action**

Morphine immediate-release oral tablets	
peak	1.1 hour
duration	<6 hours
Morphine controlled-release oral tablets	
peak	5.4 hours
duration	8–12 hours
Morphine oral solution	
peak	0.5 hours
duration	4–6 hours
Morphine rectal suppositories	
peak	1.1 hours
duration	<6 hours
Hydromorphone rectal suppositories	
peak	1 hour
duration	4–6 hours
Methadone oral tablets	
peak	not known
duration	6–8 hours
Oxycodone oral tablets and solution	
peak	3.1 hours
duration	8–12 hours

Adapted from Warren D. Practical use of rectal medications in palliative care. *J Pain Symptom Manage* 1996;11:378.

Another effective and noninvasive route for opioid administration is transdermal. Fentanyl is the only opioid currently available for transdermal administration. Transdermal fentanyl patches are indicated for management of chronic pain in patients tolerant to the respiratory depressant effects of opioids. They provide 72 hours of clinically effective CNS opioid levels in most cases, but some patients get only about 48 hours of relief from a patch. Although the patches are more expensive than oral dosage forms, they are a convenient and cost-effective alternative to parenteral opioids. Transdermal fentanyl can be used by patients unable or unwilling to use oral or rectal opioids. The patch can also be useful for patients with noncompliant behaviors, for example, patients who cannot remember to take their opioid. As mentioned previously, this dosage form can be problematic in patients who require rapid-dose titration or have rapidly changing analgesic requirements.[44,45]

Subcutaneous delivery offers a fairly easy and inexpensive mechanism to deliver opioids. The pharmacokinetics of subcutaneous delivery are quite similar to intramuscular administration for opioids, without the disadvantage of painful intramuscular injections. Subcutaneous delivery is common in hospice and palliative care, where it has been shown to provide a good alternative to the intravenous route. Subcutaneous administration should replace intramuscular administration for opioids.[5]

Intravenous opioid administration is especially useful following surgery and trauma. Intravenous patient-controlled analgesia (PCA) is routinely used in many acute settings, especially for postoperative analgesia. While intravenous opioids are warranted when gastrointestinal function is limited (e.g., postoperative ileus), the intravenous route can negatively reinforce the sick role in patients with chronic pain and those requiring end-of-life care. The major reported advantage of intravenous PCA over regularly scheduled injections is that PCA provides a sense of control for the patient. PCA offers no pharmacologic advantage over regularly scheduled oral opioids for patients able to tolerate oral medications.[46]

Spinal administration of opioids is warranted in a small number of patients. It avoids the toxicity associated with the systemic delivery of these medications. The epidural and intrathecal routes each have advantages and disadvantages. Epidural administration allows opioid placement at any dermatomal level and does not require puncturing of the dura. Larger doses, however, are required and systemic effects may occur with epidural administration, increasing the risk of adverse effects. For morphine, intrathecal doses are only 1/10 of those needed for an equianalgesic epidural dose. Intrathecal administration requires puncturing of the dura and placing the drug closer to the spinal cord receptors. Drawbacks to intrathecal use include increased potential for meningitis and risk of postdural puncture headaches. Dose-related problems associated with spinal analgesia include pruritis, urinary retention, and delayed respiratory depression. Spinal analgesia is discussed in depth in Chapter 71.

Transmucosal delivery of fentanyl is useful for managing rapidly escalating breakthrough pain. This route produces rapid serum levels of lipophilic opioids and is useful for both preoperative and preprocedural sedation as well as analgesia. Oral transmucosal fentanyl provides rapid onset because there is no submucosal fat layer in the mouth. Because of the rapid onset of action, transmucosal fentanyl may prove to be beneficial as a breakthrough medication for patients who are on time-contingent opioid regimens. Oral transmucosal forms of fentanyl is commercially available as lozenges on handles. They do not resemble lollipops and should not be referred to as such in order to minimize the risk of children assuming they are candy. This dosage form (Actiq) is indicated for breakthrough pain in cancer patients and is available in a range of strengths (See Table 58-2).

Sublingual opioid administration has been used extensively in palliative care. Advantages include ease of administration, low expense (with oral, not parenteral, solutions), avoidance of hepatic first pass, and rapid onset of action (~5 to 15 minutes). Disadvantages include relatively low bioavailability, potential for poor taste acceptance, and the need to avoid drinking anything for about 15 minutes following administration. Simple aqueous solutions are most appropriate for this route. The volume of a dose should not exceed 1 mL to minimize medication trickling down the throat. If a larger amount of medication is needed than will readily dissolve in 1 mL of water, a second dose can be given after 5 to 10 minutes. In a study of the percentage of sublingual opioid absorbed after 1 mL of an aqueous solution was held in the mouth for 10 minutes at pH 6.5, absorption was greater for lipophilic than hydrophilic opioids. Results from that study are listed in Table 58-4.[47] As the mouth pH increased, absorption increased. Opioids often taste bitter, but many patients find overly sweet solutions even less palatable. Mild citrus or bland flavors are usually most acceptable. Changes in the oral mucosa, stomatitis, increased keratinization, decreased salivary flow, and changes in salivary pH due to disease, trauma, radiation or chemotherapy, as well as the overall condition of the mouth, influence absorption from sublingual, buccal, and oral transmucosal administration.

Nebulization into the lungs, and intravaginal use of oral tablets and rectal suppositories have been reported. Nebulized morphine has been shown to be useful in the setting of dyspnea, especially in terminally ill patients.[48] However, systemic opioids may be required to effectively treat cough.[49] The use of oral and rectal morphine formulations via the vagina has been studied.[50] Because of the unpredictable bioavailability resulting from vaginal delivery, this route is not recommended. Intrastomal administration has been used with reported success by some hospice programs. Drug level data from this route have not been reported.

DRUG INTERACTIONS

Opioids interact with a variety of medications (Table 58-7). Most opioid drug interactions are a consequence of additive effects, that is, pharmacodynamic interactions. Increases in sedation can be seen when opioids are administered with alcohol, benzodiazepines, butyrophenones, phenothiazines, sedative hypnotics, and tricyclic antidepressants. Midazolam may decrease the effect of fentanyl.[51] Antinociceptive activity may be impaired by benzodiazepine administration from inhibition of the descending inhibitory control pathways.[51]

Methadone withdrawal has been precipitated by a number of agents known to induce microsomal enzymes.[52] This pharmacokinetic interaction results in an increase in the metabolism of methadone. Inhibition of methadone metabolism has also been shown with several agents, leading to increased plasma levels of methadone.

Opioids can inhibit metabolism of other agents, leading to increases in serum levels of affected drugs. Desipramine plasma levels may be increased by coadministration with methadone or morphine.[51,52]

PRINCIPLES OF OPIOID USE

A World Health Organization (WHO) Expert Committee defined five principles of opioid use in 1986 to manage cancer pain in developing countries (WHO Cancer Pain Relief 1986, 1996). Those principles have been validated numerous times in undeveloped, developing, and developed countries including the United States.[53–61] More recently, the applicability of these principles in both acute pain[5] and chronic noncancer pain has been documented.[8] These principles may be summarized as:

1. Use oral or other noninvasive routes whenever possible.
2. Individualize doses by titrating to response.
3. Select analgesics according to needs as described on the analgesic ladder.
4. Maintain effective drug levels in the body as long as there is a noxious stimulus.
5. Use indicated adjuvants.

The usefulness of this approach has been studied in over 2100 cancer patients treated over a period of 10 years for a total of 140,478 treatment days. Drugs on step 1 of the WHO analgesic ladder provided adequate analgesia for only 11% of the days, step 2 for 31% of the days, and step 3 for 49% of the treatment days. Fifty-six percent of the patients received morphine. Co-analgesics including antidepressants, anticonvulsants, and corticosteroids were used on 37% of the treatment days and drugs for other symptoms, such as laxatives, were used on 79% of the treatment days. In their final days of life, 84% of the patients rated their pain as moderate or less.[60]

A 1998 study of over 4000 cancer patients with documented daily pain who were residents in over 1400 nursing homes in five midwestern American states revealed serious underuse of opioids in managing pain. Sixteen percent received only acetaminophen or an NSAID, 32% received WHO analgesic ladder step 2 drug therapy, and only 26% received morphine. Fully 26% of these patients received no analgesia.[10] With the WHO and AHCPR guidelines on use of opioids having been available for so long, it is difficult to understand how such inadequate use of these drugs continues.

MYTHS AND MISCONCEPTIONS

Many health professionals subscribe to false beliefs about opioids. Unnecessary fears of addiction, dependence, tolerance, and toxicity often deter prescribing and taking of these important medications.

TABLE 58-7 **Clinically Important Opioid Drug Interactions**

Opioid(s)	Interacting drug(s)	Description
Codeine	Quinidine	Inhibition of conversion to morphine; decreased analgesia
Meperidine	Monoamine oxidase inhibitors (e.g., phenelzine, tranylcypromine)	Excitatory response (including seizures, arrhythmias, hyperpyrexia, and coma; potentially fatal interaction
Meperidine	Sibutramine	May induce serotonin syndrome
Meperidine	SSRIs	No evidence, but potential for serotonin syndrome should be considered
Meperidine, morphine	Cimetidine	Inhibition of opioid metabolism; Increased opioid effects
Methadone	Carbamazepine Erythromycin Phenytoin	Increased opioid metabolism; may induce withdrawal
Methadone, morphine	Desipramine	Inhibition of desipramine metabolism; toxicity possible
Opioids, (controlled-release) (e.g., MS Contin, Oramorph SR, OxyContin)	Metoclopramide	Earlier peak plasma concentration; increased sedation
Opioids (class)	Antihistamines (e.g. hydroxyzine, diphenhydramine)	Increased sedation
Opioids (class)	Butyrophenones (e.g. haloperidol)	Increased sedation
Opioids (class)	Tricyclic antidepressants (e.g. amitriptyline, desipramine doxepin, nortriptyline)	Increased sedation and potentiation of opioid Induced respiratory depression
Propoxyphene	Carbamazepine	Increased carbamazepine levels, potential for toxicity
Propoxyphene	Doxepin	Increased doxepin levels, potential for toxicity
Propoxyphene	Metoprolol, propranolol	Increased plasma levels of these beta blockers

Data from: Maurer P, Bartkowski R. Drug interactions of clinical significance with opioid analgesics. Drug Saf. 1993;8:30; Quinn D, Day R. Drug interactions of clinical importance. An updated guide. *Drug Saf* 1995;12:393. Hansten PD, Horn JR. Drug Interactions Analysis and Management. Vancouver, Wash: Applied Therapeutics, Inc.

Addiction and Dependence

Until recently, most of what was known about opioid addiction was based on the experience of drug abusers, not patients. Opioids more commonly cause dysphoria than euphoria among opioid-naive individuals. Patients in pain seek comfort, not a drug-induced high. Studies of the actual incidence of iatrogenic opioid addiction show that this phenomenon is exquisitely rare. The Boston Collaborative Drug Surveillance Program study revealed only four cases of iatrogenic addiction among 11,882 patients without prior history of substance abuse who received opioids for a broad range of indications and were followed for up to 2 years.[62] A national survey of over 10,000 burn patients without prior histories of drug abuse who received opioids for extended periods revealed no cases of addiction.[63] Only 3 of 2369 chronic headache patients, most of whom had access to opioids, abused the analgesics.[64]

Addiction is defined as the compulsive use of a substance resulting in physical, psychological, or social harm and continued use despite that harm. [65] Drug-seeking behavior does not in itself indicate addiction. Pseudoaddiction was defined over a decade ago as a drug-seeking behavior due to inadequate analgesia, not substance abuse.[66] The American Society of Addiction Medicine said in its April 1997 Public Policy Statement that ". . . individuals who have severe, unrelieved pain may become intensely focused on finding relief for their pain. Sometimes, such patients may appear to observers to be preoccupied with obtaining opioids, but the preoccupation is with finding relief of pain, rather than using opioids, *per se.* This phenomenon has been termed pseudoaddiction."[67]

Dependence is defined as a physiologic phenomenon characterized by an abstinence syndrome upon abrupt discontinuation, substantial dose reduction, or administration of an antagonist.[65] Dependence occurs predictably among patients who take opioids on a regular basis for more than a few days. It also occurs predictably among patients taking steroids and many other common drugs. Opioid dependence can usually be ended by tapering the dose over 5 to 10 days when the drug is no longer needed.[68] It should not be a barrier to use of the drugs when they are indicated. Neither dependence nor tolerance is indicative of or a predisposing factor to addiction.

Tolerance

Tolerance to opioids is widely misunderstood. Three distinct types of tolerance occur with opioids. Tolerance to the respiratory depressive effects and other manifestations of CNS depression normally occurs within 5 to 7 days of continuous, regularly scheduled opioid use. Such patients are commonly referred to as being *opioid-tolerant*. Tolerance to the constipating effects of opioids does not occur.[69] Activated μ-opioid receptors in the colon inhibit peristalsis. Stimulating laxatives, for example, senna, bisacodyl, are needed to induce colonic emptying. Stool softeners alone are not effective. Because of the risk of severe constipation and fecal impaction, prophylaxis with stimulating laxatives may be indicated when opioid therapy is started.[70]

It often is necessary to increase the opioid dose over the first few days or week of therapy while finding the effective dose. Tolerance to analgesia does not occur in most patients once the effective dose of opioid is identified and administered regularly. Neither up-nor down-regulation of opioid receptors occurs with regularly scheduled dosing. Most patients remain comfortable on a consistent opioid dose unless another variable occurs. When an otherwise stable opioid dose ceases to be effective, pseudotolerance due to increasing or new pathology, excessive physical activity after the pain decreases, drug interactions, noncompliance, or other nonpharmacologic factors should be considered.[42]

Multiple Pain Complaints

Many clinicians conclude that patients are abusing opioids when the patients complain of new pains once their initial pain complaints are controlled. In a study of 955 advanced cancer patients, 34% experienced two or more different types of pain, and 80% reported pain resulting from two or more different causes.[71] Similar findings have been reported for AIDS patients.[72] More severe pain tends to mask less intense pains. When the former is effectively treated, masked pains that require other treatment often become evident.

Save Opioids Until They Are Really Needed

A common false belief of patients is that use of opioids relatively early in the course of a progressive disease tends to render them less useful later when they may be needed more. That is not true. Pure μ opioids are effective over a broad clinical dosage range (Fig. 58-3). When pain increases, doses can be increased without loss of effectiveness.

Opioids Are Effective for All Types of Pain

Opioids are effective analgesics for most nociceptive and much neuropathic pain. But all pain is not opioid-responsive. Some pain that is opioid-responsive should not be managed with opioids, for example, constipation pain. The underlying cause of the pain should be treated before considering the sole use of opioids to control it. Examples of this include neuropathic pain for which tricyclic antidepressants, anticonvulsants, and nerve blocks may be indicated; painful infectious cysts for which incision and drainage followed by antiinfectives may be indicated; and gastrointestinal spasm for which anticholinergics may be most effective.[73]

Parenteral Opioids Are More Potent and Effective Than Oral Doses

Many patients believe that parenteral opioids are more effective than analgesics administered by oral or other noninvasive routes. As discussed earlier, this is not true. Furthermore, use of parenteral routes signals advancing disease to many patients and may be psychologically disadvantageous.

Potency is commonly misunderstood. Potency only indicates the amount of drug needed for effect. For example, 10 mg of oral morphine is approximately equal to 1.5 to 2 mg of oral hydromorphone. Hydromorphone is therefore about five times more potent, but no more effective, than morphine. When patients ask for more potent drugs, they usually mean more effective drugs.

Dose Increments Should Be Conservative

Fear of opioids causes many clinicians to use conservative dose increments. This can lead to treatment failure. Opioid doses should be increased to response. The appropriate increment is normally 50% of the dose, and this can be increased every five half-lives (twice a day for morphine). This percentage of increase applies no matter what the prior dose. When a patient knows that the opioid dose has been increased, but adequate analgesia dose not result, anxiety often increases. This increases the pain perception, which in turn increases the opioid dose requirement further. It is often better to err slightly in the direction of too much than too little opioid. Initial sedation may be advantageous when a patient is very anxious and experiencing a sleep deficit from the pain.

Opioids Prevent Safe Driving Due to Impaired Judgement and Psychomotor Function

Opioids can markedly impair judgement and psychomotor function when therapy is initiated. Similar adverse effects can occur when doses are increased. But once a patient has been continuously receiving opioids on a regular schedule for about a week, these effects usually diminish markedly. There was no significant difference in the number of motor vehicle crashes that involved 24 drivers who were taking opioids on a regular schedule for long-term pain management than among the general population of Finland.[74] A recent systematic review of the world literature confirmed this finding.[88] If the patient is experiencing no observable opioid-induced impairment and the opioid dose has been consistent for a week or more, the patient can usually drive or carry out other normal functions safely. When the dose is increased, however, the patient should refrain from those activities for about a week and until any impairment due to the increased dose resolves.

CONCLUSION

Opioids are important and commonly underused analgesic drugs. Health professionals, patients, and caregivers often harbor irrational fears about these drugs. Opiophobia has been defined as "irrational and undocumented fear that appropriate use of opioids causes addiction."[1] As a result, opioids are often underprescribed, underdosed, taken irregularly in spite of instructions to the contrary, and stopped abruptly. Inappropriate beliefs about opioids have been documented among physicians,[75] nurses,[76] and pharmacists.[77] Societal barriers to the use of opioids are now being refuted by professional organizations[8] and regulatory agencies.[9] Nevertheless, many clinicians continue to avoid opioids in their practices to the detriment of their patients. Unlike nonsteroidal anti-inflammatory drugs and even acetaminophen, long-term opioid use rarely causes end-organ toxicity.

New opioids delivery systems including oral controlled release, iontophoretic, implanted, and transdermal dosage forms are currently under development. Combination dosage forms of opioids with other drugs also are being investigated. Some of these new forms may make opioid analgesia easier. But excellent analgesia can be provided with the drugs and dosage forms currently available. All pain clinicians can and should work to overcome opioid myths and misconceptions and should encourage appropriate use of opioids when they are indicated.

REFERENCES

1. Morgan J. American opiophobia: customary underutilization of opioid analgesics. *Adv Alcohol Subst Abuse*. 1985;5:163.
2. *The Interagency Committee on New Therapies for Pain and Discomfort: Report to the White House*. US Department of Health Education and Welfare, Public Health Service, National Institutes of Health, May 1979.
3. Pinkert T. Report from the Interagency Committee on Pain and Analgesia: a Public Health Service initiative. *J Pain Symptom Manage* 1986; 1:174.
4. National Institutes of Health Consensus Development Conference. The integrated approach to the management of pain. *J Pain Symptom Manage* 1987;2:35.
5. Acute Pain Management Guideline Panel. *Clinical Practice Guideline. Acute Pain Management: Operative or Medical Procedures and Trauma*. Rockville, Md: US Dept of Health and Human Services, Agency for Health Care Policy and Research; 1992. AHCPR publication 92-0032.
6. Jacox A, Carr DB, Payne R, et al. *Clinical Practice Guideline Number 9. Management of Cancer Pain*. Rockville, Md: US Dept of Health and Human Services, Agency for Health Care Policy and Research; 1994. AHCPR publication 94-0592.
7. Portenoy RK. Opioid therapy for chronic nonmalignant pain: a review of the critical issues. *J Pain Symptom Manage* 1996;11:203.
8. Haddox JD, Joranson DE, Angarola RT, et al. Consensus Statement from the American Academy of Pain Medicine and American Pain Society. The use of opioids for the treatment of chronic pain. *Clin J Pain* 1997;13:6.
9. The Federation of State Medical Boards of the United States. Model Guidelines for the Use of Controlled Substances for the Treatment of Pain, May 2, 1998.
10. Bernabei R, Gambassi G, Lapane K, et al. Management of pain in elderly patients with cancer. *JAMA* 1998;279:1877.
11. World Health Organization. *Cancer Pain Relief and Palliative Care: Report of a WHO Expert Committee*. Technical Report Series 804. Geneva, Switzerland: World Health Organization, 1990.
12. Ferrante F. Principles of opioid pharmacotherapy: practical implications of basic mechanisms. *J Pain Symptom Manage* 1996;11:265.
13. Rushton A, Sneyd J. Opioid analgesics. *Br J Hosp Med* 1997; 7:105.
14. Singh V, Bajpai K, Biswas S, et al. Molecular biology of opioid receptors. Recent advances. *Neuroimmunomodulation* 1997;4:285.
15. Yaksh T. Pharmacology and mechanisms of opioid analgesic activity. *Acta Anaesthesiol Scand* 1997;41:94.
16. Franz D. Pharmacology of analgesic receptors. *J Pharm Care Pain Symptom Control* 1994;2:37.
17. Sabbe M, Yaksh T. Pharmacology of spinal opioids. *J Pain Symptom Manage* 1990;5:191.
18. Lipman AG, Gauthier M. Pharmacology of opioid drugs: basic principles. In: Portenoy R, Bruera E, eds. *Topics in Palliative Care.* Vol. 1. New York, NY: Oxford University Press, 1997:137–161.
19. Pasternak G. Pharmacological mechanisms of opioid analgesics. *Clin Neuropharmacol* 1993;16:1.
20. Back I, Finlay I. Analgesic effect of topical opioids on painful skin ulcers. *J Pain Symptom Manage* 1995;10:493.
21. Stein C, Pfluger M, Yassouridis A, et al. No tolerance to peripheral morphine analgesia in presence of opioid expression in inflammed synovia. *J Clin Invest* 1996;98:793.
22. Stein C, Yassouridis A. Periperal morphine analgesia. *Pain* 1997;71: 119.
23. Hare B. The opioid analgesics: rational selection of agents for acute and chronic pain. *Hosp Formulary* 1987;22:64.
24. Walker D, Zacny J. Subjective, psychomotor, and analgesic effects of oral codeine and morphine in healthy volunteers. *Psychopharmacology (Basel)* 1998;140:191.
25. Cleary J. Pharmacokinetic and pharmacodynamic issues in the treatment of breakthrough pain. *Semin Oncol* 1997;24:13.
26. Rusho W. Clinical issues and concerns in the use of extemporaneously compounded medications. *J Pharm Care Pain Symptom Control* 1996;4:5.
27. Warren D. Practical use of rectal medications in palliative care. *J Pain Symptom Manage* 1996;11:378.
28. Kaiko R, Fitzmartin R, Thomas G, Goldenheim P. The bioavailability of morphine in controlled-release 30-mg tablets per rectum compared with immediate-release 30-mg rectal suppositories and controlled-release 30-mg oral tablets. *Pharmacotherapy* 1992;12:107.
29. Korte W, Stoutz N, Morant R. Day-to-day titration to initiate transdermal fentanyl in cancer patients: short and long term experience in a prospective study of 39 patients. *J Pain Symptom Manage* 1996; 11:139.
30. Moulin D, Kreeft J, Murray-Parsons N, Bouquillon A. Comparison of continuous subcutaneous and intravenous hydromorphone infusion for management of cancer pain. *Lancet* 1991;337:465.
31. Pereira J, Bruera E. Emerging neuropsychiatric toxicities of opioids. *J Pharm Care Pain Symptom Control* 1997;5:3.
32. Christrup L. Morphine metabolites. *Acta Anaesthesiol Scand* 1997; 41:116.
33. Forman W. Opioid analgesic drugs in the elderly. *Clin Geriatr Med* 1996;12:489.
34. Sjogren P, Jensen N, Jensen T. Disappearance of morphine-induced hyperalgesia after discontinuing or substituting other opioid agonists. *Pain* 1994;59:313.
35. Glare P, Walsh T, Pippenger C. Normorphine, a neurotoxic metabolite? *Lancet* 1990;335:725.
36. Coderre T, Katz J, Vaccarino A, Melzack R. Contribution of central neuroplasticity to pathological pain: review of clinical and experimental evidence. *Pain* 1993;52:259.
37. Woolf C. Windup and central stimulation are not equivalent. *Pain* 1996;66:105.
38. Pockett S. Spinal cord synaptic plasticity and chronic pain. *Anesth Analg* 1994;80:173.
39. Twycross R. Morphine and diamorphine in the terminally ill patient. *Acta Anaesth Scand* 1984;74:128.
40. Beeton A, Upton P, Shipton E. The case for patient-controlled analgesia. Inter-patient variation in postoperative analgesic requirements. *S Afr J Surg* 1992;30:5.
41. Portenoy R, Hagen N. Breakthrough pain: definition, prevalence and characteristics. *Pain* 1990;41:273.
42. Pappagallo M. The concept of pseudotolerance to opioids. *J Pharm Care Pain Symptom Control* 1998;6:95.
43. Maloney C, Kesner R, Klein G, et al. The rectal administration of MS Contin: clinical implications of use in end stage cancer. *Am J Hospice Care* 1989;6:34.
44. Lipman AG, Ashburn MA. Titration with TTS fentanyl systems for previously uncontrolled cancer pain: in response. *Anesth Analg* 1994;79:613.
45. Ashburn MA, Lipman AG. Management of pain in the cancer patient. *Anesth Analg* 1993;76:402.
46. Kleiman R, Lipman AG, Hare B, MacDonald S. A comparison of morphine administeed by patient-controlled analgesia and regularly scheduled intramuscular injection in severe postoperative pain. *J Pain Symptom Manage* 1988;3:15.
47. Weinberg D, Inturrisi C, Reidenberg B, et al. Sublingual absorption of selected opioid analgesics. *Clin Pharmacol Ther* 1988;44:335.
48. Stein W, Min Y. Nebulized morphine for paroxysmal cough and dyspnea in a nursing home resident with metastatic cancer. *Am J Hosp Palliat Care* 1997;14:52.

49. Fuller R, Karlsson J, Choudry N, et al. Effect of inhaled and systemic opiates on responders to inhaled capsaicin in humans. *J Appl Physiol* 1988;655:1125.
50. Ostrop N, Lamb J, Reid G. Intravaginal morphine: an alternative route of administration. *Pharmacotherapy* 1998;18:863.
51. Maurer P, Bartkowski R. Drug interactions of clinical significance with opioid analgesics. *Drug Saf* 1993;8:30.
52. Quinn D, Day R. Drug interactions of clinical importance. An updated guide. *Drug Saf* 1995;12:393.
53. Takeda F. Results of field-testing in Japan of the WHO draft interim guidelines on relief of cancer pain. *Pain Clin* 1986;1:83.
54. Ventafridda V, Tamburini M, Caraceni A, et al. A validation study of the WHO method for cancer pain relief. *Cancer* 1987;59:850.
55. Walker V, Hoskin P, Hanks G, et al. Evaluation of the WHO analgesic guidelines for cancer pain in a hospital based palliative care unit. *J Pain Symptom Manage* 1988;3:145.
56. Vijayaram S, Bhargava K, Ramamani, et al. Experience with oral morphine for cancer pain relief. *J Pain Symptom Manage* 1989;4:130.
57. Giosis A, Giorini M, Ratti R, et al. Application of the WHO protocol on medical therapy for oncologic pain in an internal medicine hospital. *Tumori* 1989;75:470.
58. Schug S, Zech D, Dorr U. Cancer pain management according to the WHO analgesic guidelines. *J Pain Symptom Manage* 1990;5:27.
59. Grond S, Zech D, Schug S, et al. Validation of the World Health Organization guidelines for cancer pain relief during the last days and hours of life. *J Pain Symptom Manage* 1991;6:411.
60. Zech D, Grond S, Lynch J, et al. Validation of the World Health Organization guidelines for cancer pain relief: a ten year prospective study. *Pain* 1995;63:65.
61. Rappaz O, Tripiana J, Rapin C, et al. Soins palliatifs et traitement de la douleur cancereuse en geriatrie. Notre experience institutionnelle. *Ther Umsch* 1985;42:843.
62. Porter J, Jick H. Addiction rare in patients treated with narcotics [letter]. *N Engl J Med* 1980;302:123.
63. Perry S, Heidrich G. Management of pain during debridement: a survey of US pain units. *Pain.* 1982;13:267.
64. Medina J, Diamond S. Drug dependency in patients with chronic headache. *Headache* 1977;17:12.
65. Rinaldi R, Steindler E, Wilford B, et al. Clarification and standardization of substance abuse terminology. *JAMA* 1988;259:555.
66. Weissman DE, Haddox JD. Opioid pseudoaddiction—an iatrogenic syndrome. *Pain* 1989;36:363.
67. The American Society of Addiction Medicine. Public Policy Statement on Definitions Related to the Use of Opioids in Pain Treatment. Available at: *http://www.asam.org*. Accessed April 1997.
68. Hare BD, Lipman AG. Uses and misuses of medications in the management of chronic pain. *Prob Anesth* 1990;4:577.
69. Basta S, Anderson D. Mechanisms and management of constipation in the cancer patient. *J Pharm Care Pain Symptom Control* 1998;6:21.
70. Levy M. Pain management in advanced cancer. *Semin Oncol* 1985; 12:394.
71. Twycross R, Fairfield S. Pain in far-advanced cancer. *Pain* 1982;14: 303.
72. Breitbart W, McDonald M, Rosenfeld B, et al. Pain in ambulatory AIDS patients: pain characteristics and medical correlates. *Pain* 1996;68:315.
73. Lipman AG. Comments on Fitzgibbon and Galer [letter]. *Pain* 1995;63: 135.
74. Vainio A, Ollila J, Matikainen E, et al. Driving ability in cancer patients receiving long-term morphine analgesia. *Lancet* 1995;346:667.
75. Elliot T, Murray D, Elliot B, et al. Physician knowledge and attitudes about cancer pain management: a survey from the Minnesota Cancer Pain Project. *J Pain Symptom Manage* 1995;10:495.
76. Rankin M, Snider B. Nurses' perceptions of cancer patients' pain. *Cancer Nurs* 1984;7:149.
77. Doucette W, Mays-Holland T, Memmott H, et al. Cancer pain management: pharmacist knowledge and practices. *J Pharm Care Pain Symptom Control* 1997;5:17.
78. Hansten PD, Horn JR. *Drug Interactions Analysis and Management.* Vancouver, WA: Applied Therapeutics,Inc, updated quarterly.
79. McEvoy G, ed. *AHFS Drug Information 99.* Bethesda, Md: American Society of Health-System Pharmacists, 1999.
80. Babul N, Darke A. Putative role of hydromorphone metabolites in myoclonus. *Pain* 1993;52:123.
81. Chan G, Matzke G. Effects of renal insufficiency on the pharmacokinetics and pharmacodynamics of opioid analgesics. *Drug Intell Clin Pharm* 1987;21:773.
82. Lötsch J, Stockmann A, Brune K, et al. Pharmacokinetics of morphine and its glucuronides after intravenous infusion of morphine and morphine-6-glucuronide in healthy volunteers. *Clin Pharmacol Ther* 1996;60:316.
83. Hutchison TA, Shahan DR, eds. DRUGDEX® System MICROMEDEX, Greenwood Village, Colorado, 1997, Vol 2.
84. Mulvana D, Duncan G, Shyu W, et al. Quantitative determination of butorphanol and its metabolites in human plasma by gas chromatography-electron capture negative-ion chemical ionization mass spectrometry. *J Chromatogr* 1996;682:289.
85. Reisine T, Pasternak G. Opioid analgesics and antagonists. In: Hardman J, Limbird L, Molinoff P, et al, eds. *Goodman and Gilman's The Pharmacological Basis of Therapeutics*. New York, NY: McGraw-Hill, 1996:521–556.
86. Shyu W, Morgenthien E, Barbhaiya R. Pharmacokinetics of butorphanol nasal spray in patients with renal impairment. *Br J Clin Pharmacol* 1996;41:397.
87. Steinberg R, Gilman D, Johnson F. Acute toxic delirium in a patient using transdermal fentanyl. *Anesth Analg* 1992;75:1014.
88. Fishbein DA, Cutler RB, Rosonoff HL, Rosonoff RS. Can patients taking opioids drive safely: a structured evidence-based review. *J Pain Palliat Care Pharmacotherap* 2002;16:9–28.

CHAPTER 59 OPIOIDS FOR NONMALIGNANT PAIN: ISSUES AND CONTROVERSY

Craig L. Shalmi

INTRODUCTION

This chapter discusses the use of opioids in the treatment of chronic nonmalignant pain and focuses in on the vehement controversy that this subject continues to generate. The use of opioids has become well established for the treatment of cancer pain and acute pain.[1–3] However, opioid use for chronic nonmalignant pain has been generally regarded as unsafe and ineffective until this past decade. More recently, these views have undergone a reappraisal driven by a number of factors, including a mounting realization that pain remains drastically undertreated. Investigations into the incidence of unrelieved pain and suffering in the United States and throughout the world prompted the National Institutes of Health to designate chronic pain as one of the most significant public health problems facing medicine.[4] It is estimated to affect over 50 million Americans, and it is the presenting complaint in 80% of physician visits.[5] The cost to our society of this pain and suffering, whether measured by its deleterious effect on people's lives or in dollars and cents, is incalculable.

How is it that the strongest of painkillers, the opioids, have become so feared and stigmatized in our society. Savage has traced the U.S. experience with opioid dependence and addiction back to the 1800s when morphine was used for a variety of ailments. Those affected were predominately of the middle class, and this led to a more cautious approach with the use of opioids. The association of these drugs with sociopaths and the criminal element began after the turn of the century when large waves of immigrants crowded into American cities and opioids were used for nonmedicinal purposes as a hedge against poverty and destitution. Drug use in the United States reached epidemic proportions in the 1960s, and placed heroin on center stage with hallucinogens, marijuana, and other illicit substances. A second wave of drug use occurred in the 1980s with the introduction of PCP and crack cocaine into American society; the effect was devastating, leading to a tremendous antidrug sentiment, and out of this the War on Drugs was born.[6] More recently, there has been a proliferation of interest by physicians and other health care professionals in the care of patients with pain and terminal illnesses. The advent of a new medical specialty in pain medicine and palliative care has ushered in a renewed interest for the use of opioid medications in some patient populations. The debate concerning the role of opioids in chronic pain has its roots in the cancer literature. For use in cancer patients it has been shown, rather strikingly, that opioids can impart marked degrees of pain relief along with improvement in function and quality of life, and may do so in the absence of a significant degree of tolerance, dependence, or side effects.[1,2,7] Despite the fact that the cancer patient population differs in important ways from patients with chronic nonmalignant pain, it is certainly conceivable that these results may be observed in other patient groups.

An additional factor that has prompted a re-evaluation of opioid use is consideration of the way in which regulatory agencies, charged with the responsibility of reducing illicit drug use, have effectively curtailed legitimate prescribing practices by leading physicians who fear investigation and prosecution.[8,9]

Reluctance to Prescribe Opioid Medications

The perception that some physicians are insensitive to their patient's pain is probably rooted in a number of realities: The first of which is that chronic pain can be difficult to treat. Beyond opioids, physicians lack medications that yield a high degree of efficacy in severe pain states. So, ultimately, it is not so much the case that physicians neglect treating pain as they are reluctant to prescribe opioids. This reluctance may stem from a variety of factors. For example, many physicians believe that there is simply insufficient data to support the use of opioids outside of acute pain and cancer, while others lack the facility to prescribe these drugs in a manner that is safe and maximally effective or do not want to be involved with close monitoring that these drugs require. Many physicians avoid opioids believing that to prescribe them is to place patients at risk for dependence, tolerance, addiction, and abuse. And, as previously mentioned, the risk of regulatory scrutiny and sanctions dissuade some physicians from prescribing opioid medications, and this appears to be operant even in the case of cancer pain, where there is a clear consensus as to the indication for opioids.[10] Evidence for this trend comes directly from Drug Enforcement Administration, where a 50% decrease in the prescribing of opioids has been recorded in states using the various multiple copy prescription programs.[11] This marked decline in prescriptions has been ascribed, by some, to a reduction in illicit or inappropriate prescribing activity. However, information from the Drug Abuse Warning Network (DAWN) does not concur that these programs reduce prescription drug abuse to an appreciable extent.[12] Instead, it appears that a good deal of lawful, medically indicated prescribing of opioids and other schedule II substances is being reduced at the expense of the patients who need these medications. In essence, medical judgment and legitimate prescribing practices are being affected by regulations designed to combat substance abuse and drug addiction. This occurs despite a large body of evidence that indicates that while pain is drastically undertreated in the United States, the risk of addicting patients to opioids following their legitimate use is diminutive. This is not to say that drug abuse in the United States is not a problem when it has in fact had a devastating effect on our society. Physicians surveyed tend to agree that some regulation is important to avert improper prescribing practices; however, the message being received by physicians led many to fear investigation and prosecution even for legitimate prescribing. These fears have been borne out in a national survey of boards of medical examiners.[13] In this report, a substantial number of regulators reported that investigation of a prescriber would be warranted based on the dispensing of opioids to a patient without cancer for more than 6 months. Clearly, what is needed is a more balanced approach that provides an environment in which the legitimate prescribing of scheduled substances may proceed without fear of penalty while illicit use may be identified and dealt with. This can only occur when both regulators and physicians are working toward the same goals and have an understanding of when and how to use opioid medications.

PUBLISHED EXPERIENCE WITH OPIOIDS IN CHRONIC NONMALIGNANT PAIN

Controlled Studies

Aside from the fact that there are few controlled trials evaluating opioids in chronic pain, much of what data does appear in the literature is methodologically flawed and/or provides validity only within narrow limits. Nonetheless, there is a trend toward favorable outcomes in some of these studies. In a retrospective study, Taub reported on over 300 patients that he judged as having good overall efficacy, although 4% of these patients had developed abuse.[14] In one of the larger series, Zenz et al reported on 100 patients, most suffering either with neuropathic pain or back pain, treated with a number of opioids over a prolonged period.[15] Approximately one half achieved good pain relief as well as a functional improvement as determined by the Karnofsky Performance Status Scale. There were no cases of addiction identified. In a randomized, double-blind, placebo-controlled study, Arkinstall evaluated the efficacy of controlled-release codeine in 46 patients with chronic, nonmalignant pain.[16] Patients in the codeine group had significantly lower scores on the visual analog scale (VAS) and significant reductions when administered the Pain Disability Index, though there was also a higher incidence of nausea. Nevertheless, a marked majority of both blinded patients and investigators expressed their preference for codeine over placebo, and 93% of the patients completing the study requested long-term, open-label treatment with controlled-release codeine. In another randomized study with crossover, Moulin et al showed analgesic benefit with sustained-release morphine, and without the development of drug-seeking behaviors, but did not find any improvement in functional status.[17] Some of these studies suffer from inadequate follow-up times.

Survey Data

A good deal of survey data in the literature points to good outcomes in select populations. Still, these are not controlled trials and the information may not be generalized to specific populations. Nonetheless, some of these reports are optimistic and point toward areas that need to be carefully researched. Portenoy, Portenoy and Foley reported data on over 50 patients having a variety of diagnoses, including neuropathic pain, with about two-thirds of patients reporting either adequate or partial relief. Marked gains in functional status were considered uncommon and problems with abuse were limited to two patients who had histories of substance abuse.[18,19] Urban and colleagues used methadone to treat phantom limb pain with a duration of follow-up of 12 to 26 months. All reported pain relief in excess of 50% and no toxicity or abuse was noted. This report was particularly interesting in that it suggests efficacy in patients with neuropathic pain, an etiology that has frequently been considered to be unresponsive to opioid medications.[20] Tennant et al presented survey data on 52 patients treated with methadone for varying pain problems and reported adequate pain relief in 88% of patients, though there was a high incidence of abuse as well as side effects.[21] Many of the patients were noted to be medically ill. Kell et al presented data on 16 patients with vascular headaches treated with methadone and followed for up to 3 years. Analgesic efficacy was considered good in all patients and no adverse effects were reported.[22] These data are distinctly different from that of Brodner and Taubs, who describe four patients with chronic nonmalignant pain as having had improvement following withdrawal from opioids.[23] Improvement following discontinuation of opioids has been noted by others as well,[24] including Taylor who reported on seven patients with chronic pain who showed improvement in a number of parameters, including reports in pain diaries, mood, activity, and medication usage following detoxification from opioids, relaxation, and supportive therapy.[25] Headache studies have also reported improvement in symptoms by withdrawing the use of opioids, a phenomenon known as "drug-induced headaches."[26,27]

There are numerous reports, many from multidisciplinary pain management programs, that describe poor outcomes in the use of opioids for noncancer pain. These reports point out problems with aberrant drug behaviors, physical impairment, and failure to achieve relief of pain symptoms.[28–30] Why multidisciplinary pain management programs have had, in general, the most negative results with opioids in chronic nonmalignant pain may relate to a subset of patients that are referred to these programs. These cases are, arguably, more complex and refractory to treatment. Many of these patients have significant psychological comorbidity and/or difficult social issues. Depression, anxiety syndromes, and personality disorders are not uncommon, nor is a history or current problem with substance abuse or aberrant drug-related behaviors.

Given the great disparity of outcomes in the literature, it is not surprising that physicians are markedly divided about the appropriateness of opioids for nonmalignant pain. The degree of divergence in these studies and reports is probably best explained by the variations inherent in these patient groups. Pain patients, in particular, represent, as stated by Turk,[5] "a complex amalgam of biomedical, psychosocial ,and behavioral factors." Within a cohort of pain patients there resides a wide variety of medical and psychological disease processes. In addition, the drugs that are being tested are not uniform; these reports involve different opioids and numerous preparations at varying dosages. As previously mentioned, study design is poor with disparate follow-up times and much opportunity for observer bias. There is a tremendous need for well-conducted trials, with valid methodologies, well-defined disease processes, therapeutic endpoints, and agreement as to what constitutes a "long-term" follow-up time.

PHYSICIAN ATTITUDES AND BELIEFS IN PRESCRIBING OPIOIDS

American Pain Society Survey

The American Pain Society (APS) survey was constructed to learn more about what pain specialists think about opioids in the treatment of chronic pain.[31] It consisted of a one-page questionnaire broken down into several sections. The first part profiled the respondents with questions about time in practice and medical specialty. Other questions referred to goals of treatment, use of opi-

TABLE 59-1 **Results of the American Pain Society Survey**

1. Reported professional experience in pain management
   Ranged from 1–35 years (mean 12.3)
2. >65% of the respondents' practice consisted of non-cancer chronic pain patients
3. Average number of patients on chronic opioids per respondent was 23 (13% claimed none on opioids)
4. General agreement that opioids are underutilized in the treatment of chronic pain
5. Addiction is overemphasized but expressed concerns of tolerance and dependence
6. Rejected the notion that fear of regulatory pressure had a significant impact on their prescribing practices
7. Strong agreement that primary goal of treatment is functional improvement with improvement in symptoms less important
8. Many physicians expressed that patients do not develop significant untoward effects such as addiction, physical dependence, or tolerance[24]

oids within their practices, effect of regulatory pressure, and issues relating to tolerance, dependence, and addiction. Only 100 responses, 12% of the APS membership, were received, but within that group there was a good deal of agreement on some salient issues. First, most surveyed stated that they did treat at least some patients with chronic pain with opioids, but there were reservations expressed about this practice. Second, there was consensus that opioids are underutilized, and that fear of addiction is overemphasized, but there was concern expressed about dependence and tolerance. Third, there was strong agreement that the primary goal of therapy should be functional improvement (Table 59-1).

National Physician Survey

Two years following the publication of the APS survey, Turk et al presented the results of the National Physician Survey (NPS) in which some 7000 physicians from 7 different specialties were randomly sampled (Table 59-2). The specialties represented were family practice, internal medicine, neurology, neurosurgery, orthopedic surgery, physical medicine, and rehabilitation and rheumatology. To make the survey as representative as possible, physicians in each of the above specialties were selected from two states each out of 5 national regions (Northeast, Midwest, Southeast, Southwest, and Pacific). The questionnaire covered information concerning training, nature of practice, prescriptions for long-term opioids, concerns with prescribing such drugs, and questions about regulatory pressure.[32] A summary of the data collected is presented in Table 59-2. Although Turk reminds us that, as survey data, this information must be interpreted cautiously, there are some important similarities in the responses to these questionnaires. Pain specialists and nonpain specialists agree that improvement in function and symptomatic relief are distinct goals, and that relief of symptoms alone is not adequate justification for the use of opioids in chronic pain (surgeons were most likely to agree, and rheumatologists least likely to agree). Another important area of concurrence is that a majority of physicians will prescribe opioids for a select group of chronic pain patients. Clearly, however, physicians in the NPS do not *frequently* prescribe opioids for chronic pain. Given the large number of physicians surveyed, the overall number of patients in the category of chronic-pain-treated-with-opioids is very large, on a national basis, but the vast majority is not reported on. Of the group as a whole, we have little information.

On the question of whether regulatory pressure affects prescribing practices, here again there was agreement between the two surveys, with each group expressing that they did not feel affected by it one way or the other, although in the NPS surgeons were significantly more concerned about regulatory pressure than general practitioners. Interestingly, those physicians from states with multiple-copy prescription programs in place indicated that regulatory pressure was less of an effect than did physicians from states where no such program existed. This information is contrary to other reports in the literature (See section, Introduction), and explanations for this have been advanced.[5]

Taken together, the available data suggest that for some patients, and perhaps for groups of patients with chronic nonmalignant pain, long-term opioid therapy may confer therapeutic efficacy without negative effects such as aberrant use patterns and side effects.

TABLE 59-2 **The National Physician Survey**

1. Mean number of years practicing:	16 years
2. Number of patients with chronic pain the average respondent sees on a weekly basis:	18
3. Medical specialties grouped together due to similar reporting:	Internists and Family Practitioners Orthopedists and Neurosurgeons Neurologists and Psychiatrists Rheumatologists (kept separate)
4. Reported frequency with which various groups prescribe opioids:	Rheumatologists prescribe significantly more frequently; general practitioners second most frequent; Midwest physicians most conservative with long-term opioids
5. Views regarding negative effects (dependence tolerance, addiction)	Surgeons most concerned; rheumatologists least concerned

GUIDING PRINCIPLES IN THE USE OF OPIOIDS FOR CHRONIC PAIN

The effective use of opioids for chronic nonmalignant pain is predicated on the reduction of symptoms (pain) and functional restoration. The latter is a compilation of indices that include improved physical capacity (frequently assessed as the ability to return to work), improved psychological functioning and social interaction, as well as decreased utilization of health care resources. Presumably, if a patient has less pain, then functional status should improve as well (it is a given that most patients with chronic pain have varying degrees of dysfunction). This, however, is frequently not seen, and it raises the question, is pain relief in the absence of improved function adequate justification for long-term opioid therapy? Certainly there are individual patients for whom this may be the case; however, it is the ability of opioids to impact positively on functional restoration that leads many pain specialists to support their use in chronic pain.[14,19,28,29,33–40] Another way of looking at this is considering the chronic pain patient in whom opioid therapy does not impart pain reduction, but in whom function is improved. While this is not a common scenario, it is observed, and most clinicians would agree that here the opioid is demonstrating efficacy.

The usefulness of making functional restoration the priority of treatment resides in its shifting of responsibility for improvement from the physician back to the patient. Rather than focusing on the relief of symptoms, a passive process, the emphasis is placed on the enhanced capacity that allows for a more collaborative effort. The use of opioids becomes contingent on the patient's involvement with his care and is positively associated with graded functional improvements. Restoration of function provides more quantifiable and tangible results acting to positively reinforce and encourage further strides. Where appropriate, patients should be expected to reenter the workforce as soon as possible and perform at a level commensurate with their abilities. Some patients may not be able to return to their previous positions for a period of time, or not at all in some cases, and may benefit from retraining if available. Employment has been shown to correlate significantly with improved outcomes in patients with chronic pain,[41] and it is utilized as a functional endpoint in many studies evaluating efficacy of therapy in chronic pain. In the back pain literature, low ratings for job satisfaction were found to portend poorer outcomes, but in work where patients are able to derive a measure of satisfaction and a sense of productivity, the dividends are probably substantial.

There are conflicting data on the use of opioids and functional restoration. Some have shown that improved function actually follows withdrawal of opioids, whereas other patients make progress in rehabilitation because of the pain relief that is afforded them by opioids. Such contrary data again suggests the effect of heterogeneous patient populations and the need for standardized trials. In any case, opioids may assist in making functional restoration a more attainable goal of treatment. Nevertheless, patients with persistent pain and/or dysfunction despite well-conducted opioid trials should give the physician pause, and perhaps the patient should instead be considered for a trial of opioid taper and discontinuation. Another approach commonly utilized in more difficult cases involves a formalized agreement with the patient that continued treatment with opioids be contingent on participation in a rehabilitation program in which the patient's progress can be closely monitored.

While the techniques of opioid treatment are beyond the scope of this chapter, it should be appreciated that opioid drug trials are conducted in essentially the same way as other pharmacological trails. An opioid is introduced at low dose and titrated up until either efficacy or side effects are noted. The endpoint is an optimal balance between analgesia and improved function versus side effects. Initial doses depend mostly on whether the patient is opioid-naïve, but consideration of high-dose therapy or dose limitations is a relative issue and really depends on a patient's ability to tolerate a particular opioid.

Opioid Responsiveness

There is tremendous variation between patients and pain syndromes in the ability to achieve maximum analgesia prior to the development of dose-limiting toxicity. This variability has been coined *opioid responsiveness* and is a more specific term than *efficacy*. Portenoy states: "Opioid responsiveness indicates the probability that 'adequate' analgesia (that is, satisfactory relief without intolerable and unmanageable side effects) can be attained during dose titration."[42] Factors related to opioid responsiveness break down into three categories (Table 59-3).

The mechanism of pain is commonly observed to relate to opioid responsiveness. Bruera et al[43] has identified neuropathic pain and the presence of incident pain in cancer patients to portend inadequate analgesia. This has been confirmed by other investigators,[44,45] though more recently the former has undergone a reappraisal due to a number of reports that show response in neuropathically mediated pain.[46–48] At this time there is no evidence for opioid *nonresponsiveness* of a particular pathophysiologic pain mechanism; only that a mechanism may be somewhat predictive of degree of effect (i.e., nociceptive pain is more responsive to opioids than is neuropathic pain). Moreover, there is no clinical predictor of uniform opioid resistance that would provide reason to forgo drug trials with opioids altogether. Even the case of failure to some opioids does not necessarily imply failure with others.[42,49]

TABLE 59-3 **Factors Postulated to Contribute to Opioid Responsiveness**

Patient-Related Factors
Age
Gender
Psychological distress
Prior opioid exposure (duration and recent consumption)
Existence of cognitive impairment and other factors predisposing to opioid side effects
History of psychological dependence/addiction
Genetic factors (?)
Pain-Related Factors
Usual intensity
Existence of breakthrough pain
Rapid tempo of pain escalation
Predominant mechanism
Drug Selective Effects

Tolerance to Opioids

The phenomenon of tolerance refers to a reduction in effect of a drug with continued exposure, or the need for increasing amounts of the drug to maintain a given level of effect. Tolerance can be demonstrated in laboratory animals and humans, and explanations of its mechanistic basis have been advanced.[42(p258)] It must be borne in mind, however, that while tolerance may cause dose escalation (which is due to exposure of the drug itself), not all dose escalations, and in fact few, are due to the phenomenon of tolerance.[19,33,35] There is a significant body of literature that demonstrates constancy of dose over time in the face of a stable disease process. This being said, it follows that dose escalation should be thought of as a finding and should prompt an appropriate workup for disease progression or a change in psychological status.[3,50] Despite the widely held belief that the use of opioid drugs will inevitably lead to tolerance and compromise therapy, this has not been shown to be the case, and should not be used to justify avoidance of opioid therapy.

ADVERSE EFFECTS OF OPIOIDS

Toxicity

Studies of the long-term effects of opioids reveal no cumulative organ toxicity in patients on methadone maintenance.[51] There is, however, evidence from animal studies that opioids may be involved in an attenuating effect of the immune system.[52] Further studies are needed to determine what significance, if any, this places on the use of opioids for chronic nonmalignant pain.

Side Effects

A variety of side effects commonly occur in patients starting opioid therapy, although some frequently resolve with time. Those side effects that become persistent, such as constipation, nausea and vomiting, sedation, and cognitive dysfunction, may limit the use of adequate dosages for symptom and function improvement and thus render the treatment useless. These persistent side effects occur less frequently but may require trying different opioids or treating the side effects themselves. Constipation is the most common persistent side effect, and is probably best dealt with prophylactically. Patients should be advised about this when commencing treatment and a bowel regimen should be recommended at that time. They should also be advised on how to step up this regimen if constipation remains a problem.

Sedation commonly resolves spontaneously, and early on in treatment patients should be encouraged and reassured about this. Persistent sedation, however, can limit therapy and should be handled by changing dose and/or timing of administration (such as a smaller dose given more frequently), or substituting the present drug for a different opioid. When these measures fail, treating the sedation directly with a psychostimulant, such as methylphenidate or dextroamphetamine, is an option and has been used successfully within the cancer population. Patients that experience cognitive impairment on a persistent basis find it rather distressing. This mental clouding thereby compromises the utility of opioids unless the previous interventions, that is, dose and drug changes, bring about resolution. Fortunately, reports of persistent alterations in cognition are not commonly observed. Whether it is more prominent in subtler forms is a matter of conflicting data. Cognitive impairment surveys from multidisciplinary pain management programs[29,33] and methadone maintenance treatment programs[53] suggest that it is, but a contradictory view is offered by other data on methadone patients.[54] Many of these studies are difficult to interpret, some with poor controls for other factors that could lead to difficulty with cognition, such as poor medical condition and coadministration of other psychotropes. Further studies are needed to address this issue. For the time being, patients on long-term opioid therapy should be carefully assessed at regular intervals for cognitive impairment. If it is noted, it should be addressed, particularly in patients who need to function at a high level. Activities such as driving or working in a hazardous environment may need to be avoided until their impairment can be worked out. The literature, however, is somewhat reassuring concerning the safety of drivers who use long-term opioids. There is evidence that the driving records of these individuals are not different from age-matched controls.[55] Patients also need to know about the cumulative effects of other central nervous system depressants.

Dependence

The terms *addiction* and *dependence* are frequently used interchangeable both by health care professionals and the layman. This is particularly unfortunate in that the word addiction is strongly pejorative with the implication of psychosocial dysfunction. In contrast, physical dependence is merely a physiologic phenomenon characterized by symptoms of withdrawal (the abstinence syndrome) following abrupt discontinuation or rapid dose reduction of a μ agonist or the administration of a μ antagonist in sufficient dose to a person who has been using opioids.[56] This effect may be observed in anyone who has been using opioids repeatedly over several days, and it is an accepted risk of opioid therapy. Nevertheless, there is ample evidence that rapid dose reductions are well tolerated in patients.[36] (Moreover, there is no evidence at this time that significant physical morbidity occurs from abstinence resulting from medically indicated discontinuation of opioids.)[42] As to the question of psychological morbidity associated with abstinence, here, too, there has been no systematic evaluation, although it is commonly observed that just the possibility of dependence is enough to frighten patients away from the use of opioids. Others exhibit fear and anxiety over the prospect of running out of medication unexpectedly, while those who have actually experienced the symptoms of withdrawal relate it as a variably negative experience but do not describe it in especially traumatic terms. Schofferman describes an effect he refers to as "the pain-opioid downhill spiral.[40] This describes a scenario in which iatrogenic opioid dependence may ultimately lead to affective and neuropsychological changes along with increasing disability and subtle symptoms of abstinence. It is theorized that patients may develop a conditioned response to the abstinence that perpetuates pain symptoms and the use of opioids, and leads to aberrant drug-related behaviors. As mentioned earlier in the chapter, there are reports of patients who make functional improvement following withdrawal of opioids. Thus, if it appears that such a situation is operant, the clinician needs to carefully assess the patient and may elect to discontinue opioids during a trial period.

Addiction

The fear of addiction is the fundamental issue that drives the controversy surrounding opioid use for chronic pain. Even the definition of addiction has promoted debate in recent years owing to the incorporation of physical dependence within the definition of addiction. Given that dependence may be expected to occur with chronic opioid use in the pain population, any definition of addiction that includes physical dependence as a characteristic cannot be applied. The term addiction does not appear within the psychiatric lexicon, and the *Diagnostic and Statistical Manual of Mental Disorders*, 4th ed. (DSM-IV) uses *substance-dependence* and *substance abuse* (Table 59-4).

The most suitable definition of addiction that appears within the literature incorporates three concepts: (1) loss of control over the drug use, (2) compulsive drug use, and (3) continued use despite harm. Just how these components manifest within clinical practice can vary greatly from findings that are difficult to interpret and to behaviors that are grossly dangerous and illegal (Table 59-5). Identifying an action that is clearly associated with addiction would be straightforward in the case of a patient who intravenously injects an oral opioid preparation or who forges prescriptions, but in many cases the signs are considerably more subtle. Such is the case of a single, or very occasional, loss of a prescription, obtaining drugs from another source, or demonstrated lack of compliance with a dose regimen. Activities of this sort are not a clear indication of addiction and are not reason to withdraw therapy, but they should place the physician on alert and may suggest the need for a more structured approach. The physicians' reaction to aberrant drug-related behaviors should be commensurate with the behavior. Overreacting to a perceived problem is as inappropriate as ignoring it. Consider the patient who is reacting to a great deal of unrelieved pain. In such a case the patient may well engage in behaviors that appear suspicious but in actuality reflect attempts to relieve their distress. This is the phenomenon of *pseudoaddiction,*[57] and it is distinguished from true addiction by the resolution of the aberrant behaviors with adequate treatment of symptoms. *Therapeutic dependence* is a term that has been coined to describe the behavior of a patient who administers medication for a needed therapeutic outcome and displays variable amounts of drug-seeking behavior (fear, anxiety) at the prospect of not receiving that medication. Here, as in pseudoaddiction, the behavior is appropriate. These phenomena are part of a differential diagnosis for aberrant drug-related behaviors (Table 59-6).

TABLE 59-4 **Definition of Substance Dependence and Substance Abuse from DSM IV**

Substance dependence

A maladaptive pattern of substance abuse, leading to clinically significant impairment or distress, as manifested by three or more of the following occurring at any time in the same 12-month period.

A. Tolerance, as defined by either of the following:
   1. A need for markedly increased amounts of substance to achieve intoxication or desired effect.
   2. Markedly diminished effect with continued use of the same amount of the substance.
B. Withdrawal, as manifested by either of the following:
   1. The characteristic withdrawal syndrome for the substance
   2. The same (or close related) substance is taken to relieve or avoid withdrawal symptoms
C. The substance is often taken in larger amounts or over a longer period than was intended
D. There is a persistent desire or unsuccessful efforts to cut down or control substance use.
E. A great deal of time is spent in activities necessary to obtain the substance (e.g. visiting multiple doctors or driving long distances), use the substance, (e.g. chain smoking), or recover from its effects.
F. Important social, occasional, or recreational activities are given up or reduced because of substance use.
G. The substance use is continued despite knowledge of having a persistent or recurrent physical or psychological problem that is likely to have been caused or exacerbated by the substance (e.g. current cocaine use despite recognition of cocaine-induced depression, or continued drinking despite recognition that an ulcer was made worse by alcohol consumption).

Substance abuse

A maladaptive pattern of substance abuse leading to clinically significant impairment or distress, as manifested by one (or more) of the following, occurring within a 12-month period.

A. Recurrent substance abuse resulting in a failure to fulfill major role obligations at work school or home, (e.g. repeated absences or poor work performance related to substance use; substance related absences; suspensions or expulsions from school; neglect of children or household).
B. Recurrent substance use in situations in which it is physically hazardous (e.g. driving an automobile or operating a machine when impaired by substance use).
C. Recurrent substance-related legal problems (e.g. arrests for substance-related disorderly conduct).
D. Continued substance use despite having persistent or recurrent social or interpersonal problems caused or exacerbated by the effects of the substance (e.g., arguments with spouse about consequences of intoxication, physical fights).
E. The symptoms have never met the criteria for Substance Dependence for this class of substance.

Reprinted with permission from American Psychiatric Association, Diagnostic and Statistical Manual for Mental Disorders. 4th ed. Washington: APA Press, 1994

Reacting to aberrant drug-related behavior necessitates a measured response on the part of the physician to what is being observed. However, distinguishing between addiction, pseudoaddiction, and other psychiatric diagnoses that may account for the behavior can be quite complex. As mentioned earlier in this chapter, pain, whether as a chronic disease process or a symptom of a terminal illness, is a complex and inextricable interplay of physiologic and psychological factors. The patient with significant pain symptoms rarely presents without numerous associated findings such as anxiety, depression, loneliness, isolation, fear, work-related and economic issues, and problems related to relationships with friends and loved ones. In the effort to mitigate the risks associated with use of long-term opioids, it is the responsibility of the physician to identify and attend to psychological comorbidity that may complicate treatment, and to correctly interpret aberrant drug-related behaviors as they occur. This becomes all the more challenging as one takes into account disease-related variables and sociocultural norms. For example, what is the significance of a AIDS patient with herpes zoster who repeatedly dose escalates on his own despite instruction not to? Or the patient with severe pain from stage I complex regional pain syndrome who is out of work, appears depressed, and uses additional opioids to help with sleep? What is the appropriate response to a patient who admits to the use of "a drink or two" while on opioids or "with my medications"? The immediate goal is to limit the risk to the patient while attempting to understand the significance of the behavior. This may become apparent only over time, and for the moment the physician may need to implement measures that allow for more control. This may involve more rigid dosing or smaller prescriptions with more frequent follow-up visits, or perhaps there is a need for involving other family members or friends, urine toxicology screening, or consultation with a psychiatrist or an addiction specialist. Clearly, an indication for immediate intervention must always be a consideration in patients who are engaged in particularly dangerous activities or who present with risk of suicide or harm to others. Unfortunately, with regard to true addiction, there are no predictors that have been experimentally validated, and instead the clinician must rely on empirical data and judgement for guidance.

TABLE 59-5 **Spectrum of Aberrant Drug-Related Behaviors That Raise Concern About the Potential for Addiction**

More suggestive of addiction
- Selling prescription drugs
- Prescription forgery
- Stealing or "borrowing" drugs from others
- Injecting oral formulations
- Obtaining prescription drugs from non-medical sources
- Concurrent abuse of alcohol or illicit drugs
- Repeated dose escalation or similar noncompliance despite multiple warnings
- Repeated visits to other clinicians or emergency rooms without informing prescriber
- Drug-related deterioration in function at work, in the family, or socially
- Repeated resistance to changes in therapy despite evidence of adverse drug effects

Less suggestive of addiction
- Aggressive complaining about the need for more drug
- Drug hoarding during periods of reduced symptoms
- Requesting specific drugs
- Openly acquiring similar drugs from other medical sources
- Occasional unsanctioned dose escalation or other noncompliance
- Unapproved use of the drug to treat another symptom
- Reporting psychic effects not intended by the clinician
- Resistance to a change in therapy associated with "tolerable" adverse effects with expressions of anxiety related to the return of severe symptoms

TABLE 59-6 **Differential Diagnosis for Aberrant Drug-Related Behaviors**

Addiction

Pseudoaddiction

Psychiatric disorders associated with impulsive or aberrant drug taking

Personality disorders, including borderline and psychopathic personality disorders

Depressive disorders

Anxiety disorders

Encephalopathy with confusion about appropriate therapeutic regimen

Criminal intent

Reprinted with permission from Passik SD, Portenoy RK: Substance abuse issues in palliative care, in Berger A, Portenoy RK, Weissman D (eds): *Supportive Oncology.* Philadelphia, Lippincott-Raven, 1998; p519.

The Risk of Addiction

The true risk of addiction to patients who use opioids over the long term is unknown, but given the great numbers of patients who might be candidates for trials of chronic opioid therapy, even a small risk is significant. Some of the early literature on the subject[58–60] reported high rates of addiction stemming from prescriptions medications and also suggested that just exposure to opioids could trigger addiction in an individual.[42(p.256)] That the risk is substantive is largely backed up by data from multidisciplinary pain management programs of the 1980s, which show high rates of drug abuse (ranging from 3.2% to 33%) and aberrant drug-related behavior.[28,34,36] As discussed earlier, however, results based on patients referred to these centers may not be generalizable to other pain populations. In stark contrast to these data are other reports that show negligible addiction rates in large patient groups. For example, the Boston Collaborative Drug Surveillance Project[61] found only 4 cases of addiction in nearly 12,000 cases of hospitalized patients who did not have histories of addiction and had at least one dose of opioid. Perry and Heidrich reported on 10,000 patients treated with opioids for debridement in burn units and found no resulting cases of drug addiction.[62] Here, too, one must exercise caution in the interpretation of these results. There are important differences between the prescribing of opioids for acute pain or intermittent dosing and long-term opioid administration. Nevertheless, these reports offer an alternative view and suggest that, in patients without histories of opioid abuse and addiction, the mere exposure to opioids does not condemn significant numbers of them to addiction.

Empirical observation suggests differences in the way individuals respond to opioids, predisposing some to increased risk of addiction. It is not clear precisely what the basis of these differences are—that is, physiologic, psychological, social—or what the relative contributions of environmental, situational, and inheritable factors are. It has been noted, however, that there are some striking differences concerning exposure to opioids between drug-addicted persons and the pain population. For example, patients in pain management programs are usually withdrawn from opioids easily in contrast to the opioid addicted that tend to experience intense drug cravings.[42] There are also disparities in the mood alterations imparted by opioids; the drug addicted report euphoric effects upon exposure to opioids, in contrast to patients from the pain population who generally report no psychotropic effect or the presence of dysphoria.[63,64] The existence of individuals who use opioids and other addictive drugs on an occasional and recreational basis for long periods without developing the stigmata of drug addiction support the concept of a population that is predisposed. Robins et al performed a follow-up study of servicemen returning from Vietnam who had become drug addicted while serving in the military and found that most had given up the use of narcotics before returning home to the United States or were weaned successfully during a short period of detoxification. At the 1-year follow-up there was a sustained 95% remission rate.[65]

Taken together these data suggest that the risk of addiction may well be represented by more than just a drug's inherent properties. An individual's risk is more likely some combination of predisposing characteristics, psychological, and physiologic and social factors either inherited, acquired, or both. The collective impression, from the above data and from a large clinical experience, is that the risk of inducing iatrogenic addiction in an individual with no prior history of substance abuse is quite low. It is not zero, however, and, as previously mentioned, given the vast number of patients comprising the pain population, there will be cases of addiction that must be identified and attended to.

PATIENT SELECTION

There are no validated negative predictors that clinicians may use to exclude patients from opioid trials (patients with entirely psychological disorders are an exception), though there are characteristics that may point to who the best and poorest candidates are. A relative contraindication for opioid therapy applies to patients with histories of substance abuse and addiction. But here, too, these patients may be stratified on the basis of their current state of sobriety and clean time. For patients who are currently active in their addiction or only recently in recovery, the use of opioids and other narcotics cannot be justified if for any reason other than the patient's safety (an exception to this point would be patients with terminal illnesses). However, there is some experience with patients in stable methadone maintenance programs and with those who enjoy more substantive recovery, and the impression is that some of these patients may be managed in the short term with opioids. Stable recovery is a qualitative concept based on many factors (Table 59-7); however, none can guarantee that recidivism will not occur, and for this reason some physicians wholly proscribe long-term administered opioids as a treatment option. Other physicians will consider opioids if they find the patient is in a solid program of recovery, or if the history is quite remote or limited. Moreover, many individuals in recovery have strong feelings one way or the other about the legitimate medical use of opioids. For those willing to undergo a trial, counseling about the risks must occur prior to the initiation of therapy, and an enhanced regimen of follow-up and assessment may be in order.

Most individuals who are going to develop substance abuse problems will do so in their earlier years, and thus it can be argued that older patients presenting without histories of addiction are at lower risk. Some also contend that patients with idiopathic pain are poorer candidates than those with a precise organic basis; however this has not been proved. It has been pointed out that patients with idiopathic pain are a heterogeneous group with a higher prevalence of psychiatric comorbidity, and that it is the psychiatric component that predisposes to addiction.[42] Beyond these factors, the patient's home and social situation should be taken into consideration. Although this has not been formally examined, there is a large clinical experience that suggests patients with unstable home and social environments, as well as those with various personality disorders, have tendencies to drug-related problems. If such patients are to participate in opioid trials, psychosocial issues should be attended to initially.

Numerous researchers have published "shopping-list" guidelines for the use of opioids in chronic pain; most of them amounting to good intuitive sense (Table 59-8). They are not, however, in uniform agreement, and none has ever been experimentally validated. Portenoy has pointed out adherence to five provisions in the use of opioids for chronic pain. First, recognition that opioids are prescribed for a defined period, reversible at any time, utilizing dosage adjustments and monitoring side effects and therapeutic endpoints (e.g., symptom relief and functional status). Second, provision for either written or verbal consent during which time patients are informed of risks, side effects, and what is considered unacceptable behavior during the trial. Third, the performance of the trial be based on a working knowledge of applied opioid pharmacology with the goal of a defined titration period leading to stable dosing at which point adequate analgesia is reached and rehabilitative efforts are not compromised. Dose escalations are preceded by comprehensive reassessments of status and are deemed medically appropriate, or in cases where the clinical situation is unclear, additional consultants are called in. Fourth, opioid therapy is carried out within the context of multidisciplinary pain management where opioid therapy is considered complementary to other approaches. Fifth, a clearly defined plan shall be in place to deal with aberrant drug-related behaviors.[42] The clinician should avoid the knee-jerk response to wean and discontinue therapy and instead apply the proper controls to maximize the patient's safety until the situation is clarified.

TABLE 59-7 **Factors Associated with Stable Recovery**

Long period of relapse-free recovery (5 or more years)
Active participation in 12-step and other group self-help programs Alcoholic anonymous, narcotics anonymous, rational recovery
Use of a sponsor in 12-step programs
Stable employment
Stable home environment
No issues of current substance abuse with significant other

TABLE 59-8 **Guidelines for Chronic Opioid Therapy**

Portenoy(42 pp 274-275)

1. Should be considered only after all reasonable attempts at analgesia have failed.
2. A history of substance abuse severs character pathology, and chaotic home environment should be viewed as relative contraindications.
3. A single practitioner should take primary responsibility for treatment.
4. Patients should give informed consent before the start of therapy; points to be covered include recognition of the low risk of true addiction as an outcome, potential for cognitive impairment with the drug along and in combination with sedative/hypnotics, likeliness that physical dependence will occur (abstinence possible with acute discontinuation) and understanding by female patients that children born when the mother is on opioid maintenance therapy will likely be physically dependent at birth.
5. After drug selection, doses should be given on an around-the-clock basis; several weeks should be agreed upon as the period of initial dose titration, and although improvement in function should be continually stressed, all should agree to at least partial analgesia as the appropriate goal of therapy.
6. Failure to achieve at least partial analgesia at relatively low initial doses in the non-tolerant patient raises questions about the potential treatability of the pain syndrome with opioids.
7. Emphasis should be given to attempts to capitalize on improve analgesia by gains in physical and social function; opioid therapy should be considered complimentary to other analgesic and rehabilitative approaches
8. In addition to the daily doses determined initially, patients should be permitted to escalate dose transiently on days of increased pain; two methods are acceptable: (a) Prescription of an additional 4-6 "rescue doses" to be taken as needed during the month; (b) instruction that one or two doses may be taken on any day, but must be followed by an equal reduction of dose on subsequent days.
9. Initially, patients must be seen and drugs prescribed at least monthly. When stable, less frequent visits may be acceptable.
10. Exacerbation of pain not effectively treated by transient, small increases in dose are best managed in the hospital where dose escalation, if appropriate, can be observed closely, and return to baseline doses can be accomplished in a controlled environment.
11. Evidence of drug hoarding, acquisition of drugs from other physicians, uncontrolled dose escalation, or other aberrant behaviors must be carefully assessed. In some cases, tapering and discontinuation of opioid therapy will be necessary. Other patients may appropriately continue therapy within rigid guidelines. Consideration should be given to consultation with an addiction medicine specialist.
12. At each visit, assessment should specifically address: (a) comfort (degree of analgesia), (b) opioid-related side effects, (c) functional status (physical and psychosocial), and (d) existence of aberrant drug-related behaviors.
13. Use of self-report instruments may be helpful but should not be required.
14. Documentation is essential and the medical record should specifically address comfort, function, side effects, and the occurrence of aberrant behaviors repeatedly during the course of therapy.

Merry and colleagues[66]

1. All reasonable treatment modalities have been tried.
2. Instituted in a formalized, planned rational manner
3. Treatment should be well documented and well monitored.
4. Involve patient in decision making
5. Candidates for opioid maintenance therapy should be assessed in a multidisciplinary pain clinic

Schofferman[40]

1. Well-defined structural disease refractory to other treatments
2. Disability consistent with known structural disease
3. Psychological and social factors minimal and appropriate for known structural pathology.
4. No history of addiction

Zenz and colleagues[15]

1. Exhaustion of all therapeutic possibilities with regard to cause
2. Failure of specific therapy for specific pain
3. Exclusion of psychogenic mechanism for the pain
4. Use of surgical or non-surgical procedures
5. Use of non-opioid drugs (including psychoactive drugs when appropriate).

Clark[66]

1. There must be an identifiable organic cause that is responsible for the symptom.
2. Use of opioids must improve rather that reinforce pain behavior
3. Psychosocial complicating factors must be actively sought and managed before or at least simultaneously with the initiation of long-term opioid therapy.
4. Drugs given orally if possible.
5. Drugs prescribed regularly by-the-clock.
6. Longest acting drug should be used
7. Only one doctor prescribes
8. Adjuvants are given when required (NASAIDs, tricyclics, not barbiturates, cocaine or amphetamines).
9. Laxatives taken regularly
10. Emergence of side effects should initiate a search for overuse, additional drug use, change in pathology, affective illness, new psychosocial stressors.
11. Breakthrough pain should alert to change in pathology, depressive illness, psychosocial stressors, or inadequate dosages.

Mendelson and Mendelson[66]

1. Identify cause of pain.
2. Document that non-opioid treatment has been inadequate.
3. Obtain and document in clinical notes valid consent of patient.
4. Initially select a weak opioid combined with a non-opioid analgesic.
5. Use a more potent oral opioid if weaker agent ineffective.
6. Raise daily dosage gradually to achieve a stable maintenance dose that effectively controls the pain.
7. Monitor patient regularly (at least monthly) for sedation, motor function, and side effects.
8. Concurrently use adjuvant mediations and other pain therapies.
9. Avoid benzodiazepines, sedatives, and hypnotics.

Reprinted from 5, p 227–228

USE OF CONSENT AND AGREEMENTS

There is strong agreement that patients engaging in opioid trials should provide informed consent of the potential risks and benefits of therapy. However, the issue of treatment agreements or contracts, written or verbal, is rather controversial. Proponents of written agreements or contracts believe that they protect both the physician and the patient by clarifying the terms of treatment. It has been argued that the contract empowers the patient, giving them a stake in their therapy and encouraging participation. Many variations exist from those that are punitive and restrictive to the more lenient, but as noted by Fishman,[66] there may be legal constraints as to the conditions of a contract between a doctor and a patient in such a situation. The provisions of treatment contracts or agreements may include medication usage, prescription refills, and dose changes. Other areas that may be addressed include the terms of toxicology testing, the requirements for participation in other aspects of treatment, and clarification of action in the case of a contract violation. The risk of pregnancy while consuming opioids must always be addressed.

Those opposed to contracts note that they have the tendency to set up a nontrusting and adversarial relationship from the beginning. They also contended that there is currently no contract that has been validated for use in chronic opioid therapy. None has been correlated with improved outcome. Moreover, just as the agreement specifies certain actions on the part of the patient, so to is the physician required to hold up his end of the agreement. Failure to do so may expose the physician to liability. Some pain specialists utilize contracts only in patients with whom there have already been problems, and others do not use them under any circumstances. This of course does not preclude the use of a verbal agreement between the patient and the doctor, and in fact this is considered quite prudent.

CONCLUSIONS

Recognizing the inadequate treatment of disease-related pain and suffering has been the first major step forward in bringing about much needed change. Progress has been made on the fronts of research, patient care, and education, and indeed the word is out that this aspect of medicine is important and high in priority. The public is becoming aware that much can be done to relieve pain, treat distressing symptoms, and improve quality of life for those with chronic pain and terminal illnesses. Moreover, policy makers are in the process of appraising and revising current regulations pertaining to the treatment of pain, and in particular the use of opioids. Evidence of this is the publication by the U.S. Department of Health and Human Services of Clinical Practice Guidelines for the management of acute pain and cancer pain. This document, endorsed by the American Academy of Pain Medicine and the American Pain Society, acknowledges that narcotic analgesics are an essential part of pain management.[67] Such wording represents an important point of departure for a regulatory agency because it brings opioids into the fold of recognized and necessary treatment for those indications. At this time, however, there is no such consensus statement for the use of opioids in chronic pain. The issue remains controversial for numerous reasons, including a lack of good data, regulatory pressure, and concerns with tolerance, dependence, and addiction. Nonetheless, the bulk of available information suggests that there is a small subset of patients for whom such therapy can be used safely and effectively and without the development of untoward effects. Predicting which patients will realize these benefits is frequently difficult, necessitating that all trials must be conducted in a well-organized and controlled fashion with adherence to established guidelines. Close monitoring and follow-up is essential to detecting problems with side effects and aberrant usage. Patients need to be educated and informed of the potential risks and benefits of therapy, and the goals of treatment should be elaborated from the outset.

As the debate over the use of opioids in chronic nonmalignant pain evolves, there is an ever-greater need to generate sound, scientifically rigorous data. The information that is disseminated to the public, that which we use to educate those in health care, to make clinical decisions, and to write public policy, should be based on such data, and not on stigma, fear, and misconception.

REFERENCES

1. World Health Organization. Cancer pain relief and palliative care. Geneva, Switzerland: World Health Organization, 1990.
2. Moulin DE, Foley KM. Review of a hospital-based pain service. In: Foley KM, Bonica JJ, Ventafridda A,eds. *Advances in Pain Research and Therapy*. Vol 16. New York, NY: Raven, 1990:413–427.
3. Schug SA, Zech D, Grond S, et al. A long-term survey of morphine in cancer patients. *J Pain Symptom Manage* 1992;7:259–266.
4. National Institutes of Health. *Chronic Pain: Hope Through Research*. Bethesda, Md: National Institutes of Health, 1982. Publication 82–2406.
5. Turk DC. Clinicians' attitudes about prolonged use of opioids and the issue of patient heterogeneity. *J Pain Symptom Manage* 1996;11: 218–230.
6. Savage SR. Long-term opioid therapy: assessment of consequences and risks. *J Pain Symptom Manage* 1996;11:274–286.
7. Ventafridda V, Tamburini M, Selmi S, et al. Pain and quality of life assessment in advanced cancer patients. In: Ventafridda V, Van Dam FSAM, Yancik R, Tamburini M, eds. *Assessment of Quality of Life and Cancer Treatment*. Amsterdam, The Netherlands: Excerpta Medica, 1986:183–192.
8. Zenz M, Sorge J. Is the therapeutic use of opioids adversely affected by prejudice and the law? *Rec Results Cancer Res* 1991;121:121–43.
9. Hill CS. Influence of regulatory agencies on the treatment of pain and the standards of medical practice for the use of narcotics. *Pain Digest* 1991;1:7–12.
10. Hill CS. The negative effect of regulatory agencies on adequate pain control. *Prim Care Cancer* 1989;9:47–53.
11. United States Department of Justice, Drug Enforcement Administration. *Multiple Copy Prescription Program Resource Guide*. Washington, DC: Superintendent of Documents, US Government Printing Office, 1987.
12. Jacob TR. Multiplecopy prescription regulation and drug abuse: evidence from the DAWN network. In: Wilford BB,ed. *Balancing the Response to Prescription Drug Abuse*. Chicago, Ill: American Medical Association, 1990:205–217.
13. Joranson DE, Cleeland CS, Weissman DE, et al. Opioids for chronic cancer and non-cancer pain: a survey of state medical board members. *Fed Bull* 1992;4:15–49.
14. Taub A. Opioid analgesics in the treatment of chronic intractable pain of non-neoplastic origin. In: Kitahata LM, Collins D, eds. *Narcotic Analgesics in Anesthesiology*. Baltimore, Md: Williams & Wilkins, 1982:199–208.
15. Zenz M, Strumpf M, Tryba M. Long-term opioid therapy in patients with chronic nonmalignant pain. *J Pain Symptom Manage* 1992;7: 69–77.

16. Arkinstall W, Sandler A, Goughnour B, et al. Efficacy of controlled-release codeine in chronic nonmalignant pain: a randomized, placebo-controlled clinical trial. *Pain* 1995;62:169–178.
17. Moulin DE, Iezzi A, Amireh R, et al. Randomised trial of oral morphine for chronic non-cancer pain. *Lancet* 1996;347:143–147.
18. Portenoy RK. Chronic opioid therapy for nonmalignant pain: from models to practice. *APS J* 1992;1:285–288.
19. Portenoy RK, Foley KM. Chronic use of opioid analgesics in nonmalignant pain: report of 38 cases. *Pain* 198X;25:171–186.
20. Urban BJ, France, FD, Steinberger DL, et al. Long-term use of narcotic-antidepressant medication in the management of phantom limb pain. *Pain* 1986;24:191–197.
21. Tennant FS, Robinson D, Sagherian A. Chronic opioid treatment of intractable nonmalignant pain. *Pain Manage* 1988;Jan/Feb:18–36.
22. Kell MJ, Musselman DL. Methadone prophylaxis of intractable headaches: pain control and serum opioid levels. *AJPM* 1993;3:7–14.
23. Brodner RA, Taub A. Chronic pain exacerbated by long-term narcotic use in patients with nonmalignant disease: clinical syndrome and treatment. *Mt Sinai J Med* 1978;45:233–237.
24. Terman GW, Loeser JD. A case of opiate-insensitive pain: malignant treatment of benign pain. *Clin J Pain* 1992;8:255–259.
25. Taylor CB, Zlutnick SI, Corley MJ, et al. The effects of detoxification, relaxation and brief supportive therapy in chronic pain. *Pain* 1980;8: 319–329.
26. Blanchard EB, Applebaum KA, Jaccard J, et al. The refractory headache patient. 2. High medication consumption (analgesic rebound) headache. *Behav Res Ther* 1989;27:411–420.
27. Kudrow L. Paradoxical effect of frequent analgesic use. *Adv Neurol* 1982;33:355–341.
28. Ready LB, Sarkis E, Turner JA. Self-reported vs. actual use of medications in chronic pain patients. *Pain* 1982;12:285–294.
29. McNairy SL, Maruta T, Ivnik RJ, et al. Prescription medication dependence and neuropsychologic function. *Pain* 1984;18:169–177.
30. Maruta T, Swanson DW, Finlayson RE. Drug abuse and dependency in patients with chronic pain. *Mayo Clin Proc* 1979;54:241–244.
31. Turk DC, Brody MC. What positions do APS's physician members take on chronic opioid therapy? *APS Bull* 1992;2:1–5.
32. Turk DC, Brody, Okifuji A. Physicians' attitudes and practices regarding long-term prescribing of opioids for non-cancer pain. *Pain* 1994;59:201–208.
33. Maruta T. Prescription drug-induced organic brain syndrome. *Am J Psychiatry* 1978;135:376–377.
34. Turner JA, Calsyn DA, Fordtce WE, et al. Drug utilization pattern in chronic pain patients. *Pain* 1982;12:357–363.
35. France RD, Urban BJ, Keefe FJ, et al. Long-term use of narcotic analgesics in chronic pain. *Soc Sci Med* 1984;19:1379–1382.
36. Buckley FP, Sizemore WA, Charlton JE. Medication management in patients with chronic nonmalignant pain. A review of the use of a drug withdrawal protocol. *Pain* 1986;26:153–166.
37. Brena SF, Sanders SH. Opioids in nonmalignant pain: questions in search of answers. *Clin J Pain* 1991;7:342–345.
38. Chabal C, Jacobson L, Chaney EF, et al. The psychosocial impact of opioid treatment. *APS J* 1992b;1:289–291.
39. Fordyce WE. Opioids, pain and behavioral outcomes. *APS J* 1992;1: 282–284.
40. Schofferman J. Long-term use of opioid analgesics for the treatment of chronic pain of nonmalignant origin. *J Pain Symptom Manage* 1993; 8:279–288.
41. Dworkin RH, Handlin DS, Richlin DM, et al. Unraveling the effects of compensation, litigation, and employment on treatment response in chronic pain. *Pain* 1985;23:49–59.
42. Portenoy RK. Opioid therapy for chronic nonmalignant pain: current status. In: Fields HL, Leibeskind JC,eds. *Pharmacological Approaches to the Treatment of Chronic Pain: New Concepts and Critical Issues.* Seattle, Wash: IASP Press, 1994:256.
43. Bruera E, Macmillan K, Hanson JA, et al. The Edmonton staging system for cancer pain: preliminary report. *Pain* 1989a;37:203–210.
44. Arner S, Myerson BA. Lack of analgesic effect of opioids on neuropathic and idiopathic forms of pain. *Pain* 1988;33:11–23.
45. Kupers RC, Konings H, Adriaensen H, et al. Morphine differentially affects the sensory and affective pain ratings in neurogenic and idiopathic forms of pain. *Pain* 1991;47:5–12.
46. Mercadante S, Maddaloi S, Roccella S, et al. Predictive factors in advanced cancer pain treated only by analgesics. *Pain* 1992;50:151–155.
47. Rowbotham MC, Reisner-Kelly LA, Fields HL. Both intravenous lidocaine and morphine reduce the pain of postherpetic neuralgia. *Neurology* 1991;41:1024–1028.
48. Jadad AR, Carroll D, Glynn CJ, et al. Morphine responsiveness of chronic pain: double-blind randomised crossover study with patient-controlled analgesia. *Lancet* 1992;339:1367–1371.
49. Galer BS, Coyle N, Pasternack, et al. Individual variability in the response to different opioids: report of five cases. *Pain* 1992;49:87–91.
50. Gonzales GR, Elliot KJ, Portenoy RK, et al. The impact of a comprehensive evaluation in the management of cancer pain. *Pain* 1991;47: 141–144.
51. Kreek MJ. Medical complication in methadone patients. *Ann N Y Acad Sci* 1978;311:110–134.
52. Arora PK, Fride E, Petitto J, et al. Morphine-induced immune alterations in vivo. *Cell Immunol* 1990;126:343–353.
53. Rounsaville BH, Novelly RA, Kleber HD, et al. Neuropsychological impairment in opiate addicts: risk factors. *NY Acad Sci* 1981;362: 79–90.
54. Appel PW, Gordon NB. Digit-symbol performance in methadone-treated ex-heroin addicts. *Am J Psychiatry* 1976;133:1337–1340.
55. Gordon NB. Influence of narcotic drugs on highway safety. *Accid Anal Prev* 1976;8:3–7.
56. Martin WR, Jasinski DR. Physiologic parameters of morphine dependence in man—tolerance, early abstinence, protracted abstinence. *J Psychol Res* 1969;7:9–17.
57. Weissman DE, Haddox JD. Opioid pseudoaddiction—an iatrogenic syndrome. *Pain* 1989;36:363–366.
58. Rayport M. Experience in the management of patients medically addicted to narcotics. *JAMA* 1954;156:684–691.
59. Vallaint GE. A 20-year follow-up of New York narcotic addicts. *Arch Gen Psychiatry* 1973;29:237–241.
60. Simpson DD, Savage LJ, Lloyd MR. Follow-up evaluation of treatment of drug abuse during 1969 to 1972. *Arch Gen Psychiatry* 1979; 36:772–780.
61. Porter J, Jick H. Addiction rare in patients treated with narcotics. *N Engl J Med* 1980;302:123.
62. Perry S, Heidrich G. Management of pain during debridement: a survey of US burn units. *Pain* 1982;13:267–280.
63. Jarvik LF, Simpson JH, Guthrie D, et al. Morphine, experimental pain and psychological reactions. *Psychopharmacology* 1981;75:124–131.
64. Jaffe JH. Misinformation: euphoria and addiction. In: Hill, CS, Fields WS, eds. *Advances in Pain Research and Therapy. Drug Treatment of Cancer in a Drug-Oriented Society.* Vol. 11. NewYork, NY:Raven Press, 1989: 163–174.
65. Robins LN, Davis DH, Nurco DN. How permanent was Vietnam drug addiction. *Am J Public Health* 1974;64:38–43.
66. Fishman SM. The opioid contract in the management of chronic pain. Paper presented at: The Third Conference on Pain Management and Chemical Dependency; 1999; New York.
67. Haddox JD, Joranson D, Angarola RT, et al. The use of opioids for the treatment of chronic pain: a consensus statement from the American Academy of Pain Medicine and the American Pain Society, 1997.

CHAPTER 60 COMMON OPIOID-RELATED SIDE EFFECTS

Scott M. Fishman, Joseph Condon, and Mark Holtsman

INTRODUCTION

This chapter discusses the special set of potential opioid-related complications. Objective signs and symptoms of chronic pain are hard to ascertain, whereas opioid use is associated with concrete signs and symptoms that may act as markers for opioid side effects. Most commonly, opioids produce constipation, nausea, vomiting, sedation, and respiratory depression. Any adverse effects from opioids may significantly limit therapy, and some can present with life-threatening consequences. Unfortunately, there are few predictors of which patients will experience which side effects and which particular opioids will produce them. It is sensible to expect side effects and to take preventive action. Since not all opioid-related toxicity can be predicted or prevented, patients should be closely followed with a high level of suspicion. Effective management includes anticipation of adverse effects when possible, use of preventive measures, and choosing the best medication with the optimum method of administration. Clear communication with the patient, family, or nurse to ensure prompt recognition and response to adverse effects is of utmost importance in order to recognize and prevent possible adverse effects of opioid treatment.

CONSTIPATION

Constipation is the most common dose-dependent side effect of opioids. But unlike most other side effects, tolerance does not develop. Thus, constipation can be expected throughout the duration of opioid administration. Preventive therapy with cathartics and adequate fluid intake is a mainstay of therapy and should be offered at the time opioids are started and continued throughout opioid treatment. Stool softeners and bulking agents such as bran or psyllium derivatives alone will be inadequate because opioid-related constipation results from decreased gut motility. Therefore, active stimulating laxatives are effective and passive ones are not.

Severe constipation may respond to oral administration of naloxone, which is an opioid antagonist with specificity to bowel. Administration of oral naloxone has limited systemic bioavailability; however, it has increased concentration and efficacy in the gastrointestinal (GI) tract. Unfortunately, there is uncertainty about the dosing regimen. Opioid withdrawal has been observed when oral naloxone is administered at dosages exceeding 20% of the prevailing 24-hour morphine dose. It is suggested that initial individual oral naloxone doses should not exceed 5 mg. In our institution, we start with 1.6 mg to 2.4 mg taken orally (4 to 6 small ampules) every 4 hours until the first bowel movement, or for five doses. If ineffectual, we may try another series with a higher dose. However, constipation may be caused by factors other than opioids. Oral naloxone only works when the constipation is solely opioid-related.

Since constipation can be mitigated by direct effects of antagonists on the bowel, it is possible that opioids that are delivered without direct bowel contact induce less constipation. There is evidence that certain opioid products that are absorbed without contact to the GI tract, such as transdermal fentanyl, induce less constipation when compared with oral morphine at doses effecting the same degree of pain relief. A significant reduction in the use of laxatives has been reported. In one study of cancer patients, the incidence of constipation was reduced by up to two thirds after switching from oral morphine to transdermal fentanyl. These findings should be viewed with cautious optimism, as published studies to date have not included patients on standardized bowel care regimens. In a study by Donner et al (1996) comparing transdermal fentanyl with sustained-release morphine, the patients receiving transdermal fentanyl had a higher incidence of diarrhea. The authors speculated this occurred because 10% of the patients experienced opiate withdrawal symptoms when converting from sustained-release morphine to transdermal fentanyl. Some patients taking transdermal fentanyl continued to take laxative doses regularly as prescribed when they were previously on morphine, resulting in a sudden increase in defecation. It is unclear whether these findings apply to the other new opioid-delivery systems such as the transmucosal fentanyl system, since these products have some degree of oral absorption.

NAUSEA AND VOMITING

Although nausea and vomiting is a common early side effect of opioids, severe nausea and vomiting caused solely by opioids is rare. Addition of antiemetics or reduction of the opioid dose to the minimal acceptable level of analgesia is usually effective. A change in the route of administration may also alleviate symptoms. Fortunately, tolerance often occurs within several days of administering opioids, at which time antiemetic therapy should be discontinued. While it remains unclear why one opioid should produce nausea and vomiting and another does not, if nausea or vomiting persist, changing to a different equianalgesic opioid may reduce emetic side effects. A history of severe nausea with previous opioid treatment may prompt pretreating with antiemetic therapy. Once antiemetics are given, there is usually no need to discontinue the opioid.

Opioid-induced nausea and vomiting is thought to result from stimulation within the medullary chemoreceptor trigger zone (CTZ), a brainstem center responsible for afferent input to the emetic center. These anatomical areas are rich in neurotransmitter receptors that correspond to antiemetic agents used clinically and thus can guide therapeutic choices. These receptor systems relate to neurotransmitters and drugs such as histamine (H_1) blockers and hydroxyzine, serotonin (5-HT-3) and ondansetron, dopamine (DA-2) and droperidol, or haloperidol, anticholinergics and scopolamine, and cholinergics and low-dose metoclopramide. It is not clear whether benzodiazepine-related antiemetic effects (such as those caused by lorazepam) are caused by direct action on benzodiazepine receptors found in the CTZ or indirect action on anxiety and psychological conditioning. Risk of opioid-related nausea may be increased if a patient is ambulatory, perhaps suggesting vestibular involvement. For patients complaining of nausea associated with movement, promethazine is effective and available for oral, rectal, and parenteral administration. There are many other causes of nausea and vomiting that can concomitantly occur with, but be unrelated to, opioids. These include: chemotherapy (particularly cisplatin), radiation therapy, metastases (particularly brain and gastrointestinal), increased intracranial pressure, ulcer disease, esophagitis, gastritis, electrolyte imbalance, acid-base disorder, uremia, liver disease, infection, pregnancy, fear, or anxiety. Since the single most effective antiemetic is not always predictable, we often choose the agent that offers secondary benefits such as promotility, sedative, antipuritic, and anxiolytic or antipsychotic properties.

SEDATION

Opioid-related sedation is common and can indicate either excess drug dose or even delirium. Opioid-induced sedation is usually temporary, resolving over time as patients accommodate to a new opioid drug, and this side effect typically responds well to dose reduction. It should not be confused with delirium as discussed in more detail in a later section. In those with significant sedation, the opioid dose should be reduced to the minimal level required for adequate analgesia. In some cases where sedation occurs late in treatment, medication or metabolites may be accumulating. If so, either increasing the dose interval or changing to a different agent without active metabolites, such as fentanyl, may reduce sedation. In cases involving sedation, consider other non-opioid causes of sedation (e.g., other sedating drugs, encephalopathy, hypoxia). For unremitting sedation that limits other required therapy, stimulants such as dextroamphetamine or caffeine can reduce sedation until accommodation occurs.

PRURITUS

Pruritus is uncommon with oral opioids but a common side effect of parenterally administered opioids. Pruritus is found in the majority of patients treated with intrathecal and epidural opioids and frequently in those treated with intravenous or intramuscular opioids. Such effects often vary with dose. Usually parenteral opioids produce mild pruritus, but moderate to severe pruritus does occur infrequently. Fortunately, tolerance usually occurs quickly. Opioid-related pruritus is often localized to the face, or less often the perineum, but can become generalized. The mechanism of opioid-induced pruritus is not well understood. Suggested hypotheses include μ-receptor stimulation, 5-hydroxytryptamine-3 receptor stimulation, histamine release, local excitation of posterior horn neurons, and central migration of spinal opioids to "itch centers" in the brain.

Opioid-induced pruritus may respond to a change of opioid agents. Naloxone is effective for opioid-related pruritus from any route of administration, and used at dosages that should not interfere with analgesia (1 μg/kg IVP every 10 minutes as needed: hold for decreased analgesia). Recent studies suggest prophylaxis with nalmefene 15 μg administered intravenously at the end of surgery. It reduces the incidence of itching and nausea associated with intravenous morphine administered by a patient-controlled analgesia (PCA) pump. Antihistamines may be effective for opioid-related pruritus, except when pruritus is due to spinal opioids.

Since non-sedating antihistamines are less effective than sedating antihistamines, the antipruritic efficacy of antihistamine therapy may, in part, be related to sedation. When sedation is to be avoided, recent studies have shown that intravenous ondansetron 8 mg effectively reduces epidural morphine-induced pruritis for 5 to 7 hours. Propofol, in small dosages (1 0 mg intravenous push), is also effective for controlling some cases of pruritus due to spinal opioids. At low doses, adverse effects from propofol should be minimal.

RESPIRATORY DEPRESSION

Depressed respiration is one of the most feared opioid-related side effects. Tolerance to opioid-related respiratory depression occurs early in chronic therapy. Depression of respiratory drive may occur more rapidly when oral or intravenous opioids are combined with epidural or intrathecal opioids and their combined use should be avoided. Prevention of respiratory depression is the key. One can reduce the risk of respiratory depression significantly by looking for factors predisposing a patient to respiratory depression such as increased age, history of sleep apnea, chronic obstructive pulmonary disease, and hepatic dysfunction. For patients requiring opiate analgesics at risk for respiratory depression, one simple way to provide analgesia involves calculating the required opiate dose to decrease pain, dividing the dose by 3, and giving one third of the calculated dose until adequate analgesia or side effects occur. For example, a 60-kg woman getting 0.1 mg/kg morphine intravenously would get 2 mg of intravenous morphine every 15 minutes as needed up to 6 mg, instead of getting all 6 mg of morphine intravenously at one time. Significant acute respiratory depression can be managed with the opiate-receptor antagonist naloxone. Dosages of naloxone for treating respiratory depression are as follows: 0.1 mg intravenous push repeated every 10 to 15 minutes as needed (1/4 of the usual 0.4-mg ampule of naloxone). Although naloxone may provide a brisk response, its duration of action is short and may require frequent dosing or continuous intravenous drip. Particular care must be given to the patient taking prolonged opioids because rapid administration of naloxone can precipitate withdrawal. In special cases, reversal of opioid actions can promote pulmonary edema. This effect is likely the result of reversal of opioid-induced pulmonary vascular smooth muscle relaxation. However, this is unusual unless the patient is predisposed toward pulmonary edema (congestive heart failure, adult respiratory distress syndrome, and so forth).

TOLERANCE

Signs that a patient may be developing tolerance include a fixed dose of opioid, resulting in decreasing analgesia or increasing dosages being required to maintain a stable effect. Just like tolerance to analgesia, tolerance may also occur due to opioid side effects (i.e., nausea, pruritis) developing at different rates for different side effects. Pain in the tolerant patient can usually be treated either by changing the opioid or increasing the dose. A patient who has become tolerant to one opioid drug may respond with ample analgesia to another opioid, suggesting that cross-tolerance between these drugs may be incomplete. Owing to incomplete cross-tolerance, equianalgesic dosages are not applicable in the opioid-tolerant patient. When starting a new opioid agent in a tolerant patient, the recommended starting dose is 50% less than the equianalgesic dose and is titrated to effective analgesia. There is evidence that NMDA-receptor blockade may attenuate tolerance; however, this is not clearly established with clinically relevant drugs. Dextromethorphan has recently been used for such purposes, but at present its effective dose or clinical efficacy are not clear.

OPIOID DEPENDENCE AND WITHDRAWAL

Attempts to avoid dependency may lead to inadequate opioid dosages and undertreatment of pain. Understanding this state can help preserve the effective and humane use of opioids. Physical dependence is a pharmacologic property of opioids, implying that continuous exposure to a drug is necessary to avoid the withdrawal syndrome. Dependence reflects a biochemical adaptation from chronic exposure to opioids. Opioids inhibit cyclic adenosine monophosphate (cAMP). Sudden discontinuation of opioids or administration of an opioid antagonist can induce a rebound disinhibition of cAMP associated with symptoms of withdrawal. Physical dependence may be produced by little opiate exposure and may persist well beyond drug cessation.

Withdrawal usually occurs in a systematic progression. The least severe withdrawal symptoms typically appear earlier than the most severe. Withdrawal begins with increased irritability, restlessness, anxiety, insomnia, yawning, sweating, rhinorrhea, and lacrimation and later progresses to dilated pupils, gooseflesh, tremor, chills, anorexia, muscle cramps, nausea, vomiting, abdominal pain, diarrhea, agitation, fever, tachycardia, and other features of heightened sympathetic activity. Laboratory data may reveal leukocytosis, ketosis, metabolic acidosis or respiratory alkalosis, and electrolyte imbalance.

The withdrawal syndrome may be seen with discontinuation or antagonism of any opioid. However, sudden discontinuation of shorter acting opioids such as morphine or hydromorphone is more likely to produce withdrawal symptoms than longer acting agents such as methadone or transdermally administered fentanyl. Slow, systematic tapering of opioids at a daily rate of 15% to 20% can usually prevent the withdrawal state. Once it occurs, it may be reversed by reintroducing the opioid at dosages of 25% to 40% of the previous daily dose. Weaning bedtime doses last may help avoid sleep disturbances that are often associated with opioid cessation. Physical symptoms of sympathetic hyperactivity may be treated with sympatholytics. Effective sympatholytics include clonidine and beta blockers, although such agents can produce hypotension. Clonidine may produce sedation and its anti-withdrawal effects may be antagonized by tricyclic antidepressants.

When abrupt discontinuation of a chronic opioid is mandatory, clonidine detoxification can effectively blunt objective findings of sympathetic hyperactivity. It remains controversial whether clonidine may increase or mask subjective symptoms of withdrawal such as anxiety, insomnia, and restlessness. Such treatment often is begun at dosages of 10 to 20 μg/kg/day in 3 divided doses with subsequent adjustments to reduce signs of withdrawal while limiting hypotension. Clonidine may be maintained for 4 days for short-acting opioids and for 14 days for long-acting opioids. Tapering of clonidine can then occur over 4 to 6 days. Recently, there is increased interest in rapid opioid detoxification with intravenous naloxone and general anesthesia. Such treatment offers rapid effects but is of unproven long-term value.

DELIRIUM

Delirium is associated with fluctuating mental status and often has features of disorientation and agitation. Opioid-induced delirium is rarely due solely to an opioid and is usually multifactorial. If sedation is a prominent feature, its fluctuating pattern distinguishes it from simple drug-related sedation. Delirium induced by many various factors is thought to have an incidence in hospitalized patients of 25% to 50%, with a mortality rate of 10% to 65%.

Prominent signs of delirium include acute onset, fluctuating course, inattention, disordered thinking or speech, and altered level of consciousness. Level of consciousness is defined as "alert," which corresponds to a normal level of consciousness, "vigilant," which corresponds to a hyperalert level, "lethargy," which corresponds to a drowsy or easily arousable level, "stupor," which corresponds to a difficult to arouse level, and "coma," which corresponds to an unarousable level. The condition may include perceptual disorders such as illusions, hallucinations, sleep disorders, and abnormal psychomotor activity, which may be either increased or decreased. Life-threatening causes of delirium include Wernike's encephalopathy (thiamine deficiency: nystagmus, ophthalmoplegia, ataxia, confusion), hypoxia, hypertensive crisis, hypoperfusion states, anemia or bleeding, electrolyte imbalance (hyponatremia, hypercalcemia, hypokalemia), intracranial bleeding, edema or closed head trauma, meningitis, poisons or other drug toxicities, and withdrawal states such as from benzodiazepines. The list of medications associated with delirium is too long for this brief discussion. Drugs with anticholinergic side effects (such as found in drugs that are often co-prescribed with opioids such as tricyclic antidepressants) are among the drugs that most commonly cause delirium. Another common culprit is the class of benzodiazepine drugs. If opioids are suspected as the cause of delirium, a thorough investigation to rule out other possible causes should nonetheless be undertaken, as opioids are often incorrectly blamed for causing delirium. Treating the symptoms of delirium such as agitation or unpleasant hallucinations require use of neuroleptics. The most appropriate choice of neuroleptics is those with the least anticholinergic side effects, such as intravenous dosages of haldoperidol.

BIBLIOGRAPHY

American Pain Society. Principles of analgesic use in the treatment of acute pain and chronic cancer pain. In: *Clinical Pharmacy*. Vol. 9. 2nd ed. American Pain Society, 1990:601–611.

Borgeat A, Stirnemann H-R. Ondansetron is effective to treat spinal or epidural morphine-induced pruritis. *Anesthesiology* 1999;90:432–436.

Carr DB. Pain. In: Firestone LL, Lebowitz P, Cook C, eds. *Clinical Anesthesia Procedures of the Massachusetts General Hospital*. 3rd ed. Boston, Mass: Little, Brown, 1988:571–585.

Donner B, Zenz M, Tryba M, Stumpf M. Direct conversion from oral morphine to transdermal fentanyl: a multicenter study in patients with cancer pain. *Pain* 1996;64:527–534.

Foley KM. Controversies in cancer pain. *Cancer* 1989;63:2257–2265.

Hyman SH, Cassem NH. Pain. In: *Scientific American Medicine*. New York, NY; Scientific American 1989.

Joshi GP, Duffy L, Chehade J, et al. Effects of prophylactic nalmefene of the incidence of morphine-related side effects in patients receiving intravenous patient-controlled analgesia. *Anesthesiology* 1999;90:1007–1011.

Kendrick WD, Woods AM, Daly MY, et al. Naloxone versus nalbuphine infusion for prophylaxis of epidural morphine-induced pruritis. *Anesth Analg* 1996;82:641–647.

NIH Consensus Development Conference: the integrated approach to the management of pain. *J Pain Symptom Manage* 1987;2:35–41.

Portenoy RK. Chronic opioid therapy in nonmalignant pain. *J Pain Symptom Manage* 1990;5:S46–S62.

Sykes NP. An investigation of the ability of oral naloxone to correct opioid-related constipation in patients with advanced cancer. *Palliat Med* 1996;10:135–144.

Wall PD, Melzack R, eds. *Textbook of Pain*. 2nd ed. New York, NY: Churchill Livingstone, 1988.

Wang JJ, Ho ST, Tzeng Ji. Comparison of intravenous nalbuphine infusion versus naloxone in the prevention of epidural morphine-related side effects. *Reg Anesth Pain Med* 1998;23:479–484.

CHAPTER 61 NONSTEROIDAL ANTI-INFLAMMATORY DRUGS

Lee S. Simon

NONSTEROIDAL ANTI-INFLAMMATORY DRUGS

Nonsteroidal anti-inflammatory drugs (NSAIDs) are anti-inflammatory, analgesic, and antipyretic agents. They are used to reduce pain, decrease stiffness, and improve function in patients with osteoarthritis (OA), rheumatoid arthritis (RA), and other forms of arthritis. They are also used for the treatment of pain including headache, dysmenorrhea, and postoperative pain.[1–3] Whether their effectiveness is solely due to their anti-inflammatory or analgesic effects or other possible mechanisms is not known.[4] There are at least 20 different NSAIDs currently available in the United States (Table 61-1). In addition, cyclooxygenase-2 selective inhibitors (COX-2 inhibitors, e.g., celecoxib, rofecoxib), with similar efficacy but significantly decreased gastrointestinal (GI) and platelet effects, are available.[5–8]

NSAIDs are one of the most commonly used classes of drugs. It has been reported that more than 17,000,000 Americans use these agents on a daily basis for the relief of pain and, at times, swelling related to inflammation.[9] With the aging of the US population, the Centers for Disease Control predict a significant increase in the prevalence of painful degenerative and inflammatory rheumatic conditions and thus an increased use of NSAIDs.[9,10] Approximately 60 million NSAID prescriptions are written each year in the United States; the number for elderly patients exceeds those for younger patients by approximately 3.6-fold.[10] Aspirin, ibuprofen, naproxen, and ketoprofen are also available over the counter. At equipotent doses, the clinical efficacy and tolerability of the various NSAIDs are similar; however, individual responses are highly variable.[1,11,12] It is believed that if a patient fails to respond to one NSAID of one class that it is reasonable to try another NSAID from a different class; however, no one has studied this in a prospective controlled manner.[11,12]

Sodium salicylic acid was discovered in 1763 but more impure forms of salicylates had been used as analgesics and antipyretics throughout the previous century. Once purified and synthesized, the acetyl derivative of salicylate, acetylsalicylic acid (ASA) was found to provide more anti-inflammatory activity than salicylate alone, but at the same time increased the incidence of toxicity, particularly related to the upper GI tract. Phenylbutazone, an indoleacetic acid derivative, was introduced in the early 1950s. This drug was a weak prostaglandin synthase inhibitor, which induced uricosuria, and was rapidly found useful in patients with ankylosing spondylitis and gout. However, owing to concerns related to bone marrow toxicity, particularly in women older than the age of 60, this compound now is rarely prescribed. Indomethacin, another indoleacetic acid derivative, was subsequently developed in the 1960s to substitute for phenylbutazone. It had the potential for significant toxicity as well, and the search for safer (particularly GI safer) and at least equally effective NSAIDs ensued. Other clinical issues have driven the development of newer agents, such as once or twice daily dosing to improve compliance.

MECHANISM OF ACTION

Some of the variability in clinical response may be explained by the spectrum of inhibition of prostaglandin synthesis. Some NSAIDs appear to be potent inhibitors of prostaglandin synthesis, while others more prominently affect other nonprostaglandin-mediated biologic events.[1,2,13–16] Different responses have also been attributed to variations in the enantiomeric state of the drug or its pharmacokinetics and/or pharmacodynamics.[1,2,11,12] Although variability can be explained in part by absorption, distribution, and metabolism, potential differences in mechanism of action must be considered as possibly important to explain observed variable effects.[11,12]

The NSAIDs are primarily anti-inflammatory and analgesic by decreasing production of prostaglandins of the E series.[17] Many of these prostanoic acids are pro-inflammatory, and increase vascular permeability and sensitivity to the release of bradykinins. Decreasing the synthesis of these mediators leads to decreased pain, swelling, and edema in the peripheral tissues. In addition, there is accumulating evidence that central effects of pain modulation may be as important as the effects on the peripheral tissues. The hypothesis is that prostaglandin synthesis is upregulated in the brain with peripheral stimulation of pain particularly associated with inflammation, and those NSAIDs that are more lipophilic penetrate better into the central nervous system (CNS) and inhibit both synthesis of peripheral and central prostaglandins.[18]

NSAIDs have also been shown to inhibit the formation of prostacyclin and thromboxane, resulting in complex effects on vascular permeability and platelet aggregation in peripheral tissues, which undoubtedly contributes to the overall clinical effects of these compounds.

These prostaglandins are derived from polyunsaturated fatty acids that are constituents of all cell membranes. They exist in ester linkage in the glycerols of phospholipids and are converted through multiple enzymatic steps to prostaglandins or leukotrienes first through the action of phospholipase A_2 or phospholipase C.[17] Free arachidonic acid, released by the phospholipase from the fatty acids, acts as a substrate for the PGH synthase complex, which includes both cyclooxygenase (COX) and peroxidase. These enzymes catalyze the conversion of arachidonic acid to the unstable cyclic-endoperoxide intermediates, PGG_2 and PGH_2, which are then converted to the more stable PGE_2 and PGF_2 compounds by specific tissue prostaglandin syntheses. NSAIDs specifically inhibit COX and thereby reduce the conversion of arachidonic acid to PGG_2.

At least two isoforms of the COX enzymes have now been identified. They are products of two different genes yet share 60% homology in the amino acid sequences considered important for catal-

TABLE 61-1 **Nonsteroidal Anti-inflammatory Medications**

Medication	Proprietary (Trade) Name	Usual Daily Dose (Adults)	Serum Half-Life Hours	Approved Use*
Nonselective NSAIDS				
Carboxylic Acid Derivatives				
Aspirin (acetylsalicylic acid)	Multiple	2.4–6 g/24h in 4–5 divided doses	4–15	RA, OA, AS, JCA, ST
Buffered aspirin	Multiple	Same	Same	Same
Enteric-coated salicylates	Multiple	Same	Same	Same
Salsalate	Disalcid	1.5–3.0 g/24h bid	Same	Same
Diflunisal	Dolobid	0.5–1.5 g/24h bid	7–15	Same
Choline magnesium trisalicylate†	Trilisate	1.5–3 g/24h bid-tid		RA, OA, pain, JCA
Proponic Acid Derivatives				
Ibuprofen†	Motrin, Rufen, OTC	OTC: 200–400 mg qid Rx: 400, 600, 800, maximum: 3200 mg	2	RA, OA, JCA
Naproxen†	Naprolan, Anaprox, Naprosyn EC	250, 375, 500 mg bid	13	RA, OA, JCA, ST
Fenoprofen	Nalfon	300–600 mg qid	3	RA, OA
Ketoprofen	Orudis	75 mg tid	2	RA, OA
Flurbiprofen	Ansaid	100 mg bid-tid	3–9	RA, OA
Oxaprozin	Daypro	600–1800 mg/24h	40–50	RA, OA, pain
Tolmetin	Tolectin	400, 600, 800 mg; 800–2400 mg	1	RA, OA, JCA
Acetic Acid Derivatives				
Indomethacin†	Indocin, Indocin SR Indocin SR	25–50 mg tid or qid SR: 75 mg bid; rarely > 150 mg/24h	3–11	RA, OA, G, AS
Tolmetin	See above		1	
Sulindac	Clinoril	150, 200 mg bid to tid	16	RA, OA, AS, ST, G
Diclofenac	Voltaren, Arthrotec	50 tid, 75 mg bid	1–2	RA, OA, AS
Etodolac	Lodine	200–300 mg.bid-tid-qid maximum: 1200 mg	2–4	OA, pain
Ketorolac	Toradol	20–40 mg	2	Pain
Fenamates				
Meclofenamate	Meclomen	50–100 mg tid-qid	2–3	RA, OA
Mefenamic acid	Ponstel	250 mg qid	2	RA, OA
Enolic Acid Derivatives				
Piroxicam	Feldene	10, 20 mg q day	30–86	RA, OA
Phenylbutazone	Butazolidin	100 mg tid up to 600 mg/24h	40–80	Gout, AS
Meloxicam	Mobic	7.5–15 mg	20	OA
Naphthylkanones				
Nabumetone	Relafen	500 mg bid up to 1500 mg/24h	19–30	RA, OA
COX-2 Selective NSAIDS				
Celecoxib	Celebrex	100, 200 mg bid, 200 mg qd	11	RA, OA OA
Rofecoxib†	VIOXX	12.5, 25 mg qd 50 mg qd	17	OA Acute pain

*FDA approved.

RA = rheumatoid arthritis; OA = osteoarthritis; AS = ankylosing spondylitis; G = gout; JCA = juvenile chronic arthritis; ST = soft tissue injury.

†Available in liquid form.

ysis of arachidonic acid. The differences are primarily in their regulation and expression.[19,20] COX-1, or prostaglandin synthase H_1 (PGHS-1), regulates normal cellular (physiologic) processes and is stimulated by hormones or growth factors. It is constitutively expressed in most tissues, and is inhibited by all NSAIDs to varying degrees depending on the applied experimental model system used to measure drug effects.[21–24] It has an important role in maintaining the integrity of the gastric and duodenal mucosa, and many of the toxic effects of the NSAIDs on the GI tract are attributed to its inhibition.[25–30] It has been described as a "housekeeping enzyme."

The other isoform, prostaglandin synthase H_2 or PGHS-2 (or COX-2) is an inducible enzyme and is usually undetectable in most tissues. Its expression is increased during states of inflammation or experimentally in response to mitogenic stimuli. In monocyte/macrophage systems, endotoxin stimulates COX-2 expression; in fibroblast studies various growth factors, phorbol esters, and interleukin-1 do so.[19,31] This isoform is also constitutively expressed in the brain, specifically the cortex and hippocampus, in the female reproductive tract, the male vas deferens, in bone, and at least in some models, in human kidney.[19,20] In the brain it appears that COX-2 is upregulated with increased inflammation-induced pain inpulses; thus, the inhibition of COX-2 in the brain is thought to be an important modulator of pain in states of inflammation.[18] The expression of COX-2 is inhibited by glucocorticoids.[19,20,31] COX-2 is also inhibited by all of the currently available NSAIDs to a greater or lesser degree, and its inhibition leads to a decrease in those prostanoid products associated with increased pain and swelling.[20–23] Therefore, we have observed the effects of prolonged inhibition of COX-2 for the last 25 years as we have used traditional nonselective NSAIDs.

The *in vitro* systems used to define the actions of the available NSAIDs are based on using cell-free systems, pure enzyme, or whole cells systems.[21] Each drug studied to date has demonstrated different measurable effects within each system. As an example, it appears that nonacetylated salicylates inhibit the activity of COX-1 and COX-2 in whole cell systems but are not active against either COX-1 or COX-2 in recombinant enzyme or cell membrane systems. This suggests that salicylates act early in the arachidonic acid cascade similar to glucocorticoids, perhaps by inhibiting enzyme expression rather than direct inhibition of cyclooxygenase.

Recent accumulated evidence has demonstrated that several NSAIDs are selective and inhibit the COX-2 enzyme more so than the COX-1 enzyme. For example, *in vitro* effects of etodolac and meloxicam demonstrate primary inhibition of COX-2 compared with COX-1, at low doses.[32,33] However, at higher approved therapeutic doses this effect appears to be mitigated, as both COX-1 and COX-2 are inhibited to variable degrees. Very potent, specific COX-2 inhibitors that have no measurable effect on COX-1 mediated events at therapeutic doses are now available: celcoxib and rofecoxib.[34] Both of these COX-2 specific inhibitors (or COX-1 sparing drugs) have been shown as effective at inhibiting osteoarthritis pain, dental pain, and the pain and inflammation associated with rheumatoid arthritis as naproxen at 500 mg twice daily, ibuprofen 800 mg three times daily, and diclofenac 75 mg twice daily, without endoscopic evidence of gastroduodenal damage and without affecting platelet aggregation.[5–8,34–36] Unfortunately, because of the design of the randomized controlled trials, many of the important questions regarding the renal effects of the specific COX-2 inhibitors continue to remain unanswered.[19,20]

Other possible mechanisms of action that may explain the clinical effects of the NSAIDs include several physicochemical properties of these drugs. NSAIDs are variably lipophilic and become incorporated in the lipid bilayer of cell membranes and thereby may interrupt protein-protein interactions important for signal transduction.[13,14] For example, stimulus response coupling, which is critical for recruitment of phagocytic cells to sites of inflammation, has been demonstrated *in vitro* to be inhibited by some NSAIDs.[14] There are data suggesting that NSAIDs inhibit activation and chemotaxis of neutrophils as well as reduce toxic oxygen radical production in stimulated neutrophils.[37,38] There is also evidence that several NSAIDs scavenge superoxide radicals.[37]

Salicylates have been demonstrated to inhibit phospholipase C activity in macrophages. Some NSAIDs have been shown to affect T-lymphocyte function experimentally by inhibiting rheumatoid factor production *in vitro*. Another newly described action not directly related to prostaglandin synthesis inhibition includes interference with neutrophil-endothelial cell adherence, which is critical to migration of granulocytes to sites of inflammation. These data demonstrate that expression of L-selectins are decreased.[16] NSAIDs have been demonstrated *in vitro* to inhibit NF-kB (nitric oxide transcription factor) dependent transcription, thereby inhibiting inducible nitric-oxide synthetase.[15] Anti-inflammatory levels of ASA have been shown to inhibit expression of inducible nitric-oxide synthetase and subsequent production of nitrite *in vitro*. At pharmacologic doses, sodium salicylate, indomethacin, and acetaminophen when studied had no effect, but at suprapharmacologic doses, sodium salicylate inhibited nitrite production.[15]

Recently, it has been described that prostaglandins inhibit apoptosis (programmed cell death) and that NSAIDs, via inhibition of prostaglandin synthesis, may reestablish more normal cell cycle responses.[19,20] There is also evidence suggesting that some NSAIDs may reduce PGH synthase gene expression, thereby supporting the clinical evidence of differences in activity in NSAIDs in sites of active inflammation.

The NSAIDs have been demonstrated to have variable effects on many biologic processes; however, how important some of these effects are clinically remains unknown. Although nonacetylated salicylates have been shown *in vitro* to inhibit neutrophil function and to have equal efficacy in patients with rheumatoid arthritis,[39] clinically there is no evidence to suggest that these biologic effects are more important than prostaglandin synthase inhibition.

PHARMACOLOGY

NSAIDs are efficiently absorbed after oral administration, but absorption rates may vary in patients with altered gastrointestinal blood flow or motility. Certain NSAIDs when taken with food have decreased absorption.[1,2] Enteric coating may reduce direct effects of NSAIDs on the gastric mucosa but may also reduce the rate of absorption.

Most NSAIDs are weak organic acids; once absorbed they are >95% bound to serum albumin. This is a saturable process. Clinically significant decreases in serum albumin levels or institution of other highly protein-bound medications may lead to an increase in the free component of NSAID in serum. This may be important in patients who are elderly or are chronically ill, especially those with associated hypoalbuminemic states. Importantly, as a result of increased vascular permeability in localized sites of inflammation, this high degree of protein binding may result in delivery of higher levels of NSAIDs.

NSAIDs are metabolized predominantly in the liver by the cytochrome P450 system and the CYP 2C9 isoform, and excreted in the urine. This must be taken into consideration when prescribing NSAIDs for patients with hepatic or renal dysfunction. Some NSAIDs (e.g., indomethacin, sulindac, and piroxicam) have a prominent enterohepatic circulation, resulting in a prolonged half-life and should be used with caution in the elderly. In patients with renal insufficiency, some inactive metabolites may be re-synthesized *in vivo* to the active compound. Diclofenac, flurbiprofen, celecoxib, and rofecoxib are metabolized in the liver. These agents should be used with care and at lowest possible doses in patients with clinically significant liver disease, if used at all, including patients with cirrhosis with or without ascites, prolonged prothrombin times, falling serum albumin levels, or important elevations in liver transaminases in blood.

As noted, most of the NSAIDs and celecoxib are metabolized through the P450 CYP29 isoenzyme, whereas rofecoxib is not. The exact mechanism to explain the metabolism of rofecoxib remains unexplained.

Salicylates are the least highly protein bound NSAID: approximately 68%. Zero order kinetics are dominant in salicylate metabolism. Thus, increasing the dose of salicylates is effective over a narrow range, but once the metabolic systems are saturated, then incremental dose increases may lead to very high serum salicylate levels. Thus, changes in salicylate doses need to be carefully considered at chronic steady-state levels, particularly in patients with altered renal or hepatic function.

Significant differences in plasma half-lives of the NSAIDs may be important in explaining their diverse clinical effects. Those with long half-lives typically do not attain maximum plasma concentrations quickly and important clinical responses may be delayed. In most chronic conditions that are appropriate for the use of these drugs, the acute effects are not as important as in the treatment of headache or acute pain. Plasma concentrations can vary widely because of differences in renal clearance and metabolism. Piroxicam has the longest serum half-life of currently marketed NSAIDs: 57 ± 22 hours. In comparison, diclofenac has one of the shortest: 1.1 ± 0.2 hours (see Table 61-1). Although drugs have been developed with very long half-lives to improve patient compliance, in the older patient it is sometimes preferable to use drugs of shorter half-life so that, when the drug is discontinued, any unwanted effects may more rapidly disappear.

Sulindac and nabumetone are "pro-drugs" in which the active compound is produced after first-pass metabolism through the liver. Theoretically, pro-drugs were developed to decrease the exposure of the gastrointestinal mucosa to the local effects of the NSAIDs. Unfortunately, as was noted, with adequate inhibition of COX-1 the patient is placed at substantial risk of an NSAID-induced upper GI event as long as COX-1 activity is inhibited. This is true for drugs such as ketoralac given as an injection or by these pro-drugs when given at adequate therapeutic doses.[40]

Other pharmacologic properties may be important clinically. NSAIDs that are highly lipid soluble in serum will penetrate the central nervous system more effectively and occasionally may produce striking changes in mentation, perception, and mood.[41,42] Indomethacin has been associated with many of these side effects, even after a single dose, particularly in the elderly.

ADVERSE EFFECTS

Mechanism-based Adverse Effects

Risk for Anaphylaxis and Pulmonary Effects Many adverse reactions attributed to NSAIDs are due to inhibition of prostaglandin synthesis in local tissues (Table 61-2). For example, patients with allergic rhinitis, nasal polyposis, and/or a history of asthma, in whom all NSAIDs effectively inhibit prostaglandin synthase, are at increased risk for anaphylaxis. In high doses, even nonacetylated salicylates may sufficiently decrease enough prostaglandin synthesis to induce an anaphylactic reaction in sensitive patients.[43] Although the exact mechanism for this effect remains unclear, it is known that E prostaglandins serve as bronchodilators. When COX activity is inhibited in patients at risk, a decrease in synthesis of prostaglandins that contribute to bronchodilation results. Another explanation implicates other enzymatic pathways that utilize the arachidonate pool after it is converted from phospholipase, whereby shunting of arachidonate into the leukotrienne pathway occurs when cyclooxygenase is inhibited.[44] The leukotriene pathway converts arachidonate by 5-lipoxygenase, leading to products such as LTB_4 as well as others clearly associated with anaphylaxis. This explanation implies that large stores of arachidonate released in certain inflammatory situations lead to excess substrate for leukotriene metabolism. This results in release of products that are highly reactive, leading to increased bronchoconstriction and the risk for anaphylaxis in the right patient. Whether the main mechanism of effect is inhibition of prostaglandin synthesis or shunting of arachidonate into conversion by 5-lipoxygenase or a combination of the two, it is clear that patients who are sensitive are at great risk when NSAIDs are used. The nonacetylated salicylates as a group have been considered a safe choice for these patients because they are known to possess anti-inflammatory activity, but are relatively weak cyclooxygenase inhibitors.

Platelet Effects Platelet aggregation and thus the ability to clot is primarily induced through stimulating thromboxane production with activation of platelet COX-1. There is no COX-2 in the platelet. NSAIDs and aspirin inhibit the activity of COX-1 but the COX-2 specific inhibitors (or COX-1 sparing drugs) have no effect on COX-1 at clinically effective therapeutic doses.[19,20]

The effect of the nonsalicylate NSAIDs on platelet function is reversible and related to the half-life of the drug; whereas the effect of ASA is to acetylate the COX-1 enzyme, thereby permanently inactivating it. Since platelets cannot synthesize new cyclooxygenase enzyme after exposure to ASA, the platelet does not function appropriately for its lifespan. Therefore, the effect of ASA on the platelet does not wear off as the drug is metabolized as with the nonsalicylate NSAIDs. Patients awaiting surgery should therefore stop their NSAIDs at a time determined by 4 to 5 times their serum half-life; whereas ASA needs to be discontinued 1 to 2 weeks before the planned procedure to allow for re-population of platelets that have been unexposed to ASA.

We also have little information about the use of the COX-2 specific inhibitors in patients at risk for thrombosis.[19] The randomized clinical trials of the COX-2 specific inhibitors were not designed to address this question. Furthermore, we have little information demonstrating that the traditional NSAIDs are safer or more useful than the COX-2 specific inhibitors in this regard. Only aspirin has been studied prospectively, and low-dose aspirin (<325 mg/day) should be given concomitantly with either NSAIDs or specific COX-2 inhibitors in patients at risk for thrombosis.[45] Secondary prophylaxis of cardiovascular events with aspirin has been shown to be important. There is about a 23% to 33% decrease in atherothrombotic events in patients with a history of ischemic heart disease when they are treated with <325-mg aspirin/day.[45] There are less data about the effectiveness of low-dose aspirin in primary prophylaxis. There is little evidence that the non-aspirin NSAIDs

TABLE 61-2 **Adverse Reactions of the NSAIDs**

1. Nonspecific reactions
   - A. Rash: fixed drug eruptions, photosensitivity, exfoliative erythroderma, urticaria, Stevens-Johnson syndrome, etc.
   - B. Stomatitis
   - C. Nausea, vomiting; constipation, diarrhea
   - D. Central Nervous System
     - (1) Headaches, dizziness, confusion, depression
     - (2) Depersonalization reactions, seizures, syncope
     - (3) Hallucinations, personality change, inability to concentrate, forgetfulness, sleeplessness, irritability, paranoid ideation (particularly in the elderly)
     - (4) Tinnitus—almost always reversible, decrease in hearing may be the most prominent symptom; less likely evident at the extremes of age
     - (5) Aseptic meningitis—particularly with ibuprofen including OTC
     - (6) Ocular
       - a. toxic amblyopia
       - b. asymptomatic crystals (of drug) in cornea
   - E. Interference with response to infections
     ? Decrease in neutrophil chemotaxis and lysosomal enzyme release
   - F. Bone marrow suppression
   - G. Competition with other drugs for protein binding sites
2. Hypersensitivity reactions
   - A. Asthma/urticaria syndrome
     - (1) Triad: vasomotor rhinitis, nasal polyposis, asthma; may be seen only with history of asthma
       - a. Due to inhibition of bronchodilating prostaglandins
       - b. Due to shunting into lipoxygenase pathway
3. Platelet effects
   - A. Inhibits platelet cyclooxygenase
     - (1) ASA inhibits the enzyme irreversibly
       Needs 7–14 days to repopulate platelet population
     - (2) All others reversible but dependent on half-life of drug: 4–5×
       Short half-life: may only need 24h
       Long half-life: may need days (i.e., piroxicam may need 8 days)
4. Reversal of effects of antihypertensive drugs
   More effects on ACE inhibitors than beta blockers than diuretics
5. Renal effects
   - A. Interstitial disease and/or modify tubular function
     - (1) Occasionally observe typical hypersensitivity reaction fever, rash, eosinophilia
   - B. Glomerulopathy
     - (1) May be in association with interstitial disease
     - (2) Typically membranous in type
   - C. Rarely intratubular precipitation of either urate or drug metabolite
   - D. Modify intrinsic renal plasma flow leading to increased BUN, and serum creatinine
   - E. Modify water and electrolyte balance
6. Gastrointestinal effects
   - A. Nonspecific
     - (1) Dyspepsia, nausea/vomiting, diarrhea, constipation, anorexia
   - B. Specific
     - (1) Bleeding, gastritis, duodenitis, gastroduodenal ulcers with/without signs and symptoms
     - (2) Obstruction of small bowel
     - (3) Hepatotoxicity

have a role in primary or secondary prophylaxis of cardiovascular or cerebrovascular events. Given the additive ulcerogenic potential associated with the use of multiple NSAIDs, it would be advisable to use specific COX-2 inhibitors with aspirin when considering combination cardioprotective and anti-inflammatory therapies. In the two large bleeding trials describing the effects of celecoxib and rofecoxib, there was a statistically significant difference between the incidence of acute myocardial infarctions (MIs) with rofecoxib (0.4%) and naproxen (0.1%), whereas there was no difference in the incidence of acute MIs with celecoxib as compared with diclofenac or ibuprofen.[46,47] It is impossible to know whether these data suggest that rofecoxib induced more MIs than naproxen or whether naproxen exerted a protective effect. The study was too short with relatively too few patients to answer this question.

Gastrointestinal Tract The most clinically significant adverse effects associated with NSAIDs occur in the GI tract, affecting the GI mucosa.[48–57] These events appear to be due to local or systemic inhibition of prostaglandin synthesis. NSAIDs cause a wide range of GI problems including symptoms of intolerance such as dyspepsia, nausea, vomiting, as well as esophagitis, esophageal stricture, gastritis, mucosal erosions, hemorrhage, peptic ulceration and/or perforation, obstruction, and death.[27,48,49,58–62] The unpleasant symptoms may be observed in about 40% to 60% of patients but are not related to COX-1 inhibition in the GI mucosa.[27,28] The exact cause of these symptoms remains unknown; however, use of H_2-receptor antagonists and proton pump inhibitors typically alleviates these unpleasant effects. Erosions and ulcers as well as ulcer complications are predominantly due to the effects of NSAID-induced inhibition of COX-1, thus those prostaglandins that serve to protect the stomach mucosa from toxins. This protection consists of a mucous layer serving as a barrier, a bicarbonate gradient serving to buffer the mucosa layer from the effects of the extremely acidic lumen, developing glutathione to serve as a scavenger of superoxides, prostaglandin-mediated inhibition of gastric acid, and prostaglandin-mediated increases in mucosal blood flow. All of these effects are inhibited by the NSAIDs, which inhibit COX-1 activity. However, in an experiment with mice both COX-1 and COX-2 have to be inhibited in order for mice to have an ulcer. The exact effect of inhibiting COX-2 in this experiment is unknown, but some investigators have speculated that COX-2 plays an important role in healing of mucosal lesions.[63,64]

The mucosa of the large and small bowel may also be affected by NSAIDs. These agents in the small or large bowel may also induce stricture formation,[13,27,52–54,61–63] which may manifest as diaphragms precipitating small or large bowel obstruction, and can be hard to detect on contrast radiographic studies.

Additionally, there is evidence to suggest that NSAIDs interfere with permeability of the GI mucosa. The weakly acidic NSAIDs rapidly penetrate the superficial lining cells of the GI mucosa leading to oxidative uncoupling of cellular metabolism, local tissue injury, and ultimately cell death. This can result in local erosions, hemorrhages, and formation of clinically significant ulcers in the right patients.[13]

Endoscopic studies have clearly demonstrated that NSAID administration results in shallow erosions and/or submucosal hemorrhages that are observed in the stomach near the prepyloric area and the antrum, although they may occur at any site in the GI tract.[27] Typically, these lesions are asymptomatic, making prevalence data difficult to determine.[58] As a result, we do not know the number of lesions that spontaneously heal or which will progress to ulceration, frank perforation, gastric or duodenal obstruction, serious gastrointestinal hemorrhage, or subsequent death. Risk factors for the development of GI toxicity in patients receiving NSAIDs include age >60 years, prior history of peptic ulcer disease, prior use of antiulcer therapies for any reason, concomitant use of glucocorticoids, particularly in patients with rheumatoid arthritis, comorbidities such as significant cardiovascular disease, or patients with severe rheumatoid arthritis (Table 61-3).[25,27,48,49,64,65] Other risk factors include increasing dose of specific and singular NSAIDs.

The magnitude of risk for GI adverse events is controversial. The US Food and Drug Administration (FDA) reports an overall risk of 2% to 4% for NSAID-induced gastric ulcer development and its complications.[25,27,28] In general, based on multiple clinical trials, the relative risk is estimated to be 4.0 to 5.0 for gastric ulcer, 1.1 to 1.6 for duodenal ulcer, and 4.5 to 5.0 for clinically significant gastric ulcers with hemorrhage, perforation, obstruction, or death. The accurate absolute risk is harder to determine.

As noted, other sites in the GI tract, including the esophagus and small and large bowel, may also be affected. Exposure to NSAIDs is probably a major factor in the development of esophagitis and subsequent stricture formation.[58,59] Effects on small and large bowel have increasingly been reported.[27,53] An autopsy study on 713 patients showed that small bowel ulceration defined as ulcers >3 mm in diameter were observed in 8.4% of patients exposed to NSAIDs compared with 0.6% of nonusers of NSAIDs.[61] Ulcerations of stomach and duodenum were observed in 22% of NSAID users compared with 12% of nonusers.

Before the COX-2 selective inhibitors became available, the epidemiologic studies suggested that the nonacetylated salicylates are least likely to result in a NSAID-induced adverse GI event. Agents such as nebumatone are usually considered to be less likely to induce effects.[56,57] However, as higher doses of "safe" NSAIDs are used, then more GI damage is reported.[57] Thus at equally efficacious doses the non-selective NSAIDs all induce ulcers at variable rates, and any of these ulcers in the right patient could develop a complicated course. NSAIDs with prominent enterohepatic circulation and significantly longer half-lives such as sulindac and piroxicam have been linked to increased potential for GI toxicity attributed to prolonged re-exposure of gastric and duodenal mucosa to bile reflux and the active moiety of the drug.[27]

TABLE 61-3 **Risk Factors for NSAID-Induced Upper GI Toxicity**

1. Older than 60–65
2. History of previous GI bleed, peptic ulcer disease, or perforation or obstruction
3. History of previous NSAID-induced GI toxicity
4. Concomitant illnesses such as cardiovascular disease leading to increased disability
5. Dose of the NSAID
6. Combinations of NSAIDs
7. Concomitant glucocorticoids
8. For bleeding: concomitant warfarin
9. Concomitant need for antacids of all types
10. Independent: infection with *Helicobacter pylori*, tobacco use, and alcohol

Endoscopic data from large numbers of patients treated with COX-2 selective inhibitors strongly suggest that ulcers occur at the same rate as in patients who received placebo; whereas the traditional NSAID active comparators induced ulcers (as documented by endoscopy) in 15% (diclofenac 75 mg twice daily, ibuprofen 800 mg three times daily) to 19% (naproxen 500 mg twice daily) following 1 week of treatment in healthy volunteers and in 26% (naproxen 500 mg twice daily) of patients with OA and RA after 12 weeks of treatment.[5–8] Two large outcome trials with rofecoxib and celecoxib have now been published and have shown that rofecoxib and celecoxib both at suprapharmacologic doses (two to four times the treating doses) are associated with about two- to three-fold fewer GI complications than naproxen or ibuprofen, respectively, at standard therapeutic doses.[46,47] These data clearly show that compared with the effects of two widely used NSAIDs (ibuprofen 1.2%, naproxen 1.6%), that the COX-2 inhibitors induce bleeding complications at a lower rate (celecoxib 0.4%, rofecoxib 0.6%).[46,47] It is possible that patients with preexisting ulcer may experience delay in healing when treated with a COX-2 specific inhibitor, but only long-term outcome clinical trials will clarify if this is a risk.[63]

Approach to the Patient at Risk for NSAID-induced GI Adverse Events The approach to the patient with pain and or inflammation who is about to embark on the use of a NSAID is partly related to dose, consistency, and planned length of therapy. For most patients who will take standard doses of nonselective NSAIDs for less than 10 days, there is little risk unless they have multiple significant risk factors noted previously. However, for the patient with OA or other chronic condition at risk for an NSAID-induced GI event, the decision remains somewhat controversial. Many patients with dyspepsia or upper GI distress have superficial erosions evident on endoscopy that frequently heal spontaneously without change in therapy. Even more difficult to evaluate is whether cytoprotective agents actually alter NSAID-associated symptoms, which may or may not predict significant GI events. Although one clinical study demonstrated that >80% of patients who developed significant NSAID-induced endoscopic abnormalities were asymptomatic,[58] several prospective observational trials indicated that patients were more symptomatic with NSAID-induced toxicities than previously thought.[55]

The patient who develops a gastric or duodenal ulcer while taking NSAIDs should have treatment discontinued and therapy for ulcer disease, either H_2-antagonist or proton pump inhibitors, instituted.[27–29] If NSAIDs must be continued concomitantly, then the patient will be required to receive antiulcer therapy for longer periods.[28] Typically, most patients with uncomplicated gastric or duodenal ulcers will heal within 8 weeks of initiating H_2-antagonists. If NSAID treatment is continued, then perhaps 16 weeks of therapy may be necessary for adequate healing. Diagnostic tests to determine if the patient is *Helicobacter pylori* positive should be performed, and if the patient has positive studies, then specific antibiotic therapy to eradicate the infection should be administered.[28]

Prophylaxis to prevent NSAID-induced gastric and duodenal ulcers is more complicated. To date there has been no evidence that agents other than concomitant misoprostol therapy will prevent NSAID-induced gastric ulceration and its complications.[66–69] Although high-dose H_2-antagonists or proton pump inhibitors have been demonstrated to prevent NSAID-induced gastric and duodenal ulcers, prevention of ulceration complications has not been clearly shown. Endoscopic trials have shown that famotidine at twice the approved dose (40 mg twice daily) significantly decreased the incidence of both gastric and duodenal ulcers.[69] Similarly, an endoscopy trial demonstrated that treatment with omeprazole (a proton pump inhibitor) decreased gastroduodenal ulcers.[68] Both H_2-antagonists and proton pump inhibitors decrease dyspeptic symptoms quite effectively.

Misoprostol is a prostaglandin analogue, believed to locally replace prostaglandins whose synthesis in the gastroduodenal mucosa is inhibited by the nonselective NSAIDs.[64–66] A large prospective trial evaluated 8,843 patients with rheumatoid arthritis to determine whether misoprostol would decrease the incidence of ulcers and their complications.[64,65] Patients received various NSAIDs and were followed for 6 months either on misoprostol co-therapy or placebo. The study was powered on the basis of endoscopic observations of an 80% decrease with concomitant misoprostol therapy in endoscopically proven ulcers >0.3 to 0.5 cm in diameter in the gastric and duodenal mucosa.[66] Misoprostol successfully inhibited development of ulcer complications such as bleeding, perforation, and obstruction. There was a 40% reduction in patients treated with misoprostol as opposed to those receiving placebo.[64] Further analysis demonstrated that patients with health assessment questionnaire (HAQ) scores >1.5 (thus worse disease) had an 87% reduction in risk for a NSAID-induced toxic event if concomitantly treated with misoprostol.[65]

These data suggest that high-risk patients may benefit from concomitant misoprostol therapy if NSAID treatment is indicated. Gabriel and colleagues have demonstrated the pharmacoeconomic utility of such therapy in the high-risk patient.[70] Unfortunately, the major adverse event causing withdrawal in approximately 10% of patients was diarrhea, and 30% of patients complained of diarrhea. Therefore medications such as stool softeners and cathartics should be stopped. There are data suggesting that concomitant treatment with misoprostol once an ulcer develops will allow the ulcer to heal.[68]

Renal Adverse Effects The NSAIDs also have effects on the kidneys. The effects of the NSAIDs on renal function include changes in the excretion of sodium, changes in tubular function, the potential for interstitial nephritis, and reversible renal failure due to alterations in filtration rate and renal plasma flow.[71,72] Prostaglandins and prostacyclins are important for maintenance of intrarenal blood flow and tubular transport. All NSAIDs, except nonacetylated salicylates, have the potential to induce reversible impairment of glomerular filtration rate; this effect occurs more frequently in patients with congestive heart failure; established renal disease with altered intrarenal plasma flow including diabetes, hypertension, or atherosclerosis; and with induced hypovolemia, salt depletion or significant hypoalbuminemia.[19,71,72] Triamterene-containing diuretics, which increase plasma renin levels, may predispose patients prescribed NSAIDs to acute renal failure. NSAIDs have been implicated in the development of acute and chronic renal insufficiency, due to inhibition of vasodilating prostaglandins, thereby reducing renal blood flow.

NSAID-associated intersitial nephritis is typically manifested as nephrotic syndrome, characterized by edema or anasarca, proteinuria, hematuria, and pyuria. The usual stigmata of drug-induced allergic nephritis such as eosinophilia, eosinophiluria, and fever may not be present. Interstitial infiltrates of mononuclear cells are seen histologically with relative sparing of the glomeruli. Phenylproprionic acid derivatives, such as fenoprofen, naproxen, and tolmetin along with the indoleacetic acid derivative indomethacin, are most commonly associated with the development of interstitial nephritis.

Inhibition of prostaglandin synthesis intrarenally by NSAIDs decreases renin release and thus produces a state of hyporeninemic hypoaldosteronism with resulting hyperkalemia.[71] This effect may be amplified in patients taking potassium-sparing diuretics. Salt retention precipitated by some NSAIDs leading to peripheral edema in some patients is likely due to both inhibition of intrarenal prostaglandin production, which decreases renal medullary blood flow and increases tubular reabsorption of sodium chloride as well as other direct tubular effects. NSAIDs have also been reported to increase antidiuretic hormone effects, thereby reducing excretion of free water, resulting in hyponatremia.[71] Thiazide diuretics may produce an added effect on the NSAID-induced hyponatremia. All NSAIDs have been demonstrated to interfere with medical management of hypertension and heart failure.

All NSAIDs, including the COX-2 inhibitors with the exception of the nonacetylated salicylates, have been associated with increases in mean blood pressure in hypertensive patients but not in patients with normal blood pressure.[74] Patients receiving antihypertensive agents including beta blockers, ACE inhibitors, thiazide, and loop diuretics must be checked regularly when initiating therapy with a new NSAID to ensure that there are no significant continued and sustained rises in blood pressure.

The mechanism of acute renal failure induced in the at-risk patient treated with NSAIDs is believed to be prostaglandin mediated.[71–73] However, the role of COX-2 in maintenance of renal homeostasis in the human remains unclear. COX-2 activity is notably present in the macula densa and tubules in animals and man, and is upregulated in salt-depleted animals.[75] In humans, COX-1 is an important enzyme for control of intrarenal blood flow. It is believed that COX-2 activity importantly modulates salt and water homeostasis, whereas COX-1 activity seems important in modulating renal plasma flow. In the patient who has decreased renal plasma flow, both COX-1 and COX-2 are upregulated and therefore there is not sufficient evidence to indicate that the COX-2 specific inhibitors will be safer than traditional NSAIDs in terms of renal function. Until the appropriate clinical trials are done, any patient at high risk for renal complications should be monitored very carefully. No patient with a creatinine clearance of <30 mL/minute should be treated with either a NSAID or a COX-2 specific inhibitor.

Nonmechanism-based Adverse Events

Hepatotoxicity Elevations in hepatic transaminase levels induced by NSAIDs are not uncommon, although it occurs more often in patients with juvenile rheumatoid arthritis or systemic lupus erythematosus. Unless elevations exceed two to three times the upper limit of normal,or serum albumin falls,or prothrombin times are altered, these effects are usually not considered clinically significant.[76–78] Nonetheless, overt liver failure has been reported following use of many NSAIDs, including diclofenac, flurbiprofen, and sulindac.[77,78] Of all NSAIDs, sulindac has been associated with the highest incidence of cholestasis.[76] Therefore it is recommended that patients at risk for liver toxicity be followed very carefully. When initiating NSAID treatment, all patients should be evaluated again within 8 to 12 weeks and serious consideration given to performing a blood analysis for serum transaminase changes.

Idiosyncratic Adverse Effects Many of the toxic effects of NSAIDs are related to their mechanism of action via prostaglandin inhibition, but there are also important potential idiosyncratic effects. A typical nonspecific reaction includes skin rash and photosensitivity, which is associated with all currently available NSAIDs, particularly the phenylproprionic acid derivatives.[79] This same class of NSAID derivative may also induce aseptic meningitis, especially in patients with systemic lupus erythematosus. The underlying mechanism of action remains unknown. Ibuprofen has also been associated with a reversible toxic amblyopia.[79]

Owing to the antiplatelet effects of all NSAIDs, except the nonacetylated salicylates, concomitant therapy with warfarin (Coumadin) puts patients at greater risk for bleeding. As concomitant NSAID therapy would displace warfarin from its albumin binding sites, the prothrombin time may be prolonged. In addition, given the increased relative risk for NSAID-induced gastroduodenal ulcers and bleeding, there is an increased risk for bleeding when the NSAIDs are used concomitantly with warfarin. In that the COX-2 specific inhibitors do not cause ulcers of the GI tract, nor do they alter platelet function, the patient on warfarin would have less risk for a significant GI bleed when treated with these drugs than traditional nonselective NSAIDs. Effects such as these may also be seen with dilantin or other highly protein-bound drugs such as antibiotics.

The NSAIDs inhibit the renal excretion of lithium and should be used with caution in patients taking this drug. Cholysteramine, an anion-exchange resin, reduces the rate of NSAID absorption and its bioavailability.

The CNS side effects of NSAIDs include aseptic meningitis, psychosis, and cognitive dysfunction.[1,41,42] The latter changes are more commonly seen in elderly patients treated with indomethacin, whereas the phenylproprionic acid derivatives are more commonly associated with the development of aseptic meningitis and toxic amblyobia. Tinnitus is a common problem with higher doses of salicylates as well as the nonsalicylate NSAIDs. The mechanism is unknown. Interestingly, the young and the elderly may not complain of tinnitus but only of hearing loss. Other NSAIDs may also induce tinnitus in specific patients. Decreasing the dose usually alleviates the effect.

It has been shown that COX-2 is important for ovulation through the PPRA 1 receptor.[19] In addition, COX-2 is upregulated with implantation of a fertilized ovum or in decidualization. Although there are a few case reports of reversible infertility associated with the use of NSAIDs, given the large numbers of patients who regularly use NSAIDs there does not appear to be a generalized epidemic of infertility.[80]

Use of NSAIDs does not lead to osteoporosis.[81–82] The role of COX-1 remains unclear. Although inflammation in the joint leads to juxtaarticular osteopenia, this is the result of increased prostaglandin synthesis in the inflamed joint, which is likely directly related to increased COX-2 activity.

Some of the early available NSAIDs have been associated with an increased risk for bone marrow failure. This is particularly true of phenylbutazone and indomethacin. Strom and colleagues have described the incidence of neutropenia as a toxic effect of the NSAIDs.[83] In a case-controlled study performed using Medicaid claims data, these investigators defined that the adjusted odds ratio for neutropenia in patients treated with NSAIDs is 4.2 (confidence interval (CI), 2.0–8.7). When patients treated with either phenylbutazone or indomethacin were excluded, the odds ratio for the development of neutropenia remained quite robust: 3.5 (CI 1.6–7.6). In general, given the common use of NSAIDs, the risk of neutropenia is quite small.

There are little data documenting the effects of the NSAIDs on pregnancy or the fetus. In animal models, the NSAIDs have been shown to increase the incidence of dystocia, post-implantation loss, as well as delay of parturition and miscarriage.[80] The effect of prostaglandin inhibition may result in premature closure of the ductus arteriosus. ASA has been associated with smaller babies and neonatal bruising; however, it has been used for many years in the treatment of patients who require NSAIDs while pregnant. Typically, therapy with ASA is stopped about 8 weeks prior to delivery to decrease the risk for interfering with ductus closure. In animals, there is no evidence that ASA is a teratogen. The NSAIDs are excreted in breast milk. It is believed that salicylates in normally recommended doses are not considered dangerous to nursing infants.

SUMMARY

Although NSAIDs are known to decrease pain and inflammation and to be antipyretic, they have not been shown to decrease erosions in rheumatoid arthritis, to retard osteophyte formation in osteoarthritis, or to protect cartilage from mechanical or inflammatory injury. However, they continue to be important drugs for the palliation of pain and inflammation. Newer forms of COX-2 inhibitors are in development and are considered even better analgesics because of rapid uptake in the CNS. Time will tell the ultimate role these drugs will play as more is learned about their complex physiologic effects.

REFERENCES

1. Brooks PM, Day RO. Nonsteroidal antiinflammatory drugs: differences and similarities. *N Engl J Med* 1991;324:1716–1725.
2. Furst DE. Are there differences among nonsteroidal antiinflammatory drugs? Comparing acetylated salicylates, nonacetylated salicylates, and nonacetylated nonsteroidal antiinflammatory drugs. *Arthritis Rheum* 1994;37:1–9.
3. Abramson SB, Weissman G. The mechanisms of action of nonsteroidal antiinflammatory drugs. *Arthritis Rheum* 1989;32:1–9.
4. Simon LS. Actions and toxicities of the NSAIDs. *Curr Opin Rheum* 1996.
5. Simon LS, Lanza FL, Lipsky PE, et al. Preliminary study of the safety and efficacy of SC-58635, a novel cyclooxygenase 2 inhibitor: efficacy and safety in two placebo-controlled trials in osteoarthritis and rheumatoid arthritis, and studies of gastrointestinal and platelet effects. *Arthritis Rheum* 1998;41:1591–1602.
6. Simon LS, Weaver AL, Graham DY, et al. The anti-inflammatory and upper gastrointestinal effects of celecoxib in rheumatoid arthritis: a randomized, controlled trial. *JAMA* 1999;282:1921–1928.
7. Laine L, Harper S, Simon T, et al. A randomized trial comparing the effect of rofecoxib, a cyclooxygenase-2 specific inhibitor, with that of ibuprofen on gastroduodenal mucosa of patients with osteoarthritis. *Gastroenterology* 1999;117:776–783.
8. Hawkey CJ. COX-2 inhibitors. *Lancet* 1999;353:307–314.
9. Baum C, Kennedy DL, Forbes MB. Utilization of nonsteroidal anti-inflammatory drugs. *Arthritis Rheum* 1985;28:686–691.
10. Phillips AC, Simon LS. NSAIDs and the elderly: toxicity and the economic implications. *Drugs Aging* 1996.
11. Walker JS, Sheather-Reid RB, Carmody JJ, et al.Nonsteroidal antiinflammatory drugs in rheumatoid arthritis and osteoarthritis: support for the concept of "responders" and "nonresponders." *Arthritis Rheum* 1997;40:1944–1954.
12. Simon LS, Strand V. Clinical response to nonsteroidal antiinflammatory drugs. *Arthritis Rheum* 1997;40:1940–1943.
13. Mahmud T, Rafi SS, Scott DL, et al. Nonsteroidal antiinflammatory drugs and uncoupling of mitochondrial oxidative phosphorylation. *Arthritis Rheum* 1996;39:1998–2003.
14. Abramson SB, Leszczynska-Piziak J, Clancy RM, et al. Inhibition of neutrophil function by aspirin-like drugs (NSAIDs): requirement for asembly of heterotrimeric G proteins in bilayer phosopholipid. *Biochem Pharmacol* 1994;47:563–572.
15. Amin AR, Vyas P, Attur M, et al. The mode of action of aspirin-like drugs: effect on inducible nitric oxide synthase. *Proc Natl Acad Sci USA* 1995;92:7926–7930.
16. Díaz-González F, González-Alvero I, Companero MR, et al. Prevention of *in vitro* neutrophil-endothelial attachment through shedding of L-selectin by nonsteroidal antiinflammatory drugs. *J Clin Invest* 1995; 95:1756–1765.
17. Smith WL. Prostanoid biosynthesis and mechanisms of action. *Am J Physiol* 1992;263:F181–F191.
18. Samad TA, Moore KA, Sapirstein A, et al. Interleukin-1beta-mediated induction of COX-2 in the CNS contributes to inflammatory pain hypersensivity. *Nature* 2001;410:471–475.
19. Crofford LJ, Lipsky PE, Brooks P, et al.Basic biology and clinical application of cyclooxygenase-2. *Arthritis Rheum* 1999.
20. Dubois RN, Abramson SB, Corfford L, et al. Cyclooxygenase in biology and disease. *FASEB J* 1998;12:1063–1073.
21. Mitchell JA, Akarasereenont P, Thiemermann C, et al. Selectivity of nonsteroidal antiinflammatory drugs as inhibitors of constitutive and inducible cyclooxygenase. *Proc Natl Acad Sci* USA 1994;90:11693–11697.
22. Patrignani P, Panara MR, Greco A, et al. Biochemical and pharmacological characterization of the cyclooxygenase activity of human blood prostaglandin endoperoxide synthases. *J Pharmacol Exp Ther* 1994; 271:1705–1712.
23. Meade EA, Smith WL, Dewitt DL. Differential inhibition of prostaglandin endoperoxide synthase (cyclooxygenase) isoenzymes by aspirin and other non-steroidal anti-inflammatory drugs. *J Biol Chem* 1993; 268(9):6610–6614.
24. Laneuville O, Breuer DK, DeWitt DL, et al. Differential inhibition of human prostaglandin endoperoxide H synthases-1 and -2 by nonsteroidal antiinflammatory drugs. *J Pharmacol Exp Ther* 1994;271: 927–939.
25. Fries JP, Miller SR, Spitz PW. Toward an epidemiology of gastropathy associated with nonsteroidal antiinflammatory drug use. *Gastroenterology* 1989;96:647–655.
26. Gabriel SE, Jaaklimainen L, Bombadier C. Risk for serious gastrointestinal complications related to use of nonsteroidal antiinflammatory drugs: a meta-analysis. *Ann Intern Med* 1991;115:787–796.
27. Wolfe MM, Lichtenstein DR, Singh G. Gastrointestinal toxicity of the nonsteroidal antiinflammatory drugs. *N Engl J Med* 1999;340:1888–1899.
28. Scheiman JM. NSAIDs, gastrointestinal injury, and cytoprotection. *Gastroenterol Clin North Am* 1996;25:279–298.
29. Laine L. Nonsteroidal antiinflammatory drug gastropathy. *Gastrointest Endosc Clin North Am* 1996;6:489–504.
30. Hollander D. Gastrointestinal complications of nonsteroidal antiinflammatory drugs: prophylactic and therapeutic strategies. *Am J Med* 1994;96:274–281.
31. Charleson S, Cartwright M, Frank J, et al. Characterization of prostaglandin G/H synthase 1 and 2 in rat, dog, monkey, and human gastrointestinal tracts. *Gastroenterology* 1996;111:445–454.
32. DeWitt DL, Meade EA, Smith WL. PGH synthase isoenzyme selectivity: the potential for safer nonsteroidal antiinflammatory drugs. *Am J Med* 1993;95(suppl 2A):40S–44S.
33. Glaser K, Sung M-L, O'Neill K, et al. Etodolac selectively inhibits human prostaglandin G/H synthase 2 (PGHS-2) versus human PGHS-1. *Eur J Pharmacol* 1995;281:107–111.
34. Lipsky PE, Abramson SB, Crofford L, et al. The classification of cyclooxygenase inhibitors [editorial]. *J Rheumatol* 1998;25:2298–3003.

35. Bensen WG, Fiechtner JJ, McMillen JI, et al. Treatment of osteoarthritis with celecoxib, a cyclooxygenase-2 inhbitor: a randomized controlled trial. *Mayo Clin Proc* 1999;74:1095–1105.
36. Ehrich EW, Dallob A, De Lepeleire L, et al. Characterization of rofecoxib as a cyclooxygenase-2 isoform inhibitor and demonstration of analgesia in the dental pain model. *Clin Pharmacol Ther* 1999;65: 336–347.
37. Friman C, Johnston C, Chew C, Davis P. Effect of diclofenac sodium, tolfenamic acid and indomethacin on the production of superoxide induced by *N*-fromyl-methionyl-leucyl-phenylalanine in normal human polymorphonuclear leukocytes. *Scand J Rheumatol* 1986;15:41–46.
38. Gay JC, Lukens JN, English DK. Differential inhibition of neutrophil superoxide generation by nonsteroidal antiinflammatory drugs. *Inflammation* 1984;8:209–222.
39. Bombardier C, Peloso PM, Goldsmith CH. Salsalate, a nonacetylated salicylate, is as efficacious as diclofenac in patients with rheumatoid arthritis. Salsalate-diclofenac study group. *J Rheumatol* 1995;22:617–624.
40. Litvak KM, McEvoy GK. Ketorolace, an injectable non-narcotic analgesic. *Clin Pharm* 1990;9:921–935.
41. Saag KG, Rubenstein LM, Chrischilles EA, Wallace RB. Nonsteroidal antiinflammatory drugs and cognitive decline in the elderly. *J Rheumatol* 1995;22:2142–2147.
42. Hoppmann RA, Peden JG, Ober SK. Central nervous system side effects of nonsteroidal antiinflammatory drugs. Aseptic meningitis, psychosis, and cognitive dysfunction. *Arch Intern Med* 1991;151:1309–1313.
43. Stevenson DD, Hougham, Schrank PJ, et al. Salsalate cross-sensitivty in aspirin-sensitive pateints with asthma. *J Allergy Clin Immunol* 1990; 86:749–758.
44. Robinson DR, Skosliewicz M, Bloch KJ, et al. Cyclooxygenase blockade elevates leukotriene E4 production during acute anaphylaxis in sheep. *J Exp Med* 1986;163:1509–1517.
45. Antiplatelet Trialists Collaboration Collaborative. Overview of randomised trials of antiplatelet therapy, I: prevention of death, myocardial infarction, and stroke by prolonged antiplatelet therapy in various categories of patients. *BMJ* 1994;308:81–106.
46. Silverstein FE, Faich G, Goldstein JL, et al. Gastrointestinal toxicity with celecoxib vs nonsteroidal anti-inflammatory drugs for osteoarthritis and rheumatoid arthritis: the CLASS study-a randomized controlled trial. *JAMA* 2000;284:1247–1255.
47. Bombardier C, Laine L, Reicin A, et al. Comparison of upper gastrointestinal toxicity of rofecoxib and naproxen in patients with rheumatoid arthritis. *N Engl J Med* 2000;343:1520–1528.
48. Garcia Rodriguez LA, Walker AM, Perez Gutthann S. Nonsteroidal antiinflammatory drugs and gastrointestinal hospitalizations in Saskatchewan: a cohort study. *Epidemiology* 1992;3:337–342.
49. Griffin MR, Piper JM, Daugherty JR, et al. Nonsteroidal anti-inflammatory drug use and increased risk for peptic ulcer disease in elderly persons. *Ann Intern Med* 1991;114:257–263.
50. Garcia Rodriguez LA. Nonsteroidal antiinflammatory drugs, ulcers and risk: a collaborative meta-analysis. *Semin Arthritis Rheum* 1997; 26(suppl):16–20.
51. Bjarnason I, Thjodleifsson B. Gastrointestinal toxicity of non-steroidal anti-inflammatory drugs: the effect of numesulide compared with naproxen on the human gastrointestinal tract. *Rheumatology* 1999;38 (suppl):24–32.
52. Holt S, Rigoglioso V, Sidhu M, et al.Nonsteroidal antiinflammatory drugs and lower gastrointestinal bleeding. *Dig Dis Sci* 1993;38:1619–1623.
53. Wilcox CM, Alexander LN, Cotsonis GA, Clark WS. Nonsteroidal antiinflammatory drugs are associated with both upper and lower gastrointestinal bleeding. *Dig Dis Sci* 1997;42:990–997.
54. Wallace JL, Bak A, McKnight W, et al. Cyclooxygenase I contributes to inflammatory reponses in rats and mice: implications for gastrointestinal toxicity. *Gastroenterology* 1998;115:101–109.
55. Singh G, Ramey DR, Morfeld D, et al. Gastrointestinal tract complications of nonsteroidal antiinflammatory drug treatment in rheumatoid arthritis. A prospective observational study. *Arch Intern Med* 1996; 156:1530–1536.
56. Simon LS, Zhao SZ, Arguelles LM, et al. Economic and gastrointestinal safety comparisons of etodolac, nabumetone and oxaprozin from insurance claims data from patients with arthritis. *Clin Ther* 1998; 1218–1235; discussion, 1192–1193.
57. Agrawal NM, Caldwell J, Kivitz AJ, et al. Comparison of the upper gastrointestinal safety of Arthrtoec 75 and nabumetone in osteoarthritis patients at high risk for developing nonsteroidal anti-inflammatory drug-induced gastrointestinal ulcers. *Clin Ther* 1999;21:659–674.
58. Larkai EN, Smith JL, Lidsky MD, Graham DY. Gastroduodenal mucosa and dyspeptic symptoms in arthritic patients during chronic nonsteroidal anti-inflammatory drug use. *Am J Gastroenterol* 1987;82:1153.
59. Minocha A, Greenbaum DS. Pill-esophagitis caused by non-steroidal antiinflammatory drugs. *Am J Gastroenterol* 1991;86:1086–1089.
60. Eng J, Sabanathan S. Drug-induced esophagitis. *Am J Gastroenterol* 1991;86:1127–1133.
61. Allison MC, Howatson AG, Torance CJ. Gastrointestinal damage associated with the use of nonsteroidal antiinflammatory drugs. *N Engl J Med* 1992;327:749–754.
62. Reuter BK, Asfaha S, Buret A, et al. Exacerbation of inflammation-associated colonic injury in rat through inhibition of cyclooxygenase-2. *J Clin Invest* 1996;98:2076–2085.
63. Mizuno H, Sakamoto C, Matsuda K, et al. Induction of cyclooxygenase 2 in gastric mucosal lesions and its inhibition by the specific antagonist delays healing in mice. *Gastroenterology* 1997;12:387–397.
64. Silverstein, FE, Graham, DY, Senior, JR, et al. Misoprostol reduces serious gastrointestinal complications in patients with rheumatoid arthritis receiving nonsteroidal anti-inflammatory drugs. *Ann Intern Med* 1995;123:214.
65. Simon LS, Hatoum HT, Bittman RM, et al. Risk factors for serious nonsteroidal-induced gastrointestinal complications: regression analysis of the MUCOSA trial. *Fam Med* 1996;28:202–208.
66. Graham DY, White RH, Moreland LW, et al. Duodenal and gastric ulcer prevention with misoprostol in arthritis patients taking NSAIDs. *Ann Intern Med* 1993;119:257–262.
67. Levine LR, Cloud ML, Enas NH. Nizatidine prevents peptic ulceration in high-risk patient taking nonsteroidal anti-inflammatory drugs. *Arch Intern Med* 1993;153:2449–2454.
68. Hawkey CJ, Karrasch JA, Szczepanski L, et al. Omeprazole compared with misoprostol for ulcers associated with nonsteroidal antiinflammatory drugs. *N Engl J Med* 1998;338:727–734.
69. Taha AS, Hudson N, Hawkey CJ, et al. Famotidine for the prevention of gastric and duodenal ulcers caused by nonsteroidal antiinflammaotry drugs. *N Engl J Med* 1996;334:1435–1439.
70. Gabriel SE, Jaakkimainen RL, Bombardier C. The cost-effectiveness of misoprostol for nonsteroidal antiinflammaotry drugs-associated adverse gastrointestinal events. *Arthritis Rheum* 1993;36:447–459.
71. Schlondorff D. Renal complications of nonsteroidal anti-inflammatory drugs. *Kidney Int* 1993;44:643–653.
72. Whelton A. Renal and related cardiovascular effects of conventional and COX-2 specific NSAIDs and non-NSAID analgesics. *Am J Ther* 2000;7:63–74.
73. Bennett WM, Henrich WL, Stoff JS. The renal effects of NSAIDs: summary and recommendation. *Am J Kidney Dis* 1996;28:56–62.
74. Pope JE, Anderson JJ, Felson DT. A meta-analysis of the effects of nonsteroidal anti-inflammatory drugs on blood pressure. *Arch Intern Med* 1993;153:477–484.
75. Harris RC, McKanna JA, Aiai Y, et al. Cyclooxygenase-2 is associated with the macula densa of rat kidney and increases with salt restriction. *J Clin Invest* 1994;94:2504–2510.
76. Garcia Rodriguez LA, Williams R, Derby LE, Dean AD, Jick H. Acute liver injury asociated with nonsteroidal antiinflammatory drugs and the role of risk factors. *Arch Intern Med* 1994;154:311–316.

77. Walker AM. Quantitative studies of the risk of serious hepatic injury in persons using nonsteroidal antiinflammatory drugs. *Arthritis Rheum* 1997;40:201–208.
78. Helfgott SM, Sandberg-Cook J, Zakim D, Nestler J. Diclofenac-associated hepatotoxicity. *JAMA* 1990;264:2660–2662.
79. Simon LS, Mills JA. Drug therapy: nonsteroidal antiinflammatory drugs. *N Engl J Med* 1980;302:1179–1185, 1237–1243.
80. Nielsen GL, Sorensen HT, Larsen H, Pedersen L. Risk of adverse birth outcome and miscarriage in pregnant users of NSAIDs: population based observational study and case-control study. *BMJ* 2001;322:266–270.
81. Kawaguchi H, Pilbeam CC, Harrison JR, Raisz LG. The role of prostaglandins in the regulation of bone metabolism. *Clin Orthop* 1995; 313:36–46.
82. Pilbeam CC, Fall PM, Alander CB, Raisz LG. Differential effects of nonsteroidal anti-inflammatory drugs on constitutive and inducible prostaglandin G/H synthase in cultured bone cells. *J Bone Miner Res* 1997;12:1198–1203.
83. Strom BL, Carson JL, Schinnar R, et al. Nonsteroidal anti-inflammatory drugs and neutropenia. *Arch Intern Med* 1993;153: 2119–2124.

CHAPTER 62 ADJUVANT ANALGESICS

Steven Macres, Steven Richeimer, and Paul Duran

INTRODUCTION

Traditionally, the opioid analgesics and the nonsteroidal anti-inflammatory drugs have been the mainstay for primary analgesia. Numerous other agents, however, are available in our vast pharmacopeia that are beneficial as primary or adjuvant analgesics, particularly for chronic nonmalignant pain that is neuropathic in origin. This vast array of drugs includes the antidepressants, the anticonvulsants, systemic local anesthetics, psychostimulants, neuroleptics, autonomic drugs, calcium channel blockers, skeletal muscle relaxants, *N*-methyl-D-aspartate (NMDA) receptor antagonists, corticosteroids, capsaicin, cannabinoids, and various other miscellaneous agents (e.g., tramadol, lithium, magnesium, neuronal nicotinic acetylcholine receptor ligands, butyl-*p*-amino benzoate, bupivacaine microspheres, and SNX-111).

Classically, the nociceptive pathway consists of a three neuron chain, dual-ascending system, which can transmit pain signals from the periphery to the cerebral cortex. The cell bodies for the first-, second-, and third-order neurons reside in the dorsal root ganglion, dorsal horn, and thalamus, respectively. The dual-ascending system runs in parallel and consists of the Aδ and C fibers. The thinly myelinated Aδ fibers transmit "first pain," which tends to be sharp, stinging, and discriminatory in nature. The unmyelinated C fibers transmit "second pain," which is more diffuse, has a persistent burning quality, and carries an affective-motivational component to it. Injury to this neuronal pathway is believed to precipitate neuropathic pain. Examples of chronic neuropathic pain are listed in Table 62-1, and surgical procedures associated with neuropathic pain are shown in Table 62-2.

The pathophysiologic mechanisms that theoretically underlie neuropathic pain are numerous and may involve ectopic impulses, neurogenic inflammation, changes in protein expression associated with gene-regulated c-fos, neuropeptide changes, ephaptic connections, sympathetic dysfunction, death of inhibitory spinal neurons, peripheral and central neuronal sprouting, central sensitization, and inflammation of nervi nevorum.[1] On physical examination, patients with neuropathic pain classically display allodynia, hyperalgesia, and hyperpathia.

Attenuation of nociceptive transmission can be accomplished at various points along this pain pathway, which includes transduction, transmission, modulation, and perception. The purpose of this chapter is to discuss the numerous drugs available to achieve this. The goal is to tailor the patient's analgesic regimen by administering the appropriate drug, in the correct dose, and by the most appropriate route of administration so as to maximize analgesia and minimize side effects. Frequently, additive or even synergistic effects can be obtained by combining different types of drugs. Drug combinations may allow for the use of smaller doses and diminish side effects.

ANTIDEPRESSANTS

The use of antidepressants for the treatment of chronic pain dates back many years. Paoli et al were the first to describe the use of imipramine in the treatment of chronic pain in 1960.[2] It was not until 1964, however, that a placebo-controlled, crossover trial was performed that suggested the efficacy of amitriptyline in the treatment of migraine headache.[3] Although data from 60 controlled clinical trials[4,5] have been published since that time, suggesting the efficacy of antidepressant drugs for the treatment of chronic nonmalignant pain, controversy persists. A recent meta-analysis of 39 placebo-controlled studies by Onghena and Van Houdenhove,[5] however, revealed that antidepressants can be effective and that the "average chronic pain patient who receives an antidepressant treatment is better off than 74% of the chronic pain patients who receive placebo." The authors further conclude that the antidepressants have a direct analgesic effect independent of their antidepressant activity. Chronic pain conditions, particularly those with a neuropathic component that consists of a steady burning, lancinating, or shock-like pain, appear to benefit from a trial of antidepressants.[6,7] In the United States the commonly used antidepressants fall into several categories that include the tertiary amine and secondary amine tricyclics antidepressants, the selective serotonin reuptake inhibitors, and the atypical antidepressants.

TRICYCLIC ANTIDEPRESSANTS

The first-generation tricyclics (Table 62-3) have been the most commonly employed antidepressants for the treatment of chronic pain conditions. Amitriptyline is the prototypical tricyclic antidepressant that has been the most studied and has proved to be the most effective. Tricyclic antidepressants are most useful in the treatment of pain that is neuropathic in origin or secondary to central deafferation, particularly if it is burning or lancinating in nature. The onset of pain relief appears to be biphasic. Immediate relief is reported to occur within hours to days and is probably secondary to inhibition of catecholamine reuptake. Delayed analgesia, which occurs 2 to 4 weeks later, may be due to receptor effects of the antidepressants.[8] The tricyclic antidepressants can be considered to be coanalgesic agents that may potentiate the effects of opioids.[7,9] Several trials have described the "opioid sparing" effects of antidepressant medications, particularly in cancer pain patients with both a neuropathic and non-neuropathic component to their pain.[10,11]

Chronic pain conditions that respond well to tricyclic antidepressants include painful diabetic polyneuropathy, postherpetic neuralgia, atypical facial pain, headaches, central pain, and cancer pain. Chronic painful conditions that respond less briskly to these agents, but certainly warrant a trial, include post-laminectomy syn-

TABLE 62-1 **Examples of Chronic Neuropathic Pain**

Complex regional pain syndromes
Type 1: reflex sympathetic dystrophy (RSD)
Type 2: causalgia
Postherpetic neuralgia
Phantom limb pain
Trigeminal neuralgia
Neuroma
Entrapment neuropathy
Peripheral neuropathy
Diabetic
Alcoholic
Cancer pain components
Myelopathy
Post-traumatic
HIV

drome, phantom limb pain, stump pain, sympathetically mediated pain, post-thoracotomy pain syndrome, postmastectomy pain pain syndrome, and rheumatologic disorders.[4–7]

Pharmacokinetics

The tricyclic antidepressants have good bioavailability after oral administration. They undergo extensive first-pass metabolism in the liver and are highly protein-bound. The drugs are highly lipophilic, and as a result, the apparent volumes of distribution range from 10 to 50 L/kg. Elimination half-lives range from 20 hours for amitriptyline to 80 hours for protriptyline, which allows single daily dosing usually at bedtime.[12,13] It is noteworthy to mention that these drugs do have active metabolites. Amitriptyline and imipramine are metabolized to nortriptyline and desipramine, respectively. This is an important point to keep in mind if serum levels of the drugs are to be obtained. The serum concentration that correlates with antidepressant effects is reported to be in the range of 50 to 300 ng/mL.[13] It is unclear, however, what the therapeutic analgesic concentration should be. Watson et al[14] describe a therapeutic window for the analgesic effects of amitriptyline. Although this observation has yet to be corroborated, it appears that the effective analgesic serum level is often lower than that required for antidepressant effects.

Mechanism of Action

Traditionally, effective tricyclic antidepressant activity has been associated with the ability of the drugs to exert their action on affect through modulation of monamine neurotransmitter activity at the level of the synapse (biogenic amine hypothesis of depression). Specifically, this involves the inhibition of reuptake of serotonin and norepinephrine by the amine pump. Recent research further suggests that long-term administration of antidepressants can cause an increased sensitivity of postsynaptic α_1-adrenergic and serotonergic receptors with a concomitant decreased sensitivity of presynaptic receptors (e.g., re-regulation), resulting in normalization of neurotransmitter efficacy.[12,13] The analgesic effects of this class of drugs is independent of their antidepressant properties.[6] Norepinephrine reuptake blockade appears to make the major contribution to analgesia from the antidepressants, whereas serotonin reuptake inhibition may serve only to enhance the analgesic effects of norepinephrine reuptake inhibition.[7] Other mechanisms for analgesia that have been proposed include:

1. Direct analgesic effect[15]
   a. Inhibition of sodium channel activity[15]
   b. α-adrenergic blockade[7,8]
   c. NMDA receptor antagonism[7,17]
2. Relief of comorbid depression[5]
3. A decrease in pain-related symptoms such as insomnia[5]
4. Potentiation of opioid analgesia.[8,18]

The side-effect profile of the tricyclic antidepressants reflects their blockade of muscarinic, adrenergic, and histamine receptors. Predominant among the side effects are the anticholinergic symptoms, which include dry mouth, constipation, blurred vision, and urinary retention. Care should therefore be taken when dosing these agents in patients with a history of narrow-angle glaucoma or benign prostatic hypertrophy. Other side effects include sedation and orthostatic hypotension, so extreme care should be exercised when dosing these drugs in the elderly. Since these side effects are more prominent with the tertiary amines (e.g., amitriptyline, imipramine), prudence would dictate the use of a secondary amine (e.g., nortriptyline, desipramine), which can cause less sedation, orthostasis, and anticholinergic effects. Because these drugs can lower the seizure threshold (in particular maprotiline), they should be used with caution in patients with a seizure disorder or in combination with other medications that also lower seizure threshold (e.g., phenothiazines, tramadol). Other side effects that the patient should be cautioned about include appetite stimulation and weight gain. Side effects, which generally result in termination of therapy, include postural hypotension, tachycardia, impotence, priapism (trazodone), gynecomastia in the male, urinary retention, blurred vision, confusion, hallucinations, and excessive sedation.[12,13]

Cardiovascular side effects of concern include altered cardiac conduction with prolongation of the QT interval, tachycardia, ventricular arrhythmias, and hypotension. We recommend a baseline electrocardiogram for all patients age 40 years and older prior to the initiation of tricyclic antidepressant therapy. Prudence dictates that tricyclic antidepressants be avoided immediately following a

TABLE 62-2 **Surgical Procedures Associated with Neuropathic Pain**

Amputation
Lateral thoracotomy
Inguinal herniorrhaphy
Abdominal hysterectomy
Saphenous vein stripping
Open cholecystectomy
Nephrectomy
Mastectomy

TABLE 62-3 **Tricyclic Antidepressants**

Drug	Anticholinergic Side Effect*	Starting Dose (Adult)	Other
Tertiary Amines			
Amitriptyline	++++	10–30 mg po@hs	Very sedating
Imipramine	++	10–30 mg po@hs	
Doxepin	++	10–30 mg po@hs	
Secondary Amines			
Desipramine	+	10–30 mg po@hs	Less sedation than amitriptyline
Nortriptyline	++	10–30 mg po@hs	Less orthostasis than amitriptyline
Protriptyline	+++	5 mg po tid	May have a mild stimulative effect

*0 = none; + slight; ++ moderate; +++ high; and ++++ very high.

myocardial infarction, particularly in the presence of a bundle branch block. Consultation with the patient's cardiologist prior to initiation of therapy is recommended.

Withdrawal symptoms consistent with cholinergic rebound can occur if the drugs are not gradually discontinued over the course of 5 to 10 days. Reported symptoms include gastrointestinal distress, restlessness, and sleep disturbance.

Dosing Guidelines

Unlike the dosing regimen utilized for the treatment of depression, doses of tricyclic antidepressants for the treatment of chronic pain may be considerably less. Usually, we begin dosing at the lower end of the spectrum and titrate upward until we obtain acceptable analgesia or unacceptable side effects. A dose-response curve for analgesia with amitriptyline has been described.[19] A typical dosing regimen for amitriptyline may begin at 10 to 25 mg orally at bedtime. This can be escalated in 10 to 25 mg increments every 3 to 7 days. The dose may be gradually increased to full antidepressant levels if pain relief or significant side effects do not occur at lower levels. Should the patient experience acceptable analgesia but intolerable side effects, consider substituting a secondary amine (e.g., nortriptyline, desipramine) that has fewer anticholinergic and sedating side effects. Desipramine selectively blocks reuptake of norepinephrine and has the lowest incidence of anticholinergic side effects and sedation.[7,12,13] What constitutes the optimal analgesic dose for this class of drugs is unclear; however, if depression is associated with the patient's pain, then antidepressant doses (e.g., amitriptyline 150 to 300 mg/day) are clearly indicated.

ATYPICAL ANTIDEPRESSANTS

This category of antidepressants includes trazodone, nefazodone, bupropion, and venlafaxine (Table 62-4). Trazodone is a triazolopyridine that selectively inhibits the reuptake of serotonin by brain synaptosomes. It is well absorbed after oral administration and is extensively metabolzied in the liver. Less than 1% of the drug is eliminated unchanged in the urine. Elimination is biphasic with a terminal half-life of approximately 8 hours.[13] The drug is moderately sedating, with a potency approximately one half that of amitriptyline. It is primarily used for comorbid depression and sleep induction, and appears to have little analgesic efficacy. Although rare, the side effect of priapism should prompt discontinuation.

Nefazodone is a phenylpiperazine that is chemically related to trazodone. Unlike trazodone, however, nefazodone inhibits the reuptake of both serotonin and norepinephrine. The drug has fewer anticholiinergic side effects than the traditional tricyclic antidepressants and is less likely to cause sexual dysfunction.[13] Nefazodone may have analgesic properties since it has been shown to potentiate opioid analgesia in an animal model.[20] It is advised that nefazodone not be coadministered with either of the antihistamines astemizole or terfenadine since the plasma levels of these drugs

TABLE 62-4 **Miscellaneous Antidepressants**

Drug	Anticholinergic Side Effects*	Starting Dose (Adult)	Other
Venlafaxine	0	25 mg po tid	Associated with dose dependent increase in supine diastolic blood pressure
Trazodone	+	25–50 mg po@hs	Elevated doses associate with priapism
Bupropion	++	75 mg po bid to tid (increase dose slowly)	Increased risk of seizure @ daily doses exceeding 450 mg
Nefazodone	0/+	100 mg po bid	Structurally related to trazodone

*0 = none; + slight; ++ moderate; +++ high; and ++++ very high.

can become elevated, resulting in potentially fatal QT prolongation or torsades de pointes.[13]

Bupropion is classified as an aminoketone antidepressant and is structurally unrelated to the other antidepressants. Its exact mechanism of action is unclear at this time, but it is reported to be a weak blocker of serotonin, norepinephrine, and dopamine reuptake. Evidence of analgesic effects is sparse; however, it is marketed as a non-nicotine alternative for smoking cessation. Care should be employed when dosing the drug, since bupropion is associated with an increased risk of seizures, particularly at doses in excess of 450 mg per day. The seizure risk is decreased by dosing the drug on a three times daily schedule with each individual dose not to exceed 150 mg, which avoids high peak serum concentrations.

Venlafaxine is chemically unrelated to the other tricyclic or tetracyclic antidepressants. It may, however, have some analgesic efficacy since, like the tricyclic antidepressants, it inhibits the reuptake of both serotonin and norepinephrine at the synaptic junction. Unlike the tricyclic antidepressants, anticholinergic side effects are less bothersome. The drug can cause a sustained elevation of the supine diastolic blood pressure, particularly at doses in excess of 300 mg per day. It is recommended that the dose be lowered or the drug discontinued if elevation of the diastolic blood pressure persists.

SELECTIVE SEROTONIN REUPTAKE INHIBITORS

The newer selective serotonin reuptake inhibitors (SSRIs) include fluoxetine, paroxetine, sertraline, and fluvoxamine (Table 62-5). These drugs may be useful as adjuvant analgesics[8]; however, evidence to date suggests that serotonin reuptake blockade alone is insufficient for analgesia, but it is possible that it will enhance the analgesic effects of norepinephrine reuptake blockade.[7] These drugs have been recommended for the treatment of headaches and diabetic neuropathy,[13,21–24] chronic pelvic pain,[25] and fibrositis.[26] Common side effects with the SSRIs include insomnia, agitation, anxiety, tremor, sexual dysfunciton, and gastrointestinal distress. Fluoxetine can cause significant weight loss, especially in underweight depressed patients.[13] At present, we cannot recommend SSRIs as the primary agent for the treatment of chronic pain. Further research as to their efficacy is warranted.

ANTICONVULSANTS

The anticonvulsants are a diverse group of drugs that include phenytoin, carbamazepine, valproic acid, clonazepam, gabapentin, and lamotrigine (Table 62-6). It is widely accepted that they are effective analgesics for chronic neuropathic pain, particularly if it is lancinating and burning in nature.[15,27]

The anticonvulsants have proven to be particularly effective against trigeminal neuralgia, glossopharyngeal neuralgia, postherpetic neuralgia, and diabetic neuropathies.[27–29] The anticonvulsants may also be indicated for the treatment of cancer pain, which has a neuropathic component.[1] Carbamazepine is usually the drug of choice; however, numerous other agents are available. Unlike the other anticonvulsants, valproic acid has found some success in treating migraine headaches.[30,31] Clonazepam has proved beneficial for lancinating phantom limb pain.[32] Recently, gabapentin has been added to our pharmacopeia and there are numerous case reports that suggest efficacy in complex regional pain syndromes, radicular pain, migraine headache, postherpetic neuralgia, diabetic neuropathy, multiple sclerosis, and idiopathic peripheral neuropathies.[15,33–35] Recently, two randomized, double blind, placebo-controlled trials have been conducted and they suggest that gabapentin monotherapy may be efficacious in the treatment of pain and sleep disturbance associated with painful diabetic polyneuropathy and postheretic neuralgia.[36,37] We have personally had gratifying results with gabapentin in the treatment of phantom limb pain and syringomyelia (unpublished data in 1988 and 1989).

Pharmacokinetics

Carbamazepine is an anticonvulsant that has proved useful in the treatment of trigeminal neuralgia since the 1960s. The drug is an iminostilbene derivative, which is chemically similar to the tricyclic antidepressant. It is slowly and erratically absorbed following oral administration and is metabolized in the liver to an active 10,11-epoxide metabolite. Less than 3% of the drug is excreted unchanged in the urine. Although its initial half-life is 25 to 65 hours, this can decrease to 12 to 17 hours since the drug can induce its own metabolism.[38,39]

Although phenytoin was first synthesized in 1908, its anticonvulsant potential was not realized until 1938. The drug's pharmacokinetics are somewhat complicated. It is slowly absorbed from the small intestine and the rate and extent of its absorbtion is dependent on the product formulation. The drug is primarily metabolized in the liver to inactive hydroxylated metabolites. Less than 5% is excreted unchanged in the urine. At plasma concentrations <10 μg/mL elimination is exponential (first order) and the half-life of the drug is approximately 6 to 24 hours. At higher concentrations, however, elimination is dose-dependent and the half-life can increase to 20 to 60 hours.[38,39]

TABLE 62-5 **Selective Serotonin Reuptake Inhibitors**

Drug	Anticholinergic Side Effect*	Starting Dose (Adult)	Other
Fluoxetine	0/+	20 mg po q am	May be associated with significant weight loss. May increase TCA's serum levels.
Paroxetine	0	10 mg po q am	May be useful for chronic daily headache
Sertraline	0	50 mg po q am or @ hs	—
Fluvoxamine	0/+	50 mg po @ hs	—

*0 = none; + slight; ++ moderate; +++ high; and ++++ very high.

TCA denotes tricyclic antidepressants.

TALE 62-6 **Anticonvulsants**

Drug	Starting Dose (Adult)	Precautions
Carbamazepine	100–150 mg po bid	Monitor blood count and liver function tests periodically
Phenytoin	100–200 mg	Monitor blood count and liver function tests periodically
Valproic acid	250 mg po qd to bid	Monitor blood count and liver function tests periodically
Clonazepam	1/2–1 mg po tid (A single dose may be administered at hs)	Monitor blood count and liver function tests periodically
Gabapentin	400 mg po qd	Adjust dose in renal failure*
Lamotrigine	25–50 mg po bid	Associated with severe, potentially life-threatening rash
Topiramate	50 mg po @ hs Increase @ intervals of 50 mg po q week to a maximum dose of 200 mg po bid	Adjust dose in renal failure Increase fluid intake to decrease the risk of stone formation

*See Table 62-7.

Valproic acid is rapidly absorbed following oral administration. The drug is primarily metabolized in the liver and has a relatively short half-life of 10 hours. Very little parent drug is eliminated in the urine or feces.[38,39]

Clonazepam is a long-acting benzodiazepine, which, in addition to its anticonvulsant and anxiolytic effects, may have some utility in chronic neuropathic pain. The bioavailability of the drug is 90%. It is metabolized by the cytochrome P-450 system to the inactive 7-amino or 7-acetyl-amino derivative and has an elimination half-life of 18 to 50 hours.[38,39]

Gabapentin is a recently developed anticonvulsant that was designed as a structural analogue of γ-aminobutyric acid (GABA). It does not, however, display selectivity for GABA receptors. The bioavailability of the drug is not dose-proportional and a 400-mg dose is approximately 25% less available than a 100-mg dose. The average bioavailability is about 60% and is not affected by food. Less than 3% of the drug is bound to plasma proteins. Gabapentin does not undergo hepatic clearance, rather it is 100% eliminated by the kidney and is therefore dependent on creatinine clearance. Elimination half-life is 5 to 7 hours, which increases in the elderly and in individuals with impaired renal function (Table 62-7). Downward adjustment of the dose is therefore necessary in these circumstances. The drug is removed from plasma during hemodialysis.[38,39]

Lamotrigine is rapidly and completely absorbed following oral administration with a bioavailability of about 98%. The drug is approximately 55% protein bound and is metabolically cleared by the liver to the inactive 2-*N*-glucuronide conjugated metabolite. Approximately 10% of the drug appears unchanged in the urine and has a half-life of approximately 13 hours.[38,39]

Mechanism of Action

The pathophysiology underlying neuropathic pain may involved epileptiform discharges or spontaneous electrical activity involving ectopic foci or dysfunctional sodium channels in injured nerves.[1,15] Anticonvulsants are thought to suppress this spontaneous neuronal firing through various mechanisms.

Phenytoin, carbamazepine, valproic acid, and lamotrigine slow the rate of recovery of inactivated sodium channels, which may have a stabilizing effect on neural membranes.[38,39] In addition, valproic acid inhibits voltage-activated calcium channels and increases GABA levels by increasing synthesis and decreasing metabolism.[38] Clonazepam acts at the $GABA_A$ receptor and enhances chloride ion reflux resulting in synaptic inhibition.[38,39] The mechanism of action of gabapentin is unclear at the present time. It does not interact with benzodiazepine, glutamate, glycine, $GABA_A$, $GABA_B$, or NMDA receptors.[40] Gabapentin is reported to be similar to phenytoin and carabamazepine because it can suppress segmental and descending excitatory pain pathways yet facilitate segmental inhibitory pathways.[41] Like valproic acid, it is reported to increase brain synthesis of GABA.[40] Gabapentin is also reported to increase serotonin levels in humans.[41]

Dosing Guidelines and Side Effects

The dosing of carbamazepine in adults usually begins at 100 to 150 mg orally twice daily. This is slowly titrated upward, over several weeks, as tolerated, to a maximum dose of 1200 mg per day. Common dose-related side effects include dizziness, drowsiness, ataxia, nausea, and vomiting. Idiosyncratic reactions include aplastic anemia, liver failure, Stevens-Johnson syndrome, leukopenia, and thrombocytopenia. A baseline blood count and liver function test should be obtained prior to therapy, then monthly for 2 to 3 months, and finally every 4 to 6 months thereafter as deemed appropriate. Significant drug interactions have been reported. Coadministration of carbamazepine with fluoxetine, tricyclic antidepressants, cimetidine, diltiazem, verapamil, and propoxyphene have been reported to increase carbamazepine levels.[13(pp1832–1900)38]

Generally speaking, the average adult dose of phenytoin is 200 to 300 mg orally at bedtime. Thereafter the dose can be titrated up in 100 mg increments every 1 to 2 weeks. It is rare to exceed 400 mg orally at bedtime. Although the ideal anticonvulsant serum concentraiton is 10 to 20 μg/mL, this does not necessarily correlate with the optimal analgesic dose, which has yet to be defined. Prudence dictates that serum concentrations in excess of 20 μg/mL should not be exceeded. Since the elimination of phenytoin can be dose-dependent at higher doses, slow escalation of the dose, in 25 to 50 mg increments, is advised when dosing beyond 300 mg per day. Dose-related side effects generally involve the central nervous system and include ataxia, diplopia, nystagmus, vertigo, and confusion. Gastrointestinal side effects include nausea and vomiting. Morbilliform skin rash can occur in 2% to 5% of patients. Blood dyscrasias and hepatotoxic side effects have been reported, so baseline complete blood counts and liver function tests, with periodic monitoring, are advised. Long-term use of phenytoin can precipitate gingival hyperplasia, the incidence of which can be reduced with good oral hygiene, gum massage, and regular dental checkups.[38,39]

The usual starting dose for valproic acid for an adult is 250 mg orally once or twice a day. This can then be escalated weekly, in 250-mg increments as tolerated, to a maximum of 1000 to 2000 mg per day. The usual effective dose for epilepsy is 15 mg/kg/day. Drug-related side effects included sedation, ataxia, nystagmus, diplopia, dysarthria, confusion, and incoordination. Thrombocytopenia and abnormal coagulation indices can occur, and fatal hepatotoxicity has been reported. Platelet counts and liver function tests should be obtained prior to therapy and at frequent intervals thereafter.[38,39]

Although the recommended dosage range for clonazepam is 0.5 to 20 mg per day, dosing for neuropathic pain rarely exceeds 10 mg per day, and much lower doses can be effective. Common side effects associated with clonazepam include sedation, fatigue, dysarthria, and dizziness. The drug is therefore ideally dosed at bedtime to minimize these effects. Since the drug is a benzodiazepine, physical dependence and withdrawal symptoms consisting of restlessness, irritability, tremors, and insomnia can occur, so it is recommended that the drug be tapered and not abruptly discontinued.[38,39]

Although gabapentin can be prescribed at a dose as high as 3600 mg per day for epilepsy,[39] the ideal dose for neuropathic pain is unknown. Since the drug can cause sedation and dizziness, it is ideally dosed at bedtime during initial dose titration. A typical dosing regimen we use is 300 mg orally at bedtime, which is slowly escalated upward by 300 mg every 3 days as tolerated. If the patient does not experience significant analgesia at 1800 to 2400 mg per day, then the patient is slowly tapered off the drug over 7 days. The drug has a relatively benign side-effect profile; however, sedation, dizziness, ataxia, and confusion are common complaints, particularly if dosage escalation is too fast. Other less common side effects include headache and constipation.[38,39] Dosage adjustment is necessary in renal failure (see Table 62-7).

SYSTEMIC LOCAL ANESTHETICS

Evidence suggests that the systemic administration of a local anesthetic can effectively treat pain, particularly if it is neuropathic in nature. Early studies described successful treatment of acute pain syndromes such as postoperative pain,[42] burn pain,[43] and cancer pain.[44] Subsequent clinical reports have demonstrated the effectiveness in reducing pain associated with diabetic neuropathy,[45] postherpetic neuralgia,[46] amputation stump pain, chemotherapeutic and post-irradiation neuralgia,[47] thalamic pain syndrome,[48] radiculopathy, arachnoiditis, phantom pain, and the lightening pains of tabes dorsalis.[49] Commonly used drugs include intravenous lidocaine and the orally active agents mexiletine and tocainide. These drugs are usually third-line drugs after the patient has received a trial of an antidepressant or an anticonvulsant. Because tocainide has a greater risk of toxicity (e.g., blood dyscrasias and pulmonary fibrosis), mexiletine is our oral local anesthetic of choice.

TABLE 62-7 **Gabapentin Dosing Based on Renal Function**

Creatinine Clearance (mL/min)	Dosing Regimen Adult (mg)
>60	400 tid
30–60	300 bid
15–30	300 qd
<15	300 qod

Hemodialysis loading dose = 300–400 mg, followed by 200 to 300 mg after each 4-hour dialysis.

Pharmacokinetics

Orally administered lidocaine has poor bioavailability since 60% to 70% of the drug is metabolized by the liver before reaching the systemic circulation. The drug is dealkylated to monoethylglycine xylidide (MEGX) and glycine xylidide (GX), both of which have antiarrhythmic and convulsant properties. The elimination half-life is 1.5 to 2 hours and can increase in the event of decreased liver blood flow (e.g., congestive heart failure). Analgesic effects are usually seen at serum levels of 1 to 3 μg/ml.[50]

Mexiletine has excellent oral bioavailability. It is metabolized in the liver primarily to *N*-methylmexiletine which is less than 20% the potency of the parent drug. The mean elimination half-life is 10 to 12 hours, which can increase to 25 hours with hepatic impairment. Only 10% of the drug is excreted unchanged by the kidney, and therefore renal impairment has minimal effect on half-life.[50] Analgesic effects have been reported at mean serum levels of 0.76 μg/ml.[51]

Mechanism of Action

The exact mechanism of action of systemic local anesthetics in pain control is unknown. Analgesia has been reported at serum levels well below that necessary to block normal peripheral nerve conduction.[51] Evidence suggests that the effect may involve selective blockade of pain fibers within the spinal cord or the dorsal root ganglia.[52,53] Abram and Yaksh demonstrated that the systemic administration of lidocaine can inhibit nociception and "windup" in an experimental model.[54]

Dosing Guidelines

There are a few case reports in the literature that describe patients who experience short-term benefit from systemic lidocaine, the duration of which far exceeds the duration of the drug based on pharmacokinetic parameters.[45,55] Unfortunately, this has not been consistent. We therefore do not routinely perform lidocaine infusions unless we plan on starting mexiletine, since systemic lidocaine may be predictive of a positive repsonse to mexiletine.[51]

Before a lidocaine infusion, prudence would dictate obtaining a cardiology consultation for patients who are at risk for cardiac disease. Full cardiac monitoring should be performed and resuscitation equipment should be immediately available. Our practice is to administer 3 to 5 mg/kg of lidocaine intravenously over 30 minutes. Five minutes prior to commencing the lidocaine infusion, the patient will be receiving only normal saline. At all times the patient is blinded to the procedure and verbal analog scores are documented before the infusion and every 5 to 10 minutes thereafter. A positive response to placebo results in termination of the trial.

Dosing of mexiletine is begun at 150 mg orally at bedtime. This is slowly escalated as tolerated by 150 mg every 72 hours until there is adequate analgesia, or a maximum of 10 mg/kg/day is achieved.[56] The only absolute contraindication for the use of mexiletine is cardiogenic shock, second- or third-degree heart block, or known allergy to the medication.[50]

Side Effects

Lidocaine side effects involve the central nervous system (CNS) and cardiovascular system. At low doses initial CNS symptoms include lightheadedness and dizziness. Other symptoms include tinnitus, vertigo, blurred vision, and altered taste. Seizures occur at higher doses. Cardiovascular side effects, which occur at even higher serum concentrations, include hypotension, bradycardia, and cardiovascular collapse, which can lead to cardiac arrest.[50]

Common dose-related side effects from mexiletine include nausea, vomiting, diplopia, and tremor, hence the rationale for slowly escalating the dose. Taking the drug with a meal can decrease the gastrointestinal side effects without severely impairing absorbtion. Since mexiletine can increase atrioventricular conduction time, it is contraindicated in patients with second- or third-degree heart block.[50]

PSYCHOSTIMULANTS

Although the psychostimulants are not considered to be primary analgesics, they have proven to be beneficial adjuvant agents for both chronic malignant and nonmalignant pain. There benefits include potentiation of opioid analgesia, attenuation of opioid-related sedation and cognitive deficits and their antidepressant effect.[57,58]

The mechanism of action of the psychostimulants is thought to be related to their ability to release norepinephrine from presynaptic stores, inhibition of norepinephrine reuptake, and their dopaminergic properties.[59] Amphetamines increase arousal and maintain attention and concentration. Representative drugs include methylphenidate, dextroamphetamine, and pemoline.

Psychostimulants are rarely prescribed in our practice, and only after the patient has failed numerous other medications. The only exception to this rule, however, is the patient with cancer-related pain. A careful history and physical examination should be conducted. Care should be taken to exclude any psychiatric disorder. These drugs are contraindicated in any patient with a history of hallucinations, delirium, or paranoid disorder. The drugs are relatively contraindicated in patients with a substance abuse history. Medical contraindications include patients with hyperthyroidism, seizure disorder, arrhythmias, uncontrolled hypertension, or angina.

Usual starting doses for the psychostimulants are 5 to 10 mg of methylphenidate, 2.5 to 5 mg of dextroamphetamine, and 18.75 mg of pemoline.[58] Doses can be administered twice daily in the morning and at noon, which will avoid evening insomnia.[59]

NEUROLEPTICS

Neuroleptics are a diverse group of drugs that include the phenothiazines, thioxanthenes, butyrophenones, and the dibenzazepines. Their antipsychotic mechanism of action is presumed to involve dopamine receptor blockade. Their efficacy in pain management is suspect at best. The literature is replete with claims of efficacy for diabetic neuropathy,[60] postherpetic neuralgia,[61] trigeminal neuralgia,[61] migraine,[63] and tension headache.[64] Although these drugs have been employed in the management of pain for many years, there is no evidence from controlled trials to suggest any analgesic properties.[65]

The only indication for the use of neuroleptics in pain management is when pain is part of a psychotic disorder, or in the management of associated nausea, agitation, or delirium. Occasionally, neuroleptics can be useful in the patient with chronic pain who has problems with controlling anger. Long-term use of neuroleptics can result in tardive dyskinesia, which can be irreversible.[65]

The only neuroleptic drug that has displayed analgesic effects in controlled trials is methotrimeprazine. The drug is a phenothiazine derivative that is only available for intramuscular injection. Suggested dosing is 5 to 40 mg every 4 to 6 hours. The drug's side-effects profile includes sedation and hypotension. In the adult, 10 mg of morphine sulfate administered subcutaneously is equianalgesic to 10 to 15 mg of methotrimeprazine.[65]

ANTIANXIETY AGENTS AND THE SEDATIVE HYPNOTICS

Benzodiazepines

The benzodiazepines comprise some of the most commonly prescribed medications in our pharmacopeia. Indications for the prescribing of benzodiazepines include anxiety and sleep disorders and as anticonvulsants and antispasmotics. Unlabeled uses include irritable bowel syndrome, panic attacks, depression, premenstrual syndrome, status epilepticus, nausea and vomiting associated with chemotherapy, sedative hypnotic withdrawal syndrome, and psychogenic catatonia.[66,67] Definitive data attesting to the analgesic effects of the benzodiazepines is sparse.[68,69] Chronic pain, however, is often associated with chronic anxiety, insomnia, and muscle tension. The anxiolytic effects of the benodiazepines may underlie their ability to decrease the stress response and autonomic nervous system arousal, which can exacerbate pain. Neuropathic pain, which is lancinating in nature, appears to respond best to the benzodiazepines.[69]

Benzodiazepines potentiate the effecs of GABA throughout the central nervous system. Recent evidence indicates that there may be at least two types of benzodiazepine receptors. The BZ_1 receptor appears to mediate sleep, whereas the BZ_2 receptor is associated with memory, motor, sensory, and cognitive functions.[66,67]

Although dizepam and midazolam have proved useful in the reduction of acute postoperative pain,[70,71] their usefulness is probably secondary to their ability to decrease anxiety, tension, and insomnia. Although the efficacy of benzodiazepines for the treatment of chronic nonmalignant pain is not abundant, studies suggest that benzodiazepines may be beneficial for chronic tension headaches, temporomandibular joint dysfunction, and trigeminal neuralgia.[68,72] Other conditions that may benefit from benzodiazepines include phantom limb pain,[32] opioid-induced myoclonus,[73] paroxysmal post-laminectomy pain, and post-traumatic neuralgias.[15]

Clonazepam is our benzodiazepine of choice for neuropathic pain that is described as lancinating in nature. Since the drug has a long half-life (18 to 50 hours),[67] it can be dosed once a day, preferably at bedtime since it may cause sedation. Treatment is usually initiate at 1 mg at bedtime and titrated upward as tolerated.

The drug can be dosed three times a day if side effects are not a problem. Although the maximum recommended anticonvulsant dose is 20 mg per day, we will typically use doses of 1 to 4 mg per day for neuropathic pain.

Long-term administration of benzodiazepines for chronic pain is controversial. They can cause cognitive impairment, physical dependence, and may exacerbate underlying depression. Their use in patients with a history of substance abuse is a relative contraindication. The risk-benefit ratio must be considered when prescribing these drugs for chronic pain.

Other Antianxiety Agents

Buspirone (Buspar) is an azaspirodecanedione derivative that is chemically unrelated to the benzodiazepines. The drug has no affinity for benzodiazepine receptors and therefore does not affect GABA binding. The exact mechanism of action of the drug is unknown. The only indications for its use is as an anxiolytic and for decreasing the symptoms of premenstrual syndrome.[67]

Zolpidem (Ambien) is a nonbenzodiazepine hypnotic of the imidazopyridine class. Unlike the benzodiazepines, it appears to only bind the ω_1-benzodiazepine receptor. The only indication for the drug is for short-term treatment of insomnia. Clinical experience with the drug indicates that it infrequently produces residual daytime sedation or amnesia, which is a perceived advantage over the benzodiazepines.[66]

There is scant evidence for the analgesic benefits of the antihistamines and we never use them as a sole agent.[74] The antihistamines hydroxyzine, promethazine, and diphenhydramine are best employed as antiemetics and anxiolytics in combination with other analgesic agents. The antihistamine cyproheptadine is also serotonergic and may have some weak analgesic properties.

SKELETAL MUSCLE RELAXANTS

Drugs that are thought to reduce muscle tone are often time prescribed to patients in pain. Numerous agents exist and include carisoprodol, chlorphenesin carbamate, chlorzoxazone, cyclobenzaprine, metaxalone, methocarbamol, and orphenadrine. The exact mode of action of these drugs is unclear; however, they appear to decrease muscle tone, without impairing motor function, by depressing polysynaptic reflexes through a central mechanism. Their efficacy for acute muscle spasm is well founded; however, their use in chronic pain is of questionable efficacy.[75] The only possible exception to this may be cyclobenzaprine, which has shown some usefulness in chronic musculoskeletal disorders.[76] The widespread use of these drugs is limited by somnolence and their potential for abuse.[77,78]

Baclofen, a chemical analogue of GABA, is a unique skeletal muscle relaxant that has proved quite effective in treating neuropathic pain.[79] Although the exact mechanism of action is unclear, the drug is thought to bind $GABA_B$ receptors both presynaptically and postsynaptically. Presynaptic binding results in decreased calcium conduction, which results in a corresponding decreased excitatory amino acid release. In contrast, postsynaptic binding will increase potassium conduction, resulting in postsynaptic hyperpolarization. Overall, the drug appears to inhibit both monosynaptic and polysynaptic reflexes at the spinal cord level.[75,79,80]

Baclofen is available for both oral and intrathecal administration. It has excellent oral bioavailability and is primarily excreted by the kidney. Its half-life following oral and intrathecal administration are 4 and 1.5 hours, respectively.[80] Although the primary indication for baclofen is the painful spasticity associated with multiple sclerosis,[80] it has also been found to be quite effective in treating pain associated with trigeminal neuralgia, glossopharyngeal neuralgia, vagoglossopharyngeal neuralgia, pretrigeminal neuralgia, and opthalmic-postherpetic neuralgia.[79] The drug may also be quite effective for patients with intractable hiccup.[81]

We recommend a starting baclofen dose of 5 to 10 mg orally 3 times a day. This can be gradually increased as tolerated to a maintenance dose of 40 to 80 mg per day. Common side effects include drowsiness, weakness, and dizziness. Abrupt withdrawal of baclofen may precipitate hallucinations, manic psychosis, and seizures. It is therefore advised to taper baclofen gradually in patients who have been treated long term on high doses.

AUTONOMIC DRUGS

Sympathetically maintained pain (SMP) can occur following peripheral nerve injury, and is often time associated with chronic pain conditions such as acute shingles, postherpetic neuralgia, painful metabolic neuropathies, traumatic nerve injury, and soft tissue injury.[82] Sprouting of local α_1-adrenoreceptors is thought to underlie the mechanisms of sympathetically maintained pain, since injection of the alpha agonists norepinephrine and phenylephrine can exacerbate SMP.[82,83] On physical examination, patients will display allodynia and cold hyperalgesia. Helpful diagnostic tests include intravenous regional blockade with guanethidine, reserpine or bretylium, local anesthetic sympathetic blockade, or an intravenous administration of the alpha-adrenergic antagonist phentolamine.

The treatment of choice for SMP is sympatholysis, which can involve numerous techniques:

1. Percutaneous techniques (sympathetic ganglion blocks, peripheral nerve blocks, phenol or radiofrequency neurolysis of the sympathetic chain, and epidural administration of local anesthetic
2. Intravenous regional technique with guanethidine, reserpine or bretylium
3. Surgical sympathectomy
4. Systemic therapy with the alpha-antagonists prazosin, terazosin, or phenoxybenzamine or the α_2-agonist clonidine.[82]

Prazosin is extensively metabolized by the liver and has a half-life of 2 to 3 hours. On the other hand, terazosin undergoes minimal first-pass metabolism and has a half-life of 9 to 12 hours. Whereas prazosin is dosed two to three times a day, terazosin can be dosed just at bedtime, which can improve patient compliance. Usual doses of prazosin are 1 to 5 mg orally two to three times daily as tolerated. Starting doses of terazosin are 1 mg at bedtime, which can be titrated upward as tolerated to 5 mg at bedtime. Common side effects associated with the α_1-antagonists include first-dose syncope, nausea, nasal congestion, headache, dizziness and asthenia.[84]

The α_2-agonist clonidine is available as tablets or transdermal system. An initial oral dose is usually 0.1 mg orally twice a day in this adult. This can be titrated upward to 0.6 mg per day in divided doses as tolerated. The transdermal system is available as 0.1 mg, 0.2 mg and 0.3 mg per 24-hour patches. These are applied every 7 days. The most common side effects associated with clonidine are dry mouth, drowsiness, dizziness, sedation, and constipation. Abrupt discontinuation of the drug can cause rebound hypertension.[84]

Clonidine is also available for spinal administration, either epidurally or intrathecally, and is especially helpful for problematic neuropathic pain syndromes.[85]

N-METHYL-D-ASPARTATE (NMDA) RECEPTOR ANTAGONISTS

High concentrations of the NMDA receptors are found throughout the spinal cord in man. Putative roles for the receptor include involvement in long-term potentiation, memory, visual plasticity, rhythmic motor function at spinal levels, and seizure activity.[86] Repetitive stimulation of primary afferent C fibers at greater than 0.5 Hz can activate these receptors and cause sensitization of wide-dynamic range neurons within the spinal cord and contribute to the phenomenon of windup and the development of neuropathic pain.[87] Recent research suggests that NMDA receptor antagonists such as dextromethorphan, amantadine, and ketamine may be useful in the prevention and treatment of neuropathic pain.[87]

Dextromethorphan has not only been shown to be effective against neuropathic pain, but has also been demonstrated to attenuate the development of tolerance to morphine analgesia.[83] In addition, administering dextromethorphan before surgery may decrease postoperative pain after tonsillectomy.[89] The only drawback with the drug is that doses necessary for adequate analgesia are higher than the recommended adult antitussive dose of 120 mg per day.[90] Doses as high as 240 mg per day have been well tolerated.[91,92] However, as the dose begins to exceed this upper limit, side effects such as ataxia, slurred speech, dysphoria, and altered sensory perception may become more frequent.[90] We have dosed the drug as high as 90 mg orally four times daily (360 mg orally per day) in some patients with beneficial effect without unacceptable side effects. The drug is available in a 30 mg/5 mL liquid formulation (Delsym), and as 30 mg gel caps (DexAlone).

Amantadine, an antiviral and anti-parkinsonian agent, was shown to act as noncompetitive NMDA antagonist.[93] Unlike other NMDA antagonists, amantadine is clinically available for long-term use in humans and its level of toxicity is low. Case reports[94] and a preliminary double-blind, controlled trial[95] show that immediate administration of amantadine significantly reduces surgical neuropathic pain in cancer patients.

Ketamine is an injectable noncompetitive NMDA receptor antagonist that has been used to treat neuropathic pain.[96,97] The drug has also been successfully combined with morphine and bupivicaine in a patient-controlled epidural regimen[98] and administered preemptively to reduce postoperative narcotic requirements.[99] Psychotomimetic reactions consisting of hallucinations, vivid imagery, delirium, confusion, and irrational behavior have been reported to occur in approximately 12% of individuals receiving the drug systemically.[100] Epidural administration may minimize these reactions. Investigational NMDA receptor antagonist are currently undergoing clinical trials. MK801, an antagonist for the NMDA receptor for glutamate, has been shown to reverse mechanical hyperalgesia in streptozotocin/diabetic rats[101] and conversely to have no effect on tactile allodynia in nerve-injured rats.[102]

Activation of NMDA receptors leads to calcium entry into the cell and initiates a series of central sensitization. This sensitization may be blocked not only with NMDA receptor antagonists, but also with calcium channel blockers that prevent calcium entry into cells. A double-blind study revealed that epidural verapamil and bupivacaine reduced the amount of self administered postoperative analgesia versus epidural bupivacaine alone.[103]

MISCELLANEOUS AGENTS

Several other pharmacologic treatments that have proved beneficial in the treatment of neuropathic pain include the corticosteroids, capsaicin, and calcitonin. Corticosteroids are believed to provide long-term pain relief because of their ability to inhibit the production of phospholipase A_2 and through membrane-stabilizing effects.[104] Topical capsaicin cream (Zostrix, 0.025% and 0.075%) is a substance P depletor, and has on occasion provided relief for both herpetic neuralgia (shingles) and postherpetic neuralgia. Capsaicin is known for its selectivity for and effect on C-fiber nociceptors and heat receptors.[105] Studies have shown its ability to trigger membrane depolarization and to open nonselective cation channels,[106] which may be either reversible or lytic. Capsaicin is theorized to causae a neurotoxic celluular degeneration of primary afferent nociceptors.[107] Basically, exposure to capsaicin results in activation, desensitization, and under certain conditions, the destruction of lightly myelinated or unmyelinated primary afferent fibers.[108] Compliance may be a problem with this medication, since it needs to be applied 4 to 5 times a day for several weeks before any significant benefit is appreciated and it has intense initial burning effects.[109] A recent preliminary study proposes a clinical role for topical capsaicin at doses of 5% to 10% in patients with intractable pain.[105]

Calcitonin is a 32 amino acid polypeptide that is derived from the thyroid gland. The drug is a potent inhibitor of osteoclast-induced bone resorbtion and can decrease the pain of bone metastases. Calcitonin has also been used in Paget's disease, reflex sympathetic dystrophy (complex regional pain syndrome I) and phantom limb pain.[106] Although binding sites for the drug have been found in the pons and hypothalamus[107] and β-endorphin levels have been shown to be increased in animal models,[108] its mechanism of action remains unclear. The drug is marketed as salmon calcitonin, which is 30 times the potency of the human variety, and is available for intravenous, subcutaneous, or intranasal administration.

FUTURE DEVELOPMENTS

Agents that may soon be available for the treatment of neuropathic pain include (1) butyl-para-aminobenzoate (Butamben), an ester local anesthetic, (2) bupivacaine microspheres, and (3) ziconitide, a selective calcium channel blocker. Nicotinic acetylcholine receptor agonists such as ABT-594 are in preliminary research stages. Animal studies suggest that the intrathecal injection of neostigmine[109] or the nitric oxide synthetase inhibitor L-NG-nitro arginine methyl ester (L-NAME)[110] may effectively treat neuropathic pain. Finally, levodopa, which is a clinically available agent, is currently being investigated for the treatment of neuropathic pain.[111]

CONCLUSION

Numerous pharmacologic agents are available for the treatment of neuropathic pain. The definitive drug therapy has, however, remained elusive. Often times, triple-drug therapy with a tricyclic antidepressant, an anticonvulsant, and an antiarrhythmic is necessary. Occasionally, there is the patient who requires long-term opioid therapy in conjunction with the earlier described medications. Should the patient fail optimal systemic therapy, implantable systems such as a spinal cord stimulator or intrathecal pump are available.

REFERENCES

1. Allen RR. Neuropathic Pain: Mechanisms and Clinical Assessment. In: Payne R, Patt RB, Hill CS (eds.) *Progress in Pain Research and Management.* Vol.12, IASP Press, 1998:159–173.
2. Paoli F, Darcourt G, Corsa P. Note preliminaire sur l'action de l'imipramine don les etats douloureaux. *Rev Neur* 1960;102:503–504.
3. Lance JW, Curran DA. Treatment of chronic tension headache. *Lancet* 1964;1:1235–1238.
4. Magni G. The Use of antidepressants in the treatment of chronic pain: a review of the current evidence. *Drugs* 1991;42:730–748.
5. Onghera P, Van Houdenhove B. Antidepressant-induced analgesia in chronic non-malignant pain: a meta-analysis of 39 placebo-controlled studies. *Pain* 1992;49:205–220.
6. Watson C, Peter N. Antidepressant Drugs as Adjuvant Analgesics. *J Pain Symptom Manage* 1994;9:392–405.
7. Max MB. Antidepressants as Analgesics. In: Fields HL, Liebeskind JC (eds.). Pharmacologic approaches to the treatment of chronic pain. *IASP Press* 1994;229–246.
8. Breibart W. Pain in Aids. In: Jensen TS, Turner JA, Wiesenfeld-Hallin Z (eds). Proceedings of the 8th World Congress on Pain, Progress in Research and Management. Vol. 8, *IASP Press* 1997;63–100.
9. Jacox A, Carr D, Payne R, et al. Management of Cancer Pain. Clinical Practice Guidelines No. 14 AHCPR Publication No. 94-0592. Rockville MD: US Department of Health and Human Services, Public Health Service, Agency for Health Care and Policy Research, 1994;139–141.
10. Walsh TD. Controlled study of imipramine and morphine in chronic pain due to advanced cancer. In: Foley KM et al. (eds) Advances in Pain Research and Therapy, Vol 10 New York: Raven Press, 1986, 155–165.
11. Ventafridda V, Bonezzi C, Caraceni A, et al. Antidepressants for cancer pain and other painful syndromes with deafferentation component: comparison of amitriptyline and trazodone. *Ital J Neurol Sci* 1987;8:579–587.
12. Baldessarini RJ. Drugs and the Treatment of Psychiatric Disorders. In: Hardman JG et al, (eds). The Pharmacologic Basis of Therapeutics. Ninth Edition. McGraw Hill 1996;431–459.
13. Kastrup EK, Hebel SK, Rivard R (eds.). Drug facts and comparisons. 1998, p. 1603–1671.
14. Watson CPN. Therapeutic window for amitriptyline analgesia, *Can Med Assoc J* 1984;130:105–106.
15. Gallagher RM, Pasol E. Psychopharmacologic drugs in chronic pain syndromes. *Curro Rev of Pain* 1997;1:137–152.
16. Max MB, Culnane M, Schafer SC, et al. Amitriptyline relieves diabetic neuropathy pain in patients with normal and depressed mood. *Neurology* 1987;37:589–596.
17. Eisenach J, Gebhart G. Intrathecal amitriptyline acts as an N-methyl-D-aspartate receptor antagonist in the presence of inflammatory hyperalgesia in rats. *Anesth* 1995;83:1046–1054.
18. Botney M, Fields HL. Amitriptyline potentiates morphine analgesia by direct action on the central nervous system. *Ann Neurol* 1983;13: 160–164.
19. McQuay HJ, Carroll D, Glynn CJ. Dose response for analgesic effect of amitriptyline in chronic pain. *Anesthesia* 1993;48:281–285.
20. Pick CG, Paul D, Eison MS, Pasternak G. Potentiation of opioid analgesia by the antidepressant nefazodone. *Eur J Pharmacol* 1992;2: 375–381.
21. Diamond S, Freitag FG. The use offluoxetine in the treatment of headache. *Clin J of Pain* 1989;5:200–201.
22. Theesen KA, Marsh WR. Relief of diabetic neuropathy with fluoxetine. *DICP* 1989;23:572–574.
23. Sindrup SH, Gram LF, Brosen K, et al. The selective serotonin reuptake inhibitor paroxetine is effective in the treatment of diabetic neuropathy symptoms. *Pain* 1990;42:135–144.
24. Manna V, Bolino F, Dicicco L. Chronic tension type headache, depression and serotonin: therapeutic effects of fluvoxamine and mianserine. *Headache* 1994;34:44–49.
25. Walker EA, Sullivan MD, Stenchever MA. Use of antidepressants in the management of women with chronic pelvic pain. *Obstet Gynecol Clin North Am* 1993;20:743–751.
26. Geller SA. Treatment of fibrositis with fluoxetine. *Am J of Med* 1989;87:594–595.
27. McQuay H, Carroll D, Jadad AR, et al. Anticonvulsant drugs for management of pain: a systematic review. *BMJ* 1995;1311:1047–1052.
28. Blom S. Trigeminal neuralgia: Its treatment with a new anticonvulsant drug (G32883). *Lancet* 1962;1:839–840.
29. Calissi PT, Jaber LA. Peripheral diabetic neuropathy: current concepts in treatment. *Ann Pharmacother* 1995;29:769–777.
30. Rothrock JF. Clinical Studies of valproate for migraine prophylaxis. *Cephalgia* 1997;17:81–83.
31. Hering R, Kuritzky A. Sodium valproate in the prophylactic treatment of migraine: a double blind study versus placebo. *Cephalgia* 1992;12: 81–84.
32. Bartusch SL, Sanders BJ, D' Alessio JG, et al. Clonazpam for the treatment of lancinating phantom limb pain. *The Clin J of Pain* 1996; 2:59–62.
33. Mellick GA, Mellick LB. Reflex sympathetic dystrophy treated with Gabapentin. *Arch Phys Med Rehabil* 1997;78:98–105.
34. Houtchens MK, Richert JR, Sami A, et al. Open label Gabapentin treatment for pain in multiple sclerosis. *Multiple Sclerosis* 1997;3: 250–253.
35. Rosner H, Rubin L, Kestenbaum A. Gabapentin adjunctive therapy in neuropathic pain states. *The Clin J of Pain* 1996;12:56–58.
36. Backonja M, Beydoun A, Edwards KR, et al. Gabapentin for the symptomatic treatment of painful neuropathy in patients with diabetes mellitus. *JAMA* 1998;280:1831–1836.
37. Rowbotham M, Harden N, Stacey B, et al. Gabapentin for the treatment of postherpetic neuralgia. *JAMA* 1998;280:1837.
38. McNamara N. Drugs effective in the therapy of the epilepsies. In: Hardman JG, et al (eds). *The Pharmacologic Basis of Therapeutics.* Ninth edition. New York: McGraw-Hill 1996;461–486.
39. Kastrup EK, Hebel SK, Rivard R (eds). Drug facts and comparisons. 1998, p. 1832–1900.
40. Hill DR, Suman-Chauhan N, Woodruff GN. Localization of (3H)— gabapentin to a novel site in rat brain; autoradiographic studies. *Eur J Pharmacol* 1993;244:303–309.
41. Rao ML, Clarenbach P, Vahlensieck M, et al. Gabapentin augments whole blood serotonin in healthy young men. *J Neural Transm* 1988; 73:129–34.
42. Bartlett E, Hutaserani O. Xylocaine for the relief of post-operative pain. *Anesth Anal* 1961;40:296–304.
43. Gordon RA. Intravenous novocaine for analgesia in burns. *Can Med Assoc* J 1943;49:478–481.
44. Gilbert CRA, Hanson JR, Brown AB, et al. Intravenous use oxyflocaine. *Curr Res Anesth Analg* 1951;30:301–313.
45. Kastrup J, Petersen P, Dejgard A, et al. Treatment of painful diabetic neuropathy with intravenous lidocaine infusion. *Br Med J* 1986;292:173.
46. Hatangdi YS, Boas RA, Richards EG. Post herpetic neuralgia: Management with antiepileptic and tricycle drugs. In: Bonica JJ, Albe-Fessard D (eds). *Advances in Pain Research and Therapy.* Raven Press, New York 1976;1:583–587.
47. Tanelian DL, Brose WG. Neuropathic pain can be relieved by drugs that are use-dependent sodium channel blockers: Lidocaine, carbamazepine, and mexiletine. *Anesthesiology* 1991;74:949–951.
48. Awerbach GI, Sandyk R. Mexiletine for thalamic pain syndrome. *Int J Neurosci* 1990;55:129–133.
49. Backonja MM. Local anesthetics as adjuvant analgesics. *J of Pain Symp Manage* 1994;9:491–499.

50. Kastrup EK, Hebel SK, Rivard R (eds.). *Drug facts and Comparisons.* 1998, p. 766–842.
51. Galer BS, Harle J, Rowbotham MC. Response to Intravenous Lidocaine infusion predicts subsequent response to oral Mexiletine: A Prospective Study. *J Pain Symp Manage* 1996;12:161–167.
52. Woolf CJ, Wiesenfeld-Hallin Z. The systemic administration of local anesthetics produces a selective depression of c-afferent fibre-evoked activity in the spinal cord. *Pain* 1985;23:361–374.
53. Devor M, Wall PD, Catalan N. Systemic lidocaine silences ectopic neuroma and DRG discharge without blocking nerve conduction. *Pain* 1992;48:261–268.
54. Abram SE, Yaksh TL. Systemic lidocaine blocks nerve injury-induced hyperalgesia and nociceptor-driven spinal sensitization in the rat. *Anesthesiology* 1994;80:383–391.
55. Marchettini P, Lacerenza M, Marangoni C, et al. Lidocaine test in neuralgia. *Pain* 1992;48:377–382.
56. Dejgard A, Petersen P, Kastrup J. Mexiletine for treatment of painful diabetic neuropathy. *Lancet* 1988;2:9–11.
57. Forest W, Brown B, Brown C, et al. Dextromphetamine with morphine for the treatment of post-operative pain. *N Engl J Med* 1977; 296:712–715.
58. Bruera E, Watanabe S. Psychostimulants as adjuvant analgesics. *J Pain Symptom Manage* 1994;9:412–415.
59. Wilens TE, Biederman J. The Stimulants. Psychiatric *Clin N Am* 1992; 15:191–222.
60. Davis JL, Lewis B, Gerich JE, et al. Peripheral diabetic neuropathy treated with amitriptyline and fluphenazine. *JAMA* 1977;238:2291–2292.
61. Farber GA, Burks JW. Chlorprothixene therapy for herpes zoster neuralgia. *South Med J* 1994;67:808–812.
62. Lechin F, Vander Digs B, Lechin ME, et al. Pimazide therapy for trigerminal neuralgia. Arch Neurol 1989;9:960–962.
63. Couch JR, Diamond S. Status migrainosus: causative and therapeutic aspects. *Headache* 1983;23:94–101.
64. Hakkarainen H. Fluphenazine for tension headache: a double blind study. *Headache* 1977;17:216–218.
65. Patt RB, Proper G, Reddy S. The neuroleptics as adjuvant analgesics. *J Pain Symptom Manage* 1994;9:446–453.
66. Hobbs WR, Rail TW, Verdoom TA. Hypnotics and Sedatives; Ethanol. In: Hardman JG, et al (eds). The Pharmacologic Basis of Therapeutics, Ninth edition, McGraw Hill, 1996;361–396.
67. Kastrup EK, Hebel SK, Rivard R. *Drug facts and comparisons.* St. Louis, MO, 1998, p. 1576–1596.
68. Dellemijn PLJ, Fields H. Do Benzodiazepines have a role in chronic pain management? *Pain* 1994;57:137–152.
69. Reddy S, Patt RB. The Benzodiazepines as adjuvant analgesics. *J Pain Symptom Manage* 1994;9:510–514.
70. Singh PN, Sharma P, Gupta PK, et al. Clinical evaluation of diazepam for relief of post-operative pain. *Br J Anaesth* 1981;53:831–836.
71. Miller R, et al. Midazolam as an adjuvant to meperidine analgesia for post-operative pain. *Clin J of Pain* 1986;2:37–43.
72. Zakrzewska M. Medical Management of trigeminal neuralgia. *Br Dent J* 1990;168:399.
73. Eisele JH, Grigsby EJ, Dea G. Clonazapam treatment of myoclonic contractions associated with high-dose opioids: case report. *Pain* 1992;49:231–232.
74. Hupert C, Yacoub M, Turgeon LR. Effect of hydroxyzine on morphine for the treatment of post-operative pain. *Anesth Analg* 1980;59: 690–696.
75. Waldman HJ. Centrally acting skeletal muscle relaxants and associated drugs. *J Pain Symptom Manage* 1994;9:434–441.
76. Elenbaas JK. Centrally acting oral skeletal muscle relaxants. *Am J Hosp Pharmacy* 1980;37:131–132.
77. Littrell RA, Safe T, Miller W. Meprobamate dependency secondary to carisoprodol (Soma) use. *Am J Drug Alcohol Abuse* 1993;19:133–134.
78. Elder NC. Abuse of skeletal muscle relaxants. *Am Fam Physician* 1991;44:1223–1226.
79. Fromm GH. Baclofen as an adjuvant analgesic. *J Pain Symptom Manage* 1994;9:500–509.
80. Kastrup EK, Hebel SK, Rivard R (eds.). *Drug facts and comparisons.* 1998, p.1950–1976.
81. Walker P, Watanabe S, Bruera E. Baclofen: A treatment for chronic hiccup. *J Pain Symptom Manage* 1998;6:125–132.
82. Campbell IN, Raja SN, Selig DK, et al. Diagnosis and management of sympathetically maintained pain. In: Fields HL and Liebeskind JC, (eds). *Progress in Pain Research and Management.* IASP Press, Seattle, WA. 1994:85–100.
83. Yaksh TL. Pharmacology of the pain processing system. In: Waldman SD, Winnie AP (eds). *Interventional Pain Management.* WB Saunders, Philadelphia. 1996:19–32.
84. Kastrup EK, Hebel SK, Rivard R (eds). *Drug Facts and Comparisons.* St. Louis, MO. 1998;949–1050.
85. Eisenach JC, DeKock M, Klimscha W. Alpha-2-adrenergic agonists for regional anesthesia. A clinical review of Clonidine (1984–1995) *Anesthesiology* 1996;85:655–674.
86. Dickenson AH. NMDA Receptor Antagonists as analgesics. In: Fields HL, Liebeskind JC (eds.). *Progress in Pain Research and Management.* IASP Press, Seattle, 1994:173–187.
87. Mao J, Price DD, Hayes RL, et al. Intrathecal treatment with dextrorphan and ketamine potently reduces pain-related behaviors in a rat model of manoneuropathy. *Brain Res* 1993;5:164–168.
88. Elliott K, Hynansky A, Inturrisi CE. Dextromethorphan attenuates and reverses analgesic tolerance to morphine. *Pain* 1984;59:361–368.
89. Kawamata T, Omote K, Kawamata M, et al. Premedication with oral dextromethorphan reduces post-operative pain after tonsillectomy. *Anesth Analg* 1992;86:594–597.
90. Kastrup EK, Hebel SK, Rivard R (eds.). *Drug Facts and Comparisons.* St. Louis, MO 1998;1218–1219.
91. Bonuccelli U, Del Dotto P, Piccini P, et al. Dextromethorphan and Parkinsonism (letter), *Lancet* (UK) 1992;340:53.
92. Saenz R, Tanner CM, Albers G, et al. A preliminary study of dextromethorphan (DM) as adjunctive therapy in Parkinson's Disease. *Neurology* 1993;43:A155.
93. Kohrenhuber J, Quack G, Danysz W, et al. Therapeutic brain concentration of the NMDA antagonist Amantadine. *Neuropharmacology* 1995;34:713–721.
94. Eisenberg E, Pud D. Can patients with chronic neuropathic pain be cured by acute administration of the NMDA receptor antagonist amantadine? *Pain* 1998;74:337–339.
95. Pud D, Eisenberg E, Spitzer A, et al. The NMDA receptor antagonist amantadine reduces surgical neuropathic pain in cancer patients: a double blind, randomized, placebo controlled trial. *Pain* 1998;75:349–354.
96. Eide PK, Stubhang A, Aye I, et al. Continuous subcutaneous administration of N-methyl-d-aspartate (NMDA) receptor antagonist ketamine in the treatment of post-herpetic neuralgia. *Pain* 1995;61:221–225.
97. Takahashi H, Miyazaki M, Nanbu T, et al. The NMDA receptor antagonist ketamine abolishes neuropathic pain after epidural administration in a clinical case. *Pain* 1998;75:391–394.
98. Chia Y, Liu K, Liu Y, et al. Adding ketamine in a Multimodal Patient Controlled Epidural regimen reduces postoperative pain and analgesic consumption. *Anesth Analg* 1998;86:1245–1249.
99. Fu ES, Miguel R, Scharf JE. Preemptive ketamine decreases postoperative narcotic requirements in patients undergoing abdominal surgery. *Anesth Analg* 1997;84:1086–1090.
100. Kastrup EK, Hebel SK, Rivard R (eds.). *Drug facts and Comparisons.* 1998, p. 1804–1806.
101. Malcangio M, Tomlinson DR. A pharmacologic analysis of mechanical hyperalgesia in streptozotocin/diabetic rats. *Pain* 1998;76:151–157.
102. Wegert S, Ossipov MH, Nichols ML, et al. Differential activities of intrathecal MK-801or morphine to alter responses to thennal and mechanical stimuli in nonnal or nerve-injured rats. *Pain* 1997;71:56–64.

103. Choe H, Kim JS, Ko SH, et al. Epidural verapamil reduces analgesic consumption after lower abdominal surgery. *Anesth Analg* 1998;86: 788–790.
104. Devor M, Govrin-Lippmann R, Raber P. Corticosteroids suppress ectopic neuronal discharge in experimental neurons. *Pain* 1985;22: 127–137.
105. Robbins WR, Staats PS, Levine J, et al. Treatment of intractable pain with topical large-dose capsaicin: preliminary report. *Anesth Analg* 1998;86:579–583.
106. Dray A. Mechanism of action of capsaicin like molecules and sensory neurons. *Life Sci* 1992;Sl:1759–1765.
107. Chung JM, Paik KS, Kim JS, et al. Chronic effects of topical application of capsaicin to the sciatic nerve on responses of primate spinothalamic neurons. *Pain* 1993;53:311–321.
108. Holzer P. Capsaicin: cellular targets, mechanisms of action, and selectivity for thin sensory neurons. *Pharmacol Review* 1991;41:143–201.
109. Cottan P. Compliance problems, placebo effect cloud trials of topical analgesics. *JAMA* 1990:264:13–14.
110. Roth A, Kolaric K. Analgesic activity of calcitonin in patients with painful osteolytic metastases of breast cancer: results of a controlled randomized study. *Oncology* 1986;43:283–287.
111. Kreeger L, Hutton-Potts, J. The use of calcitonin in the treatment of metastatic bone pain (letter). *J Pain Symptom Manage* 1999;17: 2–5.
112. Lavand'homme P, Pan HL, Eisenach JC. Intrathecal neostigmine but not sympathectomy, relieves mechanical allodynia in a rat model of neuropathic pain. *Anesthesiology* 1998;89:493–499.
113. Wong CS, Cherng CH, Tung CS. Intrathecal administration of excitatory amino acid receptor antagonists on nitric oxide synthetase inhibition autonomy behavior in rats. *Anesth Analg* 1998;87:605–608.
114. Ertas M, Sagduyu, Arac N, et al. Use of levodopa to relieve pain from painful symmetrical diabetic polyneuropathy. *Pain* 1998;75: 257–259.

CHAPTER 63

PSYCHOPHARMACOLOGY FOR THE PAIN SPECIALIST

Daniel Rockers and Scott M. Fishman

A pain patient from our center recently left a series of phone messages detailing his newly discovered powers of "dolphin-sonar," and added that Elliott Ness had possession of his car. He was wondering if he could be provided with a skateboard with which to get around town. His verbal style was characterized by a bombastic manner and loose associations. Although previous conversations focused almost exclusively on his painful lower back, in these messages there was no mention of it.

This brief case sketch illustrates two important points regarding the difficulties the practitioner has in dealing with chronic pain. The first point is the high comorbidity of psychiatric diagnoses with chronic pain diagnoses. Of course, only few chronic pain patients have concomitant delusions as this patient did, but nearly all have had their lives disrupted to such an extent that a psychiatric diagnosis is highly possible. The second point has to do with the chronology of these conditions. It is often difficult to determine whether the pain caused the psychiatric diagnosis, the psychiatric condition caused the pain, or they happen to occur somewhat simultaneously. All of this suggests that a knowledge of psychopharmacology is important for a pain practitioner not only because there is a large overlap of psychiatric diagnoses with chronic pain conditions, but all of the common psychopharmacologic medication groups are also used as analgesics. Many of these agents have multiple mechanisms of action that account for their dual effects. However, the dramatic overlap of the analgesic and psychopharmacology drug arsenal suggests a significant degree of clinical homology in patients with chronic pain. Comprehensive pain management requires an understanding of basic principles of psychopharmacology. From the perspective of a non-mental health professional, it might seem fitting to ask, "Why psychopharmacology for the pain specialist?" There are several real answers to this important question:

- The majority of patients in chronic pain have comorbid psychiatric conditions, ranging from mild (anxiety, adjustment, depression) to severe (delusional, psychotic).
- Depression and anxiety are known to enhance perception of pain and may be a predominating component of some pain syndromes.
- Some psychiatric conditions manifest as pain or pain-like symptoms. For example, it has been suggested that complex regional pain syndrome (CRPS) is a conversion-like disorder.[1]
- Many psychiatric conditions are caused by, or are accompanied by, neurochemical abnormalities. These abnormalities may significantly affect the pain medications prescribed and may affect the pain condition in a significant manner. For example, serotonin is considered an important factor in pain states, as well as mood states.
- There may be malpractice suits brought against pain practitioners who do not adequately recognize or treat accompanying psychiatric conditions that affect pain states.
- Patients may often choose not to seek mental health treatment, even when instructed by the pain practitioner to do so. This may have to do with a patient's financial state, insurance coverage, or the stigma associated with seeking help for emotional difficulties.

In the following pages, several psychotropic medications and their role in pain treatment are reviewed. Antidepressants are the largest category, and this is not surprising considering the high comorbidity of depression and pain. Anxiolytics are also reviewed, as anxiety is also commonly seen in many patients suffering from chronic pain. Also, neuroleptics—medications that affect cognitive functioning, affect movement, and treat delirium—are also reviewed here.

USE OF PSYCHOPHARMACOLOGICAL AGENTS IN CHRONIC PAIN

Improving Compliance

Even the best medication may be useless if the patient does not take it as prescribed. This is a matter of special concern when utilizing psychotropic medications because some patients may get the wrong message when being prescribed psychotropic agents. Patient education about any impending treatment will help balance patient expectations and have an impact on how patients respond to and tolerate any adverse effects that may arise. For example, this is especially important with depression, a condition in which motivation and ability to focus are quite low. Many patients do not recognize that some medications require several weeks to demonstrate results. Some patients incorrectly believe that all of their medication can be taken on an as-needed basis for symptom relief. Others may not understand the difficulties associated with abrupt discontinuance. Giving the patient information about their medications offers them a sense of some control, and obviously may go a long way toward better compliance.

Ease of use of a treatment will significantly impact compliance and the simplest effective drug regimen will help ensure that the treatment will be used. Many patients are taking a long list of medications, and minimizing polypharmacy may help with compliance with essential drug regimens. Consider nonbiological treatments when they are as effective as pharmacotherapy. Minimize risk of drug–drug interactions. Establish an ongoing therapeutic relationship. By all means, get to know your patient as a person, and not just as an illness or condition.

ANTIDEPRESSANTS

Description Depression is one of the largest psychological issues comorbid with chronic pain. For example, major depression is found in 8% to 50% of patients with chronic pain, and dysthymia may be seen in greater than 75% of patients with chronic pain. In most cases of chronic pain, a patient will be prescribed an antidepressant or will already be taking one. Antidepressants often serve a dual role: treating a mood disorder as well as independently addressing pain symptoms. For these reasons, an awareness of available antidepressants as well as an understanding of their purported mechanism of action is important.

History Effective medical treatments for depression have been available since the late 1950s. The earliest forms of currently used antidepressants were tricyclic antidepressants (TCAs) and monoamine oxidase inhibitors (MAOIs), each with inhibitory actions on norepinephrine (NE) and serotonin (5-HT) reuptake. These were the drugs of choice for treating depression until the 1980s when the selective serotonin reuptake inhibitors (SSRIs) were found to possess substantial antidepressant efficacy. The SSRIs have revolutionized treatment of depression by offering efficacy with greatly reduced side-effect profiles. Over the past decade, numerous atypical antidepressants have been developed, including norepinephrine and dopamine reuptake inhibitors (NDRIs), serotonin-norepinephrine reuptake inhibitors (SNRIs), and serotonin-2 (5-HT$_2$) antagonist/reuptake inhibitors (SARIs). These newer agents are currently undergoing clinical trials to assess relative efficacy compared with standard TCAs and SSRIs.

It is notable that antidepressants are useful for many disorders other than depression, especially for anxiety disorders and neuropathic pain. Anxiolysis with antidepressants is discussed in the following sections. The history of antidepressants as analgesics began in 1960, just 2 years after imipramine was reported to be an antidepressant. When first reported to be analgesic, TCAs were thought to work by relieving the depression component of pain. It is now well known that relieving depression by any method is likely to decrease pain. Not all antidepressants, however, have independent analgesic properties.

Amitriptyline was the first TCA described to have analgesic properties that are independent of antidepressant properties (suggested to relieve migraine via vasodilatory mechanism). There is now a convincing body of controlled data as well as extensive, long-standing clinical experience supporting TCA analgesia that is independent of antidepressant actions. Although SSRIs have been suggested to be useful for pain by anecdotal reports, at present there is no controlled data to support this. The only controlled trial to date did not show independent analgesia.[2] Since reduction of depression can reduce pain, separating this antidepressant effect from other intrinsic, independent effects of these drugs is a difficult but critical part of clarifying analgesic effects.

Cyclic Antidepressants (TCAs)

Indications TCAs are approved by the U.S. Food and Drug Administration (FDA) for the treatment of major depressive disorders and secondary depression in other disorders. Other approved uses of TCAs include treating obsessive-compulsive disorder (clomipramine) and enuresis (imipramine). TCAs are also useful in treating generalized anxiety, panic disorder, agoraphobia, bulimia, attention deficit hyperactivity disorder (ADHD), and chronic pain.

Chemistry Although this class includes tricyclics and heterocyclics, they are generally referred to as tricyclics (TCAs). They are named for their three-ring structure, that is, two benzene rings connected by a double-carbon bond. The tertiary amines (amitriptyline, imipramine) have two methyl groups on the terminal nitrogen atom of the side chain. Demethylation of these results in the secondary amines nortryptiline and desipramine, respectively. In general, the secondary amines have less anticholinergic side-effects than do the tertiary amines. Table 63-1 lists the common tricyclics divided by secondary and tertiary amine groups.

Mechanism of Action There exists some question about the precise mechanism of how tricyclics combat depression. All tricyclics inhibit both serotonergic and noradrenergic reuptake; and these effects are seen early, but clinical benefits often begin 2 to 3 weeks after initiation of treatment. In other words, side effects are seen right away, whereas clinical benefits take several weeks to emerge.

This disparity raises questions about the exact relationship between NE/5-HT reuptake inhibition and the antidepressant effects of TCAs. Downregulation of β-adrenergic receptors correlates temporally with onset of action, but this is likely a marker for the role of second-messenger systems and neuronal gene regulation in the therapeutic mechanism of TCAs.

There is no dispute that relief of depression also relieves some chronic pain. Therefore, TCAs relieve pain as an antidepressant, but also may offer independent analgesia, perhaps by other mechanisms such as its blockade of sodium channels rather than by their well-described inhibitory effects on NE/5-HT reuptake. Still, some endorse the idea that because serotonin has been implicated as the major neurotransmitter in descending inhibitory tracts, TCAs relieve pain by making more serotonin available.

TCAs as analgesics rarely offer complete analgesia, and TCA side effects are common due to the antagonist effects on the cholinergic, adrenergic, and histaminergic systems. These agents are compelling analgesics, particularly with comorbid depression or insomnia. Reasonable goals for using TCAs as analgesics include decreased pain intensity from unbearable to bearable. Some mild side effects may be unavoidable in exchange for analgesia.

There are some common misconceptions about TCAs as analgesics. For instance, there probably is not a therapeutic window, whereby analgesia is diminished above and below threshold dosages. Another misconception is that analgesia requires only low

TABLE 63-1 **Tricyclic Antidepressants**

Medication	Propietary Name	Dosage Range (mg/day)
Tertiary amines		
Imipramine	Tofranil	75–300
Amitriptyline	Elavil	75–300
Clomipramine	Anafranil	75–300
Doxepin	Sinequan	75–300
Secondary amines		
Desipramine	Norpramin	75–300
Nortriptyline	Pamelor	40–200
Protriptyline	Vivactil	20–60
Amoxapine	Asendin	100–600

dosages of TCA. Evidence suggests that analgesia is maximized with increased doses as well as with time. The time course of analgesic TCAs varies between 1 and 120 days, suggesting that initial early analgesia is maximized over time. Duration of TCA analgesia also persists over time with maintenance of therapy.

Pharmacokinetics TCAs are typically lipophilic, and thus easily pass through the blood–brain barrier. They are widely distributed in major organs including lung, heart, brain, and liver. Eighty-five to 95% of the drug is protein bound, although individual differences can cause up to a four-fold variation in amount of free drug. All TCAs undergo first-pass hepatic metabolism; intermediate stages involve demethylation, oxidation, and glucuronide conjugation. As mentioned earlier, the demethylated daughter metabolites have fewer side effects. For instance, nortriptyline and desipramine have fewer anticholinergic side effects than amitriptyline and imipramine, respectively. Demethylated metabolites are usually biologically active with plasma half-lives often greater than two times that of the tertiary amine parent compound. Thus, the washout period is usually a week or more.

Because hepatic clearance involves the P450 enzyme system, drug interactions are possible. For example, P450 enzyme inhibitors, such as fluoxetine, cimetadine, and methylphenidate increase TCA plasma levels. P450 enzyme inducers such as phenobarbitol, carbamazepine, and cigarette smoking decrease TCA plasma levels. Decreased gut absorption is also a possible cause of decreased TCA plasma levels and may occur with use of common agents such as cholestyramine.

Combining TCAs with opiate agonists can lead to decreased intestinal motility, already a problem for many patients taking opioids. Additive anticholinergic and opioid effects on the bowels can lead to treatment-resistant constipation or ileus.

Phytochemical Reactions Serotonin syndrome may occur when St. John's wort is used in conjunction with TCAs (an *in vitro* study indicated that St. John's wort affected serotonin reuptake.[3] In addition, serotonin is deaminated by MAO type A, and some early studies showed that St. John's wort inhibits MAO type A.[4] Monitor the concurrent use of other phytochemicals such as kava or valerian, which function as central nervous system (CNS) depressants.

Adverse Reactions In treating depression, all TCAs are considered equally efficacious but have significantly different side-effect profiles. Thus, choosing a particular TCA can be made on the basis of side-effect profile. Some side effects such as sedation may be beneficial to some patients with insomnia.

Before initiating treatment, routine laboratory screening may include complete blood count, electrolytes, BUN, creatinine, and liver function tests. Because tricyclics have quinidine-like properties, can increase all intervals of the electrocardiogram (ECG), and are potentially proarrhythmic, ECG screening may be requested.

As previously described, TCAs interact with multiple neurotransmitter systems and as a result present with a wider side-effect profile than SSRIs. TCAs may manifest all anticholinergic symptoms including dry mucous membranes, blurred vision, constipation, urinary retention, excessive sweating, and confusion or delirium. Antagonism of histaminic receptors may result in sedation, weight gain, or confusion. Cardiovascular effects result from a combination of interactions with α_1-adrenergic, muscarinic, serotonergic, and histaminic receptors as well as IA antiarrhythmic actions of TCAs. Cardiovascular side effects include tachycardia, orthostatic hypotension, prolonged cardiac conduction, and arrhythmias. Sexual side effects are also seen with TCAs and include decreased libido, impotence, erectile difficulties, ejaculatory disturbances, and anorgasmia. As with SSRIs, TCAs may cause or exacerbate extrapyramidal symptoms. TCAs likely decrease the seizure threshold as well. Rare side effects include abnormalities in serum glucose levels, syndrome of inappropriate antidiuretic hormone (SIADH), jaundice, hepatitis, blood dyscrasias, and photosensitivity.

Rarely, patients may develop a discontinuation syndrome following abrupt cessation of the TCA. Withdrawal may manifest as anxiety, fever, sweating, myalgia, headache, nausea, vomiting, dizziness, dyskinesia, or akathesia. Overdose with TCAs can be lethal. Toxicity results from anticholinergic effects and CNS effects (including seizures and coma). The most hazardous side effect is cardiac toxicity, especially QRS complex widening. TCA overdose is a leading cause of drug-related overdose and death. Since three to five times the therapeutic dose of TCAs is potentially lethal, this low therapeutic index (ratio of toxic to therapeutic dose) must make prescribers vigilant. This is probably a large part of the reason SSRIs are chosen as first-line antidepressants over TCAs.

Dosages and Monitoring Although somewhat controversial, it is generally agreed that plasma levels may be clinically useful when using imipramine, desipramine, or nortriptyline. Plasma levels of nortriptyline may be especially useful in that a therapeutic level may exist where levels >150 may be less efficacious than lower levels. As with all antidepressants, effects are often delayed. Antidepressant effects may be seen anywhere from 2 to 6 weeks of a trial at therapeutic dosages. Following effective response, patients should continue the medication for 6 to 12 months to prevent relapse.[5] Dosage should not be decreased during the maintenance phase of treatment (Table 63-1). If a patient has had multiple recurrences of their illness, an indefinite length of treatment may be indicated.

Monoamine Oxidase Inhibitors (MAOIs)

Indications MAOIs are approved for use in major depression, double depression (dysthymia superimposed on major depression), psychotic depression, social phobia, and simple phobias and are often also used to treat anxiety, panic disorder, and obsessive-compulsive disorder. They are not considered first-line agents in the treatment of major depression due to their high incidence of side effects, dietary restrictions, and lethality in overdose. "Atypical" subtypes of depression involving mood reactivity, increased appetite, hypersomnia, leaden paralysis, and rejection sensitivity may respond better to MAOIs than other agents.

Chemistry MAOIs are divided into hydrazines and nonhydrazines. Hydrazines marketed in the United States include phenelzine (Nardil) and isocarboxazid (Marplan). The nonhydrazine is tranylcypramine (Parnate), which closely resembles the amphetamine structure.

Mechanism of Action MAOIs work by binding to the enzyme monoamine oxidase, thus inhibiting the breakdown of monamines at the synaptic junction. This results in increased concentration and availability of the neurotransmitters epinephrine, norepinephrine, and dopamine at various storage sites in the central and sympathetic nervous system. This increased availability of monoamine is what is believed to alleviate depressive symptoms. It is important to remember that MAO inhibitors block the action of MAO as well as other enzymes, thus causing alterations in the hepatic metabolism of many other drugs.[6]

MAOIs may be reversible or irreversible, though only irreversible MAOIs are available in the United States. While reversible MAOIs, known as reversible inhibitors of monoamine activity (RIMAs), are widely available outside of the United States, for our purposes, we discuss only irreversible MAOIs.

MAOIs require up to 2 weeks to achieve maximal MAO inhibition and clinical effects may not be seen for 2 to 4 weeks, although an energizing effect may occur within a few days following initiation of treatment. Table 63-2 offers some dosage guidelines for MAOIs. Another significant difference from standard TCAs and SSRIs is that MAOIs have a short half-life and require twice daily dosing. To date, there are no implications of direct analgesic effect by MAOIs. Recall that relief of depression also relieves some degree of pain.

Pharmacokinetics MAOIs are rapidly and fully absorbed from the gastrointestinal (GI) tract. They are biotransformed in the liver and excreted rapidly. Although their half-life is very short, they have long-lasting pharmacologic effects because they permanently bind to and deactivate enzymes. It takes approximately 2 to 3 weeks for the body to resynthesize monoamine oxidase; therefore, at least that long should be allowed between drug trials.

Adverse Reactions Sympathomimetic amines such as tyramine exert pressor effects on the human system; when not broken down by MAO, introduction of exogenous tyramines can set off a hypertensive crisis. For this reason, patients taking MAOIs should avoid foods high in tyramine content, such as cheeses, yeast supplements, or aged alcohols. Symptoms of a hypertensive crisis include occipital headache, neck stiffness or soreness, dilated pupils, tachycardia or bradycardia, and constricting chest pain. Because of this risk, MAOIs should be used with caution in patients with cerebrovascular disease, cardiovascular disease, or hypertension.

Although the stimulant effect of MAOIs is often helpful for some patients suffering from major depression, symptoms of insomnia, restlessness, and anxiety, they may be excessive. Other side effects include constipation, anorexia, nausea, vomiting, dry mouth, urinary retention, drowsiness, headache, dizziness, and weakness. As with SSRIs and TCAs, sexual dysfunction may occur, manifested as impotence, anorgasmia, decreased libido, ejaculation difficulties, and rarely priapism.

TCAs and SSRIs should be used cautiously with MAOIs: Fatalities have been reported from patients taking fluoxetine in concert with MAOIs. Concomitant use of MAOIs with SSRIs runs the risk of developing serotonin syndrome. Symptoms of serotonin syndrome include CNS irritability, myoclonus, diaphoresis, and elevated temperature. Severe cases may result in death. Thus, patients should discontinue MAOIs for at least 2 weeks before beginning an SSRI. Because of its particularly persistent metabolite, fluoxetine requires MAOI discontinuation for at least 5 weeks. Of course, SSRIs must be similarly discontinued for prolonged periods before starting a MAOI. These dietary restrictions should be continued for at least 10 days following discontinuation of the MAOI as a washout period.

Psychostimulants and sympathomimetics should be used cautiously, if at all, in patients taking MAOIs.Avoid using meperidine with MAOIs, as this can cause excessive serotonin concentrations resulting in excitation, sweating, hypertension, respiratory depression, coma, and vasculatory collapse. It is unclear if other opiate agonists have the same adverse pharmacodynamic effects.

TABLE 63-2 **Monoamine Oxidase Inhibitors**

Medication	Propietary Name	Dosage Range (mg/day)
Isocarboxazid	Marplan	30–50
Phenelzine	Nardil	45–90
Tranylcypromine	Parnate	20–60

TABLE 63-3 **Selective Serotonin Reuptake Inhibitors**

Medication	Propietary Name	Dosage Range (mg/day)
Fluoxetine	*Prozac*	10–80
Fluvoxamine	*Luvox*	50–300
Paroxetine	*Paxil*	10–50
Sertraline	*Zoloft*	50–200
Venlafaxine	*Effexor*	75–225

Phytochemical Reactions Any substances that act on the CNS, for example, kava kava, *Piper methysticum*, or valerian (*Valeriana officinalis*), should be carefully monitored for MAOI interactions. For the same reason, St. John's wort (*Hypericum perforatum*) should not be used with MAOIs.

Dosages and Monitoring It appears that optimal antidepressant efficacy is seen when MAOIs are given at doses that reduce MAO activity by at least 80% (see Table 63-2 for dosages). Liver function tests should be monitored periodically, as MAOIs are associated with hepatotoxicity. With long-term use, MAOIs may impair their own metabolism. Unfortunately, MAOI serum levels are not useful for guiding therapy.

Selective Serotonin Reuptake Inhibitors (SSRIs)

Since the introduction of fluoxetine (Prozac) in 1987, several other selective serotonin reuptake inhibitors (SSRIs) have been introduced and have revolutionized first-line therapy for depression (Table 63-3).

Indications Although SSRIs were initially introduced for use in major depressive disorder, the FDA has approved other indications for these agents, including panic disorder, bulimia nervosa, and obsessive-compulsive disorder. In addition, SSRIs are often used by clinicians for a variety of other conditions, including premenstrual syndrome, chronic fatigue syndrome, intermittent explosive disorder, and chronic pain management.

Chemistry SSRIs are structurally diverse.

Mechanism of Action SSRIs act via specific mechanisms in the central nervous system (CNS) and may have fewer side effects than other antidepressants as a result. The immediate effect of the SSRIs on the CNS is blockade of the presynaptic serotonin reuptake pump. This delays presynaptic reuptake of serotonin following its presynaptic release. Thus, serotonin persists in the synaptic cleft, able to exert its effects on neurotransmission for a longer duration. These effects occur almost immediately. However, clinical antidepressant response from SSRIs is usually not observed until 2 to 3 weeks following initiation of treatment. Other delayed actions, such as second-messenger effects and neuronal gene regulation, may play a role in the efficacy of SSRIs.

Although there are reports of SSRI-induced analgesia, these are anecdotal. The only controlled trial by Max et al[2] did not find these agents to possess independent analgesia. It is important to keep in mind the adage that "absence of proof is not proof of absence," and there exist those who suggest that the serotonergic mechanisms of descending inhibitory pathways are influenced by more serotonin available in the synaptic cleft.

Pharmacokinetics SSRIs are metabolized by hepatic oxidation and their use may affect serum levels of other hepatically metabolized drugs. This occurs via induction and inhibition of various cytochrome P450 enzymes. SSRIs may increase levels of tricyclic antidepressants and benzodiazepines as well as other drugs. There may also be effects on levels of carbamazepine, lithium, and antipsychotics. Other serotonergic drugs should be avoided or used with caution given the possibility of causing serotonergic syndrome. There is a report of visual hallucinations in a patient taking fluoxetine, after using dextromethorphan.[7] Dextromethorphan is metabolized by the cytochrome P450 enzyme, which is inhibited by fluoxetine. Although this is a single case report, prescribing both simultaneously may require caution.

Phytochemical Reactions As in other antidepressants or mood stabilizers, caution is advised in combining these with any phytochemicals known to affect mood, such as valerian, kava kava, or St. John's wort.

Adverse Reactions Although SSRIs have limited side effects because they have minimal effects on neurotransmitters other than serotonin, they may cause some undesirable symptoms. Possible CNS effects include headaches, stimulation or sedation, fine tremor, tinnitus, and rare extrapyramidal symptoms including dystonia, akathisia, dyskinesia, and possibly tardive dyskinesia. There are also conflicting reports regarding SSRIs lowering the seizure threshold. Cardiovascular effects are rare but there are reports of tachycardia, bradycardia, palpitations, and vasoconstriction. Gastrointestinal effects include nausea, vomiting, anorexia, bloating, and diarrhea. Rare side effects include SIADH, jaundice, hepatitis, and bleeding disorders. The limited sedation associated with these agents makes them ideal additions for patients with pain on sedating analgesics.

Lastly, approximately 10% to 15% of patients taking an SSRI will experience sexual side effects. This may manifest as decreased libido, impotence, ejaculatory disturbances, and anorgasmia. Change to another SSRI may alleviate these symptoms. However, if changing SSRIs is not effective, a switch to another class of antidepressants may or may not be necessary. Addition of adjunct agents to treat sexual side effects are often helpful. These adjuncts include amantadine, bethanacol, cyproheptadine, neostigmine, and yohimbine. Coadministration of the antidepressant bupropion (Wellbutrin), discussed in the section on Atypical Antidepressant, may also alleviate sexual side effects and provide additional antidepressant efficacy.

Dosages and Monitoring Other than to rule out a medical cause of the patient's symptoms, no initial laboratory workup is required prior to initiate treatment with SSRIs. Although plasma concentrations of fluoxetine plus norfluoxetine above 500 ng/mL seem to be associated with poorer response than lower concentrations, dosage titration is usually based on clinical response and side effects. Note that beneficial effects are usually not seen prior to 2 to 3 weeks.

When SSRIs are discontinued, the dosage should be tapered slowly to avoid withdrawal symptoms. Withdrawal is uncommon and not life-threatening, but it may be unpleasant if it does occur. Withdrawal often includes flulike symptoms including GI upset, vomiting, diarrhea, fever, diaphoresis, irritability, headache, dizziness, and arthralgia. Overdose of SSRIs alone has not been reported to cause death, and the relative safety of SSRIs in this regard contributes to their first-line status in the treatment of depression, where suicide rates may be as high as 10% to 15%. Given the incidence of depression in chronic pain patients, this relative safety offers an advantage over other antidepressants used for pain management. In the event of overdose, symptoms of toxicity include nausea, vomiting, tremor, and myoclonus. Treatment is symptomatic and supportive.

Atypical Antidepressants

Following the introduction of SSRIs, several other classes of antidepressants have been developed. These classes have been designed to target specific neurotransmitter interactions at the synaptic level. They attempt to maximize therapeutic benefits while minimizing side effects. These classes include norepinephrine and dopamine reuptake inhibitors (NDRIs), such as bupropion (Wellbutrin), serotonin-norepinephrine reuptake inhibitors (SNRIs), such as venlafaxine (Effexor), and 5-HT_2 antagonist/reuptake inhibitors (SARIs) represented by trazodone and nefazodone.

Bupropion (Wellbutrin), an NDRI, is a weak inhibitor of noradrenergic and dopaminergic reuptake pumps. However, it is metabolized to hydroxybupropion, which is a powerful inhibitor of both noradrenergic and dopaminergic pumps. This agent differs from most other antidepressants in that it has psychostimulant properties. Thus, as well as being used for depression, it may be useful for treating attention deficit hyperactivity disorder . There have been no clinical trials of its efficacy in the treatment of chronic pain; however, its stimulating properties offer advantages in treating depression in patients on sedating drugs such as opioids.

Treatment should be initiated at 75 to 100 mg once per day, starting in the morning to avoid potential insomnia. It can then be moved to twice daily dosing and gradually increased, though never above 450 mg/day or 150 mg in a single dose. A new sustained-release form is available, saving the practitioner from concern about dosage splitting. Seizures occur in approximately 0.4% of patients at dosages less than 450 mg/day. Dosages of 450 to 600 mg/day may cause seizures in 4.0% of patients. Therefore, doses above 450 mg/day should be avoided. Bupropion should also be avoided in patients with seizure disorder or those taking medications that may cause seizures. Laboratory studies are not necessary before starting bupropion and serum levels are not clinically useful. The most common adverse effects are headache, insomnia, upper respiratory complaints, nausea, restlessness, agitation, and irritability. In overdose, dosages as high as 4200 mg have been taken without death. However, bupropion should not be given with MAOIs, nor in patients with anorexia or eating disorders. Care should be taken when coadministering other drugs that are hepatically metabolized because bupropion is metabolized by the liver.

Venlafaxine (Effexor) is an SNRI that possesses no α_1, cholinergic, or histaminic inhibition. Venlafaxine has dose-related degrees of inhibition of serotonin reuptake (most potent at low doses), norepinephrine reuptake (moderate potency at higher doses), and dopamine reuptake (least potent at highest doses). Venlafaxine is indicated for major depression and possibly ADHD. Though there have been no controlled trials, some anecdotal evidence points toward efficacy in the treatment of chronic pain. Potential analgesia is suggested by its profile of dual inhibition of serotonin and norepinephrine reuptake that is similar to proven analgesic antidepressants such as imipramine, amitriptyline, and desipramine. Venlafaxine differs from these agents in its lack of anticholinergic, antiadrenergic, and antihistiminergic side effects, a difference that has unknown bearing on analgesia. Venlafaxine was approved by the FDA in 1999 for treatment of generalized anxiety disorder.

In 1997, an extended-release formulation was approved. Although in traditional form, venlafaxine is given in two or three divided daily doses beginning at 75 mg/day and increased to as high as 375 mg/day. No laboratory studies are indicated and serum levels of venlafaxine are not clinically useful. Side effects include nausea, headache, somnolence, dry mouth, dizziness, nervousness, constipation, anxiety, anorexia, blurred vision, and sexual dysfunction. No reports of fatal overdose have been reported. Venlafaxine should not be used in conjunction with MAOIs and venlafaxine may affect hepatic metabolism of other medications.

Trazodone and nefazodone are SARIs by virtue of blocking 5-HT_2 receptors as well as serotonin reuptake. These agents are used for depression and insomnia. Their usefulness in the treatment of chronic pain is undetermined, but given the incidence of insomnia in pain patients, they are likely to have at least a potential adjuvant role. Trazodone is less effective for the treatment of depression than nefazodone, though trazodone may be more sedating. Dosages should begin as low as 50 mg/day but can be increased to as high as 600 mg/day in twice daily divided doses. No laboratory studies are indicated before beginning SARIs and plasma levels are not clinically useful. Side effects include sedation, orthostatic hypotension, dizziness, headache, nausea, dry mouth, and GI upset. There are no anticholinergic effects of SARIs. Rare cases of cardiac arrhythmias have been reported. An infrequent but serious side effect is priapism (1/1000 to 1/10000), and patients should be warned of this prior to starting treatment. There have been no reported cases of death following overdose with SARIs taken alone. SARIs should not be used in conjunction with MAOIs. Also, use with astemizole or terfenadine may decrease hepatic P450 metabolism of these compounds resulting in cardiac arrhythmias. Lastly, SARIs may increase serum levels of triazolam (Halcion) and alprazolam (Xanax).

ANTIPSYCHOTICS

Description Antipsychotics are used to treat various psychoses and schizophrenia. They also are used to treat psychotic symptoms such as in paranoid disorders, schizophreniform disorder, brief psychoses, and psychoses associated with mood disorders. They have been used to treat pain as well as personality disturbances, although their potentially permanent side effect of tardive dyskinesia make such a chronic usage inadvisable.

Psychotic has many different meanings in many different contexts. Conceptually, it refers to impairment in reality testing. Early definitions (*The Diagnostic and Statistical Manual of Mental Disorders*, 4th ed. [DSM-II]) of psychotic referred to mental "impairment that grossly interferes with the capacity to meet ordinary demands of life." Across the spectrum of DSM-IV psychoses, the term refers to delusions, hallucinations, disorganized speech, and catatonic behavior. Incidence is estimated to be approximately 1 in 10,000 per year in the diagnosis of schizophrenia, schizophreniform disorder, and schizoaffective disorder. Delusional disorder prevalence estimates are around 0.03%.

History Antipsychotics, also known as neuroleptics or major tranquilizers, were introduced in the 1950s, initiating the contemporary field of psychopharmacology. Such "major tranquilizers" offered more than just sedation to patients, they helped clear cognitive processes and allowed more patients to spend less time institutionalized. Unfortunately, these new medications produced neurologic side effects that were often irreversible. For this reason they were called neuroleptics.

The experience of pain is rife with nociceptive and nonnociceptive aspects, and it is usually difficult to distinguish pain from suffering. Although neuroleptic agents possess some degree of independent analgesia, their significant and potentially irreversible side effects undermine their use in the treatment of chronic pain. However, these agents can have a role in chronic pain when used for short periods. Their potential efficacy may be further realized with the advent of new antipsychotic agents that may have greatly reduced side-effect profiles. Should the risk of tardive dyskinesia be eliminated, chronic usage of these agents may offer coanalgesia in select cases.

Some antipsychotics, including haloperidol, have a molecular structure similar to that of morphine or meperidine. Cautious and short-term use of neuroleptics in the patient in pain may be indicated when thought disorder is present or when fearfulness is not responding to other agents such as benzodiazepines. Since most analgesics can be potential culprits in the onset of delirium, it is important that the pain specialist be able to recognize delirium and treat it effectively. Treatment of delirium usually involves removing or resolving underlying causes. Neuroleptics may be invaluable for short-term management when other analgesic agents have produced delirium. Moreover, neuroleptics can be extremely useful in critical-care situations when sedation is required without either respiratory or hemodynamic depression.

Typical Antipsychotics

Indications Antipsychotics are approved to treat psychiatric symptoms and schizophrenia.

Chemistry There exists several chemical classes of neuroleptics: phenothiazines, thioxanthenes, butyrophenones, dibenzoxazepines, and dihydroindolones. The largest group—the thioxanthenes—are tricyclic, consisting of two benzene molecules connected by a sulfur and nitrogen.

Mechanism of Action Typical neuroleptics (Table 63-4) function as antipsychotics as a result of their dopaminergic antagonism, particularly at postsynaptic D_2 receptors, probably in pathways from the midbrain to the limbic system and temporal and frontal lobes. Typical neuroleptics also may affect cholinergic, α-$_1$ adrenergic, and histaminic systems. These actions are responsible for many of the considerable side effects of typical neuroleptics.

Pharmacokinetics Antipsychotic drugs are highly lipophilic and thus pass easily through the blood–brain barrier. They bind tightly to body membranes and proteins. Although plasma half-life is usually 10 to 20 hours, half-life with the central nervous system is probably longer, based on the drug's effects. Plasma serum levels are not well correlated with clinical efficacy. Antipsychotics may potentiate postural hypotension associated with antihypertensive drugs (often used for vasodilatation in reflex sympathetic dystrophy (RSD) or RPS).

Phytochemical Reactions Various phytochemicals may interact with anticholinergic medications. Those that may potentiate effects include black haw, bogbean, buchu, catsclaw, chamomile, chondroitin, deadly nightshade, and jimsonweed. Those that may depotentiate effects include jaborandi tree and pill-bearing spurge.

Adverse Reactions Antipsychotics carry risk of extrapyramidal symptoms including acute dystonia, akathisia, pseudoparkinsonism, and tardive dyskinesia; those with the least anticholinergic effects have the greatest risk. Neuroleptics also have effects on numerous hormonal systems. Prolactin may be elevated by neuroleptics with possible effects including amenorrhea, galactorrhea, and false-positive pregnancy tests in women and gynecomastia and galactorrhea in men. Neuroleptics may cause hypothalamic dysfunction (leading to SIADH and temperature regulation difficulties) or disrupt serum glucose levels. Neuroleptic malignant syndrome is a particularly serious, albeit rare, potential adverse event.

Anticholinergic activity may cause dry membranes, blurred vision, constipation, urinary retention, and confusion or delirium. Histaminic effects include sedation, cognitive impairment, and weight gain. A combination of dopaminergic, anticholinergic, and α_1-adrenergic effects may cause sexual dysfunction. In addition, neuroleptics may lower the seizure threshold, seen most in lower potency agents such as thorazine and least in high potency agents such as haloperidol. Cardiovascular effects include hypotension, tachycardia, dizziness, fainting, nonspecific CG changes, and rarely arrhythmias, including "torsades de pointes" and sudden cardiac death.

TABLE 63-4 **Typical Neuroleptics**

Medication	Proprietary Name
Phenothiazine	
Aliphatic	
chlorpromazine	*Thorazine*
Piperidine	
mesoridazine	*Senentil*
thioridazine	*Mellaril*
Piperazine	
fluphenazine	*Prolixin*
perphenazine	*Trilafon*
trifluoperazine	*Stelazine*
Thioxanthenes	
thiothixene	*Navane*
Butyrophenone	
haloperidol	*Haldol*
Diphenylbutylpiperidines	
pimozide	*Orap*
Dibenzoxazepine	
loxapine	*Daxolin, Loxitane*
Dihydroindolone	
molindone	*Moban*
Dibenzodiazepine	*Clozaril*
clozapine	

TABLE 63-5 **Atypical Neuroleptics**

Medication	Proprietary Name
Risperidone	*Risperdol*
Clozapine	*Clozaril*
Olanzapine	*Zyprexa*

Dosages and Monitoring No routine laboratory tests are necessary for the prescribing of antipsychotic agents (see Table 63-4 for dosing). Be aware of the emergence of extrapyramidal side effects—and warn patients about potential tardive dyskinesia.

Atypical Neuroleptics Atypical neuroleptics include agents such as risperidone (Risperdal), clozapine (Clozaril), and the recently released olanzipine (Zyprexa). These agents have D_2 antagonism, but to a lesser degree than typical neuroleptics. Additionally, they appear to block 5-HT_2 receptors, and to variable degrees, the D_4 receptor. Atypical neuroleptics may be more efficacious than typical neuroleptics, particularly with negative psychotic symptoms (Table 63-5). However, no controlled studies of the use of atypical neuroleptics in the treatment of chronic pain have been conducted. One advantage of atypical neuroleptics over typical neuroleptics is the lower incidence of extrapyramidal side effects.

Clozapine is a dibenzodiazepine derivative, structurally similar to loxapine. Clozapine is considered a second-line treatment for patients due to the possibility of fatal agranulocytosis in about 1% of exposed patients. Olanzapine is similar in structure and mechanism to clozapine. Olanzapine has a low drug interaction potential and reduced incidence of extrapyramidal side effects. No incidents of leukopenia have been reported for olanzepine. Risperidone also has reduced incidence of extrapyramidal side effects, and like olanzepine, is not associated with agranulocytosis. Olanzapine appears to be more sedating than risperidone; risperidone can cause insomnia.

MOOD STABILIZERS

Description Mood stabilizers are used to treat bipolar disorder, a condition that involves alternating periods and degrees of mania and depression. The mood stabilizer levels out the phasic mood fluctuations. Bipolar disorder prevalence in community samples is 0.4% to 1.6%. Cyclothymia (less severe mood fluctuations) prevalence rates are similar: 0.4% to 1%.

History Lithium is the classic agent for treating bipolar disorder. It has been used medicinally since the 1800s, but not until 1949 did the Australian Cade notice it had a calming effect on agitated psychiatric patients. Recently, however, many other agents such as anticonvulsants (valproic acid, carbamazepine, gabapentin, and clonazepam) have gained popularity in the treatment of bipolar conditions. The overlap of this group of drugs with those used to treat neuropathic pain is striking and its meaning has not yet been clarified.

While bipolar disorder is not overly common in the patient with chronic pain, it does occur and can be worsened by drugs that are commonly used in the pain arsenal. Analgesic agents that may provoke mania include antidepressants as well as steroids. However, several agents that are specifically effective against neuropathic pain also are helpful in treating bipolar disorder (i.e., carbamazepine and gabapentin) and are thus obvious choices for treatment of comorbid bipolar disorder and chronic pain.

Lithium Lithium has been used extensively for treatment of migraine and cluster headaches. However, there is no evidence of efficacy in the treatment of any other type of chronic pain. Lithium remains the most common agent used for treating bipolar disorder. A narrow therapeutic index and frequent side effects limit its use.

Anticonvulsants At present, it appears that all commonly used neuropathic analgesics are anticonvulsants in that these agents are either directly used as antiseizure agents or otherwise as antiarrhythmics or local anesthetics. Anticonvulsant drugs, including carbamazepine (Tegretol), valproate (Depakote), phenytoin (Dilantin), gabapentin (Neurontin), and clonazepam (Klonopin) are widely used for treating chronic pain, neuropathic pain in particular. This same group of drugs is being used more and more widely in treating psychiatric disorders.

Indications Valproic acid is approved for the treatment of bipolar disorder and migraine prevention. Carbamazepine is used to treat mood disorders, disruptive behavior in dementia, neuropathic pain, postherpetic neuralgia, and diabetic neuropathy.

Chemistry Lithium is an alkali metal. Gabapentin is a GABA molecule bound to a cyclohexane ring, whereas valproic acid is a simple branched-chain carboxylic acid. Carbamazepine is chemically and structurally related to the tricyclic antidepressants.

Mechanism of Action The mechanisms of action of this diverse group are understandably varied, but all are thought to act as membrane stabilizers. Phenytoin and carbamazepine both slow the rate of recovery of voltage-activated Na+ channels from inactivity. Clonazepam stimulates GABAergic pathways, valproic acid is believed to increase GABA concentrations in the brain, whereas gabapentin's action is unknown. Although it functions as a GABA analogue, gabapentin does not act at GABA receptors. The action of lithium's therapeutic effects is unknown, but postulated to be either endocrine, neurotransmission, circadian, or cellular. Lithium is not a sedative, depressant, or euphoriant.

Pharmacokinetics Lithium is absorbed almost completely from the GI tract in 8 hours, and peaks in 2 to 4 hours. Slow release preparations are available. Elimination half-life is 20 to 24 hours.

Valproic acid is absorbed almost completely from the stomach with peak concentrations in 1 to 4 hours. Almost 90% of the drug is protein bound. Half-life is about 18 hours. Periodic laboratory monitoring during use renders valproate more cumbersome to use than other neuropathic analgesics. Patients should have CBC and liver function tests before initiating treatment. Starting dosage is typically 250 mg/day, with gradual increases until therapeutic serum levels and clinical response occur. Possible side effects include blood dyscrasias (though less common than with carbamazepine) and hepatitis.

Gabapentin is rapidly absorbed and is not metabolized or protein bound; it is excreted in the urine. Half-life is about 5 to 9 hours and it is highly lipid-soluble.

Carbamazepine is absorbed slowly and erratically. Peak plasma concentrations are seen at about 4 to 8 hours; it is 75% protein bound. Half-life is 10 to 20 hours. The immediate metabolite 10,11 epoxide is as active as the parent compound. Because carbamazepine is hepatically metabolized, it may affect the metabolism of other drugs as well. In addition, there have been reports of carbamazepine-induced hepatitis. Electrolyte disturbances, especially hyponatremia and SIADH, may occur. For these reasons, follow-up laboratory studies should be conducted periodically. When beginning treatment with carbamazepine, CBC should be obtained every 2 weeks for the first 2 months of treatment and quarterly thereafter. The initial laboratory workup should include CBC, liver function tests, electrolytes, and ECG.

Although carbamazepine may be effective in the treatment of chronic pain and it is relatively safe, one may want to use it as a second-line neuropathic analgesic because of the extensive laboratory studies that are required. In addition to its usefulness as an anticonvulsant, carbamazepine is used by psychiatrists in the treatment of bipolar disorder as well as for aggressive behavioral disorders. Its mechanism of action in the treatment of mania or depression is unclear. Patients are usually started at a dose of 200 mg twice daily and the dose is gradually increased until plasma levels are therapeutic and adequate clinical response is achieved. The most concerning potential side effect is blood dyscrasia, including agranulocytosis.

Clonazepam plasma concentrations peak in about 1 to 4 hours after oral administration. It is highly lipid-soluble and binds to plasma proteins. Half-life is about 1 day; clonazepam is metabolized by nitro-group reduction.

Phenytoin absorption is slow and variable. Plasma concentrations peak anywhere from 3 to 12 hours; it is 90% plasma protein bound.

ANXIOLYTICS

Description Anxiety disorders may occur in a large percentage of patients with chronic pain. These disorders include panic disorder, generalized anxiety disorder, obsessive-compulsive disorder, and post—traumatic stress disorder. These often present with somatic symptoms including chest pain, GI upset, and neurologic symptoms (headache, dizziness, syncope, and paresthesias). Treatment of chronic pain that is comorbid with an anxiety disorder should include anxiolysis as part of the analgesic strategy.

Benzodiazepines are the most popular medication for anxiety, and in fact are the most widely prescribed medication of any type. Clonazepam is considered both a psychotropic agent (anxiolytic) and a neurologic agent (anticonvulsant). This suggests its possible usefulness in the pain clinic pharmacologic armamentarium. Why clonazepam is used over other benzodiazepines is controversial.

Indications Benzodiazepines are approved for use with anxiety disorders, alcohol withdrawal seizures, and insomnia. They have also been used to treat akathisia, agitation (including mania), depression, catatonia, and muscle spasm.

Chemistry Benzodiazepines are so named because they consist of a benzene ring connected to a seven-membered diazepine ring. Various derivatives produce similar effects.

Mechanism of Action All benzodiazepines share the same mechanism of action. Benzodiazepines depress the CNS at the levels of the limbic system, brainstem reticular activating formation, and cortex. They bind to the benzodiazepine component of the GABA receptor and facilitate the action of GABA, an inhibitory neurotransmitter. They bind tightly to plasma protein, are highly lipophilic, and resistant to removal through dialysis.

Although not primary analgesics, benzodiazepines often have a role in the analgesic regimen. Clonazepam (Klonopin) may possess special neuropathic analgesic properties; however, this has yet to be confirmed by controlled trials.

Pharmacokinetics The choice of a specific benzodiazepine is often based on onset of action and half-life (Table 63-6). In general, short-acting agents are used to treat insomnia and acute anxiety, whereas long-acting agents are used to treat chronic conditions.

Adverse Reactions The most common side effect of benzodiazepines is sedation and respiratory depression. A paradoxical reaction is also possible where a patient may become increasingly agitated and disinhibited. Although possibly difficult to recognize, if this occurs, cessation of the benzodiazepine is indicated rather than increased dosage. Rapid withdrawal from benzodiazepines can result in rebound insomnia, anxiety, delirium, or withdrawal. Severe withdrawal reactions include seizures, psychosis, and death. Therefore, it is important to discontinue dosages by gradual taper.

Dosages and Monitoring As with any medication in which tolerance develops, dosage ranges tend to be open-ended. In overdose, benzodiazepines are rarely fatal if taken alone, although they may cause respiratory depression. If taken with alcohol or barbiturates, however, benzodiazepines can be fatal, with symptoms including hypotension, depressed respiration, and coma.

Buspirone

Although not known to be efficacious for the treatment of pain, buspirone (Buspar) can be an effective anxiolytic. Buspirone does not interact with GABA receptors directly, but instead acts as a 5-HT_{1A} agonist. It is not clear how this action contributes to its anxiolytic effects. Buspirone is an especially useful anxiolytic in patients with a history of substance abuse or who may abuse benzodiazepines. In addition, buspirone may potentiate the antidepressant and anti-obsessional effects of SSRIs and is also being studied for use in post-traumatic stress syndrome. No laboratory studies are required before initiating treatment with buspirone. Patients may take 5 to 30 mg/day in divided doses, starting at 5 mg three times a day and increasing to as high as 10 mg three times daily. Unlike benzodiazepines, anxiolytic effects are not immediate, requiring 1 to 4 weeks for anxiolytic effects to appear. Fortunately, buspirone has relatively few side effects. Potential side effects include headache, dizziness, lightheadedness, fatigue, parasthesias, and GI upset, although all of these occur in less than 10% of patients. Buspirone has a low potential for abuse or addiction and it does not impair psychomotor or cognitive functions. This feature makes it a useful agent for the anxious patient in pain

TABLE 63-6 **Benzodiazepines Onset and Half Life**

Medication	Proprietary	Onset	Half-life (hours)
Alprazolam	*Xanax*	Intermediate	6–20
Chlordiazepoxide	*Librium*	Intermediate	30–100
Clonazepam	*Klonopin*	Intermediate	18–50
Clorazepate	*Tranxene*	Rapid	30–100
Diazepam	*Valium*	Rapid	30–100
Estazolam	*Prosom*	Intermediate	10–24
Flurazepam	*Dalmane*	Rapid-intermediate	50–160
Lorazepam	*Ativan*	Intermediate	10–20
Midazolam	*Versed*	Intermediate	2–3
Oxazepam	*Serax*	Intermediate-slow	8–12
Quazepam	*Doral*	Rapid-intermediate	50–160
Temazepam	*Restoril*	Intermediate	8–20
Triazolam	*Halcion*	Intermediate	1.5–5

with a history of addiction. There have been no reports of withdrawal symptoms or death from overdose. However, buspirone should be used with caution in patients taking MAOIs, as this combination may result in elevated blood pressure. Also, buspirone inhibits the metabolism of benzodiazepines and haloperidol.

SUMMARY

Treating pain often requires use of medications that affect both nociceptive and non-nociceptive processes. Without adequate familiarity of psychopharmacologic agents, the pain specialist risks limiting her or his analgesic repertoire. He or she may overlook potentially beneficial possibilities as well as potential adverse complications of polypharmacy. The ongoing revolution in development of psychoactive drugs will surely have an impact on pain management, and drugs will likely gain increased prominence in the arsenal against pain.

REFERENCES

1. Ochoa JL, Verdugo RJ. Reflex sympathetic dystrophy: a common clinical avenue for somatoform expression. *Neurol Clin* 1995;13:351–363.
2. Max MB, Lynch SA, Muir J, et al. Effects of desipramine, amitriptyline, and fluoxetine on pain in diabetic neuropathy. *N Engl J Med* 1992; 326:1250–1256.
3. Perovic S, et al. Effect on serotonin uptake by postsynaptic receptors. *Arzneimittelforschung* 1995;45:1145–1148.
4. Suzuki O, et al. Inhibition of monoamine oxidase by hypericin. *Planta Med* 1984;50:272–274.
5. Kessel JB, Simpson GM. Tricyclic and tetracyclic drugs. In: Kaplan HI, Sadock BJ, eds. *Comprehensive Textbook of Psychiatry* 6th ed. Philadelphia, Pa. Williams & Wilkins, 1995:2111.
6. Baldessarini RJ. Drugs and the treatment of psychiatric disorders: depression and mania. In: Hardman JG, Gilman AG, Limbird LE, eds. *The Pharmacological Basis of Therapeutics*. 9th ed. New York, NY: McGraw Hill, 1996:431–460.
7. Clinical Pharmacology Online, 1999. Version 1.20. [database online]. Gold Standard Multimedia Inc. Tampa, FL. Updated July, 1999.

SUGGESTED READINGS

Bezchlibnyk-Butler KZ, Jefferies JJ, Martin BA. *Clinical Handbook of Psychotropic Drugs*. 4th ed. Seattle, Wash: Hogrefe and Huber Publishers, 1994.

Bloom FE, Kupfer DJ, eds. *Psychopharmacology: The Fourth Generation of Progress*. New York, NY: Raven Press, 1995.

Cameron LB. Neuropsychotropic drugs as adjuncts in the treatment of cancer pain. *Oncology* 1992;6:65–72; discussion, 72, 77–80.

Ciraulo DA, Shader RI, Greenblatt DJ, Creelman W, eds. *Drug Interactions in Psychiatry*. 2nd ed. Philadelphia, Pa: Williams & Wilkins, 1995.

Fogel BS, Schiffer RB, eds. *Neuropsychiatry*. Philadelphia, Pa: Williams & Wilkins, 1996.

Guze B, Richeimer S, Szuba M, eds. *The Psychiatric Drug Handbook*. Boston, Mass: Mosby Year Book, 1995.

Hyman SE, Arana GW, Rosenbaum JF, eds. *Handbook of Psychiatric Drug Therapy*. 3rd ed. Boston, Mass: Little, Brown, 1995.

Hyman SE, Cassem NH. Pain. In: Scientic American Medicine. New York, NY: Scientific American, 1989.

Kaplan HI, Sadock BJ, eds. *Comprehensive Textbook of Psychiatry*. 6th ed. Philadelphia, Pa: Williams & Wilkins, 1995.

Magni G. The use of antidepressants in the treatment of chronic pain. A review of the current evidence. *Drugs* 1991;42:730–748.

Onghena P, Van Houdenhove B. Antidepressant-induced analgesia in chronic non-malignant pain: a meta-analysis of 39 placebo-controlled studies. *Pain* 1992;49:205–219.

Sindrup SH, Brosen K, Gram LF. Antidepressants in pain treatment: antidepressant or analgesic effect? *Clin Neuropharmacol* 1992;15(suppl 1, pt A):636A–637A.

Stahl SM. *Essential Psychopharmacology, Neuroscientific Basis and Clinical Applications*. Cambridge, England: Cambridge University Press, 1996.

Wall PD, Melzack R, eds. *Textbook of Pain*. 2nd ed. New York, NY: Churchill Livingstone, 1989.

Zitman FG, Linssen AC, Edelbroek PM, Van Kempen GM. Clinical effectiveness of antidepressants and antipsychotics in chronic benign pain. *Clin Neuropharmacol* 1992;15(suppl 1, pt A):377A–378A.

CHAPTER 64 ANTIEPILEPTICS FOR PAIN

Zahid H. Bajwa and Charles Ho

Antiepileptic drugs (AEDs) have been used in the treatment of chronic pain syndromes for more than 50 years.[1–4] Phenytoin, in particular, has been extensively used for the treatment of neuropathic pain during that time.[5–9] Carbamazepine was the first AED used and extensively studied specifically for the treatment of trigeminal neuralgia.[10–12] Since then a variety of neuropathic syndromes have been treated with AEDs, including diabetic neuropathy, postherpetic neuralgia, glossopharyngeal neuralgia, post-sympathectomy neuralgia, and post-thoracotomy pain syndromes.[1–4] The AEDs include the older drugs like phenytoin, carbamazepine, and valproic acid, and newer agents such as gabapentin, lamotrigine, felbamate, topiramate, vigabatrin, tiagabine, levetiracetam, zonisamide, and oxcarbazepine.

The individual AEDs are briefly reviewed here, as well as general guidelines for their use in pain control.

PATHOGENESIS OF NEUROPATHIC PAIN AND ANTIEPILEPTIC DRUG USE

Neuropathic pain is defined as pain due to dysfunction of the nervous system in the absence of ongoing tissue damage.[13] The pain typically is characterized as sharp, shooting, or burning, and is usually felt in the area of sensory deficit. It is typically worsened by mild stimuli that normally would not produce pain, such as light touch or cool air. The pain tends to be chronic and causes considerable patient discomfort. These symptoms have led to various hypotheses about the pathophysiologic mechanisms of neuropathic pain with relevance to AEDs.[14] When peripheral nerves become damaged, axons grow toward the formerly innervated area directed by an intact connective tissue sheath. If this sheath is also damaged, then axon extensions grow without any direction and become tangled into a structure called a *neuroma*. Neuromas can generate ectopic electrical impulses at the regenerating tips in the damaged primary nociceptive afferents at various levels in the nervous system, from the dorsal root ganglia to demyelinated regions of a root or nerve.[15] Since nerves have been damaged, there is a potential disruption in the balance of the excitatory (e.g., glutamate) and inhibitory (e.g., γ-aminobutyric acid, GABA) neurotransmitters. This disruption leads to hyperexcitability of the neuronal membrane sodium channels and voltage-dependent calcium channels, causing rapid ectopic firing. The AEDs have varying mechanisms of action, many of which are directed at sodium and calcium-dependent channels and GABA metabolism.

Although AEDs provide at least partial pain relief in a large percentage of patients with a variety of neuropathic pain syndromes, their use is limited by side effects in a substantial percentage of patients. In addition, older AEDs (phenytoin, carbamazepine, and valproic acid) also require monitoring of blood counts and liver function tests because of their hematologic and hepatic toxicity, leading to poor compliance. Newer AEDs (with the exception of felbamate) generally are not associated with life-threatening side effects and are easier to use.

ANTIEPILEPTIC DRUGS

Phenytoin

Phenytoin (5,5-diphenyl-2,4-imidazolidinedione) is an AED used to control generalized tonic-clonic and complex partial seizures. For years it was the most commonly used AED for the treatment of a wide variety of pain syndromes.

Phenytoin has been reported to be effective in the treatment of diabetic neuropathy, trigeminal neuralgia, neuropathic cancer pain, postherpetic neuralgia, complex regional pain syndrome (CRPS) types 1 and 2, and post-sympathectomy neuralgia.[5–9] The proposed mechanism of action is reduction of neuronal hyperexcitability by decreasing the activity of sodium channels, thereby stabilizing the neural membrane.[16]

Dilantin is supplied as 30-mg and 100-mg capsules. The recommended dose of phenytoin for epilepsy in most patients is 300 mg per day. An exact dose needed to achieve adequate analgesia has not been defined. Phenytoin use as a neuropathic analgesic should follow the guidelines for its use for epilepsy. Phenytoin has the advantage of once a day dosing and is relatively inexpensive. Absorption orally is slow and variable; peak concentrations may occur as early as 3 hours or as long as 12 hours. It is about 90% bound to plasma proteins and is metabolized primarily by the liver. Phenytoin has a half-life of 20 to 60 hours at therapeutic concentrations. However, a narrow therapeutic window and its short- and long-term side effects limit use.

Complete blood counts (CBC), liver function tests (LFTs), and serum drug levels need to be closely monitored, particularly in the first 6 months. Long-term use can result in cosmetic side effects such as gingival hyperplasia, hirsutism, coarsening of the facial features, and, rarely, cerebellar atrophy and peripheral neuropathy.

Carbamazepine

Carbamazepine (5H-dibenz(b,f)azepine-5-carboxamide) is considered to be a primary drug for partial and tonic-clonic seizures. It has structural similarities to tricyclic antidepressants, making it a particularly desirable drug for treating chronic pain syndromes. It has been widely prescribed as the drug of choice for trigeminal neuralgia,[10–12] and is considered the best neuropathic analgesic for lancinating or electric-like pain.[15] Carbamazepine is effective in other neuropathic pain syndromes such as glossopharyngeal neuralgia, diabetic neuropathy, and pain syndromes associated with multiple sclerosis.[17–20] It has also been used for the treatment of migraine headaches in pediatric populations.[21]

Carbamazepine enhances antidepressant effects and is an effective mood stabilizer. Its mechanism of action is similar to that of phenytoin in stabilizing neuronal membranes.

Carbamazepine is available as 100-mg chewable tablets, 100-mg, 200-mg, and 400-mg XR tablets, and 100 mg/5 mL suspension. The initial starting dose of carbamazepine is between 100 and 200 mg per day; the dose can be slowly increased over several weeks as needed to a maximum total dose of 1200 mg per day. It is absorbed slowly orally, and peak concentrations may be observed in 4 to 8 hours but may be delayed 24 hours. It is about 75% bound to plasma proteins. Carbamazepine is metabolized to 10,11-epoxycarbamazepine, which is an active metabolite. Its half-life is between 10 and 20 hours depending on induction of hepatic enzymes. Carbamazepine, like phenytoin, has a narrow therapeutic window. Before initiating therapy, a baseline CBC and LFTs should be obtained, with frequent monitoring thereafter, particularly in the first 6 months.

Agranulocytosis and aplastic anemia rarely occur; patients should be advised to report any episodes of fever while taking the drug so that a CBC can be checked. Other side effects of concern are hypersensitivity reactions manifesting as Stevens-Johnson syndrome with lymphadenopathy and rare cases of liver failure.

Valproic Acid

Valproic acid (*n*-dipropylacetic acid) is a broad-spectrum AED used to treat a number of epileptic syndromes. Although valproic acid has been used in the management of chronic pain,[22] it has been mainly indicated in the preventive treatment of migraine, cluster, and tension-type headaches.[23,24]

Valproic acid has several proposed mechanisms of action, including increasing GABA brain concentrations by inhibition of GABA-aminotransferase and succinic semialdehyde dehydrogenase (enzymes involved in the synthesis and degradation of GABA), selectively enhancing postsynaptic GABA responses, direct effects on neuronal membranes, and reduction of excitatory transmission by aspartate.[25] Valproic acid, like carbamazepine, is also an effective mood stabilizer.

Valproic acid is available as 250-mg capsules and 250 mg/5 mL syrup. The starting dose of valproic acid is usually 250 mg per day; it is titrated slowly upward to a maximum dose of 1000 to 2000 mg per day, usually in divided doses. Valproic acid is absorbed rapidly orally and peak concentrations are observed in 1 to 4 hours. It is about 90% bound to plasma proteins. It is metabolized hepatically with potent antiseizure metabolites. Valproic acid has an approximately 15-hour half-life.

Limitations for the use of this agent include drug interactions and drug-related side effects, such as central nervous system depression, and hepatic and hematologic toxicity. Frequent monitoring of these parameters should continue during the first year of therapy and occasionally thereafter.

Clonazepam

Clonazepam (5-(o-Chlorophenyl)-1,3-dihidro-7-nitro-2H-1,4-benzodiazepin-2-one) is a benzodiazepine that has been used successfully in providing relief for both chronic malignant and nonmalignant pain syndromes such as headaches, temporomandibular joint dysfunction, and phantom limb pain.[26–28]

Clonazepam acts by enhancing GABA-receptor-mediated chloride channels. It is particularly effective when used in combination with other neuropathic analgesics and in patients with prominent anxiety disorder and insomnia.

Clonazepam is available as 0.5-mg, 1-mg, and 2-mg tablets. The dose of clonazepam should initially be 0.5 mg at bedtime; the dose is slowly increased to 0.5 to 1 mg three times per day. Doses of up to 20 mg/day have been used in epilepsy; 1 to 6 mg per day is generally successful in treating headache and pain. It is absorbed rapidly orally with peak concentrations in 1 to 4 hours. Clonazepam is approximately 85% bound to plasma proteins. It is metabolized hepatically and has a half-life of about 24 hours.

The most common side effects are drowsiness, dizziness, fatigue, and sedation. As with other benzodiazepines, clonazepam may produce physical and psychological dependence; abrupt discontinuation is prohibited.

Gabapentin

Gabapentin (1-(aminomethyl)cyclohexanacetic acid) is one of the newer AEDs that has been approved for adjunctive treatment of partial seizures. In recently published anecdotal reports followed by multicenter, randomized, placebo-controlled studies, the drug was effective in the treatment of postherpetic neuralgia, diabetic neuropathy, refractory CRPS type 1, and migraine headaches.[29–36] The efficacy and safety of gabapentin in treating a variety of chronic pain states has renewed interest and enthusiasm in trying new and old antiepileptics in the treatment of chronic pain.

The precise mechanism of action of gabapentin is unknown. It is structurally related to the inhibitory neurotransmitter GABA, and postulated to increase the level of GABA in the nervous system. However, gabapentin does not interact with any of the GABA receptors, nor is it converted to GABA, and it does not affect the metabolism of GABA in neurons. It does not act at or bind to most receptors tested, including *N*-methyl-D-aspartate (NMDA) and kainate receptors, and does not directly act at the calcium or sodium channels.

Gabapentin is available as 100-mg, 300-mg, 400-mg, 600-mg, 800-mg capsules and 250 mg/5 mL syrup. Patients have generally reported adequate relief with gabapentin doses ranging from 900 to 2400 mg/day. It is generally well tolerated at even higher doses. Gabapentin is well absorbed orally and largely unbound to plasma proteins. It is not metabolized and is renally excreted. Gabapentin has a half-life of 5 to 9 hours.

The most common adverse effects include somnolence, diarrhea, mood swings, ataxia, fatigue, nausea, and dizziness.

Lamotrigine

Lamotrigine (3,5-diamino-6-(2,3-dichlorophenyl)-1,2,4-triazine) is a novel antiepileptic, which is chemically different from other antiepileptics. It is an adjunctive treatment for partial seizures in adults. Lamotrigine is approved for children only in the treatment of Lennox-Gastaut syndrome. There are no published placebo-controlled studies that have evaluated the efficacy of lamotrigine in treating neuropathic pain. However, there have been anecdotal reports, including a large series, of the successful use of lamotrigine in the treatment of refractory trigeminal neuralgia and facial pain[37,38] when used as adjunctive treatment with carabamazepine or phenytoin.

The precise mechanism of action of lamotrigine is unknown. It does not affect NMDA or GABA receptors directly. Lamotrigine however, is thought to stabilize neuronal membranes through the inhibition of sodium channels[39] and reduces the release of excitatory neurotransmitters such as glutamate and aspartate.

Lamotrigine is available as 25-mg, 100-mg, 150-mg, and 200-mg tablets. There are also chewable dispersible tablets in 2-mg, 5-mg, and 25-mg strengths. Lamotrigine doses range from 200 to 500 mg per day in two divided doses for epilepsy therapy, but there are no defined doses for the treatment of neuropathic pain. The starting dose of lamotrigine is 25 to 50 mg per day; it should be increased slowly to 100 mg twice per day. Caution is required when lamotrigine is used in a patient on valproic acid because the latter significantly slows the clearance of lamotrigine. The dose should be cut by at least 50% in this circumstance and should not exceed 150 mg per day. It is well absorbed after oral administration and peak serum levels are reached in 1 to 4 hours. It is metabolzied by glucuronic acid conjugation and primarily excreted in the urine. Lamotrigine is 55% protein bound and its half-life is 13 to 30 hours.

Rash is the most common side effect associated with lamotrigine and requires discontinuation of the drug. Patients should be instructed to inform their physician about any rash or hypersensitivity reaction; these can result in life-threatening complications such as Stevens-Johnson syndrome and toxic epidermal necrolysis. Patients also should be warned of the possibility of dizziness, ataxia, nausea, and vomiting, which are dose-related side effects. Long-term use of lamotrigine can lead to its accumulation and binding to melanin-rich tissues in the body, including the eye, resulting in blurred vision.

Felbamate

Felbamate (2-phenyl-1,3-propanediol dicarbamate) has been successful in controlling partial seizures in adults and the Lennox-Gastaut syndrome in children who are unresponsive to other medications.[40,41] In a neurobiologic study in rats, felbamate was found to reduce mechano-allodynia and hyperalgesia as well as heat-hyperalgesia.[42] Because of the epileptiform nature of certain neuropathic pain states, felbamate has been reported effective for controlling pain in trigeminal neuralgia.[43]

Felbamate has multiple mechanisms of action including inhibition of NMDA and AMPA/kainate receptors, potentiating GABA-receptor-mediated chloride channels, and inhibiting spontaneous discharges from the voltage-dependent sodium channels.

Felbamate is available as 400-mg and 600-mg tablets and 600 mg/5 mL suspension. Felbamate provides effective seizure control at doses of 1200 to 2400 mg per day in three divided doses.

However, felbamate is *rarely utilized* except for patients who are refractory to all other AEDs because of its association with aplastic anemia and fulminant hepatic failure. Patients taking felbamate should have frequent monitoring with CBCs and LFTs.

Topiramate

Topiramate (2,3:4,5-bis-O-(1-methylethylidene)-β-D-fructopyranose sulfamate) is a novel AED approved as adjunctive therapy for partial seizures and generalized tonic-clonic seizures. There are no published placebo-controlled trials examining the efficacy of topiramate in neuropathic pain syndromes. It has, however, been anecdotally reported to relieve pain in post-thoracotomy pain syndrome, intercostal neuralgia, headaches, and other neuropathic pain states.[44–46] Further studies are needed to define its role in the treatment of neuropathic pain and such trials are currently under way.

Pharmacologic studies postulate at least three mechanisms of action for topiramate: blocking voltage-dependent sodium channels; potentiating the action of inhibitory GABA transmission; and blocking excitatory AMPA/glutamate receptors.[47]

Topiramate is available as 25-mg, 100-mg, and 200-mg tablets. The usual starting dose of topiramate for the treatment of partial seizures is 25 to 50 mg/day; the dose can be increased to 400 mg/day in two divided doses over 8 weeks. However, the optimal dose for neuropathic pain is unknown.

Side effects of topiramate include anorexia and weight loss. Patients taking topiramate for prolonged periods may develop kidney stones due to the inhibition of carbonic anhydrase.

Vigabatrin

Vigabatrin is a novel AED reported to be effective in the treatment of complex partial seizures; it is not currently marketed in the United States.[48]

It appears to act by increasing GABA levels thorugh the inhibition of GABA metabolism in the nervous system. It causes an irreversible enzyme inhibition of GABA transaminase. Thus, like many of its predecessors that work through similar mechanisms in controlling neuropathic pain, vigabatrin can be postulated to be an effective alternative to other AEDs for patients who fail to achieve adequate analgesia.[49] The precise role of vigabatrin in pain management, however, has yet to be defined since there are currently no published randomized, controlled trials reporting its efficacy in neuropathic pain.

Vigabatrin is well tolerated in patients treated for epilepsy with minimal central nervous system side effects. Unlike the older antiepileptics, vigabatrin is not metabolized through the liver and therefore has minimal drug interactions with other medications. It is available in 500-mg tablets. Vigabatrin has been shown to be effective in controlling epilepsy in doses ranging between 1 and 4 g/day. It is rapidly absorbed orally with peak plasma concentrations in 2 hours. Vigabatrin is not extensively bound by plasma proteins and its half-life is approximately 5 to 8 hours.

Common side effects include drowsiness, tiredness, headaches, stomach upset, weight gain, and vision problems.

Tiagabine

Tiagabine ((−)-(R)-1-[4,4-Bis(3-methyl-2-thienyl)-3-butenyl]nipecotic acid hydrochloride), another new AED, is effective as adjunctive therapy for the treatment of complex partial seizures.[50]

Tiagabine increases the concentration of GABA by inhibiting the uptake catabolism pathways in presynaptic neurons and thereby prolonging the effect of this neurotransmitters.[51] This mechanism of action suggests the drug may be effective for the treatment of neuropathic pain.[52] There are some anecdotal reports that suggest its effectiveness in this role, and controlled multicenter trials are currently underway.

Tiagabine is available as 2-mg, 4-mg, 12-mg, 16-mg, and 20-mg tablets. The adult maintenance dose of tiagabine ranges from 32 to 56 mg/day in 2 to 4 divided doses for the treatment of epilepsy. It is rapidly absorbed with peak plasma concentrations occurring at approximately 45 minutes. Tiagabine is 96% bound to plasma proteins.

Side effects of tiagabine are generalized weakness, binding in the eye and other melanin-containing tissues, and rash.

Oxcarbazepine

Oxcarbazepine (10,11-dihydro-10-oxo-5H-dibenz[b,f]azepine-5-carboxamide) is a new antiepileptic, which is chemically similar to carbamazepine and may prove to be a neuropathic analgesic.[53] Oxcarbazepine is a pro-drug, which means its metabolite is the active substance. It is indicated for monotherapy or adjunctive therapy in the treatment of partial seizures.[54]

Oxcarbazepine blocks voltage-sensitive sodium channels, resulting in stabilization of hyperexcited neural membranes, inhibition of repetitive neuronal firing, and diminution of synaptic impulse propagation.[55] It may modulate high-voltage activated calcium channels and increase potassium conductance.

A small study demonstrated the efficacy of oxcarbazepine in trigeminal neuralgia.[56] Further controlled studies are under way to determine its efficacy and optimal dose in the treatment of neuropathic pain.

Oxcarbazepine is available as 150-mg, 300-mg, and 600-mg tablets. The starting dose of oxcarbazepine is 150 to 600 mg/day divided into two doses, up to a maximum of 2400 mg/day. Monitoring of hepatic enzymes or hematologic parameters is not required with oxcarbazepine to the same degree as with carbamazepine. It does not extensively undergo oxidative metabolism and has low protein binding (40%). Oxcarbazepine is metabolized to 10,11-dihydro-10-hydroxy-5H-dibenz[b,f]azepine-5-carboxamide (MHD), which is responsible for the pharmacologic effects of oxcarbazepine. The peak serum levels of oxcarbazepine and MHD are reached in 4.5 hours after oral administration. The half-life of MHD is 9 hours.

Side effects associated with oxcabazepine are primarily related to the nervous system and digestive system. The symptoms are somnolence, headache, dizziness, diplopia, ataxia, nystagmus, abdominal pain, anorexia, nausea, vomiting, and rash.

Zonisamide

Zonisamide (1,2-benzisoxazole 3-methanesulfonamide) is used for adjuvant therapy for partial seizures.[57] It is chemically classified as a sulfonamide and is unrelated to other antiepileptic agents.

Zonisamide blocks sodium channels and reduces voltage-dependent T-type calcium currents, stabilizing neuronal membranes and suppressing neuronal hypersynchronization.[58,59] It binds to the GABA-benzodiazepine receptor and facilitates both dopaminergic and serotonergic neurotransmission.

There are no published reports of its efficacy in treating headache and pain, but analgesic efficacy trials are currently under way.

Zonisamide is available in a 100-mg capsule. Its dosing is daily or twice a day. The starting dose is 100 mg/day and can be increased up to 400 to 1200 mg/day. Drug interactions with carbamazepine and phenytoin have been noted. Peak serum levels are reached in 2 to 6 hours after oral administration. Zonisamide is metabolized by the liver but does not affect cytochrome P450 metabolism. It is excreted by the kidneys. Zonisamide is 40% protein bound but does not affect protein binding of other drugs such as phenytoin, phenobarbital, or carbamazepine. Zonisamide binds extensively to erythrocytes, resulting in higher concentrations in red blood cells (RBCs) than plasma. It has a half-life in plasma of 63 hours and half-life in RBCs of 105 hours.

Zonisamide is contraindicated in patients with hypersensitivity to sulfonamides. Side effects experienced with zonisamide are anorexia, nystagmus, ataxia, abdominal pain, confusion, and fatigue. There was concern that development of nephrolithiasis was related to zonisamide but further investigation is required.

Levetiracetam

Levetiracetam ([S]-alpha-ethyl-2-oxo-1-pyrrolidine acetamide) is indicated for adjunctive therapy for partial seizures and may be useful for photosensitive epilepsy.[60,61] It was initially developed as a cognition-enhancing agent for the treatment of Alzheimer's disease. It possesses antiepileptic, anxiolytic, and cognitive-enhancing properties.

It has no significant affinity for GABA or benzodiazepine receptors. Levetiracetam appears to act via an unknown binding site in the brain. It stimulates several neurochemical systems including glutamatergic, dopaminergic, and cholinergic neurotransmission. There are no published reports of its efficacy in treating headache and pain at this time.

Levetiracetam is available in 250-mg, 500-mg, and 750-mg tablets. The recommended starting dose is 1000 mg/day divided into two doses; the maximum recommended dose is 3000 mg/day. Levetiracetam is rapidly absorbed after oral administration. Peak serum concentrations occur from 0.6 to 1.3 hours after administration. It is transformed by enzymatic hydrolysis of the acetamide group in the blood to inactive metabolite and renally excreted. Approximately 66% of levetiracetam is excreted unchanged. It is largely unbound to plasma protein and its half-life is about 6 to 8 hours.

Adverse effects include drowsiness, memory impairment, depression, nausea, and ataxia.

RECOMMENDATIONS

Despite the increase in the number of AEDs available, the rule of "old is gold" continues to be applicable in developing a general strategy to treat neuropathic pain syndromes. Phenytoin, the "grandfather" of the modern day antiepileptics, should be tried first for four major reasons:

- Availability in both oral and injectable forms, which could be helpful in providing immediate pain relief
- Lower cost
- Established safety
- Relative ease of use.

The major exception to this rule is in patients with trigeminal neuralgia, a disorder that generally has responded better to carbamazepine than to the other agents. For classic trigeminal neuralgia, carbamazepine followed by lamotrigine, topiramate, gabapentin, and oxcarbazepine should be tried either alone or in combination.

Among the newer AEDs, gabapentin appears to be the most effective and best tolerated. It probably should be considered first after dilantin for most neuropathic pain states other than trigeminal neuralgia. Gabapentin has the added advantage of easy use in combination with other AEDs that have failed as single agents since it does not interact with these agents.

Other AEDs such as valproic acid, lamotrigine, tiagabine, clonazepam, and topiramate should be tried if the above either do not provide adequate pain relief or are not tolerated. In particular, preliminary data indicate topiramate is a promising neuropathic analgesic, but results of randomized, placebo-controlled studies are not yet available. AEDs such as vigabatrin, levetiracetam, zonisamide, and oxcarbazepine have not yet demonstrated proven efficacy in controlled trials of the treatment of neuropathic pain. Felbamate should only be used as a last resort because of its association with aplastic anemia and fulminanent hepatic failure.

An important point to keep in mind is that these medications are AEDs first rather than true analgesics, and are limited by adverse effects, especially when used long term. Their use for neuropathic pain should generally follow the same dosing and monitoring guidelines used for seizure control, although in our experience, many patients benefit from low doses that are considered subtherapeutic in treating epilepsy; monitoring drug levels may not be necessary.

REFERENCES

1. Sindrup SH, Jensen TS. Efficacy of pharmacological treatments of neuropathic pain: an update and effect related to mechanism of drug action. *Pain* 1999;83:389.
2. McQuay H, Carroll D, Jadad AR, et al. Anticonvulsant drugs for management of pain: a systematic review. *BMJ* 1995;311:1047.
3. Ross EL. The evolving role of antiepileptic drugs in treating neuropathic pain. *Neurology* 2000;55(suppl 1):S41.
4. Backonja MM. Anticonvulsants (antineuropathics) for neuropathic pain syndromes. *Clin J Pain* 2000;16(suppl 2):S67.
5. Saudek CD, Werns S, Reidenberg M. Phenytoin in the treatment of diabetic symmetrical polyneuropathy. *Clin Pharmacol Ther* 1977;22:196.
6. Camtor FK. Phenytoin treatment of thalamic pain. *Br Med J* 1972;4:590.
7. McCleane GJ. Intravenous infusion of phenytoin relieves neuropathic pain: a randomized, double-blinded, placebo-controlled, crossover study. *Anesth Analg* 1999;89:985–988.
8. Chang VT. Intravenous phenytoin in the management of crescendo pelvic cancer-related pain. *J Pain Symptom Manage* 1997;13:238.
9. Ellenberg M. Treatment of diabetic neuropathy with diphenylhydantion. *N Y State J Med* 1968;68:2653.
10. Campbell FG, Graham JG, Zilkha KJ. Clinical trial of carbamzepine (Tegretol) in trigeminal neuralgia. *J Neurol Neurosurg Psychiatry* 1966;29:265.
11. Amols W. Facial pain. Treatment with carbamazepine. *N Y State J Med* 1970;70:2429.
12. Zakrzewska JM, Patsalos PN. Drugs used in the management of trigeminal neuralgia. *Oral Surg Oral Med Oral Pathol* 1992;74:439.
13. Bennett GJ. Neuropathic pain. In: Wall PD, Melzack PD, Melzack R, eds. *Textbook of Pain.* 3rd ed. Edinburgh, Scotland: Churchill Livingstone, 1994:201.
14. Woolf CJ, Mannion RJ. Neuropathic pain: aetiology, symptoms, mechanisms, and management. *Lancet* 1999;353:1959.
15. Burchiel KJ. Carbamazepine inhibits spontaneous activity in experimental neuromas. *Exp Neurol* 1988;102:249.
16. Yaari Y, Devor M. Phenytoin suppresses spontaneous ectopic discharge in rat sciatic nerve neuromas. *Neurosci Lett* 1985;58:117.
17. Rull JA, Quibrera R, Gonzalez-Millan M, Castaneda OL. Symptomatic treatment of peripheral diabetic neuropathy with carbamazepine (Tegretol): double blind crossover trial. *Diabetologia* 1969;5:215.
18. Smith PF, Darlington CL. Recent developments in drug therapy for multiple sclerosis. *Multiple Sclerosis* 1999;5:110.
19. Minagar A, Sheremata WA. Glossopharyngeal neuralgia and MS. *Neurology* 2000;54:1368.
20. Ekbom KA, Westerberg CE. Carbamazepine in glossopharyngeal neuralgia. *Arch Neurol* 1966;14:595.
21. Clancy RR. New anticonvulusants in pediatrics: carbamazepine and valproate. *Curr Probl Pediatr* 1987;17:133.
22. Guieu R, Mesdjian E, Rochat H, Roger J. Central analgesic effect of valproate in patients with epilepsy. *Seizure* 1993;2:147.
23. Norton J. Use of intravenous valproate sodium in status migraine. *Headache* 2000;40:755.
24. Rothrock JF. Clinical studies of valproate for migraine prophylaxis. *Cephalalgia* 1997;17:81.
25. Johannessen CU. Mechanisms of action of valproate: a commentary. *Neurochem Int* 2000;37:103.
26. Caccia MR. Clonazepam in facial neuralgia and cluster headache. *Eur Neurol* 1975;13:560.
27. Bartusch SL, Sanders BJ, D'Alessio JG, Jernigan JR. Clonazepam for the treatment of lancinating phantom limb pain. *Clin J Pain* 1996;12:59.
28. Harkins S, Linford J, Cohen J, et al. Administration of clonazepam in the treatment of TMD and associated myofascial pain: a double-blind pilot study. *J Craniomandib Disord* 1991;5:179.
29. Mellick LB, Mellick GA. Successful treatment of reflex sympathetic dystrophy with gabapentin. *Am J Emerg Med* 1995;13:96.
30. Mellick GA, Mellick LB. Gabapentin in the management of reflex sympathetic dystrophy. *J Pain Symptom Manage* 1995;10:265.
31. Novel Applications of AEDS: Current Research. Express report from the American Academy of Neurology 48th Annual Meeting; 1996.
32. Magnus L. Nonepileptic uses of gabapentin. *Epilepsia* 1999;40(suppl 6):S66.
33. Kanazi GE, Johnson RW, Dworkin RH. Treatment of postherpetic neuralgia: an update. *Drugs* 2000;59:1113.
34. Perez HE, Sanchez GF. Gabapentin therapy for diabetic neuropathic pain. *Am J Med* 2000;108:689.
35. Backonja MM. Gabapentin monotherapy for the symptomatic treatment of painful neuropathy: a multicenter, double-blind, placebo-controlled trial in patients with diabetes mellitus. *Epilepsia* 1999;40 (suppl 6):S57.
36. Di Trapani G, Mei D, Marra C, et al. Gabapentin in the prophylaxis of migraine: a double-blind randomized placebo-controlled study. *Clin Ter* 2000;151:145.
37. Lunardi G, Leandri M, Albano C, et al. Clinical effectiveness of lamotrigine and plasma levels in essential and symptomatic trigeminal neuralgia. *Neurology* 1997;48:1714.
38. Zakrzewska JM, Chaudhry Z, Nurmikko TJ, et al. Lamotrigine (Lamictal) in refractory trigeminal neuralgia: results from a double-blind placebo controlled cross-over trial. *Pain* 1997;73:223.
39. Brodie MJ, Richens A, Yuen AW. Double-blind comparison of lamotrigine and carbamazepine in newly diagnosed epilepsy. *Lancet* 1995;345:476.
40. Canger R, Vignol A, Bonardi R, Guidolin L. Felbamate in refractory partial epilepsy. *Epilepsy Res* 1999;34:43.
41. Jensen PK. Felbamate in the treatment of Lennox-Gastaut syndrome. *Epilepsia* 1994;35(suppl 5):S4.
42. Imamura Y, Bennett GJ. Felbamate relieves several abnormal pain sensations in rats with an experimental peripheral neuropathy. *J Pharmacol Exp Ther* 1995;275:177.
43. Chesire WP. Felbamate relieved trigeminal neuralgia. *Clin J Pain* 1995;11:139.
44. Potter D, Edwards KR. Potential role of topiramate in relieving pain in patients with clinically refractory neuropathies. *Neurology* 1998;50 (suppl):A-255.
45. Bajwa ZH, Sami N, Warfield CA, Wootton J. Topiramate relieves refractory intercostal neuralgia. *Neurology* 1999;52:1917.
46. Zvartau-Hind M, Din MU, Gilani A, et al. Topiramate relieves refractory trigeminal neuralgia in MS patients. *Neurology* 2000;55:1587.
47. Shank RP, Gardocki JF, Streeter AJ, Maryanoff BE. An overview of the preclinical aspects of topiramate: pharmacology, pharmacokinetics, and mechanism of action. *Epilepsia* 2000;41(suppl 1):S3.
48. Gidal BE, Privitera MD, Sheth RD, Gilman JT. Vigabatrin: a novel therapy for seizures disorders. *Ann Pharmacother* 1999;33:1277.
49. Alves ND, de Castro-Costa CM, de Carvalho AM, et al. Possible analgesic effect of vigabatrin in animal experimental chronic neuropathic pain. *Arq Neuropsiquiatr* 1999;57:916.
50. Gabitril package insert. Abbott Laboratories Inc.
51. Meldrum BS, Chapman AG. Basic mechanisms of gabatril (Tiagabine) and future potential developments. *Epilepsia* 1999;40(suppl 9):S2.
52. Ipponi A, Lamberti C, Medica A, et al. Tiagabine antinociception in rodents depends on GABA(B) receptor activation: parallel antinoci-

ception testing and medial thalamus GABA microdialysis. *Eur J Pharmcol* 1999;368:205.
53. Grant SM, Faulds D. Oxcarbazepine. A review of its pharmacology and therapeutic potential in epilepsy, trigeminal neuralgia and affective disorders. *Drugs* 1992;43:873.
54. Schachter SC, Vazquez B, Fisher RS, et al. Oxcarbazepine: double-blind, randomized, placebo-control, monotherapy trial for partial seizures. *Neurology* 1999;52:732.
55. McLean MJ, Schmutz M, Wamil AW, et al. Oxcarbazepine: mechanisms of action. *Epilepsia* 1994;35(suppl 3):S5.
56. Zakrzewska JM, Patsalos PN. Oxcarbazepine: a new drug in the management of intractable trigeminal neuralgia. *J Neurol Neurosurg Psychiatry* 1989;52:472.
57. Leppik IE. Zonisamide. *Epilepsia* 1999;40(suppl 5):S23.
58. Peters DH, Sorkin EM. Zonisamide. A review of its pharmacodynamic and pharmacokinetic properties, and therapeutic potential in epilepsy. *Drugs* 1993;45:760.
59. Tomlinson DR, Malcangio M, Patel J, et al. *Effects of Zonisamide on Mechanically-Induced Nociception in Rats with Streptozotocin-Diabetes*. Research supported by Elan Pharmaceuticals.
60. Patsalos PN. Pharmacokinetic profile of levetiracetam: toward ideal characteristics. *Pharmacol Ther* 2000;85:77.
61. Kasteleijn-Nolst Trenite DG, Marescaux C, Stodieck S, et al. Photosensitive epilepsy: a model to study the effects of antiepileptic drugs: evaluation of the piracetam analogue, levetiracetam. *Epilepsy Res* 1996;25:225.

CHAPTER 65 EPIDURAL STEROID INJECTIONS

John M. DeSio

CLINICAL TRIALS AND OUTCOMES OF EPIDURAL STEROID INJECTIONS

The administration of corticosteroids into the epidural space to relieve both acute and chronic pain of spinal origin has been utilized for over 40 years. In 1957 Lievre et al reported the first use of epidural hydrocortisone for the relief of back pain and sciatica.[1] Since that time numerous investigators have argued both for and against the efficacy of this technique versus alternative treatment modalities in providing significant lasting relief for patients suffering from low back and leg pain. In 1986 Benzon's review of the literature on lumbar epidural steroid injections concluded that low back pain of mechanical origin, especially accompanied by signs of nerve root irritation, may respond to epidural steroid injection.[2] In 1988 Rosen et al, performed a retrospective analysis of the efficacy of epidural steroid injections, studying 40 patients treated for low back pain and sciatica secondary to spinal stenosis or lumbar herniated disc. They concluded that 50% of the patients with radicular symptoms may receive temporary relief with epidural steroid injection (ESI); long term relief, however, occurs in less then 25% of patients treated.[3] In most studies the principal indications for administering epidural steroid injections included symptoms of low back pain or leg pain alone or in combination with varying selection criteria (e.g., previous surgery, duration of symptoms, patient age).

Most studies to date have been open trials of varying duration. There have been several investigations, however, that have attempted to control the variables that may influence the outcome and subsequently yield more accurate results regarding the efficacy of ESI. In a prospective, randomized, double-blind study, Dilke, Burry, and Grahame[4] compared patients whose cause and duration of low back pain and radiculopathy were similar, received the same steroid medication via epidural route, and had not been treated previously. They found significantly better results in the patients receiving steroid; 21 of 35 patients (60%) compared with 11 of 36 patients (31%) in the placebo group. At the 3 month follow-up, fewer patients in the steroid group had severe residual pain (1/44 vs 6/38 patients) and a greater number of patients who received placebo injections (14 vs 3 patients) were still not working.

Overall immediate success rates of ESI vary from 25% to 89%,[5–7] with long-term results falling to a mean of 80% by 6 months[8] and 56% by 2 years.[9] Ryan and Taylor found that 77% of their patients experiencing symptoms for less than 2 weeks obtained complete relief from epidural steroid injection, whereas response rates varied from 72%, 60%, and 43% for patients experiencing pain for 4 weeks, 6 weeks, and >6 weeks, respectively.[6] White et al found that epidural steroid injections were most effective in patients with nerve root irritation manifesting as radicular pain, dermatomal hypesthesia, weakness of muscle groups innervated by the affected nerve roots, decreased deep tendon reflexes, and diminished straight leg raise. They noted success rates at 6 months for 34% of their patients with acute pain and 12% of their patients with chronic pain, whereas their patients' overall success rate at 2 years was 1.3%.[10] More recently, Koes and Scholten examined 12 randomized clinical trials looking at the efficacy of ESIs for low back pain and sciatica. They found that 50% of the trials reported positive outcomes and the other half reported negative results. Additionally, they found that most of the studies involved had significant design flaws that consequently invalidated the outcomes. Subsequently, they called for additional studies, taking into account methodologic shortcomings and focusing on determining which patients would most likely respond to epidural steroid injections.[11] Watts and Silagy performed a formal meta-analysis on the same literature and concluded that there was evidence for efficacy and safety in the use of epidural steroid treatment for sciatica while acknowledging the shortcomings of meta-analysis reviews on small trials.[12] Carette et al reported a randomized, placebo-controlled trial of epidural steroids in 58 patients with documented disc herniation and found significant pain relief and improved functioning at longer follow-up intervals. As in previous similar studies, however, significant methodologic flaws, including noncomparable placebo control and inadequate study group size, likely affected outcome.[13]

There is widespread agreement that a large, randomized, blinded, placebo and active treatment-controlled trial assessing the efficacy of ESI is needed. Additionally, similar studies designed to define appropriate candidates for injection, ideal number of injections, benefit of fluoroscopic assistance versus blind technique, ideal volume and content of injectate, maximum number of injections, and amount of steroid patients should receive in a given period are also warranted (Table 65-1).

MECHANISM OF ACTION OF EPIDURAL STEROID INJECTION

The mechanism by which administering corticosteroids into the epidural space provides relief is largely thought to be by reducing inflammation. The ability of phosopholipase A_2 to induce membrane injury and produce edema has been well documented.[14] Extracts from herniated lumbar discs have been found to contain 20 to 10,000 times more phospholipase activity than those obtained from any other human source.[15] Steroids decrease inflammation by inducing the biosynthesis of a phospholipase A_2 inhibitor, which prevents prostaglandin generation.[16–17] Subsequently, epidural steroids function to inhibit the activity of phospholipase A_2 and therefore block the rate-limiting step in the production of prostoglandins and leukotrienes, which, when liberated, have been shown to sensitize small neurons and enhance pain generation.[18–19] Additionally, prostaglandins of the E series have been found to cause hyperalgesia.[20] Green et al examined intramuscular administration of dexamethasone in patients with pain from lumbar disc disease

TABLE 65-1 **Percentage of Patients with Relief from Epidural Steroids Injections**

Reference	No. of Patients	Overall Improved (%)	Criteria	Year
Rosen et al (3)	40	48	2	1988
Heyes-Moore (25)	120	62	1,2	1973
Dilke et al (4)	100	92	3	1973
Warr et al (22)	500	63	2	1972
Winnie et al (26)	20	90	2	1972
Swerdlow et al (7)	61	69	2	1970
Goebert et al (42)	113	72	2	1961

Criteria Code: (1) improvement in physical examination, (2) improvement in or relief of pain, (3) resumption of work.

From: Sandrock NG, Warfield CA: Epidural Steroids and Facet Injections. In Principles and Practice of Pain Management, 1st Ed. Warfield CA McGraw-Hill, New York, NY 1993 Pp 403.

and found that 80% of patients obtained good relief; pain returned as doses were tapered, but not to original intensity.[21] The advantages of ESI over intramuscular administration of steroid include deposition of drug into the affected area, use of a much smaller dose to achieve the desired result with lower risk of side effect, and longer duration of relief.

There has been long-standing disagreement among authors as to how many ESIs should be given in a certain period and what criteria should be used to determine continuing or withdrawing therapy. Some authors recommend performing a series of 1 to 3 injections even if no relief is obtained from the first procedure,[22] considering that some patients fail to respond initially but do receive significant lasting relief from subsequent injections. We will typically repeat an ESI even if no relief is obtained from the first injection on this basis. Should the patient fail to obtain relief from two consecutive injections, no further ESIs are offered. Likewise, if a patient experiences complete lasting relief after an initial injection, there is no need for further injections. If relief is partial, a series of up to three ESIs, each performed approximately 2 weeks apart, will be completed. At that time the patient is reassessed, remaining pain and dysfunction documented, and alternative pain management modalities considered. There is no need to give more than three consecutive injections, since additional relief has not been documented with higher numbers of injections.[23] We perform a maximum of three ESIs within a 6-month period. Should the patient's symptoms return after this time, a second series of ESIs is considered. This decision is primarily determined by the degree and duration of relief as well as improvement in function experienced after the first series of injections. Several factors have been found to be associated with a higher response rate to ESI: These include patients who have not undergone previous surgery,[24,25] patients with acute versus chronic complaints, diagnosis of nerve root inflammation, younger patients rather then older patients, and location of injection (injectate placed at the level of the affected nerve root).[26]

ANATOMY OF THE EPIDURAL SPACE

Many questions still remain regarding the anatomy of the epidural space such as distribution of fat, the extent of areas devoid of contents, the location of epidural veins, and the presence and location of fibrous structures. By nature, exploration of this area by dissection disrupts and destroys delicate tissue and septae, which disturbs the true anatomic relationships. Likewise other objective approaches to studying epidural anatomy (epiduraloscopy, magnetic resonance imaging) distort the structures by introducing contrast or air into the epidural space, or frankly do not provide the in-depth detail to answer these questions. Hogan examined epidural anatomy using cryomicrotome section with regard to influence of age, vertebral level, and disease. This technique creates minimal artifact and is therefore ideally suited to delineate details of tissue relationships in the epidural space. He found variations in epidural anatomy due to all of these factors, and concluded that they may play a role in altering the ease of epidural entry and passage of both catheters and injected solutions.[27]

The epidural space exists outside the dural sac but within the vertebral canal. It is bounded anteriorly by the vertebral bodies and intervertebral discs, posteriorly by the laminae and ligamenta flavum, and laterally by the pedicles. The posterior compartment of the epidural space is filled by a fat pad that is triangular in shape on axial section. It lies between the dura and ligamenta flavum, but it extends slightly under the caudal-most portion of the laminae above. It does not adhere to these structures, which allows movement of the dura within the canal during spinal flexion.[28–32] The lateral epidural compartment forms just medial to each intervertebral foramen and is filled with segmental nerves, vessels, and fat. The intervertebral foramen are widely patent (except in cases of severe stenosis) and allow free flow of solution injected into the epidural space. The anterior epidural space is almost entirely occupied by a nearly confluent internal vertebral plexus, from which the basivertebral vein originates as it penetrates into the vertebral body. Above the L4-5 disc level, the anterior epidural compartment is obliterated by the attachment of the posterior longitudinal ligament to each disc; below this level, the anterior epidural space widens to a capacious fat-filled cavity.[27] When performing an lumbar ESI, the needle must pierce the skin and subcutaneous tissues, as well as the supraspinous and interspinous ligaments and finally the ligamentum flavum prior to passing into the posterior epidural space (Fig. 65-1). Conversely, there is a minimal to absent interspinous ligament in the cervical vertebral column, especially above the C7-T1 interspace. At the cervical level, with negligible interspinous ligament, entry into the epidural space could be achieved without passage through either interspinous ligament or ligamenta

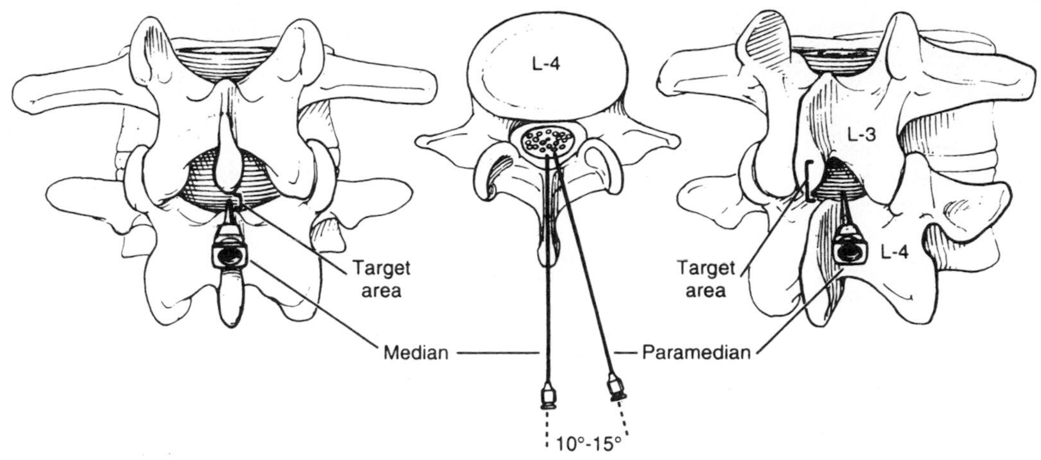

Figure 65-1 A cross–sectional anatomy of an epidural block. From Brown DL, ed. *Atlas of Regional Anesthesia.* 2nd ed. Philadelphia, Pa: WB Saunders, 1999:332.

flavum and therefore without loss of resistance. This factor, combined with the very shallow or absent posterior compartment, makes epidural needle placement especially challenging at cervical levels above C7-T1.

The epidural space behaves like a Starling resistor,[33] with pressures decreasing to a nonzero plateau after injection,[34] independent of volume.[35] As in the joint spaces and pleural cavities, the rigid enclosure of the posterior epidural space allows the tissues to generate a subatmospheric tissue fluid pressure.[36] Entrance of a needle into the epidural space further decreases epidural space pressures. Subsequently, these changes in pressure create the force that draws the hanging drop of saline into the needle hub upon entrance into the epidural space. When using a midline approach to perform both a lumbar ESI and cervical ESI in an adult, the depth from the skin to the ligamentum flavum varies from 4 to 6 cm.[37] Likewise, when drugs are injected into both the lumbar and cervical epidural spaces, they are absorbed by the epidural fat, taken up by the epidural vessels, and diffuse through the dura mater along adjacent nerve roots. Subsequently, the drug should be administered as close to the affected area as possible to maximize the amount of drug reaching the desired nerve root(s).

TECHNIQUE

Although there are many variations in technique used to access the epidural space, the rate of success is primarily dependent on the experience of the physician. Epidural injections can be safely administered in the sitting, prone, and lateral decubitus positions, with or without the assistance of fluoroscopic guidance. Additionally, confirmation of entrance into the epidural space can be achieved by loss of resistance approach, "hanging drop" technique, or administration of contrast medium yielding an epidurogram. Whichever technique is chosen, every effort should be taken to maximize patient comfort, to use the technique most familiar to the physician, and to assure proper placement of the injectate into the epidural space at the desired level. Likewise, all precautions should be taken to maximize patient safety before any invasive procedure. Typically, we will ask our patients not to eat or drink for 6 hours prior to their injections (except taking necessary medications with a sip of water) and to refrain from taking nonsteroidal anti-inflammatory drugs (NSAIDs) for at least 5 days before the scheduled procedure.

Cervical Epidural Steroid Injection

Cervical epidural steroid injections (CESIs) are most commonly indicated in patients suffering from neck and arm pain secondary to cervical disc abnormality, spinal stenosis, spondylosis, and facet arthropathy with significant foraminal narrowing, which produces nerve root irritation and resultant radiculopathy.

During the procedure, the patient is continuously monitored with electrocardiogram (ECG) and for blood pressure and O_2 saturation; a 20-gauge intravenous catheter is placed in a peripheral vein. With the patient in the sitting position and his or her elbows resting on each thigh to relax the shoulders, the neck is flexed so the chin approximates the chest with the forehead resting on a pillow support (Fig. 65-2). Taking a few moments to ensure proper positioning for the procedure in most cases allows for easy access into the epidural space and assures patient comfort. The posterior aspect of the neck is prepared and draped in usual sterile fashion and the desired interspace is identified and appropriately marked at the corresponding skin level. Next, 3 to 5 mL of 1% lidocaine is administered to the skin, subcutaneous and interspinous structures at this level, after which a 20-gauge 5-cm winged needle, or an 18-gauge 10-cm Tuohy needle, is introduced and advanced until it is firmly seated in the interspinous ligament. To use the "hanging drop" technique, the stylet of the needle is removed and preservative-free saline is used to fill the needle until a drop of saline sits above the hub of the needle. The wings of the needle are then held firmly between the thumb and index fingers while the hands rest on the patient's shoulder to ensure needle stability and a slow, smooth advance of the needle into the epidural space. When the epidural space is entered, the negative pressure within the space allows the drop of saline at the hub of the needle to be drawn into the space. Alternatively, the "loss of resistance" technique to saline or air may be used to confirm needle placement in the epidural space. After negative aspiration for blood or cerebrospinal fluid (CSF) is performed, 3 to 5 mL of preservative-free normal saline mixed with 50 mg of methylprednisolone or 80 mg of triamci-

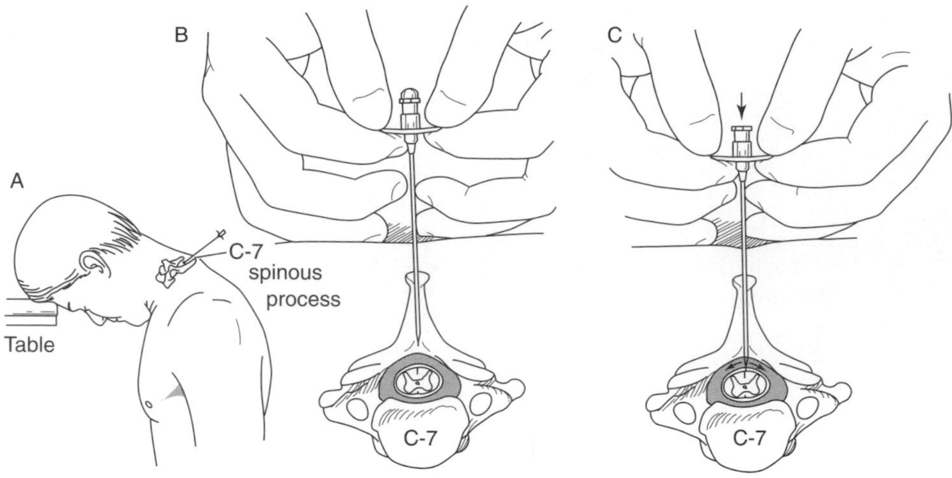

Figure 65-2 Cervical epidural steroid injection. (**A**) While in the sitting position, the patient rests his or her forehead on the edge of the table to accentuate the cervical interspinous space. (**B**) With both hands firmly resting on the back of the neck, the needle is slowly advanced until (**C**) the hanging drop is "sucked into" the needle and into the epidural space. From DeSio JM, Kahn CH, Warfield CA. Benign pain. In: Brown DL, ed. *Regional Anesthesia and Analgesia*. Philadelphia, Pa: WB Saunders, 1996:693.

nolone is injected. The needle is then flushed and withdrawn, the neck is cleaned and dressed, and the patient is brought to the post-procedure room for monitoring. Prior to discharge patients are instructed to expect some soreness at the injection site, which may last a day or two. They are also told to call the office should they experience redness or increasing tenderness at the injection site, fever or chills, or significant increase in pain lasting greater then 1 day following their procedure.

Lumbar Epidural Steroid Injection

Although a variety of positions can be used to access the epidural space at the lumbar level, concern for both patient comfort and delivery of medication to the appropriate level should be primary factors in determining how each individual procedure is performed. I prefer to use the prone position with fluoroscopic guidance; however, many times patients who have had multiple lumbar surgeries or are experiencing severe pain and muscle spasms find it impossible to maintain this position for the duration of the procedure. Likewise, some younger patients will present having had a previous bad experience when a lumbar epidural steroid injection (LESI) was attempted in the sitting position that had to be halted because of a vasovagal event. Use of fluoroscopic guidance not only ensures placement of the injectate at the desired level but also significantly reduces the duration of the procedure. Additionally, direct visualization eliminates the "poking around" some patients report having experienced on previous injections, which despite obtaining good pain relief causes anxiety and hesitation for the patient contemplating an additional injection. With continuous ECG, blood pressure, and O_2 saturation monitoring, a 20-gauge intravenous catheter is placed in a peripheral vein and the patient is placed in the prone position with pillow supports beneath his or her lower abdomen and pelvis to augment lumbar positioning for the procedure. The arms are placed overhead or hanging off the side of the table to ensure patient comfort and maintain a neutral lumbar position (Fig. 65-3). The lumbar area is prepared and draped in usual sterile fashion and fluoroscopic guidance is used to identify the appropriate interlaminar space (i.e., L4-5), which is then marked at the corresponding skin level. Next, 3 to 5 mL of 1% lidocaine is used to infiltrate the skin, subcutaneous and deeper structures, after which an 18-gauge 10-cm Tuohy needle is seated in the interspinous ligament. A 10-mL loss of resistance syringe filled with 3 to 5 mL of air or saline is attached to the needle, which is then slowly advanced under fluoroscopic assistance until the epidural space is entered, as evidenced by a positive loss of resistance. Alternatively, 3 to 5 mL of a mixture of 150 isovue and 1% lidocaine can be injected to produce an epidurogram at the desired level. We routinely use 3 to 5 mL of preservative-free saline mixed with 80 mg triamcinolone; however, a local anesthetic (1% MPF lidocaine) is occasionally used for patients who have acute low back pain with severe incapacitating symptoms. The local anesthetic is helpful in transiently decreasing the pain and spasm that typically occur during episodes of acute pain. The needle is then flushed and withdrawn, the low back is cleaned and dressed, and the patient is brought to the post-procedure room for monitoring. Before leaving, patients are given routine discharge instructions and encouraged to call should they have any questions or develop any concerns following their procedure.

MEDICATIONS

Methylprednisolone and triamcinolone are the steroid preparations most commonly employed as injectates for intraspinal and epidural injections. Methylprednisolone comes in concentrations of 40 mg/mL and 80 mg/mL; triamcinolone is available in concentrations of 25 mg/mL and 40 mg/mL. A common dose used for epidural injection is 50 to 80 mg. Each steroid preparation contains additives including polyethylene glycol, myristyl-gamma-picolinium chloride, sodium chloride, polysorbate 80, and 0.9% benzyl alcohol. Although potentially neurotoxic at higher levels, studies have supported the safety of these diluents with no documented cases of direct neurotoxicity following administration into the epidural space (Table 65-2).

Complications

For the most part complications occurring after epidural steroid injections are rare and most commonly a result of technical error (i.e., postdural puncture headache, intravascular injection of local anesthetic, increased pain due to large volume of injectate used). Vasovagal events can also occur, and in our experience are more common in younger patients at the time of first injection, when the procedure is performed in the sitting position and when ambient room temperature is increased (70° to 74° degrees vs <70°).

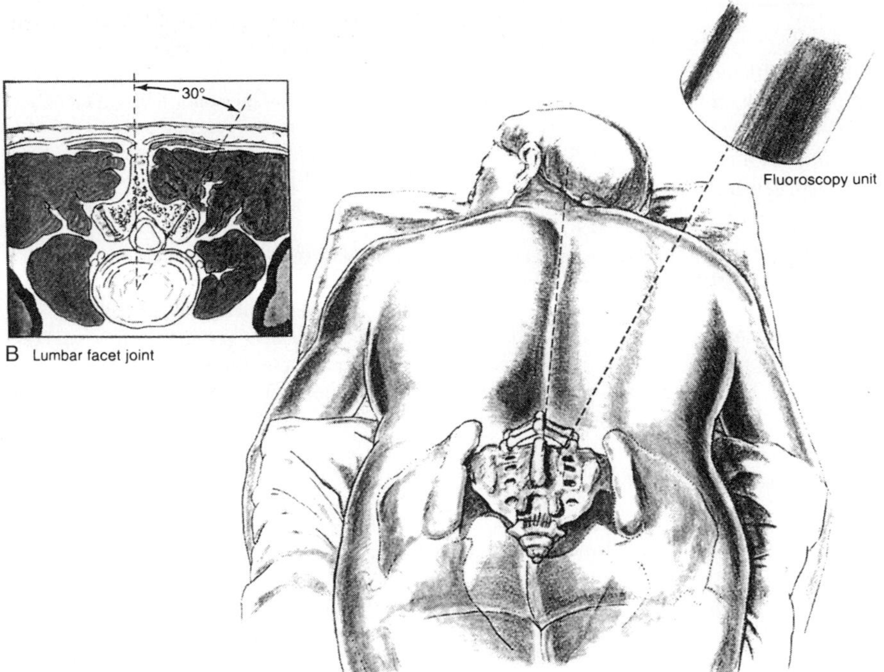

Figure 65-3 Lumbar epidural steroid injection. The patient is comfortably positioned prone on the procedure table with arms hanging at his side to maintain a neutral lumbar position for the injection. Fluoroscopic guidance is used to ensure placement of the injectate at the desired level. From Brown DL, ed. *Atlas of Regional Anesthesia*. 2nd ed. Philadelphia, Pa: WB Saunders, 1999:227.

Systemic steroid effects are rare,[38–40] although plasma cortisol suppression by epidural steroids have been observed to last up to 3 weeks after injection.[41] Subsequently, in a patient undergoing surgery within 5 weeks of receiving an ESI, exogenous steroids should be provided. Rare cases of Cushing's syndrome[38,39] have been reported, as has a case of congestive heart failure,[42] following administration of higher doses of steroids. Subsequently, a recommended maximum dose of 3 mg/kg for methylprednisolone has been determined to prevent salt and water retention.[43]

TABLE 65-2 **Steroid Preparations Used for Epidural Injection**

Depo-Medrol multidose vials			
Methylprednisolone acetate	20	40	80
Polyethylene glycol 3350	29.5	29.1	28.2
Polysorbate 80	1.97	1.94	1.88
Monobasic sodium phosphate	6.9	6.8	6.59
Dibasic sodium phosphate USP	1.44	1.42	1.37
Benzyl alcohol	9.3	9.16	8.88
Depo-Medrol single-dose vials†			
Methylprednisolone acetate	40	80	
Polyethylene glychol 3350	29	28	
Myristyl-gamma-picolinium Chloride	0.195	0.185	
Aristocort single-dose vials‡			
Triamcinolone diacetate	25	40	
Polyethylene glychol 3350	30	30	
Polysorbate 80	2	2	
Benzyl alcohol	9	9	
NACL	8.5	8.5	

- All amounts in mg/ml, †Upjohn, Kalamazoo, MI, ‡Fujisawa USA, Deerfield, IL.
- From: Abram SE, O'Connor TC: Complications Associated With Epidural Steroid Injections. Reg Anesth 21(2):149–162, 1996.

There have been several reports of neurologic sequelae following neuroaxial steroid injections, all of which have involved subarachnoid injections or attempted epidural injections in which subarachnoid placement could not be ruled out.[44] Nelson et al cited two cases of adhesive arachnoiditis among 23 patients who had undergone 83 subarachnoid injections and 1 case of aseptic meningitis developing several hours after subarachnoid administration of methylprednisolone.[45]

Several cases of epidural abscess occurring after epidural administration of both methylprednisolone[46] and triamcinolone[47] have also been reported. Simon et al[48] described a case of allergic reaction to an epidural injection of triamcinolone diacetate, which manifested as skin rash, pruritis, dyspnea, abdominal pain, and diarrhea. Repeat challenge with a small alloquot of the same drug produced a similar response that required treatment with epinephrine and antihistamine. Epidural hematoma requiring surgical decompression following repeated cervical epidural steroid injections has been reported by Williams et al.[49] This complication occurred in a patient who was taking indomethacin on a long-term basis and who had previously received 6 CESIs all without event. Additionally, intraoccular hemorrhage has been reported,[50] as a case of transient paralysis secondary to brief neurocompressive injury with spontaneous resolution within 3 hours following ESI.[51]

Other minor side effects reported include transient headache,[52] stiff neck,[53] and facial flushing and generalized erythema.[54] There appears to be little risk of serious complications associated with the use of ESI when total dose of medication given and the number of injections performed and time are kept to a minimum. Likewise, as the physician performing the procedure gains experience, those complications directly related to technique will likely diminish as well.

CONCLUSION

Epidural steroid injections can be effective in providing significant pain relief, particularly in patients experiencing low back, neck, or extremity pain secondary to nerve root irritation. The effectiveness of ESI in providing long-term relief in painful conditions as a result of bony spinal abnormalities has yet to be determined. The addition of steroid to an epidural local anesthetic or saline injection gives better results when compared with local anesthetic or saline alone.[6] The mechanism by which ESI provides relief appears to be by an anti-inflammatory mechanism secondary to the inhibition of phospholipase A_2 with resultant blockade of prostaglandin and leukotreine synthesis. A series of 1 to 3 injections is typically performed within a 6-month period, with additional injections considered after duration of relief and improvement in function have been determined. There does not appear to be a significant difference in the degree of relief provided by either methylprednisolone or triamcinolone. Plasma cortisol level is depressed following an ESI but returns to baseline within 3 to 5 weeks. ESIs are not without risk; however, the overwhelming majority of reported complications are directly related to technique with rare serious complications occurring after unintentional subarachnoid administration of steroid.

REFERENCES

1. Lievre JA, Block-Michel H, Attali P. L'injection transsacree: etude clinique et radiologigue. *Bull Soc Med* 1957;73:1110–1118.
2. Benzon HT. Epidural steroid injections for low back pain and lumbosacral radiculopathy. *Pain* 1986;24:277–295.
3. Rosen CD, Kahanovitz N, Bernstein R, et al. A Retrospective analysis of the efficacy of epidural steroid injections. *Clin Orthop Rel Res* 1988;228:270–273.
4. Dilke TFW, Burry HC, Grahame R. Extradural corticosteroid injection in management of lumbar nerve root compression. *Br Med J* 1973;2: 635–637.
5. Mount HTR. Epidural injection of hydrocortisone for the management of acute lumbar disc protrusion. In: Morley TP (ed.). *Current Controversies in Neurosurgery.* Philadelphia, Pa: WB Saunders, 1976:67–72.
6. Ryan MD, Taylor TKF. Management of lumbar nerve root pain. *Med J Aust* 1981;2:532.
7. Swerdlow M, Sayle-Creer W. A study of extradural medication in the relief of lumbosciatic syndrome. *Anaesthesia* 1970;25:341.
8. Lindholm R, Salenius P. Caudal epidural administration of anesthetics and corticosteroids in the treatment of low back pain. *Acta Orthop Scand* 1964;1:114.
9. Cappio M. Il trattemento idrocortisonico per via epidurale sacrale delle lombosciatalgie. *Reumatismo* 1957;9:60.
10. White AH, Derby R, Wynne G. Epidural injections for the diagnosis and treatment of low back pain. *Spine* 1980;5:78–86.
11. Koes BW, Scholten RJ, Mens JM, et al. Efficacy of epidural steroid injections for low back pain and sciatica: a systematic review of randomized clinical trials. *Pain* 1995;63:279–288.
12. Watts RW, Silagy CA. A meta-analysis on the efficacy of epidural corticosteroids in the treatment of sciatica. *Anesth Intens Care* 1995;23: 564–569.
13. Carette S, LeClaire R, Marcoux S, et al. Epidural corticosteroid injections for sciatica due to herniated nucleus pulposus. *N Engl J Med* 1997;336:1634–1640.
14. Vishwanath BS, Fawzy AA, Franson RC. Edema inducing activity of phospholipase A2 purified from human synovial fluid and inhibition of austocolochic acid. *Inflammation* 1988;12:549–561.
15. Saal JS et al. High levels of inflammatory phospholipase A2 activity in lumbar disc herniations. *Spine* 1990;15:674–678.
16. Fowler RJ, Blackwell GJ. Anti-inflammatory steroids induce biosynthesis of a phospholipase A2 inhibitor which prevents prostaglandin generation. *Nature* 1979;278:456–459.
17. Granstrom E. Biochemistry of the prostaglandins, thromboxanes, and leukotrienes. In: Bonica JJ, Lindblom U, Iggo A, (eds.). *Advances in Pain Research and Therapy.* Vol 5. New York, NY: Raven Press, 1983.
18. Levine LD, et al. Leukotreiene F4 produces hyperalgesia that is dependent on polymorphonuclear leukotrienes. *Science* 1984;225:743–745.
19. Levine LD, Taiwo Y. Hyperalgesic properties of 15 lipoxygenase products of arachidonic acid. *Proc Natl Acad Sci USA* 1986;83:5331–5334.
20. Ferreira SH. Prostaglandins: peripheral and central analgesia. In: Bonica JJ, Lindblom V, Iggo A, et al. *Advances in Pain Research and Therapy.* Vol 5. New York, NY: Raven Press, 1983.
21. Green LN. Dexamethasone in the management of symptoms due to herniated lumbar disc. *J Neurol Neurosurg Psychiatry* 1975;38:1211–1217.
22. Warr AC, Wilkinson JA, Burn JMD, et al. Chronic lumbosciatic syndrome treated by epidural injection and manipulation. *Practitioner* 1972;209:53–59.
23. Brown FW. Protocol for management of acute low back pain with or without radiculopathy; including the use of epidural and intrathecal steroid. In: Brown FW, ed. *American Academy of Orthopedic Surgery Symposium on the Lumbar Spine.* St. Louis, Mo: CV Mosby, 1981.
24. Green PWB, Burke AJ, Weiss CA, et al. The role of epidural cortisone injection in the treatment of discogenic low back pain. *Clin Orthop* 1980;153:121.
25. Heyse-Moore GH. A Rational approach to the use of epidural medication in the treatment of sciatic pain. *Acta Orthop Scand* 1978;49:366.
26. Winnie AP, Hartman JT, Meyers HL, et al. Pain clinic, II: intradural and extradural corticosteroids for sciatica. *Anesth Analg* 1972;51: 990–1003.
27. Hogan QH. Epidural anatomy examined by cryomicrotome section. *Reg Anesth* 1996;21:395–406.
28. Greene HM. Lumbar puncture and the prevention of postpuncture headache. *JAMA* 1926;86:391–392.
29. Smith CG. Changes in length and position of the segments of the spinal cord with changes in posture in the monkey. *Radiology* 1956;66: 259–265.
30. Reid JD. Effects of flexion-extension movements of the head and spine upon the spinal cord and nerve roots. *J Neurol Neurosurg Psychiatry* 1960;23:214–221.
31. Breig A, Marions O. Biomechanics of the lumbosacral nerve roots. *Acta Radiol* 1963;1:1141–1160.
32. Kubik S, Muntener M. Zur Topographie der spinalen Nervenwurzeln. II. Der Einfluss Des Wachstums des Duralsackes, sowie der Krummungen und der Bewegungen der Wirgelsaule auf die Verlaufsrichtung der spinalen Nervenwurzeln. *Acta Anat (Basel)* 1969;74:149–168.
33. Rocco AG, Scott DA, Boas RA, et al. The epidural space behaves as a Starling resistor and inflow resistance is elevated in a diseased epidural space [abstract]. *Reg Anesth* 1990;(suppl):39.
34. Usubiaga JE, Wikinski JA, Usubiaga LE. Epidural pressure and its relation to spread of anesthetic solutions in the epidural space. *Anesth Analg* 1967;46:440–446.
35. Paul DL, Wildsmith JA. Extradural pressure following the injection of two volumes of bupivacaine. *Br J Anaesth* 1989;62:368–372.
36. Guyton AC, Granger HJ, Taylor AE. Interstitial fluid pressure. *Physiol Rev* 1971;51:527–563.
37. Brown DL. *Atlas of Regional Anesthesia.* 2nd ed. Philadelphia, PA: WB Saunders, 1999:332.
38. Burn JM, Rao TLK, Glisson SN, et al. Epidural triamcinolone and adrenal responses to stress. *Anesthesiology* 1981;55:A147.
39. Stambough JL, Booth RE Jr, Rothman RH. Transient hypercorticism after epidural steroid injection. A case report. *J Bone Joint Surg Am* 1984;66:1115–1116.
40. Tuel SM, Mey Thaler JM, Cross LL. Cushing's syndrome from epidural methylprednisolone. *Pain* 1991;40:81–84.

41. Seghal AD, Tweed DC, Gardner WJ, et al. Laboratory studies after intrathecal steroid. *Arch Neurol* 1963;9:74–78.
42. Goebert HW, Jallo ST, Gardner WS, et al. Painful radiculopathy treated with epidural injections of procaine and hydrocortisone acetate: results in 113 patients. *Anesth Analg Curr Res* 1961;40:130–134.
43. Knight CL, Burnell JC. Systemic side effects of extradural steroids. *Anaesthesia* 1980;35:593–594.
44. Abram SE, O'Connor TC. Complications associated with epidural steroid injections. *Reg Anesth* 1996;21:149–162.
45. Nelson DA, Vates TS, Thomas RB. Complications from intrathecal steroid therapy in patients with multiple sclerosis. *Acta Neurol Scand* 1973;49:176–188.
46. Shealy CN. Dangers of spinal injections without proper diagnosis. *JAMA* 1966;197:156–158.
47. Chan ST, Leung S. Spinal epidural abscess following steroid injection for sciatica. *Spine* 1989;14:106–108.
48. Simon DL, Kunz RD, German JD, et al. Allergic or pseudoallergic reaction following epidural steroid deposition and skin testing. *Reg Anesth* 1989;14:253–255.
49. Williams KN, Jaokowski A, Evans PJD. Epidural hematoma requiring surgical decompression following repeated cervical epidural steroid injection for chronic pain. *Pain* 1990;42:197–199.
50. DeFalque RJ, McDanal JT. Retinal hemorrhage as a consequence of epidural steroid injection. *Arch Ophthalmol* 1996;114:361–362.
51. McLain RF, Fry M, Hecht ST. Transient paralysis associated with epidural steroid injection. *J Spinal Disord* 1997;10:441–444.
52. Abram SE, Cherwenka RW. Transient headache immediately following epidural steroid injection. *Anesthesiology* 1979;50:461–462.
53. Cicala RS, Westbrook L, Angel J. Side effects and complications of cervical epidural steroid injections. *J Pain Symptom Manage* 1989;4:64–66.
54. DeSio JM, Kahn CH, Warfield CA. Facial flushing and/or generalized erythema after epidural steroid injection. *Anesth Analg* 1995;80:617–619.

CHAPTER 66

SPINAL CANAL ENDOSCOPY

Dwight Ligham and Lloyd Saberski

INTRODUCTION

The epidural space was first shown to be important in radicular pain states by Lindahl and Rexed in 1950.[1] Subsequently, Goebert performed the first reported epidural steroid injection.[2] Since that time physicians have used the epidural space to gain direct access to traversing nerve roots and indirect access to the intrathecal space for medication delivery.

Anatomically, the epidural space is tubular and exists as a potential space. This tubular three-dimensional structure surrounds the dura and spinal cord. It extends from the foramen magnum to the upper sacrum. When examined in transverse plane, its external boundaries are the ligamentum flavum posteriorly, lamina and pedicles laterally, and the vertebral body and intervertebral disc anteriorly. The internal boundary is the dura.

Medication administration into the epidural space has been used to treat both acute and chronic pain. Examples include regional anesthesia for surgery, trauma, and labor. Dilute local anesthetic infusions have been used to treat postherpetic neuralgia, complex regional pain states, and cancer-related pain. Opioids and sympathomimetics have been added for synergy. Epidural steroids have been used to treat inflammatory nerve root irritation. Volumemetric injections and flouroscopically guided catheters have been used to direct medication delivery, wash away inflammatory mediators, lyse epidural adhesions, and deliver anti-inflammatory medication.

Efficacy of epidural treatment for radiculopathy is determined by multiple factors. Medical factors influencing outcome include accuracy of diagnosis, presence of nerve root inflammation, symptom duration, previous surgical intervention, patient age, and clinician ability to place the epidural steroid at the level of pathology.[3] Treatment outcome also depends on psychological and social issues. Abram delineated factors correlating with treatment failure at twice the rate expected. These factors include poor education, unemployment, pain constant in nature, sleep disturbance, nonradicular diagnosis, duration >6 months, change in recreational activities, and tobacco use.[4]

Epidural space endoscopy or spinal canal endoscopy may improve outcome by addressing some of the medical factors discussed above. The region of erythema that is likely related to inflammation is visually confirmed with the endoscope. Fluoroscopy is used to confirm the spinal level. The flexible steerable handle allows placement of medication in the lateral gutter adjacent to the nerve root. Reproduction of pain during the procedure while exploring pathology helps to confirm diagnosis.[5]

Psychological and social factors are more difficult to treat and unfortunately they are not amenable to procedural intervention. These factors cannot be ignored, however, because they are of equal or greater importance than the medical pathology.[6] Therefore attempts to address these issues by modification of behavior, structured water or land exercise programs, tobacco cessation, and improved sleep hygiene need to be made. Interventions such as targeted pharmacologic therapy to enhance restful sleep and programs to structure daily activity to enhance self-esteem are no less important. Lastly, functional goals should be set. To focus on complete pain cessation in the patient suffering from chronic pain distracts from attainable goals and ultimately is detrimental and nonproductive.

WHY SPINAL CANAL ENDOSCOPY AND WHY NOW?

One might ask the question,"Why spinal canal endoscopy and why now?" Historically, there has been no way to ensure directed delivery of medication to the area of pathology within the epidural space. Fluids flow according to physical laws of pressure and resistance. Flow of contrast solution is observed to flow from suspected pathologic sites, which are regions of low compliance toward normal higher compliance areas. We believe that all epidural solutions flow in the same manner. The technique of spinal canal endoscopy allows the operator to administer medication directly to the site of suspected pathology and is not dependent on compliance of the epidural space. This is possible because of improvements in fiberoptic technology, development of steerable catheters, and use of the caudal approach, which separates the region of procedural trauma from the suspected site of pathology. These cumulative developments culminate in the ability to examine spinal anatomy in its native state and to identify pathology that may exist there. This in itself is unprecedented and not duplicated by either surgical or radiologic technology.

HISTORY

Orthopedic surgeon Michael Burman became the first to document use of a primitive arthroscope on cadaveric spinal preparations in 1931.[7] The arthroscope's diameter (9.5 mm) was larger than the spinal canal, which severely limited its use in patients. The arthroscope's built-in light source and rudimentary optics precluded miniaturization.

Elias Stern, an anatomist at Columbia University, developed a spinascope in 1936.[8] The instrument was manufactured by American Cystoscope Makers, Inc. There is record of its clinical use in seven volunteer patients for *in vivo* examination of the neuraxis. Intrathecal anatomy was described. The scope was rigid and used direct-through-the-scope optics, which limited its use. Lighting continued to be poor. The technique was further limited by trauma at the spinal level of interest and resultant hemorrhage that obscured visualization. It was designed for intrathecal use during spinal anesthesia.

In 1942 Pool published a series of 400 myeloscopic procedures.[9,10] His myeloscope used a cannula over guide-wire technique to access the intrathecal space. Once access was confirmed, the lens and the light source were placed through the cannula and the operator observed directly through an eye piece.

Perhaps Pool's greatest achievement was his atlas of hand-drawn images of intrathecal anatomy. Unfortunately, this was also his limitation: He was technically limited by his inability to photographically record his findings.

Dr. Pool used his myeloscope to confirm a clinical diagnosis or to establish an alternative one in his clinical practice. He described and recorded neuritis, disc herniation, hypertrophied ligamentum flavum, neoplasms, varicose vessels, and arachnoid adhesions.

The literature was silent until 1969 when Yoshio Ooi published his paper on the intrathecal lumbar endoscope.[11] Miniaturization was possible in the 1970s with the advent of fiber optics and cool indirect lighting. A rigid scope continued to be used. Access continued to be at the level of interest, limiting epidural observation to a small area and increasing the risk of trauma and bleeding into the field of view. Seventy percent of the 86 patients in his series developed a post-dural puncture headache but no serious complications were reported. Photographs were obtained but they continued to be of poor quality.[12]

Rune Blomberg was the first to publish his experience with visualization of the epidural space in 1985. He described his experience both in cadaveric and living bodies.[13]

Video imaging technology became available in 1980. Koki Shimoji was the first to describe subarachnoid endoscopy using thin (0.5 to 1.4 mm) flexible epidural fiber-optic myeloscopes and used this technology in 1991.[14] Epidural visualization continued to be difficult due to the use of the lumbar paramedian approach, which required the angle of attack to be between 45 and 90 degrees. Additionally, the problem of consistent expansion of the epidural space to facilitate optics and maintain focal length remained unsolved.

Shimoji used the technique of awake pain mapping in his patients. Arachnoiditis was identified. Subarachnoid myeloscopy was possible to the cisterna magna in four of his patients. X-ray technology was used to confirm myeloscope level.

In 1991, Saberski and Kitahata solved several of the problems that had limited study and visualization of the epidural space. The caudal approach to the epidural space allowed the fiber-optic scope to be inserted distal to the area of interest, permitting inspection of native tissues free of procedural trauma.[15] This approach also solved the problem encountered with sharp attack angles: The scope could now be advanced parallel to the dura mater, which facilitated steering of the device. To further enhance steering, a disposable steering handle was developed in conjunction with Myelotec Corporation (Roswell, Ga). This steering device incorporated the port for the fiber-optic device and a separate port for fluid administration. This additional port solved the problem of maintaining a dilated epidural space needed for optical focal length and clear visualization. Lastly, the fiber-optic diameter was reduced to 0.8 mm, necessary to facilitate passage through a steering handle port and into the caudal canal. At last the technical issues limiting spinal canal endoscopy were resolved.

CLINICAL USE

New technology seems to always expand the worldview of the field that it affects and thereby expands the possibilities for clinical use. Spinal canal endoscopy is no different. Multiple factors will determine the potential use of this technology. Diagnostically, spinal canal endoscopy allows one to directly visualize the epidural space. As such, it will expand medicine's ability to make a clearer and more specific diagnosis of epidural-based pathology. Dr Pool's early myeloscopic work demonstrated this. He visually identified pathology that had never before been considered through his pioneering myeloscopic work. We can expect similar identification of new unrecognized pathology.

The ability to visually explore the epidural space opens a new world of possibilities both for treatment and for diagnosis. However, before pathology can be categorized, the normal anatomy of the *in vivo* epidural space must be categorized and understood. This process is well under way.

Currently, the spinal canal endoscope is available to practitioners under a 510 K Food and Drug Administration (FDA) market approval for diagnosis and drug delivery. The market approval was granted in September of 1996 to Myelotec Corporation (Alpharetta, Ga, unpublished data, 9/4/96 and 8/11/98). As the field grows in this technology, one may expect the indications and use of this technology to grow.

With this caveat in mind, the current use of spinal endoscopy in low back and radicular pain is limited to pain generator mapping, normal saline lavage, and visually directed delivery of anti-inflammatory medication.

INDICATIONS AND PATIENT SELECTION

The indication for this procedure is lumbar or sacral radiculopathy, either from presumed nerve root irritation without compressive lesion or minimally compressive nerve root foraminal stenosis. Spinal canal endoscopy appears to be most effective when treating inflammatory radiculopathy, with or without signs of compressive lesion in the neurologically stable patient. Signs of motor weakness, bowel, and bladder or erectile dysfunction in the acute setting or unstable neurologic picture in the chronic setting suggest the need for neurosurgic consultation and collaboration.[16]

Contraindications to the procedure include patient refusal, pathology at the site of the sacral hiatus (e.g., pilonidal cyst), active untreated infection, osteomyelitis, bleeding diathesis, lack of sacral hiatus, increased intracranial pressure, inability to tolerate the prone position, allergy to proposed medications, new motor weakness or acute bowel, and bladder or erectile dysfunction.

Relative contraindications include poorly controlled diabetes mellitus, immunocompromised states, active legal issues impacting the painful condition, and active, untreated psychiatric disorders.[17]

Patient selection based on case reports suggest better results in the subgroup of patients with an acute or subacute disc-related spinal pain syndrome who have not undergone back surgery and do not associated pain behaviors.[18,19] This subgroup of patients may be most responsive to "washout" of chemical irritants and corticosteroid anti-inflammatory effect. This subgroup of patients may also have not undergone central remodeling and secondary hyperalgesia.

At any rate, spinal canal endoscopy is indicated for radicular pain syndromes secondary to inflammation, epidural adhesion, Tarlov's cyst, post-laminectomy syndrome, and mild to moderate spinal stenosis. It is these patients who seem at this time to benefit most from this procedure.

Spinal canal endoscopy is not indicated in those patients who suffer from biomechanical pain syndromes such as lumbar facet syndrome, sacroiliac joint dysfunction, or myofascial pain syndrome.

PROCEDURE

Prior to spinal canal endoscopy, all patients must undergo a complete history and physical examination. Care should be taken to document this examination carefully, with special attention to the full neurologic examination. Imaging studies and special testing such as electromyography and nerve conduction studies should be reviewed.

Lumbosacral, flexion, extension and oblique views may be considered to rule out disease not amenable to epidural procedures. Magnetic resonance imaging of the lumbar and sacral spine should be considered to rule out compressive radiculopathy and severe spinal stenosis.

Preparation

Nonsteroidal anti-inflammatory drugs, aspirin, and other platelet inhibitors and anticoagulants should be discontinued before the procedure to allow the coagulation system to normalize.[20] This must be done with the prescribing physician's knowledge and consent to avoid possible medical complications. Appropriate laboratory studies may be ordered to document normal coagulation.

The patient is directed to use an antibacterial scrub the evening before the procedure and is directed to not eat or drink after midnight.

Equipment should be inspected and all disposables must be in place. The procedure should be scheduled with fluoroscopy, video monitor, and camera.

Preprocedure discussion with consultant anesthesiologist should include patient positioning (prone) and the need for an awake patient responsive to verbal interrogation.

Informed consent must be obtained. We use a standardized video informed consent for this procedure. This standardized informed consent process provides documentation of the content discussed.

Procedure

We advise that contact is maintained with the patient at all times during the procedure. We avoid producing severe discomfort in our patients and will frequently equilibrate the system to atmospheric pressure and administer fluids slowly.

As a prophylactic, a first-generation cephalosporin is given immediately prior to the start of the procedure.

The technique of spinal canal endoscopy follows:

1. The patient is placed prone on the fluoroscopy table with a pillow under the abdomen. Identify the sacral hiatus and mark it. Preparation is done from mid-thoracic spine to buttocks and from flank to flank. Apply drapes. Drape the fluoroscope.
2. With the fluoroscope tube directed laterally, the position of the sacral hiatus is confirmed using a radiopaque epidural needle.
3. Anesthesia is obtained by injecting a small volume of local anesthetic at the sacral hiatus. The 25-gauge 1.5-in. needle may be used as a finder to ensure proper angle of attack.
4. Insert the 17-gauge Touhy needle through the sacral hiatus to access the caudal epidural space. This can be done under real-time fluoroscopy if necessary. The loss of resistance technique to saline may help to identify the caudal epidural space.
5. The guide wire is placed through the epidural needle and followed using fluoroscopy to demonstrate easy passage through the caudal epidural space. It should pass easily without resistance. Non-ionic contrast may be used to prove needle placement within the caudal canal if the guide wire is not easily passed.
6. The fluoroscope then should be placed in the posterior-anterior (PA) position. Confirm proper threading of the guide wire. Once confirmed, the Touhy needle is removed.
7. The dilator is then passed over the wire. A No. 11 blade is used to make a vertically oriented stab incision along the wire to the level of the sacral hiatus. The dilator is then passed into the caudal canal. Some caudal canals are quite tight. The dilator is gently past several times in and out of the caudal canal. Care is taken to ensure that the guide wire continues to thread easily and is not kinked. If there is any question, fluoroscopy is used to confirm position. The dilator is removed.
8. Next assemble the dilator-sheath unit. Thread this unit over the guide wire and place the unit into the sacral canal. Ensure that the sheath is fully inserted and remove the dilator and the guide wire.
9. Flush the side arm of the introducer with 5 mL of sterile, preservative-free normal saline. Ensure that there is no cerebrospinal fluid (CSF) or blood on aspiration prior to this injection.
10. Set up the fiber-optic cable and the steering handle. Connect a 100-mL bag of sterile, preservative-free normal saline to a three-way connector using the sterile intravenous tubing supplied in the access kit. Flush the tubing. Apply the 10-mL epidural syringe to the three-way connector. Attach the three-way connector to the tubing of the steering handle and flush the system.
11. Place the fiber-optic cable through the opposite port of the steering handle. Obtain a video image and focus.
12. Advance the steering handle fiber-optic unit into the caudal epidural space. Use fluoroscopy to advance the steering handle to the site of interest. The steering handle may be placed in the same fashion as a percutaneous stimulation lead. Once the tip of the steering handle is at the desired location, gentle pulsatile saline administration may be used to dilate the epidural space, facilitating focal length and optical resolution.

It is an important practice to sustain pressure in the epidural space for no more than 2 to 3 minutes at a time. This should prevent compromise of profusion. We limit total epidural fluids to <100 mL. Most procedures last 20 to 30 minutes after saline administration and epidural viewing has begun.

After the procedure is completed, a dressing is applied and the patient is taken to the recovery area.

Post-Procedure

In the recovery room a post-procedure neurologic examination is performed. Any new deficits should be clearly detailed and followed serially. Alternatively, consultation with the neurosurgery department may be considered.

Patients are instructed not to bathe for 5 days, but showers are acceptable. Hygiene instructions are important: perineal cleaning after bowel movement should be directed away from the procedural site. The discharge instruction sheet is helpful in outlining these instructions as well as wound care and "call-for" contingencies.

The patient should be discharged with a driver and should be observed by a friend or family member for the immediate post-procedure period. A 2- or 3-day supply of post-procedural short-acting opioid such as a codeine, hydrocodone, or oxycodone preparation is appropriate.

Potential Complications

Complications attributable to the operative phase of the procedure appertain to the generation of excessive epidural pressure.[21] Excessive pressure can affect both local and more distant perfusion. Scapular or neck pain may portend retinal hemorrhage. Patient complaints of pain from small volume distention of the epidural space usually signifies a noncompliant epidural space and may transmit high pressure far from the site of fluid administration. We are careful to keep epidural fluid volumes low and to maintain contact with our patient throughout this procedure.

Other potential complications include post-dural puncture headache, epidural hematoma, infection, increased pain, and transient dysthesias. It is reassuring, however, that there has been no permanent injury reported after approximately 6000 spinal endoscopy procedures preformed throughout the world (Myelotec Inc, Alparetta, Ga, unpublished data).

OUTCOME

Hard outcome data for spinal canal endoscopy is in development. To date, there have been no randomized, controlled trials regarding the efficacy of spinal canal endoscopy or other forms of therapy both surgical and nonsurgical. However, one pre- and post-procedural survey utilizing data from 77 patients demonstrated decreased medication use and improved functional capacity up to 6 months after spinal endoscopy.

CODING FOR SPINAL CANAL ENDOSCOPY

Insurers typically cover procedures and devices that meet the following criteria: The device is medically necessary to treat the patient's condition, and the device is used according to the labeled indications approved by the FDA.

Although we offer several possible billing codes for this procedure, individual insurance companies will only honor certain ones. It is important that providers communicate with individual payers to understand their requirements.

In this complex and changing health care environment, insurance coverage is never a guarantee of payment. Insurers vary widely in the services they cover. Even among patients insured by the same insurance company, benefits may vary according to the specific plan. Some plans may be unfamiliar with spinal canal endoscopy. Educating insurers about the procedure may be necessary before a coverage decision can be made. We suggest that claims are filed manually with a complete operative report and hard copy of all supporting radiographs.

There are no available CPT codes specific to epidural diagnostic and therapeutic procedures using the spinal endoscope. Acceptable CPT codes vary from insurer to insurer. Several possible codes are listed below. As discussed, individual payers may have specific policies regarding the use of CPT codes.

Coding for Diagnosis (ICD-9-CM)

Diagnosis and the diagnostic codes must be supportive of the medical necessity for procedures and service rendered. The diagnostic codes below may be appropriate for epidural endoscopy.

353.1	Lumbosacral plexus lesions
353.4	Lumbosacral root lesions, not elsewhere classified
722.83	Post-laminectomy syndrome; lumbar region
724.4	Lumbosacral radiculitis
724.9	Other unspecified back disorder; Compression of spinal nerve root, NEC
953.2	Injury to lumbar nerve root
953.3	Injury to sacral nerve root
953.4	Injury to lumbosacral plexus

Procedure Coding

Code 64722: Decompression; unspecified nerve(s) (specify). This code requires specific identification of nerves involved. Some payers consider this code to be applicable only to "open" procedures.

Code 62289: Injection of substance other than anesthetic, antispasmodic, contrast or neurolytic solutions; lumbar or caudal epidural (separate procedure). This code is the standard epidural injection code and may be considered when injecting a steroid or multiple medications (e.g., steroid, anesthetic, opioid).

Radiographic Coding

Code 76000: Fluoroscopy (separate procedure), up to 1 hour physician time. This code may be considered for the technical component of fluoroscopy. A 26 modifier is required when billing for the professional component. Some payers do not allow for separate billing of the professional fee.

Code 62278: Injection of diagnostic or therapeutic anesthetic or antispasmodic substance (including narcotics); epidural, lumbar, or caudal, single. This code may be considered if a contrast study is performed. The report must include a radiologic review of normal and abnormal anatomy, comparison of previous studies with a discussion of any change over time, anatomic space where the contrast is injected, vertebral level of the injection and position within the space, and the extent of flow including upper and lower vertebral boundaries and any filling defects after a 5-mL contrast injection.

Code 72100-26: Radiologic examination, spine, lumbosacral; anterioposterior and lateral. This code is used for the professional interpretive component of the 62278 procedure.

Code 64999: (Unlisted procedure, nervous system).

Three Coding Scenarios

Scenario 1: Code 64722 as the primary code and 62289, 76000-26, 62278, and 72100-26 as secondary codes.

Scenario 2: Code 64999 as the solitary and primary code. Bundle the value of 64722, 62289, 76000-26, 62278, and 72100-26 into this solitary code.

Scenario 3: Code 62289-22 as the solitary and primary code. Bundle the value of 64722, 62289, 76000-26, 62278, and 72100-26 into this solitary code.

Modifiers

"A modifier provides the means by which the reporting physician can indicate that a service or procedure that has been performed has been altered by some specific circumstance but not changed in its definition or code."[22] The following modifiers are applicable to spinal endoscopy procedures:

22: Unusual Procedural Service: This modifier is used when the service provided is greater than that usually required for the procedure. It implies that additional effort was made to make a diagnosis or perform a procedure.
26: Professional Component: Appropriate for use with codes 72100 and 76000.
50: Bilateral Procedures. Medicare requires a separate port of entry for use of this modifier.
51: Multiple Procedures: This modifier may be used when multiple levels are involved.

CONCLUSION

The technology of spinal canal endoscopy has developed slowly during the 20th century. Contributions have been made by many innovators; however, only recently has this technique been developed and refined sufficiently to be used clinically.

Further study is needed to determine whether this technique holds advantages over alternative currently used techniques of medication delivery into the epidural space. Real-time direct-visual examination of epidural anatomy currently enables the identification of epidural diseases and localization of pain generators there. This ability to examine epidural pathology apart from operative trauma and to direct the delivery of medication is not duplicated by any other technique available at this time. The technology holds the promise of minimally invasive and effective therapy for both radicular and perhaps other forms of disabling back pain.

Other exciting possibilities for this technology may include removal of extra- or intradural scar tissue, cyst drainage, biopsies, studies of cell biology and inflammatory mediators, and retrieval of foreign bodies. We feel that the possibility of modifying the inflammatory process by blocking the mediators of inflammation holds the greatest promise.

Today, the technique can be used safely and effectively to deliver medication to pathology under direct vision. It opens new doors for the diagnosis and treatment of disease accessible through the epidural space.

REFERENCES

1. Lindahl O, Rexed B. Histological changes in spinal nerve roots of operated cases of sciatica. *Acta Orthop Scand* 1950;20:215–225.
2. Goebert HW, Jallo SJ, Gardner WJ, et al. Painful radiculopathy treated with epidural injections of procaine and hydrocortisone acetate: results with 113 patients. *Anesth Analg* 1991;72:820–822.
3. Sandrock NJG, Warfield CA. Epidural steroids and facet injections. In: *Principles and Practices of Pain Management*. 2nd ed. New York, NY: McGraw-Hill, 1993:401–412.
4. Abram SE. Risk versus benefit of epidural steroids. Let's remain objective. *APS J* 1994:28–39.
5. Saberski LR, Kitahata LM. Direct visualization of the lumbosacral epidural space through the sacral hiatus. *Anesth Analg* 1995;80:839–840.
6. Gatchel RJ, Turk DC, eds. Psychosocial Factors in Pain: Critical Perspectives. New York, NY: Guilford Press, 1999.
7. Burman MS. Myeloscopy or the direct visualization of the spinal cord. *J Bone Joint Surg* 1931;13:695–696.
8. Stern EL. The spinascope: a new instrument for visualizing the spinal canal and its contents. *Medl Rec (NY)* 1936;143:31–32.
9. Pool JC. Myeloscopy: diagnostic inspection of the cauda equina by means of an endoscope. *Bull Neuro Inst NY* 1938;7:178–189.
10. Pool JC. Myeloscopy: intraspinal endoscopy. *Surgery* 1942;11:169–182.
11. Ooi Y, Morisaki N. Intrathecal lumbar endoscope. *Clin Orthop Surg (Japan)*. 1969;4:295–297.
12. Saberski LR, Brull SJ. Spinal and epidural endoscopy: a historical review. *Yale J Biol Med* 1995;68(1–2):7–15.
13. Blomberg RG, Olsson SS. The lumbar epidural space in patients examined with epiduraloscopy. *Anesth Analg* 1987;68:157–160.
14. Shimiji K, Fujioka H, Onodera M, et al. Observation of spinal canal and cisternae with the newly developed small-diameter, flexible fiberscopes. 1991;75:341–344.
15. Saberski LR, Kitahata LM. Review of the clinical basis and protocol for epidural endoscopy. *Conn Med* 1995;50(2):71–73.
16. McCormack B, MacMillan M, Fessler G. Management of thoracic lumbar and sacral injuries. In: Tindall GT, Cooper PR, Barrow DI, eds. *The Practice of Neurosurgery*. 1st ed. Baltimore, Md: Williams & Wilkins, 1996:1721–1740.
17. Levin SC, Stacey BR, Cantees K. Preoperative and postoperative back pain management. In: Welch WC, Jacobs GB, Jackson GP, (eds.). *Operative Spine Surgery*. 1st ed. Stamford, Conn: Appleton & Lange, 1999.
18. Saberski LR, Kitahata LM. Persistent radiculopathy diagnosed and treated with epidural endoscopy. *J Anesth* 1996;10:292–295.
19. Saberski LR, Kitahata LM. Direct visualization of the lumbosacral epidural space through the sacral hiatus. *Anesth Analg* 1995;80:839–840.
20. Odoom JA, Sih IL. Epidural analgesia and anticoagulant therapy. Experience with 1000 cases of continuous epidurals. *Anaesthesia* 1983;38:254–259.
21. Serpell MG, Coombs DW, Colburn RW, et al. Intrathecal pressure recordings due to saline installation in the epidural space[abstract 1535]. 7th World Congress on Pain, August 1993.
22. Kirschner CG, Davis SJ, Duffy L, et al. CPT 98. Chicago,Ill: American Medical Association, 1997.

CHAPTER 67

INTRA-ARTICULAR INJECTIONS AND FACET BLOCKS

Tim J. Lamer

INTRODUCTION

The use of systemic corticosteroids for the treatment of symptomatic arthritis began shortly after the discovery and synthesis of cortisone in the 1940s.[1] Intra-articular steroid injections followed shortly thereafter. In 1951, Hollander published the results of a large series of patients treated with corticosteroid joint injections. Since then, corticosteroid injections have played an important role in the diagnosis and management of acute and chronic joint and periarticular pain problems.

INDICATIONS AND EFFICACY

Intra-articular and periarticular injections are indicated for diagnostic, prognostic, and therapeutic purposes (Table 67-1).

Diagnostic Injection

A careful history, physical examination, and supporting radiographic studies are important in the evaluation of a patient with a pain complaint, but often these three components of the evaluation fail to identify the source or sources of the patient's pain. Despite some limitations, a series of accurately performed local anesthetic injections often is the best diagnostic "test" we have to identify the pain generator(s) contributing to the patients pain problem.

Prognostic Injection

Injection techniques may help to determine if a more definitive therapeutic intervention is indicated. Pain relief following a local anesthetic injection into an arthritic joint may lead to consideration of viscosupplementation or may convince a surgeon that an operation is indicated (Fig. 67-1). The decision to perform total joint replacements or bursectomies frequently is guided by the response to one or more diagnostic injections.

Prognostic injections may help to determine if a joint denervation procedure is indicated. Chronic facet pain and discogenic pain often are treated with denervation procedures (e.g., radiofrequency). A denervation procedure is performed following a series of carefully controlled prognostic local anesthetic blocks.

Therapeutic Injection

Injections are used to treat a variety of inflammatory and noninflammatory joint and periarticular soft tissue pain problems.

Rheumatoid Arthritis Rheumatoid arthritis is a chronic systemic inflammatory disease with polyarticular involvement. Because this is a systemic disease, the principal therapeutic agents are systemic anti-inflammatory and/or immune modulating drugs. Injection of isolated joint flare-ups with local anesthetic and corticosteroid may help to quickly restore function and allow participation in physical therapy. Studies have demonstrated short-term pain relief and improved periarticular muscle strength in patients following intra-articular corticosteroid injection of a symptomatic rheumatoid joint.[3,4] For a flare-up of a single or a couple of joints, it is preferable to inject one or two joints rather than to increase the dose of systemic agents or to add an additional systemic agent.

Osteoarthritis and Other Joint Conditions The treatment continuum for osteoarthritis ranges from conservative therapy, including physical therapy and oral medications on one end, to total joint replacement on the other end. Injection therapy with corticosteroids or viscosupplementation may be used for the treatment of symptomatic flare-ups or treatment in patients who are poor surgical risks. Patients with severe bone-on-bone osteoarthritis may not respond or may have only minimal response.

Intra-articular corticosteroid injection and intra-articular viscosupplementation typically provide several weeks to months of relief.[5,6] This period can be used as a therapeutic window for an appropriate rehabilitation and exercise program. Small and non-weight-bearing joints have a longer duration of relief than large weight-bearing joints following corticosteroid injection for osteoarthritis.

Corticosteroid injection has been reported in case reports and anecdotal series to be effective in the relief of other painful joint conditions including psoriatic arthritis, lupus, crystalline arthritis (gout and pseudogout), and Reiter's disease.

Periarticular Injections

The injection of local anesthetic and corticosteroids is extremely effective in the treatment of bursitis and tendonitis. Unlike corticosteroid joint injections in which the relief tends to be short-term and temporary, symptomatic tendon and bursa inflammation typically have a longer period of relief and a significant "cure" rate if therapy is initiated early and combined with an appropriate rehabilitation program.[7,8] Table 67-2 lists the most common indications for periarticular soft tissue injections.

Contraindications

Infection in the area to be injected is the major absolute contraindication. If a joint infection is suspected clinically, a sample of synovial fluid should be aspirated and analyzed prior to performing an intra-articular injection. Documented allergy to the injectant is the only other major contraindication.

Joint injection in the presence of a coagulopathy or in patients taking systemic anticoagulants is somewhat controversial. A recent study of 32 injections and aspirations performed in patients taking therapeutic warfarin resulted in no cases of joint or soft tissue hemorrhage.[9] This was a small study but it did demonstrate that the

TABLE 67-1 **Indications for Joint and Periarticular Injection**

- Diagnostic
- Prognostic
- Reduce inflammation
- Reduce pain
- Facilitate rehabilitation

risk of significant hemorrhage was minimal after a carefully performed injection in patients taking systemic anticoagulants.

TABLE 67-2 **Common Indications for Periarticular Soft Tissue Injections**

Shoulder
- Biceps tendonitis
- Subacromial bursitis
- Rotator cuff tendonitis

Hand
- Trigger finger
- Ganglion cysts
- de Quervain's tenosynovitis

Knee
- Prepatellar bursitis
- Anserine bursitis
- Hamstring tendonitis

Hip and Pelvis
- Trochanter bursitis
- Ischial bursitis
- Iliopsoas bursitis/tendonitis
- Adductor tendonitis

Foot
- Achilles bursitis/tendonitis
- Calcaneal bursitis
- Plantar fasciitis

Elbow
- Epicondylitis
- Olecranon bursitis

INJECTION AGENTS

Corticosteroids continue to be the most commonly used therapeutic injectant. Viscosupplementation, the local injection of a viscous fluid containing hylan polymers, is commonly used to treat symptomatic osteoarthritis of the knee. Many other analgesics, anti-inflammatory, and immune modulating agents have been injected with varying success.

Corticosteroid Injection

A variety of corticosteroids are available for joint and periarticular injection. The duration of analgesic and anti-inflammatory effects is inversely related to their aqueous solubility (Table 67-3). In general, the duration of effect for triamcinolone hexacetonide, the longest duration agent, is approximately 3 to 6 weeks. Pharmacokinetic studies have shown it to be absorbed from the joint over a period of 2 to 3 weeks.[10] On the other end of the spectrum, hydrocortisone acetate has a clinical duration of less than 1 week and is completely absorbed from the joint in less than a day.

The putative mechanisms of symptomatic relief from injected corticosteroids include an anti-inflammatory or disease-modifying effect, an analgesic effect, systemic effects following systemic uptake, and a local neuronal suppressive effect.

Intra-articular steroids have been demonstrated to reduce synovial inflammation in patients with rheumatoid arthritis.[11] Similarly, they have been shown to have a favorable disease-modifying effect in osteoarthritis joints.[12] Local application of corticosteroids around damaged or inflamed nerves has been shown to suppress

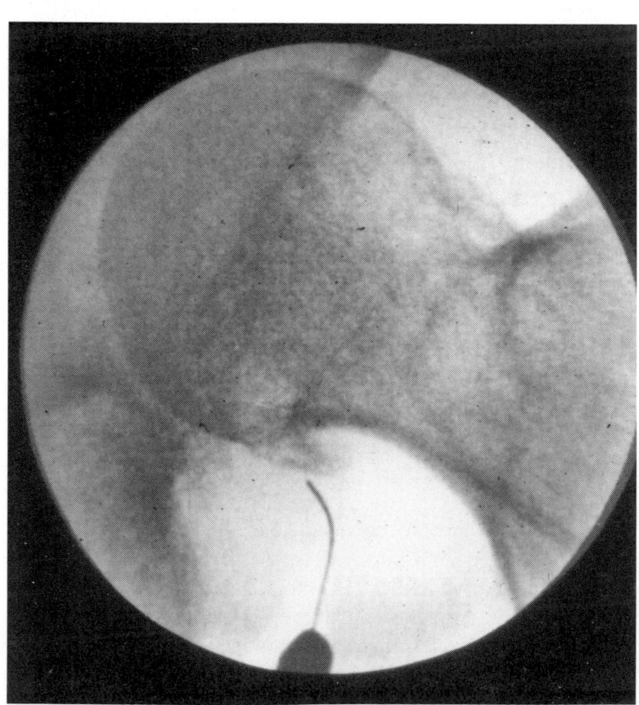

Figure 67-1 Diagnostic injection of an osteophyte on the femoral head. This was subsequently treated with surgery.

TABLE 67-3 **Relative Duration of Commonly Available Corticosteroids**

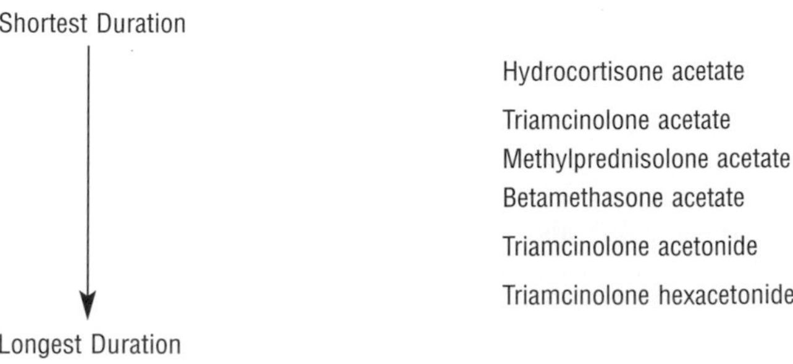

Shortest Duration

- Hydrocortisone acetate
- Triamcinolone acetate
- Methylprednisolone acetate
- Betamethasone acetate
- Triamcinolone acetonide
- Triamcinolone hexacetonide

Longest Duration

TABLE 67-4 **Relative Potency of Commonly Available Corticosteroids**

Potency	Agent	Relative Anti-inflammatory Potency
Least Potent		
	Hydrocortisone	1
	Methylprednisolone	5–6
	Triamcinolone	5–6
	Betamethasone	25–30
Most Potent		

neural discharge and symptoms of neuropathic pain.[13,14] Corticosteroids also have been shown to promote the secretion of a surface-active phospholipid into the joint, which acts as a joint "lubricant" and may contribute to improved joint mobility.[15]

Most corticosteroids are injected along with a local anesthetic to minimize the injection and post-injection pain and to provide immediate feedback regarding the effectiveness of the injection. Most local anesthetics are compatible with injectable corticosteroids; however, most manufacturers recommend the use of methylparaben-free and preservative-free anesthetics to reduce the extent of clumping or flocculation of the agent. Table 67-4 lists the relative potencies of the more commonly used agents and Table 67-5 lists dosage guidelines.

Viscosupplementation

The synovial fluid of osteoarthritic joints has been shown to be significantly less viscous than normal, at least in part due to a decreased concentration of hyaluronic acid. It is presumed that this reduces the protective function of the synovial fluid.

Viscosupplementation is the injection of hyaluronic acid derivatives into the synovial fluid of an osteoarthritic joint. Many clinical studies have demonstrated significant clinical improvement and increased synovial fluid viscosity and hyaluronic acid concentration following a series of these injections. Side effects have been minimal and typically involve a brief period of pain and swelling.

Two agents currently are approved for viscosupplementation therapy of symptomatic osteoarthritic knees. Trials involving therapy of joints other than the knee are under way. Hylan G-F 20 (Synvisc) is a viscous fluid containing hylan, which is manufactured from sodium hyaluronate, extracted from chicken combs. It is supplied in 2-mL prefilled syringes and is administered as an intra-articular knee injection 1 per week for 3 weeks.

Hyalgan also is manufactured from sodium hyaluronate from chicken combs. It is administered as an intra-articular knee injection 1 per week for 5 weeks.

Viscosupplementation has been shown to be as effective as oral nonsteroidal anti-inflammatory agents (NSAIDs).[16–18] The average duration of effect is approximately 6 months and ranges from 2 to 18 months. As this is a relatively new treatment, its role in the treatment of osteoarthritis is evolving. It may be considered as a first line of treatment in patients who cannot take NSAIDs or who do not respond to NSAIDs. It may be an adjuvant agent in patients who are taking NSAIDs.

The main difference between Hyalgan and Synvisc is the viscosity of the preparation. Synvisc has a higher molecular weight and viscosity than Hyalgan, and is very similar to that of synovial fluid. It is not known if this results in differences in efficacy as comparative studies have not been done.

Other Injectants

Injection of beta-emitting radiopharmaceutials into rheumatoid joints with active disease has been shown to produce a radiation-induced synovectomy and is effective in controlling symptoms.[19,20] The technique has not gained widespread use or acceptance because of radioactive leakage from the joint to nontarget organs. Studies are currently under way; looking at new radiopharmaceuticals that may minimize such leakage.[20]

Photodynamic therapy is a promising new therapy, which may be effective for the treatment of arthritis. Injection of hydrophobic photosensitizers may be preferentially absorbed by hypervascular inflamed synovium, which then is targeted for destruction by laser techniques. This technique is well established for the treatment of certain neoplasms, and currently is being investigated for treatment of inflammatory arthritis.[21]

Side Effects and Complications

The three major concerns with corticosteroid joint injections are infection, joint and/or periarticular tissue damage, and systemic side effects. By using sterile technique and disposable needles and syringes, the risk of infection is remote. Several large series have demonstrated the risk of infection to be 1:50,000 injections or less.[22]

Systemic absorption occurs following corticosteroid joint injection. Possible systemic side effects include virtually any side effect or untoward effect that has been reported to accompany systemic steroid administration. Practically speaking, using the lowest effective dose and limiting the number of injections minimizes the risk. Patients with diabetes may see a temporary (1 week) rise in blood glucose. Dosages >40 mg of triamcinolone may transiently suppress the hypothalamic–pituitary–adrenal (HPA) axis. Fluid re-

TABLE 67-5 **Corticosteroid Dosage Guidelines**

Structure	Triamcinolone (mg)	Methylprednisolone (mg)	Betamethasone (mg)
Large Joint	40	40	6
Small Joint	5–10	5–10	1.5
Bursa	10–20	10–20	1.5–3
Tendon Sheath	5–10	5–10	1.5

tention, weight gain, and facial flushing have been reported following corticosteroid injection.[23]

Many clinicians assume that corticosteroid injection exposes patients to a significant risk of tendon or periarticular bone or cartilage damage. Some of these concerns were initiated by anecdotal reports of "steroid arthropathy" and subprimate animal studies demonstrating bone and tendon pathology following corticosteroid injection.[24,25]

More recent human studies and primate animal studies have shown that within reasonable dosage limits, corticosteroid injections do not weaken tendons or damage bone and cartilage. In fact, recent studies have demonstrated an articular protective effect in inflammatory arthritis and steroids may actually suppress the formation of painful osteophytes in osteoarthritis.[12,26–28] The risks and benefits of joint injection can be balanced by following the dosage guidelines in Table 67-5 and limiting injections to less than 3 to 4 per joint per year.

SPECIFIC TECHNIQUES OF JOINT INJECTION

Shoulder Injections

Injection of the Shoulder Joint This injection may be performed with or without fluoroscopy. Studies of major joint injections (knee, hip, and shoulder) have shown significant rates of failure to localize the joint when fluoroscopy was not used.[29]

When performed without fluoroscopy, the patient is placed sitting or supine with the shoulder externally rotated. The point of entry is marked just medial to the head of the humerus and just below (inferolateral) the coracoid process (Figs. 67-2 and 67-3). After sterile skin preparation, the skin and subcutaneous tissues are anesthetized with lidocaine using a 27- or 30-gauge needle. Then a 22-gauge 1½- to 2½-in. needle is advanced posteriorly with a slight superolateral angle. The resistance of the joint capsule will be obvious. The needle is advanced until it "pops" through the capsule and is advanced 0.5 cm. After careful aspiration, 2 to 3 mL of anesthetic-corticosteroid suspension is injected. If pressure is encountered during injection, the needle should be repositioned slightly medially.

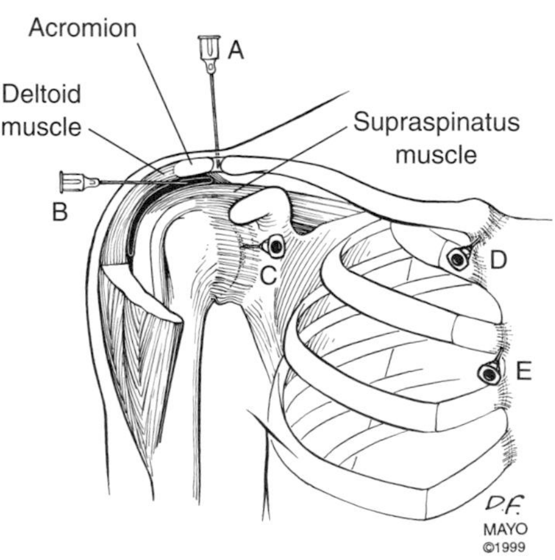

Figure 67-2 Shoulder and chest injections. Needle A–Demonstrates needle trajectory and placement for injections of the acromioclavicular joint. Needle B–Needle placement for the lateral approach to the subacromial bursa injection. Needle C– Needle placement for the anterior approach to the shoulder joint. Needle D–Demonstrates the approach to the sternoclavicular joint. Needle E–Demonstrates the approach to the costosternal joint.

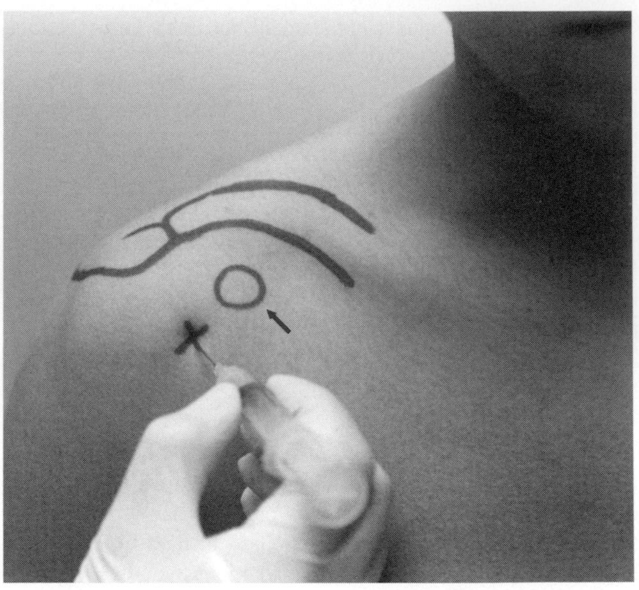

Figure 67-3 Anterior approach to intra-articular shoulder injection. Entry site is just inferior and lateral to the coracoid process (*arrow*).

Never inject any joint if resistance is encountered, as the needle ending may be in ligament, tendon, or cartilage and these structures can be damaged by mechanical disruption from a direct injection. Aspiration is important prior to injecting the agent, as it is possible for the needle to enter the axillary or subclavian vessels.

A posterior approach may also be used. The patient is in the sitting position with the arm internally rotated and adducted. This is best accomplished by having the patient place the hand of the arm to be injected on the opposite shoulder. The needle entry point is marked just under the posteroinferior border of the acromion. After sterile preparation and local anesthesia, a 22-gauge 2½-in. needle is advanced anteriorly with a slight cephalomedial angle (Fig. 67-4 and 67-5). Again, the needle is advanced 0.5 cm through the capsule and anesthetic–corticosteroid suspension is injected.

Intra-articular shoulder joint injections are used chiefly for diagnostic purposes to help determine if the shoulder joint is contributing to a patient's pain problem. There is insufficient data to determine whether or not shoulder injections have long-term therapeutic value.[30]

Injection of the Subacromial Bursa This injection can be performed using a lateral or posterior approach. Using the lateral approach, the needle entry site is marked on the lateral shoulder just inferior to the acromium. A 22-gauge 1½-in. needle is advanced toward the inferior border of the lateral acromium (see Fig. 67-2). After the needle contacts the acromium, it is "walked" inferiorly until it slips off the inferior edge of the acromium. Then it is advanced 0.5 to 1.0 cm and 2 to 3 mL of anesthetic-corticosteroid suspension is injected.

The posterior approach is the preferred approach because there is a larger space between the acromium and humeral head. The

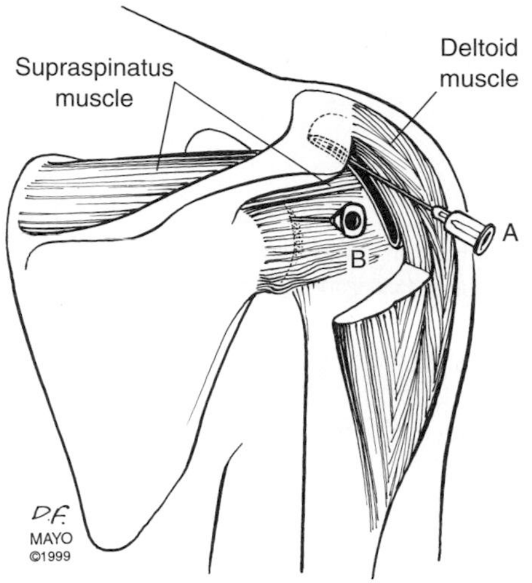

Figure 67-4 Posterior approach to shoulder injections. Needle A–Posterolateral approach to the subacromia bursa injection. Needle B–Posterior approach to injection of the shoulder joint.

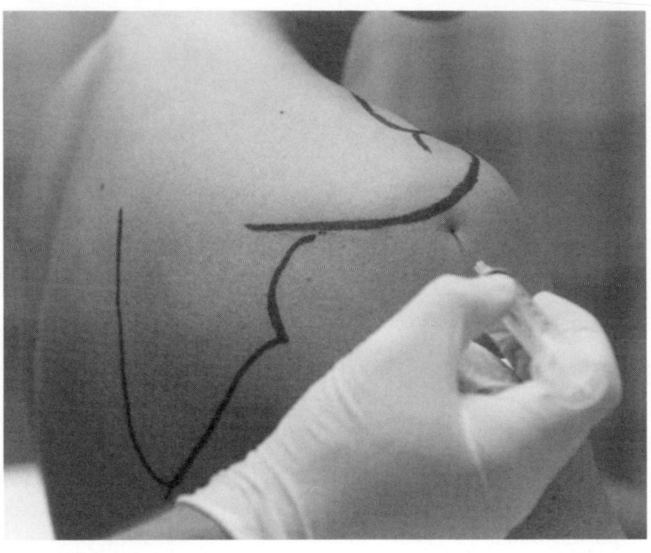

Figure 67-6 Posterolateral approach to the subacromial bursa.

point of entry is marked 1 cm below the posterior acromium, at or just medial to the angle of the acromium (Figs. 67-4 and 67-6). A 22-gauge 1½-in. needle is advanced anteriorly with a slight cephalomedial angle to contact the acromium. The needle is walked inferiorly until it slips off the inferior edge and then it is advanced 0.5 to 1 cm. If resistance is encountered during the injection, the needle should be repositioned, as the needle may be in the supraspinatous tendon. This tendon is fragile and could be damaged by an intra-tendinous injection.

Injection of the Acromioclavicular Joint The joint space is palpated as a groove or depression between the acromium and clavicle on the top surface of the shoulder. This groove is marked, and after sterile preparation and local anesthesia, a 22-gauge 1½-in. needle is advanced into the joint space (Figs. 67-2 and 67-7), then 0.5 mL of injectant is placed into the joint.

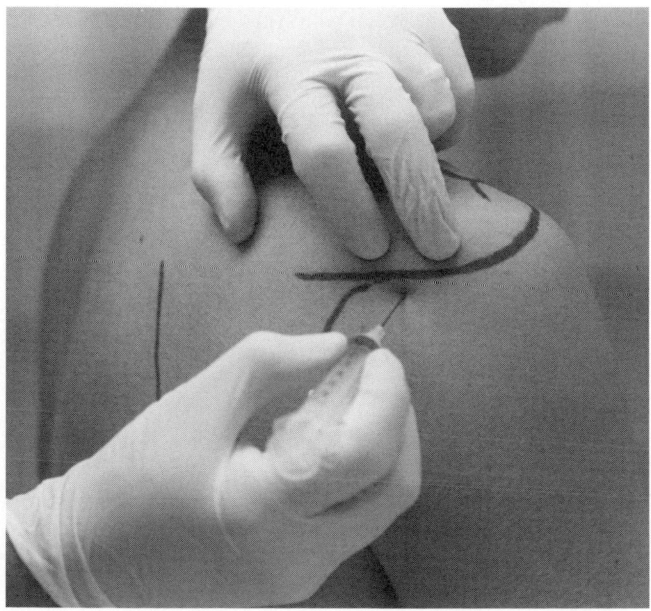

Figure 67-5 Posterior approach to the shoulder joint.

Elbow Injection

Elbow Joint Injection The elbow joint is injected using a lateral approach. The radial humeral joint can easily be palpated laterally at level of the skin crease of the elbow.

The lateral epicondyle of the humerus is the most obvious identifiable landmark. Identify this with the examining finger and then slide the finger down the epicondyle until the groove between the epicondyle and the plateau of the radius is felt. Mark this spot as the needle entry point (Figs. 67-8 and 67-9). After sterile skin preparation and cutaneous anesthesia, a 22-gauge 1½-in. needle is advanced through the needle entry point and advanced to contact the distal epicondyle. Then walk the needle distally until it slides

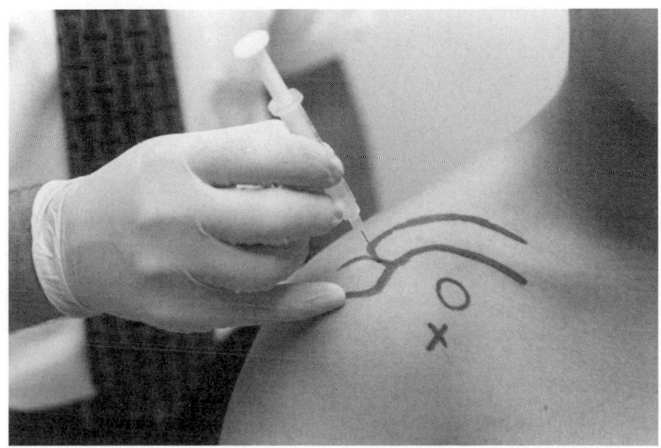

Figure 67-7 Needle approach to the acromioclavicular joint.

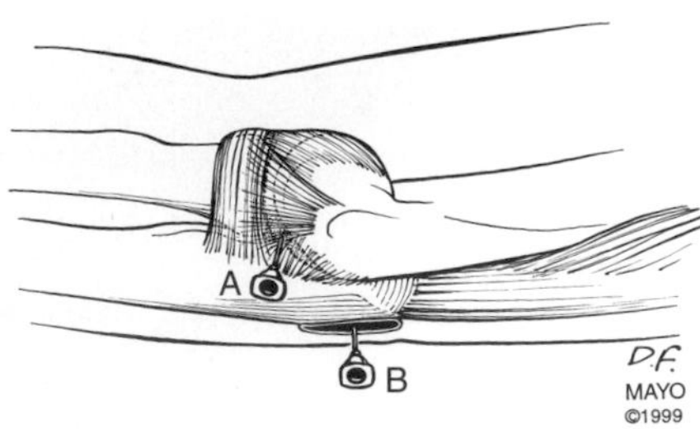

Figure 67-8 Elbow injections. Needle A–Lateral approach to the elbow joint. Needle B–Olecranon bursa injection.

off the epicondyle and into the joint space. Advance the needle 0.5 cm and inject 1 to 2 mL of injectant. If an ulnar paresthesia is elicited during this block, the needle is too dorsal and a more volar approach should be used.

Olecranon Bursa Injection The olecranon bursa is a large bursal sac between the soft tissue and the olecranon process of the ulna. After sterile skin preparation and cutaneous anesthesia, a 25-gauge 1- to 1½-in. needle is advanced in a direction perpendicular to the olecranon (see Fig. 67-8) until the olecranon surface is contacted. Then the needle is withdrawn approximately 1 to 2 mm and 1 to 2 mL of injectant is placed at the site. To avoid a subcutaneous injection, do not withdraw the needle too far after contacting the olecranon.

Hand and Wrist Injections

Finger Joint Injections The carpometacarpal (CMC), metacarpophalangeal (MCP), and interphalangeal (IP) joints commonly are affected by rheumatoid and osteoarthritis flare-ups and are amenable to injection therapy. The specific joint to be injected can

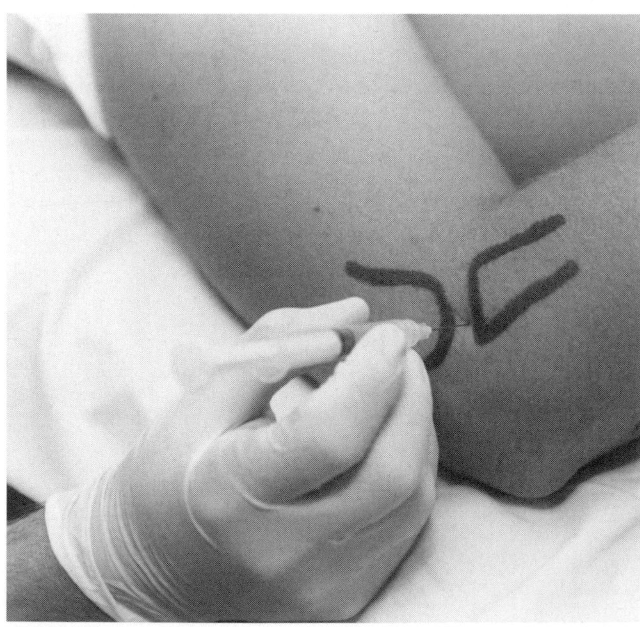

Figure 67-9 Lateral approach to the elbow joint injection.

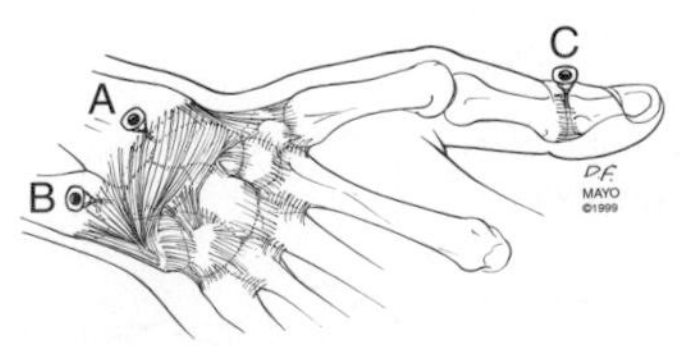

Figure 67-10 Hand and wrist injections. Needles A and B–Dorsal approach to the radiocarpal and ulnocarpal joints. Needle C–Needle approach to an interphalangeal joint.

easily be palpated. For the IP joints, a lateral or medial approach is used. For the MCP or CMC joints, a dorsal approach is used. It is best to avoid the more richly innervated volar (palmar) surface of the hand, as these injections are more painful.

A 27-gauge 1½-in. needle is advanced into the joint space. It only needs to enter the superficial joint, just through the capsule (Figs. 67-10 and 67-11). Inject 0.5 mL of anesthetic-corticosteroid solution.

Wrist Injections A dorsal approach to the radiocarpal and ulnocarpal joints is preferred. These joints can easily be palpated and the needle entry site marked (Figs. 67-10 and 67-12). Care should be taken to avoid the extensor tendons. The joint space can be "opened up" slightly by placing the wrist in 45 degrees of flexion. After sterile skin preparation and local anesthesia, a 22-gauge 1½-in. needle is advanced into the joint. Again, the needle should be advanced into the superficial joint and 1 to 2 mL of solution injected.

Hip Injections

Hip Joint Injection Intra-articular hip joint injections usually are performed diagnostically to help determine if hip arthritis is contributing to a patient's pain problem and prognostically to help determine if total hip arthroplasty would be beneficial.[31] The duration of pain relief after intra-articular corticosteroid hip injection typically is 1 to 3 months in patients with symptomatic osteoarthritis.[31,32]

The hip joint can be injected from an anterior or lateral approach. The use of fluoroscopy is highly desirable. A lateral or an-

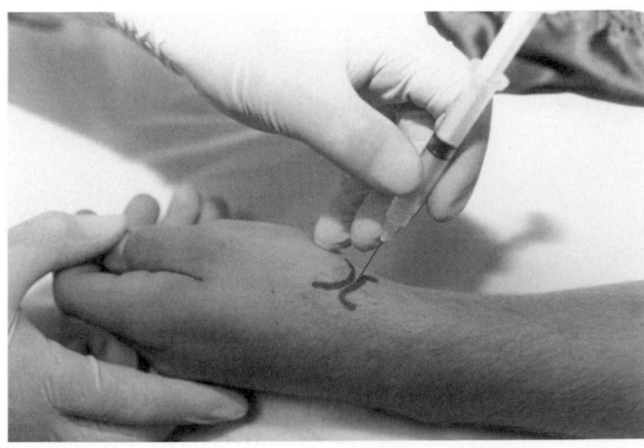

Figure 67-11 Needle approach to the carpometacarpal joint of the thumb.

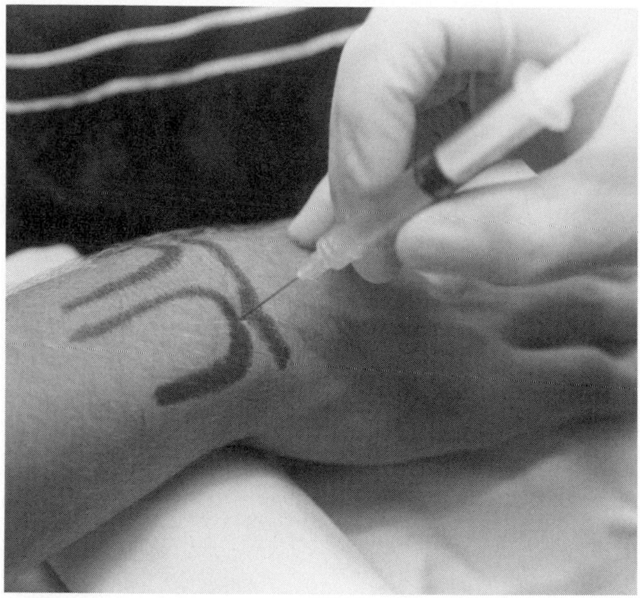

Figure 58-12 Dorsal approach to the wrist joint injection.

terolateral approach results in a more favorable needle trajectory for joint entry.

The patient is placed supine on the fluoroscopy table with the hip internally rotated (toes and knees pointed inward). The needle entry point is just anterior and cephalad to the greater trochanter (Fig. 67-13). Using fluoroscopy, the needle is directed medially and slightly cephalad (Figs. 67-13 and 67-14). The joint capsule is quite thick and easily identified with the needle. The needle is advanced just through the capsule. Aspirate to be sure the needle has not entered the femoral vessels. Two milliliters of radiopaque contrast can be injected to confirm placement. This is followed by placing 2 to 3 mL of injectant into the joint.

Trochanter Bursa Injection The trochanteric bursa is a large bursal sac located between the lateral surface of the greater trochanter

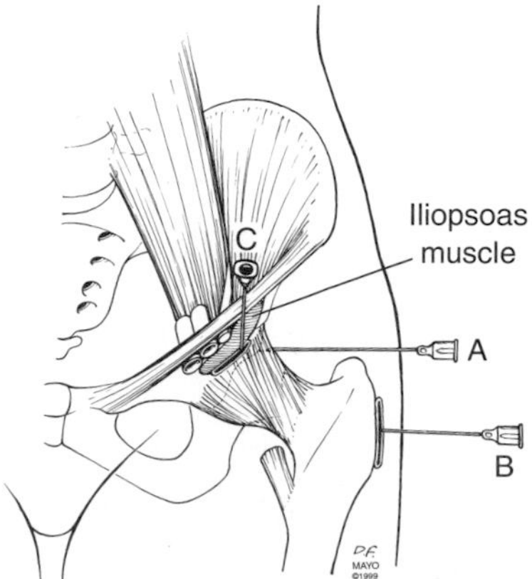

Figure 67-13 Hip injections. Needle A–Needle orientation and trajectory for lateral approach to the hip joint. Needle B–Lateral approach to the trochanteric bursa injection. Needle C – Approach to the iliopsoas bursa injection.

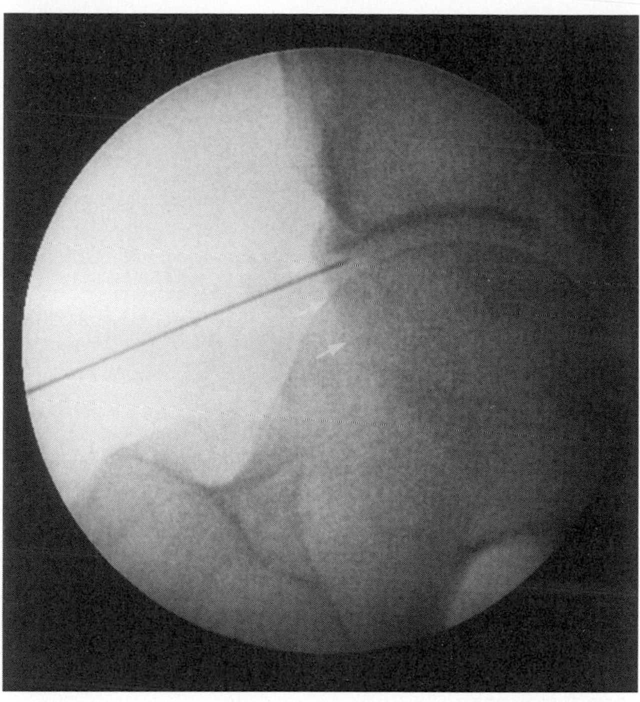

Figure 67-14 Hip joint injection. Needle placement for the lateral approach to the hip joint. The white arrows outline the margin of the acetabulum.

and the overlying iliotibial band (see Fig. 67-13). It is a common cause of lateral thigh pain and responds well to local anesthetic-corticosteroid injection.[33]

The injection is performed by placing the patient in a lateral position with the symptomatic side up (Fig. 67-15). The area of maximal trochanteric tenderness is marked. After sterile skin prepa-

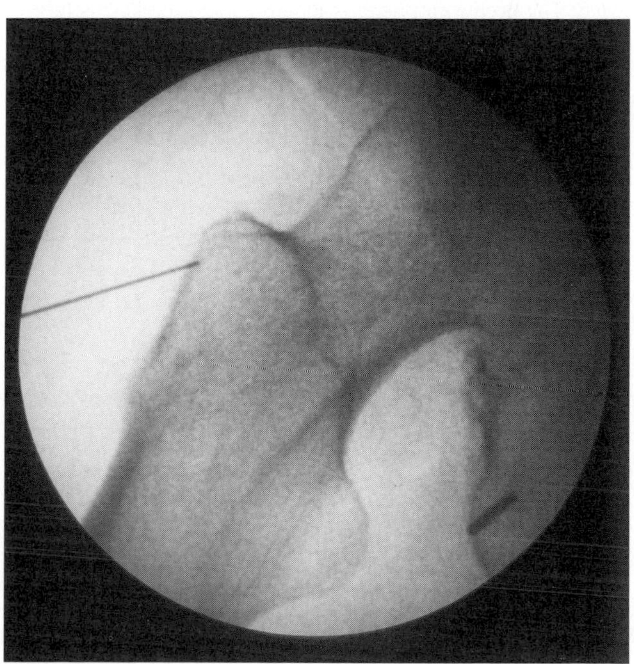

Figure 67-15 Needle approach for the trochanteric bursa injection.

ration and cutaneous anesthesia, a 22- or 25-gauge 2½- to 3½-in., needle is directed perpendicular to the trochanter and advanced until bone is contacted. Then the needle is withdrawn 3 to 5 mm and 3 to 5 mL of solution is injected.

Iliopsoas Bursa Injection The iliopsoas bursa is the largest bursa in the body and lies between the iliopsoas muscle and the anterior hip capsule (see Fig. 67-13). It is a common but often overlooked cause of groin pain.[34,35] There may be direct communication between the bursa and the joint.

The injection is performed with the patient supine. The needle entry site is just below the inguinal ligament and 1 to 2 cm lateral to the neurovascular bundle (femoral artery pulsation) to avoid needle trauma to the femoral nerve and vessels (see Fig. 67-13). After sterile skin preparation and anesthesia, a 22-gauge 3½-in. needle is advanced perpendicular to the skin and advanced until the anterior bone of the acetabulum is contacted. The needle is then withdrawn 3 to 5 mm, and after careful aspiration, 3 to 5 mL of solution is injected. If blood is aspirated, or a femoral nerve paresthesia occurs during needle placement, re-direct the needle 1 to 2 cm laterally. Be sure to check the patient for femoral nerve anesthesia prior to allowing ambulation.

Knee Injections

Knee Joint Injection Intra-articular knee joint injection can be valuable diagnostically to help determine the contribution of the joint versus periarticular structures in a patient with knee pain. It can be therapeutic in patients with rheumatoid arthritis by suppressing pain and inflammation in an acute flare-up.[36] It can provide short-term relief (2 to 4 weeks) in patients with symptomatic osteoarthritis.[37] This will allow time for affected patients to participate in an appropriate rehabilitation program.

Knee joint injection can be performed using either an anterior or a medial approach. For the more commonly used medial approach, the patient is placed supine with the leg straight or slightly flexed. The needle entry site is identified and marked as follows. The medial border of the inferior patella is identified. The needle entry site is 1 cm medial to this (Figs. 67-16 and 67-17). After skin

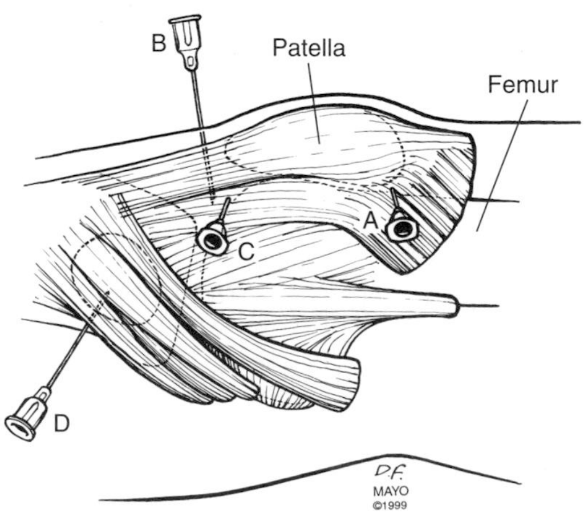

Figure 67-16 Knee injections. Needle A–Approach to the patellar bursa. Needle B–Anterior approach to intra-articular knee joint injection. Needle C–Medial approach to intra-articular knee joint injection. Needle D–Approach to the anserine bursa injection.

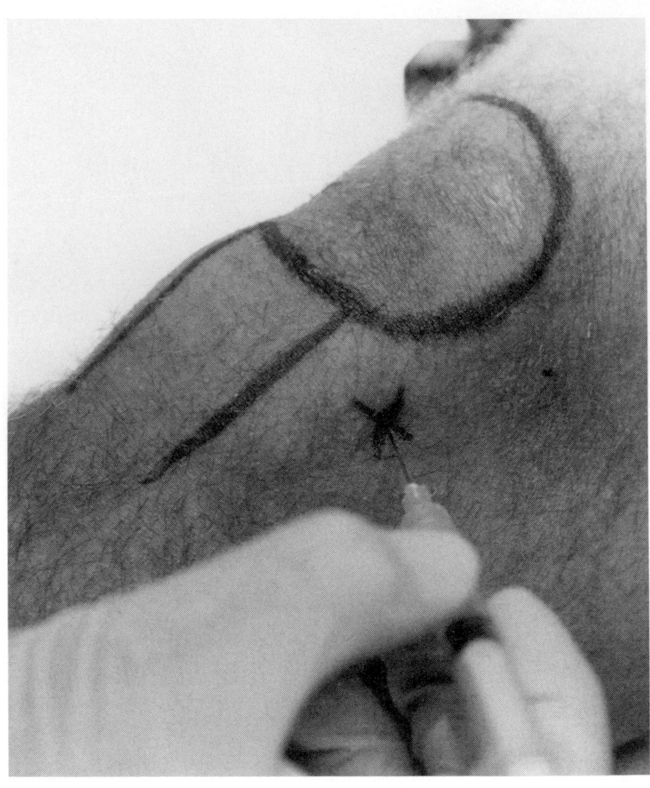

Figure 67-17 Medial approach to intra-articular knee joint injection. The marked circle outlines the patella and the lines outline the patellar tendon.

preparation and local anesthesia, a 1½- to 2-in. 22-gauge needle is advanced to contact the medial edge of the patella. Then it is walked off the patella and advanced between the patella and the medial femoral condyle and 2 to 3 mL of solution is injected.

For an anterior approach, the patient is seated with the knee flexed. The needle entry point is marked on the anterior surface of the knee as a point just below the inferior pole of the patella and just medial to the inferior patella tendon (Figs. 67-16 and 67-18). After sterile preparation and skin anesthesia, a 1½-in. 22-gauge

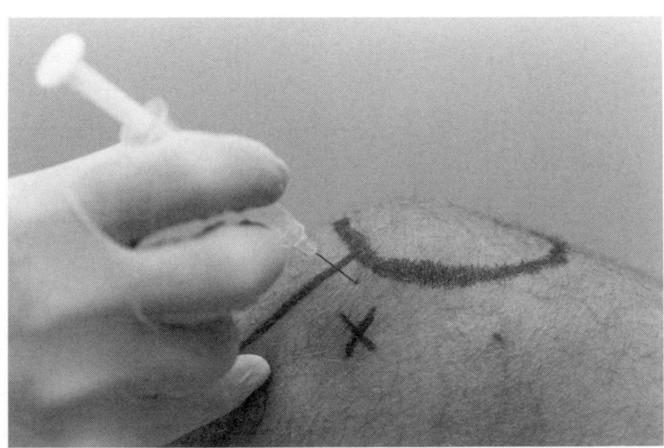

Figure 67-18 Anterior approach to knee joint injection. The "x" represents the needle entry site for the medial approach.

needle is advanced perpendicular to the skin until bone is contacted. The needle is then withdrawn 0.5 cm and 2 to3 mL of solution is injected.

Patellar Bursa Injection The prepatellar bursa lies between the patella and the overlying soft tissue. Prepatellar bursitis is a common cause of localized knee pain and responds well to local injection and rest.[38] Local injection is not much more than a trigger point injection. After skin preparation and local anesthesia, a 25-gauge needle is advanced until it contacts the patella (see Fig. 67-16). Then it is withdrawn 2 to 3 mm and 1 to 2 mL of solution is injected.

Anserine Bursa Injection The anserine bursa lies between the medial knee joint and the pes anserinus (tendons of the semitendinous, graclis, and sartorius muscles). Anserine bursitis is a common cause of medial knee pain and it responds well to injection therapy.[39]

The injection technique is quite simple and is similar to a trigger point injection. The area of maximal tenderness is identified over the medial tibial plateau and marked. After skin preparation and anesthesia, a 25-gauge 1- to 1½-in. needle is advanced until bone is contacted (see Fig. 67-16). The needle is withdrawn 2 to 3 mm and 1.0 mL of solution is injected.

Foot and Ankle Injection

Ankle Injection The ankle joint is entered from an anterior approach to enter the joint between the tibia and the talus. The patient is positioned supine with the leg-foot angle placed at 90 degrees. The point of entry is just medial to the anterior tibial and extensor hallicis longus tendons on a line drawn between the medial and lateral malleoli (Figs. 67-19 and 67-20). These tendons can be easily identified by having the patient dorsiflex the foot and great toe. After skin preparation and anesthesia, a 1-in. 22-gauge needle is advanced directly posteriorly until bone is contacted. The needle is then walked inferiorly until it slips between the tibia and talus. One to two milliliters of solution is injected. Joints between the tarsal bones are best injected by using fluoroscopic guided injection.[40]

Forefoot Injections The injection technique for metatarsal phalangeal and interphalangeal joints is exactly the same as the techniques described for the IP and MCP joints on the hand (see Fig. 67-19). Again, a lateral or dorsal approach is usually favored over the more painful plantar approach.

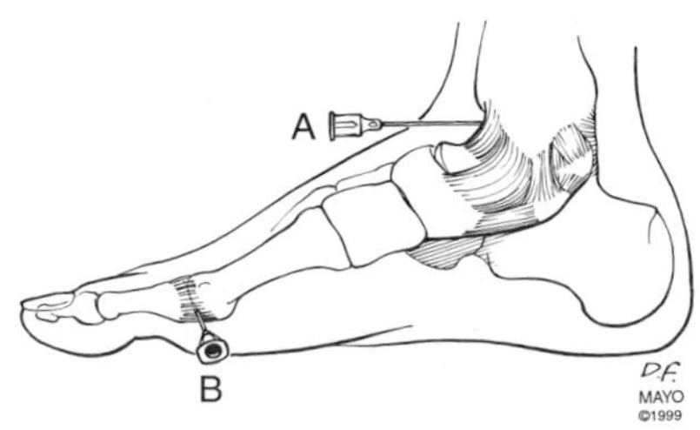

Figure 67-19 Foot and ankle injections. Needle A-Anterior approach to ankle joint injection. Needle B–Metatarsophalangeal joint injection.

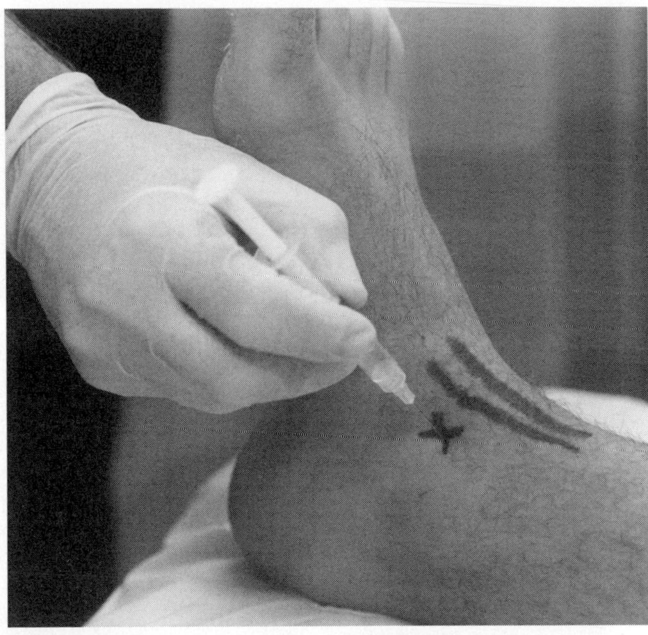

Figure 67-20 Anterior approach to ankle joint injection. The two parallel lines represent the anterior tibialis and extensor hallicus longus tendons.

Sacroiliac Joint Injection

In patients with acute spondyloarthropathies, an inflammatory sacroiliac component may be present. More often, sacroiliac joint pain occurs as a result of injury. Diagnostic sacroiliac injections are considered an important part of the diagnostic workup for mechanical low back pain because history and physical examination are notoriously unreliable.[41]

Sacroiliac joint injection can be performed with or without the use of fluoroscopy; however, when fluoroscopy is not used, there is a significant rate of failure to enter the joint. Therefore, if the block is being performed for diagnostic reasons, fluoroscopy or CT guidance should be used.

The patient is placed in the prone position. The sacroiliac joint is most accessible to injection at the most caudal or inferior portion of the joint.[42,43] Attempts to enter the synovial cavity of the joint at the middle and cranial or superior portions of the joint have a higher failure rate.

Using fluoroscopy, or by palpation, the posterior superior iliac spine (PSIS) is identified. The needle entry site is approximately 1 cm below the PSIS (Fig. 67-21A and 21B). After skin preparation and local anesthesia, a 22-gauge 2½- to 3½-in. needle is advanced through the above mentioned entry site toward the joint. The correct needle angle is typically 20 to 30 degrees laterally from the sagittal plane. Upon initial entry, the needle will traverse through the thick and tough posterior sacroiliac ligament (Fig. 67-22). The needle must be advanced through this ligament to reach the synovial joint cavity. This joint cavity may be obliterated or replaced by fibrous tissue in some patients. If fluoroscopy is used, 1 to 2 mL of radiopaque contrast can be injected to confirm an intra-articular dye patter (Fig. 67-23). This is followed by an injection of 1 to 2 mL of the diagnostic or therapeutic injectant.

If fluoroscopy is not used then a larger volume is injected in order to improve the likelihood of spread to the joint. To obtain the

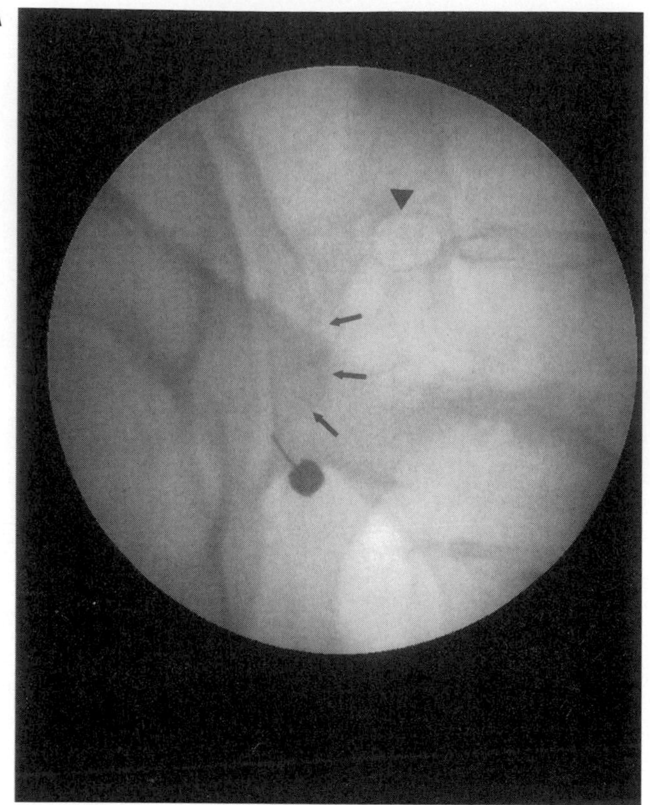

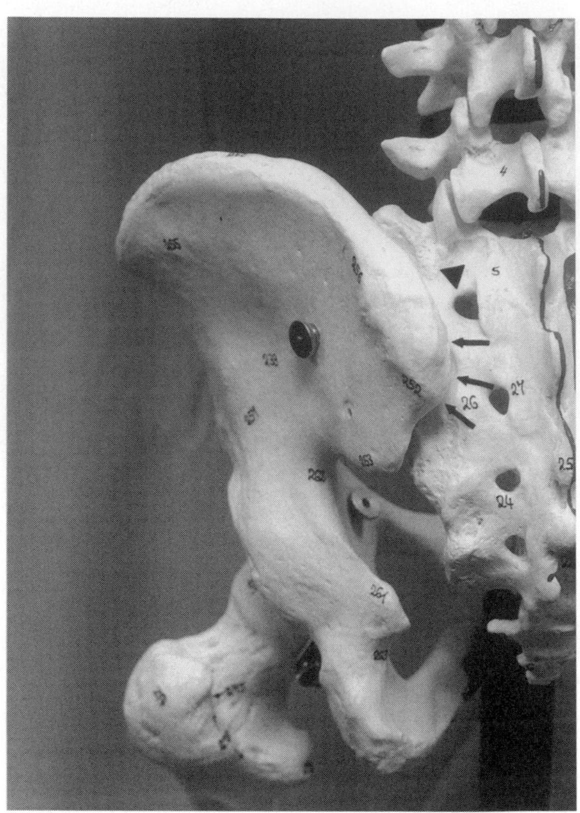

Figure 67-21 (**A**) Needle placement for sacroiliac joint injection. Small arrows outline the posterior superior iliac spine (PSIS). Large arrow is at the first sacral foramen. (**B**) Skeletal model showing corresponding landmarks. Small arrows again outline the PSIS. Large arrow is at the first sacral foramen.

greatest chance of joint entry, it is best to direct the needle down to the sacrum and then walk the needle laterally until the needle contact changes from bone to the tough ligamentous tissue. Because the injectant may spread to a variety of adjacent structures, including muscles, ligaments, and sacral nerve roots following an injection done without imaging guidance, diagnostic inferences should not be made following such a procedure.

Figure 67-22 Diagram of sacroiliac injection.

Cervical Facet Injection

Atlantoaxial Joint Injection Intra-articular cervical facet injections are performed to diagnosis and treat a variety of neck pain problems. Anatomically, the first cervical facet joint, the atlantoaxial or $C_{1\text{-}2}$ joint is markedly different from the remaining five cervical facet joints and the cervical-thoracic facet joint. This joint is responsible for the majority of axial rotation in the normal cervical spine. Accordingly, suboccipital pain with rotation of the head to the left or right often is indicative of $C_{1\text{-}2}$ joint pathology.

The $C_{1\text{-}2}$ joint may be injected using a lateral or posterior approach.[44–47] Because the vertebral artery courses along the lateral edge of the joint, the posterior approach is preferred. The patient is positioned prone on the fluoroscopy table and the fluoroscopy beam is positioned in a posteroanterior (PA) projection (Fig. 67-24). Because the teeth and jaw frequently project over the upper cervical spine, it is usually necessary to have the patient open the mouth. Once a clear view of the joint is obtained by adjusting the fluoroscopy column, the entry point is marked, sterilized, and anesthetized. Then a 3½-in. 22- or 25-gauge needle is advanced directly toward the joint with the target being the junction of the lateral one third and the medial two thirds of the joint. The needle is advanced to contact the boney edge of the joint at C_2. The needle is then walked off the bone into the joint and advanced no more than 1 to 2 mm. Intra-articular placement is confirmed by the injection of 0.25 to 0.5mL of radiopaque dye suitable for myelogra-

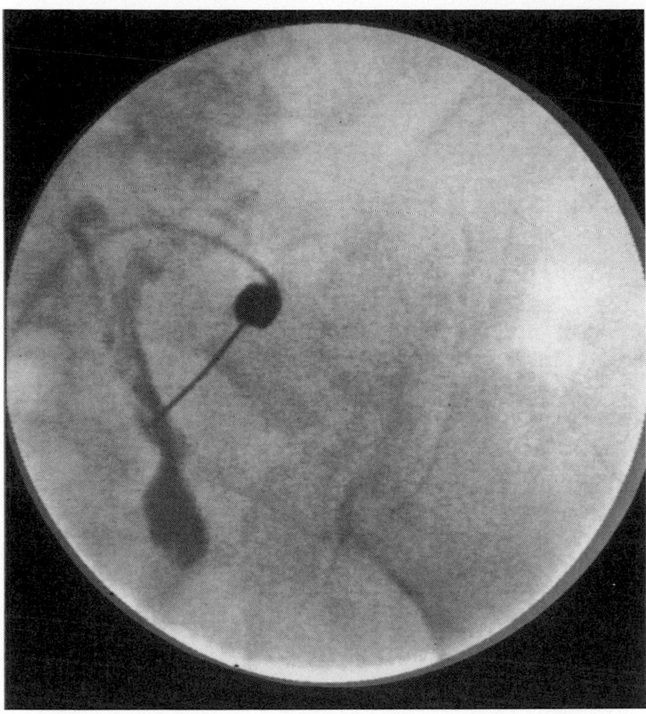

Figure 67-23 Contrast spread following sacroiliac injection.

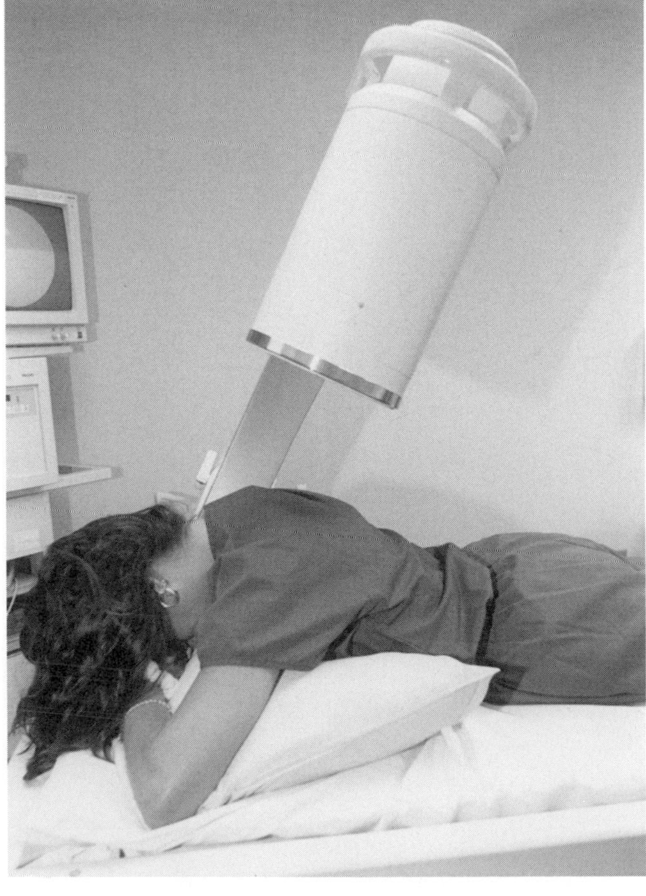

Figure 67-24 Patient positioning for posterior cervical facet joint injection.

phy (e.g., iopamidol). An appropriate arthrogram should be identifiable (Fig. 67-25) and there should not be any intravascular uptake or spread to the spinal axis This is followed by the injection of a mixture of 0.25 mL of anesthetic (recommend 1% lidocaine) and 0.25 mL of corticosteroid. The C_2 nerve root runs across the posterior surface of the joint (Fig. 67-26). If a paresthesia is obtained during needle placement, it is advisable to choose a slightly different trajectory. It is usually best to make the initial needle puncture sight slightly more caudad.

Potential complications include intravascular injection, spinal axis injection, needle trauma to the nerve root or spinal cord, and vascular injury. Since most injectable corticosteroids are particulate, it is theoretically possible for a particulate cerebral embolism to occur.

Cervical Facet Joint Injection The $C_{2\text{-}3}$ through $C_{6\text{-}7}$ joints can be injected using a posterior approach or a lateral approach.[48,49] The posterior approach is safer but technically more difficult due to the marked cephalocaudal angulation of the joints. The lateral approach is technically easier but more risky as the advancing needle can pass through the joint and into the spinal canal. This can be prevented by frequent PA and lateral fluoroscopic views.

For the posterior approach the patient is prone and the neck is slightly flexed (see Fig. 67-24). The fluoroscopy column is adjusted to identify the target joint(s). The needle entry site should be marked one level below the target joint. This will allow angulation of the needle at an angle that will facilitate entry into the cephalocaudal oriented cervical facet joints. A 3½-in. 22- or 25-gauge needle is advanced into the joint under fluoroscopic guidance. Intra-articular placement is confirmed with PA and lateral fluoroscopy by injecting 0.25 to 0.5 mL of contrast. After proper needle placement is confirmed, and following negative aspiration, a mixture of 0.25 mL of anesthetic plus 0.25 to 0.50 mL of corticosteroid is injected.

For the lateral approach, the patient may be positioned prone, lateral, or even supine. Lateral positioning usually is preferred by the patient and is convenient for the physician (Fig. 67-27). The target joint is identified and marked using fluoroscopy. Following sterile preparation and local anesthesia, a 1½- to 2½-in. 25-gauge needle is advanced to contact bone at the inferior edge of the joint.

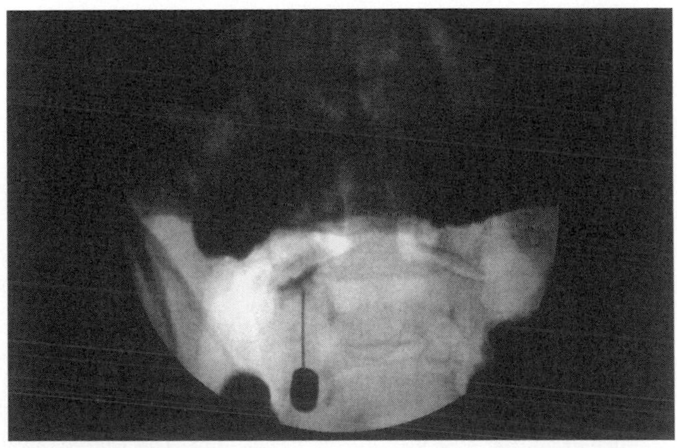

Figure 67-25 $C_{1\text{-}2}$ facet joint injection. Fluoroscopic view was obtained with the mouth wide open. The right $C_{1\text{-}2}$ joint is clearly visualized and contrast outlines the left $C_{1\text{-}2}$ joint.

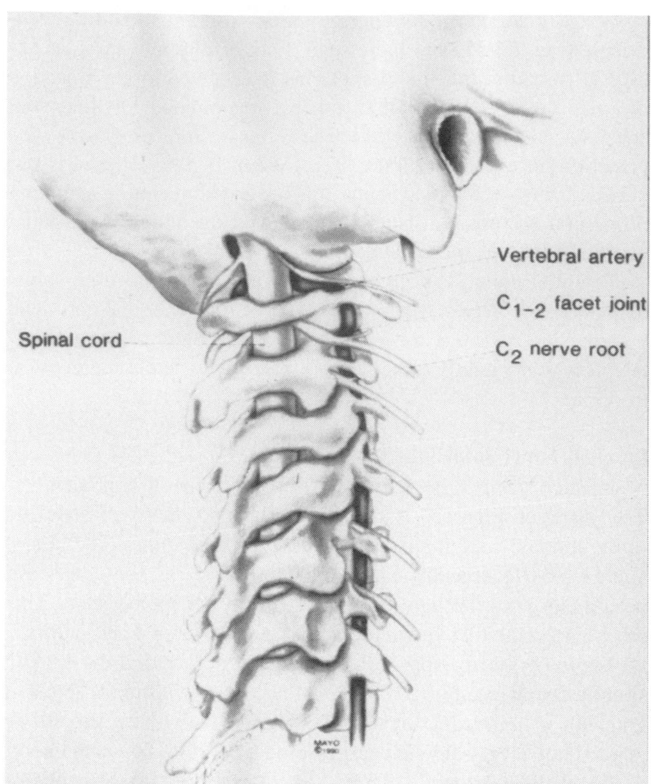

Figure 67-26 The relationship of the vertebral artery and C_2 nerve root to the C_{1-2} joint are illustrated in this oblique view of the cervical spine.

The needle is walked off the bone and advanced 2 to 3 mm into the joint (Fig. 67-28A and Fig. 67-29). Posteroanterior fluoroscopy is used to confirm that the needle is in the lateral one third of the joint (Fig. 67-28B). The needle is withdrawn slightly if the tip is beyond the lateral one third of the joint. Injection is performed as described for the posterior approach.

Complications and side effects from cervical facet blocks include intravascular injection, spinal axis injection, joint trauma, nerve root and spinal cord trauma, infection, and side effects from the injected corticosteroid.

Thoracic Facet Joint Injection

Thoracic fact joint pain is not a common clinical problem. The thoracic facet joints are not as prone to arthritic involvement as are the cervical and lumbar facet joints. The most common cause of thoracic facet pain is trauma.

Like the lower cervical facets, the thoracic facets have a marked cephalocaudal angulation. The average angle of incline from the horizontal plane is 60 degrees in the mid-thoracic region. Accordingly, the technique for thoracic facet injection is very similar to the posterior approach to the cervical facet joint.[50]

The patient is placed prone and the fluoroscopy tube is angled in order to get the best view of the target joint. The needle entry site is one to two segments below the target joint to allow angulation of the needle to facilitate joint entry (Fig. 67-30A and 30B). The remainder of the technique is as described for posterior cervical facet injection.

Lumbar Facet Joint Injection

Because of the prevalence of low back pain, lumbar facet injection is one of the most commonly performed pain management procedures. Intra-articular facet injections can be performed for diagnostic or therapeutic purposes.[51–53] Because of the oblique orientation of the lumbar facet joints, especially the lower two levels, it often is helpful to position the patient in a slightly oblique position with the side to be injected rotated up 30 to 45 degrees (Fig. 67-31).

With the patient appropriately positioned, the target joint is identified with fluoroscopic guidance and the skin is marked. It is best to identify the level by starting at the lumbosacral junction and then working up to the thoracolumbar junction. It is not unusual to have lumbosacral anomalies. To make communication between practitioners clear, it is important to specify the presence of any abnormalities and how it influences the counting and reporting of the level or levels injected.

After sterile preparation and local anesthesia, a 22-gauge needle is advanced under fluoroscopic guidance toward the target joint. A 3½-in. needle will be long enough for most patients; however, the larger patient may require a 5- or 6-in. needle. The needle is advanced until it contacts the boney edge of the facet joint. The needle is then walked off the bone to slip into the facet joint.

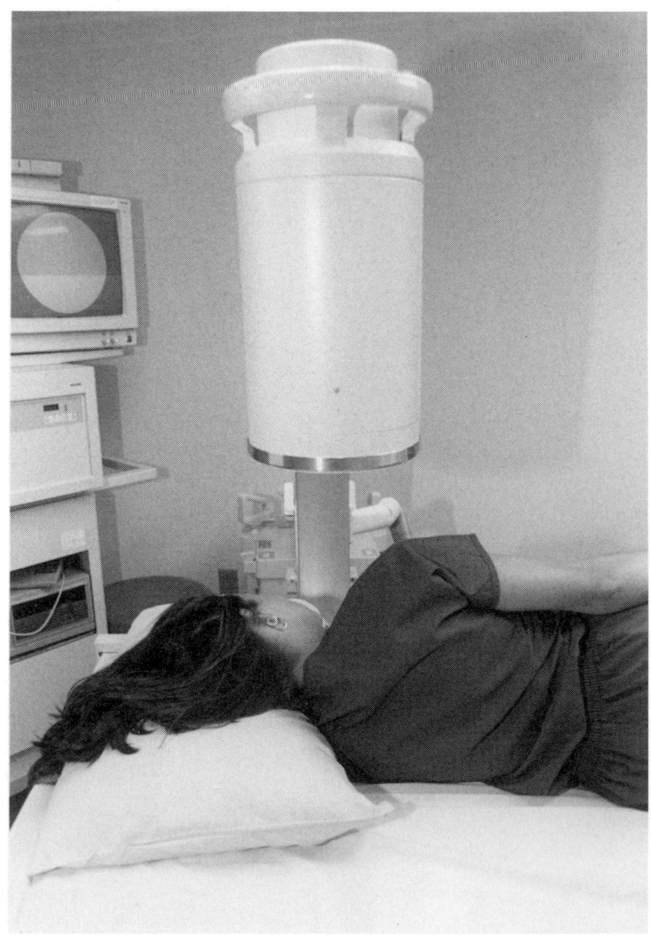

Figure 67-27 Patient positioning for lateral cervical facet joint injection.

A

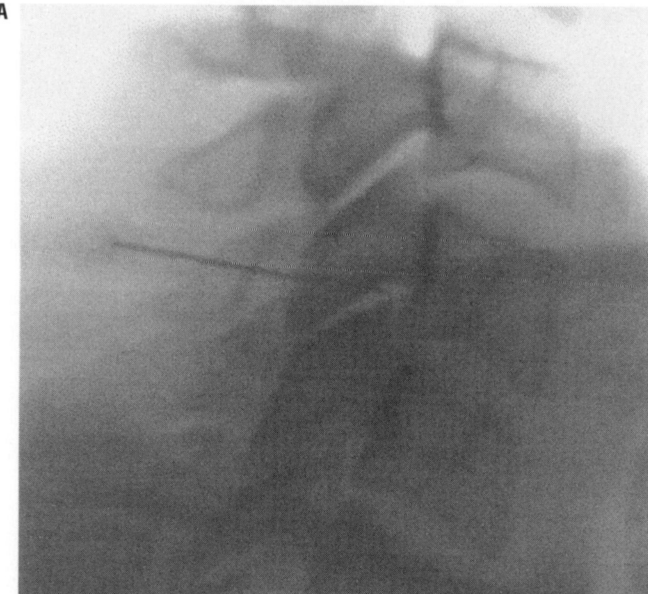

B

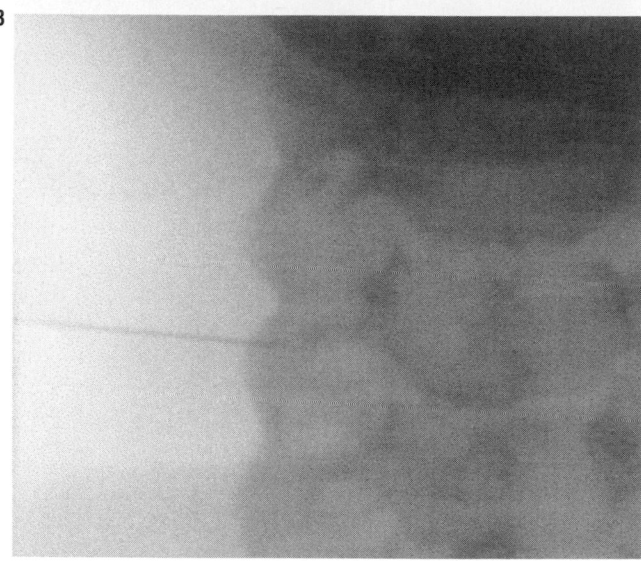

Figure 67-28 (**A**) Lateral fluoroscopic view of lateral approach to C_{4-5} facet joint. (**B**) Posteroanterior fluoroscopic view of lateral approach to the C_{4-5} facet joint. Needle is not advanced beyond the lateral one third of the joint. (Both figures: *Courtesy of the International Spinal Injection Society*).

In patients with severe osteoarthritis, the joint space may be narrowed to the point that needle entry is not possible. A periarticular injection can be performed in this situation for therapeutic purposes but a periarticular injection will be of minimal diagnostic value. Following needle entry into the joint, the needle is advanced 2 to 3 mm. Because the lumbar facet joint surfaces are curved, it is often not possible to advance more than 2 to 3 mm. Intra-articular position is confirmed by injecting 0.5 mL of contrast suitable for intrathecal injection (e.g., iopamidol). A typical lumbar facet arthrogram is shown in Figure 67-32.

It is not unusual for the facet capsule to have small fenestrations. It is possible that the injectant may spread to contiguous structures including the epidural space or intervertebral foramen. It is important to identify such spread during the contrast injection, if the injection is being used for diagnostic purposes, as spread to the epidural space or adjacent nerve root would limit the diagnostic utility of the injection. Figure 67-33 is an example of contrast spreading from the L_5S_1 facet joint to the adjacent S_1 nerve root. Arthrography is followed by the diagnostic or therapeutic injection. Typically, 0.25 to 0.50 mL of anesthetic is mixed with 0.25 to 0.50 mL of corticosteroid for each joint.

Complications following facet joint injection are uncommon and include intravascular injection, spinal injection, infection, and needle trauma to the joint or adjacent nerve root.

Costovertebral Joint Injections

The pain related to costovertebral and costotransverse joints usually is unilateral, beginning in a paravertebral location and often radiates in a banklike fashion around the thorax.[54,55] The pain is described as aching and burning, and is usually worse in the morning. It is also worsened by deep inspiration, coughing, and twisting or rotation of the torso.

The injection is performed with fluoroscopy guidance to minimize the risk of pneumothorax. The patient is placed in the prone position, and the lateral tip of the transverse process of the level

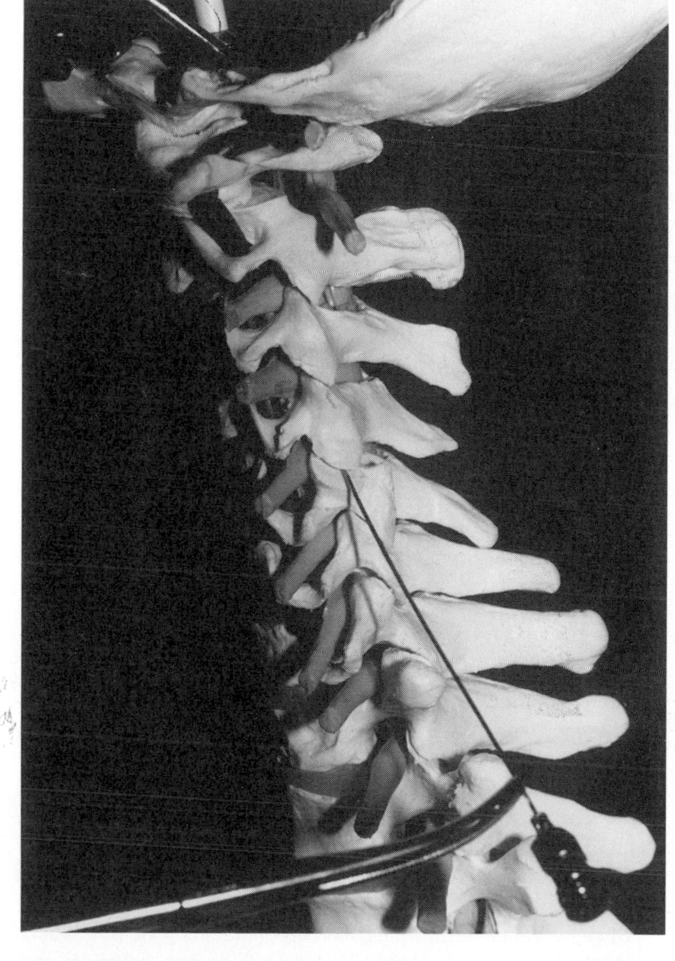

Figure 67-29 Lateral approach to the C_{4-5} facet joint.

A

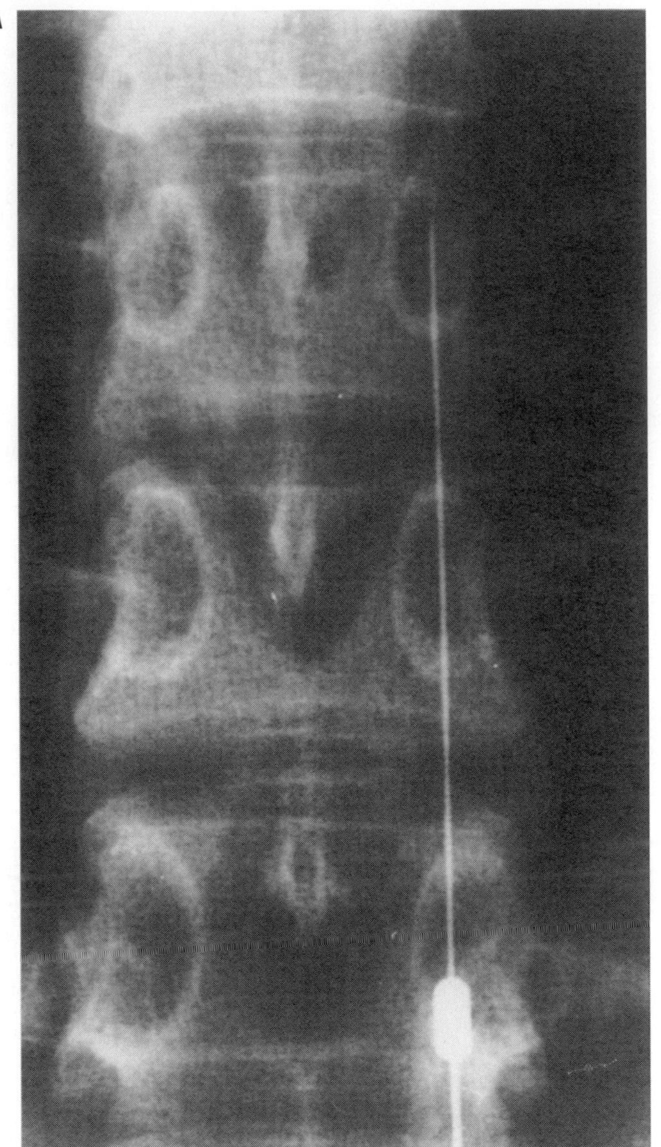

B

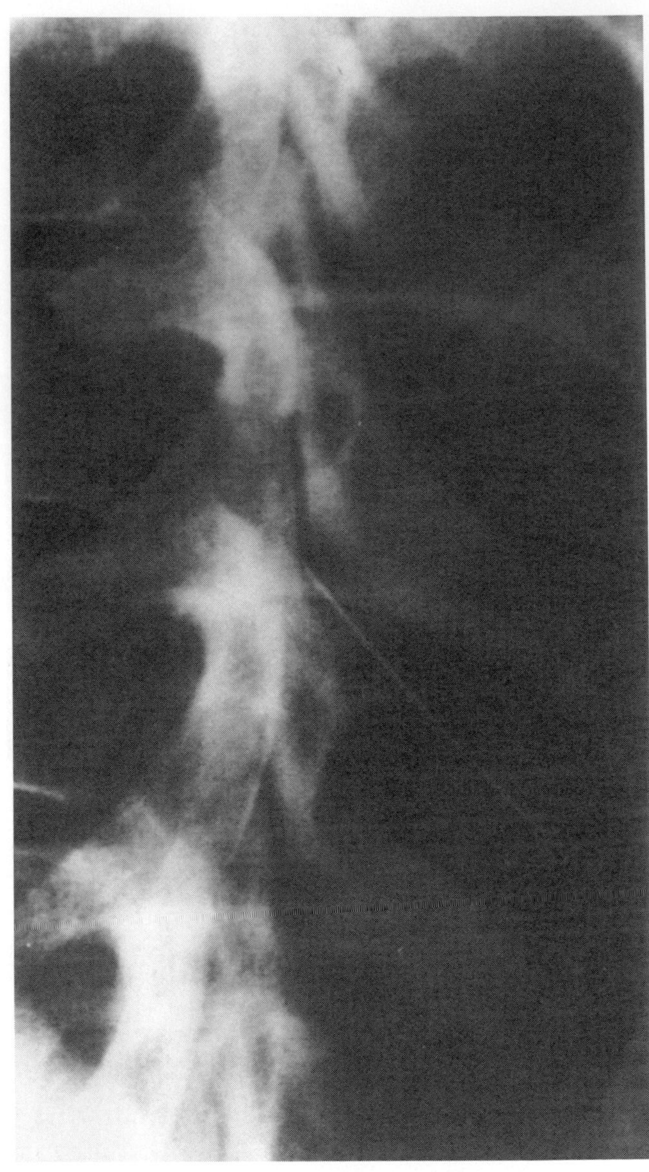

Figure 67-30 Posteroanterior fluoroscopic view of thoracic facet joint injection. (**B**) Lateral fluoroscopic view of thoracic facet joint injection. (Reproduced, with permission, from Dreyfuss P, Tibiletti C, Dreyer S. Thoracic zygapophyseal joint pain patterns: a study in normal volunteers. *Spine* 1994;9:807-811.)

in question is identified. The skin is entered just cephalad and lateral to this point, with a 25-gauge 3½-in. needle directed medially, usually approximately 3 cm from midline. The needle is advanced approximately 3 to 4 cm until contact is made with the vertebral body, which indicates that the needle tip is in the intertransverse space. The needle tip placement is then adjusted cephalad or caudad until it lies within the joint, or pierces the articular capsule. At this point, 0.5 to 1 mL of local anesthetic and/or depot steroid is injected.

Pneumothorax is the most feared complication of this block, although the incidence should be low with proper technique and fluoroscopic guidance.

Costosternal Joint Injection

Costosternal joint pain can be post-traumatic or inflammatory in nature. The costosternal joints are synovial joints; however, the joint space can be obliterated or replaced by fibrous tissue.

The patient is placed supine and the affected joint (or joints) is identified by palpation. Fluoroscopy is not helpful as the costosternal joints are not identifiable with plain x-ray films or fluoroscopy. The joint space is usually identifiable by palpating a groove between the costal cartilage and the sternum. Once identified, the affected joint is injected with 0.5 to 1.0 mL of local anesthetic and/or corticosteroid using a 25-gauge 1-in. needle (see Fig. 67-2).

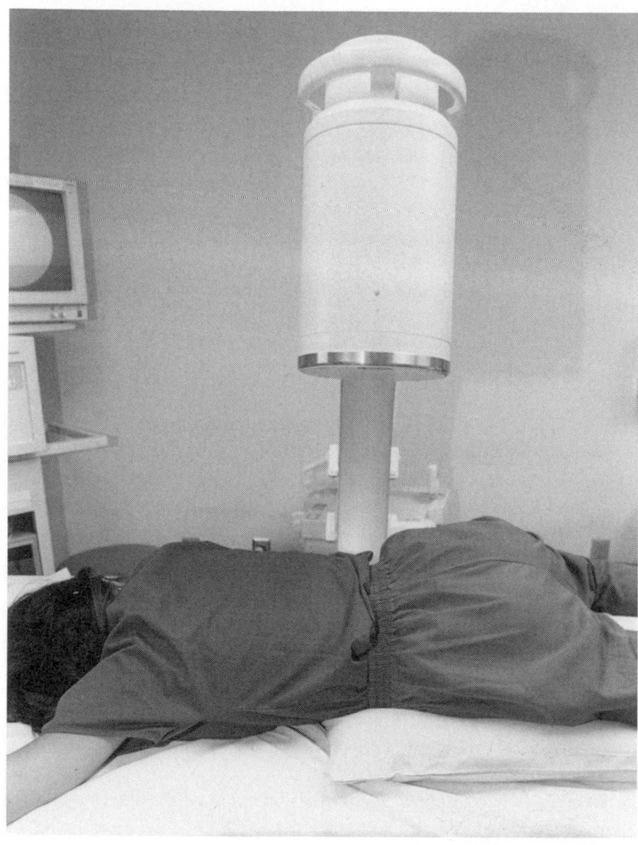

Figure 67-31 Patient positioning for lateral approach to lumbar facet injection.

Sternoclavicular Joint Injection

The patient is placed in the supine position, and the gap between the medial end of the clavicle and the sternum is palpated. The joint is entered with a 25-gauge 1-in. needle and 1 mL of local anesthetic and/or depot steroid is injected (see Fig. 67-2). There should be little resistance to injection. If resistance is encountered, the needle tip is most likely in the meniscal cartilage and should be withdrawn slightly or repositioned until the injectant flows freely.

If posterior sternoclavicular pain is suspected, the posterior ligament of the sternoclavicular joint may be injected. There are two ways to approach this ligament. With the patient in the supine position, a slightly longer 25-gauge needle may be passed completely through the joint, until ligamentous resistance is felt, and then 1 mL of local anesthetic and/or depot steroid is injected around the ligament. The alternate approach is to enter the skin above the superior aspect of the clavicle, and walk the needle off the posterior aspect of the clavicle in a slightly medial direction. Again, the injection is carried out as described above.

With both costosternal and sternoclavicular joint injections, care must be taken to have the needle enter the skin perpendicularly in order to diminish the possibility of pneumothorax. With sternoclavicular joint injections, there is also the possibility of puncture of the subclavian artery or vein with a misplaced needle. Careful attention to technique and use of short (e.g., ½ in.) needles should minimize these complications.

A

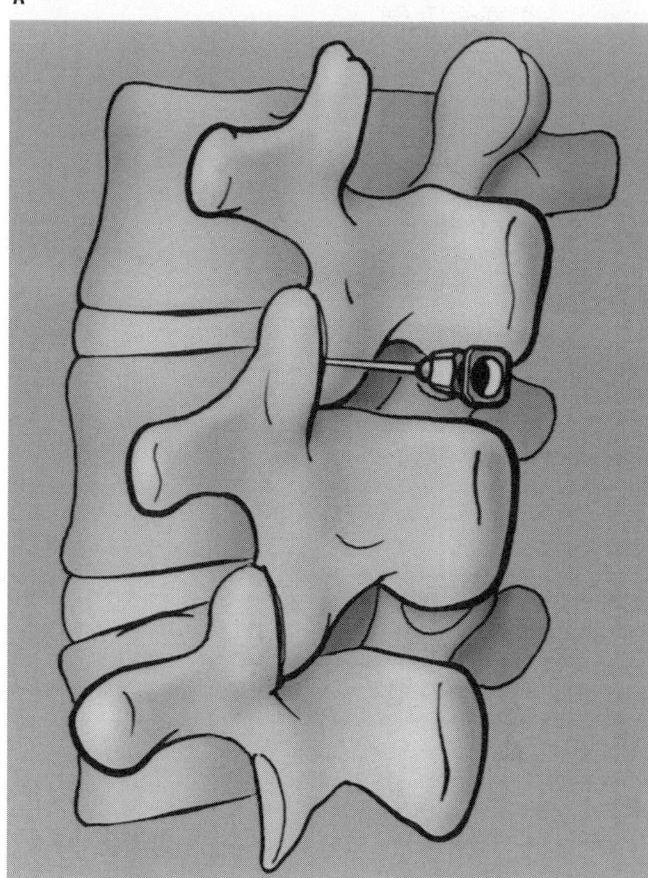

B

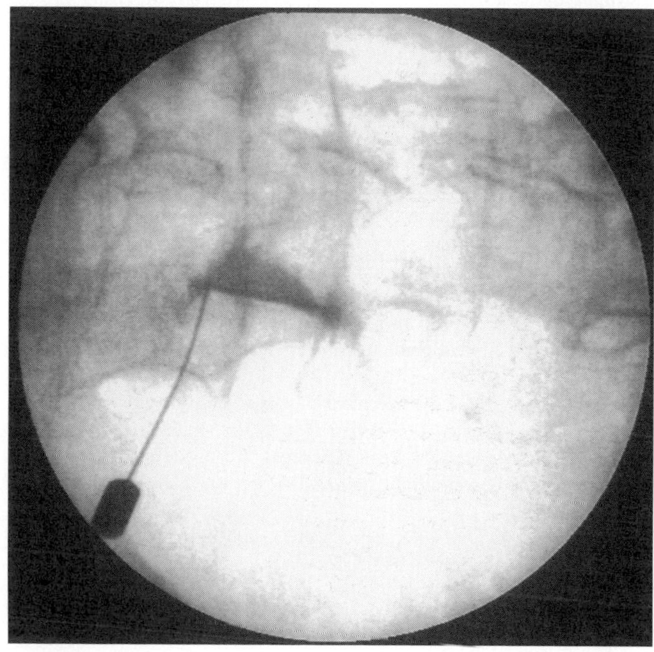

Figure 67-32 (**A**) Posterolateral approach to the lumbar facet joint. (**B**) Posterolateral fluoroscopic view of lumbar facet joint injection with contrast.

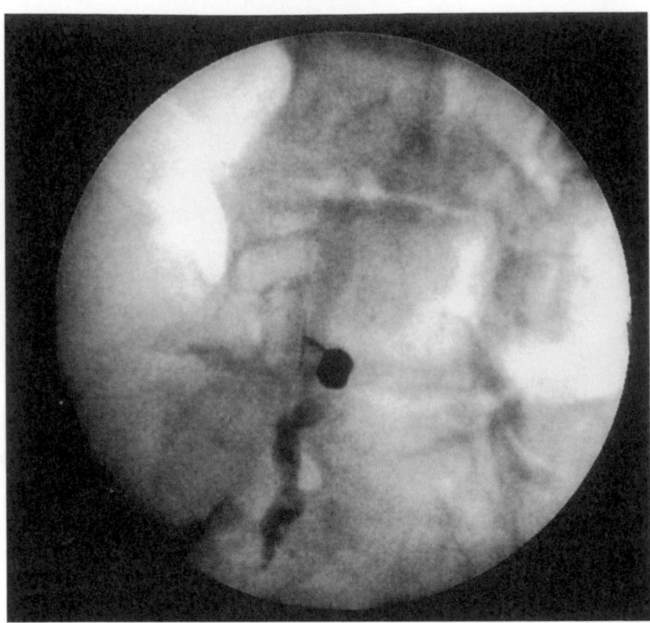

Figure 67-33 L_5S_1 facet injection with contrast. The injectant has spread beyond the ventral aspect of the joint, to surround the first sacral nerve root in this patient with previous lumbar spine surgery.

REFERENCES

1. Hench PS, Kendall EC, Slocumb CH, Polley HF. The effect of a hormone of the adrenal cortex (17-hydroxy-11-dehydrocorticosterone) and of pituitary adrenocorticotrophic hormone on rheumatoid arthritis. *Proc Staff Meet Mayo Clin* 1949;24:181.
2. Hollander JL. The local effects of compound F (hydrocortisone) injected into joints. *Bull Rheum Dis* 1951;2:3.
3. Geborek P, Monsson B, Wollheim FA, Montz U. Intra-articular corticosteroid injection into rheumatoid arthritis knees improves extensor muscle strength. *Rheumatol Int* 1990;9:265.
4. McCarty DJ. Treatment of rheumatoid joint inflammation with triamcinolone hexacetonide. *Arthritis Rheum* 1972;15:157.
5. Friedman DM, Moore ME. The efficacy of intra-articular steroids in osteoarthritis: a double-blind study. *J Rheumatology* 1980;7:850.
6. Jones A, Doherty M. Intra-articular corticosteroids are effective but there are no clinical predictors of response. *Ann Rheum Dis* 1996;54: 379.
7. Anderson B, Kaye S. Treatment of flexor tenosynovitis of the hand with corticosteroids. *Arch Intern Med* 1991;151:153.
8. Smith DL, McAfee JH, Lucas LM, et al. Treatment of non-septic olecranon bursitis: a controlled, blinded prospective trial. *Arch Intern Med* 1989;149:2527.
9. Thumboo J, O'Duffy JD. A prospective study of the safety of joint and soft tissue aspirations and injections in patients taking warfarin sodium. *Arthritis Rheum* 1998;41:736.
10. Derendorf H, Mollmann H, Grüner A, et al. Pharmacokinetics and pharmacodynamics of glucocorticoid suspensions after intra-articular administration. *Clin Pharmacol Ther* 1986;39:313.
11. Firestein FS, Paine MM, Littman BH. Gene expression in rheumatoid arthritis and osteoarthritis synovium: quantitative analysis and effect of intra-articular corticosteroids. *Arthritis Rheum* 1991;34:1094.
12. Williams JM, Brandt KD. Triamcinolone hexacetonide protects against fibrillation and osteophyte formation following chemically induced articular cartilage damage. *Arthritis Rheum* 1985; 28:1267.
13. Johansson A, Bennet G. Effect of local methylprednisolone on pain in nerve injury model. *Reg Anesth* 1997;22:59.
14. Devor M, Govrin-Lippman R, Raber P. Corticosteroids suppress neural discharge originating in experimental neuromas. *Pain* 1985;22:127.
15. Hills BA, Ethell MT, Hodgson DR. Release of lubricating synovial surfactant by intra-articular steroid. *Br J Rheum* 1998;37:649.
16. Corrado EM, Peluso GF, Gigliotti S, et al. The effects of intra-articular administration of hyaluronic acid on osteoarthritis of the knee: a clinical study with immunological and biochemical evaluations. *Eur J Rheumatol Inflamm* 1997;15:47.
17. Peyron JG. Intra-articular hyaluronan injections in the treatment of osteoarthritis: state-of-the-art review. *J Rheumatol* 1993;20:10.
18. Lussier A, Cividino A, McFarlane C, et al. Viscosupplementation with hylan for the treatment of osteoarthritis: findings from clinical practice in Canada. *J Rheumatol* 1996;23:1579.
19. Zuckerman JD, Sledge CB, Shortkroff S, Venkatesan P. Treatment of rheumatoid arthritis using radiopharmaceuticals. *Nucl Med Biol* 1987; 14:211.
20. Wang SI, Lin WY, Chem MN, et al. Rhenim-188 microspheres: a new radiation synovectomy agent. *Nucl Med Commun* 1998;19:427.
21. Trauner KB, Hassan T. Photodynamic treatment of rheumatoid and inflammatory arthritis. *Photochem Photobiol* 1996;64:740.
22. Gray RG, Tenenbaum J, Gottlieb NK. Local corticosteroid injection treatment in rheumatic disorders. *Semin Arthritis* 1981;10:231.
23. Koehler BE, Urowitz MB, Killinger DW. Systemic effects of intra-articular corticosteroid. *J Rheumatol* 1974;1:117.
24. Behrens F, Shepard N, Mitchell N. Alteration of rabbit articular cartilage by intra-articular injections of glucocorticoids. *J Bone Joint Surg* 1975;57:70.
25. Bentley G, Goodfellow JW. Disorganization of the knees following intra-articular hydrocortisone injections. *J Bone Joint Surg* 1969;518: 498.
26. Noyes FR, Grood ES, Nussbaum NS, Cooper SM. Effect of intra-articular corticosteroids on ligament properties. *Clin Orthop Related Res* 1977;123:197.
27. Gibson T, Barry HC, Poswillo D, Glass J. Effect of intra-articular corticosteroid injections on primate cartilage. *Ann Rheum Dis* 1976;36:74.
28. Balch HW, Gibson JMC, El-Ghobarey AF, et al. Repeated corticosteroid injections into knee joints. *Rheum Rehabil* 1977;16:137.
29. Partington PF, Broome GH. Diagnostic injection around the shoulder: hit and miss? A cadaveric study of injection accuracy. *J Shoulder Elbow Surg* 1998;7:147.
30. Van der Heijden G, Van der Windt D, Kleijen J, et al. Steroid injections for shoulder disorders: a systemic review of randomized clinical trials. *Br J Gen Pract* 1996;46:309.
31. Crawford RW, Gic GA, Ling RSM, Murray DW. Diagnostic value of intra-articular anaesthetic in primary osteoarthritis of the hip. *J Bone Joint Surg* 1998;80B:279.
32. Plant MJ, Borg AA, Dziedzic K, et al. Radiographic patterns and response to corticosteroid hip injection. *Ann Rheum Dis* 1997;56:476.
33. asmussen KIE, Fano N. Trochanteric bursitis. *Scand J Rheumatol* 1985;14:417.
34. Johnston CAM, Wiley JP, Lindsay DM, Wiseman DA. Iliopsoas bursitis and tendonitis. *Sports Med* 1998;25:271.
35. Toohey AK, LaSalle TL, Martinez S, Polisson RP. Iliopsoas bursitis: Clinical features, radiographic findings, and disease associations. *Semin Arthritis Rheum* 1990;20:41.
36. Menninger H, Reinhardt S, Sondgen W. Intra-articular treatment of rheumatoid knee joint effusion with triamcinolone hexacetonide versus sodium morrhuate. *Scand J Rheumatol* 1994;23:249.
37. Jones A, Doherty M. Intra-articular corticosteroids are effective in osteoarthritis but there are no clinical predictors of response. *Ann Rheum Dis* 1996;55:829.
38. ozen L, DeFond W. Prepatellar bursal neuritis: a neglected entity. *Contemp Orthop* 1994;28:237.
39. Larsson LG, Baum J. The syndrome of anserina bursitis: an overlooked diagnosis. *Arthritis Rheum* 1985;28:1062.

40. Lucas PE, Hurwitz SR, Kaplan PA, et al. Fluoroscopically guided injections into the foot and ankle: localization of the source of pain as a guide to treatment. *Radiology* 1997;204:411.
41. Dreyfuss P, Michaelson DC, Pauza K. The value of medical history and physical examination in diagnosing sacroiliac joint pain. *Spine* 1996;21:2594.
42. Ebraheim N, Rongming X, Nadaud M, et al. Sacroiliac joint injection: a cadaveric study. *Am J Orthop* 1997;26:338.
43. Maldjian C, Mesgarzadeh M, Tehranzedeh J. Diagnostic and therapeutic features of facet and sacroiliac joint injection. *Radiol Clin North Am* 1998;36:497.
44. Dreyfuss P, Michaelsen M, Fletcher D. Atlanto-occipital (AO) and lateral atlanto-axial (AA) joint pain patterns. *Spine* 1990;19:1125.
45. Lamer TJ. Ear pain due to cervical spine arthritis: treatment with cervical facet injection. *Headache* 1991;31:682.
46. Racz GB, Sanel H, Diede JH. Atlanto-occipital and atlantoaxial injections in the treatment of headache and neck pain. In: Waldman SD, Winnie AP, eds. *Interventional Pain Management*. Philadelphia, Pa: WB Saunders, 1996:220–222.
47. Busch E, Wilson P: Atlanto-occipital and atlanto-axial joint injections in the treatment of headache and neck pain. *Reg Anesth* 1989;14:45.
48. Dory MA. Arthrography of the cervical facet joints. Radiology 1983; 148:379.
49. Wedel DJ, Wilson PR. Cervical facet arthrography. *Reg Anesth* 1985;10:7.
50. Dreyfuss P, Tibilette C, Dreyer SJ. Thoracic zygapophysial joint pain patterns: A study in normal volunteers. *Spine* 1994;19:807.
51. Marks R. Distribution of pain provoked from lumbar facet joints and related structures during diagnostic spinal infiltration. *Pain* 1989;39:37.
52. Schwarzer AC, Aprill CN, Derby R, et al.The relative contributions of the disc and zygapophysial joint in patients with chronic low back pain. *Spine* 1995;20:907.
53. Schwarzer AC, Aprill CN, Derby R, et al. Clinical features of patients with pain stemming from the lumbar zygapophysial joints: Is the lumbar facet syndrome a clinical entity? *Spine* 1994;19:1132.
54. Benjamou C, Roux C, Tourliere D, et al. Pseudovisceral pain referred from costovertebral arthropathies. *Spine* 1993;18;790.
55. Raney F. Costovertebral-costotransverse joint complex as the source of local or referred pain. *J Bone Joint Surg* 1996;48A;1451.

CHAPTER 68 PERIPHERAL NERVE BLOCKS

Lance J. Lehmann

INTRODUCTION

The interruption, interference, or blockade of painful stimuli has been used in the management of pain for several decades. Acute, chronic, and postoperative pain can be diminished with various types of regional anesthesia or specific nerve blocks. In the setting of chronic pain management, various peripheral nerve blocks can be diagnostic, prognostic, or therapeutic in nature. A *nerve block* involves the injection or infusion of a short- or long-acting local anesthetic around a peripheral sensory nerve, motor nerve, or sympathetic nerve plexus. In addition to local anesthetic, a steroid preparation may be added to decrease any suspected inflammatory process. Neurolytic nerve blocks can be performed utilizing various techniques including chemical, heat, or cold. Chemical agents such as alcohol or phenol are used for the selective destruction of nerves. Pulsed radiofrequency and cryoanalgesia cause neurolysis via heat or cold lesioning. Advances in fluoroscopic imaging and computed tomography (CT) scanning allow direct visualization and targeting of specific nerves and nerve plexuses. Other improvements include the use of nerve stimulators during interscalene and axillary blocks or sensory and motor nerve stimulation performed during radiofrequency procedures to assist in accurate needle placement.

Nerve blocks are generally most useful when a specific nerve or limb is affected. Neuropathies with bilateral or multiple areas of involvement may benefit from other forms of neuromodulation including pharmacologic management, transcutaneous electrical stimulation (TENS), or spinal cord stimulation.[1,2]

Successful treatment outcomes involve numerous factors including proper patient selection, understanding the anatomy, side effects, and potential complications of each specific nerve block. A comprehensive approach to chronic pain management has been shown to produce superior outcomes.[3] Nerve blocks, when appropriate, should be considered part of the overall multidisciplinary treatment plan.

INDICATIONS FOR THE USE OF NERVE BLOCKS

Patients selected for nerve block therapy or regional anesthesia should have an accurate diagnosis for the origin of their pain. In some instances nerve blocks may aid in the diagnosis of certain acute and chronic conditions. The relief of pain comes from the interruption of nociceptive or pain sensory pathways, sympathetic blockade, or somatosensory blockade. Regional anesthesia may be used to interrupt the afferent limb of abnormal reflexes that contribute to the pathogenesis of some pain syndromes. Regional anesthesia may block efferent sympathetic outflow, which contributes to postoperative, post-traumatic, and chronic pain syndromes with sympathetic involvement such as complex regional pain syndrome (CRPS) or postherpetic neuralgia.[4]

A complete history and physical evaluation of the patient should be performed including review of laboratory studies, imaging studies, medications, and allergies. Psychiatric and psychosomatic assessment should be carried out when appropriate. Special attention should be paid to anticoagulant medications, sensory loss or motor weakness on physical examination. Complaints of sexual dysfunction, and bowel or bladder problems should also be noted. Any abnormal findings should be documented and may require further evaluation prior to any interventional nerve blocks.

The choice of local anesthetic (LA) used will affect the density of the nerve block as well as the duration. Small nerve fibers (Aδ) and unmyelinated fibers (C fibers) can be interrupted with low concentrations of LA, with minimal effect on the larger myelinated efferent fibers. The subsequent nerve block would produce analgesia without any limb weakness. In contrast, a higher concentration of LA would produce a motor block resulting in temporary limb weakness. This type of block can be therapeutic in some instances, for example, frozen shoulder, by allowing manipulation and increased range of motion.

The duration of the analgesic effect depends on the choice of LA used (For information on local anesthetics amino esters and amino amides, see Appendix C). Lidocaine has a relatively short duration of action compared with bupivicaine, which typically lasts much longer. The addition of a vasoconstrictor such as epinephrine would prolong the duration of the nerve block by decreasing the absorption of the drug into the vascular system. The choice of local anesthetic is also important when considering the anatomic site of the nerve block. For example, lidocaine may be a better choice for nerve blocks in the head and neck region. Owing to its short duration of action any possible adverse affects would be short-lived.

Finally, it can be difficult to differentiate between somatic, visceral, and sympathetic pain. There may be overlapping symptoms, for example, a peripheral nerve injury leading to sympathetic nervous system stimulation. Due to the complexity of some chronic pain syndromes, nerve blocks or regional anesthesia can be used for diagnostic, prognostic, or therapeutic purposes.[5]

NEUROPHYSIOLOGY AND PHARMACOLGY

Neuronal membranes are characterized as semipermeable, double-thickness walls composed of lipid molecules with interspaced globular proteins. Small channels allow ions such as sodium and potassium to pass between the internal and external compartments of nerve membranes. Sensory stimulation causes a sudden influx of sodium ions, which results in depolarization of the nerve membrane. Local anesthetics such as lidocaine or bupivicaine produce temporary impairment of conduction of neural impulses by blocking sodium nerve channel conductance and maintaining the nerve in a polarized state.[6] This effect on nerve membranes is temporary and reversible. The size of the nerve fiber affects its sensitivity to local anesthetics, with smaller, thinner, unmyelinated fibers being most susceptible. Peripheral nerves are composed of three types of nerve fibers:

- A fibers are the largest myelinated somatic nerve fibers. These are further subdivided into delta (δ), beta (β), and gamma (γ) fibers that transmit motor and pressure sensation. The thinner Aδ fibers transmit pain and temperature sensation.
- B fibers are myelinated preganglionic autonomic nerves. B fibers innervate vascular smooth muscle and are the most readily blocked nerve fiber. Successful blockade results in a sympathectomy, with increased warmth due to increased blood flow and decreased sweating.
- C fibers, the thinnest nonmyelinated fibers, are the slowest conducting nerve fibers. They transmit post-ganglionic pain and temperature sensation.
- The two types of pain fibers, Aδ myelinated and nonmyelinated C fibers, have slightly different functions. Aδ fibers transmit sharp pain while C fibers are responsible for the dull pain and burning sensations that accompany many chronic pain syndromes.

CLASSIFICATION OF NERVE BLOCKS

Diagnostic Injections and Nerve Blocks

Diagnostic injections and nerve blocks can help determine or differentiate:

- The anatomic location or main pain generator. Examples include trigger point injections, neuromas, or joint injections.
- Cervical or lumbar disc versus facet joint mediated pain.[7]
- Central (spinal cord or brain) versus peripheral sources of nociception.
- Local pain sources versus referred pain (i.e., facet joint pain referred into hips).
- Somatic versus visceral pain (intercostal nerve blocks will affect somatic afferent nerves in trunk wall without affecting visceral nerves).
- Sympathetic versus somatic nerve injury or dysfunction in upper or lower extremities.
- Selective nerve root blocks can help better define cervical, thoracic, or lumbar radicular pain.
- Pain that may be psychogenic in origin (i.e. differential spinal or epidural).

Prognostic Nerve Blocks

Nerve blocks can be used prognostically before a more permanent neurolytic procedure is performed. Duration of relief from the prognostic nerve block should be noted as well as any sensory or motor deficits. Several prognostic blocks may be indicated before proceeding with certain neurodestructive procedures due to possible placebo effect.[8] To aid in accuracy, these blocks should be performed under fluoroscopic or CT scan guidance.[9] Examples of prognostic blocks include:

- Cervical and lumbar medial branch nerve block prior to radiofrequency rhizotomies.
- Selective nerve root blocks prior to pulsed radiofrequency of the dorsal root ganglion.
- Intercostal blocks prior to pulsed radiofrequency.
- Celiac plexus block prior to alcohol neurolysis.
- Saddle block prior to neurolytic spinal.
- Trial spinal cord stimulation prior to permanent implantation.
- Epidural or intrathecal morphine trial prior to placement of a permanent pump.

Therapeutic Nerve Blocks

Therapeutic nerve blocks are typically performed after or in conjunction with diagnostic blocks that have established the nature and location of the pain. These blocks can be beneficial in both acute and chronic pain states. Examples include:

- Intraoperative and postoperative intercostal blocks for post-thoracotomy pain.
- Interscalene blocks followed by physical therapy for frozen shoulder.
- Continuous infusions around peripheral nerves (i.e., interpleural, intercostal, brachial plexus, or epidural catheters).
- Continuous sympathetic blockade to increase blood flow to an ischemic limb.

PRINCIPLES AND GUIDELINES FOR REGIONAL ANESTHESIA AND NERVE BLOCKS

It may be of benefit to the practitioner and patient if a set of general guidelines is followed to assure optimal outcomes prior to initiating any form of regional anesthesia or specific nerve blocks.

Patient Assessment

Chronic pain patients should always undergo a thorough evaluation before any interventional procedure. Patients may have numerous other medical problems that need to be addressed before deciding if a procedure is warranted. Examples of common medical problems include poorly controlled diabetes, asthma, or hypertension, to name a few. Elements of the patient workup and assessment should include:

- A history from the patient and any other records or diagnostic studies.
- Details of type of pain, location, duration, as well as exacerbating and relieving factors.
- Physical examination documenting any numbness, weakness, and bowel, bladder, or sexual dysfunction.
- Pain measurement tools including visual analog scale (VAS), Beck Depression Inventory, and McGill Pain Questionnaire.
- Psychological assessment and Minnesota Multiphasic Pain Inventory (MMPI).
- Medication and allergy review.

Communication and Informed Consent

Communication with the patient and family members is equally important. The description of the procedure should be discussed, including why it is being performed, alternatives to it, expected outcome, and possible side effects. The physician should also highlight possible risks prior to obtaining informed consent. Sedation, either intravenous or intramuscular, may be offered to minimize any discomfort and this may also be discussed. Finally, the post-procedure recovery period should be discussed (e.g., return to work, physical activity).

Limitations and Contraindications of Nerve Blocks

Nerve blocks can play an integral part in a comprehensive approach to pain management but may have a limited role in certain chronic pain syndromes. Diffuse musculoskeletal pain and peripheral or diabetic neuropathies will generally not benefit from specific nerve blocks. Late-stage CRPS or crush injuries may require more extensive treatments. Damaged tissue, crushed nerves, or pain covering several dermatomes will require some form of systemic treatment. Complex pain patients with no obvious neurologic abnormalities or deficits may have other factors influencing their overall condition and these factors will need to be explored as well. For example, it has been well documented that gender, psychological, cultural, and environmental factors all, or in part, can play a role in pain perception, pain behavior, and treatment outcome.[10,11]

Contraindications to Performing Nerve Blocks

Absolute contraindications are as follows:

- Infection at the proposed site of injection. This can include decubitus ulcers, fungal, or parasitic skin infections.
- Blood clotting abnormalities secondary to intrinsic disease, aspirin, warfarin, or heparin.
- LA allergy. Allergies to ester LAs (procaine, tetracaine, and chloroprocaine) are known; however these solutions are rarely used for regional nerve blocks. Amide local anesthetic allergy (lidocaine, bupivicaine, and ropivivaine) is rare. Some patients may report an allergic reaction that followed a dental procedure. Further investigation may be warranted to see if it was a true LA allergy or simply a reaction to epinephrine.
- A patient with dementia or some other form of altered mental status (i.e., drugs, alcohol, etc.).
- A patient unwilling to agree to the procedure or who does not sign an informed consent form.
- A pregnant patient if fluoroscopy is being used.

Relative contraindications include:

- Patients with systemic infection, severely debilitated, or hypovolemic individuals.
- Situations where a single or continuous nerve block may mask other pathology, such as limb ischemia from a compartment syndrome that may develop following fractures or crush injuries.

PERFORMANCE AND ASSESSMENT OF NERVE BLOCKS

The physician performing the procedure should possess the technical knowledge, experience, and expertise pertinent to the specific procedure. Knowledge of relevant anatomy, potential side effects, and complications of the procedure are essential to preventing adverse outcomes, as well as being able to deal with them should they arise. Various aids can assist accurate needle placement such as fluoroscopy, with or without contrast solutions, peripheral nerve stimulators, CT scanning, and Doppler technology have all been used.[12]

Discomfort during the procedure may be minimized by using short-acting opioids such as fentanyl. Anxiolytics or short-acting agents such as midazolam or propofol are also useful intravenous medications for minimizing anxiety or discomfort during needle placement. Excess sedation may make accurate assessment of diagnostic or therapeutic blocks difficult. For diagnostic or prognostic blocks, a small amount of LA should be used (e.g., for diagnostic medial branch nerve blocks 0.3 mL to 0.5 mL of LA would be appropriate and prevent spread to other surrounding structures). Gentle needle placement under fluoroscopic guidance and anesthetizing the skin with LA or a freezing spray (e.g.,ethyl chloride) will help to ensure patient comfort.

Before and following regional anesthesia, baseline pain measurements should be obtained. Various indicators or scales such as the visual analog scale (VAS) can be used to help document baseline pain level and response to treatment.[13] For more specific nerve blocks, additional information may be helpful. Skin temperature measurements prior to and following sympathetic nerve blockade may be recorded. An increase in temperature of the affected extremity is typically due to vasodilatation and increased blood flow following the temporary sympathectomy. For somatic nerve blocks, sensory and motor deficits should be consistent with the anticipated region or dermatome blocked.

The duration and onset of the physiologic effect of the block and its correlation with the duration of pain relief is important for several reasons. If the duration of pain relief is shorter than expected, it may indicate inaccurate needle placement, an incomplete or partial nerve block, or possibly an alternate pain source. If the duration is longer than expected, or the onset much quicker than expected, potential placebo effect should be considered. For these reasons, which can cause uncertainty in interpretation, it is advisable to repeat blocks using LAs with different durations of action.[14] Neural blockade followed by physical or occupational therapy can also assist in assessing the success of various blocks. Additional documentation can include decreased pain response or increased range of motion measurements.

Side Effects and Complications of Regional Anesthesia

Before regional anesthesia or a specific nerve block is initiated, certain issues need to be addressed. When performing the actual injection or infusion of LA, continuous monitoring of patient physiologic indices should occur as dictated by the American Society of Anesthesiology guidelines. Monitoring should include electrocardiography, blood pressure, and pulse oximetry. Verbal contact with the patient is important to detect changes in level of consciousness or sensorium. Patient monitoring after the procedure should continue for at least 30 minutes to detect any delayed complications. Examples of a delayed complication include inadvertent subdural injection following a lumbar epidural injection or a pnemothorax that can occur following intercostal nerve blocks. These complications can present with delayed hypotension and motor block in the case of a subdural injection[15] or shortness of breath with cardiopulmonary collapse in the case of a severe pneumothorax.[16]

Needle Placement and Positioning

Needle placement is not entirely risk-free and great care should be taken even when utilizing fluoroscopic guidance. Observation of the patient is important to detect increased pain during needle placement. Increased pain during needle placement may necessitate the use of more LA to anesthetize the needle trajectory, needle redirection, or repositioning of the fluoroscopy unit for a "tunnel vision view." Anterior-posterior fluoroscopic views show needle direction, whereas lateral views are required to gauge needle depth. A "heavy hand" will not be overcome by giving the patient large amounts of intravenous sedation. In addition, large amounts of intravenous sedation may cause untoward side effects including nausea, vomiting, and hypotension. Oversedation may result in unwanted patient movement due to inability to follow commands, and any altered mental status may be difficult to distinguish from LA toxicity. Nerve injury or more severe consequences can occur if the patient is unable to respond during actual needle placement or during injection of the LA solution.

Damage or irritation to neural structures can range from paresthesias during needle placement to nerve damage or paralysis.[17] Care should be taken when injecting near the neural foramen, such as during transforaminal epidural injections or when passing the neural foramen during a lumbar sympathetic block or celiac plexus block. The ulnar nerve lies superficial in the medial epicondyle and may be prone to needle injury. Cauda equina injuries or paralysis may occur following the inadvertent injection of hypertonic saline intrathecally during lysis of epidural adhesions.[18] Nerve damage or neuritis can occur from "spill over" during the injection of neurolytic substances. Therefore, small amount of phenol or alcohol should be used, except perhaps in the case of a neurolytic celiac plexus block. Finally, improper needle placement during radiofrequency neurolyis can result in neuritis of a specific nerve root.[19]

Damage to non-neural structures including bowel perforation or renal damage may also occur. These complications can be avoided or minimized by careful, gentle technique and the use of continuous fluoroscopic guidance. Complications associated with specific nerve blocks are discussed throughout the text. For some procedures, there is a small incidence of a specific complication, such as pneumothorax following intercostal blocks or supraclavicular/infraclavicular brachial plexus blocks. The incidence of discitis following provocative discography has been reported at 0.1% to 1.3% per disc.[20] The potential always exists for a needle to puncture a blood vessel resulting in bleeding or a hematoma. Hematomas can be seen following stellate ganglion blocks if the carotid artery is punctured. These usually resolve quickly on their own with minimal side effects. A hematoma within the epidual space is a rare occurrence, with potential serious side effects including paraparesis and paraplegia.[21] Discontinuing aspirin or other blood thinners, and checking coagulation studies can help avoid this serious complication. In rare instances a stroke can occur due to arterial spasm, particularly in the cervical region. Bowel perforation can occur due to poor technique following lumbar discography, lumbar sympathetic, hypogastric or impars ganglion blocks. The use of fluoroscopic guidance should be considered medically necessary in terms of standard of care and, in addition, for confirming needle placement when injecting a contrast solution.[9,22]

Local Anesthetic Effects

Local anesthetics can have a toxic effect on the central nervous system and cardiovascular system. A quick rise in LA blood level can result from inadvertent intravascular injection, rapid absorption into the circulation (e.g., intercostal blocks) or simply the use of an excessive amount of LA. Systemic effects of a LA such as lidocaine include lightheadedness or tinnitus at low concentrations (5 to 10 μg/mL plasma concentration) to seizures, respiratory arrest, and coma at higher concentrations ($>$15 μg/mL plasma concentration). Bupivicaine, another commonly used LA for nerve blocks, is four times more toxic than lidocaine and can result in ventricular arrhythmia and death from ventricular fibrillation. If epinephrine is used in the LA solution, rapid absorption or intravascular injection will result in tachycardia, hypertension, and palpitations. In general, epinephrine should be avoided, especially in patients with cardiovascular disease.

To help guard against any toxic LA effects, always aspirate prior to injection; in addition, a contrast solution can be injected to rule out intravascular needle placement or intravascular catheter migration. The dose of LA should be kept within acceptable limits (see Appendix C).

Physiologic Effects of Regional Anesthesia

Expected side effects include hypotension following sympathetic or epidural anesthesia and sensory loss or motor weakness following specific somatic nerve blocks. Unexpected effects are numerous and detailed throughout the text. Vagal reactions can occur in extremely anxious individuals, sometimes resulting in severe bradycardia or hypotension. These reactions can be quickly treated with intravenous fluids and intravenous or intramuscular ephedrine. Phrenic nerve block commonly occurs following stellate ganglion or interscalene blocks. If shortness of breath occurs in patients after intercostal nerve blocks, any potential pneunothorax should be ruled out. Patients should always be monitored closely and treated early with supportive care or more aggressive resuscitative measures if the need arises.

SPECIFIC NERVE BLOCKS

HEAD AND NECK

Trigeminal Nerve Block (Fig. 68-1).

Anatomy The trigeminal nerve consists of three divisions: the ophthalmic nerve (V1), maxillary nerve (V2), and mandibular nerve (V3). These three branches supply sensation to most of the face, excluding the angle of the jaw, which is supplied by the second cranial nerve. Trigeminal nerve blocks are used mainly to treat severe pain from trigeminal neuralgia and various malignancies affecting the face.

Gasserian Ganglion (Fig. 68-2).

Anatomy The gasserian or trigeminal ganglion lies within the medial cranial fossa across the superior border of the petrous temporal bone. The posterior two thirds is fully covered by dura matter. This posterior portion lies within a small recess called *Meckel's cave*. This invagination of the dura surrounding the posterior two thirds of the ganglion allows direct continuity with the cerebrospinal fluid.

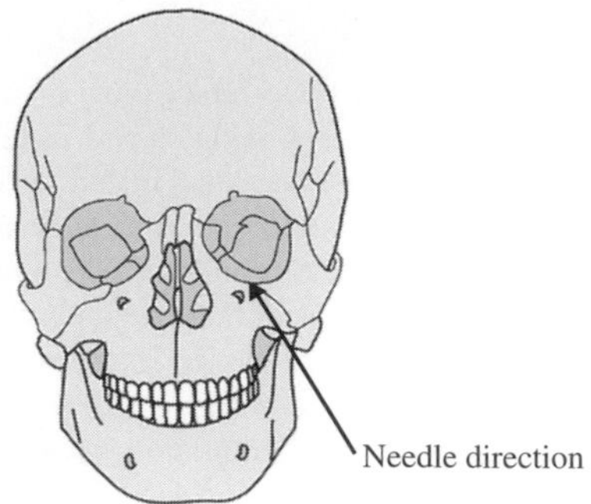

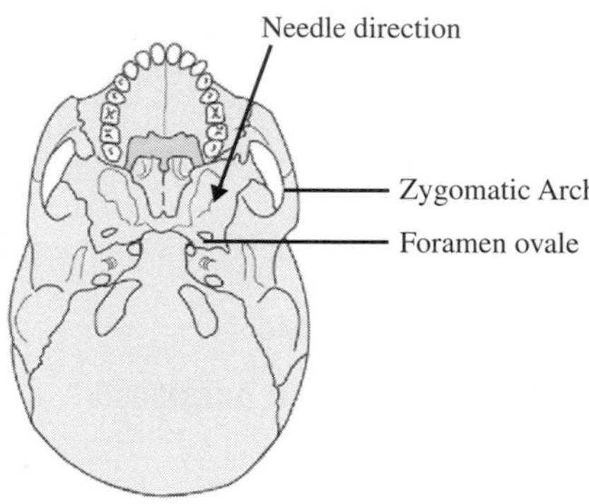

Figure 68-1 Trigeminal nerve block. (Adapted with permission from MediClip, Williams & Wilkins.)

Indications Used for intractable pain from trigeminal neuralgia (tic douloureux) or cancer after conservative treatments have failed. This type of block is recommended when more than one division of the trigeminal nerve is involved. Neurolytic solutions (alcohol, glycerol) and radiofrequency rhizotomy techniques are also used for more permanent blockade or destruction of the nerve.

Complications The major complication is corneal anesthesia leading to loss of sensation and corneal ulcers. Subarachnoid injection can cause unconsciousness or seizures.

Mandibular Nerve Block (Fig. 68-3).

Anatomy The largest of the three divisions is the third division, the mandibular nerve that exits the cranium through the foramen ovale. Below the foramen the mandibular nerve divides into a smaller anterior and larger posterior division. The anterior division innervates the muscles of mastication (lateral pterygoid, temporalis, and masseter muscles). The posterior division is mainly sensory, dividing into the inferior alveolar, lingual, and auricotemporal nerves. The mandibular nerve is both a sensory and motor nerve.

Indications Trigeminal neuralgia, malignant conditions involving the lower jaw (e.g., Ewing's sarcoma, osteogenic sarcoma) or cancer of the tongue.

Complications Neuritis if nerve is traumatized or bleeding into the cheek.

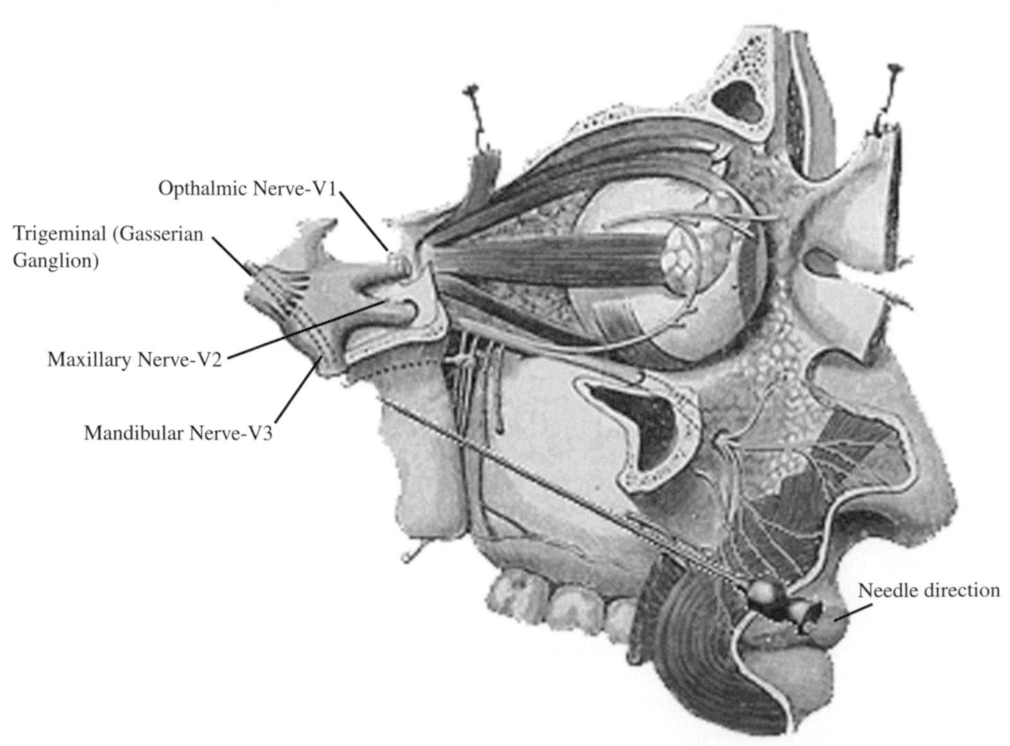

Figure 68-2 Gasserian ganglion. (Adapted with permission from MediClip, Williams & Wilkins.)

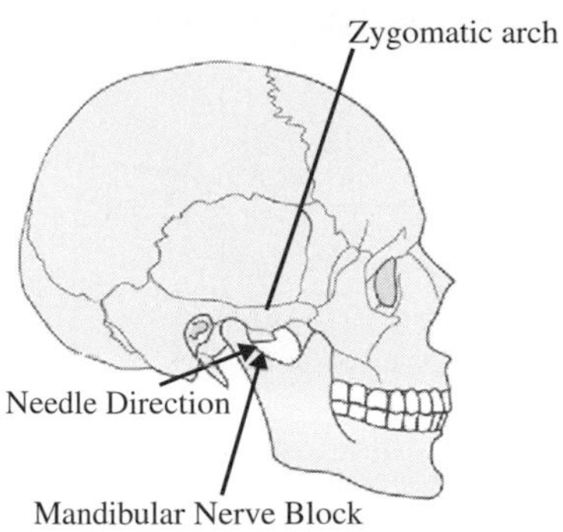

Figure 68-3 Mandibular nerve block. (Adapted with permission from MediClip, Williams & Wilkins.)

Maxillary Nerve Block (Fig. 68-4).

Anatomy After leaving the gasserian ganglion, the maxillary nerve passes along the inferior lateral border of the cavernous sinus. It then exits the middle cranial fossa through the foramen rotundum and enters the pterygopalatine fossa, where it divides into its major branches. The maxillary nerve is a sensory nerve.

Indications Trigeminal neuralgia, malignancy, or radiation damage to middle third of the face, nasal cavity, and hard palate.

Complications Bleeding due to highly vascular pterygopalatine fossa. Injections using greater the 1 mL of volume can spread into the orbit and thus affect the oculomotor and abducens nerves, resulting in visual difficulty.

Glossopharyngeal Nerve Block (Fig. 68-5).

Anatomy The glossopharyngeal nerve exits the skull through the jugular foramen located posterior to the tip of the mastoid process. The nerve then passes anteriorly between the internal jugular vein and internal carotid artery, coursing medial to the styloid process and lateral to the vagus and spinal accessory nerves. The glossopharyngeal nerve supplies sensation to the posterior one third of the tongue, the palatine tonsils, and pharyngeal wall.

Indications Glossopharyngeal neuralgia characterized by pain of the throat with possible radiation to the ear and thyroid cartilage area and pharyngeal cancer.

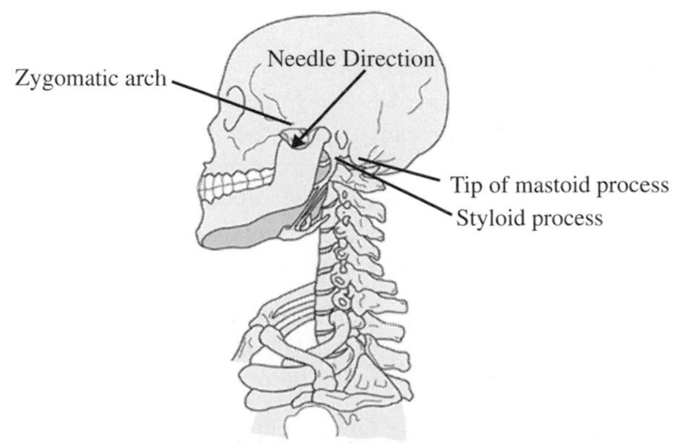

Figure 68-4 Maxillary nerve block. (Adapted with permission from MediClip, Williams & Wilkins.)

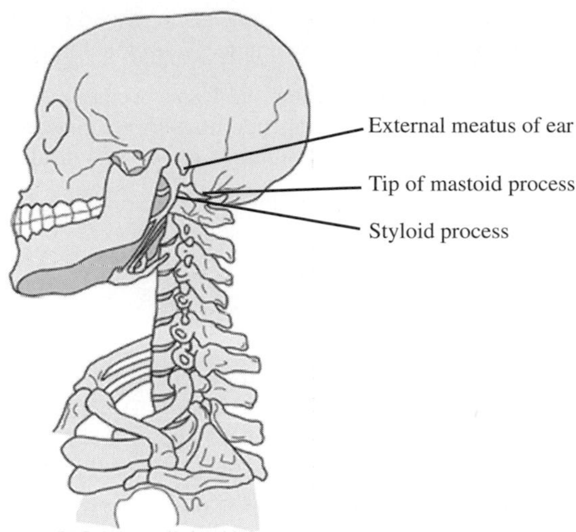

Figure 68-5 Glossopharyngeal nerve block. (Adapted with permission from MediClip, Williams & Wilkins.)

Complications Dysphagia from paralysis of the pharyngeal muscles and weakness or partial paresis of the tongue. The block should only be performed unilaterally since a bilateral block will produce complete paralysis of the pharyngeal muscles. Weakness in the trapezius muscle can also be seen due to blockade of the spinal accessory nerve.

Occipital Nerve Block (Fig. 68-6).

Anatomy The greater occipital nerve is formed from the dorsal primary ramus of the second and third cervical nerves. It supplies sensation to the medial-posterior portion of the scalp. This nerve is usually located 2 to 3 cm lateral to the external occipital protuberance and just medial to the occipital artery, which serves as a reliable landmark. The lesser occipital nerve arises from the ventral primary ramus to the second and third cervical nerves passing

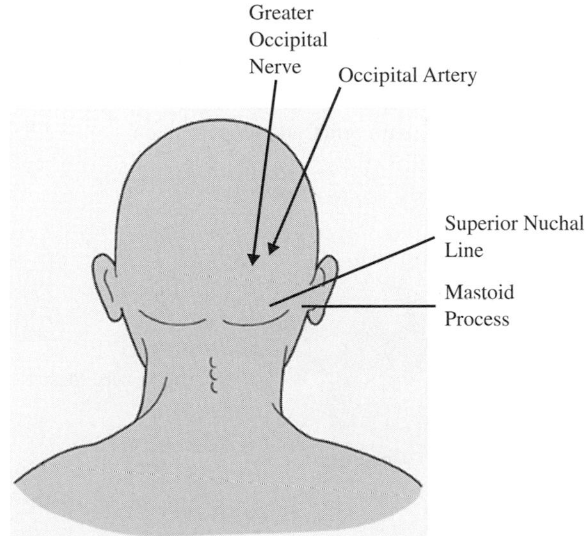

Figure 68-6 Occipital nerve block. (Adapted with permission from MediClip, Williams & Wilkins.)

along the posterior border of the sternocleidomastoid muscle. It is located approximately 2.5 cm lateral to the occipital artery.

Indications Blocking the greater and lesser occipital nerves can be used for diagnostic or therapeutic measures in managing patients with suspected occipital neuralgia or occipital headaches.

Complications Generally none. Possible seizure if large amount of local anesthetic injected into occipital artery.

Upper Extemity: Shoulder

Brachial Plexus Block (Fig. 68-7).

Anatomy The brachial plexus is formed from the ventral primary rami of the fifth (C5) , sixth (C6) , seventh (C7), and eighth (C8) cervical nerves along with the first thoracic nerve (T1). The C4 and T2 spinal nerves may also contribute to the plexus. These roots pass between the anterior and middle scalene muscles in the neck before passing into the arm. After dividing into upper, middle, and lower trunks, these nerves enter the axilla between the clavicle and first rib. The trunks then divide into anterior and posterior divisions, which in turn divide into lateral, medial, and posterior cords. Within the axilla, near the lateral border of the axilla, the cords divide into the peripheral nerves of the upper extremity.

- Long thoracic nerve contains fibers from C5, C6, and C7.
- Suprascapular nerve contains fibers from C4, C5, and C6.
- Peripheral branches of the lateral cord form the musculocutaneous nerve and lateral root of the median nerve formed from C5, C6, and C7.
- Peripheral branches of the medial cord (C8 and T1) form the medial root of the median nerve, the ulnar nerve, and the medial cutaneous branches of the arm and forearm.
- Peripheral branches of the posterior cord form the axillary, radial, and subscapular nerves.

Indications There are four approaches to blocking the nerves of the brachial plexus. The interscalene, supraclavicular, and infraclavicular approach will provide anesthesia for the entire arm including the shoulder. The axillary approach can be used for anesthesia between the hand and elbow. Continuous infusions of local anesthetic through a catheter can also be used for prolonged block of the various peripheral nerves of the brachial plexus. Indications for brachial plexus block include:

- Anesthesia for upper extremity surgery
- Postoperative pain relief and rehabilitation

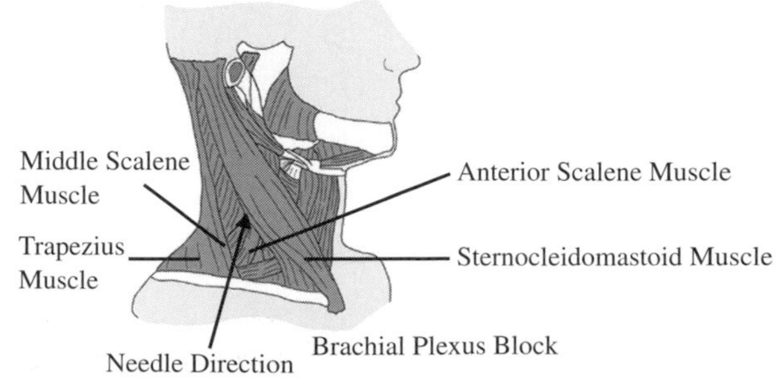

Figure 68-7 Brachial plexus block: interscalene approach. (Adapted with permission from MediClip, Williams & Wilkins.)

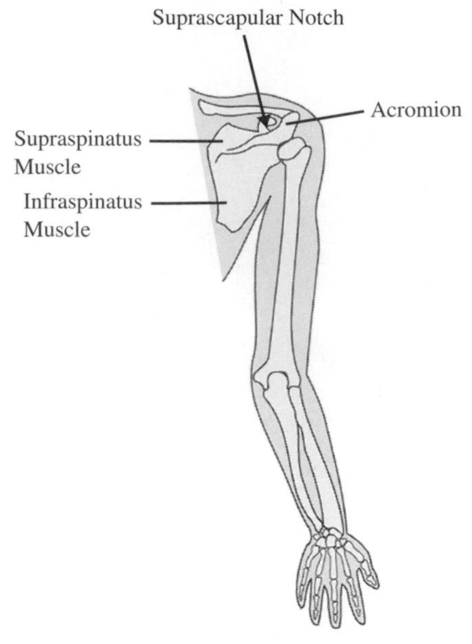

Figure 68-8 Suprascapular nerve block. (Adapted with permission from MediClip, Williams & Wilkins.)

- Differentiate sympathetic pain from peripheral nerve injury
- Manipulation of frozen shoulder or wrist injuries
- Continuous sympathetic nerve blockade to improve blood flow to the affected extremity (i.e., Raynaud's)
- Phantom limb pain
- Differentiate pain of peripheral neuralgia verses a more central origin (i.e., brachial plexus avulsion).

Complications For interscalene approach: epidural or intrathecal injection, inadvertent vertebral artery or intravenous injection, and recurrent laryngeal and phrenic nerve block.

For supraclavicular approach: phrenic nerve block, cervical sympathetic block, and 0.5% to 6.0% incidence of pneumothorax.

For axillary approach: intravascular injection with seizure incidence 1.5% and axillary artery damage.

Suprascapular Nerve Block (Fig. 68-8)

Anatomy Arises from C4, C5, and C6 contributions from the upper trunk of the brachial plexus. It passes beneath the trapezius muscle to the superior border of the scapula, where it passes through the suprascapular notch. The suprascapular nerve is the major sensory supply to the shoulder joint and motor supply to the supraspinatus and infraspinatus muscles.

Indications Used to treat arthritis or bursitis of the shoulder joint in addition to intra- and periarticular injections. Diagnostically, to confirm suprascaplular nerve irritation or entrapment.

Side Effects Paralysis of the supraspinatus and infraspinatus muscles.

Complications Pneumothorax from the needle being advanced past the upper border of the scapula. Direct nerve injury.

Upper Extremity: Elbow and Wrist

Median Nerve Block (Fig. 68-9)

Anatomy The median nerve, formed from the lateral and median roots of the brachial plexus, contains fiber from C5 through T1. There are no branches in the upper arm and it descends with the brachial artery being slightly medial to it at the elbow. It crosses the elbow anteriorly and passes between the two heads of the pronator teres. It courses through the wrist deep to the palmoris longus tendon.

Indications Used to supplement a brachial plexus block or as diagnostic and therapeutic block and the elbow or wrist (i.e., carpal tunnel).

Technique and Landmarks Medial and lateral epicondyles of the humerus and medial to the brachial artery.

Complications Direct nerve injury.

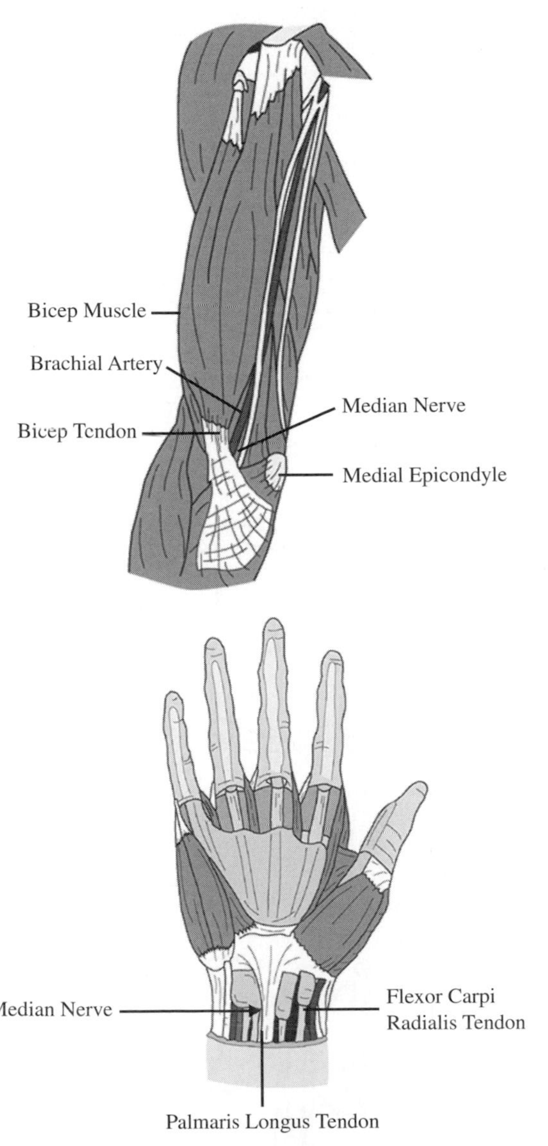

Figure 68-9 Median nerve block. (Adapted with permission from MediClip, Williams & Wilkins.)

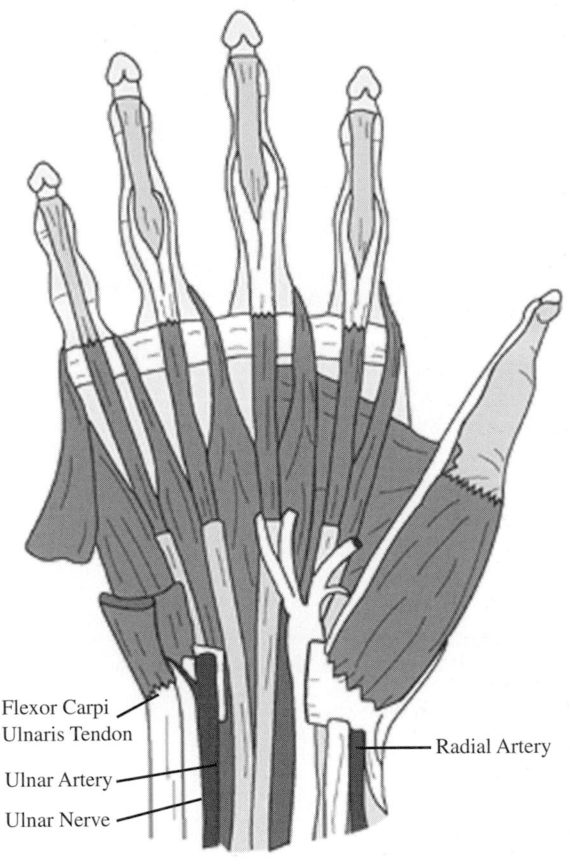

Figure 68-10 Ulnar nerve block. (Adapted with permission from MediClip, Williams & Wilkins.)

Ulnar Nerve Block (Fig. 68-10)

Anatomy The ulnar nerve is formed from the C7, C8, and T1 roots. At the elbow, it lies behind the medial epicondyle in the ulnar groove.

Indications Used to supplement brachial plexus anesthesia or as diagnostic and therapeutic block for ulnar nerve injury such as compression or entrapment neuropathies.

Complications Direct nerve injury.

Radial Nerve Block (Fig. 68-11)

Anatomy The posterior cord (C5 to T1) gives rise to the radial nerve.

Indications Used to supplement a brachial plexus block or as diagnostic and therapeutic block for radial nerve injury (i.e., humeral fracture).

Complications Direct nerve injury.

Pelvis

Ilioinguinal and Iliohypogastric (Fig. 68-12)

Anatomy The ilioinguinal and iliohypogastric nerves originate from the L1 nerve root. A small contribution from T12 can also exist. The iliohypogastric nerve courses between the transverse and external oblique abdominal musculature. It divides into lateral and anterior cutaneous branches at the level of the iliac crest. The lateral branch provides sensation to the posterolateral gluteal area.

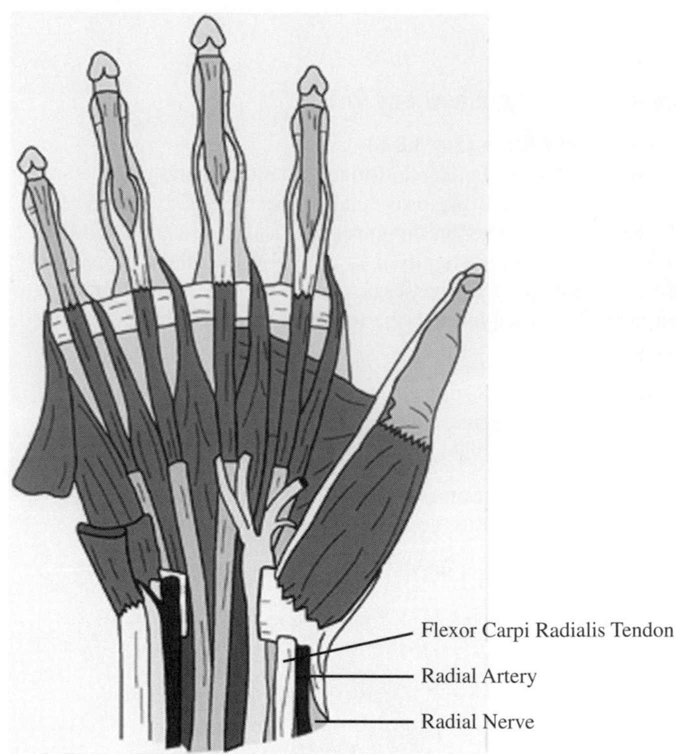

Figure 68-11 Radial nerve block. (Adapted with permission from MediClip, Williams & Wilkins.)

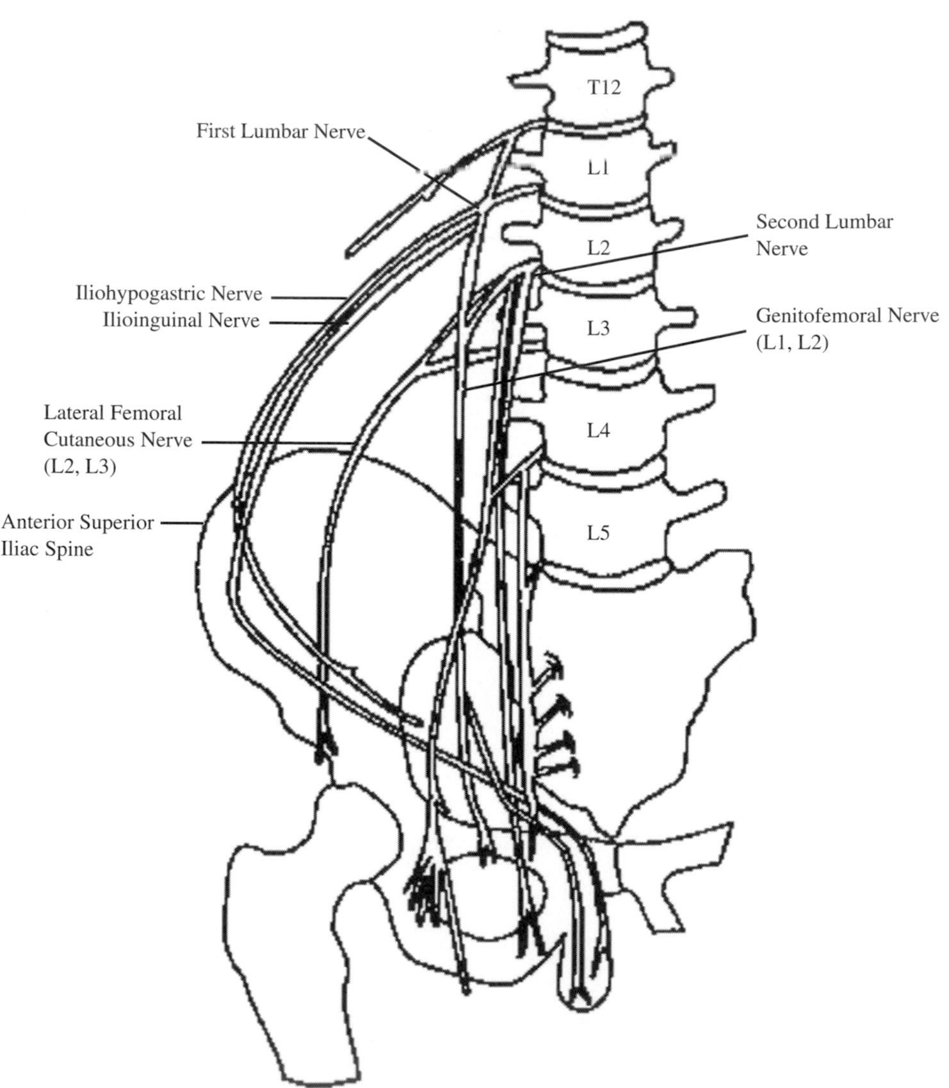

Figure 68-12 Ilioinguinal and iliohypogastric nerve block. (Adapted with permission from MediClip, Williams & Wilkins.)

The anterior branch sends sensory fibers to the skin of the abdomen around the pubis.

The ilioinguinal nerve is typically smaller. It lies slightly lateral to the iliohypogastric nerve, traversing the internal oblique muscle following the spermatic cord into the inguinal canal. Sensation is provided to the inner thigh, upper part of the scrotum in men and mons pubis and lateral labia in women.

Indications Inguinal hernia operations and to diagnose and treat postherniorrhapy nerve entrapment.

Technique Mark 1 in. medial to the anterior superior iliac spine and draw a line between this area and the umbilicus. A 25-gauge 1½—in. needle can be used to inject 8 to 10 mL of local anesthetic solution fanwise in an up and down direction.

Complications Bleeding if femoral artery or vein is punctured.

Lateral Femoral Cutaneous (Fig. 68-13)

Anatomy The lateral femoral cutaneous nerve is formed from the posterior divisions of L2 and L3 within the psoas muscle. It passes into the thigh slightly medial to the anterior superior iliac spine and beneath the inguinal ligament. It provides sensation to the anterolateral thigh and buttock.

Indications Diagnosis and treatment of meralgia paresthetica.

Technique Approximately 1 in. medial to the anterior iliac spine and just inferior to the inguinal ligament. A 25-gauge 1½-in. needle is inserted perpendicular to the skin advanced slowly until a paresthesia is obtained. Then 5 mL to 10 mL of local anesthetic solution can be injected.

Complications Bleeding if femoral artery or vein punctured. Pain at injection site.

Sciatic Nerve Block (Fig. 68-14)

Anatomy The sciatic nerve contains most of the sensory and sympathetic fibers of the leg. It is the largest nerve in the body originating from anterior divisions of L4, L5, S1, S2, and S3. This nerve leaves the pelvis through the sciatic notch below the piriforms muscle, then courses between the greater trochanter of the femur and ischial tuberosity. In the thigh it branches to the hamstring and adductor magnus muscles before dividing into the common peroneal and tibial nerves behind the head of the fibula.

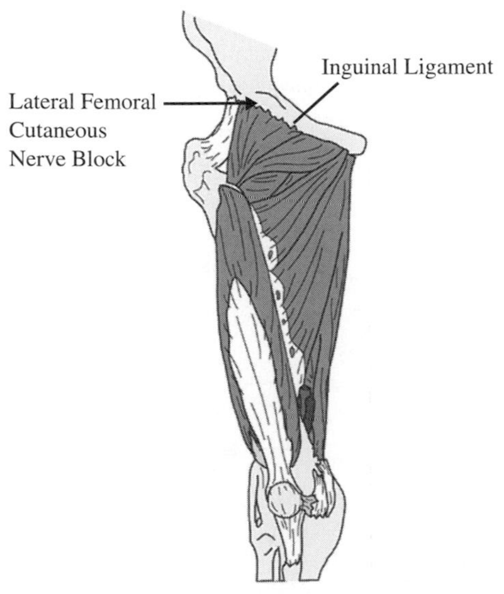

Figure 68-13 Lateral femoral cutaneous nerve block. (Adapted with permission from MediClip, Williams & Wilkins.)

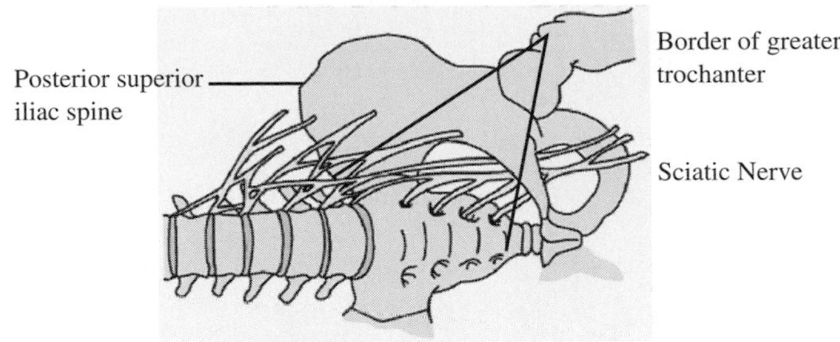

Figure 68-14 Sciatic nerve block. (Adapted with permission from MediClip, Williams & Wilkins.)

Indications For surgery or manipulation of the leg below the knee. Diagnostic and therapeutic block for sciatic nerve injury (i.e., trauma or hip fracture) piriformis syndrome.

Complications Hematoma in buttocks or nerve damage.

Femoral Nerve Block (Fig. 68-15)

Anatomy The femoral nerve is formed by the dorsal divisions of the anterior rami of the second (L2), third (L3), and fourth (L4) lumbar segments. It emerges from the psoas muscle and is primarily responsible for extension of the thigh. It passes into the thigh underneath the inguinal ligament and just lateral to the femoral artery. The femoral nerve sends branches to the sartorius, quadriceps femoris, and pectinus muscles along with sensory branches to the skin overlying anteromedial thigh. It terminates in the lower leg as the saphenous nerve, which supplies sensation to the skin on the medial aspect of the leg.

Indications Can be combined with a sciatic nerve block for surgical manipulation of the leg. Diagnosis of femoral nerve damage or entrapment.

Technique See Appendix A.

Complications Intravascular injection, or hematoma. Nerve injury.

Lower Extremity: Knee

Common Peroneal Nerve Block (Fig. 68-16).

Anatomy The common peroneal and the tibial nerve are the two major peripheral branches of the sciatic nerve. This nerve enters the lower leg behind the head of the fibula, where it then courses laterally around the neck of the fibula before dividing into the deep peroneal and superficial peroneal nerves.

Indications Generally used in combination with tibial and saphenous nerve blocks for analgesia of the lower leg.

Complications Injury to nerve adjacent to neck of fibula.

Tibial Nerve Block (Fig. 68-16).

Anatomy After branching off from the sciatic nerve, this nerve courses through the popliteal fossa into the lower leg deep between the heads of the gastronemius muscle which it supplies. This nerve becomes superficial at the ankle passing between the medial malleolus and Achilles' tendon before dividing into the lateral and me-

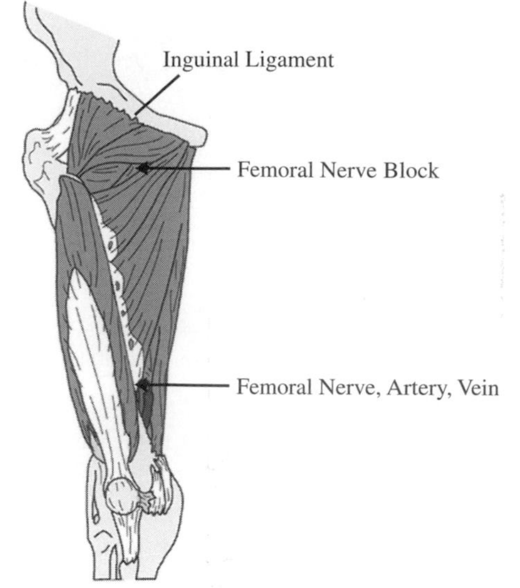

Figure 68-15 Femoral nerve block. (Adapted with permission from MediClip, Williams & Wilkins.)

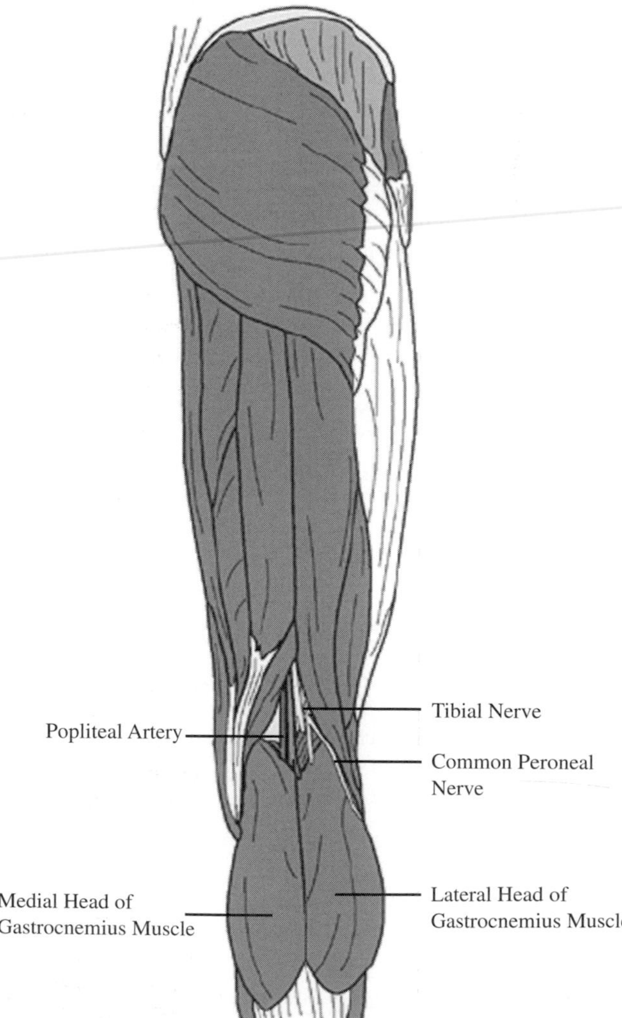

Figure 68-16 Common peroneal and tibial nerve block. (Adapted with permission from MediClip, Williams & Wilkins.)

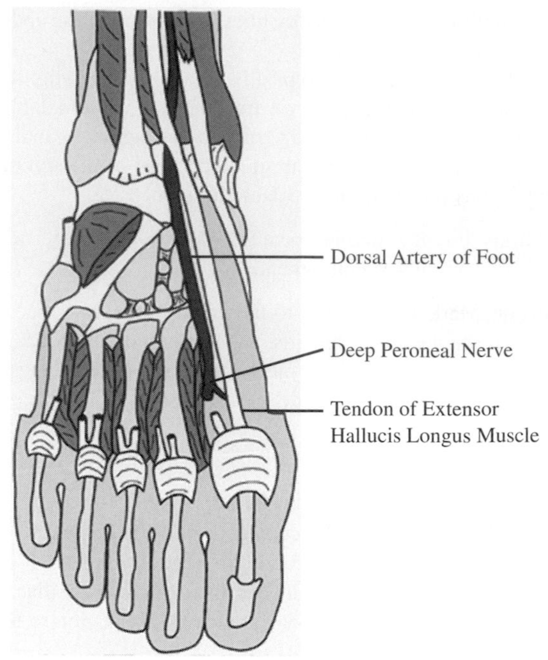

Figure 68-17 Deep peroneal nerve block. (Adapted with permission from MediClip, Williams & Wilkins.)

dial plantar nerves. It supplies sensation to the skin of the heel and medial sole of the foot.

Indications Supplement inadequate sciatic block for lower extremity interventions.

Complications Neuritis tibial nerve.

Lower Extremity: Ankle

Tibial Nerve. See previous section for discussion.

Deep Peroneal Nerve Block (Fig. 68-17).

Anatomy The common peroneal nerve branches into the deep and superficial peroneal nerves. This nerve enters the foot medial to the tendon of the hallucis longus muscle. It supplies fibers to the tarsal and metatarsal joints and the skin adjacent to first and second toes.

Indications When combined with a tibial nerve block, almost complete analgesia and sympathetic blockade of the foot is possible.

Complications Injury to nerve.

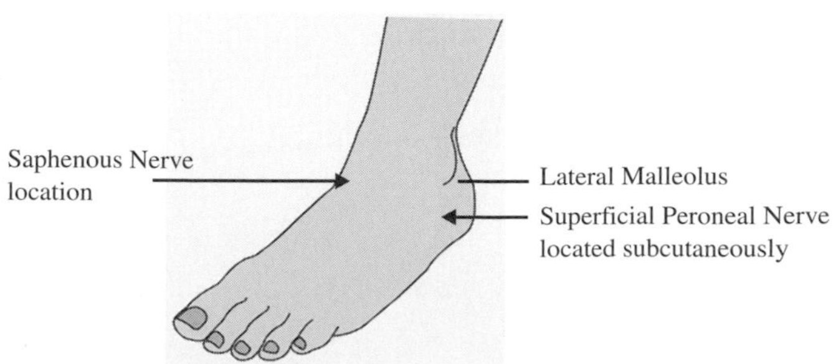

Figure 68-18 Superficial peroneal and saphenous nerve block. (Adapted with permission from MediClip, Williams & Wilkins.)

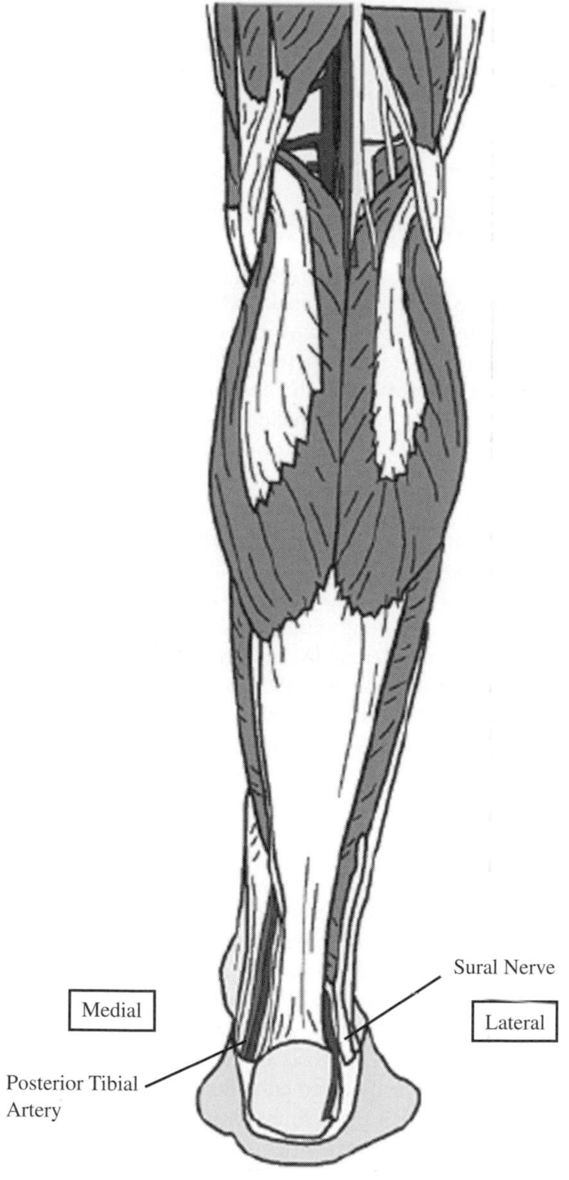

Figure 68-19 Sural nerve block. (Adapted with permission from MediClip, Williams & Wilkins.)

Superficial Peroneal and Saphenous Nerve Block (Fig. 68-18)

Anatomy After branching from the common peroneal, this nerve travels adjacent to the extensor digitorum longus muscle before dividing into terminal branches just above the ankle. It supplies sensation to the dorsum of the foot and first through fifth toes.

Indications Usually combined with other nerve blocks around the ankle for surgical anesthesia. Therapeutic interventions on foot or toes.

Complications None.

Sural Nerve Block (Fig. 68-19)

Anatomy The sural nerve branches from the posterior tibial nerve entering the foot between the lateral malleolus and the Achilles' tendon. It provides sensation to posterior lateral aspect of the lower calf, lateral side of the foot and small toe.

Indications Operative and therapeutic interventions on the foot and toes.

Complications None.

REFERENCES

1. Kumar K, Nath R, Wyant GM. Treatment of chronic pain by epidural spinal cord stimulation: a 10-year experience. *J Neurosurg* 1991;75: 402–407.
2. TerfayeS, Watt J, Benbow SJ, et al. Electrical spinal-cord stimulation for painful diabetic neuropathy. *Lancet* 1996;348:1696–1701.
3. Loeser JD. Desirable characteristics for pain treatment facilities. In: Bond MR, Charlton JE, Woolf CJ, eds. *Pain Research and Clinical Management.* Vol 4. Amsterdam, The Netherlands: Elsevier, 1991: 411–415.
4. Lilley JP, Su D, Wang JK. Sensory and sympathetic nerve blocks for postherpetic neuralgia. *Reg Anesth* 1986;11:165–167.
5. Boas RA, Cousins MJ. Diagnostic neural blockade. In: Cousins MJ, Brindenbaugh PO, (eds.). *Neural Blockade in Clinical Anesthesia and Management of* Pain. 2nd ed. Philadelphia, Pa: JB Lippincott, 1988: 885–898.
6. Butterworth JF, Strichartz GR. Molecular mechanisms of local anesthesia: a review. *Anesthesiology* 1990;72:711–734.
7. Bogduk N. International spinal injection society guidelines for the performance of spinal injection procedures. Part 1: Zygapophyseal joint blocks. *Clin J Pain* 1997;13:285–302.
8. Peck C, Coleman G. Implications of placebo theory for clinical research and practice in pain management. *Theor Med* 1991;12:247–270.
9. El-Khoury GY, Ehara S, Weinstein JN, et al. Epidural steroid injection: A procedure ideally performed with fluoroscopic control. *Radiology* 1988;168:554–557.
10. Fillingim RB, Maixner W. Gender differences in the response to noxious stimuli. *Pain Forum* 1995;4:209–221.
11. Turk DC, Flor H, Rudy TE. Pain and families. Etiology, maintenance, and psychological impact. *Pain* 1987;30:3–27.
12. Mazin E. Doppler-assisted nerve block [letter]. *Reg Anesth* 1997; 22:105.
13. Miller MD, Ferris DG. Measurement of subjective phenomena in primary care research: the Visual Analog Scale. *Fam Pract Res J* 1993; 13:15–24.
14. Buckley PF. Regional anesthesia with local anesthetics. In: Loeser JD, Butler SH, Chapman RC, et al. *Bonica's Management of Pain.* 3rd ed. Philadelphia, Pa: Lippincott Williams & Wilkins, 2001: 1893–1952.
15. Lehmann LJ, Pallares V. Subdural injection of a local anesthetic with steroids: A complication of epidural anesthesia. *South Med J* 1995;88: 467–469
16. Cory PC, et al. Post-operative respiratory failure following intercostal block. *Anesthesiology* 1981;54:418.
17. Selander D, Dhuner KG, Lundborg G. Peripheral nerve injury due to injection needles used for regional anesthesia. *Acta Anaesthesiol Scand* 1977;21:182–188.
18. Aldrete JA, Zapata JC, Ghaly R. Arachnoiditis following epidural adhesiolysis with hypertonic saline. Report of two cases. *Pain Dig* 1996; 6:638.
19. Bogduk N, et al. The cervical zygopophysial joints as a source of neck pain. *Spine* 1988;3:610–617.
20. Guyer RD, Collier R, Stith WJ, et al. Discitis after discography. *Spine* 1988;13:1352–1354.
21. Yeun EC, Layzer RB, Weitz SR, et al. Neurologic complications of lumbar epidural anesthesia and analgesia. *Neurology* 1995;45:1795–1801.
22. Renfrew DL, Moore TE, Kathol MH, et al. Correct placement of epidural steroid injections: fluoroscopic guidance and contrast administration. *Am J Neuroradiol* 1991;12:1003–1007.

CHAPTER 69 SYMPATHETIC BLOCKS

Samuel C. Sayson, Somayaji Ramamurthy

SYMPATHETIC BLOCKS

Introduction

Sympathetic blocks are widely employed for both diagnostic and therapeutic purposes. Kappis originally used paravertebral sympathetic blocks[1] as treatment for severe pain and visceral pain syndromes. Mandl[2] first introduced percutaneous interruption of the sympathetic chain in the early 20th century, and for many years thereafter it was a mainstay therapy for vascular insufficiency of the lower extremities. Current indications for sympathetic blocks include diagnosis of sympathetically maintained pain, treatment of neuropathic pain states such as acute herpes zoster, post-herpetic neuralgia, or other sympathetically maintained pain syndrome (reflex sympathetic dystrophy or causalgia, also known as complex regional pain syndrome), and management of ischemic pain. Sympathetic blocks are also used to help differentiate somatic from sympathetic pain origins. Pain syndromes responsive to initial sympathetic blocks are then treated with repeated blocks or followed up with surgical, chemical, or radiofrequency sympathectomy.

A good working knowledge of the sympathetic nervous system helps to understand how various neuraxial, plexus, and regional blocks can achieve sympathectomy. Descending autonomic projections from the hypothalamus, the oculomotor (Edinger-Westphal) complex, the locus ceruleus, and the nucleus of the solitary fasciculus terminate in the ipsilateral intermediolateral cell column in thoracic and upper lumbar spinal cord segments. Within this cell column lie the cell bodies of the preganglionic sympathetic neurons. Axons from these preganglionic cells exit the spinal cord by the anterior spinal roots and white rami communicantes to the sympathetic chain ganglia located along the left and right anterolateral margins of the spinal column. Upon reaching these paravertebral ganglia, the preganglionic sympathetic axons may synapse, pass cephalad or caudad for variable distances within the sympathetic chain before synapsing, or continue uninterrupted to a more distant ganglion or plexus, such as the celiac or hypogastic plexus. The nerves that bypass paravertebral sympathetic chain ganglia to more distant ganglia are called *splanchnic nerves*. Splanchnic nerves are the primary sympathetic fibers that innervate visceral organs. The ganglia in which they synapse are typically located near the respective organs that they innervate. Postganglionic sympathetic fibers then course along peripheral nerves or blood vessels to converge on specific organs. Once it is understood that the preganglionic sympathetics have spinal origins, and that the spread of sympathetic nerves occurs along blood vessels and peripheral nerves, it becomes easier to understand how sympathectomies can be performed not only through blockade of specific chain ganglia, but through a various number of neuraxial and regional block techniques.

Knowing the position of the sympathetic chain relative to somatic nerves helps to predict some of the side effects associated with the various sympathetic blocks. The sympathetic chain ganglia extends from the second cervical vertebra to the coccyx. In the cervical and thoracic region, these ganglia lie anterior to the base of the transverse processes or the head of the ribs; therefore they lie in close proximity to the somatic nerves. However, as the sympathetic chain courses caudally toward the lumbar region, it becomes more anterolateral to the vertebral bodies and becomes separated from somatic nerves by the psoas muscle. As a result, sympathetic blocks performed in the lumbar region become less prone to inadvertent somatic nerve blocks.

Another point to recognize is that visceromotor and nociceptive pathways course along with sympathetic fibers. The sympathetic chain receives afferent visceral fibers that conduct pain from the head, neck, abdominal and pelvic viscera, and extremities. The celiac and superior hypogastric plexi have parasympathetic and visceral nociceptive afferents; lumbar and cervicothoracic (including the stellate) ganglia have visceral nociceptive afferents as well. Therefore, sympathetic blocks are not purely sympathetic.

Patient Preparation

The patient should not be overly sedated during the procedure because verbal contact with the patient is extremely valuable. During diagnostic blocks, sedation may confound results because the sedative can affect the complex brain pathways involved with sympathetically maintained pain. Monitoring and intravenous access should be employed on the basis of the type of block performed as well as the health and mental condition of the patient. For sympathetic blocks involving the limbs, skin temperature probes are placed bilaterally on the extremities undergoing sympathetic block. The block is considered adequate if cutaneous temperature of the treated limb approaches core temperature.[3] A careful evaluation of placebo effects, systemic uptake of drug, and blockade of somatic nerves must be performed in patients who have obtained relief following a sympathetic block. As with any invasive procedure, resuscitation equipment and drugs should be readily available. Major contraindications to sympathetic blocks include coagulopathy and patient refusal.

STELLATE GANGLION BLOCKS

Anatomy

The cervical chain is composed of a superior, middle, and inferior cervical ganglion; the inferior ganglion is fused with the first thoracic ganglion, resulting in a "starlike" (stellate) appearance. It receives preganglionic sympathetic fibers via white rami communicantes from the intermediolateral cell column of T1 to T6 in the spinal cord. It is an oval-shaped structure approximately 2-cm long, 1-cm wide, and about 0.5-cm thick. The ganglion lies anterior to the first rib, extends along the C7 to T1 interspace, and may lie over the anterior tubercle of C7. It is bound inferiorly by the dome of the pleura, medially by the longus colli muscle, and laterally by the scalene muscles. It is also bound anteriorly in part by the subclavian artery and the vertebral artery, and posteriorly by the transverse processes of C7 and T1. The prevertebral fascia, which originates posterior to the sympathetic chain in the cervical region, is pierced by the chain around C7 and becomes anterior to the stellate ganglion as the fascia forms a transition from the neck to the chest. Superior to the stellate ganglion is the transverse process of the sixth cervical vertebrae, or Chassaignac's tubercle, a prominence that is easily palpable along the paratracheal region of the neck.

One must remember that while Chassaignac's tubercle is the major landmark for performing the anterior paratracheal block of the stellate ganglion, the location of the ganglion itself is inferior to the tubercle. Undoubtedly, it is the presence of Chassaignac's tubercle that has made the anterior paratracheal approach to this ganglion a popular one (compared to the lateral and posterior approaches) among pain specialists. It serves as bony protection for the vertebral artery, thus protecting the artery from unintended injection of local anesthetic and resultant seizure. It is also easily palpable, especially in the sitting position, and with adequate deep palpation, the tubercle becomes almost subcutaneous and minimizes the distance from the skin to the tubercle through which the needle must pass. Interestingly enough, ultrasonography and magnetic resonance imaging (MRI) studies suggest that local anesthetic spread to the ganglion does not occur; rather, the spread occurs anterior to the ganglion.[4,5] Other radiographic and injection studies have supported this finding as well.[6–9] This anterior spread likely relates to prevertebral fascia being in the same plane as Chassaignac's tubercle at the C6 vertebra but then becomes more anterior at the stellate ganglion, thus preventing the spread of injectate onto the ganglion. The presence of this fascia also promotes mediastinal and even contralateral spread of injectate.[5] Therefore, sympathetic neural blockade during stellate ganglion block may take place at sites other than the stellate ganglion.

Indications

The stellate ganglion block is one of the most commonly used procedures in pain management of the face and upper extremity. Painful syndromes that may benefit from stellate ganglion blocks include sympathetically maintained complex regional pain syndrome (formerly RSD or causalgia), phantom limb pain or amputation stump pain, herpes zoster and postherpetic neuralgia, frostbite, or tumor invasion of neurovascular or boney structures. Other indications include circulatory insufficiency of the arm in which thromboembolic or vasospastic events have occurred (Table 69-1).

Technique

The anterior paratracheal approach is described. It is the easiest to perform (compared to the posterior technique[10]) and involves a minimal amount of risk when performed correctly. It is also the least painful for the patient. The patient is placed in the supine position with the mouth slightly opened to relax the anterior muscles of the neck. The operator stands on the side of the neck to be blocked, palpates the cricoid cartilage, then slides his or her index and middle fingers laterally to palpate deep into the groove in the neck created by the trachea and the sternocleidomastoid muscle and major vessels of the neck. With deep, gentle palpation and

TABLE 69-1 **Indications for Stellate Ganglion Block**

Pain Syndromes of the Face and Arm
Complex Regional Pain Syndrome (RSD/Causalgia)
Phantom Limb Pain or Amputation Stump Pain
Herpes Zoster/Postherpetic Neuralgia
Frostbite
Neoplasm
Paget's Disease
CNS Lesions
Circulator Insufficiency of the Arm
Traumatic/Embolic Occlusion
Post Reimplantation
Post Embolectomy Vasospasm
Inadvertent Local Injection of α-Adrenergic Agents
Raynaud's Disease or Phenomenon
Scleroderma
Vasculitis
Miscellaneous
Hyperhidrosis
Meniere's Disease

CNS denotes central nervous system.

slight lateral retraction, the sternocleidomastoid muscle and major vessels are drawn to the side; the tubercle of the sixth cervical transverse process (Chassaignac's tubercle) can then be easily felt (Fig. 69-1). In patients with short or muscular necks, it becomes more difficult to palpate the tubercle. Placing a slight lift under the patient's back or sitting the patient up and supporting the back of the neck with the operator's other hand may help to locate the tubercle. The tubercle is then straddled by the index and middle finger.

A 2.5-cm, 22-gauge, short-beveled needle attached to an intravenous pediatric T-piece or other suitable extension tubing is connected to a syringe containing the local anesthetic injectate. The use of extension tubing allows for better control of the needle during placement, aspiration, and injection. The operator uses his or her nondominant hand to straddle Chassaignac's tubercle and manipulates the needle with the dominant hand (Fig. 69-2). The needle is advanced though the skin until the tubercle is contacted. Often the distance advanced is not more than 1.5 to 2.0 cm. An assistant aspirates for blood, then injects 1.0 mL of local anesthetic; the patient is then evaluated for inadvertent arterial or intraneural injection. Arterial injection is suggested by seizure activity immediately following injection, while intraneural injection is suspected if radiating dysethesia occurs on injection. If these observations are negative, 10 to 20 mL of local anesthetic are incrementally injected. If sympathetic block of the arm is desired, moving the patient to a sitting position as soon as the block is placed may facilitate caudal spread of the agent.

Other means to assist in appropriate needle placement include ultrasound,[4] fluoroscopy or CT guidance (Fig. 69-3). If a sympathectomy is not achieved when the stellate ganglion block is performed at Chassaignac's tubercle, a repeat block at the C7 or T1 transverse process should be considered in an attempt to inject local anesthetic on the same side of the prevertebral fascia as the ganglion. Note that a block at this level increases the risk of bra-

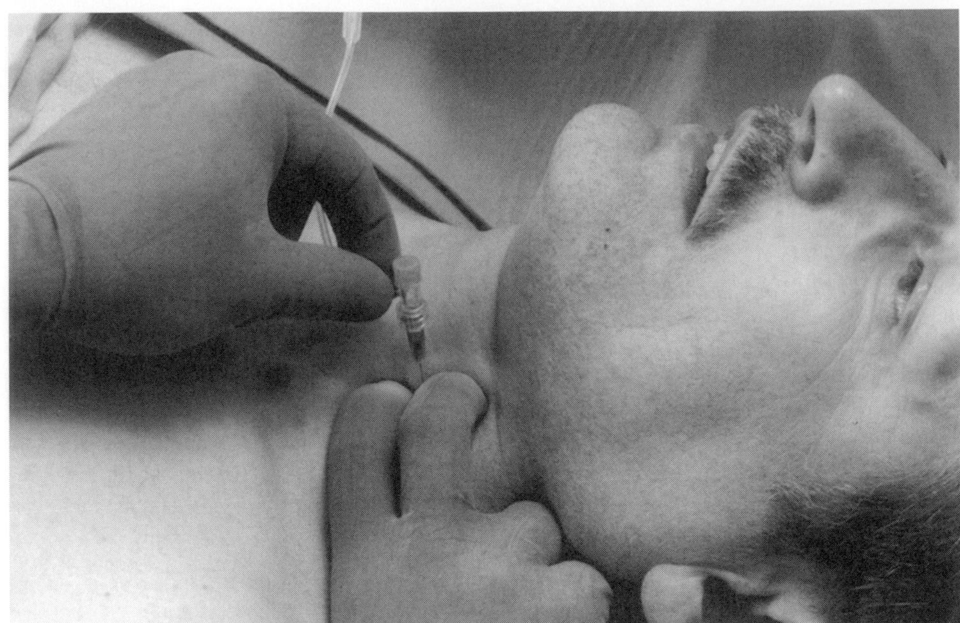

Figure 69-1 Stellate ganglion block at the level of the cricothyroid cartilage. Note that the mouth is slightly opened to relax neck musculature. Use of extension tubing with or without an assistant allows better control of the block needle during aspiration or injection.

chial plexus block; since the C7 tubercle is rather vestigial, the injectate is closer to the same plane as the brachial plexus. Occasionally, the C7 tubercle can be palpated and the needle is entered directly over this tubercle; otherwise, the needle is entered one finger breadth (1.5 to 2.0 cm) below the C6 tubercle. The risk of pneumothorax is also increased because the injection site is near the pleural dome. Larger volumes (20 mL) can improve the likelihood of a complete sympathectomy of the arm and hand (C5-T1 dermatormes)[7] but is associated with a significant incidence of hoarseness (80%), dysphagia (60%), and brachial plexus block (10%) due to spread of local anesthetic onto adjacent laryngeal nerves and cervical nerve roots.

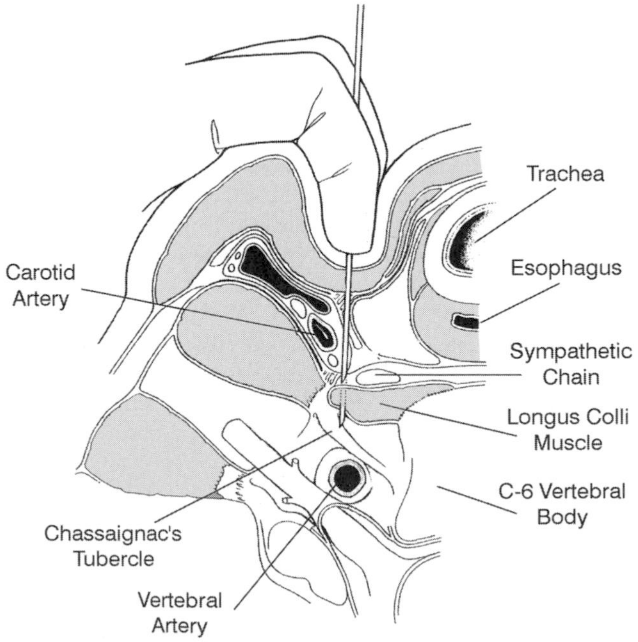

Trachea
Carotid Artery
Esophagus
Sympathetic Chain
Longus Colli Muscle
C-6 Vertebral Body
Chassaignac's Tubercle
Vertebral Artery

Figure 69-2 Stellate ganglion block: transverse section of the neck at the level of the C6 vertebrae. Note how the sternocleidomastoid and scalene muscles have been displaced laterally by the nondominant hand.

Some means to evaluate the presence of sympathectomy must be performed. While a Horner's sign (ipsilateral ptosis, miosis, anhydrosis, and conjunctival engorgement) is indicative of a sympathectomy of the head and face, it in no way suggests a sympathectomy of the arm and hand. Skin surface temperature probes placed bilaterally at the palmar thenar regions are simple yet effective. A 1.0° to1.5° C increase in the blocked side or, perhaps more specifically, an increase in temperature toward core temperature that exceeds that of the contralateral side[11,12] is strongly suggestive of a successful sympathetic block of the arm. Somatic block of the arm must also be ruled out.

Complications

Minor complications are common. Because the proximity of laryngeal nerves to the stellate ganglion, dysphagia and hoarseness are common with the anterior paratracheal approach. Following stellate ganglion block, incidental recurrent laryngeal nerve block or superior laryngeal nerve block is identified by the patient's inability to say "ee" or swallow a small amount of water or other clear liquid. The incidence of brachial plexus block is as high as 10%,[7,13] so the presence of motor or sensory block should be assessed before discharging the patient from the clinic facility.

Even without the use of imaging techniques, serious complications to stellate ganglion block are rare. Transient central nervous system (CNS) events such as seizures, aphasia, blindness, loss of consciousness, and hemiparesis can occur following injected doses as low as 15 mg of lidocaine or 2.5 mg of bupivacaine.[14–17] Because of these risks some physicians advocate placement of intravenous lines in all patients undergoing stellate ganglion blocks. Nonetheless, appropriate noninvasive monitoring and resuscitation equipment should be readily available and used as the clinical scenario dictates.

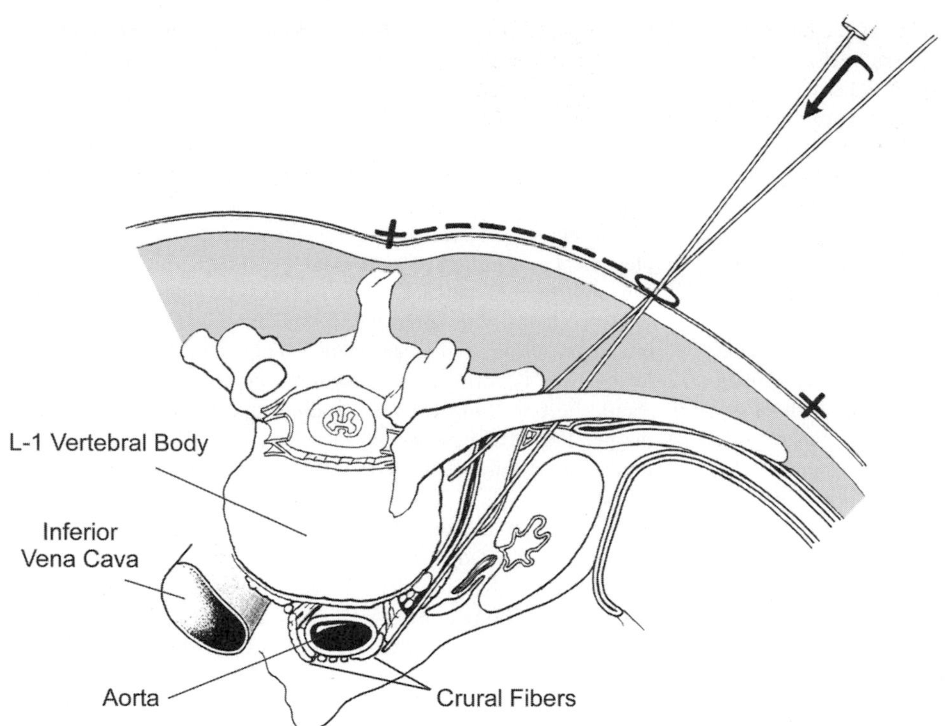

Figure 69-3 Computerized tomograph at the level of the T1 vertebrae. Injectate spread is shown to encompass the stellate ganglion.

CELIAC PLEXUS AND SPLANCHNIC NERVE BLOCKS

Anatomy

The celiac plexus is a dense matrix of diffuse nerve fibers and ganglia located around the abdominal aorta and periaortic space at the level of the T12 and L1 vertebrae. The most distinct feature of the celiac plexus are the paired semilunar ("celiac") ganglia that lie immediately superior to the pancreas in the midline and are flanked in close approximation by the adrenals. These "paired" ganglia can actually vary in number and size.[18] The aorta is surrounded by the plexus, which makes this large vascular structure an important landmark in performing the block. In fact, transgression of the aorta has been used in identifying needle placement.[19] In addition to the celiac ganglia, the components of the celiac plexus include the greater, lesser, and least (also called lowest) splanchnic nerves; there are also contributions from the aorticorenal ganglia and aortic and superior hypogastic plexus. It is important to realize that the celiac plexus is not a distinct entity but a diffuse network that varies in size, network, and position. The most consistent landmark is the celiac artery because these elements intertwine around the base of this artery.

There are sympathetic, parasympathetic, and visceral afferent contributions to the celiac plexus. The sympathetic fibers originate from the thoracic sympathetic chain via the greater and lesser splanchnic nerves, and the visceral afferents have cell bodies that originate from the dorsal root ganglion of the spinal cord and travel with the sympathetic nerves. The parasympathetics originate from the vagus nerve and sacral nerve roots. The nerves of the celiac plexus innervate most of the abdominal viscera to include the pancreas, liver, kidneys, biliary tract, spleen, adrenals, intestines, and omentum.

Indications

The celiac plexus block is indicated for patients in pain from upper abdominal tumors such as pancreatic cancer. Pain relief rates vary from 70% to 100%, with an average of 85% of patients that experience at least temporary pain relief.[20,21] Pain from these tumors can be severe, and opioid therapy is often limited by the sedation and constipation that accompany the high doses required to manage the patient's discomfort. Neurolytic celiac plexus blocks in these patients can provide superior pain relief for up to 3 to 4 months. In most patients relief will be immediate and effective. Furthermore, they can lessen the severity of opioid-induced side effects by decreasing requirements of these drugs. Gastointestinal motility is also improved by the sympathectomy caused by the block. The predictive value of a neurolytic celiac plexus block can be determined by the degree of tumor invasion. Akhan et al[22] found that the grade of tumor as measured by invasion of periaortic and paracaval fat planes was a good predictor for successful neurolytic celiac plexus block. Greater than 50% invasion of the fat planes correlated with little pain relief. Age, history of laparotomy, chemotherapy, or radiation therapy have not been shown to decrease the efficacy of neurolytic celiac plexus blocks.

Benign conditions such as acute and chronic pancreatitis may also respond to celiac plexus blocks. As with pancreatic cancer patients, acute pancreatitis is often resistant to opioid therapy; furthermore, the disease process may be improved by decreasing the ductal and sphincter spasm thought to be associated with acute pancreatitis. Addition of steroids to the local anesthetic injectate has been shown to decrease the severity of the attack.[23] Continuous catheter techniques can be effective in chronic alcoholic patients diagnosed with acute pancreatitis who were previously unresponsive to epidural analgesia. Rykowski et al[24] used 0.5% bupivacaine, 20 mL every 6 to12 hours as intermittent injection, or 0.5% bupivacaine at 6 mL per hour with good results. Using celiac plexus blocks, especially neurolytic celiac plexus blocks in chronic pancreatitis, is controversial. While 4 to 6 months of relief can be obtained from neurolytic celiac plexus blocks, a subset of alcoholic patients may view their pain-free state as an opportunity to resume their consumption of alcoholic beverages. Furthermore, because this block also interrupts the visceral afferents from abdominal organs, it may mask pain related to intraabdominal emergencies. Benefits to performing celiac plexus blocks in chronic pancreatitis patients include pain control that is superior to narcotics and an improved appetite. Often these patients are malnourished, and analgesia using celiac plexus blocks can improve their nutritional state by allowing them to eat meals without pain. The addition of steroids to the injectate has been shown to improve analgesia without the use of neurolytic agents[25] in the patient with chronic pancreatitis. Regardless of controversy, celiac plexus blocks have shown to be an effective adjunct in managing chronic pancreatitis pain.[26] Indications for celiac plexus blocks are summarized in Table 69-2.

Technique

There are a variety of techniques for approaching the splanchnic nerves or celiac plexus. In general, they can be summarized as posterior or anterior approaches. The posterolateral approach has become the most practiced and proven technique by anesthesiologists, whereas the anterior techniques using computed tomography (CT) or ultrasound guidance are preferred by invasive radiologists. In all cases, noninvasive monitoring should be used and an intravenous line should be established. Intravenous vasoactive agents, volume expanders (crystalloid or colloids), and sedative and analgesics should be made available for use as needed.

Posterolateral Approaches Posterolateral techniques allow access to both the splanchnic nerves and the celiac plexus. The posterolateral approach is one originally defined by Kappis and refined by Moore.[27] Frequently used variations of the posterolateral approach include the transcrural approach, the transaortic approach, and the retrocrural or deep splanchnic approach.

The patient is placed in a prone position with a pillow placed at the midsection of the abdomen. This minimizes the lumbar lordosis and aids in patient comfort. Occasionally, the abdominal pain can be so severe that the prone position is not tolerated, and analgesics must be used or the patient must be positioned in the lateral decubitus position. The arms are underneath behind the head or allowed to hang off the table. An intravenous line is placed to provide light sedation if necessary, and a 200 to 500 mL crystalloid bolus is administered to offset the sympathectomy-induced hypotension caused by the block. Anatomic landmarks are identified and marked in ink. Agents typically used for the celiac plexus block include 0.25% to 0.5% bupivacaine (with or without 80-mg methylprednisolone or equivalent), 6% to 10% phenol, or 50% to 100% alcohol. Volumes are described for each technique (see following sections).

TABLE 69-2 **Indications for Celiac Plexus Block**

Pancreatic Cancer
Acute and Chronic Pancreatitis
Intraabdominal Metastatic Disease
Diagnostic Test to Differentiate Between Visceral and Abdominal Wall Pain
Adjunct to Surgery*

*Data from Hamid SK, Scott NB, Sutcliffe NP, et al. Continuous coeliac plexus blockage plus intermittent wound infiltration with bupivacaine following upper abdominal surgery: a double-blind randomised study. Acta Anaesthesiology Scand 1992; 36:534.

The classic posterior approach is a two-needle technique; needle placement is similar for both sides. Landmarks include the 12th ribs and the T12 and L1 spinous processes; fluoroscopic or CT guidance helps with landmark identification and minimizes complications during needle placement and injection. A shallow isosceles triangle is formed by these three points. The lateral points should lie 6 to 9 cm from the midline and usually correspond to the junction of the paraspinal muscles and the 12h rib. After administering local anesthetic to create a skin wheal at this point, a 12- to 15-cm, 20- to 22-gauge subarachnoid needle is inserted percutaneously and angled at 45 degrees to the coronal plane and about 15 degrees cephalad. The needle is advanced until contact with the lateral body of L1 is made. This typically occurs at the depth of 8 to 10 cm; if bony contact is made at a more shallow depth than this, it is likely that the transverse process has been encountered. The needle is then withdrawn (almost subcutaneously) and the needle tip is redirected laterally an additional 10 degrees and readvanced; this next attempt should contact bone about 2 to 3 cm deeper than the previous attempt. This maneuver is repeated until the needle is "walked off" the lumbar body (Fig. 69-4). The final placement of the needle tip is 1.0 to 1.5 cm anterior to the vertebral margin. If the first needle was placed on left side, correct needle placement is confirmed by observing the needle pulsate on visual inspection and tactile analysis. Needle pulsation occurs because the final position of the needle tip is often close to the aorta. The second needle is placed on the right side using the same technique as the first; depth is guided by the final needle depth used on the left side. Fluoroscopy can be used to confirm tip placement; spread of contrast agent seen on fluoroscopy will indicate retrocrural, transcrural, transaortic, or intradiaphragmatic injection of agent (Figs. 69-5 and 69-6). If CT imaging is used, needle paths are traced from the skin to the celiac plexus to avoid injury to renal or vascular structures.

For the transcrural approach, advancing the needle tips an additional 1 to 2 cm will pierce the diaphragmatic crus and place the needle tip anterior to the diaphragm. A loss of resistance is usually felt as the crus is pierced. The anteroposterior (AP) and lateral radiographs with contrast will show a linear spread in the left lateral preaortic area. If contrast spread is predominately cephalad and appears to collect around the L1 vertebral body, the needle tip is likely to be retrocrural. Lateral radiographs can confirm that the contrast is posterior and superior to the diaphragm, also suggesting retrocrural spread. The procedure can then be performed as a deep splanchnic nerve block (see later section), or the needle is advanced to pierce the diaphragmatic crus (thus transcrural). If muscle striations are seen following contrast injection, the needle tip is likely contained within diaphragmatic muscle, and should be advanced about 1 cm. On lateral fluoroscopy, contrast agent is typically seen to spread in a cranio-caudal direction anterior to the vertebral body, but agent spread is limited to below the diaphragm (see Fig. 69-5B, contrast patttern, and Fig. 69-6B). Following negative aspiration of each needle, 15 to 25 mL of local anesthetic or neurolytic agent is injected through each needle in divided doses.

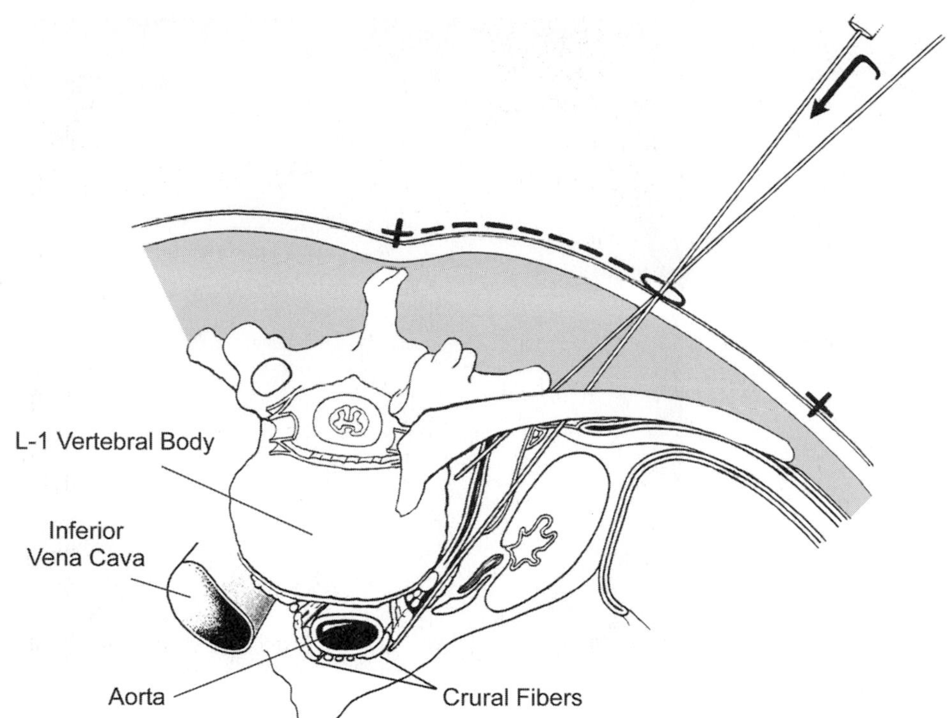

Figure 69-4 Celiac plexus block: transverse section at the level of the L1 vertebral body. The needle is "walked off" the lumbar body. Note the relationship of the needle path to the aorta and kidney.

The transaortic approach is a single needle, left-sided technique that is also transcrural.[19] The intent of this approach is to pierce the aorta with the needle to ensure that the needle tip is anterior to the aorta. Placement of the injectate anterior to the aorta can minimize the risk of neurologic complications caused by unintended spread of neurolytic agents to the lumbar plexus. Needle placement is the same as for the transcrural approach, but the needle is advanced until aortic wall penetration occurs and free-flowing blood is aspirated. The needle is then advanced further through the anterior wall of the aorta until no blood is aspirated.

A 5-mL loss of resistance syringe filled with saline can be used to identify anterior aortic wall penetration. Once blood is aspirated through the block needle, the loss of resistance syringe is attached to the needle and constant pressure is applied to the syringe plunger. A resistance to injection will be felt once the anterior aortic wall has been contacted, followed by loss of resistance once the needle tip has entered the anterior periaortic space. Following negative aspiration, contrast agent is injected and will appear anterior to the vertebral bodies (see Fig. 69-5C and Fig. 69-6A). Local anesthetic, steroid, or neurolytic agent is then injected. A smaller total volume of agent (20 to 25 mL) is used for this technique.

Anterior Approach With the anterior approach, a 12- to 15-cm, 22-gauge needle is passed through the midline epigastrium until the body of L1 is contacted. The needle is then withdrawn 1.0 to 1.5 cm and placement is confirmed using fluoroscopy, ultrasound, or CT imaging.[28,29] Patient comfort is a major advantage to this approach, especially when the patient is unable to lie prone. Only one needle is used with this technique, so there is less pain from posterior two-needle approaches. Furthermore, the risk of needle-related injury to motor nerves is significantly reduced compared to posterior approaches.

Splanchnic Nerve Blocks An alternative technique to achieve abdominal sympathectomy and visceral nerve block is the splanchnic nerve block. The splanchnic nerve block specifically interrupts the sympathetic imput to the celiac plexus without blocking the abdominal parasympathetics. The final position of the needle tip is superior to the diaphragm; the intention is to block the greater, lesser, and least splanchnic nerves before they traverse the diaphragm into the abdomen. The advantages of performing sympathectomy and visceral nerve block are multifold. Gastrointestinal

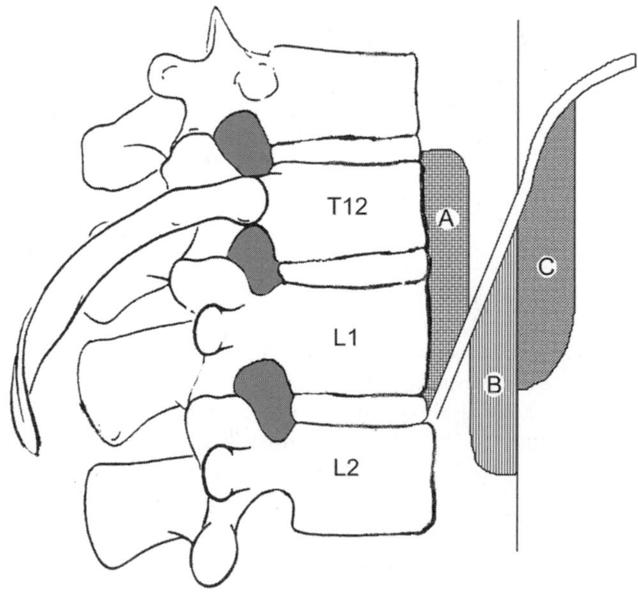

Figure 69-5 Schematic lateral view of contrast patterns for different celiac plexus block approaches. (**A**) Retrocrural or deep splanchnic block; (**B**) Transcrural block; (**C**) Transaortic block.

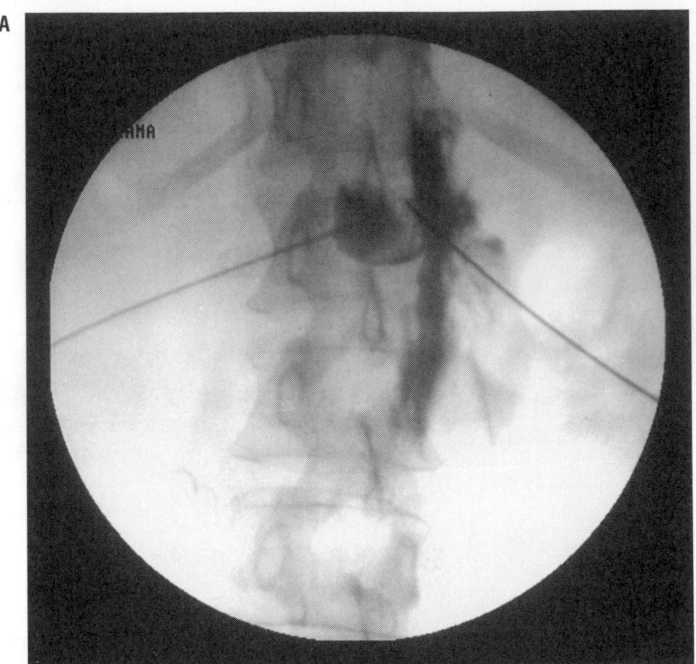

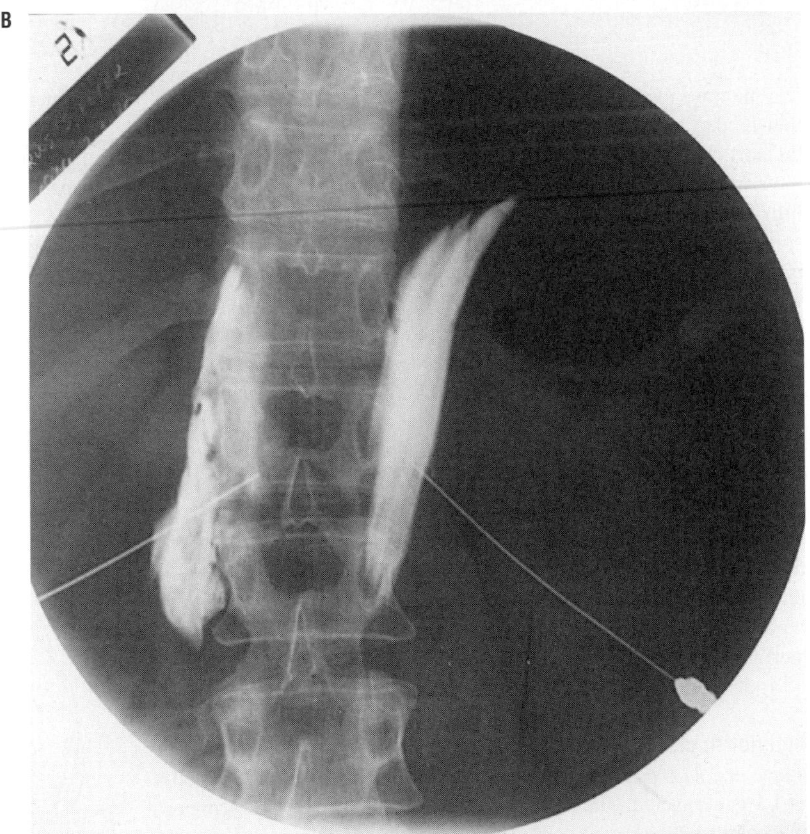

Figure 69-6 Celiac plexus block: fluoroscopic AP view of contrast patterns. (**A**) Contrast in center of radiograph is typical of transaortic injection; contrast along the left border of vertebral bodies demonstrates retrocrural spread. (**B**) Contrast on left is suggestive of transcural spread. Contrast on right demonstrates intradiaphragmatic injection. Note the striations and the smooth "feathery" appearance to the pattern.

motility is improved compared with the celiac plexus block because the parasympathetics (which join the splanchnics at the level of the celiac ganglia) are left unopposed. Also, because the lumbar sympathetics are not blocked by this technique, hypotension is decreased. Lastly, with the classic splanchnic nerve block, a smaller volume of local anesthetic or neurolytic agent can be used (3 to 4 mL per side).

For the deep splanchnic approach[30,31] (also known as the retrocrural celiac plexus block), landmarks and needle approach are similar to the transcrural celiac plexus block. The needle is walked off the vertebral body and advanced until the needle pulsates (due to the proximity of the needle tip to the aorta) on visual inspection and tactile analysis. When the block is performed correctly, 3- to 5-mL injection of contrast will remain within the retrocrural space and migrate primarily cephalad (see Fig. 69-5A). On fluoroscopic AP view, the contrast will be confined along the lateral border to the L1 vertebral body (see Fig. 69-6A). On lateral view, layering of the contrast in a narrow line along the anterior vertebral column should be seen. The procedure is then repeated on the right side. Fifteen milliliters of local anesthetic or neurolytic agent are injected through each needle. Parasympathetics and the lumbar sympathetic chain are not blocked with this technique.

The classic splanchnic nerve block is performed in a manner similar to the deep splanchnic approach, but the needle is directed toward the anterolateral margin of T12 vertebral body. A paramedian approach is used, inserting two 7- to 10-cm needles 3 to 4 cm lateral to the midline just below the 12th ribs, then directing the needle tips toward the T12 body. Radiographic contrast patterns are similar to the deep splanchnic nerve block. The disadvantages of this block relate to final position of the needle tips; compared with the transcrural and transaortic blocks, the needle tips lie posterior and cephalad to the diaphragm, which increases the risk of chylothorax and pneumothorax.

Complications

The incidence of major complications with neurolytic celiac plexus blocks is 0.15 to 1.0%.[32,33] These complications typically occur from transgression of structures during needle placement or unintentional spread of neurolytic or local anesthetic solutions. Inadvertent injury to structures can result in pneumothorax, chylothorax (secondary to thoracic duct injury), genitourinary injury, somatic nerve injury, and retroperitoneal hematoma; complications secondary to inadvertent spread of agent include sexual dysfunction, groin neuralgia, paraplegia, retroperitoneal fibrosis following repeated neurolytic blocks,[34] and pleural effusion.[35] Complications are often self-limited. In a study of 136 cases following celiac plexus block, Brown et al describes two cases of pneumothorax, neither requiring thoracostomy as therapy.[21] Renal perforation can occur, albeit typically without sequelae, especially if the block needles are placed more than 7.5 cm from midline. When inserted lateral to this point, renal impalement can occur in 10% of cases.[36] Paraplegia has been described secondary to injury to the artery of Adamkiewicz during block placement[37] and from arterial vasospasm causing anterior spinal artery syndrome.[38] Paraplegia can also occur from incorrect needle placement and subsequent injection in the subarachnoid or epidural space, or from intrapsoas muscle injection with blockade or neurolysis of the lumbar plexus. Radiographic imaging (biplanar fluoroscopy or CT) can minimize these risks.

Minor sequelae inherent to the celiac plexus block are relatively common. The most common side effects of the block include local pain (96%), hypotension (38%), and diarrhea (44%).[32] Systolic blood pressure decreases of 30 to 40 mm Hg are not uncommon and are usually seen when the patient assumes an upright or sitting position following celiac plexus block. The hypotension is caused by blood pooling in the splanchnic vessels following sympathectomy; this can be minimized by an intravenous fluid bolus at the time of block placement. Compensatory reflexes usually appear by 48 hours. Diarrhea is thought to be caused by unopposed parasympathetic activity: impairment of α-adrenergic stimulation to enterocytes that increase intestinal secretory activity as well as decrease absorptive processes may also play a role. Intractable diarrhea may respond to clonidine patches or to octreotide 0.1 mg subcutaneously twice a day.[39,40] The increase in gastrointestinal activity can be used in a therapeutic manner. Weinstabl et al used bupivacaine celiac plexus blocks to reduce the intestinal dysfunction (as measured by decreased gastric volumes) in several patients in a neurosurgical intensive care unit.[41] Nausea and vomiting can occur from the hypotension caused by the block, or from alcohol intoxication when excessive amounts of neurolytic alcohol are absorbed at the block site. Chest pain can also occur after celiac alcohol block. It usually resolves within an hour.[42]

SUPERIOR HYPOGASTRIC PLEXUS BLOCKS

Anatomy

The superior hypogastric plexus is a retroperitoneal structure located bilaterally between the level of the lower third of the fifth lumbar vertebral body and the upper third of the sacral promontory; it is inferior to the bifurcation of the abdominal aorta and in proximity to the bifurcation of the common iliac vessels. The superior hypogastric plexus along with the left and right inferior hypogastric plexus and the pelvic plexus comprise the hypogastric plexus; this network provides innervation to the pelvic viscera. The superior hypogastric plexus receives post-ganglionic sympathetic contributions from the inferior mesenteric ganglion and from the hypogastric nerves (lumbar splanchnics) that course along with the abdominal aorta.[43] Parasympathetic innervation arises from the second, third, and fourth sacral segments, and contribute to the plexus via the pelvic nerve. Finally, visceral afferents from the pelvic organs course through the hypogastric plexus and enter the spinal cord via the L1 or L2 spinal nerve roots or via the sacral segments S2, S3, or S4. Pelvic organs innervated by the hypogastric plexus include the rectum, bladder, perineum, prostate, and uterus. Pain associated with these ganglia will often cause patients to complain of pain in the lower abdominal wall around the pubic region.

Indications

Pelvic pain secondary to neoplasm can be successfully managed by superior hypogastric plexus blocks. Lee et al reported that surgical interruption of the hypogastric plexus (presacral neurectomy) can provide pain relief in various malignant and nonmalignant painful conditions.[44,45] Plancarte et al then devised a reliable means to percutaneously block nerves in this region.[46] They showed that in patients with advanced pelvic neoplasms (to include cervical, prostate, and testicular cancers) pain scores are reduced up to 90% using superior hypogastic plexus blocks and non-opioid analgesics. As with other block techniques, the superior hypogastric plexus block is performed using local anesthetic to determine efficacy, then repeated as needed using a neurolytic agent.

Superior hypogastric plexus blocks can provide pain relief in nonmalignant conditions refractory to conservative therapy. We have had considerable success using non-neurolytic superior hypogastric plexus blocks to control ilioinguinal, testicular, and scrotal pain following inguinal herniorhaphies and vasectomies. Other benign pain states that may respond to superior hypogastric plexus blocks include endometriosis, pelvic inflammatory disease, and proctalgia.

Technique

The patient is placed in the prone position with a pillow beneath the lower abdomen and hip to reduce the lumbosacral lordosis. This region is then prepared and draped in sterile fashion, and fluoroscopy is used to identify the L4-5 interspace. Skin wheals are then raised bilaterally 5 to 7 cm from the midline of the back at this level, and a 15- to 20-cm, 22-gauge subarachnoid needle is inserted through one of these skin wheals.

From a position perpendicular in all planes to the skin, the needle is oriented approximately 30 degrees caudad and 45 degrees mesiad so that the tip is directed toward the anterolateral aspect of the L5 vertebral body. The needle trajectory is in a significantly more caudal direction compared to the celiac plexus or lumbar sympathetic block (Fig. 69-7). Potential obstacles to successful needle placement include the iliac crest, the L5 transverse process, or the L5 vertebral body. Needle contact with the ilium is avoided by a more medial or superior entry site. If the L5 transverse process is encountered, redirect the needle in a more caudal direction. If the needle then contacts the L5-S1 facet, reenter the needle through a skin wheal that is 1 to 2 cm superior to the previous entry site. Once the L5 vertebral body is contacted, the needle is redirected in a less mesiad plane in an attempt to "walk off" the vertebral body. Advancing the tip 1 cm past the vertebral body may result in a loss or resistance or "pop," suggesting that the needle tip has traversed the anterior fascia of the psoas muscle (Fig. 69-8). The will typically occur at a depth of 8 to12 cm. A second block needle is inserted on the opposite side to the first, and the angles of entry and the depth of the first needle are then used as a guide. Needle tip place is confirmed by using 3 to 5 mL of water-soluble contrast dye and fluoroscopy. On lateral view, the dye is seen to spread in a smooth contour anterior to the L5 vertebral body and sacral promontory; on AP view, the contrast medium should be confined to midline. Eight to ten milliliters of 0.25% bupivacaine or 1% lidocaine is injected through each needle. Six to eight milliliters of aqueous 10% phenol should be injected through each needle if neurolysis is desired.

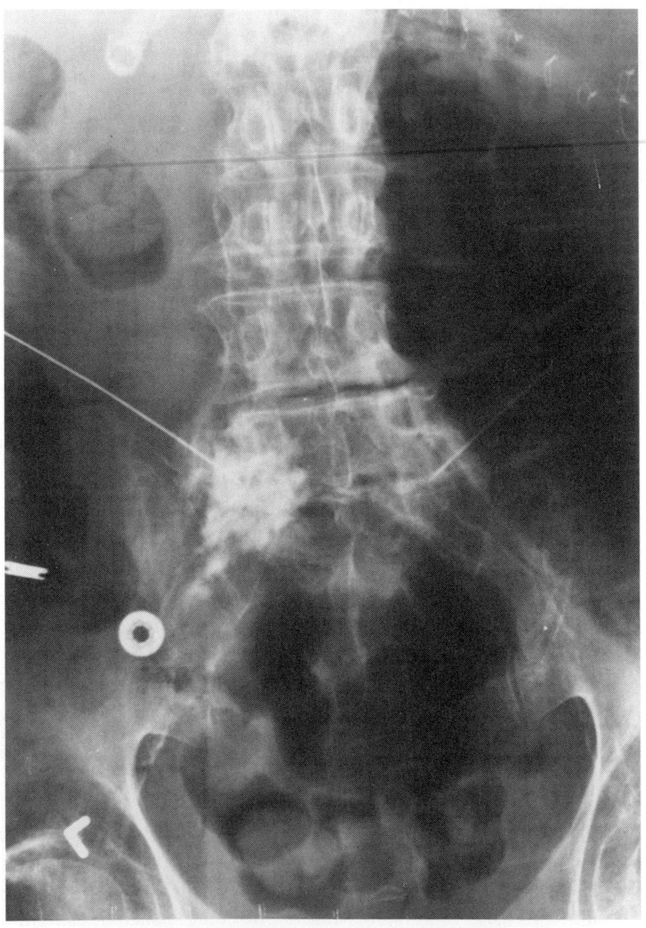

Figure 69-7 Superior hypogastric plexus block: AP radiograph illustrating proper needle placement and contrast spread.

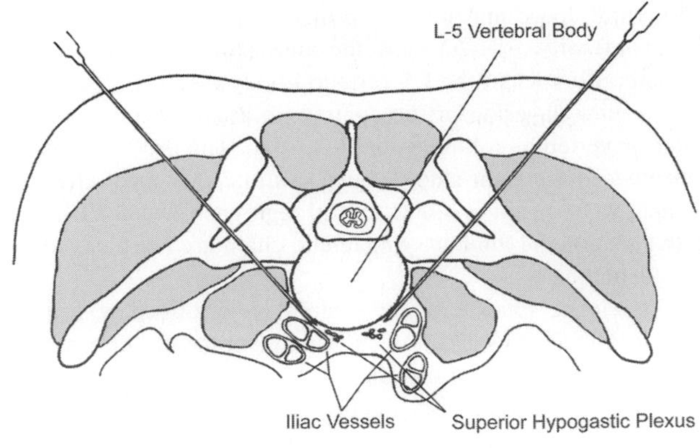

Figure 69-8 Superior hypogastric plexus block: transverse section illustrating proper needle placement and the needle position relative to the vertebral body, psoas muscle, and iliac vessels.

Variations to the above technique include a single-needle approach, a transdiscal approach, and a transarterial approach. A single-needle approach follows the same technique as thatdescribed earlier; however, only one needle is placed and a larger volume (20 to 30 mL) of local anesthetic is used. A transdiscal approach is another single-needle approach. Occasionally, the needle trajectory results in needle passage through part of the L5-S1 disk; when this occurs, the final position of the needle tip is very close to the anterior border of the disk. Confirmation of needle placement with contrast agent is performed. A discogram is seen if the needle tip remains in the intervertebral disk. When the appropriate contrast pattern is achieved, a smaller volume of local anesthetic or neurolytic solution (10 to 15 mL) is then used. The transarterial approach is employed when arterial blood is aspirated from the block needle. Aspirated blood suggests that the needle has inadvertently entered the iliac artery. The needle is then advanced until blood can no longer be aspirated. Because the iliac arteries are retroperitoneal and are in the same tissue plane as the superior hypogastic plexus, a loss of resistance technique (similar to the transaortic celiac plexus block) can then be used to confirm that the needle tip has traversed the anterior wall of the artery. Contrast dye followed by local anesthetic or neurolytic agent is then injected.

Complications

Complications are rarely serious and include hematoma from puncture of the iliac vessels, back pain and spasm from needle trauma, and intramuscular or intraperitoneal injection of local anesthetic or neurolytic solution. Other complications include inadvertent somatic block from subarachnoid or epidural injection, somatic nerve injury, and ureteral or renal puncture. According to Racz, if neurolytics are used, phenol at concentrations <6% should be used to minimize ureteral injury. He also notes that his experience in men is limited to unilateral blocks, and recommends that bilateral neurolytic blocks in men should not be performed because of the possibility of sexual dysfunction.[47] Proper technique with the use of fluoroscopy should negate these risks.

LUMBAR SYMPATHETIC BLOCKS

Anatomy

The lumbar sympathetic chain is easily blocked with few complications compared to other levels of the sympathetic chain. This is primarily because of the consistent position of the chain next to the lumbar vertebrae as well as its relative separation from somatic nerves. Once the sympathetic trunk extends into the abdomen, it assumes a prevertebral position as compared with the paravertebral position occupied in the thorax. On the right side, it lies posterior to the inferior vena cava, and on the left side, it lies lateral and slightly behind the abdominal aorta. The lumbar sympathetic chain consists of several ganglia (average three per side) between the L1 and L5 vertebral bodies.[48] The ganglia are most frequently found at the level of the lower third of the second lumbar vertebra to the middle third of the third vertebrae on both the right and left sides.[48,49] Most importantly, the psoas muscle always lays posterior to the sympathetic chain, thus separating the chain from the lumbar somatic roots. This separation of the sympathetic chain from the somatic lumbar plexus minimizes the spread of local anesthetic or neurolytic agent to these nerves during percutaneous lumbar sympathetic blocks. As a result, the untoward side effects are minimal and infrequent, making this procedure the prime means for lumbar sympathetic neurolysis.

Indications

The common indications for lumbar sympathetic blocks include compromised circulatory insufficiency, claudication, renal colic, herpes zoster, postherpetic neuralgia, phantom limb pain, amputation or stump pain, and carcinomatous invasion of nerves and plexus. A more complete list can be found in the Table 69-3. These blocks are also used to diagnose and treat complex regional pain syndrome (CRPS) of the lower extremity. They can help determine if the CRPS is responsive to sympathectomy, that is, determine whether the CRPS is sympathetically maintained or sympathetically independent. While lumbar sympathetic blocks can be used to treat pelvic and urogenital pain, bilateral blocks are often necessary to achieve satisfactory results; in these cases, superior hypogastic plexus blocks (see earlier description) are more appropriate because they do not cause temperature changes in the lower extremity as do the lumbar sympathetic blocks.

Once responsiveness to sympathetic blocks is recognized, aggressive therapy should be instituted as soon as possible. A reasonable approach to treatment involves the daily or every other day application of sympathetic blocks for 1 to 2 weeks. An alternative to administering daily injections involves the use of commercially prepared continuous infusion lumbar sympathetic block catheters. Another option is to institute continuous lumbar epidural analgesia. Initial infusion rates of approximately 6 mL/hour of 0.125% bupivacaine should suffice. Means to achieve prolonged sympathetic blockade include the use of neurolytic agents[50] and radiofrequency lesioning.[51] It is important to ensure that sympathectomy therapy of the lower (and upper) extremity is complemented by aggressive physical therapy to optimize treatment success.

TABLE 69-3 **Indications for Lumbar Sympathetic Block**

Circulatory Insufficiency of the Leg
- Arteriosclerotic Disease
- Claudication
- Rest Pain
- Ischemic Ulcers
- Diabetic Gangrene
- Following Reconstructive Vascular Surgery
- Pain Following Arterial Embolus

Pain from Other Causes
- Renal Colic
- Herpes Zoster/Postherpetic neuralgia
- Frostbite
- Sympathetically Maintained Complex Regional Pain Syndrome (CRPS)
- Phantom or Amputation Stump Pain
- Carcinomatous Invasion of Neurovascular Structures in the Head Neck and Arm

Miscellaneous
- Percutaneous Renal Procedures*
- Hyperhydrosis

*Data from Mongan PD, Strong WE, Menk EJ. Anesthesia for percutaneous renal procedures. Reg Anesth 1991;16:296.

Technique

The classic lumbar sympathetic block is performed by placing a needle at the anterolateral border of the L2, L3, and L4 vertebral bodies. Patient positioning is similar to that used in the posterolateral approach to the celiac plexus block. The patient is placed prone with a pillow beneath the lower abdomen and hip to reduce the lordosis of this region and improve identification of the L2 through L4 spinous processes. The L2 spinous process is found by identifying the tips of the 12th ribs and drawing a line between them; the midpoint typically corresponds to the L2-3 interspace. Similarly, identification of the L4-5 interspace involves locating the superior edge of the iliac crests and drawing a line between them; the midpoint of this line marks this interspace. Radiographic facilities are not required to successfully perform this block. However, fluoroscopy or CT can be used when landmarks are difficult to identify (such as in morbidly obese patients); these imaging devices can help to ensure the appropriate location of the needle tip.

A local anesthetic skin wheal is raised approximately 6 to 10 cm lateral to the spine of the second lumbar vertebrae. Needle entry can be performed medial 6 cm, but makes final placement of the needle tip at the anterolateral surface of the vertebral body more difficult. Reid et al[52] noted that needle penetration at 7 cm from midline provides easy identification of the vertebral body, yet avoids puncture of the kidney. An advantage to a more lateral approach is that the needle avoids passing through the erector spinae muscles and avoids inflicting pain and spasm in these muscles.

Ten centimeter, 22-gauge subarachnoid needles are inserted at a 45 to 60 degree angle toward midline. The transverse process may be contacted; this typically occurs at about 5 cm. The needle is then marked at 3 to 5 cm from the skin, and then repositioned inferiorly and medially to contact the vertebral body. This typically occurs at about 6 to 8 cm and is then walked off the vertebral body until it is advanced to the depth identified by the needle marker. If using fluoroscopy or CT, it is not necessary to identify the transverse process; the needle tip is advanced directly toward the anterolateral aspect of the vertebral body. As long as the needle is in the psoas muscle, there will be some resistance to injection. Using a loss of resistance technique or fluoroscopy with contrast to observe psoas tenting,[53] one can determine when the needle has advanced through the anterior surface of the psoas muscle.

Once the needle tip is positioned along the anterolateral aspect of the selected vertebral body, the needle is aspirated for cerebrospinal fluid (CSF) or blood. Contrast agent (1 to 3 mL) is then injected and a characteristic longitudinal spread of contrast dye can be seen (Fig. 69-9). Injected contrast will appear striated and spread in a diagonal pattern if the needle tip is in the psoas muscle; a "psoas stripe" can be seen (see Fig. 69-9A). This is easily corrected by advancing the needle tip an additional 0.5 to 1.0 cm; injection of contrast is then repeated. The appropriate spread is in a craniocaudal direction and appears rather thin when seen in a lateral view with fluoroscopy (see Fig. 69-9B). A 2-mL test dose of 1% lidocaine or 0.25% bupivacaine is injected and the patient is evaluated for untoward side effects. About 5 mL of local anesthetic is then injected through the needle; the procedure is then repeated at the other two (L3 and L4) lumbar sites.

Alternatively, a single-injection technique can be performed using the same approach except that once the appropriate depth is obtained, a larger volume (10 to 20 mL) of local anesthetic is injected.[54] As the ganglia are most often found at the lower portion of the second lumbar vertebral body to the middle of the third vertebral body, this area becomes the most favorable when using a single-needle technique.[48,49] The advantage of a single-needle technique is decreased post-procedure pain and muscle spasm as a result of less needle trauma through the paraspinal and psoas muscles.

Complications

Serious complications are rare and are minimized with the use of radiographic imaging. The most common sequelae is backache, typically related to needle trauma, that usually responds to conservative therapy such as short-term oral opioids, nonsteroidal anti-inflammatory drugs (NSAIDs), or ice and heat therapy. Somatic nerve block can occur from inadvertent injection of local anesthetic into the psoas muscle (psoas compartment block); it can also occur following posterior spread of local anesthetic along tendinous arches that bridge the concave sides of the lumbar vertebrae, thus blocking somatic nerves roots.[55] Hematuria occasionally occurs from needle puncture of the kidney or uterer. Although this finding usually resolves spontaneously after 2 to 3 days, the hematuria can be very distressing to the patient. Kidney puncture is avoided by limiting injections to below the L2 vertebral body.[56] Performing the block in the lateral position may also minimize the chance of puncture by theoretically allowing the kidney to fall anteriorly and out of the path of the block needle.

Genitofemoral neuralgia occurs with an incidence of approximately 20% following fluoroscopically guided neurolytic lumbar sympathetic block.[50] This incidence is decreased by using smaller volumes of neurolytic agent (thus minimizing the spread of agent to the genitofemoral nerve) and injecting cranial to the L4 vertebral body.[57] The symptoms consist of a burning dysethesia in the anteromedial area of the upper thigh; the pain is frequently severe and can last 6 to 8 weeks, but is usually controlled with transcutaneous electrical nerve stimulation (TENS) or antiepileptic medications, such as diphenylhydantoin or carbamazepine.[58]

Because incidental genitofemoral nerve block is common, it is important to consider whether the pain syndrome in question unsuspectingly involves the genitofemoral nerve or the L1 nerve root. A "diagnostic" lumbar sympathetic block that unintentionally blocks the genitofemoral nerve may yield the false diagnosis that the pain syndrome was sympathetically maintained. Such a situation may exist when a somatic pain syndrome exists in the genitofemoral or anterior thigh area and the following sequence occurs: a lumbar sympathetic block is performed to diagnose sympathetically maintained pain, an unintentional genitofemoral nerve block occurs that then alleviates the somatic pain, and the syndrome is incorrectly identified as involving sympathetic elements. Performing a sympathetic block at L2 may avoid this scenario by preferentially sparing the genitofemoral nerve.[57]

Other complications occur from inadvertent needle placement. Needle entry into the dural cuff of a somatic nerve can result in an epidural or subarachnoid block.[59] A case report of retroperitoneal hemorrhage has also been described with paravertebral blocks.[60]

ALTERNATIVES FOR REGIONAL SYMPATHETIC BLOCKS

Certain conditions preclude the pain specialist from using regional sympathetic blocks. These include coagulopathy, systemic infection, and postsurgical changes in the region of interest (such as radical neck surgery or aortic graft placement). Alternatives to regional sympathetic blocks include peripheral nerve or plexus blocks and epidural administration of local anesthetic. Options to nerve blocks include regional or systemic intravenous techniques, oral therapy, and surgical sympathectomy.

Once it has been determined that the pain syndrome is sympathetically maintained, continuous catheter techniques can be effective. Brachial plexus catheters placed in the axillae or infraclavicular region can provide continuous low-dose analgesia (e.g., bupivacaine 0.125% at 10 mL/hour) for several days. Cervical, thoracic, or lumbar epidural catheters at similar or lower infusion rates and concentrations can provide reasonable analgesia as well, although ambulation and activities of daily living may become significantly impaired. These techniques are more familiar to the practicing anesthesiologist than continuous stellate ganglion and lumbar sympathetic catheters, and are less likely to become dislodged after several days of physical therapy.

Intravenous regional sympathetic blocks have been performed using guanethidine, bretylium, and reserpine. Guanethidine inhibits the presynaptic release of norepinephrine by displacing it from storage sites in the peripheral nerve endings and preventing its reuptake. The resultant depletion of norepinephrine results in a pharmacologic sympathetic block. Bretylium produces sympathectomy by being taken up in adrenergic terminals; then it acts as a false transmitter and releases much less norepinephrine than guanethidine. Reserpine acts on the peripheral nervous system by depleting norepinephrine stores and inhibiting norepinephrine synthesis. The most widely studied agent has been guanethidine; it is no

A

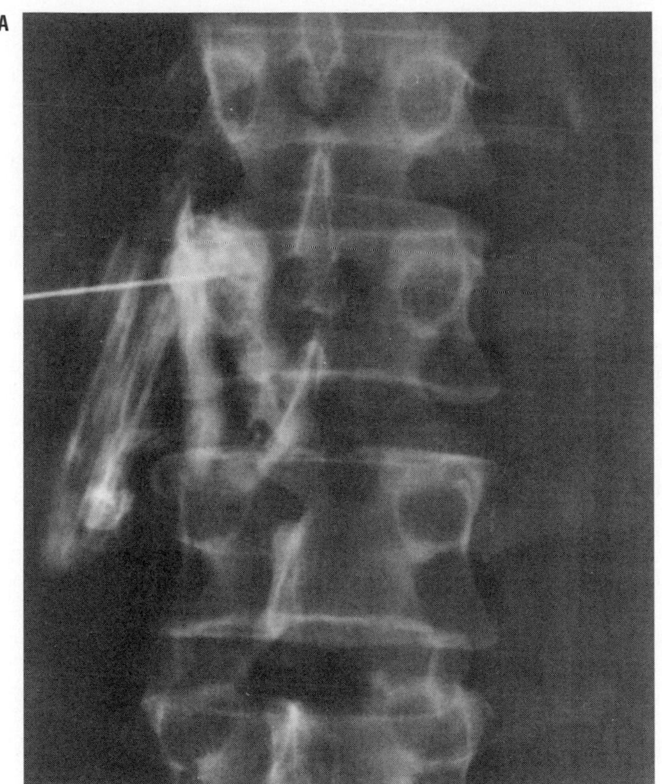

B

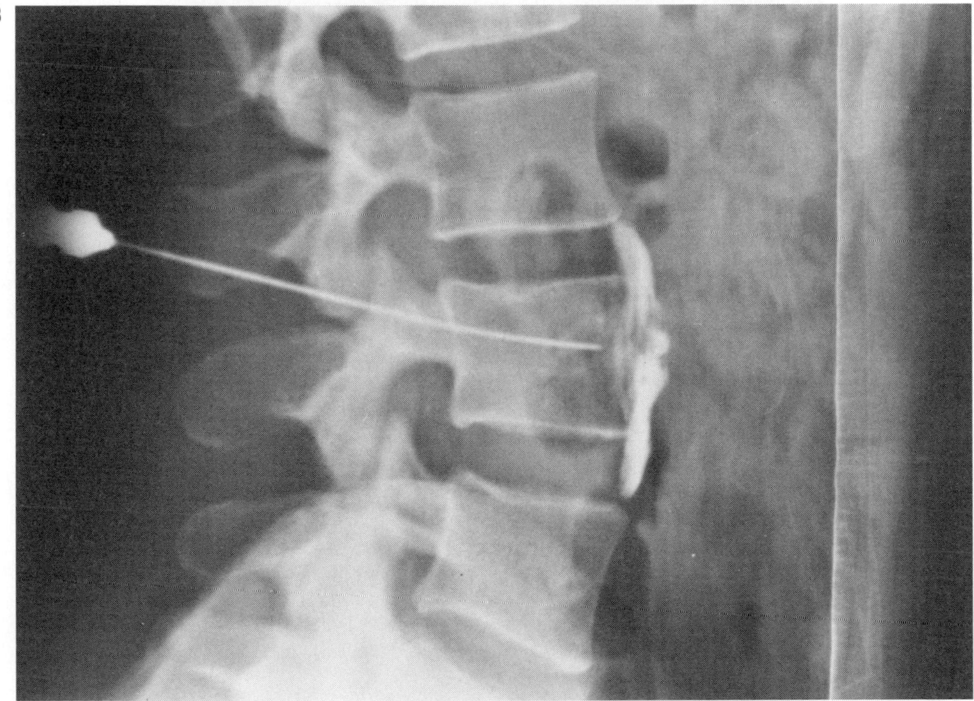

Figure 69-9 (**A**) AP radiograph of lumbar sympathetic block. Correct spread of contrast agent is along the anterolateral vertebral bodies in a cranio-caudal direction. The striated, diagonal contrast pattern also seen is a result of inadvertent injection of agent into the psoas muscle (the "psoas stripe"). (**B**) Lateral view radiograph of lumbar sympathetic block. Contrast spread is along the anterior margin of the vertebral bodies.

longer available in the United States. Twenty milliliters of guanethidine in 0.5% lidocaine (25 mL for the upper extremity, 50 mL for the lower extremity) is injected intravenously following tourniquet inflation; the tourniquet is kept inflated for 20 to 30 minutes to prevent the release of guanethidine into the systemic circulation. Lidocaine is added for patient comfort because the initial norepinephine release can be painful for the patient with CRPS; however, this practice may actually be unnecessary.[61] The procedure is repeated every 2 to 4 days for a maximum of four blocks. Reserpine 1.0 to 1.5 mg[62] and bretylium 1.5mg/kg[63] have been also used in volumes of 0.5% lidocaine as previously noted. Because the sympathectomy produced is shorter lived than with guanethidine, the regional blocks should be performed on a daily basis when these agents are used. Complications of intravenous regional sympathectomy include transient syncopal episodes with apnea,[64] orthostatic hypotension, pain with administration, nausea, and vomiting.

Varying success rates have been reported with these agents, and as a result, the use of intravenous regional sympathectomy is somewhat controversial.[61–63,65–70] In 1983, Bonnelli et al reported that in patients with reflex sympathetic dystrophy, intravenous regional guanethidine blocks provided comparable pain relief with longer duration to stellate ganglion block therapy.[68] In a 10-year follow-up study of neuralgia in the hand, Wahren noted that guanethidine therapy can provide 2 weeks to 6 months of prolonged pain relief.[69] Hord also showed in a double-blind randomized trial that intravenous regional bretylium also provided effective analgesia of reflex sympathetic dystrophy; however, a review of his data reveal that only a 30% improvement of pain relief was considered significant.[63] In contrast, randomized, double-blind studies evaluating the use of guanethidine[61,70] and reserpine[61] did not show any improvement in pain scores compared with intravenous regional therapy with placebo. A mechanism of tourniquet-induced analgesia may play a role.[61]

Phentolamine infusion has gained some popularity as an alternative to diagnosing sympathetically maintained CRPS.[71,72] Incremental dosing of intravenous phentolamine to supine patients under a monitored setting can be safely performed[73]; the total dose given over 30 to 60 minutes is 0.5 to 1.0 mg/kg. Intravenous phentolamine can help determine a responsiveness to the oral α-adrenergic blocking agents such as phenoxybenzamine. Pain relief of at least 50% or untoward effects such as hypotension, dizziness, or headache are the usual endpoints to this diagnostic test. Complications are rare, typically self-limited, and include sinus tachycardia, premature ventricular beats, or wheezing.

NEUROLYTIC AGENTS

Neurolytic agents are used to provide long-term pain relief (See also Chapter 63). Prior to injecting a neurolytic agent, a local anesthetic test block is useful to test the feasibility of a "permanent" test block. A successful test block does not always predict the outcome of a neurolytic celiac plexus block, however.

Alcohol and phenol are the two neurolytic agents most commonly used. Alcohol is used in concentrations from 50% to 100%. The mechanism of neurolysis is via extraction of cholesterol and phospholipid from neural membranes. There is also precipitation of lipoproteins and mucoproteins. Alcohol probably provides more intense nerve destruction than phenol. Alcohol diffuses more rapidly through biological tissue, thereby increasing the degree of somatic nerve damage. Of note, while no controlled studies comparing the two agents exist, there may be an increased incidence of L1 neuralgia during lumbar sympathetic block when alcohol is used versus phenol.[50] Sedation, dysphoria, and nausea and vomiting can occur from excessive systemic absorption of injected alcohol. A plasma alcohol level can be measured, but levels are highly variable and depend on concentration, volume, and metabolic rate of the patient. Phenol is usually used in concentrations of 6% to 10%. Phenol causes protein coagulation and necrosis of nerves. The higher concentrations of phenol must be made soluble in a glycerin base; as a result, the heavier viscosity makes it difficult to inject. The primary advantage of phenol is its inherent local anesthetic effect, which precludes pain on injection; in contrast, alcohol typically causes a severe, transient pain on injection. Phenol has a slower onset of action, is less efficacious, and is of shorter duration than alcohol.

REFERENCES

1. Kappis M. Weitere Erfahrungen mit der Sympthektomic. *Klin Wehr* 1923;2:1441.
2. Mandl F. Die parvertibrale Injection. J. Springer, Vienna, 1926. In: Stanton-Hicks M. Treatment of sympathetically maintained pain. *Reg Anesth* 1995;20:1.
3. Treede R-D, Davis KD, Campbell JN, et al. Plasticity of cutaneous hyperalgesia during sympathetic ganglion blockade in patients with neuropathic pain. *Brain* 1992;115:607.
4. Kapral S, Krafft P, Gosch M, et al. Ultrasound imaging for stellate ganglion block: direct visualization of puncture site and local anesthetic spread. A pilot study. *Reg Anesth* 1995;20:323–328.
5. Hogan QH, Erickson SJ, Haddox JD, et al. The spread of solutions during stellate ganglion block. *Reg Anesth* 192;17:78.
6. Lofstrom JB: Stellate ganglion block. In Ericksson E, ed. *Illustrated Handbook in Local Anaesthesia.* Philadelphia, Pa: WB Saunders; 1980:141.
7. Hardy P, Wells J. Extent of sympathetic blockade after stellate ganglion block with bupivacaine. *Pain* 1989;36:193.
8. Grodinsky M, Holyyoke EA. The fasciae and fascial spaces of the head, neck, and adjacent regions. *Am J Anat* 1938;63:367.
9. Guntamukkala M, Hardy PAJ. Spread of injectate after stellate ganglion block in man: an anatomical study. *Br J Anaesth* 1991;66:643.
10. Dondelinger TF, Kurdziel JC. Percutaneous phenol block of the upper thoracic sympathetic chain with computer tomography guidance. *Acta Radiol* 1987;28:511.
11. Hogan QH, Taylor ML, Goldstein M, et al. Success rates in producing sympathetic blockade by paratracheal injection. *Clin J Pain* 1994; 10:139.
12. Stevens RA, Stoltz A, Kao T-C, et al. The relative increase in skin temperature after stellate ganglion block is predictive of a complete sympathectomy of the hand. *Reg Anesth Pain Manage* 1998;23:266.
13. Wulf H, Maier CH. Complications of stellate ganglion blockade: results of a questionnaire. *Anaesthesist* 1992;41:146–151.
14. Korevaar WC, Burney RG, Moore PA. Convulsions during stellate ganglion block:a case report. *Anesth Analg* 1979;58:329.
15. Szeinfeld M, Laurencio M, Pallares VS. Total reversible blindness following attempted stellate ganglion block. *Anesth Analg* 1981;60:689.
16. Schot DL, Ghia JN, Teeple E. Aphasia and hemiparesis following stellate ganglion block. *Anesth Analg* 1983;62:1038.
17. Kozody R, Ready L, Basra JM, et al. Dose requirement of local anesthetic to produce grand mal seizure during stellate ganglion blockade. *Can J Anaesth* 1982;29:489.
18. Ward EM, Rorie DK, Nauss LE, et al.The celiac ganglion in man: normal anatomic variations. *Anesth Analg* 1979;58:461.
19. Ischia S, Luzzani A, Ischia A, et al. A new approach to the neurolytic block of the coeliac plexus. The transaortic technique. *Pain* 1983;16: 333.
20. Lebovits AH, Lefkowitz M. Pain management of pancreatic carcinoma: a review. *Pain* 1989;36:1.
21. Brown DL, Bulley CK, Quiel EL. Neurolytic celiac plexus block for pancreatic cancer pain. *Anesth Analg* 1987;66:869.
22. Akhan O, Altinok D, Ozman MN, et al. Correlation between the grade of tumoral invasion and pain relief in patients with celiac plexus block. *AJR* 1997;168:1565.
23. Kune GA, Cole R, Bell S. Observations on the relief of pancreatic pain. *Med J Aust* 1975;2:789.
24. Rykowski JJ, Hilgier M. Continuous celiac plexus block in acute pancreatitis. *Reg Anesth* 1995;20:528.
25. Blanchard J, Ramamurthy S, Hoffman J.Celiac plexus block with steroids for chronic pancreatitis. *Reg Anesth* 1988;13(suppl):84.
26. Bell SN, Cole R, Roberts-Thompson IC. Coeliac plexus block for control of pain in chronic pancreatitis. *Br Med J* 1980;281:1604.
27. Moore DC. Regional block. *A Handbook for Use in the Clinical Practice of Medicine and Surgery.* 4th ed. Springfield, Ill: Charles C. Thomas. 1965:145.

28. Lieberman RP, Nance PN, Cuka DJ. Anterior approach to celiac plexus block during interventional biliary procedures. *Radiology* 1988;167:562.
29. Montero MA, Vidal LF, Aguilar SJ, et al. Percutaneous anterior approach to the celiac plexus, using ultrasound. *Br J Anaesth* 1989; 62:637.
30. Singler R. An improved technique for alcohol celiac plexus nerve block. *Anesthesiology* 1982;56:137.
31. Weber JG, Brown DL, Stephens DH, et al. Celiac plexus block: retrocrural CT anatomy in patients with and without pancreatic cancer. *Reg Anesth* 1996;21:407.
32. Davies DD. Incidence of major complications of neurolytic celiac plexus block. *J R Soc Med* 1993;86:264.
33. Thompson G, Moore DC, Bridenbaugh LD, et al. Abdominal pain and alcohol celiac plexus nerve block. *Anesth Analg Curr Res* 1977;56:1.
34. Pateman J, Williams MP, Filshie J. Retroperitoneal fibrosis after multiple celiac plexus blocks. *Anaesthesia* 1990;45:309.
35. Fujita Y, Takaori M. Pleural effusion after CT-guided alcohol celiac plexus block. *Anesth Analg* 1987;66:911.
36. Moore DC, Bush WH, Burnett LL. Celiac plexus block: a roentgenographic, anatomic study of technique and spread of solution in patients and corpses. *Anesth Analg* 1981;60:369.
37. Woodham MJ, Hanna MH. Paraplegia after coeliac plexus block. *Anaesthesia* 1989;44:487.
38. Wong GY, Brown DL. Transient paraplegia following alcohol celiac plexus block. *Reg Anesth* 1995;20:352.
39. Mercadante S. Clinical note — Octreotide in the treatment of diarrhoea included by coeliac plexus block. *Pain* 1995;61:345.
40. Chan VWS. Chronic diarrhea:an uncommon side effect of celiac plexus block. *Anesth Analg* 1996;82:205.
41. Weinstabl C, Porges P, Plainer B, et al. Coeliac plexus block with bupivacaine reduces intestinal dysfunction in neurosurgical ICU patients. *Anaesthesia* 1993;48:162.
42. Abram SE, Hogan Q. Complications of nerve block. In: Benumof JL, Saidman LJ, eds. *Anesthesia and Perioperative Complications*. St Louis, Mo: Mosby-Year Book; 1992:52.
43. Crafts RC. *A Textbook of Human Anatomy*. 3rd ed. New York, NY: John Wiley and Sons; 1985.
44. Lee RB, Stone K, Magelssen D, et al. Presacral neurectomy for chronic pelvic pain. *Obstet Gynecol* 1986;68:517.
45. Frier A. Pelvic neurectomy in gynecology. *Obstet Gynecol* 1965;25:48.
46. Plancarte R, Amescua C, Patt RB, et al. Superior hypogastric plexus block for pelvic cancer pain. *Anesthesiology* 1990;73:236.
47. Raj PP, Rauck RL, Racz GB. Autonomic nerve blocks. In: Raj PP,ed. *Pain Medicine—A Comprehensive Review*. St Louis, Mo: Mosby-Year Book; 1996:227.
48. Rocco AG, Palombi D, Racke D. Anatomy of the lumbar sympathetic chain. *Reg Anesth* 1995;20:13.
49. Umeda S, Arai T, Hatano Y, et al. Cadaver anatomic analysis of the best site for chemical lumbar sympathectomy. *Anesth Analg* 1987;66:643.
50. Cousins MJ, Reeve TS, Glynn CJ, et al. Neurolytic lumbar sympathetic blockade: duration of denervation and relief of rest pain. *Anaesth Intens Care* 1979;7:121.
51. Rocco AG. Radiofrequency lumbar sympatholysis: the evolution of a technique for managing sympathetically maintained pain. *Reg Anesth* 1995;20:3.
52. Reid W, Watt JK, Gray TG. Phenol injection of the sympathetic chain. *Br J Surg* 1970;57:45.
53. Sprague RS, Ramamurthy S. Identification of the anterior psoas sheath as a landmark for lumbar sympathetic block. *Reg Anesth* 1990;15:253.
54. Hatangdi WS, Boas RA. Lumbar sympathectomy: a single needle technique. *Br J Anaesth* 1985;57:285.
55. Bryce-Smith R. Injection of the lumbar sympathetic chain. *Anaesthesia* 1991;6:150.
56. Brown VM, Kunjappan V. Single-needle approach for lumbar sympathetic block. *Anesth Analg* 1975;54:725.
57. Sayson SC, Ramamurthy S, Hoffman J. Incidence of genitofemoral nerve block during lumbar sympathetic block: comparision of two lumbar injection sites. *Reg Anesth* 1997;22:569.
58. Raskin ND, Levinson SA, Hoffman PM, et al. Postsympathetectomy neuralgia: amelioration with diphenylhydantoin and carbamazepine. *Am J Surg* 1974;28:75.
59. Gay GR, Evans JA. Total spinal anesthesia following lumbar paravertebral block. A potentially lethal complication. *Anesth Analg* 1971;50: 344.
60. Learned LO, Calhoun R. Retroperitoneal hemorrhage as a complication of lumbar paravertebral injection. Report of three cases. *Anesthesiology* 1951;12:391.
61. Blanchard J, Ramamurthy S, Walsh N, et al. Intravenous regional sympatholysis: a double-blind comparison of guanethidine, reserpine, and normal saline. *J Pain Symptom Manage* 1990;5:357.
62. Benzon HT, Chomka CM, Brunner EA. Treatment of reflex sympathetic dystropy with regional intravenous reserpine. *Anesth Analg* 1980; 59:500.
63. Hord AH, Rooks MD, Stephens BO, et al. Intravenous regional bretylium and lidocaine for treatment of reflex sympathetic dystrophy: a randomized, double-blind study. *Anesth Analg* 1992;74:818.
64. Woo R, McQueen J. Apnea and syncope following intravenous guanethidine bier block in the same patient on two different occasions. *Anesthesiology* 1987;67:281.
65. Ford SR, Forrest WH, Eltherington L. The treatment of reflex sympathetic dystrophy with intravenous regional bretylium. *Anesthesiology* 1988;68:137.
66. Hannington-Kiff JE. Intravenous regional sympathetic block with guanethidine. *Lancet* 1974;1:1019–1020.
67. Hanowell LH, Kanefield JK, Soriano SG. A recommendation for reduced lidocaine dosage during intravenous regional bretylium treatment for reflex sympathetic dystrophy. *Anesthesiology* 1989; 71:811.
68. Bonelli S, Conoscente F, Movilia PG, et al. Regional intravenous guanethidine vs. stellate ganglion block in reflex sympathetic dystrophies: a randomized trail. *Pain* 1983;16:297.
69. Wahren LK, Gordh T, Torebjork E. Effects of regional intravenous guanethidine in patients with neuralgia in the hand; a follow-up study over a decade. *Pain* 1995;62:379.
70. Ramamurthy S, Hoffman J, and the Guanethidine Study Group. Intravenous regional guanethidine in the treatment of reflex sympathetic dystrophy/causalgia: a randomized, double-blind study. *Anesth Analg* 1995;81:718.
71. Arner S. Intravenous phentolamine test: diagnostic and prognostic use in reflex sympathetic dystrophy. *Pain* 1991;46:17.
72. Raja SN, Treede RD, Davis KD, et al. Systemic alpha-adrenergic blockade with phentolamine: a diagnostic test for sympathetically maintained pain. *Anesthesiology* 1991;74:691.
73. Shir T, Cameron LB, Raja SN, et al. The safety of intravenous phentolamine administration in patients with neuropathic pain. *Anesth Analg* 1993;76:1008.
74. Hamid SK, Scott NB, Sutcliffe NP, et al. Continuous coeliac plexus blockade plus intermittent wound infiltration with bupivacaine following upper abdominal surgery: a double-blind randomized study. *Acta Anaesthesiol Scand* 1992;36:534.
75. Mongan PD, Strong WE, Menk EJ. Anesthesia for percutaneous renal procedures. *Reg Anesth* 1991;16:296.

CHAPTER 70 USE OF BOTULINUM TOXIN IN PAIN MANAGEMENT

P. Prithvi Raj and D. Sara Sangha

Botulinum toxins are potent neurotoxins produced by the bacteria *Clostridium botulinum.* The most widely studied effect of botulinum toxins is at the neuromuscular junction where they block the release of acetylcholine preventing muscle contraction and causing local flaccid paralysis (rather than rigid, or tetanic, paralysis caused by a related clostridial protein, tetanus toxin). This results in a temporary (months) chemodenervation and the loss or reduction in activity in the target organ (muscle, sweat gland, or sphincter) with minimal risk of systemic adverse effects. However, botulinum toxins work not only at the neuromuscular junction but also alter the sensory input, producing secondary changes at the central level. The broadening clinical role of botulinum toxins depends on the multiple direct and indirect effects that the toxin exerts in both the peripheral nervous system and in the central nervous system (CNS).

In 1989, the FDA approved botulinum toxin type A (BTX-A) for use in treating strabismus, blepharospasm and hemifacial spasm. In 2000–2001, both BTX-A (Allergan, Inc.) and botulinum toxin type B (BTX-B; Elan Pharmaceuticals) were FDA-approved for use in treating cervical dystonia, and in 2002, BTX-A was approved by the FDA for treatment of glabellar frown lines. Besides the FDA-approved indications, botulinum toxins have been used in a vast array of clinical problems, including achalasia; anismus; benign prostatic hypertrophy; dysphonia; dystonias; essential tremor; hyperhidrosis; kyphoscoliosis; low back pain; migraine and tension-type headache; myofascial pain; pancreatitis; pelvic floor disorders; rectal fissures; sialorrhea; spasticity; temporomandibular joint syndrome; urinary sphincter dysfunction; wrinkles; and various other movement disorders.

HISTORY AND EARLY CLINICAL DEVELOPMENT

Clostridium botulinum was first identified as a causative agent in food poisoning by Van Ermengem following a fatal outbreak in 1895.[1] In the 1920s, additional outbreaks lead to the isolation of a relatively crude form of botulinum toxin (BTX),[2] the neurotoxin responsible for food-borne botulism.

Early development of BTX began during WW II in the course of studying the nature of certain toxins, including BTX, and the means for protecting against them.[3] Although much of this initial work was carried out on BTX-A, other types of botulinum toxin were also studied, including types B, C, D, and E. The purpose was to develop a polyvalent toxoid for immunization purposes. After the war, a crystallized form of BTX-A became available and stimulated considerable scientific interest. Dr. Alan B. Scott, of the Smith-Kettlewell Eye Research Foundation, initiated efforts to study BTX in a monkey model of strabismus in the late 1960s.[4] Sufficient data was collected by 1978 to file an investigational new drug (IND) application for human clinical studies.[5] The passage of the Orphan Drug Act of 1983 and FDA approval aided clinical development of BTX-A as an orphan drug in December 1989.

PHARMACOLOGY OF BOTULINUM TOXINS

There are two types of commercial botulinum toxins presently available in the United States: Botox (Botulinum toxin type A Purified Neurotoxin Complex, Allergan, Inc., 2525 Dupont Drive, Irvine, CA) and BTX-B (Myobloc, Elan Pharmaceuticals, San Diego, CA). Botox is currently FDA-approved for the treatment of essential blepharospasm, strabismus, hemifacial spasm, cervical dystonia and glabellar frown lines in patients older than age 12 years. BTX-B was FDA-approved in December 2000 for the treatment of cervical dystonia and is presently in clinical trials for other conditions. Dysport (Botulinum toxin type A, Ipsen Ltd, Berkshire, UK) is available only in Europe.

STRUCTURE, MECHANISM OF ACTION, AND PHARMACOLOGY OF BOTULINUM TOXINS

While there are many reviews of this topic in the recent scientific literature,[6,7] the proper clinical use of BTX as a therapeutic agent rests upon a clear understanding of the relationship between its structure and mechanism of action, as well as dosing, techniques of administration, and side effects.

Structure

As the clinical uses of botulinum toxins expand, it is very important to understand the basic properties of the various serotypes (A, B, C_1, D, E, F, and G) of botulinum toxins with sequence homology amounting to approximately 50% across the serotypes. The various subtypes are most similar in regards to their larger structural features and certain functional sites, and somewhat diverse with respect to the finer details of function as well as antigenic cross-reactivity.[8] Lyophilized botulinum toxin type A supplied as a pharmaceutical agent is a bipartite protein that is synthesized in bacterial culture as a single, long-chain protein and subsequently nicked by bacterial proteases to form the free toxin. The free toxin consists of one heavy chain (H-chain; 100 kDA) and one light chain (L-chain; 50 kDA) bound together by at least one disulfide bond and additional noncovalent forces (Fig. 70-1). When secreted into culture medium by *C. botulinum,* BTX is complexed with two other proteins, a nontoxin nonhemagglutinin protein (150 kDA) and a hemagglutinating protein (600 kDA); these additional proteins greatly enhance the stability of BTX complex.[9] Most relevant to clinical use is that botulinum toxin type A appears to be the most

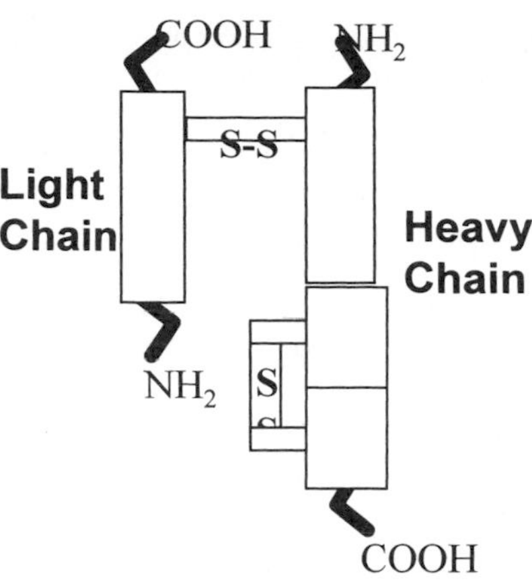

FIGURE 70-1 Diagram of botulinum toxin A free toxin. (© Allergan Inc. with permission.)

potent of the subtypes, and, when injected clinically, has the longest duration of action.[10–14] While botulinum toxin types B and F have seen limited clinical use, and others are the subject of further study, the multiple differences thus far observed suggest that the subtypes are not interchangeable.[15–18] For this reason, and because much of the preclinical and clinical literature employs BTX, this chapter presents results primarily obtained with BTX-A.

Mechanism of Action

Pharmacologic effect of BTX-A occurs in three stages, with control of each stage assignably to one of three functional units existing on either the H- or L-chain of the toxin. Each chain performs the functions associated with it in applicable model systems, even when separated from the other; however, the component chains do not block neurotransmission when applied separately.[19]

The binding of BTX-A to the motor end plate presynaptic membrane is a two-stage process, with concentration of the toxin occurring through a relatively nonspecific affinity for ganglioside-containing, lipid-rich presynaptic membrane, followed by specific binding to a protein-containing receptor.[20–22] Binding is irreversible, but not itself toxic to the neurone[23] (Fig. 70-2).

Internalization of the bound toxin occurs by receptor-mediated endocytosis.[24] Once formed, the contents of the endosome become increasingly acidic, most likely by normal cellular mechanisms. The decrease in pH within the endosome prompts a configurational change in the toxin, which then forms a channel through the membrane. The channel allows all or part of the toxin to enter the cytosol.[25–27]

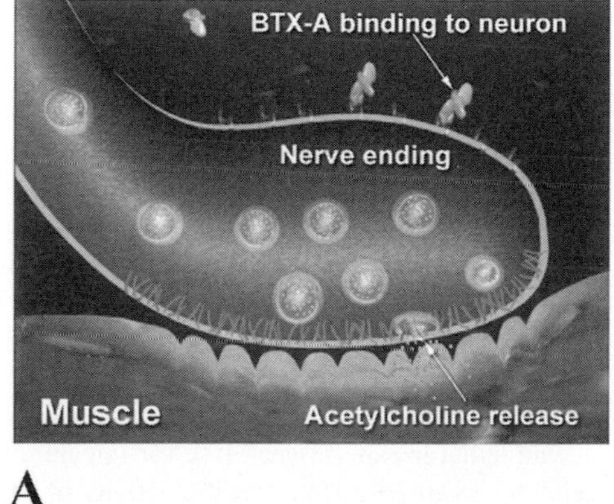

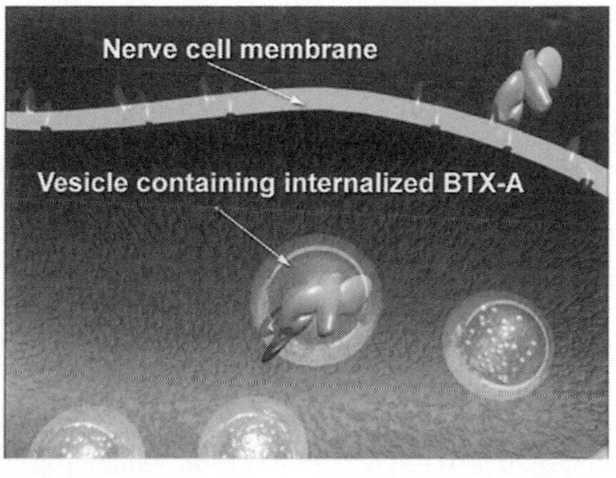

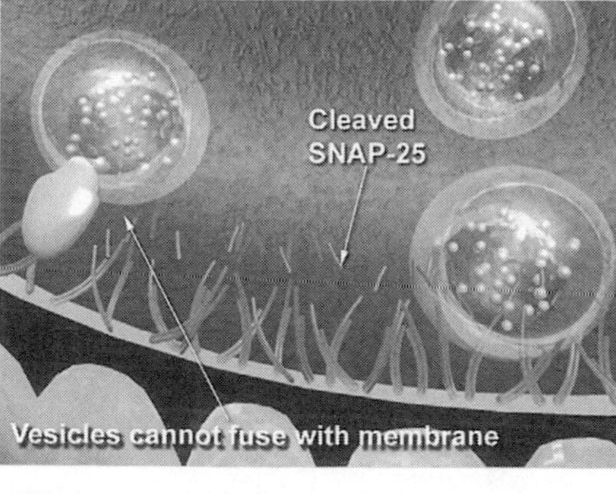

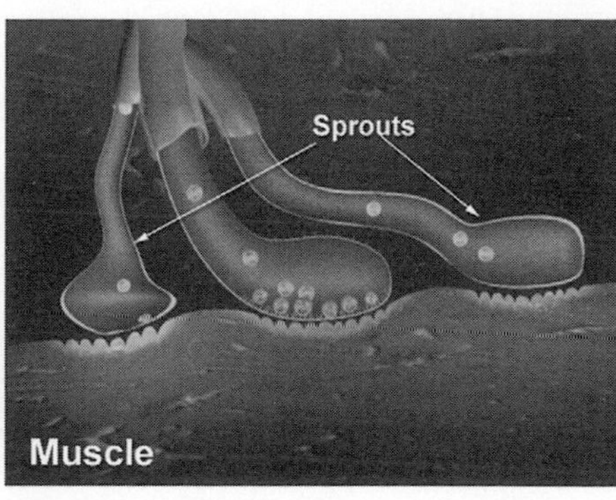

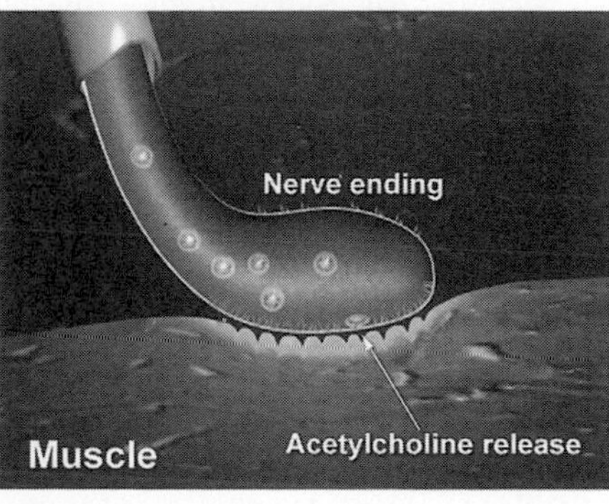

FIGURE 70-2 Representation of the sequential events that lead to the blockade of the neurotransmitter release of the neurotoxin. (**A**) The neurotoxin binds to the receptor (*arrow* on the presynaptic membrane) via the heavy chain. (**B**) Internalization of the neurotoxin, which is now in the endosome. Acidification occurs at this stage, which allows the formation of channels that allows the light chain to egress from the vesicle. (**C**) The light chain cleavages SNAP-25 (synaptosomal-associated protein, 25 kDA) by enzymatic action and does not allow the vesicle to fuse with the membrane thus the acetylcholine is prevented from release. (**D**) New sprouts of the nerve endings create new neuromuscular junction in response to the botulinum toxin action. (**E**) After return of function at the neuromuscular junction the sprouts recede and the new nerve ending is created. (© Allergan Inc. with permission.)

Once in the cytosol, the L-chain of BTX effects a long-lasting inhibition of acetylcholine (ACh) release, which current evidence suggests is accomplished by the cleavage of the SNAP-25 (synaptosomal-associated protein, 25 kDA) proteins necessary for the release of ACh by synaptosomes.[8] Although all toxin subtypes evidence a high degree of sequence homology associated with a functioning zinc-endopeptidase on the L-chain, and proteolytic activity can be found in all BTX subtypes except C_2, each toxin subtype has a characteristic specificity for cleaving a certain spectrum of proteins involved in synaptosomal function.[8]

Pharmacology

When injected intramuscularly at therapeutic doses, BTX induces a localized chemical denervation. With appropriate dose and proper localization of the target muscle, the injected muscle is only partially denervated, and therefore involuntary contracture diminishes without complete paralysis. Depending upon the underlying condition, dose and site of injection, onset of effect of BTX varies from a few days to 2 weeks. This corresponds roughly to the time it takes for the toxin to reach the cytosol of the targeted synapses and begin its enzymatically mediated cholinergic blockade. Functional denervation is observable for from 6 weeks to 6 months following injection, but typically lasts for 3 to 4 months. During peak effect, muscle histology shows evidence of atrophy and increased variation of fiber size following BTX administration. Recovery of functional innervation is associated with histological evidence of neuronal sprouting, reinnervation and enlargement of some end plates, along with the formation of new smaller end plates.[10,28,29] There is also an increase in the number of muscle fibers innervated per axon, with some fibers being innervated by more than one axon.[10] Recovery is complete after allowing sufficient time for regrowth.[30,31] Fiber size, and presumably neuromuscular function, returns to essentially normal, even after multiple cycles of injection and recovery.[32] Botulinum toxin therapy has also been reported to alleviate pain associated with various conditions with or without accompanying muscle contractions. An extensive review of the literature also indicates that BTX-A is effective in reducing pain caused by trigger points, myofascial pain, back pain, and headaches. The degree of response to BTX-A therapy in chronic pain has been variable and therefore warrants further controlled investigations. The potential mechanism of action of botulinum toxin in pain relief is discussed in the following paragraph.

Botulinum toxins (types A, B, C_1, and F) have an inhibitory effect on the *in vitro* neuropeptide release from rat embryonic dorsal root ganglia neurons and from isolated rabbit iris sphincter and dilatory muscles.[33–35] Also, BTX-A was reported to inhibit *in vitro* release of acetylcholine and substance P (but not norepinephrine) in rabbit ocular tissue.[35] Based on these in vitro and limited in vivo observations, it is hypothesized that BTX treatment reduces the local release of nociceptive peptides either from cholinergic neurons or from C- or Ad fibers *in vivo*. This reduction in neuropeptide release would prevent local sensitization of nociceptors and reduce the local perception of pain. A reduction of nociceptive signals from the periphery could result in reduced central sensitization associated with chronic pain. Preclinical investigation on the local antinociceptive effects of BTX-A was reported by Cui at the Society of Neuroscience annual meeting in 2000, and a follow-up report was submitted more recently by Aoki at the American Academy of Neurology annual meeting in 2003.[36] To investigate the mechanism of the antinociceptive effect of subcutaneous BTX-A (Allergan, Inc.), its effect on formalin-induced local glutamate release, electrophysiological activities of dorsal horn neurons and the spinal expression of c-fos, an indicator of activation of neurons, were assessed in the rat model for inflammatory pain (formalin model). Formalin (5%, 50 μL subcutaneous) OK produces prolonged distinct biphasic excitations (spikes) of dorsal horn neurons, which correspond to early (acute nociceptive) and late (tonic nociceptive) phases of the behavioral formalin pain response. Pretreatment of rats with BTX-A (1 day, sc) significantly inhibited the formalin-induced electrophysiological activities in the late phase but not in the early phase. BTX-A also dose-dependently inhibited formalin-induced glutamate release in the paw and the expression of c-fos in the dorsal horn of the spinal cord. These results demonstrate that the inhibition of neurotransmitter release from primary sensory neurons by subcutaneous BTX-A mediates, at least, some of its antinociceptive effect. Local administration of BTX-A directly inhibits the peripheral sensitization produced by local neurotransmitter release, which then results in an indirect reduction in central sensitization. Inhibition of nociceptive processing at the peripheral site and at the spinal cord level may underline the mechanism of BTX-A effect in alleviating certain chronic pain conditions. In conclusion, the preclinical (*in vitro* and *in vivo*) data, coupled with clinical observations strongly supports the theory that botulinum toxin (especially BTX-A) may have antinociceptive properties distinct from its well-documented effects on the neuromuscular junction and other cholinergic nerves.

BTX-B (Myobloc) is produced by fermentation of *C. botulinum* type B (Bean strain) as a noncovalently associated neurotoxin complex with hemagglutinin and nonhemagglutinin proteins. After the fermentation process, the neurotoxin complex is purified through a series of precipitation and chromatography steps. Myobloc is marketed as a clear to light yellow solution in 3.5 mL glass vials with 5,000 U BTX-B per mL in 0.05% human serum albumin, 0.01 M sodium succinate, and 0.1 M sodium chloride at a pH of about 5.6. Although biological activity is maintained at room temperature for 6 months; recommended storage guidelines are for refrigeration at temperatures of 2°C to 8°C, with stability maintained for 2 years. For Myobloc, one unit corresponds to the calculated median lethal intraperitoneal dose for female Swiss Webster mice weighing 18 to 20 g. The specific activity of Myobloc ranges between 70 and 130 U/ng. However, units of biological activity of BTX-B cannot be compared to or converted into units of any other BTX. Extrapolation from animal data should not be done because of differences in species sensitivity to BTX neurotoxin serotypes. Until adequate studies are done, extrapolation from human cervical dystonia dosing data to other conditions in which BTX might be used in an off-label fashion is not prudent.

The most commonly reported adverse events associated with BTX-B in clinical trials were dry mouth, dysphagia, dyspepsia, and injection site pain, with the dry mouth and dysphagia the most common reasons for discontinuation.[37] Doses up to 25,000 U were studied, but most patients received 12,500 U or less. Dysphagia increased with increasing doses injected into the sternocleidomastoid muscle. Dry mouth showed some dose-related increases with injections into the splenius capitis, trapezius, and sternocleidomastoid muscles. Additionally, dry mouth appeared to be much less of a problem with repeat dosing, even when higher doses were used.

Antibody Formation

Tsui reported on the incidence of antibody formation in 32 patients with spasmodic torticollis who received repeated injections of BTX-A.[38] Four patients (12.5%) produced antibodies after 2 to 9 months of treatment. Because the dose range used in blepharospasm is much less than that used in cervical dystonia/spasmodic torticollis, the incidence of antibody formation is far less. Based upon data from a number of studies, the incidence of antibody formation with BTX-A for the treatment of cervical dystonia is probably less than 5%.[39] It is important to note that the present Botox formulation is "cleaner" (5 ng vs. 25 ng protein) than the older formulation used in much of the published data discussing antibody formation. As a result of its lower neurotoxin complex load, current BTX-A exposes cervical dystonia patients to approximately 12 ng of protein per treatment (or 48 ng of protein per year based on treatment every 3 months) based on a mean effective dose of 236 U. Hatheway and Dang reported that an annual exposure 125 ng or less of BTX-A would result in <5% of patient population with neutralizing antibodies.[40] Based upon current data, general guidelines of keeping the dose as low as is necessary (300–600 U for BTX-A) and injecting no more frequently than every 3 months remain. The BTX-B product from Elan Pharmaceuticals contains 50 ng of neurotoxin complex per 5,000 U. As a result of this, BTX-B exposes cervical dystonia patients to ~100 ng of protein per treatment cycle based on the most effective dose of 10,000 U published in two double-blind studies.[41,42] According to the BTX-B product insert (Myobloc, US Product Insert, Elan), at 10,000 U, 18% of patients treated for 18 months developed neutralizing antibodies. There was no data on whether this neutralizing activity had any effect on efficacy. The reasons for such rapid development of neutralizing antibodies remain unclear and may be a result of previous exposure of the patients to BTX-A or the high content of protein in this product. Factors that may influence the risk of botulinum toxin antibody formation include the overall exposure to neurotoxin complex protein, protein load per effective dose of the toxin, and, most importantly, the frequency of exposure.

Because BTX-A and BTX-B display quite different chemical compositions, it has long been felt that the antibody cross-reactivity between the two is extremely small.[43] Nonetheless, concern has been expressed over the potential problem of neutralizing antibody formation with lower potency and shorter-acting BTX serotypes.[44] Preliminary data based on the amino acid sequences of botulinum neurotoxin serotypes and tetanus toxin, which provide the molecular basis for cross-reactivity, indicate that there is a molecular basis for cross-reactivity between the proteins. However, the exact clinical significance of these findings has yet to be determined.[45] Additionally, for example, although BTX-A and BTX-F have similar potency, increasing doses of BTX-F to increase duration of response to that seen with BTX-A may increase antibody formation to BTX-F. This was demonstrated in a study by Chen and colleagues, who reported that 4 of 18 (22%) cervical dystonia patients treated with BTX-F became nonresponsive to BTX-F following 12 to 66 months of treatment.[46]

PAIN ABATEMENT IN CLINICAL STUDIES WITH BOTULINUM TOXIN TYPE A

Botulinum toxin therapy has also been reported to alleviate pain associated with various conditions with or without accompanying muscle contractions. Early reports in cervical dystonia patients treated with BTX-A suggested that the pain relief was much greater than the benefits gained by decreasing excess muscle contraction.[30,41,47,48] Pain associated with myoclonus of spinal cord origin was also successfully treated with BTX-A.[49] Furthermore, tension-type headaches were also reported to improve following BTX-A therapy.[50,54] Intramuscular BTX-A administered prior to adductor release surgery in children with cerebral palsy resulted in significant antinociceptive effects. The children treated with BTX-A reported a reduced need for narcotics, were discharged earlier and had better outcomes than the placebo group. The results of this trial were so dramatic that the trial was terminated earlier than scheduled.[55] An extensive review of the literature also indicates that BTX-A is effective in reducing pain caused by trigger points, myofascial pain, back pain, and headaches. The degree of response to BTX-A therapy in chronic pain has been variable and therefore warrants further controlled investigations.

This review organizes the burgeoning number of clinical studies of BTX into a few medically useful categories into which the same or similarly classified patients have been grouped for treatment. It is thereby hoped to make evident the essential features of BTX use in a particular subcategory, while at the same time identifying principles of practice that may guide the use of BTX for neuromuscular pain in general. Considering this, the first general principle for the rational use of BTX in pain management is actually a precondition: the patient must be experiencing chronic pain of a known or highly probable etiology for which there is no curative treatment, and for which other conservative and noninvasive pain relief strategies have been considered and exhausted.

Pain related to involuntary or excessive muscle contraction can be produced by an extremely wide range of clinical conditions, some of which are associated with movement disorders, and others in which pain, spasm, and cramping are the only symptoms present. For the purpose of establishing categories among the multiple reports describing the use of BTX-A in musculoskeletal pain, one may divide case studies into categories based upon the predominance of a movement disorder, primarily the focal dystonias, or the predominance of spasticity, primarily of the CNS origin; myofascial pain syndrome can be considered in a distinct category.

Focal Dystonias with Pain

Dystonia generalized or focal, is defined as a condition of increased muscular tone that leads to abnormal fixed postures or shifting postures resulting from irregular, forceful twisting movements of the trunk and extremities. The mobile spasms of generalized dystonia are similar to those of athetosis but are usually slower and involve the larger muscle groups of the trunk, extremities and neck. Dystonic movements increase during volitional motor activity, nervousness, and emotional stress, and diminish during relaxation and sleep.[55]

Focal dystonias are more common than generalized dystonias and include such disorders as cervical dystonia, writer's cramp (occupational dystonia), blepharospasm, and spastic dysphonia. In the focal dystonias, a single area of the body is affected. Focal dystonias occur more frequently in adults than in children, remain stable over time, and rarely spread to involve other body parts.[56]
Both generalized and focal dystonias may be associated with pain, either from the extremes of posture, excessive tendon and joint tension, or from muscle contraction. The focal dystonias are more readily treated with BTX than are the generalized dystonias because of the greater number of muscles involved and consequent larger doses required in the treatment of the latter; larger doses may cause systemic toxicity and possibly lead to development of resistance. Nevertheless, if pain can be localized to one or two muscle groups, BTX may prove beneficial even in the generalized dystonias. The focal dystonias for which there is an extensive literature

detailing treatment with BTX and for which pain represents an important element of response, include cervical dystonia (spasmodic torticollis) and occupational dystonia (writer's cramp).

Cervical Dystonia Cervical dystonia is the most common focal dystonia. There are intermittent or continuous spasms of the sternocleidomastoid, trapezius, and other cervical muscles, usually more prominent on one side than on the other. Approximately 70% of patients with cervical dystonia report pain as a principle complaint. Controlled clinical trials in cervical dystonia suggest a dramatic effect of BTX injections in controlling the pain component of this syndrome; not surprisingly, objective improvements in movement were similarly improved. Supporting these findings is a survey of 19 studies in which BTX was used for the treatment of cervical dystonia.[57] The mean weighted percent of patients reporting an improvement in pain was 76% (range: 50%–100% for the 16 studies reporting pain results; N = 938 patients). Per-muscle doses of BTX ranged from 40 to 120 mU (Botox), while per-treatment doses ranged between 100 and 374 mU (Botox).

Writer's Cramp Writer's cramp, now considered a focal dystonia, is the most common form of occupational dystonia.[58] Similar disorders have been described in musicians and others whose daily work involves frequent repetitive movements of the hands.[59,60] In one large survey, the incidence of writer's cramp accounted for 25% of all focal dystonias, with an incidence of 2.7 per million population.

The syndrome typically begins with a feeling of clumsiness during writing or other fine motor activity, and there is a loss of speed and fluency of movement. The grip may be too tight, causing the hand to become quickly fatigued. Tightness and aching can extend to the forearm or shoulder and abnormal muscle contraction lead to a distortion of normal posture. In some cases, the wrist flexes or extends and the fingers curl into the palm or pull away, so that there cannot be a proper grasp, as in cervical dystonia, but it is significant in some patients. Spontaneous remission is rare and probably occurs in fewer than 5% of patients. Writer's cramp responds poorly to conventional drug, physical, and behavioral therapy.[61] Of the many pharmacotherapies tried in this focal dystonia, the most effective appear to be systemic anticholinergics. Unfortunately, these medications rarely work and must frequently be used at such high doses that the side effects become intolerable. In contrast, numerous studies of BTX in the occupational dystonias have proved effective in relieving hyperactive muscle contracture, and have provided pain relief when pain was associated with this condition.

In an early study of dystonia of diverse forms, one patient with writer's cramp showed modest motor improvement along with significant pain relief following injection with BTX.[62] A subsequent larger study showed improvement in 16 of 19 patients (84%).[63] The results of three open-label trials indicate that 83% to 92% of patients with focal hand dystonia derive at least some subjective benefit of BTX therapy the last of these showed pain abatement in all 12 subjects who reported pain as a feature of their condition.[63–67] Where patients have been observed long enough, some have continued to respond to BTX for as long as 6 years.[68]

Three published double-blind trials in writer's cramp have shown some degree of response as well; however, pain was not assessed in these studies. In one such study of 17 patients, subjective improvement was noted after 53% of the BTX injections, as compared to only one patient (7%) after placebo injection.[68] Subjective improvement lasted for 1 to 4 months in 82% of the patients following a single dose of toxin; however, objective assessments based on videotapes of patient performance failed to demonstrate a significant difference between toxin and placebo. A second double-blind study with a crossover design treated 20 patients with writer's cramp with either BTX or placebo, administered in random order. Patients were assessed subjectively and by three objective tests of pen control and writing. Of these 20 patients, 6 had subjective improvement in writing, 7 had improved writing speed, 4 had improved writing by "blinded" rating, and 12 had better pen control on quantitative testing.[69] A third study in 10 patients employed a similar double-blind, crossover design, and 80% of patients shows both a subjective and objective response.[70]

Considering that pain is relatively infrequently mentioned in studies of writer's cramp, it is interesting to note that most attempts at gauging the efficacy of BTX in this condition showed better response with subjective responses than with objective ones, even in the double-blind studies. Nevertheless, BTX-A seems to be the best treatment available at present for writer's cramp and is especially for patients who also experience pain.

Spastic Disease States with Pain

Two other subgroups of pain patients detailed in this chapter are those in whom there is a known cause of spasticity tracing its origin to either the peripheral or central nervous systems. CNS dysfunction may lead to the sometimes-painful spasticity in certain patients with cerebral palsy, multiple sclerosis, stroke, and traumatic brain injury, while peripheral lesions may cause myofascial pain syndrome.

Upper Motor Neuron Disease Syndromes and Pain Patients experiencing acute or long-standing insults and degenerative processes of the CNS may display a wide variety of signs that together constitute the upper motor neuron syndrome. Spasticity, a velocity-dependent increase in muscle tone characterized by hyperactive stretch reflexes, is but one sign. Additional positive and negative signs characterize the syndrome. Among those classed as positive are such signs as hyperactive tendon reflexes, increased resistance to passive movement, flexed posture in the arm and extension in the leg, excessive contraction of antagonistic muscles, and stereotypic movement synergies; negative signs include weakness, lack of dexterity, and paresis.[70]

Until recently, spasticity was viewed as a consequence of overactive muscle spindles or fusimotor fibers, resulting from disruption of descending inhibitory tracts, the corticospinal and corticobulbar tracts, and sensory afferents.[71] O'Brien and colleagues suggest that this view is no longer entirely accurate.[72] Spastic paresis or spastic dystonia may be better understood as an imbalance of inhibition and excitation occurring at the motor neuron level of the spinal cord, not unlike focal hypertonia with dystonic features.[73,74] The most fundamental component of this sequence is the abnormal intraspinal response to sensory input. Modulation of local spinal cord activity occurs via the descending pathways, such as the rubrospinal tract.[75,76] In general, positive symptoms such as hyperreflexia are caused by the disinhibition of local cord excitatory circuits. Negative symptoms, such as paresis or loss of dexterity, reflect dysfunction of corticospinal pathways. The positive signs of spasticity interfere with the activities of daily living, can cause fractures or contractures, increase the frequency of pressure sores, and are often associated with pain.[77] Although they can interfere with rehabilitation, they are also more amenable to clinical intervention than are negative signs.

Spasticity as described above, is a prominent clinical feature of several important afflictions of the CNS, including stroke, cerebral palsy, multiple sclerosis, Parkinson's disease, and traumatic brain injury. For chronic or degenerative states, the management of spasticity is an ongoing task, which is best begun with conservative measures and accelerated as needed.[78–81] Initially, physical therapeutic modalities should be tried, such as avoidance of noxious stimuli, passive movement exercises, thermal agents, vibratory treatment, and serial inhibitive casting.[81] Oral medications can be tried in conjunction with physical measures or alone, but neither neural depressants (e.g., oral or intrathecal baclofen, benzodiazepines, clonidine, and tizanidine) nor muscle relaxants (e.g., dantrolene) have proved very satisfactory by reason of limited efficacy and intolerable side effects.[82–84] For the more seriously affected or unresponsive patient, invasive procedures such as phenol and alcohol nerve blocks cord stimulation, rhizotomies, and intrathecal baclofen administration have been tried.[77,85–90]

The cost of prolonged care and relative lack of benefit of conservative management have lead to the suggestion that BTX be tried in the management of spasticity. BTX can be used therapeutically to produce a reversible, partial, chemical denervation when injected directly into the suggestion that BTX be tried in the management of spasticity. BTX can be used therapeutically to produce a reversible, partial, chemical denervation when injected directly into a contracted muscle. Because of its potentially pronounced paralytic action, BTX can be as effective as certain surgeries presently in use for the management of spasticity, yet it has the advantage of being reversible and generally repeatable as needed, in accord with the fluctuating state of the patient.

Quite a few preliminary studies with BTX have been reported in spasticities of varying etiology. Although the focus of this review is on pain management, it is worthwhile to note that all of these reports have shown a clinical benefit in the control of muscle tone in patients with severe spasticity. Three studies followed a randomized, double-blind, placebo-controlled design and in these studies, the results were statistically significant.

Pain is a somewhat variable feature of spasticity, depending on the degree of impairment and the specific regions of the anatomy affected. Although there are at least a dozen studies reporting the benefits of BTX in the improvement of muscle tone in spastic conditions, fewer than half include formal measures of pain relief. Even in those studies that include formal measures of pain relief, the number of patients experiencing pain at the start of study was frequently less than the total number of patients studied. There were a total of 130 patients treated in the 6 studies. Of these, 106 (82%; range: 25%–100%) had clinically significant pain at the start of study. Within the group experiencing significant pain at the start of treatment, 77% (range: 63%–90%) obtained relief. The study of Parkinson's disease patients was notable in that it contained a relatively large sample of patients similarly affected by a particularly painful lower leg cramp. In this sample, 70% of patients reported complete pain relief while the balance appeared to have obtained significant reduction in pain. Taken together, these results support the use of BTX for pain relief in all spastic conditions in which it has thus far been tested. Approximately 75% of such patients may expect to obtain pain relief.

Myofascial Pain Syndrome Chronic myofascial pain syndrome (MPS) is one of the most common findings in patients presenting at pain clinics, varying between 30% and 85% of people presenting to pain clinics, and being more prevalent in women than in men.[91] The condition is associated with regional pain and is most typically revealed by deep palpation of highly localized hyperirritable spots, which are termed trigger points. Trigger points appear as nodular masses within taut bands of skeletal muscle and cause referred pain upon palpation.

The locations of tender nodules in MPS are remarkably constant, being most frequently found at the base of the head, and in the neck, shoulders, extremities, and low back. Nodules in similar locations may be present in normal persons but are not tender (latent trigger points).

The differential diagnosis of MPS is rather critical because it can mimic the outward signs of other diseases, such as chronic headache, shoulder bursitis, or, more seriously, lumbar herniated disc with radiculopathy, angina pectoris, and appendicitis.[92]

The trigger points found in MPS should also be distinguished from the tender sites found in fibromyalgia because treatment strategies are different. The most important distinction is that the tender sites of fibromyalgia represent a widespread, nonspecific, soft-tissue pain, and when palpated, cause only local pain.[93] The nodular trigger points of MPS are thought to develop after trauma, or after overuse or prolonged spasm of muscles, and cause local and referred pain when palpated. Fibromyalgia is a systemic disease process, possibly caused by dysfunction of the limbic system and/or neuroendocrine axis and responding to a multidisciplinary treatment approach, including psychotherapy, low-dose antidepressant medication, and a moderate exercise program. The trigger points of MPS often respond to structured medical management. If there is any doubt, relief of pain by injection of local anesthetic into a suspected trigger point will relieve the pain of MPS, and confirms the diagnosis. Curiously, injection of trigger points with analgesics, saline, and even distilled water can produce temporary relief.[94,95]

In a small but carefully designed double-blind, crossover study of six patients with myofascial pain syndrome, injections of BTX-A or placebo showed a clear benefit of BTX-A.[96] Patients were selected on the basis of focal pain involving the cervical paraspinal or shoulder girdle muscles, and had discrete trigger points, which when palpated, reproduced a typical pattern of radiating pain for that patient. Patients with diffuse pain or neurological deficits were excluded. Patients were randomly injected with either BTX-A (50 mU in 4 mL normal saline) or normal saline alone on two occasions separated by at least 8 weeks. Trigger points were identically injected in the two or three sites affected on both occasions. Subjects were not told when to expect any relief, and were followed up at weekly intervals for 4 weeks and at 8 weeks after treatment. During the study, other medications for pain relief were not permitted. In addition to investigator palpation and grading of trigger points, pain was assessed both subjectively (visual analog scale) and by the application of a pressure algometer to determine pain threshold in kilograms. A positive response was defined as a reduction from baseline of more than 30% on at least two occasions. Four of six patients responded in this manner. Onset of response occurred within the first week following BTX-A injection, but not at the 30-minute observation time. Mean duration of response was 5 to 6 weeks. One subject responded to both BTX-A and saline, and one subject's pain threshold following BTX-A had not returned to baseline by the time of the placebo injection. Results between the two treatment regimens were statistically significant in favor of BTX and suggest that additional clinical testing for this indication is warranted.

The goal of treatment in MPS should be the restoration of function. Circumspect measures consisting of massage and physical therapy, preferably without using narcotic or nonnarcotic analgesics, are preferred, with the addition of lifestyle change to reduce psychosocial stressors in the home and at work where needed. If these measures fail, local anesthetics with steroids should be injected up to a maximum of three times in 6 weeks. If the pain is relieved but returns quickly, a trial of BTX injection therapy may provide longer lasting benefit. Besides providing a longer period of pain relief, this strategy may facilitate physical therapy and promote long-term improvement in quality of life.

Dosing Considerations

Once the decision is made to consider BTX for the treatment of MPS or headache, the key questions are which patient will best benefit from this therapy, what dose to administer (in what concentration and in what diluent), and how to do it. Unfortunately, the answers to these questions are still uncertain. Until more studies are performed, only general guidelines are available from the currently available literature.

Whom to Inject? As with any new therapy, especially one that is expensive, it makes sense to use BTXs only in more refractory cases until the treatment becomes established and pharmacoeconomics data is supportive. In the case of headache management, avoiding a single emergency room visit or multiple office visits, or seeing a significant reduction in expensive tripton use could easily sway the economic balance to using BTXs if the preliminary study results are confirmed in subsequent trials. In MPS, the potential for significant reduction in medication use and complete resolution of symptoms in a substantial portion of refractory cases is a strong argument in support of BTX use. In both conditions, quality of life and functional improvement can be measurably improved.

Where to Inject? With MPS, most investigators have injected active trigger points directly or used a grid pattern (Lang's method) around them to get more diffuse spread through the involved muscle.[44] Scalene or psoas compartment injections under fluoroscopic guidance can be used with success to target adjacent muscles. In the lower back, trigger points in deeper paraspinals are not as easily felt and the limited studies that have been published have either *chased tenderness or spasm* as their guide for which muscles to inject. In tension-type headache management, most investigators have *chased the tenderness* and injected posterior neck muscles (upper trapezius, levator scapulae, and suboccipitals), and, if tender, temporalis, frontalis, suboccipitals also have been injected.

How much to Inject? Cervical and VII nerve dystonia data has been used as a starting point for BTX-A dose calculations with adjustments depending upon the size of the muscle and degree of spasm. Extensive clinical experience with BTX-A supports this extrapolation to MPS/headache, but with BTX-B, it will be important to be cautious and start at a maximum of 2,500 U to 5,000 U and move upward, depending upon clinical response until data from current studies provides dose-response information.

The total maximum dose per visit for BTX (Botox) typically should not exceed 300 to 400 U (although many have gone as high as 600–700 U safely for numerous involved muscles as in diffuse spasticity/dystonia) and intervals between doses should be no less than 3 months. Following these general guidelines will reduce adverse events (primarily weakness) and antibody formation. Little data is available to help one decide on BTX-B dosing outside of cervical dystonia. It appears to be about 40 to 50 times less potent than BTX-A, with very few patients having received doses at or above 20,000 U, although these doses appear to be well tolerated. In the cervical dystonia data, BTX-B produced duration of effect between 12 and 16 weeks.

Larger volumes of injectant and doses of neurotoxin may influence the tendency for excess BTX to diffuse to nontargeted sites (adjacent muscles or remote sites). This becomes a concern especially with anterior neck injections where electromyogram guidance and low volumes of injectant (BTX-A 100 U/cc or BTX-B 5,000 U/cc) should be used. The technique of using multiple injection sites within the muscle appears to reduce unwanted side effects as does using electromyogram guidance to target motor end plates, thus allowing one to use fewer toxins.

What to Use as Diluent? Allergan recommends that only preservative-free saline (PFNS) is used as the diluent, and that once it is added to reconstitute Botox, it should be used within 4 hours because of concerns of compromised sterility and infection risk. Elan Pharmaceuticals also recommends that PFNS be used if one desires a more dilute concentration of Myobloc than 5,000 U/cc and, although the unopened toxin is stable for months at room temperature, once opened, the toxin should be used within 4 hours because of infection concern.

The use of preservative-free local anesthetic as a diluent, although outside of labeling from the manufacturers, does not denature the protein (as long as bicarbonate is not added to neutralize the acidic pH of the local anesthetic) and certainly helps to decrease local injection pain.[97] In MPS, numerous studies document that local anesthetics seem not to interfere with toxin efficacy, although studies comparing local anesthetics versus PFNS have not been done. Additionally, whether volume of diluent makes a difference in efficacy is not know, although studies are in progress to answer this question.[98]

Is Targeting of Injections Needed? The use of fluoroscopic or electromyogram guidance to identify the muscle or localize the motor end plate prior to injections appears to be a benefit in some situations (particularly in the anterior neck and the deep paraspinal muscles, and possibly to reduce unwanted remote spread by targeting motor end plates with lower toxin doses), but other clinicians have not shown that this technique is necessary when the muscles and trigger points are easily palpable.

Conclusion

BTXs appear to be a useful treatment in refractory MPS and headache. Presumably BTXs work by breaking the spasm–pain cycle, giving the patient a "window of opportunity" for traditional conservative measures to have a greater beneficial impact, but several studies suggest that a direct antinociceptive effect distinct from any reduction in muscle spasm may be at play. The major benefit of BTXs compared with standard therapies is duration of response.

We do not advocate that BTXs be used as a first-line treatment for MPS or headache. However, in refractory cases where nothing else has worked, it may offer a chance for improvement or cure not otherwise available. Data from studies presently being conducted will help us decide where to place BTX in our pain treatment continuum. For now, it remains an off-label, but increasingly accepted, approach in patients with refractory myofascial pain and headache, who, despite multidisciplinary approaches, continue to suffer.

ACKNOWLEDGMENT

We are grateful to Mike A. Royal, MD, OK for allowing us to take excerpts from his article "The use of botulinum toxins in the management of pain and headache" (*Pain Practice* 2001;1(3): 215–235).

REFERENCES

1. Van Ermengem E. A new anaerobic bacillus and its relation to botulism. *Rev Infect Dis* 1979;1:701–719.
2. Snipe PT, Sommer H. Studied on botulinus toxin. 3. Acid precipitation of botulinus toxin. *J Infect Dis* 1928;43:152–160.
3. Shantz EJ. Historical perspective. In: Jankovic J, Hallett M, eds. *Therapy with Botulinum Toxin.* New York, NY: Marcel Dekker; 1994:_ 23–36____.
4. Scott AB, Rosenbaum AL, Collins CC. Pharmacologic weakening of extra-ocular muscles. *Invest Ophthalmol* 1973;12:924–927.
5. Scott AB. Botulinum toxin injection into extra-ocular muscles as an alternative to strabismus surgery. *Ophthalmology* 1980;87:1044–1049.
6. Tsui JKC. Botulinum toxin as a therapeutic agent. *Pharmacol Ther* 1996;72:13–24.
7. Jankovic J, Hallett M, eds. *Therapy with Botulinum Toxin.* New York, NY: Marcel Dekker; 1994.
8. DasGupta BR. Structures of botulinum neurotoxin, its functional domains, and perspectives on the crystalline type A toxin. In: Jankovic J, Hallett M, eds. *Therapy with Botulinum Toxin.* New York, NY: Marcel Dekker; 1994:15–39.
9. Hesse S, Lucke D, Malezic M, et al. Botulinum toxin treatment for lower limb extensor spasticity in chronic hemiparetic patients. *J Neurol Neurosurg Psychol* 1994;57:1321–1324.
10. Sellin LC, Thesless S, Dasgupta BR. Different effects of types A and B botulinum toxin on transmitter release at the rat neuromuscular junction. *Acta Physiol Scand* 1983;119(2):127–133.
11. Sellin LC, Kauffman JA, Dasgupta BR. Comparison of the effects of botulinum neurotoxin types A and E at the rat neuromuscular junction. *Med Biol* 1983;61(2):120–125.
12. Kauffman JA, Way JF, Siegel LS, Sellin LC. Comparison of the action of types A and F botulinum toxin at the rat neuromuscular junction. *Toxicol Appl Pharmacol* 1985;79(2):211–217.
13. Schantz EJ, Johnson EA. Preparation and characterization of botulinum toxin type A for human treatment. In: Jankovic J, Hallett M, eds. *Therapy with Botulinum Toxin.* New York, NY: Marcel Dekker; 1994:41–49.
14. Sugiyama H. *Clostridium botulinum* neurotoxin. *Microbiol Rev* 1980; 44:419–448.
15. Moyor E, Settler PE. Botulinum toxin type B: experimental and clinical experience In: Jankovic J, Hallett M, eds. *Therapy with Botulinum Toxin.* New York, NY: Marcel Dekker; 1994:71–86.
16. Borodic GE, Pearce LB, Smith KL, et al. Botulinum B toxin as an alternative to botulinum A toxin: a histology study. *Ophthal Plast Reconstr Surg* 1993;9:182–190.
17. Greene P, Fahn S. Use of botulinum toxin type F injections to treat torticollis in patients with immunity to botulinum toxin type A. *Mov Disord* 1993;8:479–483.
18. Ludlow CL, Hallett M, Rhew K, et al. Therapeutic use of type F botulinum toxin. *N Engl J Med* 1992;326:349–350.
19. DasGupta BR. Structure and biological activity of botulinum neurotoxin. *J Physiol (Paris)* 1990:84:220–228.
20. Montecucco C. How do tetanus and botulinum toxins bind to neuronal membranes? *Trends Biochem Sci* 1986:11:314–317.
21. Evans DM, Williams RS, Shone CC, Hambleton P, Melling J, Dolly JO. Botulinum neurotoxin type B: its purification, radioiodination and interaction with rat-brain synaptosomal membranes. *Eur J Biochem* 1986:154:409–416.
22. Black JD, Dolly JO. Interaction of 125I-labeled botulinum neurotoxins with nerve terminals. I. Ultrastructural autoradiographic localization and quantitation of distinct membrane acceptors for types A and B on motor nerves. *J Cell Biol* 1986:103:521–534.
23. Burgen AS, Dickens VF, Zatman LJ. The action of botulinum toxin on the neuromuscular junction. *J Physiol (London)* 1949;109:10–24.
24. Simpson LL. The study of clostridial and related toxins. The search for unique mechanisms and common denominators. *J Physiol (Paris)* 1990;84:143–151.
25. Poulain B, Tauc L, Maisery EA, et al. Neurotransmitter release is blocked intracellularly by botulinum neurotoxin, and this requires uptake of both toxin polypeptides by a process mediated by the larger chain. *Proc Natl Acad Sci USA* 1988;85:4090–4094.
26. Finkelstein A. Channels formed in phospholipid bilayer membranes by diphtheria, tetanus, botulinum and anthrax toxin. *J Physiol (Paris)* 1990;84:188–190.
27. Schiavo G, Boquet P, DasGupta BR, Montecucco C. Membrane interactions of tetanus and botulinum neurotoxins: a photolabelling study with photoactivatable phospholipid. *J Physiol (Paris)* 1990;84:180–187.
28. Duchen LW, Strich SJ. The effects of botulinum toxin on the pattern of innervation of skeletal muscle in the mouse. *Q J Exp Physiol* 1968; 53:84–89.
29. Elston JS. Botulinum toxin treatment of blepharospasm. In: Fahn S, Marsden CD, eds. *Dystonia 2.* New York, NY: Raven Press; 1988: 579–581.
30. Borodic GE, Ferrante R. Histologic effects of repeated botulinum toxin over many years in human orbicularis oculi muscle. *J Clin Neuroophthalmol* 1992;12:121–127.
31. Harris CP, Alderson K, Nebeker J, et al. Histology of human orbicularis muscle Treated with botulinum toxin. *Arch Ophthalmol* 1991; 109:393–395.
32. Borodic GE, Ferrante RJ, Pearce LB, Alderson K. Pharmacology and histology of the therapeutic application of botulinum toxin. In: Jankovic J, Hallett M, eds. *Therapy with Botulinum Toxin.* New York, NY: Marcel Dekker; 1994:119–157.
33. Purkiss J, Welch M, Doward D, Foster K. Capsaicin-stimulated release of substance P from cultured dorsal root ganglion neurons: involvement of two distinct mechanisms. *Biochem Pharmacol* 2000;59: 1403–1406.
34. Welch MJ, Purkiss JR, Foster KA. Sensitivity of embryonic rat dorsal root ganglia neurons to *Clostridium botulinum* neurotoxins. *Toxicon* 2000;38:245–258.
35. Ishikawa H, Mitsui Y, Yoshitomi T, et al. Presynaptic effects of botulinum toxin type A on neuronally evoked response of albino and pigmented rabbit iris sphincter and dilator muscles. *Jpn J Ophthalmol* 2000;44:106–109.
36. Cui ML, Khanijou S, Rubino J, Aoki KR. Botulinum toxin A inhibits the inflammatory pain in the rat formalin model. Poster 246.2. Presented at the Society for Neuroscience Annual Meeting; New Orleans, LA; 2000.
37. Dekker, Inc. 1994. This is a comprehensive textbook devoted to the therapeutic uses of BTX-A and is an excellent starting place for background information. There is also a multiauthor textbook to be published by Lippincott Williams and Williams in spring 2001 by WeMOVE (Worldwide Education and Awareness for Movement Disorders), Brin MF, Jankovic J, and Hallett M, eds.
38. Racz GB. Botulinum toxin as a new approach for refractory pain syndromes. *Pain Digest* 1998;8:353–356.

39. Porta M, Perretti A, Gamba M, Luccarelli G, Fornari M. The rationale and results of treating muscle spasm and myofascial syndromes with botulinum toxin type A. *Pain Digest* 1998;8:346–352.
40. Hatheway CL, Dang C. Immunogenicity of neurotoxins of *Clostridium botulinum*. In: Jankovic J, Hallett M, eds. *Therapy with Botulinum Toxin*. New York, NY: Marcel Dekker; 1994:93–107.
41. Brin MF, Fahn S, Moskowitz C, et al. Localized injections of botulinum toxin for the treatment of focal dystonia and hemifacial spasm. *Mov Disord* 1987;2:237–254.
42. Lew MF, Adornato BT, Duane DD, et al. Botulinum toxin type B: a double-blind placebo-controlled, safety and efficacy study in cervical dystonia. *Neurology* 1997;49:701–707.
43. Abrams BM. Tutorial 36: myofascial pain syndrome and fibromyalgia. *Pain Digest* 1998;8:264–272.
44. Lang AM. Botulinum toxin for myofascial pain. In: *Advancements in the Treatment of Neuromuscular Pain*. Ch 5. Baltimore, MD: Johns Hopkins University Office of Continuing Medical Education Syllabus; 1999:23–28.
45. Atassi MZ, Oshima M. Structure, activity and immune (T and B cell) recognition of botulinum neurotoxins. *Crit Rev Immunol* 1999;19:219–260.
46. Chen R, Karp BI, Hallett M. Botulinum toxin type F for treatment of dystonia: long-term experience. *Neurology* 1998;51:1494–1496.
47. Jankovic J, Schwartz K, Donovan DT. Botulinum toxin treatment of cranial-cervical dystonia, spasmodic dysphonia, other focal dystonias and hemifacial spasm. *J Neurol Neurosurg Psychiatry* 1990;53:633–639.
48. Tsui JKC, Eisen A, Stoessl HA, et al. Double-blind study of botulinum toxin in spasmodic torticollis. *Lancet* 1986;2:245–247.
49. Polo KB, Jabbari B. Botulinum toxin A improved the rigidity of progressive supranuclear palsy. *Ann Neurol* 1994;35:237–239.
50. Porta M. A comparative trial of botulinum toxin type A and methylprednisolone for the treatment of myofascial pain syndrome and pain from chronic muscle spasm.
51. Relja M. Botulinum toxin type A in the treatment of tension-type headache. Presented at the 9th World Congress on Pain; Vienna, Austria; August 22–27, 1999, and at the International Conference 1999: Basic and Therapeutic Aspects of Botulinum and Tetanus Toxins; Orlando, FL; November 16–18, 1999.
52. Schulte-Mattler WJ, Wieser T, Zierz S. Treatment of tension-type headache with botulinum toxin: a pilot study. *Eur J Med Res* 1999;4:183–186. These data were also presented at the International Conference 1999: Basic and Therapeutic Aspects of Botulinum and Tetanus Toxins; Orlando, FL; November 16–18, 1999.
53. Smuts JA, Baker MK, et al. Botulinum toxin type A as prophylactic treatment in chronic tension-type headache. Presented at the International Conference 1999: Basic and Therapeutic Aspects of Botulinum and Tetanus Toxins; Orlando, FL; November 16–18, 1999. See also: Smuts JA, Baker MK, Smuts HM, Theta Stassen JM, Rossouw E, Barnard PWA. Prophylactic treatment of chronic tension-type headache using botulinum toxin type A. *Eur J Neurol* 1999;6(suppl 4):S99–S102.
54. Wheeler AH. Botulinum toxin A, adjunctive therapy for refractory headaches associated with pericranial muscle tension. *Headache* 1998;38:468–471.
55. Barwood S, Baillieu C, Boyd R, et al. Analgesic effects of botulinum toxin A: a randomised, placebo trial. *Dev Med Child Neurol* 2000;42:116–121.
56. Fish DR, Sawyers D, Allen PJ, Blackie JD, Lees AJ, Marsden CD. The effect of sleep on the dyskinetic movements of Parkinson's disease, Gilles de la Tourette syndrome, Huntington's disease, and torsion dystonia. *Arch Neurol* 1991;48:210–214.
57. Poewe W, Wissel J. Experience with botulinum toxin in cervical dystonia. In: Jankovic J, Hallett M, eds. *Therapy with Botulinum Toxin*. New York, NY: Marcel Dekker; 1994:267–278.
58. Sheehy MP, Marsden CD. Writer's cramp—focal dystonia. *Brain* 1982;105:461–480.
59. Hunter D. *The Diseases of Occupations*. 6th ed. London, UK: Hodder & Stoughton; 1978.
60. Gowers WR. *A Manual of Diseases of the Nervous System*. Philadelphia, PA: P. Blakiston; 1888.
61. Albanese A, Bentivoglio AR, Cassetta E, Viggiano A, Maria G, Gui D. Review article: the use of botulinum toxin in the alimentary tract. *Aliment Pharmacol Ther* 1995;9(6):599–604.
62. Cohen LG, Hallett M, Celler BD, Hochberg F. Treatment of focal dystonia of the hand with botulinum toxin injections. *J Neurol Neurosurg Psychaiatry* 1989:52:355–363.
63. Cole RA, Cohen LG, Hallett M. Treatment of musician's cramp with botulinum toxin. *Med Probl Performing Artists* 1991;6:137–143.
64. Poungvarin N. Writer's cramp: the experience with botulinum toxin injections in 25 patients. *J Med Assoc Thai* 1991;74:239–247.
65. Rivest J, Lees AJ, Marsden CD. Writer's cramp: treatment with botulinum toxin injections. *Mov Discord* 1991:6:55–59.
66. Jankovic J, Schwartz KS. Use of botulinum toxin in the treatment of hand dystonia. *J Hand Surg* 1993;18A:883–887.
67. Karp BI, Cole RA, Cohen LG, Grill S, Lou J-S, Hallett M. Long-term botulinum toxin treatment of focal hand dystonia. *Neurology* 1994;44:70–76.
68. Tsui JKC, Bhatt M, Calne S, Clane DB. Botulinum toxin in the treatment of writer's cramp: a double-blind study. *Neurology* 1993;43:183–185.
69. Cole R, Hallett M, Cohen LG. Double-blind trial of botulinum toxin for treatment of focal hand dystonia. *Move Discord*. 1995;10:466–471.
70. Young RR. Treatment of spastic paresis. *N Engl J Med* 1989:320:1553–1555.
71. Burke D. Critical examination of the case for or against fusimotor involvement in disorder of muscle tone. In: Desmedt JE, ed. *Motor Control Mechanisms in Health and Disease*. New York, NY: Raven Press; 1983:133–150.
72. Dimitrijevic MR. Spasticity and rigidity. In: Jankovic J, Tolosa E, eds. *Parkinson's Disease and Movement Disorders*. 2nd ed. Baltimore, MD: Williams and Wilkins; 1993:443–453.
73. Simpson DM, Alexander DN, O'Brien CF, et al. Botulinum toxin type A in the treatment of upper extremity spasticity: a randomized, double-blind, placebo-controlled trial. *Neurology* 1996;46(5):1306–1310.
74. Gordon J. Spinal mechanisms of motor coordination. In: Kandel ER, Schwartz JH, Jessell TM, eds. *Principles of Neural Science*. 3rd ed. Norwalk, CT: Appleton & Lange; 1991:581–595.
75. Delwaide PJ, Yoiung (Young) RR, Eds. *Clinical Neurophysiology in Spasticity*. Amsterdam, The Netherlands: Elsevier; 1985.
76. Young RR. Physiologic and pharmacologic approaches to spasticity. *Neurol Clin* 1987;5:529–539.
77. Katz RT. Management of spasticity. *Am J Phys Med Rehabil* 1988:67:108–116.
78. Gans BM, Glenn MB. Introduction. In: Glenn MB, Whyte J, eds. *The Practical Management of Spasticity in Children and Adults*. Philadelphia, PA: Lea & Febiger; 1990:1–7.
79. Mayer NH. Functional management of spasticity after head injury. *J Neurol Rehab* 1991;5:S1–S4.
80. Lehmkuhl LD, Thoi LL, Baize C, Kelley CJ, Krawcryk L, Bontke CF. Multimodality treatment of joint contractures in patients with severe brain injury: cost, effectiveness, and integration of therapies in the application of seria Vinhibitive casta. serial/inhibitive casts *J Head Trauma Rehabil* 1990;5:23–42.
81. Carthidge NE, Hudgson P, Weightman D. A comparison of baclofen and diazepam in the treatment of spasticity. *J Neurol Sci* 1974:23:17–24.
82. Whyte J, Robinson KM. Pharmacologic management. In: Glenn MB, Whyte J, eds. *The Practical Management of Spasticity in Children and Adults*. Philadelphia, PA: Lea & Febiger; 1990:201–226.
83. Chan CH. Dantrolene sodium and hepatic injury. *Neurology* 1999;40:1427–1432.

84. Reeves KD, Baker A. Mixed somatic peripheral nerve block for painful or intractable spasticity: a review of 30 years of use. *AJPM* Am J Phys Med Rehabil 1992;2:205–210.
85. Glenn MB. Nerve blocks. In: Glenn MB, Whyte J, eds. *The Practical Management of Spasticity in Children and Adults*. Philadelphia, PA: Lea & Febiger; 1990:227–258.
86. Kasdon KL, Abromovitz JN. Neurosurgical approaches. In: Glenn MB, Whyte J, eds. *The Practical Management of Spasticity in Children and Adults*. Philadelphia, PA: Lea & Febiger; 1990:259–267.
87. Albright AL, Barron WB, Fasick MP, Polinko P, Janosky J. Continuous intrathecal baclofen infusion for spasticity of cerebral origin. *JAMA* 1993;270:2476–2477.
88. Bowers DN, Averill A. Intrathecal baclofen for Intractable spasticity due to severe traumatic brain injury (abstract). *Arch Phys Med Rehabil* 1991;72:816.
89. Meythaler JM. Use of intrathecal baclofen in brain injury patients (abstract). *Arch Phys Med Rehabil* 1994;75:1036.
90. Shaari CM, Sanders I. Assessment of the biological activity of botulinum toxin. In: Jankovic J, Hallett M, eds. *Therapy with Botulinum Toxin.* New York, NY: Marcel Dekker; 1994:159–170.
91. Han SC, Harrison P. Myofascial pain syndrome and trigger-point management. *Reg Anesth* 1995;65:167–70.
92. Flax HJ. Myofascial pain syndromes—the great mimicker. *Bol Asoc Med P R* 1995;65:167–170.
93. Schneider MJ. Tender points/fibromyalgia vs. trigger points/myofascial pain syndrome: a need for clarity in terminology and differential diagnosis. *J Manipulative Physiol Ther* 1995;65:398–406.
94. Tschopp KP, Gysin C. Local injection therapy in 107 patients with myofascial pain syndrome of the head and neck. *ORL J Otorhinolaryngol Relat Spec* 1996;58:306–310.
95. Wreje U, Brorsson B. A multicenter randomized controlled trial of injections of sterile water and saline for chronic myofascial pain syndromes. *Pain* 1995;65:441–444.
96. Cheshire WP, Abashian SW, Mann JD. Botulinum toxin in the treatment of myofascial pain syndrome. *Pain* 1994;59:65–69.
97. Holz RW, Fisher SK. Synaptic transmission and cellular signaling; an overview. In: Siegal GJ, Siegel, GJ et al., eds. *Basic Neurochemistry: Molecular, Cellular and Medical Aspects*. 6th ed. Ch 10. Lippincott-Raven OK Publishers; 1999:191–212.
98. Note that because albumin is a derivative from human blood, despite effective donor screening and manufacturing processes an extremely remote risk for transmission of viral diseases and Creutzfeldt-Jakob disease exists. To date, no case of such transmission has ever been identified for albumin.

CHAPTER 71 NEURAXIAL DRUG DELIVERY

Stuart L. Du Pen and Anna R. Du Pen

The use of neuraxial analgesia for the goal of functional analgesia is the next step beyond the optimum use of oral and transcutaneous analgesia. The goal of pain relief with functional restitution should be the guiding light of all approaches of analgesia. Once a patient with acute, chronic, or cancer-related pain has been prescribed a trial of opioids and adjuvant drugs, side effects having been either treated or avoided with opioid sequential trials, then consideration should be given to alternative delivery sources. Neuraxial analgesia, with either single agent or a combination of drugs, may allow the patient to achieve relief of intractable pain when opioid analgesia alone has its limits.

The discovery of the analgesic effects of neuraxial opioids, alkaloids, and peptides has led to the expanded use of regional anesthesia in long-term analgesic delivery systems. Today the choices of analgesic agents include opioids, α_2-agonists, SNX-111, local anesthetic agents, and there are sure to be additional agents added in the future. The clinician will always be faced with a decision of when, what, and how. Patient selection, device selection, and route of delivery are and will likely continue to be the key questions.

In this chapter we approach the patient in pain with options for neuraxial analgesia. This includes discussions of drug choices and pharmacology, patient selection, and optimization of conservative therapy. Issues of delivery routes and device selection are explored, and lastly, we give the reader insights into identification and treatment of side effects and complications.

SPINAL DRUG THERAPY

Spinal opioids have been used in clinical practice routinely since the late 70s. Epidural analgesia for postsurgical, obstetric, and intractable cancer-related pain is considered standard medical care. Intrathecal opioid therapy for chronic noncancer pain has become an increasingly routine therapeutic approach over the last 10 years, although reimbursement issues continue to be problematic in some states with some payers.

Perhaps the most exciting new developments are in the area of alternative agents that are being, or may soon be, used in spinal drug delivery systems. The escalation of basic science research exploring new spinally active agents has been brisk in the last decade, and with newly committed funding for pain research at the National Institutes of Health, the next decade will surely bring an explosion of research and discovery in neuroaxial pharmacology.

There continue to be major advances in systemic opioid management, particularly the advent of long-acting oxycodone, transdermal and transmucosal fentanyl, and the soon to be released long-acting hydromorphone. These advances, and the controversy surrounding the potential link between M3G and neurotoxicity,[1] have left expert clinicians debating if morphine is still the standard drug of choice or just one of many choices for systemic therapy. There is not much debate, however, over morphine's superiority when administered spinally, particularly for chronic cancer and noncancer administration.

Morphine

It seems clear that the potency of spinally administered opioids is inversely related to its lipophilicity. Spinal concentrations of opioid after epidural administration are a result of the balance between vascular and meningeal permeability, which is influenced by lipid solubility. Although epidural morphine, with its hydrophilic profile, is up to 10 times more potent that intravenous morphine, many lipophilic agents are essentially equipotent when given either intravenously or epidurally.[2,3] In the arena of postoperative pain management, the epidural administration of lipophilic opioid alone may offer no marked clinical advantages compared with the intravenous route.[4]

The clearest advantage with spinally administered morphine is reduction of side effects associated with systemic blood levels. There is predictable vascular uptake with epidural morphine, but very little systemic impact with intrathecal morphine (Fig. 71-1). In the patient with opioid-responsive pain for whom systemic morphine provides good to excellent relief but causes unmanageable systemic side effects, epidural or intrathecal morphine will likely provide a good outcome. The hydrophilic properties of morphine allow for a long duration of action that makes it amenable to bolus dosing. These authors have taught hundreds of cancer patients to self-administer epidural morphine boluses on a scheduled basis at home. The average opioid-tolerant cancer patient will require 8 mg of epidural morphine on an every 8-hour schedule. This is generally a cost-effective way to provide epidural analgesia; however, it is only likely to succeed in those patients with nociceptive pain (i.e., no neuropathic or mixed pain character).

Bolus epidural morphine dosing can be problematic. Postoperatively, in the opioid naïve patient, the side effect that has the most potential to produce adverse outcomes with epidural morphine is delayed respiratory depression. Studies indicate that morphine's cephalad migration after a lumbar epidural bolus follows a predictable time course to the brainstem, where respiratory depression can occur.[5,6] Additionally, several authors make a good case that continuous infusion of morphine may provide better analgesia for postoperative pain management.[7–9] At least one study, however, indicated that there were significantly more dose escalations in patients treated with continuous infusion of epidural morphine versus bolus administration, leaving open the question of a differential effect for mode of administration on tolerance development.[10] Today, in managing chronic cancer or noncancer pain, this issue is rarely relevant. Patients with nociceptive pain can almost always be managed with less invasive therapy. Most advanced cancer patients requiring spinal therapy also need either local anesthetics or clonidine coadministered, which requires infusion, and most noncancer patients will likely be treated with implanted pump systems

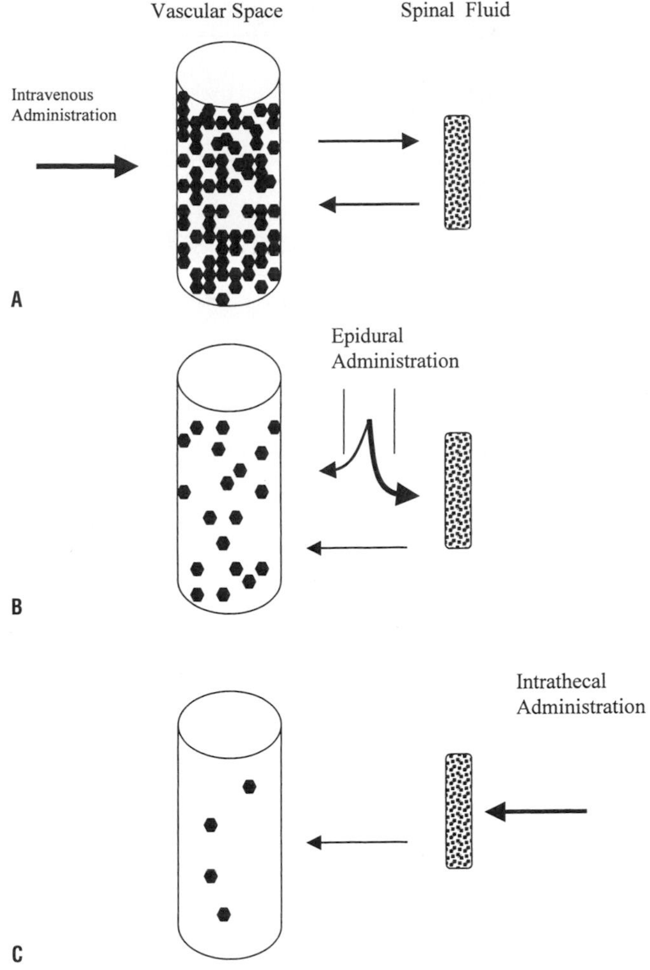

Figure 71-1 (**A**). Systemic infusion of opioids. (**B**) Epidural infusion of opioids. (**C**) Intrathecal infusion of opioids. Each example shows the diffusion and transport of drug from the site of infusion into the vascular and intrathecal spaces.

that are generally continuous infusion (intermittent dosing is possible with the computerized versions of the implanted pump systems).[11]

The choice of epidural versus intrathecal drug delivery is framed primarily around diagnosis, prognosis, severity of side effects, and cost-versus-benefit markers. Morphine is used widely both epidurally and intrathecally with internalized and externalized approaches. In the United States postoperative and terminal cancer patients have generally had epidural approaches and patients with noncancer pain syndromes have generally had implanted morphine pump systems. Over the past 5 years the European anesthesia community has increasingly published papers on the efficacy and safety of percutaneous intrathecal morphine infusions for terminal cancer patients.[12–14]

Morphine is the only Food and Drug Administration (FDA)-approved opioid for intrathecal delivery, and it is used widely in the long-term treatment of noncancer pain syndromes. A retrospective, multicenter, survey-based study reported by Paice et al examined outcomes for intrathecal morphine therapy in 429 patients (roughly two thirds noncancer and one third cancer).[15] For all patients the mean percent pain relief was 61%. Patients with somatic pain syndromes tend to have greater relief than those with neuropathic pain syndromes. Roughly 20% of the patients had bupivacaine added to the morphine. Anderson and Burchiel reported prospectively on 40 patients with severe noncancer pain that had been poorly managed on systemic medications.[11] Ten of the 40 patients failed a trial for intrathecal morphine therapy. Thirty patients had reported pain relief and were implanted with intrathecal delivery devices. Two years later, one half of the patients were still reporting at least a 25% reduction in pain as assessed by the visual analog scale (VAS).

There has been some concern about the neurologic sequelae related to high-dose morphine in the spinal canal. Cabbell and colleagues reported three cases of intrathecal granuloma formation at the spinal catheter tip, which they thought were associated with high-dose morphine (25 mg/day and up).[16] North et al previously described a case of a granulomatous mass at the tip of an intrathecal catheter causing spinal cord compression.[17] A recent survey, however, indicated that the overall incidence of this phenomenon was less than 1%.[18]

Alternate Opioids

Hydromorphone is used frequently as a second-line drug intraspinally, although it is not FDA approved for spinal use. Hydromorphone's lipid solubility is intermediate between morphine and fentanyl.[19] The rostral spread of hydromorphone in the cerebrospinal fluid (CSF) is similar to morphine after a bolus dose in the lumbar epidural space; it has a comparatively faster onset of action and shorter duration of action than morphine.[20] Halpern and associates reported no difference between morphine and hydromorphone in pain relief or in the incidence and severity of side effects.[21] Chaplan et al found the quality of analgesia with epidural morphine versus hydromorphone to be similar, but with a four-fold increase in pruritis in the morphine group.[22] Liu and coworkers studied intravenous versus epidural hydromorphone in radical prostatectomy and noted that patients in the intravenous group required twice as much drug, whereas patients in the epidural group had a greater incidence of pruritus.[23] Epidural administration did not appear to be associated with improved analgesia, patient satisfaction, or enhanced clinical outcomes when compared with the intravenous route.

Fentanyl has been used as an alternate opioid. Multiple studies have seemed to indicate no benefit for postoperative pain management for epidural versus intravenous fentanyl.[3,24,25] Epidural fentanyl has been associated with less nausea and pruritus than morphine.[26,27] Sufentanil is a highly lipophilic opioid with a high level of intrinsic efficacy that may require a relatively low-receptor occupancy. De Leon-Casasola and Lema make a strong argument for sufentanil's utility in the setting of morphine-tolerant cancer patients with severe postoperative pain.[8,28]

Local Anesthetics

Opioid-local anesthetic combinations are used widely in postoperative and cancer-related pain management, and to a lesser extent in chronic noncancer pain management. In animal studies local anesthetics and opioids have demonstrated a synergistic potentiation of antinociceptive effects.[29] Bupivacaine is the most commonly used local anesthetic in pain management, owing primarily to its long duration of action. Literally thousands of patients have successfully been treated with epidural morphine-bupivacaine combination therapy for postoperative pain. An excellent large prospective study done by de Leon-Casasola and associates reported on over 4000 patients who had received epidural morphine-bupivacaine therapy.[30] The average length of therapy was 6 days, with nausea and pruritus each occurring in 22% of patients. Respiratory depression was reported in only three patients (0.07%).

Fentanyl-bupivacaine infusions are also used extensively in acute pain management and generally may have some side effect advantages over morphine-bupivacaine.[26,27,31] The often-expected goal of reducing opioid when the bupivacaine is added may not always be achievable or may be dose-dependent. One study examined 0.1% bupivacaine as an "add-on" to epidural fentanyl in 40 patients after major abdominal surgery. The epidural fentanyl infusion of 10 μg/mL (with or without 0.1% bupivacaine) was titrated to adequate pain relief during forced inspiration. Patients reported similar median pain scores and were equally satisfied with pain relief in both groups, and the fentanyl infusion rate and plasma concentration were comparable. Respiratory and cardiovascular functions were preserved, and the incidence of nausea, pruritus, and drowsiness were similar. The investigators concluded that in low concentrations bupivacaine did not reduce the titrated dose of epidural fentanyl required for adequate pain relief during forced inspiration.[32] Sufentanil and bupivacaine are also used in combination and have been reported to provide effective analgesia during labor at reduced doses compared with either single drug alone.[33]

Epidural morphine-bupivacaine combinations are also the mainstay of cancer-related pain. Epidural bupivacaine infusions administered long term have been safely administered even with plasma bupivacaine concentrations as high as 10.8 μg/mL.[34] A combination of low-dose epidural morphine (0.5 to 1.5 mg/hour) and low-concentration bupivacaine (0.1% to 0.125%) in a 5- to 10-mL/hour volume effectively targets the most commonly seen intractable cancer pain syndromes: breast or lung carcinoma that has metastasized to the spine and is causing a severe mixed pain character syndrome. The severity of motion-related pain in these patients often causes the window between pain relief with function and side effects to be exceedingly narrow.[35] The disadvantages of using epidural bupivacaine results primarily from the sensorimotor blockade. At low to moderate concentrations of epidural bupivacaine, patients often experience cutaneous numbness in the expected dermatomal distribution. This numbness can be transient, and is often positional. Many patients that sleep on one side will awaken with "downside" numbness that will resolve with repositioning. In patients who require high concentrations of epidural bupivacaine (≥0.16%), significant sensory loss and motor dysfunction can occur. Orthostatic blood pressure can also be significant, particularly in the end-stage dehydrated cancer population.

Bupivacaine-containing solutions are also used successfully with morphine via the intrathecal route in patients with cancer and chronic noncancer pain syndromes.[35–37] Intrathecally administered bupivacaine is also limited by sensorimotor blockade or hemodynamic instability.[38,39] Clinically relevant side effects usually are not observed with doses <15 mg per day.[40]

Ropivacaine has emerged as a potential alternate to bupivacaine for pain management. Ropivacaine has sensory block advantages, providing a greater degree of dissociation between sensory and motor effects.[41] This agent may prove to be helpful in combination with epidural opioids in cancer pain management where the balance between pain relief and functionality can be narrow, particularly in patients with spinal nerve impingement from vertebral metastasis. Ropivacaine has also been used intrathecally in cancer pain management.[42]

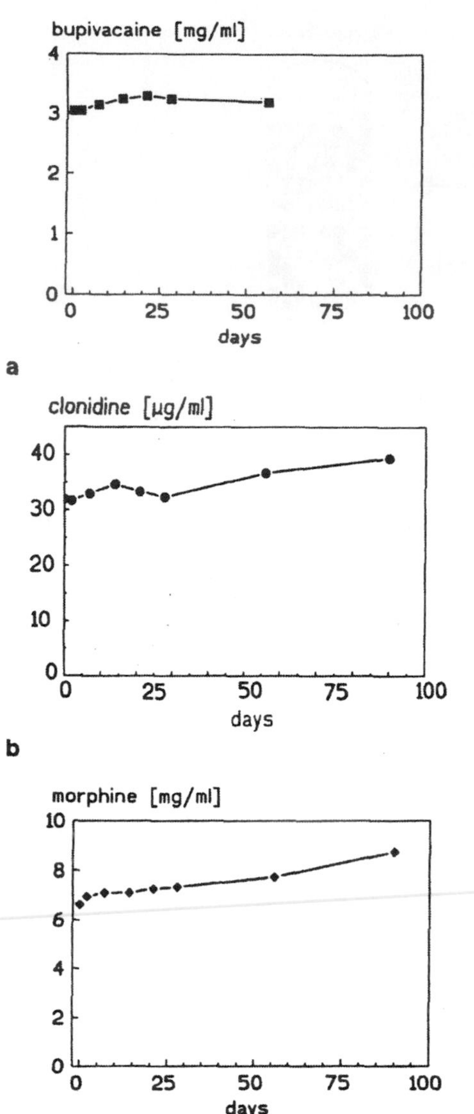

Figure 71-2 Stability of the concentration of bupivacaine hydrochloride (**A**), clonidine hydrochloride (**B**), and morphine hydrochloride (**C**) during combined storage in portable pump reservoirs. The concentration of bupivacaine after 90 days was not determined due to a technical problem with the high-performance liquid chromatography setting for bupivacaine at that time.

Pharmacy Admixture Issues

The mixing of agents together, particularly for long-term administration, raises issues of stability, compatibility, and infection control. A number of investigators have reported on laboratory experiments. Christen and coworkers looked at bupivacaine and hydromorphone.[43] Bupivacaine hydrochloride 625 and 1250 μg/mL and hydromorphone hydrochloride 20 and 100 μg/mL were mixed in 0.9% sodium chloride injection and found to be stable and compatible for up to 72 hours under fluorescent light when stored in polyvinyl chloride containers at 24°C. The physical and chemical properties of multiple drugs in solutions have also been examined.[44] Bupivacaine, morphine, and clonidine were stored in reservoir bags for up to 90 days. The bags contained (1) bupivacaine 0.75% alone, (2.) morphine 2% alone, and (3) morphine 6.66 mg/mL plus bupivacaine

3 mg/mL plus clonidine 30 μg/mL. No macroscopic or microbiologic signs of precipitation, change in color, or contamination were observed, and pH remained stable. None of the three drugs declined in concentration during the observation period. A small increase in concentration of all three drugs did occur over time, most probably due to evaporation processes (Fig. 71-2). Cook et al examined six mixtures of diamorphine-bupivacaine, representing the range of clinically useful concentrations.[45] Solutions were studied for antibacterial activity against common contaminants: *Escherichia coli*, *Pseudomonas aeruginosa*, *Enterococcus faecalis*, and a coagulase-negative *Staphylococcus* species. Challenge experiments used an inoculum or approximately 5.0 × 10^6^ cfu/mL. Mixtures were incubated at 30°C for 5 to 7 days. Viable counts of all organisms decreased with time for all the formulations tested. Formulations containing 0.5% bupivacaine were rapidly bactericidal, and increasing diamorphine concentrations increased this effect. The authors argue against frequent infusion changes. Another group of investigators combined diamorphine and bupivacaine in 100-mL bags for use with a patient-controlled analgesia pump and found no significant change in concentration of either drug over a period of 8 days.[46] Several other studies on long-term stability have been done on morphine-bupivacaine and fentanyl-bupivacaine mixtures.[47–50]

Other Spinally Active Agents

α-Adrenergic Drugs Clonidine is an α-adrenergic agonist that has been used for spinal administration in Europe for many years, but only received FDA approval in the United States in 1997.[51] Spinal clonidine has been shown to demonstrate a dose-dependent duration of analgesia in the acute setting for more than 12 hours with a dose of 450 μg.[52] There is evidence that clonidine has synergistic properties with both opioids and local anesthetics. Brunschwiler and colleagues reported that clonidine 150 μg produced a "local anesthetic sparing effect," prolonging continuous spinal anesthesia with bupivacaine significantly longer than morphine 150 μg.[53] Patients receiving 30 μg of intrathecal clonidine with 2.5 or 5 μg of sufentanil had significantly longer lasting analgesia.[54]

Clonidine has been shown to effectively impact neuropathic pain in animal models.[55,56] This is perhaps its greatest potential. Eisenach and associates did a multicenter study looking at cancer-related pain. Eight-five cancer patients were treated with patient-controlled epidural morphine with placebo or epidural clonidine (30 μg/hour). Neuropathic pain was significantly reduced in patients who received clonidine, although the frequency or quantity of morphine was not influenced. Hypotension and bradycardia were the most frequently observed side effect.[57] Rauke and associates studied epidural clonidine in the treatment of complex regional pain syndrome (CRPS).[58] Twenty-six patients received 300 μg, 700 μg, or placebo. Results showed significant analgesia within 20 minutes of injection compared with placebo. Nineteen patients went on to have clonidine administered by continuous epidural infusion; weekly VAS scores were significantly reduced to an average of 5/10 compared with 8/10 prior to clonidine therapy.

Hassenbusch and coworkers treated 32 patients with intrathecal clonidine (all but three with CRPS) in doses ranging from 480 to 900 μg/day. Fifty-six percent of patients had improvements in both their pain rating scale scores and CRPS symptoms. Systemic hypotension was observed at intermediate doses, but was eliminated at doses ≥40 μg/hour, and mostly observed with doses between 17 and 25 μg/hour.[40]

Tizanidine (often called the "son of clonidine") is another α-adrenergic drug that produces antinociception in a similar manner to clonidine but without the pronounced hemodynamic changes when administered intrathecally in animal studies.[59,60] These drugs are likely to remain an important part of neuraxial treatment of neuropathic pain.

Somatostatin Analogs Numerous investigators in the 70s and 80s published data describing the localization of somatostatin as a substance intrinsic to spinal cord interneurons in the superficial layers of the dorsal horn, displaying inhibitory effects on nociceptive neurons.[61–64] Penn and coworkers described their experience with six cancer patients using octreotide, an analog of somatostatin.[65] Patients experienced reduced pain and decreased oral opioid usage without central or systemic side effects. Somatostatin has since been isolated in the periaqueductal gray, in substantia gelatinosa of the spinal cord, and in descending modulatory systems from the brain, seeming to confirm a role in inhibition; however, two of eight patients appeared to have demonstrable histopathologic changes noted at autopsy.[66]

SNX–111 N-type calcium channel antagonists have been shown to be consistently antinociceptive in animal models.[67–69] Early results in humans have continued to show efficacy.[70,71] Staats et al reported on 102 patients treated in a double-blind, randomized, placebo-controlled trial of the efficacy and safety of SNX-111.[72] Results indicated a significant decrease in pain intensity when compared with placebo. Adverse events included dizziness, nausea, nystagmus, abnormal gait, constipation, confusion, and urinary retention.

Ketamine Spinally administered NMDA-receptor antagonists have been studied in animal models.[73,74] The relationships between opioids and NMDA antagonists continue to be explored. In a double-blind, controlled trial, one group of investigators administered doses of alfentanil and ketamine, or their combination, to normal volunteers and found no advantage of the combination over a larger dose of either drug alone in relieving pain caused by chemical stimulation.[75] These authors concluded that the opioid and NMDA-antagonist interaction was one of simple additivity and not synergy. Chia and others added ketamine 0.4 mg/mL to a standard patient-controlled epidural analgesia mixture of 0.02 mg/mL morphine, epinephrine 4 μg/mL, and 0.8 mg/mL bupivacaine in a postoperative double-blind study (N = 91). Patients in the group with ketamine had significantly lower VAS scores both at rest and with coughing and movement, and patients in the control group used more of the morphine-epinephrine-bupivacaine mixture at both the 24-hour and 48-hour assessment points.[76] Wong and associates demonstrated that ketamine coadministration with epidural morphine potentiates morphine's analgesic effect via a single bolus injection.[77] Ketamine and its oral relative dextromethorphan have failed to gain much clinical acceptance as adjuvants because of CNS side effects.

Future Development

Allan Basbaum looked to the future in a recent 25-year anniversary monograph from the International Association for the Study of Pain and noted the promise of molecular biology in "deleting" genes from the different opioid receptors.[78] He noted the ability to target drugs to the spinal cord through selective gene manipulation. One startling new discovery gives us a preview of what the future of neuraxial drug delivery could hold: orphanin FQ/nociceptin.[79] The defining of the δ-opioid receptor gene sequence in the early to mid 90s led to cloning of three receptors, μ, κ, and a previously undescribed receptor referred to as an "opioid-like orphan receptor." This orphan receptor has an endogenous ligand known as orphanin FQ/nociceptin or OFQ/N (an amino acid peptide) that is widely distributed throughout the nervous system. Investigators have reported an apparent lack of "motivational" effects,[80] indicating the lack of abuse potential and the presence of antihyperalgesic and antiallodynic effects[81] that may have efficacy for neuropathic pain.

The interesting pharmacologic aspect of this agent is that OFQ/N has potent opioid-antagonist actions in the CNS; however, at the spinal cord level, it has opioid-like activity and no anti-opioid effect. This combination of clinical properties has the potential for providing pain relief in the periphery while avoiding concurrent CNS side effects, and more importantly, avoiding centrally mediated opioid-induced hyperalgesia in the persistent pain model.

PATIENT SELECTION

The patient selection process for neuraxial drug delivery is arguably the most significant step toward achieving a successful outcome. No patient should receive an implant without having first received optimum conservative therapy. The primary goals of patient selection are to confirm the indications for implantation, evaluate the psychological stability of the patient, and estimate the patient's future responsiveness to the treatment plan. A comprehensive analgesic history should be part of the primary assessment of the patient. The comprehensive history will give the practitioner a detailed history of side effects and adverse reactions from the patient's previous exposure to oral opioids and adjuvant therapy. Oral opioids are the mainstay of treating cancer pain, and are increasingly accepted as a long-term alternative for chronic nonmalignant pain. Opioids should be aggressively titrated to pain relief or to side effects. The optimization of adjuvant analgesic drugs should precede spinal drug delivery. Nonsteroidal anti-inflammatory drugs (NSAIDs) are indicated for bone pain at any level of intensity. The tricyclic antidepressants (TCAs) and the anticonvulsants are indicated for neuropathic pain syndromes. Several of these agents can and should be given a trial in an effort to lower pain intensity. If pain intensity continues to be unacceptable despite optimum treatment with adjuvant and aggressive opioid dose escalation, the pain is considered "intractable" and the patient should be considered for alternative routes of drug delivery. These uncontrolled pain situations are generally associated with neuropathic or severe intermittent pain (i.e., pathologic fractures in the advanced cancer pain patient).

Truly unmanageable side effects from systemic opioid therapy are the most common phenomenon leading to neuraxial implant. It is typical for patients to experience some side effects of opioids, most only transiently. Persistent sedation can be managed with the use of stimulant drugs. For drug-induced nausea, the concurrent administration of an antiemetic is recommended, or sequential trials of different opioids will often result in a better efficacy to toxicity profile. The algorithm for pain management in this population is depicted in Figure 71-3.

Neuraxial opioid analgesia should not be selected solely on the basis of failed systemic opioid analgesia. Opioid intraspinal analgesia is simply another opioid delivery system, which has some advantages over oral opioids, but the quality of achievable analgesia is similar. One clear advantage is to achieve a consistent delivery modality for low-dose opioid analgesia in patients who have truly intractable dose-related opioid side effects. Morphine and nonlipophilic opioids have a distinct dose-response advantage when administered intrathecally, and are used almost exclusively for somatic pain.[82] More commonly, patients with severe nerve injury or bony destruction and neuropathic pain require the addition of local anesthetics or clonidine to achieve "functional" analgesia. Placement of the catheter tip to a specific spinal level will allow accurate delivery of local anesthetics and clonidine to the cord level of the pain processing.

Indications and Contraindications of Intraspinal Analgesia

The indications and contraindications of intraspinal analgesia are outlined in Table 71-1. There are no individual studies that indicate specific risk-factor frequency for epidural hemorrhage, hematoma formation, and other complications. The American Society of Regional Anesthesia published a consensus report in 1998 giving guidelines for epidural analgesia in the face of coagulation risk factors.[83] The individual patient's clotting factors should be close to normal before epidural catheter placement or catheter withdrawal, but it is clear from this report that there are no definable specific laboratory values that will protect the patient from adverse events.

A clear requirement for the use of these implantable techniques is the presence of support from an interested family member or significant other if the patient is to be cared for in the home. A caregiver-partner is critical for any externalized system, and the absence of a caregiver should alert the practitioner toward a fully implantable system. Although some patients may be able to manage independently in all other aspects of their lives, a partner to monitor and maintain aseptic technique, and assume accountability for intraspinal drug administration, is a prerequisite to implantation. The potential strain on this person should be discussed and factored into the decision-making process. Occasionally, family members will be reluctant to view and/or use any tubes coming out of the body. Other family members may be anxious and willing to do whatever they can to help. The caregiver should be present during the discussions of implantation and analgesic therapy initiation. Barriers to use of opioid analgesia include the attitudes of the caregivers and family. It is important for the implanting physician to understand the family dynamics before implantation. Negotiation of acceptable analgesic care includes all aspects of the device selection, implantation, drug infusion, and complications.

Home Care Issues

The home care agency or hospital pharmacy department must have a depth of experience in the nursing and pharmacy to embark on the care of a patient with an implantable device. Nurses will be asked to assess and titrate externalized infusions, and perform care of any exit site. If a device is to be implanted, special training will be required for clinic nurses to be able to refill and program the device. The pharmacy will be asked to mix infusion solutions with a variety of drug combinations, investigate drug stability and interaction information, and have necessary stock on hand. Managed

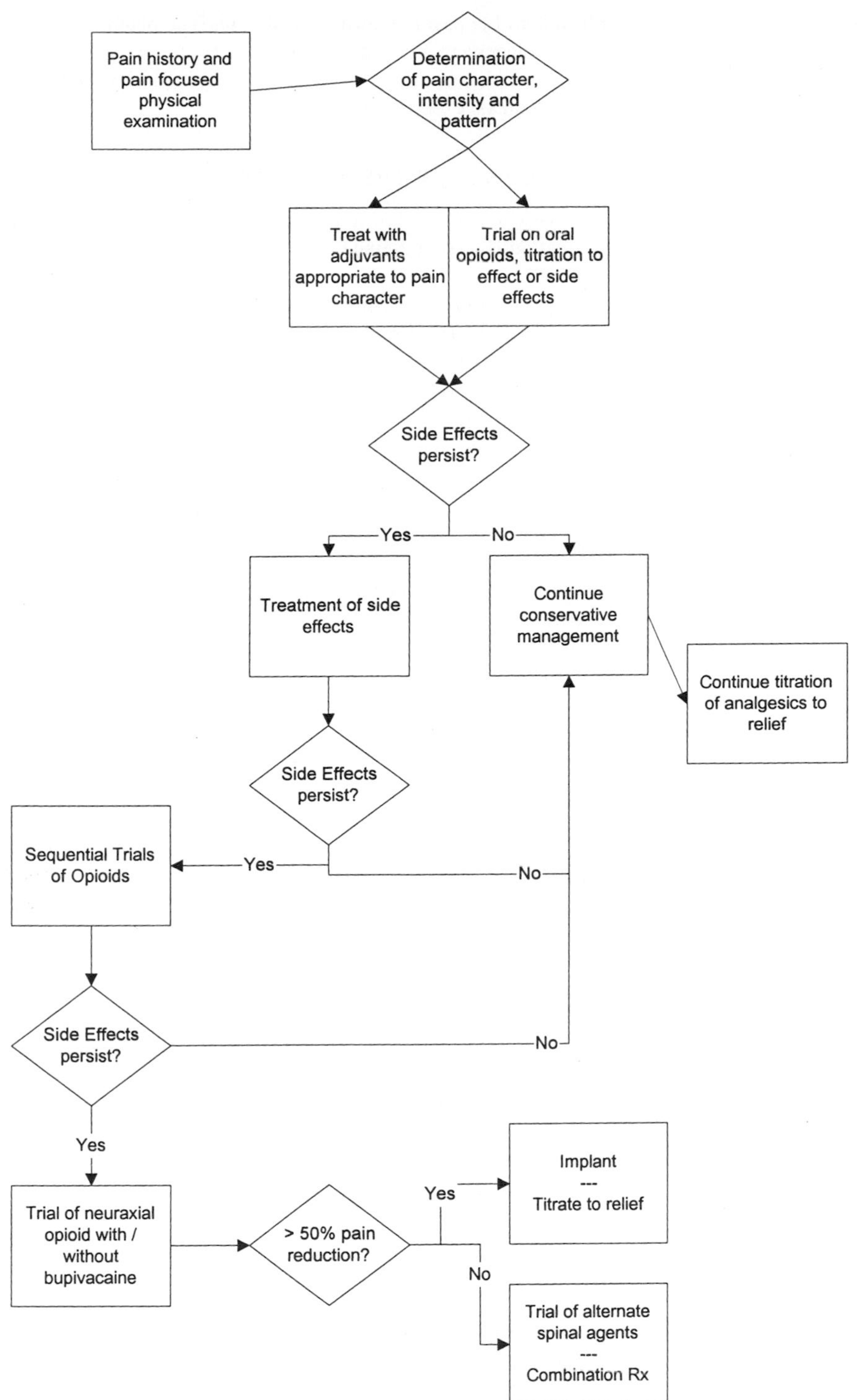

Figure 71-3 Pain treatment algorithm as developed by Du Pen and Du Pen.

care organizations and medical insurance organizations are now selecting home care and pharmacy agencies who may or may not have the skills to deliver the care required by these patients. It is important for the clinician to be constantly aware of the technical skills of the staff in agencies with whom he or she is working. This can be accomplished by having direct contact with the nursing and pharmacy staff as they interact with the patients.

The population of candidates for acute pain analgesia is the largest population of patients considered for access to a neuraxial space. Most of these patients will be experiencing postoperative pain. Also, within this class of patients are the acute trauma patients and those chronic pain patients experiencing an acute exacerbation of pain. Among the most challenging acute pain presentations involve patients with a history of drug addiction and opioid tolerance, and those who are hypersensitive to opioid side effects to the point of preferring the pain over the side effects. These patients may benefit from epidural local anesthetic with or without clonidine. Preemptive analgesic planning by clinical anesthesiologists in these difficult to treat patients will abort the postoperative crises of patients, caregivers, and the system at large.

TABLE 71-1 **Indications and Contraindications for Intraspinal Analgesia**

Indication

1. Pain greater than 6/10 after optimized oral opioid/adjuvant therapeutic trials
2. Therapy targeting causative condition exhausted/optimized
3. Persistent side effects limiting quality of life/function, despite treatment and sequential trials
4. Patient acceptance
5. Adequate support systems

Contraindications

1. Thrombocytopenia >20,000
2. Oral anticoagulation therapy
   a. Protime measurements with INR =/> 1.5
   b. Close monitoring, and no catheter movement without check of INR.
3. Active infection
4. Occlusion of epidural or subarachnoid space by tumor
5. Psychosocial issues that would make implantation untenable
6. Allergy or unmanageable side effect from anticipated treatment

Selection for Implantable Pump Systems

Patient selection for implantable pump systems differs from the selection criteria for externalized devices on the issues relating to duration of therapy and planned drug infusion. Implantable pumps are usually reserved for chronic pain and cancer patients who are expected to live and require infusion for more than 3 to 6 months. Bohme and Tryba point out the following criteria for pump implantation: pain of somatic origin, exclusion of mental diseases and psychogenic causes of pain, causal therapy is exhausted, insufficient effects of peripheral analgesics and coanalgesics, oral or transdermal opioids are insufficient despite dosages resulting in side effects, pain is sensible to opioids, and regional applications of opioids have been tested effectively before implantation.[82] The main point of their article is that implantation in a patient who does not get relief from a test on neuraxial opioid analgesia and has somatic pain will not benefit from a pump implantation. There are significant cost issues for long-term externalized infusions, where an exteriorized pump is required for infusion. Rental on pumps, cost of drug mixing, delivery, and support may be cost prohibitive for long-term infusion in the United States. The cost advantage of the subcutaneously buried intrathecal morphine pump is the lack of ongoing infusion company charges. The pumps, however, are limited in their volume capacity and therefore are difficult to use with patients who have neuropathic pain or activity-related pain and require the infusion of clonidine or local anesthetic agents. Both of these agents are not commercially available in high enough concentrations for the low-volume infusions of the subcutaneous pump systems. Pumps are used less often for the control of cancer-related pain, as the aggressive use of oral opioids and adjunctive drugs are effective in most cancer-related pain states.

Chronic nonmalignant pain patients are more often candidates for pump implantation since their use is expected to be of long duration, and their pain is often somatic in origin. Before implantation, patients in our clinic are tested for opioid responsiveness with epidural analgesia trials of 2 to 12 weeks. Psychosocial issues are evaluated with a psychological consultation. The planned location of pump placement must be addressed with the patient, particularly as it applies to activities of daily living that may cause disruption in dress, exercise, or sexuality.

Analgesic Testing before Implantation

The process of neuraxial testing before selecting a patient for pump implantation is a controversial issue. Some implanters will test the patient with a single or multiple neuraxial injections of opioid and evaluate the patient's response to determine the potential efficacy of this approach. The simple process of injection and questioning will illicite a potential placebo response. To avoid the placebo response and to determine the functional analgesia of this technique, the practitioner must evaluate the patient's response over time and in his or her own environment. We support the process of a long-term (3 to 6 weeks) epidural or intrathecal infusion of analgesic agent to determine the functional analgesia of this technique. During the long-term infusion, not only can the functional capacity be measured but the risk of continuous escalating doses can also be estimated. Patients who do achieve long-term neuraxial analgesia during this test phase will in our experience do much better after implantation.

Patient selection is a negotiation with the patient. From the patient's view this is treatment selection by the patient. Once the clinician has determined in his mind the appropriateness of the treatment plan based on the information available, the patient makes the ultimate decision. It is important for the clinician to be aware of the patient's goals, fears, and perceptions and address these as thoroughly as possible, being very clear on the amount of relief that can be anticipated and any limitations set of supplemental oral analgesics once the titration period ends. Clear communication between the patient and the physician during this phase is essential.

Selection of an Implantable Device

Selection of an implantable device is a process that is concurrent with patient selection. The decision to implant a device for drug delivery should follow an algorithmic decision process starting with the optimum use of oral opioids and adjuvant drugs and minimization of side effects. When oral and transcutaneous analgesic delivery has been maximized without functional analgesia, then patient selection and device selection of an implantable device starts.

Device selection requires an understanding of the current status of the pain generators from malignant and nonmalignant sources. In nonmalignant pain states, the specific pain generators may be identified through the use of diagnostic blocks, studies, and imaging. Surgical consultation and second opinions may be obtained to determine if additional surgery may be indicated. Once the cause of the pain is identified, the treatment aimed at the causative condition has been optimized or exhausted, conservative multimodal pain management has failed, a screening for intraspinal analgesia can begin.

Pain associated with malignancy is usually a progressive process requiring continuous reassessments and updates of the pain treatment plan. The pain-focused consultation and physical examination should include documentation of the location of original malignancy, metastatic locations, future expectations for disease spread, and future antitumor treatment options. The correlation of metastatic sights with pain sources on the pain-focused examination will not only tie the pain generator to the metastatic disease process but will also give the pain practitioner a better idea of future possible pain generators. The site of the pain generators, correlated with the pain character, pattern, and intensity, will lead to the practitioner's choice of delivery system. This is important information that will be needed in determining the choices of drug for delivery, spinal level for catheter tip location, and the method of delivery.

The presence of neoplastic spinal disease has previously been considered to be a contraindication for neuraxial drug delivery.[84] Metastatic lesions of the spine, however, account for some of the most severe pain problems, particularly when nerve root impingement occurs secondary to tumor invasion and vertebral collapse. Most of these lesions affect the vertebral bodies, leaving the posterior spinous elements and lamina relatively unaffected.[85] In nonmalignant states, trauma and/or degenerative changes may result in vertebral collapse, with extension to the epidural space, and intrathecal compression may occur. Neuropathic and activity-related pain generated from nerve root compression and disk space sources would be similar to that seen in malignant patients. When epidural space involvement is suspected, an epidurogram, magnetic resonance imaging (MRI), or contrast computed tomography (CT) scan may clarify the extent of external pressure versus epidural space-occupying lesion. Careful radiographic evaluation of vertebral involvement with identification of any current or potential epidural space compromise should be identified. When there is extensive epidural space invasion, epidural infusions may have limited efficacy due the incomplete spread of drug in the epidural space. Epidural infusions under these conditions may have a segmental effect with incomplete coverage of affected area. Intrathecal infusions may by considered both through externalized devices or subcutaneous pumps when the epidural space is compromised or when in the opinion of the practitioner the intrathecal space may have clinical advantages.

Types of Devices

Access to the neuraxial space may be achieved through several devices. Table 71-2 describes the advantages and disadvantages of intraspinal devices. The commercially available devices for epidural and intrathecal access include ports and three main categories of catheters:

TABLE 71-2 **Advantages and Disadvantages of Intraspinal Devices**

Device	Advantages	Disadvantages
Short-Term Epidural Catheter	No surgery Can be done quickly Easily replaced	Catheter externalized: ? ↑ infection risk Catheters "taped down" to the skin Restrictions on bathing/clothing Less precise tip placement Commonly requires ambulatory pump, rarely can use intermittent injections More likely to become disconnected/fall out over time requiring replacement
Permanent Epidural Catheter	Internal fixation prevents inadvertent dislodgment Physician can use radiograph control to place barium-containing catheters in best possible location No dressings on the back Catheter is larger & easier to dress/clean	Catheter externalized: ? ↑ infection risk Restrictions on bathing/clothing Commonly requires ambulatory pump, rarely can use intermittent injections Requires significant ongoing self-care and monitoring Cost of ongoing external pump lease and infusion pharmacy
Implanted Epidural Port	Catheter/port completely internal Physician can use radiograph control to place barium-containing catheters in best possible location Potential future delivery of Butamben?	Port must be accessed through the skin to administer analgesic agents: ? infection risk Commonly requires continuous infusion, rarely can use intermittent injections Care and monitoring of accessed port/needle requires careful attention to prevent dislodgment of needle Needle access discomfort Cost of ongoing external pump lease and infusion pharmacy
Implanted Intrathecal Pump System	Completely internal system - ? ↓ infection risk Can be individually programmed for bolus and continuous settings No dressings or tape with the exception of a Band-Aid after refill	More surgical considerations with creation of pump pocket "Hockey puck" size of pump Some pumps require access to special computer for refills and adjustments Cost of computerized pump and initial implantation

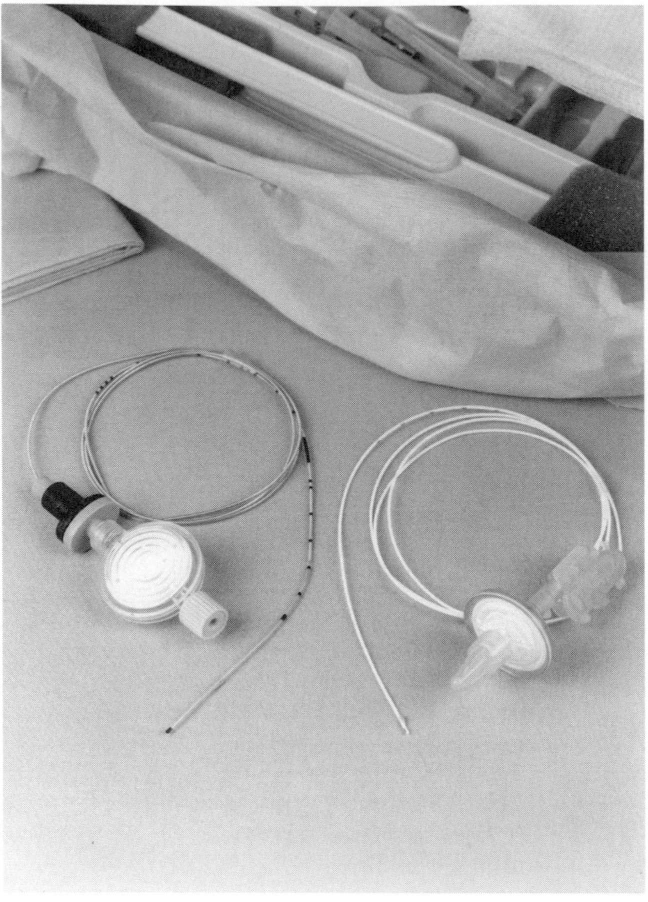

Figure 71-4 Temporary epidural catheters for use epidurally or intraspinally. (**A**) Arrow epidural catheter (Arrow International, Reading, Penn). (**B**) Abbott epidural catheter (Abbott Laboratories, North Chicago, Ill). (**C**) Braun epidural catheter (B. Braun Medical Inc, Bethlehem Pa).

1. Short-term catheters made from polyamide, polyurethane, and nylon with have friction adaptors attached to their distal end.
2. Non-kinking, wire-supported epidural catheters with friction adapters, which under ideal clinical conditions may be used for prolonged epidural access.
3. Long-term silicone rubber catheter with fixed integrated Luer-Lock adapters.
4. Implantable epidural and intrathecal ports.

Each of the short-term catheter materials differs in stiffness and tissue reactivity; some soft catheters will require a stylet for epidural placement. Figure 71-4 illustrates some of the short-term catheters on the market. Catheter stiffness, on the other hand, aids the practitioner during placement to a specific spinal level or nerve root location, when precise drug delivery to that location is desirable. Desired catheter stiffness may be obtained with soft catheters during catheter placement by the use of special wire stylets. Stiffness may play a role in catheter migration from epidural to intrathecal spaces or in the reverse direction; stiffness may also result in pressure and nerve root paresthesias. If the practitioner is concerned more about catheter kinking and obstruction than the location of the catheter tip, then the use of a wire-reinforced epidural catheter may be the best choice. Device selection is an individual choice, and the practitioner should select a device with which he is most adept and comfortable. This selection usually results in the most predictable outcomes.

Reliability is the next level of device selection. When the duration of implantation is expected to be less than 3 weeks, then the use of a temporary catheter may be the best choice; although expected duration of use is a difficult determination to make. The average short-term catheter, in the author's hands, will remain in place for an average of 2 weeks of therapy before needing replacement. The durability of the externalized catheter and catheter adapter are the weakest segment of temporary catheters. Failure of the temporary catheters usually occurs with separation of the catheter adapter and contamination of the catheter. Less commonly, the temporary catheter may break or kink. There is a gain in durability and dependability by moving from the temporary catheters to the silicone rubber catheters. The two-part catheter system with a fixed Luer-Lok adapter and the small intraspinal catheter connected to the strong externalized catheter gives the durability. This catheter system requires surgical implantation, which is a definite disadvantage over the temporary catheters that may be placed at the bedside. The silicone rubber epidural catheters are placed for expected durations of therapy in the weeks to months range. Figure 71-5 depicts the Du Pen silicone rubber epidural catheter. Although there are advantages of this system over the conventual temporary epidural catheters, there are no clinical applications that cannot be managed effectively with a temporary catheter. Patient convenience and safety may be better addressed with the permanent catheter when long-term implantation is contemplated. Catheter failure will result in loss of the infusion and added risk of infection if the continuity of the system is broken. Loss of infusion usually means an extra trip to the hospital and the resurgence of pain.

The implantable pump manufacturing companies have workshops set up around the country to teach practitioners skills needed to manage these devices, including pump implantation and fixation, dose calculation, and identification and treatment of complications associated with therapy. These are valuable instruction sessions usually taught by experienced implanters that give the practitioner a more complete understanding of the issues of patient and device selection. There are two basic types of intrathecal pumps

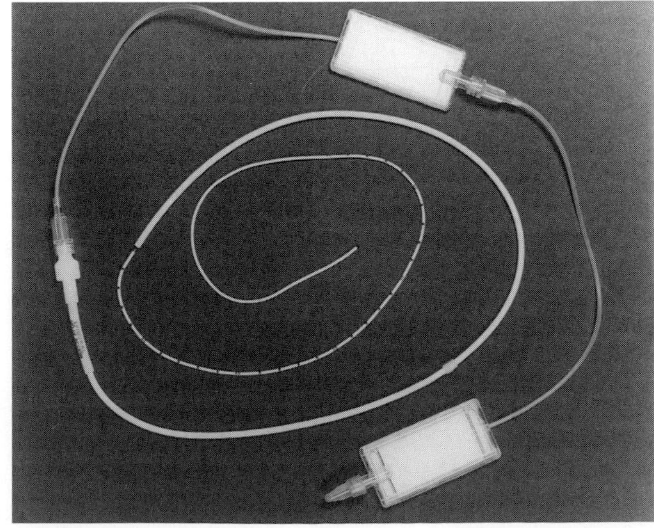

Figure 71-5 The Du Pen epidural catheter (CR Bard Access Systems, Salt Lake City, Utah).

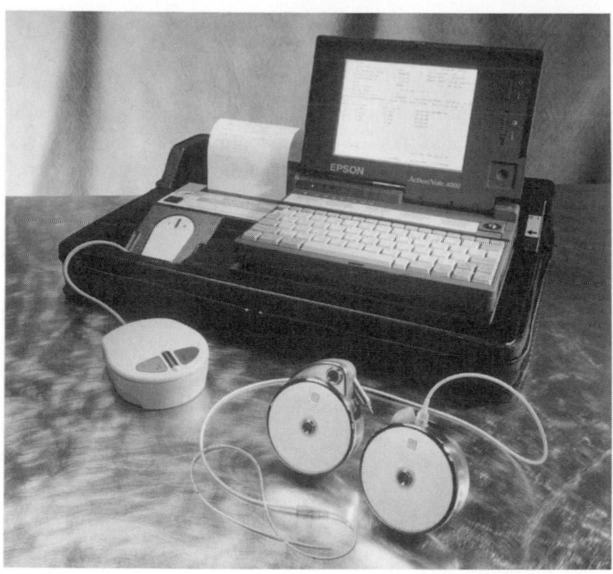

Figure 71-6 SynchroMed pump (Medtronic Neurological, Minneapolis, Minn) showing the two pump sizes and the computer.

and one intrathecal patient-activated reservoir system (still investigational) in use today. There are variable-rate, battery-powered computerized pumps and the fixed-rate, Freon gas-powered pump.

1. Medtronic SynchroMed pump (Medtronic Neurological, Minneapolis, Minn) 10 mL and 18 mL sizes with or without side ports.
2. Arrow 3000 constant flow implantable pumps (15, 30, and 50 mL sizes) with high- (1.46 to 2.0 mL/day), medium- (0.86 to 1.45 mL/day), and low-flow rates (0.5 to 0.85 mL/day).
3. The Algomed patient-activated intrathecal reservoir delivery system (Medtronic Neurological, Minneapolis, Minn, not yet approved by FDA).

Selection of an implantable pump is usually a practitioner preference issue. The two classes of pumps available on the market today were outlined earlier. The choices are between the variable-rate Medtronic pump and the Arrow fix-rate device. There are advantages to each pump type. The SynchroMed pump has a small reservoir (10 and 18 mL) but is larger in size due to its internal mechanisms (Figs. 71-6 and 71-7). Its advantages include the simple and complex infusion rates operated by the computer, adjustability by the external computer station, and its ease of reservoir and side-port accessibility. These advantages are valuable when analgesic admixtures are used that require frequent titration adjustments in infusion rates. Titration of the intrathecal analgesic does not require refilling the pump. The side-port access to the intrathecal space is protected by a screen, which can only be accessed by a 25-gauge needle.

The Arrow constant flow pump has a choice of reservoir sizes (15, 30, and 50 mL), which allows lots of flexibility in physical size and reservoir size, the rate of flow (high, medium, and low) of the pump is also selected, or a higher infusion flow model that allows for the use of local anesthetic agents. Figure 71-8 shows two of the pump sizes. The Arrow pump has a double chamber for access to the reservoir and the side port. Infusions do not require the use of a computer, allowing use in areas were the computer is not available. The low profile of the Arrow pump allows placement

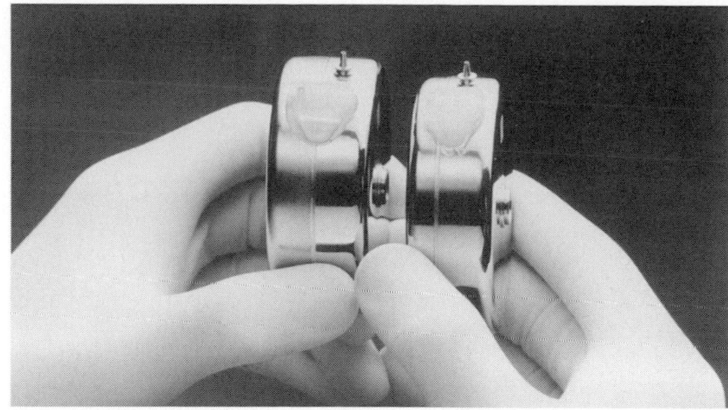

Figure 71-7 SynchroMed pumps showing the two sizes (10mL and 18mL reservoirs) in side view.

in thin patients. Its interesting to note that a heat (such as a hot tub) can increase the infusion rate, a sort of patient-controlled intrathecal analgesia effect.

The choice of implantable pump should be based on the patient's individual needs. A choice is dependent on the drug or drug combination chosen for infusion, infusion rate, need for dose titration, proximity to a pump computer, and patient choice.

The Algomed system is a patient-controlled intrathecal dose-delivery system that has no automatic or computer driven functions. The device is operated by a series of valves, which allow the patient to activate the injection chamber and administer a specified dose volume into the intrathecal space. The delay in refilling of the pump chamber determines the time allowed between doses. The Algomed system has been used in clinical studies in Europe and the United States, but has not been approved for use in the United

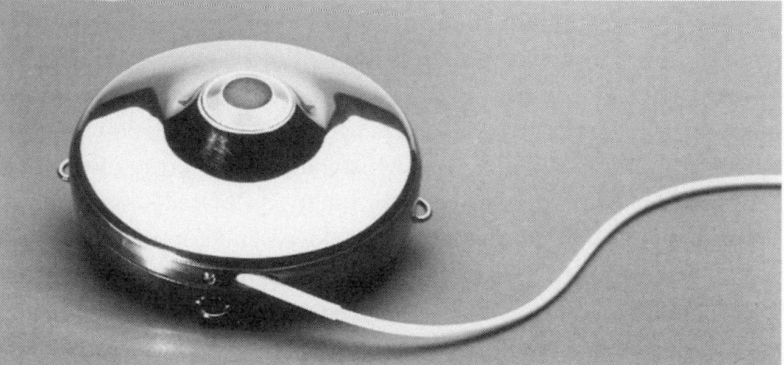

A

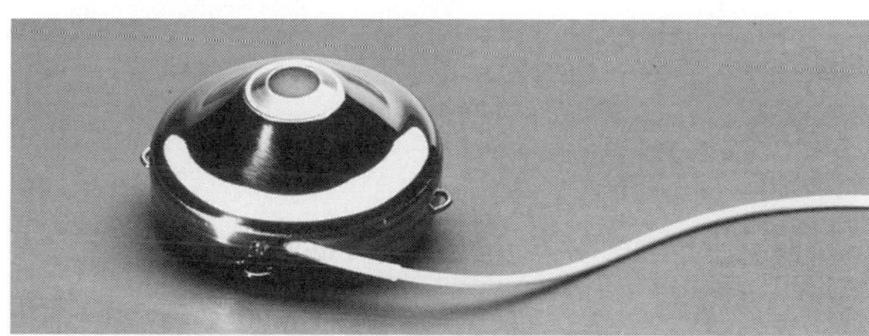

B

Figure 71-8 Arrow pumps showing the pump in two sizes: (**A**) 15 mL and (**B**) 50 mL. The pumps may be ordered in a high-, medium-, and low-flow rate.

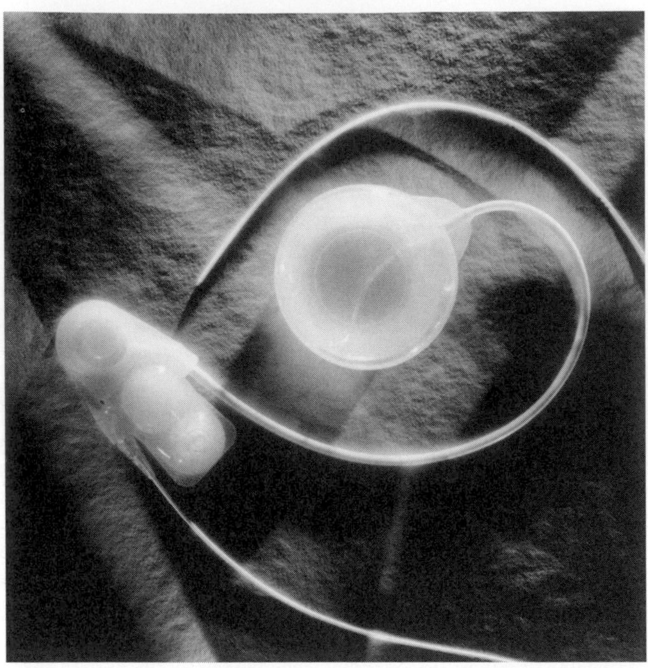

Figure 71-9 Algomed pump (Medtronic Neurological, Minneapolis, Minn). The Algomed pump is a subcutaneous intrathecal patient-controlled analgesia device.

States by the FDA at the time of this printing. Figure 71-9 shows the pump.

Ports are another alternative to accessing both the epidural and intrathecal spaces. The main attraction of the port system is the lack of externalization. This allows the patient to function normally when the port is not accessed. The pharmacokinetics of today's intraspinal analgesic therapy does not lend itself well to intermittent dosage. The practitioner has a choice of long-acting intraspinal opioids, short-acting local anesthetic agents, and α_2-agonists. The duration of injectable intraspinal opioids is from 8 to 12 hours, where the local anesthetic and α_2-agonists agents require infusion because of their short duration of action. Most patients requiring intraspinal analgesia have severe neuropathic or activity-related somatic pain. These pain states require constant infusions and continuous access of the port. The continuous access of the port effectively negates the advantages of the port system. The controversy between ports and externalized catheters for intraspinal infusion is similar to the controversy between central intravenous ports and Hickman catheters. This mode of therapy may take on a whole new utilization profile if and when we have new drugs developed that have long durations of effect.

IMPLANTATION

Implantation techniques vary from practitioner to practitioner, as there are no specific implantation standards in pain management. Individual practitioners have reported on implantation techniques, but there are no comparative studies looking at the outcomes from different techniques. There are many variables such as needle placement, location of incision, antibiotic irrigation, suture techniques, and pocket dissection. More exploratory work in this area could bring valuable information to the literature on complications.

The choice of technique depends heavily on the training and experience of the practitioner. Internally placed pumps and ports require additional technical skills. During these implantation procedures, the practitioner must be aware of and select the site of implantation, depth, and fixation. These technical differences may influence the duration of the implantation procedure, the ease of post-procedure care, patient comfort, and convenience.

Temporary Catheters

Temporary catheters of all types may be placed at the bedside into either the epidural or intrathecal space, with or without a short tunnel to add to catheter stability and possibly influence catheter track infections. Zenz et al[86] reported on the use of a single nylon catheter for more that 1[1/2] years, using a special skin fixation technique; so longer-term use is possible. These catheters may be placed under fluoroscopic guidance, when a specific location is desired, but direction of the catheter movement is difficult to control. Catheters, which have wandered along a nerve root exit, will be less effective and may result in increased neuropathic pain. Epidurograms will give the practitioner information about catheter position, patency of the epidural space, and dye flow in that space. These films may also be used as a standard for future epidurograms that the patient may require in determining the cause of failure of analgesia. Myelograms may be easily obtained to prove intrathecal catheter placement and position.

Permanent Catheters

The permanent catheters differ from temporary catheters in that their two-part construction allows for radiographic-controlled specific epidural placement with a long subcutaneous, tunneled durable catheter for stability and infection protection. There is a Dacron cuff for catheter stability and fixation and a silver-impregnated cuff as a barrier to bacterial growth along the catheter. The 33% barium content of the Du Pen catheter allows visualization with simple lumbar spine films, but does not alter the breaking strength of the catheter. Other than occasional technical problems, which may result in occlusion, the only major risk of implantation is infection. Care must be taken in all aspects of catheter management and wound care. Short-term perioperative antibiotics are commonly used for most patients receiving implanted devices. Standard therapy would include administration of a broad-spectrum antibiotic 1 hour before surgery and two doses 6 to 8 hours apart postoperatively (see section, Complications).

The procedure for epidural or intrathecal catheter implantation should be undertaken in a sterile environment and fluoroscopy should be used during the catheter placement. The patient should be placed in a lateral position, allowing access of C-arm fluoroscopy from the side away from the surgical field. The 14-gauge Hustead epidural needle is placed in the epidural space using a long paramedian approach, which avoids the sharp angle created by a midline approach and allows a smooth entry into the epidural space for accurate needle positioning.[87] The needle angle will allow the practitioner to withdraw the catheter for repositioning without a risk of catheter damage. The use of 10 to 15 mm of saline or an local anesthetic agent will not only dilate the epidural space but will give analgesia for the catheter tunneling procedure. The catheter should extend four vertebral levels above entry to ensure stability; this should be planned before the entry level is determined. The catheter should be advanced two vertebral levels above the planned catheter tip position using fluoroscopy. This allows for one vertebral segment catheter withdrawal during the process of positioning the tunneled catheter. Postoperative orders are written for an epidurogram or myelogram, postoperative antibiotics, analgesic therapy, fluids, diet, and opioid conversion. Postoperative catheter care includes daily wound cleaning and a dry 2 × 2 dressing, until the securing sutures have been removed. Orders for discharge should include comprehensive instructions on dressing care and the use of the filter system. All sutures must be removed at 10 to 14 days to avoid the added risk of infection. Activity instructions include avoidance of use of hot tubs or other possible contaminated exposure of the catheter track.

Ports

Port implantation, epidural or intrathecal, is similar to that of the permanent catheter except instead of an exit location, the catheter is connected to a subcutaneous port. The port should be placed over a bony structure to withstand the pressure required for needle access of the port. Postoperative care includes normal wound care. Care should be taken to use aseptic conditions to access the port to protect for infection. Special care should be taken if the port will be accessed for constant infusion. Under these conditions, the needle and area around the port should be constantly protected from bacterial contamination. Rotation of the needle access position and attention to health of the tissue over the port should be paramount. Dressings and skin care over the port should be optimized as long as the device is accessed.

Intrathecal Pumps

Implantation of the intrathecal pump systems requires the use of an operating suite and a full surgical setup, general or deep sedation anesthesia, and access to fluoroscopy. The patient is placed in a lateral position with access to the spine for intrathecal catheter placement and access to the lateral pelvis for pump implantation. An accomplished practitioner will have no difficulty entering the intrathecal space at any accessible level. A small 1-in. transverse incision is usually made at the L4-5 level, allowing a flat paramedian needle entry into the intrathecal space at the L3-4 or L2-3 interspace. The angle of the needle will decrease the risk of catheter damage during catheter manipulation and will avoid the risk of retrograde flow of spinal fluid along the outside of the catheter. If difficulty is encountered while attempting to enter the intrathecal space, the head of the table may be elevated to distend the dura. The intrathecal catheter is threaded into the intrathecal space; fluoroscopy may be used to ensure that the catheter remains in a central position and that it remains in the dorsal space. There are a number of devices supplied by both companies to fixate the intrathecal catheter; however, the author prefers to use a single silk suture attached to the intraspinous ligament and secured to the connection between the two catheters. This "dog leash" suture allows a gentle curvature of the catheter, but does not allow the weight of the pump to pull on the catheter.

The pump pocket location is individually selected for the greatest comfort to the patient. The incision is usually about 1 in. below the umbilicus and extends laterally about 4 in. in length. The depth of the pocket should be about 1.5 cm, but this may vary from patient to patient. Ideally, the pump is fixed to the fascia, but in most cases the layer of subcutaneous fat is too deep to allow this placement without making the pump almost inaccessible for refilling. The tunneling device is used to bring the connecting catheter from the pump to the posterior incision. After the catheters are connected and the dog leash is secured, the catheter unit is withdrawn into the tunnel, avoiding catheter kinking. Wound closure must be made watertight, as there will be a collection of fluid around the pump, and any openings will continue to "leak" until the closure is watertight.

Each company has a specific protocol to follow for the original pump filling and follow-up refills of the pump. Both companies have addressed the fear of instilling concentrated drug directly into the intrathecal space. Medtronic has a port screen, which will not allow the refill 22-gauge needle to enter the side port, whereas Arrow has a double chamber with a special bolus and refill needle.

Wound care is similar for both pumps. During the first 5 to 7 days, while the sutures are in place, the patient may shower but not use of hot tubs. In addition, providers should collaborate so that the patient is not having radiation to the site or surrounding tissues during this first week. After the sutures are removed, the patient may bathe as he or she wishes. We use an abdominal binder to support the pump for the first 3 weeks, until the scar tissue is well established and the device is fixed in place.

RADIOLOGIC STUDIES

Epidurograms are a helpful radiographic technique. The purpose of the procedure is not only to confirm epidural space location of the epidural catheter, but as a diagnostic tool to note the extent of epidural flow of dye. This information may be used to predict volume requirements or restrictions of fluid spread within the space. A baseline study may be referred to later if analgesic problem arise, which may be solved by a new epidurogram and a comparison to the baseline study. It is important to obtain the study in the radiology department to ensure reproducibility.

Pump myelograms will prove intrathecal catheter placement if fluid cannot be aspirated from the canal due to fibrosis. Pumps without side ports cannot be tested for catheter position, either by aspiration or myelography. Computed tomography and myelograms may be helpful in determining catheter position in pumps without side ports.

TREATMENT PLANNING

Treatment planning must be a flexible and continuous process. The process is based on the original assessment of the patient's pain experience and a reassessment of responses to the executed treatment plan. Responses to opioid infusions will be relatively predictable, but when neuropathic pain persists, a more complex treatment plan will likely be required. The additions of clonidine or local anesthetic agents are commonly used in epidural and intrathecal analgesia. Dilute local anesthetic solutions administered neuraxially are a comfortable therapeutic technique for the vast majority of anesthesiologists in the inpatient setting. These infusions can be easily managed at home safely with a proficient team of outpatient and home care support staff. Once stabilized, the patient can be managed with a range of infusion rate parameters for the home care nurse to titrate within. Clonidine, a relatively new entry in the field, has been extensively used for neuropathic pain states in Europe and enjoys a remarkable efficacy in some of the most intractable situations (i.e., sacral plexopathy).[51] As one might expect, clonidine requires close monitoring of blood pressure during initiation and titration. These combination infusions, opioid-local anesthetic, opioid-clonidine, and even all three together, will require close outpatient follow-up. A balance of side effects including drowsiness (opioid), skin anesthesia (local anesthetic), and clonidine (orthostatic hypotension) need to be balanced against pain relief. Most advanced cancer patients and elderly chronic pain patients are not able to come into the clinic, and hence the presence of well-trained home care nurses is essential.

The selection of an opioid for spinal administration has typically been done on a "physician's choice" basis. Some physicians are only comfortable with morphine and others prefer hydromorphone or fentanyl, perhaps because of their own experience and comfort level. Opioid selection as a part of treatment planning incorporates duration of action, efficacy and toxicity response to the opioid at screening, vertebral level site of injection, and optimum volume and concentration of injectate.[88] A patient's past history of opioid exposure will often allow the practitioner to select an opioid that has given the best performance historically for the individual.

Morphine offers the best advantage over systemic administration because of its hydrophilicity. The duration of action of bolus-administered epidural morphine is generally 6 to 10 hours when administered in the opioid-tolerant cancer population. Plummer et al in a large retrospective study looked at 313 cancer and noncancer patients treated with epidural morphine for a mean treatment period of 96 days and found that dose escalation happened less when the bolus technique was used.[89] The bolus method has implications for ease of use in the home care setting as well as cost containment. However, as the volume and sophistication of options for oral and transcutaneous opioid therapy have become widely available, the need for epidural opioid therapy alone has become almost obsolete. It is much more likely that the patient requiring neuraxial analgesia will require combinations of opioid and adjuvant drugs that make infusion therapy mandatory.

Morphine can and is still used as a sole agent by infusion both epidurally and intrathecally. In managing morphine infusions, titration to effective analgesia with minimal side effects is the method of choice in determining the ideal dose for an individual patient. Hydromorphone and fentanyl are most often found in the practitioner's second-line drug category. Either agent may be a good choice in patients where morphine has been previously efficacious without side effects; however, side effects become problematic with escalating doses. If patients seem to be very sensitive to epidurally administered morphine, switching to a second-line drug is a useful tool for ongoing treatment.

Clonidine and local anesthetic agents are added to the epidural infusion to control neuropathic pain while lowering the dose of opioid and its associated side effects. Clonidine is usually titrated to effect, starting at 10 to 20 μg//mL and working up to 30 to 40 μg/mL (Table 71-3). Blood pressure and pulse rates are monitored and treated if required. Local anesthetic agents added to the infusion may result in motor and sensory loss and postural hypotension. In our experience the use of 0.115% bupivacaine, with concentration titration between 0.1% and 0.25%, will give functional analgesia. Our method of titration is in increments of 0.005%.

TABLE 71-3 **Epidural Clonidine for Chronic Pain**

Patient Screening

- Inadequate pain relief after conservative management has been optimized.
- Baseline orthostatic blood pressure is considered acceptable.

Initiating Therapy

- Consider initiating therapy in the inpatient setting if patient has severe pain, significant side effects or orthostasis.
- Obtain baseline orthostatic blood pressure before initiating therapy.
- Plan to hydrate patient with 1 to 2 L of IV fluids if blood pressure decreases >20% after initiation of therapy; consider hydration if blood pressure decreases 10% to 20%.
- Volume of epidural clonidine infusion is based on location of pathologic condition and tip of epidural catheter. Most common concentration is 10 μg/ml at 2 to 5 ml/h; however, very high concentrations at very low infusion rates also have been used (e.g., 100 μg/ml at 0.2 to 0.5 ml/h).
- Typical epidural clonidine starting dose is 20 μg/h by continuous infusion.
- Check orthostatic blood pressure and heart rate q4h × 2, then q8h × 24 h.

Continuing Care

- Monitor pain intensity regularly (e.g., q shift or q home visit).
- Monitor orthostatic blood pressure regularly (e.g., q shift or q home visit).
- Establish a system for addressing unrelieved pain, e.g., for pain rating of 4/10 to 6/10 with stable blood pressure, increase clonidine dose (continuous infusion rate) by 5% to 10%; for pain rating >6/10 with stable blood pressure, increase clonidine dose by 10% to 20%.
- Manage blood pressure changes, e.g., for significantly decreased blood pressure or >20% decrease in orthostatic blood pressure (when patient is raised from a flat position), maximize oral fluid intake; consider initiating fludrocortisone acetate (Florinef) 0.1 mg qd to tid.
- Manage unresolved symptomatic orthostasis or signs of excessive sedation or confusion, e.g., decrease clonidine dose by 50% and reevaluate within 24 h. Add epidural or systemic opioid to control pain.
- Never abruptly discontinue epidural clonidine because this can cause life-threatening rebound hypertension. To discontinue epidural clonidine, titrate dose downward in a stepwise fashion (e.g., 30% to 50% per 24-h period). Consider using transdermal clonidine during downward titration in patients with preexisting hypertension condition.

May be duplicated for use in clinical practice. As appears in McCaffery M, Pasero C. Pain: Clinical Manual. St. Louis, MO: Mosby, Inc., 1999:315.

h, hour; L, liter; tid, three times daily; q, every; qd, daily.

Modified from DuPen S. Swedish Hospital Pain Management Service, Seattle, Wash, 1997.

COMPLICATIONS

The potential complications associated with spinal drug delivery systems, along with cost, are the biggest barriers to the widespread use of these techniques. Before considering the use of invasive devices, the practitioner must be fully aware of all the potential complications of the procedure, the devices, and the associated drugs. Complications associated with long-term spinal drug delivery systems fall into four major groups: infection, drug toxicity, practitioner errors, and mechanical problems. Physicians, patients, caregivers, and those offering home care services must be proficient in avoiding the avoidable, troubleshooting problems, and correcting or treating the complications. Practitioners who are aware of these potential problems will identify them earlier and resolve problems as they occur. The procedures themselves do not create the problems; the problems usually arise out of a misunderstanding of the implantable devices, their care, and use.

Infection

Intraspinal infections are the most feared consequence of chronic epidural and intrathecal catheterization. Epidural infections are predictable in those pain management practices that use significant long-term epidural catheters, particularly in the immunosuppressed cancer patients. Our initial infection rate with the Du Pen epidural catheter was reported at 5.4%.[90] From 1990 to 1996 the epidural infection rate within our practice has ranged between 5% and 15% in our long-term patients. Patient care provided by multiple home care agencies, multiple caregivers, and with variable filtering, tubing, and reservoir change procedures has made tracking of infection risk difficult. However, frequency of tubing and filter replacement was noted as a variable that changed over time. A protocol of changing filters weekly resulted in our previously reported 5.4% infection risk in our practice. The hospital epidemiology committee established a protocol of changing the filter and tubing every 3 days; this resulted in an increased infection rate (10% to 15%). An internal study showed no correlation between infection rate and any known factors except for duration of implantation. A colleague (William Baumgartl, MD, personal communication, July 14, 1997) reported his low incidence of epidural infections with a dual-filter system technique. He reported using two PALL epidural filters in series, the inner filter never being changed and the outer filter and pump tubing changed on a monthly basis (Fig. 71-10). The reports of intrathecal catheters used for chronic pain management from Sweden also reported a very low incidence of meningitis (0.5%). In these reports the intrathecal filters were changed once a month. There have been no studies to prove the benefits of the double-filter system or to indicate that the PALL filter is superior to other epidural filters.

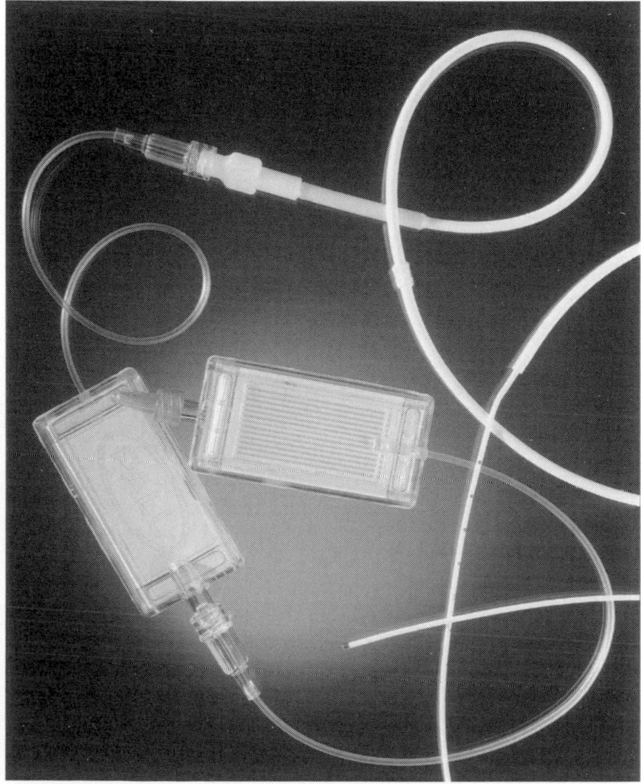

Figure 71-10 Two PALL epidural filters in series (East Hills, NY). The filter connected to the epidural or intrathecal catheter is *never* changed; the outer filter and pump tubing are changed on a monthly basis.

Identification and Treatment of Epidural Infection Early diagnosis and treatment of epidural space infections are key to a successful outcome. The most common infection occurs at the exit site. The exit site appears red, may have an exudate, and will often be painful. These infections are treated effectively with aggressive site care, often with topical antibiotic ointment, and more rarely with systemic antibiotic therapy. Of greater concern is the potential for infection inside the epidural space. The epidural infection may manifest itself from one of three sources: the drug infusate, the catheter track, or from a hematologic or local abscess source. In the 1997 calendar year, 75 permanent epidural catheters were placed at Swedish Medical Center, which is a regional pain management referral center for the northwest. Nine confirmed epidural space infections (12%) were treated in 1997. Only one of the patients presented with signs of epidural tunnel-track spread (1.3%), three patients had bowel tumors and episodic septicemia that potentially seeded hematologically (4%), and five patients had no known etiology, no exit site or track signs, and were presumed to have contaminant sources (6.6%). We adopted the double-filter protocol in 1997, and in three years we have had only four epidural infections in a total population of 145 epidural catheters, a 2.7% epidural infection rate. Clinicians should examine the potential for contamination within their institutional policies very carefully. The finding of three patients in the sample with advanced colorectal cancer suggests a higher index of suspicion in patients with bowel tumors; however, this phenomenon requires prospective clinical study.

The signs of epidural space infection include acute loss of analgesia, fever, and white blood count (WBC) elevations.[91] In the immunosuppressed cancer population, fever and WBC elevation may be delayed. Epidural space infection and catheter encapsulation present with three clinical symptoms:

1. Pain on injection
2. Retrograde flow of infusate with pooling in the paravertebral tissues
3. Loss of analgesia.

The pooling of fluid and exudate in the paravertebral tissues is the result of material tracking back out of the epidural space, often within a fibrin-like sheath surrounding the catheter. The catheter entry site through the ligamentum flavum becomes a drain, and the exudate leaks out around the catheter, causing a significant inflammatory process to occur in the soft tissues.[92]

Diagnosis is made by obtaining an epidural aspirate, Gram stain, and culture. The culture must be obtained from the epidural space. In the past, epidural catheters were immediately removed when signs and symptoms of infection were present. Catheter tip culturing was commonly used to identify infection in the epidural space and is still reported in the literature, despite being clearly problematic.[93] Bevacqua and others examined cultures from spinal catheters used for postoperative pain management (mean indwelling time, 66 hours). Cerebrospinal fluid cultures were done concurrently with removal of the catheters and culturing of the catheter tip. Semiquantitative culture methods demonstrated a relationship between the positive catheter tip cultures and contamination of the catheter that occurred on removal.[94]

Culturing of the catheter tip after removal will result in a composite culture of the epidural space, paraspinal soft tissues, catheter track, and superficial exit site. An aspirate culture from inside

TABLE 71-4 **Procedure for Epidural Culture**

Discontinue the epidural infusion.
Obtain two sterile 3-mL syringes; fill one with 2 mL of preservative-free saline.
Obtain a sterile specimen container.
Utilizing aseptic technique connect the empty 3 mL syringe directly to the luer lock of the epidural catheter. Using gentle pressure, aspirate a sample of fluid.
When an epidural infection is present there is likely to be significant fluid return, often with white particulate matter. Generally, a culture can be done on 0.5 mL or more.
If no fluid can be withdrawn, connect the saline-containing syringe to the epidural catheter and irrigate with 2 to 3 mL of preservative-free saline. Again attempt to withdraw fluid.
The specimen should be sent for STAT Gram stain with culture and sensitivity to follow.
Do not immediately remove the epidural catheter. Confirm the specimen has been received and at least the gram stain has been done.
The catheter can be used as a drain until the culture and sensitivity is confirmed. This is particularly important if there is a significant amount of fluid buildup in the epidural space.

the epidural space prior to catheter removal with subsequent identification of the organism and its sensitivity is *mandatory* for best treatment outcomes in these patients. When the volume in the epidural space is sparse and fluid cannot be aspirated, 2 mL of normal saline may be injected for sampling. Table 71-4 summarizes the procedure for performing an epidural aspirate culture.

Epidural space infections can result in accumulation of up to 20 mL of exudate in the epidural space. A syringe attached to the catheter can decompress the space of any exudate while antibiotic therapy is being initiated. Withdrawal of exudate can continue on an every 8-hour basis until no fluid can be withdrawn. This technique may help to avoid the risk of cord compression from the accumulation of fluid in the epidural space.

Epidural space infections have been treated primarily by removal of the catheter and systemic administration of antibiotic therapy directed toward the specified organism identified with the culture. Our policy, established 10 years ago in collaboration with our infectious disease staff, was that removal of the catheter (after no exudate could be withdrawn *and* culture results had been reported by the laboratory) was mandatory for complete resolution of the infection. This policy has been applied to over 70 patients with positive epidural space cultures over the last 12 years, during which time no patients had to be surgically decompressed. Appraisal of response to treatment can be done with a "wait-and-watch" approach to resolution of symptoms, or in cases where neurologic signs are present, it is best accomplished with either a MRI or a contrast CT scan.

Many clinicians have considered sterilizing the epidural catheter with epidurally infused vancomycin (with sensitive organisms) rather than removing the catheter, treating, and replacing the catheter. Hahn et al first reported a case of sterilizing an infected epidural catheter with epidurally infused vancomycin.[95] We have treated three cases of epidural infections attributed to *Staphylococcus aureus* with systemic vancomycin (1 g every 12 hours, given intravenously) for 10 days and concomitant epidural infusion of 150 μg per hour of vancomycin for 3 weeks. This treatment was done in collaboration with the infectious disease staff and with full disclosure to the patient of unknown risks. All three patients wanted to proceed with the therapy in lieu of losing their epidural catheters. In each case we followed the patients with repeat epidural cultures on a monthly basis for 3 to 6 months. In each case the epidural cultures were negative until one patient developed a second epidural infection at month 4 from a different organism. The longest time to postepidural infection was in a patient who had an epidural infusion that lasted for 1½] years without infection. There is currently no data on potential toxicity of vancomycin in the epidural space. Clearly, further examination of risk versus benefit in using this therapy is indicated. The standard of care continues to be device removal, aggressive systemic treatment, and replacement of the device after antibiotic therapy is completed.

Filters Filtering should be a standard of care for chronic intraspinal infusions. The acute pain specialist argues that filters are a site of obstruction during therapy, a barrier to aspiration of the catheter when testing for the presence of spinal fluid, and have an unproved outcome with added cost. The lack of controlled studies adds fuel to this controversy. The use of filtered epidural catheters to prevent infection in long-term epidural catheters has been generally accepted and more commercially available epidural catheter sets are now being manufactured with in-line filters. We have noted that most epidural space infections occur in the absence of exit site inflammation and negative exit site cultures. It would seem logical that the contamination is occurring through the catheter rather than alongside the catheter. Contamination occurs at the time of bag and tubing changes, and any policy that increases the incidence of those changes will increase the risk of contamination. Figure 71-10 illustrates the Du Pen epidural catheter with the double PALL epidural filter configuration.

Intrathecal Device Infections The intrathecal space may be accessed either by an externalized intrathecal catheter, port, or by placement of an intrathecal pump device. This technique has had limited use because of the fear of meningitis. Meningitis is exceedingly rare with the implanted pumps. The process of refilling the pump may result in contamination unless sterile conditions are maintained. We have had one pump-pocket infection requiring explant that was time correlated to an incident where multiple sticks were done at the time of a difficult refill. Reports of infections in implantable pumps are rare. Albright reported on infection during intrathecal baclofen therapy in children, a 5% infection rate "requiring pump removal" when utilizing the Medtronic's system.[96] Intrathecal vancomycin has been used to treat meningitis associated with pump infections,[97] and in unrelated meningitis.[98,99]

Nitescu and his colleagues at the University of Gothenburg, Sweden, have reported on the use of intrathecal exteriorized catheters to treat both chronic pain and cancer-related pain. This approach has not gained support in the US literature. The fear of meningitis has always been such a great deterrent that its use has been limited. These reports have brought a new focus to the use of intrathecal catheters. The first report described their technique in a report detailing 142 cancer patients treated with externalized spinal catheters.[100] The Portex nylon catheters were inserted at the lumbar level and tunneled paravertebrally up and over the shoulder. This first report included patients treated for 1 month using a syringe driver pump system. There were no reported cases of infection so the authors expanded the study in a second report to include another 89 patients. In this study the authors used a very low infusion rate of high concentration drug and reused CADD pump cassettes, but the cassettes were only changed or recharged on a monthly bases.[101] Again, the authors reported no infections and there was no affect on the drug concentrations when the cassettes were left in place for a full month. Nitescu et al in their report did not make a point of the reuse of the cassettes or the monthly filter changes. Their conclusions were that this is a safe and effective means of intrathecal analgesic infusion when trained nurses exchanged the cassettes and filters on a monthly basis.[102] In that same study, Nitescu, now reporting on 200 patients receiving the infusion over 7242 catheter days of use, had only a 0.5% rate of meningitis development. This low infection rate is far better than we were able to achieve during epidural infusions with filter and tubing changes every 48 to 72 hours. The only variable seems to be the frequency of "breaking into the system" or filter and tubing changes.

Another European group of investigators cited the use of externalized intrathecal systems because they were the "least costly and easiest to apply" for short periods.[103] Fifteen patients were treated with externalized intrathecal systems; 13 of the patients had the system implanted at home. No infections were reported. Devulder and colleagues studied 33 patients with tunneled intrathecal catheters connected to subcutaneous ports. Three patients developed meningitis (9+%). The authors were able to correlate the 9% infection rate to accidental disconnections in the external tubing of the pump systems with presumed contaminant events; they further recommended in-line filters.[104] Wagemans and others used externalized intrathecal catheters in 40 terminal cancer patients and reported meningitis in two patients, a 5% infection rate.[105] We have used externalized intrathecal catheters in five cancer patients over the last 3 years. These patients had no epidural space available (tumor or surgical ablation of the epidural space), or in one case the catheter was intended for epidural placement and was found postprocedure to be in the intrathecal space. One of these patients was treated for up to 1 year with no reported infections. In each case the infusion was maintained at the lowest possible infusion rate with highly concentrated drugs, to keep the infusion rates at or below 2 mL/hour. The lower infusion rates allow a single infusion bag to last several weeks, with bag changes only done by the visiting nurses. Long-term studies are needed, but there may not be a cost advantage in the United States. In the United States, pumps and infusion bags are supplied by home care agencies who rent the pump and charge for the drug preparation; these charges may exceed the expectation of the managed care organizations and providers.

Drug-related Complications

Infusion of analgesic agents into the epidural and intrathecal spaces may be associated with complications from unexpected reactions to drugs or drug combinations, drug errors, mixing errors, or infusion errors. Analgesic titration to effect or side effects is a standard of analgesic therapy. Those side effects are identified, classified for treatment priority, and treated to allow continued analgesic titration. The practitioner must be concerned about the complications of intraspinal analgesic drug therapy and how to identify, treat, and avoid drug-related complications.

Morphine appears to cause suppression of hormone production in some individual patients, resulting in endocrine alterations. Studies in animals, heroin addicts, and patients receiving long-term intraspinal morphine have demonstrated a decrease in testosterone associated with opioids.[106,107] Paice and coworkers showed a decrease in testosterone in men and a decrease in FSH in women receiving intraspinal opioids.[108] Patients exhibit decreased libido, fertility, and fatigue. Male patients may have erectile dysfunction and female patients may have amenorrhea. Testosterone and hormone replacement therapy has been successful in reversing these effects. These findings are not predictable and may be a rare occurrence. This is an area that the pain management community clearly needs to further study because sexuality can be a significant factor in our patient's lives.

Preservative content of many opioid and other drugs used for intraspinal analgesia must be watched carefully. The addition of preservatives to multidose drug preparations is common in the United States, but less common in other countries. Practitioners must be aware of the total content of any drug preparations considered for compounding into neuraxial infusions. We published a case report of a patient who received a morphine preparation containing phenol and formaldehyde in a long-term epidural infusion that was associated with neuropathic pain and the development of epidural space adhesions.[109] In this case the symptoms were reversed by removal of the preservative-containing morphine preparation. These errors may be corrected by education and information availability.

The infusion of concentrated analgesic combination into the neuraxial spaces have been studied by Yaksh, who has voiced concern over the use of untested drug combinations and concentrations and complications that may arise.[110] Neurotoxicity with high-dose intraspinal drug therapy has been reported in humans. Interestingly, two reports in the literature indicate a higher degree of risk might exist in patients with preexisting neuropathology.[111,112] Neuropathologic findings in 15 cancer patients status-post intrathecal morphine-bupivacaine therapy were reported by Sjoberg et al.[113] The majority of neuropathologic changes were cancer-related. There were changes identified within the spinal canal; however, no changes could be correlated to the cumulative dose of morphine, bupivacaine, or the oxidants contained in the formulation in this small sample. The use of subcutaneous intrathecal infusion pumps in chronic pain patients requires the use of high concentrations of the infusion drugs. Without such concentrations, the pump would require frequent access and refilling. The interventionist should maintain a high level of attention to the current literature on the neurotoxicity of concentrated drugs on the spinal cord.

Local anesthetic toxicity is rare when analgesic dose concentrations are used during epidural infusions.[34] Local anesthetic side effects include postural hypotension, skin anesthesia, and motor loss. These side effects are treated by vascular volume replacement and drug concentration adjustments. Once normovolemia is achieved, postural hypotension is rarely a problem unless the patient becomes dehydrated. High concentration local anesthetic agents have been used in intrathecal pumps; no neurotoxicity has been reported, but there have also been no controlled animal or clinical studies.

Clonidine is increasingly being used epidurally and intrathecally. Hypotension can be problematic, particularly early; however, volume replacement and slow upward titration is generally sufficient to normalize blood pressure. Intrathecal clonidine, although not approved for intrathecal use, is being used in intrathecal pumps using high concentration preparations. Yaksh has completed animal studies with concentrations as high as 6000 μg/mL (personal communication, 1998). These studies have not shown any signs of neurotoxicity. Controlled clinical trials are needed in this area to better define safety and efficacy. The more problematic issue is potential for rebound hypertension with abrupt discontinuation of spinal clonidine. Slow, downward titration of spinal clonidine, or prompt replacement with systemic clonidine, is indicated. Patients with intraspinal pumps may have mechanical failure of the pump; this unexpected failure could lead to a hypertensive crisis. Patients should be protected with an emergency kit of oral and transcutaneous clonidine.

Practical experience indicates that human error in drug administration needs to be considered. Pharmacy errors in mixing the drug for infusion have and will occur. Patients within our institution have received concentrations of drugs that were many times more or less potent than ordered, as well as the wrong drugs mixed in solution. These pharmacy errors are not predictable, so the clinician must consider these possibilities when the patient has an unexpected response to a recent refilling of the pump. When symptoms of drug withdrawal, overdose, or toxicity are noted soon after pump refills, the pump should be drained and refilled. The withdrawn solution should be saved for future analyses, if necessary. The multiple bag changes for patients receiving epidural infusions are a perfect setup for drug errors. Nursing errors in hanging the right solution for the right patient will occur, more likely in the hospital than in the home care setting. Patients within our institution have had hyperalimentation, heparin, and antibiotics inadvertently administered through permanent epidural catheters, both on the hospital floor and in the emergency room. It is important for the provider to be aware of these possibilities and to check all possible causes of any unexpected reaction and to correct the errors as they occur.

Mechanical Complications

Mechanical problems may be associated with the catheter, pump, filter, or the implanted device. One clinical dilemma associated with use of short-term epidural catheters is the failure of the adapter and connector. The connectors may become dislodged or the catheter material may become more brittle over time and break near the connector. The second most common problem is unexpected catheter withdrawal or migration outside of the epidural space. Tunneling the short-term catheter may add stability, but the durability of both catheter and connector are the major issues in maintaining the catheter for long-term use.[114] Mechanical complications of both epidural and intrathecal drug administration have been alleviated to a great extent with the advent of the permanent silicone-rubber epidural catheters.

Epidural hematoma is exceedingly rare under normal conditions.[115] Cancer patients with low platelet counts or those receiving anticoagulation therapy are, however, commonly encountered. Our policy, developed in close collaboration with the medical oncology staff, is to proceed if the platelet count is at least 20,000 *without* any signs of subcutaneous ecchymosis. Reversal of anticoagulation therapy is done on a case-by-case basis with consultation from the oncologist. This policy is consistent with the guidelines established by the consensus conference on anticoagulation and regional anesthesia organized by the American Society of Regional Anesthesia.

The most common cause of loss of analgesia encountered during epidural infusion is catheter or filter obstruction. Filter failure should be ruled out first when catheter obstruction is encountered. After catheter obstruction, failure of the externalized pump due to program input errors or an air bubble "lock" in the system is the next most common cause of analgesic failure. Utilizing aseptic technique and preservative-free saline, inject in the line above the filter and then below the filter to determine the source of the obstruction. Catheter obstruction may be further investigated by lumbar spine radiography or an epidurogram. Kinking of the catheter is easily seen on simple x-ray films. We have had one case of "crystallized" infusate in the catheter causing obstruction. This event occurred in a patient who had not been using the catheter for several months after obtaining pain relief with radiation therapy. The catheter was removed and subsequent dissection of the lumen revealed a solid mass of what was believed to be "old drug." Subsequently, our policy became to flush all unused epidural catheters with 3 mL of preservative-free saline at least once a week. Once the catheter occlusion is diagnosed, then a surgical repair or repositioning of the catheter can be accomplished. Fibrosis around the catheter in the epidural space is discussed, but in our experience this occurs only in the face of a subacute epidural space infection. A survey study of 519 implanters reported a series of patients with granulomatous catheter tip masses in the intrathecal space.[18] A second paper reports three cases of granuloma formation on an intrathecal catheter, with neurologic deficit. This a rare complication for which a cause has not been established, but infection and high concentration morphine have been suspected.[16]

Anderson and Burchiel reported that 20% of patients experience device-related complications with the implanted pump that require a repeat operation.[11] General system failure of implantable infusion devices was reported by Paice[15] and Penn as 21.6%, which is consistent with reports in the literature that vary from 10% to 40%. These system failures include catheter, pump, and connection problems. As with all multicenter, retrospective survey studies, the data are dependent on the rate of response from the implanters and the memory and recall of those clinicians.

Both external and internal pumps may be misprogrammed. It is important that two individuals check all pump programming of concentrated drugs that could endanger patient safety. A careful determination of the drug order and content of the infusion bag, pump infusion orders, and actual settings should follow any unexpected clinical outcome. In our practice, we felt the practice standards were in place, so we assumed this could not happen. We have had a major programming error event, which was corrected without sequelae; this event could have been avoided by simply having another nurse check the pump settings. The opioid-tolerant patient will tolerate most drug infusion errors, but may be placed in danger by errors of both drug concentration and infusion volume. Any abnormal patient response with signs of oversedation, neurologic deficits (not explained by tumor progress or metastatic lesions), or a combination of symptoms should alert the staff to turn down the pump significantly or stop until the cause of the symptom complex is determined. Consistent education and rational policies and procedures can minimize these human errors.

CONCLUSIONS

Interventional practitioners play an important role in facilitating analgesia where conventional techniques fail. Taking on a population of patients that requires neuraxial techniques can be a professionally and personally satisfying career decision. However, the provider must be prepared to tirelessly commit to a comprehensive approach to patient assessment, constant continuing education in spinal pharmacology, careful treatment planning, 24-hour availability, and continuous monitoring and follow-up. The basic research currently being done holds exciting promises for the future of neuraxial analgesia.

REFERENCES

1. Bruera E, Pereira J. Neuropsychiatric toxicity of opioids. In: Jensen TS, Turner JA, Weisenfeld-Hallin Z. *Proceedings of the 8th World Congress on Pain. Progress in Pain Research and Management.* Vol. 8. Seattle, Wash: IASP Press; 1997:717–738.
2. Chrubasik J, Chrubasik S, Martin E. Patient-controlled spinal opiate analgesia in terminal cancer. *Drugs* 1992;43:799–804.
3. Ellis D, Millar W, Reisner L. A randomised double-blind comparison of epidural versus intravenous fentanyl infusion for analgesia after cesarean section. *Anesthesiology* 1990;72:981–986.
4. Scholz J, Steinfath M, Koch C, et al. The pharmacologic basis of posteropative pain therapy: epidural opioid administration. *Anaesthesist* 1997;46:S154–S158.
5. Gourlay GK, Cherry DA, Cousins MJ. Cephalad migration or morphine in CSF following lumbar epidural administration in patients with cancer pain. *Pain* 1985;23:317–326.
6. Bromage PR, Camporesi EM, Durant PAC, et al. Rostral spread of epidural morphine. *Anesthesiology* 1982;56:431–436.
7. Rauck RL, Raj PP, Knarr DC, et al. Comparison of the efficacy of epidural morphine given by intermittent injection or continuous infusion for the management of post-operative pain. *Reg Anesth* 1994; 19:316–324.
8. De Leon-Casasola O, Lema J. Post-operative epidural opioid analgesia: What are the choices? *Anesth Analg* 1996;83:867–875.
9. Mercadante S. Problems of long-term spinal opioid treatment in advanced cancer patients. *Pain* 1999;79:1–13.
10. Gourlay GK, Plummer JL, Cherry DA, et al. Comparison of intermittent bolus with continuous infusion of epidural morphine in the treatment of severe cancer pain. *Pain* 1991;47:135–140.
11. Anderson VC, Burchiel KJ. A prospective study of long-term intrathecal morphine in the management of chronic nonmalignant pain. *Neurosurgery* 1999;44:289–300.
12. Gesten Y, Vainio A, Pegurier AM. Long-term infusions of morphine in the home care of patients with advanced cancer. *Acta Anaesthesiol Scand* 1997;47:12–17.
13. Nitescu P, Appelgren L, Linder LE, et al. Epidural versus intrathecal morphine-bupivacaine: assessment of consecutive treatments in advanced cancer pain. *J Pain Symptom Manage* 1990;5:18–26.
14. Sjoberg M, Nitescu P, Appelgren L, et al. Long-term intrathecal morphine and buipvacaine in patients with refractory cancer pain. *Anesthesiology* 1994;80:284–297.
15. Paice JA, Penn RD, Shott S. Intraspinal morphine for chronic pain: a retrospective, multicenter study. *J Pain Symptom Manage* 1996;11: 71–80.
16. Cabbell KL, Taren JA, Sagher O. Spinal cord compression by catheter granulomas in high-dose intrathecal morphine therapy: case report. *Neurosurgery* 1998;42:1176–1180.
17. North KB, Cutchis PN, Epstein JA, et al. Spinal cord compression complicating subarachnoid infusion of morphine: a case report and laboratory experience. *Neurosurgery* 1991;29:778–784.
18. Schuard M, Lanning, R, North R, et al. Neurologic sequelae of intraspinal drug delivery systems: Results of a survey of American implanters of implantable drug delivery systems. *Neuromodulation* 1998;1:137–148.
19. Roy SD, Flynn GL. Solubility and related physicochemical properties of narcotic analgesics. *Pharm Res* 1988;5:580–586.
20. Brose WG, Tanelian DL, Brodsky JB, et al. CSF and blood pharmacokinetics of hydromorphone and morphine following lumbar epidural administration. *Pain* 1991;45:11–15.
21. Halpern SH, Arellano R, Preston R, et al. Epidural morphine vs hydromorphone in post-caesarean section patients. *Can J Anaesth* 1996; 43:595–598.
22. Chaplan SR, Duncan SR, Brodsky JB, et al. Morphine and hydromorphone epidural analgesia. *Anesthesiology* 1992;77:1090–1094.
23. Liu S, Carpenter RL, Mulory MF, et al. Intravenous versus epidural administration of hydromorphone. Effects on analgesia and recovery after radical retropubic prostatectomy. *Anesthesiology* 1995;83:682–688.
24. Glass PSA, Estok P, Ginsberg B, et al. Use of patient controlled analgesia to compare the efficacy of epidural to intravenous fentanyl administration. *Anesth Analg* 1992;74:345–351.
25. Sandler AN, Stringer D, Panos L, et al. A randomized, double-blind comparison of lumbar epidural and intravenous fentanyl infusions for post-thoracotomy pain relief. *Anesthesiology* 1992;77:626–634.
26. Ozalp G, Guner F, Kuru N, et al. Postoperative patient-controlled epidural analgesia with opioid-bupivacaine mixtures. *Can J Anaesth* 1998;45:938–942.
27. Saito Y, Uchida H, Kaneko M, et al. Comparison of continuous epidural infusion of morphine/bupivacaine with fentanyl/bupivacaine for postoperative pain relief. *Acta Anaesthesiol Scand* 1994;38: 398–401.
28. De Leon-Casasola OA, Lema MJ. Epidural bupivacaine/sufentanil therapy for postoperative pain control in patients tolerant and unresponsive to epidural bupivacaine/morphine. *Anesthesiology* 1993;80: 303–309.
29. Saito Y, Kaneko M, Kirihara Y, et al. Interaction of intrathecally infused morphine and lidocaine in rats. Part 1: synergistic antinociceptive effects. *Anesthesiology* 1998;89;1455–1463.
30. De Leon-Casasola O, Parker B, Lema MJ, et al. Postoperative epidural bupivacaine-morphine therapy. Experience with 4,2227 surgical cancer patients. *Anesthesiology* 1994;81:368–375.
31. Berti M, Fanelli G, Casati A, et al. Comparison between epidural infusion of fentanyl/bupivacaine and morphine/bupivacaine after orthopaedic surgery. *Can J Anaesth* 1998;45:545–550.
32. Salomaki TE, Laitinen JO, Vainionpaa V, et al. 0.1% bupivacaine does not reduce the requirement for epidural fentanyl infusion after major abdominal surgery. *Reg Anesth* 1995;20:435–443.
33. Camann W, Abouleish A, Eisenach J, et al. Intrathecal sufentanil and epidural bupivacaine for labor analgesia: dose response of individual agents and in combination. *Reg Anesth Pain Med* 1998;23:457–462.
34. Du Pen SL, Kharasch ED, Williams A, et al. Chronic epidural bupivacaine-opioid infusion in intractable cancer pain. *Pain* 1992;49: 293–300.
35. Du Pen SL, Williams AR. Management of patients receiving combined epidural morphine and bupivacaine for the treatment of cancer pain. *J Pain Symptom Manage* 1992;7:125–127.
36. Krames ES, Lanning RM. Intrathecal infusional analgesia for nonmalignant pain: analgesic efficacy of intrathecal opioid with or without bupivacaine. *J Pain Symptom Manage* 1993;8:539–548.
37. Appelgren L, Janson M, Nitescu P et al. Continuous intracisternal and high cervical intrathecal bupivacaine analgesia in refractory head and neck pain. *Anesthesiology* 1996;84:256–272.
38. Berde CB, Sethna NF, Conrad LS, et al. Subarachnoid bupivacaine analgesia for seven months for a patient with a spinal cord tumor. *Anesthesiology* 1990;72:1094–1096.
39. Sjoberg M, Appelgren L, Einarsson S, et al. Long-term intrathecal morphine and bupivacaine in "refractory" cancer pain. Results from the first series of 52 patients. *Acta Anaesth Scand* 1991;35:30–43.
40. Hassenbusch SJ, Garber J, Buchser E, et al. Alternative intrathecal agents for the treatment of pain. *Neuromodulation.* 1999;2(2):85–91.
41. Markham, FD. Ropivacaine: a review of its pharmacology and therapeutic use in regional anesthesia. *Drugs* 1996;52:429–449.
42. Mercadante S, Calderone L, Barresi L. Intrathecal ropivacaine in cancer pain. *Reg Anesth Pain Med* 1998;23:621.
43. Christen C, Johnson CE, Walters JR. Stability of bupivacaine hydrochloride and hydromorphone hydrochloride during simulated epidural coadministration. *Am J Health Syst Pharm* 1996;53(2):70–173.

44. Wulf H, Gleim M, Mignat C. The stability of mixtures of morphine hydrochloride, bupivacaine hydrochloride, and clonidine hydrochloride in portable pump reservoirs for the management of chronic pain syndromes. *J Pain Symptom Manage* 1994;9:308–311.
45. Cook TM, James PA, Stannard CF. Diamorphine and bupivacaine mixtures: an in vitro study of microbiological safety. *Pain* 1998;76: 259–263.
46. Kreeger L, Cowin P, Noble-Gresty J, et al. Epidural diamorphine and bupivacaine stability study. *Palliat Med* 1995;9:315–318.
47. Tu Y, Stilles M, Allen L. Stability of fentanyl citrate and bupivacaine hydrochloride in portable pump reservoirs. *Am J Hosp Pharm* 1990; 47:2037–2040.
48. Dawson P, Bjorksten A, Duncan I, et al. Stability of fentanyl, bupivacaine, and adrenaline solutions for extradural infusion. *Br J Anaesth* 1992;68:414–417.
49. Mueller H, Biscoping J, Gips H, et al. Hygienic relations and stability of drugs in peridural long-term infusions with implanted or external pumps. *Anaesthesist* 1985;34:247–251.
50. Stiles M, Tu Y, Allen L. Stability of morphine sulfate in portable pump reservoirs during storage and simulated administration. *Am J Hosp Pharm* 1989;46:288–296.
51. Eisenach J, De Kock M, Klimscha W. Alpha-2 adrenergic agonists for regional anesthesia: a clinical review of clonidine (1984–1995). *Anesthesiology,* 1996;85:655–674.
52. Filos KS, Goudas LC, Patroni O, et al. Dose-related hemodynamic and analgesic effects of intrathecal clodidine after cesarean section. *Reg Anesth* 1993;18:18.
53. Brunschwiler M, Van Gessel E, Forster A, et al. Comparison of clonidine, morphine or placebo mixed with bupivacaine during continuous spinal anaesthesia. *Can J Anaesth* 1998;45:735–774.
54. Gautier PE, De Kock M, Fanard L, et al. Intrathecal clonidine combined with sufentanil for labor analgesia. *Anesthesiology* 1998;88: 651–656.
55. Puke MJC, Xu XJ, Wiesenfeld-Hallin Z. Intrathecal administration of clonidine suppresses autotomy, a behavioral sign of chronic pain in rats after sciatic nerve section. *Neurosci Lett* 1991;133:199–202.
56. Puke MJC, Wiesenfeld-Hallin Z. The differential effects of morphine and the alpha 2 adrenoceptor agonists clonidine and dexmedetomidine on the prevention and treatment of experimental neuropathic pain. *Anesth Analg* 1993;77:104–109.
57. Eisenach JC, Du Pen S, Dubois M, et al. Epidural clonidine analgesia for intractable cancer pain. *Pain* 1995;61:391–399.
58. Rauck RL, Eisenach JC, Jackson K, et al. Epidural clonidine treatment for refractory reflex sympathetic dystrophy. *Anesthesiology* 1993;79:1163–1169.
59. McCarthy RJ, Kroin JS, Lubenow TR, et al. Effect of tizanidine on antinociception and blood pressure in the rat. *Pain* 1990;40:333–338.
60. Kawamata T, Omote K, Kawamata M, et al. Antinociceptive interaction of intrathecal alpha 2 adrenergic agonists, tizanidine and clonidine, with lidocaine in rats. *Anesthesiology* 1997;87:436–448.
61. Hokfelt T, Elde R, Johansson O, et al. Immunohistochemical evidence for the presence of somatostatin, a powerful inhibitory peptide in some primary sensory neurons. *Neurosci Lett* 1975;1:231–235.
62. Krukoff T, Ciriello J, Calaresu F. Somatostatin-like immunoreactivity in neurons, nerve terminals, and fibers of the cat spinal cord. *J Comp Neurol* 1986;243:13–22.
63. Randic M, Miletic V. Depressant actions of methionine-enkephalin and somatostatin in the cat dorsal horn neurons activated by noxious stimuli. *Brain Res* 1978;152:196–202.
64. Murase K, Nedeljkov V, Randic M. The actions of neuropeptides on dorsal horn neurons in the rat spinal cord slice preparation: an intracellular study. *Brain Res* 1982;234:170–176.
65. Penn RD, Paice JA, Kroin JS. Octreotide: a potent new non-opiate analgesic for intrathecal infusion. *Pain* 1992;49:13–19.
66. Mollenholt P, Rawal N, Gordh T, et al Intrathecal and epidural somatostatin for patients with cancer. Analgesic effects and postmortem neuropathologic investigations of spinal cord and nerve roots. *Anesthesiology* 1994;81:534–542.
67. Bowersox SS, Gadbois T, Singh T, et al. Selective N-type neuronal voltage-sensitive calcium channel blocks, SNX-111, produces spinal antinociception in rat models of acute, persistent, and neuropathic pain. *J Pharmacol Exp Ther* 1996;279:1243–1249.
68. Chaplan SR, Pogrel JW, Yaksh TL. Role of voltage-dependent calcium channel subtypes in experimental tactile allodynia. *J Pharmacol Exp Ther* 1994;269:1117–1123.
69. Malmberg AB, Yaksh TL. Voltage-sensitive calcium channels in spinal nociceptive processing: blockade of N- and P-type channels inhibits formalin induced nociception. *J Neurosci* 1994;14:4882–4890.
70. Brose WG, Gutlove DP, Luther RR, et al. Use of intrathecal SNX-111, a novel N-type calcium channel blocker, in the management of intractable brachial plexus avulsion pain. *Clin J Pain* 1997;13:256–259.
71. McGuire D, Bowersox S, Fellman JD, et al. Sympatholysis after neuron-specific, N-type, voltage-sensitive, calcium channel blockade: first demonstration of N-channel function in humans. *J Cardiovasc Pharmacol* 1997;30:400–403.
72. Staats P, Charapata S, Presley R. Chronic, intractable neuropathic pain:marked analgesic efficacy of ziconotide. Poster presented at: The 4th International Congress of the International Neuromodulation Society; September 20, 1998; Lucerne, Switzerland.
73. Yamamoto T, Yaksh TL. Studies on the spinal interaction of morphine and the NMDA antagonist MK-801 on the hyperesthesia observed in a rate model of sciatic mononeuropathy. *Neurosci Lett* 1992;135: 67–70.
74. Yamamoto T, Shimoyama N, Mizuguchi T. the effects of morphine, MK-801, an NMDA antagonist, and CP-96,345, an NK1 antagonist, on the hyperesthesia evoked by carageenan injection in the rat paw. *Anesthesiology* 1993;78:124–133.
75. Sethna NF, Liu M, Gracely R, et al. Analgesic and cognitive effects of intravenous ketamine-alfentanil combinations versus either drug alone after intradermal capsaicin in normal subjects. *Anesth Analg* 1998;86:1250–1256.
76. Chia YY, Liu K, Liu YC, et al. Adding ketamine in a multimodal patient-controlled epidural regimen reduces postoperative pain and analgesic consumption. *Anesth Analg* 1998;86:1245–1249.
77. Wong CS, Liaw WJ, Tung CS, et al. Ketamine potentiates analgesic effect of morphine in postoperative epidural pain control. *Reg Anesth* 1996;21:534–541.
78. Basbaum A. New techniques, targets and treatments for pain: what promise does the future hold? *Celebrating 25 years*; *The International Association for the Study of Pain.* Seattle, Wash: IASP Press; 1998: 16–18.
79. Darland T, Heinricher M, Grandy D. Orphanin FQ/nociceptin: a role in pain and analgesia, but so much more. *Trends Neurosci* 1998;21: 215–221.
80. Taylor F, Dickenson A. Nociceptin/Orphanin FQ: a new opioid, a new analgesic? *Neuroreport* 1998;9:R65–R70.
81. Hao J, Xu I, Weisenfeld-Hallin Z, Xu X. Anti-hyperalgesic and anti-allodynia effects of intrathecal nociceptin/orphanin FQ in rats after spinal cord injury, peripheral nerve injury and inflammation. *Pain* 1998;76:385–393.
82. Bohme K, Tryba M. Paraspinal opioids and pump systems. *Z Arztl Fortbild Qualitatssich* 1998;92:47–52.
83. Enneking KF, Benzon HT. Oral anticoagulants and regional anesthesia: a perspective. *Reg Anesth Pain Med* 1998;23(suppl):140–145.
84. Appelgren L, Nordborg C, Sjoberg M, et al. Spinal epidural metastasis: implications for spinal analgesia to treat 'refractory' cancer pain. *J Pain Symptom Manage* 1997:13:25–42.
85. Torma T. Malignant tumors of the spine and the spinal extradural space: a study based on 250 histologically verified cases. *Acta Chir Scand.* 1987;255(suppl):1–138.
86. Zenz M, Schappler-Scheele B, Neuhans R, et al. Long-term peridural morphine analgesia in cancer pain. *Lancet* 1981;1:91.

87. Du Pen SL, Du Pen A. Tunneled epidural catheters: practical considerations and implantation techniques. In: Waldman S, Winnie A, eds. *Interventional Pain Management*. Philadelphia, Pa: WB Saunders Company; 1996.
88. Cusins MJ, Plummer JL,. Spinal opioids in acute and chronic pain. *Adv Pain Res Ther* 1991;18:457–473.
89. Plummer J, Cherry D, Cousins M, et al. Long term spinal administration of morphine in cancer and non-cancer pain: a retrospective study. *Pain* 1991;44:215–220.
90. Du Pen SL, Peterson DG, Williams AR, et al. Infection during chronic epidural catheterization: diagnosis and treatment. *Anesthesiology* 1990;73:905–909.
91. Schoeffler P, Pichard E, Ramboatiana R. et al. Bacterial meningitis due to infection of a lumbar drug release system in patients with cancer pain. *Pain* 1986;25:75.
92. Du Pen S. Implantable spinal catheter and drug delivery systems: complications. *Techniques Reg Anesth Pain Manage* 1998;2:152–160.
93. Darchy B, Forceville X, Bavoux E, et al. Clinical and bacteriological survey of epidural analgesia patients in the intensive care unit. *Anesthesiology* 1996;85:988–998.
94. Bevacqua BK, Slucky AV, Cleary WF. Is postoperative intrathecal catheter use associated with central nervous system infection? *Anesthesiology* 1994;80:1234–1240.
95. Hahn MB, Bettencourt JA, McCrea WB. In vivo sterilization of an infected long-term epidural catheter. *Anesthesiology* 1992;76:645.
96. Albright AL. Baclofen in the treatment of cerebral palsy. *J Child Neurol* 1996;11:77–83.
97. Bennett MI, Tai YM, Symonds JM. *Staphylococcus meningitis* following SynchroMed intrathecal pump implant: a case report. *Pain* 1994;56:243.
98. Abraham J, Bilgrami S, Dorsky D, et al. Stomatococcus mucilaginosus meningitis in a patient with multiple myeloma following autologous stem cell transplantation. *Bone Marrow Transplant* 1997;19: 639–641.
99. Catal'an MJ, Fernandeq JM, Vazquea A, et al. Failure of cefotaxime in the treatment of meningitis due to relatively resistant *Streptococcus pneumoniae*. *Clin Infect Dis* 1994;18:766.
100. Nitescu P, Appelgren L, Hultman E, et al. Long-term open catheterization of the spinal subarachnoid space for continuous infusion of narcotic and bupivacaine in patients with 'refractory' cancer pain. *Clin J Pain* 1991;7:143–161.
101. Nitescu P, Hultman E, Appelgren L, et al. Bacteriology, drug stability and exchange of percutaneous delivery systems and antibacterial filters in long-term intrathecal infusion of opioid drugs and bupivacaine in 'refractory' pain. *Clin J Pain* 1992;8:324–337.
102. Nitescu P, Sjoberg M, Appelgren L, et al. Complications of intrathecal opioids and bupivacaine in the treatment of 'refractory' cancer pain. *Clin J Pain* 1995;11:45–62.
103. Mercadante S. Intrathecal morphine and bupivacaine in advanced cancer pain patients implanted at home. *J Pain Symptom Manage* 1994; 9:201–207.
104. Devulder J, Ghys L, Dhondt W, et al. Spinal analgesia in terminal care: risk versus benefit. *J Pain Symptom Manage* 1994;9:75–81.
105. Wagemans MF, Spoelder EM, Zuurmond WW, et al. Continuous intrathecal analgesia in terminal cancer patients within transmural health care. *Ned Tijdschr Geneeskd* 1993;137:1553–1557.
106. Adams ML, Meyer ER, Cicero TJ. Interactions between alcohol and opioid induced suppression of rat testicular steroidogenesis in vivo. *Alcohol Clin Exp Res* 1997;21:684–690.
107. Rasheed A, Tareen IA. The effects of heroin on thyroid function, cortisol, and testosterone level in addicts. *Polish J Pharmacol* 1995;47: 441–444.
108. Paice JA, Penn RD, Ryan WG. Altered sexual function and decreased testosterone in patients receiving intraspinal opioids. *J Pain Symptom Manage* 1994;9:126–131.
109. Du Pen SL, Ramsey D, Chin S. Chronic epidural morphine and preservative induced injury. *Anesthesiology* 1987;67:987–988.
110. Yaksh TL. Preclinical models for analgesic drug study. In: Godberg AM, Zutphen LFM, eds. *Alternative Methods in Toxicology and the Life Sciences. II: The World Congress on Alternatives and Animal Use in the Life Sciences: Education, Research, Testing*. New York, NY: Mary Ann Liebert, Inc; 1995.
111. Kloke M, Bingel U, Seeber S. Complications of spinal opioid therapy; myoclonus, spastic muscle tone, spinal jerking. *Support Care Cancer* 1994;2:249–252.
112. Waters JH, Watson TB, Ward MG. Conus medullaris injury following both tetracaine and lidocaine spinal anesthesia. *J Clin Anesthesiol* 1996;8:656–658.
113. Sjoberg M, Karlsson PA, Nordborg T. Neuropathologic findings after long-term intrathecal infusion of morphine and bupivacaine for pain treatment for cancer patients. *Anesthesiology* 1992;76:173–186.
114. Ali N, Hanna N, Hoffman J. Percutaneous epidural catheterization for intractable pain in terminal cancer patients. *Gynecol Oncol* 1989;32: 22–25.
115. Geible RM, Scherer R, Peters J. Incidence of neurologic complications related to thoracic epidural catheterization. *Anesthesiology* 1997;86:55–63.

CHAPTER 72 NEUROMODULATION FOR PAIN

Jennifer A. Elliott and Thorkild Vad Norregaard

INTRODUCTION

In the past 30 years, the field of pain management has increasingly incorporated technologies of neurostimulation as part of the treatment algorithm for patients with intractable pain. These technologies include peripheral nerve stimulation, spinal cord stimulation, deep brain stimulation, sacral nerve stimulation, and trigeminal nerve stimulation. More and more patients with complex pain conditions who have failed more conservative management are finding some degree of relief through the use of these devices.

The inspiration for development of these technologies came from the landmark "gate control theory" introduced by Melzack and Wall in 1965.[1] Although this model fails to explain certain phenomena seen in painful conditions and cannot account for all of the observed effects of neurostimulation, the gate control theory remains the primary paradigm used to describe how neurostimulation acts to modify pain transmission. The gate control theory is based on the presence of cells in the dorsal horn of the spinal cord that receive afferent signals from peripheral C fibers conveying painful stimuli, as well as non-nociceptive sensory fibers. Once pain signals reach these dorsal horn interneurons, a "gate" is activated and painful impulses propagate along ascending fibers to the brain, resulting in conscious awareness of pain. Wall and Melzack proposed that the gate could be closed to the transmission of painful impulses through the selective activation of non-nociceptive fibers. Thus, the notion of using neurostimulatory devices to preferentially activate non-nociceptive fibers as a means of diminishing pain was born.

The application of neurostimulation has been increasing since C. Norman Shealy implanted the first spinal cord stimulator device in 1967. The scope of conditions amenable to these technologies has likewise expanded as they have become more widely used in varying populations of patients around the world. Current indications for the use of these devices include isolated peripheral nerve injuries, failed back surgery syndrome, peripheral vascular disease with critical limb ischemia, refractory angina pectoris, deafferentation syndromes, spinal-cord-injury–related pain, interstitial cystitis, and trigeminal neuralgia. Other applications are continuously being evaluated, including the use of spinal cord stimulation as a means to monitor evoked potentials during thoracoabdominal aneurysm repair.[2]

BEYOND GATE CONTROL: NEUROHUMORAL BASIS OF SPINAL CORD STIMULATION

Although the gate control theory seems to explain the primary mechanism by which neurostimulation works, it cannot account for some of the clinically observed effects of spinal cord stimulation. Some researchers have proposed that spinal cord stimulation inhibits transmission of painful impulses partly by inducing a differential conduction block of afferent nociceptive fibers via antidromic stimulation. That the effects of stimulation can outlast the duration of the stimulation would seem, however, to indicate this is not the only mechanism by which neurostimulation influences pain transmission. A number of investigators have speculated that neurohumoral mechanisms are also involved. Studies have been conducted to further elucidate which mediators may contribute. Substances that have been purported to be involved in the neuromodulatory effects of spinal cord stimulation include endogenous opioids, gamma (γ)-aminobutyric acid (GABA), adenosine, substance P, serotonin, calcitonin gene-related peptide (CGRP), and nitric oxide. Some of these mediators may also play a role in the sympathetic inhibitory effects of spinal cord stimulation.

Endogenous Opioids

It has been postulated by some researchers that endogenous opioid release may occur as a result of neurostimulation. There does exist evidence that transcutaneous electrical nerve stimulation (TENS) results in increased cerebrospinal fluid (CSF) levels of several types of opiate peptides. Some of these peptides appear to be μ-receptor specific, whereas others are more κ specific. The type of peptide released in response to TENS seems to depend on the frequency of the stimulation. The pain-relieving effects of low-frequency TENS appear to be reversible with naloxone, whereas those of high-frequency TENS are not.[3] There is no consistent evidence that endogenous opioid release occurs as a result of spinal cord stimulation, however; and naloxone does not reverse the effects of spinal cord stimulation. Thus, while endogenous opioid release may result from some forms of neurostimulation, it does not appear to play a significant role in spinal cord stimulation.

GABA

GABA is a major inhibitory neurotransmitter that has been shown to mediate some of the pain-relieving effects of spinal cord stimulation. GABA is able to modulate pain by controlling the release of excitatory amino acids such as aspartate and glutamate in the dorsal horn. It is believed that certain anomalies seen in chronic pain states, such as allodynia and hyperalgesia, may be caused by disrupted regulation of excitatory amino acid release in the dorsal horn.[4] This is normally kept in check by local GABA activity. Deficient GABA function as a consequence of nerve injury may result in abnormal responsiveness of wide-dynamic range neurons to tactile stimulation. The sequela of this may be the development of allodynia and hyperalgesia.

It was speculated that some of the antinociceptive actions of spinal cord stimulation are due to the ability of spinal cord stimulation to modulate GABA release in the dorsal horn. Many studies have been done to evaluate this hypothesis. In one of these studies, investigators measured GABA levels in the dorsal horn before and after initiation of spinal cord stimulation in laboratory animals exhibiting the behavioral equivalent of allodynia in humans. It was revealed that the animals that responded to the stimulation with diminished withdrawal responses to tactile stimuli indeed had enhancement of dorsal horn GABA levels after the onset of stimulation.[5] Additionally, it was noted that the animals that failed to normalize withdrawal thresholds in response to spinal cord stimulation did not have the enhanced GABA release in the dorsal horn seen in the animals that did respond to spinal cord stimulation. This prompted further study of the nonresponding animals to determine whether the use of small doses of the GABA agonist baclofen, in conjunction with spinal cord stimulation, would alter the effectiveness of the stimulation.[6] The doses of baclofen used in the study were well below those required to clinically affect withdrawal thresholds when used alone. The investigators found that the combined effects of spinal cord stimulation and low-dose baclofen resulted in diminished pain behavior in the previously nonresponding animals.

The concept of spinal cord stimulation modulating pain transmission through the effects on GABA and excitatory amino acid levels in the dorsal horn has been reinforced by a study that demonstrated that excitatory amino acid content of the dorsal horn can be diminshed during spinal cord stimulation.[7] Additional research into the role of GABA in mediating the effects of spinal cord stimulation has involved the use of GABA antagonists. The administration of the GABA antagonist Bicuculline in cats subjected to spinal cord stimulation attenuated the inhibitory effects of spinal cord stimulation on transmission of ascending impulses, as measured by a recording electrode situated over the anterolateral funiculus.[8] Thus, GABA-related functions play a critical role in the modulation of painful inputs, and it appears that spinal cord stimulation acts, in part, to alter dysfunctional GABA systems that may be present in chronic pain states.

Adenosine

The distribution of adenosine receptors in the dorsal horn of the spinal cord has led several investigators to speculate that adenosine, like GABA, may have important modulatory effects on the transmission of painful impulses. Experiments that parallel those used to evaluate the role of GABA in the allodynia-suppressing effect of spinal cord stimulation have been done using adenosine agonists and antagonists.[9–11] These studies have shown that animals with evidence of allodynic behavior that fail to respond to spinal cord stimulation alone may become responsive to spinal cord stimulation by the addition of intrathecal adenosine agonists at clinically subeffective doses. Likewise, the intrathecal administration of small doses of an adenosine receptor antagonist to animals responsive to spinal cord stimulation resulted in apparent diminution in the effectiveness of the spinal cord stimulation in abolishing allodynic behavior.

Serotonin and Substance P

Several investigators have looked at substance P and serotonin release in the dorsal horn as a consequence of spinal cord stimulation. It is thought that these mediators have an inhibiting modulatory effect on transmission of painful stimuli in the dorsal horn. It also appears that the release of these mediators during spinal cord stimulation may, in part, occur through a supraspinal loop.[12]

Calcitonin Gene-Related Peptide

Calcitonin gene-related peptide (CGRP) is another putative mediator of some of the effects of spinal cord stimulation that has been investigated. CGRP release results in a vasodilatory response, which may account for some of the beneficial effects spinal cord stimulation has been shown to have on such conditions as reflex sympathetic dystrophy (complex regional pain syndrome [CRPS I]), intractable angina, and peripheral vascular disease, and disorders in which there is a significant component of ischemia. This seems to occur by antidromic stimulation of the dorsal roots, ultimately resulting in peripheral release of CGRP and subsequent vasodilation.[13] These effects may occur through a nitric-oxide-dependent mechanism.

Nitric Oxide

As mentioned previously, it appears that nitric oxide may play some role in mediating the vasodilatory effects of spinal cord stimulation. Investigators tested this hypothesis by administering a nitric oxide synthase inhibitor in an animal model after the application of dorsal column stimulation. Vasodilation of the ipsilateral hindpaw seen during dorsal column stimulation was significantly diminished after the nitric oxide synthase inhibitor was given. Further study was done to evaluate whether these effects are mediated through the autonomic nervous system. The results seemed to indicate that the nitric oxide release may occur independently of the sympathetic nervous system outflow, since the administration of the ganglionic-blocking agent hexamethonium in an animal model did not diminish the increased cutaneous blood flow seen during dorsal column stimulation.[14]

Sympathetic Nervous System Influences

Although some of the vasodilatory effects of spinal cord stimulation appear to occur by nitric oxide and CGRP-related mechanisms, there may be some sympathetically mediated vasodilation as well. Linderoth et al examined which receptor types might be involved.[15] They administered several types of receptor antagonists to further elucidate the role of cholinergic and adrenergic activity in mediating the vasodilatory effects of spinal cord stimulation. With the administration of α_1-receptor antagonists, beta blockers, nicotinic-receptor antagonists, and the nonspecific ganglionic blocker hexamethonium, the vasodilatory effects of spinal cord stimulation were either diminished or completely abolished. Muscarinic receptor antagonists did not have these same effects. Thus, it appears that sympathetically mediated vasodilation in spinal cord stimulation occurs by stimulation of nicotinic- and adrenergic-receptor subtypes.

APPLICATIONS OF SPINAL CORD STIMULATION

While many of the mechanisms by which spinal cord stimulation exerts its beneficial effects on painful syndromes remain under investigation, the scope of conditions that are being treated with this modality is expanding. To ensure maximal efficacy of this technology, proper patient selection must be undertaken prior to implantation of these devices. This selection process depends not only on the individual to be treated but also on the condition for which it is prescribed. If all relevant information is not reviewed prior to implantation of the spinal cord stimulator, the overall chance of success with this device may be diminished. Given the increasing demand for cost containment in the current era of medical practice, the placement of such a device in an improperly screened patient is likely to result not only in patient dissatisfaction, but also in stricter regulations by third-party payers with regard to selection of appropriate candidates for these devices. The suitability of spinal cord stimulation in any given patient depends first and foremost on the condition to be treated. The most common applications of spinal cord stimulation are in peripheral vascular disease, failed back surgery syndrome, complex regional pain syndrome, and angina pectoris.

Peripheral Vascular Disease

Peripheral vascular disease ranks among the most common indications for spinal cord stimulation worldwide. Patients with advanced peripheral vascular disease that is not amenable to revascularization procedures may be candidates for treatment with spinal cord stimulation. Also, patients with other diseases resulting in limb ischemia, such as Raynaud's disease, Buerger's disease, and CRPS I may derive benefit from this treatment. Intractable pain due to peripheral vascular disease generally seems to respond well to spinal cord stimulation. Additionally, it has been noted in a number of cases that healing of ischemic ulcers appeared to be enhanced in patients in whom this modality was employed. This finding prompted further study of the use of spinal cord stimulation in peripheral vascular disease with critical limb ischemia. When groups of peripheral vascular disease patients were followed over time, those who were using spinal cord stimulation as a means of treating their pain were seen to have an increased limb salvage rate as compared with their medically treated cohort.[16,17] This effect is thought to be related to vasodilation mediated by the sympathetic nervous system during spinal cord stimulation, creating an enhanced microcirculation. The quality of life of these patients can be significantly improved through the use of spinal cord stimulation. This may not only result from decreased analgesic requirements but also from potentially delayed amputation of the affected limb. Thus, spinal cord stimulation may act to postpone disabling but necessary treatment in these individuals, in addition to treating their pain.

Failed Back Surgery Syndrome

Many patients who have undergone surgical procedures such as laminectomies to treat back pain and radiculopathy continue to experience pain postoperatively or redevelop pain at a later date. These patients may, in some cases, undergo one or more repeat operations to further treat their pain. Despite surgical interventions, a percentage of these patients will continue to be plagued by pain. When surgically remediable anatomic lesions such as herniated disks, spinal stenosis, or a suboptimal fusion have been corrected, patients may be considered for placement of a spinal cord stimulator. In addition to pain relief, outcome measures such as decreased use of analgesics, increased physical activity, loss of neurologic function, and return of the previously disabled to work have been examined in a number of studies.[18–20] These studies showed that patients who derived pain relief from spinal cord stimulation often diminished their analgesic use or discontinued it altogether. Additionally, most were be able to perform more routine daily activities, and some who had previously been unfit to work were able to gain employment. Another study has been performed to compare outcomes when patients with failed back surgery syndrome were treated with spinal cord stimulation versus re-operation.[21] In an initial series of patients, the rate of crossover from re-operation to placement of a spinal cord stimulator was much greater than the reverse. These initial results suggest that, in some patients with failed back surgery syndrome and surgically correctable lesions, spinal cord stimulation may serve as a viable alternative to re-operation in further treating pain. Traditionally, pain in a monoradicular distribution has been the most amenable to treatment by neurostimulation. With larger areas of pain, it is more difficult to adequately cover all of the pain with paresthesias, a necessary prerequisite for success in using neurostimulation. Therefore, patients with more complex pain patterns, such as bilateral radiculopathy with axial low back pain, have often been seen as less apt to respond to spinal cord stimulation. As the technology becomes more advanced, with the use of multielectrode, multichannel, and multiprogram devices, these more complex pain patterns are increasingly being viewed as responsive to spinal cord stimulation.[22–26]

Intractable Angina Pectoris

As with patients suffering from end-stage peripheral vascular disease, patients having severe coronary syndromes that are unamenable to revascularization may find relief through spinal cord stimulation. This population of patients has often undergone multiple prior coronary angioplasties or coronary artery bypass operations and is receiving maximal medical therapy with continued recurrent angina despite aggressive treatment. Most of these patients are fairly incapacitated by their symptoms and fit functional classifications III to IV of the New York Heart Association. The use of spinal cord stimulation in this group of patients with severe coronary artery disease serves not only to diminish their pain but appears to overall decrease the number of ischemic episodes as well. This is thought to be due, in large part, to a reduction of sympathetic nervous system activity induced by spinal cord stimulation. A number of studies have been done to evaluate the impact of spinal cord stimulation on myocardial ischemia. Generally, these studies have revealed that use of spinal cord stimulation in cases of intractable angina pectoris may lead to reduced episodes of angina and decreased requirements for short-acting nitrates.[27,28] It also appears that exercise tolerance is enhanced in these patients, likely due to alterations in myocardial oxygen supply-to-demand ratio and possibly through redistribution of coronary blood flow to ischemic areas. Several studies have used techniques of atrial pacing to determine how anginal thresholds are affected by spinal cord stimulation.[29–31] During these studies, patients were paced to angina before and after turning on their spinal cord stimulators. After initiating stimulation, these patients were able to tolerate pacing to higher heart rates than prior to stimulation. It was noted that these patients would ultimately still experience angina when being paced maximally. These findings are of considerable importance in this arena, as some critics have expressed concern that spinal cord stimulation may only mask the symptoms of ischemia, thereby eliminating a key warning signal for these patients. Overall, the use of spinal cord stimulation in intractable angina pectoris appears to have beneficial effects that go beyond pain relief. It may reduce the frequency of angina (i.e., ischemia) in these patients through an alteration in the dynamics of myocardial oxygen supply and demand. This may have a significant impact on the quality of life of those suffering from this disabling morbidity.[32] Given the ever-increasing number of individuals in modern society who are developing coronary artery disease, partly as a consequence of lifestyle influences, it is likely that the number of patients treated with spinal cord stimulation for refractory angina will expand in the future.

Complex Regional Pain Syndrome

Complex regional pain syndrome I, previously referred to as reflex sympathetic dystrophy, is an entity that remains somewhat of an enigma in terms of its causation. As implied by its former name, this condition appears to involve aberrant activity in the sympathetic innervation of the affected body part that results in pain and other related sequelae seen in patients with this disorder. Spinal cord stimulation has a high rate of success when used in this patient population. Many of these patients have failed to respond to more conservative measures, such as sympathetic blocks and medications, and some have failed to have full response to surgical sympathectomy. Some authors have suggested that spinal cord stimulation is preferable to surgical sympathectomy in these cases.[33] Retrospective reviews of a limited number of patients having spinal cord stimulators implanted for management of their complex regional pain syndrome have shown that patient satisfaction with this mode of therapy is quite high, with up to 90% of these individuals finding the stimulator helpful for their pain.[34,35]

Many patients may be able to discontinue opiate therapy after initiation of spinal cord stimulation. The effectiveness of this modality in treating CRPS likely relates directly to its apparent inhibition of sympathetic activity in the area of stimulation, as has been seen in other patient populations such as those with peripheral vascular disease. Control of pain in these circumstances is an important component of proper rehabilitation because patients may be significantly restricted when participating in physical or occupational therapy due to their pain. This may create a vicious cycle in which disuse of the involved extremity eventually results in irreversible atrophic changes and significant disability. Complex regional pain syndrome remains an underdiagnosed source of pain, which appears to respond favorably to spinal cord stimulation. As this condition becomes more widely recognized and understood, the application of stimulators for this phenomenon will certainly expand.

Emerging Applications

Spinal cord stimulation has been used in the management of a number of conditions aside from those previously described. These entities include phantom limb pain, post-amputation stump pain, postherpetic neuralgia, multiple sclerosis, spinal cord injury, peripheral neuropathy, and post-herniorrhaphy pain.[36] The rate of permanent implantation in some of these patient populations remains low, and thus the long-term efficacy of spinal cord stimulation has yet to be established in these cases.

SCREENING OF PROSPECTIVE CANDIDATES FOR SPINAL CORD STIMULATION

Patients who have an established pain diagnosis that has not responded to conservative therapies, such as medication trials and injections, may be potential candidates for spinal cord stimulation. Patients who are to be considered for possible implantation of spinal cord stimulators must undergo screening to determine appropriateness of this therapy for their conditions.[37] Although some individuals may technically fit diagnostic categories suitable for spinal cord stimulation, they may ultimately be considered inappropriate candidates for a variety of physical and psychological reasons. To ensure a high likelihood of success with these devices, patients should be evaluated for significant psychopathology by a qualified psychologist or psychiatrist. During this time, patients will be evaluated for the presence of significant depression, anxiety, and personality disorders. A history of drug abuse will also be explored. If any significant psychopathology is present, or if a substance abuse problem is noted, it must be determined whether these conditions are active or controlled. Any ongoing severe psychological conditions or substance abuse must be treated prior to consideration for a spinal cord stimulation trial. Additionally, there are a number of diseases and other conditions that contraindicate implantation of these devices. Absolute and relative contraindications aside from the above include concomitant pregnancy, the presence of implanted pacemakers or automatic implantable cardioverter-defibrillator devices (AICD), malignancy as the source of pain, life expectancy of less than 1 year, inability to comprehend use of the device, severe cardiac compromise, and concomitant anticoagulation therapy. Once a patient has been appropriately screened and counseled regarding expectations, a trial of spinal cord stimulation should be arranged as a prerequisite to permanent implantation.

HARDWARE AVAILABLE FOR NEUROMODULATION

A neuromodulation system consists of a contact electrode or electrodes and either a subcutaneous pulse receiver or an implanted pulse generator. Electrodes are either percutaneously implantable through a Tuohy needle or through direct surgical access, for instance, in the spinal canal by a laminotomy in which the yellow ligament is removed. Electrode systems vary from a simple percutaneous four-contact electrode to complex laminectomy-style electrodes with up to 16-electrode contacts. A subcutaneous pulse receiver with an external power unit or an implantable battery unit allow for variation in stimulation parameters such as amplitude, frequency, and pulse duration. Current equipment is manufactured by Medtronic, Inc. (Minneapolis, Minn) or Advanced Neuromodulation Systems, Inc (Allen, Tex).

A fully implanted system powered with a subcutaneous pulse generator offers higher convenience to the patient. A percutaneously powered system operating through a subcutaneous pulse receiver, which is powered by a stimulator unit that is glued to the skin, offers the advantage of broader stimulation functions and obviates the need for battery replacement. Choice of system can, in part, be influenced by information obtained during trial stimulation. If energy requirements during trial stimulation are low, an implanted power source may be a reasonable choice, whereas substantial energy requirement might lead to the choice of a percutaneously powered system.

TRIAL FOR SPINAL CORD STIMULATION

Clinical evaluation including psychological assessment helps identify patients that are suitable candidates for invasive neuromodulation therapy.[38] The preoperative evaluation does not, however, provide a guarantee for long-term effect from neuromodulation in general and spinal cord stimulation for instance in particular. Since these treatments are nonablative, a trial can therefore conveniently be performed. Trial electrodes are inserted percutaneously into the epidural space of the spinal canal. This is typically done with the patient in the prone position using fluoroscopic guidance. A strict percutaneous technique can be performed where the electrode is taped or sutured to the skin. The advantage of this approach is that the trial electrode can be removed during an office visit. If the trial leads to permanent implantation, a new electrode system will have to be implanted. Another approach is anchoring the test electrode to the superficial fascia and connecting this electrode to a percutaneous extension. If the trial is positive, this allows for keeping the trial electrode as the permanent stimulating electrode. Either one or more electrodes can be positioned during the trial procedure. The trial implantation is performed as a same-day-surgery procedure. Care should be taken to minimize tissue manipulation so that post-procedural pain does not interfere with interpretation of the test results. An unintended dural perforation can for instance also obscure the test results if significant CSF leakage occurs over the following days creating a spinal headache. The trial electrode implantation is done under local anesthesia with light intravenous sedation. When the electrode is in place, intraoperative test stimulation is performed. It is important that the patient is able to clearly understand questions and communicate with the surgeon during this part of the procedure. The subjective sensation of stimulation parasthesias, induced while stimulating, has to overlap the area where pain is felt in order to obtain pain relief.[39] After insertion of trial electrodes the patient is carefully instructed on how to perform the trial. The patient should keep a log during the trial in which pain intensity is documented when stimulating, as well as when not stimulating. In addition, consumption of pain medication and activity levels should be monitored. The trial period should be of a duration that clearly allows the patient to get a sense of the effect of stimulation. Three to eight days is a reasonable duration. Reporting at least 50% reduction in pain during the trial period without an increase in pain medication, or even better with a reduction in pain medication, is considered a positive trial and will lead to implantation of a permanent device.

A positive test trial, however, is no guarantee that spinal cord stimulation will provide long-term useful pain relief. A systematic review of the 1995 literature[19] indicated that an average of 59% of patients had greater than 50% pain relief at a mean follow-up of 16 months. Even at centers with significant experience, up to half of patients initially implanted with permanent spinal cord stimulator systems will experience long-term failure.

IMPLANTATION OF PERMANENT STIMULATION SYSTEM

A number of factors influence the choice of permanent spinal cord stimulation hardware. The choice often narrows down to whether to use a percutaneous electrode system or a laminectomy-style system for permanent stimulation. The laminectomy system requires removal of the test stimulation electrode and a direct surgical exposure of the spine. Subsequently, a laminotomy is performed, and through this spinal window, the laminectomy-style electrode is inserted. This bigger initial effort, however, is rewarded by a lower energy need for same effect, which translates into longer battery life. There is less tendency of the laminectomy-style electrode to migrate after implantation. The stimulation coverage is larger. There is less of a tendency of the stimulation to vary depending on body position. Lastly, a not infrequently seen side effect of stimulation-associated back pain is eliminated. The stimulation-associated back pain is likely to be the result of direct electrical stimulation of nociceptive fibers in the yellow ligament when using the percutaneous electrodes. The laminectomy-style electrode has a dorsal insulation, preventing stimulation of dorsally located structures.[40,41] In the cervical spine it is, however, not uncommon to have good stimulation coverage at low-energy requirement when using a percutaneous electrode. A percutaneous electrode may therefore in this setting be an appropriate electrode choice.

Permanent electrode placement using either percutaneous technique or laminectomy-style technique is again performed with the patient in a prone position resting on a fluoroscopic table. A lateral or semilateral position can be used, but anatomic interpretation of landmarks as well as fluoroscopic imagery is greatly facilitated when having the patient in a strict prone position. Using local anesthesia supplemented with intravenous sedation, any point of the spinal canal from occiput to lumbar region can be accessed. The lead placement includes fluoroscopic guidance as well as intraoperative test stimulation with patient feedback. When the proper stimulation pattern has been achieved, the lead should be secured to either yellow ligament or fascia to prevent postoperative migration.

A number of locations are possible for the implantable pulse generator or subcutaneous pulse receiver. These include lateral chest wall, abdomen, infraclavicular area, and upper gluteal area. An abdominal site often necessitates a two-step procedure; first the electrode is inserted with the patient in a prone position and, subsequently, tunneling and placement of pulse receiver or pulse generator in a lateral position. The softness of abdominal wall tissue can also pose difficulties for adequate anchoring of the subcutaneous device. The lateral chest wall can often be reached with the patient in a prone position. Placing the device over the lateral chest invariably eliminates the possibility for sleeping on the side of the implant. The pectoral or infraclavicular region can be quite suitable but may pose cosmetic issues. The gluteal area is in most instances the most suitable location. The exact positioning is important and should in general be centered approximately 7 to 8 cm below the iliac crest.

COMPLICATIONS FROM SPINAL CORD STIMULATION

The weakest mechanical link in a spinal cord stimulation system is the electrode. Electrode migration can occur, shifting stimulation coverage. As previously indicated, a laminectomy electrode reduces this risk. The increased mobility of the cervical spine increases the risk of electrode fracture secondary to metal fatigue given the amplitude of cervical spine movements. Intraspinal CSF leak following accidental dural puncture leading to spinal headache can in rare instances necessitate an epidural blood patch. Serious neurologic complications such as weakness or paralysis occur rarely. Epidural fibrosis formed around previously placed epidural stimulator electrodes can pose an additional challenge when performing revisions of such systems. Multilevel laminotomy, or even partial laminectomy, will reduce the risk of injury to the spinal cord and epidural bleeding, which otherwise can be the risk from blind sublaminar dissection of a fibrosed epidural space.

Intracranial Stimulation

Intracranial stimulation has focused on deep structures in the brain, and more recently, on the stimulation of cortical structures. Thalamic stimulation for pain was first reported in 1960.[42] Stimulation of the ventropostero lateral (VPL) nucleus of the thalamus provided relief from chronic intractable neuropathic pain. A similar effect was subsequently reported from chronic ventroposterior-medial (VPM) stimulation.[43] Stimulation of VPL and VPM is like spinal cord stimulation associated with a sensation of parasthesias of the target area. Stimulation of periaqueiductal gray matter (PAG) and periventricular gray matter (PVG)[44–46] is more efficient in treating nociceptive pain. PAG and PVG stimulation is reversible by naloxone, and therefore in part mediated by endogenous opioids. Studies in chronic pain patients have shown increased spontaneous abnormal firing pattern in VPL/VPM.[47,48] Electrical stimulation in these areas may conceivably block the abnormal bursting activity, leading to the observed pain relief. Long-term success of deep brain stimulation for nociceptive pain is in the middle 60%, whereas the effect for neuropathic pain is in the low 40%.

Implantation of deep brain stimulating electrodes require precise placement of the stimulating electrode in the intended target. The procedure is done under local anesthesia, during which a stereotactic frame is attached to the skull of the patient. Subsequently, a computed tomography (CT) scan or magnetic resonance imaging (MRI) scan is obtained with a localizing frame attached to the stereotactic base frame. The location of the anterior and posterior commeasure is determined with reference to the stereotactic frame. Assisted by a stereotactic atlas of the brain, the surgeon can with this information, locate the intended anatomic target. Intraoperatively, the anatomic target is confirmed through physiologic localization. This can include microelectrode recordings as well as micro- and macrostimulation, particularly in the thalamic targets. Stimulation in PVG or PAG is commonly associated with changes in blood pressure and heart rate. For localization of the later target, the surgeon must, however, rely primarily on anatomic landmarks. The permanent deep-brain-stimulating electrode is a quadipolar electrode (Medtronic, Minneapolis, Minn). The electrode is hooked up to a subcutaneously placed pulse generator that is placed in the subclavicular region. Since PVG/PAG stimulation is in part mediated via endogenous opioides, it is often possible to get bilateral pain relief from a single electrode inserted in the nondominant hemisphere. For unilateral pain, a contralateral PAG/PVG electrode is inserted. For VPM/VPL stimulation, effective relief of pain is only achieved from an electrode implanted in the contralateral hemisphere.

The observation of hyperactive bursting neuronal activity central to lesions in the somatosensory system prompted the concept of cortical stimulation. Stimulation of the precentral motor cortex turned out to provide pain relief as opposed to stimulation of the post-central cortex in patients experiencing post-stroke thalamic pain.[49,50] Motor cortex stimulation has also been used in the treatment of trigeminal neuropathic pain.[51] A laminectomy-style electrode is implanted into the epidural space during surgery. The location of the motor cortex is determined on the basis of anatomic landmarks as well as electrophysiologic testing. The electrode is thereafter exteriorized through a separate stab incision and test stimulation is performed for up to a week. If effective, an implantable battery unit is subcutaneously implanted in the subclavicular region and connected to the epidural lead through a subcutaneous extension. A prerequisite for effect is presence of a relatively intact motor system on clinical exam. In a study by Yamamoto et al, more than 70% of patients reported excellent pain relief by chronic motor cortex stimulation.[52] Motor cortex stimulation shows promise in treatment of these otherwise treatment-resistant conditions.

REFERENCES

1. Melzack R, Wall P. Pain mechanisms: a new theory. *Science* 1965; 150:971–978.
2. North RB, Drenger B, Beattie C, et al. Monitoring of spinal cord stimulation evoked potentials during thoracoabdominal aneurysm surgery. *Neurosurgery* 1991;28:325–330.
3. Han JS, Chen XH, Sun SL, et al. Effect of low- and high-frequency TENS on metenkephalin-Arg-Phe and dynorphin A immunoreactivity in human lumbar CSF. *Pain* 1991;47:295–298.
4. Linderoth B, Foreman RD. Physiology of spinal cord stimulation: review and update. *Neuromodulation* 1999;2:150–164.
5. Stiller CO, Cui JG, O'Connor WT, et al. Release of gamma aminobutyric acid in the dorsal horn and suppression of tactile allodynia by spinal cord stimulation in mononeuropathic rats. *Neurosurgery* 1996;39: 367–375.
6. Cui JG, Linderoth B, Meyerson BA. Effects of spinal cord stimulation on touch evoked allodynia involve GABAergic mechanisms. An experimental study in the mononeuropathic rat. *Pain* 1996;66:287–295.
7. Cui JG, O'Connor WT, Ungerstedt U, et al. Spinal cord stimulation attenuates augmented dorsal horn release of excitatory amino acids in mononeuropathy via a GABAergic mechanism. *Pain* 1997;73:87–95.
8. Duggan AW, Foong FW. Bicuculline and spinal inhibition produced by dorsal column stimulation in the cat. *Pain* 1985;22:249–259.
9. Cui JG, Sollevi A, Linderoth B, Meyerson BA. Adenosine receptor activation suppresses tactile hypersensitivity and potentiates spinal cord stimulation in mononeuropathic rats. *Neurosci Lett* 1997;223:173–176.
10. Cui JG, Meyerson BA, Sollevi A, Linderoth B. Effect of spinal cord stimulation on tactile hypersensitivity in mononeuropathic rats is potentiated by simultaneous $GABA_B$ and adenosine receptor activation. *Neurosci Lett* 1998;247:183–186.
11. Meyerson BA, Cui JG, Yakhnitsa V, et al. Modulation of spinal pain mechanisms by spinal cord stimulation and the potential role of adjuvant pharmacotherapy. *Stereotactic Funct Neurosurg* 1997;68:129–140.
12. Linderoth B, Gazelius B, Franck J, Brodin E. Dorsal column stimulation induces release of serotonin and substance P in the cat dorsal horn. *Neurosurgery* 1992;31:289–297.
13. Croom JE, Foreman RD, Chandler MJ, Barron KW. Cutaneous vasodilation during dorsal column stimulation is mediated by dorsal roots and CGRP. *Am J Physiol* 1997;272:H950–H957.
14. Croom JE, Foreman RD, Chandler MJ, et al. Role of nitric oxide in cutaneous blood flow increases in the rat hindpaw during dorsal column stimulation. *Neurosurgery* 1997;40:565–571.
15. Linderoth B, Herregodts, P, Meyerson BA. Sympathetic mediation of peripheral vasodilation induced by spinal cord stimulation: animal studies of the role of cholinergic and adrenergic receptor subtypes. *Neurosurgery* 1994;35:711–719.
16. Huber SJ, Vaglienti RM, Huber JS. Spinal cord stimulation in severe, inoperable peripheral vascular disease. *Neuromodulation* 2000;3:131–143.

17. Claeys LG. Spinal cord stimulation in the treatment of chronic critical limb ischemia: review of clinical experience. *Neuromodulation* 2000; 3:89–96.
18. North RB, Ewend MG, Lawton MT, et al. Failed back surgery syndrome: 5-year follow-up after spinal cord stimulator implantation. *Neurosurgery* 1991;28:692–699.
19. Turner JA, Loeser JD, Bell KG. Spinal cord stimulation for chronic low back pain: a systematic literature synthesis. *Neurosurgery* 1995; 37:1088–1096.
20. Wetzel FT, Hassenbusch S, Oakley JC, et al. Treatment of chronic pain in failed back surgery patients with spinal cord stimulation: a review of current literature and proposal for future investigation. *Neuromodulation* 2000;3:59–74.
21. North RB, Kidd DH, Lee MS, Piantodosi S. A prospective, randomized study of spinal cord stimulation versus reoperation for failed back surgery syndrome: initial results. *Stereotactic Funct Neurosurg* 1994; 62:267–272.
22. Alo KM, Yland MJ, Charnov JH, Redko V. Multiple program spinal cord stimulation in the treatment of chronic pain: follow-up of multiple program SCS. *Neuromodulation* 1999;2:266–272.
23. Barolat G. A prospective multicenter study to assess the efficacy of spinal cord stimulation utilizing a multi-channel radio-frequency system for the treatment of intractable low back pain. Initial considerations and methodology. *Neuromodulation* 1999;2:179–183.
24. Van Buyten JP, Van Zundert J, Milbouw G. Treatment of failed back surgery syndrome patients with low back and leg pain: a pilot study of a new dual lead spinal cord stimulation system. *Neuromodulation* 1999;2:258–265.
25. North RB, Guarino AH. Spinal cord stimulation for failed back surgery syndrome: technical advances, patient selection, and outcome. *Neuromodulation* 1999;2:171–178.
26. Oakley JC. Spinal cord stimulation for the relief of pain. Paper presented at: The 4th International Neuromodulation Society, September 16-20, 1998, Lucerne, Switzerland.
27. Jessurun GAJ, DeJongste MJL, Blanksma PK. Current views on neurostimulation in the treatment of cardiac ischemic syndromes [review]. *Pain* 1996;66:109–116.
28. Eliasson T, Augustinsson LE, Mannheimer C. Spinal cord stimulation in severe angina pectoris—Presentation of current studies, indications and clinical experience [review]. *Pain* 1996;65:169–17.
29. DeJongste MJL. Efficacy, safety and mechanisms of spinal cord stimulation used as an additional therapy for patients suffering from chronic refractory angina pectoris. *Neuromodulation* 1999;2:188–192.
30. DeJongste MJL. Spinal cord stimulation for ischemic heart disease. *Neurol Res* 2000;22:293–298.
31. Sanderson JE, Brooksby P, Waterhouse D, et al. Epidural spinal electrical stimulation for severe angina: a study of its effects on symptoms, exercise tolerance and degree of ischaemia. *Eur Heart J* 1992;13:628–633.
32. Vulink NCC, Overgaauw DM, Jessurun GAJ, et al. The effects of spinal cord stimulation on quality of life in patients with therapeutically chronic refractory angina pectoris. *Neuromodulation* 1999;2:33–40.
33. Kumar K, Nath RK, Toth G. Spinal cord stimulation is effective in the management of reflex sympathetic dystrophy. *Neurosurgery* 1997;40: 503–509.
34. Oakley JC, Weiner RL. Spinal cord stimulation for complex regional pain syndrome: a prospective study of 19 patients at two centers. *Neuromodulation* 1999;2:47–50.
35. Bennett DS, Alo KM, Oakley J, Feler CA. Spinal cord stimulation for complex regional pain syndrome I [RSD]: a retrospective multicenter experience from 1995 to 1998 of 101 patents. *Neuromodulation* 1999; 2:202–210.
36. Elias M. Spinal cord stimulation for post-herniorrhaphy pain. *Neuromodulation* 2000;3:155–157.
37. Kumar K, Nath R, Wyant GM. Treatment of chronic pain by epidural spinal cord stimulation: a 10-year experience. *J Neurosurg* 1991;75: 402–407.
38. Burchiel KJ, Anderson VC, Brown FD, et al. Prospective, multicenter study of spinal cord stimulation for chronic back and leg pain. *Spine* 1996;21:2786–2794.
39. North RB, Uewend MG, Laughton, MT, Piantadosi S. Spinal cord stimulation for chronic intractable pain: superiority of 'multichannel' devices. *Pain* 1991;44:119–130.
40. North RB, Lanning A, Hessels R, Kutchis PN. Spinal cord stimulation with percutaneous and plate electrodes: side effects and quantitative comparisons. *Neurosurgery Focus* 1997;2:xx.
41. North RB, Olin JC, Kidd DH, Sieracki JN. Spinal cord stimulation electrode design: a prospective, randomized comparison of percutaneous and laminectomy electrodes. Poster abstract at: American Association of Neurological Surgeons.
42. Mazars G, Roge R, Mazars Y. Stimulation of the spinothalamic fasciculus and their bearing on the pathophysiology of pain. *Rev Neurol* 1960;103:136–138.
43. Hosobuchi Y, Adams J, Rutkin B. Chronic thalamic stimulation for the control of facial anesthesia dolorosa. *Arch Neurol* 1973;29:158–161.
44. Richardson DE, Akil H. Pain reduction by electrical brain stimulation in man, Part 1. Acute administration in periaqueductal and periventricular sites. *J Neurosurg* 1977;47:178–183.
45. Richardson DE, Akil H. Pain reduction by electrical brain stimulation in man, Part 2. Chronic self-administration in the periventricular gray matter. *J Neurosurg* 1977;47:184–194.
46. Hosobuchi Y, Adams JE, Linchitz R. Pain relief by electrical stimulation of the central gray matter in humans and its reversal by naloxone. *Science* 1977;
47. Hirayama T, Dostrovsky J, Gorecki J, et al. Recordings of abnormal activity in patients with deafferentation and central pain: proceedings of the microelectrode meeting. *Stereotactic Funct Neurosurg* 1989;52: 120–126.
48. Lenz F, Tasker R, Dostrovsky J, et al. Abnormal single-unit activity recorded in the somatosensory thalamus of a quadriplegic patient with central pain. *Pain* 1987;31:225–236.
49. Tsubokawa T, Katayama Y, Yamamoto T, et al. Chronic motor cortex stimulation for treatment of central pain. *Acta Neurochir* 1991;52(suppl): 137–139.
50. Tsubokawa T, Katayama Y, Yamamoto T, et al. Chronic motor cortex stimulation in patients with thalamic pain. *J Neurosurg* 1993;78:393–401.
51. Meyerson BA, Lindblom U, Lindblom B, et al. Motor cortex stimulation as treatment of trigeminal neuropathic pain. *Acta Neurochir* 1993; 58(suppl):150–153.
52. Yamamoto T, Katayama Y, Hirayama T, et al. Pharmacological classification of central post stroke pain: comparison with the results of chronic motor cortex stimulation therapy. *Pain* 1997;72:5–12.

CHAPTER 73 NEUROLYTIC BLOCKS

Moris M. Aner and Carol A. Warfield

Intractable cancer pain, as well as chronic intractable benign pain, has been troublesome to the pain practitioner because of the short life span of conventional nerve blocks. Neurolytic agents have been in use since the turn of the 20th century for this particular group of pain patients for prolonged pain relief.

Neurolysis encompasses interruption of painful pathways by placement of a needle in the proximity of a nerve or plexus, either by injecting destructive chemicals or creating nerve obliteration by cold (cryotherapy) or heat energy (radiofrequency ablation).

This chapter focuses on the properties of the neurolytic agents and their clinical applications; separate chapters are dedicated to the other two techniques: cryotherapy and radiofrequency.

HISTORY

The first report of neurolysis was in 1863 by Luton, who injected subcutaneous irritant substances into painful areas and found that sciatic neuralgia was responsive to such therapy.[1] Hartel reported the first use of caustic agents on nerve roots to interrupt pain fibers in 1914,[2] and Doppler reported the use of phenol to destroy nerve tissues in 1926.[3] Putnam and Hampton, in 1936, reported the first use of phenol as a neurolytic agent for gasserian ganglion block.[4] In 1931, Dogliotti described the first use of alcohol for subarachnoid neurolysis to achieve prolonged relief.[5] The first use of phenol for subarachnoid neurolysis was reported by Maher in 1955.[6] Today, ethyl alcohol and phenol are the most widely used compounds; yet hypertonic saline, glycerol, ammonium salts, and chlorocresol have also been used.

PATIENT SELECTION

Proper selection of patients for neurolytic blocks is the key to success of these potentially harmful procedures. After successful diagnostic local anesthetic blocks, a neurolytic block can be considered with reference to the cause and localization of the pain.[7] If the patient is too debilitated, or the logistics of a procedure would not allow a trial local anesthetic block, diagnostic blocks can be combined with a neurolytic agent at the practitioner's discretion. Clear communication of alternative techniques, outcomes, complications, expectations, and disease progression with the patient and the family is important prior to a neurolytic procedure.

A multidisciplinary approach, including an aggressive trial of opioids and adjuvant medications, along with temporary nerve blocks and psychological support are the mainstays of therapy.[8] If these measures result in inadequate pain control or excessive nausea, sedation, or constipation, a neurolytic block should be strongly considered.

A thorough medical examination, including laboratory testing and imaging studies if appropriate, is necessary before performing a neurolytic block. Active infection, tumor involvement of the needle entry site, bleeding disorders, or concomitant anticoagulation therapy may be relative contraindications.

Currently, nerve stimulation techniques are widely used with all peripheral neurolytic blocks. Computed tomography (CT) or biplanar fluoroscopic guidance is common for neuroaxial and sympathetic neurolytic procedures. As in all invasive procedures, adherence to strict sterile technique is mandatory. Cardiovascular monitoring during and post-procedure with resuscitative backup play key roles in preventing adverse outcomes.

NEUROLYTIC AGENTS

Ethyl Alcohol

Ethyl alcohol is commercially available in the United States as higher-than-95% concentration, single-dose 1-mL and 5-mL ampules. Alcohol is usually used undiluted in peripheral injections. Injection of alcohol perineurally is often associated with burning dysesthesias along the distribution of the nerve. Preceding the injection with a local anesthetic can abort this significant discomfort, and may also serve as a test dose for correct placement of the needle.[9]

The neurolytic action of alcohol is by dehydration, extraction of cholesterol, phospholipids, cerebrosides, and precipitation of mucoproteins. This action results in sclerosis of the nerve fibers and the myelin sheath,[10] causing demyelination and subsequent wallerian degeneration. This nonselective process is observed in peripheral nerve injections, as well as in spinal nerve roots, after a subarachnoid injection. On histopathologic examination, patchy areas of demyelination are seen in posterior columns, Lissauer's tract, and dorsal roots. Wallerian degeneration then extends to the dorsal horn.[11] Hence, large-volume injections can result in meningeal inflammatory changes and degeneration of the spinal cord.

Alcohol is hypobaric with respect to cerebrospinal fluid, which makes it easier to use for subarachnoid neurolysis by the use of proper positioning of the patient. Concentrations of 50% to 100% have been typically employed for subarachnoid blocks. The patient is usually placed in the lateral decubitus position with the painful site up in order to utilize the hypobaric properties of alcohol. The patient is then rolled 45 degrees to place the dorsal root at the contact point of alcohol rise, the so-called lateral-prone position. A volume of 0.3 mL to 0.7 mL is injected per segment.

Absolute alcohol has been used in variable concentrations, with inconsistent results on sensory and motor differentiation. The lowest concentration of alcohol used resulting in satisfactory analgesia, with no paresis or paralysis, is as 33%.[12] Concentrations ranging from 48% to 100% have been associated with incomplete, temporary, progressive, or persistent motor paralysis. The general consensus is that, with 95% alcohol, the obliteration entails the sympathetic, sensory, and motor components of a mixed somatic nerve.

The pharmacologic properties of alcohol have important implications on clinical use:

- Alcohol, unlike phenol and glycerin, is readily soluble *in vivo*, resulting in a rapid spread from the injection site. Adequate neurolysis may require increased volume use, which may result in surrounding tissue damage.
- *In vitro* studies have associated alcohol with arterial vasospasm, which theoretically is the basis for paraplegia after celiac plexus blocks via spasm of the artery of Adamkiewicz.
- Acetaldehyde syndrome disulfiram-like effect has been described after neurolysis with alcohol on a patient treated with moxalactam, a beta-lactam type antibiotic reported to inhibit aldehyde dehydrogenase.[13] The patient experienced flushing, sweating, dizziness, vomiting, and marked hypotension for 10 minutes after an injection of 15 mL of 67% alcohol for a celiac plexus block. The pain practitioner should be cautious about patients taking agents with similar properties, such as metronidazole, chloramphenicol, the beta-lactam-type antibiotics, the oral hypoglycemic tolbutamide and chlorpropamide, and disulfiram.[14]
- Neuritis and deafferentation pain, especially with peripheral and lumbar sympathetic neurolysis, have been associated more commonly with alcohol than phenol. In the case of lumbar sympathetic neurolysis, development of genitofemoral neuralgia secondary to the degeneration of the rami communicants to the L2 nerve root has been well described.[15,16] However, this finding has not been documented in controlled studies.[17]
- After celiac plexus block with alcohol, serum ethanol levels ranging between 21 and 54 mg/dL have been reported.[18] Even though these numbers are below the levels to cause the systemic effects of alcohol intoxication, caution should be used in the setting of concurrent sedation or use of central nervous system depressants.

Phenol

Phenol is known as carbolic acid, phenic acid, phenylic acid, phenyl hydroxide, hydroxybenzene, and oxybenzene. It has a benzene ring with one hydroxyl group substituted for a hydrogen ion. Phenol is not commercially available in the injectable form, and needs to be prepared by the hospital pharmacy. At lower concentrations, phenol has local anesthetic properties, making it more tolerable than alcohol during injection for neurolysis.

Phenol is clear and poorly soluble in water and, in its pure state, forms a 6.7% solution in water. It is unstable at room temperature, and when exposed to air, undergoes oxidation turning reddish in color.[19] On the other hand, phenol is highly soluble in alcohol and other organic compounds. For clinical use, it is usually mixed with glycerin, from which it diffuses out very slowly, resulting in limited spread and highly localized tissue effect. In this form, phenol is viscous at concentrations from 4% to 10%, and hyperbaric compared to cerebrospinal fluid. The aqueous preparations of phenol also range from 3% to 10% concentrations; however, this is a more potent neurolytic. Phenol is commonly used in a contrast-material mixture to facilitate visualization under fluoroscopy.[20]

Earlier experience had led to the misconception of selective destruction of small-diameter, unmyelinated nerve fibers[21,22]—the C afferents (slow pain); Aδ afferents (fast pain); and Aλ efferents (muscle tone)—with phenol neurolysis. Later studies have proven a direct relationship between phenol concentrations and the extent of nerve destruction.[23,24] Nathan et al have demonstrated the nonselective destruction by phenol showing histopathologic and electrophysiologic proof of damage to Aα and Aβ fibers.[25]

At increasing concentrations, phenol causes a range of destructive changes on the neural tissue. Use of concentrations >5% result in protein coagulation and nonselective segmental demyelination (i.e., wallerian degeneration) similar to alcohol. Concentrations of 5% to 6% generate lysis of nociceptive fibers with minimum adverse effects. Higher concentrations result in axonal abnormalities, nerve root damage, spinal cord infarcts, arachnoiditis, and meningitis. These properties may count for the long-lasting effect of 10% phenol in sympathetic neurolytic blocks.[26,27]

Phenol in concentrations lower than 5%, when injected into the subarachnoid space produced mostly sensory blocks, as demonstrated in a study by Maher and Mehta in 1977. At higher concentrations, motor block occurred. These properties have made phenol the agent of choice for epidural neurolysis.[28]

Compared to alcohol, phenol seems to generate shorter duration and less intense blocks. In one study comparing various concentrations of alcohol and phenol, Moller et al have equated 5% phenol with 40% alcohol in neurolytic potency.[29] Degeneration with phenol takes about 14 days, and regeneration is completed in about 14 weeks.

Phenol is rapidly metabolized by liver enzymes via conjugation and oxidation and excreted by the kidney.[30] Inadvertent intravascular injection or absorption of phenol may cause transient tinnitus and flushing. Doses higher than the recommended 600- to 2000-mg range can cause convulsions, central nervous system depression, and cardiovascular collapse. Chronic toxicity may lead to hepatic and renal insufficiency.[31] Although clinical doses of 1 to 10 mL of 1% to 10% solutions are unlikely to cause serious toxicity, Boas recommends that phenol should be avoided for celiac plexus block, because of the proximity to major blood vessels, and spared for splanchnic nerve block.[32] In an nonrandomized trial of 57 cancer patients receiving peripheral neurolytic blocks with absolute alcohol or 6% aqueous phenol, Jain et al reported equal pain relief and a higher incidence of systemic side effects with phenol.[33,34]

Glycerol

Glycerol, a compound structurally related to alcohol,[35] was discovered accidentally, and quickly found to be clinically useful in the treatment of intractable facial pain.[36–38] In these studies, percutaneous retrogasserian glycerol rhizotomy for the treatment of tic douloureux is reported to be far superior to radiofrequency rhizotomy because no permanent injury to surrounding tissue is reported. Furthermore, there is preservation of facial sensation in most patients.[39,40] Potential spread to the subarachnoid space and risk of deafferentation, however, still remains a risk factor. Especially with the use of pulsed radiofrequency, well-localized, controlled lesioning still remains a preferred therapy modality. Long-term follow-up, comparing the two techniques has not been reported.[30]

Histopathologic examination after intraneuronal glycerol injection has revealed extensive myelin sheath swelling, axonolysis, and severe inflammatory response. Electron microscopy confirmed nonselective wallerian degeneration, phagocytosis, and mast cell degranulation.[19]

Ammonium Compounds

The use of ammonium salts was introduced to clinical practice in 1942 by Bates and Judovich.[41] Clinically, the action of ammonium salts is mainly on C-fiber potentials, with small effect on A fibers. Clinical information shows that at concentrations of 10%, ammonium salts preserve motor function with good analgesia.[42] Histopathology reveals acute degenerative neuropathy when these compounds are injected around a peripheral nerve, affecting all fibers. Associated adverse effects, such as nausea, vomiting, headaches, paresthesia, and spinal cord injury, have resulted in clinical abandonment of ammonia salts in clinical practice.[30]

Butamben

Butyl aminobenzoate (Butamben) is an extremely hydrophobic/lipophilic ester local anesthetic. Investigative work by Shulman and Korsten is suggestive of a potential role for this compound in the setting of chronic pain.[43,44] Both have used butamben in suspensions of 2.5% to 10% for epidural, subarachnoid, and peripheral nerve blocks for malignant and nonmalignant pain with relative selectivity and prolonged duration.

CONCLUSION

The use of neurolytic agents in different sites of innervation, with different concentrations of these agents, carries significant risks to the patient. Hence, patient selection with mutual understanding of benefits and potential adverse outcomes is of ultimate importance. However, in terminally ill patients and those with certain intractable pain syndromes, chemical neurolysis may provide comfort, along with adjuvant medications. Despite decreased need for chemical neurolysis with the development of intrathecal infusion therapies and pulsed radiofrequency techniques, the need for further research persists to provide selectively neurotoxic agents to achieve prolonged duration of action and reduced complications.

REFERENCES

1. Jain S. The role of neurolytic procedures. In: Parris WCV (ed): *Cancer Pain Management: Principles and Practice.* Boston: Butterworth-Butterworth-Heinemann, 1997;231–244.
2. Hartel F. Die Behandlung der Trigeminus Neuralgic mit Intrakraniellen Alkokoleinspritzungen. *Dtsch Z Chir* 1914;126:429.
3. Doppler K. Die Sympathike Diapttherese ander arteria femorales. *Med Klin* 1926;22:1954–1956.
4. Putnam TJ, Hampton AO. A technique of injection in the gasserian ganglion under roentgenographic control. *Arch Neurol Psychiatry* 1936;35:92–98.
5. Dogliotti AM. Traitement des syndromes douloureux de la peripherie par l'alcoolisation sus-arachnoidienne des raciness posterieures a leur emergence de la moelle epiniere. *Presse Med* 1931;39:1249–1254.
6. Maher RM. Relief of pain in incurable cancer. *Lancet* 1955;1:18–20.
7. Lipton S. Pain relief in active patients with cancer: The early use of nerve blocks improves the quality of life. *BMJ* 1989;298(6665):37–38.
8. Swerdlow M (ed): Relief of Intractable Pain, 3*rd* edition, Amsterdam, *Excerpta Medica,* 1983.
9. Raj PP, Anderson SR. Peripheral Neurolysis in the Management of Pain. In: Waldman SD (ed): *Interventional Pain Management.* Philadelphia: W.B. Saunders Company, 2001:541–553.
10. Rumbsy MG, Finean JB. The action of organic solvents on the myelin sheath of peripheral nerve tissue-II (short-chain aliphatic alcohols). *J Neurochem* 1966;13:1509.
11. Gallagher HS, Yonezawa T, Hoy RC, Derrick WS. Subarachnoid alcohol block. II: Histological changes in the central nervous system. *Am J Pathol* 1961;35:679.
12. Labat G, Greene MB: Contribution to the modern method of diagnosis and treatment of so called sciatic neuralgias. *Am J Surg* 1931;11: 435.
13. Umeda S, Arai T. Disulfiram-like reaction to moxalactam after celiac plexus alcohol block. *Anesth Analg* 1985;64:377.
14. Lyness WH. Pharmacology of neurolytic agents. In: Racz GB, ed: techniques of Neurolysis. Boston: Kluwer Academic Publishers, 1989, p.13.
15. Rocco A. Radiofrequency lumbar sympatholysis: The evolution of a technique for managing sympathetically mediated pain. *Reg Anesth* 1995;20:3–12.
16. Bogduk N, Tynan W, Wilson SS. The nerve supply to the human lumbar intervertebral discs. *J Anat* 1981;132:39–56.
17. Katz J. Current role of neurolytic agents. *Adv Neurol* 1974;4:471.
18. Sato S, Okubu N, Tajima K. Plasma alcohol concentrations after celiac plexus block in gastric and pancreatic cancer. *Reg Anesth* 1993;18:366.
19. Jain S, Gupta R. Neurolytic Agents in Clinical Practice. In: Waldman SD (ed): Interventional Pain Management. Philadelphia, W.B. Saunders Company, 2001, pp. 220–225.
20. Heavner JE. Neurolytic agents. In: Raj PP (ed): Pain Medicine: A Comprehensive Review. St. Louis: Mosby-Year Book, 1996;285–286.
21. Nathan PW, Sears TA. Effects of phenol on nervous conduction. *J Physiol* 1960;150:565–580.
22. Iggo A, Walsh EG. Selective block of small fibers in the spinal root by phenol. *Brain* 1960;83:701.
23. Nathan PW, Scott TG. Intrathecal phenol for intractable pain: Safety and dangers of method. *Lancet* 1958;1:76–80.
24. Papo I, Visca A. Phenol rhizotomy in the treatment of cancer pain. *Anesth Analg* 1974;53:993–997.
25. Nathan PW, Sears TA, Smith MC. Effects of phenol solutions on the nerve roots of the cat: An electrophysiological and histological study. *J Neurol Sci* 1965;2:7–29.
26. Wood KM. The use of phenol as a neurolytic agent: A review. *Pain* 1978;5:205.
27. de Leon-Casasola OA, Ditonto E. Drugs Commonly Used for Nerve Blocking: Neurolytic Agents. In: Raj PP (ed): *Practical Management of Pain. 3rd ed.* St. Louis: Mosby, 2000;575–578.
28. Maher RM, Mehta M. Spinal (intrathecal) and extradural analgesia. In: Lipton S (ed): *Persistent Pain: Modern Methods of Treatment.* New York: Grune & Stratton, 1977, p. 61.
29. Moller JE, Helweg-Larson J, Jacobson E. Histopathological lesions in the sciatic nerve of the rat following perineural application of phenol and alcohol solutions. *Dan Med Bull* 1969;16:116–119.
30. Anderson SR. Chemical Neurolytic Agents. In: Raj PP (ed): *Clinical Practice of Regional Anesthesia,* New York: Churchill Livingstone, 2002;229–237.
31. Churcher M. Peripheral nerve blocks in the relief of intractable pain. In: Swerdlow M, Charlton JE: *Relief of Intractable Pain. 4th ed.* Amsterdam: Elsevier, 1989, pp. 195.
32. Abram SE, Boas RA. Sympathetic and visceral nerve blocks. In: Benumof JL (ed): *Clinical Procedures in Anesthesia and Intensive Care.* Philadelphia: JB Lippincott, 1993;787–805.
33. Jain S, Kestenbaum A, Khan Y. Ethanol or phenol for peripheral neurolysis? Does it make a difference? *Pain,* 5 (Suppl.):S92, 1990.
34. Patt BR, Cousins MJ. Techniques for Neurolytic Neural Blockade. In Cousins MJ, Bridenbaugh PO (ed): Neural Blockade. In: *Clinical Anesthesia and Management of Pain.* Philadelphia, Lippincott—Raven, 1998;1007–1061.
35. Rengachary SS, Watanabe IS, Singer P, Bopp WJ. Effect of glycerol on peripheral nerve: An experimental study. *Neurosurgery* 1983;13: 681.
36. Hakanson S. Trigeminal neuralgia treated by the injection of glycerol into the trigeminal cistern. *Neurosurgery* 1981;9:638.

37. Sweet WH, Poletti CE, Macon JB. Treatment of trigeminal neuralgia and other facial pain by retrogasserian injection of glycerol. *Neurosurgery* 1981;9:647.
38. Lunsford LD, Bennett MH. Percutaneous retrogasserian glycerol rhizotomy for tic douloreux: Part I, Technique and results in 112 patients. *Neurosurgery* 1984;14:424.
39. Gentilli F, Hudson AR, Hunter D, Kline DG. Nerve injection injury with local anesthetic agents: A light and electron microscopic, fluorescent microscopic and horseradish peroxidase study. *Neurosurgery* 1980;6:263.
40. Saini SS. Retrogasserian anhydrous glycerol injection therapy in trigeminal neuralgia: Observations in 552 patients. *J Neurol Neurosurg Psychiatry* 1987;50:1536.
41. Bates W, Judovich BD. Intractable pain. *Anesthesiology* 1942;3:363.
42. Miller RD, Johnston RR, Hosbuchi Y. Treatment of intercostal neuralgia with 10% ammonium sulfate. *J Thorac Cardiovasc Surg* 1975;69: 476.
43. Korsten HHM, Hellebrekers LJ, Grouls RJE, et al. Long -lasting epidural sensory blockade by n-Butyl p-Aminobenzoate in the dog: Neurotoxic or local anesthetic effect? *Anesthesiology* 1990;73:491.
44. Shulman M. Epidural butamben for the treatment of metastatic cancer pain. *Anesthesiology* 1987;67:A245.

CHAPTER 74 CRYOANALGESIA AND RADIOFREQUENCY

Miles Day and Susan Anderson

CRYOANALGESIA

Introduction

Cryoanalgesia, that is, the use of low temperatures to provide analgesia, is a pain management technique that can be applied to a variety of painful situations. From the topical application of ice to a sprained ankle or cryoneurolysis of an intercostal nerve for postoperative pain control in a post-thoracotomy patient to cryoneurolysis of the trigeminal nerve for trigeminal neuralgia, cryoanalgesia has a multitude of uses. This chapter focuses on the application of cryoanalgesia for acute and chronic pain management.

Historical Perspectives

The first account of the use of cryoanalgesia for pain control was recorded by Hippocrates (460–377 bc). He described the use of ice and snow packs to prevent pain from surgery.[1] An 11th century Anglo-Saxon monk, Avicenna of Persia (980–1070), and Severino of Naples (1580–1656) also recognized the use of cold as preemptive analgesia for surgery.[1,2] Other historical recorders who recognized the value of cryoanalgesia include Napoleon's surgeon general, Baron Larre (1812), Dr James Arnott (1851), and Richardson (1866).[1,2]

Recently, Irvine Cooper and his colleagues (1961) developed the first prototype of a cryoprobe that could be used for analgesia.[1,3] It utilized the principle of phase change using liquid nitrogen to produce a temperature of -196°C. Several years later in 1967, Amoils developed a smaller cryoprobe that employed the Joule-Thompson principle and used carbon dioxide or nitrous oxide to produce temperatures to −50°C.[4]) Present cryoprobes use either of these two principles to produce a temperature of at least −70°C.

PRINCIPLES OF CRYONEUROLYSIS

Cryoneurolysis involves using cold to induce nerve injury, thus providing analgesia. The exact cellular mechanism of nerve injury is not known. Theories include ischemic necrosis, physical destruction by large cellular ice crystals, damage to proteins, minimal cell volume, production of autoantibodies, and membrane rupture caused by rapid water loss.[5] Cryolesioning causes a second-degree nerve injury as classified by Sunderland. A second-degree injury involves degeneration of the axon and myelin sheaths (wallerian degeneration) from the site of freezing distally to the nerve's termination.[6] The minimum temperature required is 20°C or lower.[5] The endoneurium, perineurium, and ectoneurium remain intact, thus regeneration is possible. The return of normal sensory and motor activity depends primarily on two factors: the rate of axonal regrowth (average of 1 to 2 mm per day) and the distance of the cryolesion from the end organ, although nerve conduction velocity remains only reduced to an average of 35 days.[1,7,8]

The success of a cryolesion depends on several factors: the rate of freezing and thawing, the temperature attained by the tissue in proximity to the cryoprobe, and the size of the cryolesion.[7] Evans and Gill et al showed that repeat freeze-and-thaw cycles enlarged the size of the cryolesion, improving the success of the block.[5,9] Freeze cycles are typically 1.5 to 3 minutes with a 30-second thaw period. Evans et al, using exposed rat sciatic nerves, showed that a minimum temperature of −20°C was necessary for prolonged sensory loss and that further decreases in temperature did not greatly influence the duration of sensory loss.[7] The size of the cryolesion is also important since saltatory conduction is still possible in myelinated fibers, where there are short interruptions in axonal continuity. Douglas and Malcolm in 1955 demonstrated in cats that an injury of 3 to 6 mm in length was sufficient to prevent saltatory conduction.[10]

DESIGN OF THE CRYOPROBE

The modern day cryoprobe creates low temperatures either by the expansion of a compressed gas (Joule-Thompson effect) such as nitrous oxide or carbon dioxide, or by the principle of phase change with liquid nitrogen (Fig. 74-1A and 74-1B). The expansion of a compressed gas through a small orifice can generate temperatures of −70° to −80°C and the gas most commonly used is nitrous oxide.[1,3] Liquid nitrogen cryoprobes can reach temperatures of −196°C.

The cryoprobes come in a variety of sizes and shapes. Most have a Teflon coating for insulation, and incorporate a stimulator to assist in locating the intended nerve and a thermocouple to measure core temperature. The stimulator and the thermocouple are located in the tip of the cryoprobe. The size of the freeze zone for a gas expansion cryoprobe is two to three times the probe's diameter, whereas liquid nitrogen cryoprobes create a lesion that is three to five times the size of the probe. The typical size of a cryoprobe ranges from 12 to 18 gauge (Fig. 74-2).

INDICATIONS AND CONTRAINDICATIONS

Cryoneurolysis is best suited for conditions in which the nerve to be lesioned is small and well localized. It can be done by a surgical incision, as seen with post-herniorrhaphy and post-thoracotomy pain, or closed, that is, percutaneously. The percutaneous approach is usually done for neuroma and nerve-entrapment syndromes. Specific lesions for acute and chronic pain are discussed later in this section. Contraindications include patient refusal, lesioning of a motor nerve, and the use of cryoneurolysis when a diagnostic nerve block has failed.

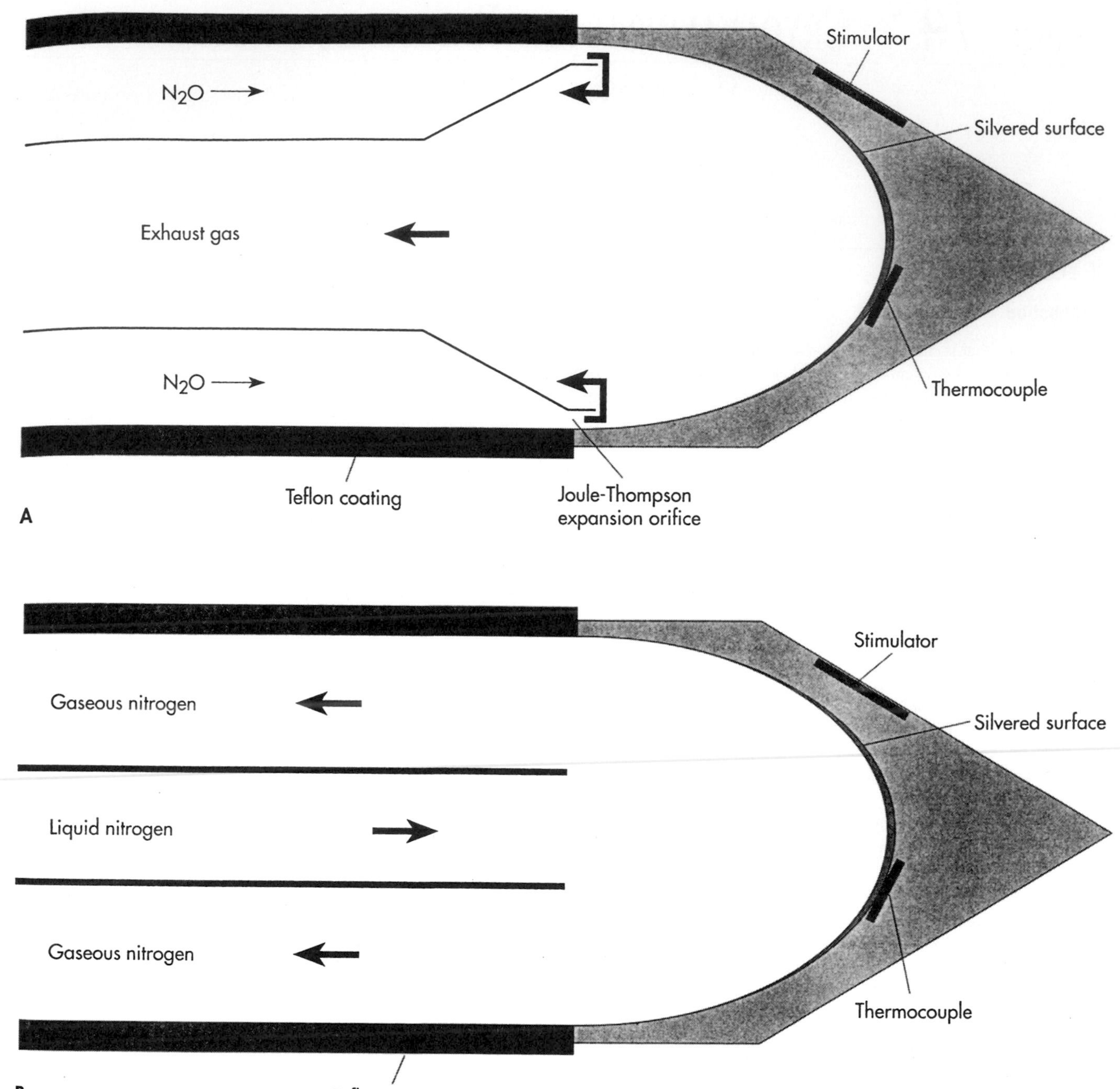

Figure 74-1 (**A**) Diagrammatic cross section of gas expansion (Joule-Thompson) and (**B**) liquid nitrogen cryoprobe tips. (From Raj, *Pain Medicine: A Comprehensive Review.* 1st ed. St. Louis, MO: Mosby; 1996;299. Used with permission.)

SPECIFIC SITUATIONS FOR WHICH CRYOLYSIS IS USEFUL

Postoperative Pain Management

Cryoneurolysis is beneficial in a variety of surgical procedures to provide postoperative analgesia. Unfortunately, clinical studies have only looked at a few such applications. Herniorrhaphy and thoracotomy are the two most common surgeries in which cryoneurolysis has been used for postoperative pain management.

Post-Herniorrhaphy Pain Herniorrhaphy provides an ideal situation in which a cryolesion could be used to provide postoperative analgesia. The ilioinguinal nerve is usually identified and retracted during the initial dissection of a herniorrhaphy. Wood et al in 1981 showed that a cryolesion of the ilioinguinal nerve after herniorrhaphy significantly decreased the amount of oral analgesics required for postoperative pain control.[11] This study compared cryoneurolysis with oral analgesics alone and paravertebral block for postoperative pain control in patients undergoing day-case herniorrhaphy patients. Prior to closure of the herniorrhaphy incision, the

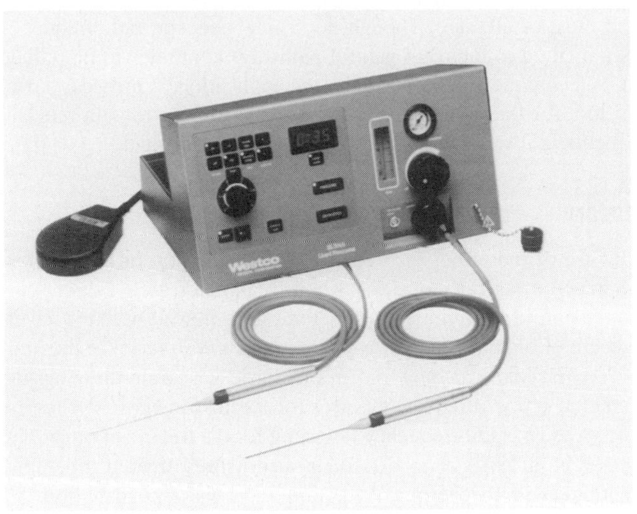

Figure 74-2 Example of a typical cryoanalgesia setup including control panel, cable, and cryoprobes.

ilioinguinal nerve was elevated and frozen until a visual lesion was noted. Not only did the patients in the cryoanalgesia group require less oral medications but they also had improved appetites, were more active, and returned to work sooner. Even though this was only a small study, it showed the benefits of cryoneurolysis in allowing patients to have less pain and enabling them to return to work earlier.

Post-Thoracotomy Pain Analgesia following thoracotomy is particularly important not only to keep the patient comfortable but also to facilitate extubation and prevent respiratory sequela via adequate pulmonary toilet. Oral analgesics have the propensity to diminish the cough reflex and to decrease respirations in the doses necessary to adequately control postoperative pain.[12] Intercoastal nerve blocks with local anesthetic generally do not provide effective long-term analgesia and frequently have to be repeated. In several studies, intraoperative cryoneurolysis of the intercostal nerves prior to closure of the thoracotomy incision has been shown to be effective in decreasing postoperative pain and the amount of oral and parenteral analgesics required post-procedure.[12–14] Before closure of the thoracotomy incision, the intercostal nerve at the site of the incision as well as the nerves two levels above and below the incision are dissected away from the intercostal vessels and cryoablated until a visual lesion is observed.

Chronic Pain Management With Cryoneurolysis

A multitude of conditions exist in the realm of chronic pain management in which percutaneous cryoneurolysis can be applied. Of note is that it should only be performed after a successful diagnostic nerve block with local anesthetic. The following section describes specific instances in which cryoneurolysis has been effective for control of chronic pain.

Facial Pain Goss in 1988 described the use of cryoneurotomy for the treatment of intractable temporomandibular joint pain.[15] In this study, six female patients who had severe temporomandibular joint pain and had failed conservative treatment with oral therapy and surgery by others underwent open cryoneurotomy of the lateral and posterior joint capsule and open cryoneurolysis of the great auricular nerve. Five of the six were pain-free for over a year. Four of the six had recurrent pain and were successfully treated with repeat cryoneurotomy. Zakrzewska and Nally studied the role of cryoneurolysis in the management of paroxysmal trigeminal neuralgia[16]; 145 patients were treated and followed up from 1 month up to 6 years. The nerves cryoablated included the infraorbital, mental, long buccal, lingual, greater palatine, and posterior-superior dental. Fifty-eight percent of 89 infra-orbital nerves treated were pain-free at 1 year, 36% of 85 mental nerves treated were pain-free after 1 year, and 66% of 23 buccal nerves treated were without pain after 1 year. Barnard and colleagues studied 21 patients with intractable facial pain, including postherpetic neuralgia, atypical facial pain, post-traumatic neuralgia, and facial pain secondary to malignant disease.[2] After cryoablation, the postherpetic neuralgia group had a median duration of pain relief of 38 days and ranged from 0 to 84 days. The other types of facial pains were grouped together and had a median duration of pain relief of 116 days and ranged from zero to 257 days. These studies indicate that cryoneurolysis has a place in the management of intractable facial pain.

Thoracic Pain Common causes of chronic thoracic pain include intercostal neuralgia secondary to a thoracotomy scar, postherpetic neuralgia, nerve root pain due to vertebral collapse, and carcinoma. Cryoneurolysis of the intercostal nerve has been shown effective in alleviating pain due to intercostal neuralgia. Jones and Murrin did a retrospective study of 70 patients from 1982 to 1984 who had intercostal pain from several causes, namely scar pain from thoracotomy and postherpetic neuralgia.[17] They found that cryoneurolysis was more effective for control of intercostal pain for patients with pain secondary to thoracotomy scar than for postherpetic neuralgia pain. This procedure is only performed when a diagnostic intercostal block with local anesthetic has given effective analgesia. Cryoneurolysis is performed percutaneously at the angle of the rib. Using aseptic technique, the skin is infiltrated with local anesthetic and an intravenous cannula (usually 12 to 14 gauge) is inserted at a 45 degree angle to the skin. The cannula is aimed at the inferior border of the rib. This can be done by palpation or under fluoroscopic guidance. The cryoprobe is then inserted through the cannula and walked under the rib. Sensory stimulation can be used to reproduce the pain. Two lesions are performed for 90 seconds, each with 30-second thaw periods. A post-procedure chest radiograph should be obtained to rule out pneumothorax.

Low Back Pain of Facet Origin Facet rhizotomy has been performed with percutaneous cryoneurolysis in patients with a facet origin of low back pain. The goal is to lesion the common branch of the posterior primary ramus as it crosses the medial portion of the transverse process near the superior pars of the facet joint. Since the facet joint is innervated by nerves from multiple levels, this procedure must also be performed one level above and one level below the facet joint in question. A positive diagnostic common branch nerve block must be obtained prior to performing this procedure. Forty-seven of 50 patients in a study done by Schuster received significant pain relief after facet rhizotomy with cryoneurolysis.[18]

Peripheral Nerve Pain Cryoneurolysis of peripheral nerves can be performed in cases of nerve entrapment or painful neuroma. Only pure sensory nerves or nerves with only a minor motor component should be cryolesioned. Precise nerve mapping should be done prior to cryoneurolysis to prevent adverse sequelae, such as lesioning a motor nerve. This can be done with diagnostic nerve blocks with local anesthetic.

Perineal Pain Entrapment of the ilioinguinal nerve with resulting neuralgia is occasionaly seen in post-herniorrhaphy patients. A diagnostic block should be performed to rule in or rule out the diagnosis. If correctly diagnosed, a percutaneous cryolesion can be performed. Racz and Hagstrom studied 25 patients with iliohypogastric and ilioinguinal nerve entrapment secondary to a variety of causes.[19] After cryolesioning, 46% reported good to excellent pain relief.

Cryoneurolysis of sacral nerve roots has been performed for cancer pain, coccydynia, and sciatic nerve pain.[3] Sciatic pain can be partially treated with S1 and S2 cryolesions, whereas bilateral S4 cryoneurolysis can help alleviate pain secondary to coccydynia and rectal cancer. Loev et al reported a novel approach to cryoablation of the ganglion impar in a 73-year-old patient with chronic anal and perineal pain secondary to surgical resection of carcinoma.[20] He and his colleagues cryoablated the ganglion impar by passing the cryoprobe through the sacrococcygeal ligament under fluorosopic guidance. The patient had 80% pain relief for 6 weeks, at which time it was repeated secondary to returning pain.

COMPLICATIONS OF CRYONEUROLYSIS

Most complications from cryoneurolysis are secondary to improper technique. If an introducer sheath is not used, frostbite can occur at the skin-entry site and cause ulceration, especially if superficial nerves, such as the supraorbital or infraorbital nerves, are cryoablated. Motor nerves can be inadvertantly lesioned if proper localization of the intended nerve is not done. Cryoneurolysis is not a permanent process and motor function will return over time. Although infrequent, there have been reports of dysesthesia following cryoneurolysis of intercostal nerves.[20]

CONCLUSION

Cryoneurolysis is a technique of prolonging analgesia without serious sequelae. It has many applications ranging from postoperative pain control to alleviation of many chronic pain states. It is a relatively safe and effective method of pain control. Data on its efficacy is however poor. Further detailed data will have to be obtained and compared with other neuroablative techniques prior to identifying it as a reliable analgesic technique.

RADIOFREQUENCY

Introduction

Interventional pain physicians continue to strive to find techniques that provide relief to chronic pain patients. The techniques sought must be percutaneous, discrete, reliable, reproducible, effective, and most of all, safe. Though not a new concept, radiofrequency as a method to interrupt painful pathways continues to be refined in its technique and broadened in its application. It provides a useful tool for the pain physician to provide long-term pain relief to patients in a safe, effective, and reproducible manner.

History

The use of radiofrequency energy for the creation of lesions may be traced to as early as 1863 when Beaunis created a direct-current lesion in the animal brain.[21] Fournie followed with the development of bipolar lesions in the animal neural tissue.[21] In the mid-1920s, Harvey Cushing did some basic research utilizing the potential of radiofrequency power for electrosurgery.[22,23] The first known use of radiofrequency lesioning for the treatment of chronic pain was in 1931 when Kirschner successfully treated trigeminal neuralgia with the thermocoagulation of the gasserian ganglion.[24,21] In 1953, William H. Sweet and Vernon Mark showed that the use of radiofrequency (RF) current for lesions production has decisive advantages over the time-tested direct current lesions that had been used for decades.[25,26] They demonstrated that the RF lesion is characterized by well-circumscribed borders that have better control of the size and shape compared with the lesion from the direct-current method[25,26] In the late 1950s, the work of Cosman and Aronow made the first commercial RF lesion generator available.[27,21]In 1960, Mundinger et al[28] emphasized the importance of monitoring the electrode temperature in RF lesion making to obtain consistent lesion size.[28,29] In 1974, Sweet and Wepsic[30] performed percutaneous retrogasserian thermal rhizotomy on 274 patients with facial pain (214 of whom had trigeminal neuralgia). Noting that touch was preserved in some or all of a trigeminal zone rendered analgesic, the authors concluded the heavily myelinated $A\beta$ fibers were more resistant to heating.[30] This was consistent with the findings of Letcher and Goldring in 1968.[31] Their study demonstrated *in vitro* the effects of RF and heat on the peripheral nerve action potential in the cat. Their demonstration that RF heat lesions block the action potentials of smaller delta and C fibers before those of the alpha-beta group of fibers formed the neurophysiologic basis for the therapeutic use of RF lesions.[31,32] Uematsu,[33] however, in 1977 described a preliminary histologic study that demonstrated the effects of RF thermocoagulation on the sciatic nerve of the cat. This study found indiscriminate destruction of both small and large myelinated fibers rather than selective destruction of the smaller myelinated fibers.[32,33] This was supported in 1981 by Smith et al[32] who studied RF lesions at 85°C in dogs. This study noted that RF lesions were not specific for unmyelinated C fibers, small myelinated fibers, or large myelinated fibers. They also demonstrated the lack of specificity for graded lesions of 45°, 55°, 65°, and 75°C.[32] Tew[34] significantly advanced the technique using a spring-loaded curved radiofrequency electrode tip that could be precisely stereotactically placed to lesion the first, second, or third branch of the trigeminal nerve.[35] The first use of RF lesioning for chronic spinal-based pain came in 1975 when Shealy performed posterior primary rami radiofrequency in the lumbar region.[36,21] In the 1980s, Sluijter advanced the applications of RF for spinal pain by refining percutaneous techniques for cervical, thoracic, lumbar, and sacral spine syndromes.[35] Sluijter and Mehta modified the existing electrode for RF, making it smaller and capable of temperature monitoring.[37] This allowed the passing of current through electrodes to reproduce the patient's pain with small-diameter RF needles. These needles were placed using local anesthesia with fluoroscopic guidance. After reproduction of the pain, a local anesthetic was placed on the targeted structure followed by painless lesioning.[35]

THERAPEUTIC MODALITIES FOR THE INTERRUPTION OF NERVE PATHWAYS IN THE TREATMENT OF CHRONIC PAIN

There are many techniques for local destruction of nervous tissue in the brain, spinal cord, or peripheral nervous system. The methods commonly used by interventional pain management specialists include[38]:

1. Chemical injection (chemical neurolysis)
2. Cryoneurolysis (freezing of the nerve)
3. Lasers
4. Radiofrequency thermocoagulation.

Chemical injection of a neurolytic such as alcohol, glycerin, or phenol can be advantageous for disruption in an area with extensive, weblike innervation, as in the sympathetic nervous system. These lesions, however, are irregular, variable in shape, and the spread can be impossible to control. This can lead to problems with reproducing an effective block at a later date. A postneurolytic neuritis from aberrant regeneration of nerve endings can be a serious, unwanted side effect in patients treated with chronic, nonmalignant pain. Cryoneurolysis is an incomplete destruction that avoids the side effect of deafferentation pain caused by RF in peripheral nerves. Therefore, in peripheral nerves, cryoneurolysis may be more appropriate than RF. However, the size of the probes (diameter >3 mm) can be of concern and may limit the spectrum of applications. The duration of effect is short: only a matter of weeks or a few months. Lasers may be used for lesioning; however, it is difficult to quantify the extent and rapidity of destruction. Also, because of the inadequate temperature monitoring, there is variability of effect, depending on tissue parameters such as blood flow and thermoconductivity.[38]

Radiofrequency thermocoagulation offers several advantages when compared to other methods of interrupting nerve pathways. The lesions from a RF needle have smooth, well-circumscribed borders. The lesion sizes may be reproducibly quantified by monitoring the temperature of the tip of the electrode. Monitoring of the temperature diminishes the risks of unwanted side effects such as boiling, charring, and sticking.[29] The target for lesioning is localized by monitoring stimulation and impedance. RF needles have different lengths (e.g., 5, 10, and 15 cm) and electrode configurations that provide suitability for different anatomic sites.[38]

GENERAL PRINCIPLES OF RADIOFREQUENCY

Radiofrequency is a high-frequency current that is applied to neural tissue through a closed circuit. The current, produced by a generator, runs *in* the active electrode (the needle, or where the lesion is made) and disperses *out* the dispersive electrode. The difference in the currents between the active electrode and the dispersive electrode is the voltage, which is monitored. The body tissue completes the circuit. The voltage generates an electric field that runs between the active (lesion) and the dispersive electrodes. This electric field causes electric force on the ions in the tissue (electrolytes move back and forth). The tissue then heats the electrode tip that in turn absorbs heat from the tissue. Therefore, an equilibration of the temperature between the tissue and the electrode tip occurs. The electrode tip temperature represents the temperature of the hottest tissue adjacent to it.[38]

The lesion size is determined by four major factors: (1) electrode size and configuration, (2) the rate of thermal equilibrium, (3) the temperature generated, and (4) local tissue characteristics.[39] The lesion size may be altered by the distance from the active electrode tip and the electrode diameter. The lesion is spheroidal around the active electrode and tapers at the tip so that minimal lesion formation occurs beyond the tip of the active electrode. In clinical practice, the placement of the active electrode should be oriented in an axis that will produce a spheroidal lesion along the desired location for neurolysis.[40,41] The lesion length is 0 to 2 mm longer than the exposed electrode tip length. The lesion diameter rises exponentially but plateaus at 30 seconds, though thermal equilibrium is reached at 60 seconds.[29] It can provide a 4- to 5-mm circumferential lesion around the radius of the length of the electrode. For example, an electrode 3 mm in length and 0.4 mm in diameter will form a lesion 5.5-mm long.[38] According to Cosman,[29] the lesion will extend 1.5 electrode diameters beyond the tip distance. For maximum lesion area, the electrode must be placed parallel to the nerve. The larger and more complete the lesion is, the longer the expected pain relief. Over time, the nerves regenerate and the pain will return. Therefore, a larger electrode will generate a larger lesion. However, it will also cause more tissue destruction on insertion, unwanted neural destruction, and larger reversible zones.[29]

Temperature monitoring creates more consistent, safer lesions. Brodkey et al established that irreversible nerve blocks occur at 45°C in the brain.[42] It is also known that at >90°C the tissue will boil, causing adherence to the probe and tearing of the tissues. Therefore, a tip temperature of >100°C must be avoided.[29] At 95°C, one might notice steam formation, charring, sticking and increased risk of hemorrhage as adherent tissues tear.[29] On the RF machine, a sudden resistance may be noted followed by a drop in current flow to zero. At these high temperatures, one may see a "popping" lesion. A rapid decrease in the current meter and an increase in the voltage meter. Gas and steam at the tip may be forced up the shaft. The electrode gives a "popping" sound. This lesion produces ragged and unpredictable damage.[29] Another advantage to monitoring the temperature is assurance that a lesion has been made.

Impedance monitoring gives independent information of the lesion process and can signal equipment failure.[43] Pre- and post-impedance changes, at a minimum, tell the operator a lesion has been made, that is, irreversible structural changes have occurred. Impedance monitoring can increase the safety of doing an RF procedure because it is an instant continuity check.[43] The RF circuit has numerous connections and wires that are vulnerable to unpredictable breakage or intermittency. The impedance monitor can alert the operator to an open-circuit problem, as well as the equally troublesome short-circuit situation.[43]

Unpredictable factors can alter the lesion size and shape. A large blood vessel near the electrode tip can serve as a heat sink, causing local cooling and irregularity of the lesion shape.[29] Cerebrospinal fluid may also act as a heat sink, drawing away the heat, and alter the lesion shape.[29]

On the histologic level, after the lesion is made, the appearance of the lesion is one of a local burn.[39] This is a neuroablative procedure. After creation of the lesion, wallerian degeneration becomes apparent. The perineurium may also be destroyed.[39] This makes RF more susceptible to neuroma formation than when cryoneurolysis is used. Though controversial, some argue there is selectivity for Aδ and C fibers with sparing of the larger Aβ fibers at lower temperatures.[39] More investigation regarding this controversy is needed.

Accurate placement of the active electrode to ensure accuracy of the lesion may be done using fluoroscopy and electrostimulation. Biplanar fluoroscopy is used to target the nerve roots, facets, disks, and sympathetic nerves. Further specificity is obtained using water-soluble, nonionic contrast dye. Electrostimulation for sensory is performed at 50 Hz. Optimal placement of the active electrode near the dorsal root ganglion is considered if there is reproduction of the patient's concordant pain at 0.4 to 0.7 V. If there is reproduction at less than 0.2 V, this may be suggestive of intraneural placement. This places the patient at greater risk for neuritis. Motor stimulation should also be tested at 2 Hz and 2 V. Fasciculation or titanic stimulation with this indicates placement near a ventral nerve root.

PATIENT SELECTION

Before deciding on RF as part of the patient's treatment algorithm, all conservative therapy must have been fully explored. This includes a thorough physical examination with appropriate diagnostic tests such as x-ray, magnetic resonance imaging (MRI), computed tomography (CT), and myelographic studies. The patient should be an active participant in a multidisciplinary pain management program that includes medical, psychological, and physical therapy evaluation and treatment. The pain should be chronic (>3 months). There should be no indication for surgical intervention and no invasive lesion at the site such as tumor or infection. A successful diagnostic block should be performed first. A prognostic block is not without its pitfalls, however. There is always concern for the placebo effect or lack of specificity of the block. Exclusion criteria includes patients with coagulopathies, psychopathology, ongoing septicemia, or neuropathic/deafferentation pain syndromes.

EQUIPMENT

For RF to remain safe, precise, and be able to yield reproducible results, the equipment must be able to[23,41]:

1. Measure impedance.
2. Stimulate a wide range of frequencies.
3. Accurately time the duration of the lesion for a precise temperature measurement in the core of the lesion tissue.
4. Accurately measure and indicate amperage and voltage.
5. Gradually increase temperature with time.

It is also imperative to check the insulation coating of the RF needle for any imperfections as "cracks" that may lead to a leakage of current into tissue and unwanted injury. Patients with a pacemaker or spinal cord stimulator must also be monitored because there can be interaction of the RF equipment.[41] As a consequence of RF lesioning, patients who have sensing pacemakers may have a period of asystole unless their pacemakers have an override. Be knowledgeable of the features of the pacemaker and use continuous electrocardiographic monitoring as indicated during procedures.[41] Though not widely documented, the possibility of current passing from the active electrode of the RF needle in the direction of the spinal cord stimulator and involving the spinal cord may exist.[41] Therefore, be sure the all spinal cord stimulators are turned off prior to initiation of the RF procedure.

TECHNIQUES FOR COMMONLY PERFORMED PROCEDURES

Stellate Ganglion

The stellate ganglion is formed by the fusion of the inferior cervical ganglion with the first thoracic ganglion. This usually lies in the front of the neck of the first rib and extends to the interspace between C7 and T1. This contains the preganglionic axons and post-ganglionic cell bodies T1 to T9. Indications for blockade of the stellate ganglion are chronic pain conditions of the head, neck, and upper extremity:

1. Complex regional pain syndrome type I (reflex sympathetic dystrophy)
2. Complex regional pain syndrome type II (causalgia)
3. Herpes zoster
4. Postherpetic neuralgia
5. Phantom limb pain
6. Hyperhidrosis
7. Vascular headaches
8. Vascular insufficiency

Complications for RF of the stellate ganglion include:

1. Intraspinal injury
2. Intravascular injury
3. Pneumothorax
4. Recurrent laryngeal nerve paralysis
5. Phrenic nerve paralysis
6. Brachial plexus injury.

Radiofrequency of the stellate ganglion block should be performed under fluoroscopic guidance after a successful diagnostic block using local anesthetic and steroid.

The patient is placed in the supine position with a pillow under his or her shoulders to extend the cervical spine. Under direct anterior-posterior (AP) fluoroscopy, the C7 vertebral body is identified. A skin wheal is raised over the ventrolateral aspect of the body of C7 with 1 mL of local anesthetic and a 25-gauge needle.[21] A 16-gauge angiocatheter is inserted through the skin wheal to contact the body of C7 in the ventrolateral aspect. This is at the junction of the transverse process and the vertebral body. Depth and direction should be confirmed in both the AP and lateral views frequently throughout the procedure. The needle tip will be positioned deep to the anterior longitudinal ligament. The longis colli will be lateral to the needle tip.[44] A 20-gauge, curved, blunt cannula with a 5-mm active tip is guided through the angiocatheter. The tip should rest at the junction of the transverse process and the vertebral body. Further confirmation of proper placement of the needle is with the injection of a water-soluble, nonionic contrast medium.

A sensory and motor stimulation trial must be performed because of the location of the phrenic nerve (lateral) and the recurrent laryngeal nerve (anterior and medial) to the lesion site.[21] A sensory trial is performed at 50 Hz and 0.9 V. A motor trial is performed at 2 Hz and 2 V. While motor stimulation is performed, the patient should phonate, saying "ee" to assure preserved motor function. If there is disruption of the phonation, the needle tip must be repositioned. A small volume of local anesthetic (0.5 mL) should be injected prior to lesioning. The lesion is instituted for 60 seconds at 80° C. The cannula is then redirected to the medial most aspect of the transverse process in the same plane.[21] Confirmation of placement in the ventral aspect must be demonstrated in the lateral view. Before lesioning, the patient must be retested for sensory and motor stimulation. A repeat dose of the local anesthetic should also be given through the cannula. A third and final lesion should be directed at the upper portion of the junction of the transverse process and the body of C7.[21,44]

Further sympathetic interruption of the upper extremity may be performed with a lesion at the T2 or T3 level. Sympathetic disruption at the thoracic level is indicated for the treatment of complex regional pain syndrome I (reflex sympathetic dystrophy), complex regional pain syndrome II (causalgia), arterial occlusions leading to ischemia, drug-resistant Raynaud's disease, Buerger's disease, and frost injuries of the upper extremities.[47] As in the stellate ganglion lesion, a diagnostic block should be performed prior to any ablative procedure. Before performing the procedure, because of the relationship of the sympathetic chain at this level and large vascular structures, a coagulopathy must be ruled out (prothrombin time, partial thromboplastin time, and bleeding time within normal limits). The patient is placed in the prone position on the fluoroscopy table. The camera is placed in the oblique view (30 degrees) to place the shadow of the body lateral to the lamina (Fig. 74-3A). A cephalocaudad view is necessary to correct for the upper thoracic kyphosis (approximately 20 degrees). A 10- to 15-cm, blunt, curved cannula with a 10-mm active tip is introduced through a 16-gauge angiocatheter that has already pierced the skin approximately 3.5 cm from the midline. A tunnel view should demonstrate the cannula advancing toward the margin of the lamina. It is advanced along the lateral body until the tip is halfway between the anterior and the posterior borders of the body (see Fig. 74-4C). Proper needle placement must be assessed with the spread of the contrast medium (water-soluble, nonionic). This should demonstrate paravertebral spread under the pedicles in the AP view without intravascular, pleural, epidural, or intrathecal uptake (see Fig. 74-4B). Sensory stimulation must be performed at 50 Hz and 0.9 V. Greater than 0.9 V will produce a deep ache. Motor stimulation at 2 Hz and 2 V must be negative. Additionally, 1 mL of a local anesthetic and steroid mix (a 50:50 mix of 0.2% ropivacaine, 2% lidocaine, and 1 mL of 40 mg/mL triamcinolone) is injected after negative aspiration. A 30-second delay should be observed before lesioning. Two lesions are performed at each level with the active tip turned cephalad for the first lesion and caudad for the second. The lesions should be made at 80°C for 90 seconds. A postoperative end-expiratory chest radiograph is taken to rule out a pneumothorax. Unfortunately, 10% to 15% of patients will suffer a postprocedure neuritis. This can last for 3 to 6 weeks.[44,46,47]

Celiac-Splanchnic Plexus

The celiac plexus lies anterior to the aorta and crux of the diaphragm at T12. It is composed of efferent preganglionic splanch-

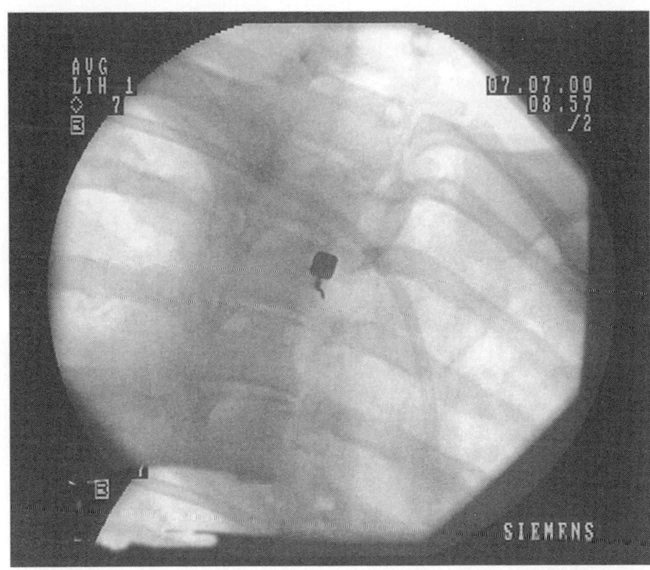

A

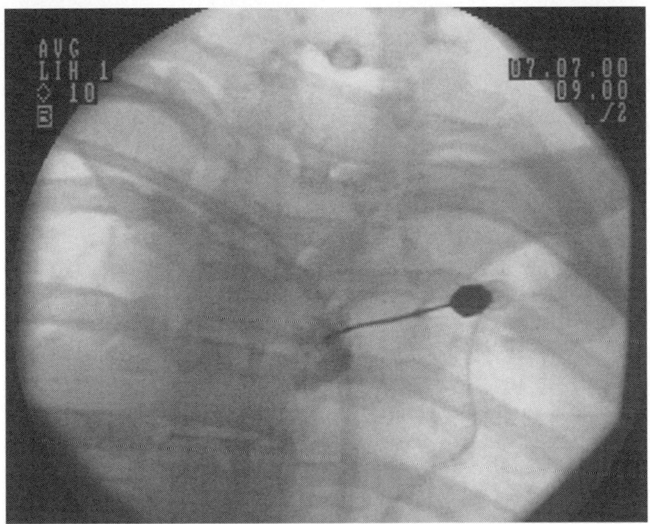

B

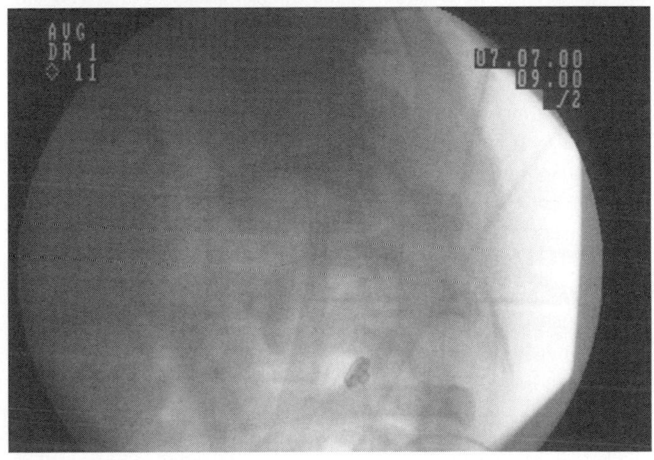

C

Figure 74-3 (**A**) Oblique view of the radiofrequency (RF) needle at the T3 level for a T2 or T3 sympatholysis. (**B**) Anterior-posterior view of the needle with contrast spread at the T3 level for the T3 sympatholysis. Note the spread remains under the pedicle. (**C**) Lateral view of the RF needle in place for the T2 orT3 sympatholysis.

nic nerves, efferent sympathetic preganglionic nerves, and afferent nerves to the viscera of the upper abdomen. This supplies visceral innervation to the pancreas, liver, gallbladder, omentum, mesentery, and alimentary tract from the stomach to the transverse colon. The RF lesioning of the splanchnic nerves prior to joining the celiac plexus allows a discrete, precise lesion from a posterior approach that avoids the risk of puncturing the aorta. The indication for a lesion of the splanchnicnerves is pain originating from the viscera innervated by the celiac plexus. Complications associated with these lesions are:

1. Hypotension
2. Paresthesia of lumbar somatic nerve
3. Vascular injury (including thrombosis or embolism)
4. Intrathecal or epidural injury
5. Paraplegia
6. Pneumothorax
7. Chylothorax
8. Intradiscal placement of the needle
9. Retroperitoneal hematoma
10. Pain during and after procedure.[48]

A diagnostic block should precede the performance of RF. The patient should be placed in the prone position on a fluoroscopy table. Using AP fluoroscopy guidance, the T12 vertebral body should be identified. The fluoroscopic view should be rotated to a 45 degree oblique view to place the shadow of the body lateral to the laminae. A caudocephalad view may be necessary to correct for the lower thoracic kyphosis (approximately 20 degrees). The edge of the diaphragm lateral to the vertebral body is viewed. Its movement during inspiration and expiration are noted. If the diaphragm shadows the T12 vertebra and its rib, then the T11 rib is identified.[48] A 10- to 15-cm blunt, curved cannula with a 10-mm active tip is introduced through a 16-gauge angiocatheter that has already pierced the skin. The target of the angiocatheter is at the junction of the rib and the vertebra.[48] A tunnel view should demonstrate the cannula advancing toward the margin of the lamina. It is advanced along the lateral body until the tip is at the junction of the anterior one third and posterior two thirds of the lateral surface of the vertebral body.[48] The patient should deeply inhale and exhale to demonstrate lack of penetration of the diaphragm in both the AP and lateral views. Proper needle placement must be assessed with the spread of the contrast medium (approximately 5 mL). This should demonstrate paravertebral spread under the pedicles in the AP view without intravascular, pleural, epidural, or intrathecal uptake. It should also flow medial to the interpleural space, above the crus of the diaphragm and anterior to the foramen.[48] Sensory stimulation must be performed as described above (50 Hz and 0.9 V). The patient may report that he or she feels stimulation in the epigastric region. This is typical and satisfactory. If the stimulation is in a girdle-like fashion around the intercostal spaces, the needle needs to be pushed anteriorly.[48] Motor stimulation must be performed and demonstrated to be negative as noted above. Additionally, 3 to 5 mL of a local anesthetic-steroid mix are injected after negative aspiration. A 1- to 2-minute delay should be observed before lesioning. Two lesions are performed with the active tip turned cephalad for the first lesion and caudad for the second. The lesions should be made at 80°C for 90 seconds. A postoperative end-expiratory chest radiography is taken to rule out a pneumothorax.

Raj et al[48] reported on a group of 22 patients with RF lesioning of the splanchnic nerves. The technique was effective for all 10 patients with cancer in this group and complication free. Of the 12 patients in the nonmalignant pain group, some required repeat lesioning at 4 months. In this group, no complications were reported.[48]

Lumbar Sympathetic Chain

The lumbar sympathetic chain lies at the anterolateral border of the vertebral bodies. The location and size of the ganglia are variable.[49] These ganglia consist of preganglionic sympathetic axons from T10 to L3 and post-ganglionic cell bodies. Classic teaching suggests the ganglia are located on the lower third of L2, upper third of L3, and mid-L4 and L5 vertebral bodies.[21] Indications for lumbar sympathetic interruption are similar to the indications for stellate ganglion block, except the location of the pain is in the lower extremity:

1. Complex regional pain syndrome I (reflex sympathetic dystrophy)
2. Complex regional pain syndrome II (causalgia)
3. Herpes zoster
4. Postherpetic neuralgia
5. Phantom limb pain
6. Hyperhidrosis
7. Cancer pain to lower extremity
8. Acute radiation neuritis
9. Post-radiation neuralgia.

As with RF of the stellate ganglion, a diagnostic block must be performed prior to lesioning of the lumbar sympathetic chain. Complications that may occur with this procedure include:

1. Vascular injury
2. Intrathecal injury
3. Nerve root injury
4. Intradiscal placement of needle
5. Renal trauma
6. Punctured ureter
7. Genitofemoral/lumbar plexus neuralgia.

Aside from the complications, there are other concerns with lumbar sympathetic interruption. One concern is incomplete sympatholysis, which can make RF lesioning of the lumbar sympathetic chain less effective than phenol neurolysis.[50] For more effective sympatholysis, at least three levels must be performed. Cllinical experience has shown a lesion at the L5 level may provide relief for foot pain.[21] The other concern is the aberrant regeneration of the sympathetic nerve fibers over time. Future studies of this phenomenon would be helpful.

For the procedure, the patient is placed on the table in the prone position. The lumbosacral area is prepared and draped in a sterile manner. Using fluoroscopic guidance, in the AP view, the desired vertebral body is identified. The operator may need to adjust the fluoroscope in a craniocaudal fashion until the disc spaces are clear. The beam is then rotated in an oblique fashion to approximately 30 degrees (Fig. 74-4A). The desired view is one where the transverse process of the vertebra in question disappears behind the body.[21] If the desired level is L2, 4, or 5, a skin wheal is raised at the inferior aspect of the transverse process at the lateral border of the vertebral body. If the desired level is L3, then the skin wheal is raised at the superior aspect of the transvese process at the lateral border of the vertebral body. A 16-gauge angiocatheter is directed through the skin wheal in "gun-barrel" fashion. A 15-cm, 10-mm active tip RF needle (a Racz-Finch curved, blunt needle

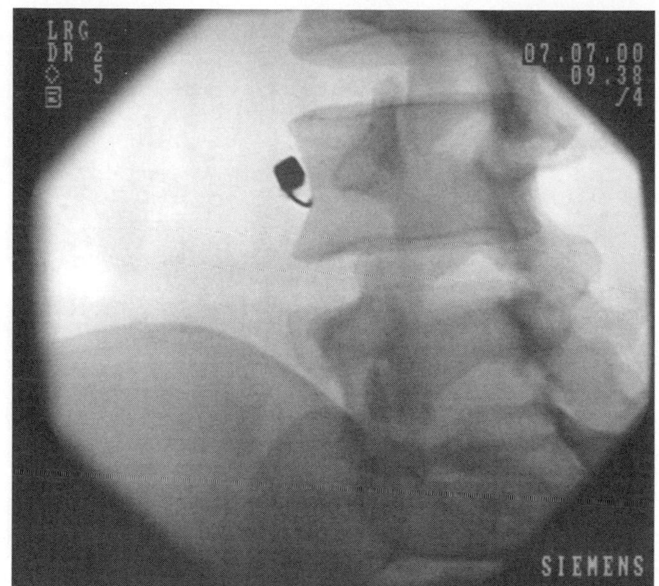

A

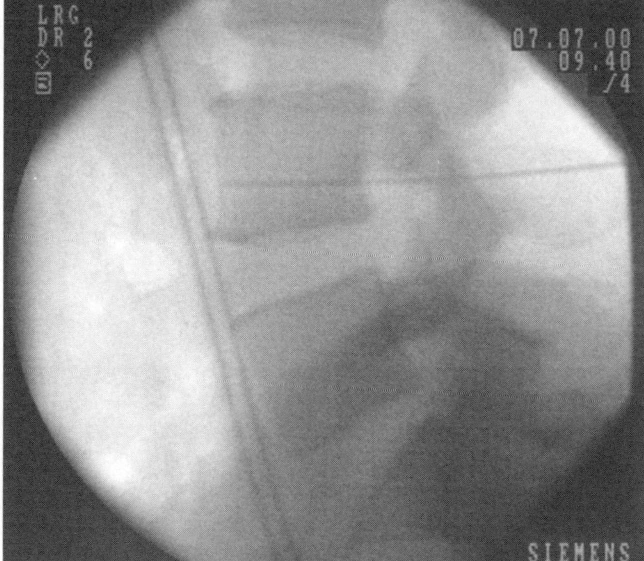

B

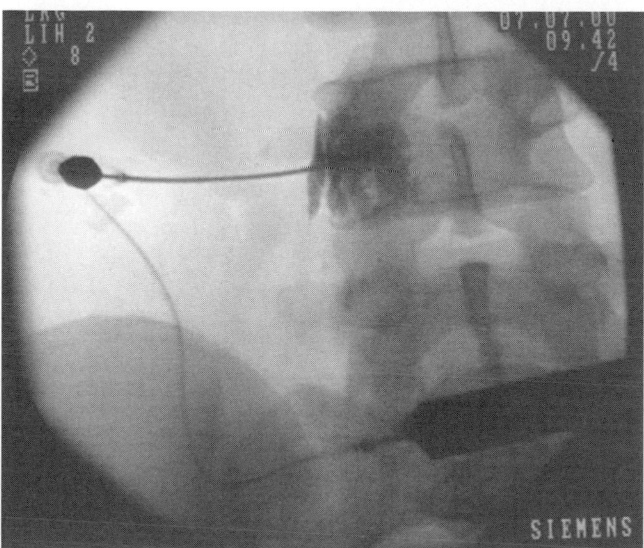

C

from Radionics is suggested) is advanced through the angiocatheter and is advanced to the anterior border of the vertebral body, as noted in lateral view (see Fig. 74-4B). Care must be taken while advancing the needle so that it "hugs" the periosteum. Confirmation of needle placement may first be noted with the spread of 1 to 3 mL of water-soluble, nonionic contrast. The spread of this dye should be hugging the anterior aspect of the vertebral bodies in the lateral view. Proper placement for the particular level is also observed in the lateral view. At the L2 level, when the needle approaches the anterior border of the vertebral body, it should be at the junction of the superior two thirds, inferior one third of the body in the craniocaudal orientation. At the L3 level, the needle should be at the superior one third and inferior two thirds. At the levels of L4 and L5, the needle should be at the junction of the superior 50% and inferior 50%. In the AP view, the spread should appear vacuolated and remain under the pedicles. There should be no observance of myoneural spread as this indicates the needle remains in the psoas major muscle. (see Fig. 74-4C) Further confirmation of proper needle placement is accomplished with sensory and motor stimulation as described above. After assurance of proper placement of the needle, 1 to 3 mL of local anesthetic/steroid (at Texas Tech, this consists of a 50:50 mix of 2% lidocaine with 0.2% ropivacaine, and 1 mL of 40 mg/mL triamcinolone) should be injected. A 45-second to 1-minute delay should follow the injection prior to lesioning at 80°C for 90 seconds. The first lesion is with the active tip turned cephalad and the second lesion is with the tip turned caudad.[21]

Radiofrequency denervation of the lumbar sympathetic chain can be an effective treatment for persistent sympathetic-mediated pain.[21] Lesioning the sympathetic chain at a single level (L3) only produces a 25% lasting response.[21,51] Performing the procedure at multiple levels results in a 75% response at 8 weeks.[21,51]

Lumbar Facets

Zygapophyseal joints have been increasingly recognized as a potentially significant source of low back pain.[53–55] The L1-4 dorsal rami form three branches—medial, lateral, and intermediate—in the intertransverse space.[56] The L1-4 medial branches curve around the root of the superior articular process and pass through a notch bridged by the mamillo-accessory ligament. This branch supplies the lower pole at the same level and the upper pole of the joint above. It also supplies the rami in the multifidus.[56–58] Each joint receives its nerve supply from the corresponding medial branch above and below the joint.[56–58] Patients who have low back pain associated with localized tenderness right over the zygapophyseal joints without other root tension signs or neurologic signs, and who respond to intra-articular joint injections or to blocks of the medial branches of the dorsal rami, can be suspected of having zygapophyseal joint pain.[59,60] Mooney and Robertson[53] demonstrated referred pain from the zygapophyseal joints to the low back region, the greater trochanter, the posterolateral thigh, the groin region, and in a few patients, pain extended down the length of the leg and foot.[53,60] These pain referral patterns were confirmed by Fukui et al.[60] Complications of denervation of the lumbar facet include:

Figure 74-4 (**A**) Oblique view of the radiofrequency (RF) needle for lumbar sympatholysis. (**B**) Lateral view of the RF needle for lumbar sympatholysis. (**C**) Anterior-posterior view of the RF needle for lumbar sympatholysis. Note the spread of the contrast under the pedicle.

1. Increased pain
2. Neuritis
3. Numbness.

For the procedure, the patient is placed in the prone position. The lumbosacral area is prepared and draped in a sterile manner. The appropriate level is identified by fluoroscopic guidance in the AP view. The camera is rotated to a 10- to 15-degree oblique view, which allows visualization of the "Scottie dog" (Fig. 74-5A). A skin wheal is raised over the "eye" of the Scottie dog. A 16-gauge angiocatheter is advanced through the skin wheal to periosteum at the inferior aspect of the superior pars (the ear of the Scottie dog). A 10-cm, 10-mm active-tip RF needle is advanced through the angiocatheter to periosteum, then walked off in the lateral superior direction. In the lateral view this should be noted to be at the level of the facet line, posterior to the foraminal line, and below the level of the disk (Fig. 74-5B). Accurate placement is determined through sensory and motor stimulation: for sensory stimulation at 50 Hz and 0.9 V; for motor stimulation at 2 Hz and 2 V. Motor stimulation at 2 Hz will ideally cause paraspinal contractions, and at 2.0 V will not cause lower-extremity fasciculations.[21] Lesioning is preceded by injection of 1.5 mL of a local anesthetic-steroid mix. After a 45-second to 1-minute delay, lesioning commences at 80°C for 90 seconds, medially and laterally, with an impedance, at less than 250 Ω.

The technique has had varying results.[53,54,61–66] Most recently, however, Van Kleef et al[67] performed a study of 31 patients with a 1-year history of chronic low back pain with positive diagnostic blocks. The patients were divided into a RF group (n = 15) and a control group (n = 16). The RF group received an 80 degree RF lesion; the control group had the same procedure but no current. The treating physician and the patients were blinded to group assignment. At 8 weeks of treatment, 10 of 15 patients in the RF group were deemed successful. There were 6 in the control group that also had pain relief at 8 weeks. However, at 3, 6, and 12 months, there were significantly more successful patients in the radiofrequency group compared with the control group.[67]

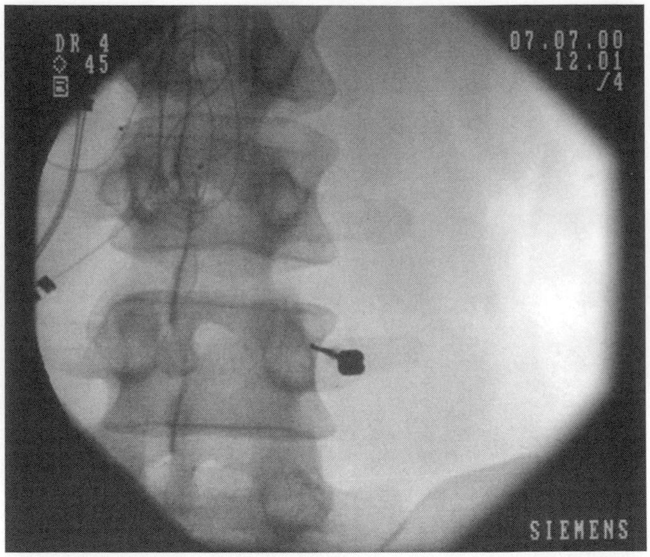

A

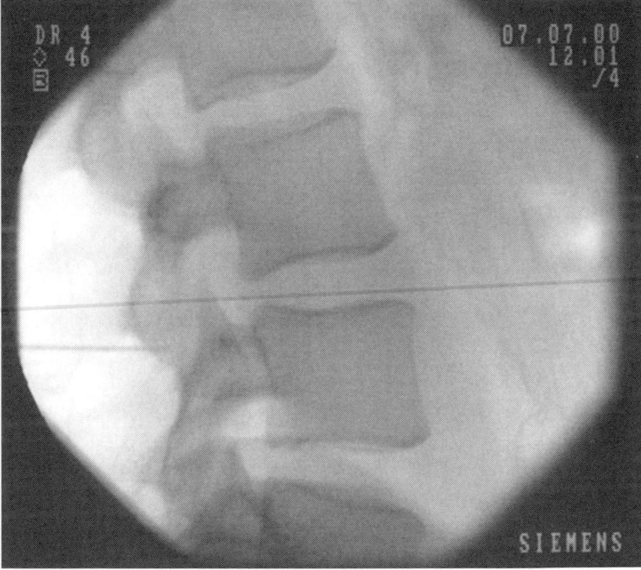

B

Figure 74-5 (**A**) Oblique view of the radiofrequency (RF) needle for lumbar facet neurolysis. (**B**) Lateral view of the RF needle for lumbar facet neurolysis. Note the tip of the needle is at the level of the facet, below the level of the disc.

Cervical Facets

There are several possible pain generators in the cervical spine—the disk, the root, the zygapophyseal joint, or the muscles. These generators may result in pain that is experienced as a headache or as neck and arm pain. Many times, there can be poor correlation between the results from CT, magnetic resonance imaging (MRI), or radiologic studies and the pain suffered by the patient.[21] A thorough history and physical examination can be helpful in the identification of pain related to the cervical zygapophysial joints. Common pain-referral patterns were established with the intra-articular injection of contrast medium.[68] Cervical disc pain often goes along with facet pain, either as a result of degeneration or as a result of trauma. This may be the result of a sensitization of the annulus fibrosis nerve roots.[21] In a study of 56 patients, 41% had both disc and facet pain, 23% had facet only, and 20% disc only.[69,21] Diagnostic facet blocks offer the most success in selecting radiofrequency candidates, with a 70% response rate.[70,21] Increasingly, the mechanism of chronic pain after whiplash injury has been deemed cervical zygapophyseal joint pain. This has been confirmed in biomechanical studies.[71–75] Postmortem studies have revealed that the joints can be affected by pillar fractures, subchondral fractures, tears of their meniscoids, and intra-articular hemorrhages.[71,75–78] It is evident that any of these findings could be associated with long-term, chronic neck pain.

To denervate the cervical facet, the anatomy must be appreciated. The cervical zygapophysial joints are innervated by articular branches derived from the medial branches of the cervical dorsal rami.[70,79] The medial branches curve medially, hugging the waists of their ipsisegmental articular pillars.[70] Articular branches arise from the medial branch as it approaches the posterior aspect of the articular pillar.[70,79] An ascending branch innervates the zygapophyseal joint above and a descending branch innervates the joint below. Consequently, each typical cervical zygapophysial joint receives dual innervation, from the medial branch above and from the medial branch below its location.[70] Owing to the anatomical differences, it is important to note that these anatomical characteristics for the techniques described hold true for C2-3 and below.

There are two different techniques described. The first technique is with the patient in the supine position and described by Wenger.[21] The level desired is identified under AP fluoroscopic guidance. The camera is then rotated to a 30-degree oblique view so the vertebral foramen may be easily visualized. The camera axis is then oriented 10 degrees caudo-cranially.[21] The posterior border of the facets is palpated and marked on the skin to assist with needle orientation. The cranio-caudad level of approach is identified by holding a clamp over the lateral neck and the cannula is inserted in this plane at the premarked posterior border of the facet. The cannula is advanced with a slight anterior angle and the bone is typically encountered in 1.5 to 2.5 cm. Cannula progress is followed in the 30-degree oblique view, taking care not to advance in the direction of the foramen. Once on bone, an AP view is taken to confirm placement at the waist of the body. Sensory stimulation is monitored for stimulation in the region of the neck and the shoulder. Motor stimulation should reveal the absence of upper-extremity motor fasciculations. An injection of 1.5 mL of a local anesthetic-steroid mix is given after negative aspiration. A delay of 45 seconds to 1 minute should occur prior to lesioning. The lesioning is then performed at 80°C for 90 seconds. Possible complications include neuritis and segmental nerve injury.[21] This resembles the technique described by Sluijter and Koetsvelt-Baart.[80]

A second technique is with the patient in the prone position and is described by Lord et al.[70] The level to be lesioned is identified in the AP view. The targeted area is the lateral margin of the articular pillar. A skin wheal is raised over the target and a 16-gauge angiocatheter is placed in gun-barrel fashion through the angiocatheter. The RF needle needs to be 10 cm with a 5-mm active tip. A needle with a curved, blunt tip is suggested for safety and ease of placement. The RF needle is advanced just medial to the lateral margin of the articular pillar until bony resistance of the back of the pillar is encountered.[70] It is imperative that bony contact be made to prevent overinsertion. After the back of the pillar is contacted, the needle is walked off laterally in small increments, until a loss of bony resistance is sensed and the needle gently slips forward, tangential to the pillar.[70] The patient is tested for motor and sensory stimulation as described earlier. Similarly, an injection of local anesthetic with steroid is given with a delay. The lesion is made at 80°C for 90 seconds, with the bevel curved cranially, then caudally.

In a study by Lord et al[81] the efficacy of denervating the cervical zygapophyseal joints was examined. In this double-blind, placebo-controlled study, patients treated with RF had a median time of 263 days of at least 50% pain relief. Of the patients receiving RF, 41% reported numbness in the area of the treated nerves, but this was not deemed a problem.[81]

Lumbar Dorsal Root Ganglion

It has been demonstrated that compression of the dorsal root ganglion by a herniated disc generates radicular pain leading to prolonged repetitive firing in sensory axons. This leads to increased mechanical sensitivity.[82] It has also been demonstrated that injury of nerve roots by chronic compression of the herniated disc, by previous surgery or by scar tissue itself, can lead to repetitive firing. Despite being compressed, stretching of these injured nerve roots leads to repetitive firing.[83] Performing a ganglionectomy can be a decision based on diagnostic nerve root blocks that suggest a monoradicular pain syndrome.[84] Ganglionectomy may be performed percutaneously by radiofrequency. The dorsal root ganglion is easily accessible by percutaneous needle. It is anatomically distinct from motor fibers and may be tested for placement with motor and sensory stimulation. A troublesome side effect of RF is neuritis. This may resolve by itself over a period of 4 to 6 weeks, or it may be treated with local anesthetic and steroid root sleeve injection. More recently, a pulsed radiofrequency technique has been advocated. While making radiofrequency lesions, the tip of the electrode is exposed to an electromagnetic field (EMF). The EMF may be the reason for the clinical effect of RF thermocoagulation. Unlike RF, EMF is not neurodestructive. Neuroablation occurs at greater than 45° C.[42] EMF is performed at 42° C. A pilot study was done to investigate the usefulness of future double-blind studies with pulsed radiofrequency adjacent to the dorsal root ganglion in patients with unilateral symptomatology. Although the mechanism remains unclear, the study demonstrated improvement in the patients, and the conclusion was that EMF may be the clinical effect. Advantages of pulsed RF over RF: (1) a virtually painless procedure, (2) no signs of neurodestruction, and (3) may be suitable for patients with neuropathic pain or peripheral neuritis.[85]

To perform the procedure, the patient is placed in the prone position. The lumbosacral area is prepared and draped in a sterile manner. Using fluoroscopy, the appropriate level is identified in the AP view. If the L2 dorsal root ganglion is the desired level, then the superior pars of the L3 vertebral body is the target site. The camera is then rotated approximately 20 to 25 degrees oblique to the ipsilateral side. The camera is then given approximately 20 degrees caudo-cranial rotation. This assists with lining the discs. A skin wheal is made over the target area, which is the superior aspect of the superior pars. A 16-gauge angiocatheter is passed in gun-barrel fashion through the angiocatheter. A 10-cm, 10-mm, active-tip RF needle is passed through the angiocatheter. (It is suggested for technical and safety reasons that the RF needle be a curved blunt tip.) It is imperative the RF needle touch periosteum at the superior tip of the superior pars. The bevel of the needle is then rotated cranially and laterally, then gently walked off the superior pars. The bevel of the needle is then immediately rotated medially. The depth is checked in the lateral view at the 6 o'clock position in the posterior aspect of the foramina and at the level of the disk. In the AP view, the tip should be no more medial than the midfacet line.[21] Sensory stimulation should be performed at 50 Hz. The patient should note a paresthesia in the distribution of the desired root between 0.3 and 0.7 V (preferentially, 0.3 to 0.5 V). If the stimulation can be felt at less than 0.3 V, there is concern for intraneural placement. If the stimulation requires more than 0.7 V, then the needle may be too far from the dorsal root ganglion. Motor stimulation should be negative at two times the sensory threshold to confirm a safe distance from the anterior motor fibers.[21] Further confirmation of placement may be done with the injection of 2 to 3 mL of water-soluble, nonionic contrast dye. This should show a distribution along the nerve root and into the epidural space. After being assured of placement of the needle, the pulsed radiofrequency may be done at 42°C for 120 seconds, a total of three cycles. No local anesthetic or steroid needs to be placed prior to the EMF. Pulsed radiofrequency offers an alternative treatment technique for patients with neuropathic pain where RF is usually a contraindication.[86] This technique needs further investigation to determine efficacy; however, case reports appear to be positive.[87]

Cervical Dorsal Root Ganglion

Pain in the neck may be related to a discogenic problem. If this is the case, pulsed RF of a cervical dorsal root ganglion may be indicated. As in all procedures, before therapy a diagnostic block with local anesthetic and steroid must be performed. The following description is for cervical roots C3 and below. The patient is placed in the supine position. The neck area is prepared and draped in a sterile manner. After identifying the appropriate level in the AP view, the camera is rotated to a 30-degree oblique view to observe the foramina. The technique is the same as for the cervical facets in the supine position; however, the 5-cm, 5-mm, active-tip RF needle is advanced to the six o'clock position into the posteriormost aspect of the vertebral canal. This dorsal-most position is used to avoid damage to the anterior vertebral artery. Frequent AP views are obtained to assure the needle does not pass medial to the midfacet line.[21] Sensory stimulation should be performed at 50 Hz and a paresthesia in the distribution of the nerve root should be illicited between 0.3 and 0.7 V. Again, the ideal stimulation would occur between 0.3 and 0.5 V. Motor stimulation is performed at twice the threshold for sensory stimulation and should be found negative. Confirmation may be done with the injection of 0.5 mL of water-soluble, nonionic contrast dye, which should be observed following the nerve root and into the epidural space. Pulsed radiofrequency is then performed at 42°C for 120 seconds for three cycles. As with pulsed radiofrequency of the lumbar dorsal root, more studies are indicated. This technique, however, appears hopeful and avoids the side effects of hypesthesia, hyposensitivity, or neuritis.

CONCLUSION

Radiofrequency provides a discrete, safe, reliable, and reproducible technique for long-term pain relief. For best outcomes, proper patient selection is critical. It is imperative that prior to the technique, a proper diagnostic block is performed. To maintain safety and reliability, the procedure must be performed under fluoroscopic guidance with proper sensory and motor stimulation prior to the lesion. In the hands of a properly trained physician, radiofrequency provides a safe and effective treatment for difficult to treat pain conditions.

REFERENCES

1. Saberski LR. Cryoneurolysis in clinical practice. In: Waldman S, Winnie A,eds. *Interventional Pain Management*. Philadelphia, PA: WB Saunders; 1996:172–184.
2. Barnard JDW, Lloyd JW, Glynn CJ. Cryosurgery in the management of intractable facial pain. *Br J Oral Surg* 1978;16:135–142.
3. Arthur JM, Racz G. Cryolysis. In: Raj PP, ed. *Pain Medicine: A Comprehensive Review*. St. Louis, Mo: Mosby; 1996:297–303.
4. Amoils SP. The Joule-Thompson cryoprobe. *Arch Ophthamol* 1967;78: 201–207.
5. Evans PJD. Cryoanalgesia. The application of low temperature to nerves to produce anaesthesia or analgesia. *Anaesthesia* 1981;36:1003–1013.
6. Sunderland S. *Nerves and Nerve Injuries*. 2nd ed. London, England: Churchill Livingstone; 1978;69.
7. Evans PJD, Lloyd JW, Green CJ. Cryoanalgesia: the response to alterations in the freeze cycle and temperature. *Br J Anaesth* 1981;53: 1121–1127.
8. Kalichman MW, Myers RR. Behavioral and electrophysiological recovery following cryogeneic nerve injury. *Exp Neurol* 1987;96:692–702.
9. Gill W, Frazier J, Carter D. Repeated freeze-thaw cycles in cryosurgery. *Nature* 1968; 219:410–413.
10. Douglas WW, Malcolm JL. The effect of localized cooling on conduction in cat nerves. *J Physiol* 1955;130:63–71.
11. Wood GJ, Lloyd JW, Bullingham RES, et al. Postoperative analgesia for day-care herniorrhaphy patients. *Anaesthesia* 1981;36:603–610.
12. Nelson KM, Vincent RG, Bourke RS, et al. Intraoperative intercostals nerve freezing to prevent post-thoracotomy pain. *Ann Thorac Surg* 1974;18:280–281.
13. Katz J, Nelson W, Forest R, Bruce D. Cryoanalgesia for post-thoracotomy pain. *Lancet* 1980;1:512–513.
14. Brynitz S, Schroder M. Intraoperative cryolysis of intercostals nerves in thoracic surgery. *Scand J Thorac Cardiovasc Surg* 1986;20:85–87.
15. Goss AN. Cryoneurotomy for intractable temporomandibular joint pain. *Br J Oral Maxillofac Surg* 1988;26:26–31.
16. Zakrzewska JM, Nally FF. The role of cryotherapy (cryoanalgesia) in the management of paroxysmal trigeminal neuralgia: a six year experience. *Br J Oral Maxillofac Surg* 1988;26:18–25.
17. Jones MJT, Murrin KR. Intercostal block with cryotherapy. *Ann R Coll Surg Engl* 1987;69:261–262.
18. Schuster GD. The use of cryoanalgesia in the painful facet syndrome. *Neural Orthop Surg* 1982;3:271–274.
19. Racz G, Hagstrom D. Iliohypogastric and ilioinguinal nerve entrapment: diagnosis and treatment. *Pain Dig* 1992;2:43–48.
20. Conacher ID, Locke T, Hilton C. Neuralgia after cryoanalgesia for thoracotomy. *Lancet* 1986;1:277.
21. Wenger CC. Radiofrequency lesions in the treatment of spinal pain. *Pain Dig* 1998;8:1–16.
22. Cosman RJ, Cosman FR. Radionics procedure technique series monographs. *Guide to Radiofrequency Lesion Generation in Neurosurgery*. Burlington, Mass: Radionics Inc; 1974.
23. Kline MT. *Stereotactic Radiofrequency Lesions as Part of the Management of Pain*. Delray Beach, Fla: St. Lucie Press; 1996:2.
24. Kirschner M. Zur elektrochirurgie. *Arch Klin Chir* 1931;147:761.
25. Sweet WH, Mark VH. Unipolar anodal electrolyte lesions in the brain of man and cat: Report of five human cases with electrically produced bulbar or mesencephalic tractotomies. *Arch Neurol Psychiatry* 1953; 70:224–234.
26. Cosman ER. Radiofrequency lesions. In: Gildenberg PL, Tasker RR, eds. *Textbook of Stereotactic and Functional Neurosurgery*. New York, NY: McGraw-Hill; 1998: 973–985.
27. Aronow S. The use of radiofrequency power in making lesions in the brain. J Neurosurg 1960;17:431–438.
28. Mundinger F, Reichert T, Gabriel E. Untersuchungen zu den physikalischen und technischen Voranssetzungeneiner dosierten Hochfrequenzkoagulation bei stereptaktischen Hirnoperation. *Z Chir* 1960;19:1051–1063.
29. Cosman ER, Nashold BS, and Ovelman-Levitt J. Theoretical aspects of radiofrequency lesions in the dorsal root entry zone. *Neurosurgery* 1984;15:945–950.
30. Sweet WH, Wepsic JG. Controlled thermocoagulation of trigeminal ganglion and rootlets for differential destruction of pain fibers. *J Neurosurg* 1974;39:143–156.
31. Letcher FS, Goldring S. The effect of radiofrequency current and heat on peripheral nerve action in the cat. *J Neurosurg* 1968;29:42–47.
32. Smith HP, McWhorter JM, Challa VR. Radiofrequency neurolysis in a clinical model: neuropathological correlation. *J Neurosurg* 1981; 55:246.

33. Uematsu S. Percutaneous electrothermocoagulation of spinal nerve trunk, ganglion, and rootlets. In: Schmidek HH, Sweet WS, eds. *Current Techniques in Operative Neurosurgery*. New York, NY: Grune and Stratton; 1977:469–490.
34. Tew JM, Keller JT, Williams DS. Application of stereotactic principles to the treatment of trigeminal neuralgia. *Appl Neurophysiol* 1978;41: 146–156.
35. Hammer M, Meneese W. Principles and practice of radiofrequency neurolysis. *Curr Rev Pain* 1998;2:267–278.
36. Shealy CN. Percutaneous radiofrequency denervation of spinal facets. *J Neurosurg* 1975;43:448–451.
37. Sluijter ME, Mehta M. Treatment of chronic back and neck pain by percutaneous thermal lesions. In: Lipton S,ed. *Persistent Pain: Modern Methods of Treatment*. Vol. 3. London, England: Academic Press, 1981:141–179.
38. Kline MT. Radiofrequency techniques in clinical practice. In: Waldman S,Winnie A, eds. *Interventional Pain Management*. Philadelpha, Pa: WB Saunders; 1996:185–217.
39. Saberski L, Fitzgerald J, Ahmad M. Cryoneurolysis and Radiofrequency Lesioning. In Raj PP, et al, eds. *Practical Management of Pain*. 3rd ed. St. Louis, Mo: Mosby; 2000:753–767.
40. Bogduk N, Macintosh J, Marsland A. Technical limitations to the efficacy of radiofrequency neurotomy for spinal pain. *Neurosurgery* 1987;20:529–535.
41. Noe CE,Racz GB. Radiofrequency In: Raj PP, ed. *Pain Medicine: A Comprehensive Review*. St. Louis, Mo: Mosby-Year Book; 1996: 305–307.
42. Brodkey JS, Miyazaki Y, Ervin FR, Mark VH. Reversible heat lesions with radiofrequency. *Curr J Neurosurg* 1964;21:49–53.
43. Cosman ER, Rittman WJ, Nashold BS, Makachinas TT. Radiofrequency lesion generation and its effect on tissue impedance. *Appl Neurophysiol* 1988;51:230–242, 1988.
44. Raj PP, Anderson SR. Stellate ganglion block. In: Waldman SD, ed. *Interventional Pain Management*. 2nd edition. Philadelphia, PA: WB Saunders; 2001.
45. Sluijter, ME. *Radiofrequency Lesions in the Treatment of Cervical Pain Syndromes*. Burlington, Mass: Radionics Inc, 1990:1–19.
46. Racz G. Techniques of Neurolysis. Boston, Kluwer Academic; 1989; 179.
47. Skabelund C, Racz G. Indications and technique of thoracic$_2$ and thoracic$_3$ neurolysis. *Curr Rev Pain* 1999;3:400–405.
48. Raj PP, Thomas J, Heavner J, et al. The development of a technique for radiofrequency lesioning of splanchnic nerves. *Curr Rev Pain* 1999; 3:377–387.
49. Rocco AG, Palombi D, Raeke D. Anatomy of the lumbar sympathetic chain. *Reg Anesth* 1995;20:13–19.
50. Haynsworth RF, Noe CE. Percutaneous lumbar sympathectomy: a comparison of radiofrequency denervation versus phenol neurolysis. *Anesthesiology* 1991;74:459–463.
51. Rocco AG. Radiofrequency lumbar sympatholysis: the evoluation of a technique for managing sympathetically maintained pain. *Reg Anesth* 1995;20:3–12.
52. Noe CE, Haynesworth R, et al. Lumbar radiofrequency sympatholysis. *J Vasc Surg* 1993;17:801–806.
53. Mooney V, Robertson J. The facet syndrome. *Clin Orthop* 1976;115: 149–156.
54. Lippitt AB. The facet joint and its role in spine pain: management with facet joint injections. *Spine* 1984;9:746–750.
55. Schwarzer AC, Aprill CN, Derby R, et al. Clinical features of patients with pain stemming from the lumbar zygapophyseal joints: is the lumbar facet syndrome a clinical entity? *Spine* 1994;19:1132–1137.
56. Bogduk N, Wilson AS, Tynan W. The human lumbar dorsal rami. *J Anat* 1982;134:383–397.
57. Bogduk N. The innervation of the lumbar spine. *Spine* 1983;8:286–293.
58. Bogduk N, Long DM. The anatomy of the so-called articular nerves and their relationship to facet denervation in the treatment of low back pain. *J Neurosurg* 1979;51:172–177.
59. Robert CM, Thomas H, Tery T. Facet joint injections and facet nerve block: a randomized comparison in 86 patients with chronic low back pain. *Pain* 1992;49:325–328.
60. Fukui S, Ohseto K, Shiotani M, et al. Distribution of referred pain from the lumbar zygapophyseal joints and dorsal rami. *Clin J Pain* 1997; 13:303–307.
61. Lora J, Long D. So-called facet denervation in the management of intractable back pain. *Spine* 1976;1:121–126.
62. Marks RC, Houston T, Thulbourne T. Facet joint injection and facet nerve block: A randomized comparison in 86 patients with chronic low back pain. *Pain* 1992;49:325–8, 1992.
63. Mehta M, Sluijter Me. The treatment of chronic back pain: a preliminary survey of the effect of radiofrequency denervation of the posterior vertebral joints. *Anaesthesia* 1979;34:768–775.
64. Ogsbury JS, Simon RH, Lehman RAW. Facet denervation in the treatment of low back syndrome. *Pain* 1977;3:257–263.
65. Shealy CN. Facet denervation in the management of back and sciatic pain. *Clin Orthop* 1976;115:157–164.
66. Silvers HR. Lumbar percutaneous facet rhizotomy. *Spine* 1990;15:36–40.
67. Van Kleef M, Barendse GAM, Kessels A, et al. Randomized trial of radiofrequency lumbar facet cenervation for chronic low back pain. *Spine* 1999;24:1937–1942.
68. Dwyer A, Aprill C, Bogduk N. Cervical zygapophysial joint pain patterns. I: a study in normal volunteers. *Spine* 1990;15:453–457.
69. Bogduk N, Aprill C. On the nature of neck pain, discography, and cervical zygapophysial joint blocks. *Pain* 1993;54:213–217.
70. Lord SM, Barnsley L, Bogduk N. Percutaneous radiofrequency neurotomy in the treatment of cervical zygapophysial joint pain (a caution). *Neurosurgery* 1995;36:732–739.
71. Bogduk N. Cervical zygapophysial joint pain and percutaneous neurotomy: an update to the Quebec Task Force Report on Whiplash-Associated Disorders. In: Gunzburg R, Szpalski M, eds. *Whiplash Injuries: Current Concepts in Prevention, Diagnosis, and Treatment of the Cervical Whiplash Syndromes*. Philadelphia, Pa: Lippincott-Raven; 1998:211–219.
72. Abel MS. Moderately severe whiplash injuries of the cervical spine and their roentgenologic diagnosis. *Clin Orthop* 1958;12:189–208.
73. Abel MS. Occult traumatic lesions of the cervical vertebrae. *CRC Crit Rev Clin Radiol Nucl Med* 1975;6:469–553.
74. Clemens HJ, Burow K. Experimental investigation on injury mechanisms of cervical spine at frontal and rear-frontal impacts. In: *Proceedings of the 16th STAPP Car Crash Conference*. Warrendale, Pennsylvania: Society of Automotive Engineers; 1972:76–104.
75. Wickstrom J. Martinez JL, Rodriguez R Jr. The cervical sprain syndrome: experimental acceleration injuries to the head and neck. In: Selzer ML, Gikas PW, Huelke DF,eds. *The Prevention of Highway Injury*. Ann Arbor, Mich: Highway Safety Research Institute; 1967: 182–187.
76. Jonsson H, Bring G, Rauschning W, Sahlstedt B. Hidden cervical spine injuries in traffic accident victims with skull fractures. *J Spinal Disord* 1991;4:251–263.
77. Taylor JR, Twomey LT. Acute injuries to cervical joints: an autopsy study of neck sprain. *Spine* 1993;9:1115–1122.
78. Taylor JR, Taylor MM. Cervical spine injuries: an autopsy study of 109 blunt injuries. *J Musculoskel Pain* 1996;4:61–79.
79. Bogduk N. The clinical anatomy of the cervical dorsal rami. *Spine* 1982;7:319–330.
80. Sluijter ME, Koetsveld-Baart CC. Interruption of pain pathways in the treatment of the cervical syndrome. *Anaesthesia* 1980;35:302–307.
81. Lord SM, Barnsley L, Wallis BJ, McDonald GJ, Bogduk N. Percutaneous radio-frequency neurotomy for chronic cervical zygapophyseal joint pain. *N Engl J Med* 1996;335:1721–1726.

82. Howe JF, Loeser JD, Calvin WH. Mechanosensitivity of dorsal root ganglia and chemically injured axons: a physiological basis for the radicular pain of nerve root compression. *Pain* 1977;3(1):25–41.
83. Benoist M, Ficat C, Baraf, Cauchoix J. Postoperative lumbar epiduro-arachnoiditis. *Spine* 1980;5:432-436.
84. North RB, Kidd DH, Campbell JN, Long DM. Dorsal root ganglionectomy for failed back surgery syndrome: a 5-year follow-up study. *J Neurosurg* 1991;74:236–242.
85. Sluijter ME, Cosman ER, Rittman WB, Van Kleef M. The effects of pulsed radiofrequency fields applied to the dorsal root ganglion—a preliminary report. *Pain Clin* 1998;11:109–117.
86. Patt RB, Cousins MJ. Techniques for neurolytic blockade. In: Cousins MJ,Bridenbaugh PO, (eds). *Neural Blockade,* 3rd ed. Philadelphia, Pa: Lippincott-Raven; 1998:1007–1062.
87. Munglani R. The longer term effect of pulsed radiofrequency for neuropathic pain. *Pain* 1991;80:437–439.

CHAPTER 75 NEUROSURGICAL TREATMENT OF PAIN

David Dubuisson and Zahid H. Bajwa

Indications for surgical interventions in the treatment of chronic pain continue to evolve as we learn more about the pathophysiology and mechanisms of chronic pain. Recent advances in technology and availability of newer and better analgesics have also helped us rely more on neuromodulation and neuroaugmentation rather than neuroablation. Establishment of multidisciplinary pain centers, formal fellowship training in pain medicine, and popularity of minimally invasive techniques has enabled clinicians from various disciplines to perform procedures that were once performed only by neurosurgeons. Surgical procedures that are used to relieve pain, and are not discussed in detail elsewhere in this book, can be divided into three major categories (Table 75-1).

I. Techniques that attempt to correct the disordered physiology of nerves without creating a lesion.
II. Destructive procedures.
   A. Procedures that transsect primary afferent fibers at the level of peripheral nerve, root, or ganglion.
   B. Operations that interrupt ascending sensory tracts in the spinal cord or brainstem.
   C. Stereotactically placed lesions of deep brain structures.
   D. Operations that inactivate a portion of the sympathetic system.
   E. Destruction of the anterior lobe of the pituitary gland.
   F. Cutting cerebral cortical structures.
III. Procedures in which a device is implanted to stimulate an analgesia-producing mechanism in the central nervous system.

PROCEDURES TO CORRECT DISORDERED NERVE PHYSIOLOGY

The first category of neurosurgical procedures for pain control includes operations designed to relieve constriction of peripheral nerves, spinal nerve roots, dorsal root ganglia, or cranial nerves. These decompressive operations are sometimes elegant and often curative. Their use is restricted to specific well-defined syndromes in which the site of disordered nerve physiology can be predicted. The prediction usually is based on radiologic studies, electromyography, nerve conduction studies, and after careful clinical examination. Most procedures of this type have high success rates. Whenever possible, they should be used in preference to destructive lesions.

The reason for the success of nerve decompression is not entirely clear since it is not always understood why pressure on a nerve causes pain. Not all sites of nerve distortion are associated with chronic pain. For example, in a large series of patients investigated for possible acoustic nerve tumors, myelograms frequently showed incidental disc protrusions. Asymptomatic lesions severe enough to distort spinal nerve roots were identified in one third of cases.[2] These well-defined disc protrusions with nerve root compression were not painful, nor were they known to the patients who had them.

From experimental studies, it appears likely that the sites of chronic nerve compression undergo demyelination and that spontaneous axonal discharges occur. These sites also become sensitive to mild mechanical distortion. Perhaps the difference between an asymptomatic site of compression and a painful one lies in the extent of demyelination, inflammation, and the amount of mechanical stress placed on the nerve during daily activities. Sometimes the relief of pain using decompression is immediate; in other cases, it may be gradual, suggesting that the initial decompression obviates the mechanical effect, and that the passage of time permits recovery from the focal loss of myelin in the afferent fibers.

Peripheral Nerve Decompression

The pain of carpal tunnel syndrome usually is amenable to decompression of the median nerve at the wrist. The procedure is done most often with local or regional anesthesia.[3] Some surgeons use a tourniquet on the forearm. The nerve is compressed by the thickened overlying flexor retinaculum of the hand, which yields as it is divided. In some cases, an additional focus of pressure is found above the wrist crease. Similar compression of the ulnar nerve may occur beneath the proximal tendinous attachment of the flexor carpi ulnaris muscle just below the elbow, causing cubital tunnel syndrome, and in other sites. In most cases, simple division of the overlying ligament suffices. Occasionally, the nerve may benefit from a minor transposition to a location where it is completely free of mechanical distortion.

Thoracic Outlet Syndromes

Chronic pain in the arm, most often in an ulnar distribution, may be accompanied by obliteration of the pulse in certain shoulder positions. This combined neural-vascular compression may be caused by fibrotic changes of the scalene muscles, cervical rib, or a fracture of the clavicle with bony callus compressing the brachial plexus.

Adequate treatment in most patients consists of decompression of the lower portion of the plexus; the exact procedure is tailored to correct the anatomic irregularity responsible. A cervical rib may be removed, a fibrous band divided, or the enlarged clavicle and surrounding scar tissue resected.

Lumbar and Cervical Radiculopathies

A common neurosurgical procedure to relieve pain is decompression of a lumbar or cervical nerve root by excision of an intervertebral disc. Few surgeons currently favor explorations of spinal nerve roots for pain alone; instead, treatment of the associated weakness, sensory loss, or sphincter disturbance assumes greater

TABLE 75-1 **Neurosurgical Techniques for Pain Relief**

Nondestructive Procedures	Carpal tunnel release Thoracic outlet decompression Root decompression Cranial nerve decompression
Destructive Procedures	
Primary afferent	Peripheral neuroectomy Excision of neuroma Glycerol injection Glangliolysis Rhizotomy Rhizidiotomy
Spinal cord or brainstem	Cordotomy Dorsal root entry zone lesions
Deep brain structures	Stereotactic lesions of thalamus, hypothalamus, or spinothalamic or spinal raticular tracts Psychosurgery
Sympathetic nerves	Thoracic sympathectomy Lumbar sympathectomy
Pituitary	Pituitary ablation
Stimulation Techniques	Peripheral nerve stimulation Vagal nerve stimulation Spinal cord stimulation Deep brain stimulation Cerebral cortical stimulation

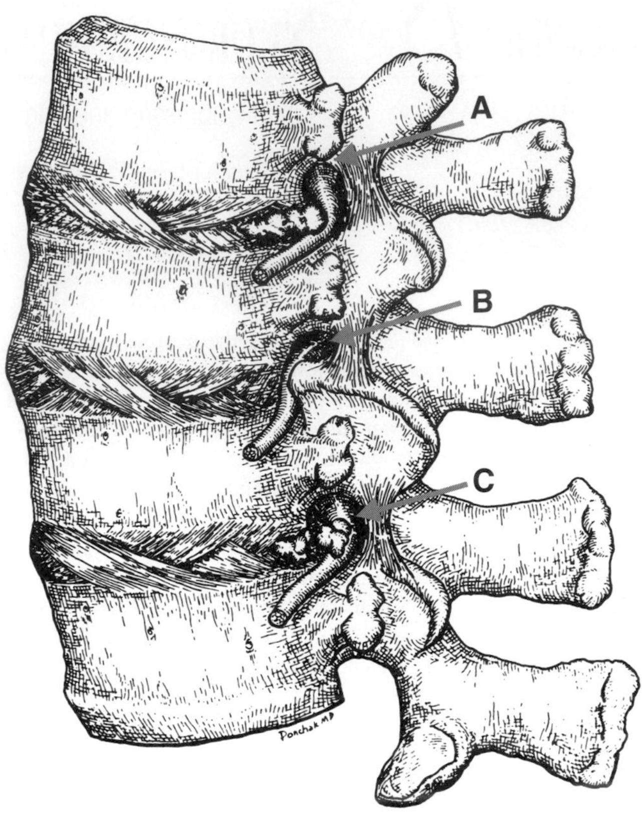

Figure 75–1 Spondylotic changes causing nerve root compression. (**A**) Disc protrusion, (**B**) facet hypertrophy, and (**C**) free disc fragment. (Illustration by Stephen Ponchak, MD.)

importance. In cases of lumbar disc disease, if a well-defined lesion is shown by myelogram, computed tomography (CT), or magnetic resonance imaging (MRI) and the appropriate neurologic signs are present, there is at least a 60% chance of relieving back and radicular pain.[4]

The cause of lumbar root compression differs from patient to patient. Often, the bulging anulus fibrosis of a degenerated disc protrudes enough to contact an adjacent root, or a firm piece of nucleus pulposus emerges through a rent in the anulus and becomes trapped in the spinal canal. However, the disorder may not be so obvious. Spondylotic changes of the facet joint and ligamentum flavum lead to joint enlargement and ligamentous thickening behind the root; bony osteophytes around the worn disc jut into the canal in front (Fig. 75-1).

These changes may require additional surgery, such as partial removal of the facet joint (facetectomy) or unroofing of the intervertebral foramen behind the compressed root (foramenotomy). When the overall dimensions of the canal are too small, all roots of the cauda equine may be compressed or their circulation impeded during erect posture. These cases of lumbar spinal stenosis require complete removal of the lamina bilaterally at every level that is narrowed significantly.

The surgical approach for lumbar disc removal is controversial. Some surgeons advocate a microsurgical approach to diskectomy, with a small skin incision and magnification of the deep structures. There is little doubt that this can be an effective means of treating a fragment of herniated nucleus pulposus; its chief advantages are reduced postoperative pain and shorter hospital stay. Major disadvantages are limitation of the surgeon's view and restricted access of instruments to the disc space itself. Not all cases of root compression consist of simple herniated nucleus pulposus. Lumbar spinal stenosis cannot be treated adequately by the microsurgical approach. It can be argued that diskectomy by a limited exposure may predispose the surgeon to retract harder on the nerve roots and aural tube. Because some of the most intractable cases of sciatica are seen after unsuccessful disc surgery, it is reasonable to ask whether certain surgical approaches may add to the previous degree of nerve root damage. Hard pressure on the root by a surgical instrument could lead to bruising, scar formation, and focal demyelination. In his discussion of the so-called battered root syndrome, Bertrand[5] advocated wider surgical exposure during discoctomy to avoid missing a hidden fragment of material that may have migrated in the epidural space and to visualize all other anatomic features that may be contributing to the patient's symptoms. In some cases, this will require a complete laminectomy. Sometimes it is necessary to explore the adjacent disc if the cause of root compression is not immediately apparent.

As a general rule, if the patient's pain does not resolve after discectomy, we should suspect that the cause of pain was not identified at the time of operation. If the pain resolves but returns in a slightly different distribution, a second disc protrusion may be present. If the pain is worse and severe numbness or dysesthesia appears, the root may have been damaged. Rarely, a patient may have a fever and severe bilateral cramps and leg spasms during the early postoperative period raising the possiblity of arachnoiditis.[6] Late recurrences of pain in the original distribution often are associated with prominent scar formation in the epidural space surrounding the nerve root. In some cases, removal of this scar tissue may be beneficial, but repeated surgery of this type is risky and often futile.

The decompression of cervical nerve roots usually is done by an anterior approach through the disc space because the roots are located directly behind the disc. Most surgeons who do cervical diskectomies fuse the interspace with a bone plug during the same operation to prevent instability and recurrence of osteophytes at that level. Two discs may be removed in this way. If more than two levels are involved, however, it is preferable to do laminectomies and decompress the nerve roots as necessary by drilling away additional bone posteriorly. In these cases of extensive cervical spondylosis, diskectomy may not be required at all provided an adequate posterior decompression of cord and roots is achieved.

Decompression of Cranial Nerves

In many instances of cranial neuralgia, there is a mechanical factor that can be corrected without sacrificing the involved nerve. Although some older procedures were directed at the peripheral portion of the nerve, as in division of the stylohyoid ligament for glossopharyngeal neuralgia, currently there is great interest in exploring the posterior cranial fossa. If the patient with typical trigeminal or glossopharyngeal neuralgia is in good enough health to undergo a craniectomy under general anesthesia, local decompression of the fifth or ninth nerve at a focus of constriction may be the definitive means of treating the neuralgia. Jannetta[7] described arteries compressing the trigeminal root near the brainstem in nearly all cases of tic douloureux. It is recognized that veins and tumors may cause similar effects, and separation of the nerve root from the compressing structure may provide long-term relief of neuralgia in 85% of patients. This procedure is termed *microvascular decompression*, or the Jannetta procedure. Jannetta and colleagues evaluated 1185 patients during a 20-year period who underwent microvascular decompression of the trigeminal nerve for medically intractable trigeminal neuralgia. Most postoperative recurrences of tic took place in the first 2 years after surgery. During the study period, 30% of the patients had recurrences of tic and 11% underwent second operations for the recurrences. Ten years after surgery, 70% of the patients were free of pain without medication for tic. An additional 4% had occasional pain that did not require long-term medication use. They determined that microvascular decompression is a safe and effective treatment for trigeminal neuralgia, with a high rate of long-term success, and even after 10 years after the procedure, the annual rate of the recurrence of tic was less than 1%.[8] The same procedure has been done successfully on the glossopharyngeal root in cases of medically refractory glossopharyngeal neuralgia.

Microvascular decompression requires a posterior fossa craniectomy under general anesthesia, with opening of the aura and retraction of the cerebellum. The procedure has a small mortality rate (>I%) and a morbidity of perhaps 3% to 5%, consisting primarily of ataxia and facial sensory loss. In cases of trigeminal neuralgia, the most common finding is an ectatic superior cerebellar artery crossing the nerve root close to the pons; this is dissected away and kept separate with a tiny plastic sponge or fragment of muscle. Other blood vessels including posterior cerebral artery, anterior inferior cerebellar artery, posterior inferior cerebellar artery, or even basilar artery is occasionally implicated in persistent and refractory trigeminal neuralgia. In approximately 10% of these patients, a compressive lesion cannot be seen. In such cases, the surgeon may have to resort to subtotal rhizotomy, although the long-term success rate of trigeminal rhizotomy is not considered very satisfactory.

DESTRUCTIVE PROCEDURES

Surgical Procedures to Interrupt Prlmary Afferent Fibers

Peripheral Neurectomy and Treatment of Neuromas Section or avulsion of peripheral nerves as a treatment of neuralgic pain has been done mainly in patients with trigeminal and occipital neuralgia. Although these procedures are simple, they have the obvious disadvantages that complete numbness will occur, and peripheral nerve fibers eventually will regenerate. In our opinion, based on clinical experience, more definitive procedures are available to treat both trigeminal and occipital neuralgia with better long-term success and no greater risk. In elderly or infirm patients, this does not necessarily require craniotomy or spinal surgery; instead, a percutaneous procedure often suffices.

Neuromas, either post-traumatic or after peripheral nerve biopsy, are difficult to treat. Usually, it is easy to detect the presence of a neuroma by palpating directly over the site of nerve injury. Neuromas are often unusually tender, and pressure directly over them is painful. Dozens of procedures have been advocated to prevent the reformation of neuromas after excision. They range from burial of the nerve end in bone or muscle to capping of the cut end with a small metal or plastic sheath. Various toxic and medicinal solutions have been painted onto the cut nerve to little avail. Most surgeons agree that simple excision of the neuroma and avoidance of pressure from surrounding tissues is a worthwhile first attempt at treatment, but if this fails, it is usually worthless to resect the neuroma repeatedly.

Although there is no proven surgical treatment of neuromas, current techniques of interest include (1) the creation of a loop by dividing the cut nerve into fascicles joined end-to-end, (2) sealing individual nerve fascicles by drawing the perineurium over the tip of each and lightly cauterizing it with microsurgical forceps, or (3) ligating each fascicle with fine suture material.[9] To the authors' knowledge, the long-term success of microfascicular anastomosis or ligation is not known. Both these procedures have at least anecdotal success, but it is wise to remember that many previous techniques to prevent neuromas have failed after brief initial enthusiasm.

Noordenbos and Wall[10] described seven patients in whom an injured nerve caused local pain and abnormal sensitivity. Resection of the damaged portion and insertion of a sural nerve graft with microsurgical technique was followed inevitably by a recurrence of pain in these patients, suggesting that the peripheral nerve injury had induced changes in the central nervous system that were not reversed by treating the injured nerve itself.

Injection of Glycerol in the Trigeminal Ganglion

Hakanson "first reported the procedure of injecting sterile 100 percent glycerol into the Meckel's cave to treat trigeminal neuralgia. He reported a 90% success rate in 100 patients with no complications and only occasional slight facial numbness.[11] Glycerol injection has been shown to cause some degree of damage to both

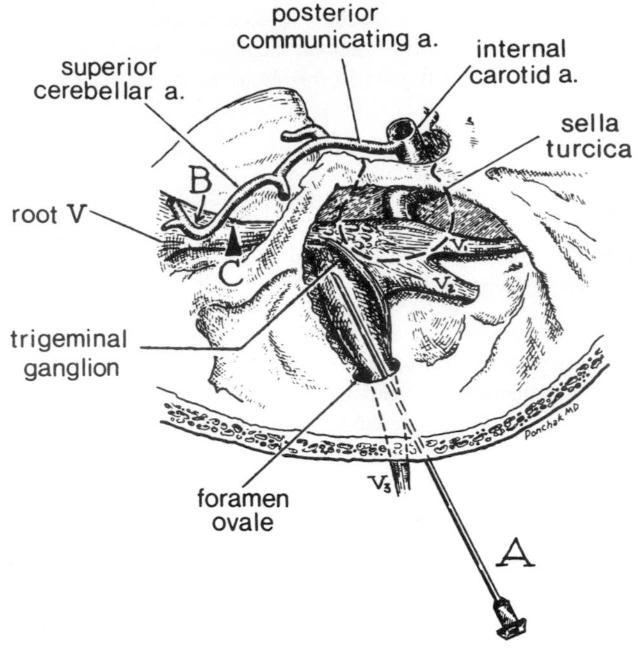

Figure 75–2 Surgical treatments of trigeminal neuralgia. The root of the trigeminal nerve is shown at left emerging from the brainstem, and the three major divisions of the nerve are at right: (**A**) Insertion of needle for thermocoagulation or glycerol injection in ganglion, (**B**) separation of vessel from root (microvascular decompression), and (**C**) subtotal root section. (Illustration by Stephen Ponchak, MD.)

myelinated and unmyelinated nerve fibers. Since its mechanism of action is still poorly understood and its aftereffects are usually slight, it might be more appropriate to consider it a means of altering peripheral nerve physiology without a lesion. Glycerol injection is considered an alternative to percutaneous thermocoagulation or radiofrequency lesioning (RFL) of the trigeminal ganglion.[12,13]

Trigeminal glycerol injection is done by passing a needle through the foremen ovale (Fig. 75-2). A 20-gauge lumbar puncture or spinal needle is suitable. The patient is given short-acting or reversible intravenous anesthetics or "conscious sedation," such as midazolam and/or fentanyl until drowsy. After anesthetizing the cheek with 1% lidocaine injection, the spinal needle is inserted 1.5-cm lateral to the corner of the mouth and directed posteriorly toward a point 2-cm anterior to the external auditory meatus and medially toward the midpupillary line. We use a C-arm fluoroscopy guidance to identify the foremen ovale. The needle tip is positioned 10 to 12 mm below the posterior clinoid processes, and with the stylet withdrawn, cerebrospinal fluid (CSF) emerges. Then the patient is placed in a seated position with the head tilted forward slightly, and 0.2 to 0.4 mL of glycerol is injected. The patient is kept upright for 45 minutes so that the glycerol does not escape rapidly from the trigeminal cistern. The amount of glycerol used determines the extent of the chemical gangliolysis; larger volumes will affect the first division of the nerve and increase the risk of corneal anesthesia and ulceration. In some cases of first division (V1) tic douloureux with a cutaneous trigger zone in the nose or upper cheek, the authors have produced excellent relief of pain with 0.25 mL of glycerol, suggesting that the primary effect was on the second division trigger zone. There was no loss of corneal sensation in those cases.

In our experience, up to 90% of patients with classic trigeminal neuralgia (TN) have either complete relief or marked improvement of their pain after an initial glycerol injection. During the following 18 months, approximately 20% return for a second injection, which is usually also successful. In cases of atypical facial pain, there has been only a 40% success rate but that is true of other neurolytic procedures also because atypical facial pain is generally refractory to many standard medical and surgical treatments.

One third of patients who undergo the procedure notice numbness or mild burning sensations in the cheek or mouth, but objective sensory testing rarely shows frank anesthesia in these areas. Careful testing with a wisp of cotton shows the corneal reflex to be blunted initially in most patients, and lubricant eye drops are prescribed. This improves during the first month in nearly all instances. Occasionally, typical cold sores of herpes simplex appear on the lips, nose, or oral mucosa during the first few days after the glycerol injection. This phenomenon may be seen in any surgical procedure on the trigeminal nerve. It is usually transient and of cosmetic importance only, but the sores can be painful, and the patient should be warned beforehand. The first author has witnessed one instance of herpetic keratitis in the ipsilateral eye that resolved promptly with treatment. No permanent complications were seen. We are not aware of any reported deaths from this procedure but use of glycerol injections has declined over the last decade for treatment of trigeminal nerve or atypical facial pain in patients that are not terminally ill.

Another percutaneous surgical treatment still widely used for medically refractory TN is radiofrequency gangliolysis (RFL) or thermocoagulation of the trigeminal ganglion. The approach is the same as that described for glycerol injection, except that a larger needle is used. The stylet is modified to also serve as a stimulation probe. With the patient moderately sedated using conscious sedation protocol, it is feasible to test before the lesion is made by passing electrical pulses through the probe to stimulate different levels of the ganglion and thereby identify the predominant division of the nerve surrounding the probe tip. The patient then is given a short-acting general anesthetic or induction agents (such as sodium thiopental or diprivan) while the lesion is made by passing radiofrequency current through the probe tip with temperature control. Diprivan is the usual agent used in the Arnold Pain Center because we try to avoid using barbiturates as much as possible for outpatient procedures. The patient is awakened to test for sensory deficit and determine whether the lesion is placed suitably. A typical radiofrequency lesion blunts pinprick but not touch in the region of pain. When the trigger zone for trigeminal neuralgia lies in a different division than the area of pain, it is helpful also to destroy the fibers serving the trigger area. Radiofrequency gangliolysis of the trigeminal ganglion relieves trigeminal neuralgia in 80% to 85% of cases in various published series. In approximately one half of all patients responding to RFL, a second lesion is required after a variable interval of 1 to 5 years; hence supporting the microvascular decompression as a more successful procedure for long-term pain relief. The second lesion is usually as successful as the first when pain returns. The mortality rate is less than 0.5%, and the rare deaths attributed to the procedure may involve misplacement of the probe with intracranial hemorrhage. The procedure itself can be painful if intravenous sedation and analgesia is not effective. There are anecdotal reports of severe arterial hypertension during the procedure with cerebral hemorrhage in elderly patients, emphasizing the need for optimal sedation and analgesia with close hemodynamic monitoring. In our experience, the procedure is not tolerated as well as glycerol injection, perhaps because in the latter, the needle is smaller, and electrical stimulation of the ganglion is not used. Moreover, the thermocoagulation lesion itself is painful; the glycerol injection usually can be done with the patient awake. Repeated positioning of the probe for accurate thermocoagulation requires extra sedation.

More cases of RFL of ganglion have been reported than of glycerol injection over the last two decades, and clinicians disagree over which procedure should be preferred. We like the glycerol technique because it is easier for the patient and it appears to have less risk of permanent facial or corneal anesthesia. We recommend using glycerol injections, particularly in patients with terminal illness and limited life expectancy. In cases of atypical facial pain, neither has the advantage, and we do not recommend microvascular decompression because the risks clearly outweigh the benefits. The percutaneous gangliolysis procedures are preferable for elderly patients or for those who cannot undergo a posterior fossa craniectomy safely. However, the recurrence rate of tic douloureux is signficantly greater, especially after the first year.[14]

Cranial Nerve Rhizotomy

When medication trials, percutaneous procedures, and microvascular decompression are unsuccessful, or when decompression is attempted but no constricting lesion can be found, a partial rhizotomy of the trigeminal root can be done with up to 80% long-term success rate for trigeminal neuralgia. Rhizotomy is believed to have a 1% to 2% mortality rate and 5% to 10% morbidity, but these figures may be overly pessimistic, given that most of the reported series were done several decades ago and the techniques of microsurgery and intraoperative and postoperative monitoring have improved. Some surgeons are reluctant to do trigeminal rhizotomies because they think that the incidence of anesthesia dolorosa is higher than with other procedures. Rhizotomy produces greater loss of facial sensation than gangliolysis or root decompression. Therefore, it is reasonable to ask whether rhizotomy has a higher incidence of severe postoperative pain than other procedures, and if not, whether the reputedly increased risk of anesthesia dolorosa is a reflection of the greater incidence of numbness in the painful area. Probably, most of the patients with this syndrome would fit the diagnostic category of atypical facial pain preoperatively rather than trigeminal neuralgia. To spare the corneal reflex, the surgeon avoids sectioning the most anterior and superior portion of the trigeminal root. Partly for this reason, some of the most refractory cases of facial pain are those involving the eye and supraorbital region.

Rhizotomy of cranial nerves IX and X remains a standard surgical treatment for glossopharyngeal neuralgia. It has a 75% to 80% long-term success rate.[15] The operation is done under general anesthesia using a posterior fossa craniectomy. Cardiovascular instability during the operation and immediately afterward is a well-recognized potential complication. The procedure therefore has a higher risk than trigeminal rhizotomy; the reported mortality rate in several series combined was reported as 5% for 166 cases.[16] Results of microvascular decompression of the lower cranial nerves[17] were not appreciably different from those of rhizotomy in cases of glossopharyngeal neuralgia, but it would seem desirable to preserve cranial nerves IX and X by decompression when a constricting lesion is present.

Spinal Rhizotomy, Ganglionectomy, and Partlal Rhizidiotomy

Pain restricted to the distribution of a few spinal nerve roots sometimes can be treated by dorsal root section or removal of the dorsal root ganglia at levels that encompass the painful area. It is desirable to do this, not only at the corresponding segmental level, but also at one or two segments above and below it as a result of the overlap of dermatomes. Rhizotomy and ganglionectomy have found their greatest use in cases of idiopathic and post-traumatic or postsurgical pain of tbe neck, trunk, and coccygeal region. The technique of selective partial rhizidiotomy attempts to spare proprioception when roots are sectioned at the level of the extremities. The basic difference between these procedures is illustrated in Figure 75-3.

Dorsal rhizotomy is done intradurally at thoracic and cervical levels; at lumbar and sacral levels, there is the option of sectioning the roots in their sheaths without exposing the spinal cord. An advantage of intradural rhizotomy is that the individual rootlets of each dorsal root (which fan out to enter the cord) can be sectioned separately, avoiding any accompanying blood vessels. With magnification, the vessels ean be separated easily and spared. Another advantage is that the ventral roots ean be avoided completely; this is not necessarily the case with extradural rhizotomies.

At thoracic levels, it is feasible to excise the dorsal root ganglia without opening tbe spinal canal. The ganglia lie beneath the most lateral portions of the laminae. Therefore, a small amount of bone removal below the transverse processes will expose them, and there is no need for laminectomies. The theoretic appeal of dorsal root ganglionectomies is that standard dorsal rhizotomy may spare some fine diameter afferent fibers that leave the dorsal root ganglion and reach the cord tbrough the sympathetic chain or the ventral roots. Although there is no anatomic proof of the existence of such afferents in humans, Hosobuchi[18] presented several cases in which dorsal rhizotomy failed but subsequent ganglionectomies succeeded in relieving truncal pain. Multiple spinal rhizotomy or dorsal root ganglionectomy has a 65% success rate in relieving pain of benign origin at thoracic levels. Reported cases include post-thoracotomy and post-traumatic intercostal neuralgia and similar idiopathic cases. The first author has done multiple thoracic dorsal root ganglionectomies in three cases of intercostal neuralgia with satisfactory long-term pain relief. In all three patients, cutaneous hypersensitivity was noticed at the upper and lower margins of the anesthetic zone, and in one, this was disturbing enough to require repeated spinal nerve blocks at the level of dysesthesia.

Intradural dorsal rhizotomy at the C1 to C3 levels provides satisfactory long-term relief of occipital neuralgia in 70% of cases, according to a large number of reported series. The first author's experience shows the procedure to be highly effective for neuralgias associated with severe arthritis or arthrosis of the C1-2 or C2-3 facet joints that impinge on the upper cervical roots as they form the greater occipital nerve. It also has been effective in post-traumatic occipital neuralgia usually resulting from severe whiplash injury. We recommend trying local anesthetic and steroid injections prior to surgical intervention since some patients may get lasting benefit from the injection therapy and may not need surgery. Surgery causes complete anesthesia in the back of the scalp, but these

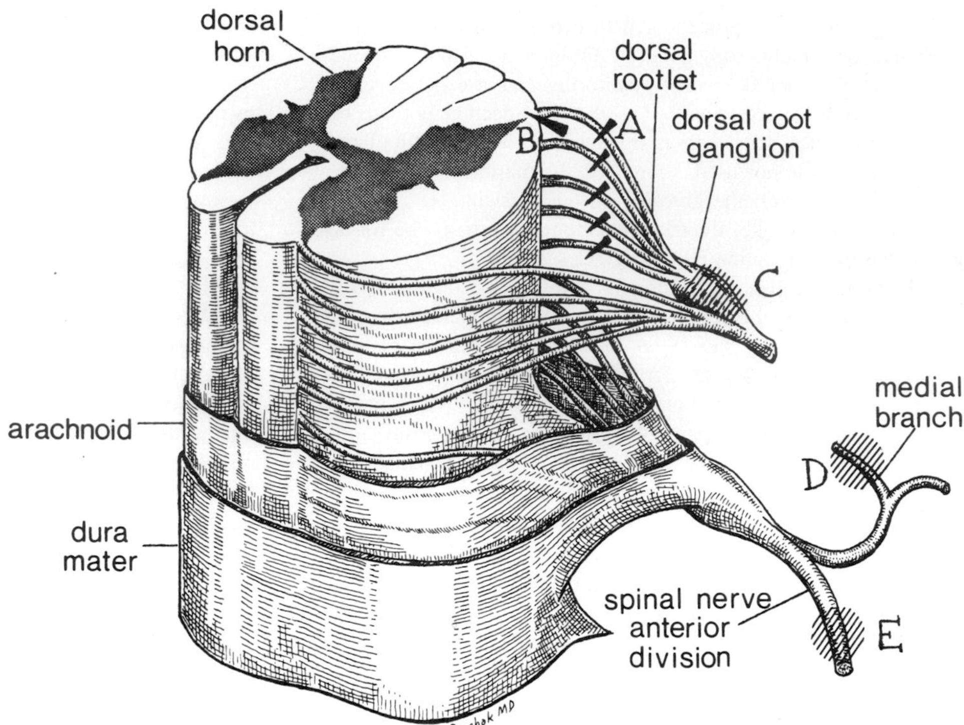

Figure 75–3 Surgical procedures at the nerve root and spinal nerve level. (**A**) Intradural dorsal rhizotomy, (**B**) selective posterior rhizidiotomy, (**C**) dorsal root ganglionectomy, (**D**) medial branch coagulation ("facet rhizolysis"), and (**E**) coagulation of spinal nerve. (Illustration by Stephen Ponchak, MD.)

patients usually are gratified by the relief of their medically refractory neuralgic pain and do not appear to be bothered by the loss of sensation.

Rhizotomy of the third sacral through coccygeal dorsal roots provided long-term relief of coccygodynia in 63% of 48 cases reported in the neurosurgical literature.[19] Sacral rhizotomy may be useful for pain caused by malignancies of the pelvis and perineal region by contrast with the relatively poor long-term success rate for pain from malignancy in the trunk, extremities, head, and neck. Dorsal rhizotomy has not been successful for treating sciatica after failed lumbar disk surgery. In 10 cases, there was a 90% long-term failure rate with the development of persistent burning or freezing dysesthesias during tbe subsequent 5 years.[5] These dysesthesias also are frequent after dorsal root ganglionectomy at single lumbar or sacral levels.

A microsurgical technique that spares some of the large diameter proprioceptive afferents in individual dorsal rootlets is known as selective posterior rhizidiotomy.[20] Because the small diameter afferent fibers tend to aggregate laterally at the root entry zone and the large fibers tend medially toward the dorsal column, it is feasible to section only the lateral portion of each rootlet. In this way, proprioception in the arm or leg can be saved. This is not the case with complete dorsal rhizotomies at the brachial and lumbosacral plexus levels. This procedure has been used successfully to treat pain of lung apex malignancies compressing or encasing cervical roots of parts of the brachial plexus.

Percutaneous radiofrequency lesioning of spinal nerves is not as selective as intradural root surgery, but it has the advantage of safety in debilitated patients, particularly those with advanced cancer. Initial rates of pain relief are 40% to 65%. The long-term success of percutaneous neurotomy is seldom discussed, but this may not be important for patients whose life expectancy is limited. Fairly heavy sedation may be required for percutaneous nerve lesions. In some cases, therefore, an alternative procedure done under general endotracheal anesthesia might have less risk of respiratory complication.

Leslons of the Spinal Cord

Open Cordotomy This category includes some surgical procedures in which a lesion is made using radiofrequency current and others in which a white matter tract is sectioned directly with a microsurgical blade (Fig. 75-4).

All have in common the goal of disrupting the neural transmission of nociceptive information from the cord or medulla to the upper brainstem and thalamus. In most instances, the limiting factor will be the proximity of descending pathways of motor control.

The prototypical procedure is anterolateral cordotomy, in which the white matter of the cord is sectioned to eliminate a large part of the ascending spinothalamic projection. Open cordotomy usually is done at the T2 or T3 level, just below the portion of the spinal cord contributing to the brachial plexus. The spinal cord is exposed by laminectomies and aural incision under general anesthesia. The dentate ligaments are identified on the lateral aspect of the cord. One of them may be sectioned to rotate the cord slightly, exposing the anterior aspect. The pial surface is cauterized lightly with fine microsurgical bipolar cautery forceps, and a small blade is inserted anterior to the dentate ligament to section the anterolateral quadrant of the cord. Bleeding usually is minimal with this procedure, and it can be stopped easily with hemostatic pledgets and microsurgical cautery.

An open T2-3 cordotomy of this sort is expected to produce a level of insensitivity to pinprick and other painful stimuli somewhere on the trunk. The level of analgesia is never as high as T2 because the ascending spinothalamic fibers gradually cross over the midline of the cord for a distance of several segments. Those from the T2-5 segments, perhaps more, have not reached the opposite anterolateral quadrant, and therefore they are not included

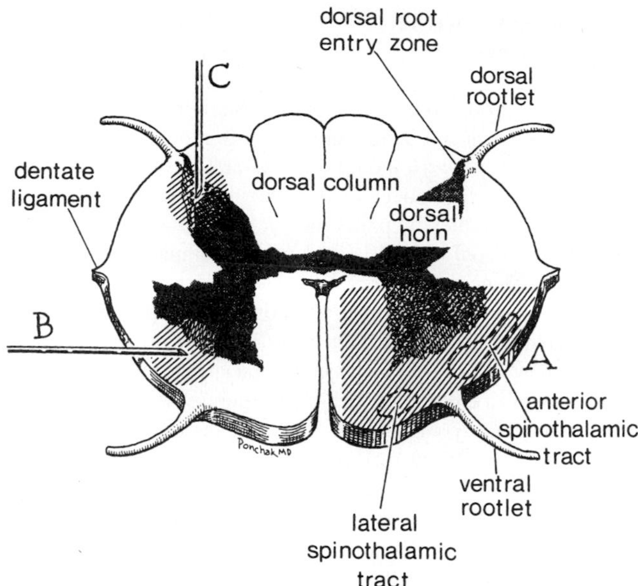

Figure 75–4 Surgical procedures at the spinal cord level. (**A**) Open anterolateral cordotomy, (**B**) percutaneous radiofrequency cordotomy, and (**C**) dorsal root entry zone {DREZ) lesion. (Illustration by Stephen Ponchak, MD.)

in the lesion. The actual level of insensitivity varies from approximately T4 to T10 level.[21] It is higher when the lesion is extended toward the midline of the cord (see Fig. 75-4). Some spinothalamic and spinoreticular tract fibers lie in the anteromedial white matter near the ventral sulcus of the cord. The anterior spinal artery is found in this sulcus and must be avoided.

Cordotomy can be a highly effective treatment for the pain of cancer in the trunk or legs.[22] The procedure can be done bilaterally, with greater risk of disrupting bowel and bladder control. The best indication for cordotomy is intractable cancer pain in one leg or one side of the pelvis. The major disadvantage of cordotomy is the tendency for pain to recur months or years later. The initial success rate in patients with cancer, that is, the chance of complete relief or mild residual pain relieved by oral medications, varies from 85% to 95% in different published series; mortality rates in recent series range from 0% to 7.5%. In patients with severe pain not caused by cancer, initial success rates were similar. Conditions amenable to cordotomy include tabes dorsalis, spinal cord and cauda equine injuries, and phantom limb pain. In all diagnostic groups, there is a disturbingly high late recurrence rate that limits long-term success to only 25% to 70%. Some recurrences are seen during the first 12 months after the procedure. It has not been possible to predict which patients are susceptible to late failure, more than 18 months, after cordotomy. Other complications of open cordotomy include weakness or paralysis of the legs, usually transient (in 3% to 15% of unilateral procedures), and persistent urinary bladder dysfunction in 2% to 10%. Fecal incontinence and impotence are also possible but the incidence is usually lower than the bladder dysfunction. The incidence of any of these complications more than doubles after bilateral cordotomies compared to the unilateral procedure. Laboratory investigations suggest several reasons why cordotomy might fail. The spinoreticular tracts and, to a lesser extent, the spinothalamic tracts are crossed only partially in primate species. Moreover, there are ascending sensory pathways in the dorsal half of the cord white matter that could assume a more significant role in nociception after disruption of the ventral tracts. Finally, the late effects of central deafferentation are not known completely, and it is tempting to speculate that some late recurrences of pain after cordotomy may be a result of the development of ectopic neuronal discharges in brainstem and thalamic neurons.

Percutaneous Upper Cervical Cordotomy A lesion similar in location, if not in extent, can be created by radiofrequency thermocoagulation of the anterolateral quadrant of the cord, using a small probe inserted through a spinal needle (see Fig. 75-4). The needle insertion is done using fluoroscopic control and an emulsion of radiographic contrast to outline the dentate ligament. Local anesthetic is injected just behind and below the mastoid process for a straight lateral approach to the cord. Electrical stimulation through the probe is used to elicit paresthesias from the ventral cord white matter to estimate the depth of insertion of the probe tip. Lesions near the cord surface just in front of the dentate ligament tend to produce analgesia in the trunk; deeper lesions affect the sacral region and leg. The patient is sedated heavily with a short-acting intravenous agent (such as methohexital or midazolam) supplemented by a narcotic while the radiofrequency lesion is made. It is feasible to do this procedure in the radiology department if equipment for induction and monitoring of general anesthesia is available. The patient is awakened to determine the extent of sensory deficit, and if necessary, the lesion may be enlarged.

The success rate of percutaneous cordotomy (as reported in several large series) was similar to that of open cordotomy with fewer complications. The percutaneous technique is valuable in debilitated patients. One drawback is the surgeon's inability to be certain of the extent of the lesion. Because there is ample evidence that the ascending sensory pathways relevant to pain are widespread in the cord and the spinothalamic tract itself is diffuse, it may be worthwhile to do an open cordotomy when the patient's general health permits and the life expectancy is long enough to make the surgical procedure and subsequent postoperative hospitalization baneficial. Of course, some patients with cancer are too ill to undergo general anesthesia for an open cordotomy, and the percutaneous procedure then may be appropriate. In many cases of this type, however, alternatives (such as an epidural morphine delivery system or continuous intravenous narcotic infusion) might be simpler.

Percutaneous cordotomy at the C1 to C2 level carries a risk of causing respiratory insufficiency from interference with the spinal axons of the respiratory neurons. The risk definitely increases with bilateral cordotomy at this level, after which there is approximately a 4% to 8% incidence of sudden respiratory arrest. This typically occurs at night when the patient is asleep. Poor performance on preoperative pulmonary function tests should be considered a relative contraindication to unilateral high cervical cordotomy and an absolute contraindication to bilateral C1 to C cordotomy.

Dorsal Root Entry Zone Lesions The technique of radiofrequency lesioning of the dorsal root entry zone was devised by Nashold. A series of small heat lesions, 2 to 3 mm apart, is created along the line of entry of dorsal rootlets in the segments corresponding to the area of pain and in adjacent segments above and below it. The lesions are made with radiofrequency current passed through a small insulated electrode at a depth of 2 mm; they should be centered in the superficial layers of the dorsal horn (see Fig. 75-4).

This procedure has been used to treat pain caused by avulsion of the brachial plexus, pain in paraplegic patients at or below the level of cord injury,[23] postherpetic neuralgia, and various other localized conditions. Nashold and Ostdahl[24] and Thomas and Jones[25] reported that approximately two thirds of patients with pain from brachial plexus avulsion had significant relief after this procedure. For pain from cord injuries or postherpetic neuralgia, the success rate is slightly less.[26,27] Complications of this operation include mild or moderate lower limb weakness, loss of proprioception in the ipsilateral leg, numbness, and paresthesias.[28] These have been reduced substantially by the use of temperature monitoring at the lesioning electrode tip using a thermocouple.

Stereotactic Lesions

With a stereotactic instrument and appropriate radiologic techniques, it is possible to place the tip of a lesioning probe in various nuclei of the thalamus and hypothalamus or in the ascending sensory tracts of the pons and midbrain. Lesions of the ventral and medial thalamus, hypothalamus, and spinothalamic or spinoreticular tracts in the brainstem disrupt ascending connections. Another variety of lesion has the rationale of blunting the patient's affective response to pain. Lesions of the frontal lobe white matter, cingulum,[30] and dorsomedial and anterior thalamus are included in this group. The latter has been termed *psychosurgery* and is practiced infrequently.

Stereotactic lesioning procedures provide an alternative to cordotomy for pain at cervical levels or in the midline of the trunk where bilateral high cervical cordotomy might be ineffective or dangerous because of its risk of respiratory complications. Currently, destructive stereotactic procedures are used less often, partly as a result of newer techniques (such as periventricular gray stimulation and implanted morphine infusion pumps). One advantage of stereotactic lesions is that they may be effective in cases of deafferentation pain where no good alternative exists. Stereotactic mesencephalic tractotomy is said to relieve deafferentation pain in 40% to 50% of cases and other types of severe chronic pain in 60% to 70% of cases.[30,31]

A typical stereotactic destructive procedure for pain relief begins by mounting the stereotactic frame on the skull, using a local anesthetic at pin insertion sites. Then a ventriculogram, and perhaps also a CT scan or magnetic resonance imaging scan of the brain, is obtained with the frame in place to locate necessary landmarks in the brain (such as the anterior and posterior commissures of the third ventricle). From these landmarks, target coordinates can be given on the frame axes for deep brain structures around the thalamus, upper brainstem, and third ventricle. Coordinates are calculated from maps of the brain in standard atlases, and adjusted according to the dimensions of the patient's brain landmarks. Lesioning of the chosen target is done with a probe inserted to reach the structure through a burr hole in the skull. If a ventriculogram was done for localization, it may be convenient to use the same burr hole. Further localization of the target can be achieved by trials of brief electrical stimulation through the probe tip and recording the patient's subjective responses and any movements produced. To do this requires the patient's attention and cooperation for some time; therefore, heavy sedation would be inappropriate. A lesion is made with radiofrequency electrical current or other means.

Stereotactic radiosurgery has been successfully tried on patients with medically refractory trigeminal neuralgia (TN). Kondziolka et al,[32] independently acquired data from 220 patients with idiopathic TN that had gamma knife radiosurgery where most patients had features of typical TN, although 16 (7.3%) described additional atypical features. One hundred thirty-five patients (61.4%) had prior surgery and patients were followed to a maximum of 6.5 years (median, 2 years). Complete or partial pain relief was achieved in 85.6% of patients at 1 year. Complete pain relief was achieved in 64.9 % of patients at 6 months, 70.3% at 1 year, and 75.4% patients at 33 months. Patients with an atypical pain component had a lower rate of achieving pain relief (P = .025). At 5 years, due to recurrence rate, only 55.8% of patients had complete or partial pain relief. The absence of preoperative sensory disturbance or prior surgery correlated with an increased proportion of patients in complete or partial pain relief over time. Ten percent of patients developed new or increased subjective facial paresthesia or facial numbness. In an other study, Brimman[33] purposes that gamma knife radiosurgery (GKS) has higher success as the primary rather than secondary management for trigeminal neuralgia. In this study 82 patients underwent GKS as their first neurosurgical intervention (group A), and 90 patients underwent GKS following a different procedure (group B). Six-month follow-up was available for 126 patients and 12-month follow up for 84 patients. Excellent (no pain and no medicine) or good (at least 50% reduction in pain and less medicine) relief was more likely to occur in group A than in group B patients 6 and 12 months following GKS for trigeminal neuralgia (P = .058). Excellent or good results were also more likely in patients with trigeminal neuralgia without multiple sclerosis (P = .042). He concluded that patients with trigeminal neuralgia who are treated with GKS as primary management have better pain relief than those treated with GKS as secondary management. Patients are more likely to have pain relief if they do not have multiple sclerosis. A study done in the Czech Republic[34] evaluated 6 men and 10 women were treated for postherpetic TN that were refractory to conservative treatment. The radiation was focused on the root of the trigeminal nerve in the vicinity of the brainstem and the median follow up was 33 months (range 8 to 34 months). The patients were divided into five groups according to degree of pain relief after treatment. A successful result (excellent, very good, and good) was reached in seven (44%) patients and radiosurgery failed in nine (56%). Pain relief occurred after a median interval of 1 month (range 10 days to 6 months). These results suggest that GKS for postherpetic TN is an other option that is safe and can be used in patients who are medically complicated.

Complications of stereotactic lesioning depend on the target, but in general, they include confusion, dysesthesias, eye movement disorders, psychic changes, and infrequent hemorrhages. There is an overall morbidity rate of approximately 10% to 40% and a mortality rate of 3% to 10%. In considering these figures, it is wise to remember that these operations usually are done as a last resort when all other treatments fail.

Sympathectomy

Procedures that interrupt the afferent and efferent axons of the sympathetic nervous system are useful for treating pain of peripheral nerve injury when causalgia or painful reflex sympathetic dystrophy is present. Recent physiologic studies of nerve injury and neuroma formation suggest that the sympathetic outflow to the damaged nerve is a factor that produces or aggravates pain, perhaps by augmenting the ectopic discharges that originate peripherally. Sympathectomy occasionally is used for painful conditions of the extremities resembling causalgia but not due to nerve trauma, if temporary sympathetic blocks repeatedly give relief. Sympathectomy has been combined with splanchnicectomy to treat pain caused by cancer of the pancreas or other upper abdominal viscera.[35]

Open sympathectomy to treat arm pain is done at the upper thoracic level. We prefer a posterior approach with removal of the head of the second rib and the corresponding transverse process; two ganglia are excised from the thoracic sympathetic chain and the caudal third of the stellate ganglion. When a true stellate ganglion does not exist, the highest thoracic ganglion is removed instead. The chain also can be approached through the axilla.[36] A percutaneous technique of radiofrequency lesions of the sympathetic chain is described by Wilkinson[37] and may be done bilaterally. Upper thoracic sympathectomy by any approach has a 70% to 75% chance of relieving arm pain resulting from causalgia or vascular disease initially. Late recurrences are not uncommon, and postoperative hyperesthesia and Homer syndrome are potential complications.

Sympathectomy for leg pain is done by an abdominal approach familiar to most vascular surgeons; the lumbar sympathetic chain is exposed and sectioned anterolateral to the vertebral prominence. Chemical lumbar sympathectomy with phenol injection is a suitable alternative.[38] This is done by lumbar paravertebral block. The use of lumbar sympathectomy for leg pain caused by vascular claudication or ischemic rest pain, causalgia, and reflex sympathetic dystrophy has an initial success rate of approximately 65% to 70%; late failures are common, possibly after progressive development of hypersensitivity to circulating catecholamines. The mortality rate for open lumbar sympathectomy is approximately 1% to 5%. Syndromes of local pain after interruption of the sympathetic nerves are described. These usually occur 7 to 12 days after the operation or injury and may be as unpleasant as the preoperative pain. Postsympathectomy neuralgia typically is felt in the anterior thighs. Sometimes, it can be relieved with carbamazepine or phenytoin.[39] Fortunately, it often remits spontaneously after several weeks or a few months.

Anterior Pituitary Ablation

Operations to ablate or destroy the anterior lobe of the pituitary gland originated from endocrine studies, suggesting that some breast and prostate carcinoma metastases may regress after oophorectomy or adrenalectomy. In many instances, there was corresponding relief of pain, which was attributed to a decrease of local pressure and swelling around the metastases, particularly in bone. More recently, as safer, simpler techniques of pituitary ablation were developed, it became clear that many patients reported pain relief almost immediately after the operation, sometimes within 30 minutes. This phenomenon, therefore, could not be explained in terms of tumor regression. There is no satisfactory explanation. One hypothesis states that an unidentified hormonal factor produced by the hypophysis or hypothalamus is disrupted by the procedure. The finding of a large concentration of β-endorphin in the pituitary aroused some interest in this regard, but circulating levels of the peptide did not correlate with pain relief. It appears that neither the extent of the anterior hypophysectomy, the extent of concomitant ventral hypothalamic damage; nor the extent of tumor regression correlates with the degree of immediate pain relief.[40]

Several techniques of pituitary destruction are available. The procedure most certain to ensure selective ablation of the adenohypophysis while sparing the neurohypophysis is transsphenoidal microsurgery.[41] Despite the extremely low morbidity and mortality of this operation in experienced hands and the quick postoperative recovery without disfigurement, patients with advanced malignancy seldom undergo the operation. The emotional barrier to surgery under general anesthesia may be related to the patient's fear of impending death from the underlying disease. Patients with cancer seem more willing to accept the idea of pituitary ablation if it is presented as a simple procedure to relieve pain rather than a major operation. Zervas[41] devised the stereotactic technique of radiofrequency thermocoagulation of the pituitary using a probe inserted through the spheroid sinus. Moricca[43] and others reported a large clinical experience with the injection of alcohol into the pituitary through a cannula inserted by the spheroidal approach. Freezing lesions also have been used. Each approach has a high rate of success and a small, but not insignificant, risk of CSF leak, meningitis, hemorrhage, hypothalamic injury, and death. Pituitary insufficiency after closed ablative procedures (such as alcohol injection) is not inevitable. In many cases, relatively normal corticotropin levels and modest thyroid-stimulating hormone levels can be maintained. Pituitary ablation is used most commonly for the pain of prostate and breast cancer, but there is good evidence that many kinds of malignancy may respond.[44] The idea that only bone metastases can be treated in this way is probably incorrect; pain due to soft tissue metastases also may subside. Published series indicate that 60% to 70% of patients have partial or complete relief of pain initially, but the long-term benefits are less. Several months of improvement are seen in most patients with cancer pain. Pituitary ablation has not been shown to increase survival, nor is it useful for pain not caused by cancer.

IMPLANTED DEVICES FOR STIMULATION

This category of neurosurgical procedures includes two devices: spinal cord stimulation units[45] and deep brain stimulation units.[46] Stimulation of the spinal cord to control pain was initially based mainly on the concept of a gate control mechanism in the dorsal horn that could be activated by stimulation of large diameter, afferent fibers in the dorsal columns of the spinal cord, but the precise mechanism of analgesia is not completely understood and is thought to be multifactorial. Electrical stimulation of the periventricular gray matter of the uppermost brainstem is thought to activate a descending analgesic/inhibitory system of neural connections that reaches the dorsal horn of the spinal cord.[47] In laboratory animals, stimulation of the central gray region causes profound analgesia by various tests.

Spinal Cord Stimulation

Electrical stimulation of the spinal cord through implanted electrodes in the epidural space or on the cord surface may provide relief of pain.[48] The precise mechanism of action of spinal cord stimulation is not known. Dorsal electrode placements probably produce volleys of afferent impulses in the dorsal columns, with effects in the dorsal horn or possibly in the brainstem.

Stimulating electrodes can be implanted temporarily by percutaneous techniques.[49] Then, if trials of cord stimulation are successful, a permanent system is installed, including a subcutaneous receiver or battery-powered pulse generator. Paresthesias should be felt in the area of pain, indicating activation of large diameter afferents in the appropriate spinal segments. Unfortunately, despite initial indications of a good result, there is considerable risk of late failure of spinal cord stimulation units. In a series of 70 such units followed for 10 years, Erickson and Long[50] reported a 95% long-term failure rate. Reasons for failure include migration or breakage of the electrodes, epidural scar formation, infection, and tolerance to the stimulation that may develop for unknown reasons even when the unit appears intact and functional. Intradural electrode placements have additional risks of cord compression and cerebrospinal fluid leakage, and therefore should be avoided.

Tasker[51] used spinal cord stimulation successfully to treat deafferentation pain syndromes and considered it to be the initial treatment of choice for this type of pain despite the late failure rate. Few effective options are available to patients in this group; therefore, improvement for 1 or 2 years might be a welcome respite.

Periventricular Gray, Internal Capsule, and Thalamic Stimulation

Electrical stimulation of deep brain structures is done by means of stereotactically implanted electrodes connected to a subcutaneous receiver or pulse generator. Stimulation in the somatosensory portion of the thalamus, in the posterior limb of the internal capsule, or medial lemniscus can be effective in suppressing deafferentation pain. Stimulation more medially in the central gray matter lining the posterior third ventricle and rostral portion of the aqueduct may activate a descending analgesia-producing system. It is useful for a wider variety of chronic pains. Opinions are divided over the long-term efficacy of central gray stimulation, and it appears that success rates initially vary from 50% to 80%. Good results in approximately 55% of patients with cancer with relatively long survivals were reported by Meyerson and colleagues.[52]

Significant relief of various types of chronic pain of peripheral origin not caused by cancer were reported in 70% to 80% of patients, including those with previously refractory low back pain after failed disk surgery.[53,54] Postherpetic facial pain can be relieved by thalamic stimulation in many cases.[55] Pain of thalamic syndrome is said to be relieved in approximately 50% of patients with stimulation near the border of the internal capsule.[56] Amputation stump pain and phantom limb pain respond favorably in more than 90% of cases.[57]

Accurate placement of deep brain–stimulating electrodes requires not only radiologic techniques but also physiologic mapping at the time of surgery. The initial phase of the stereotactic procedure consists of mounting the stereotactic frame on the patient's head. Then, deep brain landmarks are related to frame coordinates by ventriculography and CT scanning. When three-dimensional target coordinates have been calculated, the instrument is used to introduce one or more electrodes. Final targets are chosen after trials of stimulation at different depths. The author has found it useful to do stimulation trials with a probe from the tip of which a stimulating electrode emerges in a curved path. In this way, by retracting the electrode tip and rotating the probe, an area of several cubic centimeters can be explored to find an optimal site that reduces the patient's pain with minimal side effects. Periventricular electrode placements are limited by ocular side effects when the electrode tip is driven ventrally toward the midbrain. Lateral placements near the internal capsule may produce bodily movements and paresthesias.

Potential complications of deep brain stimulation include infection of the electrodes, cerebral hemorrhage, abnormal eye movements induced by stimulation, and unpleasant dysesthesias. Overall, the morbidity rate is 5% to 10%, and the mortality rate is <1%. There are recent anecdotal reports of use of vagal nerve stimulation and cortical stimulation for pain control in patients unresponsive to standard medical, anesthetic, neurolytic, and other surgical interventions.

SUMMARY

The neurosurgical approaches to the management of chronic pain are many and varied. Most commonly, they are used only after more conservative measures fail. In the past, these techniques were used only as a last resort because of a fear of untoward neurologic sequelae, but improvements in our understanding of the pathophysiology of pain and in the neurosurgical techniques themselves have resulted in a high rate of success and a low incidence of complications.

REFERENCES

1. Williams PH, Trzil KP. Management of meralgia paresthetica. *J Neurosurg* 1991;74:76–80.
2. Hitselberger WE, Witten RM. Abnormal myelograms in asymptomatic patients. *J Neurosurg* 1968;28:204–206.
3. Kuschner SH, Brien WW, Johnson D, Gellman H. Complications associated with carpal tunnel release. *Orthop Rev* 1991;20:346–352.
4. Spangfort EV. The lumbar disc herniation. *Acta Orthop Scand Suppl* 1972;142:1–95.
5. Bertrand G. The 'battered' root problem. *Orthop Clin North Am* 1975;6:305–309.
6. Auld AW. Chronic spinal arachnoiditis. A postoperative syndrome that may signal its onset. *Spine* 1978;3:88–91.
7. Jannetta P. Observations on the etiology of trigeminal neuralgia, hemifacial spasm, acoustic nerve dysfunction and glossopharyngeal neuralgia. *Neurochirurgia* 1977;20:145–154.
8. Baker FG, Jannett PJ, et al. The long-term outcome of microvascular decompression for trigeminal neuralgia. *N Engl J Med* 1996;334:1077–1084.
9. Battista AD, Cravioto H, Budsilovich GN. Painful neuroma: changes produced in peripheral nerve after fascicle ligation. *Neurosurgery* 1981;9:589–600.
10. Noordenbos W, Wall PD. Implications of the failure of nerve resection and graft to cure chronic pain produced by nerve lesions. *J Neurol Neurosurg Psychiatry* 1981;44:1068–1073.
11. Hakanson S. Retrogasserian glycerol injection as a treatment of tic douloureux. In: Bonica JJ, Lindblom U, Iggo A, et al, eds. *Advances in Pain Research and Therapy*. Vol 5. New York, NY: Raven Press, 1983:927–933.
12. Sweet WH, Poletti CE. Retrogasserian glycerol injection as treatment for trigeminal neuralgia. In: Sweet WH, Schmidek HH, eds. *Operative Neurosurgical Techniques*. New York, NY: Grune & Stratton, 1982:1107–1117.
13. Fujimaki T, Fukushima T, Miyazaki S. Percutaneous retrogasseriam glycerol injection in the management of trigeminal neuralgia: long-term follow-up results. *J Neurosurg* 1990;73:212–216.
14. Burchiel KJ, Steege TD, Howe JF, Loeser JD. Comparison of percutaneous radiofrequency gangliolysis and microvascular decompression for the surgical management of tic douloureux. *Neurosurgery* 1981;9:111–119.
15. Rushton JG, Stevens JC, Miller RH. Glossopharyngeal (vagoglossopharyngeal) neuralgia. *Arch Neurol* 1981;38:201–205.
16. Dubuisson D. Root surgery. In: Wall PD, Melzack R, eds. *Textbook of Pain*. London, England: Churchill-Livingstone, 1984:590–600.
17. Laha RK, Jannetta PJ. Glossopharyngeal neuralgia. *J Neurosurg* 1977;47:316–320.
18. Hosobuchi Y. The majority of unmyelinated axons in human ventral rootless probably conduct pain. *Pain* 1980;8:167–180.

19. Albrektsson B. Sacral rhizotomy in cases of anococcygeal pain. *Acta Orthop Scand* 1981;52:157–190.
20. Sindou M, Fischer G, Mansuy L. Posterior spinal rhizotomy and selective posterior rhizidiotomy. *Prog Neurol Surg* 1976;7:201–250.
21. White JC, Sweet WH. *Pain and the Neurosurgeon*. Springfield, Ill: Charles C. Thomas; 1969.
22. Sundaresan N, DiGiacinto GV, Hughes JE. Neurosurgery in the treatment of cancer pain. *Cancer* 1989;63(suppl 11):2365–2377.
23. Sindou M, Jeanmonod D. Microsurgical DREZ-otomy for the treatment of spasticity and pain in the lower limbs. *Neurosurgery* 1989;24: 655–670.
24. Nashold BS, Ostdahl RH. Dorsal root entry zone lesions for pain relief. *J Neurosurg* 1979;51:59–69.
25. Thomas DGT, Jones SJ. Dorsal root entry zone lesions (Nashold's procedure) in brachial plexus avulsion. *Neurosurgery* 1984;15:966–967.
26. Nashold BS, Bullitt E. Dorsal root entry zone lesions to control central pain in paraplegics. *J Neurosurg* 1981;55:414–419.
27. Friedman AH, Nashold BS. Dorsal root entry zone lesions for the treatment of postherpetic neuralgia. *Neurosurgery* 1984;15:969–970.
28. Jeanmonod D, Sindou M. Somatosensory function following dorsal root entry zone lesions in patients with neurogenic pain or spasticity. *J Neurosurg* 1991;74:916–932.
29. Hassenbusch SJ, Pillay PK, Barnett GH. Radiofrequency cingulotomy for intractable cancer pain using stereotaxis guided by magnetic resonance imaging. *Neurosurgery* 1990;27:220–223.
30. Nashold BS. Brainstem stereotaxic procedures. In: Schaltenbrand G, Walker AK, (eds.). *Stereotaxy of the Human Brain*. Stuttgart, Germany: Thieme, 1982:475–483.
31. Tasker RR. Thalamic stereotaxic procedures. In: Schaltenbrand G, Walker AK, eds. *Stereotaxy of the Human Brain*. Stuttgart, Germany: Thieme, 1982:484–497.
32. Kondziolka D, Lundsford LD, Flickinger JC. Stereotactic radiosurgery for the treatment of trigeminal neuralgia. *Clin J Pain* 2002;18:42–47.
33. Brisman R. Gamma knife radiosurgery for primary management for trigeminal neuralgia. *J Neurosurg* 2000;93(suppl 3):159–161.
34. Urgosik D, Vymazal J, Vladyka V, Liscak R. Treatment of postherpetic trigeminal neuralgia with the gamma knife. *J Neurosurg* 2000;93 (suppl 3):165–168.
35. Hardy RW. Surgery of the sympathetic nervous system. In: Sweet WH, Schmidek HH, (eds.). *Operative Neurosurgical Techniques*. New York, NY: Grune & Stratton, 1982:1045–1061.
36. Berguer R, Smit R. Transaxillary sympathectomy (T2 to T4) for relief of vasospastic/sympathetic pain of upper extremities. *Surgery* 1981; 89:764–769.
37. Wilkinson HA. Percutaneous radiofrequency upper thoracic sympathectomy: a new technique. *Neurosurgery* 1984;15:811–814.
38. Cross FW, Cotton LT. Chemical lumbar sympathectomy for ischemic rest pain: a randomized, prospective controlled clinical trial. *Am J Surg* 1985;150:341–345.
39. Raskin NH, Levinson SA, Hoffman PM, et al. Postsympathectomy neuralgia: amelioration with diphenylhydantoin and carbamazepine. *Am J Surg* 1974;128:75–78.
40. Miles J. Pituitary destruction. In: Wall PD, Melzack R, eds. *Textbook of Pain*. London, England: Churchill Livingstone, 1984:656–665.
41. Hardy J. Transsphenoidal hypophysectomy. *J Neurosurg* 1971;34:582–594.
42. Zervas N. Stereotactic, radiofrequency surgery of the normal and the abnormal pituitary gland. *N Engl J Med* 1969;280:429–437.
43. Moricca G. Chemical hypophysectomy for cancer pain. In: Bonica JJ, ed. *Advances in Neurology*. Vol 4. New York, NY: Raven Press, 1974: 707–714.
44. Tindall GT, Nixon DW, Christy JH, Neill JD. Pain relief in metastatic cancer other than breast and prostrate gland following transsphenoidal hypophysectomy. *J Neurosurg* 1977;50:275–282.
45. Spiegelmann R, Friedman WA. Spinal cord stimulation: a contemporary series. *Neurosurgery* 1991;28:6570; discussion 70–71.
46. Kumar K, Wyant GM, Nath R. Deep brain stimulation for control of intractable pain in humans, present and future: a ten-year follow-up. *Neurosurgery* 1990;26:774–781; discussion 781–782.
47. Robaina FJ, Dominiguez M, Diaz M, et al. Spinal cord stimulation for relief of chronic pain in vasospastic disorders of the upper limbs. *Neurosurgery* 1989;24:63–67.
48. Shealy CN, Mortimer JT, Resnick J. Electrical inhibition of pain by stimulation of the dorsal column: preliminary clinical reports. *Anesth Analg* 1967;46:489–491.
49. Erickson DL. Percutaneous trial of stimulation for patient selection for implantable stimulating devices. *J Neurosurg* 1975;43:440–444.
50. Erickson DL, Long DM. Ten-year follow-up of dorsal column stimulation. In: Bonica JJ, Lindblom U, Iggo A, et al, eds. *Advances in Pain Research and Therapy*. Vol 5. New York, NY: Raven Press, 1983: 583–589.
51. Tasker RR. Surgical approaches to the primary afferent and the spinal cord. In: Bonica JJ, Lindblom U, Iggo A, et al, eds. *Advances in Pain Research and Therapy*. Vol 5. New York, NY: Raven Press, 1985:799–824.
52. Meyerson BA, Boethius J, Carlsson AM. Percutaneous central grey stimulation for cancer pain. *Appl Neurophysiol* 1979;41:57–65.
53. Hosubuchi Y. The current status of analgesic brain stimulation. *Acta Neurochir Suppl (Wien)* 1980;30:219–227.
54. Plotkin R. Results in 60 cases of deep brain stimulation for chronic intractable pain. *Appl Neurophysiol* 1982;45:173–178.
55. Siegfried J. Monopolar electrical stimulation of nucleus ventroposterior medialis thalami for postherpetic facial pain. *Appl Neurophysiol* 1982;45:179–184.
56. Hosubuchi Y. Subcortical electrical stimulation for control of intractable pain in humans. *J Neurosurg* 1986;64:543–553.
57. Turnbull IM. Brain stimulation. In: Wall PD, Melzack R, eds. *Textbook of Pain*. London, England: Churchill Livingstone; 1984:706–714.

CHAPTER 76 RADIATION SAFETY FOR THE PAIN SPECIALIST

Howard S. Smith and Scott M. Fishman

INTRODUCTION

Pain management specialists who perform injections with the assistance of fluoroscopy must have a basic knowledge of radiation effects and safety. Although a complete review of this topic is beyond the scope of this chapter, the following outlines some of the most important details of working in an x-ray environment. These include basic principles of radioactivity, potential adverse effects to patients and physicians, and preventive measures for maintaining effective radiation safety.

RADIATION FUNDAMENTALS

Radiation is the process by which energy in the form of waves or particles is emitted from a source. Electromagnetic radiation (EMR) has no mass and no charge. Common types of EMR include: gamma rays, x-rays, ultraviolet visible light, infrared, radar, microwaves, and radio waves. This list is in increasing order of increasing wavelength.

X-rays are one of the most common potential radiation hazards in health care. The hazard is mainly due to potential harmful biological effects resulting from x-rays passing through matter with enough energy to remove electrons (ionizing radiation) from atoms, which can result in ionized atoms and free radicals (atoms with an unpaired electron in the outer shell). This risk of biological damage from radiation exposure can exist even with low doses. Biological effects of radiation exposure depend on two major factors: dose and duration. The greater the exposure, the greater the risk.

Radiation is both naturally occurring and man-made. It occurs all around us and cannot be completely avoided ("background" radiation.) We are also exposed to radiation through medically necessary testing (e.g., dental x-rays, nuclear medicine, and radiology procedures). Typically, the average individual is exposed to roughly 3.6 mSv per year or 360 mrem per year (see terminology in following section). This dosage is both from medical and scattered background radiation.

A BRIEF REVIEW OF RADIATION PROTECTION TERMINOLOGY

Exposure (E): is the ability of energy to ionize air (source-related). The unit is the roentgen (R), which is the amount of radiation that produces ionization of one electrostatic unit (ESU) of either positive or negative charge per cc of air at 0°C and 760 mm Hg (STP). In SI units it is coulombs (C)/kg (1R = 2.58 × 10).

Absorbed Dose (D): is a measure of the energy absorbed in a unit mass of material from radiation. It depends on the characteristics of the absorbing medium. The unit is the radiation absorbed dose or the rad (1 rad = 100 erg/g absorber). In SI units, gray (Gy) is the unit of radiation absorbed dose and is given by 1 Gy = 100 rad = 1 J/kg absorber. D = f × E (is the f-factor or roentgen-to-rad conversion factor). At diagnostic x-ray energies, the f-factor for air and soft tissues is close to 1.

Dose Equivalent (DE): is a measure of the biological damage that is likely to result from the absorbed energy. The unit is roentgen equivalents man, or rem. In SI units, the Sievert (Sv) is the unit of dose equivalent and is given by 1 Sv = 100 rem.

DE = D × QF × N

QF is the quality factor and related to linear energy transfer (LET) of the radiation in a given medium. It represents the effectiveness of the radiation to cause biological or chemical damage (X-ray QF is about 1.0).

N is the modifying factor of the radiation and related to absorption coefficient of the absorbing material (assumed to be unity).

LET is defined as the amount of energy deposited per unit length of the path by the radiation and is measured in kiloelectron volts per micrometer. LET is proportional to the square of the particle charge and is universally related to particle kinetic energy. Measure of the effectiveness of a particular radiation causing biological damage (X-rays are a low LET radiation).

Time is the amount of time a worker is exposed to radiation (should be as short as possible.)

Distance is the distance from the source (should be as far as practicable.)

Inverse Square Law is radiation exposure that varies inversely as the square of the distance. Therefore, if the distance from the source is doubled, the exposure rate is reduced by one fourth.

Shielding is the use of appropriate materials to diminish exposure from a given source. Designing shielding for radiation protection must take into account the *half-value layer* (HVL), which is defined as the amount of shielding that reduces exposure from a radiation source by one half. HVL is dependent on both the energy of the radiation and the atomic number of the absorbing material.

As a rough guideline using x-rays or fluoroscopy for the clinican, the units rad and rem are approximately equivalent (e.g., interchangeable). *Rad* refers to the radiation dose of the incident beam delivered to the air (i.e., what is coming) out of the fluoroscopy machine. *Rem* refers to the radiation dose (energy) deposited inside the patient and more closely reflects potential biological damage.

Scatter radiation is essentially any radiation other than the direct incident beam that comes out of the fluoroscopy machine.

TABLE 76-1 **Radiation Dosages Which May Produce Biological Effects Following Acute Exposure**

Target Organ	Radiation Dose, rad (Gy)	Results	Rough No. of Equivalent
Eye Lens	200 (2)	Cataract formation	10,000
Skin	500 (5)	Erythemia	25,000
Skin	700 (7)	Permanent alopecia	35,000
Whole Body	200–700 (2–7)	Death from infection due to hematopoietic failure (4 to 6 weeks)	10,000–35,000
Whole Body	700–5,000 (7–50)	Death from GI failure (3 to 4 days)	35,000–250,000
Whole Body	5,000–10,000 (50–100)	Death from cerebral edema (1 to 2 days)	250,000–500,000

INTERACTION OF X-RAYS AND MATTER

The absorption of energy from radiation in living matter may lead to molecular excitation, releasing significant amounts of energy that is capable of breaking strong chemical bonds. Ionizing radiation is generally classified as either particulate (e.g., protons, alpha particles) or electromagnetic (e.g., x-rays, gamma rays). X-rays are generally produced in an electrical device that accelerates electrons from a cathode to high energy and then stops them abruptly in a target (e.g., tungsten-anode). Part of the kinetic energy of the electrons is converted into x-rays.

The process by which x-ray photons are absorbed depends on the energy of the particular photons and the chemical composition of the absorbing material. Two major processes occur for photon energies commonly used in diagnostic radiology: the Compton process and the photoelectric process. Each of these causes a transfer of energy from photon to electron. In this way, a mark is made that can ultimately serve as an image.

BIOLOGICAL EFFECTS OF RADIATION

X-rays are scattered by the atoms of patients leading to scattered radiation. No amount of radiation can be considered safe for living matter. The maximum permissible dose (MPD) is the upper limit of radiation dose that one should be "allowed" to receive. Radiation exposure below this level probably only carries remote chances of clinically significant adverse effects.

Recall that the radiation dose from an average chest x-ray is approximately 10 to 20 mrad compared with 300 mrad for an average 2-second fluoroscopy scan. Whole body total radiation dose exceeding 1 Sv (100 rem) can lead to problems that often first affect the most rapidly multiplying cells such as mucosa, bone marrow, and skin. Common radiation-related illnesses include radiation sickness, nausea, fatigue, hematopoetic disturbances, intestinal problems, alopecia, and radiation dermatitis. The International Commission on Radiological Protection has determined that the risk of death from radiation-induced cancers or hereditary disorders of radiation is roughly 1/100 per sievert (100 rems) absorbed.

Since actively dividing cells are particularly affected by radiation, the fetus is at special risk. It is suggested that, except in emergencies, women of reproductive capacity should be x-rayed only in the first 10 days of their menstrual cycle (i.e., before ovulation has occurred—the 10-day rule). It may be most prudent to display warnings about risk to pregnancy for female patients and clinicians.

Two major long-term risks of radiation exposure are increased incidence of cancer and chromosomal abnormalities. Early effects might be a skin reaction. Patients should be informed that there have been patients who have developed skin erythema and even second-degree burns from fluoroscopy ("lead foot" practitioner). Table 76-1 lists radiation dosages that may produce biological effects following acute exposure. Table 76-2 lists recommended occupational dose limits per year from the National Council on Radiation Protection.

A major concern for those being exposed to radiation is cataract formation. A cataract is an opacification of the normally transparent lens. Dividing cells are limited to pre-equatorial region of the epithelium and progeny of these mitotic cells differentiate into lens fibers and accumulate at the equator. If dividing cells are injured by radiation, the resulting abnormal fibers are not removed from the lens but migrate toward the posterior poles. Since they are not translucent, they may evolve into a cataract. The minimum dose required to produce a progressive cataract is over 200 rad in a single exposure, with larger doses necessary in a fractionated regimen. Exposure in excess of 800 rem have been linked to induc-

TABLE 76-2 **Recommended Occupational Dose Limits per Year**

Area/Organ	Annual MPD
Thyroid	50 rem
Extremities	50 rem
Lens of the Eye	15 rem
Gonads	50 rem
Whole Body	5 rem
Pregnant Women	0.5 rem*
	To fetus*

From the National Council on Radiation Protection. MPD denotes maximum permissible dose.

ing cataracts. The latent period between irradiation and the appearance of lens opacities is dose-related but is roughly 8 years. The use of "leaded" glasses worn correctly should reduce eye exposure to minimal to nondetectable.

FLUOROSCOPY

Radiation exposure from fluoroscopy is a significant risk. Entrance skin exposure rates generally range from 1 to 10 rad/min, but can shoot up as high as 40 rad/min with continuous cine operating modes, which are commonly used in cardiology and angiography. Collimators limit the area where the beam exits. Skin dose estimates can be calculated for patients (and are required in many institutions) based predominantly on total fluoroscopy time.

The maximum NCRP limit for entrance skin exposure is 10 rad/min and should be less than 5 rad/min. Fluoroscopic systems with "high-dose" options usually have a 5 rad/min manual mode dose maximum but no limit for high-dose options. These options need special activation mechanisms that include visual and/or audible signals to indicate that the high-dose options are being used.

The skin is often a primary sign of radiation toxicity since organ doses are usually much less than skin doses secondary to soft tissue attenuation. Table 76-3 lists common radiation-induced skin injuries. Irresponsible use of high-dose fluoroscopy may produce very high doses that lead to disorders such as skin erythema or epilation. Reducing fluoroscopy time and radiation field area can minimize exposure. Additionally, whenever possible the use of "last image hold" should be employed. This "freezes" the image on the monitor after the radiation exposure has been turned off.

The maximum dose rate with conventional fluoroscopy is 10 rad/min. However, individual fluoroscopy imaging typically uses much less than this. Image quality significantly improves when increasing from 0.75 to 3 rad/minute, but beyond this, further increases do not dramatically improve image quality.

There are usually no limits placed on doses delivered in high-dose mode. High-dose mode should be used extremely sparingly and only for a few minutes at a time (e.g., to observe PTCA balloon when in place but not to just observe the catheter).

All fluoroscopy machines are not equal. Newer machines have improved safety measures. Generally, older machines yield more radiation than newer machines, which have improved changes such as tube design and image intensifier, but each system may differ markedly. Most all modern fluoroscopy machines have an image intensifier that brightens the image enough so that it can be displayed on a TV screen. Non-intensified fluoroscopy produces inferior image quality while yielding higher radiation exposures than fluoroscopy with an intensifier. Each state differs in terms of how frequently fluoroscopy machine testing (kerma rates) are required, but generally annual inspections are recommended.

TABLE 76-3 **Radiation-Induced Skin Injuries**

Skin Effects	Rads	Normal Mode (10 R/min)
Early Transient Crytherma	200	20 min
Temporary Epilation	300	30 min
Basal Cell Erytherma	600	60 min
Permanent Epilation	700	70 min
Dry Desquamation	1,000	100 min

PRACTICAL RADIATION PROTECTION

Table 76-4 lists practical tips for protecting oneself from radiation. The Nuclear Regulatory Commission and most other agencies endorse the concept of implementing the ALARA (as low as reasonably achievable) program, which states that all exposures that can be prevented should be prevented. The International Committee on Radiation Protection has recommended (1991) the maximal permissible annual dose to be 2 rem per year. This is not really a clinically significant problem for pain physicians who are careful and follow appropriate ALARA principles. Ideally, most radiation workers should not receive more than 10% of the MPD. Steps to reduce patient and physician exposure to secondary scatter radiation are:

Maximize distance from the source
Minimize time
Appropriate shielding
Minimize fluoroscopy and cine time (refers to filming time, e.g., fast sequence of images, usually in cardiology)
Use freeze frames instead of real time whenever possible.

A minimum amount of filtration is used to remove low-energy x-rays. Each system has inherent filtration to "harden" the incident beam in order to produce an incident beam of consistent energy level. This helps to diminish the amount of scatter. Generally, the scatter dose level at 1 meter from patients is roughly 0.1% of the

TABLE 76-4 **Radiation Protection Tips**

- Personnel in the fluoroscopy suite should wear lead aprons of at least 0.5 mm lead equivalent.
- During fluoroscopy, only essential workers should be in the room.
- Radiation workers should never hold a patient for a study.
- Everyone in the room should have protection before beginning fluoroscopy.
- Prior to any radiation exposure, the primary clinician should signal (e.g., "is everyone shielded, fluoro starting," etc.).
- Maintain scatter dose level at 1 meter from patients at less than 0.1% of the entrance skin dose.
- Leakage radiation from tube housing should be less than 0.1 R/h at a distance of 1 meter.
- For C-arm fluoroscopy units, it is preferable to locate the x-ray tube underneath the patient. (Radiation transmitted through the patient is usually about 5%–10% of the entrance dose.)
- Total fluoroscopy time exceeding 30 minutes may lead to radiation-induced skin injury and patients should be counseled regarding this if they are exposed to more than ½ hour.
- The lowest radiation dose and the sharpest image result from keeping the image intensifier as close to the patient as possible.
- Keep the collimators (which cover the x-rays after they are produced) "closed" to as small an exposed field size as possible (just the region of interest).

entrance skin dose (e.g., if the patient entrance skin exposure rate is 3 rad/min, the operator exposure at 1 meter would be about 3 mrad/min). Low-energy x-rays only enter and do not exit the patient. Basic protection includes minimizing time of exposure, maximizing the distance away from the source, and proper shielding (maximizing the attenuation of radiation before it reaches the skin). Physician exposure can be reduced by optimizing protective operator safety (e.g., techniques) equipment. Do not put hands in beam.

Lead aprons absorb between 90% and 95% of the scattered radiation reaching exposed fluoroscopy clinicians. Although the use of thyroid collar shields and leaded safety glasses are not required unless exposure to the thyroid or eye could exceed 5 rem per year, all physicians using fluoroscopy should wear these at all times. Additionally, when performing numerous interventional procedures with fluoroscopy, shielded surgical gloves with radiation attenuation offer further protection. Annual physical examinations should include careful thyroid examination. If exposed physicians are asymptomatic, there is no need for routine complete blood counts or thyroid function testing.

RADIATION EXPOSURE MONITORS

The Nuclear Regulatory Commission (NRC) is an independent federal regulatory agency responsible to ensure that workers and the public are protected from unnecessary or excessive exposure to radiation. If you work near radiation sources, the amount of radiation exposure that you are permitted to receive may be limited by the NRC. Additionally, employers are required to advise employees of their annual exposure. Thus, regulations must stipulate that practitioners using fluoroscopy wear radiation detection devices (RDDs).

Code of Federal Regulations (10 CFR19) require workers to receive radiation safety training, have a right to ask questions, and are required to wear RDDs if they are likely to receive more than 50 mrem/year and must receive an annual report with their exposure levels. Radiation detection devices should preferably be worn at collar level on the outside of clothes. They should not be stored in warm or humid areas, where x-ray equipment is used, and should generally be changed monthly.

Although protective garments are commonplace, it is not uncommon to find some clinicians without RDDs or radiation monitors (e.g., film badges) while performing fluoroscopic procedures. Film badges may become obsolete by the next decade, replaced by thermoluminescent dosimeters (TLD) and/or detectors of aluminum oxides. The newer RDDs are more sensitive and reliable and can be read anytime, but probably only once reliably. Without diligently wearing these monitors, and proper documentation, there is no precise way to determine how much exposure an individual has had. Some practitioners with significant exposure in the cardiac catheterization laboratory wear them inside the lead apron monitors, external monitors, and ring monitors (on their fingers). If you use fluoroscopy only rarely, a pocket dosimeter may be a convenient monitoring option; however, these must be documented by proper personnel.The question of when to be concerned (e.g., how many fluoroscopic procedures should you do) cannot be answered without the use of radiation monitors. Total fluoroscopy time per week should be kept as low as reasonably possible. Since exposure is cumulative, an effective strategy can be to limit the fluoroscopy time for each individual patient and holding all cases to less than 5 minutes.

Some clinicians attach a monitor (radiation detector device) to their personal thyroid collar shield and keep that thyroid shield in a shielded locker or any radiation protected location near the fluoroscopy suites. Of course, if your RDD is on your thyroid shield, you have to remember to wear your shield whenever you are involved with fluoroscopy or other diagnostic imaging sources of x-rays.

PATIENT INFORMED CONSENT FOR RADIATION EXPOSURE

Any procedure with known radiation exposure requires obtaining informed consent from the patient. Thus, performing fluoroscopy must include a discussion with the patient concerning the risks and benefits, as well as the alternatives, to radiation exposure from fluoroscopy. Documenting informed consent is another critical variable. Patients should be informed that radiation exposure will be kept to as low as reasonably achievable in order to properly perform the procedure. If contrast is going to be injected, the risks and benefits must be explained and documented (e.g., hypersensitivity/allergic-type reactions). Depending on the procedure and anticipated scope and duration of radiation exposure, the patient might be advised that, while it is impossible to know the exact amount of radiation exposure, it is usually somewhere between a chest x-ray and a computed tomography scan. There is less risk when a focal area is exposed versus a whole body exposure. Sine skin reaction may reflect early radiation toxicity; patients should be informed that skin erythema and even second-degree burns are possible from fluoroscopy. A separate standardized consent form for patients undergoing fluoroscopy may be useful.

SUMMARY

Maintaining safe radiation practice is a critical component of most interventional pain practices (see Table 76-4). Safe measures include practicing the basic principles of As Low As Reasonably Achievable (ALARA), Time, Distance, and Shielding. A healthy respect for EMR, continued radiation safety education, radiation monitoring, and safe "commonsense" practices will minimize the risks to patients and clinicians. Each institution should have a Radiation Safety Officer* who can offer in-depth information regarding personal protection, the safety of a particular fluoroscopic suite or machine, and how to obtain additional training or radiation safety.

SUGGESTED READINGS

Hall EJ. *Radiobiology for the Radiologist*. 4th ed. Philadelphia, Pa: JB Lippincott; 1993.

National Council on Radiation Protection and Measurements (NCRP) Report No. 100: *Exposure of the US Population from Diagnostic Medical Radiation*. Washington, DC: National Council on Radiation Protection and Measurements; 1989.

Pizarello DJ, Witcofski RL. *Medical Radiation Biology*. 2nd ed. Philadelphia, Pa: Lea & Febiger; 1982.

Sprawls P Jr. *Physical Principles of Medical Imaging*. 2nd ed. Gaithersburg, Md: Aspen; 1993.

Wolbarst AB. *Physics of Radiology*. Norwalk, Conn: Appleton & Lange; 1993.

*Note: Further information about radiation safety for your particular environment can usually be obtained by contacting the radiation safety officer (RSO) at your institution.

CHAPTER 77 COMPLEMENTARY AND ALTERNATIVE MEDICINE IN PAIN MANAGEMENT

Eric Leskowitz

INTRODUCTION

Alternative medicine is rapidly growing in popularity. In what may eventually prove to be the most frequently cited medical journal article in the postwar era, Eisenberg and colleagues demonstrated in 1993 that nearly 40% of Americans utilized alternative medical therapies, and spent more out of pocket for these approaches than they spent out of pocket for mainstream medical treatments.[1] A follow-up study in 1998 showed continued dramatic growth in these practices.[2] The National Institutes of Health (NIH) has supported an Office of Alternative Medicine since 1993, but thanks to steady increases in congressional funding, it was recently upgraded to a division within the NIH. The November 1998 issues of several of the American Medical Association (AMA)-sponsored specialty journals were devoted to the topic of complementary and alternative medicine (commonly abbreviated CAM); Micozzi's 1996 text on alternative medicine[3] was only the first of many. This rapid rise in interest to what was previously a fringe topic lends an aura of novelty to these techniques, but a cursory look at some of the most common CAM techniques (acupuncture, homeopathy, yoga) shows that these are, in fact, traditional, if not ancient, therapies. And so it should not be surprising that the most common symptom that brings people to their health care providers—pain—has a long and rich tradition of CAM interventions. This chapter outlines some of the more prominent and promising CAM approaches to pain conditions, both acute and chronic, at the same time that it outlines some fundamental similarities and differences between CAM and mainstream biomedical therapies.

To appreciate the relationship between CAM and allopathic medicine, it is helpful to consider three distinct paradigms of medical treatment. The approach taught in medical schools today, and practiced in hospitals worldwide, is known as allopathic medicine, from the Greek *allos*, meaning "other" because disease pathology is felt to be an outside force to be countered by biomedical treatment interventions. Thus, military metaphors predominate (e.g.,the "war" on cancer, our therapeutic "armamentarium") and treatments are physically focused: medications, surgery, and radiation predominate.

Over the past 30 years, as an outgrowth of Hans Selye's work on stress response systems, a second model integrating the mental and physical dimensions of health has emerged. Initially called the *biopsychosocial* model, it is now better known as *psychoneuroimmunology*, or more globally as *mind-body medicine*.[4] In this system, diseases are felt to be created when the autonomic nervous system and the endocrine system react to negative psychological, emotional inputs and inappropriately elicit the fight-or-flight reaction. Treatments focus on balancing sympathetic overdrive by using mind-body techniques such as biofeedback, hypnosis, and meditation to elicit the counterbalancing relaxation response (see Chapter 14, Psychotherapeutic Management of Chronic Pain), or by introducing new thought and behavior patterns into a person's life through cognitive-behavioral approaches.

But many of the best known techniques in CAM can clearly not be explained by either the biomedical or the mind-body paradigm, largely because they involve a somewhat mysterious phenomenon called "life energy." Known by various names in various healing traditions (*prana* in yoga, *qi* in Chinese medicine), it has no equivalent in Western medicine, and so American doctors have a difficult, if not impossible task, trying to make sense of homeopathy or laying on of hands or acupuncture as anything more than elaborate eliciters of the placebo response. Yet many strikingly successful applications of the ancient and modern CAM techniques to patients in pain behoove algologists to reconsider the possible scientific validity of this mystical-sounding concept. Although this controversy is beyond the scope of this chapter, several physicians have attempted to understand this energy using the language of biomagnetics[5] and of information theory.[6]

This chapter's discussion of CAM techniques for pain is limited to herbs, homeopathy, therapeutic touch, hypnosis, and meditation. Acupuncture, perhaps the best-known CAM technique, is discussed in detail in Chapter 78. There are several hundred treatment techniques that fall under the rubric of CAM, so space constraints obviously require significant selectivity. The scientific literature on CAM and pain is exploding: Taylor[7] alone lists 249 recent references on CAM and pain; Mauskop's text[8] is devoted exclusively to CAM and headache, and Lewith's text [9] is the European precursor to more recent American work. So it is no longer possible to provide a comprehensive review in one chapter. Rather than provide a sketchy overview of a wide range of CAM applications for pain, I have chosen to focus in more depth on the five representative CAM techniques mentioned previously. Each section that follows includes a brief historical introduction, a description of some relevant research that highlights methodologic issues, and some promising clinical applications. The interested reader is referred to the references at the end of the chapter for information on other CAM therapies.

HERBAL MEDICINE

Mainstream American medicine prides itself on the use of synthetic pharmacologically active chemicals to treat disease, seeing this as a significant advance over the more primitive use of herbal remedies by our pre-Industrial ancestors. Contemporary European physicians, however, use herbal treatments with relish, and their governments have been active in generating high-quality research in phytomedicine; Germany's Commission E report[10] is considered the bible of botanical medicine. Despite this bias, tertiary-care American hospitals in fact practice herbal medicine on a daily basis. Many well-known pharmaceuticals are actually purified preparations of naturally occurring plant compounds: the cardiac agent digitalis is derived from the foxglove plant, the antibiotic penicillin is a mold extract, and the antineoplastic agent vincristine is derived from the periwinkle vine, to name but a few.

Herbal medicines are also prominently used in the field of pain management. The opiate analgesics are all ultimately derived from the poppy plant (*Papaver somniferens*—"the bringer of sleep"). Whether the narcotic is naturally occuring (morphine, opium, or heroin) or semisynthetic (e.g., demerol, percodan, and codeine), all opiate-receptor agonists can be traced back to the poppy plant. Another mainstay in the management of less intense pain is the first nonsteroidal anti-inflammatory drug (NSAID): aspirin. Acetylsalicylic acid was originally derived from the bark of the willow tree (genus *Salix*, the Latin word from which "salicylate" derives), and all of the modern congeners are simply chemical refinements. The final herb in common use for pain control today is extracted from the chili pepper (genus *Capsicum*); the active ingredient of Zofran creme is capsaicin, which depletes substance P from preterminal afferent axons more effectively than any man-made synthetic agent. It has proven effective in controlled studies for cluster headache, postmastectomy syndrome, psoriasis, and pruritis[11]; uncontrolled reports indicate usefulness in osteoarthritis and rheumatoid arthritis, amputation stump pain, and diabetic neuropathy.[12]

Less well-known examples of herbal approaches to pain include the use of feverfew for migraine prevention,[13] ginger for arthritis,[14] and marijuana for some chronic pain conditions.[15] Definitive mechanisms of action for these botanical medicines are not known at present, but do not appear to involve the opiate receptor; feverfew is thought to effect serotonin dynamics, whereas the active ingredient of marijuana, delta-9-tetrahydrocannabinol, appears to simulate the action of an endogenous arachidonic acid derivative called *anandamide*, which binds to cannabinoid receptors in the cortex, hippocampus and cerebellum. So at least in the realm of pain management, the distinction between "modern" and "traditional" medicine is not as clear as is usually implied.

HYPNOSIS

Hypnosis is a mind-body technique that creates a state of focused attention. Hypnosis is widely misunderstood to be a process by which an all-powerful hypnotherapist manipulates the experience of a suggestible patient. In fact, all hypnosis is self-hypnosis, with the therapist functioning only as a guide to help the patient learn how to focus his or her attention in such a way as to filter out unwanted or unpleasant sensations, creating a state of receptivity to positive suggestions. This trance state of focused attention can be elicited without any external ritual, as when reading an absorbing book or when telling a story to distract a child from a painful medical procedure. Many dramatic transcultural examples of hypnotic trance for pain suppression exist: the Hindu fakir who sits on a bed of nails, the Native American warrior who endures being suspended by leather thongs that pierce his pectoral muscles, and the Polynesian firewalker all have learned to screen out nociceptive input by selective focus of attention.

Current research demonstrates that hypnosis is not simply a passive withdrawal of awareness, but rather involves an active suppression of the somatosensory cortex by the frontal cortex.[16] Measurements of somatosensory-evoked potentials and of regional cerebral blood flow show that highly hypnotizable subjects are able to activate a supervisory attentional control system of the far-frontal cortex in a topographically specific inhibitory feedback circuit that cooperates in the regulation of thalamocortical activities.[17] An important clinical point is that early intervention through hypnosis training can prevent the conversion of an acute pain syndrome into a chronic pain condition by blocking the development of "neurosignatures of pain."[18]

Acute Pain

Operative Anecdotes are widespread about the use of hypnosis to relieve operative distress. I have attended workshops in which the presenters have described successful self-hypnosis for deviated septum repair and for gallbladder removal (the most difficult part of the procedure was felt to be convincing the surgeon to proceed without medications!). I have seen a videotape of cranial trephination performed without anesthesia in rural Kenya that was so graphic that audience members fainted. But beyond these sorts of anecdotal reports is a growing scientific literature on the role of suggestion in preparing for surgery.

Recently, the use of hypnotic suggestion immediately prior to surgery under general anesthesia has been demonstrated to minimize postoperative discomfort as well as intraoperative bleeding.[19] But even 35 years ago, pre-operative encouragement and suppport (called "good bedside manner" rather than hypnotic suggestion) was known to produce similar benefits.[20] Patients now often devise their own individualized protocols for intraoperative positive suggestions that require the participation of the surgeons themselves.[21]

Injury/Trauma The classic example of using hypnotic attention to relieve acute pain is exemplified by a mother's caring hugs and kisses for an injured child. Through a combination of distraction and therapeutic touch, a child's attention may be readily refocused in a more fruitful direction. Emergency room work is in some ways ideally suited for hypnotherapeutic pain control, as the distressed patients are by definition in a state of highly focused attention and are thus more likely to be responsive to clinicians' suggestions. Ewin[22] has described a simple intervention ("I'm a doctor, and I know what to do now. Your job is to trust me by going back and remembering a time when you felt calm and relaxed.") that facilitates difficult trauma work in the emergency setting. Painful hospital procedures like wound debridement [23] can also be facilitated by the use of hypnosis.

Chronic Pain By definition, chronic pain is less responsive than acute pain to intervention. If conceived of as a learned behavior, it should be responsive to newly suggested interpretations. One chronic pain syndrome that has proved responsive to hypnosis is reflex sympathetic dystrophy (RSD), or complex regional pain syndrome (CRPS). Several workers, most notably Gainter,[24] have developed a specific hypnotherapy protocol that allows patients to access and express in symbolic form an emotional substrate that seems to have set the stage for the evolution of chronic pain even though the inciting injury is often quite trivial in nature. An informal survey of recent RSD patients seen in our inpatient pain management program shows a very high percentage with significant degrees of unacknowledged rage, either at caregivers or those responsible for the injury. This unusual degree of repressed emotion can become problematic on an inpatient milieu, either through behaviors that split staff into good versus bad, or by outright hostility and noncompliance with treatment. Psychophysiologic mechanisms may be involved in converting this intense affect into sympathetic dysfunction; high placebo response rates to test protocols in RSD (such as the intravenous phentolamine challenge) also suggest that mind-body mechanisms are crucial.[25] Adequate research in the psychotherapy of this syndrome does not yet exist.

HOMEOPATHY

In homeopathy, a symptom is considered a positive sign of the organism's vitality in throwing off a disease state. Hence, homeopathy's treatment remedies are designed to enhance this cleansing process rather than to suppress it, as in allopathic medicine. Extremely high dilutions of the active plant or mineral substance are matched with a symptom complex to provide a "healing crisis" and then a cure. The mechanism of action of homeopathy is impossible to understand via conventional biomedical dose-response pharmacokinetics, especially since remedies may be so dilute as to contain no molecules of the purported active ingredient. But the fact remains that a growing number of double-blind studies have demonstrated its efficacy for medical disorders like infantile diarrhea, asthma, and allergy. The status of its effectiveness in pain syndromes is less clear.

One of the most common applications of homeopathy in pain management is the use of *Arnica montana* for muscle bruises and soreness. Widely recommended for situations ranging from postoperative pain to exercise-induced strain, it has rarely been studied. However, one recent study from the United Kingdom is quite bold in scope. All the runners who competed in the 1997 London marathon were invited to use a standard preparation of arnica after the race, and were then assessed daily for 5 days after the race for the target symptom of muscle soreness.[26] No statistically significant differences were detected; a solid finding, given the large number of participants (N = 519).

An important conceptual and methodologic error, however, was made in this (and many other) apparently tight CAM research trials. Allopathic logic was used when all the subjects were prescribed the same remedy for an apparently identical symptom. This violated one of the key tenets of homeopathy: each individual is so unique that identical symptoms may be caused and cured by totally different remedies. Ideally, each runner in this study should have been individually prescribed one of the 60 or so specific remedies used to treat muscle soreness. Only then could results be interpreted to mean that homeopathy is ineffective for muscle soreness. Thus, recent negative results regarding the use of homeopathy in migraine prophylaxis,[27] dental pain,[28] and postoperative pain [29] must also be taken with this same grain of methodologic salt.[30]

Therapeutic Touch

Therapeutic Touch (TT) is a nursing technique based on a purported human energy field that surrounds the body,[31] much like a magnetic field surrounds a magnet. The practitioner smoothes out energy imbalances with her hands. The practice involves three steps: first the nurse calmly centers herself in the compassionate state of wishing to be of service, then she assesses the patient's energy field with her own hands to detect any abnormal areas, and then she corrects these imbalances with noncontact movements of her hands over the affected areas. Although this technique was developed and formalized in the last 25 years (to the point where it has been taught to thousands of nurses in America and worldwide), it bears striking similarities to ancient healing techniques used in China (called *external qigong*) and even to the mesmeric passes used by Franz Mesmer in animal magnetism some 200 years ago in Europe.

Methodologic Issues Research on Therapeutic Touch has addressed such pain syndromes as burn pain[32] and headache pain.[33] Findings are strongly suggestive of therapeutic benefits, especially to subjective symptoms documented both by self-report and clinician assessment. However, methodologic problems persist even when a sham treatment called mimic TT is used for double-blind testing.[34] When an experimenter duplicates the hand movements of a TT practitioner but does not first invoke a calm state of mind imbued with the intent to help, this mimic TT can serve as a valid control for TT. Patients can actually sense a subjective difference between mimic and true TT, yet even this control measure does not take into account what many researchers feel is a key ingredient in the effectiveness of many subtle energy therapies: therapist intentionality.[35]

A large literature suggests that the intent of any clinician may be as important as the particular therapy technique being used, and that the impact of intentionality may even override double-blind controls. An antibiotic can be effectively administered whether or not the researcher knows he is using active or placebo treatment. However, a standard TT session starts off with the nurse knowing and invoking this process; any process (even mimic TT) that does not include this key element cannot accurately be called TT. This is not simply semantic quibbling, because the conscious intent to help may activate the very energy mechanisms that are presumed to underlie the efficacy of TT.

This issue underlies the recent controversial publication by the prestigious *Journal of the American Medical Association* (*JAMA*)[36] of an 11-year-old schoolgirl's science fair project that allegedly debunked TT. Her finding that TT practitioners could not reliably detect the presence of the experimenter's hand was interpreted by the journal editors to mean that TT was clinically ineffective (even though no clinical outcomes were assessed). Because experimenter bias was not controlled for in this study, it would have been more accurate for *JAMA* to state that her results showed that the intent of the researcher can distort results in either a positive or negative direction.[37] Interestingly, *JAMA* has not given any space to the deluge of rebuttal letters to the editor that followed the appearance of this article.

Clinical Applications Subjective benefits have been reported for the related Chinese technique of *qi gong* with CRPD[38] and with nonspecific chronic pain.[39] Some intriguing preliminary work suggests that TT may be effective in alleviating phantom limb pain.[40] Of note is that both practitioner and patient frequently report that they are able to detect the hand of the therapist when it comes in proximity of the phantom limb. This experience cannot be reconciled with the "neuromatrix" theory of phantom sensation, which holds that cortical representations in effect create phantom sensations. This TT work suggests that there may exist a subtle energy matrix (as posited in many of the world's mystical traditions) that generates pain sensations whenever it is blocked or impeded. Because there is no innervation or neural network to transmit phantom sensation, other mechanisms of action (like subtle acupuncture meridians) must be hypothesized. If placebo and expectancy variables can be adequately controlled for, this work provides further validation for the subtle energy model underlying TT and other energy-based treatments.

MEDITATION

The ancient mystical traditions of almost all cultures describe dramatic feats of physiologic control performed by meditation masters, from voluntary stoppage of the heart, to states of prolonged suspended animation, to complete pain supression. Modern research also demonstrates the clinical effectiveness of meditation in a wide range of medical conditions, including chronic pain. These clinical applications do not require years of rigorous training. Fairly simple procedures are available. To illustrate the simplicity of the meditational process, a brief instruction in mindfulness meditation as used at Spaulding Rehabilitation Hospital follows.

Instructions: Sitting Meditation

1. Make sure you will not be distracted for the next 20 minutes. Close the door to your room and take the phone off the hook.
2. Sit in a comfortable chair, keeping your spine straight and letting your shoulders drop. Close your eyes if it feels comfortable.
3. Take a moment to let the muscles in your body relax, and then begin to pay attention to your breathe. Simply monitor the movement of your breathe in and out of your nostrils, without trying to regulate it in any way.
4. Whenever you notice that your attention has been distracted by other thoughts or concerns, simply bring your focus back to the easy rhythm of your own breathing. Do not criticize or judge yourself for getting distracted; just notice the direction of your thoughts, and return to your breathe as often as necessary.
5. When 15 minutes has passed (peek at a clock, do not use an alarm), slowly shift your attention back to the outside world, taking a good minute or two until your eyes are fully open. You are now alert and ready to move on to your next activity.

Chronic Pain Several medical centers now use meditational variants to help patients manage chronic pain. Mindfulness meditation involves a nonjudgmental moment-to-moment awareness of the contents of one's conscious awareness, without any attempt to suppress or alter the train of thought, even when it involves recognition of painful sensations. This approach, of Buddhist origin, has been used by Kabat-Zinn[41] to treat many medical disorders, including chronic pain. Outpatient instructional classes can lead to robust changes in perception of pain, with stable gains maintained over multiyear follow-up.[42] The Relaxation Response[43] is a secular variant of Transcendental Meditation, which involves focus on a regularly repeated inner sound, and has formed the foundation of Dr. Herbert Benson's work. His colleague, Dr Margaret Caudill, has integrated regular elicitation of the relaxation response with a range of cognitive-behavioral coping strategies[44] to form a comprehensive protocol for managing chronic pain. It has been shown to dramatically decrease the utilization of health care resources in one selected chronic pain population,[45] a finding of interest to insurers, given the high resource utilization of the typical chronic pain patient. A similar psychosocial intervention strategy based on meditation has effectively targeted fibromyalgia patients.[46]

SUMMARY

As I hope this survey illustrates, the field of CAM is provocative and burgeoning. A wide range of research is now being developed to answer widespread concerns about the role of placebo factors in CAM applications to pain syndromes. It is clear, though, that many treatment-specific effects are generated by CAM techniques. Mechanisms of action are often not clear, and challenge our ingrained mechanistic biomedical view of the world. But consumer interest has spurred a rising tide of research and clinical focus on this area that may potentially transform the way medicine, and pain management, is practiced in America. At least one conclusion can be definitively made at this time: CAM interventions will be a routine aspect of clinical care and pain management in the 21st century.

REFERENCES

General

1. Eisenberg DM, Kessler RC, Foster C, et al. Unconventional medicine in the United States: prevalence, costs and patterns of use. *N Engl J Med* 1993;328:246–252.
2. Eisenberg DM, Davis RB, Ettner SL, et al. Trends in alternative medicine use in the United States 1990–1997: results of a follow-up national survey. *JAMA* 1998;280:1569–1575.
3. Micozzi MS, ed. *Fundamentals of Complementary and Alternative Medicine*. New York, NY: Churchill Livingstone; 1996.
4. Borysenko J. *Minding the Body, Mending the Mind: The New Science of Mind/Body Medicine*. New York, NY: Time Warner Books; 1987.
5. Becker R. *Cross Currents: The Perils of Electropollution, the Promise of Electromedicine*. New Orleans, Louisiana: J Tarcher; 1990.
6. Rubik, B. Can Western science provide a foundation for acupuncture? *Altern Ther* 1995;1(4):41–47.
7. Taylor AG. Complementary/Alternative therapies in the treatment of pain. In: Spencer JW,Jacobs JJ, eds. *Complementary/Alternative Medicine: An Evidence Based Approach*. St. Louis, Mo: Mosby, 1999.
8. Mauskop A, Brill MA. *The Headache Alternative: A Neurologist's Guide to Drug Free Relief.* Salt Lake City, Utah: Science News Books; 1997.
9. Lewith G, Horn S. *Drug-Free Pain Relief.* Rochester, Vt: Thorsons Publishers; 1987.

Herbal Medicine

10. Blumenthal M, et al, eds. *The German Commission E Monographs—Therapeutic Guide to Herbal Medicine*. Austin, Tex: American Botanical Council, 1998.
11. Schmid G, Carita F, Bonanno G, Raiteri M. NK-3 receptors mediate enhancement of substance P release from capsaicin-sensitive spinal cord afferent terminals. *Br J Pharmacol* 1998;125:621–626.
12. Haustkappe M, Roizen M, Toledano A, et al. Review of the effectiveness of capsaicin for painful cutaneous disorders and neural dysfunction. *Clin J Pain* 1998;14:97–106.
13. Murphy JJ, Heptinstall S, Mitchell JR. Randomised double-blind placebo-controlled trial of feverfew in migraine prevention. *Lancet* 1988;2:189–192.
14. Srivastava MD, Mustafa T. Ginger (*Zingiber officinalis*) in rheumatism and other musculoskeletal disorders. *Med Hypotheses* 1992;39(4):342.
15. Doyle E, Spence M. Cannabis as a medicine? *Br J Anaesth* 1995; 74:3359–3361.

Hypnosis

16. Spiegel D, Barabasz A. Effects of hypnotic instructions of P300 event-related-potential amplitudes: research and clinical applications. *Am J Clin Hypn* 1988;31(1):11–17.
17. Crawford HJ, Gur RC, Skolnick B, et al. Effects of hypnosis on regional cerebral blood flow during ischemic pain with and without suggested hypnotic analgesia. *Int J Psychophysiol* 1993;15:181–195.

18. Crawford HJ, Knebel T, Kaplan L, et al. Hypnotic analgesia: 1. Somatosensory event-related potential changes to noxious stimuli, and 2. Transfer learning to reduce chronic low back pain. *Int J Clin Exp Hypn* 1998;46:92–132.
19. Enqvist B, von Konow L, Bystedt T. Pre- and peri-operative suggestion in maxillofacial surgery: effects on blood loss and recovery. *Int J Clin Exp Hypn* 1995;43:284–294.
20. Egbert LD, Battit GE, Welch CE, Bartlett MK. Reduction of post-operative pain by encouragement and instruction of patients: a study of doctor-patient rapport. *N Engl J Med* 1964;270:825–827.
21. Huddleston P. *Prepare for Surgery, Heal Faster: A Guide to Mind/Body Techniques*. Cambridge, Mass: Angel River Press, 1996.
22. Ewin DM. Emergency room hypnosis for the burned patient. *Am J Clin Hypn* 1986;29:7–12.
23. Patterson DR, Questad KA, deLateur BJ. Hypnotherapy as an adjunct to narcotic analgesia for the treatment of pain for burn debridement. *Am J Clin Hypn* 1989;31:156–163.
24. Gainter M. Hypnotherapy for reflex sympathetic dystrophy. *Am J Clin Hypn* 1992;34:227–232.
25. Ochoa JD, Verdugo JD. Reflex sympathetic dystrophy: a common clinical avenue for somatoform expression. *Neurol Clin* 1995;13:351–363.

Homeopathy

26. Vickers AJ, Fisher P, Smith C, et al. Homeopathic arnica 30x is ineffective for muscle soreness after long-distance running: a randomized, double-blind, placebo-controlled trial. *Clin J Pain* 1998;14:227–231.
27. Whitmarsh TE, Coleston-Shields DM, Steiner TJ. Double-blind randomized placebo-controlled study of homoeopathic prophylaxis of migraine. *Cephalalgia* 1997;17:600–604.
28. Lokken P, Straumshein PA, Tveiten D, et al. Effect of homoeopathy on pain and other events after acute trauma: placebo controlled trial with bilateral oral surgery. *BMJ* 1995;310:1439–1442.
29. Hart O, Mullee MA, Lewith G, Miller J. Double-blind, placebo-controlled, randomized clinical trial of homoeopathic arnica30c for pain and infection after total abdominal hysterectomy. *J Roy Soc Med* 1997;90:239–240.
30. Whitmarsh T. Evidence in complementary and alternative therapies: lessons from clinical trials of homeopathy in headache. *J Altern Complement Med* 1997;3:307–310.

Therapeutic Touch

31. Mulloney S, Wells-Federman C. Therapeutic Touch: a healing modality. *Cardiovasc Nurs* 1996;10(3):27–49.
32. Turner J. The effect of Therapeutic Touch on pain and anxiety in burn patients. *J Adv Nurs* 1998;28(1):10–20.
33. Keller E, Bzdek B. Effects of Therapeutic Touch on tension headache pain. *Nurs Res* 1986;35(2):68–74.
34. Meehan T. Therapeutic Touch as a nursing intervention. *J Adv Nurs* 1998;28(1):117–125.
35. Schlitz M, Braud W. Distant intentionality and healing: assessing the evidence. *Altern Ther* 1997;3(6):62–73.
36. Rosa L, Rosa E, Sarner L, Barrett S. A close look at Therapeutic Touch. *JAMA* 1998;279:1005–1010.
37. Leskowitz, E. Current controversies in Therapeutic Touch. In: Micozzi M, ed. *Current Review of Alternative Medicine*. St. Louis, Mo: Mosby, 1999.
38. Wu WH, Bandilla E, Ciccone D, et al. Effects of qigong on late-stage complex regional pain syndrome. *Altern Ther* 1999;5(1):45–54.
39. Redner R, Briner B, Snellman L. Effects of a bioenergy healing technique on chronic pain. *Subtle Energies* 1991;2(3):43–68.
40. Leskowitz, E. Phantom limb pain: subtle energy perspectives. *Subtle Energy Energy Med* 1998;7(4):1–27.

Meditation

41. Kabat-Zinn J. *Full Catastrophe Living: Using the Wisdom of Your Body and Mind to Face Stress, Pain, and Illness*. New York, NY: Delacorte Press, 1990.
42. Kabat-Zinn J, Lipworth L, Burney R, Sellers W. Four-year follow-up of a meditation-based program for the self-regulation of chronic pain: treatment outcomes and compliance. *Clin J Pain* 1987;2:159–173.
43. Benson H. *The Relaxation Response*. New York, NY: Avon Books, 1975.
44. Caudill R. *Managing Pain before It Manages You*. New York, NY: Guilford Press; 1995.
45. Caudill M, Schnable R, Suttermeister P, Benson H, Friedman R. Decreased clinic use by chronic pain patients: response to behavioral medicine interventions. *Clin J Pain* 1991;7:305–310.
46. Kaplin KH, Goldenberg DL, Galvine-Nadeau M. The impact of a meditation-based stress reduction program on fibromyalgia. *Gen Hosp Psychiatry* 1993;15:284–289.

CHAPTER 78 ACUPUNCTURE

Joseph F. Audette

INTRODUCTION

There has been growing interest in the West about the application of acupuncture to control pain since President Nixon's well-publicized trip to China in 1971. The fascination with this ancient medical modality was heightened when one of the members of the press corps, James Reston, received acupuncture during an appendectomy.

Despite the initial enthusiasm, there continues to be skepticism regarding the efficacy of acupuncture. Given the lack of definitive clinical data, some of the skepticism is warranted. Acupuncture, however, is not alone in this regard when it comes to pain treatments, and much of the standard clinical care provided by pain physicians stands on less secure ground. The publication of the National Institutes of Health (NIH) consensus statement in 1998 on the clinical applications of acupuncture was based on over 2000 scientific articles and has put acupuncture on more solid ground in the medical community (the citations are available at the web site of the National Library of Medicine).[1] Although clearly not a universal panacea for all pain syndromes, acupuncture has held up well under the last 20 years of scientific scrutiny and seems destined to continue as a viable method for the treatment of pain.

The goal of this chapter is to lay the basic theoretic and physiologic groundwork for understanding the clinical applications of acupuncture for pain. Then the current clinical data regarding the efficacy of acupuncture in various pain syndromes is discussed. Finally, a brief representation of some of the different treatment styles for common pain syndromes is outlined, and the chapter concludes by identifying further educational resources in this field.

BRIEF HISTORY OF ACUPUNCTURE

The term *acupuncture* comes from the Greek words *acus* (needle) and *punctura* (puncture) and is the English translation of *chan* in Mandarin and *hari* in Japanese.

The clinical practice of inserting needles into the body (initially stone or flint needles) occurred in China by the fifth century BC and was followed some time later, between the 2nd and 3rd century BC, by the first written medical text on acupuncture, the *Huang Di Nei Jing* or the *Yellow Emperor's Classic of Internal Medicine*.

BASIC ACUPUNCTURE THEORIES

Chinese Taoist theories of yin and yang, or the balance of opposing influences in nature, underlie the theoretical framework used in acupuncture to understand human health. Human beings are seen as an integral part of a larger macrocosm that includes all the elements of the surrounding world. These elements are seen to have varying degrees of influence on the human organism and factors such as weather, diet, and social environment are all taken to have significant effects on an individual's health. The dynamic balance of these external factors, together with the internal physical and emotional state of the organism, interact to influence health and disease. As a correlate to this holistic view of human health, Chinese medicine makes no distinction between mental and physical illness and the mind-body dualism that plagues Western medical traditions.

In this integrated framework, the workings and function of the internal organs are believed to have specific, observable effects on the external appearance of the individual. Subtle changes seen on the surface of the body are all seen to reflect accurately on the homeostasis of the internal organ system. For example, alterations in the skin color and skin texture, variations in the suppleness and flexibility of underlying muscles, the quality of arterial pulses, and the appearance of the tongue and eyes are important factors that go into making a diagnosis and treatment plan.[2]

As an outgrowth of Taoist theories of health, forces were postulated to explain how the internal and external systems interrelated. This lead to the concept of *qi*, or *vital energy*. As a means of developing treatment strategies, *qi* was postulated to flow in various channels or meridians in the body. There are 12 principal meridians, 8 extra meridians, and a total of 361 classic acupuncture points that are located on these proposed energy channels. Although an anatomical correlate to the meridians has not been found, the concept has still proved useful to help understand and treat certain patterns of symptoms seen in various disease and pain states (Fig. 78-1).

SCIENTIFIC EVIDENCE

Neurohumoral Data

Over the last 30 years, a great deal of scientific evidence has accumulated to verify that both acupuncture stimulation (AP) and electro-acupuncture stimulation (EA) has reproducible physiologic effects. There are three main lines of evidence that are presented in the following discussion. All go to the heart of the neurologic mechanisms that are currently understood to modulate and influence pain.

The evidence for the release of endogenous opioids with AP and EA derives from the seminal work done by Pomeranz[3] in animals and Mayer[4] in humans in the 1970s. Since that time, a large body of evidence has developed to show that both AP and EA lead to the release of endorphins and enkephalins into the cerebrospinal fluid (CSF). Furthermore, the release of these neuropeptides have been demonstrated to play a role in the analgesic effect of acupuncture as evidenced by opioid-receptor antagonism that can abolish the analgesia obtained with acupuncture in both human and animal models of acute pain.

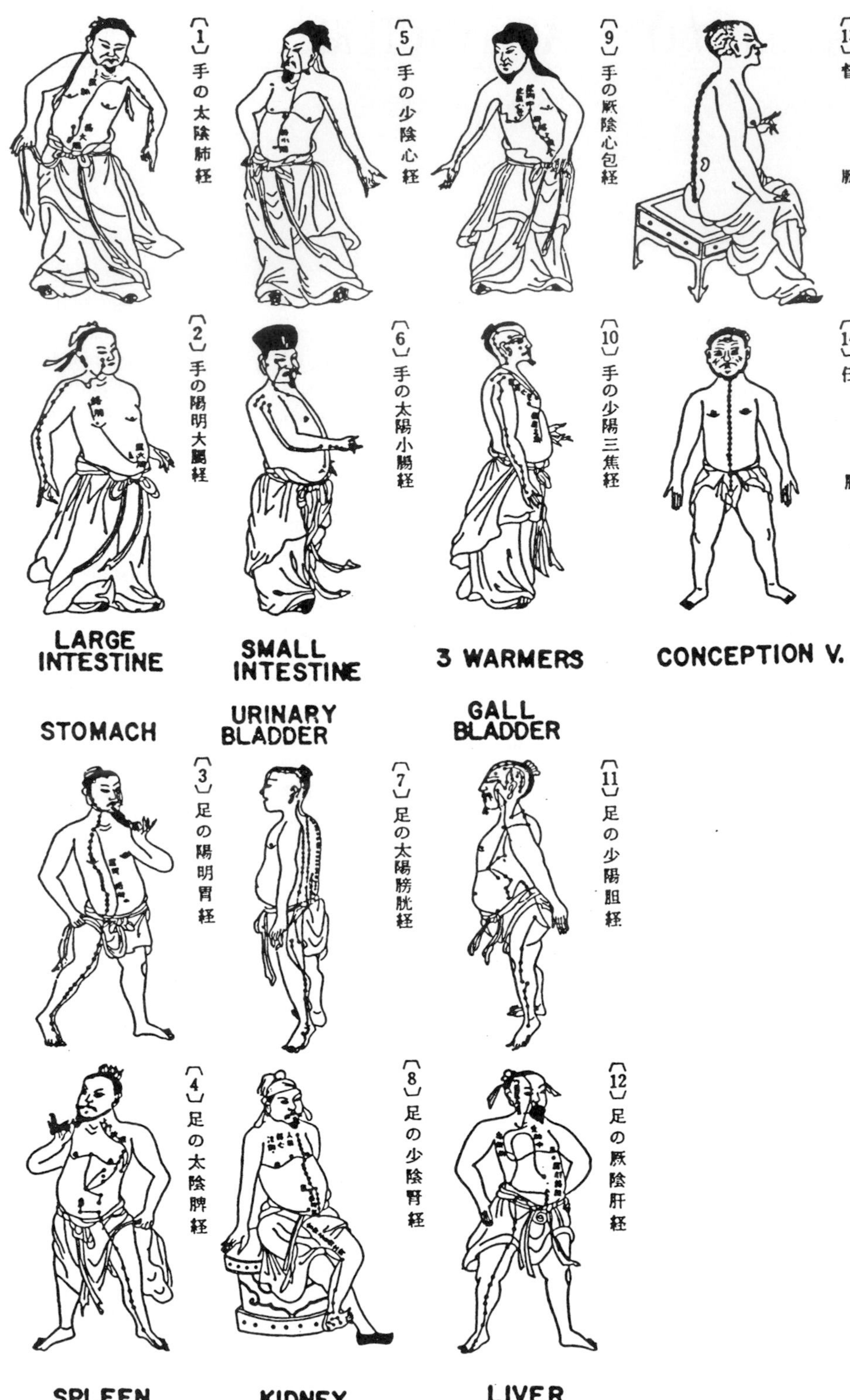

Figure 78-1 Diagrams of the 12 regular meridians and their organ correlates and two of the governing extraordinary meridians. (From Omura, Yoshiaki. Acupuncture Medicine: Its Historical and Clinical Background. Tokyo, Japan: Japan Publications Inc; 1982. Used with permission.)

Since the initial studies, both the met-enkephalin–responding neurons in the dorsal column of the spinal cord and the endorphin and enkephalin active sites in the periaquaductal gray zone of the brain have been shown to be involved in acupuncture analgesia. Both the parameters of stimulation (i.e., the intensity and frequency of EA) and the site of stimulation have significant effects on the type of chemical releases. In particular, antiserum to met-enkephalin abolished acupuncture analgesia but antiserum to dynorphin did not when a true acupuncture point was stimulated, whereas the reverse was true when a non-acupuncture or sham point was stimulated.[5]

Electro-acupuncture stimulation has also been found to elevate levels of 5-hydroxytryptamine (5-HT) in the raphe nucleus, which enhances acupuncture analgesia presumably through descending inhibitory control mechanisms. Destruction of these neurons in the raphe nucleus of the mid-brain or injection of parach† olorophenylalanine, which lowers cerebral levels of 5-HT, will attenuate acupuncture analgesia and injection of pargyline, which slows enzymatic degradation of 5-HT, enhances acupuncture analgesia.[6]

The hypothalamic–pituitary–axis and catecholamines are also influenced by EA and AP and may further influence the analgesic response to pain both through immune modulation and modulation of the sympathetic responses.

Neuroimaging Data

Recent technological advances in mapping brain activity using functional magnetic resonance scanning (fMRI) have begun to be applied to acupuncture. Comparison has been made between tactile sensation (tapping the skin with a wire at 2Hz) versus AP using a manual stimulation technique. The acupuncture stimulation used in this study involved twisting the needle at 2Hz in LI4 (a point in the first dorsal interosseous muscle of the hand). Stimulation of an acupuncture point in this manner produces a *deqi* sensation, which is a full, aching feeling at the point of the needle and is believed to be important in obtaining the clinical effect with AP. The results of unilateral AP showed bilateral neural modulation of cortical and subcortical structures. The primary action was to decrease signal intensity in the limbic region and other subcortical areas. Tactile stimulation did not produce these changes in fMRI. In addition, if the needle was placed in the point and left at rest, or placed just subcutaneously and not in the muscle, fMRI signal decrease in these deep subcortical structures was not seen. This suggests that the response of the organism to AP depends on activation of the muscle sensory afferents and not the superficial afferents in the skin.[7]

Evidence for point specificity has also been obtained in a recent study by Cho et al.[8] An acupuncture point on the lateral aspect of the small toe, Bladder 67 (B67), which is known as an influential point for vision, was stimulated and observed to cause increased fMRI activity in the occipital lobes in 12 subjects. Stimulation of the eyes directly with light caused a similar activation, whereas stimulation of a sham acupuncture point 2 to 5 cm away from B67 failed to cause occipital lobe activation.

Both of these studies are preliminary, however; they suggest that the grid of acupuncture points that has evolved over the last 2000 years may indeed represent a network of nodes in the peripheral nervous system that have profound and specific effects on modulating and regulating the activity of the central nervous system.

Neuromodulation Data

It is still an open question whether acupuncture has an influence on pain and other disease states that goes beyond the direct effect of the chemical releases previously mentioned. The early data using fMRI suggest that the sensory stimulation provided by acupuncture may have direct and selective effects on CNS function. Although the demonstration that endogenous opioids can be consistently released in both animal and human experimental models has been an important step in verifying that acupuncture analgesia has a physiologic basis, there continues to be debate about whether this effect is sufficient to explain the observed clinical benefits. One of the problems is that such humoral effects are nonspecific and short-lived and cannot explain why certain treatment methods for particular conditions would have a sustained or permanent disease-modifying result. The chemical releases observed with EA and AP may just be an epiphenomenon, indicating that there is an influence on the CNS without yet comprehending what the actual changes are. Table 78-1 lists the problems with our current understanding of acupuncture analgesia.

To give just one example of how the neurohumoral model fails to fully comprehend the clinical effect of AP, there is a recently published study using heat stimulation (moxabustion) of an acupuncture point on the fifth toe (B67) to turn breech babies after the 33rd week of pregnancy. The results of the study were profound, showing a significantly improved turning of the infants to the cephalic position at delivery compared with the control group. Of 130 fetuses in the intervention group, 98 (75.4%) were cephalic, compared with 62 (47.7%) of 130 fetuses in the control group ($P <$ .001; relative risk = 1.58; 95% CI, 1.29–1.94).[9]

One theory that may help to better explain the long-term effect of EA and AP is that by stimulating peripheral sensory afferents of the skin and muscle, sustained changes occur in the CNS through central neuromodulation. We are now just beginning to understand the basic mechanisms of pathologic neuromodulation that can lead to chronic pain. A fundamental concept that has emerged is that sustained nociceptive input can have profound effects on the CNS that cause adverse neuroplastic changes.[10] Interestingly, continuing along this line of argument, unlike transcutaneous electrical nerve stimulation (TENS), AP and EA do rely on a more "painful stimulation" of the peripheral nervous system.[11] In effect then, through controlled stimulation of peripheral nociceptors, acupuncture may be causing a *reverse neuroplasticity* in the CNS.

A clue to the neuroplastic changes that may be occurring in the CNS with EP and AP can be found in the literature looking at

TABLE 78-1 **Humoral Theories and Problems Associated with Acupuncture Analgesia**

Humoral Theory of Acupuncture Analgesia	Problems
Endogenous opioid effect	Humoral effect short-lived.
Mid-brain monoamines	Fails to explain importance of point selection and meridians.
Pituitary–hypothalamic–axis	Fails to explain disease modification and sustained analgesia obtained with acupuncture.
	Difficult to implement theory to explain effects on other nonpain-related conditions such as stroke.
	Fails to capture neuromodulating effects of acupuncture.

c-fos expression. The production of the *fos* protein in spinal cord and cerebral neurons is known to occur with painful peripheral nerve stimulation and can act as a guide to the location of neurons that have been activated by this noxious input. It is believed that the observed *c-fos* release in the CNS couples transient intracellular signals to long-term changes in the central processing of peripheral sensory input and heralds the initiation of adverse neuroplastic changes in response to nociceptive input.[12]

We now know that EP causes the expression of *c-fos* in certain cells of the CNS, but in cells that are different than those that express *c-fos* with noxious input.[13] In addition, EA has been shown to suppress *fos* expression in the spinal cord dorsal horn in response to mechanical noxious stimulation.[14] This early data with animal models suggest that some form of reverse neuroplasticity is taking place with acupuncture stimulation.

Another approach to studying the neuromodulatory effect of peripheral nerve stimulation with acupuncture on the CNS utilizes somatosensory-evoked potentials (SEP). The most fruitful of this method is the pain SEP, which is the evoked potential generated when recording over the skull with painful stimulation in the periphery. Dental pulp stimulation is the most reliable model for this technique. In a recent review, Xu presents strong arguments to suggest that AP and EA have a suppressive effect on pain SEPs and that this effect is point-specific, in that stimulation of points on unrelated meridians fail to provide a suppressive effect on the pain SEP. This argues against a purely neurohumoral acupuncture effect since one would expect that if suppression of the pain SEP depended only on the release of endogenous neuropeptides then any point would do, and that meridian-specific points would not be superior in efficacy.[15]

CORRESPONDENCE TO MYOFASCIAL TRIGGER POINTS

The previous section shows how basic research in acupuncture intersects with the current thrust of the work being done in understanding the physiology of pain. In addition, there is some evidence to suggest that EA and AP depend on stimulation of muscle sensory afferents. On the clinical side, the techniques developed for trigger-point injections and our understanding of their mechanisms of action are relevant to acupuncture techniques. Early on, Melzack demonstrated the high degree of point correlation between myofascial trigger points and acupuncture points. Recently, a connection between myofascial pain and acupuncture has been laid out in terms more relevant to practitioners of acupuncture[16,17] (Table 78-2 and Fig. 78-2).

Andersson has also recently proposed that the key element underlying the physiologic effect of AP and EA is the sensory stimulation of the low- and high-threshold mechanoreceptors in muscle tissue, which occurs with trigger-point injection methods as well.[18] One can theorize that needle stimulation of the skin afferents tends to elicit a protective pain reflex that has as its main evolutionary goal to withdraw from danger. In contrast, needle stimulation of deeper afferents in muscle and tendons, which are not normally involved in these protective reflexes, elicits a pain in-

TABLE 78-2 **Acupuncture and Myofascial Trigger Point Correlations**

Acupuncture Zone	Region of Body	Acupupoints	Muscles
Tai Yang	Dorsal Zone: Frontal region of forehead to occiput down black to lateral ankles.	B 10 SI 9–14 B 11–25, 41–45 B 53, 54 B 31, 34	Suboccipital Scapular muscles Thoracic and lumbar Paraspinals Gluteus medius Piriformis
Shao Yang	Lateral Zone: Temporalis region of head to lateral arm to wrist extensors. Down flank to lateral aspect of leg.	GB 3–6, 8 GB 16 GB 20, 21 TH 9 GB 24–28 GB 29 GB 31	Temporalis Sternocleidomastoid and scalenes Upper trapezius Finger extensors Abdominal obliques Tensor fasciae latae Iliotibial band
Yang Ming	Ventral Zone: Mouth to anterior neck, anterior chest wall down abdomen to medial aspect of leg and foot	ST 5–7 St 9,10 ST 14–18 ST 19–30 ST 31,32	Masseter Sternocleidomastoid Pectoral muscles Rectus abdominis Quadraceps muscles

Abbreviations: bladder (B); gallbladder (GB); small intestine (SI); triple heater (TH); and stomach (ST).

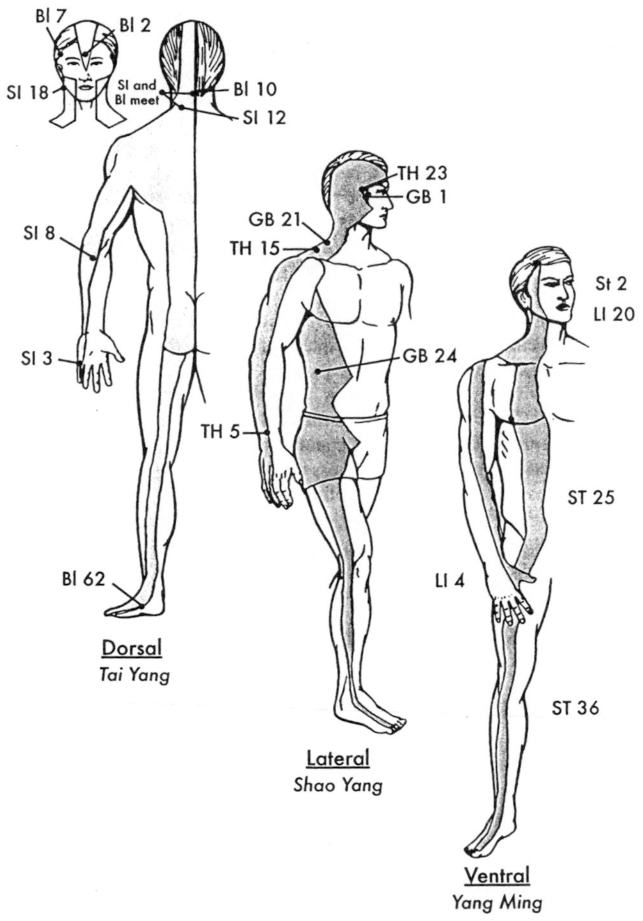

Figure 78-2 The Yang cutaneous zones are composed of the tendinomuscular, divergent, luo and regular meridians of the regions diagramed. These zones act much like myofascial maps of muscular dysfunction and help organize both diagnosis and treatment of pain syndromes. (From Seem M. Used with permission.)

hibitory rather than a pain-withdrawal reflex. Andersson makes the point that sustained, physical activity such as running also stimulates these muscle afferents, and many of the physiologic benefits of exercise might be related to the activation of the same mechanoreceptors that are stimulated with EA and AP.

Stimulation of the muscle mechanoreceptors also has distant effects on muscle tone that is not seen with cutaneous sensory stimulation. To illustrate this, EA of Large Intestine 4 and 11 (points in the first dorsal interosseous and extensor digitorum communis [EDC] muscles, respectively) has been shown to suppress the contralateral stretch reflex in the EDC, whereas painful subcutaneous stimulation in the same location had no effect.[19]

In a recent review, there have been a number of clinical trials showing that trigger-point injections and dry needling have similar efficacy, and that the type of solution injected into the trigger point is irrelevant to clinical outcome. This suggests that the most important factor in relieving the pain associated with a trigger point is the needle stimulation of the muscle sensory afferents.[20] This is supported by many of the physiologic studies of EA and AP, in which the effect was only achieved when the needle stimulation occurred in the muscle underlying the acupuncture point, again showing the convergence of clinical experience with the work on myofascial trigger-point needling.

CLINICAL RESEARCH

An exhaustive review of the acupuncture literature was performed by a panel of experts convened by NIH and their findings were published in the November 1998 edition of *JAMA*.[1] The conclusions of the review reveal that for many of the common pain conditions such as back pain, tendinitis, arthritis, headaches, and neuropathic pain, better designed studies are needed to determine scientific efficacy. A series of meta-analyses have been published by Ernst on the effect of acupuncture for the treatment of back pain, osteoarthitis and neck pain. The conclusions were similar in all cases, that in the studies that were deemed to be well-designed randomized controlled trials, acupuncture was often better than control treatments but inconsistently better than sham acupuncture treatments.[21–23] All of the studies reviewed suffered in general from small patient numbers, inconsistent use of outcome measures, and widely variable treatment strategies. Each of these methodologic problems makes it difficult to draw strong generalizations from these meta-analyses.

After reviewing data from controlled studies in which sham acupuncture was used as the control (deeply inserted needles into nonclassic locations), Lewith has proposed that these sham locations for needle insertions are not altogether inert. It is likely that sham points that are not traditionally considered true acupuncture points have some efficacy, and he estimated that there is an analgesic effect from sham point stimulation in 40% to 50% of patients in comparison to an effectiveness in 60% of patients for true acupuncture point stimulation. To sort out the relative benefits of deep-needle stimulation in classic points versus sham points, large numbers would be needed to avoid a type II statistical error (i.e., failure to reject the null hypothesis). In comparison, trials of acupuncture in which either minimal acupuncture (i.e., superficially placed needles in nonclassical locations) or mock TENS was used as a control treatment, the relative success of true acupuncture is much greater.[24] With new funding sources from the National Center for Complementary and Alternative Medicine at NIH, acupuncture research over the next decade should provide more answers to both the methodologic and clinical questions that are still largely unanswered.

There have been a number of recent clinical studies of improved methodologic quality that are suggestive of clinical efficacy. For example, in a recent review of a technique of EP called *percutaneous electrical nerve stimulation* (PENS), the authors summarize significant findings in the treatment of acute herpetic neuralgia, pain from bony metastases, migraine headaches after electroconvulsive therapy, chronic low back pain, and lumbar radiculopathy. These findings suggest that this technique can have lasting profound effects on difficult pain syndromes that allowed improved function and a reduction in the use of analgesic medications.[25]

TREATMENT PRINCIPLES

There are a number of different treatment styles of acupuncture that have influenced the practice of acupuncture in the United

States. Many of these styles herald back to pre-revolution medical traditions that were prevalent in China prior to Mao and had been exported to other Far East countries. One method commonly practiced in this country is called *acupuncture energetics*. This technique evolved in Europe based on interpretations of the classic Chinese texts and was influenced by the Vietnamese in France. With this approach, point selection for pain is governed by the pattern of pain and symptoms presented by the patient and involve palpation of the areas of pain, much as one would do for assessing the location of trigger points. Japanese techniques rely heavily on palpation of soft tissue as well, with the exception that the needling technique is not as deep, and often there is no attempt to elicit the *deqi* response.

Post-revolutions styles of traditional Chinese medicine are heavily influenced by herbal treatment strategies. During the communist revolution in China, an attempt was made to make acupuncture more systematic and uniform in technique and point location. This led to the use of diagnostic techniques developed by herbalist because it was felt by Mao at the time to be more scientific.[26] An attempt is made to diagnose the state of balance of the internal organs by asking general questions and using pulse and tongue diagnosis. Palpation of the soft tissues is less common and point selection is often directed at bringing the general state of health back into homeostasis rather than focusing on the specific local complaints of pain.

Percutaneous electrical nerve stimulation was developed in the United States and Canada. The treatment strategies are based on a neuroanatomic assessment of the pain generator rather than on traditional acupuncture theories. The pattern of pain is viewed and interpreted on the basis of which spinal segments are involved, and then EA is done along those segments (Figure 78-3).

There are numerous other treatment techniques including Korean four-needle technique, where only four needles are placed regardless of the presenting condition, and Korean hand acupuncture that represents the whole body with extra points found in the hand. Auricular acupuncture is a more widely spread treatment technique that also takes a small part of the body—the ear—and represents the whole body in that region. A special aspect of this treatment method involves the use of a point localizer that is essentially an impedance meter.[27]

Unfortunately, there is no clinical research at this time to help guide treatment type or style for particular clinical conditions. From personal clinical experience, however, failure of one techniques for a particular condition does not always imply total acupuncture failure, and there is some value in trying a few treatment techniques before labeling the acupuncture ineffective for the condition. In addition, although compared to many medical interventions, acupuncture is relatively safe, there are still some serious adverse affects that have been reported, including serious infections, vascular injury, and pneumothorax that require proper precautions to prevent.[28]

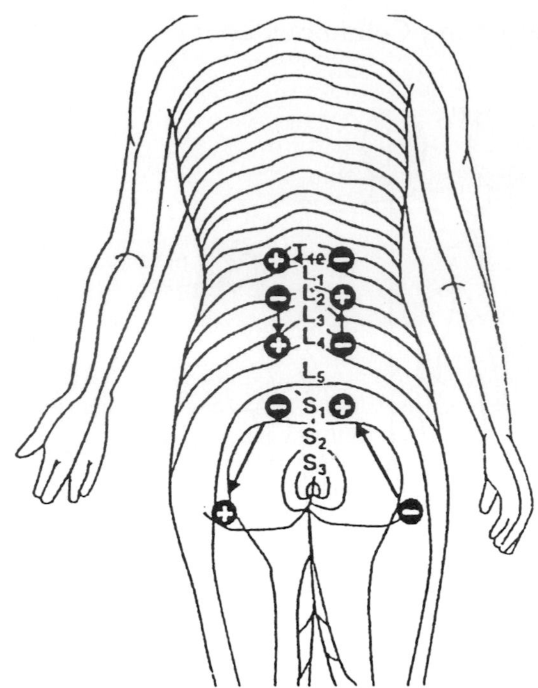

With PENS therapy, each of the five bipolar electrical stimulating leads is connected to a pair of needles, alternating the positive (+) and negative (-) positions as shown in the illustration.

Figure 78-3 Typical PENS montage used to treat low back pain organized along the dermatomes of the area of pain. (From White AR et al. Percutaneous electrical nerve stimulation: a promising alternative-medicine approach to pain management. APS Bulletin 1999; March/April:3–5. Used with permission.)

TRAINING OPTIONS

The accreditation of acupuncture educational programs is directed by the Accreditation Commission of Acupuncture and Oriental Medicine (ACAOM), formerly called the National Accreditation Commission for Schools and Colleges of Acupuncture and Oriental Medicine. The organization that credentials nonphysicians to practice acupuncture in the United States is the National Certification Commission of Acupuncture and Oriental Medicine (NCCA). The NCCA requires that candidates complete 1725 hours of formal didactics and 500 hours of clinical training in acupuncture. Candidates who meet these requirements are then eligible to sit for a national written and practical examination administered biannually. Despite these national standards, the actual practice of acupuncture is still further regulated by each individual state. Currently, 33 states and the District of Columbia license acupuncturist and most of these follow the NCCA guidelines for nonphysicians.

The regulation of the practice of acupuncture by physicians and dentists also varies from state to state. As of 1999, 35 states permit physicians to practice acupuncture within the current scope of their license without requiring additional training. There are eight states that do require some additional training and certification (anywhere from 100 to 300 hours depending on the state). Four states do not permit physicians to practice acupuncture within the scope of their license without the full training that nonphysicians are required to take (Hawaii, Montana, Rhode Island, and Vermont).[29]

For full membership in the American Academy of Medical Acupuncturists (AAMA), individuals must have an active MD or

DO license (or equivalent) to practice medicine under US or Canadian jurisdiction, have completed a minimum of 220 hours of formal training in medical acupuncture (120 hours didactic, 100 hours clinical), and have 2 years of experience practicing medical acupuncture. Currently, most physicians are able to satisfy the educational and clinical requirements demanded by any state except the four previously mentioned by completing the training offered by the Office of Continuing Medical Education at the University of California–Los Angeles (UCLA). Harvard Medical School, through the Department of Anesthesiology at Beth Israel Deaconess Medical Center, is now also offering a 300-hour course in medical acupuncture that would satisfy both the AAMA requirements and most state requirements to practice acupuncture.

The federal Health Care Financing Administration (HCFA), which is responsible with administering the Medicare program, currently denies coverage for acupuncture pending establishment of the scientific efficacy of this modality. With a showing of such efficacy, HCFA may consider acupuncture as a "reasonable and necessary" service, at which time coverage would be authorized under the federal Social Security Act 37.

CONCLUSIONS

As we move into the 21st century, the future of acupuncture for the treatment of pain is secure but still in need of better scientific validation. Acupuncture in many ways is out in front in the race to gain general scientific approval in comparison with other complementary and alternative treatment modalities. This is demonstrated by literature reviews and acceptance into many traditional western medical hospital settings. But as the older sister of a much greater family of holistic treatments, great responsibility still lies on those who are involved in this field and on those who will become involved in the future to help tear away the shroud of mystery that still clouds our view of this 2000-year-old treatment modality.

REFERENCES

1. NIH Consensus Conference. Acupuncture. *JAMA* 1998;280:1518–1524.
2. Hsu DT. Acupuncture: a review. *Reg Anesth* 1996;21:361–370.
3. Pomeranz B, Chiu D. Naloxone blockade of acupuncture analgesia: endorphins implicated. *Life Sci* 1976;19:1757.
4. Mayer DJ, Price DD, Raffii A. Antagonism of acupuncture analgesia in man by narcotic antagonist naloxone. *Brain Res* 1977;121:368.
5. Debreceni L. Chemical releases associated with acupuncture and electric stimulation. *Crit Rev Phys Rehab Med* 1993;5:247–275.
6. Pomeranz B. Scientific basis of acupuncture. In: Stux G, Pomeranz B, eds. *Basics of Acupuncture*. 2nd ed. Berlin, Germany: Springer-Verlag; 1991.
7. Hui KK, Liu J, Makris N, et al. Acupuncture modulates the limbic system and subcortical gray structures of the human brain: evidence from fMRI studies in normal subjects. *Hum Brain Mapp.* 2000;9:13–25.
8. Cho ZH, Chung SC, Jones JP, et al. New findings of the correlation between acupoints and corresponding brain cortices using functional MRI. *Proc Natl Acad Sci U S A* 1998;95:2670–2673.
9. Cardini F, Weixin H . Moxibustion for correction of breech presentation: a randomized controlled trial. *JAMA* 1998;280:1580–1584.
10. Woolf CJ, Salter MW. Neuronal plasticity: increasing the gain in pain. *Science* 2000;9:1765–1769.
11. Woolf CJ, Thompson JW. Stimulation induced analgesic: transcutaneous electrical nerve stimulation (TENS) and vibration. In: Wall PD, Melzack R, eds. *Textbook of Pain*. 3rd ed. London, England: Churchill Livingstone, 1994.
12. Morgan JI, Curran T. Stimulus-transcription coupling in the nervous system: involvement of the inducible proto-oncogenes *fos* and *jun*. *Ann Rev Neurosci* 1991;14:421–451.
13. Pan B, Castro-Lopes JM, Coimbra A. C-fos expression in the hypothalamo-pituitary system induced by electroacupuncture or noxious stimulation. *Neuroreport* 1994;5:1649–1652.
14. Lee JH, Beitz AJ. The distribution of brain-stem and spinal cord nuclei associated with different frequencies of electroacupuncture analgesia. *Pain* 1993;52:11–28.
15. Xu X, Shibasaki H, Shindo K. Effects of acupuncture on somatosensory evoked potentials: a review. *J Clin Neurophysiol.* 1993;10:370–377.
16. Seem M. *A new American Acupuncture: Acupuncture Osteopathy, the Myofascial Release of the Bodymind Holding Patterns.* Boulder, Colorado: Blue Poppy Press; 1993.
17. Seem M. *Acupuncture Physical Medicine: An Acupuncture Touchpoint Approach to the Treatment of Chronic Fatigue, Pain and Stress Disorders.* Boulder, Colorodo: Blue Poppy Press; 2000.
18. Andersson S. The functional background in acupuncture effects. *Scand J Rehab Med,* Suppl 1993;29:31–60.
19. Milne RJ, Dawson NJ, Butler MJ, Lippold OC. Intramuscular acupuncture-like electrical stimulation inhibits stretch reflexes in contralateral finger extensor muscles. *Exp Neurol* 1985;90:96–107.
20. Han S. Myofascial pain syndrome and trigger-point management. *Reg Anesth* 1997;22:89.
21. Ernst E, White AR. Acupuncture for back pain. *Arch Intern Med* 1998;158:2235–2241.
22. Ernst E. Acupuncture as a symptomatic treatment of osteoarthritis. *Scand J Rheumatol* 1997;26:444–447.
23. White AR, Ernst E. A systematic review of randomized controlled trials of acupuncture for neck pain. *Rheumatology* 1999;38:143–147.
24. Lewith G, Vincent C. Evaluation of the clinical effects of acupuncture: a problem reassessed and a framework for future research. *Pain Forum* 1995;4:29–39.
25. White PF, Phillips J, Proctor TJ, Craig WF. Percutaneous electrical nerve stimulation: a promising alternative-medicine approach to pain management. *APS Bull* 1999;March/April:3–5.
26. Andrews BJ. Acupuncture and the reinvention of Chinese medicine. *APS Bull* 1999;May/June:13–15.
27. Saku K, Mukaino Y, Ying H, Arakawa K. Characteristics of reactive electropermeable points on the auricles of coronary heart disease patients. *Clin Cardiol* 1993;16:415–419.
28. Ernst E, White AR. Acupuncture may be associated with serious adverse events. *BMJ* 2000;320:513.
29. Leake R, Broderick JE. Current licensure for acupuncture in the United States. *Altern Ther* 1999;5(4):94–96.

CHAPTER 79 PHYSICAL MEDICINE AND REHABILITATION

Donna Schramm-Bloodworth and Martin Grabois

This chapter focuses on physical therapeutics and their prescription to treat diagnoses with a significant symptom of pain. However, physical medicine and rehabilitation professionals attend or administer to persons with a wide variety of diagnoses, and they practice with a variety of allied health professions. To apprise professional services that the specialty of physical medicine and rehabilitation can offer a patient, this chapter opens with a synopsis of rehabilitation philosophy, methods, and goals. Antecedent to discussing this specialty as it applies to pain, the chapter references current review works that define the types of exercise and modalities. The chapter concludes by addressing specific diagnoses and referencing the current literature that guides the physical medicine and rehabilitation prescription.

THE SCOPE AND PHILOSOPHY OF PHYSICAL MEDICINE AND REHABILITATION

The field of physical medicine and rehabilitation spans the settings of inpatient, outpatient, and home health medicine. The philosophy of physical medicine and rehabilitation embraces an intradisciplinary approach to patient care, with not only the patient and physician working toward the patient's recovery but also a team of allied health care professionals. This team includes physical, occupational, and speech therapists, social workers, nurses, pharmacists, psychologists, recreational therapists, and vocational specialists.

The goal of physical medicine and rehabilitation interventions is the improved function of the patient, despite the presence of permanent disease or impairment. Physical medicine and rehabilitation teams treat a spectrum of diagnoses referred from medical, surgical, pediatric, and traumatic specialties. The severity and complexity of diagnoses varies from catastrophic entities such as spinal cord injury and stroke to routine soft tissue injuries, for example, shoulder impingement and shin splints. With more complex disease entities in which tissue loss or tissue death has occurred (e.g., amputation or traumatic brain injury), successful physical medicine and rehabilitation intervention compensates for impairment rather than resolves or cures the disease process.

For diagnoses with soft tissue injury (e.g., ankle sprain and shoulder impingement), physical medicine and rehabilitation interventions promote soft tissue healing. For all levels of injury, physical medicine and rehabilitation interventions aim, however, to restore function and prevent recurrent injury. Physical medicine and rehabilitation uses a team treatment approach to restore function to patients with soft tissue injury or permanent tissue loss. Tools of the field include exercise, thermal and electrical modalities, as well as education and new learning.

PHYSICAL MEDICINE AND REHABILITATION AND SPECIFIC APPLICATIONS TO PAIN TREATMENT

Except in the case of chronic pain syndrome where pain and dysfunctional behavior in response to the pain have become the impairment and disease,[1] pain is a symptom of a disease process or tissue injury. This chapter discusses the physical medicine and rehabilitation interventions for diagnoses in which pain is a complaint or symptom; these interventions involve straightforward, applied progressive exercise and education.

For the treatment of the soft tissue injuries in patients who have pain, the physician prescribes physical therapeutics, which a physical or occupational therapist administers. The treatment and improvement of the symptom of pain generally cannot be separated from the treatment and improvement of the disease process. This chapter cites available literature that notes the molecular and cellular mechanisms whereby exercise and thermal and electrical modalities may relieve pain. Physical therapeutics, which lessen pain and remedy soft tissue injury, include exercise, education, and thermal and electrical applications.

The Physical Medicine and Rehabilitation Script

The physical therapeutics at the physician's disposal for the treatment of pain and its associated soft tissue injury include stretch, range of motion, strengthening, endurance exercise, and aquatic therapy; positioning, bracing and assistive devices; transcutaneous electrical stimulation, and superficial and deep heat, and superficial cold; and learned strategies to prevent injury or simplify work (Table 79-1). When writing a prescription for soft tissue injury and pain, it is helpful to include these headings to ensure a complete script. Additional components of a prescription for physical or occupational therapy include the patient's name and contact information, the patient's diagnosis, precautions about comorbid disease processes, and goals of the treatment intervention (Fig. 79-1).

The components of exercise and thermal and electrical modalities have definitions and specific applications. When prescribing physical medicine interventions for painful conditions, the physician who trains himself to write specifically for stretch, strengthening, endurance activity, education, assistive devices and splints, and modalities should generate a complete and useful script. The following sections describe the techniques, physiology, and effects of physical therapeutics.

TABLE 79-1 **Physical Therapeutics Useful in the Treatment of Pain**

- Stretch
- Exercise
  - Strengthening
    - Isometric
    - Isotonic
      - Concentric
      - Eccentric
    - Isokinetic
  - Endurance (Aerobic)
    - Aquatic Therapy
- Modalities
  - Thermal
    - Superficial Heat
      - Hot Packs
      - Paraffin
      - Heat Lamps
    - Deep Heat
      - Ultrasound
    - Superficial Cold
      - Ice Massage
      - Ice Packs
      - Spray and Stretch
  - Electrical
    - TENS
- Bracing
  - Resting
  - Functional
- Assistive Devices
  - Mobility
  - Activities of Daily Living
- Patient Education
  - Work Simplification
  - Energy Conservation
  - Joint Conservation
  - Back Conservation

Patient's name:
Patient's contact information:

Patient's Diagnosis or impairment:
Treating discipline (OT/PT)
Precautions: (Examples: post-operative restrictions, co-morbidities)
Goals of treatment:

Stretch:
Strengthening:
Endurance:
Modalities:
Assistive devices:
Patient education:

Physician:
Follow-up interval:
Physician's contact information:

Figure 79-1 Components of a Physical Therapeutics Script

PHYSICAL THERAPEUTICS

Stretch

Stretch and flexibility are the first steps in an exercise program. Flexibility is "the ability to move a joint smoothly throughout a full range of motion."[2] Muscles, fascia, tendons, ligaments, adipose tissue, and the joint capsule affect flexibility.[3] Under normal conditions muscles and tendons and the joint capsule are the structures that most limit flexibility, but neurologic conditions with hypertonicity, and excessive adipose, when present, can also limit flexibility.[2,3]

Patients take flexibility for granted; however, stretches should comprise the initial activity in an exercise program. Participation in regular exercise without stretching does not imply that the individual is limber. It is noted that long-distance runners who do not regularly stretch have poor flexibility[3] and stretching prevents soft tissue injury.[2]

The therapist instructs clients in two types of stretch techniques: static stretch or contract-and-relax techniques.[2] The individual performs static stretch by slowly stretching the muscle to the point of discomfort and holding that position for 60 seconds.[2] Therapists utilize this technique of stretch in the first few days after injury.[2] Individuals without acute soft tissue injuries can perform contract-and-relax techniques, in which the individual maximally contracts the muscle for 10 seconds and then releases the contraction into a slow stretch while contracting the antagonist muscle group.[2] Slow, mild stretching over minutes is more beneficial than short, rapid stretches.[4] The application of heat to a joint before stretching, via ultrasound for large joints, and paraffin dips for small foot and hand joints, increases soft tissue distensibility and may be part of a script for flexibility.[3] A good review of stretches with pictured demonstrations are noted in Tollison's review article.[5]

There are special patient populations to consider when prescribing flexibility exercises. The immobile individual should receive daily range-of-motion exercises with sustained stretch at end range from a trained caregiver.[4] Range should be done over all joint groups and may conveniently accompany bathing activity. Splinting provides prolonged mild stretch and should be used on joints at high risk for functional restriction, for example, the hands, wrist, and forefoot and ankles.[4] Patients at particular risk include those with upper motor neuron lesions that result in spasticity (e.g., stroke and spinal cord injury) and patients with burns.

Caregivers and individuals should perform stretching and range of motion with caution in osteoporotic individuals since inadvertent fractures are possible. The presence of fracture, new skin grafts, and new subcutaneous lines or wires preclude stretch and range of motion. The adjuvent use of deep and superficial heat is contraindicated in the presence of low or absent sensation because burns occur. Fixed-joint contractures or heterotopic bone and myositis ossificans also preclude stretch, and orthopedic remedies should be investigated. An individual using a splint or the caregiver should, after 30 minutes of use, inspect the underlying skin for pressure areas, that is, areas of blanching redness; if redness is found, discontinue splint use until the splint can be adjusted.

Assisted range of motion, another form of stretching, is when the individual or a caregiver helps move a weakened limb through its full range of motion. The individual may use the strong contralateral limb to assist movement of the weak or painful ipsilateral limb as in stroke, where a patient interlaces the fingers and raises the weak and strong limbs overhead. After knee replacement, therapists teach patients to assist extension of the operated knee by crossing the intact ankle under the ankle of the operated side, and straightening the strong and operated knee together. Devices may assist range of motion. For example, in bicipital tendonitis, the patient learns to use an overhead pully to extend the range of the painful shoulder.

Physiologically, stretching has many effects. In animal models, cyclic stretching of animal muscle–tendon units demonstrates decreased peak muscle tension and increased muscle relaxation and increased muscle length.[6] During a cycle of 10 stretches, performed over 30 seconds, decreased muscle tension and increased length occurred primarily within the first four stretch cycles and most muscle relaxation occurred during the first 12 to 18 seconds of the 30-second cycle.[6] By contrast, in human models with a diagnosis of short or "tight" hamstrings, Halbertsma demonstrates no change in the length or elasticity of hamstrings with applied stretch, but rather increased tolerance of stretching applications.[7] Extrapolating these results to human patients, the prescriber will recommend that regional stretches occur over 20 to 30 seconds and for four to five repetitions (Fig. 79-4). Another benefit of the slowly performed stretch is that a technique which slowly stretches a muscle imposes less force on the muscle than a rapidly performed stretch.

As regards human subjects, the literature describes pain relief as well as physiologic benefit of stretching. Khalil et al describe systematic stretching applied to low back pain patients by a physical therapist.[8] These stretches include the regions of the lumbar paraspinals (Figure 79-2), the quadratus lumborum, the tensor fascia lata, the hamstrings (Figure 79-3), and the obliques. Significant benefits to the patient with low back pain included increased strength of muscle, increased maximal effort exerted, and decreased regional pain. These benefits, including pain relief, occurred in 2 weeks with the application of stretch twice a week.

Stretch
- Intensity: Slow
- Duration: Stretch over thirty seconds
- For three to five repetitions

Strengthening
- Intensity: Lift weights of medium to relatively high weight to the point of muscle fatigue
- Frequency: Three times per week
- When a weight can be easily lifted 15 to 20 times increase the weight by ten percent

Endurance
- Biking, swimming, jogging, stair-stepping, cross-country skiing
- Duration and frequency: 15 to 60 minutes, 3 to 5 times per week
- Intensity: to drive heart rate to 60 to 85% of age predicted maximum

Figure 79-2 Brief techniques and durations for stretch, strengthening and endurance activity.

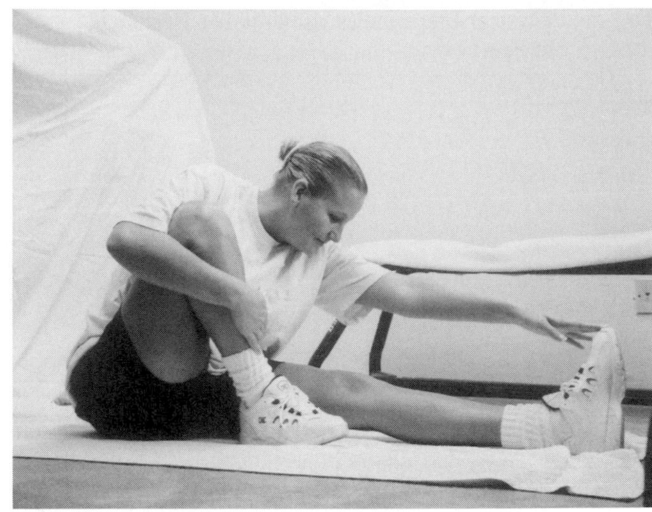

Figure 79-3 Hamstring stretch with one knee straight and one bent while reaching toward toes.

Lewit studied 244 patients with over 300 myalgic areas in a prospective but uncontrolled study.[9] Applied immediately after isometric contractions of the sore muscle, stretch provided immediate pain relief for 95% of patients.[9] To perform this technique Lewit describes first stretching the muscle passively to the point of pain and then contracting the muscle isometrically for 10 seconds and then releasing the contraction.[9] The patient is instructed to deep breathe and exhale during the release, at which time the therapist further stretches the muscle; however, the muscle is only stretched at the rate that is felt to relax and the therapist does not apply force.[9]

Strengthening

Often when the physician proposes an exercise program, the patient will state that he or she is busy all day and gets plenty of ex-

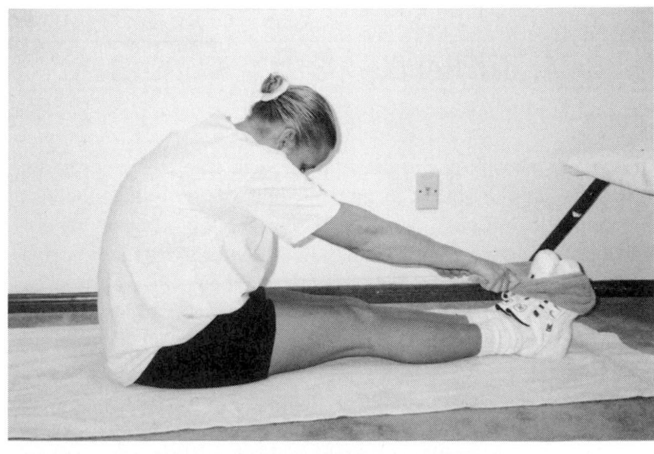

Figure 79-4 Lumbar stretch with knees straight reaching toward toes.

ercise. The literature supports intensified exercise efforts and makes clear that mundane activity does not result in adequate flexibility,[3] strength, endurance, or bone density.[10] Pollock writes that "strength refers to the ability of the muscle or muscle group to apply force. Typically, strength is defined relative to the maximal force–producing capability of a muscle."[3]

Scientists define strength as the maximal force a muscle group can generate in a single isometric contraction of unlimited duration.[3] There are three types of muscle contractions and three types of strength training: isometric, isotonic, and isokinetic. Isometric contraction, that is, where the length of the muscle does not change but is set at one length, does not have as many applications in daily activity as isotonic contraction and strength. During an isotonic contraction the muscle contracts through all or part of its normal range of motion while lifting a constant amount of weight. The classic biceps curl with a dumbbell is an isotonic example. There are two types of isotonic contractions: shortening (i.e., concentric, contractions) and lengthening (i.e., eccentric, contractions). Lastly, there are isokinetic contractions, in which the muscle contracts against a fixed torque. Many of the fixed-axis machines in exercise clubs strengthen isokinetically.

Practical examples help illustrate the difference between isometric, isotonic, and isokinetic contractions. We use isometric contractions of the finger flexors to grasp and hold a can of soda, but then we use an isotonic contraction of the biceps to lift the soda to the mouth. When lifting the can of soda to the mouth, a concentric, or shortening, isotonic contraction of the bicep occurs; when we return the can of soda to the table, it is not a passive activity of the bicep, but actually the biceps contracts eccentrically, or in a lengthening fashion, to slowly lower the can of soda in a controlled fashion to the table. If the biceps did not eccentrically control the descent of the can, it would simply slam to the table because of gravity. Isokinetic contractions do not have many practical examples. We perform an isokinetic contraction when trying to push closed a door that is on a hydraulic governor.

Strength training improves the force production of a group of muscles by any of the following mechanisms: an increase in the number of motor units activated, an increase in the rate of activation, an increase in the synchronization of motor units firing, or the hypertrophy of muscle fibers.[3,11] In the first 2 to 3 weeks of a strength-training program, strength improvements result from the synchronization of neural firing.[11] With continued strength training after 3 weeks, hypertrophy of muscle fibers causes increased force production by the muscle.

Progressive resistive training, *performed to fatigue*, strengthens muscles. DeLorme described progressive resistive training based on a 10 repetition maximum (RM), that is, the maximal amount of weight that a trainee could move 10 times through a muscle's full range of motion.[11] Following DeLorme's method, the trainee perform 10 repetitions of 10% of the 10 RM weight, followed by 10 repetitions of 20% of the 10 RM weight, followed by 10 repetitions of 30% of the 10 RM weight, and so forth, up to 10 repetitions of the full 10 RM weight. The trainee performed this regimen three to five times per week. Once a week, the new 10-repetition maximum weight for each muscle group is determined. This training method requires a large amount of time if multiple muscle groups are to be trained, and revisions of this original progressive resistive-training method exist.

Braddom's test describes an effective strength training technique in which the trainee finds a relatively high weight, one that can be lifted three to five times before fatigue or muscle failure ensues.[11] The trainee exercises each muscle group with its three to five maximal repetition weight two to three times per week; in each session the trainee lifts weights to the point of fatigue for each muscle group trained. When the trainee can lift a maximal weight 15 or more times, the weight is increased 10% (see Fig. 79-4). Usually a weight increase is indicated about every 7 to 14 days. The most important concept in strengthening is that the amount of weight lifted, very high or only moderate, is not important as long as the muscle group is exercised to the point of fatigue.[11] Using relatively lower weights to train will require more repetitions to achieve fatigue. Hickson writes that weight training of the legs to fatigue 5 days per week increased strength 40% in ten weeks.[12]

Contraindications and precautions for strength training do exist. Strengthening exercise is contraindicated in the presence of fracture; the orthopedic surgeon should prescribe the permitted activity and denote prohibited activity for a fractured limb and the contiguous joints. Strengthening exercise acutely increases blood pressure, and this vital sign needs to be monitored in patients with significant hypertension. Persons should have a "spotter" or partner when performing strengthening exercises, especially with free weights. Strengthening exercises are contraindicated in the presence of acute or unstable cardiopulmonary disease.

As noted earlier, muscle contracts in isometric, isotonic, or isokinetic fashion. Likewise, strength training, using free weights or weight machines, may be isometric, isotonic, or isokinetic. Strengthening occurs initially by neuromuscular integration and then by muscle hypertrophy. Strengthening occurs as long as exercise continues to the point of fatigue.

Endurance

The DeLorme axion states that "high weight, low repetition exercise programs build strength and low weight, high repetition exercise programs build endurance."[11] Endurance is the time that a person can maintain either a static force or a power level involving a combination of concentric and eccentric muscle actions.[2] Endurance is also defined as "the ability to continue a prescribed task in the desired manner."[11] Endurance (i.e., aerobic) exercise involves the rapidly alternating contraction of large muscle groups at low resistance for a sustained period. Examples of endurance exercises include jogging, rope skipping, skating, cross-country skiing, swimming, stair-stepping, and bicycling; strengthening exercises include weight lifting with free weights and fixed-axis machines.

While strengthening exercises increase muscle force, endurance exercises increase aerobic capacity, or maximal oxygen uptake ($V \cdot O_2$). As a result of endurance training, the number and size of mitochondria in muscle increase, the activity of mitochondrial enzymes increase, and blood flow to muscles increases because of increased numbers of capillaries and improved efficiency of blood flow shunting.[12] Adaptations in the heart and vasculature include increased stroke volume, expand blood volume, decreased resting heart rate, and decreased resting systolic and diastolic blood pressure.[12] To achieve an endurance effect, the trainee needs to participate in 15 to 60 minutes of continuous aerobic activity three to five times per week at sufficient intensity to raise heart rate to 60% to 90% of maximum[13] (see Fig. 79-4). A maximal exertion exercise treadmill test can determine maximal heart rate; however, an easy approximation of maximal heart rate for a given age is arrived at by subtraction the patient's age from 220. This level of participation, that is, increasing heart rate to 60% to 85% of maximum, will increase maximal oxygen uptake 15% to 30%.[13] However, endurance training more often than five times per week can lead to an increase in the occurrence of orthopedic injuries.[13]

As regards pain, endurance activity has been shown to increase endorphin levels. McCain summarizes these works writing that "exercise leads to a predictable increase in serum levels of beta-endorphin like immunoreactivity, ACTH, prolactin and growth hormone."[14] He continues that a state of decreased pain sensitivity, called *post-run hypoalgesia*, which is naloxone reversible, is associated with these neurohormonal and endocrinologic changes.[14] Studying elite athletes running at a submaximal level after naloxone or placebo injection, Surbey found that the athletes receiving naloxone had reduced exercise time and increased affective component of pain.[15]

Considerations for special populations of patients include short, frequent sessions of endurance exercise for markedly deconditioned patients; because frequent, short sessions of endurance activity have been shown to be as effective as equal amounts of sustained endurance activity.[13] Patients with osteoarthritis benefit from endurance exercise but require modifications including a low impact or an aquatic program. The physician should consider exercise test screening for patients who plan to participate in a moderate- to high-intensity exercise program, who are male and older than 45 years old, or female and older than 55 years old, and who have two or more risk factors for cardiac disease.[16] The risk factors for cardiac disease include positive family history of coronary disease or sudden death before age 55 years, cigarette use within the past 6 months, blood pressure elevation over 140/90 mm Hg, hypercholesterolemia with total cholesterol >200 or LDL >130, impaired fasting glucose over 110 mg/dL, or obesity with a body mass index >30 kg/m^2. Persons with known cardiovascular, pulmonary, or metabolic disease should have an exercise treadmill test prior to exercise participation. Absolute contraindications to endurance or strength training include acute and unstable cardiopulmonary, metabolic, and vascular conditions: acute electrocardiogram (ECG) changes, unstable angina, uncontrolled cardiac arrhythmias, severe symptomatic aortic stenosis, symptomatic or uncontrolled heart failure, acute pulmonary embolus of deep venous thrombosis, acute infection, suspected or known dissecting aneurysm, and acute pericarditis or myocarditis.[17]

Some additional adverse effects of endurance activity are predictable. It is possible to sustain sprains, falls, overuse injuries, or blunt injuries if exercising on busy thoroughfares. The exerciser can become dehydrated. However, one of the adverse effects of aerobic participation is not the promotion of osteoarthritis. Lane followed 30 runners with age-matched controls for 5 years to evaluate for the acceleration of arthritis due to running activity. Running did not accelerate the development of radiographic or clinical osteoarthritis of the knees.[18]

Familiarity with the types of exercise, the goals of each type, and its proper performance improve the ability of the physician to educate the patient about treatment options, and improve the ability of the physician to estimate the quality of the exercise program the patient receives from community therapy settings.

Aquatic Running

Wilder and Brennan wrote a succinct review of the techniques and benefits of aqua-running.[19] Deep water running is accomplished by floating the participant, tethered in place, in the deep end of a pool. The participant does not touch the pool bottom. Maximal heart rate and maximal oxygen carrying capacity are about 90 of those values obtained from on-land running. Maximal perceived exertion is similar for both on-land and aqua running, and both forms of training lead to increased maximal oxygen carrying capacity. Unlike on-land running there is no weight bearing but the addition of resistance from the water. The arms work harder, but the legs work less. Hydrostatic pressure may assist venous return. Body temperature during exercise is slightly lower in the aquatic setting. Aqua-running may be an alternative endurance activity for certain populations where weight-bearing exercises are painful or harmful.

Patient Education

The physician can prescribe or instruct the patient in strategies to prevent injury and promote health, such as energy and back and joint conservation; the therapist can reinforce and demonstrate these strategies. Studies discussed in reference to the specific diagnoses suggest that education may be as useful as exercise at relieving painful symptomatology.

Common sense comprises most patient education strategies. For example, patients with hip and knee arthritis are instructed to sit in higher chairs with firm seats and with arms so that the upper limbs may assist transitions to and from sitting. By contrast, plush, deep, low seating without arms make it difficult for the patient with hip and knee pain to rise from the seated position. Back conservation techniques include lifting with the arms and legs, and keeping the object lifted close to the body. Work simplification techniques, like carrying smaller packages, dressing in bed or while sitting, resting between tasks, are strategies that persons with discomfort due to dyspnea can use make activities of daily living more comfortable. Planning ahead and organizing, avoiding unnecessary trips, having all equipment available prior to starting a task, combining tasks, using lightweight tools, and resting before fatigue onsets are work simplification guidelines.[20]

Assistive Devices for Mobility and Activities of Daily Living

Assistive devices include those for mobility and those for activities of daily living (ADLs). Canes, walkers, and crutches increase balance by increasing points of contact, and thereby surface area over which the center of gravity is supported; or they function to relieve the weight from a painful or immobilized limb. A walker is the most stable among these devices, and can be self-supporting if the patient must lean on it to rest. A cane is useful because it leaves one hand free for other tasks. A properly fitting cane should be adjusted to a height so that, when used, the hook of the cane approximates the patient's trochanter. Crutches are unstable devices, and difficult to use correctly. Indications for mobility aids include lumbar and lower limb osteoarthritis, sprains, and fractures, as well as situations of weakness including stroke and lower motor neuron disease, like polio and neuropathy, and myopathic processes.

A wheelchair is also a mobility aid. It is maximally useful when the patient can propel it independently. It is useful for persons with severe lower limb weakness, knee, thigh and pelvis trauma, or dyspnea due to muscle, lung or cardiac disease. However, the chronic use of a wheelchair can predispose to muscle tightness and contracture. The prescribing of wheelchairs for persons who can otherwise ambulate but prefer to be pushed should be avoided.

Trombley catalogues devices for ADLs (Table 79-2) and other techniques to simplify ADL work.[20] Simplification techniques in-

TABLE 79-2 **Occupational Therapy Devices for ADLs**

Bathroom
Grab bars
Handheld shower head
Raised toilet seat
Long-handled devices
Reacher
Shoe horn
Inspection mirror
Bathing sponge
Dressing stick
Sock donner
Feeding
Rocker knife
Plate with sides
Hinged spoon
Weighted handles for tremor
Hinged spoon for tremor

ADLs denotes activities of daily living.

clude dressing the affected limb first, and undressing it last. Using spray deodorant is easier than using stick varieties. Using implements with short handles to feed is easier than using those with long handles. The reader treating patients with stroke, spinal cord injury, or weakness from peripheral nerve lesions can access this reference for other recommendations. Mobility and ADL devices and simplification techniques exist to make activity less painful and maximally efficient.

Electrical and Thermal Modalities

Thermal and electrical modalities are passive therapeutic interventions. Modalities that patients can apply independently at home, namely hot packs, ice packs, and transcutaneous electrical stimulation (TENS), are particularly useful. This section presents the forms, physiologic effects, contraindications, and precautions of thermal modalities and then of TENS. The proposed mechanisms of pain relief for the various physical modalities are also discussed.

Common forms of thermal therapies include superficial ice and heat and deep applications of heat (see Table 79-1). Superficial ice applications include ice packs and ice massage. Superficial forms of heat include heat lamps, hot packs, heating pads, paraffin, and hydrotherapy. Deep heat includes ultrasound and short- and long-wave diathermy.

The physiologic effects of heat are local, regional,and distant. Local physiologic effects include increased tissue histamine and prostaglandin and bradykinin release that relax vascular smooth muscle and contribute to vasodilation. At a spinal level, due to afferent thermoreceptor stimulation, decreased sympathetic tone results and further relaxes vascular muscle tone. Sufficiently warmed blood reaches the thermoregulatory hypothalamus and causes increased metabolism and preparation. At the tissue level local heating results in increased tissue elasticity and decreased viscosity.

The physiologic effects of cold include vasoconstriction, decreased edema, decreased pain possibly due to slowed nerve conduction, and decreased spasticity due to effects on the muscle spindle.[22] Ice application in the first 24 to 48 hours after acute injury is recommended to control swelling and edema. Contraindications to cold applications include cold-agglutinins, Raynaud's phenomenon, and peripheral vascular disease.

There are cognitive impairments as well as disease states that preclude the use of heat. Cognitive contraindications to hot applications include obtundation, confusion, or an infantile state. Medical contraindications to therapeutic heat include insensate skin, peripheral vascular disease, acute inflammation, tumor, and proximity to growth plates. Whirlpool immersion is contraindicated for patients while congestive heart failure.

If the patient cannot feel heat or express the perception of being burned because of inattention or peripheral nerve disorder, burns will occur. Burns can occur at home or in the therapy gym. The following examples of inadvertent burns observed over more than a decade of rehabilitation practices illustrate these concerns:

1. A paraplegic spinal-cord-injured patient with deep partial thickness to the flank after a hydrocollator pack was applied to partially cover the area below the level of injury and insensate skin.
2. A patient with traumatic brachial plexopathy who sustained full-thickness burns to the tips of the fingers when the fingers came to rest on the bottom of a paraffin unit.
3. An osteoporotic patient who sustained blisters to the back when laid on a hot pack at a therapy gym.
4. A 50-year-old woman with diabetes who sustained full-thickness burns and a subsequent below the knee amputation when she fastened an electric heating pad to her leg and fell asleep.
5. A spinal-cord-injured patient who sustained superficial to deep partial-thickness burns when the patient fell asleep on a heating pad and it slipped below the level of injury.
6. A paraplegic spinal-cord-injured person who sustained deep partial-thickness wounds to the foot when placed under a stream of hot water at home.
7. An elderly arthritic person burned on the arms and torso by flame when attempting to heat paraffin in an ordinary pan on a gas stove.

The threat of burns from external heating devices is real. Electric heating pads should be avoided or used very carefully. Absolutely never sleep with an electric heating pad. Thus, the physician should write precautions to monitor for burns when thermal modalities are prescribed.

The different types of external heating devices have various temperatures and techniques of use.[22] Hydrocollator hot packs are 71°C, and must be wrapped in six to eight layers of toweling before being applied to a patient.[22] The patient should never lay on a hot pack because the body weight and pressure on the skin impairs adequate circulation to dissipate the heat. The skin under the pack should be checked at 5 minutes; if there is excessive redness, the pack should probably be removed, or at least extra towel layers added.[22] The skin reaches maximal temperature in 8 to 10 minutes.[22]

Paraffin dips consist of paraffin wax and mineral oil; this mixture comes premixed and is heated to 47° to 54°C.[22] The hands or feet may be dipped in the mixture for eight to ten dips, or the mixture may be brushed on. Then layers of toweling are applied around the extremity for 10 to 15 minutes.[22] Common uses include various hand arthritides. To maximize the risk of flame burns, only a paraffin unit should be used to heat the paraffin-mineral oil mixture; these units can be obtained inexpensively at many department stores.

Water bottles are useful self-limited heating units but can scald if they accidentally open. Heating lamps are external heating devices prescribed by specifying the angle and distance of the unit from the patient and the minutes of use.

Heat over 45°C permanently injures living tissues and denatures proteins. At temperatures below 45°, the normal vascular response to heat with increased vasodilation limits the depth of penetration of superficial heat. The average depth of heating with superficial modalities is 0.5 cm.[22]

Ultrasound is a mode of deep heat in common use. A meta-analysis of 22 controlled studies published on the use of ultrasound for the treatment of musculoskeletal pain in human subjects found that there is no indication that ultrasound can relieve pain.[21] The technology has value, however, in the treatment of tissue distensibility, which may be a therapeutic goal.

The technology of ultrasound is passage of electric current through crystals to cause vibration and sound waves; this phenomenon is called the *piezo-electric effect*. Ultrasound penetrates to a depth of 1 to 5 cm depending on the frequency used. The most commonly used frequencies are 1 MHz, which penetrates to depth of 5 cm, and 3 MHz, which penetrates to a depth of 1 cm.[22] Ultrasound waves pass through, are absorbed, or are reflected depending on the composition of the tissue that they encounter. Tissue interfaces, such as muscle in proximity to bone, absorb more ultrasound energy and generate higher tissue temperatures.

Ultrasound requires a liquid medium to pass through because it travels poorly through air. The therapist applies ultrasound gel between the ultrasound wand and the patient, and moves the wand continuously to avoid creating hot spots.[22] Ultrasound may also be used on smaller joints, like the hand, by placing the extremity and the wand in water and moving the wand through the water about 1 cm from the extremity.[22] The prescription for ultrasound includes specifying the duration of treatment and the watts per centimeter squared, and the anatomic area of application. The desired clinical effect is the sensation of warmth in the area treated. The treatment should be discontinued immediately if the patient perceives burning. Ultrasound should not be used over artificial joints fixed by methylmethacrylate.

Superficial hot and cold and deep heat using ultrasound are common forms of thermal modalities. The patient can independently apply superficial heat and cold treatments at home, and the therapist and physician should encourage the patient to use these mediums as sprain–strain first aid to control symptoms. Cold is applied to an injury, and when swelling subsides, heat may be used. The physician should explain to the patient how to observe for burns. Patients often request ultrasound treatment, but the patient cannot utilize this modality independently, and Gam's work suggests that it has no pain-relieving effect. Prescribing ultrasound in conjunction with a stretching program under therapy management probably best serves the patient.

Transcutaneous electrical nerve stimulation is an electrically powered neuromodulating technology. A TENS unit consists of a pulse generator, an amplifier, and two to four carbon-impregnated silicone electrodes. The unit is about the size of a deck of playing cards. The pulse generated has characteristics that include configuration (for example, rectangular), pulse width in milliseconds, and frequency in hertz. The most common settings, those of conventional TENS, are a rectangular waveform of 40 to 70 Hz frequency and 0.1 to 0.5 ms pulse width, with constant current. The electrodes are placed 4 or more centimeters apart to avoid skin irritation.[23] Conventional TENS feels like vibrations; the therapist modifies the settings of the pulse to gain a deeper, broader sensation of vibration, not a stronger one. The electrodes can be placed at the area of pain or along the nerve root innervating the area.[24] TENS is not helpful in poorly localized or psychogenic pain.[25] Conventional and brief-intense TENS are not naloxone reversible, but acupuncture-like TENS is.[26]

Mannheimer reviewed the diagnoses in which TENS was helpful, including peripheral nerve injury, causaglia and reflex sympathetic dystrophy, intercostals neuritis, postherpetic neuralgia, radiculopathy, and arachnoiditis.[27] Subsequent to the publication of Mannheimer's text, the efficacy of TENS in the treatment of pain in other diagnoses has been studied. For rheumatoid arthritis, Abelson showed that TENS at 70 Hz significantly relieved hand pain and increased grip strength better than placebo, but only while the unit was on.[28]; Langley studied acupuncture-like TENS in a placebo-controlled, double-blinded design and found that neither modality was significantly better than the other but that both decreased pain and increased grip strength.[29] The efficacy of TENS to relieve pain in other diagnoses is discussed in the diagnoses-specific section of this chapter.

SUMMARY

The literature supports that stretching and endurance activity relieve pain. The mechanism for stretch is not clear but the mechanism for endurance activity may be related to changes in neurohormones. The diagnoses-specific section of this chapter discusses literature that demonstrates a pain-relieving effect of strengthening activity as well. The mechanism of this pain relief is not clear.

It is important to note that the patient does not require expensive in-home equipment or private gym memberships to participate in an exercise program. By intention, the models demonstrating the exercises and stretches in this chapter were nonprofessionals, photographed in a spare noncluttered room in a home, and they had access to no specialized equipment other than a good pair of athletic shoes.

The modalities of superficial heat and cold relieve pain, as does TENS. The mechanisms are variable and include local effects on the nerves, and modulating effects in the central nervous system. Interestingly, in a meta-analysis ultrasound has not been found to relieve pain but is useful when used in combination with stretch to relieve contracture.[21]

PHYSICAL MEDICINE AND REHABILITATION PRESCRIPTION FOR SPECIFIC DIAGNOSES

Knee Osteoarthritis

Knee osteoarthritis affects 10% of the elderly and limits the ability to use stairs, rise from a chair, and stand comfortably.[30] The literature demonstrates that patients with osteoarthritis have reduced strength, endurance, and functional performance.[30] Fisher summarizes the literature, writing that aerobic exercise for the patients with osteoarthritis increases endurance and decreases fatigue, but does not have an impact on functional capacity.[30] As regards pain, Fisher summarizes the available literature and notes that quadricep setting exercises, a form of isometric strengthening, reduce pain associated with arthritis and improves function.[30]

TENS used biweekly relieves knee pain due to arthritis.[31] Neuromuscular electrical stimulation in patients with knee arthritis increases strength, decreases swelling, increases range of motion, and decreases muscle wasting.[32,33]

A possible prescription for subacute and chronic knee osteoarthritis is as follows:

Evaluation Screen for significant contraindications to exercise; baseline ECG. The therapist is quite capable of modifying an exercise program to allow for coexistent diagnosis.

Prescription

Precautions List comorbid diagnoses.

Goals Increase knee range of motion; increase knee extension strength; and improve functional mobility.

Education Instruction in the proper sequencing of a gait with a cane; instruction in joint conservation techniques.

Stretching Sustained stretch to the hamstrings (Fig. 79-5).

Strenghtening Isometric strengthening of the knee extensors (Fig. 79-6) initially; progress to assisted and active range of motion exercise around the knee; progress to isotonic strengthening of the knee extensors. Strengthen the arm and shoulder extensors to promote joint conservation techniques.

Endurance exercise Low-impact endurance activity; or walking in a pool waist to chest deep, if available.

Modalities Ice to muscles as needed for spasm; TENS; electrical stimulation.

Frequency Physical therapy 3 days a week plus home exercise twice a day, 3 days per week.

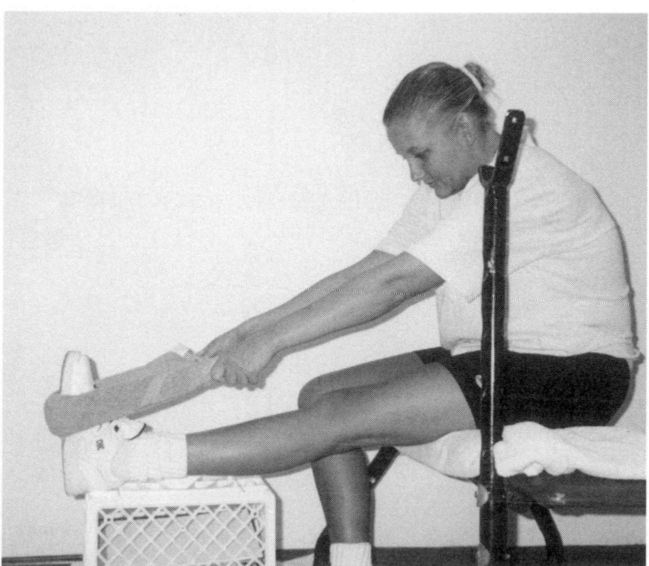

Figure 79-5 Seated hamstring stretch with the leg straight reaching toward the toes.

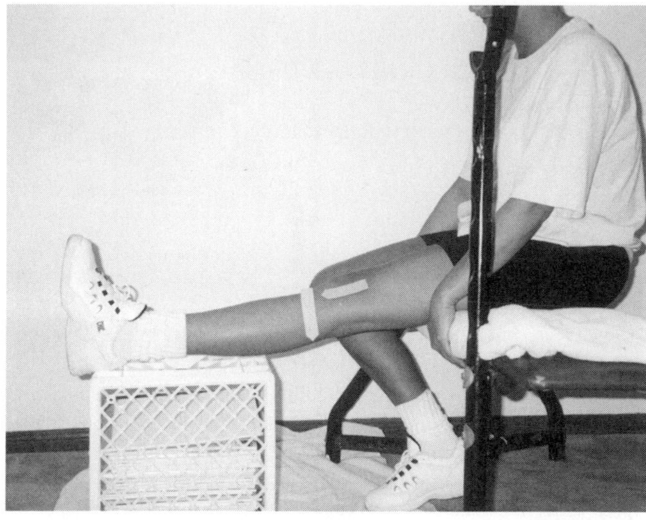

Figure 79-6 Quad set with the supported leg straight, firming the thigh muscle and pushing the leg down.

Anterior Knee Pain and Patellofemoral Syndrome

Roush describes a simple home program of modified (Muncie) straight leg arises that a randomized, controlled study showed to be significantly effective at relieving pain and improving functional impairment ratings.[34] The trainee performs the modified straight leg raise (Fig. 79-7) by sitting on the floor with the legs straight. The exercised knee is rotated out about 45 degrees, and the quadriceps muscle is set. Then the ipsilateral heel is raised 1 to 2 in. off the floor and the contraction is held for 5 seconds. This exercise is repeated 20 times twice a day.

A review article by Bourne describes phases of treatment for anterior knee pain and patellofemoral syndrome.[35] In the acute stage of pain, ice packs, massage, and patella-stabilizing bracing

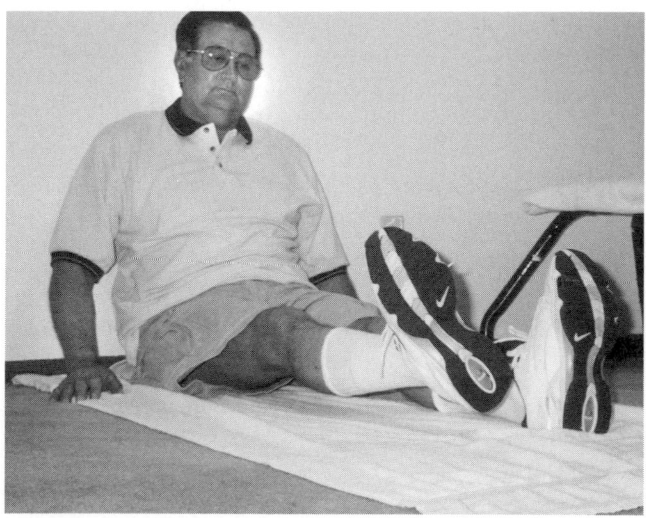

Figure 79-7 Modified straight leg raise with lifted leg straignt but externally rotated 45°.

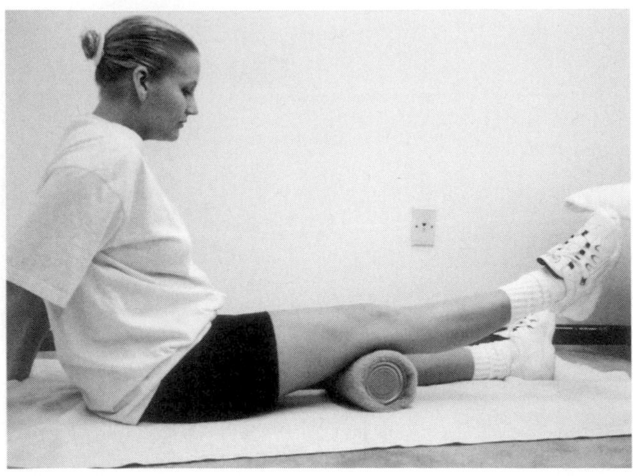

Figure 79-8 Short arc quad with can of food wrapped in a towel acting as a fulcrum under the knee while the heel is raised and lowered.

are the recommended modalities along with nonsteroidal anti-inflammatory medication. Stretching of the hamstrings (see Figs. 79-4 or 79-5) and the iliotibial band and isometric strengthening of the quadriceps and hip adductors (see Fig. 79-6 or 79-7, more difficult), and toe raises are recommended. Certain activities are proscribed, including jumping, squatting, hill running, cycling, and sitting with the knee flexed more than 40 degrees. TENS may be used for pain if ice is ineffective.

In the subacute phase, Bourne recommends exercise for 30 minutes per day consisting of multiangle isometrics quadriceps strengthening, and terminal knee extensions from 0 to 30 degrees (Fig. 79-8). In the chronic stages, one can increase the amount of weight used during the terminal extension exercises and increase the flexion moment in increments of 10 degrees until full knee range is achieved. Endurance exercises like biking, or swimming become appropriate. The trainee applies ice after activity.

A possible script for anterior knee pain (subacute and chronic) is as follows:

Evaluation Screen for significant contraindications to exercise; baseline ECG.

Prescription

Precautions List comorbid diagnoses.

Goals Decrease knee pain at rest and during functional activity; increase knee extension strength.

Stretch Exercise hamstrings and iliotibial band.

Strengthening Isometric quadricep sets, isometric hip adduction, Muncie-modified straight leg raise; terminal extension, progress to full knee range of motion.

Endurance When pain is diminished, progress to biking or swimming.

Modalities Ice after exercise for 20 minutes; TENS.

Fibromyalgia

In the treatment of primary fibromyalgia syndrome, a randomized, controlled trial demonstrates the efficacy of both exercise and education to reduce pain in tender points, physical dysfunction, and feelings of helplessness.[36] Education included information about the disease, coping and stress management, relaxation techniques, and the importance of physical activity. Physical activity included stretching and range-of-motion exercises plus walking, swimming, or cycling.

A controlled trial by McCain supported that a three times per week, 60-minute participation in cycling activity to achieve a sustained elevated heart rate resulted in improved pain thresholds of tender points and improved cardiovascular fitness.[37] Study subjects participated for 20 weeks. There was also a trend toward improvement in pain scores. The control group participated in flexibility activity only.[37] In a controlled study, Nichols showed that a less vigorous aerobic exercise program only trended toward lowered pain ratings in fibromyalgia patients. The patients walked three times per week for 8 weeks, and attempted to raise heart rate to 60% to 70% of predicted maximum.[38] Flexibility and endurance activity of vigorous to moderate intensity benefit persons with fibromyalgia.

A possible script for fibromyalgia is as follows:

Evaluation Screen for significant contraindications to exercise; baseline ECG.

Referral Psychological referral for coping and stress management.

Prescription

Precautions Contraindicated for comorbid diagnoses.

Stretching Generalized upper (Figs. 79-9, 79-10, 79-11) and lower limb flexibility (Figure 79-12 and see Figs. 79-2, 79-3)

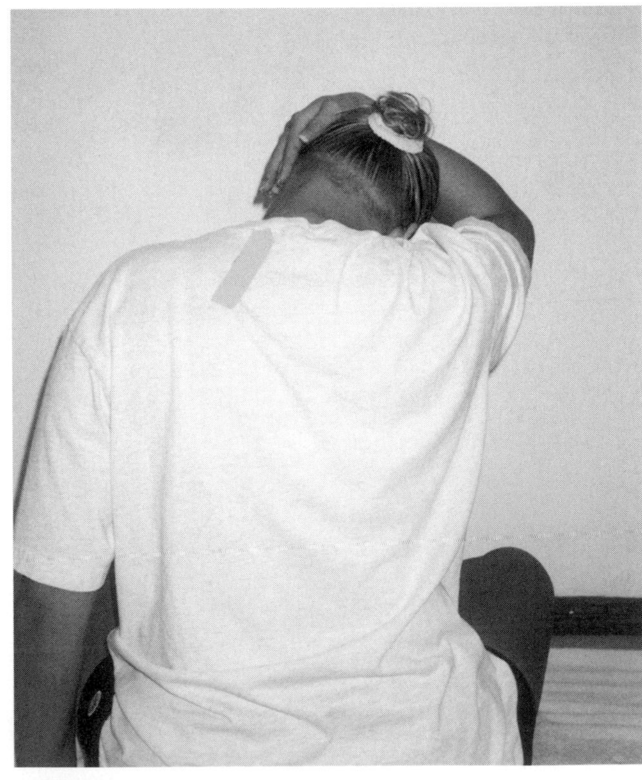

Figure 79-9 Levator scapulae stretch with head pulled forward and slightly diagonally.

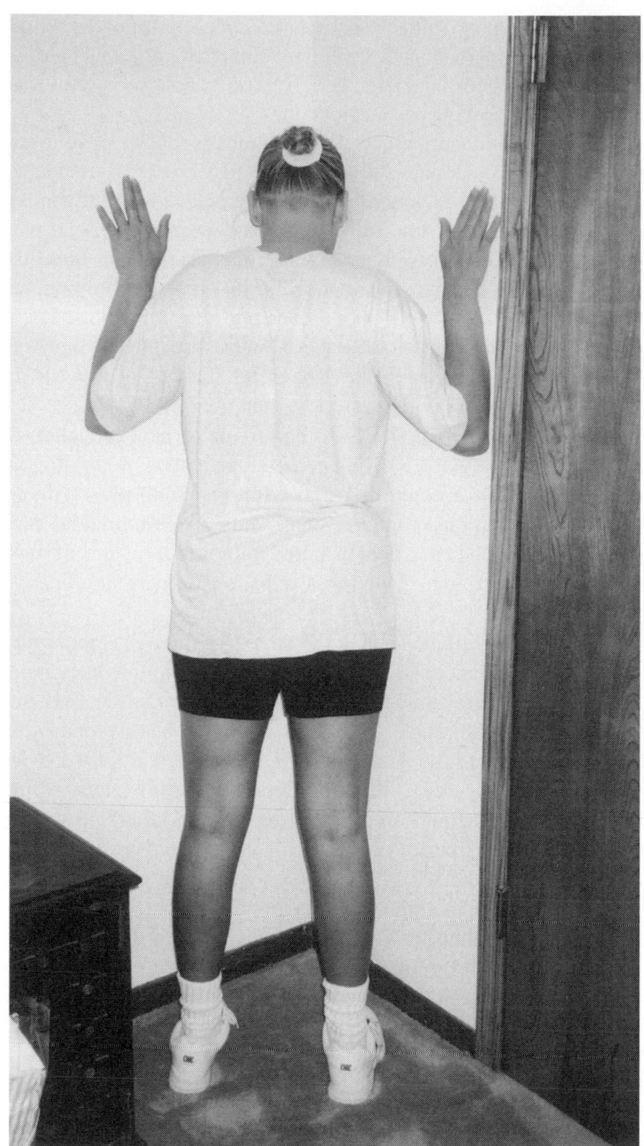

Figure 79-10 "Corner" or pectoralis stretch done with chin tucked down and hands on wall at shoulder-height while leaning into corner.

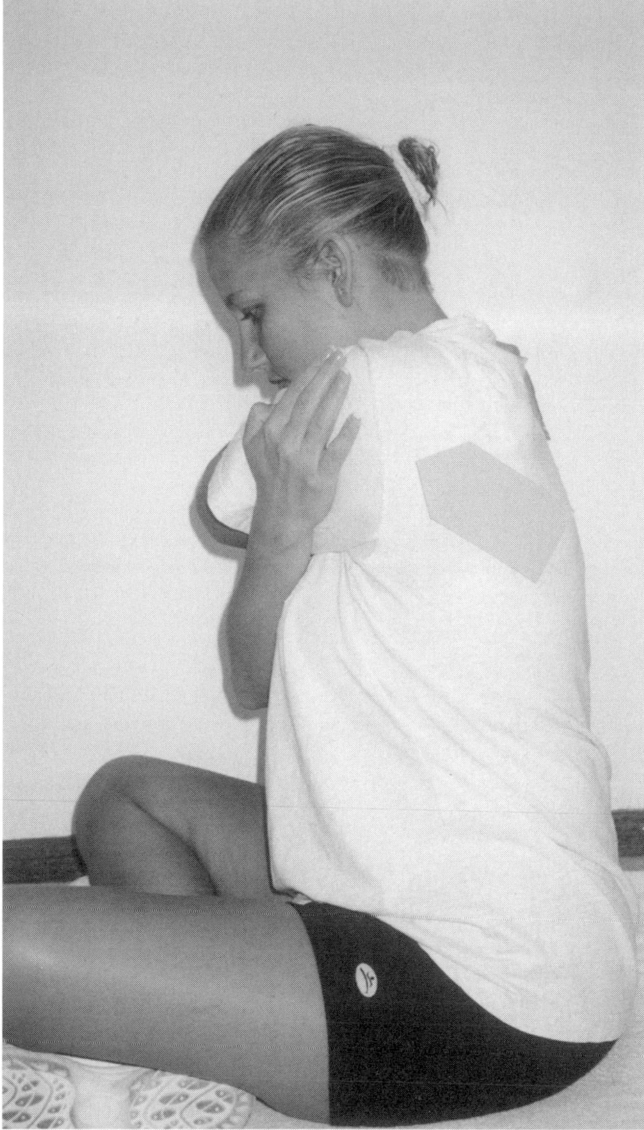

Figure 79-11 Posterior shoulder capsule stretch done by placing the hands on opposite shoulders and pulling forward.

Endurance Aerobic activity to a heart rate of >70% predicted maximum for 30 to 60 minutes.

Education Provide instruction about benefits of regular exercise.

Myofascial Pain Syndrome

Myofascial pain has seven clinical features: exquisite local tenderness, referred pain pattern, electrically quiet palpable band, perpetuation by metabolic distress, weakness and fatigability, local twitch response, and relief by stretch.[39] Thompson notes that these criteria are supported by clinical observation but have not been validated.[39] The literature does not support the utility of TENS in decreasing pain in myofascial pain syndromes.[40] Treatments that are commonly used but supported primarily by convention include spray-and-stretch techniques and trigger-point injections or dry needling followed by stretching.[39,42] Other conventional treatments include galvanic stimulation and hot pack application, massage and soft tissue mobilization techniques.[39] Aerobic exercise is probably more beneficial than stretching alone.[41] Kraus and Fischer note that in the acute state the patient may need to stretch the affected muscle group hourly.[41,42] Lewit studied 351 muscle groups in 244 patients to evaluate the effect of post-isometric relaxation techniques on pain relief and found that 94% of locations received immediate pain relief, whereas 63% of persons receiving lasting relief.[9] The study lacks control and blinding.

A possible script for myofascial pain is as follows:

Evaluation Screen for significant contraindications to exercise; baseline ECG.

Prescription

Precautions List comorbid diagnoses.

Stretching Generalized upper (see Figs. 79-9, 79-10, 79-11) and lower limb flexibility (see Fig. 79-12)

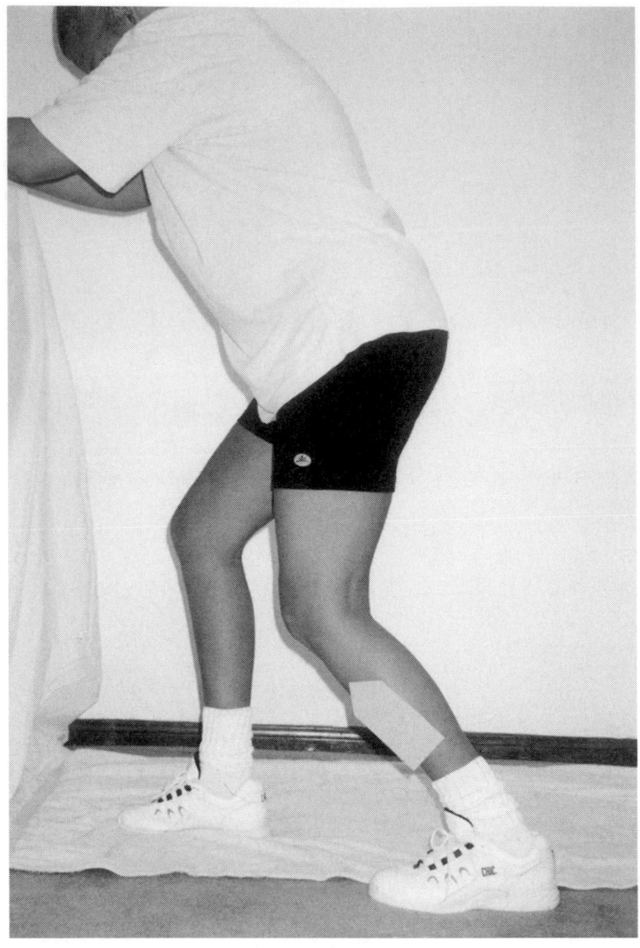

Figure 79-12 Calf stretch done with the foot flat on the ground, bending the ankle foward and flexing at the knee.

Endurance Aerobic activity to a heart rate of >60% predicted maximum for 20 to 30 minutes.

Modalities Superficial heat, spray and stretch, soft tissue massage.

Education Provide instruction about benefits of regular exercise.

Axial Low Back Pain

Axial low back pain includes diagnoses of muscular, tendonous, articular, and bony origin. The value of patient education to treat pain related to this diagnosis should not be overlooked. In a randomized, controlled study of patients admitted 3 weeks for the intradisciplinary treatment of low back pain, the researchers found that patients ranked education significantly higher than electrotherapy for overall benefit from the program. The patients ranked exercise second and electrotherapy third.[43] Sikorski prospectively studied 142 patients with low back pain, subcategorizing them into acute and chronic, and further subdividing the chronic complainants into anterior element, posterior element, movement-related, and unclassified groups.[44] He found that the patients in the chronic groups judged education to be the most valuable intervention, closely followed by exercise.[44] The acute group judged exercise to be the most valuable intervention, closely followed by education.[44] Although statistics were not compiled, all groups judged the interventions of education and exercise to be more useful than manipulation, bracing, or medication.[44]

Of interest, education and the use lumbar supports prior to experiencing low back pain were not found to decrease the incidence of low back pain.[45] A study by Walsh and Schwartz led to similar conclusions, but lost time from work was lower for workers who used a brace and received education[46]; this decrease in time lost was not true of the experimental group that received only education. The use of lumbar supports does not increase isokinetic endurance during lifting,[47] nor isometric lumbar strength and dynamic lifting capacity.[48] Bracing does not affect strength or prevent injury, but their use may decrease lost man hours.

Stretching has been shown to contribute to pain reduction in low back pain patients. Khalil studied 28 patients with myofascial low back pain in a controlled trial with stretching plus a multimodal rehabilitation program versus only the multimodal program.[8] The stretch group demonstrated improved measures of muscle function, and after 2 weeks, low back pain was significantly lowered.

Kendall and Jenkins studied the effects of three different types of strengthening exercise on patients with chronic low back pain: The regimens were lumbar extension, isometric flexion, and isotonic flexion.[49] Although all patients improved, the isotonic flexion group improved the most, but statistics were not done.[49] Davies also compared the effects of two different types of exercise of patients with back pain.[49] A control group received diathermy only, whereas the two experimental groups received diathermy plus isometric flexion exercises, or diathermy plus lumbar extension exercises.[50] All three treatment groups improved, but the extension group did better than the flexion group, who both did better than the diathermy only group.[50] However, no differences were statistically significant. A more recent randomized, controlled study showed that 149 patients with acute low back pain receiving either flexion or extension exercises did not differ in amount of improvement in reduction of disability scores or return to work; however, both groups did better than control subjects receiving no exercise.[51] There were no statistical differences. A controlled study of 123 patients with low back pain compared with 126 normal controls showed that patients with low back pain had low flexor and extensor trunk strength than normal patients, and, in addition, that extensor strength was disproportionately weaker than flexor strength in back pain patients.[52] The patients were exercised using situps (Fig. 79-13), prone trunk extensions, pelvic tilts (Fig. 79-14), and knee to chest (Fig. 79-15) stretches, and back pain decreased as strength increased.[52] The patients exercised daily for an average of about 3 months. Patients with low back pain and no identified organic lesions did better on strength gains and pain relief than patients with back pain and organic lesions (herniated disk, spondylolysis, and spondylolisthesis).[52]

The literature explores the effect of modalities on low back pain. Thorstiensson studied the placebo effect of TENS on low back pain and found that the placebo effect was similar to that noted in other double-blinded studies of medications, about 32%.[53] Marchand restudied the placebo effect of TENS in a controlled prospective study of 42 patients with low back pain.[54] He found that TENS reduced the intensity of pain more than sham-TENS but that there was no significant difference for the reduction of the unpleasantness of pain.[54] Additionally, TENS only had a significant effect in the first week but no long-term effect, and, from this observation,

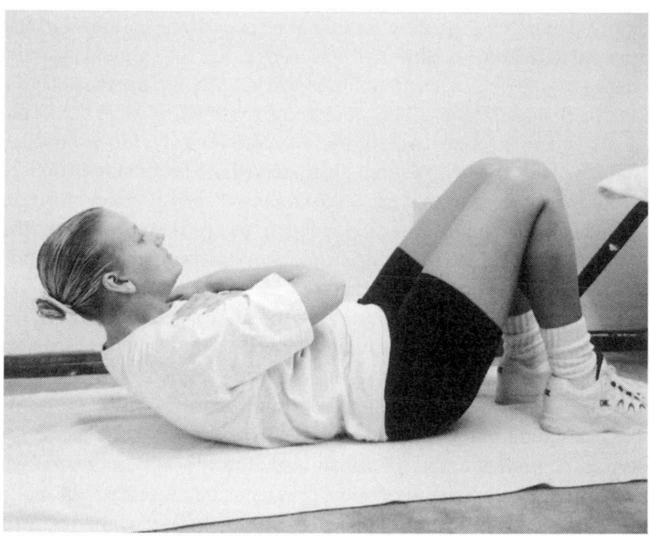

Figure 79-13 Modified situp with knees and hips flexed and heel flat on floor; arms are crossed over the chest and only the head and shoulders come up.

Marchand posited a placebo action of TENS.[54] Melzack and Jeans studied the effect of ice massage and TENS on chronic low back pain on 44 patients with chronic low back pain in a crossover, prospective study. The researchers applied TENS and ice massage to the back and the lateral malleolar area. TENS and ice massage were both reported to reduce pain levels more than 33% in about 68% of the patients, and neither modality was significantly superior to the other treatment.[55] Melzack also compared TENS to automated soft tissue massage in a double-blind study and found that TENS reduces pain significantly better than massage in low back pain patients.[56] Of the various settings for TENS, Lehmann studied conventional TENS versus electroacupuncture and found that electroacupuncture tended to improve pain better than conventional TENS or dead battery (control) TENS, but not significantly.[43] Deyo et al, in a randomized, controlled trial of TENS versus exercise and exercise plus TENS for the treatment of chronic non-operated low back pain in 144 patients, found no benefit of TENS over exercise and there was no added benefit of TENS added to exercise.[57] The

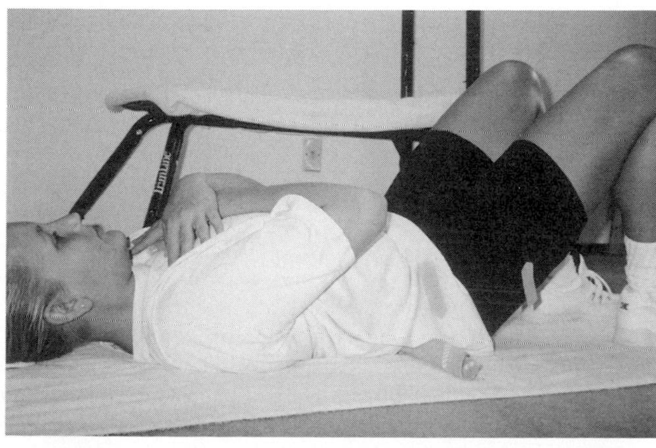

Figure 79-14 Pelvic tilt where lower abdominal muscles and gluteal muscles are contracted, rolling the lower pelvis upward.

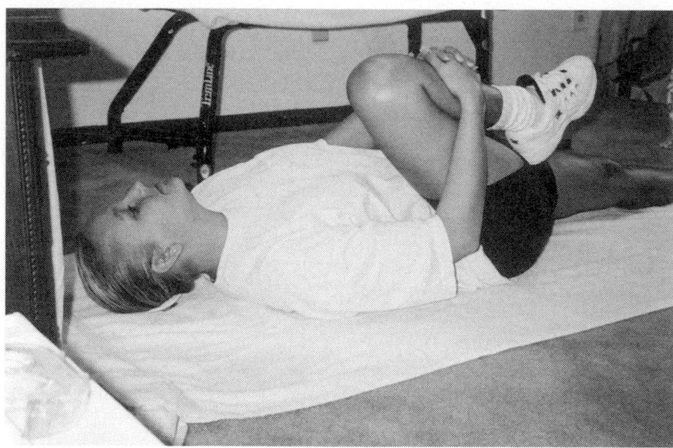

Figure 79-15 Knee to chest stretch with one knee hugged to chest, stretching gluteal muscles on that side.

exercise group improved more than the electrotherapy group, but at 2 months patients had discontinued exercises and the initial benefits were gone.

In summary, the value of education in the improvement of low back pain is considerable if not significant. Exercise, including pelvis and lumbar flexibility, and strengthening exercise including lumbar exercise with flexion and extension bias are helpful. The physician can screen for the patient's more comfortable position in the office by simply making the pelvic tilt position, crunch and prone pressup (Fig. 79-16) position part of the exam. An improved, or no-change-in pain response, is desired. Positions that increase pain should be avoided or delayed. Back bracing, except for traumatic or postoperative indications, has limited value. TENS may benefit some sufferers of low back pain, but education, flexibility, and exercise are the core components of the physical medicine and rehabilitation script.

A possible prescription for axial low back pain is as follows:

Evaluation Screen for significant contraindications to exercise; baseline ECG.

Prescription

Precautions List comorbid diagnoses.

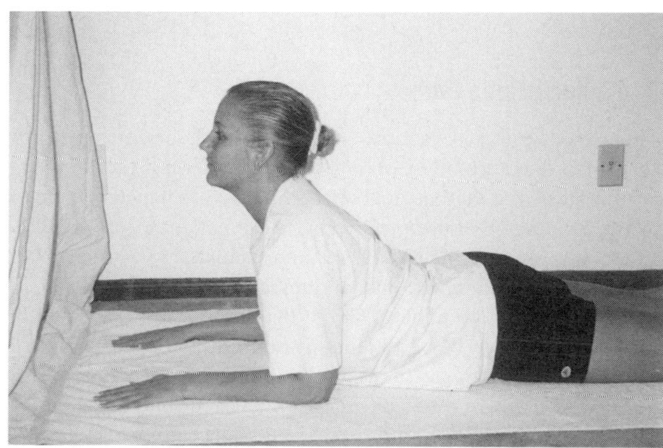

Figure 79-16 Prone press up. Bent elbows support the person arching back.

Education Back conservation and proper body mechanics, the syndrome of low back pain, its frequency and the significance or lack of significance of radiographic findings, the importance of regular exercise, and back first aid.

Stretching lumbar (see Fig. 79-2), quadratus lumborum, and lower limb flexibility, including tensor fascia lata, hamstrings (see Fig. 79-3), and gluteus (see 79-15).

Strengthening Lumbar crunches (Figure 79-13), pelvic tilts (Figure 79-14), lumbar extensions.

Modalities Superficial ice or heat for comfort.

Spondylolisthesis

Sinaki retrospectively studied the conservative treatment of spondylolisthesis.[58] Forty-eight patients participated in flexion or extension exercises for the treatment of spondylolisthesis.[58] After 3 months only 27% of the flexion troup had severe pain, but 67% of the extension group continued to have pain.[58] In the same period, 58% of the flexion group had recovered but only 6% of the extension group at recovered.[58] Exercise with flexion bias achieves pain reduction as a primary end point.

A possible prescription for spondylolisthesis:

Evaluation Screen for significant contraindications to exercise; baseline ECG.

Prescription

Precautions List comorbid diagnoses.

Education Back conservation and proper body mechanics, the syndrome of low back pain, and back first aid, the importance of regular exercise with a flexion bias (infrequently the patient will prefer the extended position).

Stretching Lumbar (see Fig. 79-3), quadratus lumborum, and lower limb flexibility, including tensor fascia lata, hamstrings (see Fig. 79-4), and gluteus (Fig. 79-15).

Strengthening Lumbar crunches (see Fig. 79-13), pelvic tilts (see Fig. 79-14).

Modalities Superficial ice or heat for comfort.

Assistive devices Bracing that blocks extension and promotes flexion radicular sciatic pain.

Radicular Sciatic Pain

The goal of physical therapy, surgery, or medicinal treatment for sciatica is the resolution of leg pain. On therapy prescriptions, physiatrists write that the goal of the exercises is the centralization of leg pain. Bed rest does not improve the patient's outcome.[59] In a randomized, controlled study Vromen evaluated 180 patients with clinical signs and symptoms of lumbar radicular disease. At 2 weeks slightly more patients in the bed rest group had less pain, but at 12 weeks 87% of patients in both groups were improved. There was no difference between the groups for functional status, medication use, absenteeism from work, or occurrence of surgery.[59] Saal and Saal completed a prospective cohort study of 64 patients with herniated lumbar disks, sciatic pain, positive electromyograms, and positive straight leg raise using the intervention of dynamic lumbar stabilization.[60] The patient could participate in the study design even if they had weakness as long as they did not have progressive weakness. Measuring a self-assessment of pain, self-assessed outcome and return to work, 85% of patients had good to excellent outcomes; 92% of patients returned to work.[60] Six patients failed to improve with the exercise regimen alone and had surgery; four of these patients had stenosis.[60] Extension exercises of lumbar stabilization were discontinued if they peripheralized or increased leg pain.[60] The appendix of the referenced article describes the exercise used in lumbar stabilization,[60] and a second reference by the one of the authors pictures the exercises.[61] Following this protocol, flexibility is the initial activity; when the strengthening exercises commence, attention to correct performance of the exercises is tantamount.

The classic McKenzie approach to evaluating and treating low back and radiating back pain first proposed the goal of exercise being the centralization of leg pain.[62] A therapist or physician, trained in the McKenzie method of spine treatment, can rapidly reduce and centralize pain of acute or chronic duration.[63] One of the interesting clinical caveats derived from McKenzie is the idea that exercises that cause centralization of the pain are to be continued and those that peripheralize or increase leg pain should cease.

A possible prescription for axial low back pain is as follows:

Evaluation Screen for significant contraindications to exercise; baseline ECG.

Prescription

Precautions List comorbid diagnoses; stop extension exercises if back pain peripheralizes or leg pain increases; stop therapy and return the patient to the physician if weakness is progressive.

Goals Centralize leg pain.

Education Provide instruction in back conservation and proper body mechanics, instruct the patient in posture maintenance, and during transitions, the importance of regular exercise, and back first aid.

Stretching Sustained stretch of the hamstrings (see Fig. 79-3), quadriceps, hip flexors (see Fig. 79-15), and calves (see Fig. 79-12).

Strengthening[64] Identify the neural position of minimal leg pain; lumbar crunches (see Fig. 79-13) 10 reps × 3 sets, pelvic tilts reps over 2 minutes (see Fig. 79-14), bridging slow reps over 3 minutes; quadriped with alternating arm and leg movements, slow reps held over 2 minutes; wall slide held 1 minute.

Endurance After leg pain is minimized and the patient can maintain standing and walking posture, treadmill walking and progress to other endurance activities.

Modalities Superficial ice or heat for comfort.

Low Back Pain After Laminectomy

The literature contains few well-designed studies that assess the utility of physical therapy with chronic low back pain after laminectomy. A randomized, controlled study by Timm of 250 patients with chronic low back pain showed that patients exercised three times a week for 8 weeks using floor set exercises and the patient group using weight-lifting equipment gained significant pain relief and lumbar range of motion compared with the patients treated with manipulation alone or those treated with modalities alone.[65]

The patients all had lumbar laminectomies and were over 1 year out from surgery.[65] The floor set exercises consisted of three sets of 10 of prone pressups and of lumbar stabilization exercises including alternating arm and leg raises in the supine and prone positions and bridging and alternating arm and leg raises in the quadruped position.[65] The patients in the exercise equipment group performed endurance and strengthening exercises; they completed 10 minutes of bicycle ergometry and then used machines to exercise the spinal flexors and extensors and rotators, and the latissimus dorsi muscle with lateral pulldowns.[65] Although these two programs were equally effective, the floor set application was less expensive to administer.[65] The modalities treatment was not effective and was the most expensive form of treatment for low back pain after laminectomy.[65]

A possible prescription for low back pain after laminectomy, 1 year out:

Evaluation Screen for significant contraindications to exercise; baseline ECG

Prescription

Precautions List comorbid diagnoses; stop exercises that peripheralize back pain or cause leg pain; contact the operating surgeon for any persistent postoperative limitations, specifically those restricting extension.

Strengthening exercises Floor exercises including prone pressups (if allowed by the surgeon) and including dynamic lumbar stabilization exercises supine and prone with supported alternating arm and leg movements; bridging exercises; quadriped exercises; lateral pull down exercises if patient has access to weight equipment.

Education Instructions in back conservation techniques with transitions.

Exercises Considerations after Discectomy

Surgeons often restrict the motion and movement of patients after spinal surgery. There is a small body of literature that supports cautious mobilization and re-examines this convention.

A small study by Kitteringham evaluated the efficacy of stretching exercises beginning in the second day after discectomy.[66] Twelve patients were studied for the effects of pulley-assisted straight leg raises after discectomy: A low-repetition group with 10 repetitions per day was compared with a high-repetition group with eight sets of 10 repetitions.[66] Compliance was poor in the high-repetition group and no significant differences were found between groups for pain or disability level or straight leg raise range in the 6-week study period.[66] There was no zero-straight-leg-raise control group because the practicing physicians believed and had demonstrated that some straight leg raises were beneficial.[66]

Carragee prospectively observed 50 patients after open discectomy for herniated lumbar who were given no postoperative restrictions, except those regarding wound healing.[67] The available literature cited by Carragee noted that patients return to work 4 to 16 weeks after back surgery.[67] In his study group, average time to return to work was 1.4 weeks. Average time to return to full duty was 3.4 weeks.[67] There were only five complications: a transient foot drop, a dural tear, one prolonged wound drainage, one antibiotic allergy, and one suprascapular nerve palsy.[67] Three reherniations (6%) occurred after 14 months.[67] The literature cited notes reherniation rates of 6% to 20%.[67] Although this study has neither control group nor randomization, the authors propose that postoperative restrictions, if unnecessary, only promote avoidance behavior and limit normal and routine spinal motion.[67] This topic merits further consideration in a randomized, controlled design.

Kjellby-Wendt studied active exercise after discectomy in a randomized, controlled study.[68] The authors note that the literature only describes therapy programs that begin more than 4 weeks after discectomy.[68] The experimental group sat the second day after surgery and were encouraged to walk.[68] The experimental group performed passive extension while lying down 5 days after surgery and flexion while lying down 3 weeks after surgery. The patient did active knee extension while lying supine with the hip flexed to 90 degrees the first day after surgery.[68] The patients in the experimental group were encouraged to do these exercises 5 to 6 times per day for the first 6 weeks.[68] In the second 6 weeks muscular strengthening exercise and spinal stabilization exercises were added and done once per day, and endurance activity like jogging and swimming was encouraged.[68] The control group only did a partial situp with the hips and knees bent once a day in the first 6 weeks; in the second 6 weeks, the control group added range-of-motion exercises for flexion and lateral flexion of the lumbar spine.[68]

Results showed that 12 weeks after surgery lumbar range of motion, especially in the extension and hamstring distension.[68] At the 6-week mark, but at no other time, more patients in the experimental group were pain-free than in the control group.[68] However, the early mobilization group had significantly less pain at 6 and 12 months than the control group.[68] Compliance for range-of-motion exercises was higher than for the strengthening exercise. At the 1 year only 11.5% of the experimental group had residual predominating leg pain, but 19% of the control group had residual predominating leg pain.[68]

These studies have difficulties including lack of control group[67] and small study size,[66] and no discussion of complication rates between groups.[68] These studies all involve the immediate postoperative period, and merit study on a larger scale with controlled design and comparison of complication rates before being implemented into conventional practice.

Prescription for Vertebral Compression Fracture in Osteoporosis

The goals of medical and exercise intervention in osteoporosis are the increase of bone mineral density, the prevention of fracture occurrence, and the relief of pain. The literature supports that exercise for osteoporosis and for vertebral compression fracture achieve these goals. Patients counseled to engage in regular exercise activity often reply that they are busy all day and get plenty of exercise. Coupland, reporting on the EPIC cohort study, noted that neither household activity (11 hours per week) nor sporting activity less than 2.5 hours per week had an effect on bone mineral density.[10] Both endurance and strengthening exercise increase bone mineral density and decrease the rate of fracture occurrence in persons with osteoporosis.

As regards endurance activity, Bemden reports that athletes have significantly higher bone mineral density than less active controls.[69] The EPIC cohort showed a significant increase in the bone mineral density of the trochanter of women who walk at a rapid pace or stair climb.[10] The duration of walking if slower did not affect bone mineral density. Other studies have shown an effect of walking duration. Smith[70] and Dalsky[71] demonstrated that walking 5 miles per week, or 30 to 60 minutes three to five times per week, increased bone mineral density. Bemden reported that women who jog, stair climb, or walk have increases of bone mineral density at the wrist hip and spine.[69] Coupland[11] cited one study that demonstrated that regular weight-bearing activity reduced fracture risk over 1 year, although the walking activity may affect balance and rates of falling, making the effect on fractures indirect.

Strengthening exercises also increase bone mineral density. Pruitt found that 9-month program for early postmenopausal women resulted in a 1.6% increase in lumbar bone mineral density but controls declines 3.6%.[72] Kerr reported that high-weight, low-repetition exercises increase bone mineral density, whereas low-load, low-repetition activity did not.[73] Sinaki in a case study demonstrated that spinal flexion bias exercises increased the rate of spinal compression fracture and increased related spinal pain, whereas extension bias exercises decreased the rate of fracture and decreased spinal pain.[74]

Precautions for women with osteoporosis, noted by Bemden[69] and Sinaki,[74] include avoiding jarring exercises like high-impact aerobics and horseback riding, abdominal flexion moments like situps and rowing, and activity that increases the risk of falling like skiing.

A possible prescription for a patient with osteoporosis alone or with spinal compression fractures:

Evaluation Screen for signs and symptoms of cardiopulmonary disease; baseline ECG.

Prescription

Education Provide instruction on back conservation; log rolling to come to sitting if needed.

Flexibility Advise corner stretches (see Fig. 79-10).

Strengthening Suggest strengthening exercises such as shoulder retractions and depressions (Fig. 79-17); prone or seated thoracic extensions (Fig. 79-18); if the patient has too much pain to mobilize from bed, supine isometric retractions and extensions (Fig. 79-19), where the patient "tries to pin the mattress with the shoulders" can be done. Patients with more skill can perform more advanced or resisted shoulder retractions with weights (Fig. 79-20).

Endurance Walking as briskly as tolerated for 30 minutes, 5 times per week.

Bracing Brace to block flexion, and hold in extension; the Jewitt brace most restricts motion. Knight, Taylor-Knight, and Cash are less restrictive braces.

Modalities TENS.

Prescription for Neck Pain

Sweeney provides instruction and review for the treatment of neck pain by cervicothoracic stabilization training.[75] The author draws initial attention to the correction of "spectator" position posture with the chin thrust forward and the head anterior to rounded shoulders. The head and neck posture, which reduces translational stress and compression of the facets and stress on ligamentous structures, is the chin-tucked position.[75] The preferred position is with the thoracic spine straight, the shoulders gently back, and the chin gently tucked toward the chest.

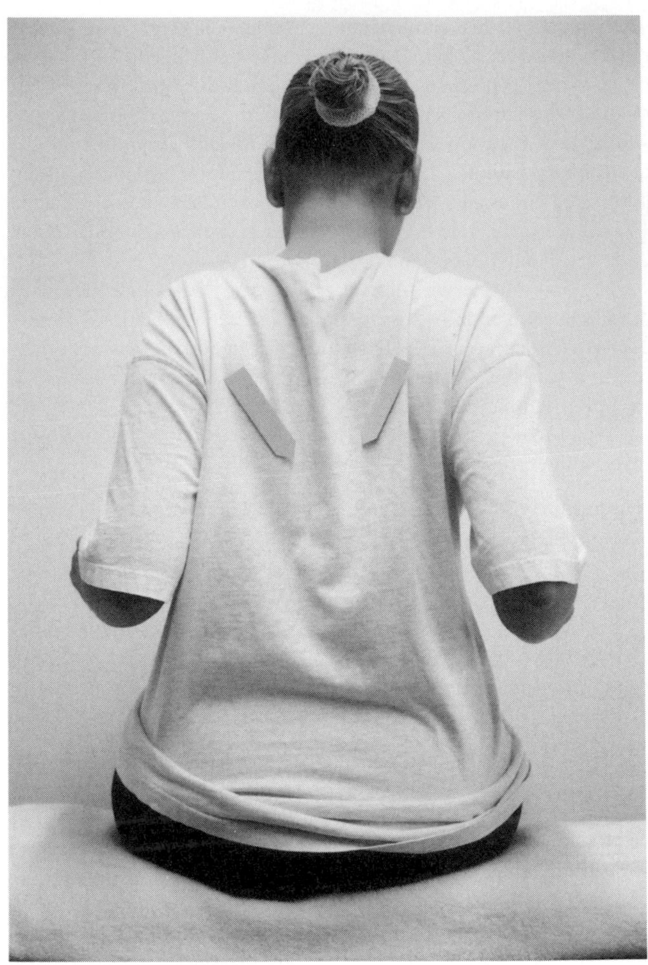

Figure 79-17 Shoulder retraction and depression, like a rowing exercise pull the scapulae and shoulders back and down.

The thoracic extensors and lumbar spine stabilizers may need to be strengthened to adequately support this head and neck posture.[75] Corner stretches (see Fig. 79-10) help stretch the rounded shoulders and thoracic spine. Patient education about posture and body mechanics, pacing activity, flexibility and strengthening, and self-applied first aid for aches and strains occurs first, followed by postural re-education using mirrors.[75] The patient learns flexibility, including range of motion in flexion, extension, and lateral flexion and rotation. Isometric strengthening in lateral and forward flexion and extension in the chin-tucked position are taught and corrected by the therapist.[75] Maintaining optimal head and neck posture through positional transitions and then during exercise round out the instruction.[75] An increase in pain, either axial or radicular, should result in reexamination of the exercise program or the technique of the participant.[75] Poor technique during exercise performance can increase pain.[75]

A possible prescription for cervical pain is as follows:

Precautions List other comorbid diagnoses; screening for signs of cardiopulmonary disease.

Goals Improved flexibility; corrected head and neck posture; maintained posture during activities; decreased pain.

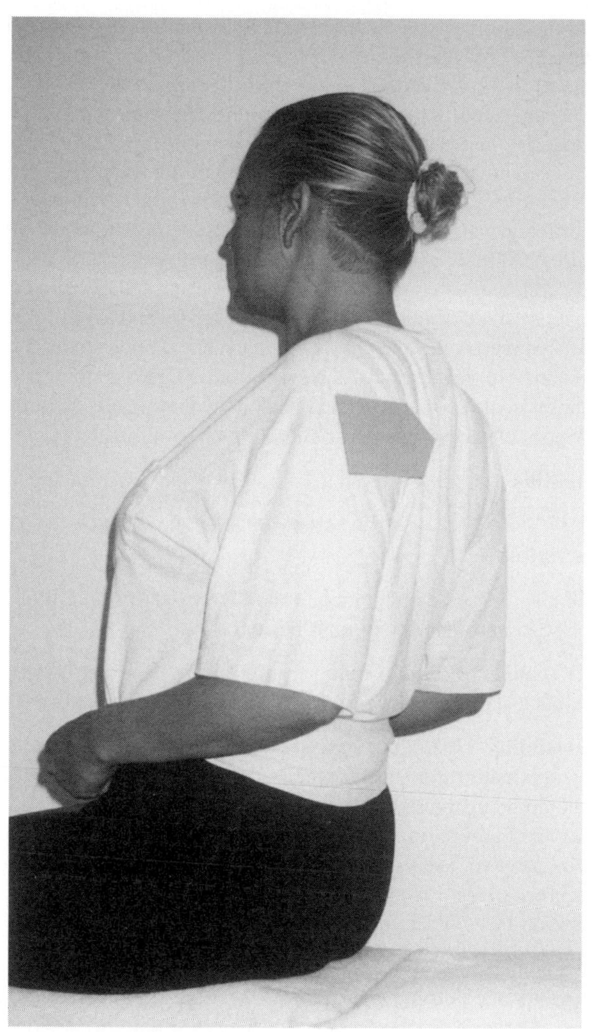

Figure 79-18 Seated thoracic extensions. The patient seated on a surface that will not flip arches the upper back and pulls back the shoulders.

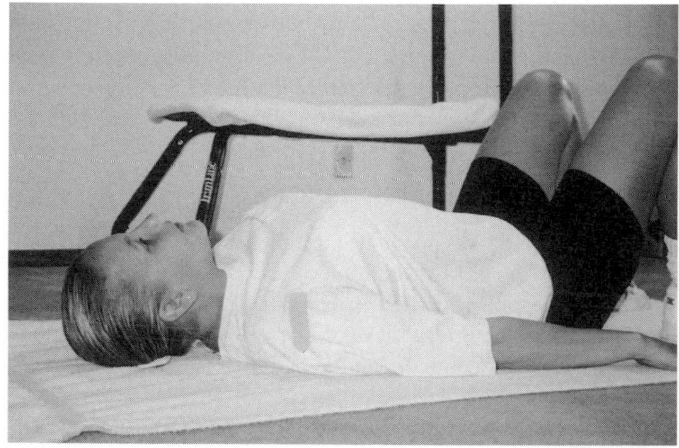

Figure 79-19 Suppine shoulder retraction done with the patient lying on a firm flat surface. The patient is asked to "push" the surface with the shoulders.

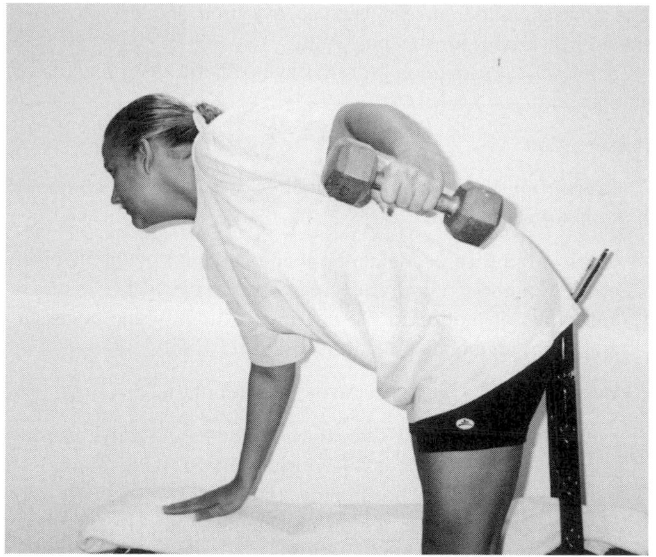

Figure 79-20 Isotonic strengthening exercise for shoulder retractors and triceps.

Education Provide instructions on optimal head and neck posture; importance of strength and flexibility; strain and sprain first aid.

Flexibility Neck and shoulder rolls ("clocks"); corner stretches; range of motion to extension, flexion, rotation, rotation with flexion and with extension.

Strengthening Thoracic extensions and lumbar stabilization; chin tucks in the flexed, neutral, laterally flexed, and extended positions.

Endurance Transition, treadmill training with attention to maintaining correct posture.

Reflex Sympathetic Dystrophy

The physiatric treatment of reflex sympathetic dystrophy remains anecdotal or weakly supported by the literature. Contrast baths of alternating hot and cold immersions of the involved limb have been suggested for "vascular exercise," but without supporting literature as one writer notes.[22] Another author advises against this treatment altogether.[76] Splinting in a functional position if tolerated may hinder contracture formation. Anecdotally, paraffin helps range of motion of nonedematous hands but should be stopped if edema occurs; heat is contraindicated if the patient has an insensate limb or sensation is diminished. Range of motion is conventionally recommended but may incite vasomotor and sudomotor instability, at which time these activities are held until medical or injection therapies can calm the syndrome. Therapy to maintain range of motion and strength at ipsilateral joints proximal to the painful extremity and in contralateral limbs as well as the cervical, thoracic, and lumbar spine should not be overlooked. By observation, these patients have weak and stiff limbs proximal to the active reflex sympathetic dystrophy. Not focusing on the patient's painful extremity and exercising other body parts may help the patient gain confidence in the treatment plan and diminish fear of pain inflicted.

The contralateral limb can become overused and the physician should be vigilant for this possibility.

A possible prescription for reflex sympathetic dystrophy (based on convention):

Prescription

Precautions Hold range of motion if sudomotor/vasomotor symptoms destabilize.

Goals Improve or maintain range of motion of the involved portion of the extremity; decreased edema; maintain strength and range of motion in the proximal extremity and contralateral limb; maintain spine posture and flexibility.

Education Pace activity; avoid "overdoing it."

Flexibility Gentle passive range of motion and active assisted range of motion of the involved extremity; passive splinting to maintain functional positioning (monitor skin for pressure areas); active range of motion and stretch of the proximal limb girdle, contralateral limb, and spine.

Strengthening Contralateral limb (Fig. 79-21) and spine.

Prescription for Chronic Pain Syndrome

Physical medicine prescription is only a portion of a multidisciplinary effort to treat chronic pain syndrome, in which pain or its report is the given reason for inactivity and withdrawal from normal social roles and functions. Persons with chronic pain syndrome are deconditioned and the focus of their treatment is conditioning or endurance activity, for example, biking, walking, or swimming.[77] Because behavior modification is the foundation of this treatment program, to reinforce desired behavior, the exercise must be relevant to the person, his or her limitations, and to the pain.[77] The activity must also be quantifiable to gauge improvement and accessible.[77] Initially, the patient and physician establish baseline activity by having the patient exercise to tolerance several days in a row.[76] When the baseline of activity is established, the therapist and physician develop a program of regular activity for the patient at or just below the baseline, and increase the activity every few days in small increments.[77,78] The patient is rewarded and reinforced for achieving goals without the display of pain behaviors.[77]

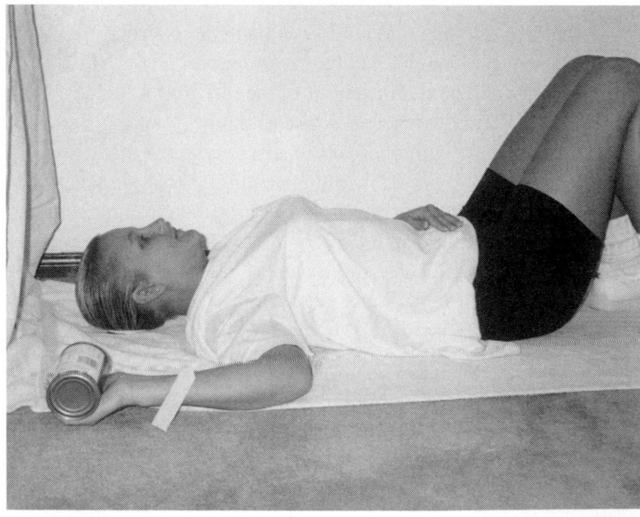

Figure 79-21 Strengthening exercise for shoulder rotators where a one-pound can is rotated from the "9 o'clock" to "3 o'clock" position while the proximal shoulder, arm, and elbow are supported.

It is important that the therapist not ask the patient about pain, and that the therapist not indulge or respond to complaints of pain by the patient. These concerns should be referred to the physician, and should not affect the progression of therapy. Obviously new and different pains, which might be indicative of cardiac or other significant illness, should be evaluated in a timely fashion.

By contrast, when the patient is having a particularly good day, the patient should be instructed to pace activity and avoid overexertion that reactivates the chronic pain cycle.[77] Patients with a preponderance of psychosocial stress, secondary gain, or psychiatric diagnoses will do less well than persons without these features.[77]

A possible prescription for chronic pain syndrome:

Evaluation Review of systems for signs of cardiopulmonary disease; baseline ECG.

Prescription

Goals Increase endurance for common activity, and diminish regression to display of pain behavior.

Education Pacing activity; resting before the onset of fatigue or pain; self-applied ice first with local ice or heat after exertion.

Flexibility Establish baseline range of motion around the symptomatic area over several days or sessions; the patient should be instructed to give effort to tolerance while establishing the baseline of flexibility; stretch to average range of motion for 4 to 5 days; increase range of stretch by two to three degrees every 4 to 5 days; at day 4 or 5 the increase range of motion takes place regardless of whether the patient is having a "good" pain day or a "bad" pain day.

Endurance activity Establish a baseline of walking activity (or other activity) to tolerance over several days or sessions of performance. Walk for the average walking time for 4 to 5 days and increase the walking time by 10% every 4 to 5 days. The increase in walking time occurs regardless of whether the patient is having a "good" pain day or a "bad" pain day on day 4 or 5. If the patient is having a particularly good day, he or she should not increase activity beyond the prescribed walking time, but perhaps enjoy some other leisure reward of limited exertion, like reading a book, relaxing outside, knitting, visiting with family or friends, eating a dessert or drinking a cup of coffee at a restaurant, or potting a small plant.

Limiting Exercise and Rehabilitation Assistance Apart from Exercise Activity

Certain disease processes like multiple sclerosis worsen with overexertion. Patients with multiple sclerosis become weaker and more symptomatic in warm weather and if they overexert while exercising or in therapy. Precautions for this population include resting the patient frequently, and avoiding exercising in a hot environment or warmed pool or whirlpool.

Up to 72% of patients with Guillain-Barré syndrome experience pain.[79] These pains include paresthesias and radicular pain, but also myalgia and arthralgia in particular shoulder pain and lumbago.[80] Movement aggravates the pain. Other rehabilitation considerations like mattress support, turning and positioning, bed cages to keep the sheets off allodynic limb, and passive range of motion may provide comfort to this population.[79] While these patients do participate in mobility therapies, moderation diminishes over exertional pain.

Forty to 64 percent of sufferers of amyotrophic lateral sclerosis (ALS) may experience pain, including skin pressure, musculoskeletal pain, and cramps.[81] Again, other considerations from the realm of physical medicine may provide comfort to this population. The caregiver can learn turning and positioning and passive range of motion. These patients also have distress and discomfort that do not fulfill the definition of pain but that rehabilitation intervention can lessen.[81] For example, a speech therapist may alleviate feeding problems and choking sensations with evaluation of swallowing, instruction in head and body positioning to facilitate swallowing, and recommendation for the appropriate consistency of the diet, for example, pureed.[81]

SUMMARY

Physical medicine and rehabilitation can provide a spectrum of services from a variety of health care professionals to address discomfort and pain that patients experience as a result of surgical, medical, traumatic, or congenital disease. Exercise prescription, including education, stretch, strength, and endurance portions, administered by physical or occupational therapists, relieves pain, improves strength and stamina and flexibility in various musculoskeletal complaints.

Physical medicine and rehabilitation strategies and personnel may also help persons with other types of discomfort or distress or dysfunction, and the physician can consult for recommendations.

REFERENCES

1. Bloodworth D, Calvillo O, Smith K, Grabois M. Chronic pain syndromes: evaluation and treatment. In: Braddom RL, ed. *Physical Medicine and Rehabilitation.* 2d ed. Philadelphia, Pa: WB Saunders; 2000:913–933.
2. Frontera WR. Exercise in physical medicine and rehabilitation. In: Grabois M, Garrison SJ, Hart ZT, et al, eds. *Physical Medicine and Rehabilitation: The Complete Approach.* Malden, Mass: Blackwell Science; 2000:487–503.
3. Pollock ML, Whilmore JH, eds. *Exercise in Health and Disease: Evaluation and Prescription for Prevention and Rehabilition.* 2d ed. Philadelphia, Pa: WB Saunders; 1990:202–237.
4. Walker WC. Retraining the neuromuscular system: biofeedback and neuromuscular electrical stimulation. In: Grabois M, Garrison SJ, Hart T, et al, eds. *Physical Medicine and Rehabilitation: The Complete Approach.* Malden, Mass: Blackwell Science; 2000:513–529.
5. Tollison DT, Kriegel ML. Physical exercise in the treatment of low back pain: Part II: a practical regiment of stretching exercise. *Orthop Rev* 1998;17:913–923.
6. Taylor DC, Dalton JD, Seaber AV, et al. Viscoelastic properties of muscle: the biochemical effects of stretching. *Am J Sports Med* 1990;18: 300–309.
7. Halbertsma JP. Stretching exercises: effect on passive extensibility and stiffness in short hamstrings of healthy subjects. *Arch Phys Med Rehabil* 1994;75:976–981.
8. Khalil TM, Asfour SS, Martincz LM, et al. Stretching in the rehabilitation of low-back pain patients. *Spine* 1992;17:311–317.
9. Lewit K, Simons DG. Myofascial pain: relief by post-isometric relaxation. *Arch Phys Med Rehab* 1984;65:452–456.
10. Coupland CA, Cliffe S, Bassey EJ, et al. Habitual physical activity and bone mineral density in postmenopausal women in England. *Int J Epidemiol* 1999;28:241–246.
11. DeLateur BJ. Therapeutic exercise. In: Braddom RL, ed. *Physical Medicine and Rehabilitation.* 2d ed. Philadelphia, Pa: WB Saunders; 2000: 392–412.
12. Hickson RC. Interference of strength development by simultaneously training strength and endurance. *Eur J Appl Phys* 1980;12:336–339.
13. Pollock ML, Wilmore JH, eds. *Exercise in Health and Disease: Evaluation and Prescription for Prevention and Rehabilitation.* 2d ed. Philadelphia, Pa: WB Saunders; 1990:91–158.
14. McCain GA. Nonmedicinal treatment in primary fibromyalgia. *Rheum Dis Clin North Am* 1989;15:73–90.
15. Surbey GD, Andrew GM, Cervenko FW, et al. Effects of naloxone on exercise performance. *J Appl Physiol* 1984;57:674–679.
16. Health screening and risk stratification. In: Franklin BA, ed. ACSM's *Guidelines for Exercise Testing and Prescription.* 6th ed. Philadelphia, Pa: Lippincott, Williams & Wilkins; 2000:22–32.
17. Pretest clinical evaluation. In: Franklin BA, ed. *ACSM's Guidelines for Exercise Testing and Prescription.* 6th ed. Philadelphia, Pa: Lippincott, Williams & Wilkins; 2000:35–56.
18. Lane NE, Michel B, Bjorkengren A. The risk of osteoarthritis with running and aging: a five-year longitudinal study. *J Rheum* 1993;20: 461–468.
19. Wilder RP, Brennan DK. Physiological responses to deep water running in athletes. *Sports Med* 1994;16:374–380.
20. Trombley CA. Retraining basic and instrumental activities of daily living. In: Trombley CA, ed. *Occupational Therapy for Physical Dysfunction.* Baltimore, Md: Williams & Wilkins; 1989:289–318.
21. Gam AN, Johanssen F. Ultrasound therapy in musculoskeletal disorders: a meta-analysis. *Pain* 1995;63:85–91.
22. Post RE, Lee SL, Syen DB. Physical agent modalities. In: Trombley CA, ed. *Occupational Therapy for Physical Dysfunction.* Baltimore, Md: Williams & Wilkins, 1989:659–673.
23. Brennen KR. The characterization of transcutaneous stimulating electrodes. *IEEE Trans Biomed Eng* BME-23 1976;4:337–340.
24. Linzer M, Long DM. Transcutaneous neural stimulation for the relief of pain. *IEEE Trans Biomed Eng BME-23* 1976;4:341–345.
25. Neilzen S, Sjolund BH, Erikkson MBE. Psychiatric factors influencing the treatment of pain with peripheral conditioning stimulation. *Pain* 1982;13:365–371.
26. Mannheimer JS, Lampe GN. Factors that hinder, enhance, and restore the effectiveness of TENS: physiologic and theoretical considerations. In: Mannheimer JS, Lampe GN, eds. *Clinical Transcutaneous Electrical Nerve Stimulation.* Philadelphia, Pa: FA Davis; 1984:63–189.
27. Mannheimer JS, Lampe GN. Differential evaluation for the determination of TENS effectiveness in specific pain syndromes. In: Mannheimer JS, Lampe GN, eds. *Clinical Transcutaneous Electrical Nerve Stimulation.* Philadelphia, Pa: FA Davis; 1984:63–189.
28. Abelson K, Langley GB, Sheppeard H, et al. Transcutaneous electrical nerve stimulation in rheumatoid arthritis. *N Z Med J* 1988;96: 156–158.
29. Langley G, Sheppeard H, Johnson M, et al. The analgesic effects of transcutaneous electrical nerve stimulation and placebo in chronic pain patients. *Rheumatol Int* 1984;4:119–123.
30. Fisher NM, Pendergast DR, Gresham GE, et al. Muscle rehabilitation: its effect on muscular and functional performance of patients with knee arthritis. *Arch Phys Med Rehabil* 1991;72:3667–3374.
31. Smith CR, Lewith GT, Machin D. Transcutaneous nerve stimulation and osteoarthritis pain. *Physiotherapy* 1983;69:266–268.
32. Godfrey CM, Jayawardena H, Quance TA. Comparison of electrical stimulation and isometric exercise in strengthening of the quadriceps muscle. *Physiother Can* 1979;31(5):1–4.
33. Gould N, Donnermeyer D, Pope M. Transcutaneous muscle stimulation as a method to retard disuse atrophy. *Clin Orthop* 1982;164:215–220.
34. Roush MB, Sevier TL, Wilson JK, et al. Anterior knee pain: a clinical comparison of rehab models. *Clin J Sport Med* 2000;10;22–28.
35. Bourne MH, Hazel WA, Scoot SG, et al. Anterior knee pain. *Mayo Clin Proc* 1988;63:482–491.

36. Burckhardtt CS, Mannerkorpi K, Hedenberg L, et al. A randomized, controlled clinical trial of education and physical training for women with fibromyalgia. *J Rheum* 1994;21:4:714–720.
37. McCain GA, Mai FM, Halliday PD. A controlled study of the effects of a supervised cardiovascular fitness-training program on the manifestations of primary fibromyalgia. *Arth Rheum* 1988;31:1135–1141.
38. Nichols DS, Glenn TM. Effects of aerobic exercise on pain perception, affect, and level of disability in individuals with fibromyalgia. *Phys Ther* 1994;74:327–332.
39. Thompson JM. The diagnosis and treatment of muscle pain syndromes. In: Braddom RL, eds. *Physical Medicine and Rehabilitation.* 2nd ed. Philadelphia, Pa: WB Saunders; 2000:943–956.
40. Han SC, Harrison P. Myofascial pain syndrome and trigger-point management. *Reg Anesth* 1997;22:585–590.
41. McCain GA. Role of physical fitness in fibrositis-fibromyalgia syndrome. *Am J Med* 1981;81(suppl 3A):73–77.
42. Kraus H, Fischer AA. Diagnosis and treatment of myofascial pain. *Mt. Sinai J Med* 1991;58:235–239.
43. Lehmann TR, Tussell DW, Spratt KF, et al. Efficacy of electroacupuncture and TENS in the rehabilitation of chronic low back pain patients. *Pain* 1986;26:277.
44. Sikorski JM. A rationalized approach to physiotherapy for low back pain. *Physiotherapy* 1985;10:571–579.
45. Van Poppel MN, Koes BW, van der Ploeg T, et al. Lumbar supports and education for the prevention of low back pain in industry. *JAMA* 1998;279:1789–1794.
46. Walsh NE, Schwartz RK. The influence of prophylactic orthoses on abdominal strength and low back injury in the workplace. *Am J Phys Med Rehabil* 1990;69:245–50.
47. Ciriello VM, Snook SH. The effect of back belts on lumbar muscle fatigue. *Spine* 1995;20:127–127.
48. Reyna JR, Leggett SH, Kenney K, et al. The use of lumbar belts on isolated lumbar muscle. *Spine* 1995;20:68–73.
49. Kendall PH, Jenkins JM. Exercises for backache: a double blind controlled trial. *Physiotherapy* 1968;54:154.
50. Davies JE, Gibson T, Tester L. The value of exercises in the treatment of low back pain. *Rheumatol Rehabil* 1979;18:243.
51. Detorri JR, Bullock SH, Sutlive TG, et al. The effects of spinal flexion and extension and their associated postures in patients with acute low back pain. *Spine* 1995;20:2103–2313.
52. Takemasa R, Yamamoto H, Tani T. Trunk muscle strength in and effect of trunk muscle exercises for patients with chronic low back pain. *Spine* 1995;20:2522–2530.
53. Thorsteinsson G, Stonnington HH, Stillwell GK, et al. The placebo effect of transcutaneous electrical stimulation. *Pain* 1978;5:31–41.
54. Marchand S, Li J, Chenard J-R, et al. Is TENS purely a placebo effect? A controlled study on chronic low back pain. *Pain* 1993;54: 99–106.
55. Melzack R, Jeans ME, Monks RC. Ice massage and transcutaneous electrical stimulation: Comparison of treatment for low back pain. *Pain* 1980;9:209–217.
56. Melzack R, Vetere P, Finch L. Transcutaneous electrical nerve stimulation for low back pain. A comparison of TENS and massage to pain and range of motion. *Phys Ther* 1983;64:489–493.
57. Deyo RA, Walsh NE, Martin DC, et al. A controlled trial of transcutaneous electrical nerve stimulation (TENS) and exercise for chronic low bak pain. *N Engl J Med* 1990;322:1627–1634.
58. Sinaki M. Lumbar spondylolisthesis: retrospective comparison and three year follow up of two conservative treatment programs. *Arch Phys Med Rehabil* 1989;70:594–598.
59. Vroomen PC, De Krom MC, Wilmink JT, et al. Lack of effectiveness of bed rest for sciatica. *N Engl J Med* 1999;340:418–423.
60. Saal JA, Saal JS. Nonoperative treatment of herniated lumbar intravertebral disc with radiculopathy: an outcome study. *Spine* 1989;14: 130–137.
61. Saal JA. Dynamic muscular stabilization in the nonoperative treatment of lumbar pain syndromes. *Orth Rev* 1990;19:691–700.
62. McKenzie RA. *The Lumbar Spine: Mechanical Diagnosis and Therapy.* Waikanae, New Zealand: Spinal Publications; 1981.
63. Donelson RG. The McKenzie approach to evaluating and treating low-back pain. *Orthop Rev* 19:681–686.
64. Saal JA. The new back school prescription: stabilization training part II. *Occup Med: State of the Art Rev* 1992;7(1):33–41.
65. Timm KE. A randomized-control study of active and passive treatments for chronic low back pain following L5 laminectomy. *JOSPT* 1994; 20(6):276–286.
66. Kitteringham C. The effect of straight-leg-raise exercises after lumbar decompression surgery-a pilot study. *Physiotherapy* 1996;82(2):115–123.
67. Carragee EJ, Helms E, O'Sullivan GS. Are post-operative activity restrictions necessary after posteroir lumbar discectomy? *Spine* 1996;21: 1893–1897.
68. Kjellby-Wendt G, Styf J. Early active training after lumbar discectomy. *Spine* 1998;23:2345–2351.
69. Bemben DA: Exercise intervention for osteoporosis in postmenopausal women. *J Okla State Med Assoc* 1999;92(2):66–70.
70. Smith EL, Reddan W. Physical activity: a modality for bone accretion in the aged. *AJR* 1976;126:1297.
71. Dalsky GP, Stocke KS, Ehsani AA, et al. Weight-bearing exercise training and lumbar done mineral content in postmenopausal women. *Ann Intern Med* 1988;108:824–828.
72. Pruitt LA. Weight training effects on bone mineral density in early postmenopausal women. *J Bone Miner Res* 1992;7:179–185.
73. Kerr D. Exercise effects on bone mass in postmenopausal women are site-specific and load dependent. *J Bone Miner Res* 1996;11:218–225.
74. Sinaki M, Mikkelson BA. Postmenopausal spinal osteoporosis: flexion versus extension exercised. *Arch Phys Med Rehabil* 1984;65:593–596.
75. Sweeney T. Neck school: cervicothoracic stabilization training. *Occup Med: State of the Art Rev* 1992;7(1):43–54.
76. Schutzer SF, Gossling HR. The treatment of reflex sympathetic dystrophy syndrome. *J Bone Joint Surg* 1984;66-A(4):625–629.
77. Grabois M. Chronic pain. In: Goodgold J, ed. *Rehabilitation Medicine.* St. Louis, Mo: CV Mosby; 1988:663–674.
78. Fordyce WE. *Behavioral Methods for Chronic Pain and Illness.* St. Louis, Mo: CV Mosby; 1976.
79. Pentland B, Donald SM. Pain in the Guillain-Barré syndrome: a clinical review. *Pain* 1994;89:159–164.
80. Ropper IH, Shahani BT. Pain in Guillain-Barré syndrome. *Arch Neurol* 1984;41:511–514.
81. Oliver D. Terminal care. In: Williams AC, ed. *Motor Neuron Disease.* London, England: Chapman and Hill; 1994:281–293.

PART VII

PAIN, ADMINISTRATION, AND THE LAW

CHAPTER 80 THE ROLE OF PAIN CLINICS

Gerald M. Aronoff

HISTORICAL DEVELOPMENT

In the past 30 years, pain centers have revolutionized the management of complex chronic pain problems. Before discussing important clinical issues, a brief history is presented to give the reader background and perspective.

Several factors contributed to the development of the multidisciplinary pain center. One common observation was need for a facility for the vast group of patients who did not respond to conservative treatment measures and were not appropriate for, or did not respond to, interventional approaches. These patients had chronic pain syndromes with concomitant poor coping, dysfunctional pain behaviors, excessive health care utilization, self-limitations in activity level, medication dependency problems, emotional disturbance, work loss, and global life disruption. (I have emphasized for many years that the term *chronic pain syndrome* is not a diagnosis, but a descriptive term having some or all of the foregoing noted characteristics.) Another observation was the increasing recognition of the importance of psychosocial factors in the development and maintenance of chronic pain syndrome. This clinical observation made by Beecher[1] in 1959 was strengthened further through theoretic formulations.[2]

In the 1950s, our methods for treating chronic pain consisted primarily of bed rest, medication, nerve blocks, or surgery. Currently, bed rest generally is thought to be contraindicated for most chronic nonmalignant pain syndromes. Opioids, often the medications of choice during the 1950s, then fell into disfavor through the 1980s. They are now again being used selectively to treat nonmalignant pain with the recognition that opioids may provide adequate analgesia to maintain high-activity level and prevent work loss and disability.[3] The indications for nerve blocks and surgery are being redefined and used more selectively. Whereas pain centers once were considered treatments of last resort, currently this is often the judgment reserved for invasive treatments. Concepts regarding the treatment of chronic pain changed dramatically, as has the health care system generally in the United States. Health care providers have recognized that early patient referrals may eliminate needless or multiple surgeries, reduce health care costs, and promote the patient's return to productivity, and earlier referral to pain centers appeared to be more commonplace. Insurance carriers ultimately benefit from chronic pain programs when successful outcomes reduce health care costs. Ineffective surgical procedures, multiple physician visits, medication dependency, iatrogenic complications, and lost workdays may be reduced.[4,5]

Throughout the 1960s, pain centers were rare in the United States and even less common outside this country. These facilities were on the fringes of medical acceptability even during the early 1970s. Patients who had multiple surgeries or numerous nerve blocks were not considered to have been treated radically, and yet, patients treated in pain programs with operant conditioning, biofeedback, psychotherapy, and rehabilitation often caused many raised eyebrows.

In 1976, *Medical World News* listed approximately 30 major comprehensive pain centers distributed throughout the United States. By 1979, this number had grown to 278 (according to a questionnaire survey conducted by the American Society of Anesthesiologists). By 1983, the number of alleged pain programs had grown to more than 1000.[6] These numbers represent questionnaire surveys, and there has been no attempt to validate the accuracy of the information provided. Although it is suggested that there are differences in methods, program content, and delivery systems in these various facilities, details regarding their efficacy are not available. In recent years, clinicians are hanging up signs, advertising in local publications, or advertising on the Internet, claiming to be pain programs or specialists without prior experience in the treatment of pain or any specific pain credentials. It is estimated that there are now 1500 to 2000 pain treatment programs in the United States.[7]

The first multidisciplinary pain centers were founded separately by Drs John Bonica and Benjamin Crue. Although different in structure and conceptual framework, both radically changed the treatment of patients with chronic pain syndrome and served as prototypes for the pain centers that followed. As pioneers in the pain movement, both Drs. Bonica and Crue advocated the multidisciplinary team approach to manage intractable chronic pain syndromes. Despite this, there were some fundamental differences in regard to the role of invasive treatments in their pain programs. Dr. Bonica, an anesthesiologist, more frequently used nerve blocks diagnostically or therapeutically. Dr. Crue, a neurosurgeon, viewed chronic nonmalignant pain more as a psychosomatic process, rarely used invasive techniques, and advocated a more behavioral-biopsychosocial and physical rehabilitative approach. Despite these different viewpoints, both programs were successful. Even now, more than 45 years after the inception of these programs, it is unclear whether one approach is preferred over the other. We do not have adequate statistical data to condemn or support one type of pain program over another, but, rather, we are learning that the crucial factor is more likely to depend on the type of pain problem, type of patient, and experience of the treating physicians and support team; we need to accumulate better data to improve specificity of treatments. In my opinion, this is part of the problem.

Throughout the development of the multidisciplinary pain centers (MPC), there has been a move away from the model that treats chronic pain as an extension of acute pain. Over time, there has been increasing importance placed on central factors in the cause and maintenance of chronic pain and associated suffering. Current treatment approaches offer strategies for peripheral management of pain but evaluate the impact of central factors.[8]

By 1979, the American Pain Society, in an attempt to get a better understanding of the status of formal pain management programs in the United States, established a special committee, chaired by this author, to investigate the problem and develop guidelines for classifying pain treatment facilities. The following represents the most complete classification of pain programs currently available. The types and descriptions of these pain programs has not changed significantly and include:

1. Unidisciplinary programs having one discipline and including either MDs or non-MDs.
2. Interdisciplinary programs including at least one physician in an interactional system with nonphysicians as part of the treatment team.
3. Multidisciplinary programs including two or more physicians and nonphysicians.
4. Pain clinics in which pain treatment teams are organized in an outpatient setting.
5. Pain units that specialize in inpatient programs localized in a separate geographic area specifically for the management of pain.
6. Comprehensive pain center that has a program with an inpatient and outpatient pain clinic, facilities for pain research, and teaching programs. Generally treats a heterogeneous population of patients.
7. Syndrome-oriented programs that are specific to certain types of pain (such as cancer, arthritis, back pain, fibromyalgia, or headaches).
8. Modality-oriented pain programs, based on the method used, ranging from transcutaneous electrical nerve stimulation (TENS) to acupuncture, physical therapy, psychotherapy, and biofeedback clinics. The types of modality-oriented programs possible are almost endless. Although some of these programs may offer legitimate services, it also was thought that others may use fringe therapies that border on quackery.

In 1982, the American Pain Society established a committee on Standards for Pain Treatment Facilities, which I was also privileged to chair. Our charge was to gather information and develop guidelines to establish national standards for pain facilities in the United States. It was decided, at that time, that since the American Pain Society was a scientific organization, it would not be involved in on-site surveys or directly participate in the accreditation process. Concurrently, the Commission on Accreditation of Rehabilitation Facilities (CARF) convened a national advisory committee that met in Chicago in July 1982 to develop standards for chronic pain and multidisciplinary inpatient and outpatient programs. The committee accomplished its task, and by January 1983, these standards were published. Throughout the development and implementation of these standards, CARF solicited the assistance of the American Pain Society and the American Academy of Pain Medicine (AAPM). I served as the liaison member from the Board of Directors of APS and AAPM to CARF, and believe that the standards developed reflect the national advisory view that nonphysicians, especially nurses, psychologists, and physical therapists, are often the essential team members in MPCs.

The CARF Standards from 1983 to 1998 were for multidisciplinary and interdisciplinary chronic pain management programs. At the 1998 CARF National Advisory Committee meeting, it was decided to modify the standards for programs now referred to as Interdisciplinary Pain Rehabilitation Programs. The standards can be obtained directly from CARF. In the program description CARF states that "an Interdisciplinary Pain Rehabilitation Program provides outcomes-focused, coordinated, goal-oriented interdisciplinary team services to measure and improve the functioning of persons with pain and encourage their appropriate use of health care systems and services. The program can benefit persons who have limitations that interfere with their physical, psychological, social, and/or vocational functioning. Information about the scope of the services and the outcomes achieved is shared by the program with stakeholders."[9]

In the 1980s and early 1990s it appeared that the aforementioned changes represented an

improvement in meeting the needs of an unfortunate population, who for years became invalids within the health care system. Managed care has unfortunately changed that, and most patients find that their insurers are reluctant to pay for interdisciplinary pain care despite accumulating data that demonstrate its clinical usefulness and cost effectiveness.[10–12] Unfortunately, changes in the health care system brought about by managed care currently threaten the survival of the MPC concept.

In 1990, the International Association for the Study of Pain published desirable characteristics for pain treatment facilities. In doing so, they defined pain treatment facilities as multidisciplinary pain centers, multidisciplinary pain clinics, pain clinics, and modality-oriented pain clinics. Their guidelines included recommendations for staffing, represensation of various specialties, and communications among these health professionals, credentials of the director or coordinator, and services that should be offered. They also made recommendations regarding space, record keeping, support staff, licensing, protocols, and educational programs.[13]

NATURE OF THE POPULATION SERVED

Patients with chronic pain, in their desperate search for the elusive cure, often "chase windmills" and convince their doctors to do many invasive tests and procedures. As a result of their pain behavior, many have iatrogenic complications, suffering, and disability. Those involved in the treatment of these patients must find improved ways to detect this highly susceptible population, establish a therapeutic alliance, and short circuit their pain careers. Our health care system cannot rely solely on the traditional methods of medical and surgical approaches often used with this population.

We should not ask people to live with pain if there is an acceptable treatment to alleviate it and if the potential benefits outweigh the potential risks and side effects. Therefore, I believe that, in all pain treatment facilities, the assessment must begin with a review of the patient's medical status, past medical records, especially those pertaining to prior pain evaluations and treatments, prior pharmacologic trials, and an updated physical examination. This investigation should be done by those experienced in the evaluation of chronic pain. Through the years, I have been distressed by the many clinical recommendations offered by inexperienced consultants. When seeing a patient with chronic pain syndrome, they frequently order extensive diagnostic studies and invasive therapies, whereas more experienced consultants follow a more conservative course. As pain clinicians, our goal should be to develop and provide the most effective therapies for the various pains we treat. Clinical research on the spectrum of pain disorders may help us delineate not only the treatments of choice but also the methods involved in their implementation.[14,15]

TREATMENT VARIABLES

Regarding the patient's educational level, their average education ranged from a sixth grade level or less in a rural environment at the University of Virginia Pain Clinic[16] to more than 12 years of education in the predominantly urban population at the Boston Pain Center[17] to a more mixed population at the Charlotte-based Presbyterian Center for Pain Medicine.[18]

Back pain was the primary site of pain in most MPCs; this was consistent with chronic pain complaints in the general population.[19] At the Boston Pain Center, 45% of recent patient admissions were for back pain; this figure was 50% at the University of Virginia. Murphy[20] reported that back and headache together accounted for two thirds of patients at the University of Washington. Some MPCs focus exclusively on patients with back pain.[21]

Based on a review of more than 1000 pain center patients who had one or more prior spinal surgeries and persistent back pain, I recommended criteria for patients who should have a second opinion before elective surgery (Table 80-1).

Because low back surgeries are being done more selectively and less frequently, pain centers should be viewed as a positive alternative for treatment, not only by concerned physicians and health care providers but also by cost-conscious insurance carriers and employers.[14]

Despite some evidence indicating that narcotic addiction in medical patients is low,[22] many patients with chronic pain have been described as dependent on narcotic medications when admitted to MPCs.[23] Carron and Rowlingson[16] reported that 85% of their admissions had received narcotic analgesics. At the Boston Pain Center,[17] 55% of patients were admitted to the program while they were taking narcotic medication; this figure was 43% at the University of Washington.[20] After narcotic medications, benzodiazepines were administered most frequently. Carron and Rowlingson[16] reported that 85% of their patients had received benzodiazepines, resulting in a 60% drug dependence that necessitated incorporation of detoxification as a part of treatment. In other programs, the percentage of patients taking sedative-hypnotics was substantially lower, with 9% of patients at the Boston Pain Center admitting to having received benzodiazepines. At the University of Washington, 15% of patients had been taking diazapam.

Studies from MPCs, however, have often provided conflicting data regarding the use of opioid analgesics for nonmalignant pain.[24–31] It must be noted, however, that much of these data were uncontrolled, anecdotal, and without adequate information provided to reach definitive conclusions. For example, patients were queried about opioid use. Generally this involved short-acting opioids with an analgesic half-life of 3 to 4 hours. Yet the opioids were often prescribed every 6 to 8 hours. Patients were asked whether they had sustained benefit, significant functional improvement, or improved ability to cope with pain. Generally the responses were not affirmative, and it was concluded that opioids were ineffective for their chronic pain.

I suggest that the conclusions were unwarranted, misleading, and often reflective of inadequate or inappropriate opioid prescribing without adequate attention to pharmacodynamics or pharmacokinetics. As some of the patients responded to an interdisciplinary pain center approach, this further reinforced the conclusion that opioids should not be used in chronic pain. As recently as 12 years ago, one of the outcome measures for a successful multidisciplinary pain center was the percentage of patients "successfully" tapered from opioids during the treatment program and maintained off of opioids during follow-up. In retrospect, I can say that many of these patients had not done well prior to their admissions when they were taking opioids and therefore justification of the medication taper was not difficult. With 20/20 knowledge in hindsight, however, I suspect that many of us may have done a disservice to a small group of patients, "detoxified" or treated for "drug dependence," who might have benefited from long-term opioid treatment but for whom we dogmatically refused to prescribe opioids.[16,32] We now know that controlled-release opioids have a significant role in a carefully selected subgroup of chronic pain sufferers.

In terms of surgical treatment, many patients admitted to MPCs have had previous surgery. Murphy[20] reported that 40% of admissions have had one or more pain-related surgeries (average, 2.4 procedures). Gottlieb and coworkers[21] reported an average of two surgical procedures. At the Boston Pain Center,[17] a survey indicated an average of 1.29 surgeries, although our previous study of 104 consecutive admissions revealed an average of 1.8 pain-related surgeries per patient.[33] Crue and Pinsky[34] found that 60% of their patients had had one or more surgical procedures (average, just under two per patient).

Vocational status is an important consideration when dealing with these patients because the presence of chronic pain syndrome may interfere markedly with vocational functioning. Seres and colleagues[35] reported that 40% of their admissions were "disabled" by pain. At the Boston Pain Center (BPC), more than 50% of admissions were labeled unemployed due to pain. The average time out of work was 29.4 months.[17]

Most patients at the BPC (1976–1994) and at the Presbyterian Center For Pain Medicine (PRCPM)(1994–1999) were involved in pain-related litigation from work injuries and personal nonindustrial accidents. A pilot study[36, 37] at the BPC included a retrospective review of 50 patients who had been discharged between 1985 and 1987 and had returned for follow-up (all had received workers' compensation). The study suggested that, for those who sustain work-related injuries late in their careers and in whom limited education decreases their retraining potential, secondary gain factors may compromise improvement and return to a functional state. Other factors believed to adversely influence return to work included (1) being out of work more than 1 year, (2) negative treatment course and poor mastery of pain, (3) poor work history with little incentive to return to work; (4) major psychopathology, (5) narcotic dependency, (6) primary, secondary, and tertiary gain, (7) litigation, and (8) delay in return to work after discharge from the pain center.

Our policy at the BPC, which continued at the PRCPM, was that only motivated patients without major conscious secondary

TABLE 80-1 **Criteria for Second Opinion before Elective Surgery**

Two or more pain-related surgeries without beneficial results.
One or more pain-related surgeries with negative findings.
Attorney-referred patients involved in pain-related litigation.
Known or highly suspected major psychopathology.
History of unjustified overuse of health-care system.

Adapted from Aronoff GM. Chronic pain and the disability epidemic. *Clin J Pain* 1991;7:333.

gain or suspected malingering were admitted to the pain program. At the BPC we often recommended to patients who had litigation pending that they resolve these issues and if their pain problem persisted, they could then contact us to structure a treatment program for them at that time. The attrition rate after claims closure and litigation resolution was high.[14] This policy has been reconsidered as we have found that there are many industrially injured patients with chronic pain syndrome who through no fault of theirs, having been compliant with treatment recommendations, nonetheless have ongoing pain and suffering in need of treatment. We now believe that they should not be denied treatment because of having unresolved workers' compensation issues or personal injury litigation if the patient is motivated to participate in the full treament program.

Malec and associates[38] found that no patients were employed or in training at the time of admission. Vasudevan and colleagues[39] reported that only 19% of their patients were employed when admitted.

In general, the typical MPC admission may be described as a patient in his or her mid-40s, with slightly less than a high school education, working most probably in a skilled or unskilled occupation but no longer able to work as a result of back pain. The average patient probably is receiving short-acting narcotic analgesics at admission and has had more than one surgical procedure.

PSYCHOLOGICAL CHARACTERISTICS

Because chronic pain has such disruptive effects on people's lives and physical functioning, it is not surprising that psychological and social functioning also is affected. The psychosocial aspects of pain have been reviewed elsewhere in this volume, and many books have covered this topic.[19,40–44] Herein the discussion is confined to delineating the psychological characteristics of patients admitted to MPCs. Keep in mind that patients seen in private practice settings may differ from these patients with regard to their psychological characteristics. Chapman and colleagues[45]compared depression and so-called illness behavior in patients treated in pain clinics or private practices. They found that those treated in private practices were significantly less depressed and showed less conviction of disease, bodily preoccupation, and hypochondriasis. They had less affective disturbance.

Typically, the patient with chronic pain admitted to a MPC is not psychologically minded and has little understanding of the role that psychological issues play in the pain problem. The patient often vehemently denies that there is any psychological component to the pain problem and can be rigidly defensive, using most often denial and repression (an unconscious mechanism wherein psychological issues and conflicts are kept out of the patient's awareness). Emotional conflicts often are expressed through somatic symptoms and are discharged in autonomic, vascular, or neuromuscular responses. They have been described as alexithymic.[46]

Patients may share some or all of the following characteristics: (1) preoccupation with pain, (2) strong needs for dependency and nurturance that may be denied directly and sought through so-called pain behavior, (3) feelings of loneliness and isolation, (4) self-defeating behavior patterns, (5) anger, and (6) hostility.

Seres and coworkers[35] reported that 70% of their patients had hysterical features, and more than 50% were depressed. Gottlieb and colleagues[21] found that virtually all (71 of 72 patients in their study) had moderate to severe psychopathologic disorders (indicated by significant deviations on standardized psychological tests).

Research using the Minnesota Multiphasic Personality Inventory (MMPI) showed that patients treated in MPCs (and patients with chronic pain in general) achieve significantly elevated scores on the hypochondriasis, depression, and hysteria scales of that test.[47] This profile has been referred to as the *neurotic triad* and suggests a high level of depression, denial of emotional conflicts, and a tendency toward the expression of needs through somatic symptoms. Some investigators suggest that this pattern reflects premorbid neurotic symptoms that contribute to the development of the pain syndrome; others view the pattern as reflecting the emotional problems that result from the chronic pain experience.[48] In support of the latter interpretation, there is evidence to suggest that patients with chronic pain cannot be differentiated from those with chronic disease on the basis of their MMPI profiles.[49]

In looking at the backgrounds of chronic pain admissions, some similarities are found. Some of these were addressed by Engel[50] in his classic treatise on the so-called pain-prone patient. They have been updated by Blumer and Heilbronn.[51] These latter authors proposed the term *pain-prone disorder* to identify a distinct subgroup of patients with characteristic clinical, psychodynamic, biographic, and genetic features. Some of these features are: continuous pain of obscure origin, hypochondriac preoccupation, desire for surgery, denial of conflicts, prepain workaholism, idealization of self and family relations, and depression. In the family history, there is a high incidence of alcoholism, depression, and relatives with chronic pain. Past abuse by a spouse and sexual abuse by a parent or sibling also may occur. This author believes that many such patients who later in life develop even a minor illness or injury that becomes chronic are indirectly telling us that they are tired of not getting their needs met. Their symptoms are their way of saying, "Now it's my turn to be taken care of."

It has been this author's belief that many patients consulting primary care physicians or specialists with headaches, back pain, diffuse myalgias, abdominal pain, and other symptoms such as fatigue and nonrestorative sleep have underlying depression and somatization. Through physical symptoms, they are communicating that their life hurts and they are unable to deal with multiple stressors.[52] (Yet this somatization is generally not diagnosed because most pain clinicians do not take an adequate psychosocial or developmental history.) Instead, patients develop a socially acceptable symptom and get a socially acceptable treatment: analgesics, muscle relaxants, benzodiazepines "to relax muscles," a variety of sleeping pills, and so forth. But the stressors continue, and frequently act as perpetuating factors in the chronic pain process. Vague symptoms, overinterpretation of mild diagnostic test "abnormalities" (which more likely represent normal variations), and subjective complaints of tenderness by overly aggressive and inexperienced (at working with chronic pain patients) physicians result in iatrogenically disabled patients who develop invalid lifestyles not because of their condition but as a result of the treatment.

Whether the psychological dysfunction preceded or followed the onset of the pain problem, by the time the patient is admitted to a MPC, there is often global life disruption. Addison[53] states that characteristics common on evaluation include ". . . the perception of one's life being out of one's own control, or a lack of contingencies based on individual behaviors, a sense of helplessness in intervening in one's own behalf is most often the general overlay to all other psychological and emotional changes."

STRUCTURE OF PAIN CENTERS

During the past decade, MPCs have coalesced into similar forms, with common underlying philosophies, assumptions about treatment, and organization.[54,55] A major characteristic is the integration and interdependency of their components.[56] This interdependency means that, despite the diversity of disciplines represented in a MPC, patients are given a message about the nature of their problem and the proposed treatment that is consistent with the philosophy and assumptions of the center as a whole.

The BPC and PRCPM treatment programs focused on several major patient problem areas, including:

- Clarification of the etiology of the pain
- Clarification of the reasons to or not to pursue further diagnostic evaluation or interventional approaches
- The pain–depression–insomnia cycle
- Medication use and abuse issues
- Pain-related physical dysfunction
- Psychosocial factors affecting the pain syndrome
- The distinction between impairment and disability
- Early return to work, school, or other productive activity
- Quality of life issues.

It is crucial to the effective functioning of the MPC that staff are aware of these treatment objectives and can convey the appropriate messages to patients. If a new staff member or consultant arrives whose orientation differs from that of the program, the nature of the treatment milieu changes. For instance, a common goal of many MPCs is medication reduction. I believe this emphasis is appropriate if the medication cannot be demonstrated to bring about therapeutic efficacy but not for medications felt to be of benefit. Pain center consultants must be made aware of the team treatment philosophy or the integrity of the MPC message may be compromised, even if the recommendations are not implemented. Inconsistency in communication fosters division of staff (splitting) and may interfere with effective MPC treatment.

Assumptions Underlying MPC Treatment

An assumption of virtually all MPCs is that chronic pain syndrome always involve psychological, social, biologic, and medical factors.[57] This assumption is inherent in the gate control theory[2] and has been accepted widely throughout the community of pain clinicians. Crue[58] as early as the 1960s made the statement that, although accurate, was inflammatory to many medical and surgical audiences. Namely, that chronic pain is always psychosomatic. He was not implying that there was not underlying pathophysiology, but that chronic pain not only affected organs systems but also affected people, their personalities, and their social systems. Aronoff[59] emphasized that "any treatment program designed for pain patients must be holistic in its orientation if it is to be effective" (Table 80-2). This assumption does not mean that psychosocial factors are only sequelae to a more fundamentally biologic or medical malady, nor does it mean that patients treated in a MPC have primarily psychogenic pain. The prevalence of pain disorders associated with psychological factors (only) in MPCs is remarkably low. However, the prevalence of pain disorders associated with psychological factors and a medical condition is much higher.[60] We must recognize the complex relationship between chronic pain,

TABLE 80-2 **Pain Center Goals**

I. Clarify the diagnosis. Review medical records and the need for additional diagnostic studies or invasive procedures.

II. Improve pain control (eliminate pain if possible) through physical therapies:
   A. Help the patient to be more comfortably active, with a return to a functional and productive life.
   B. Promote the use of alternative noninvasive pain-control therapies other than potent medications.
   C. With individually structured exercise programs, reduce the patient's fear of reinjury.
   D. Teach proper body mechanics and postural awareness.
   E. Evaluate limitations and restrictions.

III. Improve psychological functioning:
   A. Define and address psychosocial issues influencing chronic pain syndrome.
   B. Relieve drug dependency.
   C. Treat depression and its frequently associated insomnia.
   D. Address primary and secondary gains from pain.
   E. Assess family system.
   F. Strengthen support network (e.g., personal, family and community).

IV. Provide access to occupational and vocational rehabilitation and any other significant healthcare personnel and resolve disability when possible.

V. Communicate with the patient's referring physician by discharge summary, telephone, or personal meetings to obtain any information that will assist in the continued management of the patient.

VI. Reduce inappropriate use of the health-care system.

VII. Decrease the cost of medical care associated with chronic pain syndrome.

Adapted from Aronoff GM, McAlary PW. Pain centers: treatment for intractable suffering and disability resulting from chronic pain. In: Aronoff GM, ed. *Evaluation and Treatment of Chronic Pain.* 2nd ed. Baltimore: Williams & Wilkins; 1992:417.

life stressors, and psychopathology. Chronic pain changes people's lives. Some adapt better than others. For some, the stress of chronic pain is overwhelming and activates or reactivates previously quiescent emotional-behavioral disorders. Our goal must be "above all do no harm. . . ." Our treatments should be geared to improving quality of life.

Pain Center Goals

I. Clarify the diagnosis. Review medical records and the need for additional diagnostic studies or invasive procedures.
II. Improve pain control (eliminate pain if possible) through biopsychosocial therapies:
   A. Help the patient to be more comfortably active, with a return to a functional and productive life.
   B. Promote the use of alternative noninvasive pain-control therapies other than potent medications when possible.
   C. With individually structured exercise programs, reduce the patient's fear of reinjury.
   D. Teach proper body mechanics and postural awareness.
   E. Evaluate limitations and restrictions.
III. Improve psychological functioning:
   A. Define and address psychosocial issues influencing chronic pain syndrome.
   B. Evaluate drug-seeking behaviors and treat substance problems if present.
   C. Treat depression and its frequently associated insomnia.
   D. Address primary, secondary, and tertiary gains from pain.
   E. Assess family system.
   F. Strengthen support network (e.g., personal, family, and community).
   G. Define and treat cognitive distortions contributing to dysfunctional pain-disability behaviors.
IV. Provide access to occupational and vocational rehabilitation and any other significant health care personnel and resolve disability when possible.
V. Communicate with the patient's referring physician by discharge summary, telephone, or personal meetings to obtain any information that will assist in the continued management of the patient.
VI. Reduce inappropriate use of the health care system.
VII. Decrease the cost of medical care associated with chronic pain syndrome.

Adapted from Aronoff GM, McAlary PW. Pain centers: treatment for intractable suffering and disability resuiting from chronic pain. In: Aronoff GM, (ed.). Evaluation and Treatment of Chronic Pain. 2nd ed. Baltimore, Md: Williams & Wilkins, 1992:417.

The staff in MPCs generally view the pain syndrome itself as the focal point of treatment, not only as a symptom of some underlying pathophysiologic process. Thus, legitimate directions of treatment are to reduce pain behaviors, life disruption, inappropriate medication usage, and secondary gain; and to increase activity level, physical functioning, and improve vocational status.

The focus on the syndrome of chronic pain in MPCs can be in opposition to the expectation of patients. It is common for patients to expect that pain itself will be the focus of treatment, or perhaps that they will receive another extensive diagnostic evaluation to discover the underlying cause of pain. This discrepancy between patient expectations and MPC orientation needs to be resolved during treatment (as patient and staff come to a common conceptualization of the nature of the pain problem).[42] However, for treatment to be successful, they must believe that they have been appropriately evaluated; that is, what should have been done, has been done.

Another assumption shared by MPCs is the emphasis on the advantages of patients' taking an active role in their rehabilitation. Although research regarding the influence of the so-called locus of control on rehabilitation is equivocal, it is believed that this may reflect difficulties in operationalizing the concept of active responsibility rather than problems with the concept itself.

Active responsibility and independence are orientations shared by many chronic disease specialities, and they differ markedly from those of acute medical care. Patients also may dislike the emphasis placed on independence, seeing this as inadequate caretaking by the staff, who are seen as not understanding the nature of their problem. This discrepancy often is based on patients' (and some clinicians') failure to differentiate acute from chronic pain problems.

A related assumption is that "curing" pain (in the sense of alleviating the cause of nociception) is not always possible. Crue and Pinsky[34] take a centralist, rather than a peripheralist, point of view and argue that, in its chronic form, pain does not require continued nociceptive input. These authors state, "We regard chronic pain syndrome as a result of central nervous system phenomena without the need for an ongoing peripheral nociceptive arm to complete the clinical picture." Not all MPC staff share the centralist viewpoint that cure (in the acute care sense) is not the ultimate focus for treatment of pain syndromes.

Stafflng of a Multidisciplinary Pain Center

The core specialities represented at MPCs are usually similar. This similarity occurs because the assumptions are operationalized.[54,55] Also, CARF has delineated staffing guidelines that often are followed by pain centers, not only because of clinical efficacy but also as a result of the importance of certification in some regions.

Conformity with CARF guidelines for inpatient MPCs requires the services of a physiclan, psychologist or psychiatrist, physical therapist, specialized nursing care, access to a dietician's services, and social services. In addition, many pain centers have occupational therapy and/or vocational services as an integral part of the program.

Medical Director

As noted in the CARF guidelines,[9] the medical director of the pain program does not need to be the clinical director, although frequently the same person serves in both capacities. Current guidelines are as follows:

A. Qualifications for medical director include:
   1. Board certification in his or her specialty area.
   2. Certification as a Fellow of the Royal College of Physicians and Surgeons of Canada or a certificate of the Canadian College of Family Physicians(Canada).
   3. Certification as a specialist by the National Board of Health and Welfare(Sweden).
B. Demonstrating the equivalent of two years' full-time post-residency experience in an interdisciplinary pain rehabilitation program.
C. Membership in a regional or national multidisciplinary pain society.

D. Participation at least annually in continuing medical education in pain rehabilitation that is accredited by the Accreditation Council for Continuing Medical Education (ACCME) or the American Osteopathic Association (AOA).
E. Participation at least annually in continuing medical education in pain rehabilitation.

I believe that the medical director should have adequate clinical skills in the evaluation and treatment of pain to allow for the formulation and implementation of an appropriate treatment plan for the given patient population. With these patients, who are at risk for iatrogenic complications, it is as important (perhaps more so) for the physician to know when not to request additional invasive diagnostic studies and procedures than when to request them. Although this clinical decision often is difficult, it must be emphasized that if we pursue the diagnostic evaluation past a certain point, it often is counterproductive, contraindicated, and may contribute to iatrogenic impairment and disability. Defining that certain point involves combining the science and art of medicine.This point is emphasized because in a fee-for-service health care system frequent use of interventional approaches carries a significant financial incentive. This author has been in the field long enough to have evaluated many patients exemplifying excessive use of these procedures for marginal clinical indications. This has damaged the credibility of the field of pain medicine with those who pay for health care as well as patients with poor outcomes from unnecessary treatments.

Services Offered at Pain Centers

A similarity of services is also common in MPCs. These usually consist of medical services (including evaluation, supervision, and medication monitoring) and speciality consultation. Psychological services include evaluation and testing, and group, individual, and family psychotherapy. The psychologist also can be involved in program development, research, and program management.

Physical therapy is a crucial component to any MPC. Often a good physical therapy examination can reveal problems that have been overlooked previously. These include biomechanical dysfunctions, myofascial restrictions, diminished endurance, and functional status in relation to the patient's daily vocational and/or leisure activities. Methods offered by physical therapy range from more traditional acute pain treatments (such as heat or cold packs, whirlpool, and ultrasound) to TENS and strengthening, flexibility, and endurance exercises. Some pain centers, in an attempt to emphasize functional improvement and independence, limit physical therapy involvement to evaluation and active exercise programs; others use active and passive modalities as needed. In recent years with diminishing reimbursement for health care, this author has been dismayed to find many programs utilizing lesser experienced or trained therapists or therapy assistants who are woefully inadequate to deal with this difficult population.

Systematic relaxation training and biofeedback are common features of MPCs because environmental stressors and elevated emotional tension are prevalent in patients with pain and can exacerbate painful conditions. There appears to be little difference in the efficacy between biofeedback and general relaxation training (such as progressive muscle relaxation or autogenic training).[61,62] Both biofeedback and general relaxation training are more effective in pain reduction than no treatment. Biofeedback methods include electromyography (EMG), temperature, and electrodermal response (EDR). Cognitive-behavioral treatments have demonstrated significant improvement in treatment outcome when combined with other types of pain management.

The nature of the nursing care often can be the most important way of communicating treatment assumptions to patients, especially if the nursing component in the MPC is strong. Sample and colleagues[63] state: "The Pain Unit nurse is a unique practitioner. As in all hospitals, the nurse has a major responsibility for the total well-being of the patient. She must exercise accurate clinical judgment and have understanding of pain mechanisms, psychosocial aspects of the chronic pain syndrome, operant conditioning, and behavior modification."

The role of social services in pain programs often is to provide family counseling and educate patients and their families about the impact of chronic pain on family functioning.[64,65] Interventions, in general, assume that chronic pain affects the entire family, not just the patient, and that family members can provide either strong support for behavioral change and necessary life modifications or they can sabotoge treatment goals. It is essential to assess the patient's interactions with his or her significant other as part of the evaluation and treatment process.

Vocational services are offered by an increasing number of MPCs as return to work or other productive activity becomes a more integral aspect of the patient's rehabilitation. The extent of services varies widely, from referral to state vocational rehabilitation agencies to comprehensive vocational evaluation, job analysis or work-hardening programs, and job placement as part of the MPC program. Several professional specialties may take part in MPC vocational services; these include certified vocational counselors, social workers, occupational therapists, and physical therapists.

A formalized educational program also is common in MPCs. Topics are offered that are relevant to patients with chronic pain (and their significant others) and include discussion about medications, depression, body mechanics, the role of psychological factors in pain, the importance for the person in pain to take an active role in the "getting well" process and in making decisions about his or her future rather than taking a victim role. More formalized stress management and assertiveness training programs often are included. The goal of educational programs is to give these patients information that they can use to move out of a position of helplessness[66] to one where they can feel more in control of their lives, with their pain syndrome and its sequelae assuming a less dominant position in their lives.

Although perhaps not accurately considered a service, the milieu and therapeutic community atmosphere is a crucial aspect of treatment in many MPCs. The supportive and sometimes confrontational atmosphere of other patients who also have problems with pain often is one of the most powerful factors in promoting change to a more productive and less pain-focused life. Group interaction is encouraged and activities are managed to maximize socialization among patients and promote group cohesiveness. Unfortunately, the therapeutic milieu has becoming a casualty of the many changes in the MPC brought about by managed care and other current changes in health care reimbursement.

REFERRAL PROCESS

Although physicians generally are beginning to recognize the pain center as an important community resource, it is equally important to understand which patients may be appropriate for a referral to the MPC. Usually a referred patient has a chronic nonmalignant pain syndrome that has been unresponsive to conventional therapy and is associated with significant life disruption. Often the patient has tried physical therapy, psychological therapy, and medication sporadically, all without significant or sustained benefit.

Most comprehensive MPCs treat a heterogeneous population of patients with chronic pain who have problems including intractable headache syndromes, neuropathies, complex regional pain syndrome I (CRPS, also known as reflex sympathetic dystrophy), CRPS II (causalgia) chronic low back pain, rheumatologic, phantom limb, thalamic, facial, gastrointestinal, and other nonmalignant pains. Many therapeutic techniques used in the management of chronic nonmalignant pain syndromes also may be effective in chronic cancer pain syndromes. Generally, however, these patients are treated in separate programs because of our recognition of the distinct diagnostic and therapeutic challenges in each group.

Pain can disrupt the patient's life, causing prolonged unemployment, medication dependency, or depression. When asked directly, these patients often deny depression, but this can be assessed through questions regarding their vocational, marital, or financial disruptions; possible recent deaths of significant others in their lives; decreased concern about personal appearance; changes in sleeping or eating habits; and the presence of social isolation.

It often may be appropriate to refer a patient to a MPC if there is excessive pain behavior during consultation or examination, pain complaints in excess of that expected from the physical findings, pain that has persisted despite extensive evaluation or treatment, and pain for which surgery or nerve blocks are not believed to be treatments of choice. Despite the ubiquity of psychosocial and economic dysfunction, these patients' chronic pain is real (with the exception of malingering), and they should not be given the impression that you, as their physician, believe it is not. Many patients believe that referral to a pain center means that their pain is "all in their heads." For instance, one patient said he was referred to the BPC because ours was a place for people who "think they have pain."

Treatment at a pain center begins with the referral. Ideally, referring physicians indicate to their patients, positively and supportively, that they would like to try a new approach to the management of the patient's chronic pain. The referring physician then explains that, because the pain clearly is a complex process that does not seem to be resolving adequately, a comprehensive pain center would provide a better setting in which to deal with the many complicated medical, psychological, and social factors that have become intertwined. Many patients may think that, if either medical or surgical intervention has not helped them, then their pain must be imaginary. Reassurance that this is not the case can contribute to a more positive attitude toward pain rehabilitation. The following are criteria for patients appropriate for referral to a pain center:

- Patient has been adequately evaluated.
- Pain is refractory to conventional treatments.
- Significant life disruption
- Associated psychosocial difficulties
- Pain-related medication problems or substance abuse
- Significant pain behavior or poor coping
- Patient is motivated to change.
- Resolution of the pain problem is more important to the patient than maintaining secondary gains and/or disability.

It is important that physicians tell their patients that the pain center treatment program generally is not primarily involved in looking for a cure for pain through new diagnostic procedures. Although MPCs offer medical evaluation and diagnostic services, these should generally be performed prior to the treatment program. Otherwise, many referred patients expect these to be either the only services offered or those that are emphasized most. Patients who expect to have their previous diagnostic evaluations repeated often express considerable anger and hostility when it is not forthcoming; this, in turn, may interfere with rehabilitation. Therefore, in general, diagnostic evaluations should be done prior to MPC treatment. That is not to say that the treatment program may not involve consultations with appropriate medical subspecialists and result in further diagnostic testing; however, it must be emphasized that this is not the primary reason for the admisssion.

Finally, it is essential that the patient leave the referral meeting with some sense of hope. Patients are discouraged by the prospect of having to "learn to live with it." They are aware that, for them, treatment has failed, and they often feel discouraged and depressed. Patients may be more hopeful if they realize that, despite previous treatment failures, they can be helped at a pain center equipped to address the complexities of their pain problems.

When determining appropriate candidates for referral, the importance of the patient's motivation cannot be overemphasized. Poorly motivated patients sometimes respond to the pain center milieu, but they often resist demands to participate fully in the active treatment regimen. A patient strongly motivated to return to an active and productive life has a better prognosis for success in a MPC.

Most of this discussion applies to both outpatient and inpatient programs. Having evaluated and treated thousands of patients with chronic pain, Aronoff and McAlary[67] concluded that most of these patients can be treated effectively in a structured outpatient day program. Patients traveling a great distance can be housed in a nearby hotel. This avoids costly hospitalization and more realistically simulates typical activities of daily living. For many patients, this is an easier transition from the treatment program back to their usual lives.

It is my belief that treatment for those with difficult chronic pain problems should be based on a wellness model, recognizing that generally pain does not make them "sick" (in the acute medical sense of the word) but rather that it interferes with their optimal functioning in various areas of their lives. These patients generally do not require around-the-clock medical or nursing care.

Recommendations for In-Hospital Pain Treatment

Currently, recommendations for in-hospital treatment include the following:

- Patients requiring diagnostic testing best provided in a hospital
  - Those with unstable medical illness requiring inpatient monitoring and around-the-clock nursing or medical supervision
  - Those who are not ambulatory or independent in activities of daily living
- Patients with major medication dependency, especially with a substance abuse disorder (some of these patients are best treated in chemical dependency centers; others who are highly motivated may be treated as outpatients)
- Those who are acutely suicidal or have unstable major psychiatric disorders (some are best treated in a psychiatric unit)

- Those who previously have been unsuccessful with outpatient pain center treatment (assuming the patient was motivated, and the center was credible).

At present, because hospitals must respond to the economic and administrative pressures of maintaining their patient census, the option of inpatient versus outpatient pain treatment unfortunately may be influenced as much (or more) by these factors as by the best interest of the patient.[5]

If I were to subdivide the chronic pain population I have worked with at the BPCand PRCPM, approximately one third of the patients truly desire to be involved actively in their health care, with the goal of suffering less with pain, using less medication, and returning to a more active productive life than was the case at the time of their admission. This group generally is reasonably self-motivated and eagerly awaits training in new techniques to help them live better with pain and suffer less. Another one third of this population consists of those who have learned to be patients with pain; that is, they have developed goal-directed conditioned pain behaviors (learned helplessness), often maintaining these unconsciously. Nonetheless, these patients are "stuck," and investigation has revealed patterns of self-defeating behaviors. Although somewhat more defensive than those in the first group, these patients are at least receptive to participating in a structured program designed to maximize function and minimize dysfunction and to replace maladaptive coping with more adaptive techniques. They can learn not to be disabled by pain. Generally, these two segments of the chronic pain population do well in multidisciplinary pain programs. We have had a major impact on the quality of their lives and also serve society by returning to it more functional members. It is the remaining one third of this population that is the greatest concern. Although this group tends to be the most "abused" by the health care system, it is also the group that abuses the health care system and society.

Increasingly, it appears that there are some patients who cannot be helped, who at some time may not want to be helped, and whose agenda of being enmeshed in the health care system has nothing to do with receiving health care but, rather, with receiving benefits. We must identify this segment of the population more efficiently and not treat them. Regardless of a patient's complaints, after we have established that the tools at our disposal are unlikely to ameliorate their symptoms, we should establish a series of recommendations, and if the patient is unable or unwilling to consider these, at this point the system may have fulfilled its responsibility adequately to the patient and should no longer attempt to treat them.[5,68]

We should not underestimate the importance of a physician's authoritative guidance; this can be offered as supportive paternalism or maternalism. Patients will either live up to our expectations that they need not be disabled or, conversely, become invalids unnecessarily through learned helplessness. It is our ethical responsibility to improve a patient's health whenever possible. Their physical, emotional, social, and spiritual well-being is more likely to be realized with the self-esteem that results from feeling useful (often from gainful employment) rather than from disability (which frequently is preventable).

Survival of the MPC

Despite the increasing recognition of the efficacy of MPC in treating motivated pain patients with refractory pain associated with dysfunctional pain behaviors, deconditioning from limiting ADLs, and associated life disruption, the survival of the MPC concept is a serious concern of pain medicine physicians and has become a dominant focus for discussion at meetings of the AAPM, APS, and other national and regional pain meetings.

With blatant disregard for extensive research supporting clinical and cost efficacy of the MPC concept in the management of chronic pain and associated suffering and disability, access to care and adequate pain treatment is extremely limited (by payers) for most chronic pain sufferers. Despite more than three decades of evolution advocating the importance of treating pain as a biopsychosial process, often health care reimbursement and the structure of many managed care systems prevent or discourage this. As a result, many excellent MPC treatment programs have had to either close, reinvent themselves as "occupational medicine functional restoration" programs, or significantly reduce the services they provide. While philosophically we have progressed from the Cartesian dualistic concept that viewed illness as being either physical or emotional, in reality many of those who pay for health care have compartmentalized reimbursement so that "mental health" benefits are handled from a different payer than physical medicine benefits, imposing further disincentives for interdisciplinary pain treatment programs.

Kulich has commented on the crisis facing MPC programs in Massachusetts, where many health care professionals refuse to treat injured workers because of poor reimbursement (personal communication, report to the American Chronic Pain Foundation). He says, "Because the reimbursement fee schedule for injured workers was so low, patients could only access treatment in large hospital settings where costs could be shifted, while many pain facilities closed due to this issue. . . ." Currently, no interdisciplinary pain center can treat this patient population, as the reimbursement rates now fall so far below costs.

The American Chronic Pain Association, a patient advocacy group, indicates that "education of people with chronic pain is being threatened at a time when support of health-related and general education is being strengthened." Cowan notes that reduced funding has caused the elimination of many MPCs, limiting access to care by a population in great need (personal communication). She adds, " Witholding the important services available through MPCs is equivalent to withholding education from our children or withholding education dollars from other disease-prevention programs proven to be effective. . . . Therefore, instead of being threatened, MPCs should be supported through managed care programs as an important source of providing people with education and support. Through such services, unncessary, costly care is avoided; people learn to manage their pain; and quality of life is enhanced."

Chapman,[71] in a recent article addressing problems facing MPCs states, "One frequently hears of programs closing down or modifying their treatment protocols to meet their own survival needs rather than meeting the needs of the patients they serve. . . ." He discusses fundamental problems within the managed ("mangled") care systems and workers' compensation systems adversely affecting the survival of MPCs and a reimbursement system that rewards procedural interventions preferentially to pain rehabilitation or the use of cognitive-behavioral techniques geared toward functional restoration. He concludes, "The present danger lies in the fact that a major subset of patients whose lives and function have been the most pervasively affected by pain are losing the opportunity to participate in the precise mode of treatment (i.e., comprehensive interdisciplinary pain rehabilitation) that has been proven to be the most effective in helping them to improve their ability to function and their productivity. Unfortunately, the reasons for this have more to do with politics, profit, and the structure of current insurance than with evidence-based quality care."

Steig et al,[72] in an article titled "Roadblocks to Effective Pain Treatment" states that "the new stewards of American health care (the payers, government, managed care organizations, and countless other intermediaries) have created administrative barriers that affect access to care for pain patients and beleaguered physicians who try to care for them. . . ." The authors discuss the multiple social and political issues that create roadblocks, including organized medicine's failure to meet the needs of people in pain. In their conclusion, they discuss the burden on primary care physicians of treating patients with complex chronic pain that requires the expertise of a pain specialist. They state," Whenever possible, early referral to a recognized pain specialist may help to prevent the vortex of events that often leads to permanent disability. The primary care physician must recognize, however, the difference between specialists who offer palliative care (pain management), such as anesthesiolgists who specialize in nerve blocks, from those who are trained to evaluate and treat all of the medical and social issues associated with chronic pain (pain medicine). While there is compelling evidence that referral to pain medicine clinics improves the quality of life of chronic pain suffers, the risk of caring for this population has been gradually shifting unfairly from payers to health care professionals. . . ."

The National Pain Foundation (NPF) is a nonprofit educational organization created to address chronic pain as a major public health problem. Created by leaders in pain management, the NPF serves as an objective and easily accessible resource for the growing population of pain patients, their health providers, and insurers. The NPF will establish an extensive network of information regarding proven, integrated approaches to pain management that will draw from traditional, alternative, and behavioral approaches to pain management. The NPF is built on the belief that early intervention with appropriate pain management can change the course of people's pain and their lives. The mission of the NPF is to create a highly accessible information network that will empower individuals to make optimum use of available resources to manage chronic pain. I am currently chairing a committee that is addressing issues related to access to care in an attempt to increase public and political awareness of this crisis in health care.

CONCLUSION

My career has been the full-time practice of pain medicine for the past 25 years. Most of that time, I was medical director of the Boston Pain Center, a large interdisciplinary inpatient and outpatient program in Boston, Massachusetts. In more recent years, I have been medical director of a primarily outpatient pain program (in Charlotte, NC) with inpatient capability for patients meeting the criteria mentioned earlier in this chapter. I have participated in the pain treatment of more than 13,000 chronic pain sufferers, and have observed the remarkable transition of many individuals whose lives revolved around pain and suffering, disability, and learned helplessness and were enmeshed in the health care system to regaining control of their lives and again becoming functional and productive members of society as a result of the MPC treatment they received. I applaud their efforts and those of my very capable staffs.

Unfortunately, many MPCs have become casualties from the multiple forces described above. For many of the survivors, the vitally important therapeutic milieu has become extinct. Clinicians who remain in the field are often being asked to compromise their professional integrity to provide services that are cost effective, although it is less clear that they are clinically effective. They are often being asked (or forced) to work with physicians, nurses, therapists, and others with little or no training in chronic pain mangement. Those with PhDs are being sacrificed for MA level therapists, RNs for LPNs, registered PTs for PT assistants or exercise physiologists. In so doing, the qualtity of care rendered to the populations being served is compromised.

Our hospital has recently closed the MPC as a result of reimbursement issues. Fortunately, we have a strong anesthesia pain clinic staffed by physicans with an understanding in the concepts of pain medicine and I continue to work closely with them as a consultant. When faced with the complex chronic pain syndrome patient not appropriate for an interventional approach, not having responded to an interventional approach or requiring a pain rehabilitation approach, they do not hesitate to refer the patient. Many of them are now seen in my office without the benefit of a support team of therapists or a therapeutic milieu. Often, in addition to my treatments, I will coordinate, as best I can, other treatment with therapists or physicians. I rarely, if ever, see these consultants and there is no opportunity to have interdisciplinary meetings to benefit patient care. The real casualties in this process are the chronic pain patients, many of whom will never realize what they are missing, what is possible for them, and all that we should be able to offer them but cannot. They are rapidly losing access to optimal chronic pain care.

REFERENCES

1. Beecher HK. *Measurement of Subjective Responses: Quantitative Effects of Drugs*. New York, NY: Oxford University Press, 1959.
2. Melzack R, Wall PD. Pain mechanisms: a new theory. *Science* 1965; 50:971–979.
3. Aronoff GM. Opioids in chronic pain management: is there a significant risk of addiction? *Curr Rev Pain* 2000;4:112–121.
4. Aronoff GM, McAlary PW, Witkower A, et al. Pain treatment programs: do they return workers to the workplace? *Spine State Art Rev* 1987;2(1):123–126.
5. Aronoff GM, McAlary PW. Pain centers: treatment for intractable suffering and disability resulting from chronic pain. In: Aronoff GM, (ed.). *Evaluation and Treatment of Chronic Pain*. 2nd ed. Baltimore, Md: Williams & Wilkins, 1992:417–420.
6. Aronoff GM, Crue BL, Seres J. *Pain Centers: Help for the Chronic Pain Patient, Mediguide to Pain*. New York, NY: Della Corte, 1983:1–5.
7. Steele-Rosomoff R. The pain patient. *Spine* 1991;5:417–427.
8. Hardy PA, Hill P. A multidisciplinary approach to pain management. *Br J Hosp Med* 1990;43:45–47.
9. *Standards Manual for Facilities Serving People with Disabilities*. Tucson, Ariz: Commission on Accreditation of Rehabilitation Facilities, 2000:131–149.
10. Fishbain DA, Cutler RB, Rosomoff HL, Rosomoff RS. Status of chronic pain treatment outcome research. In: Aronoff GM, (ed.). *Evaluation and Treatment of Chronic Pain*. 3rd ed. Baltimore, Md: Lippincott Williams & Wilkins, 1999:655–670.
11. Turk, DC, Okifuji A. Efficacy of multidisciplinary pain centers: an antidote to anecdotes. *Bailliere's Clin Anesthesiol* 1998;12:103–119.
12. Turk DC. Efficacy of multidisciplinary pain centers in the treatment of chronic pain. In: Cohen JM,Campbell JN, (eds.). *Pain Treatment Centers at a Crossroads: A Practical and Conceptual Reappraisal*. Seattle, Wash: IASP Press, 1996: 257–273.

13. *Desirable Characteristics for Pain Treatment Facilities*. Seattle, Wash: International Association for the Study of Pain, 1990.
14. Aronoff GM. *The disability epidemic*. Editorial. *Clin J Pain* 1985; 1:1–3.
15. Aronoff GM. Chronic pain and the disability epidemic. *Clin J Pain* 1991;7:331–333.
16. Carron H, Rowlingson JC. Coordinated outpatient management of chronic pain at the University of Virginia Pain Clinic. In: Ng LKY, (ed.). *New Approaches to Treatment of Chronic Pain: A Review of Multidisciplinary Pain Clinics and Pain Centers*. Rockville, Md: National Institute on Drug Abuse, 1981.
17. Aronoff, GM, Evans WO. Evaluation and treatment of chronic pain at the Boston Pain Center. In: Aronoff, GM, (ed.). *Evaluation and Treatment of Chronic Pain*. Baltimore, Md: Urban & Schwartzenberg, 1985: 495–510.
18. Aronoff GM, Feldman JB. Preventing disability from chronic pain: a review and reappraisal. *Int Rev Psychiatry* 2000;12:157–169.
19. Aronoff GM. Psychological aspects of non-malignant chronic pain: a new nosology. In: Aronoff GM, (ed.). *Evaluation and Treatment of Chronic Pain*. 2nd ed. Baltimore, Md: Williams & Wilkins, 1992; 399–408.
20. Murphy TM. Profiles of pain patients, including chronic pelvic pain: University of Washington Clinical Pain Service. In: Ng LKY, (ed.). *New Approaches to Treatment of Chronic Pain: A Review of Multidisciplinary Pain Clinics and Pain Centers*. Rockville, Md: National Institute on Drug Abuse, 1981.
21. Gottlieb H, Strite L, Koller R, et al. Comprehensive rehabilitation of patients having chronic low back pain. *Arch Phys Med Rehabil* 1977; 58:101–108.
22. Porter J, Jick H. Addiction rate in patients treated with narcotics. *N Engl J Med* 1980;302:123.
23. Murphy TM, Anderson S. Multidisciplinary approach to managing pain. In: Benedetti C, Chapman CR, Moricca G, (eds.). *Advances in Pain Research and Therapy*. Vol. 7. New York, NY: Raven Press, 1984.
24. Buckley FP, Sizemore WA, Charlton JE. Medication management in patients with chronic nonmalignant pain. A review of the use of a drug withdrawal protocol. *Pain* 1986;26:153–166.
25. Finlayson RD, Maruta T, Morse BR. Substance dependence and chronic pain: profile of 50 patients treated in an alcohol and drug dependence unit. *Pain* 1986;26:167–174.
26. Finlayson RD, Maruta T, Morse BR, Martin MA. Substance dependence and chronic pain: experience with treatment and follow-up results. *Pain* 1986;26:175–180.
27. Maruta T. Prescription drug-induced organic brain syndrome. *Am J Psychiatry* 1978; 135:376–377.
28. Maruta T. Problems with the use of oxycodone compounds in patients with chronic pain. *Pain* 1981;11:389–396.
29. Maruta T, Swanson DW, Finlayson RE. Drug abuse and dependency in patients with chronic pain. *Mayo Clinic Proc* 1979;54:241–244.
30. Ready LB, Sarkis E, Turner JA. Self-reported vs actual use of medications in chronic pain patients. *Pain* 1984;18:169–177.
31. Turner JA, Calsyn DA, Fordyce WE, Ready LB. Drug utilization pattern in chronic pain patients. *Pain* 1982;12:357–363.
32. Aronoff GM, Wagner JM, Spangler AS Jr. Chemical interventions for pain. *J Consult Clin Psychol* 1986;54:769–775.
33. Aronoff GM, Evans WO. Evaluation and treatment of chronic pain at the Boston Pain Center. *J Clin Psychiatry* 1982;43:4–9.
34. Crue BL, Pinsky JJ. Chronic pain syndrome—four aspects of the problem: New Hope Pain Center and Pain Research Foundation. In: Ng LKY, ed. *New Approaches to Treatment of Chronic Pain: A Review of Multidisciplinary Pain Clinics and Pain Centers*. Rockville, Md: National Institute on Drug Abuse, 1981:138.
35. Seres JL, Painter JR, Newman Rl. Multidisciplinary treatment of chronic pain at the Northwest Pain Center. In: Ng LKY, (ed.). *New Approaches to Treatment of Chronic Pain: A Review of Multidisciplinary Pain Clinics and Pain Centers*. Rockville, Md: National Institute on Drug Abuse, 1981.
36. Aronoff GM, McAlary PW, Witkower A, et al. Pain treatment programs: do they return workers to the workplace? *Spine* 1987;2:123–136.
37. Aronoff GM, McAlary PW, Witkower A, et al. Pain treatment programs: do they return workers to the workplace. *J Occup Med* 1988; 3:123–136.
38. Malec J, Cayner JJ, Harvey RF, Timming RC. Pain management: long term following of an inpatient program. *Arch Phys Med Rehabil* 1981; 62:369–372.
39. Vasudevan SV, Lynch NT, Abram S. Effectiveness of an ambulatory chronic pain management program [abstract]. *Pain* 1981;1(suppl): S294.
40. Sternback RA. *The Psychology of Pain*. New York, NY: Raven Press, 1978.
41. Barber J, Adrian C. *Psychological Approaches to the Management of Pain*. New York, NY: Brunner/Mazel, 1982.
42. Turk D, Meichenbaum D, Genest M. *Pain and Behavioral Medicine: A Cognitive Behavioral Perspective*. New York, NY: Guilford, 1983.
43. Aronoff GM. Psychodynamics and psychotherapy of the chronic pain syndrome. In: Aronoff GM, ed. *Evaluation and Treatment of Chronic Pain*. 3rd ed. Baltimore, Md: Lippincott Williams & Wilkins, 1999: 283–290.
44. Aronoff GM. Psychiatric aspects of nonmalignant chronic pain: a new nosology. In: Aronoff GM, ed. *Evaluation and Treatment of Chronic Pain*. 3rd ed. Baltimore, Md: Lippincott Williams & Wilkins, 1999: 291–300.
45. Chapman CR, Sola AR, Bonica JJ. Illness behavior and depression compared in pain center and private practice patients. *Pain* 1979;6:1–7.
46. Sifneos PE. The prevalence of 'alexithymic' characteristics in psychosomatic patients. *Psychother Psychosom* 1973; 22:255–262.
47. Sternbach RA. *Pain Patients: Traits and Treatment*. New York, NY: Academic Press, 1974.
48. McCreary C, Turner J, Dawson E. The MMPI as a predictor of response to conservative treatment for low back pain. *J Clin Psychol* 1979;35:278–284.
49. Naliboff BD, Cohen MJ, Yellen AN. Does the MMPI differentiate chronic illness from chronic pain? *Pain* 1982;13:333–341.
50. Engel GL. 'Psychogenic' pain and the pain-prone patient. *Am J Med* 1959; 26:899–918.
51. Blumer D, Heilbronn M. Chronic pain as a variant of depressive disease. The pain-prone disorder. *J Nerv Ment Dis* 1982;170:381–394.
52. Aronoff GM, Tota-Faucette M, Phillips L, Lawrence CN. Are pain disorder and somatization valid diagnostic entities? *Curr Rev Pain* 2000; 4:309–312.
53. Addison RG. Treatment of chronic pain: The Center for Pain Studies, Rehabilitation Institute of Chicago. In: Ng LKY, (ed.). *New Approaches to Treatment of Chronic Pain: A Review of Multidisciplinary Pain Clinics and Pain Centers*. Rockville, Md: National Institute on Drug Abuse, 1981:17.
54. Aronoff GM, Wagner JM. The pain center: development, structure and dynamics. In: Burrows GD, Elton D, Stanley GV, (eds.). *Handbook on Chronic Pain Management*. Amsterdam, The Netherlands: Elsevier, 1987.
55. Aronoff GM, McAlary PW. Organization and function of the multidisciplinary pain center. In: Aronoff GM, (ed.). *Pain Centers: A Revolution in Health Care*. New York, NY: Raven Press, 1988:55–74.
56. Rowlingson JC, Hamill RJ. Organization of a multidisciplinary pain center. *Mt Sinai J Med* 1991;58:267–272.
57. Melzack R. *The Puzzle of Pain*. Harmondsworth, England: Penguin; 1973.
58. Crue BL, Pinsky JJ, Agnew DC, et al. Observations on the taxony problem in pain. In: Crue BL, (ed.). *Chronic Pain*. New York, NY: SP Publications, 1979:13–28.
59. Aronoff GM. A holistic approach to pain rehabilitation: the Boston Pain Unit. In: Ng LKY, (ed.). *New Approaches to Treatment of Chronic Pain: A Review of Multidisciplinary Pain Clinics and Pain Centers*. Rockville, Md: National Institute on Drug Abuse, 1981:34.

60. Fishbain DA, Goldberg M, Meagher BR, Steele R, Rosomoff H. DSM-III diagnosis in chronic pain patients. Paper presented at the meeting of the America Pain Society; October 1985, Dallas, Texas.
61. Turner JA, Chapman CR. Psychological interventions for chronic pain: a critical review, 1: relaxation training and biofeedback. *Pain* 1982; 12:1–21.
62. Tan SY. Cognitive and cognitive-behavioral methods for pain control: a selective review. *Pain* 1982;12:201–228.
63. Sample S, Burgess-Page M, Hayes M. Chronic pain management: the nurse's role. In: Aronoff GM, (ed.). *Evaluation and Treatment of Chronic Pain*. Baltimore, Md: Urban & Schwartzenberg, 1985:565.
64. Hayes MA, McAlary PW, Popovsky J, et al. Alteration in comfort of chronic pain: a nursing challenge. In: Aronoff GM, (ed.). *Evaluation and Treatment of Chronic Pain*. 2nd ed. Baltimore, Md: Williams & Wilkins, 1992;455–464.
65. Goldberg P. The social worker, family systems, and the chronic pain family. In: Aronoff GM, (ed.). *Evaluation and Treatment of Chronic Pain*. 2nd ed. Baltimore, Md: Williams & Wilkins, 1992;465–474.
66. Seligman MEP. *Helplessness*: *On Depression, Development, and Death*. San Francisco, Calif: Freeman, 1975.
67. Aronoff GM, McAlary PW. Multidisciplinary treatment of intractable pain syndromes. In: Liptons, Tunks E, Zuppi M, (eds.). *Advances in Pain Research and Therapy*. Vol 13. New York, NY: Raven Press, 1990:267–277.
68. Aronoff GM. What is happening to medicine? [editorial]. *Clin J Pain* 1988;4:65–66.
69. Chapman SL. Chronic pain rehabilitation: lost in a sea of drugs and procedures? *APS Bull* 2000;10(3):1–9.
70. Steig RL, Lippe P, Shepard TA. Roadblocks to effective pain treatment. *Med Clin North Am* 1999;83:3.

CHAPTER 81 SETTING UP A PAIN TREATMENT FACILITY

Steven D. Waldman

INTRODUCTION

Over the past several years there has been considerable interest in expanding the role of the pain management specialist as an integral member of the health care team. This interest has been stimulated in part by the increased availability of health care professionals with a special interest and advanced training in pain medicine and in part by the unprecedented economic pressures of our rapidly evolving health care system. These economic pressures have forced many pain management specialists to explore new avenues of revenue generation as well as to examine new strategies to help improve the efficiency and cost-effectiveness of the care they provide.

The purpose of this chapter is to serve as a guide for the pain management specialist who may be considering setting up a pain treatment center or expanding the scope of services currently offered. Although many of the concepts presented are basic, failure to take them into consideration may lead to high levels of professional frustration and dissatisfaction, damage to the professional image of the pain management specialist, economic loss, and increased exposure to malpractice liability.

BASIC CONSIDERATIONS

Should Pain Management Services Be Offered?

There is no question that there is a huge demand for quality pain management services. The Nuprin Pain Report, which to date is the only comprehensive evaluation of pain in the United States, reveals that there are four billion work days lost due to pain in America alone.[1] Seventy-three percent of the patients interviewed reported one or more headaches that interfered with their ability to work; 50% of the people interviewed reported back pain, which limited their ability to work; 46% reported abdominal pain, which limited their ability to work. The Nuprin Pain Report further noted that 43% of Americans saw a physician at least one time in the year preceding the statistical analysis and, surprisingly, 29% of those patients surveyed sought the help of a physician for pain four or more times in the year proceding statistical analysis. Of great interest to our specialty is that of those patients who sought medical attention for more than an occasional pain, 58% saw their family physician; 18% saw a chiropractor; 12% sought help from their pharmacists; and 9% percent sought help from dentists or other health care professionals. Only 3% sought the advice and help of a pain management specialist. From these data, it is obvious that there are a huge number of patients who could potentially benefit from quality pain management services and, equally obvious, is that our specialty has a problem with recognition and identity.

Interfacing Pain Management Services With Existing Services

The first question that must be asked when considering the implementation or addition of new pain management services is how the addition of this new service will interface with existing professional activities. One must take into account the impact of such new services on existing care. The addition or expansion of pain management services requires a high level of commitment from *all* members of the health care team. Even if additional professional staff is added to provide pain management services, consideration must be given to such issues as call responsibilities, vacation coverage, and so forth.

As with all health care endeavors, there must be sufficient expertise to provide an ongoing level of quality care. One would not implement an open heart surgery program or start a burn unit without adequate expertise or additional training. Pain management requires the same level of training, expertise, and commitment. In addition to the clinical expertise required to provide quality pain management services, there must be the administrative expertise if the endeavor is to be economically viable. This is especially important when setting up a pain treatment facility under the managed care paradigm.[2]

Are There Adequate Personnel To Provide Quality Care?

When setting up a pain treatment facility it is important that the pain management specialist recognize the high level of commitment in terms of the time and energy essential to provide quality pain management services. For this reason, the pain management specialist must ensure that there are adequate personnel to provide high-quality coverage for any new services that are contemplated or to cover the expansion of existing services.

There is a common misconception that pain management can be done at the convenience of the pain management specialist. This is simply not the case. This approach can only lead to high levels of dissatisfaction from both patients and referring physicians. Today's patient, or what has become affectionately known as today's "health care consumer," is unwilling to wait for extended periods in order to receive care. During implementation of a new pain management facility or an expansion of an existing one, a realistic appraisal of the time required to provide the proposed care must be undertaken to assure the provision of care in a timely manner. Just as there must be an adequate number of health care professionals to provide high-quality pain management services, there must also be a high level of motivation in order for the pain facility to ultimately succeed.[3] All members of the health care team must be committed to quality and compassionate provision of pain management services. A lone pain management specialist, no matter how motivated and caring, can do little to make up for the uninterest and lack of support of the remainder of the pain management team. This statement applies not only to the clinical personnel but to the administrative personnel as well.

Is The Support Staff Adequate?

When setting up a pain treatment facility, care must be taken to be sure that the practice infrastructure is adequate to support a busy and growing pain management service. If the pain management specialist's existing billing office is unable to keep up with the volume of work generated from existing activities, the addition of billings from new or expanded pain management service may throw the entire office into disarray and adversely affect cash flow. Obviously, additional help can be added to alleviate this situation, but this should be done in a prophylactic manner.[4]

Services Offered

Prior to setting up a new pain treatment facility, the first decision that needs to be made is the decision as to which specific services (e.g., evaluation, neural blockade, drug management and detoxification, etc.) should be offered. To adequately delineate these services, the pain management specialist must take into account his or her existing expertise, experience, and preferences as well as those of other health care professionals providing pain management services within the group practice. The availability of support services such as physical therapy, occupational therapy, psychiatry, and radiology support services, such as computed tomography (CT) scanning, magnetic resonance imaging, and biplanar fluoroscopy must also be considered. Under the managed care paradigm, some services may not be reimbursed at levels adequate to justify their use from a purely economic viewpoint.

It is important to clearly define to the patient as well as the referring physician what a new pain treatment facility can and cannot offer. Too often a pain management specialist with limited experience and training tries to hold himself or herself out as a specialist in all areas of pain management. This is not only academically dishonest but often leads to high levels of patient and referring physician dissatisfaction.[5] It may also place the pain management specialist, and those with whom he or she practices with, in a potentially serious medicolegal situation. Services should not be advertised that are not available or cannot be provided with sufficient expertise to keep complications to a minimum.

Types of Patients Seen

The second decision that needs to be made is delineating the types of patients that the pain management specialist feels are appropriate for the scope of pain management services he or she has chosen to offer at the new facility. The pain management specialist should determine if he or she is comfortable treating cancer pain, headache and facial pain, chemical-dependent problems, acute and postoperative pain, and so forth. The pain management specialist must also determine whether he or she will accept patients who are involved in workers' compensation claims and patients who are involved in litigation. Third, the pain management specialist must decide whether he or she will accept self-referred patients or if he or she will require patients to be evaluated and then referred by another physician (see section on physician referral). Finally, the pain management specialist will also have to decide whether he or she will accept primary responsibility for patients who are admitted to the hospital. This decision has specific implications that must be carefully thought out from a quality-of-care viewpoint, because some pain management specialists may be incapable or unwilling to deal with the many medical problems that may occur while the patient is hospitalized under their care. Political issues as to the appropriateness of a pain management specialist providing primary care may also have to be addressed.[6,7]

Financial Considerations

The following issues must be handled according to each pain management specialist's existing financial situation, current policies, prior contractual agreements with the hospital and/or third-party carriers, as well as his or her own philosophical and ethical viewpoints on providing indigent care. To ignore these variables when starting a pain treatment facility is to ensure economic disaster.

For the pain management service to remain on a strong economic footing in this period of ever-decreasing revenues, financial considerations must be carefully considered.[8] Some pain management specialist's have chosen to provide pain management services on a cash-only basis. While this may work in some affluent communities, by and large, in view of the high cost of many of the modalities offered, this represents an impractical approach for most pain management specialists.

A decision must be made as to the desirability of accepting Medicare assignment as well as other third-party assignments of insurance benefits. Participation in managed care plans should also be carefully weighed.[2] Obviously, local factors have to dictate the variables to be taken into account when making this decision. The pain management specialist must also decide what provisions will be made for the indigent patient who has Medicaid or who is solely responsible for the payment of his or her health care costs. The pain management specialist is likely to be approached by attorneys who desire care to be rendered on a contingency basis. The economic impact of these decisions cannot be overstated.

Availability

It has been said that there are three "As" of a successful practice of pain management: ability, amiability, and availability. Obviously from a patient-care viewpoint, ability is the most important issue. From a practice management viewpoint, however, there is no question that availability is the most important. When starting a pain treatment center, it is imperative that the clinical and administrative staff all agree on the appropriate levels of availability if the facility is to succeed. Most patients expect to see the same physician at each visit, and this fact has specific impact on call schedule issues, for example, days off after call, vacation scheduling, afternoons off. If *all* members of the pain management care team are not motivated to facilitate the provision of quality pain management services, it is impossible for a single member of the team to make the pain management service successful. This statement also applies to the administrative staff. If the administrative staff refuses to work in additional patients or limits the hours of operation of the pain treatment facility, adverse economic consequences will often result.

Additional issues that need to be determined when setting up a pain treatment facility include the hours of operation for the pain management center. The availability of evening hours has become increasingly important and is increasingly expected by the health care consumer in today's competitive market. Weekend coverage and holiday coverage must be also clearly defined for both the patient and referring physician. Expectations of the pain management specialist who is covering these periods should also be delineated to avoid friction between members of a group pain management practice and to assure appropriate availability from all members of the pain management care team. A clear protocol for how emergency referrals will be handled is mandatory in order to assure quality, compassionate care with a high level of satisfaction for both patient and referring physician.

How patient phone calls are handled will also have an impact on the ultimate success of the pain management specialist. Calls from referring physicians, the pharmacy, and patients, as well as support services including laboratory, radiology, physical therapy, and occupational therapy are the rule rather than the exception. Again, it must be clearly defined as to how these call will be handled by all members of the pain management care team in order to provide consistent, quality care and avoid lost revenues through missed consults or unavailability. The use of answering machines and voice mail as a way to avoid dealing with patients and referring physicians is to be avoided, and may require careful monitoring by the pain treatment facility management team.

Coupled with the need for the prompt returning of phone calls is the timeliness in which outpatient appointments and inpatient consultations are handled. Although specific times may vary from community to community, seeing inpatient consults (other than emergencies) within 24 hours of being called works well in most situations. Any consult requested on an emergency basis should be seen as soon as possible. Seeing all routine consults that are received before 4:00 PM on that same day (this includes Saturdays, Sundays, and holidays) projects a strong message that the pain patient will not suffer needlessly while waiting for pain management service to be implemented. The same reasoning applies to the availability of outpatient consultation. When setting up a pain treatment facility, immediate appointments should be available on a same-day basis for patients with acute pain problems and pain emergencies. Such appointments should allow appropriate screening and triage for such patients without disrupting the flow of previously scheduled patients.

This approach also makes good sense from a time management viewpoint. As the pain treatment facility grows busier, if inpatient and outpatient consultations are put off, a large backlog of patients waiting to be seen may result. Given the competitive nature of pain management services in most geographic areas, such delays will result in significant lost revenues and high levels of patient and referring physician dissatifaction.

Support Staff Availability

Tandem to the issue of physician availability is the issue of support staff availability. How consultations and phone messages for the pain management service are to be handled is of paramount importance to the ultimate success of the pain practitioner. In many hospital-based pain treatment facilities, all scheduling activities have been made the responsibility of the hospital secretarial staff. Oftentimes this simply does not work, both in terms of efficiency as well as motivation, when applied to the pain management service. The hospital employee may not be willing or able to provide prompt and courteous handling of phone calls from referring physicians as well as patients. Messages may get misplaced or lost. Generally the 7:00 AM to 3:30 PM staffing patterns of the hospital do not meet the needs of the referring physician who is often in his or her office until 5:00 or 5:30 at night. For this reason it is desirable as well as cost-effective to hire a high-quality secretary whose prime responsibilities are the administrative aspects of the pain management service. This will ensure that the phone is answered courteously and promptly, that phone messages are handled appropriately, that patient records are readily available, and that there is an appropriate level of motivation to work in add-on and emergency patients.

The pain management support staff must be available during regular clinic hours. The overuse of an answering machine and voice mail is strongly discouraged because most busy referring physicians are unwilling to make several calls trying to reach the pain management physician to discuss or schedule a patient. Provisions for phone coverage during lunch and break periods by the pain management support staff is mandatory.

Physician-Referred versus Self-referred Patients

Pain management specialists have traditionally felt that physician-referred patients are desirable. In fact, many practitioners will not accept self-referred patients. There are distinct advantages and disadvantages to this philosophical viewpoint as outlined in Tables 81-1 and 81-2.

The physician-referred patient *may* be appropriately worked up and carry a correct diagnosis. Conversely, the pain specialist has limited control over the appropriateness and quality of the evalua-

TABLE 81-1 **Physician-Referred Patients**

Advantages

1. The patient *may* be appropriately worked up.
2. The patient's condition *may* be appropriately diagnosed.
3. The patient *may* be familiar with pain management services and the reason that they have been sent to the pain center.
4. The referral *may* be appropriate for the services and expertise of the pain center.
5. Patient acquisition is low cost relative to advertising for self referred patients.

Disadvantages

1. The pain specialist has limited control over the appropriateness of the evaluation and treatment.
2. The patient may be inadequately worked up, which puts tremendous medicolegal responsibilities on the pain management physician to complete the evaluation.
3. The patient may be sent to the pain management specialist carrying the wrong diagnosis.
4. The patient may be an inappropriate referral to the pain clinic relative to the services being offered.
5. The pain management physician may inherit a patient who has been inappropriately treated by a referring physician and assume significant medical liability if he continues this treatment.

TABLE 81-2 **Self-Referred Patients**

Advantages

1. The pain management specialist may control the evaluation and treatment.
2. The pain management specialist may choose consultants needed to help him make the diagnosis that are of a higher quality than those chosen by the referring physician.
3. The pain management specialist has control over treatment and the use of prescription medication (especially controlled substances)
4. The pain management physician may exercise a choice in diagnostic imaging facilities or for hospitals should admission for further evaluation be necessary.

Disadvantages

1. The pain management specialist has sole responsibility for the evaluation and treatment.
2. The pain management specialist assumes the role of primary care physician.
3. Once the patient is under the care of the pain management specialist, transfer of the patient to a more appropriate specialist may be difficult should a problem arise.
4. Cost of patient acquisition is high relative to physician-referred patients if advertising is used.

tion and treatment of the physician-referred patient. The patient may be inadequately or inappropriately evaluated, which puts tremendous medicolegal responsibilities on the pain management physician to complete the evaluation. These problems can be magnified under the managed care paradigm since the managed care plan may want to save money by limiting diagnostic testing. Furthermore, the patient referral may not be appropriate for the services and expertise available at the pain treatment facility chosen by the referring physician or managed care plan.

Advantages of the self-referred patient include pain management specialist control over the evaluation and treatment and the choice of consultants needed to help him make the diagnosis, these consultants may be of a higher quality than those utilized by some referring physicians. The pain management specialist has control over treatment and the use of prescription medication (especially controlled substances) when providing care for the self-referred patients. Furthermore, the pain management specialist may exercise a choice in diagnostic imaging facilities or for hospitals should admission for further evaluation be necessary. As an increasing number of patients under managed care have out-of-network or point-of-service benefits as part of their managed care contract, such patients can choose the pain management physician and/or pain treatment facility in spite of the dictates of the managed care plan.[9,10] Such patients can represent a significant source of revenue for a pain treatment facility, and care should be taken to identify patients with such benefits before assuming they cannot be seen at a pain treatment facility.

Disadvantages of self-referred patients include the fact that the pain management specialist and pain treatment facility has sole responsibility for the evaluation and treatment, essentially assuming the role of primary care physician. Once the patient is under the care of the pain management specialist and facility, transfer of the patient to a more appropriate specialist or facility may be difficult should a problem arise.

The pain management specialist and the pain treatment facility must weigh these variables to determine the best course to follow. Should a pain management specialist decide to accept self-referred patients, he or she must recognize that in essence one is assuming the role of primary care physician. Incumbent to this role is an increase in responsibility with its attendant nighttime phone calls, emergencies, talking with family members, and so forth. Regardless of the pain management specialist's ultimate decision, it is the author's strong belief that the physician-referred patient requires the same level of vigilance and quality of evaluation that a self-referred patient does, especially under the managed care paradigm.

Hospital-Based Versus Free-Standing Facilities

As hospital administrators, government, managed care plans, and third-party payers seek to exert greater control over hospital-based physicians, pain management specialists have sought to limit their vulnerability to this situation, for example, the opening of surgical centers, affiliating with rehabilitation centers, and so forth.[11] An additional option is the development of a freestanding pain treatment facility. By developing such a facility, the pain management specialist may avoid the "label" associated with a given hospital. This can be good or bad depending on the public perception of a specific hospital. It should be remembered that these perceptions can change over time and what may be a desirable hospital to practice in at one point may represent a negative practice location at another.

An additional advantage of starting a freestanding pain treatment facility is that the pain management specialist may choose its geographic location. This is advantageous if the pain management specialist's primary hospital practice is located at a less desirable geographic area of the city.[12] A freestanding pain treatment facility can use advertising to great advantage when seeking to increase market penetration at a new geographic location.[13]

In some localities, it is possible for the pain management specialist to bill not only for his or her professional fees but also for the drugs, trays, radiology services, laboratory services, and block room and recovery room charges. Some third-party carriers in specific geographic locations in the United States (e.g., the East Coast) allow the pain management specialist to charge 150% of his or her professional fee to cover the cost of drugs, trays, and room charges. In other areas, local or state law as well as policies of the third-party carriers may require that the facility be licensed and accredited as an ambulatory surgery center in order for a facility fee to be paid. At the time of this writing, Medicare is considering paying the pain management physician a higher professional fee if he or she provides care in an office setting rather than an ambulatory surgical center or hospital-based pain treatment facility. This may lead to a shift in where pain management services are provided in the future.

In the freestanding pain treatment facility, the pain management specialist will have greater control of the space, staffing, hours of operation, capital expenditures, and utilization review–quality assurance activities. Obviously with this added control and flexibility, there comes an added measure of responsibility and risk.[14]

TABLE 81-3 **Hospital-Based Pain Center**

Advantages

1. The rent is free.
2. The personnel are free.
3. The equipment is free.
4. There is high visibility to referring physicians.
5. There is a high level of convenience for inpatients.
6. There is excellent emergency support should problems arise.
7. There is high-technology equipment readily available.
8. Support services (such as physical therapy, occupational therapy etc.) are available.

Disadvantages

1. There may be a lack of adequate designated space.
2. The pain management specialist does not have control of staffing.
3. The hospital administration may be very unwilling to provide the capital expenditure necessary to provide appropriate diagnostic and therapeutic equipment.
4. If the hospital develops a negative perception in the community, this will be carried over to the pain management services.
5. The pain management specialist will be subject to hospital utilization review and quality assurance activities.
6. The pain management specialist is subject to medical staff rules that may limit his ability to use operating room facilities, admit patients, etc.
7. The pain management specialist receives no portion of the revenues from the facility, laboratory, radiology, and support service fees generated.

TABLE 81-4 **Freestanding Pain Centers**

Advantages

1. The pain management specialist can avoid the "label" of a specific hospital.
2. The pain management specialist can choose the location of the freestanding pain center.
3. The pain management specialist may bill for drugs, trays, radiology services, laboratory services, and block room and recovery charges.
4. The pain management specialist can control the space, staffing, hours of operation, capital expenditures, and utilization review–quality assurance activities.

Disadvantages

1. Cost.
2. The pain management specialist assumes the added liability of the facility.
3. The pain management specialist assumes the added liability of the staff.
4. There is not a built-in referral source of patients.
5. There is no back up for emergencies.
6. There may not be high-technology equipment available to perform some procedures.

The major disadvantage of the freestanding pain treatment facility is cost. The pain management specialist can anticipate a large capital expenditure to provide adequate space, equipment, and personnel to implement pain management services at a freestanding location. In addition, the pain management specialist assumes the added liability and cost of malpractice insurance of the facility as well as the liability for professional services offered. The pain management specialist also inherits the liability for the actions of his or her staff. The advantages and disadvantages of the hospital-based pain management practice versus the freestanding pain center are summarized in Tables 81-3 and 81-4.

SUMMARY

Starting a pain treatment facility is a significant undertaking both in terms of time as well as tangible expense. While the risks are great, so can be the rewards if done properly. By addressing the previously mentioned issues as an integral part of the planning process, the pain management specialist will be better able to determine if setting up a pain treatment facility is the right decision.

REFERENCES

1. Saper J. A review of the Nuprin Pain Report. *Top Pain Manage* 1987;2:2–4.
2. Waldman SD. Joining a managed care plan: a guide to the pain management specialist. *Am J Pain Manage* 1992;2:215–218.
3. Waldman SD. Motivating the pain center employee. *Am J Pain Manage* 1993;3:114–117.
4. Waldman SD. Hiring employees for the pain center. *Am J Pain Manage* 1992;2:164–166.
5. Waldman SD. Tottal quality management for the pain center—an idea whose time has come. *Am J Pain Manage* 1993;3:38–41.
6. Waldman SD. The antitrust implications of medical staff credentialing–Part I. *Am J Pain Manage* 1997;7:22–27.
7. Waldman SD. The antitrust implications of medical staff credentialing–Part II. *Am J Pain Manage* 1997;7:66–69.
8. Waldman SD. Reimbursement for chronic pain management service—The cloud's silver lining. *Reg Anesth* 1993;18:227–228.
9. Waldman SD. Any willing provider laws—paradox or panacea. Part I. *Am J Pain Manage* 1996;6:54–61.
10. Waldman SD. Any willing provider laws—paradox or panacea. Part II. *Am J Pain Manage* 1996;6:93–96.
11. Waldman SD, Ford NA. Selling your medical practice–Part I. *Am J Pain Manage* 1998;8:23–28.
12. Waldman SD, Ford NA. Selling your medical practice–Part II. *Am J Pain Manage* 1998;8:53–60.
13. Waldman SD. Advertising pain management services. *Am J Pain Manage* 1993;196–200.
14. Waldman SD. The new OSHA regulations: implications for the pain management specialist. *Am J Pain Manage* 1993;3:85–87.

CHAPTER 82 HOW TO MANAGE A PAIN PRACTICE

Edgar L. Ross

INTRODUCTION

A well-managed pain management center is more than an economically successful pain clinic; it provides high-quality multidisciplinary care that meets the changing needs of today's health care environment.

Pain management centers have had long-standing credibility issues with payers.[1–5] Costs of care, narrowly focused specialty specific care, seemingly endless treatment without endpoints, along with unsubstantiated subjective outcomes have resulted in chronic pain management programs being placed under increasing scrutiny. Meanwhile, numerous studies have documented that multidisciplinary pain management centers have better outcomes. These studies have shown that multidisciplinary pain management centers provide improved care, are cost-effective, and have improved long-term outcomes.[2–4] Anesthesiology as a specialty is expanding beyond its traditional role in the operating room to provide leadership in the treatment of chronic pain.[5] Anesthesiologists have an opportunity to participate in the development of, and provide leadership in, the development of multidisciplinary pain management centers of excellence. To succeed in this role, anesthesiologists must recognize the complexity of chronic pain.[6,7]

The successful treatment of chronic pain requires the understanding that chronic pain is a multifaceted problem. Chronic pain is not only a sensory complaint but it has profound impacts on a patient's affect, social circle, vocational pursuits, and cognitive abilities. Pain management centers of excellence understand the unique needs of each of their patients and provide cost-effective care based on those needs. The characteristics of a well-managed pain management that set it apart are:

- The recognition that chronic pain is multifactorial problem that requires specialized care delivered by a team of specialized providers with a full-time commitment to the treatment of chronic pain.
- The organization of the pain management center administration is set up to recognize that different patient groups are affected by chronic pain.
- Specific emphasis on accessibility and customer-focused initiatives that enhance treatment outcomes and facilitate referrals.
- Recognition and planning for outcome measures that understand and trace the specific outcome important to specific payer classes.
- Creation of a network of mutually beneficial relationships that sustain the center's growth with the center's various customers including hospital administration and payers.
- Innovative products and services to help patients recover all aspects of their lives, as part of a continuum of care.
- The commitment to increase the visibility and viability of pain management as a discipline within the health care environment.

Single-modality pain management centers that emphasize procedures and short-term relief that these blocks produce do not meet the previously mentioned characteristics. An overemphasis on procedures for short-term relief serves only to enhance the perception of disability and does little for the long-term pain management problems that need to be solved for enhanced patient function. Well-managed pain management centers are organizations that are equipped to manage all aspects of chronic patient disability. A broad focus such as this requires long-term commitments toward multidisciplinary team and program development.

Formulating a strategy is key for successful program development. Separating a multidisciplinary pain management center into smaller elements or key components can facilitate the developmental process. These elements are:

- Organizational structure and administration
- Physical facilities
- The medical treatment continuum
- Service lines
- Practice infrastructure
- Trained interdisciplinary team
- Key patient groups
- Information and outcomes management
- Fiscal management and business planning.

KEY COMPONENTS OF A PAIN MANAGEMENT CENTER OF EXCELLENCE

In the following sections each of these elements is examined; strategies are suggested that will lead an organization through the different stages of growth toward a pain management center of excellence.

Organizational Structure and Administration

Chronic pain management centers are under constant pressure to perform, as well as being viewed by many skeptical payer organizations as a large financial burden without appropriate returns. Yet chronic pain remains one of this country's primary public health problems. Centers of excellence provide the leadership and advocacy necessary to influence the attitudes of the local community about pain management services.

This component recognizes that the organizational foundation of a pain management practice is important to achieve these objectives. These objectives are achieved through the following:

1. Mission statement developed by the interdisciplinary team.
2. Showing a complete commitment to the discipline of pain management with full-time staff and board certification such as the added qualifications in pain offered by the American Board of Anesthesiology.

3. Developing key relationships with affiliated institutions and working toward complete integration of pain management services.
4. Development of a governing body that includes members from various interest groups that are representative of patient groups treated by the pain center.
5. Formation of a dedicated organization provides the foundation from which a pain management center can build.

The pain management center must initially make the needed alliances to ensure that the appropriate resources are available. This can be in the form of informal professional contacts, to forming actual contractual links with pertinent organizations such as drug-addiction treatment centers or vocational rehabilitation organizations. Developing an appropriate continuum of care requires not only considerable effort to identify appropriate personnel who have an interest in treating chronic pain but it also requires some ongoing interactions with referral sources and payers to determine the necessary resources needed to fund this treatment continuum. Determining the type of treatment to be included in the treatment continuum requires an understanding of the needs of the referral sources as well as the patients being sent to the pain center. Understanding this requires the tracking of outcomes as well as determining demographics that are seen within a pain management center.

Intensive training in advances in pain management and allied interests, such as enhancing return to work rates, research on adaptive appliances for disability, must be ongoing. This training also lends itself to team building, which is a vital component of a multidisciplinary center. The synergism that occurs during team building will improve outcomes and enhance customer satisfaction. Developing a pain management center of excellence requires a substantial investment in time and personnel to develop the needed resources as previously described to treat chronic pain.

The Physical Facility

Process of care for chronic pain requires team interactions. The physical facility should be developed to enhance interdisciplinary team interaction.[8] In addition, as the practice grows, the facility must have enough space that can be allocated to facilitate the integration of medical management services, various psychotherapies, and individual and group as well as rehabilitative therapies in one contiguous building. This integration of services or interdisciplinary treatment approach will have positive impact on patient outcomes. Tight coordination will exist among the disciplines for patient conferences and team interaction. The facility should be designed to enhance patient comfort and confidentiality as well as convenient and accessible for patients with disabilities. The physical facility should have enough space for family conferences, so they can also participate in the rehabilitation process.

The Medical Treatment Continuum

As the pain management center grows, clinical problems tend to increase in complexity. There becomes a need to customize a treatment plan for each patient. Rational customizing of treatment plans requires a framework to classify patients into similar groups and develop an understanding of their unique needs. The emphasis on treatment being both cost-effective and efficient must lead to an understanding of how to optimize the treatment to these groups of patients.[9] Treatment of chronic pain requires a triad of therapies: medical management, behavioral, and physical rehabilitation. The assessment of a chronic pain patient must lead to an understanding of the patient's needs in each of these areas. This assessment could then lead to the classification of the pain syndrome using a combination of various tools available today. The International Association for the Study of Pain (IASP) taxonomy of pain provides both an axis tool and a list of chronic pain diagnoses that can provide a framework for the optimization of treatment plans. Since psychological factors often figure prominently in chronic pain diagnosis, additional understanding of patient subgroups requires a means of stratifying the IASP diagnostic groups.[10] The SF-36 (Short Form-36) is a useful evaluation tool that evaluates impact of disease on the patient's physical and psychological functioning. Using this multidimensional approach allows further subclassificaiton of patients.[11] The data collected allow efficient customization of an individual patient plan, as well as the accumulation of data along with outcome data that facilitates quality-improvement activities.

Service Lines

A service line is a list of needed services that are required in the order of occurrence that they are required in order to perform clinical evaluations and treatment. This list becomes a blueprint upon which these clinical processes can be developed. Service lines are useful concepts that can be used to evaluate outcomes and facilitate internal quality-improvement initiatives. Multidisciplinary teams enhance chronic pain management outcomes. But these multidisciplinary teams add greatly to the complexity of determining cost-effectiveness or treatment outcomes as well as determining best practices. Effective treatment requires that the patient be evaluated and treated systematically. This process can become complex to analyze when the many different individualized encounters are considered for the unique needs of each chronic pain patient. Yet, in order to achieve the efficiency and outcomes demanded by today's health care environment, these processes must be thoroughly understood, documented, and evaluated. Service lines facilitate the identification of the processes and systems that are used to treat patients. This identification process must involve the entire staff. Service lines lend the pain management center a valuable tool to understand the complex processes that must occur for a chronic pain patient to be successfully treated. A service line with a list of processes breaks the treatment continuum into manageable parts and allows analysis to occur that will optimize treatment outcomes. Service lines are used to track all the clinical activities of the pain management center. The processes involved that support the clinical activities, as well as the clinical activities themselves, are listed in flow diagrams that allow the staff to understand the necessary activities to treat a patient. These flow charts are then used to form a framework to measure key outcomes that reflect the needs of referral sources, and the values of the organization as articulated in the mission statement.

For example, a service line such as Evaluation and Assessment could be used to measure the speed that a new referral patient is seen. Managed care places a premium on customer service and the importance of rapid response to patient concerns. Pain management centers working with managed care organizations could use the service line Evaluation and Assessment to understand the barriers to timely intervention and improve performance. Other service line examples are:

1. Limited Service Line is used to describe patients who need treatment plans with a smaller focus.

2. Comprehensive Pain Management Program used to describe treatment plans that require comprehensive treatment such as returning a long-standing disabled worker to work.
3. Research Service Line can be used to track the research activities of a pain management center. Integration of a clinical trial's center can be a useful tool to enhance expertise in the clinical staff, improve the image of expertise of the pain management center, and develop important referral sources.
4. Follow-up and Referral service line is used to track long-term outcomes of patients after they have left the active treatment program.

Service lines can be used to formulate outcomes as well as treatment costs that will allow the pain center to engage in creative managed care contracting, which gives the pain center a potentially competitive edge. Data using performance measures of these processes are used for quality-improvement activities directed toward meeting specific needs of the pain management center's patients, referral sources, and payers. The data that are collected allow the pain center to become a strong advocate for its patients and their unique needs.[12]

Practice Infrastructure

The multidisciplinary nature of chronic pain management treatment requires extensive interaction and team building on an ongoing basis to achieve optimal outcomes. This at times can make team building difficult, but this must occur nonetheless. In addition, the rapidly changing health care market demands that an organization be versatile, communicate effectively, and be able to innovate quickly and effectively. Regular meetings within the pain management center personnel to identify issues as they occur and create solutions are a vital component of the success or failure of any pain management center. Meetings such as those devoted to performance improvement or customer service are just two examples of important skills that pain management centers must have. Other subcommittees may be formed within a pain management center to keep the organization vital; these can include a managed care committee, quality assurance, and various ad hoc committees to address new program development as the opportunities become apparent. By having these meetings on a regular basis, all personnel within the pain management center begin to understand the intricacies and nuances of the varied professional backgrounds of the multidisciplinary team. This helps to strengthen the team and also understand the broad range of services that the pain management center can offer. The need to move away from modality-based services such as repeated epidural steroid injections in the case report described earlier to more comprehensive outcome functionally orientated treatment plans should be apparent. Functionally oriented treatment plans are increasingly being demanded by managed care. The continuing case report in this section illustrates this.

TRAINED INTERDISCIPLINARY TEAM

An interdisciplinary team forms the foundation of treatment of any chronic pain management center.[3,4,9] The primary goal of any treatment plan is to provide for the unique needs of each individual. Patient satisfaction has been used to provide insight to treatment effectiveness.[13] Patients who report high satisfaction with their treatment are less likely to miss appointments,[14] show better treatment compliance,[15] and adopt a more active role in the treatment plan.[16] These are all important success criteria for chronic pain management treatment plans. In addition, high patient satisfaction correlates with successful treatment outcomes.[17] Payers are also increasingly looking for providers with consistently high patient satisfaction results to form relationships with.

The foundation of successful outcomes begins when a patient makes an appointment. The professional interaction of the interdisciplinary team conveys trust and facilitates the transference that will lead to patient trust to change behavior. Chronic pain management treatment plans often require multiple visits and intensive treatment regimens. Patient satisfaction and the resulting transference will provide the needed motivation for patients to radically depart from the norms they have come to rely on. Ingrained behaviors such as long-term disability are difficult to change.

High customer satisfaction means performing pain management center services in a manner that patient's view as highly valid and appropriate. Pain at times can be overwhelming for a patient; accessibility and convenience are important elements of a customer-service-driven organization. In today's health care market, price for service seems to be the only criterion upon which one is evaluated. Customer satisfaction can be a key positioning point when negotiating for new referral sources. To achieve uniform high customer satisfaction ratings, the entire organization must be dedicated to that goal with a passion that is equaled only by the passion for high-quality care. It is important to understand that what a health care professional may determine is important for customer satisfaction is not necessarily the same for varied groups of patients that receive their treatment in a pain management center. Customer satisfaction means much more than timeliness of office appointments. Customer satisfaction may mean having services in a convenient location, where a person may not need to miss work, and varied services that will support patient needs such as letter writing to employers, disability evaluations, and general efficacy for a patient who has chronic pain.

Key Patient Groups

A pain management center's influence should extend beyond the walls of the clinic. The roots of relationships that link the pain management center to the community are critical for survival. Focused efforts to enhance these relationships will result in an ongoing positive image in these areas. External relationships are necessary to track patients and to cultivate local, regional, and national referral sources. In addition, these interactions can help to improve reimbursement and generate community support and good will. Identification of key patient groups is very important in determining needs, patient treatment satisfaction, and successful outcomes.[18]

High-quality pain management services are recognized as a right in today's health care environment. However, providing these services effectively demands an appropriate referrals and reimbursement. Relationships to address these concerns are vital. Positive internal relationships are imperative to keep the team, administration, and referral sources abreast of all new program development in the pain management center. External key customer relationships between a pain management center should include payers, referral sources, vendors of medical equipment, pain management center users (such as patients and case managers), and other health care institutions within the community with which the pain management center must interact. These entities can support the patient referrals, medical education, latest technology, reimbursement, and their external consultations that a pain management center needs in order to survive. Strong relationships with these entities are essential to development and success of a pain management center.

Marketing is also another activity that is placed in this key component. Marketing not only involves activities to increase the visibility of the pain management center but it is also used to identify specific patient needs, which may lead to restructuring of the pain management center described in earlier key components. For example, marketing for workers' compensation programs requires an understanding of what services are highly valued and will enhance the care for patients from these referral sources. For example, this may involve developing a seamless continuum of care, which brings a patient through a pain management center that engages in specific rehabilitative needs and is able to refer immediately to a vocational training program so that back-to-work rates are optimized. Regular round table discussions with referral sources will be helpful to focus the pain management centers efforts and provide the necessary understanding to customize programs.

Information and Outcomes Management

Ensuring the delivery of consistent high-quality medical care along with patient satisfaction has to become part of the culture of the pain management center. Activities have to be focused on achieving these goals. Concurrent program evaluation and identification of areas needing improvement leading to the design of new systems and processes are the key to reaching and maintaining consistent high-quality care. This evaluation, leading to innovation followed by implementation, is a constant cycle in any organization that is focused on becoming a center of excellence. All activities included in the pain center have to be understood by the team in the minutest detail, and evaluation systems put into place by the people who are responsible for these tasks. Appointing an "overseer" to run these activities can quickly destroy effective teamwork and lead to deterioration in morale, decreased staff effectiveness, and decreased customer satisfaction. Performance goals that are set by the team are much more meaningful and lead to more rapid improvement in quality of care. Continuous quality improvement is part of everyone's job. Appropriate outcomes for chronic pain management are often discussed. Examples such as back-to-work rates, perceived helpfulness, and physical activity scores are all used to define value of chronic pain management programs. Increasingly pain management programs are being called upon to justify expenditures and to control costs.[1] Determining program costs, cost-effectiveness, and cost-benefits of a program requires a thorough and complete understanding of the pain management center processes used to deliver care. Payers will require appropriate financial analysis (*give examples*) of pain management center treatment.[22] Evidence-based algorithms are the foundation for determining cost of care and calculating cost-effectiveness of treatment.[23] Algorithms should be diagnosis-specific, evidenced-based, and inclusive enough to achieve pain center physician consensus. Algorithms are then used to standardize treatment for each specific diagnosis, thus permitting financial analysis and disease-specific outcome analysis. Using this structure, a center of excellence will be able to accumulate data to permit informed analysis of the entire treatment continuum for chronic pain management.

Fiscal Management and Business Planning

In general all managers must have the appropriate information to manage, and pain management centers should have access to theirs as well. Knowing the monetary impact a pain center can have on an institution's bottom line is vital. This is extremely important for success in negotiations with the institution. These financial reports should provide the pain management center with the necessary information to develop reimbursement strategies, and search for new business opportunities that are ever developing in this rapidly changing health care environment. Meetings with payers to discuss their needs and develop new services along with them can provide valuable new insights and ensure successful program development. Appropriately structured pain management centers can provide services in a fiscally responsible manner and still achieve excellent patient outcomes. This perspective not only comes from the hospital itself but also from payers and referral sources. Chronic pain has a devastating impact on a significant number of people in the United States.

Any successful enterprise requires the development of a clearly written business plan. Although this will not guarantee that your practice will be a success, most successful businesses are based on well-developed business plans that are revised as required for changing conditions. The purpose of a business plan is to document in writing a brief description of the business, the market niche served by that business, as well as the infrastructure that is required to become a successful practice. Financial resources required to start, sustain, and staff the clinic as well as an outline of a marketing plan are also vital components of a business planning process. Developing a comprehensive outline and understanding of the reimbursement climates under which the pain center exists, including governmental managed care insurance companies, and patients is vital. This can only occur in an accurate fashion when a pain management center develops the solid internal and external relationships as described in an earlier key component.

CHANGING HEALTHCARE ENVIRONMENT

Managed care has become the most important force driving the health care market in the United States. Different areas of the country are in various stages of managed care penetration. For ease of description, managed care penetration has been placed in four stages. Each stage of change requires adaptations in the delivery of health care services to meet this challenge. These are known as the evolving stages of value.[24] Pain management centers are part of this evolving health care market and therefore must identify the stage of the local area in which they are operating. The evolving stages of value in the health care market describe four levels:

- Stage 1, or the unstructured stage, describes a market with independent hospitals and physicians, few unsophisticated purchasers, and >10% penetration of managed care. The organizational source of value comes from its hard assets, and quality is defined internally while reimbursement is fee-for-service. Examples of chronic pain management care in this environment would be the intensive 6- to 8-week inpatient programs, with very little program customization for individual patient needs.

TABLE 82-1 **Matrix of the Characteristics Key Components Through the Five Stages of Change**

Key Components	Stage 1 Product-Focused Practice	Stage 2 Customer-Focused Practice	Stage 3 Market-Segment-Focused Practice	Stage 4 Opportunity-Focused Practice	Stage 5 Pain Management Center of Excellence
Organizational Structure/Administration	• Create mission statement • Make commitment to become a pain center • Educate key relationships about pain management	• Build relationships with key advisors • Educate advisors on chronic pain and total quality management as it applies to pain	• Set up systems to expand and new service lines • Revisit mission statement • Establish and educate board	• Add administrative capability to support larger patient base • Expand relations with board	• Maintain strong active board • Build structure to allow rapid growth • Revisit mission statement
Physical Facilities	• Facility shared with other services	• Space dedicated to chronic pain services	• Offer inpatient and outpatient facilities • Offer transportation to pain center from other system locations • Design work areas that encourage interaction	• Maintain central treatment facility • Establish basic services in satellite locations	• Expand services in satellite locations • Facility reflects regional reputation
Medical Treatment Continuum	• Limited pain treatment offered • Broaden knowledge of chronic pain management • Build physician network to ensure full diagnosis • Begin collection of outcomes data • Offer patient education	• Commit to full treatment continuum • Establish basic treatment protocols • Execute contracts with external providers • Expand patient education	• Offer full range of medical treatments • Expand and refine treatment protocols • Analyze processes for better outcomes • Test patient education	• Able to treat all types of pain problems • Develop critical pathways • Develop protocols for different venues of care • Improve treatment processes • Institute follow-up care	• Offer full treatment continuum • Refine critical pathways • Continuous refinement of treatments for enhanced outcomes • Integrated patient education
Service Lines	• Basic chronic pain treatment offered • Broaden professional expertise • Essential feedback loops in place	• Identify basic service lines • Support service lines with documentation systems	• Design multidisciplinary service lines • Offer 24-hour service • Strengthen infrastructure • Ensure consistency of care	• Discover opportunities for new service lines • Customize service lines for payers and patients	• Create service line and extensions for niche markets • Create seamless delivery of health care for chronic pain • Essential customer feedback loops in place

Practice Infrastructure	• Establish regular team communication • Keep team focused and motivated	• Regular team meetings • Team building • Activities begin	• Team focused on patient assessment • Regularly scheduled team-building activities • Cross training is begun	• Activities to promote cohesive team • Continuous training for cohesive team	• Conduct ongoing team building
Trained Interdisciplinary Team	• Identify members of the core team	• Add to core team as required	• Team dedicated solely to pain management	• Full team in place	• Maintain strong team communication
Key Patient Groups	• Identify patient customer groups • Measure patient satisfaction	• Expand efforts to attract customers • Expand patient satisfaction surveys • Begin patient-orientated market research • Begin community education efforts	• Expand marketing efforts • Communicate with patients regularly • Establish clinic-wide customer service policies • Begin community education	• Attract patients from wider service radius • Work toward exceeding customer expectations • Continue community education efforts	• Develop the ability to customize all aspects of patient care • Gather continuous customer feedback • Increase COE visibility • Broaden reputation
Information/Outcomes Management	• Establish basic record-keeping systems • Develop basic patient treatment outcome parameters	• Expand patient treatment outcome parameters • Measure and report patient satisfaction • Educate team on continuous quality improvement	• Develop and track outcome studies • Create databse • Implement continuous improvement cycles • Establish nonthreatening management systems	• Team proactively improves processes • Streamline information exchange • Work across department boundaries	• Team committed to strive for perfection • Management removes barriers for team improvement • Quality, not quantity, is measure of success
Fiscal Management/ Business Planning	• Create business plan • Conduct informal market research • Establish financial reporting systems	• Develop individual and team goals/action plans • Conduct market research for business planning • Develop a budget	• Conduct feasibility studies for new ventures • Create dedicated financial reports • Negotiate managed care contracts	• Create tactical plans • Conduct S.W.O.T. analysis • Maintain managed care links and contracts	• Team empowered to change workplace • Apply CQI to management systems • Management serves as advisors and facilitators

Data from Ross G, Kay M. Toppling the Pyramids; Redefining the Way American Companies Are Run. New York, NY: Times Books, 1994.

- Stage 2, or the loose framework stage, is characterized by a growing presence of managed care, decreasing profit margins, and eroding hospital bottom lines. With the emphasis on outpatient care, hospitals have excess inpatient capacity. Joint ventures are beginning to form between the medical staff and health care facilities. Quality increasingly is defined by the near-term cost of care. Chronic pain management treatment plans in this environment require customization of treatment plans specific to each patients needs, with an increasing emphasis on outpatient care and day programs.
- Stage 3, or the consolidation stage, is defined by the development of large health care systems and increasing emphasis on developing a complete integrated health system. Quality is defined by customer satisfaction, along with cost of care. Managed care is an important part of the market, with penetration now up to 50%. This stage is found in most major population centers in the United States. Pain management centers existing in this environment must also reengineer themselves to reflect these changes. Internally, the pain center must focus on outcomes, understand the needs of their referral sources, and design programs that address these needs. Pain management centers that work toward becoming part of an integrated delivery system will find many opportunities in this environment.
- Stage 4, or managed competition, is characterized by employer coalitions, which drive the market toward the formation of strategic alliances and the shifting of risk to the health care provider. The focus of these organizations on health status and quality is now defined by the health status of populations or covered lives. Health care systems are driven to provide the highest customer value, and the most important source of value comes from capability of the organization and its image. Capitation is an important reimbursement mechanism in this stage. Specific disease-state-management initiatives are developed for high cost or high volume diagnoses. Chronic pain in this stage has now become a real cost that must be effectively and appropriately treated.

Using the components and health care stages described in the preceding sections, five stages can be described that allow pain management centers to set goals and respond to the changes of the health care market. Table 82-1 presents a matrix of the key components as well as characteristics of each of these five stages.

Health care is changing from a product-focused practice (fee-for-service reimbursement) where reimbursement encourages utilization, to much more sophisticated reimbursement schemes that emphasize outcomes. Capitation is an example of the focus being shifted to outcomes rather than reimbursement plans based purely on volume of services.

It is important to note that as a pain management center begins to work itself through the stages of change, as outlined earlier, all nine key components must be coordinated to achieve progress. Planning time frames of years can be needed to achieve desired results. Only with total and complete commitment of the pain management staff can the pain center evolve into a center of excellence. The stages described are fluid, and changes in personnel and health care reimbursement strategies may cause the pain center to regress. A commitment for ongoing process improvement as described earlier will allow a pain management center to achieve and maintain leadership in the community. The key to achieving a center of excellence reputation is the full-time commitment of the medical staff. Pain management should not viewed as opportunity to earn supplementary income by providing procedure-orientated services. Reviewing Table 82-1, along with the previously described stages, will give a comprehensive understanding of the planning process that must take place for success to occur. Understanding these stages of change[25] and using them as a framework for a methodical planning process and breaking the planning process into the key components described earlier will lead to a strong and dedicated organization with a passion to succeed and an ability to achieve the goal of becoming a well-managed pain management center known as a *pain management center of excellence*.

REFERENCES

1. Taricco A. Perils of payers: a pain center paradigm. In: Cohen MJM, Campbell JN, eds. *Pain Treatment Centers at a Crossroads: A Practical and Conceptual Reappraisal.* Seattle, Wash: ISAP Press, 1996: 109–116.
2. Turk DC. Efficacy of multidisciplinary pain centers in the treatment of chronic pain. In: Cohen MJM, Campbell JN, eds. *Pain Treatment Centers at a Crossroads: A Practical and Conceptual Reappraisal.* Seattle, Wash: ISAP Press, 1996:257–273.
3. Kames LD. Effectiveness of an interdisciplinary pain management program for the treatment of chronic pelvic pain. *Pain* 1990;41:41–46.
4. Flor H. Efficacy of multidisciplinary pain treatment centers: a meta-analytic review. *Pain* 1992;49:221–230.
5. Taricco A. *Medical Issues of Fraud and Abuse in Workers' Compensation.* Hiroshima, Penn: LRP Publications; 1995.
6. Greene NM. The 31st Rovenstein lecture: the changing horizons in anesthesiology. *Anesthesiology* 1993;79:164–170.
7. Jacobson L, et al. Beyond the needle. *Anesthesiology* 1997;87:1210–1218.
8. Loeser JD. *Desirable Characteristics for Pain Treatment Facilities.* Seattle, Wash: Washington International Association for the Study of Pain, 1990.
9. Turk DC. Interdisciplinary approach to pain management: philosophy, operations, and efficacy. In: Ashburn MA, (ed.). *The Management of Pain.* New York, NY: Churchill Livingstone, 1998:235.
10. Merskey H, Bogduk N, (eds.). *Classification of Chronic Pain: Descriptions of Chronic Pain Syndromes and Definitions of Pain Terms, 2nd ed.* Seattle, Wash: ISAP Press.
11. Turk DC. Strategies for classifying chronic orofacial pain patients. *Anesth Prog* 1990;37:155–160.
12. Bonica JJ. Interdisciplinary, multimodal pain management programs. In: Bonica JJ, (ed.). *The Management of Pain, 2nd ed.* Philadelphia, Pa: Lea & Febiger; Section G: 1990;2104–2120.
13. Hall JA, Milburn MA, Epstein AM. A causal model of health status and satisfaction with medical care. *Med Care* 1993;31:84–94.
14. Hertz P, Stamps PL. A re-evaluation of appointment-keeping behavior. *Am J Public Health* 1977;67:1033–1036.
15. Attkisson CG, Stegner BL. Assessment of patient satisfaction: development and refinement of a service evaluation questionnaire. *Eval Prog Plan* 1983;6:299–314.
16. Ware JE Jr, Davies AR. Behavioral consequences of consumer satisfaction with medical care. *Eval Prog Plan* 1983;6:292–297.
17. McCraker LM, et al. Assessment of satisfaction with treatment for chronic pain. *J Pain Symptom Manage* 1997;14:292–299.
18. Nelson EC, Larson C. Patients' good and bad surprises: how do they relate to overall patient satisfaction? *QRB* 1993, (March) 89–94.
19. Chapman SL, Jamison RN, Sanders SH. Treatment helpfulness ques-

tionnaire: a measure of patient satisfaction with treatment modalities provided in chronic pain management programs. *Pain* 1996;68:349–361.

20. McNeill JA, Sherwood GD, Starck PL, Thompson CJ. Assessing clinical outcomes: patient satisfaction with pain management [abstract]. *J Pain Symptom Manage* 1998;16:29.
21. Huber MR. The evolving medical marketplace. In: *Measuring Medicine: An Introduction to Health Status Assessment and a Framework for Application*. Vol. 2. Faulkner & Gray's Medical Outcomes and Practice Guidelines Library, Washington, D.C. pgs. 1–8.
22. Grady ML, Weis KA, eds. Identifying health technologies that work searching for evidence. In: *Conference Proceedings, Cost Analysis Methodology for Clinical Practice Guidelines*. Rockville, Md: US Dept of Health and Human Services, Agency for Health Care Policy and Research; March 1995; AHCPR publication 95-001.
23. Brent CJ, et al. Management by fact: what is CPI and how is it used? In: Horn SD, Hopkins DSP, (eds.). *Clinical Practice Improvement: A New Technology for Developing Cost-effective Quality Health Care*. Vol 2. Faulkner & Gray's Medical Outcomes and Practice Guidelines Library, Washington, D.C. pgs. 39–54.
24. Kauer R, Berkowitz UE. Stages of managed care. *Physician Exec* 1997; Nov/Dec.
25. Ross G, Kay M. *Toppling the Pyramids; Redefining the Way American Companies Are Run*. New York, NY: Times Books, 1994.

CHAPTER 83 CERTIFICATION IN PAIN MEDICINE

Honghui Feng and Howard S. Smith

In the last decade, management of acute and chronic pain has attracted significant attention on both the patient and professional level. The need of qualified personnel to supply services for the patients who have pain has increased. Pain medicine as a subspecialty has been well recognized by the public. Therefore, several organizations offer credentialing and certification.

Pain syndromes often involve exceedingly complex issues and no single, traditional, established specialty can simply and effectively cover all aspects of pain-related problems. Pain management is truly a multidisciplinary medical practice that involves application of a wide variety of techniques to which no single currently existing specialty can lay sole claim. Pain management still exists as a division of a larger department throughout most parts of the country—and not as a department of its own. Pain medicine has not been established as a generally accepted teaching course in medical schools even though some pioneer medical schools offer elective introduction courses to medical students. Medical school education in pain is usually minimal. In the first 2 years of formal lectures, it is common for coverage of this field to be limited to 1 to 2 hours. During the second 2 years of clinical rotations, students often receive additional informal education; however, little if any of this education is provided by experts in the field. Some medical schools (including Harvard Medical School) have started to offer didactic sessions as well as elective rotations in pain centers for senior students. These rotations can vary from 1 day to 1 month. Overall, however, medical school education in pain medicine remains minimal. Postgraduate training is mainly affiliated with other pain-related subspecialties or as part of training in such subspecialties. A distinct residency program in pain management has not been accepted. Additionally, the overwhelming majority of pain fellowship programs are affiliated with various primary specialty programs: mostly anesthesiology. The number of anesthesiology pain management fellowship programs, however, has increased significantly in the past 10 years. The Accreditation Council for Graduate Medical Education (ACGME) also expects the anesthesiology residency programs to provide some pain management training in a pain clinic setting.

There are several different pain management certifications offered currently. The American Board of Anesthesiology (ABA) took the first step. The ABA, founded in 1941, first notified the American Board of Medical Specialties (ABMS) of their intention to subcertify physicians in pain management in 1989, and then held discussions with other ABMS member boards interested in certifying physician in pain management. On September 26, 1991, the ABMS agreed with the ABA to issue a pain management certificate. The first subspecialty pain certificate to the qualified ABA diplomates was issued in 1993.[1] Five years later, with the support of the American Board of Anesthesiology, the American Board of Physical Medicine and Rehabilitation (ABPM&R), and the American Board of Psychiatry and Neurology (ABPN) submitted a joint proposal to offer subspecialty certification in pain management. The first certification of subspecialty in pain management was issued in 2001 by ABPM&R and ABPN. Diplomates from other member boards of the American Board of Medical Specialties may also be allowed to apply for certification to the ABPM&R or ABPN if they meet the criteria.

The three member boards of the American Board of Medical Specialties (the American Board of Anesthesiology, the American Board of Physical Medicine and Rehabilitation, and the American Board of Psychiatry and Neurology) formed a joint committee with representatives from each specialty. There is a 3-year term for the question authors in the committee. The three boards adopt a single set of credentialing criteria. With assistance of the ABPM&R and the ABPN, the ABA will be responsible to administer a computer-based examination covering the various content areas of pain management and determine the passing standard. The test will be the same for all three boards. This pain certification examination will be monitored for quality assurance by the National Board of Medical Examiners (NBME). Only diplomates from the ABA can apply for the certification through the ABA boards. Diplomates from the ABPM&R and the ABPN will apply through their respective boards. However, diplomates from other ABMS member boards can apply through either the ABPM&R or the ABPN boards if they meet the requirements.

Requirements for admission to examination in the subspecialty of pain management[2,3]:

1. Be a diplomate of one of the ABMS boards. (Only a diplomate of ABA may apply for the ABA pain specialty certification.) Pain Management candidates who hold general certification from an ABMS member board other than the ABPM&R, the ABPN, or the ABA must provide documentation of permission from their original certifying board to pursue subspecialty certification in Pain Management.
2. Hold a current, valid, and unrestricted license to practice medicine or osteopathy in a US licensing jurisdiction of Puerto Rico, or licensure in Canada.
3. Fulfill the education requirement for subspecialization in Pain Management.
4. Satisfy the pain management examination requirement for Pain Management sub-specialization.

The education requirement is slightly different for ABA from ABP&R and ABPN.

The continuum of education in Pain Management for ABA consists of[4]:

1. Completion of 12 months of full-time, non-interrupted training in acute, chronic, and oncology pain management, which must be in an anesthesiology pain management program in the United States or its territories accredited by the ACGME.

2. The pain management training must follow the completion of the anesthesiology training. Exception may be made with special approval of the Credentials Committee of the ABA.

Currently, the ABA certification examination in Pain Management consists of 200 questions given in one half-day session.

The continuum of education in Pain Management for ABP&M and ABPN consist of:

1. Completion of 12 months of ACGME-approved pain management training program
2. Temporary criteria before 2003:

Satisfactory completion of residency training for primary certification by an ABMS member board prior to September 1, 2000 (prior to September 1, 1998 if apply for ABP&R) and one of the following:

(a) Completion of 12 months of formal training in pain management, OR
(b) Completion of 24 months of full-time equivalent pain management practice. The practice has to take place during the 8 years immediately preceding the deadline for receipt of application to take examination, OR
(c) The credit for the combination of practice and education could be granted on individual basis.

Beginning in 2004, only candidates who complete 12 months of pain management fellowship training will be eligible for Pain Management subspecialization.

All the three boards require recertification examination every 10 years.

Pain management programs will consider anesthesiologists as well as non-anesthesiologists as candidates for pain management fellowship programs. If a pain management fellowship program already exists for an institution, then that program will continue as the institution's pain management training program. An institution can only have one pain management fellowship training program.

The process of finding fellowship training is not yet standardized. Anesthesiology leads the way with a listing of available programs published by the American Society of Regional Anesthesia (ASRA). The Association of Anesthesiology Pain Program Directors (AAPPD) is currently recognized as a committee of ASRA, and has worked to develop updated listings of anesthesiology-based fellowship programs. This same organization has proposed that interviews should be completed in the fall months and that candidates should be offered positions at the end of December. Many programs, however, still do not follow this proposed time schedule. Non-anesthesiology programs are more difficult to identify, and there have been no such efforts to identify the fellowship programs and organize the recruitment process.

Anesthesiology offers most of the postresidency fellowships with clear training guidelines but there are a few other specialties that offer formal fellowships of 12 or more months' duration (1999–2000):

- Anesthesiology based: 97 programs = 292 positions
- Neurology/Neurosurgery based: 13 programs = 29 positions
- Physiatry: 6 programs = 13 positions.

The American Academy of Pain Medicine (AAPM) was organized in 1983 with the initial name of the American Academy of Algology. It was the first national physician organization dedicated to the specialty of pain medicine. As such, it continues to be involved in education, training, advocacy and research in the field of pain medicine.

The American Board of Pain Medicine (ABPM) was started by a group of members of the American Academy of Pain Medicine and it offers certification to pain specialists with a process similar to that of the American Board of Anesthesiology. It was founded in 1991 as the American College of Pain Medicine as the certifying body for the American Academy of Pain Medicine (AAPM). The first annual examination for credentialing was given in 1992. To obtain the recognition of pain management as one of the member boards of ABMS as a primary medical specialty, like the other traditional medical specialties, the name of the American College of Pain Medicine was changed to American Board of Pain Medicine in 1994. ABPM is hoping that pain management will be officially recognized as a primary medicine specialty by the ABMS.

The requirements to be certified by the American Board of Pain Medicine are[5]:

1. Must have a current valid, unrestricted license to practice medicine or osteopathy in the United States or its territories or possessions or a branch of the United States Uniformed Services, or one of the provinces or territories of Canada.
2. Must have completed an ACGME-approved residency training program that included pain management.
3. Must be currently certified by American Board of Anesthesiology, the American Board of Neurological Surgery, the Board of American Psychiatry and Neurology, or the American Board of Physical Medicine and Rehabilitation,

   OR

   Must be board certified by other member boards of the American Board of Medical Specialties with documentation of identifiable training in pain management in an ACGME-accredited training program.
4. Must have a minimum of 2 years of postresidency practice experience in pain management (Fellowship training time in pain management can be included).
5. Must have a minimum of 50 category I CME credits in the past 2 years.
6. Must pass the certification examination of the American Board of Pain Medicine.

Recertification is required every 10 years to those who hold the certificate awarded after January 1, 1999. The process of recertification is still under the construction.

There are total of 400 multiple-choice questions in the certification examination and it is given in two half-day sessions over the course of one full day. All the questions are developed by the ABPM Examination Council a group of ABPM diplomates. The examination question pool is updated every year to catch up with the current updated knowledge and technology.

The American Academy of Pain Management (AAPM) is another pain organization and should not be confused with the American Academy of Pain Medicine (also AAPM). This organization credentials both physicians and nonphysicians.

There are three levels of credentialing offered by the AAPM:

1. *Diplomate*: for the candidates who hold a doctorate degree in a related health care field and who have a minimum of 2 years of clinical pain management practice experience.
2. *Fellow*: for the candidates who hold a master's degree in a related health care field with a minimum of 2 years of clinical pain management experience.

3. *Clinical Associate*: for the candidates who holds a bachelor of arts degree, or its equivalent, in an appropriately related health care field with 5 years of clinical pain management experience.

Board certification certificates originally required very little verification of qualifications, but now all candidates have to pass the credentialing examination to be a credentialed pain practitioner with the American Academy of Pain Management. The examination contains 100 multiple-choice questions given in a period of 2 hours. "Grandfathered" certificates were offered to members of the American Academy of Pain Management at an early time before the examination was established.

The American Association of Nurse Anesthetists (AANA) also announced its proposal to receive the certification in pain management in conjunction with AAPM.[6]

The American Society of Pain Management of Nursing is planning to establish a certification system for nurses who practice in pain management fields. Further information can be obtained from its web site and contact address, which is in the following list.

Contact Information

1. The American Board of Anesthesiology
   4101 Lake Boone Trail
   Suite 510
   Raleigh, NC 27607-7506
   Tel: (919) 881-2570
   Fax: (919) 881-2575
   Web site: www.abanes.org
2. The American Board of Physical Medicine and Rehabilitation
   Norwest Center, Suite 674
   21 First Street SW
   Rochester, MN 55902
   Tel: (507) 282-1776
   Fax: (507) 282-9242
   Web site: www.abpmr.org
3. The American Board of Psychiatry and Neurology
   500 Lake Cook Road, Suite 335
   Deerfield, IL 60015
   Tel: (847) 945-7900
   Web site: www.abpn.com
4. The American Academy of Pain Medicine
   4700 W. Lake Avenue
   Glenview, IL 60025
   Tel: (847) 375-4731
   Fax: (847) 734-8750
   E-mail: aapm@amctec.com
5. American Academy of Pain Management
   13947 Mono Way #A
   Sonora, CA 95370
   Tel: (209) 533-9744
   Fax: (209) 533-9750
6. The American Board of Pain Medicine
   4700 W. Lake Avenue
   Glenview, IL 60025-1485
   Tel: (847) 375-4726
   Fax: (847) 375-6326
   Web site: www.abpm.org
7. American Society of Pain Management of Nursing
   7794 Grow Drive
   Pensacola, FL 32514
   Tel: (888) 342-7766
   Web site: www.aspmn.org

REFERENCES

1. Still A. *ASA Newsletter* 2000; (11).
2. American Board of Physical Medicine and Rehabilitation. Web site: *www.abpmr.org.*
3. American Board of Psychiatry and Neurology. *Information for Applicants for Certification in the Subspecialty of Pain Management*. Deerfield, Ill: American Board of Psychiatry and Neurology, 2001.
4. American Board of Anesthesiology. *Booklet of Information*. Raleigh, NC: American Board of Anesthesiology, November 2000.
5. American Board of Pain Medicine. *Certification Examination in Pain Medicine. Bulletin of Information*. Glenview, Ill: American Board of Pain Medicine, 2000.
6. American Association of Nurse Anesthetists. *News Bulletin* 2000, June.

CHAPTER 84

DISABILITY ASSESSMENT OF PAIN-IMPAIRED PATIENTS

Joseph Audette and Michael Schaufele

OVERVIEW

Approximately one third of all Americans have a chronically painful condition; 50% to 60% of these individuals are partially or totally disabled. Cost estimates in the United States run as high as $79 billion a year in direct and indirect expenses, with 40 million physician visits annually due to chronically painful conditions.[1] Much of these costs are related to the disability process including workers' compensation, litigation, personal indemnity, lost productivity, and Social Security Administration (SSA) payments. There has been a 73% increase in workers' compensation costs as a percentage of payroll in the period from 1980 to 1994, and in the same period, the medical costs in compensation cases rose 1.5 times faster than did general health care costs in the United States.[2] Although from 1988 to 1996 the length of disability on workers' compensation decreased by 60.9% and the average cost per claim decreased by 41.4%, this likely reflects state policy changes with more aggressive case management.[3] Given that during this same period applications for SSI and SSDI rose by greater than 40% in 1992, one can assume that there may have been a shift from workers' compensation to federal compensation. Interestingly, pain was a factor in 40% to 60% of these SSA claims.[4] The reasons for this dramatic increase are multifactorial: increased social and vocational demands, and change in work ethics may have contributed. Health care professionals themselves may be a significant cause of this change. In one study, using the Health Care Providers' Pain and Impairment Relationship Scale (HC-PAIRS), community health care providers had much lower expectations regarding the functional performance of patients with chronic low back pain than health care professionals who treated these patients with a functional restoration approach.[5] Perhaps we demand too little from our chronic pain patients, therefore contributing to increased disability.

One question that is often raised is, what distinguishes those individuals with chronically painful conditions that are disabled from those that are not. Ideally, one would expect that there would be major differences in disease severity that could be assessed with the use of standard clinical methods. What is frustrating for many physicians dealing with the question of impairment and disability in chronic pain is that there are no generally accepted standards to assess these differences. The pain field lacks the tests and examination techniques that rise to the level of a gold standard to which all other clinical methods can be compared for validation. To illustrate the difficulty, it is all too common for a patient with severe congenital scoliosis who has undergone spinal fusion with instrumentation at multiple levels to have no pain and little in the way of functional limitations. Contrast this to another typical patient with a remote history of low back injury, minimal findings on examination and imaging studies, and yet, who has, by self-report, severe disabling pain. Many of the instruments used to predict outcome that utilize the self-report of the patient in various domains of pain, function, and psychological distress have to be used with caution in a disability assessment recognizing that "prediction of failure to return to work would be used as a predictor of certification of inability to work."[6]

We begin by analyzing the current definitions of impairment and disability and point out where these definitions break down when it comes to occult conditions such as chronic pain. We then present the advances that have been made in this field over the last 10 years and propose a pragmatic, systematic approach to the functional evaluation of pain-impaired patients.

DEFINITIONS OF IMPAIRMENT, DISABILITY, AND HANDICAP

The terms *impairment*, *disability*, and *handicap* are commonly used in daily medical practice. Significant confusion, however, exists about the appropriate use of these terms. In addition to the well-known International Classification of Diseases (ICD), the World Health Organization (WHO) published the International Classification of Impairments, Disabilities, and Handicaps (ICIDH) in 1980.[7] Because of dramatic demographic changes and technological advances, medical care in industrialized countries has had to address the increasing prevalence of chronic diseases and this has led to a change from a disease- to an illness-consequence focus. This shift required an internationally accepted, common language outside the traditional medical model to serve the needs of people with disabilities. It is no longer sufficient to record the occurrence of a disease and its consequences solely in terms of complete recovery or death.[8] Many conditions, such as chronic pain, result in long-term, functional limitations that are nonfatal and which call for a different theoretical framework. Since its introduction, the ICIDH has been a widely accepted framework for understanding the consequences of a disease for a person at the structural, individual, and societal level (Fig. 84-1).

Impairment is defined as "any loss or abnormality of psychological, physiological or anatomical structure or function." Examples of impairments are decreased range of motion or loss of strength. Disability that results from an impairment is "any restriction or lack of ability to perform an activity in the manner or within the range considered normal for a human being" and is represented by activity limitations such as difficulties with community ambulation, inability to perform activities of daily living (ADLs), or disturbances in appropriate social behaviors. A handicap is caused by an impairment or disability that "limits or prevents the fulfillment of a role that is normal (depending on age, sex, and social and cultural factors) for that individual." For example, the inability to meet social obligations or fulfill occupational requirements may be a result of an impairment or disability.[9]

In summary, impairment is the result of an injury or disease at the level of the organ, that is, decreased range of motion or poor endurance. Disability describes the possible effects of an impair-

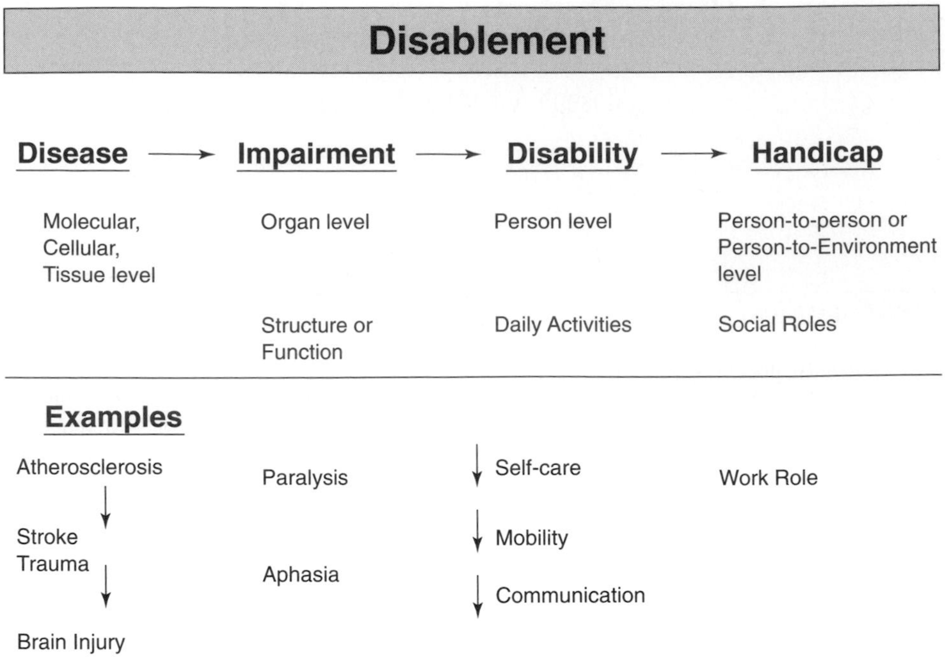

Disablement

Disease →	Impairment →	Disability →	Handicap
Molecular, Cellular, Tissue level	Organ level	Person level	Person-to-person or Person-to-Environment level
	Structure or Function	Daily Activities	Social Roles

Examples

Atherosclerosis ↓ Stroke	Paralysis	↓ Self-care	Work Role
Trauma ↓ Brain Injury	Aphasia	↓ Mobility ↓ Communication	

Figure 84–1 Schematic of the progression from a disease process to a disability and handicap.

ment at the level of the individual such as the inability to walk or lift. A handicap characterizes the consequences of impairment and disability at the level of the environment and society, that is, the work role.

Since the introduction of the ICIDH, the World Health Organization has worked on a revised version of the ICIDH, which is due to be released in the near future. It will put greater emphasis on presenting handicap as a description of the circumstances that people encounter due to the interaction between their impairment or disability and their physical and social environment. Disability will be defined as an activity limitation rather than inability and handicap as a participation restriction. One of the goals of the revised ICIDH is to provide a framework for functional diagnoses for persons with chronic limitations, similar to the medical diagnoses that comprise the ICD.[8] This is a concept that may be particularly helpful in addressing the problems of chronic pain patients with occult impairments by focusing on the functional effects rather than the disease.

AMA AND SSA GUIDELINES

While the goal of the ICIDH is the maximization of societal participation and improvement in the quality of life of people with disabilities and changes in social practices at the international level, the American Medical Association (AMA) uses impairment evaluations as a medicolegal tool to guide physicians to assess, report on, and communicate information about the impairments of human organ systems.[10] The purpose of the AMA evaluations is to estimate the severity of a person's impairment, for example, to assist in the settlement of workers' compensation cases, and therefore has entirely different implications than the ICIDH. Although the AMA definition of impairment closely parallels the WHO definition, one of the major criticisms of the AMA guidelines is that the rating of impairment is done in isolation without reference to the greater social context of potential disability and handicap. Physicians using the AMA guidelines determine impairment, but the matter of interest in medicolegal cases is disability or the patient's work capacity. Although the AMA guidelines recognize that an impaired individual is not necessarily disabled (i.e., a surgeon who loses his leg is impaired but not disabled from performing his job as a surgeon if fitted with an appropriate prosthesis), the impairment rating system breaks down when there is a paucity of impairments with severe disability such as is often seen in chronic pain states.

The Social Security Administration (SSA) regulations define disability as an "inability to engage in any substantial gainful activity by reason of any medically determinable physical or mental impairment which can be expected to result in death or which has lasted or can be expected to last for a continuous period of not less than 12 months.[11] For the purposes of SSA, pain is a symptom not an impairment, and so must be corroborated by medical signs or laboratory or imaging findings. In addition, chronic pain has been deemed not sufficient to demonstrate a mental impairment. As a result, what is assumed with the AMA guidelines is more overtly stated by the SSA, that disability is causally linked to impairment, and the greater the impairment found, the greater the disability.

An illustration of how the inference from impairment to disability can break down is well illustrated in the spinal cord injury (SCI) population. Up to 75% of SCI patients suffer from chronic pain with the intensity of pain being positively associated with greater disability, greater perceived stress, and lower measures of well-being. This is true despite the fact that greater pain intensity and disability in SCI has been shown to be negatively correlated with the degree of physical impairment as measured by accepted standards.[12]

We must keep in mind that disability determination is not in any straightforward way based solely on medical factors. Even from state to state the environment in which disability is determined will vary markedly. For example, the court determined percent disability for a man with low back pain will vary on average from 9.4% in New Hampshire to 27% in Tennessee.[2] Ultimately, disability is inevitably tied to the incentives, values, and goals of both the patient and the society in which he or she lives.

CONTRADICTIONS OF DISABILITY DETERMINATION IN CHRONIC PAIN

As can be seen from the previous discussion, the current medical paradigm is not ideally suited for the assessment and determination of disability in patients with chronic pain. The problem is further complicated by the medicolegal construct, in which the identification of disability is meant to be static. Defining a certain level of disability may convey the message to the patient that the rehabilitation effort has ended and will be of no further benefit despite functional limitations that are quite effort-dependent in chronic pain conditions.[13] Identification of impairments with a level of disability may erroneously give the patient the idea that the disability is considered fixed, and therefore will weaken the patient's motivation for recovery. Even in other catastrophic medical illnesses (such as stroke, myocardial infarction, and others) functional recovery, disability, and impairment are based both on the fixed lesions and on factors that are alterable such as patient motivation, family support, cultural and environmental background, and the medical and social commitment of resources to rehabilitation. Hence, a disability determination may be countertherapeutic in a chronic pain patient if it negatively affects these alterable factors.

On the other hand, a disability rating that results in the settlement of a workers' compensation or a personal liability case may be necessary from a psychological point of view before a chronic pain patient gives his or her full effort to reach maximal functional improvement in a rehabilitation program. In this setting, secondary gain issues, whether conscious or unconscious, may be impeding the positive outcome of rehabilitation.[14]

In many cases, physicians end up sanctioning or reinforcing disability inappropriately, especially in cases in which the patient complains of pain and functional limitations and there has been a history of major pain-related surgery such as with *failed back syndrome*. This group of chronic pain patients is at high risk for becoming disabled. The data are abysmal with high re-operation rates (17% to 20% in an industrial setting), and low return to work rates (only 23% to 43% return to work after disk surgery and up to 51% of patients will still be on disability 3 years following spinal fusion). In this setting physicians tend to "over-medicalize" the patient (repeat surgeries, overmedication, repeated invasive injection procedures) in an attempt to relieve pain because the pain report is generally believed, given the history of structural damage. This tends to lead the treating physician to sanction the reported disability of the patient since at least there is "objectively" something wrong with the patient's spine and none of the applied treatments have diminished the pain.[5] However, this inevitable path to permanent disability can be significantly reversed if the patient is given an aggressive functional restoration program that includes behavioral as well as physical treatment. The return to work rates for this group of *failed back* patients can be as high as 87% despite no change in the structural impairments.[15]

FUNCTIONAL ASSESSMENT METHODS IN PAIN PATIENTS

Disability assessment should be viewed as an attempt to determine the behavior or performance of an individual in a specific context.[16] Loss of a specific function such as the *inability* to bend to pick up a 15-lb box at work may coexist with the *ability* to bend and pick up a 30-lb, 3-year-old child. This functional dissonance can exist without conscious malingering because of the powerful differences between the absolute inability to perform a task versus the inability to perform a certain task comfortably in a specific environmental context. This makes the differentiation between those who cannot work from those who do not want to work quite difficult. Pain is subjective and is influenced by environmental factors. Impairments and disabilities may fluctuate depending on the situation in which a chronic pain patient finds himself.

There are a wide range of functional assessment methods available, which vary from simple range-of-motion measurements that can be easily performed in the office setting, to sophisticated, 2-day functional capacity evaluations that require expensive equipment and trained personnel. The most commonly used methods are pain measurement tools, functional assessments (by patient report or examination), psychological measurements, and information about the general health status. The use and combination of these different methods depends largely on the goal of the assessment. These goals may be a medicolegal disability rating in a workers' compensation case, identification of limitations to direct the patient to an appropriate therapy program, or for research purposes. Table 84-1 gives an overview of the different categories and frequently used assessment methods in pain patients. The most widely used measurements are discussed in the following paragraphs.

Pain Intensity

Since pain is a multidimensional experience and is private and subjective in nature, it may be the most difficult measurement to perform in health assessment. Its results often do not follow the ba-

TABLE 84-1 **Categories and Examples for Commonly Used Assessment Methods in Pain Patients**

Impairment Level
Pain Intensity
Visual Analog Scale
Verbal Rating Scale
Numerical Rating Scale
Pain Drawing
Functional Tools
Standardized Assessment of Flexibility, Strength, Lifting, and Endurance
Psychological Measures
Minnesota Multiphasic Personality Inventory (MMPI)
Beck Depression Index (BDI)
Symptom Checklist 90 (SCL-90)
Illness Behavior Questionnaire (IBQ)
Pain Management Inventory (PMI)
Disability Level
Oswestry Low Back Pain Disability Questionnaire
Functional Capacity Evaluations
Medical Rehabilitation Follow Along
Pain Disability Index (PDI)
Waddell Disability Instrument
Multidimensional, General Health Status, and Quality-of-Life Measures
Short-Form Health Survey (SF-36)
Sickness Impact Profile (SIP)

sic requirements of psychometric measurement, that is, reliability and validity. Pain measurement can capture two dimensions of the pain experience; namely, the sensory aspects of the pain and the person's emotional reaction to the pain. Although most clinical applications use fairly simple intensity scales, newer measurement methods are starting to evolve. Based on sensory decision theory, these methods attempt to distinguish the stimulus strength from the subjective response. It has been demonstrated, for example, that a placebo works as an analgesic primarily by reducing the respondent's tendency to label an experimental stimulus as "painful" rather than by altering the person's ability to feel it. Thus, the placebo seems to alter the affective response, not the perception of the stimulus.[17]

Most pain measurement methods can be divided in the following categories: pain questionnaires that record verbal or written responses to pain; behavioral measurements of pain that depend on observed pain behaviors of the subject; and analog methods, commonly used in laboratory studies, in which the respondent compares his pain with an experimentally induced pain stimulus of known intensity.[18] However, these different approaches measure different aspects of pain, and there appears to be little correlation between them.

The most commonly known and widely accepted questionnaires are the different subtypes of the visual analog pain rating scales. They provide a simple way to record a subjective estimation of pain intensity. Several types have been used, but the original scale, popularized by Huskisson, consisted of a straight line, 10-cm long, that represented the range of pain to be rated.[19] The visual analog scale (VAS) has been studied extensively, showing excellent reliability and adequate validity. In the comparison of different types of pain rating scales, it has been demonstrated that the numerical ratings are preferable to the verbal rating scales. For children and illiterate patients, a version showing faces is available. Overall, the VAS provides a robust, sensitive, and reproducible method of expressing pain severity that is applicable to a wide age range (children age 5 and older to adults that are cognitively intact) and is easily applied in a clinical setting.

Melzack's McGill Pain Questionnaire (MPQ) is the most commonly used measurement to describe the diverse dimensions of pain. The MPQ was initially presented in 1975 as a preliminary method. However, the questionnaire continues to be used in its original form and is considered the gold standard against which other, newer instruments are compared.[18] An attempt to address three major dimensions of pain—sensory-discriminative, motivational-affective, and cognitive-evaluative—are represented on the MPQ. The complete MPQ includes the patient's history and diagnosis, drug regimen, symptoms, and the effects of pain on the patient. The most commonly used section, however, is the 102-word questionnaire in which the patient has to mark pain attributes (i.e., sharp, burning, lancinating, punishing), pain intensity, accompanying symptoms (i.e., headache, dizziness), sleep, food intake, activity, and time course. It also includes a dermatomal pain drawing.

Four different scoring methods have been described by Melzack. The reliability of the MPQ is only weak, and the validity is adequate. There have been considerable discussions whether the selection and grouping of words reflect the dimensions he proposed.[20] Nevertheless, the importance of the MPQ is demonstrated by the incorporation of certain of its sections into several other scales and its use in many study protocols. The questionnaire takes about 15 to 20 minutes to administer, and is therefore probably too long for a routine office visit, but it may be helpful for an initial evaluation.

Functional Impairment

Limitations at the impairment level can be easily measured with the addition of a small number of functionally oriented examination techniques. Determining physical parameters such as range of motion, strength, lifting, and endurance can be incorporated in routine office visits or evaluation protocols and enables numeric documentation of structural impairment. Waddell studied the correlation between physical examination findings and self-reported disability in low back pain patients, demonstrating that total lumbosacral flexion measured at the T12-L1 interspace explained the greatest proportion of variance in disability scores when compared with any other physical examination test performed to assess chronic low back pain.[21] Once impairments are identified, treatment can focus on improvement of these functions rather than pain reduction. This becomes increasingly important in chronic pain patients, in which a pain elimination treatment approach is rarely successful.

Inclinometer techniques have become increasingly popular, especially in the physical assessment of back pain patients, since they are easy to apply.[22] They have become standard measurements in functional restoration programs for chronic back pain. Total lumbosacral flexion and extension can be assessed by placing a single inclinometer over the T12-L1 spinous processes. Straight leg raising can be tested by using the inclinometer placed on the tibial tuberosity. Suggested normal range of motion values for lumbosacral mobility are a minimum of 100 degrees of flexion and 25 degrees of extension, and for straight leg raising, a minimum of 75 degrees. Recorded measurements can be documented on graphs for quick reference (Fig. 84-2). Initial measurements in pain patients are likely to be influenced by psychological issues as well as physical tolerances, since patients may be inhibited by emotional distress, fear of injury, and pain. Therefore, although measurements may not represent true physiologic abilities, they still provide a numeric measure of the patient's psychophysical status and a meaningful starting point for treatment decisions.

The testing of strength, lifting, and endurance can be performed in a number of ways. None of the strength measure methods (isometric, isotonic or isokinetic) is superior in this setting, since all provide quantification of strength impairments. One relatively inexpensive method of lower back extension strength testing was developed using a standard back extension unit found in many fitness facilities (Fig. 84-3).[23] The testing protocol determines the maximum amount of weight that a subject can lift for four repetitions. Testing weight is begun at 9 kg. The endpoints for the test are psychophysical (subjective maximum), form (poor performance), or safety (more than 120% of the body weight). Based on normative data, the trunk extensor strength for a non-impaired person should be around 100% to 110% of ideal body weight.[23] Chronic back pain patients typically have an isometric extension strength that shows an approximate 50% reduction compared with non-impaired persons. Although other measurements of impairments have been described in the literature, this method illustrates the basic concept that the effects of pain on physical performance rather than solely the pain intensity itself should be measured. Similar strategies should be adopted for other pain syndromes not related to the spine.

The role of functional capacity evaluations (FCEs) has considerably increased over the last several years. They are used for work injury prevention and in rehabilitation to define an individual's functional abilities or limitations. By asking the patient to perform

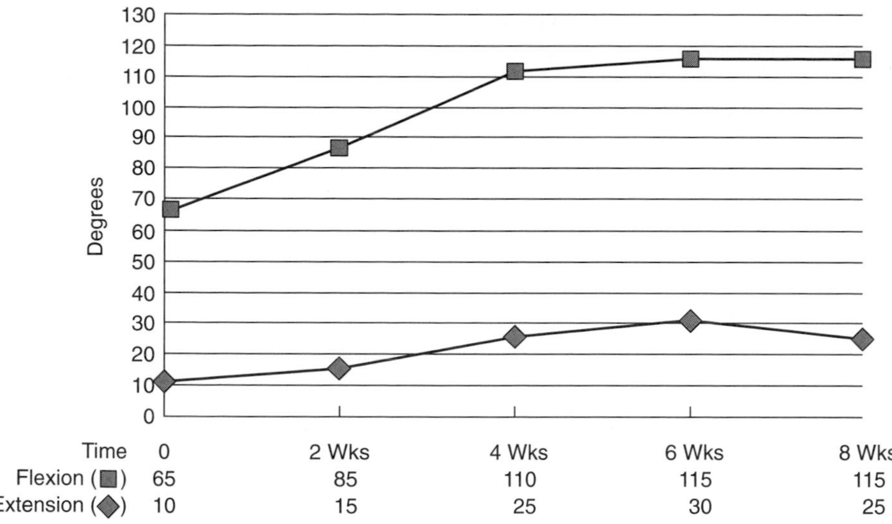

Figure 84–2 Graph for lumbosacral flexion and extension measured with the single inclinometer technique.

a set of certain test activities, the individual's ability to meet the required work demands can be assessed. FCEs are increasingly used to determine a patient's ability to return to his workplace, for pre-employment screening, for disability determinations, and to assist in determining case closure in medicolegal cases.[24] Although all systems share the common goal of attempting to measure work-related functional performance objectively, considerable differences in length of assessment, psychometric evaluation, costs, and standardization exist. Research to justify the use of FCEs for disability determination is sparse and the testing measures of consistency should not be inappropriately used to make a determination of possible malingering.

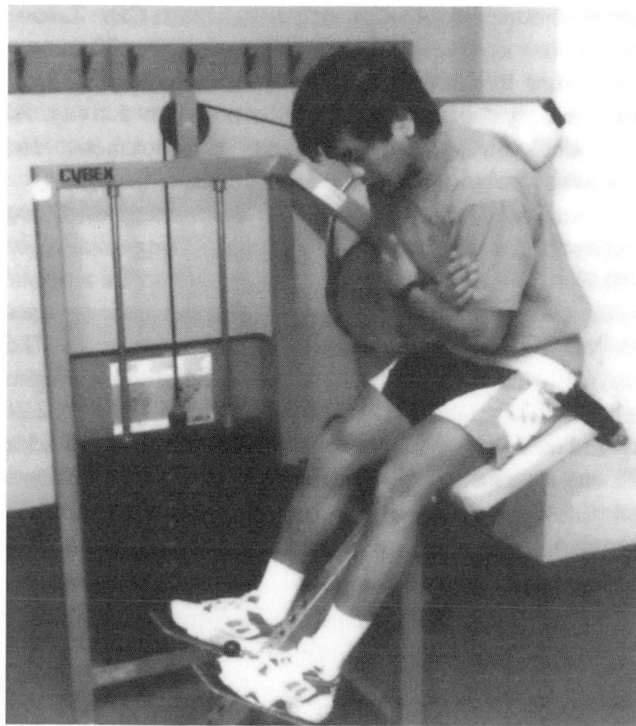

Figure 84–3 Lower back-extension strength testing with a standard back extension unit.

DIAGNOSTIC STUDIES

There has been a marked increase in the use of diagnostic imaging over the last 10 years. Recent analysis of the data from the National Low Back Pain Study found that men receiving disability compensation were much more likely to have both computed tomography (CT)-myelogram and magnetic resonance imaging (MRI) when compared with those with a comparable diagnosis who were not receiving compensation.[25] One possible explanation is that this overuse of imaging techniques in compensation patients is driven by the goal to find a structural abnormality to justify the degree of reported disability, since either imaging test alone would normally be sufficient to rule out serious injury or need for surgery.

The perception that references to structural abnormalities necessarily increases objectivity in disability assessment is not supported by the literature. There is very poor correlation between objective structural deficits seen with various diagnostic studies and pain or functional loss. In a recent study of MRI findings of the lumbar spine in pain-free individuals, only 36% of asymptomatic individuals had a normal study.[26] Up to 70% of asymptomatic individuals have degenerative disk disease demonstrable on plain films.[27] The objective function of the spine, as measured by isokinetic trunk muscle strength for patients with chronic low back pain, has been shown to be independent of the degree of degenerative changes seen on CT scans.[28] Conversely, the absence of findings on diagnostic testing of a patient with pain does not prove in any way that the pain syndrome lacks a physical cause. There are numerous conditions that have a paucity of objective findings on the diagnostic tests commonly available but, nevertheless, have accepted diagnostic criteria based on clinical examination techniques. Examples include myofascial pain, fibromyalgia, and complex regional pain syndromes. Should we then call all of these conditions *behavioral disorders* as has been recommended for nonspecific low back pain by the International Association for the Study of Pain (IASP) Task Force on Back Pain in the Workplace?[29]

Attempts to overcompensate for the lack of clear structural deviations in chronic pain patients by excessive diagnostic testing to find something "objective" only reinforces illness behavior. Even when a test is positive for some abnormality, the anatomic finding may have nothing to do with the functional losses observed, given the low specificity of most tests. Use of less common testing procedures such as thermograms and quantitative sensory testing are even less sensitive and specific and offer no help. In a survey of 80 pain specialist asked to rank the utility of various tests and procedures used to evaluate pain patients in order to develop a weighted ranking, the top seven ranked methods of evaluation were clinical examination procedures: examination of the nervous system, gait, spinal mobility, muscular function, soft tissue, and joint mobility were all ranked higher than any imaging or laboratory test.[30] The same authors have developed a total index of pathology (Medical Examination and Diagnostic Information Coding System, MEDICS) using 17 biomedical procedures commonly used to evaluate chronic pain conditions.

ILLNESS BEHAVIOR AND SECONDARY GAIN

The progression from acute to chronic pain can be viewed to occur in three stages[31]:

Stage 1: Onset of pain produces individual emotional reaction to pain.

Stage 2: After pain persists more than 2 to 4 months, there is an increase in the emotional, behavioral, and physical maladaptation to the pain.

Preexisting psychosocial and socioeconomic factors may weigh heavily at this stage. Increased somatization and symptom magnification is probable for someone who is premorbidly hypochondriacal or who may have conscious or unconscious secondary gains from being disabled.

Stage 3: Patient adopts a sick role and becomes accustomed to being relieved from normal responsibilities, social obligations, and financial responsibilities.

Attempts to develop a systematic approach to quantifying illness behavior in spine patients have been well established by Waddell (Table 84-2). A high Waddell score is defined as 3/5 positive signs and has been associated with poor performance on functional capacity evaluations, poor outcomes in surgery, and is often used as an indication that a mental health consult is necessary. There is a less clear picture with regard to its prognostic relevance in determining degree of disability. There have been a number of well-designed studies showing that there was no predictive value in using the Waddell signs when looking at return to work, work retention, or post-treatment health care utilization following an intensive functional restoration program.[32] Others have found some utility in using the Waddell scores in screening of those who will do well in an intensive work-hardening rehabilitation program that did not have a behavioral treatment component.[33]

Does compensation status influence disability in pain patients? Table 84-3 illustrates some of the socioeconomic factors that are predictive of disability. The majority of well-designed studies have demonstrated that patients receiving or seeking financial compensation exhibit greater levels of psychological distress and depression, higher levels of pain severity, and perceived disability.[14,34,35] In these studies, pain severity and perceived loss of function were independent of physical impairments. Is this all due then to problems of conscious secondary gain? Arguing against this is that these factors do not tend to be predictive of subsequent employment or health care utilization in prospective studies where an appropriate rehabilitation intervention has been applied.[36] Following the rehabilitation process, measures such as improved strength and range of motion were correlated with reduced levels of pain and depression in both the compensation and noncompensation groups. In general, a traumatic onset of pain and lack of employment have been associated with higher levels of emotional distress and perceived disability, and are likely playing an independent role in compensation cases.

TABLE 84-2 **Waddell's Assessment Tools for Illness Behavior and Exaggerated Symptoms**

Assessment Methods	Normal Illness Behavior	Abnormal Illness Behavior
Pain Drawing	**Localized with Appropriate Neuroanatomical Features**	**Magnified, Covering Diffuse Regions of Body**
Pain Adjectives	Sensory	Affective, evaluative
Symptoms		
Pain	Localized	Whole leg pain
Numbness	Dermatomal	Whole leg
Weakness	Myotomal	Whole leg giving away
Time Pattern	Varies with time	Never free of pain
Response to Treatment	Variable benefit	Intolerance of treatments, frequent ER visits
Signs		
Tenderness	Localized	Superficial, nonanatomical
Axial Loading	No lumbar pain	Lumbar pain
Straight leg raise	Limited on distraction	Improves with distraction
Sensory	Dermatomal	Regional
Motor	Myotomal	Jerky, give away weakness
Tenderness	Appropriate pain	Overreaction

TABLE 84-3 **Data from National Health and Nutrition Epidemiologic Survey of 5,202 disabled persons aged 24–70**

Factors Associated with Disability	Comments
Demographic	
Age 55–65	Sharp rise in prevalence from 45–55 age group
Low Income	Disability 4 times higher in <$7000/y group than in >$25,000 income group
Limited Education	Highest rates with maximum 8-years' education, 5 times that of college educated
Widowed or Divorced	Married individuals with lowest rates of disability
Socioeconomic	
Adverse Work Environment	Employees exposed to unpleasant conditions, 2 times as likely to be disabled

Data from Cats-Baril WL, Frymoyer JW. Demographic factors associated with the prevalence of disability in the general population: analysis of the NHANES I database. Spine 1991;16:671–674.

Unfortunately, both Waddell signs and questions of increased emotional distress with exaggerated ratings of pain severity and disability have been attributed to malingering or conscious secondary gain. This is not, however, a medical determination, and is better left to a court of law. Ultimately, short of a surveillance videotape, we must rely on patient reports of pain and dysfunction and cannot make determinations of conscious falsification of the data based on observed pain behaviors or seemingly exaggerated complaints. Fishbain points out that the concept of secondary gain is confused in any case, and does not help distinguish between true physical pathology from purely psychological pathology since both can have secondary gain issues.[37] The reality is that many of the secondary gains, conscious or not, are more than compensated for by the secondary losses related to chronic pain, and thus the lack of utility in using this concept for predicting disability outcome. This is demonstrated by ample case experiences of patients whose cases are finally settled and who will still exhibit continued heightened pain behaviors and signs of emotional distress if not treated for their pain issues. Multiple signs on Waddell testing by Waddell's own analysis are not a test of credibility or malingering but rather indicate the need for further psychological assessment.[38]

PSYCHOLOGICAL ASSESSMENT

It is well accepted that a number of psychosocial factors contribute to poor functional outcomes in pain. These include attitudes, beliefs, cultural norms, moods, focus of attention, motivation, and personality traits. Although most chronic pain patients are depressed and anxious, they seldom have a history of long-standing psychiatric problems. Rather, most of their symptoms reflect their current condition. Although chronic pain patients may exhibit certain personality traits that potentially contribute to their inability to cope with a chronic condition, rarely are these traits suggestive of significant psychopathology.[39] Certain psychosocial risk factors have been identified that are more likely to result in poor treatment outcomes and the development of disabling pain if left untreated (Table 84-4). In New Zealand, comprehensive guidelines for the treatment of low back pain were designed to assist health care professionals in recognizing these patients early and to ensure timely mental health referrals (Table 84-5).[47]

Nevertheless, the role of psychological assessment is still poorly understood by many pain specialists. The traditional notion that the lack of an easily identifiable physical or "organic" cause of pain implies that the pain must be psychogenic or "nonorganic" and deserves a mental health referral is erroneous logic. This type of faulty reasoning does the patient and society a disservice at many levels. By embracing such a dualistic view of the body where there is an attempt to compartmentalize the painful sensations reported by a patient either into the body or the mind is wrong both philosophically as well as physiologically and therapeutically. The perception and interpretation of pain is just as important as the nociceptive input. The notion that we can come to a firm conclusion about the objective origins of a pain experience based on diagnostic testing, examination, and/or various diagnostic and therapeutic invasive treatments is not founded on science.[26,48] That a patient does not respond to treatment as expected often means we have not taken into sufficient account the myriad of psychosocial, socioeconomic, and physical factors that are influencing the patient's pain experience. The presence of emotional distress, anxiety, depression, and anger is often present in the chronic pain state, even in the absence of work disability, and does not signify the absence of nociceptive input. Functionally oriented treatment of chronic pain patients even with elevated scores of hypochondriasis, depression, and hysteria as measured by the MMPI, has been shown to be successful, and typically the post-treatment scores on these three scales drop significantly.[49] This indicates that it is not a fixed personality trait that predisposes patients to chronic pain but the pain itself that may underlie the emotional distress.

The value of a systematic psychological assessment is to try to determine those factors that, if left untreated, will ultimately lead to prolonged loss of function and disability. In a study of pain severity by Von Korff,[50] four grades of disability scores were developed from a population survey of a large HMO in Washington state:

Grade I: Low Disability score, Low Pain Intensity score
Grade II: Low Disability score, High Pain Intensity score
Grade III: Moderately Limiting, High Disability score
Grade IV: Severely Limiting, High Disability score

The disability score was based on days missed from work over a 6-month period and degree of limitation and pain severity determined by self-report. Pain severity was not included in the grading of grades III and IV since these individuals uniformly reported elevated pain intensity. What is of interest is knowing what the differences were between individuals in the transition from grade II to III. These groups by definition had significant differences in degree of disability (3 days off work versus on average 23 days off work in last 6 months) but no discernible differences in pain scores, per-

TABLE 84-4 **Factors Shown to Influence Poor Disability Outcome in Low Back Pain (LBP) and Rheumatoid Arthritis (RA)**

Domain (study reference)	External Factors	Internal Factors
Socioeconomic		
LBP (Cats-Baril[40])	Physical demands of job (heavy labor vs sedentary)	Perception of compensable nature of injury
	Occupation	Job satisfaction or unpleasantness
	Benefits policy	Perception of fault
	Educational lLevel	
	Past hospitalizations	
LBP (Lehmann[41])	Litigation status	
	Workers' compensation case status	
LBP (Gatchel[42])	Female	
	Workers or personal injury case status	
RA (Wolfe[43])	Education level	
Psychosocial		
LBP (Gatchel[42])		Pain severity
		Perceived disability
LBP (Dionne[44])		Somatization
		Depression
LBP (Sanders[45])	Low activity	Elevated hysteria
	Elevated pain behavior	Negative beliefs about pain and activity
		Depression
Upper Extremity Pain (Burton[46])	Previous history of psychopathology	Depressed mood
	Previous history of substance abuse	Pain severity
	Anxiety or borderline disorder	Perceived disability
	Hx of child abuse	
RA (Wolfe[43])		Perceived disability
		Pain severity

sistence of pain, or recency of onset of pain. The largest differences turned on behavioral variables such as reported functional limitations, unemployment status, and health care utilization rather than differences in psychological variables such as depression and health status. Grade IV patients did show significantly higher levels of depression.[50] This suggests a gradient of dysfunction in chronic pain, where many individuals may be disabled due to nonadaptive reinforcing patterns of behavior rather than overt emotional distress or psychological impairment. Psychological referral is appropriate both in cases of overt psychopathology and when the problem is more due to dysfunctional patterns of illness behavior.

TABLE 84-5 **Psychosocial Risk Factors for Chronic Back Pain**

- Maladaptive attitudes and beliefs concerning back pain
- Frequent display of pain behaviors
- Reinforcement of pain behavior by family members
- Heightened emotional reactivity
- Lack of social support
- Job dissatisfaction
- Compensation issues

Data from National Advisory Committee on Health and Disability. Guide to Assessing Yellow Flags in Acute Low Back Pain. Wellington, NZ: Ministry of Health; 1997.

BASIC SET OF INFORMATION FOR DISABILITY EVALUATION

In clinical practice, a screening method to quantify the three important areas of physical functioning, pain, and psycho-affective well-being is needed. A quick overview of these three areas could help the clinician in prescribing therapies for problems that most significantly affect the patient based on the degree of disability found. One approach, based on Internet technology is the Medical Rehabilitation Follow Along (MRFA). This interactive tool has been designed to assist in patient screening, resource allocation, and outcome assessment for pain patients in the outpatient setting. The MRFA was developed by using major concepts from the Functional Assessment Screening Questionnaire (FASQ), the Oswestry Scale, the short form of the McGill Pain Questionnaire, and the Brief Symptom Inventory.[51]

The administration of the self-report questionnaire takes approximately 15 minutes and can be filled out prior to every office visit. The scores of eight subcategories are summarized in the areas of physical functioning, pain experience, driving, and affective well-being. With the use of computer technology, the results are available to the treating physician within minutes. This allows the physician to tailor the treatment plan according to the results. The patient's profile can be compared with other patients from the database, especially during follow-up visits when the effectiveness of a therapy plan is assessed. Differences from a "normal" recovery process are recognized immediately, allowing immediate changes in the treatment strategies. This may permit identification of problematic patients early on in the recovery process, allowing intervention before disability develops from chronic pain.

Another strategy was developed as part of the recognition by the SSA of the growing problem with pain-related disability. The Commission on the Evaluation of Pain was formed, and together with the Institute of Medicine, a predictive tool was developed called the Multiperspective Multidimensional Pain Assessment Protocol (MMPAP). Like the MRFA, the MMPAP combines a number of recognized instruments (the McGill Pain Questionnaire, the Multidimensional Pain Inventory, and the Oswestry Pain Inventory) together with a structured functional assessment by the examining physician to rate patient's pain behavior, medical status, and rehabilitation potential. The MMPAP has been tested and validated with good interrater reliability when rehabilitation medicine specialists were given training in the use of the tool. Findings support that the individual's ability to adapt or cope with pain is a significant determinant of disability. The analysis also indicates that functionally oriented physician assessments can be predictive of future disability risk if properly trained (Table 84-6).[4]

CONCLUSION

Recent estimates reported in *Business Week* (March 1, 1999) of the costs for the treatment of pain are now rising to $100 billion dollars a year in the United States with 515 million work days lost each year. Last year, Congress voted to allocate $102 million to the National Institutes of Health for pain research, a 15% jump from the prior year. Despite this, chronic pain continues to grow, and as physicians, we must shift our attention from trying to *cure* these patients

TABLE 84-6 **From Analysis of Social Security Administration Applicants' Subsequent Employment and Pain Status Using Data from the MMPAP**

	Assessed by MD	Patient Report
Predictive Factors		
Subsequent Employment Status		
Frequency of Pain	+	+
Degree to which Patient Verbalizes about Pain	+	+
Length of Pain-Free Periods		+
Unpleasantness of Pain when Severe		+
Hopelessness, Depression		+
States "Will never work again"		+
Difficulty with Relationship with Significant Other		+
Gait Abnormalities	+	
Joint Deformities	+	
Functional Limitations with ADLs	+	
Perception that FCE would require Extreme Effort	+	
Estimation of Level of Treatment Needed	+	
Subsequent Pain Intensity		
Functional Limitations with ADLs	+	+
Estimation of Level of Treatment Needed	+	
Perception that Pain Complaints were Exaggerated	+	
Nonpredictive Factors		
Subsequent Employment Status		
Functional Limitations with ADL's		+
Social Support Network		+
Subsequent Pain Intensity		
Pain Intensity		+
Unpleasantness of Pain		+
Depression, Hopelessness		+
Social Support Network		+

From Rucker KS, Metzler HM. Predicting subsequent employment status of SSA disability applicants with chronic pain. Clin J Pain 1995;11:22–35.

MMAP denotes Multiperspective Multidimensional Pain Assessment Protocol; FCE, functional capacity evaluations.

TABLE 84-7 **Basic Contents of a Pain Evaluation**

1. Pain-Related Medical History
   - Description of pain localization, quality, intensity, time course
   - Medications (past/current)
   - Diagnostic procedures
   - Therapies
   - Procedures
   - Surgeries
   - History of similar pain problems
   - Ever-pain free?
   - Pain improved by
   - Pain worsened by
   - Pain drawing
   - Visual analog scale (VAS)
2. Functional/Occupational History
   - Occupation
   - Education
   - Level of physical activity prior to onset of pain
   - Current level of activity: difficulties with
     - personal care (washing, dressing)
     - lifting real life objects (groceries, small children)
     - walking distance
     - sitting time
     - standing time
     - traveling
   - Work-related or traumatic accident?
   - Job satisfaction?
   - Could you do your last job today?
   - If not, what type of jobs could you do now?
3. Psychosocial History
   - Marital status
   - Who lives with you?
   - Current social activity level (or desired level)
   - Primary social role (i.e., work, education, homemaking)
   - Current social role activity level (or desired level)
   - History of childhood abuse, family dysfunction
   - Depressive, Anxious symptoms
   - History of psychological/psychiatric problems
   - Pain-related fears
   - Financial problems
   - General life satisfaction?
4. Physical Examination
   - General medical examination
   - Neurological examination
   - Musculoskeletal examination including assessment of muscular function (tone, mass, strength), joint motion, and soft tissue
   - Gait
   - Spinal mobility using inclinometer technique (or similar)
   - Dynamic strength examination (e.g., lifting of several predetermined weights)
   - Waddell signs (axial loading, straight leg raise, sensory, motor, tenderness)

to finding ways of limiting loss of function and disability. To do this, the complex multidimensional nature of pain must be accepted as part of the territory. Physical, psychosocial, and socioeconomic factors must be included in the assessment to avoid being more a part of the problem than part of the solution. We end by offering a minimal guide of the four domains of assessment that should be included in any pain evaluation (Table 84-7).

REFERENCES

1. Bonica JJ. General Considerations of chronic pain. In: Bonica JJ ed. *The Management of Pain*. Vol 1. Philadelphia, Pa: Lea & Febiger; 1990.
2. Durbin D. Workplace injuries and the role of insurance: claims costs, outcomes, and incentive. *Clin Orthop Rel Res* 1997;336:18–32.
3. Hashemi L, Webster BS, Clancy EA. Trends in disability duration and cost of workers' compensation low back pain claims (1988–1996). *J Occup Environ Med* 1998;40:1110–1119.
4. Rucker KS, Metzler HM. Predicting subsequent employment status of SSA disability applicants with chronic pain. *Clin J Pain* 1995;11: 22–35.
5. Rainville J, Bagnall D, Phalen L. Health care providers' attitudes and beliefs about functional impairments and chronic back pain. *Clin J Pain* 1995;11:287–295.
6. Carey TS. Disability: how successful are we in determining disability? *Neurol Clin North Am* 1999;17(1):167–178.
7. World Health Organization. *International Classification of Impairments, Disabilities, and Handicaps*. Geneva, Switzerland: WHO; 1980, 1993.
8. Thuriaux MC. The ICIDH: evolution, status and prospects. *Disabil Rehabil* 1995;17:112–118.
9. deKleijn-deVrankrijker MW. The International Classification of Impairments, Disabilities, and Handicaps (ICIDH): perspectives and developments (Part 1). *Disabil Rehabil* 1995;17:109–111.
10. *Guides to the Evaluation of Permanent Impairment*. 4th ed. Chicago, Ill: American Medical Association; 1995.
11. Social Security Act 42 USC, Section 423 as amended by Social Security Disability Reform Act of 1984, PL 98-460.
12. Rintala DH, Loubser PG, et al. Chronic pain in a community-based sample of men with spinal cord injury: prevalence, severity, and relationship with impairment, disability, handicap, and subjective well-being. *Arch Phys Med Rehabil* 1998;79:604–614.
13. Sullivan MD, Loeser J. The diagnosis of disability: Treating and rating disability in a pain clinic. *Arch Intern Med* 1992;152:1829–1835.
14. Rainville J, Sobel JB, Hartigan C, et al. The effect of compensation involvement on the reporting of pain and disability by patients referred for rehabilitation of chronic low back pain. *Spine* 1997;22:2016–2024.
15. Mayer TG, McMahon MJ, Gatchel RJ, et al. Socioeconomic outcomes of combined spine surgery and functional restoration in workers' compensation spinal disorders with matched controls. *Spine* 1998;23:598–605.
16. Fordyce WE. On the nature of illness and disability: An editorial. *Clin Orthrop Rel Res* 1997;336:47–51.
17. Clark WC, Yang JC. Application of sensory decision theory to problems in laboratory and clinical pain. In: Melzack R, ed. *Pain Measurement and Assessment*. New York, NY: Raven Press; 1983:15–25.
18. McDowell I, Newell C. *Measuring Health: A Guide to Rating Scales and Questionnaires*. 2nd ed. New York, New York: Oxford University Press; 1996.
19. Huskisson EC. Measurement of pain. *J Rheumatol* 1982;9:768–769.
20. Turk DC, Rudy TE, et al. The McGill Pain Questionnaire reconsidered: confirming the factor structure and examining appropriate uses. *Pain* 1985;21:385–397.
21. Waddell G, Somerville D, et al. Objective clinical evaluation of physical impairment in chronic low back pain. *Spine* 1992;17:617–628.
22. Rainville J, Sobel JB, Hartigan C. Comparison of total lumbosacral

flexion and true lumbar flexion measured by a dual inclinometer technique. *Spine* 1994;19:2698–2701.
23. Rainville J, Sobel JB, Hartigan C, et al. Decreasing disability in chronic back pain through aggressive spine rehabilitation. *J Rehabil Res Dev* 1997;34:383–393.
24. King PM, Tuckwell N, Barrett TE. A critical review of functional capacity evaluations. *Phys Ther* 1998;78:852–866.
25. Ackerman SJ, Steinberg EP, et al. Patient characteristics associated with diagnostic imaging evaluation of persistent low back problems. *Spine* 1997;22:1634–1641.
26. Jenson MC, Brandt-Zawadzki MN, et al. Magnetic resonance imaging of the lumbar spine in people without back pain. *New Engl J Med* 1994;331:69–73.
27. Hadler NM. Regional musculoskeletal diseases of the low back. *Clin Orthop* 1987;221:33–41.
28. Keller A, Johansen JG, Hellesnes J, Brox JI. Predictors of isokinetic back muscle strength in patients with low back pain. *Spine* 1999;24: 275–280.
29. Teasell RW, Merskey H. Chronic pain disability in the workplace. *Pain Forum* 1997;6(4):228–238.
30. Rudy TE, Turk DC, Brena SF, et al. Quantification of biomedical findings of chronic patients: development of and index of pathology. *Pain* 1990;42:167–182.
31. Gatchel RJ, Gardea MA. Psychosocial Issues: Their importance in predicting disability, response to treatment, and search for compensation. *Neurol Clin North Am* 1999;17(1):149–166.
32. Polatin PB, Cox B, Gatchel RJ, Mayer TG. A prospective study of Waddell signs in patients with chronic low back pain: when they may not be predictive. *Spine* 1997;22:1618–1621.
33. Werneke M, Harris D, Lichter R. Clinical effectiveness of behavioral signs for screening chronic low-back pain patients in a work-oriented physical rehabilitation program. *Spine* 1993;18:2412–2418.
34. Cassisi, JE, Sypert GW, et al. Pain, disability, and psychological functioning in chronic low back pain subgroups: myofascial versus herniated disc syndrome. *Neurosurgery* 1993;33:379–385.
35. Turk DC, et al. Perception of traumatic onset, compensation status and physical findings: impact on pain severity, emotional distress, and disability in chronic pain patients. *J Behav Med* 1996;19:435–453.
36. Wright A, Mayer TG, Gatchel RJ. Outcomes of disabling cervical spine disorders in compensation injuries. A prospective comparison to tertiary rehabilitation response for chronic lumbar spine disorders. *Spine* 1999;15:178–183.
37. Fishbain DA, Rosomoff HL, Cutler RB, et al. Secondary gain concept: a review of the scientific evidence. *Clin J Pain* 1995;11:6–21.
38. Main CJ, Waddell G. Behavioral responses to examination. A reappraisal of the interpretation of 'nonorganic signs'. *Spine* 1998;23:2367–2371.
39. Jamison RN. Psychological factors in chronic pain: assessment and treatment issues. *J Back Musculoskel Rehabil* 1996;7:79–95.
40. Cats-Baril WL, Frymoyer JW. Identifying patients at risk of becoming disabled because of low-back pain: The Vermont Rehabilitation Engineering Center predictive model. *Spine* 1991;16:671–674.
41. Lehmann TR, Spratt KF, et al. Predicting long-term disability in low back injured workers presenting to a spine consultant. *Spine* 1993; 18:1103–1112.
42. Gatchel RJ, Polatin PB, Mayer TG. The dominant role of psychosocial risk factors in the development of chronic low back disability. *Spine* 1995;20:2702–2709.
43. Wolfe F, Hawley DJ. The longterm outcomes of rheumatoid arthritis: work disability: a prospective 18 year study of 823 patients. *J Rheumatol* 1998;25:2108–2117.
44. Dionne CE, Koepsell TD, Von Korff M, et al. Predicting long-term functional limitations among back pain patients in primary care settings. *J Clin Epidemiol* 1997;50:31–43.
45. Sanders SH. Risk factors for the occurrence of low back pain and chronic disability. *Am Pain Soc Bull* 1995;5:1–5.
46. Burton K, Polatin PB, Gatchel RJ. Psychosocial factors and the rehabilitation of patients with chronic work-related upper extremity disorders. *J Occup Rehabil* 1997;7;139–153.
47. National Advisory Committee on Health and Disability. *Guide to Assessing Yellow Flags in Acute Low Back Pain*. Wellington, New Zealand: Ministry of Health; 1997.
48. North RB, Kidd DH, Zahurak M, Piantadosi S. Specificity of diagnostic nerve blocks: a prospective, randomized study of sciatica due to lumbosacral spine disease. *Pain* 1996;65:77–85.
49. Barnes D, Gatchel RJ, Mayer TG, et al. Changes in MMPI profiles of chronic low back pain patients following successful treatment. *J Spinal Disord* 1990;3:353–355.
50. Von Korff M, Ormel J, Keefe FJ, Dworkin SF. Grading the severity of chronic pain. *Pain* 1992;50:133–149.
51. Baker JG, Granger CV, Ottenbacher KJ. Validity of a brief outpatient functional assessment measure. *Am J Phys Med Rehabil* 1996;75:356–363.
52. Cats-Baril WL, Frymoyer JW. Demographic factors associated with the prevalence of disability in the general population: analysis of the NHANES I database. *Spine* 1991;16:671–674.

CHAPTER 85 MEDICAL-LEGAL CONSIDERATIONS IN PAIN MANAGEMENT

Sarah H. Hines and John H. Eichhorn

Physicians involved in pain management should be aware that there are many legal issues involved in the practice of pain management. Some patients who present to pain management centers may be involved in litigation or compensation cases. The impact of these issues on patient outcome is controversial. Patients with pain often are labeled "difficult" because of their responses to the stress of their pain. Furthermore, there is a widespread perception that anesthesiologists working in pain management centers are at a greater risk of being sued for malpractice than those working in the traditional operating room setting.

The available information, however, does not support this perception. For example, during the period 1971 to 1982 in Washington State, of 192 malpractice claims against anesthesiologists, 56 involved regional anesthesia, but only one (for a pneumothorax during stellate ganglion block) involved pain management.[1] Data from the claims files of the Risk Management Foundation of the Harvard Medical Institutions shows only one anesthesia pain management claim during a recent 10-year period. In this claim, a man received a corticosteroid injection for meralgia paresthetica. Shortly after leaving the hospital, approximately 50 minutes after receiving the injection, he became dizzy. He returned to the pain clinic and fell, allegedly sustaining a back injury that caused permanent residual pain. The claimant alleged a failure to obtain informed consent and that the physician did not advise him to remain for observation for adverse reactions. The claim was resolved without a lawsuit.

The database of the American Society of Anesthesiologists Closed Claims Project shows that while the proportion of anesthesia malpractice claims involving nonoperative pain management is fairly low, it is increasing over time, from 2% of all claims in the 1970s to 8% of all claims in the 1990s. In a review of the database of closed claims, the most common injuries were pneumothorax, nerve damage, headache, and back pain. Claims for very serious complications such as brain damage or death represent a small but not insignificant fraction (10%) of the claims. The median payment for operative claims was much higher than the payment for nonoperative pain management claims ($100,000 vs $16,250). The likelihood of payment for a claim was similar between the two groups, as was reviewer judgment of appropriateness of care.[2]

Exposure to the risk of a malpractice claim will vary with the degree of a physician's involvement with pain management and the type of procedures performed. The greatest risk for major claims appears to be associated with the administration of ablative nerve blocks.[3–5]

One moderate-sized pain management center in a university teaching hospital doing approximately 1000 procedures (nearly all injections) annually had the following distribution of case mix: lumbar epidural steroids, 66%; epidural narcotic catheters, 1%; transcutaneous electrical nerve stimulation (TENS), 2%; stellate ganglion, 6%; facet, 3%; and blood patch, 1%. Only a few blocks performed during this period were neurolytic. Therefore, this pain center, and other pain centers performing similar procedures, are most likely to be at a relatively low risk for major claims for complications from procedures.

THE PHYSICIAN AS A WITNESS

Physicians may be involved as a witness in a malpractice case as either a fact witness or an expert witness. A physician involved in a patient's care may be forced to testify (by deposition or subpoena) as a fact witness by the plaintiff or the defense. When pain management physicians are subpoenaed as a routine fact witness, involvement of the physician's own attorney is usually unnecessary. An expert witness renders an opionion (usually for a fee) on the facts of the case.

STANDARDS OF CARE

Pain management practitioners are physicians, not technicians who do procedures "ordered by" referring physicians. It is inappropriate for an orthopedic surgeon, neurosurgeon, or other physician to "order" procedures, such as an epidural corticosteroid injection or stellate ganglion block. It is equally inappropriate (and legally inadvisable) for the anesthesiologist to follow blindly such an order.

The pain management physician becomes a fully responsible provider when the patient is accepted. As an independent practitioner, the pain management physician takes note of the information accompanying the patient but, functionally, must start his or her evaluation from the beginning as any physician does with a new patient. In the event of a complication or unfortunate result, it is no protection to state that one was acting on the suggestion or even "orders" of another physician. A thorough comprehensive medical history and a complete physical examination are absolutely necessary. When indicated, appropriate diagnostic tests must be done. It is insufficient to focus only on the pain problem. Doing so might cause failure to diagnose some previously undiscovered causal or associated condition that is a threat to the patient. Overlooking this underlying problem (such as a pathologic fracture from a metastatic lesion) represents poor quality medical care and exposes the pain management physician to a potential malpractice claim when the overlooked condition is discovered later.

THE PHYSICIAN-PATIENT RELATIONSHIP

The physician-patient relationship is a consensual agreement, rarely taking the form of an express or written contractual agree-

Portions of this chapter reprinted with permission from Danner D. *Medical Malpractice: A Primer For Physicians*. Rochester, NY: The Lawyers Co-operative; 1986:4–7.

ment. The relationship, however, is implied readily when the physician begins treating a patient, and the patient accepts the physician's services and advice.

A physician must have a duty to the patient that is created by the existence of a physician-patient relationship before a physician can be found liable for medical malpractice.

Once a physician has undertaken the care and treatment of a patient, this does not imply an unlimited right to terminate the relationship at will. The relationship may be terminated in one of the following ways: (1) the patient no longer requires the physician's services, (2) the patient initiates termination of the relationship, or (3) the physician terminates the relationship by giving the patient a reasonable period of notice of termination so that the patient may arrange for alternative services. However, the physician must remain available for consultation until an alternate provider is obtained. It is not clear from case law whether making an appointment (such as with a pain management unit) constitutes a relationship or whether the patient actually must be seen by the physician.

The physician may be liable for abandonment if notice of termination of the relationship is not given in a reasonable and timely fashion. This occurs when the physician does not meet the obligation to provide medical services. Physicians who withdraw from a physician-patient relationship while a need for medical services exists, and without proper notice, may also be found liable for breach of contract. If the patient can prove that some harm resulted from the abandonment, the physician may be liable for malpractice as well.

When the physician wishes to withdraw from the care of a patient, the patient should be notified in writing by registered mail of the intent to terminate the relationship. The physician should indicate willingness to provide medical records to subsequent treating physicians and to see the patient for urgent problems that may arise before services of another physician are secured. The reasonableness of the time between notice and termination depends on factors including the patient's condition, availability of alternative providers, and the patient's resources. Although a physician has obligations after a relationship with a patient is established, the physician is not obliged to see every patient seeking an appointment.

RECORD KEEPING

After the patient is accepted and a relationship established, it is critical that a complete medical record be kept. Clinics or units that are part of a larger facility (such as a hospital or medical center) usually keep separate charts in the individual unit rather than trust intermittent entries in the large master medical record of the institution. Many malpractice attorneys claim that the medical record is the single most important factor in determining the outcome of a medical malpractice case. A thorough, objective, concise, unaltered record might deter a plaintiff attorney from filing a suit.

The medical record of any treating physician may be subpoenaed ("is discoverable") by one or both sides in a legal case. It is imperative to keep inflammatory speculation out of the patient's medical record and document only the actual facts.

All patient interactions (including telephone calls) should be recorded on the physician's clinic or office record. Problems can arise when there are questions about undocumented telephone conversations in which treatment recommendations are made to the patient. Furthermore, all telephone calls with the patient's pharmacy must be documented, especially in the event that telephone orders for new medications or refills for current medications are authorized.

All procedures should be documented with a procedure note or, better, on a preprinted graphic record designed for pain treatment. This record should include patient background data, patient positioning for the procedure, technique used, preparation, type of needle used, paresthesias, solution injected over what period of time, responses, vital signs throughout, and patient condition and disposition at the end of the procedure. The recovery period needs a similarly complete record. All follow-up telephone calls and visits to the patient should be recorded. Even the smallest details of care can take on great importance in a malpractice suit.

In one case,[6] a patient with chronic pain in the left shoulder and back pain received an injection of 10 mL of a solution of hydrocortisone, lidocaine, and tetracaine. She immediately complained of chest pain and was advised to lie down because she was "probably just upset about the injection." She did not feel better but was sent home with a prescription for diazepam to calm her. The patient later was admitted to the hospital with a diagnosis of iatrogenic pneumothorax. Her suit alleged that the injection caused the pneumothorax. The defendant's physician said he gave the injection with a 5/8-in., 25-gauge needle, which all experts agreed probably would not have caused a pneumothorax. However, the plaintiff expert testified that, because the solution would not flow through a 25-gauge needle, a 19-, 20-, or 21-gauge needle was needed, and that it would be able to penetrate to the pleura. The defendant physician did not remember the details of the injection given and had not recorded the size of the needle used. He could testify only to what he thought he would have done. Both plaintiff and defense expert testimony tended to discount the possibility of spontaneous pneumothorax. Therefore, because the defendant could not remember with certainty the size of the needle and had not documented the procedure thoroughly, the question of causation became simply a competition among various expert witnesses.

An inadequate medical record can render a malpractice case difficult to defend. The medical record and memory of the witnesses are all that can be used to counter the plaintiff's recollection of care rendered. A good medical record can refresh the physician's memory of a particular case and provide precise details of the history, findings, treatment plans, consent process, procedures done, outcome, and follow-up. Even if the medical record is inadequate, incomplete, or misleading, it is absolutely vital that physicians (or anyone) never alter a record after it has been created. If there is need to amend or explain something in the record, this must be done in a later separate entry that is dated and timed appropriately. Any suggestion that the record has been falsified or tampered with makes a case essentially indefensible. Any problem or uncertainty about the record can cloud the issue. In one case,[7] the defendant physician did a disk injection. The plaintiff subsequently complained of numbness; this progressed to paraplegia. One available hospital record stated that an injection of betamethasone and bupivacaine was done under x-ray control. However, the circulating nurse's operative record, on which the drugs were recorded, was missing from the chart. The physician later testified during two depositions that he believed he used betamethasone and bupivacaine. Four years later, the plaintiff's counsel discovered that, instead of these drugs, the defendant mistakenly had injected colchicine, a potentially neurotoxic medication that may have caused the paraplegia. After this discovery of discrepancies in the records, the claim was settled for $1 million.

Hospital records and private office records frequently are requested by patients and plaintiff attorneys. Generally, hospital records are accessible to patients and their authorized representatives when written authorization from the patient is obtained. The laws regarding patient requests for physician office records vary from state to state. In all cases, patient medical information should not be released without the express written authorization of the patient. When medical records are requested properly by the patient, the patient's attorney, or by subpoena, copies of the records should be given to the requesting party. The original files should be retained by the responsible physician or institution.

When prescribing controlled substances to a patient, a number of issues must be addressed in the patient's medical record to document the validity of prescribing these medications to the patient. These issues include[8]:

1. Medical history and physicial examination including past treatments for the pain problem, history of substance abuse, affects of the pain on physical and psychological function, and a diagnosis that is an indication for the use of controlled substances.
2. Periodic reassessment of the patient, including progress toward treatment goals.
3. A written treatment plan, including an outline of therapeutic courses and changes of treatment direction; including objectives to be used for treatment success (such as improved physical function).
4. Referral to other consultants, as needed.
5. An ongoing relationship established with the patient's pharmacist; the patient should receive controlled substances from only one physician and only one pharmacist, if at all possible.
6. Periodic reassessments of addictive behavior; a written agreement between the physician and the patient may be necessary ("narcotic contract") to delineate patient responsibilities for the continued prescription of controlled substances.
7. Documentation that risks, benefits, and alternatives to narcotics were discussed.
8. Documentation that treatment with non-narcotic medications have failed.

INFORMED CONSENT

Obtaining true informed consent for proposed treatment is an important aspect of pain management. The doctrine of informed consent is based on the recognition of the individual's right to self-determination. For a patient, a nonmedically trained individual, to make an informed decision about whether or not to undergo a proposed course of therapy, the physician must explain and inform the patient fully in language that can be understood. After the patient is informed fully, consent can be given that will help protect the physician from liability exposure for failing to advise the patient fully of potential material risks, benefits, and alternatives to treatment.

Complete informed consent generally requires disclosure of the following elements:

1. Explanation of the diagnosis or condition that requires treatment.
2. Nature and purpose of the treatment.
3. Probable outcome without treatment.
4. Known benefits and material risks of proposed treatment.
5. Explanation of reasonable alternative treatments, including material risks and benefits.
6. The probability of success of the treatment.

The definition of true informed consent is changing. At one time, there was a so-called professional standard[9] that required disclosure of risks in a manner customarily used by physicians in the local community. The concept of materiality has, in general, now replaced the concept of professional standard.[10] A material risk "is one which the physician knows or ought to know [what] would be significant to a reasonable person in the patient's position of deciding whether or not to submit to a particular medical treatment or procedure."[11] The *Harnish v Children's Hospital Medical Center*[12] case showed the importance of disclosing all material risks. If all material risks are not disclosed, then the consent is not fully informed. This decision created many questions about the necessity of disclosing even very rare complications. An important later decision[13] qualified the original materiality requirement by stating that it is not necessary to disclose every incredibly rare complication for which the chances are "negligible."

Attempting to disclose every complication, even those that are extremely rare, was felt to cause unrealistic and unnecessary burdens on practitioners. This decision emphasized the balance that is necessary between full disclosure and fairness for those doing the disclosing. There is no case law defining how rare a complication has to be for it to be negligible.

Individual pain management physicians must evaluate which risks are negligible and which are material and then decide on a case-by-case basis exactly what to disclose in obtaining informed consent. It may be difficult to decide what information will be the most material to an individual patient. Whether all patients receiving blocks should be told that there are remote risks of permanent neurologic damage, or even death, still remains an individual decision. In all cases, careful thought must go into the process of risk disclosure.[14] It is especially difficult when a jury, looking in retrospect at an injured plaintiff, feels that a particular undisclosed risk is material to a supposed informed-consent decision that may have occurred years before. The informed-consent process must be documented carefully, and it is important to distinguish between obtaining the consent and documenting it. Although asking a patient to sign a preprinted form with a long list of potential complications can be one way to document obtaining the consent, the signing per se is not informed consent. Informed consent is an ongoing process that depends on discussion and understanding between patient and physician.[15] After this is achieved and the patient gives consent for treatment, then the consent must be documented. Having the patient sign a form or even countersign the physician's note in the medical record is useful to show the contents of the discussion that occurred and that the patient consented. It is valuable to explain to the patient that signing does not constitute a release from liability (which it does not under any circumstance) and does not limit the patient's rights, but it does serve as a memorial of the conversation that took place. It is desirable that the patient receive a copy of the form to reinforce the information disclosed.

Neurolytic blocks demand the most careful attention to consent. Independent of associated factors (such as advanced metastatic cancer with a bleak short-term prognosis), the gravity and permanence of this type of intervention must be made clear to the patient. Careful explanation of the maximum deficit possible is required.

A printed form for neurolytic blocks in general should contain basic information on potential complications of any anesthetic or related procedure. Then, in addition, the form could list the following risks: increased pain; hyperesthesia; paresthesias; temporary or permanent paralysis of the affected area or a greater area;

temporary or permanent loss of sensation in the affected or greater area; temporary or permanent impairment of autonomic function; bladder, bowel, or sexual dysfunction; loss of skin at the injection site; organ or tissue injury from the needle; and for certain central blocks, blindness, seizures, or coma. Such a comprehensive list is not meant to frighten the patient. Patients can be told that it is expected that none of these untoward things will happen, and that the printed form is intended to encourage discussion and disclosure of information.

POINTS OF LAW: NEGLIGENCE

Virtually all malpractice actions against physicians allege negligence. Negligence, in general, means failure to exercise reasonable care. However, the legal elements of negligence are specific. For an act to be negligent, four elements must be established: duty, breach, causation, and damage.

Duty

The element of duty has two aspects. It first must be proved that the physician owed a duty to the person who was harmed. Second, the scope of the duty owed must be established. Generally, the physician owes a duty of reasonable care to those with whom a physician-patient relationship has been established. Reasonable care, often called "standard of care," is the care that usually is given by practitioners who are qualified by training and experience to perform a similar service under similar conditions.

Breach

The plaintiff must prove that the physician did not meet the standard of care, and therefore "breached" the duty owed to the patient; that is, that the physician did not meet the standard of care. The claimant must establish (almost always by expert testimony) what the owed standard of care is and then prove that the defendant physician deviated from that standard by omission (that is, by not doing a required act) or commission (that is, doing something that should not have been done).

Causation

The plaintiff must prove that there was a reasonably close causal relation between the breach of duty (or deviation from the standard of care) and the harm suffered by the plaintiff. This is generally the most difficult element of negligence to prove.

Damage

Finally, the plaintiff must prove that an actual loss or damage was suffered. The harm alleged can be physical, financial, or emotional.

IF YOU ARE SUED

Good medical practice and strong patient-physician relationships should help prevent claims of medical malpractice. However, malpractice suits cannot be prevented completely. There are many things to be remembered if you are sued. A noted medical malpractice defense attorney offered many of the following suggestions.[16] Unless instructed otherwise by your defense attorney and/or insurance company representative:

1. Do not panic when served a summons. Notify your institution (if any), insurance company, and attorney immediately.
2. Do not alter your records in any way.
3. Do not transfer your assets.
4. Do not discuss the case with anyone except your claims representative and defense attorney.
5. Do not talk to the plaintiff, their family, and their friends, or the plaintiff's attorney.
6. Do not talk to the media about the suit.
7. In your frustration, do not be hostile to your insurance claims representative and defense attorney. They are on your side.
8. Do not expect that a counterclaim against the plaintiff will get the suit dropped or be successful.
9. Do keep the suit in perspective compared with the entirety of your professional and personal life.
10. Do cooperate fully and quickly with the insurance claims representative and defense attorney.
11. Do gather all relevant records regarding the plaintiff. This includes office records, hospital records, correspondence with the patient, financial records, and results of diagnostic tests.
12. Dictate or write as soon as possible a summary of all that you know about the incidents and parties involved and share it with your claims representative and defense attorney.
13. Be prepared to educate your defense attorney and claims representative about the medical aspects of the case.
14. If a suit has not been brought yet and the patient requests a meeting, consult with your claims representative before discussing the case with the patient.
15. If the patient's lawyer requests medical records, supply a copy or written summary of your care and treatment after notifying your insurer and attorney. Do not send original records. Also, be sure you have received authorization to release the patient's records. Once your insurer has been notified, your claims representative and defense attorney will be in contact with you to discuss your case and advise you further.

PAIN MANAGEMENT IN PATIENTS WITH PENDING LITIGATION

Some patients referred for treatment in a pain management clinic will be involved in workers' compensation cases, disability determination cases, or malpractice suits against other physicians. Physicians may choose not to see such patients. This is permissible as long as there has not been the prior clear establishment of a physician-patient relationship. If this relationship has been established, patients may charge abandonment by the physician who refuses to see them. It is more appropriate to exercise this judgment during the prescreening process. An appointment request from a patient's attorney or compensation board makes the situation clear. Often, the letter from the referring physician will contain information relative to this point; or an inquiry can be made to the referring physician. The use of a medical history questionnaire to be completed by the potential patient before the first appointment is common. Included, if desired, can be the question, "Are you involved in a compensation case or medical malpractice suit related to your pain condition?" In situations in which a prescreening questionnaire is used, the question of exactly when a physician-patient relationship is established may arise. It is not clear from case law whether making an appointment constitutes a relationship or whether the patient actually must be seen by the physician. For those sufficiently concerned on this point, having the patient complete and return a questionnaire before being given an appointment would seem to be the most logical course.

Workers' Compensation

The American system of workers' compensation was developed to help relieve the financial impact of a work-related injury. It is an alternative to tort litigation and was developed as a no-fault system. Benefits may include medical care and rehabilitation as well as cash payments. There has been some concern that the workers' compensation system encourages malingering. In some studies, when return to work time after a work-related injury in US workers was compared with similarly injured patients in other countries, the time of return to work was longer in the US workers. Such factors as job satisfaction, stress, and amount of compensation may also have an impact on return to work status.[17]

Tort Litigation

Tort litigation is a negligence-based and fault-based system. In the current American system of tort litigation, patients can recover damages for alleged injuries, which may include pain and suffering in addition to economic damages. Subjective pain and suffering are difficult to quantitate or determine when the patient might be fabricating or exaggerating his or her pain. It may be difficult to determine when the patient is misleading the physician. Jury awards for these types of damages have fluctuated widely in amount, and have produced huge awards in some cases.[17]

Outcome

Whether pending litigation has an impact on outcome is controversial. Some practitioners recommend caution in treating these patients, believing that improvement with treatment is reduced in these individuals. Since permanent injuries tend to be compensated with larger awards than temporary injuries are, this may present some incentive to prevent rehabilitation. Some studies have shown much higher costs in treating comparable injuries in those patients having pending compensation issues, compared with those who do not. It has historically been presumed that pending litigation or disability compensation for pain-related injury encourages functional impairment and compromises rehabilitation effort.

Some authors speculate that patients do not want to admit to experiencing improvement in their pain problem after being involved with litigation or disability claims, in fear that they will be admitting fraud, or that they will be accused of fraud. Others may be concerned that their benefits might be reduced if their case is reviewed in the future and they have shown improvement.[18]

In one study, patients with chronic low back pain were entered into a multidisciplinary pain management program. This program involved exercise therapy, cognitive restructuring, relaxation therapy, and coping skills. Measures of impairment (measured by flexibility, pain, and muscle endurance) and disability (measured by exercise fitness) were improved in the group as a whole. However, handicap (measured by sickness impact profile scores) were much higher in the patients involved in litigation. The authors speculate that, while the litigant group had improved impairment and disability, the factor of ongoing litigation impedes the restoration of function to their lives.[19]

Patients' perceptions about the cause and treatment of their pain may influence their response to treatment. In one study, perception of fault was evaluated in patients with chronic pain. Patients who felt that their pain was someone else's fault (employer, physician, etc.) had more current distress, less expected improvement from treatment, and a higher incidence of worsened condition from a previous treatment. These negative effects were highest in those patients who felt that their employer was at fault.[20]

Some authors feel that evidence of the philosophy that compensation and litigation promotes poorer outcome with treatment is somewhat controversial. In reviews of the literature on the effect of the compensation and litigation on low back pain and pain secondary to whiplash injury, the findings are somewhat equivocal, depending, in part, on the patient population studied and the oucome critieria. The type of compensation and litigation may influence return to work status. Some studies have shown that litigation affects return to work in workers' compensation claimants but not in other insurance claimants.

In one study that evaluated litigation status in patients with whiplash injury, litigation status (current versus postlitigants) was not predictive of employment status. The authors speculate that their results (which are different from several other studies) may be different because of study design. Only one type of pain problem was studied, and only one type of litigation was involved (tort litigation).[21]

OPIOIDS AND THE LAW

Clinicians who provide medical care to patients who suffer from chronic pain, especially nonmalignant pain, must recognize that legal issues are an important part of the prescription process for controlled substances. Not only must prescribers be familiar with the medical indications for the use of opioids and other scheduled drugs, they must also be familiar with the regulatory restrictions that may impede their ability to prescribe such substances.[8]

Physicians may be concerned about these legal implications of prescribing controlled substances for their patients, and this may contribute to undertreatment of pain, especially in some patient populations. A 1994 study found that noncancer patients receive less adequate pain treatment than patients with cancer-related pain. Women, elderly, and minority patients are more likely than others to receive inadequate pain treatment.[22] In one study, 75% of cancer patients reported suffering pain, with 40% to 50% reporting moderate to severe pain and 25% to 30% reporting severe pain. Over two thirds of nursing home residents experience serious chronic pain. In one California survey of physicians, 69% reported that concern over the possibility of disciplinary action tended to make them more conservative in prescribing opioids for pain. These physicians reported that their own patients might be suffering from untreated pain.[23]

The use of opioids in pain management is influenced by physicians' fear of legal consequences—investigation by the state medical board, the Drug Enforcement Administration, or some state agency that regulates controlled substances. Some physicians may be concerned that they will be investigated or disciplined even if they are treating the patient's pain appropriately. Some state medical boards may use only length of treatment and dosage of opioids as criteria for inappropriate prescribing of controlled substances; some do not understand the difference between drug abusers who are psychologically dependent on a drug and patients who take opioids for pain management who are physically, but not psychologically, dependent on a drug.[22]

Even the definition of "proper prescribing" of opioids can be controversial. For example, when the Minnesota Board of Medical Examiners evaluated physicians' philosophies about proper prescribing of narcotics, they found that there were significant variations in physicians' philosophies: between those who prescribed according to textbook standards and those who prescribed on the basis of their own practice experience; based on practice locale (rural versus urban); and type of practice (primary care specialist versus other specialists).

Approximately 30% of the physicians were less willing to prescribe opioid analgesics for chronic nonmalignant pain than cancer pain. Only 25% of the family practitioners and 30% of the internists were willing to accept new patients who required prescriptions for controlled substances.[8]

Both federal and state laws are involved in regulating prescriptions written for opioids. The Comprehensive Drug Abuse Prevention and Control Act was passed in 1970, which developed a classification system for drugs with the potential of being abused. This system groups these drugs into five groups on the basis of the potential for physical or psychological dependence. Drugs in schedule V are felt to have low potential for abuse. Drugs in schedule I are felt to have the highest potential for abuse. Drugs in schedule II have less abuse potential than those in schedule I, and so on.

There are also federal laws requiring pharmacists to monitor the prescription process. Pharmacists may be penalized if they fill prescriptions that are not considered to be following standard treatment, or are not issued for a legitimate medical purpose. Therefore, physicians must remember that pharmacists evaluate the behavior of both the patient *and* the physician when they fill prescriptions for controlled substances.[8]

States have their own individual regulations and statutes that govern the prescription of controlled substances. Many of these are patterned after federal laws. For example, many states have laws which define the monitoring role of the pharmacist in the prescription process. Physicians should always be aware of the laws and regulations that are in effect where the physician practices, because there are some variations in these laws among the different states.[8]

The Project on Legal Constraints to Access to Effective Pain Relief (a research project of the American Society of Law, Medicine, and Ethics) developed the proposed Pain Relief Act, in an effort to encourage and improve state regulations concerning pain management and the use of controlled substances. It is hoped that patients will have access to better pain management if health care professionals feel less threatened by disciplinary actions. The Pain Relief Act proposes that if a physician can show that their practice is in compliance with an accepted guidline on pain management, the prescription of controlled substances for relieving intractable pain should not lead to disciplinary action. The Pain Relief Act was also developed to encourage states to adopt similar guidelines. If legislation of this type is adopted, it could be used in litigation to help define standard of care for the treatment of patients with chronic pain. State regulations and guidelines could also address other issues, such as informed consent or record keeping.[24]

Recently, the Federation of State Medical Boards of the United States developed some guidelines for health care agencies and state medical boards for use in regulating the use of controlled substances. These guidelines encouraged the development of consistent standards throughout the medical community to facilitate the adequate and effective control of pain. These guidelines assured physicians that they would not be disciplined for the appropriate prescription of controlled substances if these medications are for a legitimate medical purpose. The guidelines also encouraged the evaluation of appropriateness of controlled substance prescription to be based on the patient's medical condition, instead of the quantity and chronicity of the dispensing of these medications.[25]

Since more guidelines have been developed for pain management, in the future courts may include these guidelines to determine standard of care for pain management. For example, the US Department of Health and Human Services Agency for Health Care Policy and Research has released *Acute Pain Management Guidelines* and *Cancer Pain Management Guidelines*. These may be used, along with state guidelines and legislation, the Pain Relief Act, and institutional pain management policies to evaluate standard of care issues. Some states' statutes recognize guidelines of this type to be admissible in malpractice cases to help determine whether a physician was meeting the standard of care. Increased public recognition of the importance of pain management will broaden liability exposure of health care providers who mismanage pain. In a 1990 lawsuit, for the first time, a health care provider was found liable for inappropriate treatment of pain. A nurse delayed or withheld analgesics from a patient with metastatic prostate cancer on the basis that she felt that he was "addicted to morphine." The jury verdict was for $15 million on the basis of physical pain and suffering and emotional and mental anguish for this untreated pain.[24]

Health care institutions can decrease liability risk for inadequate pain management by educating their caregivers about proper pain control and developing pain-management policies that address issues such as physical versus psychological addiction, pain assessment, and treatment of side effects.[26]

SUMMARY

Physicians involved in pain management have an ethical obligation to treat pain as effectively as possible. In the past, chronic pain has often been undertreated due to concerns about legal or disciplinary action for prescribing controlled substances. The development of guidelines dealing with the use of controlled substances for pain management should reduce fear of disciplinary action for prescribing these substances, and lead to more effective pain management. The pain management physician can keep liability risks at a minimum by well-documented medical records, adherence to complete informed consent for all procedures, and familiarity with the risks and possible complications of a procedure. The pain management physician should be aware of what procedures he or she would be comfortable performing, and be willing to refer the patient to another physician to perform those procedures that the pain physician is unfamiliar with. Adherence to the recommendations in this chapter should help to keep the pain management physician's liability to a minimum.

REFERENCES

1. Solazzi RW, Ward RJ. The spectrum of medical liability cases. In: Pierce EC, Cooper JB, (eds.). *Analysis of Anesthetic Mishaps*. Boston, Mass: Little, Brown, 1984:43–59.
2. Kalauokalani DAK, Posner KL, et al. Malpractice claims associated with non-operative pain management. *Anesthesiology* 1998;89:A1077.

3. Bridenbaugh PO, Wedel DJ. Complications of local anesthetic neural blockade. In: Cousins MJ, Bridenbaugh PO, eds. *Neural Blockade*. Philadelphia, Pa: Lippincott; 1998:639–661.
4. Charlton JE, Macrae WA. Complications of neurolytic neural blockade. In: Cousins MJ, Bridenbaugh PO, eds. *Neural Blockade*. Philadelphia: Lippincott, 1998:663–672.
5. Abram SE, Hogan QH. Complications of nerve blocks. In: Benumof JL, Saidman LJ, (eds.). *Anesthesia and Perioperative Complications*. St. Louis, Mo: Mosby–Year Book; 1992:52–76.
6. *Earlin v Cravetz*, 399 A2d 783 (Pa Super 1979).
7. *Henman v DeLuca*, Harris County (Tex) No. 83-14149. Reported in North Carolina Hospital Association Trust Fund Risk Review 1986; 4(6):8.
8. Clark HW, Sees KL. Opioids, chronic pain, and the law. *J Pain Symptom Manage* 1993;8:297–305.
9. *Natanson v Kline*, 168 Kan 393, 350 P2d 1093, 1106 (1960).
10. *Canterbury v Spence*, 464 F2d 772 (DC Cir), *cert denied*, 409 US 1064 (1972).
11. Peters JD, Feinberg KS, Kroll DA, Colins V. *Anesthesiology and the Law*. Ann Arbor, Mich: Health Administration Press, 1983:23.
12. *Harnish v Children's Hospital Medical Center*, 387 Mass 152 (1982).
13. Curran WJ. Informed consent in malpractice cases: a turn towards reality. *N Engl J Med* 1986;314:429–430.
15. President's Commission for the Study of Ethical Problems in Medicine and Biomedical and Behavioral Research. In: *Making Health Care Decisions: The Ethical and Legal Implications of Informed Consent in the Patient-Practitioner Relationship*. Washington, DC: US Government Printing Office, 1982.
16. Gutheil TG, Bursztajn H, Brodsky A. Malpractice prevention through the sharing of uncertainty: informed consent and the therapeutic alliance. *N Engl J Med* 1984;311:49–51.
17. Danner D. *Medical Malpractice: A Primer for Physicians*. Rochester, NY: Lawyer's Co-operative, 1986:4–7.
18. Weintraub MI. Chronic pain in litigation. What is the relationship? *Neurol Clin* 1995;13:341–349.
19. Bellamy R. Compensation neurosis, financial reward for illness as nocebo. *Clin Orthop Rel Res* 1997;336:94–106.
20. Blake C, Garrett M. Impact of litigation on quality of life outcomes in patients with chronic low back pain. *Ir J Med Sci* 1997;166:124–126.
21. DeGood De, Kiernan B. Perception of fault in patients with chronic pain. *Pain* 1996;64:153–159.
21. Swartzman LC, Teasell RW, et al. The effect of litigation status on adjustment to whiplash injury. *Spine* 1996;21:53–58.
22. Hyman CS. Pain management and disciplinary action:how medical boards can remove barriers to effective treatment. *J Law Med Ethics* 1996;24:338–343.
23. Johnson SH. Disciplinary actions and pain relief: analysis of the pain relief act. *J Law Med Ethics* 1996;24:319–327.
24. Shapiro RS. Health care providers' liability exposure for inappropriate pain management. *J Law Med Ethics* 1996;24:360–364.
25. Federation of the State Boards of the United States, Inc. *Model Guidelines for the Use of Controlled Substances for the Treatment of Pain*. Adopted as policy by the House of Delegates of the Federation of State Medical Boards of the United States, May 1998.
26. Shapiro RS. Liability issues in the management of pain. *J Pain Symptom Manage* 1994;9:146–152.

CHAPTER 86 END-OF-LIFE ETHICS

Edward Lowenstein

INTRODUCTION

Why is a chapter on end-of-life ethics included in a textbook of pain treatment? After all, this topic was not included in the previous edition. There are at least two major reasons: first, pain is common at end of life; second, many have contended that most suffering at end of life is due to pain, and that most requests for assistance in dying or hastening death would disappear if adequate pain relief were provided. Both these reasons raise many ethical issues. The emerging field of biomedical ethics is influencing the approach to pain treatment and to dying. This brief essay will be confined to familiarizing the reader with specific, limited ethical aspects regarding the present status of pain treatment and some ethical considerations having an impact on end-of-life care.

CHANGES IN SOCIETY AND MEDICINE

With the expansion of the concept of autonomy to patients and the erosion of the authority of physicians over the past generation, dramatic changes have occurred in the way the public (and part of the medical profession) view the process of dying.[1,2] At the end of the 20th century (or at the threshold of the 21st) we are the recipients of more than a century of scientific and biomedical progress. This has changed the expectations of physicians and the public alike. Only a few decades ago the ability of medical practitioners to diagnose and cure was exceedingly scant. When illness struck, physicians would attempt to reduce fever and relieve pain. A large proportion of their practice was to comfort patients and families. The famous portrait of "The Doctor" by Fildes accurately portrays the impotence of the physician to cure (Fig. 86-1). It depicts the physician in the home, providing a bedside vigil of a sick, perhaps dying, child with the parents present in the background. In the past half century, as "cure" became the norm, specific diagnosis the expectation, specialization accepted, and hospitalization the standard, a progressive distancing of the physician from the patient-family unit occurred.

Nowhere has this distancing been more dramatic than at the end of life. Whether from a feeling of failure, a belief that further expenditure of effort would be wasteful, or simply the discomfort of the physician with death, patients who could not be cured often became ignored or abandoned. At the same time, until the conclusion was reached that further effort was futile, no measure was overlooked. This sometimes led to prolongation of dying and increased suffering.

THE RIGHT TO DIE

One of the consequences of these changes has been the growth of the right-to-die movement. The tenets of this are that when an individual rationally decides that his or her suffering outweighs the benefits of living, that decision should be honored.[3,4] Only the person who experiences suffering can know its nature, its magnitude, and whether or not it is tolerable for him or her. Different individuals faced with identical situations may come to different conclusions. The judgments are undoubtedly affected by personal, cultural, and social values and mores. Furthermore, physicians and other health care providers bring their own cultures, views, and biases to the situation, and these may conflict with those of the patient and/or the family, as well as with other health care providers.

LEGAL PRINCIPLES

Several relevant legal principles have been established unequivocally. One is that patients may refuse initiation of treatment.[5] A second is that patients have a right to stop treatment that has been initiated, even if stopping the treatment will harm them, importantly including the harm of dying.[5] While these principles are legally established, barriers to implementation may be put in the way. A hospital or provider may seek to have the patient declared incompetent on a number of grounds. An incompetent patient may be assigned a surrogate, who may not adhere to the wishes of the patient. Physicians may pressure patients or surrogates to accept treatment or may simply disregard their wishes. One basis for the latter is "paternalism," another is that the physician is merely making a decision about technical matters (such as inserting an endotracheal tube and initiating mechanical ventilation). Despite these types of exceptions, these legal principles have been largely accepted.

HASTENING DEATH

Taking what are considered active measures to produce or hasten death, or to relieve intolerable suffering, is far more controversial. Physician-assisted dying, physician-assisted suicide, and voluntary active euthanasia and involuntary euthanasia have each gained a varying amount of acceptance. In physician-assisted suicide, the physician provides the means for the patient to end his or her own life, but the patient takes the actual actions leading to death. Several jurisdictions (New South Wales, Australia; Oregon) have passed laws enabling physician-assisted suicide of competent patients, though Oregon is the only one with a functioning law at present.[6] The Netherlands has the greatest documented experience with physician-assisted suicide and the most published data.[7,8] Though physician-assisted suicide is illegal in the Netherlands, there is a societal agreement that the physician will not be prosecuted if he or she adheres to certain procedures and safeguards. Thus, it is tolerated by governmental authorities rather than being strictly legal.

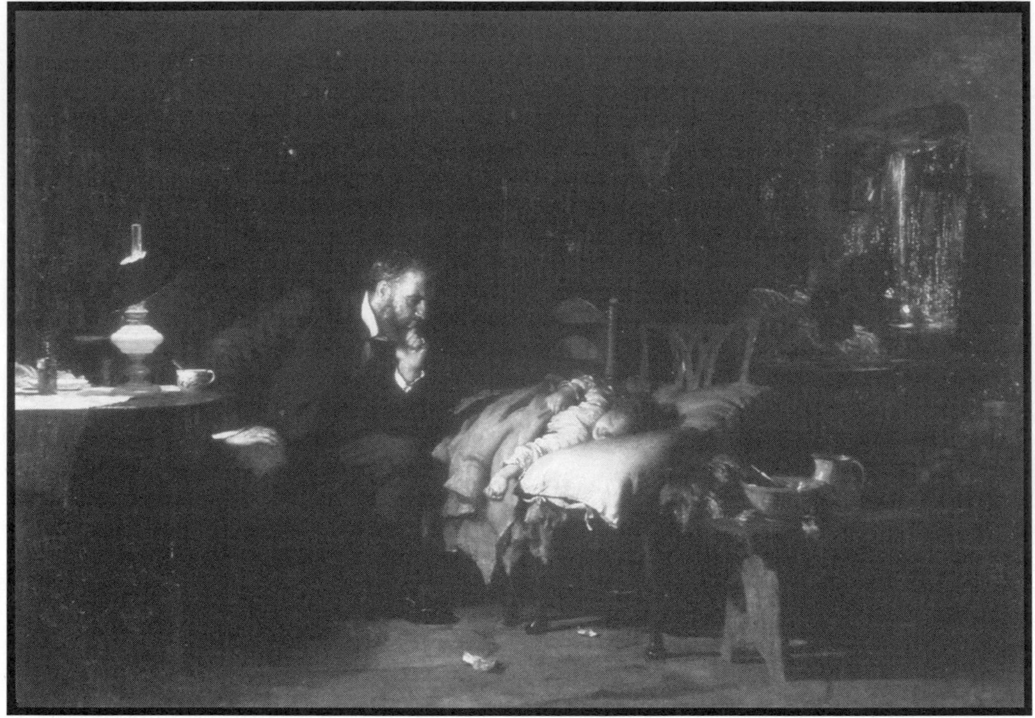

Figure 86–1 "The Doctor" by Fildes portrays a physician keeping a bedside vigil with his young patient's parents.

Voluntary active euthanasia occurs when the euthanist (physician or not) takes action to end the life of a person who has requested it. This has similar standing to physician-assisted suicide in the Netherlands. Involuntary euthanasia is not condoned by any government, to the knowledge of this author, considered murder by most, and is considered morally reprehensible.

ADEQUACY OF PAIN RELIEF

That pain treatment is inadequate in many circumstances has been documented frequently in the past and again recently. The SUPPORT study reported that 50% of conscious ICU patients who subsequently died experienced moderate or severe pain at least half the time during the last 3 days of life.[9] The intervention of having a dedicated nurse to both point out the presence of pain and suggest possibilities for effective treatment to those providing care was ineffective (i.e., it did not result in decreasing the reported incidence or severity of pain).[9] This was true despite the recent development and dissemination of simple and effective regimens for pain relief.[10] Sadly, this appears to be the rule rather than the exception. That there is both a professional and a moral failure in this is merely stating the obvious.

The reasons for inadequate pain relief are legion. However, one crucial reason from an ethical point of view is the fear of being the agent who hastens death, which many physicians, other health care providers, and, of course, members of the lay public consider ethically unacceptable.

THE DOCTRINE OF DOUBLE EFFECT

The doctrine of double effect is an ethical principle which states that effects which are morally impermissible if caused intentionally are morally permissible if foreseen but unintended.[11] The palliative care community, many gerontologists, primary care physicians, intensivists, oncologists, and others have accepted the doctrine of double effect as a satisfactory method to deal with the dilemma that providing sufficient medication to relieve pain may also create the hazard of hastening death. The doctrine of double effect arose from Roman Catholic moral theology, and was originally utilized to provide moral justification for undesirable effects associated with a just war. It has been applied in medical practice since approximately the late 19th century ad.

The doctrine of double effect has four conditions:

1. The act must be morally good (or at least morally neutral);
2. The good effect rather than the bad effect must be intended, whereas the bad effect may be foreseen but not intended;
3. The bad effect must not be the means to the good effect;
4. The good effect must outweigh the bad effect (i.e., proportionality).

Deficits of Double Effect in End-of-Life Decisions

Shortcomings of the doctrine of double effect have been eloquently articulated by Quill et al.[11] They include the complexity and ambiguity of intent, the doctrine's inapplicability to the practice of terminal sedation or "slow euthanasia" where death is the inevitable end point, the withdrawal of mechanical ventilation from a patient known to be dependent upon it, the rejection by individuals and groups in our multicultural society of the thesis that death is a moral evil when intolerable suffering exists, and a number of others.

An additional shortcoming that has not received attention is the practice of claiming the doctrine of double effect when knowingly intending death. Perhaps the most dramatic example of this is Dr. Jack Kevorkian's recent lethal injection of Thomas Youk, a patient with amyotrophic lateral sclerosis.[12] Youk requested the aid of Dr. Kevorkian, who at that time had claimed to help 130 patients commit suicide. He was charged with murder for this act. The interpretation of the jury was that intent was irrelevant to the admitted (and videotaped) fact that Dr. Kevorkian's act of injecting the compound led to Mr. Youk's death. Despite any request Youk had made, the jury ruled that killing of an innocent person constitutes murder and convicted Dr. Kevorkian. Curiously, the verdict was second degree murder, which is defined as without premeditation. The defendant has stated he will appeal the conviction.[12]

Alternatives to Double Effect

Dr. Kevorkian had stated he was merely trying to relieve the patient's suffering rather than intend the patient's death, perhaps unsuccessfully invoking the doctrine of double effect. The ethical argument (though perhaps not the legal argument) might have been quite different if Dr. Kevorkian had stated that the only way he could relieve the suffering was to kill (not murder) the patient, and he therefore intended both. He could have claimed the doctrine of double effect by contending that proportionality was adhered to since the moral hazard of not relieving the suffering outweighed that of killing the patient. His actions,however, appear unequivocal evidence that he intended to kill. He could perhaps have successfully drawn a distinction between killing and murder. The former sometimes morally justifiable; the latter never.

Edward Pellegrino, a staunch opponent of hastening death, has espoused in different circumstances that a system which promotes lying by physicians will cause irreparable harm to the profession and the individual physician.[13] A solution might be a system in which a physician openly states intent whenever he or she intends to "hasten death" (a euphemism for kill) at the durable request of a competent patient. This is quite different from the doctrine of double effect and accepts the apparent truth that some suffering is worse than death. This "truth," of course, is not accepted by many. The sole determinant of whether suffering is tolerable or intolerable must always be the patient's (i.e., candidate for dying). Safeguards and justifications might likely be more frequently adhered to than is probably the case at present, though reliable statistics regarding their present status are not available. Surveys have established that many physicians and nurses have knowingly and actively hastened death, both with and without explicit durable requests.

Billings and Block have defined an act they term "slow euthanasia."[14] In this, the intent is to hasten or assure death of a terminally ill patient by not decreasing or increasing the dose of medication (often morphine) despite relief of pain or other physical distress. This seemingly relieves many physicians of moral agency, doubt, and guilt. Yet the end result is the same as a lethal injection resulting in proximate death, though the time frame is different.

INTOLERABLE SUFFERING DESPITE PAIN RELIEF

Recent data from the first year of experience under the Death with Dignity Act of the state of Oregon, which permits physician-assisted suicide, strongly reinforces previous studies indicating pain is not the principal reason for requesting physician-assisted suicide, and that relieving pain will not abolish requests for physician aid in dying. Only 1 of 15 patients expressed concern about pain at the end of life as a principal cause for the request.[15] This is consistent with a large body of evidence from anonymous surveys[16] and from the Netherlands[7] documenting that unrelieved or unrelievable pain is infrequently the sole or even the principal reason given for the request of aid in dying. This has important implications in light of the decision of the United States Supreme Court that a constitutional right to physician-assisted suicide does not exist, though encouraging experiments by individual states.[17,18] The decision has been interpreted as a mandate for effective palliative care, seemingly on the erroneous premise that if only pain were relieved, requests for aid in dying would eventually disappear.[19] However, many other causes of suffering exist. Up to one quarter of hospice patients reported their dyspnea as "unbearable" in the last week of life.[20] Weakness, fatigue, and dependence, the most commonly cited reasons for wanting physician-assisted death, are frequently irremediable. Such suffering can be alleviated by terminal sedation, that is, sedation to unconsciousness, often accompanied by cessation of nutrition and hydration.[21] A distinction between this and slow euthanasia is difficult to appreciate, perhaps because it does not exist.[14]

SUMMARY

End-of-life care is replete with ethical ramifications and moral dilemmas for care providers and patients alike. Much pain can be relieved, but the knowledge to accomplish this is applied far less frequently than the need. There is no adequate moral justification for this lack of pain relief; it is an ethical responsibility of physicians and other health care providers to attain and apply existing knowledge. However, unrelieved or unrelievable pain, though important and distressing, is not the major factor associated with requests for assistance in ending life.

The American value of autonomy has been accorded a strong place in the hierarchy of principles governing medical ethics. This has led to a progressively greater role of patients in medical decision making. Federal and state courts have granted the right of patients and surrogates to refuse and/or discontinue treatment. The US Supreme Court reversed two appellate court decisions affirming the existence of a constitutional right to physician-assisted suicide. The Supreme Court decision appeared to be based on fear that condoning a role in hastening death by physicians would constitute the beginning of a "slippery slope" leading to voluntary active euthanasia and involuntary euthanasia,[22] and a belief that effective palliative care would diminish or even abolish the need for physician assistance in ending life. They felt that greater experience applying existing knowledge of pain relief at end of life was required before establishing a new constitutional right.

The doctrine of double effect is at present used by many physicians as a morally justifiable way to relieve pain and suffering of terminal patients with full knowledge that the methods employed may hasten death. Though a requirement of the doctrine of double effect in these circumstances is that death may be foreseen but is not intended, sometimes death is clearly intended. A dramatic example concerns Dr. Jack Kevorkian's lethal injection of Thomas Youk, who suffered from amyotrophic lateral sclerosis, but anonymous surveys have established that many deaths were intended.

Dr. Kevorkian unsuccessfully claimed intent to relieve suffering rather than kill the patient, a distinction the jury that convicted him of second degree murder did not accept. Recognition of the limitations of medicine to alleviate suffering in some patients short of causing death may in the future permit more widespread moral acceptance of the concept of providing competent patients who experience unrelievable, intolerable suffering the means to cause their own death. The doctrine of double effect would seem to have severe limitations in the justification of decisions at end of life. Clearer ethical principles guiding end-of-life treatment are needed.

REFERENCES

1. Beauchamp TL, Childress JF. *Principles of Biomedical Ethics*. London, England: Oxford University Press, 1994.
2. Jackson DL, Youngner S. Patient autonomy and "death with dignity": some clinical caveats. *N Engl J Med* 1979;301:404–408.
3. Wanzer SH, Adelstein SJ, Cranford RE, et al. The physician's responsibility toward hopelessly ill patients. *N Engl J Med* 1984;310:955–959.
4. Wanzer SH, Federman DD, Adelstein SJ, et al. The physician's responsibility toward hopelessly ill patients: a second look. *N Engl J Med* 1989;320:844–849.
5. President's Commission for the Study of Ethical Problems in Medicine and Biomedical and Behavioral Research. *Deciding to Forego Life-Sustaining Treatment: A Report on Ethical, Medical and Legal Issues in Treatment Decisions*. Washington, DC: US Government Printing Office;1988.
6. Oregon Death with Dignity Act, Oregon Revised Statute 1994;127.800-127.897.
7. Van der Maas PH, van Delden JJM, Pijnnenborg L. Euthanasia and other medical decisions concerning the end of life: an investigation performed upon request of the Commission of Inquiry into the Medical Practice concerning Euthanasia. Health Policy 1992:22 (1 & 2): special issue. Amsterdam, The Netherlands: Elsevier, 1992:57–69.
8. Pijnenborg L, Van der Mass PJ, van Delden JJM, et al. Life-terminating acts without explicit request of patient. *Lancet* 1993;341:1196–1199.
9. The SUPPORT Principal Investigators. A controlled trial to improve care for seriously ill hospitalized patients: the Study to Understand Prognoses and Preferences for Outcomes and Risks of Treatments (SUPPORT) [correction published in *JAMA* 1996;275:1232]. *JAMA* 1995;274:1591–1598.
10. Jacox A, Carr DB, Payne R, et al. *Clinical Practice Guideline Number 9. Management of Cancer Pain*. Rockville, Md: US Department of Health and Human Services, Agency for Health Care Policy and Research; 1994. Publication 94-0592.
11. Quill TE, Dresser R, Brock DW. The rule of double effect—a critique of its role in end-of-life decision making. *N Engl J Med* 1997;337:1768–1771.
12. Belluck P. Kevorkian is found guilty of murdering dying man. *New York Times*. March 27, 1999:1.
13. Pellegrino ED. Managed care at the bedside: how do we look in the moral mirror. *J Kennedy Inst Ethics* 1997;7:321–330.
14. Billings JA, Block SD. Slow euthanasia. *J Palliat Care* 1996;12:21–30.
15. Chin AE, Hedberg K, Higginson GK, et al. Legalized physician-assisted suicide in Oregon—the first year's experience. *N Engl J Med* 1999;340:577–583.
16. American Law Institute. *Model Penal Code and Commentaries*. Philadelphia, Pa: American Law Institute; 1985:229–241(Section 2.02).
17. *Washington v Glucksberg*, 117 S.Ct. 2258;1997.
18. *Vacco v Quill*, 117 S.Ct. 2293;1997.
19. Burt RA. The Supreme Court speaks; not assisted suicide but a constitutional right to palliative care. *N Engl J Med* 1997;337:1234–1236.
20. Ingham J, Portenoy R. Symptom assessment. In: Cherny NI, Foley KM, (eds.). *Hematol Oncol Clin North Am* 1996;10:21–39.

CHAPTER 87

ETHICAL ISSUES AND PROBLEMS OF TRUST IN THE MANAGEMENT OF CHRONIC PAIN

Steven H. Richeimer and Gretchen A. Case

INTRODUCTION

The ethics literature regarding pain management has typically focused on end-of-life issues involved with the treatment of patients experiencing terminal pain. But many if not most of the problems that arise with pain treatment involve problems with the treatment of chronic nonmalignant pain. A large portion of these problems can be traced to underlying problems with the ability of the physician to trust the patient. In this chapter I describe some of these ethical dilemmas, examine the underlying problems with trust, then propose how reconceptualizing some of the pain clinic treatment systems might serve to diminish some of the ethical problems.

Consideration of the ethical issues involved in pain management typically conjures up images of the terminally ill patient. The literature and research dealing with care at the end of life is extensive; however, there is a remarkable void of literature and research considering the common ethical issues that arise on a daily basis with the care of patients with chronic nonmalignant pain. These issues tend not to receive much of our attention; however, the problems are real and frequent. It is my hope that by focusing on these issues, we can start to clarify the nature of the underlying problems, and perhaps start to institute systems to minimize their frequency.

The following cases do not represent single individuals, but condensations of several cases from discussions of the monthly Ethics Round Table meetings at the University of California Davis Medical Center Pain Clinic. After reviewing a case history, we examine the ethical issues and later develop a methodology for building trust. We then apply this methodology to additional cases.

We have employed a case-study format for discussion because it is common practice in both medical and ethics education and best affords the reader concrete examples of potential clinical and ethical dilemmas.

BACKGROUND

Ethical deliberation usually consists of the application of basic ethical *theories* that support and guide ethical decision making. Such philosophical theories, or models of deliberation, provide different approaches for analyzing basic ethical *principles* and how such principles are to be judged in relation to others. English[1] states that "an ethical theory attempts to achieve a general applicability to considerations of moral behavior, with as few exceptions as possible. Important characteristics of a theory include universalizability, comprehensiveness, and consistency." As this is a chapter devoted to ethical issues in chronic pain management, the reader should be aware of the relevant and predominant ethical theories that exist to guide them in ethical analysis. Of the three theories subsequently listed (there are many more), we have adopted a more casuist approach for this chapter.

Utilitarianism

Utilitarianism, identified most closely with Jeremy Bentham (1748–1832) and John Stuart Mill (1806–1873), is the theory whereby the rightness of an act is judged by its ability to bring about the greatest good or benefit. Therefore, utilitarians judge actions by their consequences. In medicine, a physician is to maximize the benefits to their patients while minimizing the burdens of treatment.

Deontology

Deontology is the study of duties that persons have toward one another. The most prominent of the classic deontologic theories is that developed by Immanuel Kant (1724–1804). Considered duty-based, as opposed to action-based utilitarians, deontologists judge actions by the intent behind them instead of their consequences (however, consequences can be taken into account in decision making).

Casuistry

Casuistry was an influential ethical theory in medieval and early modern philosophy. "Rather than concentrate on rules and general principles that may be applied to specific cases, casuists insist that moral judgment must emerge from particular cases, or better still, from experience with a number of cases that can be compared to one another in various ways." Casuists regard ethics as a set of practices that arise from human moral experience.[1]

As mentioned earlier, there are many methodologies for analyzing clinical ethical dilemmas. Fins[3] and Loewy[4] have argued persuasively that a problem-solving approach—similar to developing a medical diagnosis and treatment plan—is more useful than the application of predetermined ethical principles. Their arguments apply primarily to the approach to each individual clinical-ethical problem. However, when examining a group of problems in an effort to search for common themes and possible solutions, it may still be useful to apply the template or framework of primary ethical principles. Most clinical ethical dilemmas involve a conflict between two or more of the following basic or primary ethical principles:

1. Respect for persons, which includes respect for the autonomy, or self-determination, of the patient and the need to protect those patients with diminished autonomy
2. Beneficence, which includes the obligation to maximize possible benefits while minimizing the risks, and the requirement to do no harm (nonmaleficence)
3. Justice, which includes the need to provide fair access to medical care and fair allocation of scarce resources.[3]

Solutions to such dilemmas begin with a basic understanding of these concepts and the clinician's ability to incorporate these principles into their everyday clinical practice.

CASE EXAMPLES

Case 1

A 41-year-old man is seen for a 3-month history of complex regional pain syndrome (CRPS, also known as RSD, reflex sympathetic dystrophy) of his left foot. He reports debilitating pain. Examination reveals classic features of CRPS, including severe allodynia. The patient's past medical history is significant for heroin abuse. He has not abused any drugs for the past year. For the last 2 months his primary care physician has prescribed acetaminophen with codeine (30 mg), one tablet three times per day. The patient reports that this does not touch his pain. The physician refuses to provide more or stronger narcotics. The pain clinic consultant develops a treatment plan. Many of the treatments yield slow and uncertain results. Meanwhile, in spite of concerns regarding potential drug abuse, the consultant establishes a pain medication contract with the patient for the use of long-acting oral morphine: 15 mg, two times per day. Five days later, the patient calls the clinic and reports that the new narcotic prescription is better, but still inadequate. The consultant feels that she has increased the narcotic dose by a large amount and is not willing to increase it further at this time. She tells this to the patient.

Discussions with the consultant reveal that she is uncomfortable with a number of aspects of this case. She recognizes that her opinion regarding an appropriate drug dose is influenced by the patient's prior history of drug abuse. This history suggests that the patient may be at higher risk of developing an addiction, but this history does not have a direct impact on how much pain the patient is experiencing. She finds herself uncertain about whether the patient is accurately reporting his pain levels. Furthermore, the physician notes that the patient appears to be adopting a defensive attitude, as if he needs to justify his pain and his need for treatment. Finally, upon introspection, the consultant realizes that if this patient were suffering with pain from a malignancy, she would be more aggressive with her prescribing of analgesics; yet she knows that the pain of CRPS can be more intense than the pain associated with malignancy.

Analysis

Within the framework of the basic bioethical principles described earlier, we can see that the scenario in case 1 describes an infringement of the obligation to respect the patient, or more specifically to respect the autonomy of the patient. The consultant is assuming a paternalistic attitude—which typically is considered to be contrary to the principle of autonomy–and determines for the patient what is the appropriate amount of medication. However, according to English,[1] there are circumstances in which the initial status of respect for autonomy (of the patient) is overruled by, among other reasons, the concept of *professional autonomy* (a professional is not obliged to act against personal or professional ethical convictions). Given the complicating factor of prior drug use in this case, it is possible that the consultant, concerned that this patient is at higher risk for developing another addiction that would be harmful, *could* employ the concept of professional autonomy to justify at least a prudent delay in prescribing more or increasing the dose of narcotics. Such concerns and reasoning should also be shared with the patient so that they may understand the physician's concern for his or her best interest, especially with regard to the patient's risk of developing another addiction. However, had this patient no prior history of drug abuse, the principle of professional autonomy would not be as applicable. The physician likely feels that her drug limits are required by the principle of nonmaleficence, since she feels that higher doses of narcotic medication significantly increases the risk of addiction. In her efforts to do no harm, however, the physician may not be following the other half of the principle of beneficence; that is, the requirement to maximize the potential benefits while minimizing the risks. Finally, this case may also demonstrate a violation of the principle of justice. By virtue of a previous medical problem (heroin addiction), the patient is now not receiving medication for the relief of pain equal to what would be prescribed for a patient without such a history. If this is the result of prejudice, as opposed to a considered assessment of the involved risks to the patient, then this would represent unfair limits on the access to medical resources (i.e., medications). Similarly, if the patient would receive more analgesic medication if the underlying cause of his pain was cancer, and if the reason for more medication was simply a reflection of societal attitudes regarding cancer pain versus nonmalignant pain, then this too may reflect an ethically unjustifiable limit on the provision of medical care.

Without exploring the causes that underlie these dilemmas, resolution will be difficult. The physician is stuck trying to balance the potential benefits and risks of higher doses of narcotics. She knows that the history of prior addiction and the diagnosis of chronic nonmalignant pain do appropriately affect the treatment decisions, but she has a difficult time being sure that societal or personal prejudices are not also affecting her decisions. The consultant wishes that she could rely on the patient to make these judgments for himself, but she realizes that she does not trust that the patient is capable of this.

Trust is, in fact, the critical element that underlies all of these problems. It is commonly recognized that we ask our patients to trust us—their physicians. Somerville[5] takes the medical profession to task for expecting the blind trust of our patients rather than earning their trust. However, as noted by Sass,[6] there is another side to the equation: ". . . medicine necessarily will have to shift attention from physician ethics toward patient ethics and a partnership in health care. From the perspective of trust-based communication and trust-based cooperation, it is only logical to strengthen the other side of the partnership and make difficult cases of clinical decision making an issue for trust-based decision making in partnership." Sass is not suggesting that we increase our blind trust in our patients, but rather that we enable our patients to earn our trust, and that such earned trust "safeguards all expert-lay interactions."[6]

On reexamination of the ethical problems in Case 1, we see that each of these problems is triggered by a problem with trust, or more specifically with a problem of the patient not having earned the trust of the physician. In all cases involving the treatment of chronic nonmalignant pain, the clinician must rely on the subjective reports of the patient. The physician has no means of entering or examining the reality of the patient. Scarry[7] notes that "to be in pain is to have certainty, while hearing about pain is to have doubt." Therefore, there is an automatic or basic lack of trust: Is the patient accurately reporting his or her experience of pain? In this particular case, the lack of trust is exacerbated by the patient's history of prior drug abuse. Because of this lack of trust, the consultant feels that she cannot rely on the patient's autonomy and his ability to accurately determine his own need for medication; she therefore acts in a paternalistic fashion and determines her own limits for the medications. Similarly, because she feels that she cannot rely on the patient's reports of his pain, she has no gauge for judging when she has provided maximal benefit. Without the ability to judge the degree of benefit, it is natural to rely more heavily on the obligation to minimize risk and harm. Finally, lack of trust may often underlie the tendency to treat nonmalignant pain less aggressively than cancer-related pain. Vrancken[8] gives a telling description of the attitude of many pain physicians regarding cancer pain patients. "They really have something, it is also recognized by everybody that they really have something. Their problems are also very real which makes it more easy for doctors as well as patients to face psychosocial factors too." Vrancken is telling us that cancer pain patients are trusted more than patients with nonmalignant pain. There is nothing inherent about nonmalignant pain that makes its sufferers less trustworthy; therefore, problems with trusting patients with nonmalignant pain may lead to encroachments on the ethical principle of justice.

Pappagallo and Heinberg[7] raise another point in regard to chronic pain patients with a past history of addiction, which is that they may not want opioids to manage their pain for the fear of relapse. Considering both potential responses from such patients, Pappagallo and Heinberg give further treatment suggestions for reducing the risk of relapse in dealing with chronic pain patients with a past history of addiction. They recommend:

1. The distinction between physical dependence, which is to be expected, and addiction, which should be avoided, should be clarified for the patient.
2. The patient should be encouraged to join or increase involvement in a recovery program or in individual psychological care in order to garner support and develop and bolster relapse prevention strategies.
3. A behavioral contract should be made, to provide the patient with a clear definition of problematic use, misuse, and abuse behaviors.
4. Close supervision should be provided by the physician, including frequent follow-up appointments, the use of only one prescribing physician and dispensing pharmacy, and toxicology screenings.
5. Long-acting opioids, or around-the-clock dosing, may be helpful in reducing the reinforcing, and therefore addictive, properties of these medications.

From such suggestions, one can develop an ethical and clinically sound standard of practice for such patients, and help move the burden of decision making solely from the physician to the patient-physician team.

Two additional cases are presented to illustrate how the method of analyzing trust may underlie potential infringements of basic bioethical principles as the lack of trust creates an unethical barrier to appropriate, unbiased treatment.

Case 2

A 24-year-old woman is referred to the chronic pain clinic. The patient reports constant, severe, mid-pelvic pain. She is unable to concentrate on her graduate school work. She has seen numerous specialists and has had extensive evaluations including laparoscopy, all without result. After the laparoscopy, a new, burning pain developed in her left labia and inguinal area. The patient's gynecologist reported generalized vulvar and pelvic tenderness, with more exquisite pain responses with light touch of the left labia. The pain consultants felt that this newer pain is suggestive of an ilioinguinal neuralgia. There is no apparent cause for the original pelvic pain. Even narcotics have not helped. During the clinic evaluation, the patient reveals a childhood history of sexual abuse. Her affect is depressed and angry. She is very frustrated by all the previous failed diagnostic and therapeutic efforts, and their apparent complications. The patient asks the pain clinic physicians to please do nerve blocks. The physicians are concerned about the patient's psychological health. They explain the potential for interaction between physical and emotional distress. They tell the patient that they will consider nerve block techniques for the left inguinal and labial pain, but she should first undergo psychological evaluation and treatment. The patient states that she is unwilling to do this. Efforts to address her concerns about the treatment plan fail. The patient continues to insist that nerve blocks be performed. The clinic physicians explain that they provide a comprehensive treatment plan, and that they cannot proceed with only one element (the blocks) without the other elements (the psychotherapy). The patient is upset and leaves the clinic.

Case 3

A 33-year-old man is being seen in the pain clinic for a 1-year history of incapacitating low back pain. The primary care doctor, the orthopedic surgeon, and the pain consultant are all unable to establish a cause for the patient's pain. Magnetic resonance imaging of the lumbar region reveals mild disk bulges, which would not be expected to cause the degree of discomfort that the patient reports. A psychological evaluation reveals mild depression and somatic preoccupation, findings common to most patients with chronic pain. Nerve conduction studies are normal. The patient reports that the pain interferes with his ability to concentrate, his relationships with colleagues, and his ability to maintain prolonged sitting or standing positions. Because of this he has been unable to return to work. The workers' compensation insurance company now insists on a report on whether the pain clinic agrees with the patient's claim that he is totally disabled.

Analysis

In Case 2, the primary concern is regarding autonomy. The physicians were concerned that acceding to the patient's requests for nerve blocks, without prior psychotherapy, carried an unacceptably high risk of harm. Respect for autonomy requires that patients' decisions regarding care be made without coercion; however, the consultants verged on coercion by telling the patient that they would only consider providing the treatment she desired (nerve blocks) if she accepted a treatment that she did not want (psychotherapy). As noted by Whedon and Ferrell,[10] pain patients may be exceptionally susceptible to subtle coercion, since they are so vulnerable to any offered possibility of relief. This situation is based on a lack of trust. The physicians did not trust the patient's judgment and insight. They felt that she did not recognize her own psychopathology and how this psychopathology was interacting with her experience of both pain and medical treatment.

In Case 3, the clinician faces a dilemma. The patient may be malingering; however, this cannot be determined simply on the basis that there is a lack of objective data. A report of disability may reinforce unconscious pain behaviors and diminish healthy, productive behaviors. Therefore, such a report may not be in the patient's best interests, yet a failure to report disability may cause the loss of the patient's only potential income. The bases and rationale for determining disability are complex and beyond the scope of this paper; however, here too, the core of the problem is a lack of trust. The clinicians recognize that the possibility of monetary gain may be consciously or unconsciously influencing the patient. Since they cannot enter the patient's reality, they look for objective evidence that might explain the patient's pain. When they cannot find such evidence, the concerns regarding the trustworthiness of the patient are heightened.

BUILDING TRUST

Problems with trust underlie many of the ethical problems that arise in the treatment of chronic nonmalignant pain. Trust is the overriding principle and virtue that establishes and safeguards all expert-lay interactions, particularly in the clinic.[6] With this understanding, we can reexamine our interactions with our patients. We can enable more of our patients to earn our trust, and thereby prevent ourselves from having to blindly and perhaps foolishly trust some of our patients.

Techniques with potential for trust building are already widely utilized; however, the full potential of these techniques are not realized because they are not explicitly thought of in terms of trust building, but rather in terms of contracts or patient compliance. Reframing the ideas of patient treatment agreements, monitoring of compliance and progress, and patient education are three approaches that may enable more patients to earn our trust and enable clinicians to more clearly recognize those patients that have not earned our trust.

Patient treatment plan agreements are commonly used tools for educating our patients about the treatments that will be provided, the expectations regarding their participation, and the operating rules of the pain clinic. Our patient treatment plan establishes:

1. The anticipated duration of treatment
2. Which treatments are likely to be provided
3. Goals for increased function
4. Requirements
   - **a.** for clinic attendance
   - **b.** for use of medications
   - **c.** for drug testing
   - **d.** for compliance with all treatment modalities
   - **e.** for having a primary physician to assume care when the treatment is completed.

Such treatment plan agreements are valuable, and when properly used, they may help to promote trust. The discussion might start with an explanation that pain treatment programs rely heavily on the ability of the clinicians to trust the patients. That it would be nice to blindly trust all patients, but this is not possible in a setting that involves the treatment of subjective complaints with potentially dangerous drugs and procedures and decisions regarding impairment and disability. Therefore, we give all of our patients the opportunity to earn our trust, while at the same time working to earn theirs. The discussion would continue with explanations showing how the Treatment Plan Agreement gives the patient an opportunity to demonstrate his or her compliance and motivation to pursue multiple treatment modalities (e.g., physical therapy, psychotherapy, and medication use). Effort and dependability are considered signs of trustworthiness. Failure to earn our trust signals that we are unlikely to be able to help the patient.

Pain logbooks or diaries may also help to establish that the patient is a trustworthy reporter of his pain. Patients who report maximal pain levels without variation are unlikely to be accurate and trustworthy reporters.

Upon reanalysis of case 2, we can see the potential value of explaining to the patient that all our patients need to establish that they are trustworthy in terms of their judgment and insight before we can rely on such insight to help us make treatment decisions. Such a discussion might have failed; the patient might still have left upset. Such a discussion, however, would have clarified the universal need of the clinic for patients to earn trust and might have minimized any coercive aspects in the interaction.

In case 3, it is critical to provide the patient the opportunity to demonstrate her efforts to get better. It would be valuable to discuss that it is impossible to clearly establish disability based on subjective complaints. However, the patient can earn our trust over a 4- to 6-month period by demonstrating her effort and compliance with a carefully tailored but demanding physical therapy and psychotherapy program (including homework assignments).

A potential pitfall must be noted. It is reasonable to expect patients to be compliant and to demonstrate effort, but it is not reasonable to demand that patients get better. Treatment failure does not establish that the patient is not trustworthy; rather it may imply misdiagnosis or the need for alternative treatments.

TRUST MUST BE MUTUAL

Patients are much more likely to accept our suggestions and treatment plans if they trust the physician. Failure to comply with treatment does not necessarily mean that the patient is not trustworthy, but may indicate that the patient did not find the physician to be trustworthy. Chronic pain patients may be particularly prone toward mistrusting their caregivers since they have typically been through extensive, failed therapeutic efforts. *Business & Health* reported on what patients endure before referral to a comprehensive pain management center: the percentage of patients with litigation, 20%; on workers' compensation, 50%; not working, 75%; who are depressed, 55%; those taking medication, 90%; and have had at least one surgery, 58%.[11] Furthermore, when treatment efforts fail the patient is then often been treated in a dismissive manner.

Physicians can and must earn the trust of the patient by : (1) being there (within boundaries), (2) attempting to understand the problem, (3) being respectful, (4) pursuing the best interests of the patient (ignoring self-interests), (5) avoiding harm, (6) providing nonprejudicial care, and (7) maintaining knowledge and expertise.

Pursuing the best interests of the patient rather than professional self-interests means that caregivers must carefully analyze their own motives to ensure that they are not affected by potential "secondary gains" such as financial reward, research benefits, the acquisition of experience, or the avoidance of anxiety regarding liability or legal regulations.

SUMMARY

Problems with trust underlie many of the daily ethical dilemmas that are seen in pain clinics. Reconceptualizing and refocusing the processes of patient education and treatment plan agreements may provide more patients the opportunity to earn our trust. In addition to monitoring levels of pain and function, now the clinician can also monitor the parameter of earned trust. We like to think that patients are our partners in the treatment process, but in fact this is not always true. Attention to the parameter of earned trust may provide the clinician with a firmer basis for difficult treatment decisions.

REFERENCES

1. English Dan C. *Bioethics: A Clinical Guide for Medical Students.* New York, NY: WW Norton & Company; 1994.
2. Ahronheim JC, Moreno J, Zuckerman C. *Ethics in Clinical Practice.* New York, NY: Little, Brown and Company; 1994.
3. Fins JJ, Bacchetta MD, Miller FG. Clinical pragmatism: a method of moral problem solving. *Kennedy Inst Ethics J* 1997;7:129–143.
4. Loewy EH. Suffering as a consideration in ethical decision making. *Cambridge Q Healthcare Ethics* 1992;1(2):135–142.
5. Somerville MA. Death of pain: pain, suffering, and ethics. In: Gebhart GF, et al, (eds.). *Proceedings of the 7th World Congress on Pain, Progress in Pain Research and Management.* Seattle, Wash: IASP Press, 1994.
6. Sass HM. The clinic as testing ground for moral theory: a European view. *Kennedy Inst Ethics J* 1996;6:351–355.
7. Scarry E. *The Body in Pain, the Making and Unmaking of the World.* New York, NY: Oxford University Press, 1985.
8. Vrancken MAE. Schools of thought on pain. *Soc Sci Med* 1989; 29:435–444.
9. Pappagallo M, Heinberg L. Ethical issues in the management of chronic nonmalignant pain. *Semin Neurol* 1997;17:203–211.
10. Whedon M, Ferrell BR. Professional and ethical considerations in the use of high-tech pain management. *Oncol Nurs Forum* 1991;18:1135–1143.
11. Special Report. *Business & Health,* Fall 1996.

SUGGESTED READINGS

Cain JM, Hammes BJ. Ethics and pain management: respecting patients' wishes. J Pain Symptom Manage 1994;9:160–165.

The National Commission for the Protection of Human Subjects of Biomedical and Behavioral Research. *The Belmont Report: Ethical Principles and Guidelines for the Protection of Human Subjects of Research.* Washington, DC: US Government Printing Office; 1979.

GLOSSARY

Accommodation The property of a nerve by which it adjusts to a slowly increasing strength of stimulus so that the strength at which excitation occurs is greater than it would be were the strength to have risen more gradually

Acroparesthesia Paresthesia of an extremity or an extreme degree of paresthesia

Adynamia Weakness

Afferent Bringing to or into as in nerves transmitting information to the spinal cord

Alexithymia A state of restricted cognitive and affective characteristics that are common in patients with psychosomatic disorders

Algesia A state of increased sensitivity to pain

Algodystrophy Sympathetic dystrophy

Allesthesia (Allaesthesia) A form of allochesthesia in which the sensation of a stimulus in one limb is referred to the opposite limb

Allocheiria (Allochiria) Allesthesia

Allochesthesia A condition in which a sensation is referred to a point other than that to which the stimulus is applied

Allodynia Any stimulus that results in pain

Alloesthesia (Alloaesthesia) Allesthesia

Analgesia Loss of sensibility to pain

Analgesia Algera Anesthesia dolorosa

Anesthesia (Anaesthesia) Total loss of all forms of sensation

Anesthesia Dolorosa Spontaneous pain in a part, associated with loss of sensibility

Antidromic Propagation of an impulse along a nerve in a direction the reverse of normal

Arthrodesis The stiffening of a joint by operative means

Arthrosis A trophic degeneration of a joint

Asymbolia Loss of the power of appreciation by touch of the form and nature of an object

Auriculotherapy A form of acupuncture in which points in the ear are stimulated

Axonotmesis Interruption of the axons of a nerve without severance of the supporting structure

Biofeedback A training technique used to gain voluntary control over autonomic functions

Blepharospasm Spasmodic winking of the orbicularis muscle

Bruxism Grinding together of the teeth

Capsaicin A pungent alkaloid found in red peppers

Causalgia Sustained burning pain after a traumatic nerve lesion combined with vasomotor or sudomotor dysfunction and late trophic changes

Central pain Spontaneous pain and painful overreaction to objective stimulation resulting from lesions confined to the substance of the central nervous system

Cholecystokinin A peptide first described as a gastrointestinal hormone. It is also a potent analgesic

Coccydynia (Coccygodynia) (Coccygalgia) (Coccyodynia) Pain in the coccygeal region often caused by a disorder of the sacrococcygeal joint

Commissural Fibers A bundle of nerve fibers passing from one side to the other in the brain or spinal cord

Cordectomy Excision of a part of the spinal cord

Cordotomy (Chordotomy) Division of tracts of the spinal cord by various techniques

Cortectomy Excision of part of the cortex

Cryalgesia Pain caused by cold

Cryesthesia Sensitiveness to cold

Cryoanalgesia Pain relief by cold, commonly by freezing nerves with a probe

Deafferentation A loss of sensory nerve fibers from a portion of the body

Dermatome The area of skin supplied by a single afferent nerve fiber from a single dorsal root

Dynorphin One of three classes of opioid peptides. The others are β-endorphin and enkephalins

Dysesthesia A condition in which a disagreeable sensation is produced by ordinary stimuli

Dysnosognosia A psychopathologic state of abnormal illness behavior

Dystonia A state of abnormal tonicity in any of the tissues

Efferent Conducting outward

Electrogenesis A generation of a neural impulse

Endorphin One of a family of opioid-like polypeptides

Enkephalin A pentapeptide that binds to some pain-related opiate receptors

Fibromyalgia An ambiguous term often used to refer to myofascial syndrome

Fibrositis An ambiguous term often used to refer to myofascial trigger points

Gangliolysis The dissolution of a ganglion, e.g., by radiofrequency

Ganglionectomy Excision of a ganglion

Glossodynia (Glossalgia) Pain in the tongue

Heterotopic Pain Referred pain

Hypalgesia Decreased sensitivity to pain

Hyperalgesia (Hyperalgia) An increased sensitivity to painful stimuli with a lowered threshold to painful stimuli

Hyperesthesia (Hyperaesthesia) An increased response to pain and tactile and temperature sense with a lowered threshold to painful stimuli

Hyperpathia Unpleasant long-lasting pain sensation with delay in its appreciation after stimulation and a continued after sensation when the stimulus is ended, usually associated with a raised threshold to stimulation

Hypesthesia (Hypoesthesia) A diminution of sensation

Hypoesthesia (Hypoaesthesia) Hypesthesia

Mydriasis Dilatation of the pupil

Myelotomy Any incision of the spinal cord

Myofascial Syndrome Pain and/or autonomic phenomena referred from active myofascial trigger points with associated dysfunction

Myofibrositis A term often used to refer to myofascial syndrome

Myosis (Miosis) Contraction of the pupil

Myositis Inflammation of a muscle

Myotome Those muscles innervated by a single spinal segment

Nerve Block Interruption of nerve conduction wholly or in part, temporarily or permanently

Nervus Intermedius A sensory nerve forming the sensory portion of the facial nerve

Neuralgia Pain of a severe, throbbing, or stabbing character in the course or distribution of a nerve

Neurectomy Excision of a portion of a nerve

Neuritis Inflammation of a nerve

Neuroma A neoplasm of a nerve or a proliferative mass (not neoplasm) of Schwann cells and neurites that may develop at the proximal end of a severed or injured nerve

Neuropathy Any disease of the nervous system

Neuropraxia A state of a nerve in which conduction is blocked across a point but is present above and below the lesion

Neurotmesis Complete division of a nerve

Nociceptors A peripheral nerve organ or mechanism for the appreciation and transmission of painful stimuli

Odontalgia Toothache

Operant Conditioning A technique of increasing the frequency of a specific desired response by pairing it with a reinforcer

Oxyesthesia Hyperesthesia

Pacinian Corpuscles Pressure-sensitive neural structures in the fingers, mesentery, tendons, and elsewhere

Panalgesia Pain in the entire body

Paresthesia Crawling, burning, tingling, or pains-and-needles feelings that arise spontaneously

Percutaneous Through unbroken skin

Pes Cavus An exaggeration of the normal arch

Pes Valgus Eversion of the foot

Pes Varus Inversion of the foot

Proenkephalin Precursor of an opioid peptide

Radiculitis Inflammation of a spinal nerve root

Radiculopathy Disease of the spinal nerve root

Radiofrequency Radiant energy of a certain frequency; often used to create a heat lesion

Referred Pain Pain perceived as coming from an area remote from its actual origin

Reflex Sympathetic Dystrophy A painful syndrome associated with autonomic dysfunction but not preceded by major nerve trauma

Rhizidiotomy A selective microsurgical technique of rhizotomy that spares the large diameter proprioceptive afferents

Rhizotomy Sectioning of the spinal nerve roots

Sciatica Neuralgia of the sciatic nerve usually caused by a herniated lumbar vertebral disk but occasionally by sciatic neuritis

Sclerotome All tissues of embryonic mesodermal origin (muscle, fascia, and connective tissue) innervated by a single spinal segment

Somatic Parietal; relating to the wall of the body cavity

Somatization The conversion of anxiety into physical symptoms

Somatostatin A peptide that inhibits the release of growth hormone but also seems to have effects similar to opiates

Spondylolisthesis Forward movement of the body of one lower lumbar vertebra on the vertebrae below it

Spondylolysis Breaking down or dissolution of the body of a vertebra

Spondylosis Vertebral ankylosis; this term also is applied often nonspecifically to any lesion of the spine of a degenerative nature

Substance P A polypeptide in brain and intestine that may be a neurotransmitter of nociceptive sensory afferents

Substantia Gelatinosa Area of the posterior horn of the spinal cord with large amounts of opiate

Sudek Atrophy Bony atrophy associated with sympathetic dystrophy

Sympathalgia Pain occurring after sympathectomy

Sympathetic Dystrophy Group of autonomic dystrophies that includes causalgia and reflex sympathetic dystrophy

Synesthesalgia (Synaesthesialgia) Painful synesthesia

Synesthesia A condition in which a stimulus, in addition to exciting its usual sensation, gives rise to a subjective sensation of different character or localization

Telalgia Referred pain

Thigmanesthesia Loss of light touch

Topoanesthesia Loss of tactile localization

Tractotomy The operation of severing or incising a nerve tract

Transcutaneous Percutaneous

Trichoanesthesia Loss of sensation on stimulation or movement of the hairs

Trigger point A focus of hyperirritability in a tissue that, when compressed, causes referred pain

William's Exercises A group of exercises aimed at strengthening back and abdominal muscles and used in the treatment of low back pain

Xerostomia Dryness of the mouth

Abbreviations

AIB	Abnormal illness behavior
AIP	Acute inflammatory polyneuropathy
CDH	Chronic daily headache
CIBPS	Chronic intractable benign pain syndrome
CRPS	Complex regional pain syndrome
CRPS	Chronic regional pain syndrome
CT	Computed tomography
DAS	Drug administering system
DJD	Degenerative joint disease
DREZ	Dorsal root entry zone
DRG	Dorsal root ganglion
EBP	Epidural blood patch
ECG	Electrocardiography
EEG	Electroencephalography
EHL	Extensor hallucis longus
EMAS	Endorphin-mediated analgesia system
EMG	Electromyography
ESI	Epidural steroid injection
GABA	γ-Aminobutyric acid
IBQ	Illness behavior questionnaire
IDET	Intradeical electrothermocoagulation
It	Intrathecal
IVRB	Intravenous regional block
LLD	Leg length discrepancy
MMPI	Minnesota multiphasic personality inventory
MPQ	McGill pain questionnaire
MRI	Magnetic resonance imaging
NMDA	N-methyl D-aspartate
NSAIDs	Nonsteroidal anti-inflammatory drugs
OA	Osteoarthritis
PCA	Patient-controlled analgesia
PDN	Painful diabetic neuropathy
PHN	Post-herpetic neuralgia
PID	Pelvic inflammatory disease
POEA	Postoperative epidural analgesia
PRI	Pain rating index
PSPI	Psychosocial pain inventory
RFL	Radiofrequency lesioning
RSD	Reflex sympathetic dystrophy
SCL	System check list
SCS	Spinal cord stimulate
SG	Substantia gelatinosa
SI	Sacroiliac
SLR	Straight leg raising
SPA	Stimulation-produced analgesia
TCAD	Tricyclic antidepressant
TENS	Transcutaneous electrical nerve stimulation
TGN	Trigeminal neuralgia
TMJ	Temporomandibular joint
TPI	Trigger-point injection
VAS	Visual analog scales
WHO	World Health Organization

APPENDIX A

NERVE BLOCKING TECHNIQUES

The following is a guide to the performance of some common techniques used in a pain management practice. For other blocks, the reader is referred to any standard textbook of regional anesthesia. Although not specifically mentioned, the anesthesiologist should use their own discretion regarding such details as whether intravenous placement before the block is necessary, whether the patient should be maintained with an empty stomach for several hours before the injection, and whether resuscitative equipment is needed at the bedside.

The complications and side effects mentioned are those specific to the particular nerve block discussed. Other potential complications inherent in any injection technique include intravascular injection, hematoma formation, and infection, the seriousness of which will be determined by the particular site of injection. The anesthesiologist is advised to keep these potential complications in mind when attempting to perform any block.

I. STELLATE GANGLION BLOCK

Technique

The patient lies supine with the neck hyperextended and a thin pillow under the shoulders. The carotid artery is palpated, the trachea identified, and using two fingers, the transverse body of C6 (Chassaignac tubercle) is palpated (block at C7 is associated with a higher incidence of pheumothorax). This is the most prominent of the cervical transverse processes and lies at the level of the cricoid cartilage. A skin wheal is raised and a 22-gauge 1½-inch needle is advanced between the carotid and cricoid perpendicular to the skin until it contacts the transverse process. The needle then is pulled approximately 2 mm back, the syringe is aspirated, and a 1-ml test dose is given. Assuming there is no untoward reaction, the remaining solution is injected. This volume will spread along the fascial plane, typically from the middle cervical ganglion to T4 or T5 ganglion, thus affecting the sympathetic supply to structures of the head and neck, upper extremity, and chest.

Drugs

Use 8 to 20 ml of lidocaine 0.5% to 1%, or bupivacaine 0.25% to 0.5%, or procaine 1%.

Tips

1. Patient should be informed to expect a Horner syndrome, hoarseness, and warmth.
2. Success of block is confirmed by a Horner syndrome (miosis, ptosis, and anhidrosis) and more importantly, a skin temperature of the arm of at least 2°F greater than the contralateral arm.
3. The patient should be cautioned not to swallow or talk during the procedure but should be instructed to communicate paresthesias by raising a hand.
4. Avoid bilateral blocks.
5. Meticulous aspiration for blood or cerebrospinal fluid should be done before and during the procedure.
6. After the block is completed, the patient should be instructed to sit up to avoid undue edema of the airway and promote caudad spread of the drug to the nerve of Kuntz.

Complications and Side Effects

1. Vertebral or carotid artery injection with central nervous system toxicity.
2. High spinal or epidural injection.
3. Pneumothorax.
4. Vocal cord paralysis.
5. Vasovagal syncope.
6. Orthostatic hypotension.

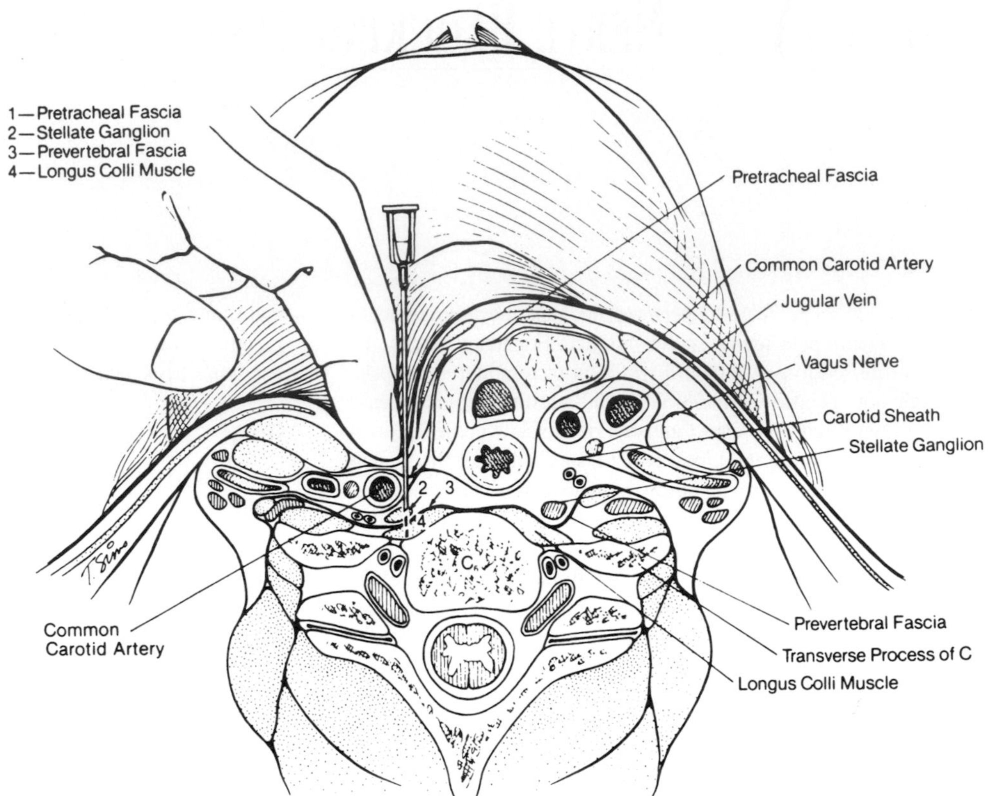

Figure A-1 Stellate ganglion block, paratracheal approach. Transverse section at the level of C6, showing the needle medial to the finger retracting the carotid vessel laterally. (Reproduced with permission from Raj PP, ed. *Handbook of Regional Anesthesia*. New York: Churchill Livingstone; 1985.)

II. LUMBAR SYMPATHETIC BLOCK

Technique

The patient is positioned prone with a pillow under the hips. At the lateral edge of the paravertebral muscle opposite to the L2 spinous process, a skin wheal is made and the deeper tissues are infiltrated with a local anesthetic. A 20-gauge 6-inch needle is directed medially at a 45° angle under x-ray control. The vertebral body generally is encountered at a depth of approximately 4 in. The anteroposterior and lateral view of the L2 vertebra is important in verifying the depth and location of the needle tip. The position of the needle tip will be satisfactory if it is close to the anterior aspect of the L2 vertebral body. To determine if the needle is still in the psoas sheath, a small 2 to 3-ml injection of normal saline or local anesthetic is attempted. As long as the needle is in muscle, there will be some resistance to injection. The needle then is advanced slowly until it pierces the fascia when a sudden loss of resistance will be felt. (If a needle smaller than 20 gauge is used, this loss of resistance may be missed.) The correct placement of the tip of the needle is verified repeatedly by aspirating with a dry syringe for the presence of blood or spinal fluid. If a permanent chemical sympathectomy is planned, 1 to 2 ml of contrast media is injected, and radiographic evidence of the spread is verified by taking an x-ray to localize the position of the tip of the needle.

For routine diagnostic or therapeutic lumbar sympathetic blocks, radiologic facilities are helpful but not required. The block can be done safely only with the anatomic landmarks described. If the transverse process is encountered (usually at a depth of approximately 2 in, the needle should be redirected caudad to about twice this depth. After correct placement of the needle and after aspiration with a syringe, a 2-ml test dose of local anesthetic solution is injected. After waiting a few minutes to observe for untoward effects, 15 to 20 ml of local anesthetic is injected.

Drugs

1. Local anesthetic of 12 to 20 ml of lidocaine 1% or bupivacaine 0.25%.
2. Neurolytic of 10 to 15 ml of phenol in saline 6%.

Tips

1. Block at L2 alone is usually sufficient to provide sympathectomy to the entire leg; may alternatively be performed at L3. Some prefer individual blocks at L2, L3, and L4, especially for neurolysis since a smaller volume can be used.
2. If a neurolytic procedure is done, a permanent copy of the x-ray confirming correct needle position should be retained.

Complications and Side Effects

1. Orthostatic hypotension.
2. Spinal or epidural injection.
3. Injury to kidney, ureter, or renal pelvis.
4. Genitofemoral block.

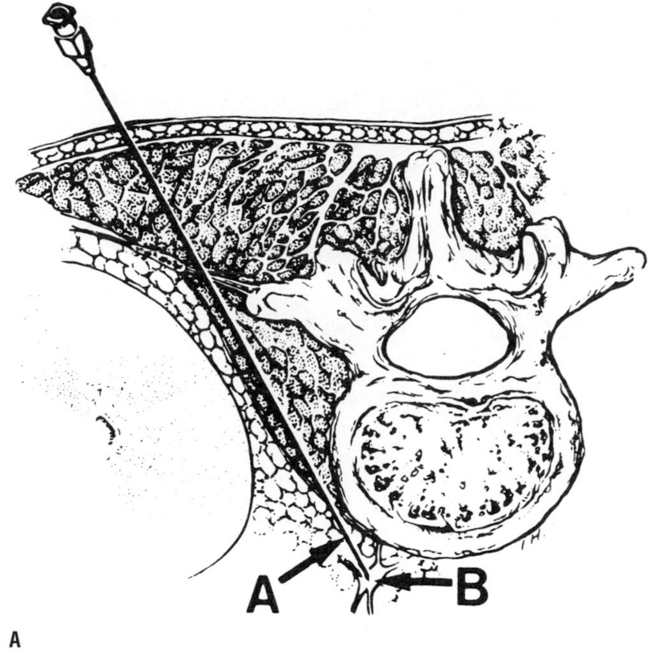

A

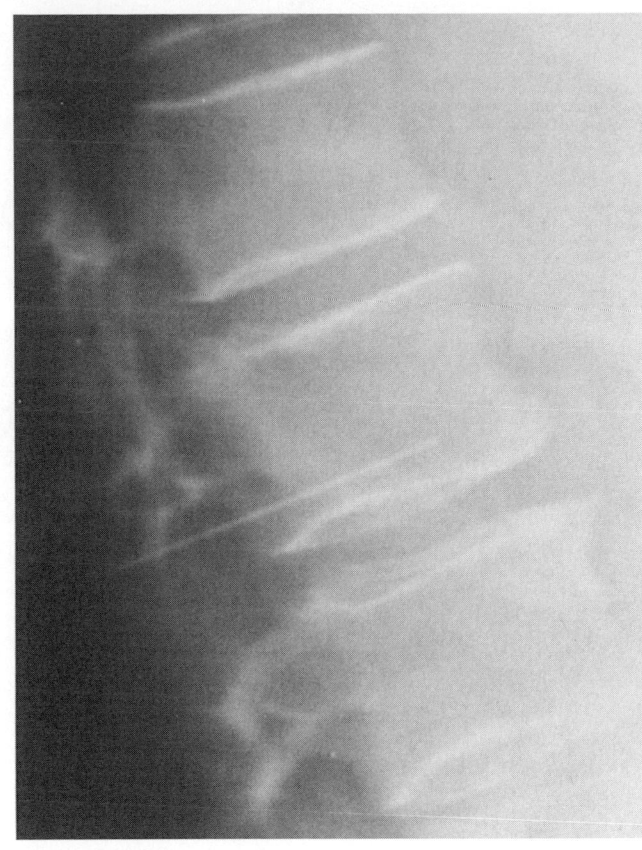

B

Figure A-2 *(a)* Lumbar sympathetic block. Anatomic drawing showing the relationship of the needle (A) to the sympathetic chain (B) at the L2 level. (Reproduced with permission from Carron H, Korbon GA, Rowlingson JC. *Regional Anesthesia: Techniques and Clinical Applications.* Orlando, FL: Grune and Stratton; 1984.) *(b)* Lumbar sympathetic block. Lateral x-ray view. (Courtesy of S. Jain, M.D.)

III. CELIAC PLEXUS BLOCK

Technique

With the patient in the prone position and a pillow under the abdomen, the T12 and L1 spinous processes and the 12th rib are palpated and marked. The position is confirmed by fluoroscopy if possible. A triangle is drawn using the inferior portion of each spinous process and the third point 7 to 8 cm lateral at the inferior edge of the 12th rib. A skin wheal of local anesthetic is raised at the lateral apex of the triangle, and deeper infiltration along the path is done.

Using a 6-in 20- or 22-gauge needle, the needle is advanced at approximately a 45° angle from the apex, under the inferior edge of the 12th rib toward the body of L1. In an average-sized person, this will approach a depth of approximately 10 to 12 cm. After bony contact is made, the position can be confirmed by fluoroscopy. After this is done and a note is made of the angle and depth of the needle, the needle is redirected so that it ultimately lies 1 to 2 cm beyond the anterolateral edge of the body of L1. Fluoroscopic examination can confirm the position, and aspiration should be done to exclude the possibility of blood, cerebrospinal fluid, or urine aspirate. At this point, a small test dose is given before injection of the usual 20 ml of solution. The same procedure then may be done on the contralateral side.

Drugs

1. Local anesthetic of 15 to 20 ml of lidocaine 1% or bupivacaine 0.5%. (A unilateral block with a large volume (50 ml) should provide bilateral anesthesia.)
2. Neurolytic of 15 to 20 ml of alcohol 50% to 95% or phenol 6% (phenol 10% in Renografin 76 is useful for observing dispersion of the injection).

Tips

1. Patient should be well hydrated before the block.
2. Because the left ganglion is usually lower than the right, needle placement on the left should be two-thirds of the way down L1 and, on the right, 1 cm above L1.
3. Fluoroscopy with a permanent spot film to confirm needle placement may be desirable for a neurolytic procedure.

Complications and Side Effects

1. Orthostatic hypotension.
2. Aortic or venacaval puncture with retroperitoneal hematoma.
3. Pneumothorax.
4. Puncture of liver, spleen, kidney, pancreas, or ureter.
5. Neurolytic blocks may result in neuritis, sensory and motor loss, skin sloughing, and alcohol intoxication.

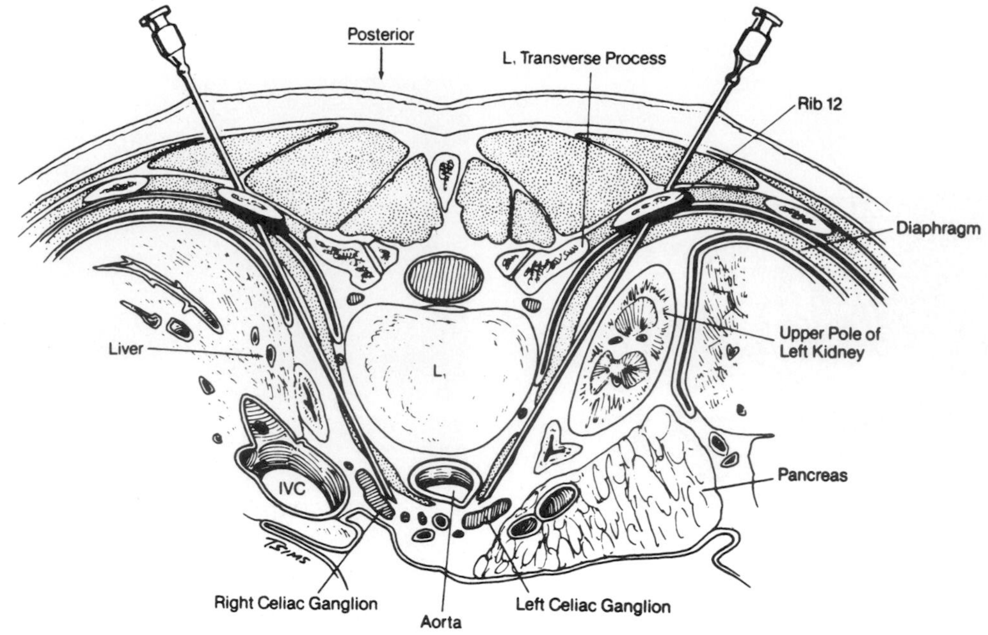

A

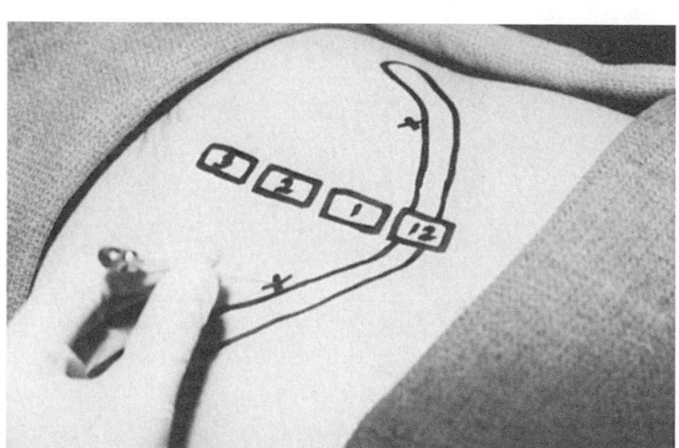

B

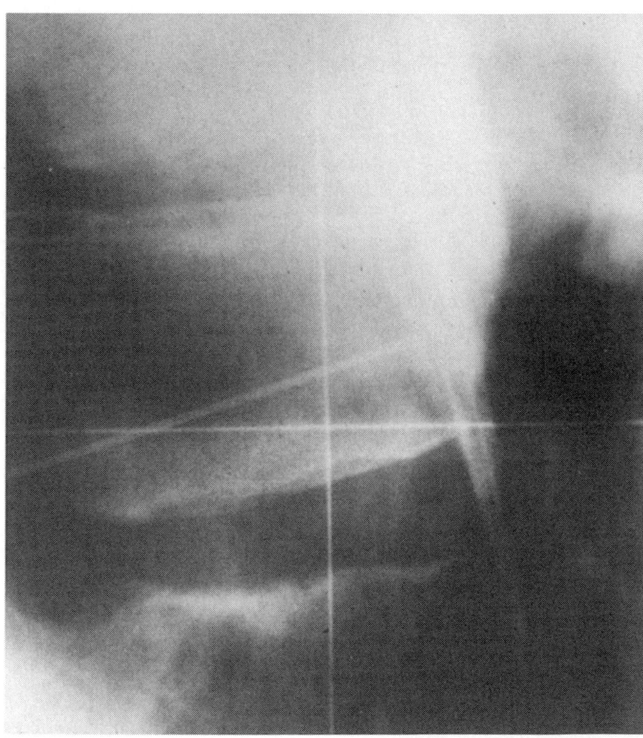

D

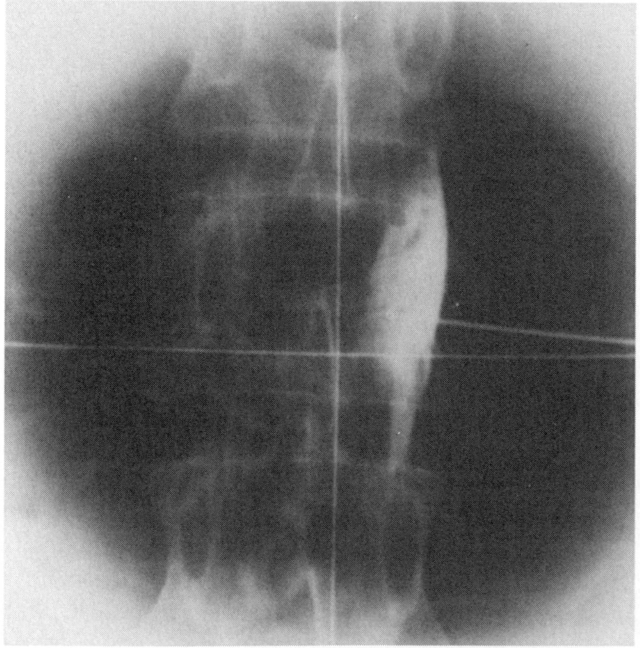

C

Figure A-3 *(a)* Transverse section at the level of L1 showing entry of 6-in 20-gauge needles bilaterally to the celiac plexus. (Reproduced with permission from Raj PP, ed. *Handbook of Regional Anesthesia.* New York: Churchill Livingstone; 1985.) *(b)* X marks point of entry of needle for celiac plexus block. *(c and d)* AP *(c)* and lateral *(d)* views of needle in position for left celiac plexus block. Contrast dye further confirms position.

V. EPIDURAL CORTICOSTEROID INJECTION

Technique

The patient is positioned in the lateral decubitus position with the painful side down. Standard sterile precautions are observed, and local anesthesia of the injection site is obtained by infiltration. A 17- to 20-gauge Tuohy needle is used, and the epidural space is identified with loss of resistance to air or saline. After the solution is injected slowly, the needle is cleared with 1 ml of a local anesthetic or saline. The patient should remain in the lateral decubitus position for 15 min.

Drugs

1. 50 to 100 mg of triamcinolone diacetate in 5 to 10 ml of lidocaine 1% or bupivacaine 0.5%.
2. 80 to 120 mg of methylprednisolone acetate also has been used.

Tips

1. Injection should be made at the involved level.
2. A paramedian approach may be useful for patients who cannot flex and is mandatory for patients with previous posterior spinal fusion.

Complications and Side Effects

1. Immediate: high spinal injection.
2. Late: spinal headache, exacerbation of symptoms for 24 to 48 h, epidural hematoma, arachnoiditis, adrenal suppression, Cushing syndrome, and neurologic deficit.

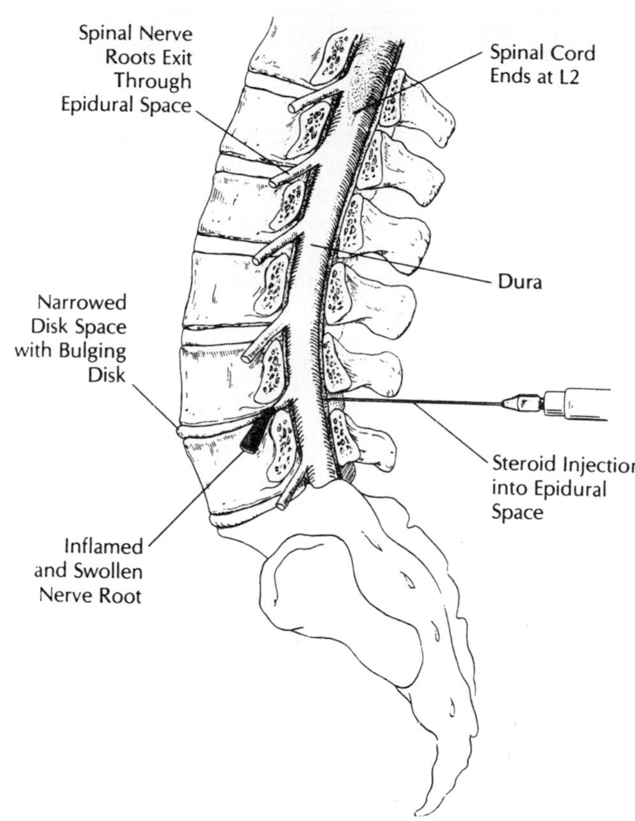

Figure A-4 Because root compression in diskogenic disease occurs most commonly in the epidural space, epidural injection of corticosteroids is the preferred procedure. Injection is given at the level of the affected nerve root. (Reproduced with permission from *Hosp Pract* 1985; 20:32k. Illustration by Pauline Thomas.)

VI. FACET JOINT INJECTION

Technique

The patient is positioned prone on a radiolucent table with a pillow under the hips. Under fluoroscopic control, the appropriate vertebral level is located in the anteroposterior direction. The image intensifier (or patient) then is rotated until the facet joint space is seen clearly. A skin wheal is raised where an imaginary line from the center of the image intensifier intersects the skin. A 22-gauge 3½-in needle is advanced at right angles to the image intensified under fluoroscopic guidance until it enters the joint.

Drugs

Use 1 to 2 ml of lidocaine 1% or bupivacaine 0.5% followed by 20 to 25 mg of triamcinolone diacetate.

Tips

To confirm needle placement, rotate the patient or image intensifier after the needle is in the joint. The needle should continue to appear to be in the joint regardless of the angle of view.

Complications and Side Effects

1. Spinal anesthesia.
2. Neurologic deficit.

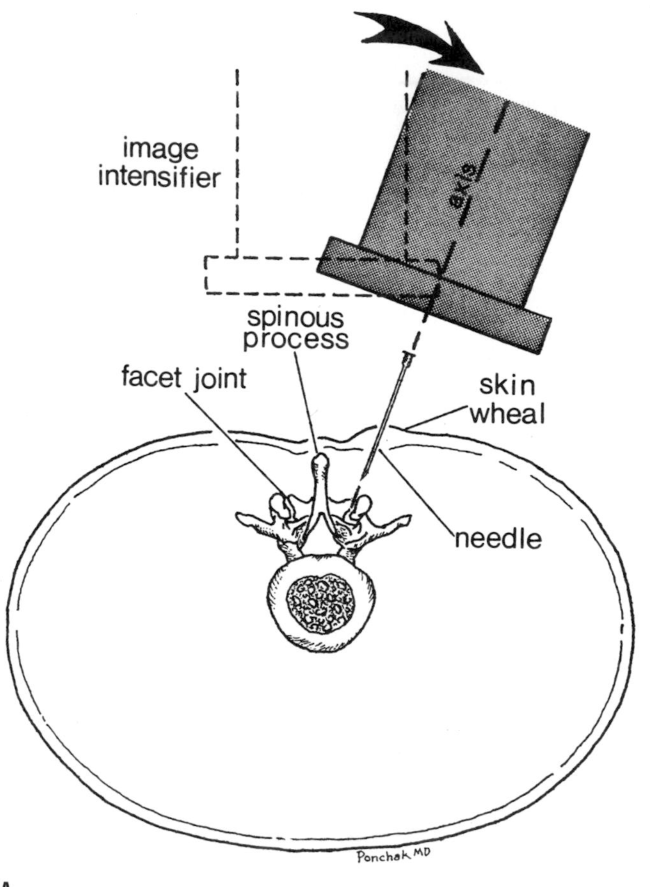

A

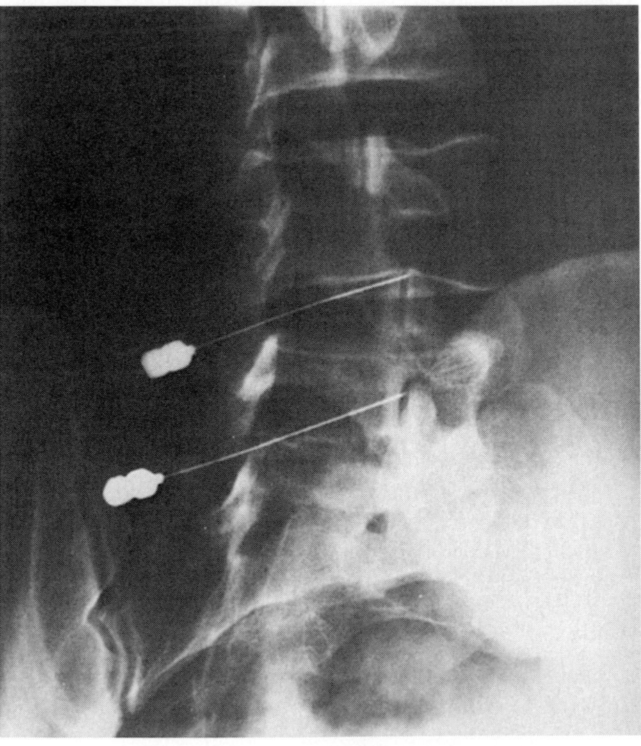

B

Figure A-5 *(a)* The image intensifier (or patient) is rotated until the joint space is seen clearly. A skin weal is raised where an imaginary line from the center of the image intensifier intersects the skin. Under fluoroscopic control, a 22-gauge, 3-in needle is advanced into the facet joint along this axis. (Illustration by Steven Ponchak, M.D.) *(b)* X-ray indicating correct needle position in the L4,5 and L5S1 facet joints.

VII. PARAVERTEBRAL SOMATIC BLOCK

Technique

With the patient in the prone position, a skin wheal is raised, and a 22-gauge 3½-in needle is inserted 3 cm lateral to the cephalad end of the dorsal spinous process of the vertebral level to be blocked. It is directed perpendicular to the skin to meet the corresponding transverse process. The needle then is redirected so that it lies approximately 3 cm medial and caudad to the transverse process. The aim is to have the tip of the needle close to the intervertebral foramen, where the corresponding nerve emerges. Paresthesias may or may not be elicited.

Drugs

Use 10 ml of lidocaine 1%, bupivacaine 0.5%, or procaine 1%.

Tips

When a paresthesia is elicited, less local anesthetic (6 to 8 ml) will be needed.

Complications and Side Effects

1. Subdural, epidural, and subarachnoid block.
2. Pneumothorax.
3. Hypotension from sympathetic block.

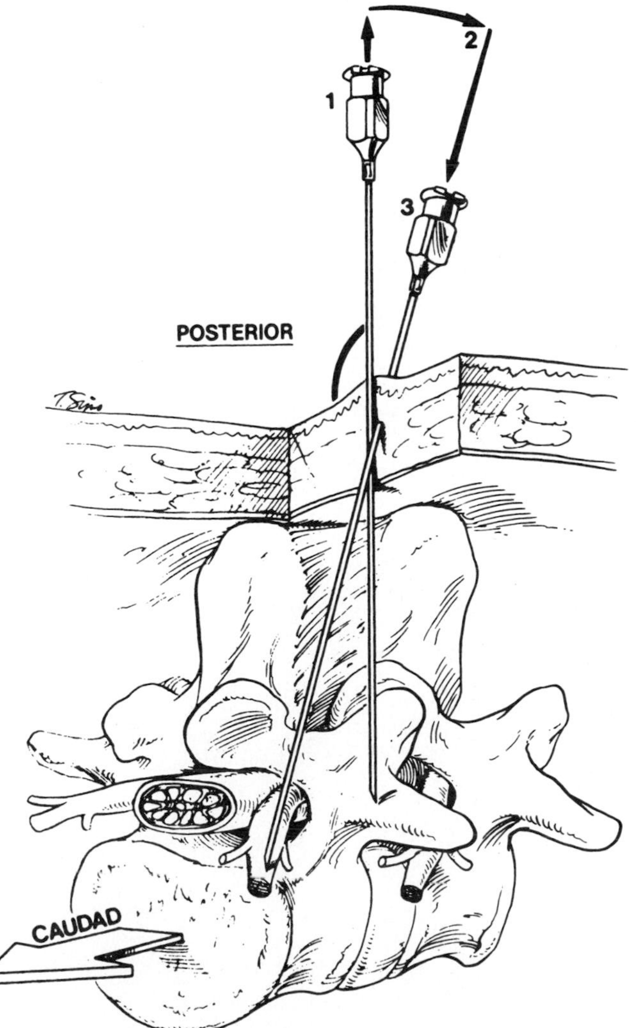

Figure A-6 Lateral view of the lumbar nerve roots, showing point of entry and direction of the needle for lumbar somatic block. (Reproduced with permission from Raj PP, ed. *Handbook of Regional Anesthesia.* New York: Churchill Livingston; 1985.)

VIII. PERMANENT INTRASPINAL CATHETER IMPLANTATION

Technique

The following implantation technique for permanent intraspinal narcotic catheters has been used successfully at the Beth Israel Hospital in Boston:

> "After informed consent is obtained, the patient is given a dose of an anti-staph antibiotic, is positioned in the lateral decubitus position and the back, flank and lower lateral abdominal wall are prepped and draped. After infiltration with local anesthetic a three centimeter paraspinous incision is made at the appropriate lumbar level. A Tuohy needle is introduced through the incision and the epidural space identified via a paraspinous approach with a loss of resistance technique. The epidural catheter is then threaded six to eight centimeters past the tip of the needle. The needle is removed, the catheter is aspirated and a test dose of local anesthetic is injected to rule out entry into the subarachnoid space or vessel. Local anesthetic is then injected through the catheter in a dose and volume adequate to not only confirm positioning within the epidural space but also to provide anesthesia for the tunneling procedure (20cc 3% chlorprocaine, for example). The catheter is secured with a purse string suture. The catheter is then tunneled subcutaneously around the flank to the lower abdominal wall and is connected either to an externalized catheter, a subcutaneous injection port, or a subcutaneous continuous infusion device. The wounds are then closed."

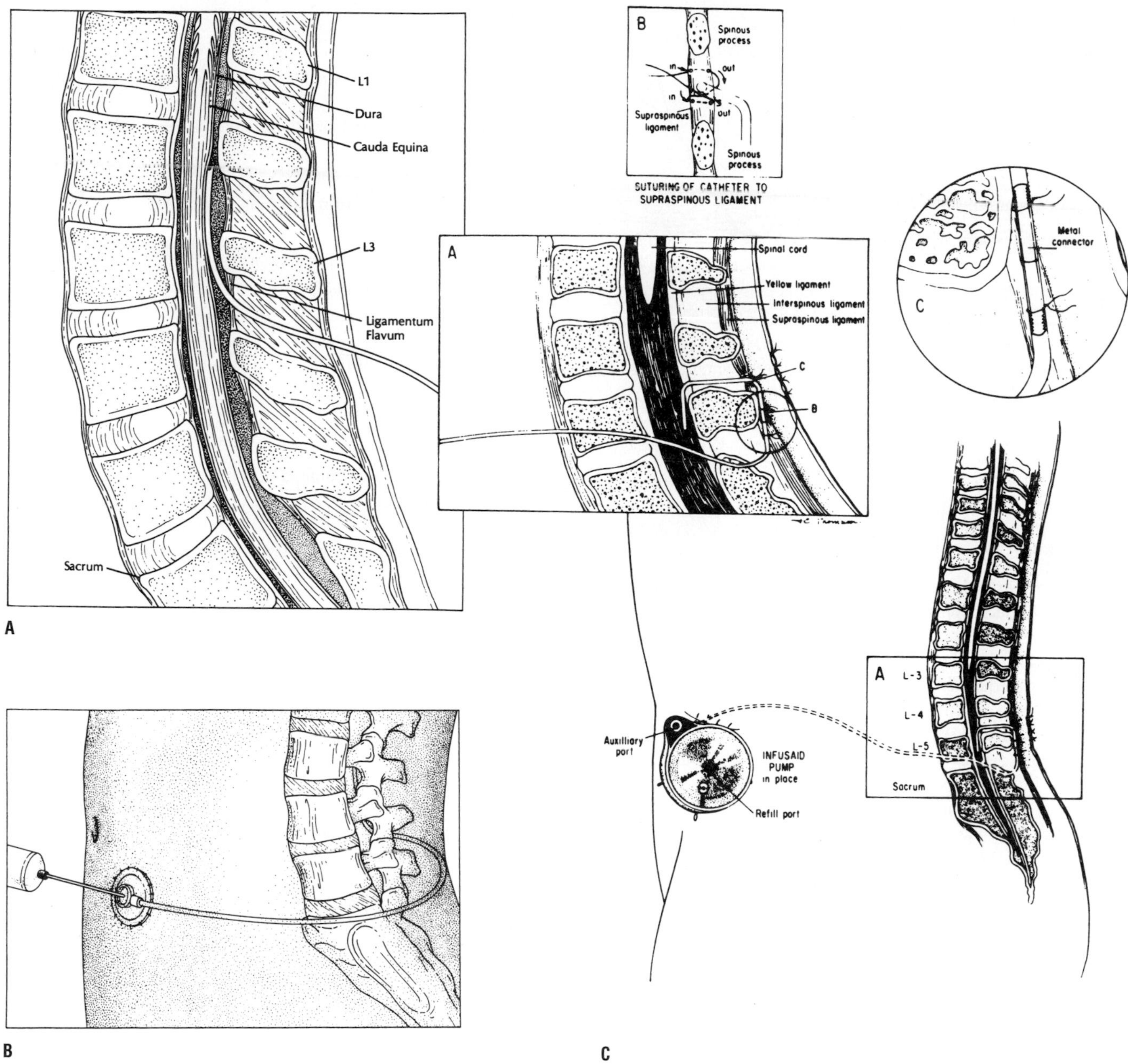

Figure A-7 *(a)* Position of the epidural catheter after it has been tunneled subcutaneously through the lower abdominal wall for long-term use. *(b)* Narcotics can be injected through a subcutaneous port as shown or infused continuously. *(c)* Continuous-infusion pump is located in a subcutaneous pocket on the abdominal wall and anchored to the underlying fascia with heavy nonabsorbable sutures at four quadrants. Either an intrathecal or epidural catheter placement can be selected; only the former is shown to emphaize the spinal anchoring technique. The joined catheters wrap around the flank in a subcutaneous tunnel. (A) Close-up perspective of the catheter entrance into the spine. (B) Close-up of the suture technique used to anchor the catheter firmly to the supraspinous ligament to discourage dislodgement. A figure eight is placed before introducing the Tuohy epidural needle, thus eliminating the risk of needle injury to the spinal catheter. When snugged down, the figure eight will reduce the leakage of cerebrospinal fluid along the catheter and forestall hygroma formation. (C) Close-up of the fixation technique to bond the two catheters together over a straight metal connector. (Figures *(a)* and *(b)* reproduced with permission from *Hosp Pract* 1989; 24:44–48, illustrations by Susan Tilberry. Figure *(c)* reproduced with permission from Coombs D. *Continuous Intraspinal Morphine Analgesia for Relief of Cancer Pain.* Norwood, MA: Intermedics Infusaid; 1981:5.)

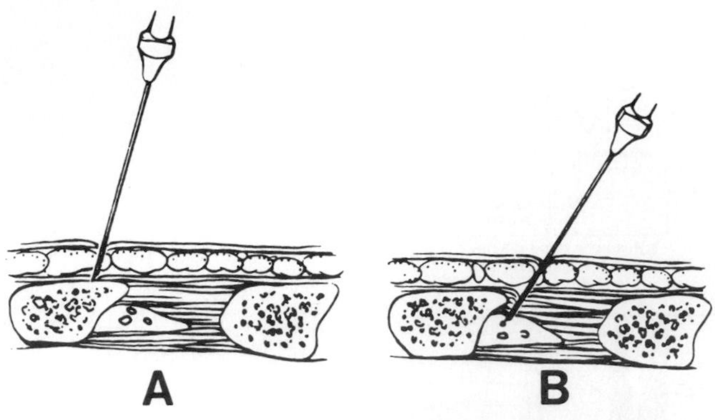

Figure A-8 Intercostal nerve block. Anatomic drawing showing (A) step I and (B) step II. (Reproduced with permission from Carron H, Korbon G, Rowlingson J. *Regional Anesthesia.* Orlando, FL: Grune and Stratton; 1984.)

IX. INTERCOSTAL BLOCK

Technique

The injection may be made at the angle of the ribs; at the lateral border of the sacrospinalis muscle; or at the posterior, mid, or anterior axillary line as indicated. With the patient in the lateral or prone position with the arms abducted overhead, the rib is palpated and the skin retracted slightly upward. A 25-gauge 1½-in needle is introduced through a skin wheal until it contacts the rib. It then is "walked off" the inferior edge of the rib and advanced approximately 2 mm. After a negative aspiration, 3 to 5 ml of local anesthetic are injected, and the needle is removed. This procedure is repeated at each of the levels to be blocked. Control of the needle at all times is of the utmost importance in this procedure, and the hand must at all times stabilize its position.

Drugs

Use 3 to 5 ml of lidocaine 1%, bupivacaine 0.5%, or procaine 1%.

Tips

1. A 25-gauge needle is associated with a low incidence of pneumothorax, but breath sounds should be checked and documented after the block.
2. A large dose of local anesthetic may provide a block of several interspaces.

Complications and Side Effects

1. Local anesthetic toxicity from rapid intravascular absorption.
2. Pneumothorax.
3. Epidural or spinal block.

X. LATERAL FEMORAL CUTANEOUS BLOCK

Technique

With the patient lying supine, a skin wheal is raised 2 to 3 cm medial to and 2 to 3 cm caudad to the anterior superior iliac spine. A 22-gauge 3½-in needle is inserted at right angles to the skin until a "pop" is felt when it passes through the fascia. Then 10 to 15 ml of a local anesthetic is injected as the needle is moved in and out of the fascia in a lateral and medial fan-like direction.

Drugs

Use 10 to 15 ml of lidocaine 1%. (When this block is used to treat meralgia paresthetica, 40 mg of methylprednisolone acetate or triamcinolone often are added to the local anesthetic.)

Tips

Because this is actually a field block, the fanning motion during injection is critical.

Complications and Side Effects

Femoral nerve block with resultant temporary motor loss may occur.

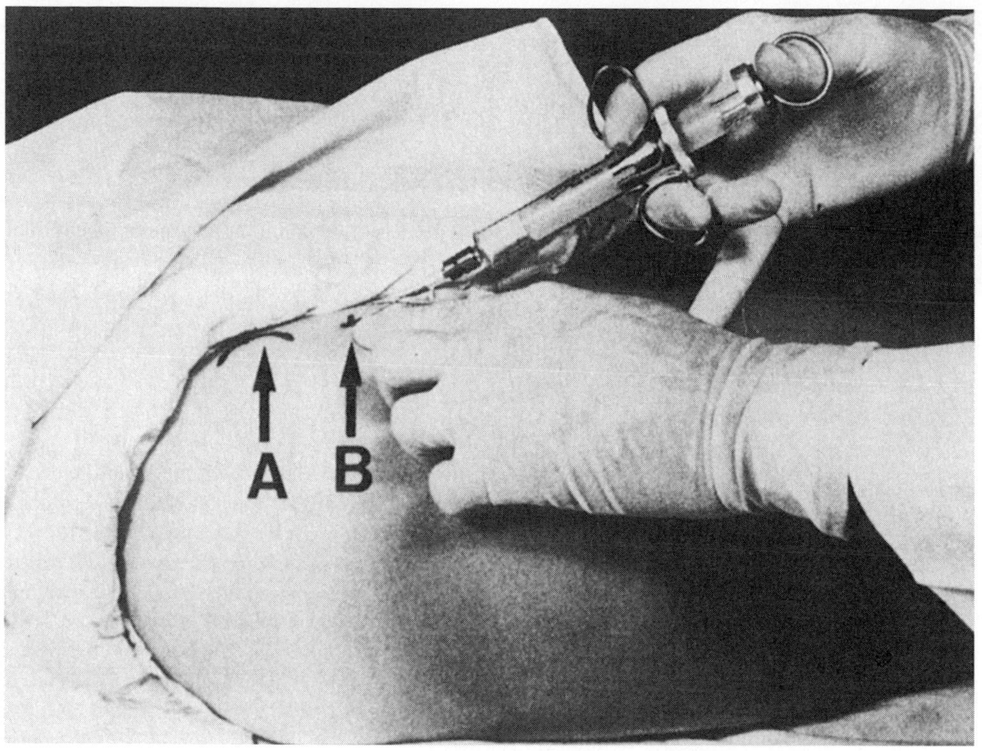

A

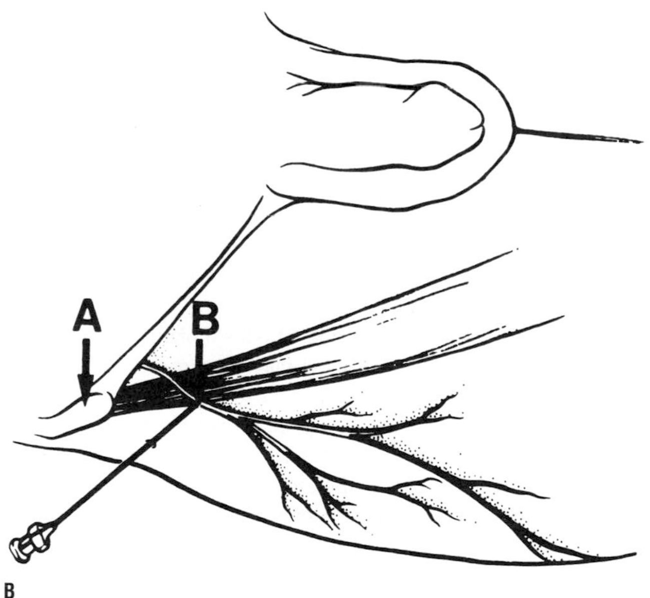

B

Figure A-9 *(a)* Lateral femoral cutaneous nerve block. Landmarks: (A) indicates the anterior superior iliac spine. Needle entry point (B) is 2 cm medial and 2 cm caudad to point (A). *(b)* Lateral femoral cutaneous nerve block. Anatomic drawing showing relationship to the anterosuperior iliac spine (A) to the nerve (B). (Reproduced with permission from Carron H, Korbon G, Rowlingson J. *Regional Anesthesia.* Orlando, FL: Grune and Stratton, 1984.)

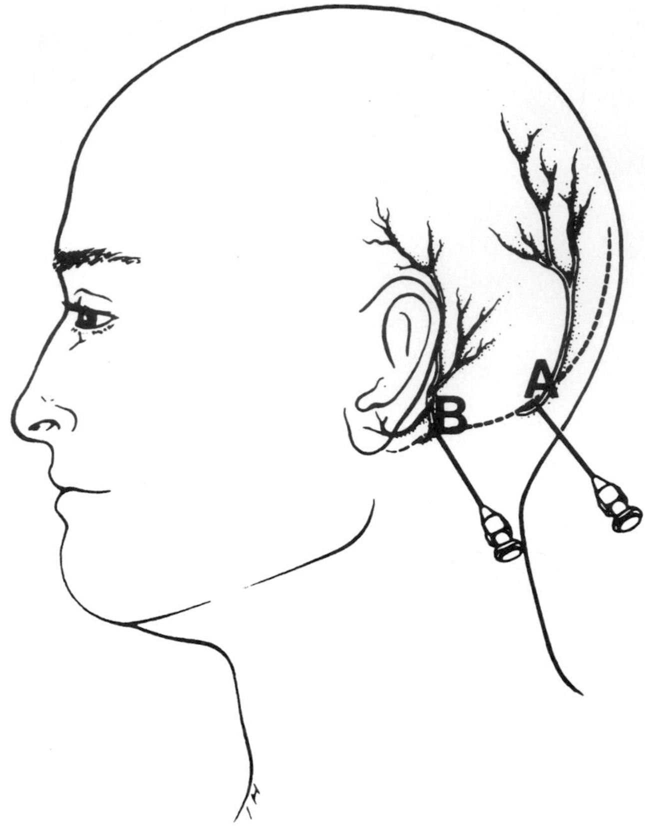

Figure A-10 Occipital nerve block. Anatomic drawing showing relationships and distribution of the greater (A) and lesser (B) occipital nerves. (Reproduced with permission from Carron H. *Relieving Pain with Nerve Blocks.* Cleveland, OH: Modern Medicine Publications; 1978:50.)

XI. GREATER OCCIPITAL NERVE BLOCK

Technique

With the patient seated and their head flexed, a skin wheal is raised just caudad to the superior nuchal line at the lateral edge of the insertion of the trapezius muscle. This point is midway between the mastoid and the midline. A 22- to 25-gauge 1½-in needle then is inserted in a cephalad direction until bone is contacted. After negative aspiration, 3 to 5 ml of a local anesthetic is injected.

Drugs

Use 3 to 5 ml of lidocaine 1% or bupivacaine 0.5%. (Methylprednisolone or triamcinolone 20 to 40 mg sometimes are added to the local anesthetic in the treatment of occipital neuralgia.)

Tips

In a patient with occipital neuralgia, the greater occipital nerve often is tender, and therefore, the most tender spot along the superior nuchal ridge will provide the location for injection.

Complications and Side Effects

1. Accidental occipital artery injection may produce seizures.
2. Injection into the foramen magnum may produce a cisternal block or damage to the brainstem.

XIII. INTRATHECAL NEUROLYSIS

Technique

The patient is positioned at a 45° angle with the painful side uppermost for alcohol and downward for phenol. Under fluoroscopic control, a 22-gauge spinal needle for alcohol, or 20-gauge for phenol, then is inserted into the subarachnoid space at the level of the most painful segment. The needle is withdrawn until cerebrospinal fluid just flows. Then 0.2 ml of solution is injected, and pain relief is assessed. The table is tilted as necessary to confine the flow, and additional 0.1-ml increments of solution are injected at 3-min intervals as needed. The patient's position is maintained for 45 min.

Drugs

1. 0.2 to 0.5 ml of phenol 5% in glycerin or
2. 0.2 to 0.5 ml of alcohol 95% ± 0.1 to 0.2 ml of absorbable contrast medium.

Tips

1. Bilateral block should not be done at the same time because it is associated with a higher incidence of paresis.
2. A permanent spot film should be obtained for later confirmation of needle position.
3. The injection is made at the level corresponding with the spinal cord segment involved; this may be above the level corresponding with root exit.
4. Alcohol is more painful on injection than phenol, and the patient must be warned of this. Some practitioners use local anesthetic to ablate the pain and confirm positioning before neurolysis. Others believe this interferes with the patient's feedback regarding pain relief.
5. Saddle block for rectal pain may be performed with the patient sitting and a 20-gauge spinal needle placed at L5S1. Phenol 5% in .5 ml increments is injected. Bowel and bladder dysfunction are possible.

Complications and Side Effects

1. Motor weakness.
2. Neuritis.
3. Tissue necrosis.
4. Bowel and bladder dysfunction.

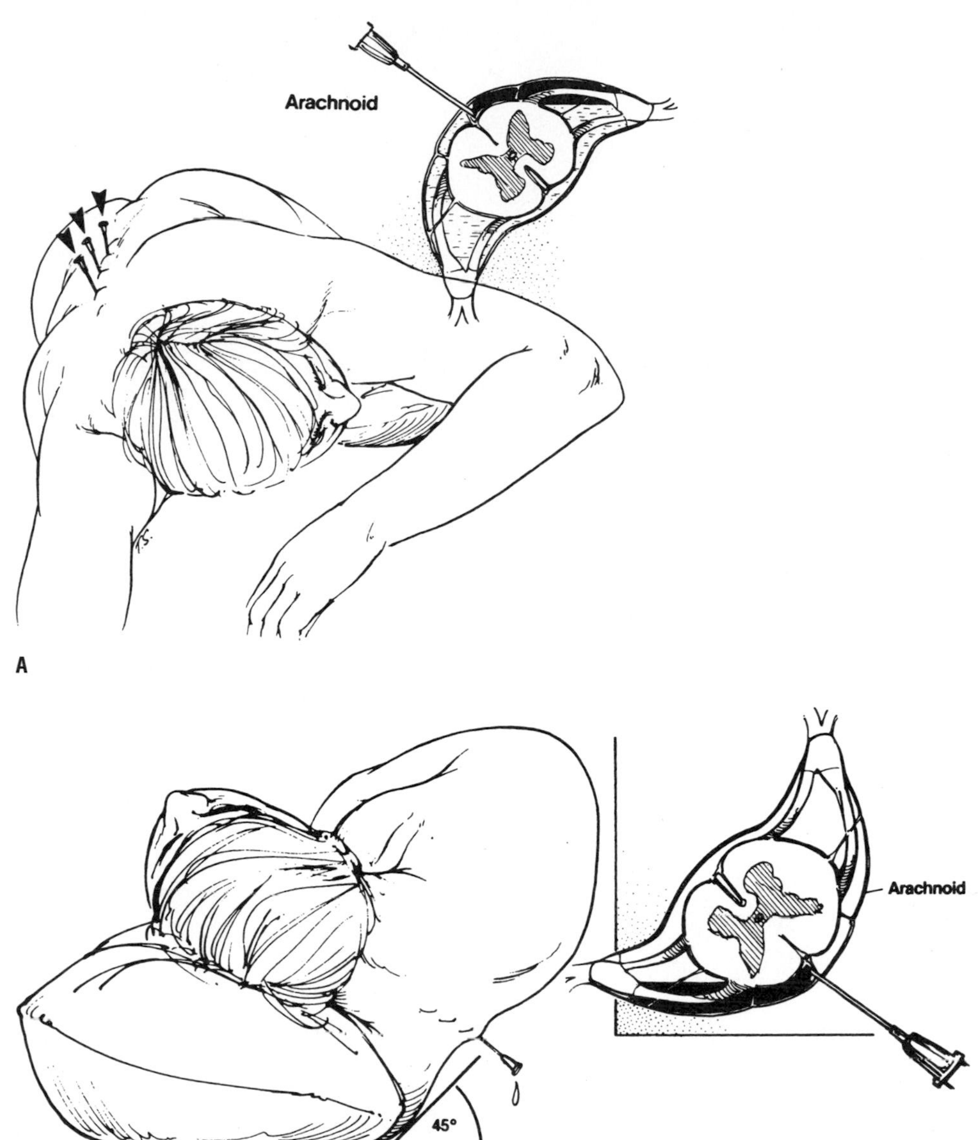

Figure A-11 *(a)* Technique of alcohol neurolysis in the subarachnoid space. The painful part is uppermost, and the angle is 45° to position the posterior nerve roots uppermost. *(b)* Phenol neurolysis in the subarachnoid space. The painful part is lowermost, and the angle is 45° to position the posterior nerve roots lowermost. (Reproduced with permission from Raj PP, ed. *Handbook of Regional Anesthesia.* New York: Churchill Livingstone; 1985.)

APPENDIX **B1**

Beth Israel Deaconess Medical Center

Boston, MA 02215

patient label

Arnold Pain Management Center

PROCEDURE RECORD

DATE OF SERVICE: ________/________/________

ATTENDING: ______________________ (print) FELLOW: ______________________ (print)

NURSE: ______________________ (print) MEDICAL STUDENT: ______________________ (print)

CHIEF COMPLAINT:

STATEMENT OF MEDICAL NECESSITY:

MEDICATIONS:

Aspirin	☐ Yes	☐ No	☐ PT
Warfarin	☐ Yes	☐ No	☐ PTT
NSAIDs	☐ Yes	☐ No	☐ INR
Heparin	☐ Yes	☐ No	
Low Molecular Weight Heparin	☐ Yes	☐ No	

ALLERGIES:

INTERVAL HISTORY & PHYSICAL EXAM:

NO CHANGES SINCE ______/______/______

AGE ________	HT ________	WT ________	Temp ________	O_2 Sat ________
HR ________	RR ________	BP ________	PAIN SCORE Pre ________	
NPO ________	ESCORT ________		Post ________	

APPENDIX B2

DIAGNOSIS:	PROCEDURE:

☐ Consent   Position: ☐ Sitting ☐ Lying   ☐ Sterile Prep & Drape   ☐ Fluoro

Needle Size: ☐ 17g Tuohy ☐ 20g Weiss ☐ 22g spinal ☐ 25g spinal ☐ 25g ☐ 27g ☐ 30g
☐ 22g Regional Block ☐ Other

Needle Length: ☐ 1" ☐ 1.25" ☐ 1.5" ☐ 2" ☐ 3.5" ☐ 4.5" ☐ 5" ☐ 6" ☐ Other ____________

EPIDURAL STEROIDS

Level: ______________________________

Steroid (name): ______________________________

______________ mg IN ______________

Loss of Resisitance:	☐ Saline	☐ Air
Paresthesia:	☐ Yes	☐ No
CSF:	☐ Yes	☐ No
Heme:	☐ Yes	☐ No

TRIGGER POINTS

Medication:

____

OTHER PROCEDURE:

TREATMENT PLAN:

SEEN BY: ______________________________
Fellow/Resident

ATTENDING NOTE: ☐ I personally performed the procedure.
☐ I was present for the key portions of the procedure.

____
Attending M.D. Signature

Distribution: White Copy- Medical Records, Pink Copy - Pain Center

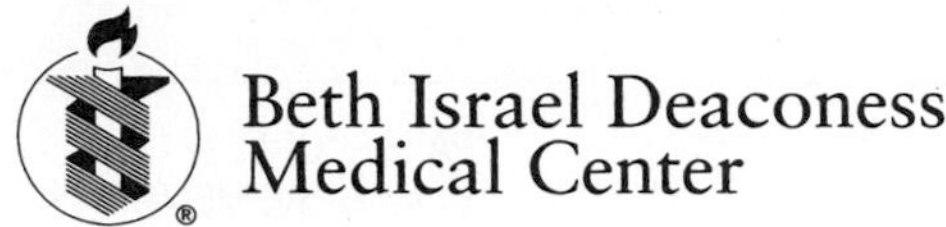

Arnold Pain Management Center

EVALUATION RECORD

DATE OF SERVICE: ________/________/________ TYPE OF VISIT: ☐ NEW ☐ F/U ☐ WORKER'S COMP.

REFERRED BY: ______________________ PCP: ______________________ INTERPRETER: ☐ YES

CHIEF COMPLAINT:

HISTORY

HISTORY OF PRESENT ILLNESS (location, quality, severity, duration, timing, context, modifying factors, signs & symptoms)

MVA – Date ______/______/______ OCCUPATION LAST DAY WORKED______/______/______

PAST MEDICAL HISTORY: no change since______/______/______

MEDICATIONS:

ALLERGIES:

LABS/XRAYS:

FAMILY HISTORY: no change since______/______/______

SOCIAL HISTORY: no change since______/______/______

ALCOHOL/DRUGS: SMOKING:

(*New evals only) Do you ever feel afraid in any of your relationships? ☐ YES ☐ NO

Have you ever been emotionally, physically or sexually hurt by your partner or someone close to you? ☐ YES ☐ NO

(if yes to either of the above questions, refer to nursing)

REVIEW OF SYSTEMS

Constitutional	☐ normal ☐ abnormal	GI/Abdominal	☐ normal ☐ abnormal	Psychiatric	☐ normal ☐ abnormal
Head/Eyes	☐ normal ☐ abnormal	Genitourinary	☐ normal ☐ abnormal	Endocrine	☐ normal ☐ abnormal
ENT, Mouth, Neck	☐ normal ☐ abnormal	Musculoskeletal	☐ normal ☐ abnormal	Hematologic/Lymphatic	☐ normal ☐ abnormal
Cardiovascular	☐ normal ☐ abnormal	Skin	☐ normal ☐ abnormal	Allergic/Immunologic	☐ normal ☐ abnormal
Respiratory	☐ normal ☐ abnormal	Neurological	☐ normal ☐ abnormal	**ALL ELSE NEGATIVE**	☐

NOTE ANY ABNORMAL ROS FINDINGS HERE:

MC 1318

APPENDIX **B4**

EXAM

AGE:	HT:	WT:	TEMP:	PAIN SCORE:
HR:	BP:	RR:	O_2 SAT:	% IMPROVEMENT:

Constitutional	☐ normal	☐ abnormal	Cardiovascular	☐ normal	☐ abnormal	Genitourinary	☐ normal	☐ abnormal
Head/Eyes	☐ normal	☐ abnormal	Respiratory	☐ normal	☐ abnormal	Lymphatic	☐ normal	☐ abnormal
ENT, Mouth, Neck	☐ normal	☐ abnormal	GI/Abdominal	☐ normal	☐ abnormal	Skin	☐ normal	☐ abnormal

NOTE ANY ABNORMAL EXAM FINDINGS HERE:

MUSCULOSKELETAL:	Range of Motion	Muscle Strength & Tone	Inspection & Palpitation	Stability
• Upper extremities:	______________	☐ 5/5 bilaterally		
• Lower extremities:	______________	☐ 5/5 bilaterally		
• Head & Neck:	______________	☐ normal		

OTHER MUSCULOSKELETAL EXAM FINDINGS:

NEUROLOGIC:

• Cranial nerves ☐ II-XII intact

• Sensation ☐ normal light touch

☐ finger to nose normal bilaterally

• Straight leg raise L________ ° R________ °

• Deep tendon reflexes ☐ Babinski normal

Left Lower Extremities______ Right Lower Extremities______

Left Upper Extremities______ Right Upper Extremities______

OTHER NEUROLOGIC EXAM FINDINGS:

PSYCHIATRIC:

DIAGNOSIS:

TREATMENT PLAN:

SEEN BY: ______________________________

Fellow/Resident

ATTENDING NOTE: ☐ I personally performed the evaluation.

☐ I was present for the key portions of the evaluation.

HISTORY:

EXAM:

DIAGNOSIS:

TREATMENT PLAN:

LEVEL OF VISIT: ______________

____

Attending MD Signature

DISTRIBUTION: WHITE COPY - MEDICAL RECORDS, YELLOW COPY - PAIN CENTER

APPENDIX C LOCAL ANESTHETICS

Local Anesthetics

			Concentration (%)						
								Maximum Dose [mg]	
Drugs	**Latency**	**Duration**	**Infiltration**	**Peripheral Nerve**	**Epidural**	**Spinal**	**Topical**	**with Epi**	**without Epi**
Esters									
Procaine (Novacain)	Immediate	Short (30–45 min)	1	—	2	2	—	800	500
Chloroprocaine (Nesacaine)	Fast	Short (45–60 min)	1	—	2	2	—	700	600
Tetracaine (Pontocaine)	Slow	Long (2–3 h)	0.1–0.2	0.1–0.2	—	1	0.5–1	100	75
Cocaine	Slow	Intermediate (60–120 min)	—	—	—	—	4–10	—	150
Amides									
Lydocaine (Xylocaine)	Fast	Intermediate (60–120 min)	0.5–1	1–1.5	1–2	5	4	500	200
Mepivacaine (Carbocaine)	Fast	Intermediate (60–120 min)	1	1–1.5	1.5–2	—	—	500	200
Dibucaine (Nupercainal)	Slow	Very long (3–4 h)	—	—	—	0.5	—	—	50
Bupivacaine (Marcaine)	Intermediate	Very long (4–8 h)	0.25–0.5	0.25–0.5	0.5–0.75	0.5	—	250	150
Prilocaine (Citanest)	Slow	Intermediate (60–120 min)	0.5–1	1	2–3	—	—	600	400
Etidocaine (Duranest)	Fast	Very long (4–8 h)	0.5	0.5–1	1–1.5	—	—	400	300
Ropivacaine (Naropin)	Fast	Very long	.5–.75	0.5–0.75	0.5–1	—	—	250	150
Levobupivacaine (Chirocaine)	Slow	Very long	0.25–0.5	0.25–0.5	0.5–0.75	0.5	—	300	200

INDEX

Note: Page numbers followed by f indicate figures; those followed by t indicate tables.

D

J

K

M

O

P

Q

R

S

T